Treatment of Cancer

Treatment of Cancer

Fourth Edition

Edited by

PAT PRICE MA, MD, FRCP, FRCR
Professor of Radiation Oncology,
Christie Hospital,
Manchester, UK

and

KAROL SIKORA MB, PhD, FRCP, FRCR
Visiting Professor of Cancer Medicine,
Imperial College School of Medicine,
Hammersmith Hospital, London, UK

ARNOLD

A member of the Hodder Headline Group
LONDON   NEW YORK   NEW DELHI

First published in Great Britain in 1982 by
Chapman & Hall, London, UK
Second edition 1990
Third edition 1995
also by Chapman & Hall, London, UK

This fourth edition published in 2002 by
Arnold, a member of the Hodder Headline Group,
338 Euston Road, London NW1 3BH

http://www.arnoldpublishers.com

Distributed in the United States of America by
Oxford University Press Inc.,
198 Madison Avenue, New York, NY10016
Oxford is a registered trademark of Oxford University Press

British Library Cataloguing in Publication Data
A catalogue record for this book is available from the British Library

Library of Congress Cataloging-in-Publication Data
A catalog record for this book is available from the Library of Congress

ISBN 0 340 75964 X

1 2 3 4 5 6 7 8 9 10

Commissioning Editor: Joanna Koster
Development Editor: Tim Wale
Production Editor: Rada Radojicic
Production Controller: Iain McWilliams
Cover Designer: Terry Griffiths

Typeset in 10/12 pt Minion by Charon Tec Pvt. Ltd, Chennai, India
Printed and bound in Great Britain by the Bath Press

What do you think about this book? Or any other Arnold title?
Please send your comments to feedback.arnold@hodder.co.uk

Contents

Contributors

Andreas Adam MB BS, FRCP, FRCR, FRCS
Department of Radiology, First Floor, Lambeth Wing,
St Thomas' Hospital, Lambeth Palace Road,
London SE1 7EH, UK

Roshan Agarwal BSc, MRCP
Section of Medicine, Haddow Laboratories,
Institute of Cancer Research, Cotswold Road,
Sutton, Surrey SM2 5NG, UK

Helen Anderson BhB, MB ChB, FRACP
Vancouver Cancer Centre, 600 West 10th Avenue,
Vancouver, B.C., Canada

Amit K. Bahl MD, MRCP, FRCR, FFR RCSI
Bristol Haematology and Oncology Centre,
Horfield Road, Bristol BS2 8ED, UK

Hugo R. Baillie-Johnson FRCR, FRCP
Department of Oncology, Norfolk and Norwich Hospital,
Brunswick Road, Norwich, Norfolk NR1 3SR, UK

Ronald Beaney MD, MB ChB, FRCP, FRCR
Guy's and St Thomas' Hospital Cancer Centre, St Thomas'
Hospital, Lambeth Palace Road, London SE1 7EH, UK

Richard H.J. Begent MD, FRCP, FRCR, FMedSci
Department of Oncology, Royal Free and University
College Medical School, University College London,
Royal Free Campus, Rowland Hill Street,
London NW3 2PF, UK

Irving S. Benjamin BSc, MD, FRCS (Glas & Eng)
Academic Department of Surgery, Guy's, King's and
St Thomas' School of Medicine, King's College Hospital,
Denmark Hill, London SE5 9RS, UK

John Bingham FRCP, FRCR
Department of Radiology, Guy's and St Thomas' NHS
Trust, Lambeth Palace Road, London, SE1 7EH, UK

Peter Blake BSc, MD, MB BS, FRCR
Gynaecology Unit, The Royal Marsden Hospital,
Fulham Road, London SW3 6JJ, UK

Mark Bower PhD, MRCP
Department of Oncology, Chelsea and Westminster
Hospital, Fulham Road, London SW10 9NH, UK

Jill A. Bullimore MB BS, FRCR, MRCP
Bristol Oncology Centre, Bristol Royal Infirmary,
Bristol, UK

Anna M. Cassoni BSc, FRCP, FRCR
The Meyerstein Institute of Oncology, The Middlesex
Hospital, UCL Hospitals NHS Trust, Mortimer Street,
London W1N 8AA, UK

David Chao BM, BCh, MRCP, DPhil
Department of Oncology, Royal Free Hospital,
University College Medical School, Rowland Hill Street,
London NW3 2PF, UK

Sunil Chopra MRCP
Royal London Hospital, Whitechapel Road,
London E1 1BB, UK

Anthony C. Chu FRCP
Faculty of Medicine, Imperial College of Science,
Technology and Medicine, Hammersmith Hospital,
Du Cane Road, London W12 0NN, UK

Justin P. Cobb FRCS
Department of Orthopaedics, The Middlesex Hospital,
UCL Hospitals NHS Trust, Mortimer Street,
London W1N 8AA, UK

Rory Collins MB BS, MSc
Clinical Trial Service Unit and Epidemiological Studies
Unit, University of Oxford, Oxford, UK

Christopher H. Collis MB, BChir
Department of Radiotherapy, Royal Free Hospital, School
of Medicine, Rowland Hill Street, London NW3 2PF, UK

Bernard J. Cummings MB ChB, FRCPC, FRCR, FRANZCR
Department of Radiation Oncology, Princess Margaret
Hospital, 610 University Avenue, Toronto,
Ontario M5G 2M9, Canada

Roger G. Dale MSc, PhD, C.Phys, FInst.P, FIPEM
Hammersmith Hospital NHS Trust and Imperial College
School of Medicine, Department of Radiation Physics
and Radiobiology, Charing Cross Hospital,
Fulham Palace Road, London W6 8RF, UK

Angus Dalgleish BSc, MB BS, MD, FRCPath, FRCP, FRACP
Department of Oncology, Gastroenterology,
Endocrinology and Metabolism, Division of Medical
Oncology, St George's Hospital Medical School,
Cranmer Terrace, London SW17 0RE, UK

Rosy Daniel BSc, MB BCh
The Oncology Department, The Harley Street Clinic,
81 Harley Street, London, W1G 8PP, UK

Thomas F. DeLaney MD
Department of Radiation Oncology, Massachusetts
General Hospital, Boston, MA, Harvard Medical School,
Boston, MA 02114, USA

Stanley Dische MD, FRCR, FACR
Marie Curie Research Wing, Mount Vernon Hospital,
Northwood, Middlesex HA6 2RN, UK

H. Jane Dobbs MA, FRCP, FRCR
Guy's and St. Thomas' Cancer Centre, St. Thomas' Hospital,
Lambeth Palace Road, London SE1 7EH, UK

Ros A. Eeles MA, MRCP, FRCR
Department of Cancer Genetics, Institute of Cancer
Research and Royal Marsden Hospital, Downs Road,
Sutton, Surrey SM2 5PT, UK

Edward J. Estlin PhD, MRCP
Oncology Department, Royal Manchester Children's
Hospital, Hospital Road, Pendlebury,
Manchester M27 4HA, UK

Jeffry Evans MB BS, MD, MRCP (UK), FRCP (Glasgow)
CRC Department of Medical Oncology, West of Scotland
Clinical Trials Unit, Beatson Oncology Centre, E Block,
Western Infirmary, Glasgow G11 6NT, UK

Kate Fife MD, FRCR
Addenbrooke's Hospital, Hills Road,
Cambridge CB2 2XZ, UK

Annabel B.M. Foot MB ChB, FRCPCh, FRCP
Department of Paediatric Oncology, Bristol Royal Hospital
for Children, Upper Maudlin Street, Bristol BS2 8BJ, UK

John M. Goldman DM, FRCPath
Department of Haematology, Imperial College School of
Medicine, Hammersmith Hospital, Du Cane Road,
London W12 0NN, UK

Martin E. Gore PhD, FRCP
Department of Medical Oncology, The Royal Marsden
Hospital, Fulham Road, London SW3 6JJ, UK

Richard Gray MA, MSc
University of Birmingham Clinical Trials Unit,
Somerset Road, Edgbaston, Birmingham B15 2RR, UK

R. Kate Gregory MD, MB BS, MRCP
Department of Medicine, Royal Marsden Hospital,
Fulham Road, London SW3 6JJ, UK

Ashley B. Grossman BA, BSc, MD, FRCP, FMedSci
Department of Endocrinology, St Bartholomew's Hospital,
West Smithfield, London EC1A 7BE, UK

Rajinish Kumar Gupta BSc, PhD, FRCP, FRCPI
The Cancer Strategy Department, Regional General
Hospital, Dooradoyle, County Limerick, Ireland

Jeffrey W. Hand PhD, DSc, FIPEM, FIEE, FInstP
Department of Imaging, Hammersmith Hospitals NHS
Trust and Imperial College School of Medicine,
Du Cane Road, London W12 0HS, UK

Clive Harmer FRCP, FRCR
Department of Radiotherapy, The Royal Marsden NHS
Trust, Fulham Road, London SW3 6JJ, UK

David C. Harmon MD
Department of Radiation Oncology, Massachusetts
General Hospital, Boston, MA, Harvard Medical School,
Boston, MA 02114, USA

Corinne Hayes MA, MB BS, MRCP, MRCPCH
Royal Devon and Exeter Hospital, Exeter EX2 5DW, UK

Robert Heddle MB BS, FRCS, MRCS, LRCP
Department of Surgery, Kent and Canterbury Hospital,
Ethelbert Road, Canterbury, Kent CT1 3NG, UK

Anne P. Hemingway MB BS, FRCP, MCRP, MRCS, RCP, FRCR
Department of Diagnostic Radiology, Hammersmith
Hospital, Du Cane Road, London W12 0NN, UK

Alan Horwich PhD, MRCP, FRCR
Academic Radiotherapy Unit, The Institute of Cancer
Research, The Royal Marsden Hospital, Cotswold Road,
Sutton, Surrey SM2 5PT, UK

Robert Huddart PhD, MRCP, FRCR
Academic Radiotherapy Unit, The Institute of Cancer
Research, The Royal Marsden Hospital, Cotswold Road,
Sutton, Surrey SM2 5PT, UK

John L. Hungerford FRCS, FRCOphth
Ocular Oncology Service, Department of Ophthalmology,
St Bartholomew's Hospital, West Smithfield,
London EC1A 7BE, UK

Philip J. Johnson MD, FRCP
Institute of Cancer Studies, The University of Birmingham,
Vincent Drive, Edgbaston, Birmingham B15 2TT, UK

Bleddyn Jones MA, MD (Cantab), MSc, FRCP, FRCR (Lond)
Department of Clinical Oncology, Imperial College
School of Medicine, Hammersmith Hospital,
London W12 0HS, UK

Philip H. Jones MA, PhD, MRC
CRC Department of Oncology, University of Cambridge,
Hutchinson/MRC Research Centre, Addenbrooke's Hospital,
Hills Road, Cambridge CB2 2XZ, UK

Ajay K. Kakkar BSc, PhD, FRCS
Department of Gastrointestinal Surgery, Imperial College
School of Medicine, Hammersmith Hospital,
Du Cane Road, London W12 0NN, UK

Hemant M. Kocher MS, FRCS
Academic Department of Surgery, King's College Hospital,
London SE5 9RS, UK

Hannah E. Lambert MB BS, FRCOG, FRCR
Department of Clinical Oncology, Hammersmith Hospital,
Du Cane Road, London W12 0HS, UK

Tanya Levine MA, PCDipPath (Cyto), MRCPath
Department of Histopathology, Royal Free Hospital,
Pond Street, London NW3 2PF, UK

Adam A.M. Lewis FRCS, FRCSE
Department of Clinical Oncology, Royal Free Hospital
School of Medicine, Rowland Hill Street,
London NW3 2PF, UK

T. Andrew Lister MD, MB BChir, FRCP, MRCP, MRCS, LRCP, FRCPath
Department of Medical Oncology, St Bartholomew's
Hospital, West Smithfield, London EC1A 7BE, UK

Stephen P. Lowis PhD, MRCPCH
Department of Paediatric Oncology, Bristol Royal Hospital
for Children, Upper Maudlin Street, Bristol BS2 8BJ, UK

R. Hugh MacDougall FRCS, FRCR, FRCP
Directorate of Clinical Oncology and Haematology,
The Edinburgh Cancer Centre, Western General Hospital,
Crewe Road, Edinburgh EH4 2XU, UK

Srinivasan Madhusudan MRCP
Bristol Haematology and Oncology Centre, Horfield Road,
Bristol BS2 8ED, UK

E. Jane Maher MB BS, FRCR, FRCP
Mount Vernon Centre for Cancer Treatment, Mount Vernon
Hospital, Northwood, Middlesex HA6 2RN, UK

Henry J. Mankin MD
Orthopaedic Oncology, Massachusetts General Hospital,
Fruit Street, Boston, MA 02114, USA

Anthony Maraveyas PhD, MRCP
Academic Department of Oncology, The Princess Royal
Hospital, Saltshouse Road, Hull HU8 9HE, UK

Trevor J. McMillan PhD
Department of Biological Sciences, Institute of
Environmental and Natural Sciences, Lancaster University,
Lancaster LA1 4YQ, UK

Graham M. Mead DM, FRCP, FRCR
Department of Medical Oncology, Royal South Hants
Hospital, Brinton's Terrace, off St Mary's Road,
Southampton SO14 0YG, UK

Gillian Mitchell MRCP, FRCR
Department of Cancer Genetics, Institute of Cancer
Research and Royal Marsden Hospital, Downs Road,
Sutton, Surrey SM2 5PT, UK

Tariq I. Mughal MB, MD, MRCP, MRCS, FACP
CRC Department of Medical Oncology, Royal Preston
Hospital, Sharoe Green Lane North, Preston PR2 4QF, UK

Alastair J. Munro MB, FRCP(E), FRCR
Department of Radiation Oncology, Ninewells Hospital
and Medical School, Dundee DD1 9SY, UK

Guy F. Nash MB BS, FRCS
Department of Gastrointestinal Surgery, Imperial College
School of Medicine, Hammersmith Hospital,
Du Cane Road, London W12 0NN, UK

Anne Naysmith FRCP
Pembridge Palliative Care Centre, St Charles Hospital,
Exmoor Street, London W10 6DZ, UK

Marianne C. Nicolson BSc, MD, FRCP
Anchor Unit, Aberdeen Royal Infirmary, Foresterhill,
Aberdeen AB25 2ZN, UK

Mary E.R. O'Brien MD, MRCP
Department of Medicine, Royal Marsden Hospital,
Downs Road, Sutton, Surrey SM2 5PT, UK

J. Roger Owen MB BS, FRCP, FRCR
GI Oncology Centre, Cheltenham General Hospital,
Sandford Road, Cheltenham GL53 7AN, UK

Hardev S. Pandha PhD, MRCP, FRACP
Division of Medical Oncology, St George's Hospital
Medical School, Cranmer Terrace, London SW17 0RE, UK

Richard T. Penson MD, MRCP
Department of Haematology–Oncology,
Massachusetts General Hospital, Blossom Street,
Boston, MA 02114, USA

Sir Richard Peto FRS, Hon MRCP
Clinical Trial Service Unit and Epidemiological Studies
Unit, University of Oxford, Oxford, UK

P. Nicholas Plowman MA, MD, FRCP, FRCR
Department of Radiotherapy, St Bartholomew's Hospital,
West Smithfield, London EC1A 7BE, UK

Vanessa A. Potter BSc, MRCP, PhD
CRC Department of Clinical Oncology, Nottingham City
Hospital, Hucknall Road, Nottingham NG5 1PB, UK

Christopher G.A. Price MD, FRCP
Bristol Haematology and Oncology Centre, Horfield Road,
Bristol BS2 8ED, UK

Pat Price MA, MD, FRCP, FRCR
Academic Department of Radiation Oncology,
Christie Hospital, Wilmslow Road, Withington,
Manchester M20 4BX, UK

Roy Rampling PhD, FRCR, FRCP, MB BS
Beatson Oncology Centre, Western Infirmary,
Dumbarton Road, Glasgow G11 6NT, UK

Graham Read MA, MRCP, FRCR
Royal Preston Hospital, Sharoe Green Lane North,
Preston PR2 9HT, UK

Gareth J.G. Rees FRCP, FRCR
Bristol Haematology and Oncology Centre, Horfield Road,
Bristol BS2 8ED, UK

Andrew E. Rosenberg MD
Massachusetts General Hospital, Boston, MA,
Harvard Medical School, Boston, MA 02114, USA

Daniel Rosenthal MD, FACR
Harvard Medical School, Cambridge Street,
Boston, MA 02114, USA

Tarun Sabharwal MB BCh, FRCSI, FRCR
Department of Radiology, First Floor, Lambeth Wing,
St Thomas' Hospital, Lambeth Palace Road,
London SE1 7EH, UK

Diana Samson BSc, MD, FRCP, FRCPath
Department of Haematology, Imperial College School of
Medicine, Hammersmith Hospital, Du Cane Road,
London W12 0NN, UK

Michele I. Saunders MD, FRCP, FRCR
Marie Curie Research Wing, Mount Vernon Hospital,
Northwood, Middlesex HA6 2RN, UK

Michael J. Seckl PhD, MRCP
Department of Medical Oncology, Charing Cross Hospital,
Fulham Palace Road, London W6 8RF, UK

Karol Sikora MB, PhD, FRCP, FRCR
Imperial College School of Medicine, Hammersmith
Hospital, Du Cane Road, London W12 0NN, UK

Maurice L. Slevin MD, FRCP
Department of Medical Oncology, St Bartholomew's
Hospital, West Smithfield, London EC1A 7BE, UK

Howard M. Smedley MB BS, Kibd, FRCR
Department of Clinical Oncology, Kent and Canterbury
Hospital, Ethelbert Road, Canterbury, Kent CT1 5NG, UK

W. Pat Soutter MSc, MD, FRCOG
Department of Obstetrics and Gynaecology, Imperial
College Faculty of Medicine, Hammersmith Hospital,
Du Cane Road, London W12 0HS, UK

James F. Spicer MRCP
The Breakthrough Tony Robins Breast Cancer Research
Centre, Institute of Cancer Research, Mary-Jean Mitchell
Green Building, Chester Beatty Laboratories,
Fulham Road, London SW3 6JB, UK

Ira J. Spiro* MD
Formerly Department of Radiation Oncology,
Massachusetts General Hospital, Boston, MA,
Harvard Medical School, Boston, MA 02114, USA

Nicholas D. Stafford MB, FRCS
Academic Surgical Unit, University of Hull School of
Medicine, Alderson House, Hull Royal Infirmary,
Anlaby Road, Hull HU3 2JZ, UK

Herman D. Suit MD, DPhil
Department of Radiation Oncology, Massachusetts
General Hospital, Boston, MA 02114, USA

Diana M. Tait MD, FRCP, FRCR
Department of Radiotherapy, The Royal
Marsden Hospital, Downs Road, Sutton,
Surrey SM2 5PT, UK

Denis C. Talbot BSc, MA, PhD, FRCP
ICRF Medical Oncology Unit, The Churchill Hospital,
Old Road, Headington, Oxford OX3 7LJ, UK

Nicholas Thatcher MB BChir, PhD, FRCP, MRCP, DMRT, DCH
CRC Department of Medical Oncology,
Christie CRC Research Centre, Christie Hospital
NHS Trust, Wilmslow Road, Withington,
Manchester M20 9BX, UK

Hilary Thomas MA, PhD, MB BS, MRCP, FRCR
St. Luke's Cancer Centre, Royal Surrey County Hospital,
Egerton Road, Guildford, Surrey GU2 5XX, UK

Paul A. Vasey MSc, MD, MRCP
CRC Department of Medical Oncology, West of Scotland
Clinical Trials Unit, Beatson Oncology Centre, E Block,
Western Infirmary, Glasgow G11 6NT, UK

Clare C. Vernon MA, FRCR
Department of Clinical Oncology, Hammersmith Hospital,
Du Cane Road, London W12 0NN, UK

Louiza Vini MD, FRCR
Radiotherapy Department, Diavalkaniko Medical Centre,
Askipiou 10, Pylaia, 570 01, Thessalonika, Greece

Jonathan Waxman BSc, MD, MB BS, FRCP
Department of Cancer Medicine, Faculty of Medicine,
Imperial College of Science, Technology and Medicine,
Hammersmith Campus, Du Cane Road,
London W12 0NN, UK

Paula Wells PhD, MRCP, FRCR
Department of Clinical Oncology, St Bartholomew's
Hospital, West Smithfield, London EC1A 7BE, UK

Keith Wheatley DPhil
University of Birmingham Clinical Trials Unit,
Somerset Road, Edgbaston, Birmingham B15 2RR, UK

Jeremy S. Whelan MD, MRCP
The Meyerstein Institute of Oncology, The Middlesex
Hospital, UCL Hospitals NHS Trust, Mortimer Street,
London W1N 8AA, UK

Robin C.N. Williamson MD, FRCS
Department of Gastrointestinal Surgery,
Imperial College School of Medicine,
Hammersmith Hospital, Du Cane Road,
London W12 0NN, UK

Penella J. Woll MB BS, PhD, BMedSc, MRCP, JCHMT, FRCP
CRC Department of Clinical Oncology, University of
Nottingham, City Hospital, Hucknall Road,
Nottingham NG5 1PB, UK

John Yarnold MRCP, FRCR
Department of Radiotherapy, The Royal Marsden NHS Trust,
Downs Road, Sutton, Surrey SM2 5PT, UK

*Deceased.

Historical foreword

Cancer has been present since time immemorial, before man himself had developed; sarcomas have been seen in bones of dinosaurs and of our predecessor *Pithecanthropus erectus*. We have feared cancer especially after it was first recognized by Hippocrates (*c.* 460–370 BC), and named by Galen of Pergamon (AD 129–216).

Surgery was the natural first treatment, and was usually extensive and often mutilating, even more so after anaesthesia came into use in the nineteenth century; but, unfortunately for the patient, recurrence was frequent. The many drugs and medicines available were of little avail, even when caustics were applied. Then X-rays were discovered in 1895, and radium in 1898, and soon each began to be used with some success. Nevertheless the energy of the rays was low, in kilovolts only, and their use in cancer treatment was of lasting benefit against no more than basal and squamous cell skin cancers. Radium, however, was soon found to have remarkable value when inserted into tumours of the uterus and when implanted into superficial and accessible cancers. Replication of treatments necessarily required definition and measurement of units – the röntgen, rad and gray for dose; and the curie and becquerel for activity. Methods and results were steadily improved up to the 1930s. Therapy units had then become available to produce X-rays of energy as high as 500 kV, and two of these were constructed in series to make the first million volt machine, installed in St. Bartholomew's Hospital in 1938; 'Megavoltage X-ray therapy' had begun, but only in one privileged centre.

The Second World War intervened for six long years, from 1939 to 1945, with peace coming in the Far East only after the atomic bombs were dropped. Artificial radioactive isotopes then became freely available, not only those such as iodine-131 and phosphorus-32 but more importantly cobalt-60, emitting megavoltage γ-rays. Sources were constructed with activities of tens and hundreds of curies, far more than even the largest radium 'bombs'. These were, first of all, placed into teleradium housings, with great benefit, and soon into purpose-built 'cobalt units', operating at 80 or 100 cm source–skin distances. In 1952 an even better unit arrived – the linear accelerator, operating at 4 Mev or more. This was truly revolutionary – with the help of wedge filters and good planning one could now treat deep tumours anywhere within the body; there was also no skin reaction, which had long been an unpleasant side-effect limiting prescribed dosage. The 'LA', as it became known, had also been achieved as a result of wartime research – at the heart of the linear accelerator was a high-power electron source, the magnetron, which had been developed at the Malvern Telecommunications and Radar Establishment for use in radar equipment. Within a few years megavoltage treatment became available everywhere.

One other revolutionary discovery had also come from the war: nitrogen mustard had been shown to be sensationally effective against Hodgkin's disease in about 1948, and then bleomycin in 1972 against squamous carcinoma. More drugs followed, together with more hormones, particularly tamoxifen. They began to be used in combinations, and chemotherapy joined surgery and radiotherapy as another ally against cancer.

The first edition of *Treatment of Cancer* was published in 1982, at this time it was sorely needed. After the Second World War, two texts had been published, from David Smithers in London in 1946 describing X-ray therapy, and Ralston Paterson in Manchester in 1948 (second edition in 1963) comprehensively covering both X-ray and radium treatment. These were followed in 1955 by Rock Carling, Windeyer and Smithers' *British practice in radiotherapy*, and Ronald Raven's *Cancer* in 1960. By the 1970s these were beginning to become out of date. I began planning my own book in 1977. The first edition was well received and a second edition was requested after I had retired and had begun work for 2 years in Hong Kong. Karol Sikora kindly took over as joint editor for the second edition, published in 1990, bringing in molecular biology, oncogenes, sensitizers, hyperthermia and AIDS. Pat Price joined him as editor for the third edition in 1995, by which time cost-efficiency, genetics and audit needed further space.

Yet more is to come, I am looking forward with much pleasure to the publication of the fourth edition.

Keith Halnan, FRSE

Preface

Cancer is an increasingly common problem: by the year 2020, it is likely that one in two of the global population will develop the disease at some time. This striking increase is mainly due to an increasingly ageing population. The treatment of cancer is therefore a vital component of modern healthcare provision.

Oncology crosses the traditional boundaries in which medicine is taught, researched and practised, thereby providing a great challenge for those involved in its treatment. It is a truly multidisciplinary subject. One of the current dogmas, almost a cliché, is the importance of integration and teamwork between those involved in its management: surgeons, radiotherapists, medical oncologists and a myriad of other organ-based specialists. But the most exciting discoveries of the past two decades have been in the laboratory. Our understanding of the process of growth control and its deregulation has gone through a remarkable transformation, with the discovery of oncogenes, tumour suppressor genes and their encoded products. Coupled with the tremendous advances in imaging and the likely explosion in our understanding of the genome, we are set for a dramatic improvement in cancer therapy over the next decade.

This book attempts to synthesize in one place scientific discoveries together with the best of current practice. Tumours of all kinds, common and esoteric, are considered so that authoritative help on how best to manage an individual patient can be found rapidly. Our authors come from many disciplines, to paint as broad a canvas as possible of oncological knowledge. Many are associated in some way with the Hammersmith Hospital, but we have also invited colleagues from the UK and abroad to share with us their special expertise. In many cases we have teamed a surgeon with an oncologist to give a complete overview of the management of an individual tumour type.

The book is divided into three parts. The first section considers the principles of cancer treatment and the likely developments that will take place over the next decade. The contributors here are active participants in current research programmes in their area. The second and main part – practice – is an extensive series of chapters covering every individual class of tumour. They represent the distillation of considerable experience from senior clinicians. For many tumours, such as early carcinoma of the larynx, treatment has become standardized as well as successful. For others, such as breast cancer, there is considerable controversy. We have given more space to those tumours where controversy reigns, for it is here that difficulties in management are most likely to arise. We have used some diplomatic editing, with the agreement of the authors, to make their management plans widely applicable. In this way we hope the book will provide sufficient guidance to point the way to the best contemporary treatment protocols for individual patient care throughout the world.

The final section – management – gives further essential detail on the general problems of caring for the cancer patient. Here we consider medical problems that commonly arise, and also the development of continuing care philosophies which have revolutionized the management of those patients for whom no cure is yet available. We consider radiotherapy planning techniques as well as new developments in conformal planning. We review medical audit and clinical trials, both essential tools of progress in an emerging discipline. We also consider complementary medicine and cancer, for the first time, we believe, in an orthodox oncology text.

We have been greatly helped by the expertise of our contributors, who have produced such excellent manuscripts. We are indebted to Sandie Coward for her skilled assistance in co-ordinating and organizing the chapters, as well as her secretarial expertise. We hope that this multiauthor text will pave the way for this exciting branch of medicine as we enter the new millennium.

Pat Price
Christie Hospital, Manchester

Karol Sikora
Hammersmith Hospital, London

Acknowledgement

The editors gratefully acknowledge the invaluable guidance given by Dr Keith Halnan in planning this edition and for his insight as the originator of this book.

Radiation units

SI (Système Internationale) units have been in use in Britain since 1986. Their introduction in the European Economic Community (EEC) had been authorized since 1978. In many other parts of the world, such as the USA, there are no plans yet for change. A table of conversion is given below.

Measurement	Name unit and symbol	In other SI units	Old unit and symbol	Relationship old to new units
Exposure	–	C/kg	röntgen (R)	$1\,R = 2.58 \times 10^{-4}\,C/kg$
Absorbed dose	gray (Gy)	J/kg	rad (rad)	$1\,rad = 0.01\,Gy$
Dose equivalent	sievert (Sv)	J/kg	rem (rem)	$1\,rem = 0.01\,Sv$
Activity	becquerel (Bq)	s^{-1}	curie (Ci)	$1\,Ci = 3.7 \times 10^{10}\,Bq$

The table below gives the prefixes to be used with SI units.

Multiples			Sub-multiples		
Factor	Prefix	Symbol	Factor	Prefix	Symbol
10^{18}	exa	E	10^{-1}	deci	d
10^{15}	peta	P	10^{-2}	centi	c
10^{12}	tera	T	10^{-3}	milli	m
10^{9}	giga	G	10^{-6}	micro	μ
10^{6}	mega	M	10^{-9}	nano	n
10^{3}	kilo	k	10^{-12}	pico	p
10^{2}	necto	h	10^{-15}	femto	f
10^{1}	deca	da	10^{-18}	atto	a

Principles

Introduction

KAROL SIKORA

This book is written by many authors around one common theme – the optimal treatment of cancer. The problem at first seems relatively simple. There are about 10^{13} cells in the human body. From the fertilized egg to death in old age, a human being is the product of 10^{16} cell divisions. Like all complex systems, growth control can go wrong, resulting in the loss of normal territorial restraint, producing a family of cells that can multiply indefinitely. But it is not just the local growth of tumour cells that makes them so lethal. It is their spread, directly through invasion and by metastases to other sites of the body. Tumours that remain localized can usually be cured by surgery or radiotherapy, even when enormous. Patients with large, eroding basal cell skin cancers, for example, can be treated successfully, as these tumours seldom invade deep into the skin or spread to lymph nodes. Yet a breast lump less than 1 cm in diameter, which causes the patient no problems and is picked up in a screening clinic, can be lethal if metastases have already arisen from the primary site. It is this spread that provides the plethora of clinical problems that arise. Just as no two individuals are alike, no two tumours behave in exactly the same way, although we can make some broad generalizations from clinical experience. The physical and psychological interaction of a patient with a growing cancer, requires careful analysis and action by those involved in their care.

Cancer is not universally fatal. Tremendous advances have been made in the treatment of leukaemia, lymphoma, testicular cancer, choriocarcinoma and several other rare tumours, where cure of even widespread disease is now common. Even with lung cancer, the most common single tumour type throughout the world, about 8 per cent of patients will survive for many years to die of other causes. Although there are some pointers, we do not understand why this 8 per cent should be spared. If they can be cured, why not the rest?

Vast sums of money are currently spent worldwide on research, and yet for most common tumours there has been little change in overall cure rates over the past 30 years. As an intellectual problem to the scientist, malignant disease has always appeared eminently soluble. After all, it would seem a relatively straightforward task to identify the differences between normal and malignant cells and devise a selective destruction process. Yet we still do not know with any precision the first biochemical step that takes a cell down the road to neoplasia. The recent advances in molecular biology seem poised to rectify this and give us new avenues for clinical exploitation. But we have to treat our patients now – providing for them the best of today's technology with the skill of the caring physician.

EPIDEMIOLOGY

The global incidence of cancer is soaring due to rapidly ageing populations in most countries. By the year 2020, there will be 20 million new cancer patients each year. Seventy per cent of them will live in countries that, between them, will have less than 5 per cent of the resources for cancer control (Table 1.1). We have seen an explosion in our understanding of the disease at a molecular level and are now poised to see some very significant advances in prevention, screening and treatment.

Dramatic technological change is likely in surgery, radiotherapy and chemotherapy, leading to increased cure rates, but at a price (Imperial Cancer Research Fund, 1995). The completion of the human genome project will almost certainly bring sophisticated genetic risk assessment methods requiring careful integration into existing screening programmes (Holtzman and Shapiro, 1998). Preventive strategies could considerably reduce the global disease burden at low cost; and palliative care to relieve pain and suffering should be a basic right of all cancer patients. The next 25 years will be a time of unprecedented change in the way in which we will control cancer. However, the optimal organization of prevention and detection programmes, as well as treatment services, is a universal problem in all economic environments.

The world is in a health transition. Infection as a major cause of suffering and death is giving way to new epidemics of non-communicable disorders such as cardiovascular disease, diabetes and cancer (WHO, 1998a). Different countries are in different stages of this transition, depending on their age structure and economy. Some countries are faced with a double burden with increasing infection problems compounded by surging cancer rates. This is fuelled in part by the globalization of unhealthy lifestyles (Murray and Lopez, 1996).

Cancer is often thought to be the problem of rich countries. The 1998 WHO *World Health Report* (WHO, 1998b) provides life expectancy data for 1997 and World Bank data on per capita gross national product expressed in US dollars (pcGNP US$) are available for 155 countries. *Cancer in Five Continents* (Parkin *et al.*, 1997) and the *Electronic database for cancer* (IARC/WHO, 1998) provide incidence figures for 1990 and those predicted for 2020. The incidence for men and women were analysed separately. The ratio of cancer incidence per 100 000 population in 2020 to 1990 can be compared and correlated to wealth.

Longevity and wealth

Figure 1.1 examines the relationship between life expectancy at birth for both men and women and wealth of the 155 countries. There is a clear relationship between increasing GNP and longer life. There are relatively large gains for small increases in pcGNP US$ in the poorer countries, reflecting reduced infant and childhood mortality. Above a pcGNP US$ of 1000, the proportional gain in longevity is markedly reduced. This almost certainly reflects the importance of basic measures such as vaccination, good water supply, improved health education and access to simple medical care. After this, longevity continues to increase with wealth, but increasingly slowly, reflecting the biological determinants that cause disease and death in all human populations.

There are two interesting clusters (Table 1.2). The first is of those countries where longevity is significantly less than expected for their relative wealth, with a pcGNP US$ above 2000 but a longevity of less than 60 years. These are three African countries – Namibia, Botswana and Gabon. The high level of HIV-related disease is the responsible factor (WHO, 1998b). The second cluster is of those states with a higher than expected longevity, of greater than 65 years, but a pcGNP US$ of below 1000. These 20 countries are listed in Table 1.2. Common factors are efficient public health systems, low infant and childhood mortality and an integrated primary care system: a further confounding factor is the relatively recent reduction in pcGNP US$ in these countries, caused by external factors and political change. Clearly, there is a long incubation period between the factors responsible for longevity and the outcome. Major changes over the past decade will have considerable impact over the next 25 years.

Table 1.1 *The global cancer burden*

- Current population 6 billion
  10 million new cancer patients – 6 million deaths
  50% in developing countries with 5% resources

- 2020 population 8 billion
  20 million new cancer patients – 12 million deaths
  70% in developing countries

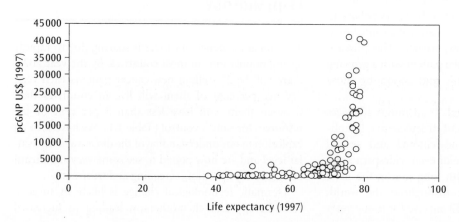

Figure 1.1 *Longevity and wealth.*

Wealth and cancer incidence

Figure 1.2 shows the relationship between wealth and cancer. There is a clear correlation between increasing wealth and cancer incidence. This is almost certainly due to the influence of tobacco and dietary factors as well as other more complex lifestyle factors, together with increased longevity of the population. Exceptions include a cluster with a pcGNP US$ of greater than 5000 and a cancer incidence of less than 150 per 100 000. These are all Arabian Gulf states (Table 1.3). This almost certainly reflects the benefit of the traditional lifestyle maintained by the majority of the population. The second cluster is of the former socialist countries of Europe, certain former Soviet Republics and South

Africa, where the cancer incidence exceeds 250 per 100 000 but the pcGNP US$ is less than 5000. This reflects increased longevity due to good public health and efficient healthcare systems, a Western lifestyle and, again, a reduction in real pcGNP US$ due to political factors.

Figure 1.3 shows the ratios of cancer incidence in 2020:1990 correlated to relative wealth. The largest changes in incidence are clearly predicted for poorer countries, with a good correlation between poverty and greatly increased incidence. Countries with the greatest increase will have the least facilities to deal with the healthcare problems posed by the disease. In many parts of the world, patients usually present with late-stage disease, not amenable to simple surgery.

Table 1.2 *Longevity and wealth*

Longevity lower than expected: pcGNP US$ >2000, longevity <60 years	Longevity higher than expected: pcGNP US$ <1000, longevity >65 years
Namibia Botswana Gabon	Egypt, Trinidad, Honduras, Nicaragua, Vietnam, Mongolia, Indonesia, China, Surinam, Kyrgistan, Sri Lanka, Tajikstan, Turkmenistan, Uzbekistan, Armenia, Georgia, Azerbaijan, Albania, Macedonia, Solomon Islands

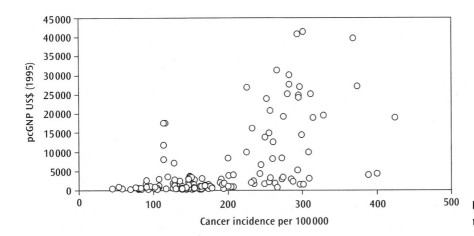

Figure 1.2 *Cancer incidence and wealth.*

Table 1.3 *Cancer incidence and wealth*

Lower incidence than expected: pcGNP US$ >5000, incidence <150 per 100 000	Higher incidence than expected: pcGNP US$ <5000, incidence >250 per 100 000
Kuwait, Quatar, Saudi Arabia, Bahrain, United Arab Emirates	Bulgaria, Czech Republic, Hungary, Poland, Romania, Russian Federation, Kazakstan, Belarus, Slovakia, Ukraine, Estonia, Croatia, South Africa, Albania

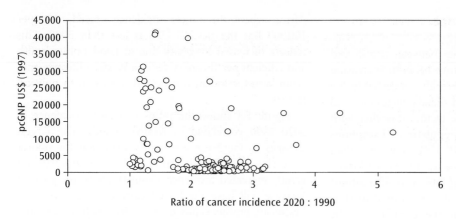

Figure 1.3 *Change in cancer incidence by 2020.*

PREVENTION

Tobacco

Optimal use of current knowledge could reduce the overall cancer incidence by at least 3 million. Tobacco control is the most urgent need (Doll and Peto, 1985). We need to look for long-term solutions here. The politics of tobacco is a complex conspiratorial web of industrialists, farmers, manufacturers, politicians and the pensions business, all looking after their own interests (Taylor, 1984). Reduce cigarette consumption in many countries and the economy simply collapses. Governments are naturally cautious. In democracies they are subject to intense lobbying. In less democratic societies corruption, using the massive profits generated by the industry, usually achieves the desired end point. Advertising blatantly exploits the young of the developing world, associating images of sex, success and wealth with cigarettes as a lifestyle marker. The solutions are complex and require considerable political will. But with forceful and concerted international action against cigarette promotion, we could reduce cancer incidence by 20 per cent by the year 2020.

Diet

Dietary modification could result in a further 30 per cent reduction across the board. The problem is in refining the educational message and getting it right in different communities. Changing our current high-fat, low-fibre diet, with its low fruit and vegetable intake, is a common theme for cancer prevention. But many features of the modern Western diet are now being adapted globally as branded fast food makers seek out new markets. Again, political will is necessary to reduce the costs to the public of healthy foods. We need to get more data so that we can make firmer recommendations. The European Prospective Investigation into Cancer and Nutrition (EPIC) study currently in progress is a good example, where painstaking data and serum collection from 400 000 Europeans could, over the years, provide a vast resource for investigating

Table 1.4 *Common dietary guidelines for cancer prevention*

- Avoid animal fat
- Increase fibre intake
- Reduce red meat consumption
- Increase fruit and vegetable intake
- Avoid obesity and stay fit

prospectively the complex interrelationships between diet and cancer (Riboli and Kaaks, 1997). Cancer incidence varies enormously across Europe, providing an excellent natural laboratory for such studies. Interventional epidemiology using rigorously controlled studies could produce the evidence that could lead to major changes. The current problem is the difficulty in making dietary advice specific and, in some countries, affordable. Although several groups have produced guidelines, there are so far few data about their uptake or significance in large populations. Table 1.4 provides a summary of the main consensus from several sources.

Infection

Infection causes around 15 per cent of cancer worldwide and is potentially preventable (Table 1.5). This proportion is greater in the developing world, where an estimated 22 per cent of cancer has an infectious cause (Pisani *et al.*, 1997). Hepatitis B immunization in children has significantly reduced the incidence of infection in China, Korea and West Africa. Shortly we will see if it has reduced the incidence of hepatoma, which begins in endemic regions by the third decade of life. The unconfirmed trends are already encouraging (Chang *et al.*, 1997). Cancer of the cervix, the most common cancer of women in parts of India and South America, is clearly associated with certain subtypes of human papillomavirus. Vaccines are now becoming available and entering trial (Monsonego and Franca, 1996). *Helicobacter pylori* is associated with stomach cancer. Here, without any intervention, there has been a remarkable downward

Table 1.5 *Infection and cancer*

Infection	Associated cancer
Hepatitis B virus (HBV)	Hepatoma
Human papillomavirus (HPV)	Cervix, anus
Helicobacter pylori	Stomach
Epstein–Barr virus (EBV)	Lymphoma, nasopharynx
Human immunodeficiency virus (HIV)	Kaposi's sarcoma, lymphoma
Schistosomiasis	Bladder
Liver fluke	Cholangiocarcinoma

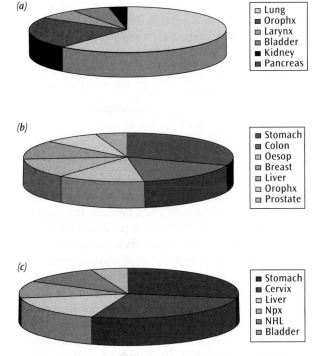

Figure 1.4 *Global causes of cancer: (a) tobacco; (b) diet; (c) infection. Orophx, oropharynx; Oesop, oesophagus; Npx, nasopharynx; NHL, non-Hodgkin's lymphoma.*

cancer-causing factors which, between them, are responsible for 7.5 out the 10 million new patients annually. Targeted prevention programmes are very cost effective and can be shared by different countries with similar cancer patterns. Countries with limited resources need not keep reinventing the wheel. Prevention packages can be tailored and adapted widely. To do this we need good data of incidence in relation to geography. Descriptive epidemiology provides a fertile hunting ground for patterns of carcinogenesis. Relating genetic changes in cancer to their cause and geography – the emerging discipline of molecular epidemiology – will complete the circle and point the way to specific interventions. The future of prevention will almost surely be about using such techniques to carefully target preventive strategies to those who would benefit most. In the post-genomic era it is likely that cancer prevention programmes, at least in developed countries, will be completely individualized – a combination of environmental and lifestyle data will be used to construct very specific personalized messages.

SCREENING

Cancer screening is one of the great controversies of medicine. At the interface between public health and specialist care, economics create tensions between professional groups, politicians and the public – a screening test may be cheap, but applying it to a population (with rigorous quality control and effective processing of patients with abnormal results) creates a huge workload and therefore cost. Screening can also have psychological effects on individuals with false-positive results who require investigation but are eventually found not to have cancer.

Unless screening can be shown to reduce the mortality from a specific cancer, the money used is better spent on improving care, and this has led to a disparity in screening recommendations between countries. The human genome project is likely to provide new approaches to cancer risk assessment and will bring new challenges to this complex area. Cancer screening is defined as the systematic application of a test to individuals who have

trend in incidence worldwide. Dissecting out the complex factors involved, including food storage, contamination, preparation and content, is a considerable challenge. Other cancer-causing infections are schistosomiasis, the liver fluke, the human T-cell leukaemia virus and the ubiquitous hepatitis B virus. Although geographically localized, their prevention by lifestyle changes and vaccination programmes are realistic short-term goals. Clearly the effectiveness of any infection control or immunization programme at reducing the cancer burden will depend on many factors and requires careful research and field evaluation.

Targeting

The key to success in cancer prevention is careful targeting. Figure 1.4 shows estimates of the three main reversible not sought medical attention because of symptoms. It may be opportunistic (offered to patients consulting their doctor for another reason) or population-based (covering a predefined age range, with elaborate call and recall systems). The risk of dying from a cancer increases with its degree of spread, or stage; thus, the aim of screening is to detect cancer in its early, asymptomatic phase. The problem is that many screening tests are relatively crude, and cancers may have metastasized before they are detected.

Sensitivity varies between tests. A 100 per cent sensitive test detects all cancers in the screened population. The most rigorous means of calculating sensitivity is to determine the proportion of expected cancers not presenting as interval cases between screens. Good cancer registration is essential when making this calculation. *Specificity* is the proportion of negative results produced by a test in individuals without neoplasia. A 100 per cent specific test gives no false-positive results. Investigation of patients without cancer is a major factor in the cost of screening.

Advantages and disadvantages of screening

The advantages and disadvantages of screening (Table 1.6) must be considered carefully; they vary between cancers and tests. The three main problems in assessing the benefit of any screening test for cancer are lead-time bias, length bias and selection bias, all of which impair the effectiveness of screening as a method of reducing cancer mortality. *Lead-time bias* advances the diagnosis but does not prolong survival, as occurs when the disease has already metastasized although the primary tumour is still small – patients die at the same time as they would have if the disease had not been detected early. *Length bias* results in diagnosis of less aggressive tumours. Rapidly growing cancers with a poorer prognosis present in the screening interval, reducing the value of the screening process. *Selection bias* occurs even in the best-organized healthcare systems. Worried but healthy individuals (who would present with cancer symptoms early) comply with screening, whereas less well-educated and socially disadvantaged individuals do not. In the UK NHS breast cancer screening programme, compliance rates vary between communities, depending on their relative deprivation.

Developing a screening programme

Rational decision-making about cancer screening requires a detailed analysis of factors that may vary between populations (Sikora, 1999). The cancer should be common and its natural history should be properly understood. This allows a realistic prediction of the proposed test's likely value. The test should be effective (high sensitivity and specificity) and should be acceptable to the population. Cervical smears, for example, are difficult to perform in many Islamic countries where women prefer not to undergo vaginal examination, and the take-up rate for colonoscopy is low in asymptomatic individuals because it is uncomfortable and sometimes unpleasant. The healthcare system must be able to cope with patients who produce positive results and require investigation. This may be a particular problem at the start of a population-based study. Ultimately, screening must improve the survival rate in a randomized controlled setting. The natural history of many cancers (including incidence and mortality) may change over time for reasons that are poorly understood. In Europe, the incidence of stomach cancer has decreased dramatically over the past few decades, whereas breast cancer deaths reached a peak in the UK in 1989 and have decreased slightly each year since.

Lobby groups often exercise political pressure to implement screening programmes (even when their effectiveness is undemonstrated), and manufacturers of equipment or suppliers of reagents may exercise commercial pressure. In a fee-for-service-based provider system, there is a financial inducement for doctors to investigate because doing nothing earns no money. The launch of the NHS breast screening service by the UK government in 1989 was viewed by many as a pre-election vote-winning exercise rather than a rational public health intervention, and there are now similar pressures to introduce prostate cancer screening, though uncertainty remains about the management of men with slightly elevated prostate-specific antigen (PSA).

Many groups (e.g. governmental organizations, medical charities, health maintenance organizations, professional

Table 1.6 *Advantages and disadvantages of screening*

Advantages	Disadvantages
Better outcome	Longer morbidity if prognosis unaltered
Less radical therapy	Overtreatment of borderline abnormalities
Reassurance for those with negative results	False reassurance for false positives
Psychological benefit to population	Unnecessary investigation
Attractive to politicians	Risks of screening test
Savings because therapy is less complex	Resource costs of screening system

bodies) have produced guidelines on cancer screening. These guidelines vary widely between countries, reflecting bias in interpretation of evidence and cultural values in the practice of medicine; for example, annual PSA testing and digital rectal examination in men over 50 years of age are recommended by the American Cancer Society, but are not advocated in most other countries. The incidence of a particular cancer in a particular country and the economics of screening must be considered carefully – the cost of the technology required must correspond with the gain. Low-cost, direct inspection techniques for oral and cervical cancer by non-professional health workers seem attractive in achieving tumour downstaging and hence better survival results, but cervicoscopy programmes in India and China have shown surprisingly poor overall effectiveness (Sankaranarayanan et al., 1998). It remains to be seen whether intra-vital staining with acetic acid can enhance specificity at little extra cost. A major cost in instituting any screening procedure is informing the public and then developing the logistics, often under difficult geographical conditions. Cultural barriers may be insurmountable without better education, particularly of girls, who as mothers will become responsible for family health.

Low-technology tests have low specificity: as a result, hard-pressed secondary-care facilities are inundated with patients with non-life-threatening abnormalities. Detailed field assessment, preferably in a randomized setting, is essential before firm recommendations can be made, but political factors often interfere with this process (Goodman et al., 1946). The well-meaning charitable donation of second-hand mammography units to some African countries has led to haphazard introduction of breast screening in populations in which the incidence of breast cancer is low and where there are few resources to deal with abnormal results.

Assessing the benefits of screening programmes

The ultimate measure of success in a screening programme is a demonstrable reduction in mortality in the screened population. This requires large numbers of individuals, however, and at least 10 years' assessment in most of the common cancers. Although randomized studies may show conclusive benefit, it must be remembered that the expertise and professional enthusiasm available to a study population may be considerably greater than that achievable under subsequent field conditions. Quality of mammography interpretation and investigation of breast abnormalities are good examples of this, and may explain the relatively disappointing results of breast screening in practice. Case-control studies using age-matched individuals from the same population and non-randomized comparison between areas providing and not providing screening may give useful indicators, but are not as conclusive as randomized trials.

Surrogate measures of effectiveness can be used to assess a programme with relatively small numbers of patients soon after its implementation, but are insufficient to prove that screening saves lives. When a population is first screened, a higher than expected incidence of cancer should be seen because screening is detecting cancer that would not present with symptoms for several years. Subsequent rounds of screening are less productive. Tumour downstaging is a second measure of impact. An increase in early stage cancer detection and, consequently, reduction in advanced disease are expected over 3–5 years. The third, short-term evaluation is a comparison of the survival of screen-detected patients with that of those presenting symptomatically. Success in terms of these three indices may not necessarily be translated into a useful screening programme. In the 1970s, a study of routine chest radiography and sputum cytology to detect lung cancer showed a 5-year survival of 40 per cent in screen-detected patients compared with an overall figure of 5 per cent, but a reduction in mortality from lung cancer in large populations has not been seen.

DIAGNOSIS

Cancer presents with a myriad of symptoms depending on the site, size and growth pattern of the tumour. Although some symptoms alarm patients more than others, there is tremendous variability in the speed at which cancer can be diagnosed. A lump can be biopsied, but many deep-seated tumours present late, long after they have already spread. Most patients have actually been harbouring the cancer for several years before it becomes apparent.

Trying to speed up the diagnostic process and to get on with definitive treatment makes good sense. But delays plague all healthcare systems. In Britain the current obsession is to get all patients with cancer-related symptoms seen within 2 weeks. This was a politically inspired to show something could be achieved quickly. The problem is defining what constitutes a cancer-related symptom – there are just so many. Studies show that having two queues for entry into the hospital system – one urgent and one not – leads to either excess system capacity or serious delays in the slow queue. Forming a unified entry system and shortening it makes more sense. A far bigger problem is getting a complex series of investigations performed with a reasonable start time for definitive therapy. Attempts to do this have been hampered by the poor information technology systems, which are fragmented, non-communicative and primitive. In an age when a WAP cellphone can be used to instantly book a complex travel itinerary, including hotels and opera tickets, it is a huge indictment that a GP in many parts of the world cannot fix a hospital appointment for a potential cancer patient without posting a letter.

The two drivers of the improvement of cancer diagnosis are imaging and biomarkers. The past two decades have seen a massive rise in the use of computed tomography (CT) and magnetic resonance imaging (MRI) scans to outline beautifully and in great detail the anatomy of a cancer and its surrounding normal structures. Positron emission tomography, in which a molecule is labelled with a radioactive marker, allows us to examine the living biochemistry of the body. The future of imaging lies in coupling high-definition structural information with real-time functional change. In this way the precise effects of a drug or other treatment can be monitored in three dimensions. It is also likely that the telecom revolution will produce new devices for examining the interior compartments of the body without causing distress to the patient.

Biomarkers are biochemical changes produced by the presence of a cancer. They may be synthesized directly by the cancer, such as prostate-specific antigen (PSA), or represent a complex change in an organ system, such as abnormal liver function tests caused by liver metastases. As we understand more about the molecular abnormalities that lead to cancer, through the science of genomics and proteomics, novel biomarkers will be identified. These will not only give us the ability to diagnose cancer at an earlier stage but also to predict the likely natural history of the cancer – whether it will spread rapidly or invade neighbouring structures. This information will be essential for planning optimal care. The basic tests are likely to be converted to kits sold in pharmacies. It is possible that a cancer screening kit for the four major cancers will be on sale within the next decade. Already there is great variation in the practice of cancer screening in different countries. It is likely that the availability of commercial kits will increase consumerism. There will be a rise in cancer screening and prevention clinics in the private sector, almost certainly attached to the 'cancer hotels' of the future.

Looking further forward, it is likely that continuous monitoring for potentially dangerous mutations will be possible. Up-market car engines have systems to measure performance against baseline, sending a signal to the driver if a problem arises. Implanted devices to identify genomic change and signal abnormalities to a home computer may well allow the detection of cancer well before any metastasis. It will be essential to carry out careful outcome research on such new diagnostic and screening techniques to validate their benefits.

SURGERY

Cancer surgery has been a dramatic success. Effective cancer surgery began in the late nineteenth century, when it was realized that tumours could be removed along with their regional lymph nodes. This enhanced

Table 1.7 *Future of surgery*

- Organ conservation
- Minimally invasive surgery
- Robotic surgery
- Distance surgery
- Tailored adjuvant approaches
- Biopsy only for many cancers
- All fast tracked – next day service

the chances of complete cure, as it had the greatest possibility of avoiding any spread of the cancer. Surgery still remains the single most effective modality for cancer treatment. Increasingly it has become far more conservative, able to retain organs and structures and, in turn, maintain good function in many parts of the body. Breast cancer is an excellent example. The radical mastectomy performed until 30 years ago left women with severe deformity of the chest wall. This was replaced, first, by the less-mutilating simple mastectomy and, now, by simple excision followed by radiotherapy. The breast remains fully intact. New technology permits minimally invasive (keyhole) surgery for many cancer types. The science of robotics will allow completely automated surgical approaches with enhanced effects and minimal damage to surrounding structures. Ultimately, it is likely that surgery will disappear as an important treatment and become confined simply to biopsy performed under local anaesthetic with image guidance to check that the correct sites are biopsied (Table 1.7).

RADIOTHERAPY

Radiotherapy was first used for cancer treatment over 100 years ago. Originally, crude radium was used as the radiation source, but now we have a variety of sophisticated techniques. Modern linear accelerators – the workhorse for radiotherapy – allow precise dose delivery precisely to the shape of the tumour. Conformal therapy aims to deliver a high dose, just to the tumour volume, in three dimensions, killing the cancer cells and avoiding sensitive normal surrounding tissue. Novel computer-based imaging techniques have revolutionized our ability to understand the precise anatomy of cancer in a patient and therefore to deliver far more effective radiotherapy. The future of radiotherapy is about further computerization, with multimedia imaging and optimized conformal planning. We have also learnt to understand the biological differences between different tumours in patients and can begin to plan individualized treatment courses to optimize selective destruction. And with remarkable technological changes in imaging and computerization, continued development is essential (Table 1.8). In many parts of the world radiotherapy is the Cinderella of cancer care.

Table 1.8 *Future of radiotherapy*

- Multimedia imaging
- Robotic set-up
- Optimized conformal planning
- Biological optimization
- Designer fractionation

Table 1.9 *Chemotherapy – the current position*

High CR, high cure	High CR, low cure	Low CR, low cure
HD	AML	NSCLC
ALL	Breast	Colon
Testis	Ovary	Stomach
Choriocarcinoma	SCLC	Prostate
Childhood cancers	Sarcoma	Pancreas
BL	Myeloma	Glioma

CR, complete response; HD, Hodgkin's disease; ALL, acute lymphoblastic leukaemia; BL, Burkitt's lymphoma; AML, acute myeloid leukaemia; SCLC, small cell lung cancer; NSCLC, non-small cell lung cancer.

CHEMOTHERAPY

Chemotherapy began after the sinking of an American battleship in Bari Harbour, Italy in 1943. It was noticed the white blood count of many of the injured soldiers and sailors fell. Although shrouded in secrecy at the time, a chemical warfare agent was being carried on the battleship. This led naval physicians to treat patients with lymphoma and leukaemia who had a rising abnormal white count with the same chemical agent – nitrogen mustard. In 1946, 67 patients were reported as having had good, but brief, responses to injections of this drug (Goodman *et al.*, 1946). A new era of cancer care had begun.

The current position of chemotherapy for advanced cancer is shown in the Table 1.9. Essentially there are three groups of cancers, the first in which we can achieve a high complete response rate and a high cure rate. These include diseases such as Hodgkin's disease, childhood leukaemia and testicular cancer. Unfortunately, this group of successfully treated cancers represents less than 5 per cent of the global cancer burden. At the other end, we have a group with a low complete response and low cure rate, such as lung cancer, colon cancer and stomach cancer. So far chemotherapy has made few inroads into their treatment, although some useful palliation and prolongation of survival, sometimes for months, can be achieved. In the middle, we have a group of diseases with a high complete response but a low cure rate. These cause problems to those involved in rationing cancer care. The use of taxanes in breast and ovarian cancer is a classic example. Here high-cost drugs can achieve extension of life by several months for many patients. When deciding on priorities we have to assess how much we are willing to pay for a month of reasonable-quality life.

We are at the beginning of a revolution in cancer care. The pharmaceutical industry has taken on the new challenge and is now going through a massive transition from an era of classical chemotherapy drugs – not too dissimilar to nitrogen mustard – discovered by screening programmes for their potential to destroy cells, to a molecular targeted approach. Currently there are over 500 molecules in clinical development by 43 pharmaceutical companies. It is likely that fewer than 30 will actually make it to the marketplace, and fewer than five will make a big impact on cancer care. Increasing consolidation in the industry has resulted in a shrinking of the total number of key players in cancer drug development.

However, there has been a dramatic increase in research on molecular therapies. The Human Genome Project has created a dictionary of the genome. But we can now interrogate it through sophisticated bioinformatic systems. Not only do we have the library but we have the search tools. We can now predict the three-dimensional structural biology of many proteins and create images of drugs *in silico*, using computers to design small molecules which then can be synthesized in the laboratory to check their activity. A platform approach to drug discovery is creating a massive increase in new candidate molecules for cancer therapy.

Currently, one of the problems is the large numbers of targets that have been identified in the cell to which new drugs can be developed. These targets include growth factors, cell-surface receptors, signal transduction cog molecules, transcription factors, apoptosis stimulating proteins and cell cycle control proteins. Which one to target and to invest research funds into is a difficult decision. The total cost of bringing an anti-cancer drug to market exceeds £300 million. Well-defined targets are the starting point on the road to our future treatments. It is likely that classical cytotoxic drugs will continue to be used for the next 25 years, although they will have a declining share of the total marketplace. By 2015 successful molecular targeted approaches will overtake cytotoxics and transform cancer medicine (Fig. 1.5). These new drugs will be individualized, chosen on the basis of molecular measurements on the patient's tumour and normal cells, and taken orally for long periods of time.

The classical way in which we develop cancer drugs is split into three phases. In phase I, maximally tolerable doses are determined by gradually escalating the dose in patients with cancer. From this we can determine a workable dose that patients can tolerate and yet is likely to have a therapeutic effect based on animal studies. We then carry out phase II studies, in which a series of patients with cancers that can be easily measured by X-rays or photographs are given the drug to see what effect it has on their cancer. This allows us to determine the response rate. Phase III is the last and longest phase. Here patients are randomized to receive either the new drug or the best available treatment and their long-term survival determined.

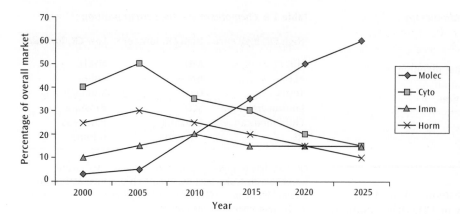

Figure 1.5 *Predicted cancer drug use: Molec, molecular targeted therapies; Cyto, cytotoxic chemotherapy; Imm, immunological approaches; Horm, hormonal agents.*

This traditional approach may not be appropriate for many of our new agents. Toxicity may be minimal and effectiveness may be greatest well below the maximally tolerated dose. Furthermore tumours may not actually shrink but just become static, so no responses are seen. As our new agents have been discovered by measuring their effect on a specific molecular target in the laboratory, it should be feasible to develop the same assay for use in patients. This gives us a short-term pharmacodynamic end point and tells us that we are achieving our molecular goals in a patient. Genomic technology has come to our aid. Gene chips allow us to examine the expression of thousands of genes simultaneously before and after administration of the drug. If a second biopsy can be obtained for the tumour, then we can compare gene expression patterns in both tumour and normal cells in the same patient after exposure to a new drug. This enables us to get the drug to work in the most effective way. A particularly intriguing approach for the future is to use gene constructs, which signal tiny light pulses when their molecular switches are affected by a drug.

We would also like to get information about how a drug becomes distributed within the body and ideally get a picture of the changes it causes in a tumour. Functional imaging allows us to do just this. The aim is to understand the living biochemistry of a drug in the body. Here we label the drug with a radioactive tracer and then image it using positron emission tomography. Such techniques promise to revolutionize our ability to understand drug activity and to select and improve on the way in which we choose anti-cancer drugs for further development.

The next decade is likely to be a new golden age for cancer drug discovery, with many novel targeted molecules coming into the clinic. These agents will eventually transform cancer care forever.

CONCLUSION

Cancer care, like the much of medicine, is in transition. The boundaries of state and individual responsibility for health are blurred. The majority of health service infrastructure is already completely privatized – the finance to build new hospitals, the cleaning, catering and security services. The remainder is highly state regulated with constant buffeting by the winds of political change. Only increasing consumerism can empower patients to make choices for their future.

We are going through a technological explosion which will allow us to prolong survival way beyond the dreams of our ancestors. The aim of medicine must now be not only to add years to life but life to years. We must strive for compressed morbidity, by which older people retain function – physical, mental and spiritual – right up to the end of their lives. Achieving good-quality life for the majority of people with cancer is on the horizon. All of us – patients, carers, politicians, healthcare professionals and the industry – have to work together to avoid the potential for financial meltdown unless careful investment is made. Ultimately it will be the patient that chooses the options and how to pay for them. We all need to work together to develop mechanisms to cope with the technological revolution going on around us.

REFERENCES

Chang, M.-H., Chen, C.J., Lai, M.S. *et al.* (1997) Universal hepatitis B vaccination in Taiwan and the incidence of hepatocellular carcinoma in children. Taiwan Childhood Hepatoma Study Group. *N. Engl. J. Med.* **336**, 1855–9.

Doll, R. and Peto, R. (1985) *The causes of cancer.* Oxford: Oxford University Press.

Goodman, L., Wintrobe, M., Dameshek, W., Goodman, M., Gilman, A. and McLennan, M. (1946) Nitrogen mustard therapy. *JAMA* **132**, 126–32.

Holtzman, N.A. and Shapiro, D. (1998) Genetic testing and public policy. *BMJ* **316**, 852–6.

IARC/WHO (1998) *Cancer in five continents. Electronic database for cancer.* Lyon: International Agency for Research on Cancer/WHO.

Imperial Cancer Research Fund (1995) *Vision 2020 for cancer*. London: Imperial Cancer Research Fund.

Monsonego, J. and Franca, E. (1996) *Cervical cancer control. General statements and guidelines.* Paris: EUROGIN.

Murray, C.T. and Lopez, A.D. (1996) *The global burden of disease.* Boston: Harvard University Press.

Parkin, D., Whelan, S., Ferlay, J., Raymond, L. and Young, J. (1997) *Cancer in five continents*, Vol. VII. Lyon: International Agency for Research on Cancer, Scientific Publications.

Pisani, P., Parkin, D.M., Munoz, N. and Ferlay, J. (1997) Cancer and infection: estimates of the attributable fraction in 1990. *Cancer Epidemiol. Biomarkers Prev.* **6**, 387–400.

Riboli, E. and Kaaks, R. (1997) European Perspective investigation into cancer and nutrition. *Int. J. Epidemiol.* **26**(suppl. 1), 6–14.

Sankaranarayanan, R., Wesley, R., Somanthan, T. *et al.* (1998) Visual inspection of the uterine cervix after the application of acetic acid in the detection of cervical carcinoma and its precursors. *Cancer* **83**, 2150–6.

Sikora, K. (1999) Developing a global strategy for cancer. *Cancer Screen. Med.* **27**, 35–9.

Taylor, P. (1984) *Smoke ring – the politics of tobacco.* London: Bodley Head.

WHO (1998a) *WHO Executive Board, EB 102.* World Health Organisation, Geneva, 1998.

WHO (1998b) *The World Health Report.* World Health Organisation, Geneva, 2000.

2

Molecular biology

KAROL SIKORA

INTRODUCTION

The past two decades have given us remarkable insights into the biology of cancer. The fine dissection of the molecular cogs that control cell growth represents a tremendous global achievement. Cancer is now recognized as a genetic disease where mutations in genes, inherited or acquired, result in the transition from a normal to a malignant growth pattern. These discoveries have come from the study of many biological systems as diverse as the fruit fly, the worm and yeast, as well as rats and mice. The pace of acquisition of genetic knowledge is now firmly on an exponential curve, due to the combination of sophisticated high-throughput tools for genetic analysis and the computational ability to retain and organize this information. The recent completion of the human genome sequence has provided a remarkable repository of information which is now being used to aid the understanding of an increasingly wide range of biological processes in both health and disease.

This remarkable dataset will further enhance the identification of proteins encoded by cancer cells, which represent novel targets for a new generation of cancer therapeutics. These newly identified molecules may be functioning as oncogenes, tumour suppressor genes, components of the cell cycle, regulators of apoptosis, cell senescence and tumour angiogenesis, or play a role in the progression of disseminated disease. Genomics, target identification and validation, assay development and computerized structure-based design will advance dramatically

in the next few years, creating a plethora of logically constructed molecules for entry into clinical trials.

The dramatic increase in the pace of discovery of new molecules with potential clinical benefit will require novel approaches for their development in the clinic. Tumour profiling, based on genetic changes, will be needed to identify those patients likely to respond to specific, logically based novel therapies. This will require integrated molecular solutions for the stratification of patients in addition to conventional histopathological criteria.

To enhance the speed of development, it will be essential to identify surrogate end points to validate the effectiveness of a potential drug. In the short term, such assays will determine the activity on a specific molecular target *in vivo* and allow the construction of dose–response curves, often in healthy volunteers. This is a radical departure from cytotoxic drug development and will require close interaction with clinical pharmacology. This approach will replace the current phase I dose-escalation schedules by which the maximum tolerated dose of a drug is determined. Once the maximally effective dose has been identified, further surrogate end points of effectiveness to halt tumour progression will be required. Such markers may include the release of specific tumour DNA fragments into serum, the quantification of novel tumour markers or the identification of downstream effects of tumour growth delay, such as apoptosis, necrosis or the interaction with local blood vessels. Biochemical markers will be sought but other approaches, such as positron emission tomography, nuclear magnetic spectroscopy and a range of innovative non-invasive imaging systems, may well provide interesting data. It is conceivable that genetic indicator systems, introduced by direct injection into tumours, could provide useful information on both the effect of the drug locally and the response of cancer cells to it. Such techniques will enhance the speed of early candidate selection dramatically and reduce the risk of later failure. They will almost certainly form part of future regulatory packages. Classical measurement of the healthcare benefit of future cytostatic agents may take several years to collect. Short-term assessment of tumour response, time to treatment failure or time to disease progression may well become inappropriate, as trials will increasingly involve patients earlier in the evolution of the natural history of their cancer. Long-term survival comparisons, together with effective quality-of-life assessment, will still be essential. Surrogate end points will accelerate the initial phases of cancer drug development and bring confidence to commercial decision-making processes prior to embarking on long-term studies.

Currently over 500 compounds are undergoing clinical trial for cancer. The past 5 years has seen a definite trend to develop drugs acting on known molecular targets, rather than the older blunderbuss approach characterized by our current therapeutic armamentarium.

THE TECHNOLOGY

Genes

Genetic information in normal and diseased cells is coded by the sequence of nucleotides within the DNA of the cell's nucleus. Genes have two functions. The first is to replicate themselves precisely. The complementary base pairing of adenine–thymine and guanine–cytosine provides the specificity required to produce identical copies of each of the single strands of a segment of DNA. DNA replication is a complex process, requiring the presence of several enzymes and cofactors. The most important of these is DNA polymerase, which induces the polymerization of the deoxyribonucleoside triphosphates. In addition to the synthetic machinery there are also 'proof reading' mechanisms to ensure fidelity of reproduction (Lindahl, 1982). These are vital functions to maintain the stability of the genome. The second function of the gene is to produce messenger RNA (mRNA), a process called transcription. The mRNA, in turn, produces protein by its translation on ribosomes.

In mammalian cells DNA is arranged in a complex structure coupled to a set of proteins; these are the histone and non-histone proteins. These proteins structure DNA into packets called nucleosomes which are, in turn, coiled up to form the chromosome (McGhee and Felsenfeld, 1980) (Fig. 2.1). Most of the DNA in a human cell is not involved in information transfer directly. It has been estimated that there are 3×10^9 base pairs in the

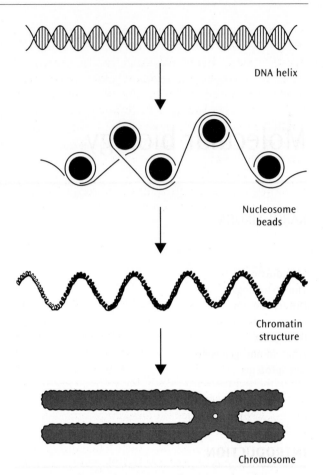

Figure 2.1 *Chromatin structure, demonstrating the remarkable packaging of DNA within chromosomes.*

genome of a human cell, of which only 10^7 are transcribed at any one time into functional mRNA. Some of the apparently redundant sequences are involved in holding the expressed sequences in the correct position for transcription and its associated control mechanisms. Some sequences may represent genetic 'junk', acquired through the millennia of evolution and locked in by the continual process of replication. These pieces of DNA may be preserved purely by maintaining a correct sequence for self-preservation: so-called 'selfish DNA' (Orgel and Crick, 1980).

There are five techniques vital to the elucidation of the biology of genes in health and disease: restriction enzyme digestion, gene cloning, polymerase chain reaction, DNA sequencing and nucleic acid hybridization. These techniques are the essential ingredients of the recombinant DNA technology. In addition, there are several techniques to measure gene expression, the most important of which is gene array hybridization – often called gene chip technology (Abbott, 1996).

Restriction enzymes

Many bacteria make enzymes that can cleave DNA at defined sites. Such enzymes recognize specific sequences

4–6 nucleotides in length and make a cut. These enzymes protect bacteria from phage infection by destroying injected phage DNA that contains the recognized sequences. Over 200 restriction enzymes have now been isolated, and can be used to identify specific sequences in any piece of DNA (Smith, 1979). By using a combination of different restriction enzymes, followed by the separation of the resultant fragments by electrophoresis on agarose gels, pieces of DNA can be compared (restriction mapping). Simple restriction enzyme digestion followed by electrophoresis can discriminate between DNA from patients with sickle-cell anaemia and their normal relatives (Orkin *et al.*, 1982).

Gene cloning

Fragments of DNA can be amplified by inserting them into a plasmid or bacteriophage vector, and growing such vectors in their bacterial hosts – a process called gene cloning. A variety of tricks is used to increase the chances of obtaining the correct clones. These include the use of antibiotic resistance markers in the vector. A marker for antibiotic resistance within the site for insertion of the piece of DNA to be cloned will allow the recombinant vectors to be identified by their sensitivity to the antibiotic.

After selection of bacterial clones containing the vector, large amounts of DNA can be collected and isolated by restriction enzymes (Fig. 2.2). A gene library consists of a large number of different clones, isolated by taking restriction fragments of a complex piece of DNA; for example, the entire human genome (Cohen, 1980). If large enough, such libraries will contain all the genes present in the DNA from which they were derived. The problem is how to index them for function. Some, of course, will be those involved in mRNA production; other clones in the library will have a control function, and yet others will be genetic junk.

An alternative strategy is to begin the cloning process by selecting only those DNA sequences that are transcribed into mRNA. Messenger RNA is extracted using an affinity column composed of cellulose linked to oligo-deoxythymidine (oligo-dT). The oligo-dT binds to the polyadenylated chains that mark the end of functional messages. Messenger RNA can be copied using the enzyme reverse transcriptase to produce cDNA ('c' stands for complementary). Single-stranded cDNA molecules can be converted into double-stranded DNA by DNA polymerase, inserted into vectors, and cloned. Using such techniques, the human genes for several protein hormones, such as insulin, somatostatin and growth hormone, have been cloned. Furthermore, by modifying the vector so that it can transcribe functional messages with its bacterial host, production of the protein can be induced in the bacteria. Genetically engineered human interferons, interleukins and various marrow support growth factors are now made in this way.

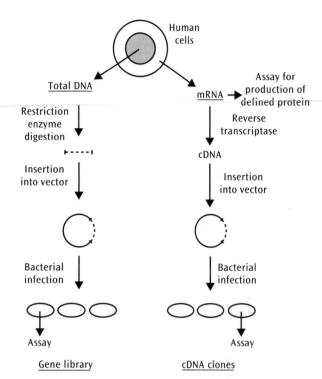

Figure 2.2 *Gene cloning by preparation of a gene library and by reverse transcription of mRNA into cDNA.*

Polymerase chain reaction

The polymerase chain reaction (PCR) was invented in the mid-1980s and has proved to be useful for a very wide range of techniques involving the manipulation of DNA. The reaction requires a double-stranded template DNA molecule, relatively high concentrations of two primers which are short (about 20 bases) DNA oligonucleotides, the four nucleotides (ATCG) and the DNA polymerase enzyme. The reaction depends on cycles of high and low temperature which dissociate the strands of the template DNA and then allow annealing (binding) of the short primers. The enzyme then catalyses the 'filling-in' of the remainder of each strand, creating a copy of the template between the two primers. This reaction is repeated up to 40 times, giving a vast amplification of the selected region of the original template. The reaction is so sensitive that a single DNA molecule may be amplified fairly readily from a cell. The technique has been used for gene cloning, detection of mutations, gene mapping, DNA fragment assembly and in many other creative and imaginative ways.

DNA sequencing

The nucleotide sequence of cloned DNA fragments can be determined simply and quickly (Sanger, 1981). We now have the precise sequence of nearly the full set of 30 000 human genes. The application of minicomputers has become an essential part in the matching of overlapping DNA sequences, obtained by analysing many clones from

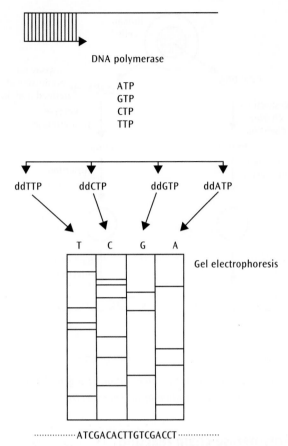

Figure 2.3 *DNA sequencing using the dideoxynucleotide method. The dideoxynucleotide stops chain elongation at the position of the relevant nucleotide.*

a single long piece of DNA (Fig. 2.3). It is now easier to sequence the amino acids in a protein by first sequencing its gene and using the genetic code as a dictionary to work back to the protein sequence.

Hybridization techniques

Once a purified piece of DNA has been isolated by cloning, the presence of complementary sequences can be detected in any other DNA source, using hybridization techniques. DNA is denatured by heating or increasing the pH. The strands fall apart, but by slowly cooling or bringing the pH back to neutral they renature or hybridize. Under appropriate conditions, hybridization can be made base-pair specific, i.e. adenine combining with thymine, or guanine with cytosine. By making a piece of cloned DNA radioactive – by using ^{32}P, for example – probes can be obtained which will identify specific sequences in mixtures of restriction fragments separated by electrophoresis.

Let us say we have a cloned probe for insulin, produced by making cDNA from mRNA obtained from pancreatic islet cells. If we now take a restriction enzyme digest of total human DNA and run this on an agarose gel the insulin gene will be located in one or more of the fragments.

By using a nitrocellulose filter we can make a replica of the gel by simple blotting. The blot can be denatured by heating, making the DNA single stranded. The radioactive probe is now added under renaturing conditions, and after a suitable time any excess probe is washed off the filter (Fig. 2.4). The position of the probe, and hence the insulin gene sequences in the original DNA sample, can be identified by autoradiography (laying a photographic film on to the filter to detect the position of the radioactivity). This technique is often called Southern blotting, after its inventor, Ed Southern. Hybridization can also be carried out to RNA immobilized on filters – Northern blotting. Specific DNA sequences can be localized within chromosomes using *in situ* hybridization. Here, the radioactive probe is added directly to squashed, fixed chromosomes in which the DNA has been denatured by exposure to high pH. Using this technique, the precise chromosomal location of a number of genes has now been determined.

Messenger RNA

The process of transcription – the production of functional messenger RNA – is a key to understanding the changes that occur when a normal cell becomes malignant. In mammalian cells, three RNA polymerases appear to be involved in the process of transcription. A specific DNA sequence – the promoter – signals where RNA synthesis is to begin. The polymerase then moves along the DNA strand, producing RNA in a 5′ to 3′ direction. A further specific DNA sequence provides the termination signal, causing the RNA to be released together with the polymerase enzyme.

There are many unanswered questions about transcription in eukaryotic cells, mainly due to the complex organization of DNA within nucleosomes. Furthermore, the primary messenger produced is modified in several ways before emerging through the nuclear membrane. The first modifications occur at either ends of the new message. At the 5′ end a 7-methyl guanosine residue is linked via a triphosphate. This cap will provide a binding site for the ribosomal proteins, enabling the message to be locked on to the ribosome (Perry, 1981). At the 3′ end a further enzyme, poly(A) polymerase, adds 100–200 residues of adenylic acid. The signal for this polymerase molecule to operate is provided by the short sequence AATAAA found 50–60 nucleotides upstream from the site of adenylation. The primary transcript, modified both at its 5′ and 3′ ends, is now processed. This entails the removal of large chunks of RNA sequence, which are not required for protein synthesis, from the centre of the molecule (Chambon, 1981). Such RNA splicing uses a series of enzymes and ribonucleoprotein to remove the non-coding, intervening sequences, or introns. The existence of a splicing apparatus seems, at first sight, a wasteful use of a cell's resources. However, its main advantage is genetic flexibility. Changes in the splicing patterns can occur

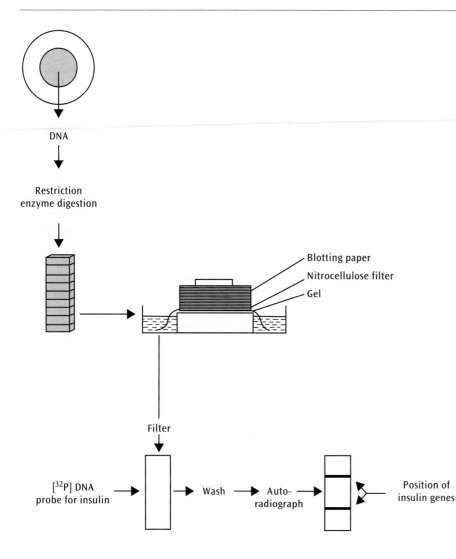

Figure 2.4 *Detection of insulin genes in a restriction enzyme digest of total human DNA using a ^{32}P-labelled cDNA insulin probe and Southern blotting.*

during differentiation, allowing several different related proteins to be produced from a single piece of genome.

Gene chips

The analysis of gene expression has been revolutionized by the development of gene expression microarrays, often called gene chips. This technology could well revolutionize biology in the same way that transistors revolutionized electronics. Basically, solid-phase systems are used to analyse patterns of gene expression. Such patterns can then be related to clinically important factors, such as the natural history of a tumour or its response to therapy. Techniques such as laser capture microscopy allow the collection of specific cell types from a heterogeneous tumour. In this way, detailed patterns of expression can be studied in pure cell populations (Emmert-Buck, 1996; Bonner, 1997).

Proteins

The complex machinery of the ribosome translates the sequence encoded in mRNA into the amino acids found in proteins. New techniques have been devised recently with which to characterize the small numbers of diverse proteins found within a cell. These include new electrophoretic techniques, such as two-dimensional gels separating first on the basis of charge and secondly on the basis of molecular size. In addition, monoclonal antibodies have provided tools of remarkable specificity to identify these end products of gene expression. Molecular biology now has the methods to look at each stage in the production of a protein and its subsequent post-translational modification by cleavage and glycosylation. We can now examine how this technology can be used to look at the differences between cancer cells and their normal counterparts.

DIFFERENTIATION

One of the remarkable features of a multicellular organism is the difference in structure and function found between cells in different tissues. The reasons for differentiation must reside in the accumulation of different sets of proteins. Each cell possesses the same DNA content; but, in differentiation, genes are expressed in varying amounts. Although the control of gene expression is well understood in bacteria, in eukaryotes the coordination of the complex series of switches that occurs in producing a muscle or brain cell remains a mystery. There are, however, three significant observations that concern the oncologist.

First, a fully differentiated cell nucleus can revert under certain circumstances to its less differentiated ancestor. Perhaps the best example is the insertion of a fully differentiated frog cell nucleus from intestinal epithelial cells into a frog egg from which the nucleus has been removed. A normal tadpole will result, indicating that the fully differentiated nucleus possessed all the information required for the production of tissues of all differentiation types (Gurdon, 1968). Other examples include the repair of limbs by invertebrates, and the strange differentiation patterns seen in teratocarcinoma in man. Although certain gene blocks are normally switched on during the process of differentiation, reversion to a less differentiated state is clearly possible.

The second observation is that control of gene expression in eukaryotes is at the level of transcription. The best evidence for this comes from comparing mRNA populations in different tissues, using hybridization techniques. Totally different populations are found, indicating that differentiation results in the production of different sets of mRNA molecules. In cancer, there is a reversion to a more primitive, or less differentiated, mRNA pattern.

A third finding of importance is that differentiation results from the planned switching on of gene blocks by gene regulatory proteins in a coordinated manner. The best experimental example of this comes from the homeotic mutations found in *Drosophila* – the fruit fly. Here, certain point mutations can cause a leg to be made instead of an antenna. This mutation occurs in a major control site, which triggers the set of genes to produce limb proteins instead of antenna proteins. The bizarre differentiation states found in human teratocarcinoma and its benign counterpart, teratoma, are further examples of control in differentiation by combinatorial gene regulation.

CANCER CELLS

Cancer cells differ from their normal counterparts by their ability to grow, divide and invade, without the normal restraining forces operating. In many ways, cancer cells resemble undifferentiated cells, which exhibit similar properties during normal embryogenesis. We can obtain a partial understanding of the reasons behind the changes by applying the techniques outlined above to examine cancer cells.

Cell surface

The cell surface is a vital component for both the recognition and behavioural control of the cell. It is composed mainly of a fluid lipid structure in which a large number of complex glycoproteins are floating. These proteins have external domains, which can be recognized by ligands and the immune system from outside the cell. Internally, many of these molecules connect with multiple downstream signalling pathways. Other proteins act as pumps for ions, metabolites and molecules. Cancer cells have been known for many years to have aberrant expression of many surface molecules. However, the relationship of these changes to abnormal growth pattern is not so clear.

The study of cell surface components now has considerable therapeutic relevance. Export pumps, such as the p180 glycoprotein, have been found to be responsible for one type of drug resistance, simply by increasing the extrusion rate of a cytotoxic drug from within the cell. Growth factor receptors, such as the epidermal growth factor receptor, bind to their cognate ligand and send signals for increased growth to the nucleus of the cell. Cancer cells may have a mutated receptor – switching on growth even in the absence of ligand – and may also have increased quantities of receptor, which in turn stimulate abnormal growth. In both cases, specific drugs have been developed to block signal transduction.

The immune system has been used for many years to identify molecules on the surface of tumour cells that differ in quantity from those present on normal cells. Although there is considerable evidence that the immune system is able to recognize tumour cells, the complexity of the interaction has so far precluded detailed analysis. The advent of monoclonal antibodies (MCAs), and lines of cloned T lymphocytes with defined specificity, now allows the immune system to be dissected into its individual components. We can use MCAs to detect circulating tumour markers precisely, and to target radioactive isotopes to tumour cells in patients. Extensive studies are now being pursued to see if drugs, toxins or high specific-activity radionuclides can be coupled to MCAs to effect tumour destruction in patients. The selectivity is supplied by the monoclonal antibody, while the drug or toxin provides the killing mechanism. The availability of human MCAs may produce exciting clinical results. Already three antibodies against cell surface components are licensed for therapy: Herceptin®, which binds to the erbB2 protein in breast cancer; Rituximab®, which binds to the CD20 glycoprotein in non-Hodgkin's lymphoma; and Campath®, which recognizes another lymphoma-specific antigen.

Perhaps more important in the long term is the use of these precise tools to identify differences between tumour cells and normal cells that can be exploited in other ways. By defining molecules on the cell surface using immunological tools, we can then use gene cloning to understand fully the reasons for these differences.

The cytoskeleton

The behaviour of a cell is determined not only by its surface properties but also by the cytoplasmic network of microfilaments in microtubules that forms the cytoskeleton. This cytoskeleton influences a cell's shape, motility, adhesion and division – properties that are known to change with transformation. Cytoskeletal disruption is a common observation in malignant cells, although its cause remains unknown. The construction of human genomic DNA probes for cytoskeletal proteins, such as tropomyosin, provides a starting point to examine the reasons for this disruption. Cloned genes for these proteins can be inserted into transformed cells and the effects of behaviour in the recipient cells studied. Specific cytoskeletal defects in malignant cells can be analysed and mechanisms determined to reduce these defects.

The genome

Although the cell surface and cytoskeleton are altered in malignancy, the ultimate source of any change during the development of cancer must reside in the genome. Genetic rearrangements can now be studied directly in DNA extracted from biopsy samples of human tumours. Restriction enzymes that cleave DNA at specific sites can map changes occurring within any gene for which a probe is available. Using the hybridization techniques described above, rearrangements, deletions and additions to the genome in a cancer cell can be determined. Certain segments of DNA have been found to have oncogenic potential in the transfection assay (Weinberg, 1982). In this assay, DNA is prepared from human tumour cells, precipitated with calcium phosphate and incubated with a mouse fibroblast cell line. These fibroblasts normally grow as confluent monolayers in a culture. After exposure to oncogene-containing DNA, these cells may exhibit features of malignancy, such as the ability to form clumps of cells and grow into soft agar.

Subsequent analysis has shown that in the process of transfection, donor DNA is taken up into the nuclei of the fibroblast cells and incorporated there. By combining the techniques of genetic engineering and the transfection assay, oncogenes from human tumours can now be isolated and characterized.

Cell communication

So far, we have considered how the information in the gene is converted into the differentiation pattern of a cell. In addition, elaborate communication systems exist to keep different tissues informed of events occurring at distant sites. Such communication systems are clearly essential for the survival of any multicellular organism.

Cell communication occurs at three levels (Fig. 2.5). The first is the gap junction. This is a tightly bonded region

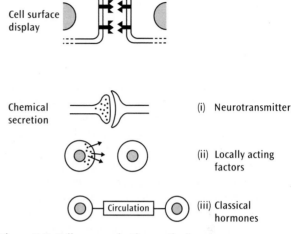

Figure 2.5 *Cell communication methods.*

occurring in the plasma membranes of two adjacent cells, which permits the transmission of ion fluxes and other cytoplasmic signals. This is clearly only important in communication between adjacent cells; for example, in an epithelium lining the small intestine. A second, and poorly documented, method of communication is by the interaction of molecules attached to the cell surface. When cells bearing such interacting molecules meet, a defined response occurs. Such effects are difficult to investigate experimentally, as the surface-bound molecules are in low concentration and difficult to solubilize. Finally, cells communicate by the secretion of chemicals. Specialized neurotransmitters, such as acetylcholine, are released locally and mediate their effects at high concentrations within the enclosed environment of a synaptic junction. Substances such as histamine and prostaglandins also interact locally at relatively high concentration. Finally, there are hormones which, on secretion, can bring about their actions at great distances from their cell of origin. Such molecules must operate at high dilutions in the order of 10^{-8} M. Their chemical nature varies: peptides, glycoproteins, steroids and modified amino acids all function as hormones binding to receptors.

ONCOGENES

Observations on the mutagenicity of carcinogens, the presence of damaged and translocated chromosomes in malignant cells and the recognition of families with an inherited predisposition to the development of cancer, led to the belief that the key to understanding the differences between normal and malignant cells lay in the study of the genome. It was predicted that genetic changes took place in small discrete sequences of DNA termed oncogenes. The problem lies in the complexity of the human genome. With 30 000 functional genes buried within thousands of kilobases of non-coding sequences, where should the search begin?

Viral oncogenes

Although techniques were not initially available to search the human genome for putative oncogenes, the study of the genetics of tumour viruses became feasible by virtue of their relative simplicity. Segments of viral genome could be readily cloned and sequenced by the new recombinant DNA techniques. Tumour viruses are categorized into two groups, the DNA and the RNA viruses. DNA viruses showed early promise with the demonstration of a conditioned mutation that affected the ability of polyoma virus to transform cells in culture. Unfortunately, their cytopathic effect and complex overlapping coding sequences made their study difficult. The RNA tumour viruses, on the other hand, were found to possess only three or four non-overlapping genes, replicated freely without destroying the host cell and, of particular interest, some were capable of rapidly inducing malignancy within days after infection, making them the most potent carcinogens known.

The first RNA virus was described by Peyton Rous, in 1911, as a filterable agent inducing sarcomas in chickens. Subsequently, over 40 have been characterized, producing several tumour types in a variety of species, including rats, mice, chickens and cats. Although they can cause tumours in primates, they are not a major cause of human tumours – with the leukaemia induced by human T-cell lymphotrophic virus (HTLV1) being the only well-defined example. The structure of these viruses is remarkably similar. There are three genes coding for proteins essential for viral replication, flanked by sequences acting as transcription promoters. *Pol*, the reverse transcriptase gene, converts viral genomic RNA into DNA, which then integrates into the host's genome. The other two genes, *gag* and *env*, code for proteins that package nascent viral RNA. The host's cellular machinery is subverted by the virus to manufacture fresh virus particles which are then released to infect further cells. When fully sequenced, RNA viruses capable of rapid induction of tumours were found to have extra coding sequences spliced into their genome. This often destroys their ability to replicate independently; 'helper viruses' are necessary to provide the machinery for replication.

The element of the virus genome that was found to be responsible for the rapid transforming capability was termed the viral oncogene (v-*onc*). Each of these genes has been given a three-letter code, depending on the species and/or tumour it caused. The necessity of this gene for transformation was demonstrated by deleting it. This causes the virus to lose its transforming capacity. Furthermore, temperature-sensitive mutants were shown to maintain the transformed phenotype only at the permissive temperature. Mild heating returns infected cells to their non-malignant form. This phenomenon could be mapped to changes in the v-*onc* gene.

Cellular oncogenes

A knowledge of viral oncogene sequences allowed the generation of gene probes that could recognize similar sequences in the cellular genome by DNA hybridization (Table 2.1). The discovery of homologous genes in cells that had not been infected by virus was first a great surprise. The significance of this observation was underlined by the detection of these sequences in species as diverse as yeast, fruit fly and man, with remarkable evolutionary conservation. This suggested that they are essential to basic cellular functions.

These genes have been termed proto-oncogenes to emphasize that they are only potentially oncogenic. There are a number of important differences between viral oncogenes and their cellular homologues. There are small changes in nucleotide sequences. Intervening non-coding sequences (introns) divide proto-oncogenes into several pieces that are later spliced together by post-transcriptional processing.

It would appear then that, far from being viral, oncogenes are cellular in origin. The illegitimate recombinant events that must occur to transduce a cellular oncogene into a RNA virus are rare. The presence of a v-*onc* is a survival disadvantage to the virus as these viruses may be replication defective. For this reason, epidemics of acute retrovirus-transformed animal tumours have never been seen. They are best understood as rare events which, although a poor model for human carcinogenesis, have led us to begin to detect cellular genes that are involved in cancer through other mechanisms.

Table 2.1 *Examples of viral oncogenes and their cellular homologues*

Oncogene	Origin	Tumour	Human gene
v-*src*	Chicken	Sarcoma	c-*src*
v-*ras*	Rat	Sarcoma	c-*ras*
v-*myc*	Chicken	Leukaemia	c-*myc*
v-*fes*	Cat	Sarcoma	c-*fes*
v-*sis*	Monkey	Sarcoma	c-*fes*
v-*erbB*	Chicken	Erythroblastosis	c-*erbB*
v-*myb*	Chicken	Myeloblastosis	c-*myb*
v-*fins*	Cat	Sarcoma	c-*fms*
v-*abl*	Mouse	Leukaemia	c-*abl*
v-*fos*	Mouse	Osteosarcoma	c-*fos*

Transfection

Most proto-oncogenes so far identified have been found through their homology to a v-*onc*. A very different approach has been to use transfection assays to detect genes that can directly convey the malignant phenotype. DNA extracted from tumour cell lines or fresh tumour biopsies can be cleaved with restriction enzymes and precipitated with calcium phosphate (Shih *et al.*, 1981). In this form, certain mouse fibroblasts (NIH 3T3 cells) can take up foreign DNA and incorporate a proportion of it into their genome and subsequently express the genes involved – a process termed transfection. As a consequence, some cells develop the characteristics of malignancy, with loss of contact inhibition causing colonies to pile up and then grow as tumours in nude mice. The analysis of these transformed cells shows mainly mouse, but some human DNA. By successive rounds of transfection, the amount of human DNA can be whittled down to the gene responsible for transformation.

Experiments of this type first demonstrated that DNA from a human bladder carcinoma, responsible for transformation in the transfection assay, was an oncogene of the c-*ras* family. Indeed, most of the oncogenes detected by this assay are of the c-*ras* type. This is probably due to the constraints of the system rather than the c-*ras* gene being the gene most frequently responsible for human cancer. However, the transfection of NIH 3T3 cells by c-*ras* from a variety of tumours has yielded fascinating information about mutations at defined sites within the gene that are tumorigenic. Most of the mutated genes isolated so far contain single base-pair changes at positions corresponding to either the 12th or 61st amino acid from the N-terminus. This implies that these two sites are vital in maintaining the proper control of the molecule. The switch of a single amino acid can clearly result in changes that subvert the cell to malignancy. Further analysis has shown that about one-fifth of all human tumours contain point mutations in the c-*ras* gene.

Methods of oncogene activation

There are two models for the activation of a proto-oncogene. The first is the quantitative model, where transformation occurs as a result of abnormally high levels of expression of an intact gene. There is also a qualitative model, where a gene undergoes mutation to make a product with a cellular activity that differs from its normal counterpart. Almost certainly, both mechanisms operate in the production of human tumours.

To assess these possibilities, functionally modified or unmodified oncogenes have been tested in the NIH 3T3 transfection assay. With few exceptions, molecularly cloned cellular oncogenes fail to transform cells. Furthermore, phage or plasmid vectors, carrying copies of the c-*src* gene, fail to transform normal diploid cells.

The enhanced transcription of c-*myc* in retroviral lymphomas in chickens is an argument advanced for the quantitative model, but this does not explain the 20 per cent of retroviral lymphomas where *myc* is not activated. Translocation of c-*myc* sequences in Burkitt's lymphoma was thought to cause enhanced transcription due to promoter sequences associated with the immunoglobulin loci. But even after exhaustive study there is no consensus as to whether c-*myc* expression is enhanced in Burkitt's lymphoma when compared with normal cells (Erikson *et al.*, 1983). Efforts to relate elevated expression of some oncogenes with neoplastic transformation has failed to show positive correlations. Finally, oncogenes are frequently active in normal untransformed cells and particularly so during embryogenesis, liver regeneration or wound repair. Genes such as c-*raf*, c-*ras* and c-*myc* are expressed at different levels in various tissues throughout embryogenesis.

Evidence that qualitative changes in oncogenes can generate malignancy is persuasive. Most v-oncogenes identified are altered by point mutation and deletion when compared with their cellular precursors. Furthermore, the gene product is frequently a fusion protein derived from both viral and cellular sequences. Comparison of the *src* gene of Rous sarcoma virus (RSV) and its cellular prototype demonstrates scattered point mutations amounting to 1–2 per cent of the sequence. Both ends of the v-*src* gene include small regions that are not related to essential retroviral genes and are not contiguous with c-*src* sequences. In an attempt to identify which changes in the *src* gene are crucial to its transforming potential, a number of variants of the virus have been developed. If RSV is constructed to express c-*src* rather than v-*src*, such viruses cannot induce transformation in chicken cells. Even when c-*src* is expressed at very high levels by the insertion of an active promoter sequence, the morphological transformation of the cells does not extend to growth in nude mice. Experiments with a variety of constructed c-*src* genes suggest that loss of the C-terminal amino acids leads to oncogenic activation.

WHAT DO ONCOGENES DO?

The control of cell growth and development is a complex process. Oncogenes have been shown to be involved at each level of this process and it can be seen that alterations to this finely balanced system could result in unregulated cell growth – transformation (Waxman and Sikora, 1989).

Growth factors

These are extracellular proteins that act as growth modulators. They have several properties that indicate an involvement in carcinogenesis. Some growth factors will transform normal cells *in vitro*. Conversely, in some systems the induction of cell transformation can result in an increased production of growth factor. The observation that growth factors can both initiate and be a product of transformation suggests the possibility of self-perpetuating positive feedback loops, with unregulated cell division as the consequence. This phenomenon, termed autocrine secretion, has been implicated in various situations involving rapid growth, such as wound repair and embryogenesis as well as malignant transformation. Both transformation and growth factor stimulation result in similar biochemical changes, such as increased tyrosine phosphorylation and altered cellular lipid metabolism. One human oncogene, c-sis, has been shown to code for a protein with marked sequence homology with a known growth factor – platelet-derived growth factor (PDGF).

Growth factor receptors

Several oncogene-coded proteins form part of a cell surface receptor. The presence of the appropriate growth factor switches the receptor 'on', with a resultant increase in tyrosine kinase activity within the cell, stimulated via the transmembrane section. The kinase can also be regulated by an internal regulatory region, allowing responses to intracellular events. The consequences of the increased kinase activity are, at present, unknown, but such activity is a hallmark of transformed cells.

Small alterations in the receptor can produce defects in the regulation of tyrosine kinase activity. An example of this is c-erbB, which codes for the cellular receptor of epidermal growth factor receptor (EGFR). The equivalent viral gene, v-erbB, which has transforming activity, encodes for a receptor with a truncated external receptor. In addition, there are alterations in the regulatory region internally. Transformation can occur by the viral gene product assuming a 'locked-on' configuration, tricking the cell into rapid growth (Rozengurt, 1999).

A second mechanism is alteration in tyrosine kinase activity. An example of this is the fms oncogene which codes for the receptor for the colony-stimulating factor, CSF-1, in differentiating macrophages. The transforming viral gene, v-fms, possesses enhanced kinase activity compared with its cellular counterpart.

Intracellular messengers

The best candidate for oncogene involvement at this level is the ras family of genes (Lemoine et al., 1989). The gene products have structural similarities to proteins termed G- and N-proteins, which control adenylate cyclase activity. Ras-coded products have also been shown to have guanosine triphosphatase (GTPase) activity. These proteins are all thought to be important in the 'second messenger' system and thus provide a link between events at the cell membrane and the nucleus.

Nuclear-acting oncogenes

Several oncogenes, such as myc, myb and fos, code for nuclear-associated proteins. At present their precise localization and function are unknown; a working hypothesis would be that these oncogenes may be involved in control of gene expression, acting to initiate the production of growth factors, for example.

Tumour suppressor genes

In the examples described above, the gene product behaves in a dominant manner, i.e. the presence of one abnormal gene is sufficient to produce transformation. Recently it has become apparent that certain genes are involved in oncogenesis due to the loss of their activity. These genes are not oncogenes, in that their products do not themselves transform cells. It has been postulated that the normal function of these genes is to switch off growth – thus functioning in opposition to dominant oncogenes which stimulate growth and development. Abnormalities at both alleles are necessary for the development of malignancy. The gene for familial polyposis coli fits this model. The gene maps to chromosome 5 and the heterozygote develops multiple benign polyps. Further mutation to homozygosity at this site results in the progression to frank adenocarcinoma. Mutations at the same site are present in at least 40 per cent of sporadic colorectal carcinomas, suggesting that this mechanism may be of importance in a large proportion of cancers.

The gene for retinoblastoma is also of great interest. Inherited cases carry an abnormal gene on chromosome 13, termed RB. As in the above example, mutation to homozygosity at this site results in the development of the tumour. Patients with inherited, but not sporadic, retinoblastoma also have an increased incidence of osteosarcoma and soft-tissue sarcomas. They do not, however, have an increased incidence of, for example, epithelial malignancies. This suggests that the RB gene may be of importance in 'switching off' growth in a variety of mesenchymal, but not epithelial, tissues.

Other examples of tumours associated with recessive oncogenes include Wilms' tumour and acoustic neuroma. It seems likely that further example of growth-suppressing genes will come to light, and this mechanism may prove of fundamental importance to the understanding of growth control.

Mutator genes

Many of the oncogenes described above are activated in human tumours by mutation. Recently it has been found that genes involved in DNA repair, or in fidelity of DNA replication, may also be altered in tumour cells. Damage to these genes allows the occurrence of more frequent 'fixation' of mutations in DNA. Examples of these are the *MSH2* and *MLHI* genes, which are normally involved in DNA repair. These genes have been found to be mutated in patients with hereditary non-polyposis colorectal cancer. Loss of efficient function of these types of genes is sometimes manifest by 'minisatellite instability'. This is where short, highly repetitive DNA sequences, which are scattered along the chromosomes, are copied incorrectly, giving rise to chromosomes that have different numbers of repeats. It is assumed, however, that the important targets to be affected are the dominant oncogenes.

Another enigmatic gene often found to be mutated in human tumours is the *p53* gene. It is thought that this, in some way, monitors damage to DNA caused by radiation or chemicals, and prevents cell division occurring until this is repaired. It is hypothesized that mutation of *p53* itself may make this restraint less effective, allowing cells to cycle more freely and to incorporate mutation more frequently. More genes of these types may be found, and certainly more research needs to be done to understand their functions and importance in human cancer.

ONCOPROTEINS

Genes exert their activity through the production of proteins. These are the executive molecules of the cell through their structural, enzymatic and regulatory functions. The isolation and characterization of oncoproteins is in its infancy. The conservation of oncogene sequences throughout vertebrate evolution points to a pivotal role for their resulting proteins in normal cell development. Cancer genes are clearly not unwanted guests but essential constituents of the cell's genetic apparatus. They betray the cell only when their structure or control is disturbed.

The evidence implicating oncoproteins in growth control is strengthened by the determination of the function of several oncogene products (Burgess, 1985) (Table 2.2). The c-*sis* gene product, p28 c-Sis, has been shown to have homology to 109 amino acids of platelet-derived growth factor. This important protein is involved in wound healing and the control of growth. It binds to a receptor

Table 2.2 *The evidence that oncogenes are involved in human cancer*

Existence of c-*onc* in humans
Transfection studies
Chromosomal aberrations
Amplification and mutation of c-*onc*s
Oncogene product function
    c-*sis*: platelet-derived growth factor
    c-*erbB*: epidermal growth factor receptor
    c-*fms*: colony-stimulating factor receptor
    c-*erbA*: steroid receptor
    c-*myc*: nuclear acting transcription factor

on the cell surface and subsequently activates a biochemical cascade culminating in increased cellular activity. A second oncogene, c-*erbB*, has been found to have homology to epidermal growth factor receptor. This large transmembrane structure consists of two components. The receptor itself is on the outside of the cell membrane and is associated with an internal component, a structure with protein kinase activity, having a molecular weight of 70 kDa. When epidermal growth factor binds to its receptor it activates the protein kinase on the inside of the cell, so culminating in growth potentiation. Presumably, aberrant production of the internal portion in a 'locked-on' position could result in growth without the requirement for exogenous epidermal growth factor. Indeed, the c-*erbB* gene codes for this internal portion. A third oncogene implicated in growth control is c-*myc*. This 62 kDa protein binds in a curious way to the matrix of cell nuclei. It has a very short half-life of 20 minutes and has been implicated in cell-cycle control. The level of c-*myc* mRNA increases when cells are stimulated into division.

In order to examine the relevance of oncoproteins, molecular flags for them have been constructed by making monoclonal antibodies. As the genes have been cloned, their DNA sequence can be determined. The recently devised technique of peptide immunization has been used to construct such antibodies. Using a genetic dictionary, the DNA sequence of the gene is converted into the amino acid structure of the oncoprotein. Peptides of between 10 and 20 amino acids long are then synthesized. The regions chosen for synthesis and immunization are those predicted to be exposed within the intact molecule. This prediction is made using computer plots of the relative hydrophilicity and hydrophobicity of different parts of the amino acid sequence. Mice are then immunized to produce polyclonal and monoclonal antibodies. In this way, antibodies suitable for a variety of clinical uses can be developed.

CLINICAL APPLICATIONS

A variety of techniques have been used to explore the molecular biology of these genes and their proteins. Techniques such as Southern blotting, polymerase chain reaction, DNA sequencing, dot blot hybridization, Western blotting and immunohistology have allowed the analysis of DNA, RNA and protein in clinical samples from patients with a variety of neoplasms. A major problem is that the reagents for such exploration are, in many cases, only just becoming available. Monoclonal antibodies constructed against a variety of oncogene products are now commercially available. It is likely that over the next few years, reagents will allow the dissection of the full catalogue of 40 or more genes.

Already, there are hints that the information provided can give us a molecular blueprint for a cell and allow the prediction of the likely course of disease in an individual patient. The temporal and spatial expression of these genes produce the molecular keyboard on which the destiny of the tumour, and hence the patient, is to be played. They also provide novel targets for pharmacological and immunological attack.

DNA

Karyotypic abnormalities were noted in various cancers several decades ago. A wide range of molecular techniques has now been developed to detect the amplification of specific genes within tumour biopsies. These include the use of *in situ* hybridization and comparative genome hybridization, which are sensitive detection methods for increased copy number of a gene. Table 2.3 lists genes that have been found to be amplified in certain tumours. For some tumours there is a clinical correlation between amplification and clinical outcome. The best correlation is in neuroblastoma (Table 2.4) where disease-free and

Table 2.3 *Oncogene alterations in human tumour biopsies*

Gene	Tumour	Amplification	Rearrangement
c-*myc*	Breast	+	
	Burkitt's		+
	Stomach	+	−
N-*myc*	Neuroblastoma	+	−
	Retinoblastoma	+	−
	APML	+	−
	Breast	+	−
	Lung	+	−
c-*abl*	CML		+
c-*myb*	AML		+
	Colon	+	
c-*erbB*	Breast	+	
	Glioma	+	
c-*erbB2*	Breast	+	

APML, acute promyelocytic leukaemia; CML, chronic myeloid leukaemia; AML, acute myeloid leukaemia.

Table 2.4 N-myc *gene amplification in neuroblastoma (reproduced with permission from Seeger* et al., *1985)*

Stage	
I	0/8
II	2/16
III	13/20
IV	19/40
IVS	0/15
DFS at 18 months	
N-*myc* copies	
1	70%
3–10	30%
>10	5%

DFS, disease-free survival.

absolute survival are strongly correlated to amplification of the N-*myc* gene (Seeger *et al.*, 1985). A weaker, but equally interesting, correlation has been observed between *erbB* and c-*myc* in breast cancer (Cline *et al.*, 1987). Related to *erbB*, which codes for the internal domain of the receptor for epidermal growth factor, is another gene – c-*erbB2*. It has structural homology to c-*erbB* but codes for a different receptor. Its ligand has yet to be identified. Amplification and expression of this gene may correlate with prognosis in breast cancer (Venter *et al.*, 1987; Zeillinger *et al.*, 1989). Studies are in progress to evaluate the long-term prognostic significance of these abnormalities. Why gene amplification should result in a change in the physiology of the cell remains unclear. The main problem is that the function of the proteins coded for by these genes is not known. A good example is c-*ras*. Here mutations around the 12th and 61st position within the amino acid chain codes for a 21 kDa protein which is less able to bind to GTP. Although GTP binding is one of the functions of Ras, its other functions remain a mystery (McCormick *et al.*, 1985).

Specific chromosomal translocation is a common feature of certain tumours. An example is Burkitt's lymphoma, which almost invariably carries a translocation involving chromosome 8;14. The break point in chromosome 8 is at the site of the c-*myc* oncogene. In the more common follicular lymphoma, translocations between chromosome 14 and 18 have been noted. The break point region has been cloned and designated *bcl-2*. This region may well be an oncogene (Weiss *et al.*, 1987). The Philadelphia chromosome in chronic myeloid leukaemia is a chromosome 9;22 translocation. Here c-*abl* proto-oncogene related to the v-*onc* of the murine Abelson leukaemia virus is moved from chromosome 9 into a fragmented segment of chromosome 22. Examination of the break point shows that it always occurs within a 5.8 kb segment designated *bcr* (break point cluster region). An mRNA transcript has been detected in chronic myeloid leukaemia (CML) cells that is a fusion product of the c-*abl* and *bcr* regions. Furthermore, the protein product of this message has a molecular weight of 210 kDa and has tyrosine kinase activity (Kurzrock *et al.*, 1987). By constructing antibodies against this protein, new diagnostic and, possibly, therapeutic agents may become available (Li *et al.*, 1989).

RNA

Over the past 10 years an intensive investigation of oncogene transcription in clinical samples has been carried out. Large numbers of tumours have been collected, RNA isolated and the number of copies present per cell estimated using hybridization. The simplest and most commonly used method has been dot blotting. Problems abound, however. First, RNA degrades very rapidly, even from the time of surgical clamping. Furthermore, RNA is difficult to process because of its instability. Dot blotting techniques can be tremendously variable and critically depend on the quality and length of the specific probe used. For these reasons, much of the literature is difficult to reproduce and the results must be viewed with some scepticism. The biggest single series was of 54 tumours probed with 15 different oncogene probes (Slamon et al., 1984). No obvious pattern of gene expression to any specific tumour or particular aggressive state of the tumour was obtained. Correlations between outcome have been claimed for c-myc and c-ras in colorectal and breast cancer. Careful study of DNA, RNA and protein in the same tumour samples is badly needed to clarify the problems (Sikora et al., 1987).

Protein

In order to examine the relevance of oncoproteins, antibodies have been constructed to synthetic peptides. Such peptides are chosen from hydropathic plots of the predicted amino acid sequence of the oncogene product. The hydrophilic sequences are likely to be on the outside of the molecule and therefore to constitute antigenic determinants. Polyclonal and monoclonal antibodies are now available to several oncoproteins. These reagents can be used in immunohistology and Western blotting. Correlations between prognosis and gene expression have been made for c-myc, N-myc, c-ras, c-erbB and c-erbB2 in several tumours (Chan et al., 1987).

Although histology is good for giving geographical information about the distribution of oncoproteins in normal and malignant tissues, it is bad for quantification. Sensitive flow-cytometric assays have been developed to quantify precisely oncoproteins in nuclei isolated from wax-embedded tumours. Correlations can now be made between differentiation state and clinical outcome and the levels of p62 c-Myc and other proteins in lung, colonic, testicular and cervical cancer (Watson et al., 1987).

Tumour markers

Sera from patients with various tumours have been found to contain circulating oncoproteins at a higher level than normal. Unfortunately, the results in one large series are not clear-cut. This study looked at proteins immunologically related to c-ras, c-sis, c-src gene products in the urine of patients with several tumour types (Niman et al., 1985). More recently, p62 c-Myc levels have been found to be elevated in patients with colorectal and breast cancer (Chan et al., 1987). Such antibodies have also been used for immunoscintigraphy. Tumour localization has been obtained successfully using antibody against c-Myc in small cell lung cancer, and against epidermal growth factor receptor in gliomas. There is little evidence that such scans are any more sensitive than conventional radiological procedures, but they may be of value in finding out more about a tumour's response to drugs or radiation, and thus have clinical utility.

Risk prediction

Restriction fragment length polymorphism analysis (RFLP) has been used successfully for the diagnosis of genetic disorders from trophoblast samples in the early stages of pregnancy. It is also the basis of genetic fingerprinting: a technique that has recently resulted in successful criminal convictions. Briefly, it involves taking a sample of DNA from a patient, usually from peripheral blood lymphocytes, cleaving it with restriction enzymes at defined sites, running the DNA in an electrophoretic gel and probing with a relevant probe. DNA sequence differences will produce different patterns and probe binding. The recognition of polymorphic patterns in populations after restriction enzyme digestion is the basis of RFLP analysis. RFLPs have been observed to occur round the c-ras gene locus. Certain patterns are found to be more likely associated with leukaemia, lung and colon carcinoma (Krontiris et al., 1985). Here, it is the perfectly normal genome of the individual that has sequences that make them more vulnerable. It is conceivable that in the not too distant future, RFLP analysis will enable prediction of high cancer risk.

New therapies

The discovery of oncogenes has clearly given tremendous impetus to the understanding of the biology of cancer. It also provides new targets for developing pharmacological agents (Table 2.5). Growth factors, growth factor agonists and antibodies to the receptors for growth factors are clearly fruitful areas for new drug design. Furthermore, nucleoside analogues of guanosine triphosphate may successfully inhibit the Ras protein, even though its function is as yet undefined. Many oncogene products, such as tyrosine kinases, exert their effects by phosphorylating tyrosine and other proteins. Several agents are available that can block this activity. The most

Table 2.5 *Oncogene products and cancer therapy*

Gene product	Agents
Growth factors	Agonists
	Antagonists
	Antibodies
Receptors	Downregulators
	Signal interference
Protein kinases	Suicide peptides
GTP binders	Nucleoside analogues
Nuclear oncoproteins	Analogues
	Blockers
	Partition shifters

promising are the small molecular weight inhibitors which compete with adenosine triphosphate (ATP) at its binding site on the internal domain. Two such drugs, Iressa and Tarceva, will be licensed for clinical use in different indications during 2002. There is also a humanized monoclonal antibody – C225 – that binds to the external domain reducing activation. The interesting feature of the small molecule inhibitors is their synergy with chemotherapy and the lack of correlation between the level of epidermal growth factor receptor as detected by immunohistochemistry and subsequent response (Robinson *et al.*, 2000).

Gene therapy

Over the past few years gene therapy has come to be accepted as a realistic approach to the treatment of several human diseases. Cancer is one of the most promising areas, as in many cases no other effective therapies are available, yet the nature of the causal changes at the level of the DNA is unknown. The concepts can be divided into two broad areas: *ex vivo* and *in vivo* approaches. *Ex vivo* gene therapy essentially consists of placing a new gene into normal cells (such as T cells) or into tumour cells cultured outside the body, and then reintroducing them back into the patient. Most approaches of this type seek to improve the efficiency of recognition of tumour cells by the immune system, either by making the T cells more active or the tumour cells more immunogenic. Several clinical trials of these strategies are currently under way.

The second approach of *in vivo* therapy employs various methods to introduce recombinant DNA into tumour cells *in situ*. Vectors include viruses, liposomes or physical methods such as direct injection of DNA. The end result of these strategies is to make the tumour cells more immunogenic or more sensitive to drug treatments by expression of drug metabolizing enzymes. Despite the complex nature of these new concepts, this is currently a very active area of research.

USING MOLECULAR BIOLOGY TO DEVELOP NEW CANCER DRUGS

Over the next 5 years a large number of novel, mechanistically targeted drugs will enter clinical trial for cancer. Our remarkable progress in understanding the molecular biology of cancer has provided an enormous range of validated targets for drug discovery. Following lead optimization and suitable pharmaceutical formulation these compounds have undergone rapid screening in pre-clinical models. Innovative methods of clinical development are now essential to ensure optimal dose determination and scheduling. This requires the imaginative use of biomarkers to determine the pharmacodynamics of target effect, the stratification of potential responders by molecular profiling and surrogate endpoints for clinical efficacy. A greater investment in obtaining information at an early stage of drug development will be required as these compounds may not produce classical tumour responses but convert cancer into a chronic, controllable disease. The selection of the correct dose by determination of the maximal effective dose will be necessary, before beginning costly and time-consuming randomized pivotal studies. The discovery of novel surrogates for efficacy is essential in this fast moving area and requires imaginative partnerships between academic groups and the pharmaceutical industry. Such surrogates will herald a new era in the search for effective cancer-preventive agents.

Cancer drug development is entering a remarkable new phase. Recent developments in molecular biology have led to a host of new validated targets. *In silico* drug design allows the construction of thousands of virtual compounds, the most promising of which can be rapidly synthesized. This complements robotic high throughput screening of well organized chemical and natural compound libraries (Garrett and Workman, 1999). This has led to a platform approach to drug discovery – the creation of specific inhibitors for each member of a gene family such as the protein kinases (Robinson *et al.*, 2000). This approach has been remarkably successful and a range of small molecules are now available which affect processes as diverse as cell cycle control, mitotic spindle separation, apoptosis, signal transduction, angiogenesis and tumour invasion. Over the last 5 years there has been a shift away from the search for new cytotoxic drugs to drugs acting through defined molecular mechanisms known to be aberrant in cancer. There are currently over 500 molecules undergoing clinical study and this may well reach 1000 by 2005. Clearly, new methods to identify the most promising candidates are necessary as there are only limited resources to take these compounds into expensive and time-consuming phase III studies.

The traditional approach to cytotoxic drug development is not appropriate for many of these new agents for several reasons. Firstly, as their precise molecular mechanism is known it should be possible to develop a pharmacodynamic assay for their molecular effectiveness in patients. This can be used to determine the maximally effective dose for use in further studies (Evans and Relling, 1999). This approach will replace the classical phase I study which in the past has been used to evaluate the maximal tolerated dose. Secondly, it may not be possible to rely on tumour response in phase II as a guide to survival benefit. Many of the new agents will cause disease stabilization and not shrinkage. Thus it will be necessary to commit to expensive randomized phase III studies without having the confidence generated by a successful phase II programme. The key to success in this mechanistically based future will be the collection of far more data in the early phase of drug development by the use of surrogates of both molecular target effects and clinical efficacy.

Definitions

There is a lack of consistency in how certain terms are used despite several attempts to formalize definitions. A *surrogate endpoint* is defined as a substitute measurement of benefit (derived from Latin – surrogare – to substitute). Tumour shrinkage is an effective surrogate for clinical efficacy as measured by long-term survival. The complete disappearance of tumour on an X-ray image carries a better prognosis than only a minor effect after giving chemotherapy or radiation. Similarly, the generation of data showing a long average time to disease progression with therapy can in some cases be a surrogate for long-term survival. In addition, the decline of a serum biochemical tumour marker suggests a tumour response that may lead to a better outcome. Although some tumour markers are reliable surrogates for ultimate outcome (HCG in choriocarcinoma and testicular teratoma), changes in others such as PSA or CEA are less tightly correlated to subsequent survival.

A *biomarker* can be defined as a biological marker of target effect. By definition, it will always be a surrogate for the effect of a drug on its molecular target. In certain cases it may also be a surrogate for tumour response and subsequent prolonged survival, although this will need to be verified. A biomarker may be biochemical or reflect a physiological by-product such as the production of hypotension or platelet aggregation. It may involve a complex imaging process such as positron emission tomography or the genomic analysis of tumour biopsies before and after therapy. Tumour markers are just a subset of biomarkers that are sometimes useful in predicting prognosis. Biomarkers are commonly used outside oncology to monitor the effectiveness of a therapy. Serum cholesterol, glycated haemoglobin and blood pressure are biomarkers for statin therapy, control of diabetes and anti-hypertensive treatment respectively. They are also effectiveness surrogates for the likely long-term consequences of the relevant disease. Unfortunately, we currently lack such tightly correlated biomarkers which will become essential as cancer becomes a chronic illness.

Functional imaging can be defined as the imaging of a biological process. Recent advances in technology have made it possible to begin to visualize mitosis, apoptosis, inflammation, receptor targeting and blood flow as well as the structural changes associated with tumour regression. Novel computer technology can integrate structural and functional images giving detailed information on drug effects (Anderson *et al.*, 2001).

A *predictive marker* allows the stratification of patients by their likelihood of response to an agent. It may be determined by immunohistology such as the presence of hormone receptors or HER2 expression, or by some more complex interactive assay to determine the effect of an agent on a clinical sample such as the SF2 assay for radiosensitivity. Predictive markers are particularly feasible when the precise molecular mechanism of a drug is known and its target variably expressed across the spectrum of cancer. The regulatory label for a drug may restrict its use to patients with tumours that express a specific marker. Examples include Herceptin and erbB2 over-expressing breast cancer; Glivec and the bcr-abl translocation in chronic myeloid leukaemia and the expression of CD20 in non-Hodgkin's lymphoma for the use of the monoclonal antibody – Rituximab.

Molecular profiling is the holistic profiling of a tumour using several technologies to determine its likely natural history and optimal therapy. The beginnings of such correlations have been used in assays for the expression of specific gene products in increased, reduced or mutated form. Examples include *erbB*1, *erbB*2, *ras* and *p*53 (Scherf *et al.*, 2000). The emerging technologies of genomics, proteomics and metabonomics can produce enormous datasets to correlate with tumour behaviour patterns and response to different therapies. Eventually such technologies are likely to result in *personalized medicine* for cancer.

A toolkit for early cancer drug development

Biomarkers, surrogate endpoints, functional imaging and predictive markers can be developed to form an essential toolkit for early drug development. The target molecules for novel anti-cancer agents can be grouped by their biological function. In this way a set of biomarkers can be developed for each function (Table 2.6).

The practical value of each component can be evaluated in cell lines and animal tumours to determine its effectiveness in producing accurate dose–response information – a pre-requisite for determining pharmacodynamic endpoints. For safety, an escalating dose scale will still be necessary when a compound first enters the clinic. However, the toolkit can be used to avoid the need to determine the maximal tolerated dose (MTD).

Conventionally the safe starting dose is one tenth of the LD10 in the most sensitive of three species. This can then be increased using an accelerated titration method until the maximal molecular effect can be obtained on the drug's target (Simon *et al.*, 1997). This dose may produce no toxic effects whatsoever. Choosing the correct dose based on pharmacodynamic data permits proof of principle studies to proceed with confidence. It reduces the number of patients required for a phase I, speeding up this phase and avoiding many patients receiving a sub-therapeutic dose. Furthermore, it reduces the risk of operating at a dose higher than peak effectiveness if the effect of the drug peaks at a certain concentration. It also avoids a later potential commercial disaster if the drug priced for a high dose close to toxicity is demonstrated to work just as well at a much lower one.

For most novel agents the toolkit for measuring biomarkers of cell function can be validated in healthy volunteer subjects. This is a radical departure for trials of

Table 2.6 *A molecular toolkit for developing cancer drugs*

	Mitosis	Apoptosis	ST inhibitors	Angio	Invasion	Differentiation
Biomarker	+	+	+	+	+	+
Surrogate	−	−	−	+	+	+
Functional imaging	+	+	−	+	−	−
Predictor	−	−	+	−	−	+

Biomarkers are needed for each class of agent. Surrogate endpoints of efficacy are particularly important for agents that do not necessarily cause tumour shrinkage such as anti-angiogenics and invasion inhibitors. Functional imaging is necessary where the timing of drug administration is critical. Predictors of response are useful for drugs that inhibit signal transduction (ST) pathways.

cancer agents and an area where oncologists traditionally have no expertise. This enhances the speed of data acquisition by forward planning and avoiding the need to identify cancer patients in real time as stacking for a defined future timepoint would be unethical given the likely progress of the disease.

The different components of the early development toolkit have different costs, risk and potential information yield. The investment payback will depend on how critical the information is to the successful development of drugs against a defined target. Thus biomarkers of molecular effect are a requirement for all drugs. Surrogate endpoints of clinical benefit are particularly important for drugs whose long-term administration is necessary to achieve either tumour stabilization such as anti-angiogenic agents or prevention of metastasis where the cost in both time and effort of pivotal studies is immense. Success is achieving surrogate benefit here gives the confidence to commit long-term financial resource by effectively reducing the risk of failure. Functional imaging studies are particularly helpful where optimizing the effect of a drug requires precise scheduling – cell cycle inhibitors and pro-apoptotic agents. By obtaining real-time images of mitosis and apoptosis in patients, logical decisions about enhancing selectivity can be made more easily.

It currently takes an average of 10 years for a cancer drug to reach the market from the identification of the lead compound. The sheer number of drugs now becoming available will require a rigorous selection process during the early phase of clinical development. Over the next decade systematic programmes of cancer risk assessment will be established and cancer preventive agents will enter into clinical trial. Novel surrogate endpoints will be essential to determine their benefit without waiting for a further generation of cancer patients. Molecular biology will continue to remain one of the main drivers of progress in this exciting area.

CONCLUSIONS

The study of oncogenes provides a fascinating insight into the mechanisms by which cell growth is controlled. Abnormalities in this process appear to be of major importance in the generation of malignant disease. Future advances in this field hold great promise for yielding new approaches to the diagnosis, staging and treatment of cancer.

SIGNIFICANT POINTS

- The basic tools of molecular biology:
  - DNA sequencing:
    amplification by polymerase chain reaction (PCR)
    cloning
    hybridization – Southern blotting
    transfer into cells;
  - RNA transcription assays:
    sequencing
    reverse transcription
    PCR
    hybridization – Northern blotting;
  - Protein sequencing
    antibody recognition – Western blotting
    gel analysis.
- Cell communication:
  - gap junctions
  - cell surface interaction
  - cell adhesion molecules
  - growth factors
    autocrine
    paracrine
  - cytokines
  - hormones.
- Oncogene–tumour suppressor gene changes:
  - mutations
    germ line
    somatic
  - translocation
  - deletion
  - amplification
  - loss of control.

KEY REFERENCES

Cancer genome anatomy project (2000) www.ncbi.nlm.nih.gov/ncicgap/

Cooper, N.C. (ed.) (1994) *The human genomeproject*. Mill Valley: University Science Books.

Gabra, H. (1999) Molecular approaches to sporadic ovarian cancer. *Cancer Topics* **15**, 10–14.

Ramsay, G. (1998) Gene chips: state of the art. *Nat. Biotechnol.* **16**, 40–44.

Strausberg, R., Dahl, C. and Klausner, R. (1999) New opportunities for uncovering the molecular basis of cancer. *Nat. Genet.* **21**, 25–32.

REFERENCES

Abbott, A. (1996) DNA chips intensify the sequence search. *Nature* **379**, 392–4.

Anderson, H., Price, P., Blomley, S. *et al.* (2001) Measuring changes in human tumour vasculature in response to therapy using functional imaging techniques. *Br. J. Cancer* **85**, 1085–93.

Bonner, R. (1997) Laser capture microdissection. *Science* **278**, 1481–3.

Burgess, A. (1985) Oncogenes and growth factors. *Immunol. Today* **6**, 107–21.

Chambon, P. (1981) Split genes. *Sci. Am.* **244**, 6071.

Chan, S., Gabra, H., Hill, F., Evan, G. and Sikora, K. (1987) The detection of a 40K c-*myc* related protein in cancer patients' sera. *Mol. Cell Probes* **1**, 73–82.

Cline, M.J., Battifora, H. and Yododa, J. (1987) Proto-oncogene abnormalities in human breast cancer: correlations and anatomic features and clinical course of disease. *J. Clin. Oncol.* **5**, 999–1006.

Cohen, S.N. (1980) The manipulation of genes. *Sci. Am.* **243**, 102–7.

Emmert-Buck, M. (1996) Laser capture microdissection. *Science* **274**, 998–1001.

Erikson, J., Arrushdi, A. and Drwinga, H. (1983) Transcripted activation of the translocated c-*myc* oncogene in Burkitt's lymphoma. *Proc. Natl. Acad. Sci.* **80**, 820–7.

Evans, W. and Relling, M. (1999) Pharmacogenomics: translating functional genomics into rational therapeutics. *Science* **286**, 487–91.

Garrett, M. and Workman, P. (1999) Discovering novel chemotherapeutic drugs for the third millennium. *Eur. J. Cancer* **35**, 2010–30.

Gurdon, J.B. (1968) Transplanted nuclei and cell differentiation. *Sci. Am.* **219**, 24–35.

Krontiris, T.G., Dimartinon, A., Colb, M. and Parkinson, D.R. (1985) Unique allelic restriction fragments of the human H-*ras* locus in leucocyte and tumour DNAs of cancer patients. *Nature* **313**, 369–73.

Kurzrock, R., Shtalrio, M., Romero, P. and Gutterman, J.U. (1987) Abnormal c-*abl* protein product in a Philadelphia positive acute lymphotrophic leukaemia. *Nature* **325**, 631–3.

Lemoine, N.R., Mayall, E., Wyllie, F. *et al.* (1989) High frequency of ras oncogene activation in all stages of human thyroid tumorigenesis. *Oncogene* **4**, 159–64.

Li, W., Dreazen, O., Kloetzer, W., Gale, R.P. and Arlinghaus, R.B. (1989) Characterisation of *bcr* gene products in haemopoietic cells. *Oncogene* **4**, 127–38.

Lindahl, T. (1982) DNA repair enzymes. *Ann. Rev. Biochem.* **51**, 61–88.

McCormick, F., Clark, B.F., la Cour, T.F. *et al.* (1985) A model for the tertiary structure of p21, the product of the *ras* oncogene. *Science* **230**, 78–82.

McGhee, J.D. and Felsenfield, G. (1980) Nucleosome structure. *Ann. Rev. Biochem.* **49**, 1115–26.

Niman, H.L., Thompson, A.M.H., Yu, A. *et al.* (1985) Anti-peptide antibodies detect oncogene related protein in urine. *Proc. Natl Acad. Sci.* **82**, 7924–9.

Orgel, L.E. and Crick, F.H.C. (1980) Selfish DNA: the ultimate parasite. *Nature* **284**, 604–7.

Orkin, S.H., Little, P.F., Kazazian H. *et al.* (1982) Improved detection of the sickle mutation by DNA analysis. *N. Engl. J. Med.* **307**, 32–6.

Perry, R.P. (1981) RNA processing comes of age. *J. Cell. Biol.* **91**, 28–38.

Robinson, D., Wu, Y. and Lin, S. (2000) The protein tyrosine kinase family of the human genome. *Oncogene* **19**, 5548–57.

Rozengurt, E. (1999) Autocrine loops, signal transduction and cell cycle abnormalities in the molecular biology of lung cancer. *Curr. Opin. Oncol.* **11**, 116–22.

Sanger, F. (1981) Determination of nucleotide sequences in DNA. *Science* **214**, 1205–10.

Scherf, U., Ross, D., Waltham, M. *et al.* (2000) A gene expression database for the molecular pharmacology of cancer. *Nature Genetics* **24**, 236–44.

Seeger, R.C., Brodeur, G.M. and Sather, H. (1985) Amplification of N-*myc* in human neuroblastoma correlates with advanced disease stage. *N. Engl. J. Med.* **313**, 1111.

Shih, C., Padhy, L.C., Murray, K. and Weinberg, R.A. (1981). Transforming genes of carcinomas and neuroblastomas introduced into mouse fibroblasts. *Nature* **290**, 261–4.

Sikora, K., Chan, S., Evan, G. and Watson, J. (1987) C-*myc* oncogene expression in colorectal cancer. *Cancer* **59**, 1289–95.

Simon, R., Friedlin, B., Rubinstien, L. *et al.* (1997) Accelerated titration designs for phase I trials in oncology. *J. Nat. Cancer Inst.* **89**, 1138–44.

Slamon, D.J., Dekernion, J.B., Verma, I.M. and Cline, M.J. (1984) Expression of cellular oncogenes in human malignancies. *Science* **224**, 256–62.

Smith, J. (1979) Nucleotide sequence specificity of restriction endonucleases. *Science* **205**, 455–62.

Venter, D.J., Tuzi, N.L., Kumar, S. and Gullick, W. (1987) Over expression of the c-*erbB2* oncoprotein in human breast carcinomas: immunological assessment correlates with the gene amplification. *Lancet* **2**, 69.

Watson, J., Stewart, J., Cox, H., Evan, G. and Sikora, K. (1987) Flow cytometric quantitation of the c-*myc* oncoprotein. *Mol. Cell Probes* **1**, 151–8.

Waxman, J.W. and Sikora, K. (eds) (1989) *Molecular biology of cancer.* Oxford: Blackwell Scientific Publications, 1–134.

Weinberg, R.A. (1982) Use of transfection to analyse genetic information and malignant transformation. *Biochim. Biophys. Acta* **651**, 25–35.

Weiss, L.M., Warnke, R.A. and Sklar, J. (1987) Molecular analysis of the t14–18 chromosomal translocation in malignant lymphomas. *N. Engl. J. Med.* **317**, 1185.

Zeillinger, R., Kury, F., Czerwenka, K. *et al.* (1989) HER amplification, steroid receptors and epidermal growth factor receptor in primary breast cancer. *Oncogene* **4**, 109–14.

3

Molecular radiobiology

TREVOR J. McMILLAN

INTRODUCTION

The past few years have seen enormous leaps in our understanding of how cells respond to ionizing radiation and hopefully we will now see this has an impact on medicine in diagnostics, therapy and cancer incidence. The genetics and biochemistry that have been uncovered can now be set against a wealth of information on the whole-animal, tissue, cellular and subcellular effects of ionizing radiation. While modern techniques reveal aspects of the cellular radiation response which were not evident previously, a major aim of this area has to be to explain cellular phenomena which have been demonstrated to be critical in the cytotoxic and mutagenic effects of radiation.

THE FIVE 'Rs' OF RADIOBIOLOGY

Variation in patient response to radiotherapy, both within and between tumour types, is evident clinically. A simple view of this is that the success of the treatment will be determined by how many tumour cells are killed by a given sequence of dose fractions, within the constraints laid down by normal tissues irradiated at the same time. Thus we need to consider what determines the number of tumour cells that are killed. Clinical observation and experimental radiobiology have identified five factors that are clearly influential in the determination of

the outcome of a course of fractionated radiotherapy. These are the five 'Rs' of radiobiology (Fig. 3.1) and they form the fundamental basis for the application of our molecular knowledge.

Recovery

Recovery is the decrease in the effectiveness of radiation when exposure is prolonged or fractionated (the term sublethal damage recovery, SLDR, is often used). In addition, cells held in a non-proliferating state after irradiation show a reduced sensitivity compared to proliferating cells. This is potentially lethal damage recovery, PLDR. Both of these processes are believed to be a consequence

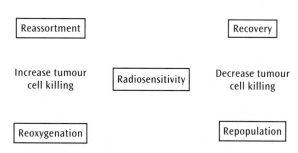

Figure 3.1 *The five 'Rs' of radiobiology. Radiosensitivity can be considered as the base line from which the other Rs increase or decrease the number of cells which survive radiation.*

of the repair of radiation damage to DNA. However, SLDR and PLDR are apparently not controlled by the same processes, since they have differing effects on the number of gene mutations that are induced by radiation (Thacker and Stretch, 1983). The molecular dissection of these processes is still in its infancy but there are data to link the gene *TP53* to PLDR (Schwartz *et al.*, 1999). Of recent interest is the finding that clonogenic cell survival curves may have a steep component at low doses and that some radioprotective processes might be induced by radiation. This could have important implications for cellular recovery in different fractionation regimes and attempts are being made to exploit this in the clinic (*see* below).

Reoxygenation

Low oxygen levels render cells relatively resistant to ionizing radiation, largely because of a decreased induction of DNA damage. In some tumours, and to a minor extent in normal tissues such as cartilage, vascular supply is inadequate to maintain good oxygen supply to all regions, so there are cells that are hypoxic and therefore resistant to radiation. Clinically this has been demonstrated to limit the success of therapy (Overgaard, 1989) but its influence is reduced when the radiation is fractionated, due to the process of reoxygenation. The death of some tumour cells may lead to improved oxygen supply to others, and thus to an increase in their radiosensitivity. Furthermore, the opening and closing of blood vessels in a tumour is a dynamic process, so that cells adjacent to a closed vessel at the time of one fraction may be oxygenated at the next fraction if the vessel has opened. The effect of a subpopulation of resistant cells at each treatment time may be quite small in some cases, but when amplified over a multiple fraction regime it can result in a significant reduction in the theoretical tumour curability (Tannock and Hill, 1998). The control of angiogenesis in tumours is a major area of research and clinical interest at present and it will be important to consider whether this can be combined with radiotherapy to beneficial effect.

Reassortment

Cells vary in their radiosensitivity as they progress through the cell cycle. For example, cells in mitosis have been found to be approximately twice as sensitive as cells in the latter part of the DNA synthesis phase. Radiation therefore exerts selective effects in favour of cells in the resistant phases of the cell cycle. If there were no cell-cycle progression, then a second radiation treatment would be less effective than the first. The effect of cells progressing through the cell cycle in between treatments is that cells that survive the first treatment because of their presence in a resistant phase move into a more sensitive phase before the next fraction is delivered.

Importantly, one of the key cellular responses to DNA damage is the triggering of cell-cycle checkpoints towards the end of G_1 and in G_2. These have been examined extensively in relation to cellular radiosensitivity (*see* Section 3.10) but their influence on cell-cycle reassortment during radiotherapy has not been well characterized. In the context of fractionated radiotherapy, the important determining factors are the time between fractions, the length of the delay and the degree of synchrony of the cell population when cells resume proliferation. There has been much interest over a long period in the possibility of utilizing cell synchronization to exploit the high sensitivity of cells in some cell-cycle phases. This has generally proved to be an unfruitful approach because synchronization is not very strong and it is difficult to apply this approach to fractionated radiotherapy, but with an increased understanding of cell-cycle control and the potential for more specific cell-cycle blocking agents there may be scope for the resurrection of a modification of this approach.

Repopulation

Proliferation of tumour cells during a course of radiotherapy is potentially a major obstacle to the success of treatment. It is apparent that the proliferation of tumour cells can be faster in a treated tumour than in an untreated tumour, and this 'accelerated-repopulation' appears to have a significant bearing on the efficacy of radiotherapy (Withers *et al.*, 1988). Acceleration may partly be due to physical effects, i.e. the removal of dead cells may lead to an improved nutrient supply to surviving cells. If depopulation within the tumour leads to reduced cell loss, then survivors may proliferate with a doubling time that approaches the 'potential doubling time', a process that has been described as the 'unmasking' of the high proliferation rate of clonogenic tumour cells.

Radiosensitivity

It is intuitively reasonable to expect that the inherent radiosensitivity of tumour cells can be a significant factor in the overall level of cell killing induced by radiation. The clinical radioresponsiveness of tumours of different histological origins correlates strongly with radiosensitivity of cells taken from those tumours (Deacon *et al.*, 1984). To take this one step further, the radiosensitivity of tumour cells from cervix carcinomas has been demonstrated to be predictive of local tumour control (West *et al.*, 1993). In cervix cancer it therefore appears that cellular sensitivity is a major determinant of the overall response. Not all studies have shown this relationship in other tumour types, and there is still work to be done to determine whether these results are a true reflection of a varied influence of inherent sensitivity or whether technical problems in the assay systems have blurred the situation.

VARIATION IN NORMAL TISSUE RESPONSE

It has been recognized for some time that individuals vary in the sensitivity of their normal tissues to radiation (Burnet *et al.*, 1996). At its extreme this is seen in the syndrome ataxia telangiectasia, where all the normal cells are so sensitive that patient radiation tolerance doses are less than 30 per cent of those of the general population. In addition, there is some evidence that the inherent sensitivity of connective-tissue cells is related to the extent of clinical normal tissue response in apparently normal patients (Burnet *et al.*, 1992). However, as with tumour cells, not all studies have found this. A widely held view is that some variation in the sensitivity of normal cells does exist in the non-syndromic population, and that this will affect the normal tissue response. However, while the variation may be enough to be a significant factor, it is small enough to make reliable measurement of it very difficult with current methods. An important aim for molecular radiobiology is to resolve this debate.

INITIAL PHYSICAL AND CHEMICAL EVENTS: THE STARTING POINT FOR BIOLOGY

Figure 3.2 shows the sequence of events that follow irradiation of a cell. Ionizing radiation transfers energy to the molecules with which it interacts. At this stage, many of the biological effects of irradiation can be determined because the amount of energy transferred depends to a large degree on the type and energy of the radiation. The extent and nature of damage inflicted by different qualities of radiation depends to a large extent on their density of ionization. Densely ionizing radiations (i.e. α-particles, heavy ions, etc.) have a much greater biological effectiveness than sparsely ionizing radiations such as X- or γ-rays.

Interaction of radiation with an atom causes the ejection of one or more electrons, which may have a high energy and therefore cause secondary ionizations: these cause the subsequent chemical changes that lead to biological damage. The principal product of this process in water is an ionized water molecule, H_2O^+ which interacts with a neighbouring water molecule to form OH^- radicals which are very strongly oxidizing species with very high reactivity. Highly reactive reducing species ($H\cdot$ and e^-_{aq}) are also formed. The major target for these reactive species in terms of eventual biological effects is the DNA.

Radiation damage to DNA is separated into direct and scavengable effects which arise from energy deposited in water molecules surrounding DNA. It is now clear that the use of the term 'indirect damage' is not satisfactory, since the close proximity of water molecules may result in electrons produced in the DNA-associated water directly causing ionizations within the DNA. Therefore ionizations occurring directly in the DNA and outside the DNA may ultimately result in the same reactive centres within the DNA. The early chemical processes leading to DNA damage are well reviewed by O'Neill and Fielden (1993).

There are many substances that can modify the cellular response to irradiation by interfering with free-radical processes. Oxygen is the most obvious one. Oxygen sensitizes cells to the effect of radiation and the most plausible explanation of this is that free radicals formed in DNA react rapidly with oxygen to form peroxyradicals. This reaction, which is irreversible, competes effectively with a chemical repair process in which hydrogen atoms can be transferred from thiol-containing compounds to the free radicals on the DNA. As will be discussed below, the level of thiols and oxygen within a cell can therefore influence the efficacy of radiation treatment.

DNA DAMAGE INDUCTION

The level and type of DNA damage is established within seconds of irradiation, so that at this point cell signalling pathways are triggered and the biological repair pathways can recognize the problem they have to deal with. The nature and level of initial damage therefore has important implications for the overall biological effects of radiation.

Types of damage

A variety of lesions are produced in DNA by ionizing radiation, including base or sugar damage, DNA single-strand and double-strand breaks, DNA–protein crosslinks and DNA–DNA crosslinks (Table 3.1). For most cells it appears that the DNA double-strand break (dsb) is the critical lesion, causing cell death by ionizing radiation (reviewed in Iliakis, 1991). For example, in yeast and mammalian cells it can be demonstrated that DNA double-strand breaks induced by other methods (e.g. restriction

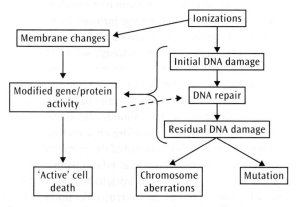

Figure 3.2 *The sequence of events from irradiation to biological effect.*

Table 3.1 *Radiation-induced DNA damage*

Type	Number per Gy per cell
DNA double-strand breaks	40
DNA single-strand breaks	1000
DNA–protein crosslinks	150
DNA–DNA crosslinks	30
Base damage	2000
Sugar damage	1500

endonucleases) lead to cellular inactivation, and in mammalian cells they produce similar types of chromosome damage and cytotoxicity to ionizing radiation. However, dsbs are not a uniform category of lesion. They may vary by virtue of the termini on the free ends of the molecule, also the proximity of other lesions. It has been suggested that a significant number of double-strand breaks will have other types of DNA damage nearby. These lesions have been termed clustered damage or local multiply damaged sites, and they may be particularly significant for radiation cell killing. It is hypothesized that the complexity of these clusters will increase with increasing linear energy transfer (LET) of the radiation. The potential significance of these is that they are formed by single tracks and that they will be more difficult to repair as the complexity of the cluster increases (Goodhead, 1994). At the present time we are unable to distinguish these different kinds of dsbs experimentally, however the reparability of dsbs is known to decrease with an increase in LET (Jenner *et al.*, 1993).

One consequence of the recent explosion in molecular radiobiology is that the importance of other types of DNA damage is being re-explored. It is clear that in some cell types the 'straightforward' physical breakage of chromosomes is only one of the ways in which they die. The process of apoptosis (described below) is a form of 'programmed cell death' that can be triggered by many types of DNA damage, including single-strand breaks for example. Thus it now needs to be considered that such 'lesser' types of damage might be important in cell death in some situations.

Variation in damage induction between cells

There have been several reports that cells can differ in the amount of damage that is detected immediately after irradiation ('initial damage'). Although these need to be assessed carefully because of the inadequacies of some of the DNA damage assays currently available, initial damage needs to be considered as a likely determinant of radiosensitivity in some situations. Radford (1990) proposed that the level of initially induced DNA double-strand breaks is directly related to radiosensitivity in a number of situations, including cell-cycle variation and differences in radiosensitivity between cell lines. Several

authors have also found such differences in human tumour cell lines, using a variety of assays (Whitaker *et al.*, 1995).

Although the energy deposition in critical cellular targets for a given radiation should be identical in all cells, this stage is followed by the chemical reactions that may modify the amount of damage inflicted in DNA. Exogenously applied thiol-modifying compounds can modify radiosensitivity, an effect that is especially large when cells are irradiated in hypoxic conditions. For example, the thiol-containing compounds cysteamine, WR-1065 or WR-255591 can show confer considerable radioprotection on cells (Murray *et al.*, 1991). This effect is reduced under oxic conditions because the kinetics of damage fixation by oxygen are significantly more favourable than those of chemical repair/scavenging by thiols. Nevertheless, such an effect does happen under oxic conditions, so that these chemical repair pathways have the potential to influence inherent cellular radiosensitivity as normally measured.

The effects of oxygen on free radicals are described above. In the absence of thiols, oxygen does not significantly modify the amount of DNA strand breaks. However, fixation of DNA damage by oxygen in the presence of thiols results in an increased induction of damage following irradiation compared to hypoxic conditions (i.e. before biological repair processes can take place). Oxygen therefore leads to an increase in cell killing. The oxygen enhancement ratio is similar for survival and damage induction, suggesting that the modification of damage induction is the main cause of the oxygen effect. There may be a slight effect of oxygen on repair processes, but this is less well understood.

Control of damage induction

The main cellular protection against radicals, their secondary reactants and peroxide is provided by cellular glutathione (GSH), GSH peroxidase, GSH transferase (GST) and catalase enzymes. GSH amounts to almost 90 per cent of the non-protein thiols in a cell. Studies on patients with 5-oxoprolinuria, who are glutathione synthetase deficient and have a very low GSH level, have shown a reduced oxygen enhancement ratio for both single-strand break (ssb) induction and survival, and these individuals have a slightly increased sensitivity (in terms of cell survival) to irradiation under oxic conditions (Debieu *et al.*, 1985). However, cells exhibiting a tenfold increase in πGST protein had the same radiation survival as those of the parent cell line (Chelon *et al.*, 1992). Thus the relationship between levels of these enzymes and radiosensitivity is not straightforward.

In addition to the soluble scavenging factors present in cells it is now clear that the protein components of chromatin play a major role in protecting DNA from the effects of radiation. Removal of histones and/or non-histone proteins from DNA has been demonstrated to greatly increase the amount of DNA damage inflicted (Mateos *et al.*, 1998a) to the point where an 80-fold increase in DNA damage results when naked DNA is compared to intact cells. Thus the constituents and structure of chromatin (i.e. the normal DNA–protein complex) is of increasing interest and importance in studies of the control of damage induction in cells, since there are some indications that the magnitude of these different levels of protection can vary between cells (Mateos *et al.*, 1998b).

GENE INDUCTION BY IONIZING RADIATION

It is well recognized that ionizing radiation alters the activity of specific genes and proteins in mammalian cells. This area of study has progressed from broad comparisons of overall mRNA from irradiated and non-irradiated cells in which a number of polypeptides were recognized as being induced by radiation (e.g. Boothman *et al.*, 1989) to the analysis of specific genes and the biological implications of the changes. In particular, it is now recognized that critical cell-signalling pathways can be triggered by radiation and that this may influence radiation sensitivity. The effects that can be conferred by transmembrane growth factor receptor tyrosine kinases, G-proteins and cytoplasmic serine/threonine kinases demonstrate how critical the signalling pathways are in the determination of radiosensitivity.

Two of the key responses are those relating to the cell cycle and apoptosis (discussed on pp. 40–42). In addition, a number of growth factors and cytokines are known to be induced by ionizing radiation in mammalian cells. These include tumour necrosis factor-α, interleukin-1 (IL-1), fibroblast growth factor (FGF), platelet-derived growth factor (PDGF-α) and transforming growth factor-β (TGF-β). The significance of this covers a wide area, including possible explanations of normal tissue-damaging effects of ionizing radiation. PDGF-α and basic fibroblast growth factor (bFGF) are released from vascular endothelial cells following radiation exposure. They have therefore been implicated in the proliferation of smooth muscle and endothelial cells observed in smaller arterioles after irradiation. Transforming growth factor (TGF-β) has been shown to be associated with pathological changes of late radiation damage in normal hepatocytes. The relative levels of TGF-β in irradiated hepatic tissue correlate with the extent of hepatic fibrosis. It has also been demonstrated that TGF-β secretions increase from monocytes in irradiated lung tissue, implying that TGF-β may be associated with the pathogenesis of the late effects of radiation in this tissue.

Although there are well-characterized inducible damage–response pathways in bacteria, which improve survival after ionizing radiation treatment, there is limited evidence for them in mammalian cells (reviewed in Joiner, 1994). What information there is comes from three areas:

1 An 'adaptive response' is seen when chromosome aberrations are counted in cells irradiated following a small priming dose: the number of chromosome aberrations is less when a priming dose has been given.
2 Cells irradiated with small doses prior to infection with irradiated virus can repair the virus more efficiently. This has been termed 'enhanced reactivation' and in some situations it has been found to be reduced in ataxia telangiectasia cells.
3 The slope of the clonogenic survival curve of irradiated mammalian cells has been shown to be initially very steep but is then shallower after doses of >1 Gy. This change in slope has been suggested to be due to an inducible radioprotective process that may be repair. Although the precise mechanism underlying this steep initial slope is yet to be elucidated the prediction of an increase in efficacy of fractionated radiotherapy when very small fraction sizes are used is beginning to be explored, with some encouraging early results.

DNA REPAIR

Once damaged, a primary aim for a cell has to be to restore as accurately as possible the structural and functional integrity of the DNA. The way in which this is done for DNA double-strand breaks (dsbs) in mammalian cells was virtually unknown 10 years ago but now the repair pathways have been characterized in some detail.

Rejoining of strand breaks

The disappearance of DNA dsbs induced with low LET radiation generally follows biphasic kinetics, with a half-time ($T_{1/2}$) of the fast component in the region of 20–40 minutes and a slow phase with a $T_{1/2}$ of several hours. These parameters can vary slightly between cells and the rate of repair has been correlated with radiosensitivity in some studies of human tumour cells (Schwartz *et al.*, 1988; Nunez *et al.*, 1996). In addition, there is some variation in the final level of breaks remaining (e.g. at 24 hours after treatment) and, again, these can be shown to relate to cell killing in some cell types (e.g. fibroblasts). At the extreme, however, are a number of mutants of hamster cell lines (e.g. *xrs* mutants) that show large reductions in the extent of dsb rejoining (e.g. 40 per cent repaired at 4 hours compared with 80 per cent repaired in the parental cell line, after 20 Gy; Whitaker and McMillan, 1992).

Studies of 'residual DNA damage' are hampered by a lack of sensitivity of the available assays, especially for those detecting dsbs. To overcome this problem some studies have utilized low dose-rate irradiation as a tool that can evaluate the extent of repair. Decreasing the dose-rate at which radiation is delivered results in a decrease in its efficacy of cell killing. This is believed to be the result of repair occurring during the protracted irradiation. Blöcher *et al.* (1991) used this to detect an increased level of damage in ataxia telangiectasia homozygotes and heterozygotes relative to control cells. Similarly, Cassoni *et al.* (1992) have identified differences in the amount of damage present after low dose-rate irradiation in four cell lines derived from human lung carcinomas, in such a way that the residual damage correlated well with radiosensitivity. The mechanistic basis of these correlations is, however, difficult to evaluate, since we have found that altering the dose rate within a single cell line does not seem to modify the final level of damage detected (Ruiz de Almodovar *et al.*, 1994). This may mean that the only lesions that were detected after a repair time at all dose rates are the severe lesions formed by single events which cannot be repaired at any dose rate. Alternatively, the lesions detected may be quantitatively similar but qualitatively different at each dose rate.

The accuracy of repair

Most of the damage assays used to assess repair are only able to measure the amount of DNA strand break rejoining. They are not able to assess the accuracy with which the repair process occurs, and this is obviously crucial to the subsequent gene function. This is not an easy factor to assess, but the investigation of radiation-induced mutations can shed some light on this (*see* p. 40). A more precise, but more artificial system involves the assessment of the ability of a cell to repair a foreign DNA molecule that has been damaged before being inserted into the cell in question.

One way in which this has been achieved is by cutting a plasmid with restriction endonucleases prior to transfection. The dsbs are placed within a gene that confers resistance to growth in a selective medium, e.g. mycophenolic acid (MCA). The repair of plasmid can therefore be analysed by growth in MCA. This method was used to demonstrate reduced repair fidelity in ataxia telangiectasia compared with normal fibroblasts. Repair deficiencies have also been detected in sensitive human tumour cell lines (Powell *et al.*, 1992, 1998). Such experiments have shown that repair of DNA can result in significant loss of genetic material, which suggests that even simple dsbs produced by restriction endonucleases can be converted into large deletions, either as a consequence of endonuclease activity or by the process of recombination.

DNA repair pathways for strand breaks

As stated earlier, ionizing radiation induces complex lesions, including both single-strand and double-strand breaks. Obe *et al.* (1992) sequenced DNA fragments after exposure to ionizing radiation and found that a large proportion had deletions of nucleotide sequence. This demonstrated that repair of strand breaks first requires processing of the damaged termini in order to leave clean ligatable ends. This is achieved by enzymes, including those with phosphodiesterase activity and kinase activity.

Single-strand breaks are protected by the abundant nuclear protein poly(ADP-ribose) polymerase-1, known as PARP1 (Lindahl and Wood, 1995). Although PARP has no clear role directly in single-strand break repair, it interacts with Xrcc1 (Masson *et al.*, 1998), which in turn interacts with DNA polymerase β and DNA ligase III (Caldecott *et al.*, 1996; Nash *et al.*, 1997). Binding of PARP to single-strand breaks can therefore lead to the recruitment of the gap-filling polymerase β and the ligase required to seal the resulting nick. The Xrcc1, DNA polymerase β and DNA ligase III proteins are also required to complete the process of base excision repair following removal of damaged bases (reviewed by Lindahl *et al.*, 1995). Xrcc1 was, in fact, the first gene to be isolated directly by virtue of its ability to modify cell sensitivity to ionizing radiation, since it corrects the radiosensitivity of the EM9 mutant of Chinese hamster ovary (CHO) cells which have a deficiency in single-strand break repair (Caldecott *et al.*, 1992).

In the case of DNA dsbs the scenario cannot be so simple. Even once the termini are clean, a straightforward ligation would lead to a change in sequence because the damaged bases will have been removed. Two main pathways are important for dsb repair. These are non-homologous end joining (NHEJ) and homologous recombination repair (HRR). NHEJ is critical in this context, as demonstrated by the extreme radiosensitivity and inadequate dsb rejoining in the hamster *xrs* cells and cells from severe combined immune deficient (*scid*) mice, both of which are now known to be defective in this process and the process of V(D)J recombination (reviewed by Jeggo *et al.*, 1995). An outline of this process is given in Figure. 3.3. The first stage involves the binding of the Ku heterodimer to the ends of the break. This dimer is made up of Ku80, an 80 kDa protein that is encoded by the *XRCC5/Ku80* gene (this is defective in *xrs* cells) and Ku70, a 70 kDa protein, encoded by the *XRCC6/Ku70* gene. The exact role of Ku is not known, but it is likely to be involved in recognizing DNA damage, protecting the ends of the DNA from nucleolytic degradation and pulling together the two DNA ends. Once bound to the DNA, Ku can recruit the catalytic subunit of the DNA-dependent protein kinase (DNA-PK$_{cs}$) to the DNA ends, resulting in a stimulation of the kinase activity. DNA-PK$_{cs}$ is the enzyme that is defective in radiosensitive *scid* mice, so it clearly has a role in the radiation response. DNA-PK phosphorylates many different proteins *in vitro*, but it is not clear which are its important cellular targets. With this function it may be an important signalling molecule (though the decrease in its activity by

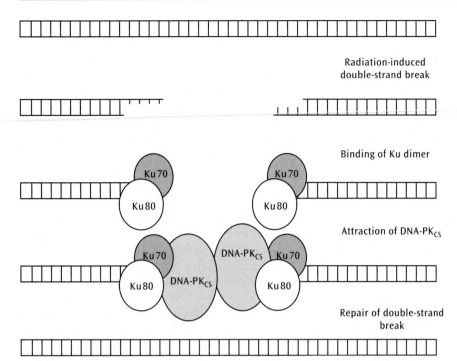

Radiation-induced
double-strand break

Binding of Ku dimer

Attraction of DNA-PK$_{CS}$

Repair of double-strand
break

Figure 3.3 *An outline of the initial stages of the repair of DNA double-strand breaks by non-homologous end rejoining.*

autophosphorylation reduces the possibility of this) or it may provide a marker for key repair proteins to locate to the break. These may include the Nbs1/Mre11/Rad50 complex (required for nucleolytic processing of damaged DNA) and DNA ligase IV and XRCC4 (required for ligating ends in NHEJ).

Homologous recombination repair (HRR) is the dominant dsb repair process in yeast. Since it needs extensive regions of DNA sequence homology, it is largely limited to the late S- and G$_2$-phase of the cell cycle in mammalian cells. However, the increased radiosensitivity of hamster cells defective in this process (e.g. *irs1* and *irs1SF* that are defective in XRCC2 and XRCC3, respectively), demonstrates the significance of the process in mammalian cells (Thacker, 1999). HRR has been largely characterized in bacteria and yeast but the recent isolation of human genes with sequence similarity to the critical yeast genes means that progress is likely in the characterization of human pathways. Once the DNA is broken, it appears that the human RAD52 protein binds to the ends of the DNA and may then recruit proteins required for homologous recombination, including Rad51 and possibly Xrcc2 and Xrcc3 (Van Dyck *et al.*, 1999). Rad51 protein is known to bind to DNA to form a nucleoprotein filament which is then able to initiate a search for homologous DNA molecules (Benson *et al.*, 1994; Baumann *et al.*, 1996). Rad51 can then catalyse pairing and strand exchange between homologous molecules to form heteroduplex DNA. Intact DNA molecules can then be generated following the action of a polymerase, a resolvase and a ligase to synthesize the new DNA, unravel the complex and ligate the DNA ends.

At least some of the proteins required for homologous recombination are involved in the repair of dsbs by the single-strand annealing (SSA) pathway. This has a requirement for the presence of repeat regions either side of the dsb. Resection of the 5′ ends reveals complementary DNA sequences which can then be annealed. Subsequent processing of intermediates by structure-specific endonucleases and ligases results in generation of products in which the sequence between the repeats is deleted.

RADIOSENSITIVE SYNDROMES

A small number of human inherited syndromes are associated with an increased radiosensitivity. These include ataxia telangiectasia and Nijmegen breakage syndrome, and these are proving valuable in elucidating aspects of the cellular response to DNA damage.

Ataxia telangiectasia

Ataxia telangiectasia (A-T) is an autosomal recessive human disorder that is associated with severe neurological problems, immunological deficits, an increase in T-cell leukaemias and lymphomas, and a greatly increased sensitivity to ionizing radiation. This radiosensitivity has been known for over 30 years and several cellular features of the syndrome have been identified, including a decrease in rejoining of dsbs, a decrease in the fidelity of dsb rejoining and defective cell-cycle checkpoints (at the G$_1$/S boundary, within S-phase and at the G$_2$/M transition). Many attempts were made to bring these features under a unifying hypothesis, but it now appears that some of the checkpoint defects can be separated from the radiosensitivity, so that A-T may be a dual repair/checkpoint defect (Jeggo *et al.*, 1998). The genetic mutation in A-T cells was identified in 1995 and the gene involved was labelled as the *ATM* gene ('AT mutated'; Savitsky *et al.*, 1995). ATM belongs to a family of kinases that includes proteins involved in DNA repair (DNA-PK$_{cs}$), meiotic recombination (mei41), control of telomere length (TEL1) and cell-cycle checkpoints (MEC1 in *Saccharomyces cerevisiae*, RAD3 in *S. pombe*) The ATM kinase has been shown to phosphorylate p53 in response to DNA damage, linking it directly to a role in the G_1/S damage checkpoint, and also to phosphorylate the single-strand-binding protein, RPA, which is required for dsb repair.

There has been considerable interest in the significance of A-T heterozygotes in the human population, since they may be present at a frequency of around 1 in 200. A suggestion that these individuals have an increased predisposition to breast cancer has been suggested by some studies, although a less convincing effect has been seen by others (Shayeghi *et al.*, 1998). Of particular relevance to breast cancer predisposition is the recent finding that ATM phosphorylation of the Brca1 protein in response to DNA damage is required for the function of Brca1 in dsb repair (Cortez *et al.*, 1999). Of relevance to radiotherapy is the suggestion that A-T heterozygotes may have a modest increase in cellular radiosensitivity, and that this may be at the root of some of the cases of extreme normal tissue damage after radiotherapy, although this needs to be investigated in detail.

Nijmegen breakage syndrome

Nijmegen breakage syndrome (NBS) is a rare autosomal recessive chromosome instability disorder that is associated with a cellular sensitivity to ionizing radiation and an abnormal S-phase cell-cycle checkpoint (like A-T it demonstrates so-called radioresistant DNA synthesis). The individuals suffer growth retardation, immunodeficiency, microcephaly and a predisposition to lymphoid malignancies. NBS cells do not show any gross defect in the repair of DNA dsbs, but the recent cloning of the gene defective in these individuals, *NBS1* (Varon *et al.*, 1998), and the characterization of the encoded protein (named nibrin or p95), has linked this syndrome to DNA repair. It is now evident that nibrin associates with Mre11 and RAD50 at the sites of DNA dsbs (Dong *et al.*, 1999) and that this is important in dsb repair.

THE NATURE OF RADIATION-INDUCED MUTATIONS

Overall, low-LET radiation is a rather poor mutagen because of its high lethality. However, the quantification of ionizing radiation-induced mutations has obvious significance in the study of carcinogenesis. In addition, mutation has been a useful tool in mechanistic studies analysing the molecular basis of radiosensitivity. As described earlier, Thacker and Stretch (1983) showed that potentially lethal damage repair and sublethal damage repair affected mutation frequencies to different degrees. Thus, what had been seen in cell survival studies to represent an increase in clonogenic cell survival in each case was suggested to be a consequence of different processes.

It is well recognized that radiation mainly produces fairly large deletions, rather than simple point mutations. For example, it was found that radiation increased mutation to 6-thioguanine resistance but not to ouabain resistance (Thacker *et al.*, 1978). This appears to be because the enzyme that needs to be mutated for resistance to 6-thioguanine is the *hgprt* gene, which is nonessential and therefore can be removed completely. On the other hand, the target for ouabain is a membrane ATPase that is essential for cell viability. Only a small base change within the ouabain binding site can result in a viable cell that is resistant to ouabain. Any more drastic change in this enzyme leads to loss of cell function. To support this, the assessment of marker loss along chromosomes has shown that significant areas of chromosome can be lost after irradiation within a single cell (Yandell *et al.*, 1990).

More detailed investigations of specific genes have revealed that radiation-induced mutations are randomly induced within a particular sequence and, in a majority of mutants, complete genes are lost. Smaller deletions and insertions of genetic material are also commonly detected (Breimer, 1988). These results contrast with spontaneous mutations that involve large deletions much less frequently. Direct DNA sequencing of the mutations has demonstrated that the two ends of a deletion commonly contain direct and inverted repeats, which may pair erroneously to result in an illegitimate recombination (Morris and Thacker, 1993). This suggests that a single break may be converted into a deletion by a recombination event between two similar sequences around the break, which fits with what is now known about repair pathways (*see* above).

DNA DAMAGE AND THE CELL CYCLE

The sequential completion of the various phases of the cell cycle and the avoidance of DNA damage are essential features of effective cell proliferation. Cell-cycle checkpoints have been recognized that monitor the cell cycle at various points to ensure the completion of the preceding phases (Dasika *et al.*, 1999). Such pathways also recognize damaged DNA, and so ionizing radiation, like other DNA-damaging agents, is known to result in cell-cycle delays, when the cell recognizes that it is damaged and so stops progression through the cycle. Two main points of arrest/delay are observed in irradiated cells – at the G_1/S boundary and at the G_2/M boundary – with a third checkpoint leading to a slowing of the DNA synthesis phase. These arrests have presumably evolved to allow repair to take place before the cell tries to replicate a damaged template or condense and separate damaged chromatids.

The importance of the G_2/M checkpoint in the radiation response is demonstrated very well in yeast *rad9* mutants that do not undergo a cell-cycle delay at the G_2/M boundary and are much more sensitive to ionizing radiation than the parental strains. In mammalian cells the significance of this checkpoint has been less easy to prove. The transfection of normal cells with the *ras* gene plus *myc* gene increases the G_2/M delay and causes an increase in radioresistance (McKenna *et al.*, 1991), and agents such as caffeine, which push cells through the checkpoint, do sensitize cells. It does appear, therefore, that this checkpoint is a significant determinant of the killing effect of radiation.

Cyclin B levels are reduced after irradiation, especially when cells are irradiated in S-phase (Muschel *et al.*, 1992) and p34^{cdc2} H1 kinase activity is also decreased in irradiated cells (Lock and Ross, 1990). Since the function of the cyclin–cdc2 complex appears to be essential for progression of cells through the G_2/M checkpoint the effects on cyclin production may well explain at least some of the observed changes in cell-cycle progression after radiation treatment.

Central to the checkpoint at the G_1/S boundary is the p53 protein. In response to DNA damage, p53 protein becomes less labile and increases in concentration in the cell. This increases its activity as a transcription factor, with one of its notable targets being the p21$^{cip1/waf1}$ protein that is a cyclin-dependent kinase inhibitor (CDKI). The role of CDKIs is to regulate cyclin/CDK complexes, which are the molecules that drive the cell cycle. Thus the increase in activity of p21$^{cip1/waf1}$ turns off various cyclin/CDK complexes so that the cycle is arrested. Of particular importance at the G_1/S boundary is the effect on cyclin D/CDK4 or 6, which exerts its effect through phosphorylation of the retinoblastoma protein Rb (Fig. 3.4). Despite this effect on cell-cycle progression, it is important to note that an absence of p53 does not lead to an increased radiosensitivity, rather, in many cases, it has been shown to lead to radioresistance. The explanation of this resistance is that, as well as stopping the cell cycle, the increase in p53 can lead to the onset of apoptosis (*see* below), so that a death pathway which is important in some cells is removed. However, these data do suggest that p53 is not involved in protection against the lethal effects of radiation, but the possibility of it protecting against mutation is raised. This is supported by the work of Kemp *et al.* (1994) who showed that p53-deficient mice are indeed more susceptible to radiation-induced tumours as well as spontaneous tumours.

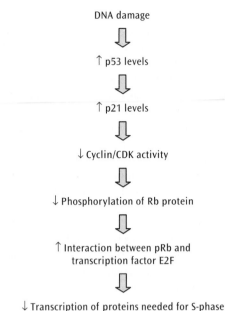

Figure 3.4 *An outline of the core pathway linking DNA damage to a cell-cycle arrest at the G_1/S boundary.*

APOPTOSIS

Apoptosis is the most well studied of the 'programmed cell death' pathways. It is characterized by distinct morphological changes in the cell (condensation of the chromatin, cell shrinkage, blebbing of the cell surface) and the fragmentation of chromatin at the linker regions between nucleosomes by a specific endonuclease. It is seen in cells that are lost during embryonic development, T- and B-cell maturation and endocrine-induced atrophy (Kerr *et al.*, 1972). Apoptosis has been implicated for a considerable time in the radiation response of some cells. For example, the extreme radiosensitivity of some cells of the crypts in the small intestine is believed to be related to a propensity to apoptosis, a process which is probably vital for the control of crypt size and function (Potten *et al.*, 1994). Several cell types have also been shown *in vitro* to undergo apoptosis following treatment with ionizing radiation. These include thymocytes, a human medulloblastoma cell line and a number of solid transplantable murine tumours.

The biochemical pathways involved in apoptosis and their genetic control have been increasingly well characterized (Budihardjo *et al.*, 1999). The activation of a variety of enzymes (caspases) that degrade cellular components is at the heart of this process, and it is recognized that this is initiated by proteins such as p53, which appears to be required for apoptosis to take place after irradiation (Clarke *et al.*, 1993). p53 seems to influence this process by controlling the levels of proteins such as Bcl-2 and Bax that are involved in regulating the permeability of the mitochondrial membrane. This, in turn, controls the juxtaposition of cytochrome *c* (a primary activator of caspases) and caspase precursors, so that apoptosis is regulated. The significance of apoptosis in clinical radiotherapy is still not clear. Studies looking at the relationship between apoptosis levels and radioresponsiveness have not demonstrated a relationship, and studies on cell lines in culture have not demonstrated any significance. However, in the latter case it is possible that cell lines are not the best subject for these studies as the mere fact that they are established in culture may mean that their apoptotic machinery is not functioning normally. It has been demonstrated in mouse models that inactivation of p53 function can increase the radioresistance of tumours (Lowe *et al.*, 1994) and Pirollo *et al.* (1997) have sensitized cells by the addition of wild-type p53. Thus, since p53 is mutated in a high proportion of cancers, this may be an important factor weighing against a desirable therapeutic index.

WHAT WILL THE ONCOLOGIST DO WITH THIS INFORMATION?

Predict sensitivity of normal and tumour cells

There is likely to be significant clinical advantage in predicting the inherent cellular sensitivity of tumour or normal cells. In the case of the tumour cells, this may aid any decision where there is a choice between radiotherapy and other modalities, and should provide useful information for the evaluation of trials of new treatment regimes. This latter point comes with the realization that modifications to treatment aimed at counteracting the effects of proliferation or hypoxia may only show advantages in tumours where the cells have a sensitivity in the middle of the range (Tucker and Chan, 1990). For normal cells, the identification of patients at the sensitive end of a spectrum may, in extreme cases, allow a reduction in dose, so that very severe side-effects are avoided. For those at the resistant end of the spectrum an increase in dose could be considered.

Any predictive test used in this way should be rapid, and molecular end points have an advantage over cellular end points in this regard. The use of gene expression as a reliable indicator of radiosensitivity will be difficult, as there are likely to be too many genes that can influence the level of radiosensitivity, unless a particular process dominates within a particular tumour type. For example, if a particular cell type is prone to apoptosis, then a specific set of genes could be analysed. Recent studies have confirmed this conclusion in that, for example, the activity of DNA-PK does not correlate with radiosensitivity in a range of human fibroblast cell lines (Kasten *et al.*, 1999). Clearly, advances in DNA array technology will increase the chances of success with this approach. DNA damage end points still have a potential role in this regard since they may directly reflect, or indeed cause, cell killing. The empirical approach that the level of damage induced, the rate of repair or the level of damage after 1 hour (presumably reflecting the combined effect of the first two) are possible predictive parameters. As we learn more about the nature and biological effects of specific types of damage, and we develop better assays to measure them, then better end points will be identified (McMillan and Peacock, 1994).

Identification of some cancer-prone individuals

There have been suggestions that chromosomal aberration end points following irradiation can detect a large spectrum of inherited syndromes which predispose to cancer, including Gardner's syndrome and xeroderma pigmentosum (Knight *et al.*, 1993), but the reliability and reproducibility of this still needs to be examined. A-T patients can be identified by radiation-induced chromosomal aberrations and DNA damage assays. However, in most cases it is probably not necessary to use radiation in such individuals as A-T is likely to be obvious, unless testing is done on a fetus or extremely young baby. The ethical questions associated with this are clear. Perhaps more importantly, there is one study suggesting that A-T heterozygotes can be identified using DNA dsb measurement after low dose-rate irradiation (Blöcher *et al.*, 1991). In addition, it is apparent in mice that the carriers of mutations in the *BRCA1* or *BRCA2* genes that predispose to breast and other cancers have a defect in dsb processing. This raises the possibility that both high and low (but not insignificant) cancer risks might be detectable if there is a broad relationship between radiation response and cancer proneness. As the methodology for screening large numbers of genes is developed and perfected, it may be argued that a role for radiation response in this context will become less. However, radiation still holds the promise of an almost universal probe that removes the need for translation of genetic changes into cellular phenotypes.

The design of new approaches to radiosensitization

A knowledge of controlling factors in the determination of the cellular response to radiation will allow the design of novel methods to modify cellular sensitivity. Several approaches are theoretically possible. Proteins may be inactivated by appropriately designed pharmacological agents, while gene expression and translation may be modified by so-called gene therapy approaches, and there are clear candidate genes for use in such protocols, e.g. *ATM* and *DNA-PK*.

The thought of being able to increase the sensitivity is obviously exciting and this could reduce tumour cure doses to achievable levels in a greatly increased number of patients. However, as with all gene therapy approaches, problems of delivery and the stability of the new phenotype have to be considered carefully. In radiotherapy this has to be looked at in relation to the limitations of fractionation that are dictated by normal tissue response. In a simple analysis, even the 18 Gy needed to cure a 1 g tumour in which *all* cells have been sensitized to a SF_2 (surviving fraction at 2 Gy) of 0.1 will need some fractionation, and this requires a stable sensitization. Once the conversion frequency is reduced to currently achievable levels, this is even more evident. It is possible to calculate the expected outcome if 10 per cent of the cells are stably sensitized and compare it with a situation where 10 per cent of the viable cells are sensitized before every fraction. If hypoxia is ignored and constant uptake of sensitizing agent into the viable cell population is assumed, such calculations suggest that the majority of the population will need to be sensitized with a stable agent (10 per cent is certainly not enough), or a sensitization procedure that allows sensitization of a constant proportion of cells before each treatment should be used. If these are satisfied, then important benefits could be achieved with these approaches. However, it is apparent that consideration will need to be given to the fractionation regime used in the context of genetic radiosensitization in order to exploit fully the characteristics of the sensitizing agent.

The search for gene targets for sensitization have been focused largely on the effect of oncogenes and tumour suppressor genes on radiation response, as this provides an obvious increase in specificity. For example, restoring p53 function to tumour cells has been demonstrated to provide a marked increase in radiosensitivity that is reflected in an increase growth delay in experimental tumours (Pirollo *et al.*, 1997). In addition, a knowledge of the biochemical pathways involving oncogenes has provided novel targets. Bernard *et al.* (1998) have used an approach that involves inhibitors of the process of prenylation, which is a chemical modification that is essential for the membrane localization of the Ras oncogenic protein, which in turn is necessary for Ras activity. As mentioned previously, increased *ras* expression can increase radioresistance, so that inhibiting its function leads to a sensitization.

An alternative approach uses the information that we now have about radiation-induced modification of the expression of some genes, and it is the controlling elements (promoters) of these genes that are instrumental in this. As an example of this, Chung *et al.* (1998) have demonstrated that this might be used for benefit in cancer therapy, by applying an idea published by Weichselbaum in 1991. They linked a gene coding for a toxic protein (in the report of Chung *et al.* this was tumour necrosis factor-α) to the promoter region from a radiation-inducible gene.

In this way the toxin is only produced when the radiation dose is sufficient to trigger the radiation-inducible gene promoter. Thus, if the DNA construct is inserted into the patient's cells the accuracy of radiotherapy means that selectivity towards the tumour is achieved. This approach is very attractive, although the release of a highly toxic molecule from the cells is a two-edged sword. On the one hand, it leads to a bystander effect within the tumour (i.e. tumour cells that do not incorporate the gene are also killed), but some of the selectivity is lost because of diffusion into the surrounding normal tissues.

FINAL REMARKS

There has been much development in our understanding of the molecular basis of the radiation response. Repair pathways are identified and rapid progress is being made in elucidating the elements of the pathways and how they fit together. Control of gene expression and oncogenic pathways are now known to impinge on the radiation response. Since radiation is the most effective non-surgical anti-cancer therapy, the application of molecular radiobiology to clinical situations has the potential to have a large overall benefit in the treatment of cancer.

SIGNIFICANT POINTS

- Radiotherapy and radiation biology have posed a great many questions which can now be approached using modern molecular techniques.
- An understanding of the physics and chemistry of radiation action suggests that the DNA damage induced by ionizing radiation is complex and modifiable by the quality of the radiation and oxygen.
- DNA double-strand breaks (dsbs) are believed to be the most critical form of radiation-induced damage, but they are highly heterogeneous and, for some cell types, other damage types may induce important pathways, including apoptosis.
- The level of DNA damage induced can be modified by scavengers of free radicals and can vary between cells of different sensitivity.
- DNA double-strand breaks are repaired by direct ligation, homologous recombination repair and, most importantly, non-homologous end rejoining.

- The extent and rate of disappearance of DNA dsbs has been correlated with radiosensitivity, as has the fidelity of repair.
- Radiation induces changes in expression of a large number of genes, including those involved in the control of cell growth, the cell cycle and apoptosis.
- A knowledge of the molecular basis of radiosensitivity will allow the prediction of tumour and normal tissue responses, identify some cancerprone individuals and the design of new approaches to radiosensitization/radioprotection.

KEY REFERENCES

Burnet, N.G., Wurm, R., Nyman, J. and Peacock, J.H. (1996) Normal tissue radiosensitivity – how important is it? *Clin. Oncol.* **8**, 25–34.

Jeggo, P.A., Tacciolo, G.E. and Jackson, S.P. (1995) Ménage à trois: double strand break repair, V(D)J recombination and DNA-PK. *Bioessays* **17**, 949–57.

Joiner, M.C. (1994) Induced radioresistance: an overview and historical perspective. *Int. J. Radiat. Biol.* **65**, 79–84.

Lindahl, T. and Wood, R.D. (1999) Quality control by DNA repair. *Science* **286**, 1897–905.

Nunez, M.I., McMillan, T.J., Valenzuela, M.T., Ruiz de Almodovar, J.M. and Pedraza, V. (1996) Relationship between DNA damage, rejoining and cell killing by radiation in mammalian cells. *Radiother. Oncol.* **39**, 155–65.

O'Neill, P. and Fielden, E.M. (1993) Primary free radical processes in DNA. *Adv. Radiat. Biol.* **17**, 53–120.

Thacker, J. (1999) A surfeit of RAD51-like genes? *Trends Genet.* **15**(5), 166–8.

REFERENCES

Baumann, P., Benson, F.E. and West, S.C. (1996) Human Rad51 protein promotes ATP-dependent homologous pairing and strand transfer reactions *in vitro. Curr. Genet.* **30**, 461–8.

Benson, F.E., Stasiak, A. and West, S.C. (1994) Purification and characterization of the human Rad51 protein, an analogue of *E. coli* RecA. *Hum. Genet.* **94**, 705–7.

Bernhard, E.J., McKenna, W.G., Hamilton, A.D. *et al.* (1998) Inhibiting Ras prenylation increases the radiosensitivity of human tumor cell lines with activating mutations of ras oncogenes. *Cancer Res.* **58**, 1754–61.

Blöcher, D., Sigut, D. and Hannan, M.A. (1991) Fibroblasts from ataxia telangiectasia (AT) and AT heterozygotes show an enhanced level of residual DNA double-strand breaks after low dose-rate gamma-irradiation as assayed by pulsed field gel electrophoresis. *Int. J. Radiat. Biol.* **60**, 791–802.

Boothman, D.A., Bouvard, I. and Hughes, E.N. (1989) Identification and characterization of X-ray-induced proteins in human cells. *Cancer Res.* **49**, 2871–8.

Breimer, L.H. (1988) Ionising radiation-induced mutagenesis (review). *Br. J. Cancer* **57**, 6–18.

Budihardjo, I., Oliver, H., Lutter, M., Luo, X. and Wang, L. (1999) Biochemical pathways of caspase activation during apoptosis. *Annu. Rev. Cell Dev. Biol.* **15**, 269–90.

Burnet, N.G., Nyman, J., Turesson, I., Wurm, R., Yarnold, J.R. and Peacock, J.H. (1992) Prediction of normal-tissue tolerance to radiotherapy from *in-vitro* cellular radiation sensitivity. *Lancet* **339**, 1570–1.

Burnet, N.G., Wurm, R., Nyman, J. and Peacock, J.H. (1996) Normal tissue radiosensitivity – how important is it? *Clin. Oncol.* **8**, 25–34.

Caldecott, K.W., Tucker, J.D. and Thompson, L.H. (1992) Construction of human XRCC1 minigenes that fully correct the CHO DNA repair mutant EM9. *Nucleic Acids Res.* **20**, 4575–9.

Caldecott, K.W., Aoufouchi, S., Johnson, P. and Shall, S. (1996) XRCC1 polypeptide interacts with DNA polymerase beta and possibly poly (ADP-ribose) polymerase, and DNA ligase III is a novel molecular 'nick-sensor' *in vitro. Nucleic Acids Res.* **24**, 4387–94.

Cassoni, A.M., McMillan, T.J., Peacock, J.H. and Steel, G.G. (1992) Differences in the level of DNA double-strand breaks in human tumour cell lines following low dose-rate irradiation. *Eur. J. Cancer* **28A**, 1610–14.

Chelon, A., Giaccia, A.J., Lewis, A.D., Hickson, I. and Brown, J.M. (1992) What role do glutathione s-transferases play in the cellular response to ionising radiation? *Int. J. Radiat. Oncol. Biol. Phys.* **22**, 759–63.

Chung, T.D., Mauceri, H.J., Hallahan, D.E. *et al.* (1998) Tumor necrosis factor-alpha-based gene therapy enhances radiation cytotoxicity in human prostate cancer. *Cancer Gene Ther.* **5**, 344–9.

Clarke, A.R., Purdie, C.A., Harrison, D.J. *et al.* (1993) Thymocyte apoptosis induced by p53 dependent and independent pathways. *Nature* **362**, 849–52.

Cortez, D., Wang, Y., Qin, J. and Elledge, S.J. (1999) Requirement of ATM-dependent phosphorylation of brca1 in the DNA damage response to double-strand breaks. *Science* **286**, 1162–6.

Dasika, G.K., Lin, S.C., Zhao, S., Sung, P., Tomkinson, A. and Lee, E. (1999) DNA damage-induced cell cycle checkpoints and DNA strand break repair in development and tumorigenesis. *Oncogene* **18**, 7883–99.

Deacon, J., Peckham, M.J. and Steel, G.G. (1984) The radioresponsiveness of human tumours and the initial slope of the cell survival curve. *Radiother. Oncol.* **2**, 317–23.

Debieu, D., Deschavanne, P.J., Midander, J., Larsson, A. and Malaise, E.P. (1985) Survival curves of glutathione synthetase deficient human fibroblasts: correlation between radiosensitivity in hypoxia and glutathione synthetase activity. *Int. J. Radiat. Biol.* **48**, 525–43.

Dong, Z., Zhong, Q. and Chen, P.L. (1999) The Nijmegen breakage syndrome protein is essential for Mre11 phosphorylation upon DNA damage. *J. Biol. Chem.* **274**, 19513–16.

Goodhead, D.T. (1994) Initial events in the cellular effects of ionising radiations: clustered damage in DNA. *Int. J. Radiat. Biol.* **65**, 7–17.

Iliakis, G. (1991) The role of DNA double strand breaks in ionising radiation-induced killing of eukaryotic cells. *Bioessays* **13**, 641–8.

Jeggo, P.A., Taccioli, G.E. and Jackson, S.P. (1995) Ménage à trois: double strand break repair, V(D)J recombination and DNA-PK. *Bioessays* **17**, 949–57.

Jeggo, P.A., Carr, A.M. and Lehmann, A.R. (1998) Splitting the ATM: distinct repair and checkpoint defects in ataxia-telangiectasia. *Trends Genet.* **14**, 312–16.

Jenner, T.J., de Lara, C.M., O'Neill, P. and Stevens, D.L. (1993) Induction and rejoining of DNA double strand breaks in V79-4 mammalian cells following γ- and α-irradiation. *Int. J. Radiat. Biol.* **64**, 265–73.

Joiner, M.C. (1994) Induced radioresistance: an overview and historical perspective. *Int. J. Radiat. Biol.* **65**, 79–84.

Kasten, U., Plottner, N., Johansen, J., Overgaard, J. and Dikomey, E. (1999) Ku70/80 gene expression and DNA-dependent protein kinase (DNA-PK) activity do not correlate with double-strand break (dsb) repair capacity and cellular radiosensitivity in normal human fibroblasts. *Br. J. Cancer* **79**, 1037–41.

Kemp, C.J., Wheldon, T. and Balmain, A. (1994) p53-deficient mice are extremely susceptible to radiation-induced tumorigenesis. *Nat. Genet.* **8**, 66–9.

Kerr, J.F.R., Wyllie, A.H. and Currie, A.R. (1972) Apoptosis: a basic biological phenomenon with wide-ranging implications in tissue kinetics. *Br. J. Cancer* **26**, 239–57.

Knight, R.D., Parshad, R., Price, F.M., Tarone, R.E. and Sanford, K.K. (1993) X-ray-induced chromatid damage in relation to DNA repair and cancer incidence in family members. *Int. J. Cancer* **54**, 589–93.

Lindahl, T. and Wood, R.D. (1999) Quality control by DNA repair. *Science* **286**, 1897–905.

Lindahl, T., Satoh, M.S., Poirier, G.G. and Klungland, A. (1995) Post-translational modification of poly(ADP-ribose) polymerase induced by DNA strand breaks. *Trends Biochem. Sci.* **20**, 405–11.

Lock, R.B. and Ross, W.E. (1990) Possible role for p34cdc2 kinase in etoposide-induced cell death of Chinese hamster ovary cells. *Cancer Res.* **50**, 3767–71.

Lowe, S.W., Bodis, S., McClatchey, A. *et al.* (1994) p53 status and the efficacy of cancer therapy *in vivo*. *Science* **266**, 807–10.

Masson, M., Niedergang, C., Schreiber, V., Muller, S., Menissier-de Murcia, J. and de Murcia, G. (1998) XRCC1 is specifically associated with poly(ADP-ribose) polymerase and negatively regulates its activity following DNA damage. *Mol. Cell. Biol.* **18**, 3563–71.

Mateos, S., Peacock, J.H., Steel, G.G. and McMillan, T.J. (1998a) Study of DNA double-strand break induction in different chromatin substrates of radioresistant and radiosensitive human tumour cell lines. *Biomed. Lett.* **58**, 7–18.

Mateos, S., Steel, G.G. and McMillan, T.J. (1998b) Differences between a human bladder carcinoma cell line and its radiosensitive clone in the formation of radiation-induced DNA double-strand breaks in different chromatin substrates. *Mutat. Res.* **409**, 73–80.

McKenna, W.G., Iliakis, G., Weiss, M.C., Bernhard, E.J. and Muschel, R.J. (1991) Increased G2 delay in radioresistance cells obtained by transformation of primary rate embryo cells with the oncogenes H-*ras* and v-*myc*. *Radiat. Res.* **125**, 283–7.

McMillan, T.J. and Peacock, J.H. (1994) Molecular determinants of radiosensitivity in mammalian cells. *Int. J. Radiat. Biol.* **65**, 49–55.

Morris, T. and Thacker, J. (1993) Formation of large deletions by illegitimate recombination in the HPRT gene of primary human fibroblasts. *Proc. Natl Acad. Sci.* **90**, 1392–6.

Murray, D., Prager, A., Altschuler, E.M. and Brock, W.A. (1991) Effect of thiols on micronucleus frequency in gamma-irradiated mammalian cells. *Mutat. Res.* **247**, 167–73.

Muschel, R.J., Zhang, H.B., Iliakis, G. and McKenna, W.G. (1992) Effects of ionising radiation on cyclin expression in HeLa cells. *Radiat. Res.* **132**, 153–7.

Nash, R.A., Caldecott, K.W., Barnes, D.E. and Lindahl, T. (1997) XRCC1 protein interacts with one of two distinct forms of DNA ligase III. *Biochemistry* **36**, 5207–11.

Nunez, M.I., McMillan, T.J., Valenzuela, M.T., Ruiz de Almodovar, J.M. and Pedraza, V. (1996) Relationship between DNA damage, rejoining and cell killing by radiation in mammalian cells. *Radiother. Oncol.* **39**, 155–65.

Obe, G., Johannes, C. and Schulte-Frohlinde, D. (1992) DNA double-strand breaks induced by sparsely ionising radiation and endonucleases as critical lesions for cell death, chromosomal aberrations, mutations and oncogenic transformation. *Mutagenesis* **7**, 3–12.

O'Neill, P. and Fielden, E.M. (1993) Primary free radical processes in DNA. *Adv. Radiat. Biol.* **17**, 53–120.

Overgaard, J. (1989) Sensitization of hypoxic tumour cells – clinical experience. *Int. J. Radiat. Biol.* **56**, 801–11.

Pirollo, K.F., Hao, Z., Rait, A. *et al.* (1997) p53 mediated sensitization of squamous cell carcinoma of the head and neck to radiotherapy. *Oncogene* **4**,1735–46.

Potten, C.S., Merritt, A., Hickman, J., Hall, P. and Faranda, A. (1994) The characterisation of radiation-induced apoptosis in the small intestine and its biological implications. *Int. J. Radiat. Biol.* **65**, 71–8.

Powell, S.N., Whitaker, S.J., Edwards, S.M. and McMillan, T.J. (1992) A DNA repair defect in a radiation-sensitive clone of a human bladder carcinoma cell line. *Br. J. Cancer* **65**, 798–802.

Powell, S.N., Mills, J. and McMillan, T.J. (1998) Misrepair of DNA strand breaks in radiosensitive human tumour cells. *Br. J. Radiol.* **71**, 1178–84.

Radford, I.R. (1990) The level of induced DNA double-strand breakage correlates with cell killing after X-irradiation. *Int. J. Radiat. Biol.* **48**, 45–54.

Ruiz de Almodovar, J.M., Bush, C., Peacock, J.H., Steel, G.G., Whitaker, S.J. and McMillan, T.J. (1994) Dose-rate effect for DNA damage induced by ionising radiation in human tumor cells. *Radiat. Res.* **138**, S93–S96.

Savitsky, K., Bar-Shira, A., Gilad, S. *et al.* (1995) A single ataxia telangiectasia gene with a product similar to PI-3 kinase. *Science* **268**, 1749–53.

Schwartz, J.L., Rotmensch, J., Giovanazzi, S., Cohen, M.B. and Weichselbaum, R.R. (1988) Faster repair of DNA double strand breaks in radioresistant human tumour cells. *Int. J. Radiat. Oncol. Biol. Phys.* **15**, 907–12.

Schwartz, J.L., Rasey, J., Wiens, L., Jordan, R., and Russell, K.J. (1999) Functional inactivation of p53 by HPV-E6 transformation is associated with a reduced expression of radiation-induced potentially lethal damage. *Int. J. Radiat. Biol.* **75**, 285–91.

Shayeghi, M., Seal, S., Regan, J. *et al.* (1998) Heterozygosity for mutations in the ataxia telangiectasia gene is not a major cause of radiotherapy complications in breast cancer patients. *Br. J. Cancer* **78**, 922–7.

Tannock, I.F. and Hill, R.P. (1998) *The basic science of oncology.* New York: McGraw-Hill.

Thacker, J. (1999) A surfeit of RAD51-like genes? *Trends Genet.* **15**(5), 166–8.

Thacker, J. and Stretch, A. (1983) Recovery from lethal and mutagenic damage during postirradiation holding and low dose rate irradiations of cultured hamster cells. *Radiat. Res.* **96**, 380–92.

Thacker, J., Stephens, M.A. and Stretch, A. (1978) Mutation to ouabain-resistance in Chinese hamster cells: induction by ethyl methanesulphonate and lack of induction by ionising radiation. *Mutat. Res.* **51**, 255–70.

Tucker, S.L. and Chan, K.S. (1990) The selection of patients for radiotherapy on the basis of tumor growth kinetics and intrinsic radiosensitivity. *Radiother. Oncol.* **18**, 197–211.

Van Dyck, E., Stasiak, A.Z., Stasiak, A. and West, S.C. (1999) Binding of double-strand breaks in DNA by human Rad52 protein. *Nature* **401**, 403.

Varon, R., Vissinga, C., Platzer, M. *et al.* (1998) Nibrin, a novel DNA double-strand break repair protein, is mutated in Nijmegen breakage syndrome. *Cell* **93**, 467–76.

Weichselbaum, R.R. (1991) Possible applications of biotechnology to radiotherapy. *Eur. J. Cancer* **27**, 405–6.

West, C.M.L., Davidson, S.E., Roberts, S.A. and Hunter, R.D. (1993) Intrinsic radiosensitivity and prediction of patient response to radiotherapy for carcinoma of the cervix. *Br. J. Cancer* **68**, 819–23.

Whitaker, S.J. and McMillan, T.J. (1992) Pulsed-field gel electrophoresis in the measurement of DNA double-strand break repair in xrs-6 and CHO cell lines: DNA degradation under some conditions interferes with the assessment of double-strand break rejoining. *Radiat. Res.* **130**, 389–92.

Whitaker, S.J., Ung, Y.C. and McMillan, T.J. (1995) DNA double-strand break induction and rejoining as determinants of human tumour cell radiosensitivity. A pulsed-field gel electrophoresis study. *Int. J. Radiat. Biol.* **67**, 7–18.

Withers, H.R., Taylor, J.M.G. and Maciejewski, B. (1988) The hazard of accelerated tumour clonogen repopulation during radiotherapy. *Acta Oncol.* **27**, 131–7.

Yandell, D.W., Dryja, T.P. and Little, J.B. (1990) Molecular genetic analysis of recessive mutations at a heterozygous autosomal locus in human cells. *Mutat. Res.* **229**, 89–102.

4

Clinical radiobiology

STANLEY DISCHE AND MICHELE I. SAUNDERS

INTRODUCTION

In the care of patients with cancer, the oncologist seeks to obtain a high level of tumour cure but with a low level of treatment-related morbidity. Essential to the good and safe practice of radiation therapy is a knowledge of the biology of tumours and of normal tissues, together with an understanding of the way in which they are affected by ionizing radiation. Topics most important to clinical practice will be considered in this chapter.

INHERENT CELLULAR RADIOSENSITIVITY

In most normal tissues and in most tumours careful histological study in the first few days after beginning a course of conventional radiotherapy reveals no obvious change; however, in all tissues irradiated, changes in the DNA are induced and these lead to damage that affects reproductive ability of the cells. This may not be manifest until mitosis is attempted; in some circumstances several cell divisions follow before cell death occurs, while other cells survive but lose the ability to reproduce. These are the effects which are important to the cure of tumours and to the appearance of late change in the normal tissues. There are, however, tissues that show immediate effects: after radiotherapy to the bone marrow or to the salivary glands evidence of apoptosis or intermitotic death may become apparent within hours following treatment and may be associated with steep falls in lymphocyte counts or steep rises in the serum amylase concentration as early as 24 hours after administration of doses as low as 2 Gy.

Tumour cells

Initially the inherent radiosensitivity of cells derived from animal and human tumours, as measured in the laboratory by the survival of clonogenic cells after high radiation doses, did not appear to differ greatly from that of cells derived from normal tissues. However, Fertil and Malaise (1981) demonstrated in cell lines derived from animal tumours that the surviving fraction of cells irradiated using a clinically relevant dose of 2 Gy (SF2) did differ widely from each other and from that of normal cells, and that the results could, in broad terms, predict the radio-curability, as determined when the tumour cells were implanted in mice. With human tumour cell lines grown in nude mice, the sensitivity shown in the laboratory broadly reflected that observed clinically (Steel and Adams, 1989).

Assays of the SF2 have been performed prior to radiotherapy to determine its value as a predictor of radiosensitivity and curability. West *et al.* (1997) showed that in carcinoma of cervix there was a close correlation between the SF2 and tumour control and survival. However, no correlation has been demonstrated in head and neck tumours (Brock *et al.*, 1992). The demonstration of a relationship between inherent sensitivity and tumour response in one common tumour in humans is important in radiobiology, but so far it does not offer a useful method of prediction because over 4 weeks must elapse before the results of an assay can be read.

Following radiotherapy, micronuclei can be seen in radiation-damaged cells and this has been related quantitatively to intrinsic radiosensitivity. Chromosomal damage can be determined quantitatively by fluorescence *in situ* hybridization (FISH) (McMillan and Steel, 1997). However, neither of these techniques lend themselves to practical clinical application at this time.

Normal cells

It has long been known that patients who have inherited ataxia telangiectasia show an extreme sensitivity to radiation, which appears to be at a level severalfold greater than that of normal people. Patients with Cockayne's, Gardner's, Down's and basal cell naevoid syndromes, and those with Fanconi's anaemia, may also show unusually severe reactions. Some patients with dermatomyositis and other collagen diseases have also shown a marked hypersensitivity. Cultures of fibroblasts taken from the skin of subjects with ataxia telangiectasia have been shown to possess a high radiosensitivity and this has also been shown in some patients who have produced severe reactions after receiving conventional courses of radiotherapy (McMillan, 1997).

However, such patients only account for a fraction of 1 per cent of all those presenting for consideration of treatment. It is a common observation that, among a normal population, there is a range of sensitivity: among a group of patients receiving identical treatment there are those where reactions, both early and late, are minimal, while others show considerable effects. Some correlation has been obtained between the radiosensitivity of human fibroblasts cultured *in vitro* and the radiosensitivity of the normal tissues, determined when previously they have been given a course of radiotherapy. The technique remains a demanding one, requiring a month to complete, and so remains a research tool. There is also interest in the radiosensitivity of peripheral blood lymphocytes because they can easily be obtained; however, there is no consensus as to the value of studies of lymphocyte sensitivity as predictors of radiation response (Begg, 1997).

The determination of the inherent radiosensitivity of tumours and of normal tissues has a potentially wide application in clinical oncology. There are case descriptions that report a similar high sensitivity of the tumour in the sensitive patients, but it is yet to be shown whether this is so generally. Those individuals shown to have a high degree of normal-tissue radiosensitivity might be best channelled to alternative methods of treatment. If patients whose normal tissues are particularly sensitive to radiation are excluded, then it may be possible to increase radiation doses to the remainder of the patients, and hence increase tumour control without significantly increasing overall morbidity (Denekamp and Hirst, 1992). The field is therefore a potentially important one, but progress has been slow and no technique is currently available to help make decisions in the management of human tumours.

DOSE–RESPONSE RELATIONSHIPS

Careful analysis of data derived from work with animal models and clinical studies has yielded important knowledge concerning the relationship between radiation dose and, on the one hand, tumour control and, on the other, the incidence of post-radiation change in normal tissues (Bentzen, 1997).

Gamma values

Dose–response curves have a sigmoid, or S, shape with a threshold level before the curves significantly depart from the base line (Fig. 4.1). In normal tissues there is generally a higher threshold dose but a steeper dose–response relationship. The steepness of the dose–response curve is given by the 'gamma value' (Brahme, 1984). This measure gives the increase in response in percentage points for a 1 per cent increase in dose. The commonly demonstrated

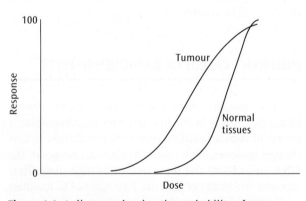

Figure 4.1 *A diagram showing the probability of tumour control and the incidence of late effects in the normal tissues. The actual curves in an individual case will depend upon the characteristics of the tumour and of the normal tissues irradiated, as well as the regime of radiotherapy.*

gamma values for squamous cancer of the head and neck region are in the range 1.5–2.5. With a gamma value of 2, a 10 per cent increase in dose can be expected to increase the tumour cure probability by 20 per cent; this may mean an elevation from 60 to 80 per cent. Animal tumour models usually show much higher gamma values – they commonly exceed 10. The greater heterogeneity of human tumours and inhomogeneities of radiation dose, together with inevitable inaccuracies in staging and inadequacies in follow-up, probably account for the much lower values found in the human situation.

At dose levels high in the therapeutic range, the gamma values for severe late reactions in normal tissues show greater values, and emphasize the importance, in the planning of radiotherapy, of avoiding maximum doses to significant areas in excess of that prescribed to the tumour.

We can conclude that the gamma values observed for both tumours and normal tissues in humans indicate that in clinical radiotherapy there is a relatively steep response gradient, and that therefore small variations in dose may have a critical effect upon the outcome.

Acute and late responses

Much knowledge has accumulated in the animal model and in the human concerning the responses to radiation seen acutely and in the long term, in different normal tissues. Commonly, tissues are divided into the 'acutely responding', showing reactions during and immediately after a course of treatment, and the 'late responding' tissues, which show little evidence that they have been irradiated until a number of months have passed following treatment. Among the former are the skin and the mucosa of the upper digestive and the lower digestive tract, while subcutaneous tissues, fat, liver, kidney and spinal cord are examples of late responding tissues. Early responding tissues may also show late changes, but these may be secondary to effects in the supporting connective tissue.

Whole- or part-organ irradiation

The effect of part- or whole-organ irradiation differs according to the tissue concerned. Loss of a considerable portion of the liver, or part (even the whole) of one kidney, may lead to little functional disability and be an acceptable consequence of radiotherapy if the clinical situation justifies it. With other structures, such as the intestine and the central nervous system, loss of, or severe damage to, a small part may have a vital effect.

Normal tissue tolerance

A broad guideline as to normal tissue tolerance, based upon the work of Rubin (1989), is shown in Table 4.1. Considerable variations will occur with different dose fractionation regimes of radiotherapy and when treatment is combined with other modalities, such as cytotoxic chemotherapy. None of the tolerance dose levels given should be applied without careful consideration.

The acceptable risk of morbidity of any measure of treatment must be related to the purpose for which treatment is being given and the result likely to be achieved. The functional loss of a considerable portion of a lung will give some disability which could well be justified in the control of an advanced bronchial carcinoma; on the other hand, any impairment of respiratory function is not acceptable following radiotherapy given after lumpectomy for an early carcinoma of the breast in a young patient.

Table 4.1 *Guide to organ tolerance: fractionated radiotherapy in 2 Gy daily doses (based on Rubin, 1989)*

Organ	Tolerance to partial-organ irradiation (Gy)		Tolerance to whole-organ irradiation (Gy)		Common severe complications
	5% severe morbidity in 5 years	50% severe morbidity in 5 years	5% severe morbidity in 5 years	50% severe morbidity in 5 years	
Lens	–	–	6	12	Cataract
Ovary	–	–	6	10	Sterility
Bone marrow	35	45	2	10	Aplasia
Liver	35	40	35	40	Liver failure
Stomach	–	–	50	55	Ulceration
Intestine	50	65	45	55	Ulceration/stricture
Brain	–	–	50	60	Necrosis
Spinal cord	50	60	–	–	Myelitis
Heart	55	60	45	50	Peri- and pancarditis
Lung	30	50	20	30	Pneumonitis/fibrosis
Kidney	–	–	23	28	Nephrosclerosis

Even in the management of advanced and inoperable tumours, levels of risk must be low in certain vital tissues because of the dire consequences that may follow, which can be as distressing as uncontrolled tumour growth. An example here would be radiation myelitis leading to paraplegia, where a risk greater than 1 per cent can rarely be justified.

CELL CYCLE AND RADIOSENSITIVITY

It has long been recognized that the phase in mitosis at the time of therapy may significantly affect radio- and chemosensitivities (Tubiana *et al.*, 1990). With ionizing radiation the maximum resistance is in S-phase and the greatest sensitivity in M and late G_2: there may be a factor of two in the relative sensitivity. Cytotoxic drugs show a number of patterns, but generally S-phase is the most sensitive period. However, with some drugs, resting-phase cells have been reported to be more sensitive than those that are proliferating.

The initial treatment in a fractionated course of radiotherapy may, after the period of mitotic arrest, lead to cell-cycle synchrony and, if the next treatment is given when the cells are in a sensitive phase of the cycle, an increase in cell kill may occur. So far, these experiments have been confined to the laboratory and there is no immediate application in clinical radiotherapy. With the multifraction techniques employed for cure in the clinic, it is difficult to see synchrony maintained beyond a second treatment. This makes it improbable that a manipulation of the cell cycle can be employed to improve the results of radiotherapy.

REPAIR OF SUBLETHAL INJURY

Sublethal injury

After exposure to radiation, some of the damage sustained within the cell can be repaired. The rate of repair falls in an exponential fashion, and in laboratory models the time for the rate to fall to half has been calculated to range from 30 to 120 minutes. Some variation is seen from one tissue to another, and two or more components of repair with different half-times may be present (Joiner, 1997a).

When more than one treatment is given each day, the duration of time between fractions must be chosen with care in order to allow as much repair as possible to occur in the normal tissues. It is important to note that the proportion of damage that is recoverable is smaller in tumours and in acutely responding tissues, such as skin and mucosa, than in the late responding tissues, such as kidney and connective tissue.

Clinical experience

In the 1980s inter-fraction intervals between 2 and 8 hours were employed in pilot studies of hyperfractionation in compromises between gaining the maximum amount of repair but coping with the practical problems associated with the organization of treatment more than once a day. Nguyen *et al.* (1985) employed the shortest recorded inter-fraction interval – 2 hours – and encountered a very high and totally unacceptable incidence of post-radiation morbidity, which exceeded 50 per cent in some groups. In a Radiation Therapy Oncology Group (RTOG) study of twice-daily treatment in head and neck cancer, it was noted that those cases where the inter-fraction interval was less than 4.5 hours showed a higher early and late morbidity than those where this interval was longer (Cox *et al.*, 1991). Bentzen *et al.* (1996) suggested that the half-times for repair in human normal tissues may be longer than those originally suggested.

Neural tissue and repair of sublethal injury

In the pilot study of continuous, hyperfractionated accelerated radiotherapy (CHART), five cases of radiation myelitis were observed when the maximum spinal cord dose, given in 36 treatments over 12 days with a 6-hour inter-fraction interval, ranged from 45 to 49 Gy (Dische and Saunders, 1999). Applying the linear quadratic equation and assuming practically complete repair at the end of 6 hours, radiation doses in excess of 60 Gy ought to have been tolerated without risk of myelitis. This led to considerable review and new laboratory experiments. Evidence emerged to suggest that repair times for neural tissue may be considerably longer than those in other tissues. In animal models half-times for recovery may exceed 4 hours, compared with 30–120 minutes for other tissues. From 1989, the permitted radiation dose to the spinal cord using the CHART regime was set at 40 Gy, with a maximum of 44 Gy in exceptional circumstances. With this reduction, no further cases of radiation myelitis have presented, with approaching 2000 cases treated worldwide. The situation demonstrates the difficulties that may present in the translation of laboratory data to the clinic, and the need for careful clinical observation so that unpredicted problems can be detected at the earliest possible time.

Half-time of repair in humans

Further analyses of the CHART trial data have now provided good evidence that, generally, the half-time of repair of sublethal injury in the human is probably of the order of 4 hours (Bentzen *et al.*, 1999). This accounts for the level of late morbidity seen in the CHART study where, although it was below that of conventional radiotherapy, it was not as markedly reduced as was predicted on the radiobiological evidence available when the regime was devised. Extrapolating from the animal data, the half-time of repair of neural tissue in humans may be close to 8 hours. Such a half-time would fully account for the unexpected myelopathy seen with CHART.

Knowledge of half-time of repair in human tissue is most important for the future design and refinement of altered fractionation regimes.

FRACTION SIZE

Fractionation formulae

In the early years of radiotherapy, benefit in terms of increased tumour control, with acceptable tissue morbidity, was achieved by moving from a single, or a few, large dose fractions to small doses given daily over a number of weeks. To achieve this benefit it was found that the total dose given in many small fractions needed to be increased. When, for example, treatment was changed from one single to 30 daily treatments over 6 weeks, the total dose needed to be multiplied by a factor of three.

Strandqvist (1944) proposed a mathematical formula to relate total dose and overall time to skin tolerance. Subsequently it was found that the effects of fraction number and overall time needed to be separated; this was an important contribution made by Ellis (1969). The Ellis formula was widely employed and helpful in clinical practice. However, it later became apparent that, when the number of fractions was reduced below 12, there was a greater incidence of late normal tissue effects than predicted (Thames and Hendry, 1987).

Linear quadratic formula

In 1982, the linear quadratic formula (LQ) was proposed as more widely applicable when dose fractionation regimes were being compared (Barendsen, 1982). It has been shown that, at clinically relevant doses, tumours and early reacting tissues respond to ionizing radiation, dominantly with a linear relationship between dose and effect – the α or linear element. In the late reacting tissues, however, an important element is related to the square of the individual dose – the β or quadratic element. The important implication of this linear quadratic model is that, by giving radiotherapy in many small doses, there should be further sparing of the damage in late reacting tissues but little alteration in the response of the early reacting normal tissues and, most particularly, of the tumour.

Clinical experience with LQ

Support for the appropriateness of the linear quadratic model has been gained from clinical experience. Reports

have appeared of levels of late tissue injury in spinal cord, skin, bowel, bone, pericardium and mediastinum after the use of a large dose per fraction that have been greater than that expected from the Ellis formula but could have been predicted by LQ (Joiner and van der Kogel, 1997). The reduced severity of late normal tissue injury with the use of a small dose per fraction has been confirmed in clinical trials where, by giving doses of 1.15–1.2 Gy twice daily to total doses of 74–81.6 Gy, the late normal tissue changes were no greater than when using a conventionally fractionated course of radiotherapy of 2 Gy daily for 7 weeks to a total dose of 70 Gy; with these higher doses greater tumour control was achieved (Horiot et al., 1998; Fu et al., 2000).

The study performed by the British Institute of Radiology, which compared five and three fractions per week and incorporated a reduction in total dose for the three fractions of 11–13 per cent, appeared to show a 'null' effect, with the reduction in the number of fractions giving similar tumour control and late morbidity (Rezvani et al., 1989; Wiernik et al., 1990). However, this trial, like its companion, which compared long and short durations, was conducted at an early stage in the development of the methodology of clinical trials and had a low sensitivity. The margins, although they did not reach statistical significance, were in favour of the concept that fraction size was important in determining late tissue injury and that benefit could be improved by the use of hyperfractionation.

Low dose per fraction

The long-term follow-up of patients in the CHART pilot study and in the randomized trial has given confirmation of the sparing of late change because of low dose per fraction together with lower total dose (Dische et al., 1997). However, the marked reduction in acute and late change in skin was not anticipated by the radiobiological evidence used to design the protocol. Since then, support for reduction in skin reaction with short overall time has come from one study of the tolerance of pig skin. The result may be due to a completion of all radiation prior to the onset of cellular proliferation, which can occur without inhibition by continued irradiation. Alternatively, the process of cellular proliferation in the skin may be less efficient when treatment is prolonged. Confirmation, in the randomized trial, of the observation made first in the pilot study is of importance for the use of this accelerated regime with tumours which, for their treatment, require irradiation of skin to full dose (e.g. skin in areas that are particularly radioresponsive, such as the perineum) (Dische and Saunders, 1999).

The sparing of late effects achieved with a low dose per fraction has important implications for clinical radiotherapy. In the pursuit of tumour cure, the highest tolerable doses must be achieved, but when there are sensitive

Table 4.2 *Schedules of radiotherapy employed at the Mount Vernon Cancer Centre and their calculated biological units of late effect*

	No. of fractions	Dose per fraction (Gy)	Total dose (Gy)	Overall duration (days)	Effect on late tissue (units of effect)
Definitive treatment for cure	33	2.0	66	45	112
	30	2.0	60	40	100
	20	2.6	52	33	97
	36	1.5	54	12	81
Postoperative treatment	25	2.0	50	33	83
	15	2.7	40	19	76
Palliation	10	3.0	30	12	60
	6	5.0	30	18	80
	2	8.5	17	8	65
	1	12.0	12	1	60

tissues in the volume for treatment, in which late injury must be kept to a minimum, the fraction size should be no greater than 2 Gy. Further advantage may be gained by a reduction of individual doses down to the level of 1 Gy.

Low-dose hyper-radiosensitivity

Until recently there was no reason for clinicians to be interested in radiation doses below 1 Gy, but with the development of new techniques, research into radioresistant cell lines, initially carried out at the Gray Laboratory, has shown an excess of cell kill at doses below 1 Gy relative to that predicted by the LQ model. This phenomena is termed 'low-dose hyper-radiosensitivity' (LDHRS) and has been shown to be present in many human tumour cell lines; its effect being generally greater in those that are radioresistant (Saunders *et al.*, 1999). LDHRS has been demonstrated using single and multiple fractions of treatment in cell culture and in xenografts. The effect can be demonstrated in rodent normal skin and kidney but not in spinal cord. Modelling the effects of LDHRS suggests that there may be an increase in the therapeutic ratio for tumour cell kill to normal tissue effects. A therapeutic gain factor of 1.9 has been calculated in a comparison of glioma cell lines to normal skin, and 2.7 comparing glioma cell lines to normal rat spinal cord. The prospect of treating two or three times daily for periods of 5–6 weeks is a daunting one; however, if the promise is sustained, then a remarkably improved radiation response may be obtained in highly resistant tumours, such as gliomas, where it has been difficult to progress with any form of non-surgical treatment in recent years.

Fractionation in clinical practice

It is important to recognize that there are many circumstances in radiotherapy where a larger dose per fraction may be employed safely. These will include those situations in treatments for cure when only a small volume

of normal tissue with a high tolerance for late effect is included, or where a reduction in overall time, by reducing time for tumour cell proliferation, allows a lower total dose to be set. When postoperative radiotherapy is administered, where there is a low tumour cell burden, a lower total dose is needed and this may be given in larger doses per fraction while keeping risks of morbidity low. In palliation, where relatively low total doses need to be given, large doses per fraction are best, for fewer attendances bring obvious advantages to the patient and reduce the burden upon the facilities for treatment.

In a centre of oncology, a whole range of dose fractionation regimens should be available to deal with all the clinical situations that present (Table 4.2) (Dische, 1993). Laboratory and clinical research has provided good evidence to support these practices.

TUMOUR CELL PROLIFERATION

Doubling times

When there is an opportunity to observe the natural progression of a carcinoma or sarcoma, several months may pass before the tumour doubles its size. When serial observations have been possible, volume doubling times have ranged from 30 to over 300 days, with median values often over 100 days (Steel, 1997a). These observations, together with knowledge that there is a period of mitotic arrest after exposure to ionizing radiation, led radiotherapists to the view that growth during a course of radiation therapy lasting 4–7 weeks was not likely to be important in influencing the result. Advances in knowledge have caused this opinion to be revised.

Tumour cell kinetics

In the past it was only possible to study the cell kinetics of human tumours by administering tritiated thymidine.

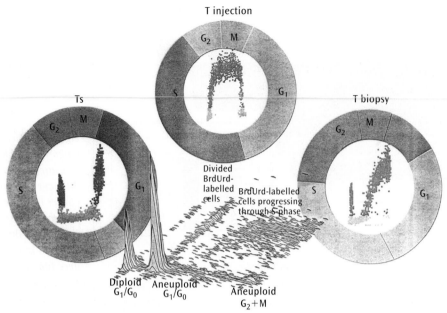

T injection

G_2 M

Ts

G_2 M

S G_1

S G_1

T biopsy

M

G_2

S G_1

Divided
BrdUrd-
labelled
cells

BrdUrd-labelled
cells progressing
through S-phase

Diploid
G_1/G_0

Aneuploid
G_1/G_0

Aneuploid
G_2+M

Figure 4.2 *Measurement of potential doubling time (Tpot) by flow cytometry. The distribution of bromodeoxyuridine (BrdUrd)-labelled cells immediately after an injection of BrdUrd shows a uniform distribution throughout S-phase. At the time of biopsy, some cells have divided and reside in G_1 while the others are progressing towards G_2. At Ts, all cells have either divided or now reside in G_2. Assuming that the progression of BrdUrd-labelled cells through S-phase is uniform, the Ts can be computed using the method described by Begg* et al. *(1985). The inset shows a three-dimensional dotplot obtained from a carcinoma of the tongue removed 5 hours after an injection of BrdUrd. In this aneuploid tumour, the Ts was 12.8 hours, the LI (the number of cells incorporating BrdUrd, corrected for cell division) was 11.7 per cent in the aneuploid population. This gave a Tpot of 3.6 days.*

As the radioactive burden of this technique is considerable, only patients with advanced disease could be investigated. Further, the procedure is a complex one, requiring autoradiography and many weeks to complete a study (Denekamp, 1982).

By giving an injection of a small dose of bromodeoxyuridine (BrdUrd) and performing a biopsy 4–6 hours later, Begg and his colleagues (1985) were able to determine the cell kinetics of a tumour and to obtain a result in 24 hours. With use of a cell sorter, the proportion of cells preparing for division (the labelling index) and the duration of S-phase could be determined (Fig. 4.2). From these values the potential cell doubling time was calculated. This is a measure of the proliferative activity of tumour cells, taking into account the presence of dividing and non-dividing cells, but assuming the absence of cell loss.

A wide range of values has been obtained in over 1000 human tumours using this technique. In squamous cell cancer in the head and neck region and in the uterine cervix median values lie between 4 and 5 days, while median values a little higher are seen in other tumours (Fig. 4.3). Spontaneous cell loss, due to apoptosis, nutritional deprivation and differentiation, accounts for the 10- to 20-fold differences between cellular doubling times and volume doubling times observed clinically.

With an immunohistochemical technique, the cells that have taken up the BrdUrd can be seen clearly under the

microscope and considerable variation in the proportion of labelled cells can be observed from field to field. At the growing edge of many squamous cell carcinomas up to 60 per cent of the cells may appear to contain BrdUrd and therefore be in DNA synthesis (Bennett *et al.*, 1992). The advantage of the immunohistochemical technique over flow cytometry is that tumour cells can be readily differentiated from normal cells. This is particularly important in diploid tumours where it is not possible, using the flow cytometer, to separate them. In squamous cell cancers in the head and neck region the labelling indices determined by immunohistochemistry have been combined with the duration of S-phase determined by flow cytometry to calculate the potential doubling time. When the maximum labelling index, as seen microscopically, is used, half the tumours show potential cell doubling times of less than 2 days (Bennett *et al.*, 1992).

Kinetics after initiating treatment

When tumour cells are destroyed by radiotherapy or cytotoxic chemotherapy, it is likely that the pattern of cell division and loss will be altered considerably. It is most probable that the high spontaneous cell loss occurring in the unperturbed tumour will be greatly reduced, and the surviving tumour cells will realize their full reproductive

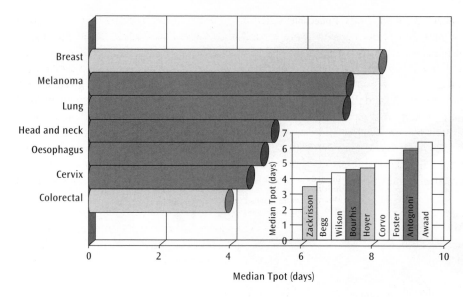

Figure 4.3 *Median values for potential doubling time (Tpot) measured in a variety of different tumours at the Gray Cancer Institute (data provided by George Wilson). The inset shows published data from different groups for head and neck tumours only.*

potential. It is even possible that cellular division may be accelerated with an increased growth fraction of the surviving tumour cells, and the cell-cycle time may be reduced so that repopulation occurs at a rate even faster than that suggested by the cell kinetics performed prior to treatment.

Evidence to support the view that repopulation is an important factor in determining the result of a course of radiotherapy has been derived from analyses of clinical data. Prolongation of a course of radiotherapy has been shown to result in the reduction of the probability of tumour cure at a number of sites, including head and neck, uterine cervix and breast. The prolongation of overall duration of treatment for head and neck cancer by 1 week may reduce tumour cure rates by 13 per cent (Maciejewski *et al.*, 1983; Fowler and Lindstrom, 1992). Most of this work is the result of retrospective analysis of consecutively treated patients, where treatment may have been prolonged for many reasons. The most convincing data have been obtained from the results of a randomized trial of split-course therapy in head and neck cancer (Overgaard *et al.*, 1988).

Control of the cell cycle

Recent research in molecular biology has revealed the complexity of control mechanisms for tumour growth (Milas *et al.*, 1998). Knowledge of the time of onset of repopulation after tumour cell destruction by radiotherapy or cytotoxic chemotherapy is of importance for exploitation of cellular repopulation. In normal tissues there is a considerable variation in the time of repopulation after cellular depletion: in the bone marrow this will occur within 24 hours, but only after 14 days in the skin (Denekamp, 1982). A relationship between the time of repopulation in a tumour and in the normal structure from which it is derived is a reasonable, but unproven hypothesis.

Onset of repopulation

In different animal tumour models the time to commencement of repopulation has shown a wide range of intervals (7–21 days have been reported). Withers *et al.* (1988) researched the literature reporting the results of radiotherapy in head and neck cancer and derived 59 sets of data where they were able to estimate the dose required to achieve 50 per cent local tumour control, normalizing to express the dose given as if it had been applied in all series in 2 Gy dose fractions. They found evidence that repopulation of squamous cell cancer in the head and neck region may begin after a lag period of 3–5 weeks after initiation of radiotherapy. However, further analysis of the same material by Bentzen and Thames (1991) has failed to show a lag before repopulation commences.

We know that in the head and neck region squamous cell carcinoma may have a cell loss factor exceeding 90 per cent. At the end of the first week of a conventional course of radiotherapy, using 2-Gy fractions daily, 95 per cent of the tumour cells may be destroyed. It seems unlikely, in these circumstances, that the pretreatment cell loss factor persists at the previous high level and that, at least in some tumours, repopulation does commence within 2 weeks of the initiation of treatment. The intensity of the course of treatment may also be a factor modifying the time of onset of repopulation. In a number of analyses of clinical data it has been calculated that, when repopulation does commence, an extra dose of the order of 0.6 Gy is required each day to overcome it, and this is consistent with a 4-day clonogen doubling time (Withers *et al.*, 1988).

Molecular markers

Several proteins appear to be expressed in proliferating, but not in quiescent, cells. Antibodies have been developed to these proteins and can be used to assess proliferation by immunohistochemical or flow cytometric methods. If, with such markers, tumour cell kinetics can be determined on routine biopsy material, or even archival sections, drug administration will be avoided and it will be unnecessary for further biopsies to be performed.

Ki67, MIB1, PCNA, p53 and cyclins A and B are among the markers that have been studied. Some appear to give, to a greater or lesser extent, the proportion of cycling cells (growth fraction) but do not, of course, give the rate of progression through the cell cycle as obtained with BrdUrd. Other markers may relate to alterations in tumour progression through phases of the cell cycle. They may give further knowledge concerning the progress of malignancy and relate quantitatively to the response to treatment and to the prognosis.

Kinetics and prediction of response

There was considerable interest in the possibility that the tumour cell kinetics of an individual tumour would be predictive of its response to conventional radiotherapy (Begg et al., 1998). Initially correlations were observed; however, with the accumulation of larger numbers, the potential cell doubling time determined using BrdUrd has not been correlated significantly with the response of head and neck tumours treated by conventional radiotherapy. Of course, the proliferative characteristics of the tumour during radiotherapy are most important, and they may not be closely related to the characteristics determined in the unperturbed tumour. There is, unfortunately, no way of determining kinetics once treatment has commenced. Failure to relate the potential cell doubling time to the result in an individual case does not nullify the general observations that have been made and the great advance in knowledge that has come from studies of tumour cell proliferation.

MODIFICATION OF RADIOTHERAPY PROGRAMMING

Over the past 25 years many pilot studies of altered fractionation have been performed and some have proceeded to randomized controlled clinical trial. The greatest amount of knowledge has been gained in the management of squamous cell cancer in the head and neck region, but important studies have been carried out in the management of other tumours.

Squamous cell cancer in the head and neck region

HYPERFRACTIONATION

Hyperfractionation, the employment of an increased number of fractions without alteration in overall time,

was tested in hypopharyngeal tumours in a randomized controlled clinical trial (EORTC 22791) which included a total of 358 cases between 1980 and 1990. A radiation dose of 1.15 Gy given twice daily resulted in a total dose of 80.5 Gy, which was compared with 70 Gy given in 2-Gy fractions. There was a significant improvement in local tumour control (61 per cent compared with 42 per cent at 5 years), while the incidence of moderate and severe late effects was equal; a clear benefit was therefore achieved (Horiot et al., 1998). This regime was also tested in RTOG 6492. A first report on the trial, which included over 1000 cases, indicates that this approach gave significantly better local tumour control, with 2-year figures of 54.4 per cent, versus 46 per cent for the conventionally treated group (Fu et al., 2000). So far no significant increase in late sequelae has been observed.

ACCELERATION

Acceleration – reduction in the overall duration of a course of radiotherapy, in order to minimize the time during which cell proliferation can take place – has been tested in a number of pilot studies. To keep the fraction size to 2 Gy or below, it is necessary to give the radiotherapy on more than one occasion each day. Working with a range of head and neck tumours, early attempts by Italian groups to reduce the overall duration of treatment without modification of the conventional 2 Gy dose led to unacceptable late morbidity, even though the total dose, given in thrice-daily treatments over two working weeks, was reduced to between 54 and 56 Gy (Peracchia and Salti, 1981; Olmi et al., 1990). An interfraction interval of 4 hours was commonly used, and this does complicate the interpretation, but most importantly, tumour control did not appear to be improved.

HYPERFRACTIONATION USING A SPLIT COURSE

Work at Leuven in the late 1970s showed that, despite a reduction of the individual dose to 1.6 Gy when treating three times a day to accelerate treatment, reactions in patients with head and neck tumours early in the third week prevented continuation of therapy. In further work, after intensive treatment over 2 weeks, patients were given a 4-week rest period before completion of therapy, in an overall period of 7 weeks. An EORTC multicentre study which followed, however, showed no benefit (Van den Bogaert et al., 1986) and the experience suggested that it was most important that the overall duration of therapy be reduced. Wang et al. (1985), using a similar approach but reducing the overall time to 6 weeks, reported highly significant improvements in retrospective comparisons at all the main sites of head and neck. The scheme of accelerated treatment was one of three experimental arms in RTOG 6492. First analyses reported in 2000 suggested no advantage in local tumour control over conventional radiotherapy, and similar levels of morbidity (Fu et al., 2000).

In a further EORTC trial, the overall duration was reduced to 5 weeks and a short rest period incorporated early in the second week. A significant improvement in local tumour control was demonstrated, but this was achieved at the expensive of a significant increase in serious late effects (Horiot et al., 1998).

Although the second EORTC trial did show significant improvement, the morbidity encountered has discouraged its application. It seems unlikely that accelerated hyperfractionation using a split course will be further explored in the management of head and neck cancer.

CONCOMITANT BOOST

A boost to the area of known disease is given as a second treatment in the day during part of the main course of therapy, instead of following it as in normal practice. It was found, however, that the boost was best given during the closing weeks of the main course of treatment. In a pilot study in oropharyngeal carcinoma, locoregional control was achieved in 86 per cent of 200 cases (Morrison et al., 1999) – an exceedingly good result considering that 62 per cent were T3 or T4 or N+ – and this regime was incorporated in RTOG 6492. The first report indicates that the concomitant boost regime gave significantly better local tumour control, with 2-year figures of 54.5 per cent versus 46 per cent for the conventionally treated group (Fu et al., 2000). So far, no significant increase in late sequelae has been observed.

SIX FRACTIONS PER WEEK

In the Danish Head and Neck Cancer Study (DAHANCA) 5 and 6, the overall treatment time was reduced from 6.5 to 5.5 weeks by giving an extra treatment each week, either on the Saturday or as a second treatment after at least 6 hours on a Friday. All other conditions of treatment were similar in both arms of the study. In this large, randomized, controlled trial, which also included over 1000 cases, a significant improvement in locoregional control (at 3 years, 62 per cent against 54 per cent, $P = 0.001$) and in overall survival was achieved without any apparent increase in morbidity (Overgaard et al., 1998). This fractionation is now standard for management of squamous cancer of the head and neck region in Denmark.

CONTINUOUS HYPERFRACTIONATED ACCELERATED RADIOTHERAPY

Continuous hyperfractionated accelerated radiotherapy (CHART) was devised at Mount Vernon Hospital with the objective of combining the greatest chance of eradicating all tumour by acceleration, with the minimization of late effects in normal tissues by employing hyperfractionation. All treatment is given in 12 days, so that the acute reactions which present in the head and neck region using accelerated radiotherapy do not appear until

after the course is completed. During most of the period of the pilot study, which was commenced in January 1985, an individual dose fraction of 1.5 Gy was given three times a day at 6-hourly intervals, so that in 12 days a total dose of 54 Gy (minimum tumour dose) was achieved (Saunders, 1998).

By March 1990, 168 patients with head and neck cancer had been treated using this regime. In T3 and T4 tumours, there appeared to be a significant improvement in primary tumour control when comparison was made with previously treated cases. This, combined with the reduced level of morbidity, was the indication for a randomized controlled multicentre trial which was completed in March 1995 when 918 patients had been included. Overall there was no significant improvement in locoregional control but subgroup analysis suggested that those patients with differentiated, as opposed to undifferentiated, tumours derived benefit and, further, that advanced tumours, particularly those of the larynx, also gained benefit (Dische et al., 1997).

CONTINUOUS DAILY TREATMENT

With continuing daily treatment through the weekends, Maciejewski and his colleagues achieved a total dose of 70 Gy using conventional 2-Gy fractions in 5 instead of 7 weeks. The group reported locoregional control rates of 68 per cent compared with 22 per cent in their conventional group at 2 years, but also a significant and unacceptable level of morbidity. The fraction size has now been reduced to 1.8 Gy and it is reported that control rates have been maintained while morbidity levels have been reduced to that of the control group (Skaladowski et al., 2000).

THE CURRENT POSITION WITH REGARD TO ALTERED FRACTIONATION

There can be no doubt that repopulation is an important factor influencing the response to radiotherapy of squamous cell cancer in the head and neck region. We can conclude from the CHART trial that 54 Gy gives similar tumour control in 12 days to 66 Gy given over 45 days. If repopulation commences towards the end of the fourth week, then 0.6 Gy is employed each day just to overcome this repopulation in the remaining portion of a conventional course of radiotherapy. This figure is very similar to that which has been calculated from the retrospective studies of the effect of unplanned prolongation of conventional therapy.

There is some evidence to suggest that poorly differentiated tumours have lost the ability to accelerate their proliferation in response to depletion, but we can conclude that for the bulk of squamous cancers in the head and neck region overall treatment time should never be prolonged, and a reduction in overall time can lead to improved control.

This evidence-based medicine should be applied in routine care, but the exact form of accelerated treatment to be employed in the radiotherapy of head and neck cancer is less clear. In North America, the concomitant boost seems to be favoured over hyperfractionation, even though both gave similar results in the recent RTOG study. The practical difficulties of giving 70 treatments compared with 47 probably influences this view. In Denmark, six treatments per week are standard for head and neck cancer.

It is important to recognize that improvements in tumour control must be measured against any alteration in late morbidity. Time is needed for observations to be continued and full assessments made. The CHART study has shown a significant reduction in late change and this has been maintained in follow-up. However, with overall equal locoregional control, the regime is not favoured for routine treatment. The low morbidity encountered, however, does encourage its further use, particularly in postoperative radiotherapy where rapid proliferation may occur even before radiotherapy commences, and a randomized controlled trial has now commenced. A slightly modified regime (CHARTWEL), in which treatment is not given at the weekends, is being employed. It is important in this trial, as in all those that have been completed, for long-term follow-up and careful observation of morbidity to be continued and reported. Further results of the seven-day-a-week regime are awaited. New studies are being planned incorporating concurrent cytotoxic chemotherapy and further shortening of overall time. In these the control arms will be the successful experimental arm of the previous studies.

Intrathoracic tumours

SMALL CELL CARCINOMA

Small cell carcinoma has long been recognized as one of the most rapidly progressive tumours and, in some cases, advance in tumour bulk can be detected on a week-to-week basis. On histological examination, a high mitotic rate is observed. With such a tumour, it must be expected that acceleration of radiotherapy, and indeed acceleration of all treatment, should be advantageous.

Twice-daily regimes of radiotherapy and concurrent or closely related courses of chemotherapy have been the subject of study. A recent randomized trial has given evidence to support the view that accelerated radiotherapy should be employed in the management of the primary tumour. A significant increase in survival at 2 years (47 per cent vs. 41 per cent) was observed in patients given 45 Gy in 21 days, compared with those given a similar dose in 35 days respectively (Turrisi et al., 1999).

NON-SMALL CELL LUNG CANCER

In a hyperfractionation study performed by the RTOG, in which twice-daily treatment was given to cohorts of patients to rising total doses, no benefit in terms of survival was achieved above a total dose of 69.6 Gy (Cox et al., 1990). This hyperfractionated schedule of radiotherapy has been further explored in combination with chemotherapy, but in a randomized controlled clinical trial has shown no benefit over daily radiotherapy with chemotherapy (Curran et al., 1999). In Australia, a standard regime of 60 Gy in 2-Gy fractions given over 6 weeks was compressed into 3 weeks. A modification of the CHART regimen, CHARTWEL (CHART without weekends), has been piloted with a dose escalation to 60 Gy without a significant increase in morbidity; neo-adjuvant chemotherapy has also been added and has been shown to be feasible. Further studies with concomitant chemotherapy are underway. In a four-arm study, the regime was tested with and without chemotherapy. A total of 200 patients were included. No significant advantage of either chemotherapy or of acceleration was observed (Ball et al., 1999). There was some increase in morbidity but this did not reach a significant level.

In the randomized controlled trial of CHART in non-small cell lung cancer, a highly significant improvement in survival was observed, and this was associated with improved primary tumour control (Saunders et al., 1997). Benefits seem to extend to all stages and subgroups. Squamous cell cancer accounted for 82 per cent of the patients and, when this group was examined alone, survival beyond 3 years was doubled in the CHART patients. Based on this evidence, CHART has been recommended in the United Kingdom as standard treatment for advanced, inoperable non-small cell lung cancer. The survival advantage of 9 per cent in the overall study can be compared with 4 per cent observed in the overview of the addition of cytotoxic chemotherapy when only the effective cisplatin-containing regimes were analysed. The combination of CHART with chemotherapy is the logical next step.

OESOPHAGEAL CANCER

Accelerated regimes of radiotherapy have been applied to the management of carcinoma of the oesophagus. Acute reactions do not appear to be significantly increased and so there seems value in the quick completion of all treatment. The combination of CHART with an intra-cavitary application did give a high level of palliation but a significant level of stricture formation. Accelerated radiotherapy such as CHART combined with chemotherapy would seem logical here.

Altered fractionation regimes in other sites

BRAIN

There have been many studies of altered fractionation in the management of brain tumours, but no clear picture has emerged. On the whole, results have been disappointing. When multiple treatments are given each day, the long half-time for repair in neural tissues may prejudice the result, as in many cases it is difficult to separate late sequelae due to radiation from recurrence of tumour.

GASTROINTESTINAL TRACT

Accelerated regimes of radiotherapy have been attempted cautiously in the management of gastrointestinal tumours. The inevitable irradiation of radiosensitive and fast-proliferating normal tissues in the gut has reasonably led to a cautious approach and the area remains one for clinical trial (Glynne-Jones *et al.*, 1999).

CARCINOMA OF CERVIX

It is probable that accelerated radiotherapy would be of value in the management of carcinoma of the cervix, but there is little clinical corroboration of this. There is evidence to suggest that the interval between external-beam therapy and the subsequent intra-cavitary treatment should be kept as short as possible, for prolongation may lead to an increased rate of failure.

SOFT-TISSUE SARCOMAS

Twice-daily treatment has been employed, but we have no firm evidence that it is of advantage. It is likely that the soft-tissue sarcomas will present a very wide range of proliferation rates and a selection process is required if accelerated treatment is to advance care. Because of the nature of the normal tissues which are usually related to such tumours, acute and late morbidity may not present problems in the management of these tumours.

HYPOXIA

The relationship between oxygen tension and radiation response has long been recognized in radiobiology. Mottram (1935) gave a clear account of the importance of radioresistance due to hypoxia, and it was his colleague, Hal Gray, who gathered the evidence together and brought it to wide attention (Gray *et al.*, 1953). There is good evidence to show that hypoxia exists commonly in human tumours and that hypoxic tumour cells are resistant to radiotherapy. A process of reoxygenation has been shown to occur in tumours during a fractionated course of radiotherapy: as sensitive oxic tumour cells are destroyed, hypoxic ones move to take over the blood supply released and so become sensitive. There is good circumstantial evidence, however, to suggest that this process is incomplete in some tumours, and that hypoxia is a cause for failure to achieve cure (Dische and Saunders, 1998).

Among the many methods that have been introduced in order to make these hypoxic tumour cells sensitive are:

1 breathing 100 per cent oxygen or carbogen (95 per cent oxygen: 5 per cent carbon dioxide);
2 hyperbaric oxygen at 3 atmospheres absolute;
3 use of chemical sensitizing agents systemically and by intra-tumoral injection;
4 administration of cytotoxic agents, such as mitomycin C, which have a greater effect upon hypoxic compared with oxic tumour cells.

Of 15 randomized trials performed with hyperbaric oxygen, three showed significant therapeutic benefit; six others showed a margin of benefit which did not reach statistical significance, essentially because the numbers included were too few. The benefit, however, had to be balanced against some increase in normal tissue effects.

The large majority of randomized controlled clinical trials performed using chemical sensitizers of radiotherapy showed no benefit. Studies in oropharyngeal and supraglottic tumours performed by the Danish group have, however, been an exception. With misonidazole there was a significant improvement in local tumour control and this benefit was later achieved in a subsequent trial with another chemical sensitizer, nimorazole, which, unlike misonidazole, did not induce peripheral neuropathy.

Overview

Overgaard and his colleagues have performed an overview of trials of methods employed clinically to overcome the resistance associated with hypoxia, and have gathered data concerned with over 10 600 patients. A margin of 5 per cent of improvement in locoregional control ($P < 0.0001$) was demonstrated, and with it a 3 per cent improvement in survival ($P = 0.04$) (Horsman and Overgaard, 1997).

The overview is important in that it demonstrates that there is an oxygen effect and that methods of overcoming it can be successful. However, the margin is small and it is obvious that the normal process of reoxygenation, which occurs during radiotherapy, is commonly successful.

The use of nimorazole in the treatment of oropharyngeal and supraglottic carcinomas has been clearly established in the DAHANCA 5 study, and so in Denmark it is now standard best therapy. Unfortunately, the long time-scale in development in this area, combined with difficulties of supply of an orphan drug unsupported by a drug company, have hindered its more widespread adoption.

Tumours where hypoxia is important

The identification of tumours where hypoxia is a major factor determining the result seemed to be indicated, to identify those patients likely to benefit from methods for hypoxic cell radiosensitization. Many studies have been performed, and these have included methods to measure oxygen tension using sophisticated probes, radiolabelled nitroimidazoles to identify hypoxic areas and measurements of vascular perfusion, often using MR techniques, besides many other approaches. All these investigations have demonstrated hypoxia in the majority of human tumours, but they have all shown great complexity and variety of pattern from one tumour to another, even when they are of the same type and in an identical site. This research has been important for the development of our understanding of human tumours, but has not, so far, yielded a technique that can be readily applied to identify patients where hypoxia is a major problem and where a method to overcome it is indicated (Dische and Saunders, 1998).

Wider importance of hypoxia

Studies in molecular biology have shown that hypoxia can cause a wide range of genetic changes, which influence not only new vessel formation but also the potential for cells to metastasize.

Transient hypoxia

Evidence has accumulated to show that in addition to the chronic hypoxia that has been described, there is transient or acute hypoxia due to temporary occlusion of small vessels. Such a process may lead to radioresistance of a proportion of the tumour cells during the several minutes of a daily radiation treatment. Vasoactive drugs, such as pentoxifylline and nicotinamide, have been introduced to overcome this problem.

ARCON (accelerated radiotherapy, carbogen and nicotinamide)

It seems likely that a tumour that is rapid in proliferation is also one that outgrows its vascular supply to become hypoxic. The ARCON concept brings together carbogen to overcome chronic hypoxia, nicotinamide to overcome transient hypoxia and acceleration to deal with cellular proliferation (Dische and Saunders, 1998).

Pilot studies with ARCON, using a variety of schedules of acceleration, have given a range of results. The result of a pilot study in laryngeal cancer performed at Nijmegen has been outstanding. Here, with relatively advanced disease, long-term tumour control has been attained in 86 per cent of cases (Kaanders *et al.*, 1998) and, in bladder cancer, retrospective comparison showed marked improvement in local tumour control compared with previously treated cases (Hoskin *et al.*, 1999). Randomized controlled clinical trials are now under way.

Hypoxic cytotoxicity

The work to develop hypoxic cell radiosensitizers has also produced compounds which are in themselves cytotoxic to hypoxic cells. A drug developed by the Stanford group, tirapazamine, has shown promise in phase I/II clinical trials (Brown, 1993). Such a drug needs to be given in combination with radiotherapy or cytotoxic chemotherapy, so that the oxic component of the tumour can be dealt with. The drug may also enhance the cytotoxic effect of *cis*-platinum, and remarkably good results have recently been reported from a small pilot study of the combination in advanced head and neck cancer. Randomized trials of the use of tirapazamine are now awaited.

ANAEMIA

Clinical experience

In 25 papers reporting the clinical experience of radiation response and anaemia, 23 reported an adverse radiation response in anaemic patients. The interpretation of retrospectively derived data of this sort must always be made with caution (Dische, 1991). There is no doubt that there is, in many tumour sites, an association between anaemia and advancement of disease. Even taking this into consideration, however, the evidence does suggest a real association between anaemia and response to radiation. A randomized controlled clinical trial of the use of blood transfusion in carcinoma of the cervix showed an improvement in primary tumour control when the haemoglobin was brought to 125 g/L or above, compared with the control group where the haemoglobin level lay between 100 and 125 g/L during therapy (Bush *et al.*, 1978). However, in the Danish head and neck cancer sensitizer and fractionation studies a subrandomization to test the value of transfusion showed only a small margin of advantage, which was not of statistical significance (Overgaard, personal communication, 1999).

Implications for radiotherapy

Taking all the evidence, anaemia does seem of importance and the implication for clinical practice is that in the curative situation the haemoglobin level should be brought to normal levels before radiation therapy is commenced. It is noteworthy that in the Danish studies in which anaemia was associated with impaired response in head and neck tumours, the level of haemoglobin chosen to divide the cases was 9 mmol (144 g)/L for men and 8 mmol (128 g)/L for women – levels in the lower part of the range of normality (Dische, 1991). The demands upon a blood transfusion service to achieve this in clinical practice may be considerable. Attention is now being given to the stimulation of bone marrow function using erythropoietin which can, in moderately anaemic patients, bring the haemoglobin concentration to within normal levels in 10–14 days. The effectiveness of erythropoietin in elevating the haemoglobin level of patients with cancer selected for radiotherapy has clearly been shown (Lavey and Dempsey, 1993), but so far we have no evidence that worthwhile benefit will be attained, and the results of randomized controlled clinical trials are awaited.

RADIOPROTECTORS

Radioprotectors were developed out of the efforts in the United States to develop compounds that might give some protection in atomic warfare; the compound that has reached clinical testing in oncology is amifostine (WR-2721).

The initial work in the laboratory with amifostine suggested that the drug does not accumulate in tumours; however, the total reliability of this remains uncertain. The progress of this drug in clinical trial has been extremely slow (Kligerman, 1988) but its use in head and neck patients with a view to reducing late effects upon salivary gland function has yielded a highly significant benefit, and the drug is now marketed for this purpose (Brizel et al., 1999). Amifostine may have value in combination with cytotoxic drugs, such as cyclophosphamide, for protection of the bone marrow, as has been demonstrated in clinical trials.

NEUTRONS

The efficiency of any ionizing radiation increases with the density of the ionization along its track. X- and γ-rays are sparsely ionizing radiations, but neutron beams and heavy-ion beams have densities that may be several hundred times greater per unit length. The relative biological effectiveness (RBE) is normally determined by comparison with 250 kV X-rays. Values between 2 and 10 may be obtained, according to the energy of neutron beam, and, importantly, the size of dose per fraction, for there is an inverse relationship between dose per fraction and RBE.

The biological advantages rest upon a lessened influence of oxygen tension and the position in the mitotic cycle, together with, in animal models and human tumour transplants, a more uniform response among tumour types (Joiner, 1997b). The results of phase II and phase III clinical trials have been difficult to interpret because of case selection, unusual dose fractionation regimes, a variable handling of morbidity and, in some trials, the use of a combination of photons and neutrons. A place was suggested in the management of squamous cancer in the head and neck region but was not confirmed in further trials (Duncan and Arnott, 1979). With evidence based on small numbers, there may be a particular advantage in advanced parotid and prostatic carcinoma (Wambersie et al., 1994). It can, however, be concluded that the considerable resources needed to pursue neutron therapy might give a greater benefit if employed in other ways to advance radiotherapy.

CHARGED PARTICLES

The ion beams of charged particles increase their rate of energy emission as they slow down, finally stopping and releasing energy in an intense burst of ionization (the Bragg peak). The beam produced may be used to deliver high doses to small areas and spare adjacent sensitive structures, so bringing advantages over photon therapy: an example would be the treatment of tumours in the base of skull. When employed clinically, photon and helium ion beams have a similar LET to photons and 250 kV X-rays and present, therefore, only the advantage of dose distribution. The beams of the heavier ions, such as carbon, neon and argon, combine the biological advantage of high LET with those of dose distribution (Joiner, 1997b).

If deeply placed tumours are to be treated with proton beams, high-energy cyclotrons are required. The cost and complexity of the apparatus required for production of a heavy-ion beam are even greater than with neutrons (Joiner, 1997b). The advantage of proton ion beams has, however, been well demonstrated in the treatment of tumours closely related to the spinal cord and brainstem (Suit et al., 1982) and a strong justification has been made for the establishment of national centres where such therapy may be available for those patients likely to benefit.

BRACHYTHERAPY

Biological advantages of low dose rate

Interstitial and intra-cavitary applications of radioactive sources have an important place in radiotherapy. A high cure rate is obtained with accessible, well-defined tumours of small or moderate size, and such techniques may also be used to give a boost to the area of gross tumour after external-beam treatment. With the original low-activity sources, applications were for 1–7 days and the dose rates were commonly less than 1 Gy/h. This can be compared with conventional external-beam therapy, when 2 Gy may often be given in 1–2 minutes.

Sublethal injury is important in determining the late effects of external-beam therapy using photons, but it has now been shown in the laboratory that there is complete recovery of all sublethal injury at the low dose rates used for brachytherapy (Steel, 1997b). This does accord with the excellent normal tissue tolerance with limited late changes associated with brachytherapy. There is a further advantage in that, with overall treatment times in brachytherapy ranging over 1–7 days, treatment is accelerated compared with conventional external-beam therapy and little or no time is allowed for repopulation. Finally, it has also been shown in the laboratory that the oxygen enhancement ratio is considerably reduced and that reoxygenation appears to be very effective under low-dose therapy, even though overall times are relatively short (Tubiana *et al.*, 1990). In addition to the considerable biological evidence to support the efficacy of brachytherapy, there is the well-localized dose distribution (Tubiana, 1988).

Afterloading and high dose rate

The hazard of radiation exposure to staff has led to the introduction of hollow applicators and subsequent afterloading of the radioactive sources; this is most safely performed mechanically. However, the long period of exposure to radiation with traditional brachytherapy techniques is difficult to reproduce with machines for afterloading. With the advent of small, high-intensity sources, high dose-rate techniques have been introduced and exposure times reduced from days to less than 30 minutes. The dose rate thus becomes similar to that of conventional external-beam therapy and we must therefore expect similar biological characteristics. As one or a few large doses are commonly given, there is not the benefit of multiple fractions usually associated with conventional external-beam therapy. Reductions in dose have been made, but in some centres these were initially inadequate and morbidity was considerably increased. Fractionated brachytherapy is obviously a useful approach, easier to achieve with a boost rather than with definitive therapy. Treatment units have now been constructed to allow introduction of very high activity sources for a few minutes every hour. Calculations based upon laboratory experiments have suggested that this approach will allow safe brachytherapy with biological effects similar to those of continuous low dose-rate techniques (Brenner *et al.*, 1991). A cautious clinical exploration will be required before this technique can be considered safe.

THE COMBINATION OF CHEMOTHERAPY WITH RADIOTHERAPY

The combination may be employed to enhance tumour control within the irradiated volume and/or deal with occult disease elsewhere. The combination of local effect may be due to a simple addition of cell kill or to a true radiosensitization – processes often difficult to separate (Steel, 1997c).

The giving of combined therapy concurrently, or with only a few days separation, does commonly lead to an enhancement of effect upon the tumour; this may also be seen in the normal tissues. Reduction in total radiation

dose may be necessary, and this complicates the interpretation of results. When chemotherapy and radiotherapy are separated, an increased effect in normal tissues is not often demonstrated (Stewart and Saunders, 1997). However, the administration of actinomycin D, even following an interval of some years after irradiation, can lead to a recall of radiation reaction in the skin. With growing awareness that cellular repopulation may occur in gaps between treatments, whether they be surgery, radiotherapy or chemotherapy, the trend has been for concurrent radiotherapy and chemotherapy. Considerable margins of benefit have been demonstrated in the management of anal and oesophageal cancer, where the combination therapies have become standard. In head and neck and non-small cell lung cancer, margins have been smaller and overall results variable. Overviews have demonstrated small but certainly significant gains, concurrent therapies appearing more successful. These have led to fairly wide adoption of combination chemotherapy in these conditions; however, there must be concern with late morbidity for overviews are relatively insensitive in evaluating morbidity. There is the necessity for large, randomized trials, where tumour effects and those in normal tissues are given equal priority in order to assess overall benefit.

TUMOUR VOLUME AND CLONOGENIC TUMOUR CELL NUMBER

A tumour mass will contain normal and necrotic tissue, as well as tumour cells. Among patients with tumour masses of similar size there may therefore be a great variation in the number of viable tumour cells contained within them. There is, again, a variation in the proportion of those tumour cells which are clonogenic. In some neoplasms, such as the lymphomas, it is believed that the number of clonogenic cells is relatively few in number, thus accounting, in part, for their relative radiosensitivity (Tubiana *et al.*, 1990).

The clonogenic tumour cell burden is an important parameter in determining the response and this has been clearly shown in laboratory experiments. We can expect in humans that in any one type of tumour, the number of clonogenic cells within a nodule 5 mm in diameter may be 1000 times fewer than the number within a mass 5 cm in diameter (Tubiana *et al.*, 1990). Given standard conditions of radiotherapy, very different total doses are required to give a 90 per cent probability of elimination of all tumour cells. In the postoperative state, such as after a neck dissection for metastatic squamous carcinoma of neck nodes, or after lumpectomy for primary carcinoma of breast, where any nodule of residual tumour is unlikely to be greater than a few millimetres in diameter, a total radiation dose of 46–50 Gy given in 2-Gy fractions may be adequate to achieve a high degree of probability of elimination of all tumour. For a primary squamous cell carcinoma of 20 mm diameter in the head and neck region, the dose given in 2-Gy fractions may need to be elevated to 66 Gy to give an equal probability of cure; with a big tumour mass of 5 cm diameter, however, 75 Gy may not give even a 50 per cent local cure rate. Other factors such as hypoxia, inherent radiosensitivity and proliferation characteristics will all modify and complicate the situation. Nevertheless, the tumour cell burden is, itself, an important biological parameter and justifies the use of a range of doses in clinical practice (Steel, 1997a).

PRECISION IN DOSIMETRY AND ITS BIOLOGICAL SIGNIFICANCE

Because of the steepness of the curve relating dose to tumour eradication, an elevation or depression of dose of 5 per cent at the 50 per cent control point can be expected to elevate or depress tumour control in the human situation by approximately 10 per cent.

In clinical practice there is commonly a 10 per cent variation in dose across the target volume at the centre of the fields of treatment, and when a three-dimensional view is taken, variations up to 15 per cent or even 20 per cent may be encountered. These dose variations within the area irradiated will also have important biological implications for the normal tissues (Dische, 1993). Where the total dose is lowered, normal tissue effects will be diminished further by the lower dose per fraction. On the other hand, where the dose is elevated, the effect will be increased further by the higher dose per fraction. Using a conventional 2-Gy increment and a 66 Gy total dose, an increase of 10 per cent in part of the irradiated volume is likely to lead to a 13 per cent increase in biological effect, because of the increase in dose per fraction. This has been described by Rodney Withers as 'double trouble'.

CONCLUSIONS

Laboratory and clinical research have greatly extended our knowledge of the processes that influence tumour control and normal tissue injury after radiotherapy. Brachytherapy and the fractionation of external-beam therapy, which have largely been built upon a continued process of clinical trial and observation, have now been given a firm scientific basis.

Modification of the fractionation has now given guidance as to how the benefit of radiotherapy can be enhanced by reprogramming treatment for the management of tumours in certain clinical situations.

The complexity of the biology of human tumours, varying from site to site and tumour to tumour, combined with the many interacting factors that influence the result of a course of radiotherapy, add to the clinician's burden as he attempts to give the individual patient the most appropriate treatment. The complexity has to be recognized and tackled by high-standard research, which must be interpreted carefully and applied to the individual case. The chosen schedule will only be successful if there is good planning and delivery of treatment.

In every aspect of clinical research to improve the results of treatment the importance of observation of the normal tissue effects, particularly in the long term, must be emphasized and are essential to the evaluation of any approach to improve the care of patients by radiotherapy.

Clinical oncologists should keep in close contact with their laboratory colleagues and understand the tumour biology and radiobiology important to their work. A high standard of clinical science must then be brought to the bedside so that advances originating in the laboratory can be exploited to the benefit of the patient with cancer.

SIGNIFICANT POINTS

- A knowledge of the biology and radiobiology of tumours and that of normal tissues is essential to the best practice of radiation oncology.
- The tumour and the normal tissues must be observed and responses recorded with equal care.
- The number of tumour cells capable of dividing, their proliferation characteristics, the inherent radiosensitivity and hypoxia will be important to the outcome. Also important will be the size of the individual dose fraction, the total dose and its overall duration.
- As many factors may influence the result of a course of radiotherapy, manipulating just one may not give benefit; all must be considered when designing a protocol.
- Research into the fractionation of treatment has advanced patient care, and further work continues. Areas of current activity that may influence practice in the future include the determination of inherent radiosensitivity, hypoxic cell sensitization and the interaction with biological modifiers and cytotoxic agents.
- Differences in physical dose across the tumour lead to even greater biological variations in effect. Radiation planning and delivery of high quality are essential.
- Future advances depend on a close collaboration between laboratory and clinic. To test a new concept fully, a high standard of clinical science is needed at the bedside.

KEY REFERENCES

Denekamp, J. and Hirst, D.G. (eds) (1992) Radiation science – of molecules, mice and men. *Br. J. Radiol.* (suppl. 24). London: British Institute of Radiology.

Overgaard, J. (1991) Tumour hypoxia. Proceedings of a Consensus Meeting organized by the EORTC Cooperative Group for Radiotherapy, Leuven, Belgium, December 1989. *Radiother. Oncol.* **20**(suppl. 1).

Steel, G.G. (1997) *Basic clinical radiobiology* (2nd edn). London: Arnold.

Steel, G.G. and Adams, G.E. (1989) *The biological basis of radiotherapy* (2nd edn). Amsterdam: Elsevier.

REFERENCES

Ball, D., Bishop, J., Smith, J. *et al.* (1999) A randomised phase III study of accelerated or standard fraction radiotherapy with or without concurrent carboplatin in inoperable non-small cell lung cancer: final report of an Australian multicentre trial. *Radiother. Oncol.* **52**, 129–36.

Barendsen, G.W. (1982) Dose fractionation, dose rate and iso-effect relationships for normal tissue responses. *Int. J. Radiat. Oncol. Biol. Phys.* **8**, 1981–97.

Begg, A.C. (1997) Individualisation of radiotherapy. In Steel, G.G. (ed.), *Basic clinical radiobiology* (2nd edn). London: Arnold, 234–6.

Begg, A.C., Haustermans, K., Hart, A.A.M. *et al.* (1998) The value of pretreatment cell kinetic parameters as predictors for radiotherapy outcome in head and neck cancer: a multicenter analysis. *Radiother. Oncol.* **50**, 13–23.

Begg, A.C., McNally, N.J., Shrieve, D.C. and Karcher, H.A. (1985) A method to measure the duration of DNA synthesis and the potential doubling time from single sample. *Cytometry* **6**, 620–6.

Bennett, M.H., Wilson, G.D., Dische, S. *et al.* (1992) Tumour proliferation assessed by combined histological and flow cytometric analysis: implications for therapy in squamous cell carcinoma in the head and neck. *Br. J. Cancer* **65**, 870–8.

Bentzen, S.M. (1997) Dose–response relationship in radiotherapy. In Steel, G.G. (ed.), *Basic clinical radiobiology* (2nd edn). London: Arnold, 78–86.

Bentzen, S.M. and Thames, H.D. (1991) Clinical evidence for tumor clonogen regeneration: interpretations of the data. *Radiother. Oncol.* **22**, 161–6.

Bentzen, S.M., Ruifrok, A.C.C. and Thames, H.D. (1996) Repair capacity and kinetics for human mucosa and epithelial tumors in the head and neck: clinical data on the effect of changing the time interval between multiple fractions per day in radiotherapy. *Radiother. Oncol.* **38**, 89–101.

Bentzen, S., Saunders, M. and Dische, S. (1999) Repair halftimes estimated from observations of treatment-related morbidity after CHART or conventional radiotherapy in head and neck cancer. *Radiother. Oncol.* **53**, 219–26.

Brahme, A. (1984) Dosimetric precision requirements in radiation therapy. *Acta Radiol. Oncol.* **23**, 379–91.

Brenner, D.J., Huang, Y. and Hall, E. (1991) Fractionated high dose-rate versus low dose-rate regimens for intracavitary brachytherapy of the cervix: equivalent regimens for combined brachytherapy and external irradiation. *Int. J. Radiat. Oncol. Biol. Phys.* **21**, 1415–23.

Brizel, D.M., Wasserman, T.H., Strnad, V. *et al.* (1999) Final report of a phase III randomized trial of amifostine as a radioprotectant in head and neck cancer. Proceedings of the American Society for Therapeutic Radiology and Oncology 41st Annual Meeting. *Radiat. Oncol. Biol. Phys.* **45**(suppl. 3).

Brock, W.A., Brown, B.W., Goefpert, H. and Peters, L.J. (1992) *In vitro* radiosensitivity of tumor cells and local tumor control by radiotherapy. In Dewey, W., Edington, M., Fry, R., Hall, E. and Whitmore, G. (eds), *Radiation research: a twentieth century perspective.* San Diego: Academic Press, 696–9.

Brown, J.M. (1993) SR 4233 (tirapazamine): a new anticancer drug exploiting hypoxia in solid tumours. *Br. J. Cancer* **67**, 1163–70.

Bush, R.S., Jenkin, R.D.T., Allt, W.E.C. *et al.* (1978) Definitive evidence for hypoxic cells influencing cure in cancer therapy. *Br. J. Cancer* **37**, 302–6.

Cox, J., Azarnia, N., Byhardt, R. *et al.* (1990) A randomized phase I/II trial of hyperfractionated radiation therapy with total doses of 60.0 Gy to 79.2 Gy: possible survival benefit with >69.6 Gy in favorable patients with Radiation Therapy Oncology Group stage III non-small-cell lung carcinoma: report of Radiation Therapy Oncology Group 83-11. *J. Clin. Oncol.* **8**, 1543–55.

Cox, J.D., Pajak, T.F., Marcial, V.A. *et al.* (1991) Astro plenary: interfraction interval is a major determinant of late effects, with hyperfractionated radiation therapy of carcinomas of upper respiratory and digestive tracts: results from Radiation Therapy Oncology Group protocol 8313. *Int. J. Radiat. Oncol. Biol. Phys.* **20**, 1191–5.

Curran, W. Jr, Scott, C., Langer, R. *et al.* (1999) Phase III comparison of sequential vs concurrent chemoradiation for patients with unresected stage III non-small cell lung cancer (NSCLC): initial report of Radiation Therapy Oncology Group (RTOG) 9410. (Proceedings of ASCO) *Lung Cancer* **18**, 484a.

Denekamp, J. (1982) *Cell kinetics and cancer therapy.* Springfield, Illinois: CC Thomas.

Denekamp, J. and Hirst, D.G. (eds) (1992) Radiation science – of molecules, mice and men. *Br. J. Radiol.* (suppl. 24). London: British Institute of Radiology.

Dische, S. (1991) Radiotherapy and anaemia – the clinical experience. *Radiother. Oncol.* **20**, 35–40.

Dische, S. (1993) What do we know concerning fractionation in radiotherapy? *Clin. Oncol.* **5**, 330–2.

Dische, S. and Saunders, M.I. (1998) Hypoxic cell radiosensitisation – clinical relevance in 1998. In Kogelnik, H. and Sedlmayer, F. (eds), *Progress in radio-oncology VI*. Bologna: Monduzzi Editore, 205–21.

Dische, S. and Saunders, M. (1999) The CHART regimen and morbidity. *Acta Oncol.* **38**, 147–52.

Dische, S., Saunders, M., Barrett, A. *et al.* (1997) A randomised multicentre trial of CHART versus conventional radiotherapy in head and neck cancer. *Radiother. Oncol* **44**, 123–36.

Duncan, W. and Arnott, S.J. (1979) Results of the clinical application with fast neutrons in Edinburgh. *Eur. J. Cancer* (suppl.), 31–6.

Ellis, F. (1969) Dose, time and fractionation: a clinical hypothesis. *Clin. Radiol.* **20**, 1–7.

Fertil, B. and Malaise, E.P. (1981) Inherent cellular radiosensitivity as a basic concept for human tumor radiotherapy. *Int. J. Radiat. Oncol. Biol. Phys.* **7**, 621–9.

Fowler, J.F. and Lindstrom, M.J. (1992) Loss of local control with prolongation in radiotherapy. *Int. J. Radiat. Oncol. Biol. Phys.* **23**, 457–67.

Fu, K.K., Pajak, T.F., Trotti, A. *et al.* (2000) A Radiation Therapy Oncology Group (RTOG) phase III randomized study to compare hyperfractionation and two variants of accelerated fractionation to standard fractionation radiotherapy for head and neck squamous cell carcinomas: first report of RTOG 9003. *Int. J. Radiat. Oncol. Biol. Phys.* **48**(1), 7–16.

Glynne-Jones, R., Saunders, M.I., Hoskin, P. and Phillips, H. (1999) A pilot study of continuous, hyperfractionated, accelerated radiotherapy in rectal adenocarcinoma. *Clin. Oncol.* **11**, 334–9.

Gray, L.H., Conger, A.D. and Ebert, M. (1953) The concentration of oxygen dissolved in tissues at the time of irradiation as a factor in radiotherapy. *Br. J. Radiol.* **26**, 638–48.

Horiot, J.C., Bontemps, P., Begg, A. *et al.* (1998) New radiotherapy fractionation schemes in head and neck cancers. The EORTC trials: a benchmark. In Kogelnik, H. and Sedlmayer, F. (eds), *Progress in radio-oncology VI*. Bologna: Monduzzi Editore, 735–41.

Horsman, M.R. and Overgaard, J. (1997) The oxygen effect. In Steel, G.G. (ed.), *Basic clinical radiobiology* (2nd edn). London: Arnold, 132–40.

Hoskin, P., Saunders, M. and Dische, S. (1999) Hypoxic radiosensitizers in radical radiotherapy for patients with bladder carcinoma. Hyperbaric oxygen, misonidazole and accelerated radiotherapy, carbogen and nicotinamide. *American Cancer Society* **86**(7), 1322–8.

Joiner, M.C. (1997a) Modelling of radiation cell killing. In Steel, G.G. (ed.), *Basic clinical radiobiology* (2nd edn). London: Arnold, 52–7.

Joiner, M.C. (1997b) Particle beams in radiotherapy. In Steel, G.G. (ed.), *Basic clinical radiobiology* (2nd edn). London: Arnold, 173–83.

Joiner, M.C. and van der Kogel, A.J. (1997) The linear-quadratic approach to fractionation and calculation of iso-effective relationships. In Steel, G.G. (ed.), *Basic clinical radiobiology* (2nd edn). London: Arnold, 106–22.

Kaanders, J., Pop, L., Marres, H. *et al.* (1998) Accelerated radiotherapy with carbogen and nicotinamide (ARCON) for laryngeal cancer. *Radiother. Oncol.* **48**, 115–22.

Kligerman, M.M., Turrisi, A.T., Urtasun, R.C. *et al.* (1988) Final report on phase I trial of WR-2721 before protracted fractionated radiation therapy. *Int. J. Radiat. Oncol. Biol. Phys.* **14**, 1119–22.

Lavey, R.S. and Dempsey, W.H. (1993) Erythropoietin increases hemoglobin in cancer patients during radiation therapy. *Int. J. Radiat. Oncol. Biol. Phys.* **27**, 1147–52.

Maciejewski, B., Preuss-Bayer, G. and Trott, K.R. (1983) The influence of the number of fractions and overall treatment time on local control and late complication rate in squamous cell carcinoma of the larynx. *Int. J. Radiat. Oncol. Biol. Phys.* **9**, 321–8.

McMillan, T.J. (1997) In Steel, G.G. (ed.), *Basic clinical radiobiology* (2nd edn). London: Arnold, 70–7.

McMillan, T.J. and Steel, G.G. (1997) In Steel, G.G. (ed.), *Basic clinical radiobiology* (2nd edn). London: Arnold, 58–67.

Milas, L., Ang, K.K. and McBride, W. (1998) Growth factors and cytokines: implications for radiotherapy. In Kogelnik, H. and Sedlmayer, F. (eds), *Progress in radio-oncology VI*. Bologna: Monduzzi Editore, 15–23.

Morrison, W.H., Garden, A.S., Ang, K.K. and Peters, L.J. (1999) Long term results of the concomitant boost fractionation schedule for treatment of oropharyngeal carcinoma. Proceedings of the American Society for Therapeutic Radiology and Oncology 41st Annual Meeting. *Int. J. Radiat. Oncol. Biol. Phys.* **45**(suppl. 3), 197.

Mottram, J.C. (1935) Annual Report of the Mount Vernon Hospital and Radium Institute, Northwood, UK.

Nguyen, T.D., Demange, L., Froissart, D. *et al.* (1985) Rapid hyperfractionated radiotherapy. Clinical results in 178 advanced squamous cell carcinomas of the head and neck. *Cancer* **56**, 16–19.

Olmi, P., Cellai, E., Chiavacci, A. and Fallai, C. (1990) Accelerated fractionation in advanced head and neck cancer: results and analysis of late sequelae. *Radiother. Oncol.* **17**, 199–207.

Overgaard, J., Hansen, H., Overgaard, M. *et al.* (1998) Importance of overall treatment time for the outcome of radiotherapy in head and neck carcinoma. Experience from the Danish Head and Neck Cancer Study. In Kogelnik, H. and Sedlmayer, F. (eds), *Progress in radio-oncology VI*. Bologna: Monduzzi Editore, 743–52.

Peracchia, G. and Salti, C. (1981) Radiotherapy with thrice-a-day fractionation in a short overall time: clinical experiences. *Int. J. Radiat. Oncol. Biol. Phys.* **7**, 99–104.

Rezvani, M., Alcock, T.J., Fowler, J.F. *et al.* (1989) A comparison of the normal tissue reactions in patients treated with either 3 F/wk or 5 F/wk in the BIR (British Institute of Radiology) trial of radiotherapy for carcinoma of the laryngopharynx. *Int. J. Radiat. Biol.* **56**, 717–20.

Rubin, P. (1989) The radiation tolerance of human tissues. In Vaeth, J.M. and Meyer, J.L. (eds), *Radiation tolerance of normal tissues.* Basel: Karger, 1–32.

Saunders, M.I. (1998) CHART: the results and the relevance to clinical practice. In Kogelnik, H. and Sedlmayer, F. (eds), *Progress in radio-oncology VI.* Bologna: Monduzzi Editore, 753–66.

Saunders, M., Dische, S., Barrett, A. *et al.* (1997) Continuous hyperfractionated accelerated radiotherapy (CHART) versus conventional radiotherapy in non-small-cell lung cancer: a randomised multicentre trial. *Lancet* **350**, 161–6.

Saunders, M.I., Shah, N. and Joiner, M.C. (1999) Low dose hyper-radiosensitivity – is it a clinical reality and can it influence the radiation schedules used in the treatment of gliomas? Proceedings of the American Society for Therapeutic Radiology and Oncology 41st Annual Meeting. *Int. J. Radiat. Oncol. Biol. Phys.* **45**(suppl. 3), 267–8.

Skaladowski, K., Maciejewski, B., Golen, M. (2000) Randomised clinical trial on 7-day-continuous accelerated irradiation (CAIR) of head and neck cancer – report on 3-year tumour control and normal tissue toxicity. *Radiother. Oncol.* **55**, 101–10.

Steel, G.G. (ed.) (1997a) *Basic clinical radiobiology* (2nd edn). London: Arnold, 8–13.

Steel, G.G. (ed.) (1997b) *Basic clinical radiobiology* (2nd edn). London: Arnold, 163–72.

Steel, G.G. (ed.) (1997c) *Basic clinical radiobiology* (2nd edn). London: Arnold, 184–94.

Steel, G.G. and Adams, G.E. (1989) *The biological basis of radiotherapy* (2nd edn). Amsterdam: Elsevier.

Stewart, F.A. and Saunders, M.I. (1997) In Steel, G.G. (ed.), *Basic clinical radiobiology* (2nd edn). London: Arnold, 195–202.

Strandqvist, M. (1944) Studien Uber Die Kumulative Wirkung Der Rontgenstrahlen Bei Franktionierung. Erhfahrungen Aus Dem Radiumhemmet An 280 Haut Und Lippenkarzinomen. *Acta Radiol.* (suppl. 55), 101–4, 108–9, 120–1, 287–92.

Suit, H., Goitein, M., Munzenrider, J. *et al.* (1982) Evaluation of the clinical applicability of proton beams in definitive fractionated radiation therapy. *Int. J. Radiat. Oncol. Biol. Phys.* **8**, 2199–205.

Thames, H.D. and Hendry, J.H. (1987) *Fractionation in radiotherapy.* London: Taylor and Francis.

Tubiana, M. (1988) Repopulation in human tumors – a biological background for fractionation in radiotherapy. *Acta Oncol.* **27**, 83–8.

Tubiana, M., Dutreix, J. and Wambersie, A. (1990) *Introduction to radiobiology.* London: Taylor and Francis.

Turrisi, A.T., Kim, K., Blum, R. *et al.* (1999) Twice-daily compared with once-daily thoracic radiotherapy in limited small-cell lung cancer treated concurrently with cisplatin and etoposide. *N. Engl. J. Med.* **340**, 265–71.

Van den Bogaert, W., van der Schueren, E., Horiot, J.C. *et al.* (1986) The EORTC randomized trial on three fractions per day and misonidazole (trial no: 22811) in advanced head and neck cancer: long-term results and side effects. *Radiother. Oncol.* **35**, 91–9.

Wambersie, A., Richard, F. and Breteau, N. (1994) Development of fast neutron therapy worldwide. *Acta Oncol.* **34**, 261–74.

Wang, C.C., Blitzer, P.H. and Suit, H. (1985) Twice-a-day radiation therapy for cancer of the head and neck. *Cancer* **55**, 2100–4.

West, C.M., Davidson, S.E., Roberts, S.A. and Hunter, R.D. (1997) The independence of intrinsic radiosensitivity as a prognostic factor for patient response to radiotherapy of carcinoma of the cervix. *Br. J. Cancer* **76**, 1184–90.

Wiernik, G., Bates, T.D., Bleehen, N.M. *et al.* (1990) Final report of the general clinical results of the British Institute of Radiology fractionation study of 3 F/wk versus 5 F/wk in radiotherapy of carcinoma of the laryngo-pharynx. *Br. J. Radiol.* **63**, 169–80.

Withers, H.R., Taylor, J.M.G. and Maciejewski, B. (1988) The hazard of accelerated tumour clonogen repopulation during radiotherapy. *Acta Oncol.* **27**, 131–46.

5

Mathematical modelling and its application in radiation oncology

ROGER G. DALE AND BLEDDYN JONES

INTRODUCTION

There are occasions when clinical experience and knowledge of the results of clinical trials can provide little more than tentative guidance on how to manage a difficult clinical problem. Although the available treatment options may be well understood by the prescribing physician, it is useful to have a quantitative assessment of their likely clinical impact. The use of well-founded radiobiological models is one way in which difficult cases can be formally assessed: by a numerical appraisal of the likely biological outcomes the best available option can be selected and, if necessary, modified in a direction compatible with safety of outcome.

The amount of mathematics required for simple radiobiological assessments is well within the grasp of radiation oncologists, who should have a basic understanding of radiation effect models, their usefulness and limitations. Although computers are necessary for more advanced modelling, a wide range of clinically relevant calculations may be performed using a pocket calculator.

Radiation oncology is concerned with dose–effect relationships and their clinical optimization. With so many controllable variables (overall time, dose fractionation, choice of modalities, etc.) and inter-patient variations (in the biological parameters that influence outcomes), predictive models are likely to become an essential supplement to clinical judgement. The only practical alternative is to perform a series of randomized clinical trials, which would inevitably be complex and may be impossible to implement for a variety of reasons.

Modelling assessments are already invaluable in special circumstances, e.g. treatment delivery errors (under- or overdosage) or if treatment is unintentionally interrupted. Where higher than usual doses of radiation are used, dose gradients assume increased significance and modelling offers a valuable aid in the assessment of the resultant biological effect. Also, in the reporting of clinical data that comprise multiple different fractionation schedules, the quantification of the expected biological effect provides a method for inter-patient and inter-departmental comparisons. Modelling can be used to:

- identify and modify dangerous treatment schedules;
- provide a standard way of reporting clinical data;
- optimize radiotherapy treatment outcomes;
- analyse clinical results;
- aid in the design of better clinical trials; and
- assist in the testing of medico-legal issues.

This chapter begins by examining the application of radiobiological models to a range of practical problems. The last part of the chapter considers more advanced aspects of modelling which have the potential to improve the design of future radiotherapy schedules (henceforth a fractionation or brachytherapy schedule will be referred to simply as a 'schedule'). Modelling assessments are illustrated throughout by a number of worked examples.

THE BASIS AND ROUTINE APPLICATION OF RADIOBIOLOGICAL MODELS

Types of model

Earlier radiobiological models were based on logarithmic power law formulations, similar in form to those used to predict the behaviour of gases under adiabatic conditions. Such models were empirical and significant deviations from the predicted results have been observed when they are applied at doses (or fractional doses) that lie outside the range of values from which the empirical relationships were originally derived. Thus, at very low and high doses per fraction, errors were found. Additionally, when power laws were first introduced, there was still only limited awareness of the fact that acute-reacting tissues behaved differently from late-reacting tissues, although tissue-specific line fitting did overcome this problem to a limited extent.

No further discussion is required here about power law models, but practising oncologists should be aware that, until quite recently, many patients received treatments which had been calculated using the Ellis, cumulative radiation effect (CRE) or time, dose, fractionation (TDF) formulations. A full description of the historical development of these models has been given by Thames and Hendry (1987).

More reliable radiobiological models have been derived from consideration of the biophysical events that govern radiation effects. Multi-target and multi-hit models were initially developed, but the nature of the targets was undefined and the mathematics awkward. Currently the best and most commonly used radiobiological model is the linear-quadratic (LQ) formulation, which can be derived from consideration of physical lesions in double-stranded DNA and their repair and mis-repair (Barendsen, 1982; Dale, 1985; Thames, 1985). In LQ methodology, lethal radiation damage consists of two components, A and B. Type A lethal damage is caused by a single ionizing event, the amount increasing linearly with dose with a proportionality constant of α(unit: per Gy). Type A damage is not influenced by changes in the pattern of fractionation. Type B lethal damage is a consequence of there being an interaction between two sublethal damage components, each created in different ionizing events with an overall proportionality constant of β(unit: per Gy^2). Unlike Type A damage, the amount of Type B damage is dependent on the pattern of fractionation and on the dose rate. For radiation fractions delivered in short irradiation times, the Type B damage is proportional to the square of the dose per fraction.

Thus, for a single acute fractional dose of d (Gy), the total effect may be written as the summation of the Type A and Type B components:

$$\text{Effect } (E) = \text{Type A} + \text{Type B} \tag{5.1}$$

i.e.:

$$E = \alpha d + \beta d^2 \tag{5.2}$$

For n such fractions, delivered several hours apart, both types of damage are n times greater, i.e.:

$$E = n\alpha d + n\beta d^2 = n(\alpha d + \beta d^2) \tag{5.3}$$

It is clear from the dose-squared terms in Equations 5.2 and 5.3 that high doses per fraction create proportionately more effect than lower doses per fraction, the extent of this effect being governed by the relative magnitude of the β parameter. The LQ formulation is reliable over the range of dose per fraction encountered in conventional radiotherapy, but there are indications that it is less accurate at very large (>6 Gy) and low values (<1.8 Gy).

The concept of biologically effective dose

The biologically effective dose (BED) is a useful measure of biological effect which allows easy comparison of different radiation schedules. The BED (in units of Gy) for a conventional course of fractionated radiotherapy is found by dividing both sides of Equation 5.3 by α and re-arranging, i.e.:

$$\text{BED} = \frac{E}{\alpha} = n\left[d + \frac{\beta d^2}{\alpha}\right]$$

i.e.:

$$\text{BED} = nd\left[1 + \frac{d}{\alpha/\beta}\right] \tag{5.4}$$

The bracketed term in Equation 5.4 is called the relative effectiveness per unit dose (RE) and is a factor that converts physical dose to biological dose. The α/β ratio is the inverse of the fractionation sensitivity and is a measure of how a particular tissue will respond to changes in fractionation or dose-rate, thus any calculated BED is also tissue specific. BEDs calculated via use of a specified fractionation sensitivity value are normally written with the α/β factor as a suffix to the dose unit, e.g. a BED of 100 Gy derived using an α/β value of 3 Gy is written as 100 Gy_3, etc.

As the product nd in Equation 5.4 is the total physical dose (TD) delivered by the treatment, then, in words:

Biological dose (BED) = Total physical dose (TD)
$$\times \text{ Relative effectiveness (RE)} \tag{5.5}$$

The relationship summarized in Equation 5.5 is of general application and applies also to radiotherapy that does not involve well-spaced fractions and to brachytherapy. In such cases, the form of the RE factor is more complex.

What does the BED represent? BED is the (hypothetical) dose required for a given biological effect when delivered by the most gentle form of radiotherapy, i.e. using very small doses per fraction or, in the case of continuous irradiation, very low dose-rates. To understand this, consider Equation 5.3 in situations where d is progressively decreased, but with n correspondingly increased in order to maintain an iso-effect. The βd^2 term then becomes very small relative to αd and $E \cong n\alpha d \cong \alpha D$, where D is the total physical dose. Thus, the BED (i.e. E/α)

corresponds to the iso-effective physical dose when delivered using very low dose per fraction or very low dose rate.

The strength of the BED concept is that it can be calculated for any practical situation in radiotherapy, and a particular BED value may be achieved by a wide variety of schedules. Thus, the biological effects of quite different schedules can be compared using this single radiobiological yardstick. Also, because BED is tissue specific, it is a 'one-number' representation of either tumour or normal tissue response at the point of calculation. Finally, it should be noted that BEDs are additive, thus a single BED can be used to represent a radiotherapy schedule consisting of two or more components (e.g. external radiotherapy plus brachytherapy).

Two fractionation schedules of total doses D_1 and D_2 and dose per fractions of d_1 and d_2, respectively, are said to be iso-effective on a particular tissue if:

$$D_1\left[1 + \frac{d_1}{\alpha/\beta}\right] = D_2\left[1 + \frac{d_2}{\alpha/\beta}\right] \qquad (5.6)$$

Equation 5.6 may thus be utilized to design a fractionated treatment which is iso-effective to a first, or it may be used to estimate α/β ratios if parameters D_1, D_2 and d_1, d_2 are already known from existing iso-effect treatments which are similar in their effects on a specific tissue.

(α/β) ratios

These may be derived from data sets where different fractionation schedules have been used to achieve a common clinical end point. Typical α/β value ranges are 10–30 Gy for squamous cell carcinomas and 4 Gy for breast cancer (Joiner and van der Kogel, 1997). There is a continuing debate about the value of α/β in prostate cancer; the value may be as low as 1.5 Gy (Duchesne and Peters, 1999; King and Fowler, 2001). In the case of melanoma it may also be small (Thames and Hendry, 1987). A generic value of 10 Gy is often used for the tumour α/β when the exact value is not known, but a range of realistic values should be used wherever possible.

Normal tissue α/β ratios are generally smaller (1–4 Gy) than those for experimental cancers and many human tumours. A generic value of 3 Gy is often used, but it is sometimes prudent to select lower values for situations

where normal tissue tolerance may be compromised due to age, concomitant medical conditions, etc. A case in point is spinal cord, for which the fractionation sensitivity is around 2 Gy (Joiner and van der Kogel, 1997). Generic values of α/β derived from animal studies may not be representative for clinical use because of natural variation in α and β values in humans. Even for tumours of similar histology, radiosensitivity variations in heterogeneous clinical data are a potentially significant factor affecting the reliability of BED-based predictions. It is clear that fractionation sensitivities need to be determined more accurately in a wider range of human tumours and normal tissues.

WORKED EXAMPLE 5.1

What are the tumour and late-responding BEDs associated with a dose of 45 Gy/25 fractions? Using generic α/β values of 10 Gy for tumour and 3 Gy for late-responding normal tissue we have:

$$\text{BED}_{\text{tumour}} = 45 \times \left[1 + \frac{1.8}{10}\right] = 53.1 \text{ Gy}_{10}$$

and:

$$\text{BED}_{\text{late}} = 45 \times \left[1 + \frac{1.8}{3}\right] = 72 \text{ Gy}_{10}$$

The fact that BED_{late} is greater than $\text{BED}_{\text{tumour}}$ does *not* mean that the late-responding tissue is receiving a greater biological dose than the tumour. Rather, the two numbers represent how much dose would be required for the same respective effects on the two tissues if a very gentle treatment (very low dose per fraction) could be used.

Table 5.1 gives some examples of how a selection of disparate fractionation schedules can be summarized and compared in terms of BED values. In the left hand column the schedules are ranked in order of their total physical dose. In columns 2, 3 and 4 are listed the respective later-responding BEDs corresponding to α/β values of 2, 3 and 4 Gy. The numbers in bold show, for each value of α/β, the BED late-effect rankings of each of the schedules.

Table 5.1 *Fractionation schedules summarized and compared in terms of BED values (modified from Fowler (1989), with permission)*

Schedule	BED$_2$	BED$_3$	BED$_4$
(a) 68 fractions $\times$ 1.2 = 81.6 Gy	130.6 (**4**)	114.2 (**3**)	106.1 (**1**)
(b) 35 fractions $\times$ 2.0 = 70 Gy	140.0 (**2**)	116.7 (**1**)	105.0 (**2**)
(c) 30 fractions $\times$ 2.0 = 60 Gy	120.0 (**5**)	100.0 (**5**)	90.0 (**5**)
(d) 20 fractions $\times$ 2.8 = 56 Gy	134.4 (**3**)	108.3 (**4**)	95.2 (**4**)
(e) 36 fractions $\times$ 1.5 = 54 Gy	94.5 (**6**)	81.0 (**6**)	74.3 (**6**)
(f) 16 fractions $\times$ 3.38 = 54.1 Gy	145.5 (**1**)	115.0 (**2**)	99.8 (**3**)

The table illustrates two important points relating to radiobiological assessments. First, total dose alone is a poor predictor of radiobiological effect, as evidenced in particular by schedule (f). Second, the 'hotness' ranking is influenced by the particular α/β selected to perform the BED calculation. Thus, where specific values are not known, it is prudent to use two or more α/β values in order to obtain a more balanced view.

The consequences of tumour repopulation

Tumour cells born during treatment reduce overall treatment efficacy and need to be accounted for in calculations. If repopulation occurs at a continuous (exponential) rate throughout treatment, then the net effect is dependent on the treatment duration (T) and the effective tumour doubling time t_{eff} (in units of days). The consequence of this is that the expression for biological effect (E) in Equation 5.3 is modified to:

$$E = n(\alpha d + \beta d^2) - 0.693 \frac{T}{t_{eff}} \qquad (5.7)$$

To express this in terms of BED, it is necessary to divide E by α, as occurred in the derivation of Equation 5.4, i.e.:

$$BED = nd\left[1 + \frac{d}{\alpha/\beta}\right] - 0.693 \frac{T}{\alpha t_{eff}} \qquad (5.8)$$

If the subtractive repopulation factor in Equation 5.8 is simply referred to as RF, the aide-mémoir for calculating BED (Eqn 5.5) is then changed to:

$$BED = TD \times RE - BRF \qquad (5.9)$$

where the biological repopulation factor, BRF (units of Gy), is a measure of the total biological dose that is 'wasted' in combating repopulation during treatment. It will be noted from Equation 5.8 that inclusion of an allowance for repopulation in the calculation of a tumour BED requires a value for α to be assumed. This potential disadvantage may be overcome by use of a clinically derived value for the repopulation rate, e.g. in head and neck tumours the average daily repopulation may be equivalent to as much as 0.6 Gy/day, i.e. over a 6-week (42-day) treatment the RF factor (i.e. the 'wasted' dose) is $42 \times 0.6 = 25.2$ Gy. These clinically-estimated figures are referred to as K-values, where $K = 0.693/(\alpha t_{eff})$.

WORKED EXAMPLE 5.2

Comparison of tumour and late-normal tissue BEDs delivered by three schedules:

(a) total dose of 60 Gy in 2 Gy fractions over 40 days;
(b) total dose of 50 Gy in 2.5 Gy fractions over 26 days;
(c) total dose of 52.5 Gy in 2.625 Gy fractions over 26 days.

Assumed tumour parameters:
$\alpha/\beta = 10$ Gy, $\alpha = 0.35$/Gy, $t_{eff} = 5$ days.

The assumed α/β for the normal tissue (which is assumed to receive the same dose schedule as the tumour) is 3 Gy. The results of applying Equations 5.5 and 5.8 are summarized in the table:

Schedule	Tumour BED (Gy$_{10}$) (via Eqn 5.8)	Normal tissue BED (Gy$_3$) (via Eqn 5.5)
(a) 60 Gy/30 fractions/40 days	$72.0 - 15.8 = 56.2$	100.0
(b) 50 Gy/20 fractions/26 days	$62.5 - 10.3 = 52.2$	91.7
(c) 52.5 Gy/20 fractions/26 days	$66.3 - 10.3 = 56.0$	98.4

The table indicates how biological effects are governed by dose per fraction and duration as well as total dose. Particularly noteworthy is the fact that schedules (a) and (c) are closely identical in terms of their effects on both tumour and late-responding tissue, yet the total dose delivered in the latter schedule is 7.5 Gy (12.5 per cent) less than in the former.

Delayed repopulation

For some tumours (e.g. well-differentiated squamous cell cancers), there is an apparent time delay before significant repopulation is detectable (Withers et al., 1988). To allow for this, a simple time-delay factor (T_K) can be incorporated into the LQ equations, i.e. Equation 5.8 becomes:

$$BED = nd\left[1 + \frac{d}{\alpha/\beta}\right] - 0.693 \frac{(T - T_K)}{\alpha t_{eff}} \qquad (5.10)$$

Clearly the repopulation factor in Equation 5.10 is only required in cases where $T_K < T$. T_K values of 21–28 days are frequently recommended. Because the average K-value over an entire treatment for head and neck tumours is equivalent to around 0.6 Gy/day this implies that the figure to use after the 28-day lag period is even higher, and head and neck K-values as high as 1.2 Gy/day have been derived (Roberts and Hendry, 1999). A working value of 0.9 Gy/day may be appropriate for general calculation purposes (Fowler and Harari, 2000; Fu et al., 2000) but it is stressed that the K and T_K values are not known with certainty and will likely change in the light of continuing research.

Loss of control with extended treatment time – the effect of unscheduled treatment interruptions

Tumour repopulation during treatment effectively wastes a significant amount of the delivered dose. It follows that, for rapidly growing tumours, the presence of unintended gaps in the treatment schedule will have the effect of wasting even more dose. It has been estimated that, for head and neck tumours, the loss of control amounts to 1–2 per cent per day of treatment extension (Fowler and Lindstrom, 1992). This figure, however, is from datasets that included a wide range of parameter variations within the treated population and may seriously underestimate the loss of control that occurs in individual patients. Tumour loss of control with increasing time is critically dependent on the expected tumour cure probability (TCP) and is most significant when the TCP is in the middle range, for example between 30 and 60 per cent. In such situations, the values may be as high as 5 per cent per day for individuals.

The potential seriousness of unscheduled gaps in treatment is such that the Royal College of Radiologists (RCR) has issued guidelines on how to deal with the issue (Royal College of Radiologists, 1996). There are many technical, clinical and social reasons why individual patients might miss one or more fractions part-way through a prescribed course of treatment. It is important to appreciate that the gap in treatment is less of a problem if the prescribed treatment can still be completed within the originally stipulated treatment time. The bigger radiobiological problems arise if it is necessary to extend the overall treatment time. Essentially three methods may be employed to offset the effects of an unscheduled treatment gap once it has occurred:

1 Maintain the original prescription time by treating the 'missing' fractions at weekends and using the prescribed dose per fraction.
2 Maintain the original prescription time by employing twice-daily fractionation (using the prescribed dose per fraction) with a minimum of 6-hour intervals between daily fractions.
3 Devise a radiobiological compensation employing altered fractional doses.

Methods 1 and 2 (either individually or in combination) are the preferred options as they maintain the number of fractions and dose per fraction as originally prescribed. However, if the unscheduled gap occurs late in the schedule it can be impossible to effect a compensation without increasing the treatment time, and in cases such as this, method 3 must be invoked.

WORKED EXAMPLE 5.3

A patient prescribed a schedule of 60 Gy in 30 fractions over 6 weeks misses the whole of the second week of treatment (five fractions). How can this unscheduled gap be compensated for?

Answer: After the gap, i.e. at the beginning of the third week of treatment, there are still 25 fractions to

be delivered. If weekend working is possible, then the 'lost' fractions can be treated on five of the six remaining weekend days, the rest of the treatment proceeding as prescribed. If treatment cannot be performed at weekends, then, on five of the remaining treatment days, two fractions per day should be delivered, with a minimum 6-hour gap between those particular fractions.

WORKED EXAMPLE 5.4

A patient prescribed a schedule of 60 Gy in 30 fractions over 6 weeks misses the whole of the final 2 weeks treatment (10 fractions). How can this unscheduled gap be compensated for?

Answer: This is much more difficult case to resolve as it is impossible to treat the 'lost' fractions without overrunning the orginally prescribed treatment time. If it is not possible to treat at weekends, then in order to restrict the 'overrun' as much as possible, the only viable possibility is to treat twice daily on Monday to Friday of the week after the unscheduled break, taking the overall treatment time to 7 weeks (46 days).

If the average dose-equivalent of daily repopulation (K-value) is 0.5 Gy/day, the generic BEDs expected form the treatment as prescribed are:

$$BED_{tumour} = 60 \times \left[1 + \frac{2}{10}\right] - 0.5 \times 39 = 52.5 \ Gy_{10}$$

$$BED_{late} = 60 \times \left[1 + \frac{2}{3}\right] = 100 \ Gy_3$$

The extra dose required to offset the repopulation in the 1 week extension of treatment time is $7 \times 0.5 = 3.5$ Gy, and this is the amount by which the tumour BED will be reduced if no compensation is made, i.e. BED_{10} will be $49 \ Gy_{10}$ rather than the expected $52.5 \ Gy_{10}$. Increasing the dose per fraction can restore the BED_{10} but at the cost of a BED_3 which is greater than that prescribed. Delivery of more than 10 fractions, with a view to decrease dose per fraction, might seem a possible solution, but this will take the treatment into the eighth week and require more dose to offset yet more repopulation. This is the essential dilemma involved in difficult cases and the inevitable result is that there must be some compromise to the therapeutic ratio. The prescribed late BED can only be respected at the cost of a reduced tumour BED; achievement of a tumour BED which is close to that expected from the uninterrupted treatment can only be attained with some increase in the late BED. Usually it is necessary to consider several possible scenarios in order to identify the most acceptable compromise.

Methods of presenting modelling results: the equivalent dose delivered in 2 Gy fractions

Several methods exist for presenting the results of modelling assessments, e.g. comparison of BED values or their derived TCPs or normal tissue complication probabilities (NTCPs). However, for day-to-day clinical application the results can be summarized in a form that relates directly to the prescribing practice of the radiation oncologist. It is possible to stipulate any treatment in terms of a 2 Gy/fraction equivalent. This concept is easy for most clinicians – the calculated equivalent dose can be related to previous clinical experience of treating with 2 Gy fractions to form a judgement of both tumour control and normal tissue complication risk.

WORKED EXAMPLE 5.5

A treatment prescription for 50 Gy in 25 fractions includes the optic chiasm. Suppose there is an inhomogeneity which results in a 10 per cent increase in dose across the target volume. What does this dose increase imply?

For an α/β ratio of 2 Gy (applicable to the optic chiasm, a fractionation-sensitive structure) the prescribed BED is:

$$50 \times \left[1 + \frac{2}{2}\right] = 100 \text{ Gy}_2$$

Because of the 10 per cent increase, the fractional dose is $2 \times 1.1 = 2.2$ Gy, instead of the prescribed 2 Gy. Over 25 fractions the total dose will be $25 \times 2.2 = 55.0$ Gy. The true BED is then:

$$55.0 \times \left[1 + \frac{2.2}{2}\right] = 115.5 \text{ Gy}_2$$

Thus, although the dose increase is 10 per cent, the resultant increase in BED_2 is 15.5 per cent. What does this mean in clinical terms? This can be assessed by calculating how many 2-Gy fractions would give a similar increase in BED.
To find the equivalent total dose given in N fractions each of 2 Gy, solve:

$$N \times 2 \times \left[1 + \frac{2}{2}\right] = 115.5$$

leading to $N = 28.9$, which is rounded up to 29 fractions, i.e. the 10 per cent dose increase is equivalent to delivering four extra 2-Gy fractions. The equivalent total dose in 2-Gy fractions is approximately $29 \times 2 = 58$ Gy.

Brachytherapy

For high dose-rate brachytherapy the LQ equations to use are essentially the same as those required for teletherapy. For low or medium dose-rate continuous radiation the situation is different, for the following reason. If the delivery of a radiation dose is protracted, such that the time of delivery takes more than a few minutes, then there is an opportunity for sublethally damaged cells to repair during the course of radiation delivery. The amount of lethal damage caused by interaction between sublethally damaged entities is thus reduced. Specifically, there is a smaller amount of Type B (β-mediated) lethal damage than occurs in acute radiation delivery. For a given dose the overall treatment time is determined by the dose-rate, and the Type B damage calculation must include an allowance for this. Type A damage, because it is caused only by instantaneous lethal events, is unaffected by extension in irradiation time and is therefore independent of dose-rate.

A realistic radiobiological assessment of brachytherapy applications is always more difficult than in the case of teletherapy, principally because of the non-homogeneous doses and the rapid fall of dose with distance from the source(s) (Dale and Jones, 1998). In particular, it should be remembered that the critical normal tissue may receive a lower dose than that prescribed to the tumour and this should be allowed for in the calculation of the normal-tissue BED. Also, the dose gradients within any tissue that contains sources causes the effective BED to that tissue volume to be higher than that calculated at the reference isodose surface. This point is returned to in the section on brachytherapy dose-gradients on p. 77.

BED calculations in brachytherapy

For fractionated high dose-rate (FHDR) brachytherapy the relevant equations to use to calculate BED values are Equations 5.4 or 5.8, the latter being required in cases where it is necessary to include an allowance for tumour repopulation.

For continuous low dose-rate (CLDR) brachytherapy the required equation is:

$$\text{BED} = RT\left[1 + \frac{2R}{\mu(\alpha/\beta)}\right] \qquad (5.11)$$

where R is the dose-rate (Gy/h) and T (h) is the duration of brachytherapy, μ is the DNA sublethal damage repair rate constant, related to the repair half-life via:

$$\mu = \frac{0.693}{T_{1/2}}$$

Equation 5.11 is a simplified form of a more complex equation (Dale, 1985), but is nevertheless reliable in most cases where the CLDR treatment time is greater than around 12 h.

WORKED EXAMPLE 5.6

A CLDR gynaecological treatment delivers to Point A a dose of 40 Gy in 48 h. If an FHDR treatment involving six fractions is to be used instead, what total dose is required in order to maintain the normal tissue iso-effect?

As Point A represents a normal-tissue dose-limiting site, it will be assumed that α/β is 3 Gy and the repair half-life is 1.5 h, i.e. $\mu = 0.693/1.5 = 0.46/h$.

The dose-rate (R) at Point A is $40/48 = 0.83$ Gy/h, therefore, from Equation 5.11:

$$BED_3 = 40 \times \left[1 + \frac{2 \times 0.83}{0.46 \times 3}\right] = 88.1 \text{ Gy}_3$$

To match this BED value with six FHDR fractions requires a dose per fraction of d Gy, where:

$$6 \times d \times \left[1 + \frac{d}{3}\right] = 88.1$$

i.e.:

$$2d^2 + 6d - 264.3 = 0$$

i.e. the required dose per fraction (d) is 5.3 Gy.

In cases where brachytherapy is combined with teletherapy, the individual BEDs for each component may be summed to obtain a measure of the total biological effect, i.e.:

$$BED \text{ (total)} = BED \text{ (external beam)} + BED \text{ (brachytherapy)} \quad (5.12)$$

WORKED EXAMPLE 5.7

A pelvic teletherapy regime of 45 Gy/25 fractions is combined with an FHDR brachytherapy regime of 2×7 Gy prescribed to Point A. The bladder and rectum each receives 100 per cent of both the teletherapy dose and the brachytherapy dose. What is the BED for the bladder/rectum, assuming an α/β value of 3 Gy?

$$BED = 45 \times \left[1 + \frac{1.8}{3}\right] + 14 \times \left[1 + \frac{7}{3}\right] = 118.7 \text{ Gy}_3$$

If geometrical sparing of the bladder/rectum during brachytherapy reduces the dose from that component to 80 per cent of the prescribed Point A dose, what is the new BED?

$$BED = 45 \times \left[1 + \frac{1.8}{3}\right] + 14 \times 0.8 \times \left[1 + \frac{7 \times 0.8}{3}\right]$$
$$= 104.1 \text{ Gy}_3$$

In general, the severe side-effects associated with pelvic radiotherapy manifest after BED values which significantly exceed 110 Gy$_3$ (Leborgne et al., 1997). This example therefore demonstrates how, in principle, a modest reduction of the brachytherapy dose and dose per fraction to the critical organ can bring about a reduction in the likelihood of serious toxicity.

Amelioration of an incorrectly delivered radiotherapy treatment

It is sometimes said that no amount of radiobiological manipulation will correct a treatment which is incorrectly prescribed or executed. While this is correct in cases involving a geometrical miss or significant over- or underdosing, there are occasions where changes in time–dose-fractionation may significantly ameliorate the potential damage, although it may be necessary to accept a reduction in control probability if total dosage has to be reduced. The problem is essentially one of obtaining the best benefit/risk ratio in a particular set of circumstances.

WORKED EXAMPLE 5.8

A patient has received an overdose of 15 per cent to the spinal cord. The error is detected after six fractions have been given in a treatment course prescribed as 46 Gy in 23 fractions. How can the overdose be corrected over the remaining treatment course if the dose per fraction is reduced to 1.8 Gy?

Intended spinal cord BED assuming $\alpha/\beta = 2$ Gy:

$$46 \times \left[1 + \frac{2}{2}\right] = 92 \text{ Gy}_2$$

In the first six fractions, the BED actually delivered is:

$$6 \times 2 \times 1.15 \times \left[1 + \frac{2 \times 1.15}{2}\right] = 29.7 \text{ Gy}_2$$

The remainder of the treatment course will thus require to give a BED$_2$ which should not exceed $92.0 - 29.7 = 62.3$ Gy$_2$. At 1.8 Gy per fraction, the number of fractions (n) required to deliver this 'residual' BED$_2$ is found by solving:

$$n \times 1.8 \times \left[1 + \frac{1.8}{2}\right] = 62.3$$

From which $n = 18.2$. It is therefore decided to give 18 fractions of 1.8 Gy.

If the tumour α/β value is 15 Gy, how is the tumour BED affected by the change to the schedule?

The prescribed tumour BED was:

$$46 \times \left[1 + \frac{2}{15}\right] = 52.1 \, Gy_{15}$$

whereas the true value will be:

$$6 \times 2 \times 1.15 \times \left[1 + \frac{2 \times 1.15}{15}\right]$$
$$+ 18 \times 1.8 \times \left[1 + \frac{1.8}{15}\right] = 52.2 \, Gy_{15}$$

which is scarcely different from that prescribed. Thus, the treatment error has been effectively overcome by the altered fractionation and use of a lower (and hence, more forgiving), dose per fraction.

WORKED EXAMPLE 5.9

A patient is treated to a tolerance dose equivalent to 70 Gy in 35 fractions by:

1 initial wide-field radiotherapy of 39.6 Gy in 22 fractions; followed by
2 reduced field sizes to a further 16 Gy in 8 fractions; and then
3 focal radiotherapy given in 4 fractions.

Calculate the dose per fraction (d) required for the focal therapy (assume $\alpha/\beta = 2$ Gy).
   The total BED will be:

$$70 \times \left[1 + \frac{2}{2}\right] = 140 \, Gy_2$$

The following condition must hold:

$$BED_{phase\ 1} + BED_{phase\ 2} + BED_{phase\ 3} = 140 \, Gy_2$$

and:

$$39.6 \times \left[1 + \frac{1.8}{2}\right] + 16 \times \left[1 + \frac{2}{2}\right]$$
$$+ 4 \times d \times \left[1 + \frac{d}{2}\right] = 140$$

So that:

$$75.2 + 32 + 4d + 2d^2 = 140$$

i.e.:

$$d^2 + 2d = 16.4$$

$$d = 3.2 \, Gy$$

MORE ADVANCED CONSIDERATIONS

Thus far the discussion and examples in this chapter have focused on what might be called general modelling;

the parameters used are intrinsically assumed to apply throughout individual tumour volumes and throughout whole patient populations. For example, use of the radiosensitivity factor α assumes a uniform radiosensitivity throughout the tumour, i.e. in hypoxic and oxic zones, and also inclusive of clones which in reality may possess variations in intrinsic radiosensitivity. Likewise, the T_{eff} value is generalized, being a one-figure representation of a more complex pattern of repopulation throughout very heterogeneous tumours. Even the ubiquitous α/β ratios are averages which probably incorporate the effects of multiple radiobiological processes, such as reoxygenation (in the case of tumours), cell-cycle redistribution and repopulation. Thus, although the LQ model has a sound biophysical basis, the variations inherent in the critical parameters place a limit on how accurate modelling can be in individual cases.

The alternative approach is to attempt to model the processes in greater detail while accepting the associated drawback that multiple parameter assumptions are necessary. Some more advanced approaches are discussed briefly below.

Estimation of tumour cure probabilities (TCPs) from BEDs

If the number (C) of clonogenic cells is known, then the Poisson model may be used to estimate TCP:

$$TCP = \exp[-C \exp(-\alpha \times BED)] \qquad (5.13)$$

The slope of the dose response generated by the Poisson distribution (i.e. TCP plotted against BED or total dose) is much steeper than found in datasets obtained from large numbers of patients. This is to be expected because, as the Poisson distribution reflects the probability of achieving a cure from the elimination of all cells in a single tumour, it is essentially useful only for individual tumours. The alternative logistic function is applicable to population data and has a less steep dose–response curve.

WORKED EXAMPLE 5.10

A particular tumour has an average K-value of 0.5 Gy/day and consists of 10^8 clonogens. It is treated with 60 Gy/30 fractions over 6 weeks (39 days). What is the expected TCP? Assume $\alpha/\beta = 10$ Gy.
   From Equation 5.8:

$$BED = 60 \times \left[1 + \frac{2}{10}\right] - 0.5 \times 39 = 52.5 \, Gy_{10}$$

In order to calculate TCP from Equation 5.13, it is necessary to assume a value for α. If this is taken to be 0.35/Gy, then:

$$TCP = \exp[-10^8 \times \exp(-0.35 \times 52.5)]$$
$$= 0.35\ (35\ \text{per cent})$$

If the tumour is treated without weekend breaks, i.e. is treated with 2 Gy fractions on 7 days of each week, the overall time falls to 29 days. The BED then increases to:

$$BED = 60 \times \left[1 + \frac{2}{10}\right] - 0.5 \times 29 = 57.5\ \text{Gy}_{10}$$

For this BED the associated TCP is:

$$TCP = \exp[-10^8 \times \exp(-0.35 \times 57.5)]$$
$$= 0.83\ (83\ \text{per cent})$$

This example clearly demonstrates how overall treatment time can have a strong influence on TCP in individual patients.

Optimization

Clinically effective radiotherapy requires a balance to be maintained between a number of potentially conflicting requirements. For example, use of small fractional doses is more likely to minimize NTCP, but this may require the use of so many fractions that treatment time is greatly extended, thereby allowing more tumour repopulation, and hence, a reduced TCP. As the LQ model includes such effects, there exists the possibility of extending the model in order to identify schedules which are optimized for a given set of circumstances. By consideration of how tumour cell kill varies with changes in dose per fraction and overall time, calculus may be used to derive an optimum dose per fraction which maximizes the TCP while respecting any given normal tissue effect (Jones *et al.*, 1995). In conjunction with accurate predictive assays, this development could be an important step towards 'tailored' radiotherapy.

Incorporation of cell-loss factors

An alternative explanation for the apparent appearance of delayed acceleration is that tumour repopulation rates are initially small but progressively increase during the course of treatment. When analysing the effect in a range of datasets such a phenomenon could easily be mistaken for a two-component process (Fig. 5.1). An explanation for an asymptotically increasing repopulation rate may be developed from consideration of the role of the potential doubling time (T_{pot}) and the cell-loss factor ϕ, which is the probability that newly born cells will die due to causes such as hypoxia and insufficiency of nutrients and growth factors. The cell-loss factor is likely to decrease during radiotherapy due to improved tumour

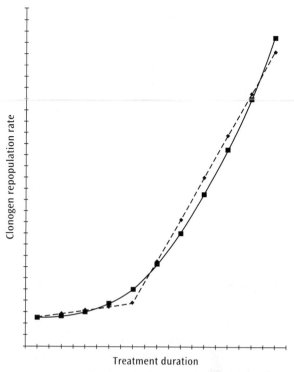

Figure 5.1 *A schematic representation demonstrating how a continuously increasing repopulation process (solid line) can be mistakenly interpreted as a two-component linear process with accelerated repopulation beginning part-way through treatment (dashed line).*

microvascular perfusion. The probability that new born cells will survive can be represented by $(1 - \phi)$, and Jones and Dale (1995) have developed an equation that allows for BED to be assessed when there is a slow exponential reduction in ϕ due to improved blood perfusion during treatment.

The problem with closely spaced fractions

The delivery of an acute dose of radiation results in the creation of both lethal and sublethal damage. By definition, the lethal damage is unrepairable, but the sublethal damage component is able to repair pseudo-exponentially with a repair half-time typically in the range 0.5–3 h. When the fractional doses are well spaced (e.g. as 24-h gaps) the residual sublethal damage after any particular fraction is effectively fully repaired before delivery of the next fraction and therefore does not have any influence on the ultimate biological outcome.

If, however, the fractions are delivered at much closer intervals, then any unrepaired sublethal damage remaining after any one fraction can be compounded to extra lethal damage by fractions delivered later in the schedule. The amount of extra damage so created is dependent on several factors, but clearly the inter-fraction intervals and the repair rates are of prime importance and, within the LQ formulation, the extra damage due to closely spaced fractions appears in the form of a modified β term in Equation 5.2 (Thames, 1985). Any increased damage due to this effect is obviously beneficial in a tumour, but will be of major concern if it occurs in a critical normal tissue.

The equations for dealing with closely spaced fractions are complex but, using a table provided in both Thames and Hendry (1987) and Joiner and van der Kogel (1997), a simpler alternative may be used. The table provides values of an incomplete-repair factor, h_M which allows for different numbers of treatments per day, repair half-times and inter-fraction intervals. When h_M is incorporated into the basic BED equation, the latter is modified to:

$$BED = nd\left[1 + \frac{d(1 + h_M)}{\alpha/\beta}\right] \qquad (5.14)$$

WORKED EXAMPLE 5.11

60 Gy is to be delivered in 30 fractions (2 Gy per fraction) over 10 consecutive days by treating three fractions per day at 4-hour intervals. Assuming the DNA sub-lethal damage repair half-time is 1.5 hours and $\alpha/\beta = 3$ Gy, what is the late-responding BED?

From Table 6.3 of Thames and Hendry (1987), $h_M = 0.2265$; therefore, from Equation 5.14:

$$BED = 30 \times 2 \times \left[1 + \frac{2 \times (1 + 0.2265)}{3}\right] = 109.1 \text{ Gy}_3.$$

The BED_3 for 60 Gy delivered as daily fractionation is 100 Gy$_3$. Therefore three fractions per day increases this figure by approximately 9 per cent.

New models of repair

Most radiobiological models assume that sublethal damage repair is a mono- or multi-exponential process, the latter being required when there is the apparent presence of separate fast and slow repair rates. A quite different description of the repair process has been suggested by Fowler (1999). *In-vitro* DNA repair data is consistently better fitted by assuming that the fraction of unrepaired breaks decreases in proportion to the reciprocal of the time elapsed (t) since their production, i.e. proportional to $1/(1 + zt)$, where z is an appropriate constant. This postulation of a 'reciprocal-time' pattern of repair is consistent with the view that there is total saturation of repair enzymes at clinically relevant doses. The practical advantage is that the observed presence of separate components of fast and slow repair in some cell lines can be covered by an equation involving only one rate constant (z), rather than several exponential rate constants.

The reciprocal-time model may be incorporated into the LQ model, in which form it predicts the breakdown in tissue tolerance when the CNS is irradiated by three fractions per day. This is in contrast with bi-exponential models of repair, which cannot satisfactorily explain the clinical problems which were observed in the early CHART trials. The implications of this new model of repair are yet to be fully explored, but early predictions are that:

- Repair in normal tissues may remain incomplete for much longer intervals of time, such as 18–24 hours, than had previously been thought.
- It is only over a weekend 'gap' that late-reacting normal tissue repair may be complete.
- For long exposures, as occur in LDR brachytherapy, the apparent rate of repair after irradiation appears to be slower for longer irradiation times. These issues have been examined in depth by Dale *et al.* (1999).

Allowance for RBE effects

The standard formulations for calculating BED inherently assume that the radiation involved has a low linear energy transfer (LET) and thus possesses a relative biological effectiveness (RBE) of unity. High-LET radiations (e.g. neutrons, protons and those emitted by some brachytherapy radionuclides) have RBE > 1 and produce greater biological damage (i.e. higher BEDs) for a given physical dose. A potential complication is that RBE is itself dependent on fraction size, being greatest when dose per fraction is very small. Despite this, allowance for the RBE effect for all fraction sizes may be achieved through a simple change to the formulae used to calculate BED. This is effected by replacing the unity factor in the relevant RE equations by RBE_{max}, where RBE_{max} is the maximum RBE observed when small fraction sizes are employed (Joiner and Field, 1988). Thus, for example, Equation 5.4 would be changed to:

$$BED = nd\left[RBE_{max} + \frac{d}{\alpha/\beta}\right] \ldots \qquad (5.15)$$

The α/β value to use in formulae for calculating high-LET BEDs is the same as is conventionally used, i.e. it is the α/β ratio appropriate to *low*-LET radiations. This combination of the RBE_{max} value with the low-LET α/β ratio ensures that calculated low- and high-LET BED values may be directly compared one with another (Dale and Jones, 1999; Jones and Dale, 2000).

Limitation in the scope of BED intercomparisons

Examples 5.1–5.4 demonstrate how the BED parameter may be used to intercompare existing treatments or to design a new treatment which is iso-effective to an existing treatment. It is nevertheless important to appreciate that, as conventionally used, BED is a measure of radiobiological effect at one particular point within the treated volume. BED intercomparisons thus lose much of their usefulness if they are used to compare treatments in which the geometrical details (e.g. field shapes, number of applied fields, irradiated volumes, etc.) of the compared treatments are not held constant. Indeed, the application of LQ methodology in cases where these conditions are not met may produce some very misleading results. This point also needs to be borne in mind when using BED calculations to assess retrospectively the results of clinical trials for which the various treatment schedules do not share common geometrical field arrangements, or where there are significant dose inhomogeneities.

The particular problem caused by brachytherapy dose-gradients

For brachytherapy the above observations are all the more important, principally because of the non-homogeneous doses and the rapid fall of dose with distance from the source(s) (Dale and Jones, 1998). The radiobiological significance of brachytherapy dose gradients has been discussed in detail elsewhere (Dale et al., 1997), from which some general guidelines have been established. In cases where there is a continuous dose gradient from the reference (or prescription) surface (at which the dose is prescribed) to the sources, as occurs in most gynaecological treatments and line-source applications, the effective BED throughout the volume enclosed by that surface can be derived using tabulated multiplying factors (MFs). The BED at the surface is first calculated using the simple equations outlined earlier and then corrected by an MF appropriate to the particular treatment set-up. In the case of an FHDR brachytherapy application, the MF value will be mostly dependent on the number of fractions and the dose per fraction, but only marginally so on the radiobiological factors (α, α/β, etc.). The treatment geometry (e.g. line source, point source) also has little influence. For CLDR applications the MFs are mostly influenced by total dose and dose-rate.

WORKED EXAMPLE 5.12

An FHDR gynaecological treatment involves delivering 6 fractions of 5 Gy to Point A. What is the effective BED to the tissues within the isodose surface which contains Point A?

First, the BED_3 is calculated in the usual manner:

$$BED_3 = 6 \times 5 \times \left[1 + \frac{5}{3}\right] = 80 \text{ Gy}_3$$

From Table 7 of Dale et al. (1997), the appropriate MF value for this particular combination of dose per fraction and fraction number is 1.185, hence the effective BED throughout the enclosed volume is $80 \times 1.185 = 94.8 \text{ Gy}_3$.

Tumour volume changes during radiotherapy

Tumour regression generally follows a negative exponential function. In such cases, if V_0 and V_t are the tumour volumes at times 0 and t, respectively, then

$$V_t = V_0 e^{-zt}$$

where z is the regression rate coefficient. Consequently, if the regression rate is measured accurately one can predict the volume at a future time point. This information may be used to plan additional treatment, such as conformal therapy, where the reduced volume allows a higher radiation dose to be delivered.

WORKED EXAMPLE 5.13

Serial imaging during the first part of a course of radiotherapy shows that a tumour, originally of volume 95 cm^3, has a volume regression rate of 3 per cent per day. Estimate the volume of tumour 28 days after completion of a 35-day course of treatment.

$$V_t = 95 \cdot e^{-0.03 \times 63} = 14.4 \text{ cm}^3$$

The volume effect and difficulties in relation to normal tissues

Although it is clinically well established that large volumes of normal tissue will tolerate less radiation than small volumes (the so-called 'volume effect'), accurate modelling of the effect is a difficult and controversial issue. One reason for this is that the volume effect is strongly influenced by variations in tissue physiology and anatomical location, yet attempts at formulating the phenomenon tend to concentrate almost exclusively on physical and radiobiological considerations. A further difficulty is that the changes in radiation tolerance with treatment volume are often modelled empirically using clinical dose–response data of limited usefulness. The result is that most of the existing NTCP models have little biological basis; thus the use of simpler BED iso-effect calculations backed by clinical judgement is reasonable until better predictive models are found.

Intercomparison of treatment alternatives on the basis of their net costs

The net costs of treatment can be estimated by inclusion of the fixed costs (treatment planning, treatment delivery, etc.) together with the notional costs associated with treatment failure. The former costs can take account of the treatment complexity, whereas the latter are based on the cost of additional medical/surgical care in the event of failure to control the primary tumour. For a given set of radiobiological parameters, cost-optimized treatments will often differ from radiobiologically optimized treatments, this being especially true of those more complex treatments which offer relatively small gains in TCP. Such modelling may have a useful role to play in identifying the situations in which the more complicated (and hence, more costly) methods of treatment can be most effectively employed (Dale and Jones, 1996; Jones and Dale, 1998).

Radiotherapy combined with other modalities

For concomitant chemoradiotherapy or the use of chemotherapy in close temporal approximation to radiotherapy, it can be assumed that repopulation is absent due to the cytostatic effect on dividing cells – an easy method which can also be applied for biological cytostatic therapies. The alternative is to allow a particular cell kill per exposure; this is difficult to quantify but can be estimated from reported clinical trials. Sensitization of the radiotherapy is another method – where the dose per fraction is enhanced by a factor of 1.2–1.5 or more. (For further discussion of modelling gene therapy see Wheldon *et al.*, 1998; Jones and Dale, 1999.)

Serum tumour markers

The serum marker concentration is assumed to reflect the total number of cells present and, although marker levels fall during or after therapy, the absolute levels during a period of such change do not reflect the absolute number of cells. If the half-life ($T_{1/2}$) of the marker is known, then the tumour marker production rate (TMP), which will better represent the absolute number of cells, can be calculated as in the equation of Price *et al.* (1990),

$$TMP = C_2 - C_1 \cdot e^{-\frac{0.693(t_2 - t_1)}{T_{1/2}}}$$

where C_1 and C_2 are the marker concentrations at times t_1 and t_2 respectively.

WORKED EXAMPLE 5.14

Consider a pre-treatment situation where the marker is slowly rising, so that in 14 days, the level changes from 95 to 100 units. If $T_{1/2}$ is 12 hours (0.5 days), the average TMP, expressed as units per day, in this period is:

$$TMP = 100 - 95 \cdot e^{-\frac{0.693(14)}{0.5}} = 100 - 0 = 100/day$$

Now if, in a 2-day interval near to the completion of radiotherapy, the levels fall from 75 to 60, then the new marker production rate falls to:

$$TMP = 60 - 75 \cdot e^{-\frac{0.693(2)}{0.5}} = 60 - 4.69 = 55.3/day$$

Commercial software packages for radiobiological bioeffect planning

Despite the advances radiobiological understanding, treatment planning in radiotherapy continues to be based on the computation and assessment of physical dose distributions. Where radiobiological features are available on commercial systems, two approaches have been adopted. The first is to transform physical dose distribution to a BED distribution, a method which, in principle, allows the biological effects of various radiation treatments, e.g. external-beam therapy and brachytherapy, to be added graphically. The second approach is to produce estimates of TCP and NTCP in specific volumes of interest. TCP calculations are based on clonogenic cell survival and may take into account non-uniform dose delivery. NTCP calculations are based on models of normal tissue functional organization in which the subunits are not regarded as independent for response purposes. Despite the growing acceptance of the potential importance of bioeffect planning, progress in this area remains generally slow because of difficulties in identifying user requirements, limitations of the models and concern relating to the clinical interpretation of results.

WORKED EXAMPLE 5.15

If a high-LET radiation with an RBE_{max} of 1.4 is used in place of conventional (low-LET) photons, what high-LET dose is equivalent, in terms of late effects, to 30×2 Gy?

Assume that the low-LET α/β is 3 Gy for late effects and that the high-LET dose also is to be delivered in 2 Gy fractions.

From Equation 5.4 the low-LET BED is:

$$BED_{low} = 30 \times 2 \times \left[1 + \frac{2}{3}\right] = 100 \text{ Gy}_3$$

Equation 5.15 is used to calculate the number (n) of high-LET 2 Gy fractions required:

$$n \times 2 \times \left[1.4 + \frac{2}{3}\right] = 100 \text{ Gy}_3$$

i.e. $n = 24.2$.

Thus, when both schedules are delivered in 2 Gy fractions, 48.4 Gy with the high-LET radiation is equivalent to 60 Gy at low-LET. Note that this high-LET dose is greater than is calculated by simply dividing the low-LET dose (60 Gy) by RBE_{max} (1.4); use of Equation 5.15 properly allows for the effect of fraction size and the α/β ratio to be included in the calculation.

CONCLUSION

Radiobiological models can provide a useful complement to clinical judgement in a variety of circumstances. In the routine practice of radiotherapy there are many factors that can prompt a review of patient management (e.g. geometrical difficulties, dosimetric errors, treatment interruptions, etc.) and modelling can allow compensatory treatment schedules to be suggested.

The necessary caveats have been mentioned throughout the chapter. However, even with these caveats, modelling can often guide or inform clinical judgement, e.g. by means of ranking a series of alternative treatments in order to reject the less satisfactory options. For radiation oncologists in training, the teaching value of being familiar with the simpler methods of quantifying radiobiological effect should not be underestimated. Even simple radiobiological estimates can provide a useful assessment of disparate treatments. In research and development, quantitative appraisal of proposed new techniques or clinical trials should always be the subject of a modelling review. Similarly, in order to allow quantitative comparisons between new and existing treatment schedules, all published works should record at least the generic BEDs associated with the treatments which are being described.

Technological developments presently abound in radiation oncology. However, while some technological advances (e.g. the ability to reduce irradiated normal tissue volumes through use of conformal techniques and intensity-modulated radiotherapy (IMRT)) provide seemingly obvious benefits, the full potential of modern radiotherapy will be realized only if commensurate attention is given to the radiobiological aspects that determine treatment outcome. Radiation oncology thus faces an interesting future, with radiobiological modelling providing more pivotal guidance on how to make optimal use of the emerging technology.

SIGNIFICANT POINTS

- Biological effect is not related solely to the total physical dose delivered in a radiotherapy treatment – factors such as dose per fraction and dose-rate are also fundamentally important.
- Modern radiobiological models take account of a range of practical and radiobiological factors which are known to influence treatment outcome.
- Simple radiobiological assessments can provide a useful supplement to clinical judgement in a variety of ways.

- More advanced modelling ideas, when coupled with the results of reliable predictive assays, will allow more appropriate use of the emerging technologies.
- Radiobiological models already have an important role to play in the teaching and understanding of clinical radiotherapy.
- In order to facilitate easier comparison between clinical studies, reports and publications should routinely record the BEDs, etc. associated with the treatments under discussion.

KEY REFERENCES

Dale, R.G. (1985) The application of the linear quadratic dose–effect equation to fractionated and protracted radiotherapy. *Br. J. Radiol.* **58**, 515–28.

Fowler, J.F. (1989) The linear quadratic formula and progress in fractionated radiotherapy. *Br. J. Radiol.* **62**, 679–94.

Joiner, M.J. and van der Kogel, A.J. (1997) The linear-quadratic approach to fractionation and calculation of isoeffect relationships. In Steel, G.G. (ed.), *Basic clinical radiobiology*. London: Arnold, 106–22.

Thames, H.D. and Hendry, J.H. (1987) *Fractionation in radiotherapy*. London: Taylor and Francis, 148–63.

REFERENCES

Barendsen, G.W. (1982) Dose fractionation, dose rate and iso-effect relationships for normal tissue responses. *Int. J. Radiat. Oncol. Biol. Phys.* **8**, 1981–97.

Dale, R.G. (1985) The application of the linear quadratic dose–effect equation to fractionated and protracted radiotherapy. *Br. J. Radiol.* **58**, 515–28.

Dale, R.G. and Jones, B. (1996) Radiobiologically-based assessments of the net costs of fractionated radiotherapy. *Int. J. Radiat. Oncol. Biol. Phys.* **36**(3), 739–46.

Dale, R.G. and Jones, B. (1998) The radiobiology of brachytherapy. *Br. J. Radiol.* **71**, 465–83.

Dale, R.G. and Jones, B. (1999) The assessment of RBE effects using the concept of biologically effective dose. *Int. J. Radiat. Oncol. Biol. Phys.* **43**, 639–45.

Dale, R.G., Coles, I.P., Deehan, C. and O'Donoghue, J.A. (1997) Calculation of integrated biological response in brachytherapy. *Int. J. Radiat. Oncol. Biol. Phys.* **38**, 633–42.

Dale, R.G., Fowler, J.F. and Jones, B. (1999) A new incomplete-repair model based on a 'reciprocal time' pattern of sub-lethal damage repair. *Acta Oncol.* **38**, 919–29.

Duchesne, G.M. and Peters, L.J. (1999) What is the α/β ratio for prostate cancer? Rationale for hypofractionated high dose-rate brachytherapy. *Int. J. Radiat. Oncol. Biol. Phys.* **44**, 747–8.

Fowler, J.F. (1989) The linear quadratic formula and progress in fractionated radiotherapy. *Br. J. Radiol.* **62**, 679–94.

Fowler, J.F. (1999) Is repair of DNA strand break damage from ionizing radiation second-order rather than first-order? A simpler explanation of apparently multiexponential repair. *Radiat. Res.* **152**, 124–36.

Fowler, J.F. and Harari, P.M. (2000) Confirmation of improved loco-regional control with altered fractionation in head and neck cancer. *Int. J. Radiat. Oncol. Biol. Phys.* **48**, 3–6.

Fowler, J.F. and Lindstrom, M.J. (1992) Loss of local control with prolongation in radiotherapy. *Int. J. Radiat. Oncol. Biol. Phys.* **23**, 457–67.

Fu, K.K., Pajak, T.F., Trotti, A. *et al.* (2000) A Radiation Therapy Oncology Group (RTOG) Phase III randomised study to compare hyperfractionation and two variants of accelerated fractionation to standard fractionation radiotherapy for head and neck squamous cell carcinomas: first report of RTOG 9003. *Int. J. Radiat. Oncol. Biol. Phys.* **48**, 7–16.

Joiner, M.C. and Field, S.B. (1988) The response of mouse skin to irradiation with neutrons from the 62MV cyclotron at Clatterbridge, UK. *Radioth. Oncol.* **12**, 153–66.

Joiner, M.J. and van der Kogel, A.J. (1997) The linear-quadratic approach to fractionation and calculation of isoeffect relationships. In Steel, G.G. (ed.), *Basic clinical radiobiology*. London: Arnold, 106–22.

Jones, B. and Dale, R.G. (1995) Cell loss factors and the linear quadratic model. *Radiother. Oncol.* **37**, 136–9.

Jones, B. and Dale, R.G. (1998) Radiobiologically based assessments of the net costs of fractionated focal radiotherapy. *Int. J. Radiat. Oncol. Biol. Phys.* **41**, 1139–48.

Jones, B. and Dale, R.G. (1999) Inclusion of molecular bio-therapies with radical radiotherapy: modelling of combined modality treatment schedules. *Int. J. Radiat. Oncol. Biol. Phys.* **45**, 1025–34.

Jones, B. and Dale, R.G. (2000) Estimation of optimum dose per fraction for high LET radiations: implications for proton radiotherapy. *Int. J. Radiat. Oncol. Biol. Phys.* **48**, 1549–57.

Jones, B., Tan, L.T. and Dale, R.G. (1995) Derivation of the optimum dose per fraction from the linear quadratic model. *Br. J. Radiol.* **68**, 894–902.

King, C.R. and Fowler, J.F. (2001) A simple analytic derivation suggest that prostate cancer α/β ratio is low. *Int. J. Radiat. Oncol. Biol. Phys.* **51**, 1–3.

Leborgne, F., Fowler, J.F., Leborgne, J.H., Zubizarreta, E. and Chappell, R. (1997) Biologically effective doses in medium dose-rate brachytherapy of cancer of the cervix. *Radiat. Oncol. Invest.* **5**, 289–99.

Price, P., Hogan, S.J. and Horwich, A. (1990) The growth rate of metastatic non-seminomatous germ cell testicular tumours measured by marker production doubling time – I. Theoretical basis and practical application. *Eur. J. Cancer* **26**, 450–3.

Roberts, S.A. and Hendry, J.A. (1999) Time factors in larynx tumour radiotherapy: lag times and intertumour heterogeneity in clinical datasets from four centres. *Int. J. Radiat. Oncol. Biol. Phys.* **45**, 1247–57.

Royal College of Radiologists (1996) *Guidelines for the management of the unscheduled interruption or prolongation of a radical course of radiotherapy.* Document BFCO(96)4. London: Royal College of Radiologists.

Thames, H.D. (1985) An 'incomplete-repair' model for survival after fractionated and continuous irradiations. *Int. J. Radiat. Biol.* **47**, 319–39.

Thames, H.D. and Hendry, J.H. (1987) *Fractionation in radiotherapy.* London: Taylor and Francis, 148–63.

Wheldon, T.E., Mairs, R.J., Rampling, R.P. and Barrett, A. (1998) Modelling the enhancement of fractionated radiotherapy by gene transfer to sensitize tumour cells to radiation. *Radiother. Oncol.* **48**, 5–13.

Withers, H.R., Taylor, J.M.G. and Maciejewski, B. (1988) The hazard of accelerated tumour clonogen repopulation during radiotherapy. *Acta Oncol.* **27**, 131–46.

6

Hyperthermia in the treatment of cancer

CLARE C. VERNON AND JEFFREY W. HAND

INTRODUCTION

All cancer treatments aim to exploit the differences between normal and malignant cells, and hyperthermia is no exception. The first use of heat in cancer therapy dates back to around 3000 BC, when the Edwin Smith papyrus describes the use of a 'fire drill' in a patient with breast cancer. A more validated account of tumour regression following whole-body hyperthermia can be seen in W. Busch's report in 1866 of a neck sarcoma, which regressed after an erysipelas-induced fever (Busch, 1866). However, it was not until the 1960s that a systematic investigation of the anti-cancer effects of hyperthermia began, by a variety of experimental and clinical studies and including analysis of a vast literature of anecdotal reports. The results confirmed that hyperthermia did have an anti-tumour effect and led to the development of a rationale for its clinical use. Techniques for heating tumours and raising temperature *in situ* were improved and the overall interest and effort in this field increased dramatically – the past few years have seen great advances in clinical areas. From preclinical data, it was expected that the addition of hyperthermia to radiotherapy would improve local tumour control, without enhancing radiation toxicity, and such results have now been demonstrated in randomized clinical trials.

The local control of cancer has an important impact on quality of life and survival of patients with cancer (Suit, 1982; *see also* Table 6.1), and hyperthermia is one method of improving this. An increase in temperature by only a few degrees has profound effects on cellular and body functions. Heat has been used in past times as cautery for superficial tumours and, more recently, as laser therapy, but neither of these methods delivers controllable heat. Hyperthermia, as used today in the clinical setting, refers to the heating of localized tumours to a temperature of 41–43°C or whole-body heating to 40–42°C. There is now a firm biological rationale for using heat in this range of temperatures, which seeks to exploit weaknesses of the tumour compared to the normal tissues and attempts to combine heat with irradiation or chemotherapy, in such a way that these modalities become more cytotoxic than they would be alone.

RATIONALE FOR THE CLINICAL USE OF HEAT

The vasculature and blood supply in tumours is generally different and inferior to that of normal tissues, which leads to areas of abnormal perfusion within the tumour (Reinhold and Endrich, 1986). This has a number of consequences:

1 Some tumours, or regions within tumours, will have poorer cooling capacity than normal tissues and may thus become hotter than normal tissues in a localized treatment field.
2 Deficiencies in tumour vasculature results in the development of cells which are:
   (a) hypoxic, which (in contrast to X-rays) seems not to affect their response to hyperthermia markedly;
   (b) at low pH and/or nutrient deficient, both factors making cells substantially more sensitive to heat.
3 Cells in the DNA synthetic phase of the cell cycle are particularly sensitive to heat but relatively resistant to

Table 6.1 *Estimated incidence, mortality and sites of failure of the most common types of cancer in the United States in 1995*

| Organ | Cases/year | Deaths/year | L-R only | Distribution of failures (deaths) | | | Total deaths L-R tumour |
				Combination L-R and DM	DM only		
Lung	157000	142000	49700	49700	42600		99400
Colon and rectum	155000	60900	6090	14225	39585		21315
Breast	150900	44300	6645	26580	11075		33225
Prostate	106000	30000	4500	19500	6000		24000
Uterus*	46500	10000	2000	5000	3000		7000
Oral, pharynx, larynx	42800	12100	6050	3630	2420		9680
Bladder	49000	9700	2910	2425	4635		5335
Lymphomas	54800	28700	5740	5740	17220		11480
Pancreas, biliary	42700	36900	7380	22140	7380		29520
Oesophagus, stomach	33800	23200	6960	11600	4640		18560
Leukaemia	27800	18100	7240	7240	3620		14480
Ovary	20500	12400	11160	620	620		11780
Brain, CNS	15600	11100	10711	278	111		10989
Total	902400	439400	127086	169678	142636		296764 (68%)

L-R, local–regional tumour; DM, distant metastases.
Data from American Cancer Society, *Cancer facts and figures, 1995.*
*Cervix, invasive and endometrium.

X-rays, so that a combined treatment with hyperthermia and radiotherapy might be advantageous in some circumstances.

4 Combining heat with chemotherapeutic drugs may enhance the therapeutic affect either by increasing drug uptake or by enhancing sensitivity to the drugs.

5 It has been suggested that neoplastic cells may be intrinsically more sensitive than the normal cells at risk.

There are profound differences between the vessels in most normal tissues and those in tumours. In particular, 'tumour vessels' are longer and more tortuous and lack smooth muscle. High interstitial pressure, resulting from lack of lymph drainage, will increase the probability of vascular (capillary) occlusion.

The influence of regions of poor perfusion in tumours will be very important for a variety of anti-cancer techniques. Reduced Po_2 will reduce the effectiveness of radiotherapy but can increase the sensitivity to certain drugs (bioreductive compounds). Poor perfusion will limit the penetration of anti-cancer drugs, but result in higher temperatures on local or regional heating. Reduced rate of removal of waste products, in particular lactate, will lead to reduced pH, which will alter the effectiveness of certain drugs, increase tissue sensitivity to hyperthermia and decrease the development of thermotolerance. There is, therefore, considerable therapeutic potential for manipulation of blood flow.

Vasoactive agents can potentially be used in hyperthermal treatments, and of particular importance to hyperthermia are compounds that selectively reduce flow in tumours, e.g. hydralazine which acts on smooth muscle, therefore increasing flow to normal tissues and 'stealing'

blood from the tumour. Administration of hydralazine has been shown to decrease blood flow in transplanted tumours and increase sensitivity to hyperthermia (Dewhirst *et al.*, 1990).

Clearly, a greater knowledge of effects of modifiers of blood flow can result in the design of treatment methods that take advantage of differences in vasculature between tumours and normal tissues. Some of the tools necessary for human studies of tumour blood flow and metabolism, i.e. positron emission tomography or magnetic resonance spectroscopy, are now available.

RESPONSE OF CELLS AND TISSUES TO HYPERTHERMIA

Cellular response

Temperatures of around 41°C or greater can be lethal to mammalian cells, and the cause of cell death after irradiation is damage to DNA as cell die when they attempt to divide. Cell death after hyperthermia occurs far more quickly and affects cells at all stages of the cell cycle. The exact target for heat-induced damage is not fully understood and more than one mechanism may be involved. Following hyperthermia there is chromosomal damage and cellular membranes lyse, and this may be due to the denaturing of a membrane protein, repair enzyme or even a chromosomal protein. Many tissues, especially those that are slowly dividing (or even post-mitotic), respond to hyperthermia far more quickly than to ionizing radiation.

Pathology

Superficially there is acute oedema and cellular infiltration, and this may be compared to damage caused by a thermal burn produced by any other means (Fajardo, 1984). Depending on its severity, hyperthermia may be followed by oedema, focal haemorrhage, granulocytic infiltration and even necrosis within the first day or so. Compression and occlusion with haemorrhage, stasis and leakage of the blood vessels is also seen. If there is no necrosis at the acute stage, then there are unlikely to be any long-term effects and all should heal satisfactorily. However, if damage has been severe acutely, then late-stage necrosis and fibrosis occurs. Clinically, hyperthermia is usually combined with radiation, which also produces similar effects, and it is difficult to separate the two effects. When used correctly with radiation, hyperthermia should not increase normal skin or deep-tissue reaction, either in the short or long term.

Thermotolerance

Survival curves after heat are similar in shape to those following irradiation, the curves becoming less steep with decreasing temperatures. There is normally a transition at about 42.5°C, above which a change in temperature of 1°C is equivalent to a change in heating of a factor of 2. Small differences in tissue temperature are very likely to occur in clinical treatments, and therefore may lead to marked variations in biological responses. Below 42.5°C and as the heating time increases, the curves flatten out, resulting in a resistant tail. This transition is thought to result from the induction of thermotolerance, i.e. resistance to subsequent heating, which is known to be reduced or abolished by low pH. This can have a substantial effect, altering the cell survival curve by a factor of 15. The effect is transient, the time course depending on the particular cell type or tissue.

Almost all cells and tissues show this type of thermotolerance, the maximum extent varying between an increase in heating time of a factor between 2 and 4.5. There are no consistent indications that thermotolerance is less in tumours than in normal tissues, despite the regions of lower pH.

Both the extent of the maximum thermotolerance and its timing have been shown *in vitro* and *in vivo* to be related to the effectiveness of the first treatment. Thus the greater the effectiveness of the first (or primary) heat dose, the greater is the extent of thermotolerance and the longer it takes before the maximum is reached. A model of thermotolerance was proposed by Li and Hahn in 1980, which discusses three separate phases: induction or 'trigger', which can occur at any temperature; development phase, which can only occur at temperatures below about 42°C and decay.

The molecular basis for thermotolerance is not well understood, but there are numerous reports that hyperthermia results in the synthesis of a specific set of proteins (heat stress or heat-shock proteins) and there is evidence to suggest that these proteins are a protective mechanism produced by the cell. It appears that thermotolerance is related to one such protein with molecular weight 65–70 kDa. By assaying these proteins it would be possible to watch the decay of thermotolerance and decide the best and most effective time to give the second dose of hyperthermia. At the present time it would appear to be sensible to avoid the problem of thermotolerance in the clinical situation by giving hyperthermia on a weekly basis, which allows most thermotolerance to decay.

The maximum differential might be achieved by heating at relatively low temperatures for long times. Unfortunately, this may not be very practical clinically.

In clinical practice, combined heat and radiation are normally given in fractionated schedules. It is therefore important to determine whether or not thermotolerance influences the enhancement of radiation damage by subsequent heat treatments. This problem has been studied by a number of authors and the majority of the results indicate that prior hyperthermia does reduce the radiosensitizing effect of a subsequent heat treatment, i.e. values for thermal enhancement ratio (TER) are reduced. However, the effect is less dramatic than that for direct thermal damage. The development of thermotolerance will obviously influence the response to heat and radiation given in fractionated regimes, but at the present stage of knowledge the effect is difficult to predict.

Step-up and step-down sensitization

Cellular sensitivity to heat can be altered during a fractionated course, depending on the different temperatures used. Step-up heating, which is not useful clinically, refers to the situation where a second higher temperature is less effective. Step-down heating occurs when a brief exposure to a temperature greater than 43°C is followed by a lower temperature which becomes more effective than it might have been when given alone. It may be related to the inhibition of thermotolerance and might be useful clinically.

INTERACTION BETWEEN HEAT AND IONIZING RADIATION

The improvement in tumour kill seen with the combination of radiation and hyperthermia over radiation alone can result from two independent mechanisms. Heat can cause direct injury to the cells which would be in addition to that caused by radiation, and which would work at a complementary time in the cell cycle and give an improved kill for hypoxic, nutritionally deprived cells at a low pH. It can also sensitize the radiation effect by reducing the capacity of the cell to repair sublethal and potentially lethal cell damage, and this would appear as a reduction in the size of the shoulder of the cell survival curve, i.e. reduction in D_0, the dose required to reduce a cell population from 100 per cent to 37 per cent. For the latter effect, hyperthermia should be given after the radiation.

In general, direct thermal injury is observed at times before radiation damage is expressed. Mild heat treatments, which cause no measurable effect, may enhance the response of cells or tissues to ionizing radiation, the response to the combined treatment being qualitively similar to that following radiation. The effect of heat in enhancing the radiation response can be expressed as a TER, defined as the dose of radiation required to cause a given response in the absence of hyperthermia divided by the radiation dose required to cause the same response in combination with hyperthermia.

The TER increases with the magnitude of the heat treatment. It becomes greater than 1 for heat treatments of approximately 41°C for 60 minutes or equivalent, up to maximum TER values of 3 or 4, beyond which the hyperthermia begins to cause direct thermal injury.

A crucial question is whether the TER for tumours is likely to be greater than that for normal tissues. The rationale for expecting greater destruction of tumours by heat alone is not, however, the same for the combined treatment, for example:

1 Studies *in vitro* indicate that when heat is used to enhance radiation response, pH is far less important than for direct heat cytoxicity.
2 It appears that the oxygen enhancement ratio for ionizing radiation (about 3 for photons) does not change significantly for the combination of heat and radiation. As a result, heat enhances radiation injury to hypoxic and oxic cells approximately equal.
3 Only if the tumour becomes hotter than the surrounding normal tissues will the combined treatment give a therapeutic advantage.

Sequencing of heat and radiation

The greatest TER is obtained when the two modalities are used simultaneously, utilizing both the direct injury and the radiosensitization effects of the hyperthermia. However, this applies for both the tumour and the normal tissue – thus there is no therapeutic gain, unless hyperthermia can be applied preferentially to the tumour, as in interstitial therapy.

As the separation between the two modalities is increased, the enhancing effect decreases. If heat is given after X-rays, the data indicate that the interaction is reduced to zero when the interval is 3–4 hours, or greater. With this type of treatment regime the two treatment modalities thus act independently and the heat damage to tumour would be expected to be greater than that to normal tissues. By separating the two in time, the

enhancing effect of the radiation is reduced, and indeed lost by about 8 hours after irradiation. Used in this way, the optimal dose of radiation can be used without increasing the side-effects. This is important, as there is no advantage in using hyperthermia with irradiation if the same result could be obtained by merely using a higher dose of radiotherapy. An even greater therapeutic gain will be seen if the tumour is heated preferentially, due to abnormal tumour vasculature which will decrease cooling and alter the microenvironment.

Re-treatment of previously irradiated tissue

Hyperthermia is frequently used clinically when a tumour recurs following a radical course of radiotherapy, when it would not be possible to give a further full course of treatment. The addition of hyperthermia to a smaller dose of irradiation in this situation does not appear to increase the side-effects, over those which would be expected from the radiation alone, although the response rate is increased considerably.

THERMAL DOSE

The response of tumours to heat depends on time of heating at a given temperature, not on energy deposition as in radiation therapy. The concept of dose for heat, which is disputed, is therefore a difficult one as there are many variables. If the temperature were fixed and constant, time of heating at the raised temperature would be a reasonable method of defining a thermal dose. However, the temperature in hyperthermia is not fixed, and in clinical practice is certainly far from constant.

Sapareto and Dewey (1984) proposed that 43°C should be used as a reference temperature and that all treatment be described as equivalent minutes of heating at 43°C. This has become known as the thermal isoeffect dose (TID). Despite problems, the TID has been used clinically and results can be compared with this measurement. The Dewey formula is a method of calculating this:

$$t_2/t_1 = R^{(T_1 - T_2)}$$

where t_1 and t_2 are the heating times at temperatures T_1 and T_2 to produce equal biological effects. R is a constant equal to 2 below the break point of 42.5°C and 6 above 42.5°C.

These considerations, however, apply to hyperthermia given at a constant temperature. In particular, it takes some time to reach the required temperature, which is then subject to considerable variations. This problem may be dealt with in practice by integration of the equation over the whole treatment time to produce an accumulated thermal dose. However, variations in temperature can have a marked effect in determining the overall biological response. For example, either thermotolerance or

Table 6.2 *Prognostically significant thermal parameters in radiotherapy and hyperthermia parameters correlating with response*

Thermal parameters correlating with response	Reference	Number of evaluable patient sites	Response criteria
1. Minimum tumour temperature	Dewhirst and Sim (1984)	117	CR (for 1 month)
	Kapp *et al.* (1987)	15 (31)	CR (at 3 weeks after
	van der Zee *et al.* (1986)	33 (44)	completion of treatment)
2. Minimum equivalent time at 43°C	van der Zee *et al.* (1986)	112	CR + PR (for duration of at least 1 month)
3. Lowest average tumour temperature	Luk *et al.* (1984)	33	CR (initial)
4. Average tumour temperature	Kapp *et al.* (1985)	31	CR (at time of maximum tumour regression)
5. Number of satisfactory heat sessions	Sapozink *et al.* (1986)	112	CR + PR (at 1–2 months)
	Dunlop *et al.* (1986)	116	CR at 3 months

CR, complete remission; PR, partial remission.
[a] Large animal spontaneous tumours.

'step-down sensitization' may be induced. Clearly, these effects have the potential to invalidate the above equation. However, the range of times and temperatures seen clinically are not great and the formula has been shown to hold true experimentally over the ranges commonly seen.

Tumour response is most likely to correlate with the minimum tumour TID (Dewhirst and Sim, 1984) and complications relate better to the maximum normal tissue temperature recorded. TIDs are not usually added from individual treatments in a treatment course to give a total for that course. Significant thermal parameters correlating with complete response are shown in Table 6.2.

The parameters of R and the break point are not well known for human tumours, which could have marked effects on the TID, and for these reasons not all researchers would recommend its use in clinical studies. The Sapareto–Dewey formula provides a practical and reasonable method of comparing hyperthermal treatments under conditions likely to be met in practice, i.e. moderate variation about a fairly steady temperature. However, the formula does not apply for large variations in temperature resulting in a significant effect of step-down sensitization, nor does it account for absolute differences in sensitivity between tissues, nor does it address the problem of varying sensitivity throughout a course of fractionated heat treatments.

Throughout the whole history of clinical applications of hyperthermia, the technical difficulties of applying heat to the body and measuring the temperature have been major limiting factors to its progress.

HYPERTHERMIA PHYSICS

Delivery of hyperthermal therapy in a predictable and efficacious manner and monitoring of the resulting temperature field present significant technical challenges. However, considerable progress has been made in these areas in recent years and the quality of treatments available today is considerably greater than was the case a decade ago.

Heating techniques

Heating techniques for clinical hyperthermia may be grouped into three broad categories: whole body, regional and localized. In whole-body hyperthermia, the temperature of the patient's entire body is raised for a period of a few hours. Heating is achieved either through irradiation of the body with infrared or radiofrequency radiations, invasively by perfusion with extracorporeally heated blood via a femoral arterial–venous shunt or by peritoneal irrigation, or by direct contact between the skin and heat source (e.g. molten wax, hot water, water blanket). In all cases, heat loss is minimized by thermally insulating the patient. Although a relatively uniform temperature distribution can be achieved within deep-seated tumours, the maximum tolerated temperature is in the range 41.8–42.0°C, the limit being set by function and thermal damage of critical organs such as heart, lungs, liver and brain. Techniques for whole-body hyperthermia have been reviewed by Bull (1995).

In contrast, in regional and local hyperthermia, techniques are designed to achieve temperatures typically in the range 42–45°C. In regional hyperthermia, large volumes of the trunk or whole limbs are heated, and often a difference between perfusion of the tumour and normal tissues is relied upon to produce a temperature differential. Non-ionizing (radiofrequency, RF) electromagnetic (EM) fields are usually employed in this approach, although in some cases (e.g. regional hyperthermia of limbs) the blood is heated extracorporeally. In local hyperthermia, a smaller volume of tissue local to the tumour is heated by electromagnetic fields (radiofrequency or microwave) or ultrasound (around 1 MHz, i.e. at frequencies slightly lower than those used for diagnostic purposes). Local hyperthermia may also be induced using devices implanted into tissue or inserted into body cavities. A variety of interstitial implants, including radiofrequency, microwave, or ultrasound sources or simple hot sources that rely on thermal conduction (e.g. implants heated by magnetically induced currents, DC electric currents or hot water), may be used. Most interstitial techniques are compatible with brachytherapy methods.

In view of the variety of tumour sizes, shapes, perfusions and locations encountered, several types of hyperthermia system have been developed. The following paragraphs summarize the techniques available for superficial, deep body and interstitial hyperthermic treatments.

SUPERFICIAL HYPERTHERMIA

Early hyperthermia systems relied upon use of a single applicator and so could not counter spatial variations in temperature that arose from tissue heterogeneity and variations in perfusion. More recent systems offer greater flexibility; and, by using arrays of applicators, larger fields may be treated and a good degree of spatial control of the power deposition pattern is possible. In some circumstances (e.g. for treatment of neck nodes) the constructive interference of fields from several applicators driven coherently can lead to a modest improvement in the depth at which effective heating is achieved. Further details of electromagnetic applicators for superficial treatments can be found in Fessenden and Hand (1995), Lee (1995), Rossetto et al. (1998) and Rossetto and Stauffer (1999).

Multi-transducer ultrasound systems, usually driven at a frequency in the range 1–3 MHz, which offer spatial control of energy deposition, are also commercially available. Scanned focused ultrasound (see below) at 1–4 MHz has been used to deliver high-quality hyperthermia treatments of recurrent tumours covering extensive areas on the chest wall. Local pain is by far the most commonly reported toxicity with ultrasound-induced hyperthermia, although the policy at some institutions is to administer analgesics and to treat at tolerable levels of pain. Summaries of ultrasound-induced local hyperthermia are given by Hand (1998) and Diederich and Hynynen (1999).

There is also a trend in developing equipment that allows the delivery of hyperthermia simultaneously with external radiotherapy, in order to achieve radiosensitization at temperatures of approximately 41°C (Straube et al., 2001).

DEEP-BODY HYPERTHERMIA

So-called capacitive applicators usually employ two electrodes, approximately 20–25 cm in diameter, with integral water boluses positioned above and below the patient. In this way, the electrodes are separated by a distance comparable with, or smaller than, their diameter, and

so might be expected to produce sufficiently high levels of absorbed power throughout the region between them. Whereas these systems appear attractively simple at first sight, disadvantages of the method include excessive power deposition in subcutaneous fat (the orientation of the electric field is predominantly perpendicular to adipose tissue boundaries) and the lack of control over the distribution of absorbed power within the tissues. Capacitive systems with three electrodes offer some control over power deposition patterns during treatment.

Significant power deposition deep within the patient may be achieved through the use of one or more radiative sources arranged to produce a field aligned along the patient's longitudinal axis. Devices using this principle include annular arrays of aperture sources or dipoles and the so-called TEM applicator. A degree of control over the absorbed power distribution can be achieved with this class of device, either by electronic means or by moving the patient within the applicator.

The induction of deep-body hyperthermia by means of focused ultrasound beams, produced using single sources having curved radiating surfaces, lenses or reflectors, or from electronically controlled multiple transducers (so-called phased arrays) has been investigated (Diederich and Hynynen, 1999; Lin et al., 1999). Since the focal volume associated with such systems is inherently small compared with tumour volumes, methods of delivering ultrasound energy over the whole target volume are required. This may be achieved by mechanically scanning the small focal volume around a predetermined trajectory within the target volume, a technique that has been applied successfully in the treatment of bulky tumours in the breast and other superficial sites. Electronically controlled ultrasound phased arrays offer very flexible methods of heating. In addition to 'spot scanning', the electronic analogue of mechanical scanning described above, phased arrays also offer the possibility of synthesizing complex heating patterns directly, without the need for scanning. Focused ultrasound has the potential for delivering treatment in which the thermal dose achieved is more spatially uniform.

INTERSTITIAL HYPERTHERMIA

By implanting the energy source(s), many of the problems associated with unwanted heating of normal tissues are avoided. Microwave, radiofrequency and ultrasound sources have been used in these approaches but recent developments, particularly with the latter two types, have concentrated on the ability to control spatially energy deposition and therefore temperature (Stauffer et al., 1995).

At 27 MHz, capacitive coupling from source to tissue through the wall of a plastic catheter is possible, and multi-electrode systems that offer spatial control of specific absorption rate (SAR) on a scale of about 1 cm have been developed (Crezee et al., 1999). At around 915 MHz, applicators based on dipole, spiral and sleeved antennas have been designed for insertion into catheters. The heating associated with these antennas has greater radial penetration than the RF types but it is more difficult to control SAR distribution along the antenna, and heating patterns can also be dependent upon the depth to which the antenna is inserted into the tissue.

Ferromagnetic seeds consist of thin cylinders or wires of ferromagnetic material. The seeds are heated by subjecting to a radiofrequency magnetic field (typically 100–200 kHz) which induces eddy currents within them. Two classes of seed are available: constant power seeds, in which the heating power depends upon the frequency and strength of the magnetic field and is essentially independent of its temperature; and constant temperature seeds, which are produced from material whose Curie temperature (the temperature above which spontaneous magnetization of ferromagnetic material vanishes) is close to the desired operating temperature (Van Wieringen *et al.*, 1996; Kotte *et al.*, 1998).

An alternative interstitial technique that can provide good spatial control of heating involves the use of small ultrasound sources (Diederich *et al.*, 1996; Deardorff *et al.*, 1998; Lee *et al.*, 1999).

Temperature measurement

The principles of the various thermometers used in clinical hyperthermia and the requirements for adequate thermometry have been discussed by Waterman (1995). Although many clinical treatments still involve invasive measurement, significant advances have been made towards the goal of non-invasive temperature measurement (Bolomey *et al.*, 1995). In particular, temperature-dependent magnetic resonance (MR) parameters, especially chemical shift, are proving to be of practical use (Wlodarczyk *et al.*, 1998, 1999; Craciunescu *et al.*, 2001). Investigations of ultrasonic methods for non-invasive measurement of temperature are also under way (Seip *et al.*, 1996).

Treatment planning

There has been significant progress in the development of hyperthermia treatment planning systems (Gellerman *et al.*, 2000; Lagendijk, 2000; Van de Kamer *et al.*, 2001). In general, these consist of three major parts:

1 an anatomical model of the patient;
2 a routine for calculating the electromagnetic (or ultrasound) field within this model; and
3 a routine for predicting the resulting temperature distribution.

Excellent discussions of the relative merits of the approaches used for (1) and (2) are given by Paulsen *et al.* (1999) and Wust *et al.* (1999).

In most cases, the transport of heat within tissues is dominated by blood flow. The presence of large vessels and the heterogeneous nature of perfusion are the usual causes of the variations in temperature observed during hyperthermic treatments. There has been progress in understanding and modelling heat transport processes within tissues in recent years. Although the conventional bioheat transfer equation continues to be used for many purposes, the strengths and weakness of other models based on more realistic descriptions of vascular effects on heat transport are now understood (Arkin *et al.*, 1994; Van Leeuwen *et al.*, 1998, 2000). Numerical algorithms for the practical application of such models to the prediction of spatially accurate temperature and thermal dose distributions are now available and will have a significant impact on hyperthermia treatment planning.

Quality assurance

The need for quality assurance in hyperthermia was highlighted by the difficulty in interpreting studies where quality assurance was lacking (Perez *et al.*, 1989). Subsequently, guidelines that outline criteria for selecting equipment and for its safe and effective use were proposed. These recommendations, together with useful comments on their practical implementation, have been reviewed by Visser and Van Rhoon (1995). More recently, guidelines have been drawn up specifically for deep-body hyperthermia (Hornsleth *et al.*, 1997; Lagendijk *et al.*, 1998). The use of phantom materials is a necessary part of all quality assurance programmes. Recent phantom materials have been discussed by Schneider *et al.* (1995a) and Craciunescu *et al.* (1999). Methods for measuring electric field directly may be used to check phases and amplitudes of annular arrays (Schneider *et al.*, 1995b).

Summary of hyperthermia physics

Advances in controlling the spatial distribution of energy deposition and tissue temperature, in non-invasive measurement of temperature, in treatment planning and in quality assurance are all contributing to the ability to deliver improved hyperthermia.

CLINICAL ASPECTS

Although the biological rationale has been well established for some time, clinical application has lagged behind, mainly due to technical difficulties in producing controllable and uniform heating of human tumours. However, in the last few years, major advances in both heat delivery and temperature measurement have been seen.

Prognostic factors

Response to hyperthermia does not appear to be strongly related to histology, unlike radiotherapy or chemotherapy, but it does depend on the microenvironment, i.e. pH, and the vasculature. Several factors influence hyperthermic treatment approach and outcome.

TUMOUR VOLUME

Large tumours are more difficult to control by the combined modalities of irradiation and hyperthermia. Valdagni *et al.* (1988) treated N3 metastatic neck nodes and observed complete responses (CRs) of 75 per cent with nodes <6 cm, but only 36 per cent with larger nodes. Van der Zee *et al.* (1986) had similar results and also showed that minimum thermal doses tended to decrease with increasing volume, while the maximum and mean temperatures increased with volume. However, the negative effect of volume is even greater for irradiation alone (Dewhirst and Sim, 1984) and this is probably due to the fact that larger tumours have a relatively higher percentage of poorly perfused, hypoxic cells at low pH, which have a higher sensitivity to hyperthermia. Thus size is less important for the combined treatments than for irradiation alone (*see also* Table 6.3).

TUMOUR DEPTH AND TEMPERATURE

The tissue absorption characteristics of microwave and ultrasound radiation with therapeutically useful wavelengths dictate that heating to depths greater than 2–3 cm requires multiple and/or focused sources, either fixed or scanning, or in special lower frequency EM techniques. The limitation of power penetration is routinely observed in the clinic. Single-point temperature measurements are not representative of temperature distributions through a tumour and correlate poorly with response. Perez *et al.*

(1989) found that the minimum temperatures in tumour are the most important variable overall in predicting complete response. The duration of complete response also correlates with the average measured minimum tumour temperature for all treatment in a course and is inversely correlated with the percentage of measured intra-tumoral temperatures less than 41°C (Hand *et al.*, 1997).

SELECTION OF APPLICATORS

No differences in response have been noted to the modality of heat delivery, but the physical method of inducing hyperthermia will determine the power distribution in tissue and therefore tissue temperature, and will also affect patient tolerance to treatment, e.g. ultrasound in bone causes greater patient discomfort than others, forcing power reduction during therapy sessions. Tumour accessibility or heat-sensitive structures, such as the lens, can be a problem, and attempts to design special applicators to overcome some of these problems are under way.

Problems include limited field volumes, and approaches to overcome this have included mechanical scanning of microstrip and antenna arrays, or the use of stationary arrays of multiple microstrip antennas or arrays of ultrasound transducers. Curved surface areas with tumour involvement, e.g. the extremities or chest wall, have presented difficulties. Microwave blanket arrays have been developed for the treatment of such lesions.

The optimum utilization of applicators for hyperthermia requires a detailed knowledge of intra-tumoral and adjacent normal tissue temperatures. Most operators aim to keep the temperatures below 41°C for normal tissue. The number of temperature probes required will be

Table 6.3 *Prognostic significance of tumour size in trials of radiation therapy and hyperthermia*

Reference	Number of evaluable patients (sites)	Response criteria	Tumour size	XRT + HT (%)	XRT alone (%)
Dewhirst and Sim (1984, 1986)[a]	227	CR (of 1 month duration)	<1.8 cm^3	76	60
			1.8–8.4 cm^3	54	60
			8.4 cm^3	48	15
Hiraoka *et al.* (1984)	36 (40)	CR (at time of maximum response)	<4 cm	100	ND
			4–10 cm	55	ND
			>10 cm	0	ND
Luk *et al.* (1984)	133	CR (initial)	<3 cm	61	ND
			>3 cm	44	ND
Dewhirst *et al.* (1985)	43[b]	CR	<2 cm^3	86	50
			2–10 cm^3	86	0
			>10 cm^3	57	13
Perez *et al.* (1986, 1991)	48 (XRT plus HT), 116 (XRT alone)	Local control (in field)	1–3 cm	79	48
			>3 cm	65	28
Kapp *et al.* (1987)	18 (38)	Local control (in field)	<5 cm^3	81	ND
			>5 cm^3	25	ND

[a] Large animal spontaneous tumours.
[b] Malignant melanomas only.
CR, complete response; XRT, radiation therapy; HT, hyperthermia treatment; ND, not done.

a function of the tumour size and complexity, and the larger tumour, the greater the number of probes needed. In general, for superficial tumours a temperature probe should be placed intra-tumorally at the location expected to be at the lowest temperature and other probes should be placed at the normal–normal tissue junction. Additional sensors should be placed to monitor any areas of normal tissue or tumour at risk for overheating, e.g. skin folds, scar or necrotic regions.

NUMBER AND FREQUENCY OF HYPERTHERMIA TREATMENTS

Most workers (Kapp et al., 1987; Alexander et al., 1987) found that one hyperthermia treatment per week is as effective as two – this due to thermotolerance, which must be allowed to decay. There is also evidence that a small number of good treatments are as effective as a larger number, e.g. two versus four (Dunlop et al., 1986).

Theoretically, hyperthermia will be most effective immediately after irradiation, and if tumours can be selectively heated (as in interstitial hyperthermia) simultaneous or immediate treatment will produce the greatest cell kill. However, for most treatments the reaction of normal tissues must also be considered, and delaying hyperthermia until 2–4 hours after the irradiation decreases normal tissue reaction more so than tumour, compared to immediate treatment (Overgaard and Overgaard, 1987) as the potentiation by hyperthermia of the inability to repair potentially lethal damage appears to last longer for tumours. Thus sequential treatments with time intervals of more than 2–3 hours can increase therapeutic gain. Further results can be seen in Table 6.4.

Interesting results were achieved with continuous low-temperature hyperthermia and interstitial hyperthermia (Armour et al., 1993), but this technique is difficult practically and has not been taken up by other groups.

RADIATION DOSE AND FRACTIONATION

A strong correlation exists between radiation dose and response – Valdagni et al. (1988) reported no CRs with doses of 10–29 Gy, a 50 per cent CR rate with 30–39 Gy and a 67 per cent CR rate with doses of 44–49 Gy.

TOXICITIES

Experimentally, it is known that radiation damage to normal tissues is enhanced by hyperthermia, but in most clinical situations the normal tissue damage does not appear to have occurred in significantly greater numbers following the combined treatments than for irradiation alone. Toxicities may be due to either potentiation of radiation effects or the direct effects of hyperthermia alone. Certain direct effects due to sub-acute toxicities have been attributed to hyperthermia; these are superficial burns or blisters, which are usually asymptomatic and heal within 2–5 days, deeper burns which require longer periods to heal but are relatively uncommon, and ulceration developing in treated tumours and on normal tissue which can persist for weeks but are usually asymptomatic additionally. Acute toxicities do appear to be indicative of long-term toxicity and are relatively uncommon. Ben-Josef and Kapp (1992) found that the average of maximum measured intra-tumoral temperatures was higher in fields that developed complications (45.9°C) compared with those that did not (44.6°C).

Overall, the majority of patients have not had excessive skin reactions from the combination, beyond that which might have been expected from the radiation alone; these have depended upon a variety of factors, including the average of the maximum measured intra-tumoral temperatures and the number of treatments, the timing of the two treatments, the irradiation dose used, the coupling of the applicators on irregular surfaces of the body, and whether or not active skin cooling has been used. This is also confirmed by late skin-reaction studies, with some minimal increase in fibrosis or induration particularly when high doses of irradiation have been used (Ben-Josef and Kapp, 1992).

Therefore these studies would suggest that attempts should be made to use the minimum number of hyperthermia treatments and to limit extremely high temperatures in tumours during treatment. Most workers attempt to keep the skin temperature below 41°C.

Clinical results

In the early years, a large number of non-randomized clinical trials were carried out and research was aimed

Table 6.4 *Prognostically significant thermal parameters in trials of radiation therapy and hyperthermia correlating with duration of complete response*

Reference	Number of evaluable patient (sites)	Thermal parameters correlating with duration of complete response
Dewhirst and Sim (1984)	117	Non-site specific average minimum equivalent minutes at 43°C
Kapp et al. (1987)	29 (85)	Average minimum temperatures over all treatments. Average (%) of temperature less than 41°C for all treatments (negatively correlated). Average of average temperatures over all treatments

mainly at the development of systems with which tissue temperatures could be increased to a therapeutic level. In these studies, many patients were included who had failed standard therapies, and hyperthermia was given in addition to relatively low-dose re-irradiation. The clinical results observed in these patients were encouraging, with results higher than those that might be expected from radiation alone. Superficial malignancies, which included skin nodules, melanomas, head and neck tumours and chest-wall recurrences were studied.

Somewhat more convincing results were reported from experience with 'matched pairs of lesions' in patients with multiple lesions – some of these being treated with radiotherapy alone and others with the combination treatments. The addition of hyperthermia results, overall, in about a doubling of the response rates. (van der Zee et al., 1998). The enthusiasm of the 1970s and 1980s waned when the first randomized trials from the USA (Perez et al., 1991) failed to show the promised beneficial effect from additional hyperthermia. However, in retrospect, the negative results of these trials were explained by the fact that these early applications of hyperthermia were premature, because they were performed using inadequate heating and thermometry techniques that existed at the time, and in effect these tumours did not receive hyperthermia. A sub-analysis of the tumours superficial enough to be heated sufficiently showed a beneficial effect for hyperthermia.

In contrast to these early studies, there have now been nearly 30 randomized clinical trials demonstrating a marked improvement with the addition of hyperthermia. The important ones are listed in Tables 6.5–6.7, and are discussed below.

HYPERTHERMIA ALONE

This has a response rate of approximately 50 per cent, with a CR rate of 10 per cent, which is usually of short duration. Hyperthermia can stimulate the immune system and part of the response may be due to this. Melanomas in a distant part of the body to that undergoing hyperthermia have been seen to resolve. It can be recommended in the palliative situation, where it may be of use to control bleeding or give pain relief – for both it is remarkably effective. Both local and whole-body hyperthermia have been used for this purpose.

Hyperthermia alone has also been used intraoperatively for the treatment of biliary and brain tumours, but neither have been investigated extensively. Some benign diseases, such as benign prostatic hypertrophy (Stawartz et al., 1991), menorrhagia (Prior et al., 1991), psoriasis, cardiac arrhythmias, sinusitis and acute lung injury may also benefit from hyperthermia.

RESULTS FROM HYPERTHERMIA AND RADIATION

Many studies have been performed, mainly in Europe, in the USA and in Japan, on patients with both superficial and deep-seated tumours. Most studies have involved the use of microwaves to induce heat, and most have used invasive thermometry placed with local anaesthesia. Commonly, temperatures of 42–44°C for 30–60 minutes, following a wide variety of radiotherapy schedules, once or twice weekly have been used.

Superficial

Tumours less than 3 cm from the surface have provided the greatest experience with tumour response to hyperthermia. Recent technical development provided microwave applicators with large effective field diameters, and arrays of microwave and ultrasound applicators are being developed that provide increasingly broader field sizes and segmental control of applicator power, for greater temperature homogeneity, improved power of delivery to areas of limited access, the ability to avoid sensitive adjacent normal tissues, greater conformity to curved treatment surfaces and improved patient comfort during treatment.

The first of the numerically large studies to be published was the ESHO (European Society for Hyperthermic Oncology) melanoma phase III trial. Here a total of 134 metastatic or recurrent lesions in 70 patients were randomly assigned to receive radiotherapy alone (three fractions of 8 or 9 Gy in 8 days) followed by hyperthermia. The addition of hyperthermia led to significant improvements in both complete response rate and local control at 2 years. For patients receiving the combined treatments, a complete response was achieved in 62 per cent of patients with a 2-year local control rate of 46 per cent, whereas patients receiving radiotherapy alone had complete response rates of 35 per cent and local control rates of 28 per cent at 2 years.

Cox multivariate regression analysis showed the most important prognostic variables to be hyperthermia (odds ratio for 2-year local control 1.73 (95 per cent CI, 1.07–2.78) $P = 0.023$), tumour size (odds ratio 0.91 (95 per cent CI, 0.85–0.99) $P = 0.05$) and radiation dose (odds ratio 1.17 (95 per cent CI, 1.01–1.36)). The addition of hyperthermia did not increase acute or late radiation reactions in the subgroup of 23 patients in whom all known disease was controlled, 38 per cent survived 5 years compared to those 47 patients with persistent disease whose 5-year survival was 10 per cent. Thus successful treatment of patients with a single or few metastatic melanomas may have curative potential (Overgaard et al., 1995).

A larger study was the MRC/ESHO/PMH locally advanced and recurrent breast carcinoma study (Vernon et al., 1996). This trial was the combination of five similar trials comparing radiotherapy alone to radiotherapy plus hyperthermia, and closed in 1993 with 308 patients. Patients were eligible if they had advanced primary or recurrent breast cancer, and where local radiotherapy was indicated in preference to surgery. The end point for the trial was local complete response. Most of these patients had already failed radiation, hormones and chemotherapy.

Table 6.5 *Hyperthermia in combination with radiotherapy: phase III studies*

Reference/ name of trial	Tumour entity (stage)	Type of trial	Number of patients	Results of control arm (RT only)	Results of hyperthermia arm RT and HT	Significance of results ($P < 0.05$)
Perez et al. (1989, 1991) RTOG 81-04	Head and neck (superficial measurable tumour)	Prospective, randomized, multicentre	106	34% CR	34% CR	–
Datta et al. (1990)	Head and neck (untreated locoregional tumour)	Prospective, randomized	65	32% CR 19% DFS at 1.5 years	55% CR 33% DFS at 1.5 years	+ +
Valdagni et al. (1988) Valdagni and Amichetti (1994)	Head and neck (N3 locoregional tumour)	Prospective, randomized	41	41% CR 24% LRFS 0% OS at 5 years	83% CR 68% LRFS 53% OS at 5 years	+ + +
Overgaard et al. (1995) ESHO-3	Melanoma (skin metastases or recurrent skin lesions)	Prospective, randomized, multicentre	70	35% CR 28% LRFS at 5 years	62% CR 46% LRFS at 5 years	+ +
Vernon et al. (1996) MRC/ESHO-5	Breast cancer (local recurrences or inoperable primary lesions)	Randomized, multicentre	306	41% CR c. 30% LRFS c. 40% AS at 2 years	59% CR c. 50% LRFS c. 40% AS at 2 years	+ + –
Van der Zee et al. (2000)	Rectal cancer	Prospective, randomized, multicentre	143	15% CR 22% OS at 3 years	21% CR 13% OS at 3 years	– –
	Bladder cancer		101	51% CR 22% OS at 3 years	73% CR 28% OS at 3 years	+ –
	Cervical cancer		114	57% CR 27% OS at 3 years	83% CR 51% OS at 3 years	+ +
Sneed et al. (1998)	Glioblastoma (postoperative)	Prospective, randomized	79	15% OS at 2 years	31% OS at 2 years	+

AS, actual survival; CR, complete remission; DFS, disease-free survival; HT, hyperthermia; LRFS, local relapse-free survival; OS, overall survival; RF, radiofrequency electric currents; RT, radiotherapy.

Table 6.6 *Hyperthermia combined with chemotherapy (from Falk and Issels, 2001)*

Reference	Tumour entity (stage)	Type of trial	Number of patients	Type of chemotherapy	Results
Li and Hou (1987)	Oesophageal cancer (preoperative)	Phase II	32	CDDP + Bleo + Cyc	8 CR/13 PR (65% RR)
Sugimachi et al. (1992)	Oesophageal cancer (preoperative)	Phase III	20	CDDP + Bleo	1 CR/5 PR/4 MR (50% RR); FHR (41.2%)
			20	CDDP + Bleo	0 CR/5 PR/0 MR (25% RR); FHR 18.8%
Kakehi et al. (1990)	Stomach cancer	Phase II	33	Mitomycin + 5FU	3 CR + 10 PR (39% RR)
	Pancreatic cancer		22	Mitomycin + 5FU	3 CR + 5 PR (36% RR)
Falk et al. (1986)	Pancreatic cancer	Phase II	77	Mitomycin + 5FU ± immunostimulation	27.3% survival at 1 year
Issels et al. (1990)	Sarcomas (pretreated with chemotherapy)	Phase II (RHT 86) Follow up	38 65	VP16 + IFO VP16 + IFO	6 pCR + 4 PR + 4 FHR (37% RR) 9 pCR + 4 PR + 8 FHR (32% RR)
Issels et al. (1993, 1998)	High-risk soft-tissue sarcomas	Phase II (RHT 91)	59	VP16 + IFO + ADR	1 CR/6 pCR + 8 PR + 13 MR (47%); OS: 46% at 5 years
Issels (1995)	High-risk soft-tissue sarcomas	Phase III (EORTC 62961)	112	VP16 + IFO + ADR	(08/00)
Eggermont et al. (1996)	Soft-tissue sarcomas	Phase II	55	TNF + IFN + L-PAM	10 CR/35 PR (82% RR)
Wiedemann et al. (1994)	Sarcomas/teratomas (metastatic)	Phase I/II	19	IFO + CBDCA	6 PR (32% RR)
Wiedermann et al. (1996)	Sarcomas (metastatic)	Phase II	12	IFO + CBDCA + VP16	7 PR (58% RR)
Robins et al. (1997)	Refractory cancers (advanced or metastatic)	Phase I	16	L-PAM (dose-escalation)	1 CR/2 PR (19% PR)
Romanowski et al. (1993)	Paediatric sarcomas	Phase II	34	VP16 + IFO + CBDCA	12 NED ('best response'), 7 CR; duration: 7–64 months
Wessalowski et al. (1998)	Paediatric non-testicular germ cell tumours	Phase II	10	CDDP + VP16 + IFO (=PEI)	5 CR + 2 PR (70% RR); 6 patients alive without evidence of tumour (10–33 months)
Rietbroek et al. (1997)	Cervical cancer	Phase II	23	CDDP (weekly)	2 pCR/ICR + 9 PR (52% RR)
Takahashi et al. (1994)	Rectal cancer (Dukes' C preoperative)	Phase II	27 35	Mitomycin C Mitomycin C	3 LR 13 IR

ADR, Adriamycin, doxorubicin; Bleo, bleomycin; CDDP, cisplatin; 5FU, 5-fluorouracil; IFN, interferon-γ; IFO, ifosfamide; P, intraperitoneal hyperthermic perfusion; l-PAM, Melphalan; TNF, tumour necrosis factor-α; VP16, etoposide; WBH, whole-body hyperthermia. CR, complete remission; FHR, favourable histological response >75%; LR, local recurrence; MR, minor response; NED, no evidence of disease; p, pathohistological; PR, partial remission; RR, response rate.

Table 6.7 *Hyperthermia combined with radiotherapy (from Falk and Issels, 2001)*

Reference	Tumour entity (stage)	Type of trial	Number of patients	Type of radiochemotherapy	Results
Hou et al. (1989)	Oesophageal cancer	Phase III	23	40 Gy + Bleo + CDDP (4 weeks)	CR + PR (94% RR); 2-year survival: 48%
Ueo and Sugimachi (1990)	Oesophageal cancer (resectable)	Phase II/III	62	30 Gy + Bleo (3 weeks)	14 pCR (23%) 2-year survival: 50.4%
Ueo and Sugimachi (1990)	Oesophageal cancer (not-resectable)	Phase II/III	31	30 Gy + Bleo (3 weeks) 46.9 Gy + Bleo (5 weeks)	14 pCR (12%) 2-year survival: 15.5%
Sugimachi et al. (1992)	Oesophageal cancer (preoperative)	Phase III	83 53	Gy + Bleo (5 weeks) 32 Gy + Bleo (3 weeks)	2-year survival: 1.2% 7 pCR (26%) with RHT (n = 27) 2 pCR (8%) without RHT (n = 26)
Ohno et al. (1997)	Rectal cancer	Phase II	36 52	30 Gy + 5FU (3 weeks) 30 Gy + 5FU (3 weeks)	5-year survival 91% 5-year survival 64%
Rau et al. (1998)	Rectal cancer (preoperative)	Phase II	37	45 Gy + 5FU/Lv (4 weeks)	5 pCR (14%) + 17 PR (46%); 3-year survival: 86%
Bornstein et al. (1992)	Breast cancer (recurrences)	Phase I/II	29	30–60 Gy + CDDP (3–6 weeks)	15 CR (53% RR)
Amichetti et al. (1993)	Head and neck (N2/N3)	Phase I/II	18	70 Gy + CDDP (7 weeks)	13 CR + 3 PR (89%)

Bleo, bleomycin; CDDP, cisplatin; 5FU, 5-fluorouracil; LHT, local hyperthermia; RHT, regional hyperthermia; Lv, leucovorine; p, pathohistological; CR, complete remission; PR, partial remission; RR, response rate.

Radiotherapy doses were 50–70 Gy in 2–3 Gy fractions given five times weekly for patients who had not received previous radiotherapy, and for those who received previous radiotherapy (the majority) the radiotherapy dose was 28–32 Gy in fractions of 1.8–4 Gy given 2–5 times per week. The number of hyperthermia sessions varied from 2 to 8. Although the different groups used different radiation and hyperthermia schedules, the overall result for all groups was highly significant, with a 41 per cent complete response rate for radiation alone and a 59 per cent complete response rate for the addition of hyperthermia to radiation.

This gave, after stratification by trial, an odds ratio of 2.3. In the multiple logistic regression analysis, stratified by trial and adjusted for the baseline characteristics that were individually prognostic for complete response (maximum diameter, tumour area and systemic disease), the benefit of hyperthermia was confirmed and enhanced, with an odds ratio of 3 (95 per cent CI, 1.7–5.1, $P = 0.0001$). The greatest effect was observed in patients with recurrent lesions in previously irradiated sites, where further radiotherapy was extremely limited. Again the addition of hyperthermia to radiotherapy did not significantly enhance early or late radiation reactions. The difference in local control was maintained after 8 years of follow-up, but no effect on overall survival was seen.

A third study was first published by Valdagni et al. (1988) and this compared the results of radiotherapy alone versus radiotherapy plus hyperthermia in 41 patients with squamous cell carcinoma (SCC) of the head and neck, metastatic to cervical lymph nodes. Radiotherapy was conventional radical treatment to a total dose of 64–70 Gy with twice-weekly hyperthermia. The complete response rates were 82 per cent for the combined arm versus 37 per cent for radiotherapy alone, with similar toxicities. The medical records (1993) were reviewed 5 years later to evaluate long-term control and toxicity. The complete response rates continued to be large and significant, with 83 per cent for the combined modalities maintaining complete response, versus 41 per cent for radiotherapy alone. The difference in early local control was maintained at 5 years – 69 per cent for the combined treatments versus 24 per cent for radiotherapy alone. The actuarial survival was also significantly better ($P = 0.02$) in the combined arm (53 per cent) versus 0 per cent in the radiotherapy arm.

Deep-seated tumours

The heating of deep-seated tumours is technically more difficult and limiting side-effects have included systemic heating, pain at bone interfaces when focused ultrasound is used and preferential fat heating when capacitance methods are used. The placement of catheters for temperature measurement can be a problem and is usually done under CT control. Limiting side-effects have mainly been due to systemic heating, which can be minimized by a variety of techniques.

Tumours studied have included pelvic and abdominal, as well as some brain tumours. The most commonly used techniques have involved capacitance methods with large electrodes or annular arrays. Focused ultrasound has been less frequently used, but theoretically is an attractive idea. Studies involving the annular array system have been conducted more recently – again, side-effects have not been a major problem.

A third randomized trial, published in 2000, is the Dutch locally advanced pelvic tumour trial, which closed in 1996 (Van der Zee et al., 2000). In this trial 363 patients with T3 and T4 bladder tumours, IIB and IV cervical tumours and inoperable or recurrent rectal tumours were randomized to radical standard radiotherapy (including brachytherapy for the cervical tumours), versus radiotherapy with the addition of hyperthermia.

Hyperthermia was given weekly during the radiotherapy for 60 minutes, and three different hyperthermia systems were utilized. Analysis was performed on intention to treat with a median follow-up time of 21 months, and the results show a significant improvement in durable local control ($P = 0.005$) for the addition of hyperthermia. The initial complete response rates were 39 per cent for radiotherapy alone and 56 per cent for the combined arm. The addition of hyperthermia also improved overall survival ($P = 0.0014$) and, at 3 years' follow-up, this was 24 per cent for radiotherapy and 31 per cent for the combined arm.

The greatest effect of hyperthermia was seen in the patients with cervical carcinoma ($n = 115$), where the complete response rate was 57 per cent for radiotherapy and 83 per cent for radiotherapy and hyperthermia, and overall survival improved from 27 per cent to 52 per cent at 3 years. In bladder cancer the difference in local control was lost after 4 years and did not result in improved survival. For rectal cancer where 114/143 had recurrent disease, there was no difference in local control, although good palliation appeared to be obtained with the additional of hyperthermia. In The Netherlands, it is now standard therapy to offer hyperthermia with radiotherapy to all patients with locally advanced cervical cancers.

Interstitial hyperthermia

Interstitial hyperthermia, like interstitial radiotherapy, offers a method for providing uniform heating to a small volume below the skin surface, and tumours that have been studied include brain, breast, cervix and head and neck, and techniques include radiofrequency, microwaves, hot-water sources and ferromagnetic seeds. Experience is more limited than with external applicators and no randomized studies have been completed. Most phase I/II studies have reported complete response rates in the order of 55–65 per cent for recurrent or persistent tumours.

One randomized trial that has been completed utilizing interstitial hyperthermia is from UCSF (Sneed et al., 1996). In this study patients with newly diagnosed, focal supra-tentorial glioblastoma multiforme were registered postoperatively and treated with partial brain radiotherapy to 59.4 Gy with oral hydroxyurea. Those patients whose tumours were implantable after external-beam radiotherapy, were randomized to a brachytherapy boost (60 Gy) without or with hyperthermia for 30 minutes immediately before and after the brachytherapy.

Eighty patients were randomized and, when analysed by intention to treat, time to progression and survival from date of diagnosis were significantly better for those patients treated with hyperthermia. The median survival for patients treated with hyperthermia was 85 weeks, versus 76 weeks for the radiotherapy-alone arm. The 2-year survival in the combined arm was 31 per cent and in the brachytherapy-only arm, 15 per cent. Again, toxicity was acceptable.

Intracavity hyperthermia

Transrectal or transurethral hyperthermia for benign prostatic hypertrophy is increasingly popular and symptomatic relief is reported in the order of 65–70 per cent, but few reports are available of treatment of malignant disease. Intracavity heating has been attempted for rectal tumours (Qing-Shan *et al.*, 1993, with percentage survival at 5 years of 73.7 per cent for 40 Gy plus heat; 58.8 per cent for 40 Gy alone and 42.9 per cent for 30 Gy plus heat for 122 patients), and prostatic, cervical, bronchial and oesophageal tumours.

RESULTS FROM HYPERTHERMIA AND CHEMOTHERAPY WITH OR WITHOUT IRRADIATION

Hyperthermia and chemotherapy have been most usefully combined in regional, perfusion studies and whole-body hyperthermia and, to a lesser extent, in local hyperthermia. The interpretation of results and technical problems are even greater in this group. Certain drugs are more effective with used in combination with hyperthermia, but this is a variable response and several mechanisms may be responsible (Dahl and Mella, 1990).

Much of the present interest in the interaction of chemotherapeutic agents and hyperthermia results from work done by Hahn and others in the late 1970s and early 1980s. The thermal interactions of most chemotherapeutic drugs are complex and far from being completely understood.

Thermal enhancement is influenced by pH, O_2 tension, nutrient supply and rate of heating, and all these influence the development of thermal tolerance, which affects drugs as well as hyperthermia. As cytotoxicity from both hyperthermia and chemotherapy is related to the damage they cause at the DNA level, it is not surprising that they have important interactions (Table 6.8).

Certain drugs combine usefully with hyperthermia and will show an additive effect, and these include the vincas and the antimetabolities (methotrexate, 5-fluorouracil (5-FU)). True thermal enhancement is seen with the alkylating agents, and the anti-tumour antibiotics, although the degree may vary between the different members of the group. In most, the degree of thermal enhancement will increase with temperature above a threshold temperature.

Table 6.8 *Chemotherapeutic drugs and hyperthermia*

Supra-additive effect, i.e. 1 + 1 = 3
Mustine effect
Thiotepa
Cyclophosphamide
Melphalan
Mitromycin C
Nitrosureas
Cisplatin
Ifosfamide
Anthracyclines
Bleomycin
Etoposides
Taxols
Misonidazole
Interferon
Lonidamine
Additive effect, i.e. 1 + 1 = 2
Vincas
Methotrexate
5-FU
Less than additive 1 + 1
AMSA
Ara-C

Ara-C, cytosine arabinoside; 5-FU, 5-fluorouracil.

Time sequencing of the hyperthermia affects these drugs, and hyperthermia must be given simultaneously with the drug to achieve the maximum cytotoxic effect. Prolonged heating, as in whole-body hyperthermia, can lead to inactivation of these drugs. Some drugs may be modified by heat, e.g. misonidazole and 5-thio-D-glucose, and both these drugs show increased cytoxity to hypoxic cells at hyperthermic temperatures. Other drugs, e.g. ethanol, amphotericin B, cysteamine, etc., are cytotoxic only at elevated temperatures. Both interferon (Lienard *et al.*, 1992) and *Corynebacterium parvum* show thermal enhancement of non-specific immunostimulation.

Theoretically, regional perfusion allows blood to be used as the vehicle to transport and distribute both heat and drugs, as well as allowing biochemical analysis of the effects of hyperthermia. Body extremities can be heated by isolating major arteries and veins; this closed-circuit system is then perfused with extracorporeally heated blood and drugs. Technically there are many problems, but there have been some very encouraging results. Suitable sites include melanomas and sarcomas of the limbs as well as primary and metastatic tumours of the liver and other organs.

A variety of phase II trials have shown significant advantages in both disease-free and actuarial survivals for patients treated in this way (Cavaliere *et al.*, 1983; Krementz, 1983). The first randomized trial was performed by Ghussen and co-workers in 1984, when over 100 patients with stage I–III malignant melanomas, Clark levels of more than IV and tumour thicknesses of greater than 1.5 mm were studied. Half received conventional surgery only and half received hyperthermic limb perfusion and melphalan. This trial was terminated early as the combined treatment group was found to have a highly significant disease-free survival advantage over the surgery-only arm.

Regional hyperthermia for limb sarcomas using etoposide and ifosfamide (Issels *et al.*, 1990) has shown an overall response rate of 37 per cent, with 6/38 complete remissions (CRs) and four partial remissions (PRs) for pretreated locally advanced tumours. Similar results were also obtained by the same group for pelvic tumours. Based on this study, a randomized EORTC/ESHO trial has recently commenced and is expected to randomize 300 patients. Additionally there are a number of phase II studies which are also being extended to phase III because of encouraging results, e.g. the groups of Sugimachi for preoperative oesophageal carcinoma, Wiedermann for metastatic sarcomas, Romanowski for paediatric tumours and Rietbroek for recurrent cervical carcinomas (*see* Table 6.6).

Hyperthermic infusion has also been tried with metastatic liver tumours and advanced bladder tumours – the former with disappointing results and the latter, which also included irradiation, with more 'promising' results.

Nature's hyperthermia, fever, is one of the body's defences against infections and, no doubt, involves stimulation of the immune system, and likewise it is probable that whole-body hyperthermia has a similar effect. Whole-body hyperthermia can be achieved in several ways, as described earlier. Most are elaborate and require intensive patient monitoring systems, as the patient needs to be under heavy sedation and often general anaesthesia for temperatures greater than 41.5°C. They all require measurement of core temperature with oesophageal and rectal thermometers, and careful fluid replacement. Cardiovascular stress is a major problem, with pulse rate and cardiac output frequently doubling, and therefore pulmonary catheterization may be required to monitor right pulmonary atrial pressure, pulmonary capillary wedge pressure and cardiac output (Bull, 1995). Thermal enhancement of drugs certainly occurs, and although this is likely to be beneficial in most cases, it is also possible to enhance drug toxicity.

Despite these problems, a number of patients with advanced disease have been treated with whole-body hyperthermia. Certainly, the idea that cancer is a whole-body disease and should be treated as such makes the procedure more attractive. However, it is difficult to draw sensible conclusions from the studies so far performed, as most are complicated by a large number of variables, including the type and stages of diseases studied, the specific drugs and the dosages used, and the degree and duration of heat employed.

Promising phase II studies were completed by Bull *et al.* (1992), who treated 17 patients with resistant sarcomas with whole-body hyperthermia and BCNU (1,3-*bis* (2-chloroethyl)-1-nitrosurea) (two PRs, four objective responses), and Engelhardt (1988), who treated 15 patients with small cell lung cancer with whole-body hyperthermia

and Adriamycin®, cyclophosphamide and vincristine (CR + PR 15/22 in the hyperthermic arm and CR + PR 8/22 for the normothermic arm).

Most other studies have concentrated on tumours which are thought to be resistant to more conventional therapies, such as unresectable tumours of the gastrointestinal tract, e.g. pancreas, stomach and oesophagus, and lung tumours other than oat cell tumours. In addition, tumours that have failed standard therapy and have disseminated, e.g. lymphomas, sarcomas, leukaemias and breast cancers, have also been studied. Although most of these studies have reported a low CR rate (less than 10 per cent), many have reported substantial regressions (approximately 30 per cent), especially with regard to pain relief. This, in itself, may be considered remarkable, remembering that patients had advanced disease, thought untreatable in most cases.

Other potential uses for whole-body hyperthermia include the treatment of disseminated disease (alone or with chemotherapy) or as an adjuvant with chemotherapy for micrometastatic disease.

When the normal tissue tolerance has been reached for radiotherapy, the combination of hyperthermia and chemotherapy has been found to be useful in a number of studies, despite the fact that the vascular damage caused by the irradiation may limit the concentration of the drug reaching the tissues. Two trials have compared the effects of chemotherapy alone to chemotherapy plus hyperthermia. Chemotherapy (Adriamycin® or bleomycin) and hyperthermia have also been usefully combined for the treatment of head and neck tumours.

Trimodality trials

A prospective randomized trial was reported by Sugimachi *et al.* (1992) on 53 patients treated with trimodality therapy using bleomycin given preoperatively for carcinoma of the oesophagus, and a significant difference was found in those receiving hyperthermia. Herman *et al.* (1982) have reported on the treatment of 24 patients using hyperthermia, radiation and *cis*-platinum and have shown a 25–67 per cent CR (depending on the dose of *cis*-platinum used).

Specific sites

OESOPHAGEAL, STOMACH AND PANCREAS

Local persistence and progression still remain as major problems in these diseases. Reports on oesophageal and stomach carcinomas treated with hyperthermia mainly come from the Far East, and the best results are from trimodality therapy. Despite the fact that information is somewhat limited, these results warrant further investigation.

SOFT-TISSUE SARCOMAS AND BONE TUMOURS

The largest series has come from the excellent group in Munich headed by Issels, where hyperthermia is combined with etoposide and ifosfamide, and this now a phase III EORTC study. Preoperative hyperthermia with radiation has been used in the Duke University Radiation Oncology Department, and locoregional control was 94 per cent at 10 years. Whole-body hyperthermia (achieved with the reinfusion of extracorporeal heated blood) combined with ifosfamide and carboplatin for patients with refractory sarcomas and teratomas was used by Wiedemann et al. (1994), and six partial responses were seen.

PAEDIATRIC TUMOURS

The German Society of Paediatric Oncology and Haematology has investigated the use of hyperthermia with several drug combinations for refractory paediatric tumours (Romanowski et al., 1993), and has seen encouraging results.

CERVICAL CARCINOMA

In addition to the excellent results obtained in the Dutch pelvic study (van der Zee, 2000) for hyperthermia and irradiation, encouraging results have also been seen from Holland for the use of hyperthermia and chemotherapy. Rietbroek et al. (1997) investigated the use of hyperthermia with cis-platinum for recurrent cervical carcinoma, and found a response rate of 52 per cent with a median duration of response of 9.5 months and a 1-year survival of 42 per cent. For locally advanced carcinomas of the cervix, hyperthermia is now routinely recommended in The Netherlands.

RECTAL CARCINOMA

A number of studies have shown improved results in phase II studies and the results of ongoing phase III studies are awaited.

BREAST CANCER

It is in the treatment of recurrent breast cancer that the use of hyperthermia has been most convincingly demonstrated, and here the treatment of these patients should routinely include hyperthermia. Treatment of large primary breast carcinomas is now under investigation using neoadjuvant chemotherapy and hyperthermia.

HEAD AND NECK CANCERS

Both treatments with hyperthermia and radiotherapy, and hyperthermia and chemotherapy, appear to produce impressive results in phase III studies.

THE FUTURE

There is still a challenge for physicists and engineers to develop better heating systems and non-invasive thermometry. The vast majority of studies so far carried out show an advantage for hyperthermia and radiation over radiation alone, and randomized phase III studies are now appearing in press with significantly positive results. Hyperthermia is an effective treatment modality for cancer, and can lead to improved local control and better overall survival, without increased toxicity. Future randomized trials will need to be multi-institutional to recruit sufficient number of patients quickly, and it is vital that strict quality assurance guidelines are adhered to.

Although modern megavoltage radiotherapy has significantly improved the cure rate, there is still an unacceptable rate of failure of local control. Viable cells in the residual tumour at the primary site will lead to the spread of metastases and ultimately death. Probably one-third of all cancer deaths follow lack of local control in the primary (Suit, 1982) and if local control were improved, it is probable that cure rates would be increased.

The technical application of local–regional hyperthermia or whole-body hyperthermia is feasible, safe and effective. Clinical studies (phase II/III) on regional hyperthermia with radiotherapy, chemotherapy or radiochemotherapy have shown impressive results at clinically relevant temperatures in locally advanced tumours of different entities in terms of objective response rates, local tumour control and relapse-free survival. This is especially so in well-defined tumour entities, e.g. breast, melanoma, head and neck tumours, cervical tumours and glioblastomas, where the addition of hyperthermia to radiotherapy significantly improves response and survival. These can be considered proven therapy, but for other situations, hyperthermia as an adjunct should be tested in randomized clinical trials.

The greatest advantage for hyperthermia in combination with radiation at the present time appears to be in combination with radiation, for the treatment of cancers where local control is a problem. These cancers are certain breast, head and neck, cervical and brain tumours. The results from the re-irradiation of recurrent breast/chest wall disease indicate that where re-irradiation is to be used, that it should be combined with hyperthermia. In The Netherlands the addition of hyperthermia to irradiation is now standard for locally advanced cervical tumours.

With technology improving constantly, it is expected that there will be more phase III studies in the more deep-seated tumours, where failure of local control is an even greater problem. It is likely that studies will also continue with metastatic lesions, but here the aim will be palliation, and the answers will be of a more scientific nature regarding the interaction of the two treatment modalities. As yet we do not really know what kind of temperature distribution is optimum to achieve the best clinical results, and nor how many hyperthermia treatments are required.

Phase III studies for whole-body hyperthermia in combination with chemotherapy are under way and tumours with a high growth fraction, e.g. small cell lung carcinomas or perhaps some high-grade non-Hodgkin's lymphomas, are suitable. There is also considerable interest in treating patients with AIDS with whole-body hyperthermia.

It is possible that one day we might gain insight into thermotolerance by its relationship to heat-shock proteins, and then a rapid assay of heat-shock proteins would tell us when to treat to get the best result.

There is no doubt that hyperthermia holds great promise for the future as a cancer treatment in selected sites, as an adjunct to both radiation and chemotherapy, but it is time-consuming and needs a dedicated team to perform it efficiently and safely. Ideally hyperthermia units should be placed in regional referral centres to maximize their efficiency and to perform economically.

SIGNIFICANT POINTS

- Hyperthermia is defined as the elevation of tumours to 41–44°C to increase the response rate of tumours to radiotherapy and chemotherapy.
- There is a well-established biological rationale for the understanding of the effectiveness of hyperthermia.
- Hyperthermia may be applied superficially (4 cm), deep (>4 cm), to the whole body, or as an interstitial or intracavity treatment, or as regional perfusion.
- Heat may be delivered using microwaves, ultrasound or radiofrequency – all appear to have the same effect biologically for the same temperature reached.
- Development of thermal tolerance suggests that once-weekly treatments are optimum.
- Separation of hyperthermia and radiation in time allows better recovery of normal tissues and reduces toxicity.
- Thermal isoeffect dose (TID), as used at the present time, appears to be the best measure of dose.
- Hyperthermia is well tolerated with a low rate of toxicity and complications.
- Randomized clinical trials are now showing convincing evidence that hyperthermia is a successful and safe modality of treatment.

KEY REFERENCES

Field, S.B. and Hand, J.W. (eds) (1990) *An introduction to the practical aspects of clinical hyperthermia*. London: Taylor and Francis.

Seegensmiedt, M.H. and Sauer, R. (eds) (1993) *Interstitial and intracavity hyperthermia (IHT) in oncology*. Medical Radiology. Berlin: Springer-Verlag.

Seegenschmiedt, H.M., Vernon, C.C. and Fessenden, P. (1996) *Principles and practice of thermoradiotherapy*, vols I and II. Medical Radiology. Berlin: Springer-Verlag.

REFERENCES

Alexander, G.A., Nervi, D. and Civavdalli, A. (1987) Problems of sequence and fractionation in the clinical application of combined heat and irradiation. *Cancer Res.* **15**, 959–72.

Amichetti, M., Griaff, C., Fellin, G. *et al.* (1993) Cisplatin, hyperthermia, and radiation (trimodal therapy) in patients with locally advanced head and neck tumors: a phase I–II study. *Int. J. Radiat. Oncol. Biol. Phys.* **26**, 801–7.

Arkin, H., Xu, L.X. and Holmes, K.R. (1994) Recent developments in modeling heat transfer in blood perfused tissues. *IEEE Transactions on Biomedical Engineering* **41**, 97–107.

Armour, E.P., McEachern, D., Wang, Z., Corry, P.M. and Martinez, A. (1993) Sensitivity of human cells to mild hyperthermia. *Cancer Res.* **53**, 2740–4.

Ben-Yosef, R. and Kapp, D.S. (1992) Persistent and/or late complications of combined radiation and hyperthermia. *Int. J. Hyper.* **8**(6), 733–47.

Bolomey, J.C., LeBihan, D. and Mizushina, S. (1995) Recent trends in noninvasive thermal control. In Seegenschmiedt, M.H., Fessenden, P. and Vernon, C.C. (eds), *Thermo-radiotherapy and thermo-chemotherapy*, vol. 1. Heidelberg/Berlin: Springer, 361–79.

Bornstein, B.A., Zouranjian, P.S., Hansen, J.L. *et al.* (1992) Local hyperthermia, radiation therapy, and chemotherapy in patients with local-regional recurrence of breast carcinoma. *Int. J. Radiat. Oncol. Biol. Phys.* **25**, 79–85.

Bull, J.M.C. (1995) Whole-body hyperthermia: new dimensions. In Seegenschmiedt, M.H., Fessenden, P. and Vernon, C.C. (eds), *Thermo-radiotherapy and thermo-chemotherapy*, vol. 2. Heidelberg/Berlin: Springer, 303–22.

Bull, J.M.C., Cronau, L.H., Mansfield-Newman, B. *et al.* (1992) Chemotherapy resistant sarcoma treated with whole body hyperthermia (WBH) combined with 1-3-*bis*(2-chloroethyl)-1-nitrosurea (BCNU). *Int. J. Hyperthermia* **8**(3), 297–304.

Busch, W. (1866) Verhandlungen ärtlicher Gesellschaften. *Berl. Klin.Wochenschr.* **3**, 245–6.

Cavaliere, R., Mondovi, B., Moricca, G. *et al.* (1983) Regional perfusion hyperthermia. In Storm, F.K. (ed.),

Hyperthermia in cancer therapy. Boston: Hall Medical, 369–99.

Craciunescu, O.I., Howle, L.E. and Clegg, S.T. (1999) Experimental evaluation of the thermal properties of two tissue equivalent phantoms. *Int. J. Hyperthermia* **15**(6), 509–18.

Craciunescu, O.I., Das, S.K., McCauley, R.L., MacFall, J.R. and Samulski, T.V. (2001) 3D numerical reconstruction of the hyperthermia induced temperature distribution in human sarcomas using DE-MRI measured tissue perfusion: validation against non-invasive MR temperature measurements. *Int. J. Hyperthermia* **17**, 221–39.

Crezee, J., Kaatee, R.S.J.P., van der Koijk, J.F. and Lagendijk, J.J.W. (1999) Spatial steering with quadrupole electrodes in 27 MHz capacitively coupled interstitial hyperthermia. *Int. J. Hyperthermia* **15**(2), 145–56.

Dahl, O. and Mella, O. (1990) Hyperthermia and chemotherapeutic agents. In Field, S.B. and Hand, J.W. (eds), *An introduction to the practical aspects of clinical hyperthermia*. London: Taylor and Francis, 108–42.

Datta, N.R., Rose, A.K. and Kapoor, H.K. (1987) Thermoradiotherapy in the management of carcinoma cervix (IIIB): a controlled clinical study. *Indian Med. Gazette* **121**, 68–71.

Datta, N.R., Bose, A.K., Kapoor, H.K. and Gupta, S. (1990) Head and neck cancers: results of thermoradiotherapy versus radiotherapy. *Int. J. Hyperthermia* **6**, 479–86.

Deardorff, D.L., Diederich, C.J. and Nau, W.H. (1998) Air-cooling of direct-coupled ultrasound applicators for interstitial hyperthermia and thermal coagulation. *Med. Phys.* **25**(12), 2400–9.

Dewhirst, M.W. and Sim, D.A. (1984) The utility of thermal dose as a predictor of tumour and normal tissue responses in combined radiation and hyperthermia. *Cancer Res.* **44**(Suppl.), 4772s–80s.

Dewhirst, M.W. and Sim, D.A. (1986) Estimation of therapeutic gain of clinical trials involving hyperthermia and radiotherapy. *Int. J. Hyperthermia* **2**(2), 165–78.

Dewhirst, M.W., Sim, D.A., Forsyth, K., Grochowski, K.J., Wilson, S. and Bicknell, E. (1985) Local control and distant metastases in primary canine malignant melanomas treated with hyperthermia and/or radiotherapy. *Int. J. Hyperthermia* **1**(3), 219–34.

Dewhirst, M.W., Prescott, D.M., Clegg, S. *et al.* (1990) The use of hydralazine to manipulate tumour temperatures during hyperthermia. *Int. J. Hyperthermia* **6**, 971–83.

Diederich, C.J. and Hynynen, K. (1999) Ultrasound technology for hyperthermia. *Ultrasound Med. Biol.* **25**(6), 871–87.

Diederich, C.J., Khalil, I.S., Stauffer, P.R. *et al.* (1996) Direct-coupled interstitial ultrasound applicators for simultaneous thermobrachytherapy: a feasibility study. *Int. J. Hyperthermia* **12**(3), 401–19.

Dunlop, P.R.C., Hand, J.W., Dickinson, R.J. and Field, S.B. (1986) An assessment of local hyperthermia in clinical practice. *Int. J. Hyperthermia* **2**, 39–50.

Eggermont, A.M.M., Koops, H., Liénard, D. *et al.* (1996) Isolated limb perfusion with high-dose tumor necrosis factor-α in combination with interferon-γ and melphalan for nonresectable extremity soft tissue sarcomas: a multicenter trial. *J. Clin. Oncol.* **14**, 2653–65.

Engelhardt, R. (1988) Summary of recent clinical experience in whole-body hyperthermia combined with chemotherapy. *Recent Results Cancer Res.* **107**, 200–4.

Fajardo, L. (1984) Pathological effects of hyperthermia in normal tissues. *Cancer Res.* **44**(Suppl.), 4826s–35s.

Falk, M.H. and Issels, R.D. (2001) Hyperthermia in oncology. *Int. J. Hyperthermia* **17**(1), 1–18.

Falk, R.E., Moffat, F.L., Lawler, M., Heine, J., Makowka, L. and Falk, J.A. (1986) Combination therapy for resectable and unresectable adenocarcinoma of the pancreas. *Cancer* **57**, 685–8.

Fessenden, P. and Hand, J.W. (1995) Hyperthermia therapy physics. In Smith, A.R. (ed.), *Radiation therapy physics*. Heidelberg/Berlin: Springer, 315–63.

Gellermann, J., Wust, P., Stalling, D. *et al.* (2000) Clinical evaluation and verification of the hyperthermia treatment planning system hyperplan. *Int. J. Radiat. Oncol. Biol. Phys.* **47**, 1145–56.

Ghussen, F., Kruger, I., Groth, W. and Stutzer, H. (1984) The role of regional hyperthermic cytostatic perfusion in the treatment of extremity melanoma. *Cancer* **61**, 654–9.

Hand, J.W. (1998) Ultrasound hyperthermia and the prediction of heating. In Duck, F.A., Baker, A.C. and Starritt, H.C. (eds), *Ultrasound in medicine*. Bristol/Philadelphia: Institute of Physics, 151–76.

Hand, J.W., Machin, D., Vernon, C.C. and Whaley, J.B. (1997) Analysis of thermal parameters obtained during phase III trials of hyperthermia as an adjunct to radiotherapy in the treatment of breast cancer. *Int. J. Hyperthermia* **13**(4), 343–65.

Herman, T.S., Zukoski, C.F., Anderson, R.M. *et al.* (1982) Whole-body hyperthermia and chemotherapy for treatment of patients with advanced refractory malignancies. *Cancer Treat. Rep.* **66**, 259–65.

Hiroaka, M., Jo, S., Takashashi, M. and Abe, M. (1984) Clinical results of radiofrequency hyperthermia combined with radiation in the treatment of radioresistant cancers. *Cancer* **54**, 2898–904.

Hornsleth, S.N., Frydendal, L., Mella, O. *et al.* (1997) Quality assurance for radiofrequency regional hyperthermia. *Int. J. Hyperthermia* **13**(2), 169–85.

Hou, B.S., Xiong, Q.B. and Li, D.J. (1989) Thermo-chemo-radiotherapy of esophageal cancer, a preliminary report on 34 cases. *Cancer* **64**, 1777–82.

Issels, R.D. (1995) Soft tissue sarcomas – What is currently being done. *Eur. J. Surg. Oncol.* **21**(suppl.), 471–4.

Issels, R.D., Prenninger, S.W., Nagele, A. *et al.* (1990) Ifosamide plus etoposide combined with regional hyperthermia in patients with locally advanced sarcomas: a phase II study. *J. Clin. Oncol.* **8**(11), 1818–29.

Issels, R.D., Bosse, D., Abdel-Rahman, S. *et al.* (1993) Preoperative systemic etoposide/ifosfamide/ doxorubicin chemotherapy combined with regional hyperthermia in high-risk sarcoma: a pilot study. *Cancer chemotherapy pharmacol.* **31** (suppl. 2), S233–7.

Issels, R.D., Abdel-Rahman, S., Salat, C. *et al.* (1998) Neoadjuvant chemotherapy combined with regional hyperthermia (RHT) followed by surgery and radiation in primary and recurrent high-risk soft tissue sarcomas (HR-STS) of adults (updated report). *J. Cancer Res. Clin. Oncol.* **124** (suppl.), R105.

Kakehi, M., Ueda, K., Mukojima, T. *et al.* (1990) Multi-institutional clinical studies on hyperthermia combined with radiotherapy or chemotherapy in advanced cancer of deep-seated organs. *Int. J. Hyperthermia* **6**, 719–40.

Kapp, D.S., Samulski, T.V., Fessenden, P. *et al.* (1987) Prognostic significance of tumour volume on response following local-regional hyperthermia (HT) and radiation therapy (XRT). Thirty-fifth Annual Meeting of the Radiation Research Society, Atlanta, Georgia, 21–26 February, 17.

Kotte, A.N.T.J., Van Wieringen, N. and Lagendijk, J.J.W. (1998) Modelling tissue heating with ferromagnetic seeds. *Phys. Med. Biol.* **43**(1), 105–20.

Krementz, E.T. (1983) Chemotherapy by isolated regional perfusion for melanoma of the limbs. In Schwemmle, K. and Aigner, K. (eds), *Vascular perfusion in cancer therapy.* Berlin/Heidelberg/New York: Springer, 193–203.

Lagendijk, J.J.W. (2000) Hyperthermia treatment planning. *Phys. Med. Biol.* **45**, R61–76.

Lagendijk, J.J.W., van Rhoon, G.C., Hornsleth, S.N. *et al.* (1998) ESHO quality assurance guidelines for regional hyperthermia. *Int. J. Hyperthermia* **14**(2), 125–33.

Lee, E.R. (1995) Electromagnetic superficial heating technology. In Seegenschmiedt, M.H., Fessenden, P. and Vernon, C.C. (eds), *Thermo-radiotherapy and thermo-chemotherapy*, vol. 1. Heidelberg/Berlin: Springer, 193–217.

Lee, R.J., Buchanan, M., Kleine, L.J. and Hynynen, K. (1999) Arrays of multielement ultrasound applicators for interstitial hyperthermia. *IEEE Trans. Biomed. Eng.* **46**(7), 880–90.

Li, G.C. and Hahn, G.M. (1980) A proposed operational model of thermotolerance based on the effects of nutrients and the initial treatment temperature. *Cancer Res.* **40**, 4501–8.

Li, D.J. and Hou, B.S. (1987) A preliminary report on the treatment of esophageal cancer by intraluminal microwave hyperthermia and chemotherapy. *Cancer Treatment Reports* **71**, 1013–19.

Lienard, D., Ewalenko, P., Delmotte, J.-J., Renard, N. and Lejeune, F. (1992) High-dose recombinant tumor necrosis factor alpha in combination with interferon gamma and melphalan in isolation perfusion in the limbs for melanoma and sarcoma. *J. Clin. Oncol.* **10**(1), 52–60.

Lin, W.L., Chen, Y.Y., Lin, S.Y. *et al.* (1999) Optimal configuration of multiple-focused ultrasound transducers for external hyperthermia. *Med. Phys.* **26**(9), 2007–16.

Luk, K.H., Pajak, T.F., Perez, C.A., Johnson, R.J., Corner, N. and Dobbins, T. (1984) Prognostic factors for tumour response after hyperthermia and radiation. In Overgaard, J. (ed.), *Hyperthermic oncology.* London: Taylor and Francis, 353–6.

Ohno, S., Tomoda, M., Tomisaki, S. *et al.* (1997) Improved surgical results after combining preoperative hyperthermia with chemotherapy and radiotherapy for patients with carcinoma of the rectum. *Diseases of the Colon and Rectum* **40**, 401–6.

Overgaard, J. and Overgaard, M. (1987) Hyperthermia as an adjuvant to radiotherapy in the treatment of malignant melanoma. *Int. J. Hyperthermia* **3**, 483–502.

Overgaard, J., Gonzalez-Gonzalez, D., Hulshof, M.C.C.M. *et al.* (1995) Randomised trial of hyperthermia as adjuvant to radiotherapy for recurrent or metastatic melanomas. *Lancet* **345**, 540–3.

Paulsen, K.D., Geimer, S., Tang, J. and Boyse, W.E. (1999) Optimization of pelvic heating rate distributions with electromagnetic phased arrays. *Int. J. Hyperthermia* **15**(3), 157–86.

Perez, C.A., Kuske, R.R., Emami, B. and Fineberg, B. (1986) Irradiation alone or combined with hyperthermia in the treatment of recurrent carcinoma of the breast in the chest wall: a non randomized comparison. *Int. J. Hyperthermia* **2**, 179–87.

Perez, C.A., Gillespie, B., Pajak, T. *et al.* (1989) Quality assurance problems in clinical hyperthermia and their impact on therapeutic outcome: a report by the Radiation Therapy Oncology Group. *Int. J. Radiat. Oncol. Biol. Phys.* **16**, 551–8.

Perez, C.A., Pajak, T., Emami, B. *et al.* (1991) Randomised phase II study comparing irradiation alone or combined with hyperthermia in superficial measurable tumours. Final report by the RTOG. *Am. J. Clin. Oncol.* **2**,133–41.

Petrovich, Z., Langholtz, B., Gibbs, F.A. Jr (1989) Regional hyperthermia for advanced tumours: a clinical study of 353 patients. *Int. J. Radiat. Oncol. Biol. Phys.* **16**, 601–7.

Prior, M.V., Phipps, J.H., Roberts, T. *et al.* (1991) Treatment of menorrhagia by radiofrequency heating. *Int. J. Hyperthermia* **7**, 213–20.

Qing-Shan, Y., Rui-Zhi, W., Guang-Qi, S. *et al.* (1993) Combination preoperative radiation and endocavitary hyperthermia for rectal cancer: long-term results of 44 patients. *Int. J. Hyperthermia* **9**(1), 19–24.

Rau, B., Wust, P., Hohenberger, P. *et al.* (1998) Preoperative hyperthermia combined with radiochemotherapy in locally advanced rectal cancer. A phase II clinical trial. *Annals of Surgery* **227**, 380–9.

Reinhold, H.S. and Endrich, B. (1986) Tumour microcirculation as a target for hyperthermia. *Int. J. Hyperthermia* **2**, 111–37.

Rietbroek, R.C., Schilthuis, M.S., Bakker, P.J.M. *et al.* (1997) Phase II trial of weekly locoregional hyperthermia and cisplatin in patients with a previously irradiated recurrent carcinoma of the uterine cervix. *Cancer* **79**, 935–42.

Robins, H.I., Rushin, D., Kutz, M. *et al.* (1997) Phase I clinical trial of melphalan and 41.8°C whole-body hyperthermia in cancer patients. *J. Clin. Oncol.* **15**, 158–64.

Romanowski, R., Schött, C., Issels, R. *et al.* (1993) Regionale Hyperthermie mit systemischer Chemotherapie bei Kindern und Jugendlichen: Durchführbarkeit und klinische Verläufe bei 34 intensiv vorbehandelten Patienten mit prognostisch ungünstigen Tumorerkrankungen. *Klinische Pädiatrie* **205**, 249–56.

Rossetto, F. and Stauffer, P.R. (1999) Effect of complex bolus-tissue load configurations on SAR distributions from dual concentric conductor applicators. *IEEE Trans. Biomed. Eng.* **46**(11), 1310–19.

Rossetto, F., Stauffer, P.R., Manfrini, V. *et al.* (1998) Effect of practical layered dielectric loads on SAR patterns from dual concentric conductor microstrip antennas. *Int. J. Hyperthermia* **14**(6), 553–71.

Sapareto, S.A. and Dewey, W.C. (1984) Thermal dose determination in cancer therapy. *Int. J. Radiat. Oncol. Biol. Phys.* **10**, 787–800.

Sapozink, M.D., Gibbs, F.A. Jnr and Egger, M.J. (1986) Regional hyperthermia for clinically advanced deep-seated pelvic malignancies. *Am. J. Clin. Oncol.* **9**, 162–9.

Schneider, C.J., Olmi, R. and van Dijk, J.D.P. (1995a) Phantom design: applicability and physical properties. In Seegenschmiedt, M.H., Fessenden, P. and Vernon, C.C. (eds), *Thermo-radiotherapy and thermo-chemotherapy*, vol. 1. Heidelberg/Berlin: Springer, 381–97.

Schneider, C.J., Kuijer, J.P., Colussi, L.C. *et al.* (1995b) Performance evaluation of annular arrays in practice: the measurement of phase and amplitude patterns of radio-frequency deep body applicators. *Med. Phys.* **22**, 755–65.

Seip, R., van Baren, P., Cain, C.A. and Ebbini, E.S. (1996) Noninvasive real-time multipoint temperature control for ultrasound phased array treatments. *IEEE Trans. Ultrason. Ferroelect. Frequency Control* **43**(6), 1063–73.

Sherar, M., Lui, F.-F., Pintilie, M. *et al.* (1997) Relationship between thermal dose and outcome in thermoradiotherapy treatments for recurrences of breast cancer; data from a phase III trial. *IJROBP* **39**(2), 371–80.

Sneed, P.K., Stauffer, P.R., Diederich, C.J., McDermott, M.W., Lamborn, K.R. and Weaver, K.A. (1996) Results of a study comparing radiotherapy alone vs radiotherapy combined with interstitial hyperthermia in patients with glioblastomas. *Int. J. Radiat. Oncol. Biol. Phys.* **36**, 159.

Sneed, P.K., Stauffer, P.R., McDermott, M.W. *et al.* (1998) Survival benefit of hyperthermia in a prospective randomised trial of brachytherapy boost (hyperthermia for glioblastoma multiforme). *Int. J. Radiat. Oncol. Biol. Phys.* **40**, 287–95.

Stauffer, P.R., Diederich, C.J. and Seegenschmiedt, M.H. (1995) Interstitial heating techniques. In Seegenschmiedt, M.H., Fessenden, P. and Vernon, C.C. (eds), *Thermo-radiotherapy and thermo-chemotherapy*, vol. 1. Heidelberg/Berlin: Springer, 279–320.

Stawarz, B., Smiegielski, S. and Petrovich, Z. (1991) A comparison of transurethral and transrectal microwave hyperthermia in poor surgical risk benign prostatic hyperplasia patients. *J. Urol.* **146**, 353–7.

Straube, W.L., Klein, E.E., Moros, E.G., Low, D.A. and Myerson, R.J. (2001) Dosimetry and techniques for simultaneous hyperthermia and external beam radiation therapy. *Int. J. Hyperthermia* **17**, 48–62.

Sugimachi, K., Kitamura, K., Baba, K. *et al.* (1992) Hyperthermia combined with chemotherapy and irradiation for patients with carcinoma of the oesophagus – a prospective randomized trial. *Int. J. Hyperthermia* **8**(3), 289–95.

Suit, H.D. (1982) Potential for improving survival rates for cancer patients by improving efficiency of treatment of primary lesion. *Cancer* **50**, 1227–34.

Takahashi, M., Fujimot, S., Kobayashi, K. *et al.* (1994) Clinical outcome of intraoperative pelvic hyperthermochemotherapy for patients with Dukes' C rectal cancer. *Int. J. Hyperthermia* **10**, 749–54.

Ueo, H. and Sugimachi, K (1990) Preoperative hyperthermochemoradiotherapy for patients with esophageal carcinoma or rectal carcinoma. *Seminars in Surgical Oncology* **6**, 8–13.

Valdagni, R. and Amichetti, M. (1994) Report of long term follow-up in a randomised trial comparing radiation therapy and radiation therapy plus hyperthermia for to metastatic neck nodes in stage IV head and neck patients *Int. J. Radiat. Oncol. Biol. Phys.* **28**, 163–9.

Valdagni, R., Amichetti, M. and Pani, G. (1988) Radical radiation alone versus radical radiation plus microwave hyperthermia for N3 (TNM-UICC) neck nodes: a prospective randomized clinical trial. *Int. J. Radiat. Oncol. Biol. Phys.* **15**, 13–24.

Van de Kamer, J.B., De Leeuw, A.A., Hornsleth, S.N. *et al.* (2001) Development of a regional hyperthermia treatment planning system. *Int. J. Hyperthermia* **17**, 207–20.

van der Zee, J., van Putten, W.J.L., van den Berg, A.P. *et al.* (1986) Retrospective analysis of the response of tumours in patients treated with a combination of radiotherapy and hyperthermia. *Int. J. Hyperthermia* **2**(4), 337–49.

van der Zee, J., Gonzalez-Gonzalez, D., Vernon, C.C. *et al.* (1998) Therapeutic gain by hyperthermia added to radiotherapy. *Progress in Radio-Oncology* **VI**, 137–45.

van der Zee, J., Gonzalez-Gonzalez, D., van Rhoon, G., van Dijk, J., van Putten, W. and Har, A. (2000) Comparison of radiotherapy alone with radiotherapy plus hyperthermia in locally advanced pelvis tumours: a prospective randomised, multicentre trial. *Lancet* **355**, 1119–25.

Van Leeuwen, G.M.J., Kotte, A.N. and Lagendijk, J.J.W. (1998) A flexible algorithm for construction of 3-D vessel networks for use in thermal modeling. *IEEE Trans. Biomed. Eng.* **45**, 596–604.

Van Leeuwen, G.M.J., Kotte, A.N.T.J., Raaymakers, B.W. and Lagendijk, J.J.W. (2000) Temperature simulations in tissue with a realistic computer generated vessel network. *Phys. Med. Biol.* **45**, 1035–49.

Van Wieringen, N., Van Dijk, J.D.P., Nieuwenhuys, G.J. *et al.* (1996) Power absorption and temperature control of multi-filament palladium-nickel thermoseeds for interstitial hyperthermia. *Phys. Med. Biol.* **41**(11), 2367–80.

Vernon, C.C., Hand, J.W., Field, S.B. *et al.* (1996) Radiotherapy with or without hyperthermia in the treatment of superficial localised breast cancer – results from 5 randomised controlled trials. *Int. J. Radiat. Oncol. Biol. Phys.* **35**, 731–44.

Visser, A.G. and Van Rhoon, G.C. (1995) Technical and clinical quality assurance. In Seegenschmiedt, M.H., Fessenden, P. and Vernon, C.C. (eds), *Thermo-radiotherapy and thermo-chemotherapy*, vol. 1. Heidelberg/Berlin: Springer, 453–72.

Waterman, F.M. (1995) Invasive thermometry techniques. In Seegenschmiedt, M.H., Fessenden, P. and Vernon, C.C. (eds), *Thermo-radiotherapy and Thermo-chemotherapy*, vol. 1. Heidelberg/Berlin: Springer, 331–60.

Wessalowski, R., Kruck, H., Pape, H., Kahn, T., Willers, R. and Göbel, R (1998) Hyperthermia for the treatment of patients with malignant germ cell tumors. A phase I/II study in ten children and adolescents with recurrent or refractory tumors. *Cancer* **82**, 793–800.

Wiedemann, G.J., d'Oleire, F., Knop, E. *et al.* (1994) Ifosfamide and carboplatin combined with 41.8°C whole-body hyperthermia in patients with refractory sarcoma and malignant teratoma. *Cancer Res.* **54**, 5346–50.

Wiedemann, G.J., Robins, H.I., Gutsche, S. *et al.* (1996) Ifosfamide, carboplatin, and etoposide (ICE) combined with 41.8°C whole-body hyperthermia in patients with refractory sarcoma. *Eur. J. Cancer* **32A**, 888–91.

Wlodarczyk, W., Boroschewski, R., Hentschel, M. *et al.* (1998) Three-dimensional monitoring of small temperature changes for therapeutic hyperthermia using MR. *J. Magn. Reson. Imaging* **8**(1), 165–74.

Wlodarczyk, W., Hentschel, M., Wust, P. *et al.* (1999) Comparison of four magnetic resonance methods for mapping small temperature changes. *Phys. Med. Biol.* **44**(2), 607–24.

Wust, P., Nadobny, J., Seebass, M. *et al.* (1999) Influence of patient models and numerical methods on predicted power deposition patterns. *Int. J. Hyperthermia* **15**, 519–40.

7

Principles of chemotherapy and drug development

PAUL A. VASEY AND JEFFRY EVANS

BASIC PRINCIPLES

Chemotherapy drugs are developed for their potential to cause a greater proportion of cell death among neoplastic as opposed to normal cells. Differences exist between normal and malignant cells which result in the latter being more susceptible to anti-cancer drugs by virtue both of their biological and proliferation characteristics.

Cancer cell kinetics

CHARACTERISTICS OF THE TUMOUR CELL

The proliferation of tumour cells is not entirely autonomous and there is increasing evidence of local control by autocrine and paracrine factors produced by the tumour cells and the stroma. The rate of proliferation during the lifetime of a tumour is not constant (Fig. 7.1). In experimental tumours in the early stages, growth is exponential and the growth fraction is high. As the tumour enlarges, the growth rate slows and the growth fraction falls. Deceleration of growth is commonly observed for transplantable tumours in animals and is probably as a result, in part, from decreasing tumour vascularity and cellular nutrition, leading to slowing of cell proliferation, and also as a result of cell loss due to death or differentiation. The smallest tumour that is likely to be clinically detectable (either by physical or radiological assessments) will be approximately 1 cm in diameter and will contain 10^8–10^9 tumour cells, depending on the contribution of stroma and other elements to tumour bulk, and growth

of these small, clinically detectable tumours follows a Gompertzian pattern (Fig. 7.1). Such a tumour will have undergone approximately 30 doublings in cell number if it is clonally derived from a single transformed cell, and will usually weigh about 1 g. Growth to a potentially lethal mass of 1 kg of tumour requires only a further 10 doublings of cell number. Thus the period of tumour growth that is clinically apparent is only a relatively short period in the total life history of a tumour and, clearly, the potential exists for micrometastases to develop before detection of the primary tumour.

The effect of chemotherapy on a tumour is influenced by some of the features of its growth pattern:

- response to chemotherapy is proportional to the number of cells synthesizing DNA;

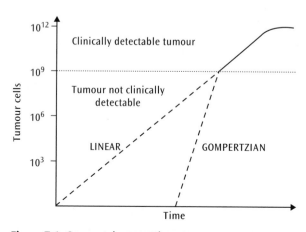

Figure 7.1 *Gompertzian growth curve.*

- the shorter the doubling time at the onset of treatment (i.e. the more rapid is tumour growth), the better the response to chemotherapy since more cells will be synthesizing DNA;
- as the tumour grows, the disease becomes less easy to cure;
- as the tumour shrinks with treatment, the growth rate increases because of the Gompertzian growth pattern.

CELL CYCLE

All proliferating cells go through a series of events that comprise the cell cycle (Fig. 7.2). The division of the cell cycle into discrete phases followed the demonstration that DNA synthesis took place during a defined time interval, rather than continuously during interphase. After mitosis (M), the cell spends a variable resting period (G_1), during which DNA synthesis does not occur but RNA and protein are produced. Entry to the S-phase is heralded by an increase in RNA synthesis followed by doubling of the DNA content. The G_2-phase follows as DNA synthesis ceases, and is followed by mitosis.

The total duration of the cell cycle depends mainly on the duration of the G_1-phase which may be 0–30 hours. The duration of the S-phase (6–8 hours), M-phase (less than 1 hour) and G_2-phase (2–4 hours) are fairly constant in both normal and malignant cells. Consequently, the cycle of a malignant cell may last between 9 and 43 hours. For aggressive, highly proliferative tumours the cell cycle will be at the shorter end of the time span, but for more indolent low-grade tumours the cell cycle will be significantly longer. The mean cycle time of cells within human tumours is typically much shorter than the mean volume doubling time of the tumours for two main reasons: a high rate of cell death, and a high rate of non-proliferating cells. The term G_0 is applied to cells which are out of cycle. The proportion of cells within a population that is undergoing active proliferation in the cycle is termed the growth fraction. Estimates of growth fraction, calculated by comparing the measured proportion of cells in S-phase with that predicted from the phase distribution of cycling cells, are consistently of the order of 20–30 per cent. This is particularly relevant as most anti-cancer drugs do not cause cell death during the G_0-phase. Furthermore, although higher proportions of S-phase cells are found in some rapidly growing tumours, such as high-grade lymphomas, most tumours do not have a higher proportion of S-phase cells than some normal highly proliferative tissue, such as bone marrow and intestinal crypt cells.

Mathematical models have been developed to describe the interaction of cytotoxic chemotherapy and tumour growth kinetics and may be used to evaluate hypothetical strategies for cancer treatment (Birkhead *et al.*, 1987).

ANTI-CANCER DRUGS AND THE CELL CYCLE

Cytotoxic chemotherapy agents have traditionally been classified as phase- or non-phase-specific, depending on the effect on the cell cycle (Table 7.1). *In vitro* models demonstrate that phase-dependent drugs kill cells exponentially at lower doses but reach a plateau when given at a higher dose because they are only able to kill cells in a specific part of the cell cycle. Non-phase-dependent drugs kill cells exponentially with increasing dose, and are equally toxic for both cycling cells and those in G_0. The practical value of this classification is somewhat limited, in that chemotherapy regimens designed on kinetic principles have so far shown no advantage over those derived empirically.

SKIPPER HYPOTHESIS FOR CELL KILL BY CYTOTOXIC AGENTS

In the early 1960s, Skipper *et al.* (1964) formulated some principles of tumour cell kill on the basis of experiments using the L1210 murine leukaemia model:

1. The survival of an animal is inversely related to the tumour burden.
2. A single leukaemic cell is capable of multiplying to kill the host.

Table 7.1 *Cytotoxic drugs and the cell cycle*

Predominantly non-phase-specific agents	Predominantly phase-specific agents
Nitrogen mustards	Methotrexate
Cyclophosphamide	Cytosine arabinoside
Melphalan	6-Mercaptopurine
Chlorambucil	6-Thioguanine
Busulfan	Vincristine
Thiotepa	Vinblastine
5-Fluorouracil	Bleomycin
Doxorubicin	Etoposide
Mitomycin C	Procarbazine
Dacarbazine	
Actinomycin D	

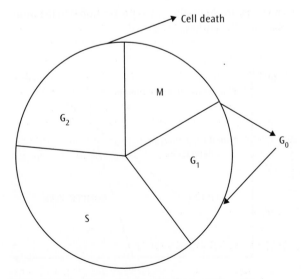

Figure 7.2 *The cell cycle. M, mitosis; S, DNA synthesis.*

3 For most drugs there is a clear relationship between dose of drug and eradication of tumour cells.

4 Cell destruction by anti-cancer drugs follow log kill kinetics. That is, a given dose of drug kills a constant fraction of cells and not a constant number. Thus, if a particular dose of an individual drug kills 3 logs of cells and reduces the tumour burden from 10^{10} to 10^7 cells, the same dose used at a tumour burden of 10^5 will reduce the tumour burden to 10^2 cells. The cell kill is therefore proportional regardless of tumour burden.

These principles established that there is an inverse relationship between cell number and curability and implies that tumours are best treated when they are small in volume. Furthermore, if drug treatment is discontinued as soon as the tumour is no longer clinically detectable, at least 10^9 tumour cells remain and relapse is inevitable. However, these observations should be considered in the context of the growth differences between this murine leukaemia model and human cancers. For example, L1210 leukaemia is a rapidly growing tumour, with a high percentage of cells in S-phase, and a growth fraction of 100 per cent, giving a consistent and predictable cell cycle. In contrast, the cell cycles of human tumours are heterogeneous, prolonged and with a smaller growth fraction.

Overall the evidence favours a Gompertzian growth pattern with a growth fraction that is not constant and with an exponential decrease in growth as the tumour enlarges. Nevertheless, Gompertzian kinetics also supports the notion that chemotherapy is more likely to be effective in eradicating a small tumour burden. When the tumour burden is small (such as when no longer clinically detectable), its growth fraction would be at its largest, and the proportional cell kill would be larger. This is one of the principles that forms the basis of adjuvant chemotherapy strategies.

NORTON–SIMON HYPOTHESIS

In tumours that show Gompertzian-type growth curves, the rate of regrowth increases as the tumour shrinks with therapy. Thus, the level of treatment necessary to initiate a regression may be insufficient to maintain the regression and produce cure. Norton and Simon (1977) hypothesized that to overcome the slowing rate of regression in a tumour responding to therapy, it was necessary to increase the intensity of treatment as the tumour became smaller. This can be achieved in one of two ways:

1 increase the dose intensity of the chemotherapy agents used to induce remission; and
2 switch to alternative cytotoxic agents in an aggressive schedule.

Dose intensity is commonly used in leukaemia, where agents such as cytosine arabinoside are used in high-dose pulses after the induction of remission. In addition, high-dose chemotherapy with bone marrow transplantation or peripheral blood stem-cell harvesting with growth factor support is another means of achieving dose intensity. The concept of dose intensity is discussed more fully in Section 7.1.2.

Alternatively the use of alternative cytotoxic agents in hybrid regimens, such as MOPP–ABVD for Hodgkin's disease (Glick et al., 1998), not only exposes the tumour to drugs different from those used to achieve induction or remission, but also targets residual populations of cells which are biochemically resistant to the initial combination of drugs.

GOLDIE–COLDMAN MODEL

Spontaneous mutation is a basic property of DNA. There is also evidence that tumour cells may be more genetically unstable than normal cells. In 1979 Goldie and Coldman proposed a model to explain the genetically determined resistance to cancer chemotherapy based on this principle (Goldie and Coldman, 1979). They proposed that populations of cells within a tumour are capable of randomly mutating and becoming resistant to the cytotoxic agents. These spontaneous mutations occur at population sizes of less than 10^6 tumour cells, which is less than the clinically detectable level. As such mutations occur at frequencies of 10^{-6} or higher, then a clinically detectable tumour of 10^9 cells is likely to have several drug-resistant clones. However, the absolute number of resistant cells would be relatively small and these tumours would probably respond initially to treatment with a complete or partial remission, only to relapse and re-appear when the resistant clone(s) expand, a clinical picture that is familiar in oncology practice. Some tumours are resistant to cytotoxic chemotherapy agents even when they present with a relatively small tumour volume. However, such slow-growing tumours may have considerable cell loss through cell death, up to 90 per cent of the tumour volume. Therefore what appears to be an early tumour may have gone through many more cell doublings than expected in order to compensate for cell loss in achieving that size. Consequently, these cells may have undergone a higher frequency of spontaneous mutations, leading to a tumour that consists predominantly of drug-resistant clones.

However, there are many other mechanisms of drug resistance, including decreased uptake due to changes in drug-specific transport mechanisms, decreased activation of pro-drugs, alterations in cellular metabolism and repair mechanisms, increased inactivation of drugs, target alterations and acquisition of a multi-drug resistance phenotype. Drug resistance is discussed more fully in Chapter 8.

Principles of treatment

ROUTE OF ADMINISTRATION

The route of administration of a cytotoxic drug is determined by the stability, size, molecular charge and sclerosant characteristics of that drug. Traditionally, the oral route has been used infrequently because of the unpredictability of patient compliance and variable absorption of the drug. However, the desire to move cancer treatment from a predominantly hospital-based, inpatient system into the ambulatory setting, together with a growing body of information showing higher anti-tumour activity or lower systemic toxicity with dosing regimens that produce prolonged exposure to some cancer agents, suggests that oral cancer chemotherapy may be increasingly of interest in the future. This has already led to the evaluation of oral administration of anti-cancer drugs that have been available for many years (e.g. etoposide, idarubicin) as well as novel strategies for oral use of anti-cancer drugs traditionally given intravenously, for example the oral fluoropyrimidines (McLeod and Evans, 1999). Subcutaneous and intramuscular routes are rarely employed because large volumes of diluent are frequently required to dissolve the drug or because, once dissolved, they are often highly toxic to tissues in the extravascular compartments.

For the majority of cytotoxic drugs, the intravenous route is the optimal means of delivery for most indications, and they can be administered by bolus injection, short infusions or protracted venous infusion, usually through an indwelling central venous catheter in the latter case (*see* p. 107). Other routes of administration that can be used for specific indications include the intrathecal administration of non-sclerosant water-soluble drugs such as methotrexate or cytosine arabinoside to palliate or prevent meningeal disease; intra-arterial administration of drugs via the hepatic artery to achieve high doses of drug to be delivered locally or in chemo-embolization strategies; intra-arterial administration in isolated limb perfusion in melanoma or sarcoma; intravesical administration in reducing recurrence rates of superficial bladder cancers; and intraperitoneal administration to small tumour nodules on the peritoneal surface.

COMBINATION CHEMOTHERAPY

Based on the cancer cell kinetics data, it is reasonable to assume that even small tumours, when clinically detectable, already have resistant clone(s) of cells. The use of cytotoxic agents of different groups in combination should give a broader range of cover of resistant cell lines in a heterogeneous tumour population, and prevent or slow the development of new resistant cell lines, thereby giving maximum cell kill not possible with a single-agent regimen.

There are four general principles which guide the selection of drugs for use in effective combination chemotherapy regimens:

1 Each drug should have activity against the tumour when used alone, with those drugs with maximal efficacy most preferable.

2 Drugs should have different mechanisms of action.
3 Drugs should have minimal overlapping toxicities. When several drugs of a class are available, a drug should be selected with minimal overlapping toxicity, which, although leading to a greater range of side-effects, decreases the risk of potentially life-threatening cumulative toxicity to the same organ system.
4 Each drug in a combination should be used in its optimal dose and schedule.

However, it should also be noted that omission of a drug from an effective combination may allow overgrowth of a cell line that is sensitive to that drug alone and resistant to the other drugs in the combination. Conversely, adding too many drugs to a regimen with the aim of increasing efficacy may reduce the doses of some, or all, of the component drugs of the combination below the threshold of efficacy, thereby decreasing activity of the regimen.

DOSE AND DOSE INTENSITY

Within experimental systems it is easy to demonstrate the dose–response effect of anti-cancer drugs on cancer cells. This relationship is more difficult to demonstrate and quantify in patients due to the heterogeneity of tumour responses and also because of the variability of drug absorption, binding, distribution, metabolism, excretion and delivery of the drug to the tumour. Nevertheless, a positive dose–response relationship has been demonstrated in retrospective studies (Hryniuk and Levine, 1986), and also in prospective studies in advanced ovarian, breast and colon cancers, and in the lymphomas (DeVita *et al.*, 1987; Hryniuk, 1987; Levin and Hryniuk, 1987; Kaye *et al.*, 1992).

In experimental models, the dose–response relationship is a steep linear relationship and the principles of chemotherapy include exploiting the differences between the dose–response curves of normal and tumour tissue. Reduction of doses in this linear phase of the dose–response curve in experimental models results in a decreased cure rate before there is a reduction in the response rate. Although complete remissions are still observed in these animal tumours, a few residual cells will not be killed and ultimately repopulate, leading to relapse. It has been suggested that in these experimental models, a dose reduction of 20 per cent will lead to a loss in the cure rate in excess of 50 per cent (Skipper, 1986; DeVita *et al.*, 1987). Conversely, in high growth-fraction tumours, a twofold increase in dose often leads to a tenfold increase (1 log) in tumour cell kill. This not only reinforces the desire to minimize the reductions in recommended doses, but also justifies efforts to increase dose to aim for increased cure rates in chemosensitive tumours. The principal restriction to dose escalation is toxicity of normal tissues. When myelosuppression is the dose-limiting toxicity, this can be overcome by use of recombinant bone-marrow growth factors such as g-csf, by bone marrow transplantation, or by haemopoietic support using peripheral blood progenitor cells. Ultimately, dose escalation of these agents (and those agents which have non-bone-marrow dose-limiting toxicities) will be restricted by toxicities to tissues such as myocardium, lungs and kidneys, for which there is no currently available means to overcome toxicity. Consequently, the number of drugs that can be used in dose-escalation strategies are few, as are the tumour types that demonstrate a dose response to these agents.

SCHEDULING OF CYTOTOXIC CHEMOTHERAPY

The concentration of a cytotoxic agent in plasma or in tissue does not depend on total dose only but also on the schedule of administration, that is, it is believed that 'drug exposure' as measured by the area under the concentration–time curve (AUC) is a crucial determinant of drug activity in many situations. In a series of classical experiments with the L1210 murine leukaemia model, Goldin and Schabel (1981) demonstrated that methotrexate was more effective and less toxic when administered to mice in an intermittent rather than a daily regimen, and this observation has also been noted in clinical practice.

Scheduling is also a determinant of achieving dose intensity. Hryniuk and colleagues have defined dose intensity as the amount of drug delivered per unit time, expressed as mg/m^2 per week (Levin and Hryniuk, 1987). Relative dose intensity is the amount of drug delivered per unit time relative to an arbitrarily chosen standard single drug, or, for a combination regimen, the fraction of the ratio of the test regimen to the standard regimen. In this way, treatment delays are given equal consideration to dose reductions when calculating dose intensity. Clearly, if the time interval between successive courses of chemotherapy is too prolonged, then this can allow repopulation of cancer cells which may well have acquired resistance to the cytotoxic agents to which they have been exposed. If the time interval is too short, then toxicity in normal tissues may be unacceptable. Consequently, scheduling may influence outcome by affecting toxicity, allowing greater doses to be administered over the same time frame. In this regard, accurate scheduling is also required to rescue normal tissues from the toxic side-effects of certain chemotherapy drugs; for example, higher doses of methotrexate can be administered to patients during 24 hours when a sufficient flow of alkaline urine is maintained and by rescue of normal tissues by giving folinic acid titrated to the plasma concentration of methotrexate. Similarly, scheduling of individual cytotoxic agents can enhance response rates, e.g. when 5-FU (5-fluorouracil) is given as a continuous intravenous infusion rather than by intermittent boluses (Lokich *et al.*, 1989; Anderson, 1993), and also in exploiting potential interactions between cytotoxic drugs to achieve optimal synergistic effects.

DRUG DEVELOPMENT

Although many of the agents currently in use were developed by a combination of science and serendipity, the acquisition and evolution of novel agents is generally the result of both carefully thought-out screening processes, and the exponentially increasing knowledge of the molecular basis of carcinogenesis and cellular metabolism. Figure 7.3 outlines the steps involved in anti-cancer drug development. Criteria for selecting new anti-cancer drugs can include:

- novel chemical entity
- novel mechanism of action
- selective for solid tumours
- *in vivo* activity in solid tumour models
- evidence for a positive therapeutic index
- feasibility of supply.

The serendipitous discovery of active anti-cancer agents has accounted for many important drugs. In the

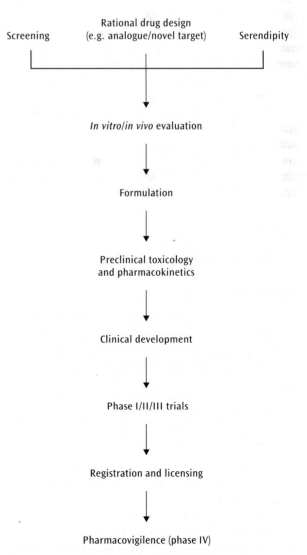

Figure 7.3 *Steps in anti-cancer drug development.*

mid-1960s, Rosenberg was studying the effects of electric currents on the growth of bacterial cultures. He noted that the application of an alternating voltage reduced the growth rate of the bacteria, and that this effect was due to the formation of platinum complexes in the growth medium due to dissolution of platinum from the electrodes. Neutral platinum complexes exhibited a relatively selective effect on rapidly dividing bacterial cells, and therefore these compounds were tested as anti-cancer agents. Platinum was thus found to have significant anti-tumour activity in these tests and subsequently also on a wide variety of animal models.

Another way in which new agents are appropriated is by chemically modifying an existing active agent that may otherwise have restricted utility because of toxicity. The term 'structure–activity relationship' describes the link between varying specific chemical substructures on the parent compound and differential anti-tumour activity. Analogue development is aimed primarily at producing:

1 a drug either as effective as the parent compound, with significantly less toxicity;
2 a more potent drug; or
3 one with a different spectrum of anti-tumour activity.

Examples of successful analogues are epirubicin (from doxorubicin), carboplatin (from cisplatin), topotecan or CPT-11 (from camptothecin).

It is expected that more active agents will be developed as a result of the increasing understanding of the biochemical and biological behaviour of cancer cells. Certainly, focusing on a defined molecular target and using computers to design and construct molecules that would interact and antagonize these targets would increase the potential selectivity for such an agent. However, empirical drug screening for novel agents will continue to play a major role into the twenty-first century.

Acquisition of drugs

SCREENING

Large-scale, empirical screening for the discovery of new anti-cancer agents was initiated by the National Cancer Institute (NCI) of the United States in 1955. During the next 20 years, nearly half a million potential anti-cancer agents of natural or synthetic origin were screened, producing over 50 per cent of all clinically useful agents. This screen used a tumour panel with two models being used primarily – murine leukaemia L1210 and P388. In the mid-1980s it was decided to change this leukaemia-based strategy because:

1 not many drugs were discovered with broad activity against common solid tumours;
2 agents inactive against P388 were often active in other preclinical models, and vice versa; and
3 many active agents, e.g. bleomycin, were inactive against P388.

The NCI disease-oriented *in vitro* screen has been used regularly since 1991. Here, human tumour cell lines derived from seven common cancers have been selected and maintained for use as a test-bed for novel agent sensitivity. Such a screen could theoretically speed up the process of clinical development for agents found to be differentially sensitive to a particular tumour type. Secondary *in vitro* studies may be used in order to examine the effects of schedule, exposure and potential mechanisms of action. Finally, *in vivo* testing is carried out, generally using the most sensitive human tumour cell line as a subcutaneous xenograft in a nude mouse.

FORMULATION

An intravenous formulation is generally preferred for preclinical studies, in order to exclude variations in bioavailability and to enable promising drugs to be used at their maximum tolerated dose (MTD). Solubility is also very important, as limited solubility is regularly a reason to discontinue overall development of an agent. Various approaches and experimental methods for solubilization are being used, in addition to techniques such as liposomal encapsulation, conjugation to polymers and other delivery systems which could empower the clinical evaluation of a promising agent. However, these means of solubilizing the drug may alter the toxicity profile and/or the anti-tumour efficacy.

Toxicological and pharmacological testing

Unlike other drugs in clinical use, cytotoxic agents have very narrow therapeutic windows, i.e. the most biologically active doses are often close to the lethal doses. It is therefore necessary to try to predict the potential toxic effects, and also to define a safe (but still potentially active) starting dose prior to human studies. Animal studies are often done using two species. In Europe, an accepted method for obtaining the safe dose for human clinical trials is defined as one-tenth the dose which is lethal to 10 per cent of mice (called the LD_{10}), providing this dose is safe in another species, e.g. rat. However, it is important to note that animal toxicities do not always predict for similar toxicity in humans. It is rarely necessary to perform additional tests on larger animals (e.g. dogs, monkeys), although some data suggest that these species are more able to predict certain human toxicities. Additional toxicological studies are undertaken in order to evaluate more fully any organ toxicity demonstrated in the animals, and to investigate any relationships with dose, schedule and whether any documented effects are potentially reversible. Single-dose and multiple-dose studies are undertaken, in order to mimic more accurately the anticipated human trial protocols. Finally, pharmacological studies derive knowledge about bioavailability, metabolism, route of excretion, etc., and allow rational schedule design for the clinical testing of the agent.

Clinical testing

For many anti-cancer drugs a dose–response relationship is observed in preclinical studies, and this knowledge is subsequently integrated into the design of the initial clinical studies. There are three stages (phases) of clinical studies used for the evaluation of a novel compound.

PHASE I TRIALS

Phase I studies are concerned with the first exposure of a novel agent to humans. The primary objective is to establish the MTD by an escalating dose protocol, and to document the toxicity profile of the agent at the chosen dose, schedule and route of administration. However, one of the goals of preclinical studies is to try and predict a phase I starting dose close to the agent's therapeutic window. Despite this, it has been noted that clinical response rates in phase I trials are less than 5 per cent overall. This raises ethical dilemmas, particularly with respect to informed consent. However, these studies are conducted in a patient population deemed to have disease that is refractory to standard chemotherapy, or have disease for which there is no known effective treatment. Anti-cancer efficacy is therefore necessarily a secondary end point, and the first patients are often unfortunately treated at subtherapeutic doses. Research on study designs that decrease the number of patients treated at subtherapeutic doses is ongoing, and include the accelerated titration design and continual reassessment method (CRM). The former design allows for one patient per dose level in the early stages, provided no significant toxicity is encountered. CRM allows for intra-patient dose escalation. Both designs may be useful, provided that data on toxicity are always as up to date as possible. In most trials, however, patients (generally three) are treated at the first dose level, and monitored for toxicity. Subsequent patients are entered at the next dose level (cohort) and so on, until significant toxicity is encountered. Historically, the degree of dose escalation is based on a modified Fibonacci scheme (e.g. dose level 2 is twice dose level 1; level 3, 67 per cent of level 2; level 4, 50 per cent of level 3). Some studies have used a pharmacokinetically guided scheme, using target AUCs. All studies incorporate pharmacokinetic and pharmacodynamic studies, and assessments of biological end points are often included (e.g. inhibition of a target enzyme). Dose-limiting toxicities (DLTs) are defined, and once the MTD has been reached at a particular dose level, the previous lower dose level is generally expanded to a larger cohort of patients and becomes the recommended dose for further studies. Any anti-tumour activity documented may also be useful in planning subsequent phase II studies.

PHASE II TRIALS

These studies are conducted using the dose and schedules from phase I studies considered to be optimal in terms of pharmacology and therapeutic index (i.e. near to the MTD). The stated objective of phase II trials is to determine a level of efficacy for the drug in question, and therefore patients with measurable disease are selected. In addition, patients are less heavily pretreated, in order to select a patient population with the best chance of demonstrating anti-tumour activity, if it exists. Phase II studies may be directed towards specific tumour types, based upon any responses seen in phase I studies, or a well-defined spectrum of preclinical activity. Further information on drug toxicity is gathered, and specific data on cumulative toxicity are acquired, because more patients are likely to receive multiple cycles of treatment. Phase II trials are designed to allow early study termination if a drug is proving to have no or minimal efficacy. Designs such as the Gehan two-stage model allow a number of patients to be accrued (generally 14), and if one or more response is documented, recruitment proceeds to a total of 25 patients. If no responses are documented in these first 14 patients, the trial terminates. A response rate of 20 per cent may be considered worthy of further evaluation; however, this should relate to the patient population being tested. If performed in patients with a relatively chemoresistant malignancy, pretreated with 'standard' chemotherapy, the likelihood of detecting activity may be prejudiced. Another design is to randomize patients to the experimental treatment and a drug with known activity in the disease (e.g. the parent compound of a novel analogue), or even to another experimental agent. Such studies will not be powered to determine efficacy differences, but may give a baseline response rate for the patient population being selected. Finally, new active agents are often subsequently added to other standard therapies in two-, or three-drug combination regimens. These need to be piloted as feasibility/phase I type studies to ensure that toxicity is neither additive nor synergistic.

PHASE III TRIALS

The next stage of testing for a novel agent is to compare against the existing standard therapy. The most scientifically valid method is by a prospective, randomized clinical trial, in which patients eligible for the protocol are randomly assigned to one of the treatment arms. Suitable end points for a phase III study include progression-free survival (PFS), overall survival (OS) and overall response rate (ORR). Data on quality of life and comparative toxicities are also collected, in order to determine the overall clinical benefit of a treatment. Stratification for known prognostic factors is carried out to ensure that the arms of the study are statistically balanced. Such procedures do not ensure that the study will include a representative sample of the general population with the disease, but can provide evaluation of the relative merits of the treatments being compared. Variations on the simple randomized study format include:

1 the crossover design, which allows patients relapsing on one treatment to receive the other drug, therefore using the patient as his/her own control; and
2 the 2×2 factorial design, wherein the first factor may be a comparison between two treatments (e.g. the novel agent versus standard therapy), and the second factor two interventions consequent on the first factor (e.g. maintenance treatment or not).

Phase III trials are generally large, consisting of hundreds of patients, because the differences between treatments may be small and therefore increasing sample size increases the chance of small differences in outcome being statistically significant.

CLASSIFICATION OF CYTOTOXIC DRUGS, MODE OF ACTION, TOXICITIES AND CLINICAL UTILITY

Historically, anti-cancer agents have been divided into groups according to the mechanism of cytotoxicity. However, the increasing number of new drugs, and their diverse and novel mechanisms of action, make such divisions increasingly difficult and arbitrary (Table 7.2).

DNA alkylators

The alkylating agents were the first compounds identified to have activity against neoplastic diseases, and have been in use now for over 50 years. Early studies used the nitrogen mustard mechlorethamine, following on from observations from the mustard gas chemical warfare programme that soldiers exposed to this agent developed aplasia of the bone marrow. Mechlorethamine was subsequently found to induce significant tumour regression in patients with lymphoma in clinical trials.

Mechlorethamine is ideally suited to illustrate the chemistry of alkylation, having the simplest structure of the class (Fig. 7.4). The $-CH_2CH_2Cl$ linked to nitrogen is labelled the mustard group, and in the case of mechlorethamine there are two such groups, thus giving the term 'bifunctional nitrogen mustard'. Following administration, the drug undergoes an internal cyclization reaction and loses a chloride ion to form an electron-deficient, positively charged aziridinium ion. These highly reactive species are able to react and form covalent bonds ('adducts') with electron-rich (nucleophilic) sites in DNA, such as the 7-nitrogen group of guanine on the major groove. Other biological macromolecules, e.g. proteins, are also targeted, but it is the reactions involving the nitrogenous bases in DNA which are critical for the anti-cancer action of the alkylating agents. Adduct formation

Table 7.2 *A classification of chemotherapy agents*

Class	Examples
Alkylators	Mechlorethamine
	Melphalan
	Chlorambucil
	Cyclophosphamide
	Ifosfamide
	BCNU/CCNU
	Busulfan/treosulfan
	Thiotepa
	Mitomycin C
	Dacarbazine
	Hexamethylmelamine
	Procarbazine
	Cisplatin/carboplatin/oxaliplatin
Antimetabolites	Methotrexate
	Raltitrexed
	5-Fluorouracil
	UFT
	6-MP/6-TG
	Cytosine arabinoside
	Gemcitabine
Antibiotics	Doxorubicin/daunorubicin/epirubicin
	DaunoXome™/Caelyx™
	Mitoxantrone
	Bleomycin
	Actinomycin D
Plant-derived	Vincristine/vinblastine/vindesine/ vinorelbine
	Paclitaxel/docetaxel
	Topotecan/irinotecan
	Etoposide
Miscellaneous	L-Asparaginase
	Hydroxyurea
	Bryostatin
	Ecteinascidin 743
	Aplidine

BCNU, 1,3-*bis*(2-chloroethyl)-1-nitrosurea; CCNU, 1-(2-chlorothyl)-3-cyclohexyl-1-nitrosurea; UFT, uracil/Tegafor; 6-MP, 6-mercaptopurine; 6-TG, 6-thioguanine.

with two separate bases on the DNA, especially across the two antiparallel strands – the inter-strand crosslink – is thought to be the most lethal interaction. The results of DNA alkylation involve interference with the fidelity of replication and transcription by abrogating the functions of DNA and RNA polymerases. It follows that alkylating agents are most toxic to rapidly cycling cells; tumours with a high fraction of cells in S-phase are more vulnerable, possibly as they have less damage-repair time. In addition, adduct formation leads to structural lesions, which include ring opening and base deletions. Cellular repair processes attempt to restore the integrity of the DNA, but if incomplete can result in further damage, such as the creation of apurinic sites or strand breaks. Furthermore, it appears that these repair processes may be able to

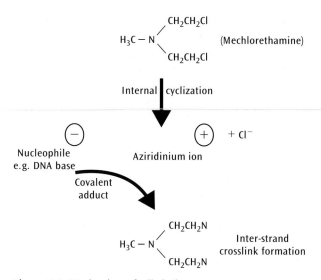

Figure 7.4 *Mechanism of alkylation.*

be saturated by higher doses of alkylating agents, thus providing a rationale for extending the use of these agents into high-dose chemotherapy techniques.

MECHLORETHAMINE (NITROGEN MUSTARD, MUSTINE)

Mechlorethamine is administered intravenously, and has a half-life of approximately 3 minutes due to rapid hydrolysation. It is has extremely vesicant properties, and may also cause severe phlebitis and sclerosis of the vein used. A usual dose is 6 mg/m^2, and the major use is in the treatment of Hodgkin's disease, as part of the combination MOPP (nitrogen mustard, vincristine, procarbazine and prednisolone). It is also occasionally administered by direct intra-cavity infusion for the treatment of malignant effusions.

MELPHALAN

Melphalan is another bifunctional alkylating agent, and is a phenylalanine derivative of mechlorethamine. It is active against a broad cross-section of tumours (lymphomas, breast and ovarian cancers, multiple myeloma) and can be administered orally, intravenously or intraperitoneally. Although the oral bioavailability is variable, with 20–50 per cent being excreted in the stool, the ease of oral administration makes this the most common route employed. It routinely causes myelosuppression, with nadir counts occurring at 4–5 weeks following a short 7-day oral course. Doses require to be adjusted according to the level of myelosuppression, and 10 mg daily is a usual starting dose. It is also used in high-dose chemotherapy regimens for haematological malignancies and multiple myeloma, due to exponential cell killing demonstrated in cell culture. Occasionally, it is used intraperitoneally for relapsed ovarian cancer, although efficacy data are not well established.

CHLORAMBUCIL

This bifunctional alkylating agent is a benzene butanoic derivative of mechlorethamine, and is also a close structural congener of melphalan. It is almost completely absorbed when given by the oral route, and is used either continuously or intermittently for long periods in low-grade lymphoma, chronic lymphocytic leukaemia and multiple myeloma. It can also be given to elderly patients with ovarian cancer who are unable to tolerate more aggressive chemotherapy. Doses are usually 5–10 mg daily, and the toxicity is a predictable myelosuppression, which makes dose adjustments fairly straightforward. However, stem-cell damage is cumulative and irreversible, leading to problems of severe myelosuppression with subsequent cytotoxic drug use. Longer-term use (e.g. >1 year) has been associated with pulmonary toxicity and the development of second malignancies.

OXAZAPHOSPHORINES (CYCLOPHOSPHAMIDE AND IFOSFAMIDE)

Cyclophosphamide differs from the previously described alkylating agents in that it is a pro-drug, requiring activation to develop cytotoxicity. It undergoes a complex multistep activation process, initially being metabolized by the cytochrome P450 system in the liver and eventually converted to a variety of active metabolites, of which phosphoramide mustard is thought to be the major cytotoxic derivative. One of the main metabolites, acrolein, is excreted in the urine and can cause a chemical (haemorrhagic) cystitis in up to 10 per cent of patients. Adequate hydration and the concurrent administration of sodium-2-mercaptoethane (MESNA), which inactivates acrolein in the urine, can prevent this toxicity. Cyclophosphamide has good oral bioavailability of around 90 per cent and therefore is often utilized by this route. The main toxicity is myelosuppression, with the nadir occurring 10–21 days after intravenous administration. Oral doses are usually 100 mg/m^2 daily, but the intravenous dose varies widely, depending on the situation. Doses of 750 mg/m^2 are common in regimens like intravenous CMF (cyclophosphamide, methotrexate and 5-fluorouracil), whereas doses as high as 10 g/m^2 may be given as part of high-dose stem-cell transplantation. Such high doses can lead to problems such as hyponatraemia, haemorrhagic carditis, cardiomyopathy and pulmonary fibrosis. Like all alkylating agents, there is a risk of developing second malignancies. The major use of cyclophosphamide is as a component of combination regimens for cancers of the breast, bladder, lung and haematological malignancies. The CMF regimen is still one of the mainstays of chemotherapy for breast cancer, with variations existing which deliver different dose intensity and toxicity. It has recently fallen out of favour in ovarian cancer treatment, with the introduction of newer, more active combinations.

Ifosfamide is a structural analogue of cyclophosphamide, which exhibits a similar spectrum of activity but different pharmacological properties and toxicity profile. It is generally administered as prolonged infusions, with concurrent MESNA and hydration, due to a higher incidence of urothelial toxicity. In addition, ifosfamide can cause a severe but reversible neurological syndrome, characterized by altered mental state, cerebellar dysfuction, cranial neuropathies and epileptiform seizures. Risk factors for the development of neurotoxicity are impaired renal or hepatic function. Both ifosfamide and cyclophosphamide can cause impairment of gonadal function. The usefulness of ifosfamide is evidenced by its incorporation into chemotherapy regimens which have been shown to be curative in germ-cell malignancies. It is also used in the treatment of sarcomas and lymphomas and has demonstrated activity in ovarian cancer. As part of the 'ICE' regimen (ifosfamide, carboplatin and etoposide) or with vincristine given midcycle – 'VICE' – it is commonly utilized as first-line chemotherapy in small cell lung cancer.

NITROSUREAS (BCNU, CCNU)

BCNU (1,3-*bis* (2-chloroethyl)-1-nitrosurea, carmustine) and CCNU (1-(2-chlorothyl)-3-cyclohexyl-1-nitrosurea, lomustine) are important agents in that they exhibit only partial cross-resistance with the other alkylating agents. They are highly lipid-soluble and easily cross the blood–brain barrier. Clinical activity has been observed in lymphoma, melanoma, myeloma and malignant glioma. Major toxicities are emesis and delayed myelosuppression, which can be severe. BCNU is given intravenously, whereas CCNU can be administered orally.

ALKYLAKLANE SULPHONATES (BUSULFAN, TREOSULFAN)

Busulfan is an orally available bifunctional alkylating agent which, when hydrolysed, binds extensively to nucleophilic sites on DNA to form crosslinks. It is used mainly in haematological malignancies, and is an integral component of many high-dose chemotherapy regimens preceding stem-cell transplantation. Myelosuppression can be severe and long lasting after excessive dosing. Other notable toxicities include 'busulfan lung', a form of interstitial pulmonary fibrosis, and increased pigmentation in an Addisonian distribution. Treosulfan was synthesized in 1961 as dihydroxybusulphan and is a bifunctional alkylator, structurally related to busulfan. It is a pro-drug, activated to the reactive epoxide in a non-enzymatic, first-order, pH-dependent process. It has demonstrated specific activity in ovarian cancer, and is available in intravenous and oral form. The predominant toxicity is mild-to-moderate myelosuppression.

AZIRIDINYL DRUGS (THIOTEPA, MITOMYCIN C)

Thiotepa, (N,N',N''-triethylenethiophosphoramide), is a complex drug that acts as a monofunctional DNA-alkylating agent. It is thought to act as a pro-drug, being metabolized to highly reactive aziridine moieties via hydrolysis, following diffusion into the cell. It is delivered by the intravenous or intra-cavity route and readily crosses the blood–brain barrier. It has a role in the palliation of refractory ovarian cancer as an intraperitoneal agent, and recently there has been a resurgence of interest in its use as part of high-dose chemotherapy due, to its relative lack of non-myelogenous toxicity.

Mitomycin C is related to the anthracycline antitumour antibiotics, being derived from *Streptomyces* species, but differs substantially in that it is the prototype bioreductive agent, undergoing preferential activation in the hypoxic environment found in solid cancers. Once activated, mitomycin C performs bifunctional alkylation, crosslinking DNA with the adduct in the minor groove, and causing strand breaks. The utility of mitomycin C is limited by delayed myelosuppression, similar to that of the nitrosureas, and it is generally dosed at 10 mg/m^2 in combination regimens. Other notable toxicities include renal failure and cardiomyopathy, both related to the total cumulative dose of mitomycin C administered. The elucidation of the mechanism of action of mitomycin C has invoked great interest due to the potential of tumour selectivity through preferential reductive activation in hypoxic solid tumour masses. A range of aziridinyl agents, including E09, have been developed and are undergoing clinical evaluation.

N-METHYLTRIAZINES AND MELAMINES

Dacarbazine (DTIC) was initially thought to function as an antimetabolite, given that its genesis was as an analogue of 5-amino-imidazole-4-carboxamide, a purine precursor. However, it is now thought to be hepatically activated to function as an alkylating agent. It is decomposed by exposure to light, and is administered by intravenous infusion. It is active against a broad spectrum of tumours, but the main clinical utility is in the treatment of malignant melanoma, lymphoma and sarcomas.

Hexamethylmelamine has an uncertain mechanism of action, but is likely to act as a DNA-methylating agent, with crosslink formation. However, it is incompletely cross-resistant with classical alkylating agents such as cyclophosphamide. It is administered by the oral route, but bioavailability is erratic due to variable first-pass metabolism. It is used in the treatment of ovarian cancer, but emesis can be problematic. In addition, it can produce neurological toxicity in some patients.

Procarbazine is metabolically activated in the liver microsomes into a DNA-methylating species. It is generally administered orally in the treatment of Hodgkin's disease, and is also useful in the treatment of brain tumours due to its ability to penetrate well into the cerebrospinal fluid. Doses are usually 100 mg/m^2 daily. Side-effects are usually not severe, but care should be taken with co-administration of other drugs, due to procarbazine having an inhibitory effect on monoamine oxidase.

PLATINUM ANALOGUES

Platinum is a transition metal in the third row of the periodic table of elements. It possesses eight electrons in its outer d shell, which are highly polarizable and able to form covalent bonds. Cisplatin is a square planar molecule, which has two chloride and two ammonia ligands in the *cis*-configuration. This stearic conformation is important for anti-tumour effect, as the *trans*-isomer has no activity. The pharmacological behaviour and activation to a cytotoxic species is determined by the aquation reaction (Fig. 7.5), in which a chloride ion is replaced by a water molecule. This reaction mainly occurs in the cellular cytoplasm, as the low chloride ion concentration favours driving the formation of the active species. Once in the cell, platinum complexes are able to react with nucleophiles, such as DNA bases, RNA and proteins, to form adducts. These adducts can bridge the strands of DNA in a similar way to the crosslinks formed by melphalan and chlorambucil. The actual pathway from DNA damage to cell death has not been fully elucidated, but involves many steps, resulting ultimately in apoptosis or programmed cell death.

Cisplatin is generally given intravenously, and has an initial half-life of 40 minutes and a terminal half-life of greater than 24 hours. It is highly protein-bound, and renally excreted. This results in nephrotoxicity, due to a mechanism thought to be related to persisting adducts in renal tissue DNA. Large volumes of fluid are required to abrogate this renal damage, but significant cumulative doses of cisplatin invariably lead to an irreversible reduction in glomerular filtration rate. Renal wasting of magnesium and potassium can occur, and therefore supplementation is provided during the hydration phases. In addition, cumulative cisplatin dosing produces neurotoxicity, which usually manifests as a sensory peripheral neuropathy or hearing loss. No interventions are known to abrogate this toxicity, and when present it is thought to be only partially reversible over many months or years. Other significant toxicities include emesis, which is routinely managed by prophylactic use of $5HT_3$ antagonists in addition to corticosteroids. Myelosuppression is mild to moderate.

Cisplatin has a wide spectrum of activity against solid tumours, and is an integral component of curative regimens for testicular and ovarian cancer. It is also used in the treatment of upper gastrointestinal cancers, head and neck cancer, cervical and endometrial cancer, lung cancer (non-small cell and small cell), bladder cancer and osteosarcomas. Intraperitoneal cisplatin has been utilized in malignancies such as ovarian cancer and gastrointestinal cancer, with demonstrated activity and a decreased frequency of systemic toxicity. However, optimal pharmacokinetic and pharmacodynamic considerations mean that intraperitoneal tumour masses of >1 cm are required to ensure adequate delivery of drug to target.

Carboplatin is a cisplatin analogue which is less potent but more stable, with a longer half-life (Fig. 7.6). Mechanistically, the ultimate reaction products of carboplatin are thought to be chemically identical to that of cisplatin, and the drugs have similar if not identical spectra of activity. However, toxicity profiles are different, with carboplatin being much less nephrotoxic and neurotoxic, but causing more bone-marrow suppression. Clearance of carboplatin is also renal, with the majority of the administered dose appearing in the urine during the first 24 hours. Dosing is most accurately performed using the Calvert formula, wherein the required area under the curve (AUC) is chosen, and the dose in milligrams calculated by: (glomerular filtration rate + 25) × desired AUC. Carboplatin has virtually replaced cisplatin in combination chemotherapy for ovarian cancer, having demonstrated equivalent efficacy in prospective, randomized trials. However, carboplatin has been shown to be less effective than cisplatin in testicular cancer, therefore cytotoxic equivalency extrapolations between tumour types is not recommended.

Oxaliplatin is a third-generation platinum analogue, from the 1,2-diaminocyclohexane (DACH) platinum family. Preclinical studies have demonstrated at least equivalent potency when compared with cisplatin but, more interestingly, a degree of non-cross-resistance with other platinum compounds. In addition, data from the US National Cancer Institute (NCI) COMPARE program – a screen for functional families of cytotoxics – identified DACH platinum compounds as mechanistically different to cisplatin and carboplatin. Although oxaliplatin engages DNA in a similar way to the other platinum compounds, it seems likely that the specific cellular target and exact mechanism of action is different.

Tumour types sensitive to oxaliplatin include ovarian cancer and colorectal cancer, and there is evidence for synergy with 5-fluorouracil. Doses as a single agent are

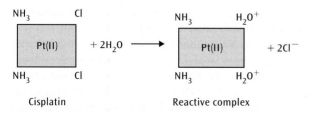

Cisplatin

Reactive complex

Figure 7.5 *Cisplatin – aquation reaction.*

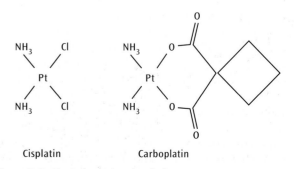

Cisplatin

Carboplatin

Figure 7.6 *Cisplatin and carboplatin.*

$130 \, \text{mg/m}^2$ as a 2-hour infusion. An unusual type of peripheral neurotoxicity has been documented, mainly characterized by reversible paraesthesias or cold-related dysaesthesias. Haematological toxicity is mild.

Antimetabolites

Antimetabolites interfere with key steps in normal cellular metabolism due to their similarity of structure with certain RNA and DNA precursors. They can act as substrates for key enzymes, or inhibit enzymic reactions crucial to the synthesis of RNA and DNA, and are therefore S-phase specific.

ANTIFOLATES

Methotrexate primarily inhibits dihydrofolate reductase (DHFR), an enzyme that functions to catalyse the conversion of dihydrofolate to tetrahydrofolate, which, in turn, is converted to a variety of co-enzymes involved in reactions where the carbon atom is transferred in the synthesis of thymidylate, purines, methionine and glycine. By abrogating thymidylate monophosphate synthesis, methotrexate inhibits RNA and DNA synthesis. Folic acid (also known as leucovorin), given orally or intravenously, is converted to the tetrahydrofolate co-enzymes that are needed for the function of thymidylate synthase (TS). This is able to bypass the blocking activity of methotrexate to prevent systemic toxicity. It can also be given locally as a mouthwash or as eye drops.

Methotrexate is well absorbed orally at low doses, but higher doses are given parenterally. An initial fast half-life is followed by a prolonged phase of renal excretion, and a long terminal half-life. This is responsible for methotrexate toxicity to the bone marrow, mucous membranes and gastrointestinal tract – areas of high cell turnover and active DNA synthesis. Because methotrexate can accumulate in third spaces and be slowly released into the circulation, its use should be avoided in patients with effusions because of the risk of severe toxicity. Methotrexate also penetrates the blood–brain barrier at high doses ($>1.5 \, \text{g}$), and can be given intrathecally for meningeal disease at doses of $10 \, \text{mg/m}^2$. With high doses, adequate diuresis should be obtained. It is also 50 per cent albumin bound and can be displaced by other protein-bound drugs, leading to higher systemic levels of free methotrexate and increased toxicity. However, it is generally well tolerated, with few side-effects unless the risk factors are not taken into account. Severe toxicity is manifested by myelosuppression, oropharyngeal ulceration and diarrhoea, with renal and hepatic failure and pneumonitis seen less commonly. Indications for use are as part of combination regimens in breast cancer, haematological malignancies, osteosarcoma and choriocarcinoma.

Methotrexate is also known to act partly through inhibition of TS, which catalyses the methylation of deoxyuridylate (dUMP) to thymidylate, which is then incorporated into DNA. More specific inhibitors of TS have been developed, which target the folate-binding site of the enzyme. Raltitrexed (Tomudex^{TM}) acts as a direct and specific TS inhibitor which, once transported into cells, is extensively polyglutamated to chemical entities which are even more potent inhibitors of TS. Such polyglutamation increases the duration of TS inhibition, which in theory could improve anti-tumour activity. MTA (LY231514, Eli Lilly and Co.) targets TS, but also inhibits dihydrofolate reductase and glycinamide ribonucleotide formyl transferase (GARFT), folate-dependent enzymes involved in purine synthesis. Again, once inside the cell, MTA is an excellent substrate for folylpolyglutamate synthase. Both agents are the subject of ongoing clinical evaluation as single agents and as components of combination regimens.

FLUOROPYRIMIDINES

5-Fluorouracil (5-FU) is an analogue of uracil which is converted by multiple alternative biochemical pathways to several cytotoxic forms. 5-FU is converted to 5-fluoro-2′-deoxyuridine (FUDR) by the enzyme thymidine phosphorylase, and subsequent phosphorylation by thymidine kinase results in the formation of 5-fluoro-deoxyuridine monophosphate (FdUMP). In the presence of reduced folate, FdUMP forms a stable covalent complex with TS, which is also a key enzyme in the *de novo* synthesis of the pyrimidine deoxynucleotide, deoxythymidine triphosphate (dTTP), a direct precursor for the synthesis of DNA. This inhibition of TS is considered to be the main mechanism for the action of 5-FU, although nucleotides of 5-FU can also be incorporated directly into both DNA (5-fluoro-2′-deoxyuridine-5′-triphosphate, FdUTP) and RNA (fluorouridine triphosphate, FUTP). The TS–FdUMP complex is slowly dissociable, with a half-life of 6 hours, and the expression of TS is cell-cycle dependent, with high activity during the S-phase. Also, as the presence of reduced folate is critical for TS–FdUMP complex formation, depletion of intracellular reduced folates impairs the maintenance of TS inhibition. Co-administration of leucovorin has been shown to increase the duration of TS inhibition, and enhance the cytotoxic effect of 5-FU.

The pharmacology of 5-FU is complex and characterized by erratic oral bioavailability, non-linear elimination pharmacokinetics and significant intra/inter-patient variability. Clearance is rapid, especially when given by bolus injection, with a half-life of 15 minutes. Several randomized trials have demonstrated the advantage of continuous infusion over bolus injection, but this is at the expense of considerable patient inconvenience (with the requirement of an indwelling central venous catheter) and increased cost. The main uses are in the treatment of breast and gastrointestinal cancers. Toxic effects include nausea, diarrhoea, mucosal inflammation and moderate myelosuppression. Infusional schedules also increase the

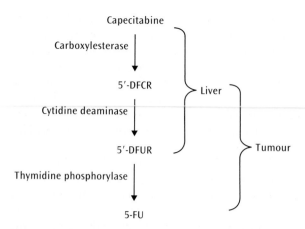

Figure 7.7 *Bioactivation of capecitabine. 5'-DFCR, 5'-deoxy-5-fluorocytidine; 5'-DFUR, 5'-deoxy-5-fluorouridine; 5-FU, 5-fluorouracil.*

incidence of plantar-palmar erythrodysaesthesia ('hand–foot syndrome').

The development of oral fluoropyrimidines is proceeding apace, with the aim to deliver optimal 5-FU to the tumour in a convenient and controlled fashion, while minimizing the variability and clearance. Capecitabine (Xeloda™) is a new orally available tumour-selective fluoropyrimidine carbamate. Following administration, it is bioactivated to 5-FU by a cascade of three enzymatic reactions (Fig. 7.7). After oral administration it passes unchanged through the gastrointestinal tract and is metabolized in the liver by carboxylesterase to 5'-deoxy-5-fluorocytidine (5'-DFCR). Then it is converted to 5'-deoxy-5-fluorouridine (5'-DFUR) by cytidine deaminase in liver and also tumour tissues. Further metabolism of 5'-DFUR occurs selectively within tumours by thymidine phosphorylase (dThdPase) to 5-FU, thus minimizing the exposure of normal tissues to systemic 5-FU. Side-effects resemble that seen with infusional 5-FU and are reversible; severe (grade III/IV) toxicities were shown to be infrequent and manageable with subsequent dose-modification. The most frequent events observed were diarrhoea, nausea, hand–foot syndrome, vomiting, fatigue and stomatitis. Clinical development is proceeding quickly, with expected utility in gastrointestinal and breast cancer.

The enzyme dihydropyrimidine dehydrogenase (DPD) is the rate-limiting step for the catabolism of 5-FU, and converts over 85 per cent of clinically administered 5-FU into inactive metabolites. It is primarily responsible for the high systemic clearance and short half-life of this drug, and therefore limits the amount of 5-FU available for conversion to the most active cytotoxic metabolite, 5-FUTP. DPD is found in many human tumours, but also in normal tissues, including the liver and the intestines, where it is largely responsible for the erratic bioavailability of 5-FU. Pharmacological inhibition of DPD may therefore increase the therapeutic index and efficacy of oral 5-FU, by allowing consistent dose delivery,

eliminating hepatic clearance and producing more predictable drug clearance through the renal tract. Such a strategy leads to the exciting possibility of dosing 5-FU according to glomerular filtration rate, in a similar fashion to carboplatin administration. In addition, overexpression of DPD in tumour cells may result in rapid intracellular fluoropyrimidine destruction and increased resistance to 5-FU. It is theoretically possible that the oral administration of fluoropyrimidines together with DPD inhibitors may overcome clinical drug resistance.

In contrast to capecitabine, which is absorbed as an inactive pro-drug, other novel oral fluoropyrimidine formulations are co-administered with inhibitors of DPD in order to produce an improved pharmacokinetic profile for 5-FU. Compounds currently in clinical trials include UFT (uracil/Tegafur), eniluracil, S-1 and BOF-A2. These novel agents all deliver a therapeutic advantage from DPD modulation, and permit safe and effective 5-FU administration (Vasey, 1999).

PURINE ANALOGUES

6-Mercaptopurine (6-MP) is an analogue of the natural purine base hypoxanthine. It is converted by the enzyme hypothine–guanine phosphoribosyl transferase to the active nucleotide 6-mercaptopurine ribose phosphate, which inhibits *de novo* purine synthesis. The triphosphate nucleotides also incorporate into DNA causing strand breakage. 6-MP is absorbed well orally, and broken down by hepatic xanthine oxidase to inactive metabolites, with half the dose excreted within 24 hours. Allopurinol can inhibit this enzyme, and therefore care is needed if both drugs are co-administered, in order to reduce the risk of increased toxicity. Doses of 50–100 mg/day are common, and 6-MP is generally limited to haematological cancers. Toxicity includes emesis, myelosuppression and a hepatic toxicity characterized by cholestatic jaundice.

6-Thioguanine (6-TG) is an analogue of guanine and has a similar mechanism of action to 6-MP. However, xanthine oxidase is not involved in its metabolism, and therefore there is no interaction with allopurinol. Again, oral administration is used, and the main indications are in haematological cancers.

PYRIMIDINE ANALOGUES

Cytarabine (cytosine arabinoside; Ara-C) is an analogue of deoxycytidine isolated from the sponge *Cryptothethya crypta*. It follows the same metabolic pathways of its physiological counterpart, and thus requires to be transported to the cell for activation. Cytarabine triphosphate (ara-CTP) is the cytotoxic metabolite of cytarabine, and acts via inhibition of DNA replication and repair, and by incorporation into the DNA. Because of this, it is considered as an S-phase-specific drug, although it is active at other phases of the cycle. The main use is in the treatment of lymphoma and leukaemia, and it is given by intravenous injection because it is affected by first-pass metabolism if given orally. Intrathecal cytarabine is administered in the treatment of meningeal leukaemia and carcinomatosis. Toxicities include myelosuppression, emesis and diarrhoea. Syndromes of pulmonary toxicity and neurological toxicity occur rarely.

Gemcitabine (2′,2′-difluorodeoxycytidine) is a new pyrimidine analogue structurally similar to cytarabine. The metabolism differs in that accumulation of its active cytotoxic metabolite is higher than ara-CTP, and its elimination is much more prolonged. The mechanism of activity is similar, consisting of incorporation into DNA and inhibition of DNA synthesis. However, gemcitabine can also be incorporated into RNA. Toxicity is relatively low, consisting of myelosuppression, lethargy, flu-like symptoms and a skin rash. A rare pulmonary toxicity is also thought to be implicated. Gemcitabine is active in many preclinical solid-tumour models, and has demonstrated clinical activity against ovarian, gastrointestinal, and non-small cell lung cancers. Furthermore, preclinical evidence for synergism has been demonstrated with several other cytotoxic agents, including cisplatin, etoposide and mitomycin C, and clinical trials of combinations are ongoing in various tumour types.

Antitumour antibiotics

ANTHRACYCLINES

Doxorubicin hydrochloride (Adriamycin®, Fig. 7.8) is probably the most globally ubiquitous anti-cancer drug, and has the broadest spectrum of activity of all chemotherapeutic agents. Daunorubicin was first isolated from *Streptomyces* in the 1960s, and was found to have activity against a variety of cancers. Mutations of *Streptomyces* led to a new strain from which doxorubicin was isolated. These two first-generation anthracyclines differ structurally by a single hydroxyl group, which results in a considerable difference in their anti-tumour activity. The mechanism of action has not been completely determined, but seems to involve DNA intercalation, free-radical formation, covalent DNA binding and inhibition of the enzyme topoisomerase II.

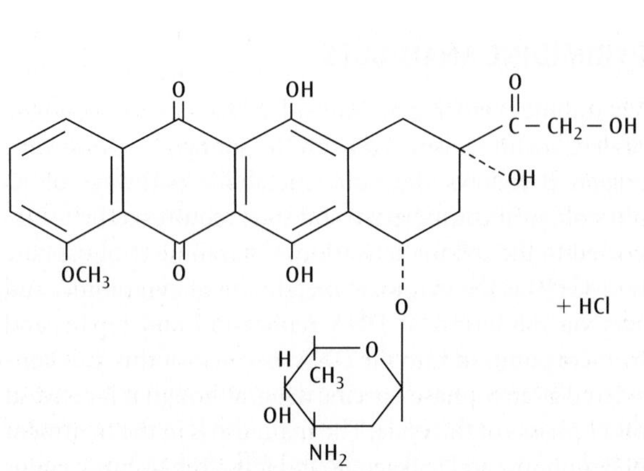

Resistance to anthracyclines (and other agents derived from natural products such as etoposide, vinca alkaloids and the taxanes) is primarily through 'multi-drug resistance' or MDR. MDR tumour cells generally demonstrate an energy-dependent efflux of cytotoxic agents linked to the expression of an approximately 170 kDa membrane protein, termed the P-glycoprotein (P-gp), that is present in higher levels of the resistant compared to the parental lines. Furthermore, the development of resistance to one drug results in cross-resistance to other drugs, without the cell being exposed to them. One strategy used to overcome tumour cell drug resistance is to employ small molecule inhibitors that block the efflux activity of P-gp. When used *in vitro*, these P-glycoprotein modulating agents lead to increased cellular accumulation of cytotoxic agents and can restore drug sensitivity to previously drug-resistant tumour cells. Small molecule modulators have been identified which bind with high affinity to P-gp and demonstrate potent *in vitro* reversal activity against MDR human tumour cell lines. Overcoming MDR is one of the 'holy grails' of cancer medicine.

Daunorubicin is mainly used for the treatment of acute non-lymphocytic leukaemia, whereas doxorubicin has a much wider spectrum of activity and is particularly used in the treatment of lymphomas, small cell lung cancer, breast cancer, upper gastrointestinal cancer, sarcomas and ovarian cancer. Doxorubicin is administered by the intravenous route, and is rapidly metabolized by the liver, to be excreted in bile. Caution must be used in hepatic dysfunction, and it (and all anthracyclines) are highly vesicant. Other toxicities include emesis, myelosuppression, oropharyngeal ulceration, diarrhoea and alopecia. The major long-term complication is a cumulative, dose-limiting cardiotoxicity which is irreversible and may be fatal. Doses are usually up to 75 mg/m² as a single agent every 3 weeks, but cardiotoxicity becomes increasingly frequent at cumulative doses of >450 mg/m². 'Cardioprotectors' such as bisdioxopiperazine have been developed in an attempt to circumvent this cardiotoxicity, and are thought to work by chelating iron required by doxorubicin to produce the free radicals proposed to initiate the membrane damage evident in cardiac cells.

Developmental chemistry has produced over 1000 structural anthracycline analogues in an attempt to either increase activity of the drug, or decrease toxicity, especially cardiac. Most do not proceed to clinical testing, and many get to trials only to demonstrate no clear advantage over doxorubicin or different toxicities. Epirubicin was synthesized in 1975, and has a similar spectrum of activity to doxorubicin while exhibiting less chronic cardiotoxicity. Idarubicin was shown to have a high affinity for lipids, and therefore can be administered effectively by the oral route.

PK1 is a polymeric drug-delivery system which consists of doxorubicin complexed to HPMA [*N*-(2-hydroxypropyl) methacrylamide] copolymer by a peptidyl linker. This macromolecular construct enters tumour cells by

Figure 7.8 *Doxorubicin hydrochloride.*

pinocytosis, where the linker is cleaved intracellularly, allowing intratumoural drug release. Preclinical work has demonstrated radically altered pharmacokinetics compared to free doxorubicin, and significant activity in animal tumours. Decreased cardiotoxicity has been demonstrated in early trials, and activity appears to be maintained (Vasey *et al.*, 1999a). Pharmacokinetic studies showed that PK1 has a prolonged distribution $t_{1/2}$ and is cleared 1000 times slower than free doxorubicin.

Liposomal drug-delivery systems (e.g. daunorubicin encapsulated by distearoylphosphatidylcholine/cholesterol, DaunoXome™, and polyethylene glycol (PEG)-coated liposomal encapsulation of doxorubicin, Caelyx™) have been extensively investigated as carriers for anticancer agents. Both DaunoXome™ and Doxil™ have longer half-lives, higher AUCs and lower clearances than either free daunorubicin or doxorubicin, and also appear to be free of significant cardiotoxicity, and generally have decreased anthracycline-like toxicities. However, myelosuppression is still an important feature of both formulations at recommended doses (DaunoXome™, 40–60 mg/m²; Caelyx™, 25–40 mg/m²), with neutropenia occurring at grade III/IV in 50–60 per cent of patients. In addition, plantar-palmar erythrodysaesthesia was noted to be dose-limiting at higher cumulative doses of Caelyx™. Liposomal drug delivery systems have been found to be especially useful in the treatment of AIDS-associated Kaposi's sarcoma (AIDS-KS), as conventional treatment with anthracyclines tends to be limited by cumulative toxicities (especially cardiac) preventing prolonged courses of chemotherapy.

MITOXANTRONE

Mitoxantrone is a relative of the anthracyclines, and is based on the anthracenedione structure. It is completely synthetic and was designed with the aim of retaining anthracycline anti-tumour activity with less toxicity. It undergoes DNA intercalation, in a similar fashion, and also inhibits topoisomerase II. It is given by intravenous injection, and has a long terminal half-life of up to 40 hours. Doses are 10–14 mg/m² every 3 weeks and it is used in leukaemia, breast cancer and in combination regimens for the treatment of lymphomas. The reduced toxicity profile makes it an attractive drug to use in the elderly breast cancer patient. In addition, cardiac toxicity is less than that due to doxorubicin, probably as a result of its decreased free-radical production.

BLEOMYCIN

Bleomycin is a mixture of low molecular weight glcopeptides isolated from the fungus *Streptomyces verticullus*, and has both antibacterial and anti-cancer activity. The mechanism of cytotoxicity appears to relate to DNA binding and the production of strand breakage, with ferrous iron being essential to this mechanism. It is administered by parenteral injection, and is renally excreted with an initial half-life of 30 minutes, and a later elimination phase of 2–9 hours. Doses are usually 10–20 units/m² given weekly, although this needs to be reduced in renal impairment. It is generally administered either by intravenous infusion or intramuscular injection, and also has utility via the intra-cavity route to control pleural or pericardial effusions. It has virtually no myelosuppressive toxicity or gastrointestinal side-effects. Chronic administration can produce pneumonitis, which can lead to an irreversible and occasionally fatal interstitial fibrosis. Fevers, chills and flu-like symptoms are common, and prolonged administration also leads to skin pigmentation. It is used mainly in combination regimens for the treatment of germ-cell tumours and lymphomas, but also has been used against cervical, vulval, vaginal, skin, non-small cell lung and oesophageal cancers.

ACTINOMYCIN D

This compound is also isolated from *Streptomyces*, and acts in a similar fashion by DNA intercalation and the induction of strand breaks. It is eliminated almost unchanged in the bile and urine. Actinomycin D is usually administered intravenously at doses between 10 and 15 mg/kg per day for 5 days. It is active against choriocarcinoma, Wilms' tumour, Ewing's sarcoma, embryonal rhabdomyosarcoma, and, to a lesser extent, testicular cancer, lymphoma and Kaposi's sarcoma. The main toxicities are myelosuppression, mucositis, diarrhoea and alopecia. In addition, drug extravasation can lead to severe tissue necrosis. Actinomycin D appears to inhibit DNA repair after radiation damage, and therefore the combination of both modalities enhances the risk of toxicity.

Plant-derived agents

In the USA approximately two-thirds of commercially available drugs are of natural origin. Overall, these compounds are usually more potent than agents derived synthetically.

VINCA ALKALOIDS

Compounds with marked anti-tumour activity have been extracted from the periwinkle plant. Vinblastine and vincristine have been widely used, both as single agents and in combination with other drugs. Vinca alkaloid analogues have been prepared either by functional transformation (vindesine, desacetylvinblastine-amide) or, more recently, by hemisynthesis (vinorelbine, 5'-noranhydrovinblastine). Although these compounds are all chemically related, differences have been observed in anti-tumour activity and toxicity. The mode of action of vinca alkaloids is yet to be completely understood, but they act as mitotic spindle poisons which impair chromosomal segregation during mitosis. Microtubules are essential for normal cellular function, and are involved in the maintenance of cell shape, mobility, adhesion and intra-cellular integrity, as well as having a role in formation of the mitotic spindle during proliferation.

Vinblastine is active in haematological cancers, and testicular and breast cancer. Vincristine is also active in these tumours, in addition to Wilms' tumour, Ewing's sarcoma, neuroblastoma, hepatoblastoma and embryonal rhabdomyosarcoma. The anti-tumour activity of vindesine is similar to that of vinblastine and vincristine, whereas vinorelbine is particularly active in non-small cell lung cancer, breast cancer, ovarian cancer and Hodgkin's disease. Vincristine and vindesine administration can cause neurological toxicity characterized by a decrease in the deep tendon reflexes, paraesthesias, constipation, myalgias, muscle weakness and paralytic ileus. Vinblastine generally produces haematological toxicities. Vinorelbine neurotoxicity is usually very mild, with only rare cases of paraesthesia or paralytic ileus being reported. Experimental evidence suggests that this may be due to the capacity of vinorelbine to bind to mitotic microtubules, rather than axonal microtubules. Clinical pharmacokinetics of vinca alkaloids are characterized by large distribution volume, high systemic clearance, and long terminal half-life, although there are significant differences between analogues. A major obstacle to effective cancer chemotherapy with vinca alkaloids is MDR.

TAXANES

Paclitaxel (Taxol^{TM}) is a chemically complex molecule first isolated from the bark of the Pacific Yew tree *Taxus brevifolia* in the early 1970s. Its unique mechanism of action was not elicited for almost a decade and its importance as a major advance in the treatment of malignant disease was not recognized until 1989. Paclitaxel interferes with cell division by manipulating the molecular regulation of the cell cycle. In the presence of paclitaxel, polymerization of the α- and β-subunits of tubulin occurs, and the formed microtubules resist disassembly, thus shifting the equilibrium toward microtubule formation (Figs 7.9 and 7.10). Disruption of this equilibrium interferes with cell division and normal cellular activities involving microtubules.

The pharmacokinetic behaviour of paclitaxel has been studied during the early phase I trials in the 1980s. These studies used infusional schedules of between 1 and 24 hours and optimally modelled the concentration/time profile using a triphasic model, with half-life parameters of: α, 10 minutes; β, 2 hours; and γ, 15 hours. In general, administered dose was proportional to the area under the time/concentration curve (AUC). However, shorter infusions of paclitaxel (=3 hours) seem to demonstrate non-linearity, and the important implication for this feature is that small dose de-escalations may result in a disproportionate lowering of the AUC, with subsequently decreased anti-tumour activity. Paclitaxel is >90 per cent bound to plasma proteins, but this is readily reversible and results in rapid elimination of the drug. Renal excretion is negligible, and no renal metabolites have been identified. There may be significant hepatic metabolism, and various studies are in progress to look at the effects that other drugs that use the cytochrome P450 pathway may have on the pharmacological behaviour of paclitaxel.

Administration of paclitaxel is associated with allergic hypersensitive reactions ranging from acute anaphylaxis and hypotension to flushing, rashes and urticaria. Indeed, development of this agent was almost halted in the early stages due to the severity of these reactions. However, the instigation of a premedication regimen consisting of corticosteroids and H_1/H_2 blockers has significantly reduced the incidence of allergic reactions from 20 per cent to <3 per cent. Although the formulation of paclitaxel in Cremophor EL® (due to its limited aqueous solubility) may be responsible for the hypersensitivity phenomena, some contribution of paclitaxel itself is possible, as hypersensitivity reactions also occur with the semisynthetic analogue, docetaxel, formulated in Tween-80.

Leukopenia is the dose-limiting toxicity, and thrombocytopenia is rare. Myelosuppression occurs early, and is associated with a rapid recovery, allowing treatment to proceed on a 3-week cycle. Neurotoxicity occurs with higher cumulative doses of paclitaxel, and with higher doses per course. This is mainly a sensory neuropathy and manifests in a 'glove and stocking'-type distribution. It is at least partially reversible with time. Many cardiac arrythmias have been reported with paclitaxel administration, ranging from asymptomatic bradycardia to various degrees of heart block and atrial/ventricular tachyarrythmias. However, the relationship between these events and paclitaxel was frequently uncertain and routine cardiac monitoring is unnecessary. Other frequently reported toxicities include alopecia (universal), fatigue and arthralgia/myalgia. Indications for use include breast cancer (anthracycline-pretreated) and ovarian cancer.

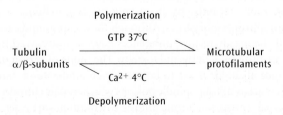

Figure 7.9 *Mitotic spindle formation.*

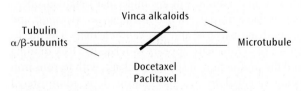

Figure 7.10 *Taxanes – mechanism of action.*

Docetaxel (Taxotere™) is a new member of the taxoid family and is currently licensed in the UK and USA for the treatment of relapsed breast cancer. There is preclinical evidence to suggest that docetaxel may be superior to paclitaxel. Docetaxel has been shown to be more potent (up to fivefold) *in vitro* than paclitaxel with regard to the promotion of tubulin polymerization and inhibition of depolymerization. In a direct comparison with paclitaxel in a large number of freshly explanted tumours (including breast, ovarian, lung, colorectal tumours), docetaxel was found to have at least equivalent cytotoxicity, but with incomplete cross-resistance. Docetaxel also had a longer residence time, accumulated at higher concentrations within cells and demonstrated a superior therapeutic index *in vivo*. Clinical studies have confirmed the presence of incomplete cross-resistance with paclitaxel, reporting activity for docetaxel in paclitaxel-resistant metastatic breast cancer. In addition, docetaxel has proved superior to doxorubicin in a direct comparison in metastatic breast cancer patients, whereas paclitaxel has failed to do so.

Docetaxel pharmacokinetics following a 1-hour infusion, demonstrate that the plasma elimination at the highest doses follows a triphasic decay, with a terminal half-life of 13.5 hours and a plasma clearance of approximately $21 \, l/h$ per m^2. The AUC increases linearly with the dose and correlates with the percentage decrease of neutrophils. Less than 10 per cent of the administered dose is excreted unchanged in the urine. The recommended dose as a single agent is $100 \, mg/m^2$ given as a 1-hour intravenous infusion. Patients that have been heavily pretreated or have abnormal hepatic function should receive a reduced $dose/m^2$. The most frequent toxicity is an early, reversible, non-cumulative neutropenia, which is associated with a low rate of concurrent infections. Anaemia has also been observed. Hypersensitivity reactions occurred in 25 per cent of patients that were un-premedicated with corticosteroids, and that these generally occurred on the first course, within a few minutes of the start of the infusion. Premedication with corticosteroids has reduced the incidence of hypersensitivity reactions to less than 5 per cent. Cutaneous reactions occur, characterized by a rash, occurring mainly on the extremities (but also localized eruptions on arms, face or thorax), and were occasionally associated with pruritis. These were usually transient and had resolved prior to the next course of treatment. Less frequently, desquamation was observed. Nail changes (onycholysis, hypo/hyperpigmentation) were also seen. A fluid retention syndrome, characterized by asymptomatic weight gain and/or oedema (and less often pleural, peritoneal or pericardial effusions), has been observed. This generally starts in the lower extremities and at cumulative doses of $>400 \, mg/m^2$. The pathogenesis of this condition is incompletely understood (capillary leak syndrome?) but appears reversible on cessation of docetaxel treatment, and can be significantly reduced by premedication with

dexamethasone. Mild degrees of this syndrome can be treated adequately by diuretic therapy, but it is recommended that patients with severe oedema should not continue with docetaxel. Clinically significant cardiac events occurred in less than 2 per cent of all patients treated, and was not clearly related to docetaxel administration. Other significant toxicities encountered were alopecia, hepatotoxicity (mild, reversible transaminase elevations), mucositis, diarrhoea, arthralgia/myalgia and peripheral neuropathy (sensory and motor). Emesis was generally mild and easily treated with $5HT_3$ antagonists. Ongoing clinical trials will hopefully define the place of both paclitaxel and docetaxel in cancer chemotherapy (Vasey, 1997; Vasey *et al.*, 1999b).

TOPOISOMERASE I AND II INHIBITORS

DNA topoisomerase I and II are enzymes that bind to supercoiled DNA, forming a 'cleavable complex' and, through strand breakage, passage and religation, allow a wide variety of essential DNA metabolic reactions, including replication and repair, to take place. These enzymes are functionally related, work together, and appear to be essential to maintain cellular viability throughout the cell cycle. Since it was shown in the 1980s that the cleavable complex could be stabilized by known cytotoxic drugs such as doxorubicin, etoposide and camptothecin, resulting in interference with the strand breakage–religation catalytic cycle and subsequent cell death, much research has taken place into the development of agents that exploit this novel nuclear target. Established inhibitors of topoisomerase II include the anthracycline antibiotics (e.g. doxorubicin) and the epipodophyllotoxins (etoposide), which were not developed on the basis of rational drug design against this specific cellular target, and are in fact not 'pure' topoisomerase II inhibitors. The only specific topoisomerase I inhibitors with anti-tumour activity are the heterocyclic alkaloid camptothecin, and its analogues.

Isolated in 1966 from the tree *Camptotheca acuminata*, early studies with camptothecin demonstrated unpredictable and severe toxicity with limited efficacy. However, the development of water-soluble synthetic/semi-synthetic analogues of camptothecin, such as irinotecan (CPT-11) and topotecan, and the discovery that topoisomerase I levels were higher in some tumours compared to normal tissues, has led to renewed interest in the topoisomerases as important targets for anti-cancer agents. Drugs that are able to inhibit both topoisomerase enzymes are in clinical trials (Twelves *et al.*, 1999); however, combining specific inhibitors of topoisomerase I and II together appears to be associated with significant myelotoxicty, although there is evidence that this may be schedule dependent (Vasey and Kaye, 1997).

Topotecan exerts its cytotoxic effects by stabilizing the covalent DNA–topisomerase I cleavable complex, thus blocking DNA repair. When DNA replicates in the presence of this complex, double-strand breaks occur and the resulting DNA fragmentation causes cell death. The major side-effect of topotecan is myelosuppression, which can be severe, is schedule dependent and may be associated with infectious complications. Currently, a d1–5 intravenous bolus schedule of 1–1.5 mg/m^2 per day every 3 weeks is considered standard. Oral formulations are in development, although more diarrhoea has been observed in early studies. Thrombocytopenia and anaemia are also common, and non-haematological toxicities are otherwise mild – emesis, diarrhoea, oropharangeal ulceration and alopecia. Significant activity has been observed in refractory ovarian cancer, small cell lung cancer, breast cancer, lymphoma, and head and neck cancer. It has only modest activity against gastrointestinal tumours, unlike CPT-11 (irinotecan). Combination studies of topotecan with other cytotoxic agents, including platinum and paclitaxel, are ongoing, but myelosuppression is dose limiting, generally requiring dose reductions of both agents. Optimal combination schedules need to be defined, as does the role of this compound in first-line therapy.

CPT-11 was developed in Japan, and has recently been licensed in the UK for the treatment of 5-FU-relapsed colorectal cancer. In addition to colorectal cancer, activity has been observed in ovarian cancer, lung cancer (small cell and non-small cell) and cervical cancer. It is converted by hepatic carboxylesterases to a major metabolite, SN-38, which is up to 2000-fold more effective at topoisomerase I inhibition than the parent compound. Like topotecan, the formation of a cleavable complex effects damage to the DNA through double-strand breaks. After intravenous infusion, CPT-11 concentrations decline in a multiexponential manner, with a mean terminal half-life of 6 hours, whereas the equivalent SN-38 half-life is 10 hours. SN-38 is much more highly protein-bound than CPT-11. The schedule of intravenous administration is usually either 300–350 mg/m^2 every 3 weeks, or 125 mg/m^2 weekly for 4 weeks with 2 weeks' rest. The main toxicities are myelosuppression, which can be severe, and diarrhoea. CPT-11 can induce both early and late diarrhoea, which appears to be mediated by different mechanisms. Early diarrhoea (within 24 hours) is cholinergic in nature and can be abrogated by atropine administration. Late diarrhoea can be prolonged and severe, and requires prompt instigation of loperamide as it can quickly lead to dehydration and electrolyte imbalance.

ETOPOSIDE

Podophyllin and podophyllotoxin are derived from the mandrake root, and act as mitotic poisons in a similar fashion to vinca alkaloids. Early clinical trials were stopped because of significant toxicities, and researchers looked at analogue development as a way of proceeding. VP-16 (etoposide) is an epipodophyllotoxin analogue which is not only less toxic, but has a different mechanism of action from the parent compound. It interferes with the religation of topoisomerase II, causing stabilization of DNA–topoisomerase II complexes which are cleavable and result in DNA strand breaks. Another possible contributory mechanism of cytotoxicity is the generation of free radicals.

Oral VP-16 bioavailability is approximately 50 per cent (range 17–100 per cent), and approximately 50 per cent of the VP-16 dose is eliminated as unchanged drug or glucuronide within 24 h of administration. Protein binding is approximately 90 per cent. VP-16 clearance appears to be related to renal clearance, and therefore increased toxicity may be expected in patients with poor renal function. Bone-marrow and gastrointestinal toxicity predominate the side-effect profile, but other common side-effects include alopecia, nausea, vomiting and diarrhoea. VP-16 is active in small cell lung cancer, germ-cell tumours, ovarian cancer, choriocarcinoma and haematological cancers. Dosing schedules generally involve intravenous administration, but many studies have demonstrated that chronic oral dosing is feasible and safe.

Miscellaneous agents

AGENTS DERIVED FROM MARINE ORGANISMS

Marine organisms have survived for up to 700 million years through natural selection and the release of potent chemicals which offer protection in a hostile milieu without the need for bioactivation. It follows that there is extraordinary potential among these toxic chemicals for anti-tumour specificity. Over the past 10–15 years a wide range of potent chemicals with different cellular targets has been isolated. Many are now undergoing clinical trials, and some are listed briefly here.

Bryostatin 1 is the prototype of a novel class of structurally related compounds isolated from the marine bryozoan, *Bugula neritina*. It is a macrocyclic lactone which exhibits many biological effects mediated through modulation of protein kinase C, a family of enzymes crucial in cellular signalling pathways controlling proliferation and differentiation. It has demonstrated broad-spectrum preclinical anti-tumour activity, and has also been shown to induce differentiation, enhance the immune response and inhibit the production of members of the matrix metalloproteinase family thought to be essential for angiogenesis.

Dolastatin 10 was isolated from a herbivorous mollusc in the Indian Ocean, and acts by abrogating microtubule assembly. Exceptional potency has been described in preclinical models, and it is rapidly and extensively metabolized, with high protein binding.

Ecteinascidin 743 (ET-743) was isolated from Caribbean tunicate in 1990, and forms covalent adducts with DNA in the minor groove, with sequence specificity. In addition, effects on the microtubular spindle are postulated, and downregulation of transcription factors.

A broad spectrum of preclinical anti-cancer activity has been demonstrated, in addition to a lack of cross-resistance with other agents, including anthracyclines, taxoids and platinum. Target organs for toxicity are the liver and bone marrow.

Aplidine is a potent cyclic depsipeptide isolated from a Mediterranean marine truncate, *Aplidium albicans*. The mechanism of action is not completely understood, but studies are in progress to identify the potentially unique target involved in its anti-tumour activity.

NEW TARGETS AND FUTURE DIRECTIONS

The development of new anti-cancer therapies in future is likely to be reliant on exploiting our increasing understanding of the molecular basis of cancer. The identification of putative molecular targets, allied to high-throughput screening strategies of potential compounds, and utilizing the advances in biotechnology (particularly in the field of drug delivery) gives rise to the exciting possibility of a raft of novel therapies, many of which are already undergoing preclinical and even early clinical evaluation. However, the preclinical and early clinical evaluation of these novel therapeutic strategies targeted to specific molecular pathways presents new challenges which will require an integrated approach from both laboratory and clinical scientists. Preclinical evaluation will require demonstration of reproducible biological effects in experimental systems at concentrations of drug comparable to that which can be achieved in the clinic. In addition to the conventional end points of toxicity and pharmacokinetics, early clinical evaluation will also require demonstration of desired biological activity, which is likely to be particularly pertinent in those agents which are likely to have a cytostatic effect, in order to determine the optimal biologically active dose for subsequent clinical trials. Furthermore these agents may not have objective evidence of anti-tumour activity by classical tumour response criteria in patients with bulk disease, which usually make up the patient population in whom new agents are evaluated. Consequently evaluation of these agents will require identification of appropriate candidate patients (e.g. presence of molecular target in biopsy material), demonstration of desired biological effect, usually in tumour biopsy material or by assessment of surrogate biological end points, and identification of the appropriate clinical scenario for evaluation, e.g. as maintenance therapy after 'debulking' chemotherapy, or as adjuvant therapy for agents with a proposed cytostatic effect.

One of the most prominent examples of the development of anti-cancer drugs based on the specific molecular abnormality present in a human cancer is STI-571, a specific inhibitor of the BCR-ABL tyrosine kinase. The characteristic genetic abnormality of chronic myeloid leukaemia (CML) is the Philadelphia chromosome, which results from a reciprocal translocation between the long arms of chromosomes 9 and 22 (Rowley, 1973). The molecular consequence of this translocation is the generation of the fusion protein BCR-ABL, a constitutively-activated tyrosine kinase, which is present in virtually all patients with CML. *In vitro* studies and studies in animal models have established that BCR-ABL alone is sufficient to cause CML, and mutational analysis has established that the tyrosine kinase activity of this protein is required for its oncogenic activity (Daley *et al.*, 1990; Heisterkamp *et al.*, 1990; Kelliher *et al.*, 1990; Lugo *et al.*, 1990).

STI-571, identified by *in vitro* screening for tyrosine kinase inhibitors, functions through competitive inhibition at the ATP-binding site of the enzyme, which leads to the inhibition of tyrosine phosphorylation of proteins involved in BCR-ABL signal transduction. It shows a high degree of specificity for BCR-ABL, the receptor for platelet-derived growth factor, and c-kit tyrosine kinases. On the basis of its anti-leukaemic activity in preclinical models, it has been evaluated in patients with CML in whom treatment with interferon-alpha had failed (Druker *et al.*, 2001a). This study demonstrated that STI-571 is well tolerated and complete haematological responses were observed in 53 of 54 patients treated with daily doses of 300 mg or more, and typically occurred in the first four weeks of therapy. Furthermore, STI-571 also has substantial activity (response rate = 55%; n = 38) in the myeloid-blast-crisis phenotype of CML and in Philadelphia-chromosome positive acute lymphoblastic leukaemia (Druker *et al.*, 2001b). Thus, the goal of developing novel anti-cancer agents by exploiting the molecular basis of cancer can be achieved.

Differentiation agents

Included amongst the newer strategies in oncology practice is the evaluation of a number of agents designed to induce differentiation in tumour cells, thereby leading to inhibition of cellular proliferation and apoptosis. The most prominent of these so-called differentiation agents are the retinoids and vitamin D analogues.

RETINOIDS

Vitamin A and its biologically active derivatives, retinal and retinoic acid, together with a large repertoire of synthetic analogues, are collectively referred to as retinoids. Naturally occurring retinoids regulate the growth and differentiation of a wide variety of cell types and play a crucial role in the physiology of vision and as morphogenic agents during embryonic development.

Retinoids exert most of their effects by binding to specific receptors and modulating gene expression. The nuclear retinoid receptors are members of the steroid/thyroid hormone superfamily of receptors (Evans, 1988) with which they share common structural and functional properties. The diversity of retinoid-induced signalling pathways is mediated by at least six retinoid receptors which fall into two subfamilies, retinoic acid receptors (RARs) α, β and γ, and the retinoid X receptors (RXRs) α, β and γ (Chambon, 1995). The mechanism of action of retinoid receptors, and the cellular consequences of retinoid stimulation, has been reviewed extensively (Evans and Kaye, 1999a). Briefly, the RARs bind all-*trans* retinoic acid (ATRA) with high affinity (Giguere *et al.*, 1987; Petkovich *et al.*, 1987) whereas the stereoisomer 9-*cis* retinoic acid is a bifunctional ligand which can bind to and activate both RARs and RXRs (Mangelsdorf *et al.*, 1992; Allenby *et al.*, 1993). Despite these similarities, the RXRs belong to a subgroup of nuclear receptors distinct from the RARs (Laudet *et al.*, 1992), suggesting that these two groups of retinoid receptors have distinct roles in retinoid signalling. Both negative and positive effects on transcription can occur in the absence of ligand and these biomodal transcriptional properties of retinoid receptors are mediated, in part, by the ability of these receptors to associate with various co-activators and co-repressors such as SMRT and N-CoR (Chen and Evans, 1995; Kurokawa *et al.*, 1995; Horwitz *et al.*, 1996). Transcriptional regulation by receptors would therefore seem to be controlled by selective recruitment of co-activators and co-repressors in response to hormone, and in turn, control of activity of a target promoter. It may be that the role of ligand binding is to cause a conformational change in the receptor, and as a result of this a co-repressor protein is dissociated from the receptor and a co-activator binds to the receptor, thereby initiating transcription (reviewed in Perlmann and Evans, 1997).

The diversity of dimer complexes that can occur increases the complexity of retinoid signalling mechanisms. Both RARs and RXRs can bind response elements as homodimers, albeit at high concentrations, although heterodimerization of RARs and RXRs enables high-affinity binding of RARs to response elements. Furthermore, RXRs also serve as promiscuous partners in a multitude of other hormonal response systems, including vitamin D signalling pathways (Kliewer *et al.*, 1992). Therefore a large number of different receptor complexes can be formed, controlling distinct pathways (Nagpal *et al.*, 1992). Consequently, a range of possible effects is possible by disruption of these pathways by pharmacological agents.

At the cellular level, activation of the retinoid receptors can inhibit cell proliferation, induce differentiation and induce apoptosis in normal and transformed cells in tissue culture. Although there is a difference between various cell-line models in the receptor which mediates these processes, it appears in some models that activation of RARs alone is sufficient to induce differentiation, but activation of RXRs is essential for induction of apoptosis (Nagy *et al.*, 1995). Numerous putative mechanisms have

been proposed for the induction of apoptosis by retinoids, including activation of the AP-1 complex for which activation of the receptors is not necessary (Schadendorf *et al.*, 1996) but the exact mechanism remains unknown. However, retinoids can cause growth regression in *in vivo* xenograft models of experimental cancer (Schadendorf *et al.*, 1996) as well as having antipromotion activity in several animals models of carcinogenesis (reviewed in Lotan, 1996). Most of the clinical trials of retinoids as chemoprevention agents focus on individuals at an increased risk of developing cancer, such as patients with premalignant lesions or patients who have been treated successfully for an early-stage carcinoma and have a high risk of developing a second primary cancer. None of these studies has, as yet, demonstrated significant chemopreventive effect with acceptable toxicity than can be maintained after retinoid withdrawal, which could justify routine use in clinical practice (Evans and Kaye, 1999a).

The most prominent example of retinoids as differentiating agents in oncology practice is the remarkable activity of all-*trans* retinoic acid in patients with acute promyelocytic leukaemias (APL). Numerous phase II studies have confirmed that ATRA induces complete remission in the vast majority of patients, with rapid resolution of the characteristic life-threatening coagulopathy (Huang *et al.*, 1988; Castaigne *et al.*, 1990; Chen *et al.*, 1991; Warrell *et al.*, 1991; Fenaux *et al.*, 1992; Ohno *et al.*, 1993; Frankel *et al.*, 1994; Kanamaru *et al.*, 1995). The duration of remission with ATRA alone is usually brief and post-remission chemotherapy is required to diminish the likelihood of relapse. A randomized study has confirmed that ATRA as induction or maintenance treatment improves disease-free and overall survival as compared with chemotherapy alone, and should be included in the treatment of APL (Tallman *et al.*, 1997). The increasing understanding of retinoid-induced signalling pathways should lead to the design of combination therapies with other agents acting on steroid hormone receptors, agents which inhibit intracellular signalling pathways, and raises the intriguing possibility of enhancing the sensitivity of tumours to cytotoxic agents and of overcoming drug resistance by adjusting the apoptotic set point (Evans and Kaye, 1999a).

VITAMIN D ANALOGUES

In addition to its role in calcium homeostasis, vitamin D can also promote cellular differentiation, inhibit proliferation and induce apoptosis in cancer cells, as well as inhibiting tumour-induced angiogenesis (Majewski *et al.*, 1993) and inhibiting the invasive potential of breast cancer cells *in vitro* (Hansen *et al.*, 1994). Vitamin D mediates its action through the activation of the vitamin D receptor, where the receptor–ligand complex functions as a transcription factor and binds with DNA by interacting with vitamin D response elements, leading to either activation or suppression of target gene transcription (Carlberg, 1995).

Vitamin D_3 is limited in its potential clinical application because of the induction of hypercalcaemia at therapeutic doses. A number of analogues have been synthesized with the aim of decreasing this calcaemic effect and enhancing its antiproliferative actions. MC903, as a topical application can stabilize locally advanced and cutaneous metastatic breast cancer (Bower *et al.*, 1991). EB1089 can induce regression of colon and breast cancers in animal models without causing significant hypercalcaemia (James *et al.*, 1994; Akhter *et al.*, 1997) and has been evaluated in a phase I study in breast and colon cancer (Gulliford *et al.*, 1998). Although no objective responses were seen in this early clinical study, it is reasonable to expect that differentiation agents such as this are unlikely to have any measurable effect on the advanced disease seen in the typical phase I population. However, the possibility remains that they may have some activity in early stage disease or in patients with minimal disease states.

Angiogenesis and its inhibitors

The inhibition of angiogenesis is considered to be one of the most promising approaches that might lead to the development of novel anti-cancer strategies. Like most biological processes, angiogenesis is regulated through a balance of stimulators and inhibitors. The mechanisms of new blood vessel formation and its role in malignant transformation, tumour growth and metastasis are discussed in Chapter 13.

There are many attractive features of these angiogenesis mechanisms which can be exploited therapeutically (Twardowski and Gradishar, 1997):

1 Endothelial cells in normal adult tissues have an extremely slow turnover rate (up to hundreds of days) compared to that of approximately 4 days in endothelial cells engaged in active tumour angiogenesis. Therefore its likely that agents that selectively block endothelial cell proliferation would be relatively non-toxic. Moreover, as endothelial cells have a low mutation rate, the risk of developing drug resistance would be low.

2 New blood vessel formation by tumours creates access to the circulation and facilitates metastases. Potentially, inhibition of new blood vessel formation may block haematogenous dissemination of cancer cells.

3 Endothelial cells have a growth-stimulating paracrine effect on malignant cells, and inhibition of angiogenesis may decrease the proliferation of some tumour cells.

A number of experimental approaches have been evaluated as inhibitors of angiogenesis (Augustin, 1998; Gasparini, 1999). These include:

1 Naturally occurring inhibitors of angiogenesis such as the plasminogen fragment, angiostatin; the collagen XVIII fragment, endostatin; platelet factor 4, which inhibits endothelial cell proliferation.

2 Specific inhibitors of endothelial cell growth such as TNP-470, an analogue of the antibiotic fumagillin which inhibits endothelial cell migration and proliferation; thalidomide; and interleukin-12.

3 Agents neutralizing angiogenic peptides or their receptors, such as fibroblast growth factor (FGF), vascular endothelial growth factor (VEGF), suramin.

4 Agents that interfere with vascular basement membrane and extracellular matrix, such as matrix metalloproteinase inhibitors (*see* below).

5 Anti-adhesion molecules, such as antibodies to the $\alpha v/\beta 3$ integrin, which consequently induce endothelial cell apoptosis.

Additionally, vascular targeting is aimed at using specific molecular determinants of angiogenic endothelial cells for the delivery of a biological or pharmacological substance that will then act locally either as an angiogenesis inhibitor or in a tumoricidal manner (e.g. directing suicide genes to proliferating endothelial cells by using endothelial cell-specific promoters).

MATRIX METALLOPROTEINASE INHIBITORS

Matrix metalloproteinases (MMPs) are a class of structurally related enzymes that function in the degradation of extracellular matrix proteins that constitute the pericellular connective tissue and play an important role in both normal and pathological tissue remodelling. Increased MMP activity is detected in a wide range of cancers and seems to be correlated to their invasive and metastatic potential. Consequently MMPs are an attractive target for therapies.

The activity of MMPs is usually controlled by the latency of the secreted enzymes as well as by naturally occurring inhibitors (reviewed in Denis and Verweij, 1997). In cancer, there is an imbalance between the levels of activated enzymes and their inhibitors, which results in a breakdown of extracellular matrix, thus facilitating the direct expansion and local invasion of the primary tumour, the movement of tumour cells across the vascular basement membrane, and the local growth and invasion of any secondary tissue. However, other proteases, such as urokinase-type plasminogen activator, may also be involved in these processes in certain tumours.

The naturally occurring inhibitors are likely to be limited in their use as therapeutic agents by their low oral bioavailability. However, numerous synthetic MMP inhibitors have been developed and have shown encouraging activity in preclinical evaluation, and are now in clinical trials (Denis and Verweij, 1997). Again, as cytostatic agents, these agents are unlikely to achieve objective tumour regression in advanced, bulky disease, as is usually the case in a typical phase I population.

As such, randomized phase III trials are in progress to evaluate their efficacy as 'maintenance' therapy after initial debulking with cytotoxic chemotherapy.

Growth factors and growth-factor signalling

Signalling pathways that drive cell proliferation are closely associated with malignancy. The components of these signalling pathways include the platelet-derived growth factor (PDGF)-like ligand Sis, the tyrosine kinases Src and HER2/c-Neu, and the GTP-binding switch Ras. Growth factor receptors comprise an extracellular domain containing the ligand-binding site, a single trans-membrane α-helix and a cytoplasmic domain which includes a tyrosine kinase (TK) region. Binding by ligands such as PDGF, epidermal growth factor (EGF), EGF-like ligands (e.g. Tgf-α) or insulin-like growth factor (IGF), leads to receptor dimerization and the autophosphorylation of several tyrosine residues which then specifically bind the Src homologous domains SH2 of effector or adaptor proteins, initiating a cascade of protein–protein interactions. Signalling enzymes (e.g. Grb2, Shc) serve as a molecular scaffold from which subsequent signals emanate. For example, the guanine nucleotide exchange factor Sos binds to Grb2, which then activates the Ras protein and consequently the microtubule-associated protein (MAP) kinase cascade. Several components of this complex array of intracellular circuits have been implicated in tumorigenesis and are putative targets for developing anti-cancer agents (Corda and D'Inalci, 1997; Gibbs, 2000).

GROWTH FACTOR RECEPTORS

Unlike other members of the EGF receptor family, HER2 has no known ligand. HER2 is overexpressed in 25–30 per cent of breast cancers and predicts for a worse prognosis, as measured by shorter disease-free survival and overall survival (Slamon et al., 1989; Seshadri et al., 1993; Press et al., 1997). Antibodies directed to the extracellular domain of HER2 can inhibit the growth of tumour xenografts and transformed cells that express high levels of this receptor (Drebin et al., 1985; Stancovski et al., 1991). The recombinant humanized anti-HER2 antibody, herceptin, has a cytostatic growth inhibitory effect against breast cancer cells expressing HER2 and can also enhance the anti-tumour activity of doxorubicin and paclitaxel against human breast cancer xenografts overexpressing HER2/neu (Baselga et al., 1998). Clinical activity of herceptin has been demonstrated in breast cancer (Baselga et al., 1996) and subsequent trials have led to Food and Drug Administration (FDA) approval.

Therapeutic antibodies have also been developed against the EGF receptor (Fan and Mendelsohn, 1998; Yang et al., 1999). Other approaches include inhibition of the intracellular tyrosine kinase domain of the EGF receptor (Moyer et al., 1997), and inhibiting PDGF receptor kinase activity (Eckhardt et al., 1999).

INHIBITION OF RAS SIGNALLING PATHWAYS

The ras family of oncogenes is one of the most frequently activated groups of dominant transforming genes in both human and experimental cancers (Bos, 1989). The ras family of genes encode highly similar proteins with molecular weights of 21 kDa, which are thought to play a key role in signal transduction (Barbacid, 1987). One strategy for regulating ras gene expression is by the use of an antisense oligonucleotide directed against H-ras expression (Holmlund et al., 1999). An alternative approach is by inhibiting protein farnesylation. Ras proteins carry an essential lipid moiety – a farnesyl group – at their COOH termini. Inhibition of Ras farnesylation blocks Ras localization to the plasma membrane, and as a consequent Ras fails to interact with regulatory and effector molecules (Lowy and Willumsen, 1993). Inhibition of farnesyl transferase is currently in early clinical trials (Gibbs, 2000). However, it has been suggested that farnesyl transferase inhibitors (FTIs) act at a level beyond that of suppressing Ras function (Lebowitz and Prendergast, 1998).

Ras activation results in a series of protein phosphorylation events within the cell. The first key step is the direct binding of the Raf protein kinase to Ras-GTP. Raf in turn phosphorylates and activates MAP/ERK kinase (MEK), which in turn phosphorylates and activates MAP kinase (Gibbs, 2000). Potential anti-cancer strategies targeted to this pathway are at an early stage of development and include an antisense oligonucleotide to Raf (Holmlund et al., 1999), Raf protein kinase inhibitors (Hall-Jackson et al., 1999) and MEK inhibition (Sebolt-Leopold et al., 1999).

Cyclin-dependent kinases and the cell cycle

Cyclin-dependent kinases (CDKs) regulate the transition from one cell-cycle phase to the next by phosphorylating key structural and regulatory substrate molecules. This activity is regulated by the orderly appearance of cyclins, prompted by environmental cues and by post-translational modification of CDKs through phosphorylation of key stimulating and inhibitory sites in the catalytic subunit. Furthermore, endogenous inhibitors of CDK activity have been identified, including p16, p21 and p27. The biochemical events involved in cell-cycle progression have been reviewed in detail (Pines, 1995; Sherr, 1996; Morgan, 1997). Altered expression of CDK components have been demonstrated in malignant cells with consequent loss of regulation of cell-cycle progression, and as such are targets for developing novel therapeutic strategies. These can be considered as direct CDK inhibitors, that is agents which inhibit the function of an activated CDK; or indirect inhibitors, that is agents which alter the activation state of CDK.

DIRECT CDK INHIBITION

Early clinical trials with CDK modulators have evaluated flavopiridol (Senderowicz et al., 1998) and UCN-01 (Sausville et al., 1998). Preclinical studies have demonstrated that flavopiridol inhibits CDKs 1, 2 and 4, although it may have mechanisms of actions other than on the cell-cycle regulatory mechanisms (Carlson et al., 1996). UCN-01, a staurosporine derivative, has also entered clinical evaluation. Other putative inhibitors include purine analogues such as roscovitine (Meijer et al., 1997), and peptides that mimic the function of endogenous CDK inhibitors such as p21 (Ball et al., 1997). However, these agents have not yet entered clinical evaluation.

INDIRECT CDK INHIBITORS

Drugs that cause decreased expression of cyclin D genes, or altered efficiency of cyclin D translation leading to a decrease in cyclin D protein levels, can indirectly inhibit CDK activity, e.g. rapamycin (Hashemolhosseini et al., 1998). Moreover, a number of compounds, including the differentiation agents (retinoids and vitamin D analogues), can increase the expression of p21, an endogenous CDK inhibitor. Finally, altering CDK checkpoint control in the presence of DNA-damaging agents, e.g. by UCN-01 (Bunch and Eastman, 1996), may enhance the cytotoxicity of these DNA-interacting agents.

The telomerase structure and the telomerase enzyme

Telomerase is a ribonucleotide which, although thought to be required during development, is largely repressed in adult somatic tissues (Harley and Villeponteau, 1995). Telomerase replicates the terminal sequences of eukaryotic chromosomes, namely the telomere (Morin, 1997). The absence of telomerase activity from normal somatic cells has led to the proposal that telomere shortening may be a molecular clock which contributes to the onset of cellular senescence in normal cells (Harley and Sherwood, 1997). Conversely, the reactivation or expression of telomerase may be a major mechanism by which cancer cells overcome normal cellular senescence (Kim, 1997; Parkinson et al., 1997). Indeed, telomerase activity may be present in more than 80 per cent of tumour biopsies, yet absence or reduced in normal somatic tissues (Shay and Bacchetti, 1997). The realization that activation of telomerase can co-operate with a limited number of other 'genetic hits' leading to malignant transformation (Weitzman and Yaniv, 1999), allied to the high levels of expression of the telomerase enzyme in specific cancers, reinforces the notion that the telomerase enzyme and the telomeric structure are exciting targets as potential

anti-cancer strategies. Numerous potential therapeutic strategies have been proposed including telomerase-interactive compounds (peptide nucleic acids, antisense oligonucleotides, ribozymes, reverse transcriptase inhibitors) and telomere-interactive compounds, such as the G-quartet interactive agents (Sharma et al., 1997). One potential drawback of these strategies is the 'phenotype lag', that is the number of cell divisions necessary before inhibition of telomerase leads to sufficient shortening of the telomerase to give rise to a phenotypic effect, suggesting that these agents are likely to be active in minimal disease states.

Genes, vaccines and drug delivery

Strategies to target the underlying genetic lesions of the cancer cell are often considered under the umbrella of 'gene therapy', and include antisense oligonucleotides, recombinant vaccines as immunotherapy (Evans and Kaye, 1999b), transducing a drug-resistance gene into bone-marrow stem cells to protect the bone marrow during chemotherapy, and the use of expression vectors to convert an inactive pro-drug into active drugs (Roth and Cristiano, 1997). These approaches are discussed more fully in Chapters 12 and 14. Many of the existing vectors for gene delivery and expression have limitations (Roth and Cristiano, 1997) and improvement in drug-delivery mechanisms and vector design remains a crucial area in order to increase the efficiency of expression, the precision of targeting, and to reduce toxicity. The possibility of specific gene targeting, and possible synergy with other, existing cancer therapeutics is a promising goal for future development.

SIGNIFICANT POINTS

- Smaller tumours have more rapid growth rates and are more likely to be responsive to chemotherapy; cure rates are likely to be higher with a small tumour burden.
- Route of administration of a cytotoxic drug is determined by the stability, size, molecular charge and sclerosant characteristics of the drug.
- Combination chemotherapy aims to prevent or slow the development of resistant tumours; drugs used in such regimens have activity as single agents, different mechanisms of action and minimal overlapping toxicities.
- Acquisition of novel anti-cancer drugs is usually by either serendipitous discovery, large-scale empirical screening, analogue

development from an existing agent or based on knowledge of a defined molecular target.

- Clinical drug development takes many years and consists of a logical sequence of trials: phase I (toxicity), phase II (activity) and phase III (comparative activity compared with standard treatments).

- Anti-cancer drugs can be grouped by mode of action, e.g. alkylators, antimetabolites, anti-tumour antibiotics; although the increasing number of new drugs with novel mechanisms of action makes such divisions difficult and arbitrary.

- In the twenty-first century, the development of new agents with novel mechanisms of action will require additional clinical end points, such as demonstration of the desired biological activity.

KEY REFERENCES

American Society of Clinical Oncology. (1997) Critical role of Phase I clinical trials in cancer treatment. *J. Clin. Oncol.* **15**, 853–9.

Grever, M.R. and Chabner, B.A. (1993) Cancer drug discovery and development. In de Vita, V.T., Hellman, S. and Rosenberg, S.A. (eds), *Principles and practice of oncology*. Philadelphia: Lippincott.

Ratain, M., Mick, R., Schilsky, R. *et al.* (1993) Statistical and ethical issues in the design and conduct of phase I and II clinical trials of new anti-cancer agents. *J. Natl Cancer Inst.* **85**, 1637–43.

Winograd, B. (1995) New drug development. In Peckham, M., Pinedo, H.M. and Veronesi, U. (eds), *Oxford textbook of oncology*. Oxford: Oxford University Press.

REFERENCES

Akhter, J., Chen, X., Bowrey, P. *et al.* (1997) Vitamin D analog, EB1089, inhibits growth of subcutaneous xenografts of the human colon cancer cell line, LoVo, in a nude mouse model. *Dis. Colon Rectum* **40**, 317–21.

Allenby, G., Bocquel, M.-T., Saunders, M. *et al.* (1993) Retinoic acid receptors and retinoid X receptors: interactions with endogenous retinoic acids. *Proc. Natl Acad. Sci. USA* **90**, 30–4.

Anderson, N.R. (1993) 5-Fluorouracil: a re-appraisal of optimal delivery in advanced breast cancer. *J. Infus. Chemother.* **3**, 111–18.

Augustin, H.G. (1998) Anti-angiogenic tumour therapy: will it work? *Trends Pharmacol. Sci.* **19**, 216–22.

Ball, K.L., Lain, S., Fahreus, R. *et al.* (1997) Cell cycle arrest and inhibition of CDK4 activity by small peptides based on the carboxyl terminus of p21^{WAF1}. *Curr. Biol.* **7**, 71–80.

Barbacid, M. (1987) *ras* genes. *Ann. Rev. Biochem.* **56**, 779–827.

Baselga, J., Tripathy, D., Mendelsohn, J. *et al.* (1996) Phase II study of weekly intravenous recombinant humanized anti-p185^{HER2} monoclonal antibody in patients with HER2/neu overexpressing metastatic breast cancer. *J. Clin. Oncol.* **14**, 737–44.

Baselga, J., Norton, L., Albanell, J. *et al.* (1998) Recombinant humanized anti-HER2 antibody (Herceptin™) enhances the anticancer activity of paclitaxel and doxorubicin against HER2/neu overexpressing human breast cancer xenografts. *Cancer Res.* **58**, 2825–31.

Birkhead, B.G., Rankin, E.M., Gallivan, S. *et al.* (1987) A mathematical model of the development of drug resistance to cancer chemotherapy. *Eur. J. Cancer Clin. Oncol.* **23**, 1421–7.

Bos, J.L. (1989) Ras oncogenes in human cancer: a review. *Cancer Res.* **49**, 4682–9.

Bower, M., Colston, K.W., Stein, R.C. *et al.* (1991) Topical calcipotriol treatment in advanced breast cancer. *Lancet* **337**, 701–2.

Bunch, R.T. and Eastman, A. (1996) Enhancement of cisplatin induced cytotoxicity by 7-hydroxy staurosporine (UCN-01), a new G2 checkpoint inhibitor. *Clin. Cancer Res.* **2**, 791–7.

Carlberg, C. (1995) Mechanisms of nuclear signalling by vitamin D3. Interplay with retinoid and thyroid hormone signalling. *Eur. J. Biochem.* **231**, 517–27.

Carlson, B.A., Dubay, M.M., Sausville, E.A. *et al.* (1996) Flavopiridol induces G1 arrest with inhibition of cyclin-dependent kinase (CDK) 2 and CDK4 in human breast carcinoma cells. *Cancer Res.* **56**, 2973–8.

Castaigne, S., Chomienne, C., Daniel, M.T. *et al.* (1990) All-trans retinoic acid as differentiation therapy for acute promyolocytic leukaemia. Clinical results. *Blood* **76**, 1704–9.

Chambon, P. (1995) The molecular and genetic dissection of the retinoid signalling pathway. *Recent Prog. Horm. Res.* **50**, 317–32.

Chen, J.D. and Evans, R.M. (1995) A transcriptional co-repressor that interacts with nuclear hormone receptors. *Nature* **337**, 454–7.

Chen, Z., Zue, Y., Zhang, R. *et al.* (1991) A clinical and experimental study on all *trans* retinoic acid treated acute promyelocytic leukaemia patients. *Blood* **78**, 1413–19.

Corda, D. and D'Inalci, M. (1997) Cell signalling and cancer treatment. *Ann. Oncol.* **18**, 429–33.

Daley, G.Q., Van Etten, R.A. and Baltimore, D. (1990) Induction of chronic myelogenous leukemia in mice by the P210bcr/abl gene of the Philadelphia chromosome. *Science* **247**, 824–30.

Denis, L.J. and Verweij, J. (1997) Matrix metalloproteinase inhibitors: present achievements and future prospects. *Invest. New Drugs* **15**, 175–85.

DeVita, V.T., Hubbard, S.M. and Longo, D.L. (1987) The chemotherapy of lymphomas: looking back, moving forward. The Richard and Hinda Rosenthal Foundation Award Lecture. *Cancer Res.* **47**, 5810–24.

Drebin, J.A., Link, V.C., Stern, D.F. *et al.* (1985) Down-modulation of an oncogene protein product and reversion of the transformed phenotype by monoclonal antibodies. *Cell* **41**, 695–706.

Druker, B.J., Talpaz, M., Resta, D.J. *et al.* (2001a) Efficacy and safety of a specific inhibitor of the BCR-ABL tyrosine kinase in chronic myeloid leukaemia. *New Engl J Med.* **344**, 1031–7.

Druker, B.J., Sawyers, C.L., Kantarjian, H. *et al.* (2001b) Activity of a specific inhibitor of the BCR-ABL tyrosine kinase in the blast crisis of chronic myeloid leukemia and acute lymphoblastic leukemia with the Philadelphia chromosome. *New Engl J Med.* **344**, 1038–42.

Eckhardt, S.G., Rizzo, J., Sweeney, K.R. *et al.* (1999) Phase I and pharmacologic study of the tyrosine kinase inhibitor SU101 in patients with advanced solid tumours. *J. Clin. Oncol.* **17**, 1095–104.

Evans, R.M. (1988) The steroid and thyroid hormone superfamily. *Science* **240**, 889–95.

Evans, T.R.J. and Kaye, S.B. (1999a) Retinoids: present role and future potential. *Br. J. Cancer* **80**, 1–8.

Evans, T.R.J. and Kaye, S.B. (1999b) Vaccine therapy for cancer – fact or fiction? *QJM* **92**, 299–307.

Fan, Z. and Mendelsohn, J. (1998) Therapeutic application of anti-growth factor receptor antibodies. *Curr. Opin. Oncol.* **10**, 67–73.

Fenaux, P., Castaigne, S., Dombret, H. *et al.* (1992) All trans reinoic acid followed by intensive chemotherapy gives a high complete remission rate and may prolong remissions in newly diagnosed acute promyelocytic leukaemia: a pilot study on 26 cases. *Blood* **80**, 2176–81.

Frankel, S.R., Eardley, A., Heller, G. *et al.* (1994) All trans retinoic acid for acute promyolcytic leukaemia. *Ann. Intern. Med.* **120**, 278–86.

Gasparini, G. (1999) The rationale and future potential of angiogenesis inhibitor in neoplasia. *Drugs* **58**, 17–38.

Gibbs, J.B. (2000) Anticancer drug targets: growth factors and growth factor signaling. *J. Clin. Invest.* **105**, 9–13.

Giguere, V., Ong, E.S., Segui, P. and Evans, R.M. (1987) Identification of a receptor for the morphagen retinoic acid. *Nature* **330**, 624–9.

Glick, J.H. *et al.* (1998) MOPP/ABV hybrid chemotherapy for advanced Hodgkin's disease significantly improves failure-free and overall survival: the 8-year results of the Intergroup Trial. *J. Clin. Oncol.* **16**(1), 19–26.

Goldie, J.H. and Coldman, A.J. (1979) A mathematical model for relating the drug sensitivity of tumours to the spontaneous mutation rate. *Cancer Treat. Rep.* **63**, 1727–33.

Goldin, A. and Schabel, F.M. (1981) Clinical concepts derived from animal chemotherapy studies. *Cancer Treat. Rep.* **65**(suppl. 3), 11–19.

Gulliford, T., English, J., Colston, K.W. *et al.* (1998) A phase I study of the vitamin D analogue EB1089 in patients with advanced breast and colorectal cancer. *Br. J. Cancer* **70**, 6–13.

Hall-Jackson, C.A., Geodert, M., Hedge, P. and Cohen, P. (1999) Effect of SB203580 on the activity of c-*Raf* *in vitro* and *in vivo*. *Oncogene* **18**, 2047–54.

Hansen, C.M., Frandsen, T.L., Brunner, N. *et al.* (1994) 1α 25-dihydroxyvitamin D3 inhibits the invasive potential of human breast cancer cells *in vitro*. *Clin. Exp. Metastasis* **12**, 195–202.

Harley, C.B. and Sherwood, S.W. (1997) Telomerase, checkpoints and cancer. *Cancer Surv.* **29**, 263–84.

Harley, C.B. and Villeponteau, B. (1995) Telomeres and telomerase in ageing and cancer. *Curr. Opin. Genet. Dev.* **5**, 249–55.

Hashemolhosseini, S., Nagamine, Y., Morley, S.J. *et al.* (1998) Rapamycin inhibition of G1 to 2S transition is mediated by effects on cyclin D1 mRNA and protein stability. *J. Biol. Chem.* **273**, 14424–9.

Heisterkemp, N., Jenster, G., ten Hoeve, J., Zovich, D., Pattengale, P.K. and Groffen, J. (1990) Acute leukaemia in bcr/abl transgenic mice. *Nature* **344**, 251–3.

Holmlund, J.T., Monia, B.P., Kwoh, T.J. and Dorr, F.A. (1999) Towards antisense oligonucleotide therapy for cancer. ISIS compounds in clinical development. *Curr. Opin. Mol. Ther.* **1**, 372–85.

Horwitz, K.B., Jackson, T.A., Rain, D.L. *et al.* (1996) Nuclear hormone receptor co-activators and co-repressors. *Mol. Endocrinol.* **10**, 1167–77.

Hryniuk, W.M. (1987) Average relative dose intensity and the impact of design on clinical trials. *Semin. Oncol.* **14**, 65–74.

Hryniuk, W. and Levine, M.N. (1986) Analysis of dose intensity for adjuvant chemotherapy trials in stage II breast cancer. *J. Clin. Oncol.* **4**, 1162–70.

Huang, M., Ye, Y., Chen, S. *et al.* (1988) Use of all trans retinoic acid in the treatment of acute promyelocytic leukaemia. *Blood* **72**, 567–72.

James, S.Y., Mackay, A.G., Binderup, L. *et al.* (1994) Effects of a new synthetic vitamin D analogue EB1089, on the oestrogen-responsive growth of human breast cancer cells. *J. Endocrinol.* **141**, 555–63.

Kanamaru, A., Takemoto, Y., Tanimoto, M. *et al.* (1995) All-trans retinoic acid for the treatment of newly diagnosed acute promyelocytic leukaemia. *Blood* **85**, 1202–6.

Kaye, S.B., Lewis, C.R., Paul, J. *et al.* (1992) Randomised study of two doses of cisplatin with cyclophosphamide in epithelial ovarian cancer. *Lancet* **340**, 329–33.

Kelliher, M.A., McLaughlin, J., Witte, O.N. and Rosenberg, N. (1990) Induction of a chronic myelogenous leukemia-like syndrome in mice with v-abl and BCR/ABL. *Proc. Natl Acad. Sci. USA* **87**, 6649–53.

Kim, N.W. (1997) Clinical implications of telomerase in cancer. *Eur. J. Cancer* **33**, 781–6.

Kliewer, S.A., Umesono, K., Mangelsdorf, D.J. and Evans, R.W. (1992) Retinoid X receptor interacts with nuclear receptors in retinoic acid, thyroid hormone, and vitamin D_3 signalling. *Nature* **355**, 446–9.

Kurokawa, R., Soderstrom, M., Horlein, A. *et al.* (1995) Polarity-specific activities of retinoic acid receptors determined by a co-repressor. *Nature* **377**, 451–4.

Laudet, V., Hanni, C., Coll, J., Catzeflis, F. and Stehelin, D. (1992) Evolution of the nuclear receptor gene superfamily. *EMBO J.* **11**, 1003–13.

Lebowitz, P.F. and Prendergast, G.C. (1998) Non-*ras* targets of farnesyltransferase inhibitors: focus on Rho. *Oncogene* **17**, 1439–45.

Levin, L. and Hrynuik, W.M. (1987) Dose intensity analysis of chemotherapy regimens in ovarian carcinoma. *J. Clin. Oncol.* **5**, 756–7.

Lokich, J.J., Ahlgren, J.D., Gullo, S.J. *et al.* (1989) A prospective randomised comparison of continuous infusion fluorouracil with a conventional bolus schedule in metastatic colorectal carcinoma. A Mid-Atlantic Oncology Program Study. *J. Clin. Oncol.* **7**, 425–32.

Lotan, R. (1996) Retinoids in cancer chemoprevention. *FASEB J.* **10**, 1031–9.

Lowy, D.R. and Willumsen, B.M. (1993) Function and regulation of *ras. Ann. Rev. Biochem.* **62**, 851–91.

Lugo, T.G., Pendergast, A.M., Muller, A.J. and Witte, O.N. (1990) Tyrosine kinase activity and transformation potency of bcr-abl oncogene products. *Science* **247**, 1079–82.

Majewski, S., Szmurlo, A., Marczak, M. *et al.* (1993) Inhibition of tumour-cell induced angiogenesis by retinoids, 1,25-dihydroxyvitamin D3 and their combinations. *Cancer Lett.* **75**, 35–9.

Mangelsdorf, D.J., Borgmeyer, U., Heyman, R.A. *et al.* (1992) Characterisation of three RXR genes that mediate the action of 9-cis retinoic acid. *Genes Dev.* **6**, 329–44.

McLeod, H.L. and Evans, W.E. (1999) Oral cancer chemotherapy: the promise and the pitfalls. *Clin. Cancer Res.* **5**, 2669–71.

Meijer, L., Borgne, A., Mulner, O. *et al.* (1997) Biochemical and cellular effects of roscovitine, a potent and selective inhibitor of the cyclin dependent kinases cdc2, cdk2, and cdk5. *Eur. J. Biochem.* **243**, 527–36.

Morgan, D.O. (1997) Cyclin dependent kinases: engines, clocks and microprocessors. *Annu Rev. Cell Dev. Biol.* **13**, 261–91.

Morin, S.G. (1997) The implication of telomerase biochemistry for human disease. *Eur. J. Cancer* **33**, 750–60.

Moyer, J.D., Barbacci, E.G., Iwata, K.K. *et al.* (1997) Induction of apoptosis and cell cycle arrest by CP-358, 774, an inhibitor of epidermal growth factor receptor tyrosine kinase. *Cancer Res.* **57**, 4838–48.

Nagpal, S., Saunders, M., Kastner, P. *et al.* (1992) Promoter context – and response element-dependent specificity of the transcriptional activation and modulating functions of retinoic acid receptors. *Cell* **70**, 1007–19.

Nagy, L., Thomazy, V.A., Shipley, G.L. *et al.* (1995) Activation of retinoid X receptors induces apoptosis in HL-60 cell lines. *Mol. Cell. Biol.* **15**, 3540–51.

Norton, L. and Simon, R. (1977) Tumour size, sensitivity to therapy and design of treatment schedules. *Cancer Treat. Rep.* **61**, 1307–17.

Ohno, R., Yoshida, H., Fukutani, H. *et al.* (1993) Multi-institutional study of all trans retinoic acid as a differentiation therapy of refractory acute promyelocytic leukaemia. *Leukaemia* **7**, 1722–7.

Parkinson, E.K., Newbold, R.F. and Keith, W.N. (1997) The genetic basis of human keratinocyte immortalization in squamous cell carcinoma development: the role of telomerase reactivation. *Eur. J. Cancer* **33**, 727–34.

Perlmann, T. and Evans, R.M. (1997) Nuclear receptors in Sicily: all in the famiglia. *Cell* **90**, 391–7.

Petkovich, M., Brand, N., Krust, A. and Chambon, P. (1987) A human retinoic acid receptor which belongs to the family of nuclear receptors. *Nature* **330**, 444–50.

Pines, J. (1995) Cyclins and cyclin dependent kinase: a biochemical view. *Biochem. J.* **308**, 697–711.

Press, M.F., Bernstein, L., Thomas, P.A. *et al.* (1997) HER-2/neu gene amplification characterized by fluorescence *in situ* hybridisation: poor prognosis in node-negative breast carcinomas. *J. Clin. Oncol.* **15**, 2894–904.

Roth, J.A. and Cristiano, R.J. (1997) Gene therapy for cancer: what have we done and where are we going? *J. Natl Cancer Inst.* **89**, 21–39.

Rowley, J.D. (1973) A new consistent chromosomal abnormality in chronic myelogenous leukemia identified by quinacrine fluorescence and Giemsa staining. *Nature* **243**, 290–3.

Sausville, E.A., Lush, R.D., Headlee, D. *et al.* (1998) Clinical pharmacology of UCN-01 initial observations and comparison to pre-clinical models. *Cancer Chemother. Pharmacol.* **42**, S54–S59.

Schadendorf, D., Kern, M.A., Artuc, M. *et al.* (1996) Treatment of melanoma cells with the synthetic retinoid CD437 induces apoptosis via activation of AP-1 *in vitro* and causes growth inhibition in xenografts *in vivo. J. Cell Biol.* **135**, 1889–98.

Sebolt-Leopold, J.S., Dudley, D.T., Herrera, T. *et al.* (1999) Blockade of the MAP kinase pathway suppresses growth of colon tumours *in vivo. Nat. Med.* **5**, 810–16.

Senderowicz, A.M., Headlee, D., Stinson, S.F. *et al.* (1998) Phase I trials of continuous infusion flavopiridol, a novel cyclin-dependent kinase inhibitor in patients with refractory neoplasms. *J. Clin. Oncol.* **16**, 2986–99.

Seshadri, R., Firgira, F.A., Horsfall, D.J. *et al.* (1993) Clinical significance of HER-2/neu oncogene amplification in primary breast cancer. The South Australian Breast Cancer Study Group. *J. Clin. Oncol.* **11**, 1936–42.

Sharma, S., Raymond, E., Soda, H. *et al.* (1997) Preclinical and clinical strategies for development of telomerase and telomere inhibitors. *Ann. Oncol.* **8**, 1063–74.

Shay, J.W. and Bacchetti, S. (1997) A survey of telomerase activity in human cancer. *Eur. J. Cancer* **33**, 781–91.

Sherr, C.J. (1996) Cancer cell cycles. *Science* **274**, 1672–7.

Skipper, H. (1986) Data and analyses having to do with the influence of dose intensity and duration of treatment (single drugs and combinations) on lethal toxicity and the therapeutic response of experimental neoplasms. Southern Research Institute Booklets 13, 1986, and 2–13, 1987.

Skipper, H.E., Schabel, F.H., Wilcox, E.S. *et al.* (1964) Experimental evaluation of potential anticancer agents XII: on the criteria and kinetics associated with 'curability' of experimental leukaemia. *Cancer Chemother. Rep.* **35**, 1–11.

Slamon, D.J., Godolphin, W., Jones, L.A. *et al.* (1989) Studies of the HER-2/neu proto-oncogene in human breast and ovarian cancer. *Science* **244**, 707–12.

Stancovski, I., Hurwitz, E., Leitner, D. *et al.* (1991) Mechanistic aspects of the opposing effects of monoclonal antibodies to the erbB-2 receptor on tumour growth. *Proc. Natl Acad. Sci. USA* **88**, 8691–5.

Tallman, M.S., Andersen, J.W., Schiffer, C.A. *et al.* (1997) All-trans retinoic acid in acute promyelocytic leukaemia. *N. Engl. J. Med.* **337**, 1021–8.

Twardowski, P. and Gradishar, W.J. (1997) Clinical trials of anti-angiogenic agents. *Curr. Opin. Oncol.* **9**, 584–9.

Twelves, C.J., Gardner, C., Flavin, A. *et al.* for the CRC Phase I/II Committee (1999) Phase I and pharmacokinetic study of DACA (XR5000): a novel inhibitor of topoisomerase I and II. *Br. J. Cancer* **80**(11), 1786–91.

Vasey, P.A. (1997) Paclitaxel and Docetaxel in breast and ovarian cancer. *Drug Ther. Bull.* **35**(6), 43–6.

Vasey, P.A. (1999) The role of oral fluoropyrimidines in the treatment of breast and colorectal cancers. http://www.medscape.com/Medscape/oncology/Treatmentupdate/1999/tu01/public/toc-tu01.html

Vasey, P.A. and Kaye, S.B. (1997) Combined topoisomerase I/II inhibition – is this a worthwhile/feasible strategy? (Editorial). *Br. J. Cancer* **76**(11), 1395–7.

Vasey, P.A., Kaye, S.B., Morrison, R. *et al.* (1999a) Phase I clinical and pharmocokinetic study of PK1 (HPMA Co-polymer doxorubicin): first member of a new class of chemotherapeutic agents – drug–polymer conjugates. *Clin. Cancer Res.* **5**(1), 83–94.

Vasey, P.A., Coleman, R., Eggleton, S.P.H. *et al.* (1999b) Is docetaxel–carboplatin an alternative to paclitaxel–carboplatin in ovarian cancer? *Br. J. Cancer* **80**(S2), 2.13.

Warrell, R.P., Frankel, S.R., Miller, W.H. *et al.* (1991) Differentiation therapy of acute promyelocytic leukaemia with tretinoin (all-trans retinoic acid). *N. Engl. J. Med.* **324**, 1385–93.

Weitzman, J.B. and Yaniv, M. (1999) Rebuilding the road to cancer. *Nature* **400**, 401–2.

Yang, X.D., Jian, X.C., Corvalan, J.R.F. *et al.* (1999) Evaluation of established tumors by a fully human monoclonal antibody to the epidermal growth factor receptor without concomitant chemotherapy. *Cancer Res.* **59**, 1236–43.

8

Drug resistance

PHILIP H. JONES AND DENIS C. TALBOT

Despite the notable advances in cancer management over recent decades, drug resistance remains the most important reason for treatment failure, with the result that cancer remains the second most common cause of death in the Western world. In clinical practice, drug resistance results in two types of tumour behaviour. In the first category, an initial response to cytotoxic chemotherapy is followed by relapse. The recurrent tumour is often resistant to treatment with drugs that are chemically unrelated to those used in first-line treatment. Tumours that demonstrate induced resistance to treatment include small cell lung cancer, acute myeloid leukaemia and lymphoma. The second category is typified by melanoma and non-small cell lung cancer. These tumours do not usually respond to first-line treatment, owing to intrinsic drug resistance. The patterns of response that typify different tumour types are set out in Table 8.1.

There are numerous models of mechanisms of drug resistance. Several of these derive from insights into the biology of solid tumours, while others come from studies on cancer cell lines. Validating these models in human tumours is often difficult; the biology of human tumours differs significantly from that of cancer in animal models, it is not safe to assume that such data have a direct bearing on drug resistance in the clinical setting. It is likely that there are multiple reasons why solid tumours resist chemotherapy, with several mechanisms operating in parallel in a given patient being treated with a particular chemotherapy regimen.

The major advance in understanding drug resistance in the past 5 years has been in gaining insight into the molecular mechanisms by which cytotoxic chemotherapy leads to cell death. This has revealed new insights into drug resistance, which may offer hope for overcoming clinical drug resistance in the future. This chapter describes the progress in understanding mechanisms of resistance to common cytotoxic drugs, focusing on those which are implicated in resistance in human tumours and which

Table 8.1 *Types of clinical drug resistance*

Clinical behaviour of tumour	Tumour type	Type of drug resistance	Treatment outcome
Responds completely to chemotherapy	Burkitt's lymphoma Choriocarcinoma Hodgkin's disease Acute leukaemia Teratoma	None	Curable with chemotherapy
Initial response, but later relapses do not respond	Ovarian cancer Breast cancer Gastrointestinal cancer Non-Hodgkin's lymphoma	Induced resistance	Chemotherapy gives symptomatic improvement or short increase in length of life, but not curable
Resistant	Melanoma Pancreatic cancer	Intrinsic resistance	Chemotherapy usually ineffective

Table 8.2 *Causes of cytotoxic drug resistance and their clinical implications*

Mechanism of resistance	Clinical implication
Genetic instability	Basis for combination chemotherapy and high-dose chemotherapy
Cytokinetic resistance	Altered administration schedules for phase-specific drugs, e.g. etoposide, infusional 5-fluorouracil
Tumour microenvironment – hypoxia	Development of hypoxically activated drugs, e.g. tirapazamine
Privileged sites	Radiotherapy to brain or testis in leukaemia
Multiple drug resistance	Development of P glycoprotein inhibitors
Resistance to chemotherapy-induced apoptosis	Development of gene therapy approaches, e.g. p53 repair, BCL2 inhibition
Decreased drug uptake	Development of trimetrexate
Increased detoxification	Clinical trials of buthione sulphoxide to overcome low glutathione levels in cisplatin resistance
Increased DNA repair	Use of DNA repair inhibitors

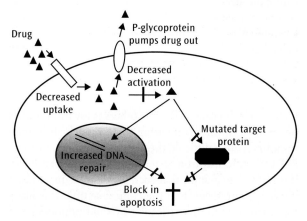

Figure 8.1 *Cellular mechanisms of resistance.*

have implications for therapy (*see* Table 8.2 and Fig. 8.1). Strategies to overcome drug resistance, including new approaches in clinical development, are also discussed.

GENETIC INSTABILITY

A universal characteristic of all cancers is genetic instability. Cancer cells undergo mutation at a far higher rate than normal cells, resulting in an unstable genome in which genes are rearranged and amplified (Cahill *et al.*, 1999). Mutations that favour cell growth and survival are acquired and preserved as the population of cancer cells increases. Once a tumour is clinically detectable, the single clone of cells that was present in the earliest stages of carcinogenesis has diversified into numerous, genetically distinct populations of cells. These genetic differences underlie the variation in the degree of differentiation and proliferation, both between cells within a primary tumour and between primary and metastatic tumours.

The Goldie and Coldman hypothesis proposes that genetic instability is the basis of induced resistance to chemotherapy. At the stage when most cancers are treated with primary chemotherapy, a few of the many different subpopulations of cells in the tumour are likely to possess mutations that make them resistant to treatment (Goldie and Coldman, 1984). The clones that are sensitive to the drug are rapidly eliminated, while those that are resistant persist and continue to proliferate. After an interval, the resistant clones present as a clinical relapse unresponsive to treatment. The genetic diversity of tumours is the rationale for the use of combination chemotherapy, discussed below.

Combination chemotherapy

The Goldie–Coldman hypothesis offers a rational basis for combination chemotherapy (Goldie and Coldman, 1984). If 1 in 10^3 cells has intrinsic resistance to one agent and 1 in 10^5 resistance to another drug, only 1 in 10^8 cells will have resistance to a combination of both agents. In chemosensitive tumours, such as leukaemia, lymphoma and germ-cell malignancies, combining drugs that have shown activity as single agents has led to the development of combinations with far greater anti-tumour activity than any single drug. It is the use of drugs in combination that has resulted in curative therapy for such tumours. In palliative chemotherapy for intrinsically resistant tumours, such as non-small cell lung cancer, the benefits of combination treatment are less clear cut. Combinations produce slightly higher response rates than the most active single agents, but the benefits may be outweighed by increased side-effects (Lilenbaum *et al.*, 1998).

Not all clinical data support the Goldie–Coldman hypothesis, which predicts that at relapse after primary chemotherapy tumour cells would be genetically resistant to repeat challenge with the same drugs as used in initial treatment (Fennelly *et al.*, 1998). Patients who developed metastatic breast cancer a year or more after adjuvant cyclophosphamide, methotrexate and 5-fluorouracil (CMF) have a response rate of over 50 per cent to repeat CMF (Valagussa *et al.*, 1986). Similarly, repeated treatment with platinum-based chemotherapy in patients with ovarian cancer who relapse more than 18 months after primary therapy may produce responses (Gore *et al.*, 1990).

High-dose chemotherapy

Whereas some cancer cell lines and tumours display absolute resistance towards some agents, showing no response however high a concentration of drug is used, in most cases tumour response is dose dependent (Goldie and Coldman, 1986). It has been argued that tumours that respond to chemotherapy given at conventional doses, such as advanced breast and ovarian cancer, might be cured if chemotherapy was given at significantly higher doses. The most common dose-limiting toxicity associated with chemotherapy is myelosuppression; this can be overcome by use of haemopoietic growth factors, re-infusing haemopoietic stem cells harvested from the patient prior to chemotherapy, or bone-marrow allografting.

Several large, randomized trials comparing standard treatment with high-dose therapy have been completed in breast cancer. Interpretation of such trials is made more difficult because different high-dose regimes and different control 'conventional' treatment arms have been used. The two largest studies of high-dose adjuvant therapy in poor-prognosis disease showed no 3-year survival benefit from high-dose therapy. Similarly, for patients with metastatic disease, the only study including over 100 patients showed no survival benefit following high-dose chemotherapy (Livingston and Crawley, 1999). Long-term follow-up is needed in these studies and more trials are ongoing, but at present there is no evidence to justify high-dose therapy in breast cancer outside of ongoing clinical trials (Antman, 1999; Hortobagyi, 1999). Phase III studies of high-dose schedules are being conducted in testicular tumours, non-Hodgkin's lymphoma and ovarian cancer (Herrin and Thigpen, 1999; Morrison and Peterson, 1999; Sobecks and Vogelzang, 1999). The role of high-dose therapy will only be clarified once these large randomized trials are completed and long-term follow-up data, including that on the late toxicity of both treatment arms, is available.

CYTOKINETIC RESISTANCE

Early in evolution, all tumours acquire mutations favouring cell proliferation (Cahill *et al.*, 1998). There is a broad relationship between the rate at which tumours proliferate and the probability of cure by chemotherapy. Many curable tumours, such as lymphomas, have a high proportion of cycling cells, whereas in tumours that are relatively unresponsive to chemotherapy, such as melanoma and gastrointestinal cancer, only 2 or 3 per cent of the cells are proliferating (Tannock, 1978). There is a considerable range in the proportion of cycling cells among tumours of the same histological type and site of origin. Variation

can also be seen between different regions within a single tumour mass. This probably reflects both the genetic differences between cells and the poor blood supply of some parts of the tumour, which deprives cells of nutrients and halts their proliferation (Tannock, 1968; Brown and Giaccia, 1998).

Some drugs, such as cytosine arabinoside, methotrexate and the vinca alkaloids are toxic only to proliferating cells, sparing cells out of the cell cycle in the G_0-phase. Other drugs are only cytotoxic for cells in certain phases of the cell cycle. For example, 5-fluorouracil (5-FU) and the anthracyclines are phase specific for cells in S-phase. If cells have a prolonged cell-cycle time, a short period of exposure to a S-phase-specific drug will result in a far smaller proportion of cell kill than when cells are cycling rapidly.

Overcoming cytokinetic resistance

One way to overcome cytokinetic resistance may be to alter the schedules of chemotherapy administration. Traditionally, chemotherapy has been given as a bolus or a short infusion. For drugs that are phase specific, administration of the drug using a prolonged schedule would be predicted to be more effective than bolus dosing. Provided the concentration of drug is kept above the threshold required for cytotoxicity, a higher proportion of tumour cells will be exposed to the drug during the vulnerable phase of the cell cycle with the use of a more protracted schedule. The clearest clinical demonstration of this effect has been with the topoisomerase II inhibitor, etoposide, which acts in the late S- and early G_2-phase of the cell cycle. In a study of etoposide therapy for patients with small cell lung cancer, patients were randomized to receive a 24-hour infusion of 500 mg or five 2-hour infusions on successive days (Slevin *et al.*, 1989). Pharmacokinetic monitoring was carried out to demonstrate that the area under the concentration versus time curve (AUC) in the patients was the same in both schedules. The response rates differed dramatically (10 per cent in the single-infusion arm and 89 per cent in the 5-day-treatment arm), despite each arm of the study receiving the same AUC. Although it cannot be proved that the difference in response rate is due to the cytokinetic benefit of the longer schedule, these results are consistent with overcoming cytokinetic resistance.

The S-phase-specific drug, 5-FU, is often used in the first-line treatment of colorectal cancer. Several randomized trials have compared the effectiveness of prolonged infusion of 5-FU with bolus administration of the drug (de Gramont *et al.*, 1997; Meta-analysis group in cancer, 1998). A meta-analysis of the available trials suggested that continuous infusion significantly improved tumour response rates and resulted in a small, but significant, increase in survival over bolus 5-FU (Meta-analysis group in cancer 1998). The pattern of toxicity differed between the two schedules; infusional therapy gave rise to an increased incidence of hand–foot syndrome but less haematological toxicity. Without pharmacokinetic monitoring it is impossible to know if the AUC between different schedules was equivalent, but again these observations may be explicable on a cytokinetic basis.

TUMOUR MICROENVIRONMENT

Whereas cells in normal tissues live in a finely regulated homeostatic environment, there is a wide variation in the physiological conditions to which cancer cells are exposed between different areas in a given solid tumour. There is evidence that some factors in the tumour microenvironment contribute towards drug resistance.

Hypoxia

The partial pressure of oxygen within a single solid tumour varies widely; cells furthest from the tumour vasculature may be significantly hypoxic. Data from animal tumour models suggests many cytotoxic drugs are less effective under hypoxic conditions. Cyclophosphamide, for example, has 40-fold less cytotoxic activity under hypoxic conditions in experimental models (Teicher and Frei, 1998). Preclinical data also suggest that hypoxia increases cancer cell resistance to radiotherapy. Clinical trials of radiotherapy in combination with agents that improve tumour oxygenation suggest that correcting hypoxia can improve treatment outcome (Overgaard et al., 1998).

Clinical studies to investigate the relationship between hypoxia and the effectiveness of chemotherapy have yet to be performed, but drugs designed to overcome resistance due to tumour hypoxia have been developed based on preclinical evidence. The goal of this research is to produce agents that are activated under hypoxic conditions, to generate cytotoxic metabolites. This would enhance effectiveness of drugs in regions of tumours that would otherwise be resistant to conventional chemotherapy (Brown and Giaccia, 1998).

Tirapazamine is a cytotoxic pro-drug that is metabolized by an enzyme in the cell nucleus to form a highly reactive metabolite that causes DNA strand breaks. Oxygen converts the active metabolite back into tirapazamine. Hence high concentrations of the toxic metabolite are only generated under hypoxic conditions. In experiments on cell lines, tirapazamine shows a 20- to 300-fold increase in cytotoxicity under hypoxic conditions compared with aerobic culture. In combination therapy in preclinical studies, tirapazamine was found to be synergistic with cisplatin (Brown and Giaccia, 1998). In phase I/II clinical trials, tirapazamine in combination with cisplatin has been well tolerated. Two large-scale randomized trials have been conducted to determine if tirapazamine is synergistic with cisplatin in non-small cell lung cancer. The CATAPULT I trial compared tirapazamine plus cisplatin with cisplatin alone. Patients who had the tirapazamine and cisplatin combination treatment had significantly longer survival and greater response rate than those who received cisplatin alone (Von Pawel et al., 2000). The CATAPULT II trial, is a randomized comparison of tirapazamine plus cisplatin with etoposide plus cisplatin in non-small cell lung cancer. Follow-up of over 500 patients is ongoing and the results of this trial will confirm whether tirapazamine is of benefit when added to a standard chemotherapy schedule in non-small cell lung cancer (Gatzemeier et al., 1998). Another drug activated by hypoxia, the topisomerase inhibitor AQ4N, is now entering early phase clinical trials.

Extracellular matrix

The extracellular matrix proteins secreted by both normal and malignant cells do far more than simply act as scaffolding to hold the tissue together. Signals from matrix proteins regulate cell differentiation and proliferation and inhibit apoptosis. A study of small cell lung carcinoma (SCLC) has shown that human tumours secrete an extensive stroma of matrix proteins such as fibronectin and collagen (Sethi et al., 1999). SCLC cell lines similarly secrete matrix proteins. When the cell lines are allowed to adhere to collagen, laminin or fibronectin, the degree of apoptosis following treatment with etoposide or cisplatin is substantially reduced. The extracellular matrix proteins also promote tumour cell growth. The receptors that the tumour cells use to bind to matrix proteins are proteins of the integrin family. Drugs that regulate integrin function are under development and may provide a new means to enhance the effectiveness of cytotoxic drugs in tumours such as SCLC.

Privileged sites and resistance

One reason for treatment failure in highly chemosensitive diseases, such as childhood leukaemia and lymphoma, has been that tumour cells in certain body sites, such as brain or testis, are not exposed to sufficient concentrations of cytotoxic drugs. Curative treatment schedules need to include intrathecal chemotherapy or radiotherapy to ensure that otherwise sensitive cells do not escape therapy by virtue of being in a privileged site.

CELLULAR MECHANISMS OF RESISTANCE

Many mechanisms of acquired drug resistance have been characterized through the study of cancer cell lines. It is important to identify which of these are important in drug resistance in the clinical setting. Several examples of cellular changes that correlate with observations made in human tumours are discussed below, and given in Figure 8.1 and Table 8.2.

Decreased drug uptake

If a drug enters the cell by a specific active transporter protein, cells can become resistant if the activity of the transport system is decreased. This mechanism of resistance operates in tumour cell lines that have become resistant to the antimetabolite methotrexate. Methotrexate enters cells via the reduced folate transporter protein. In cell lines in which the function of the protein is defective a 250-fold higher concentration of methotrexate is required for equivalent cell killing compared with cell lines with normal transporter function. The resistant cells are able to use a second folate transporter protein that does not bind methotrexate to maintain their supply of folates.

The use of a fluorescent analogue of methotrexate has allowed this mechanism of drug resistance to be demonstrated directly in leukaemic blast cells freshly isolated from patients with acute lymphoblastic leukaemia. Of 30 untreated patients, 28 had high folate transporter activity, but in treated patients with clinical methotrexate resistance only 30 per cent of patients had retained the ability to transport folate at the normal level (Gorlick et al., 1997).

Trimetrexate is a lipophilic analogue of methotrexate that does not use the reduced folate transporter protein. Trimetrexate has activity in breast cancer, non-small cell lung cancer and head and neck cancer, and is under evaluation in a phase III trial. It is not known if trimetrexate will prove clinically superior to its parent drug (Gorlick and Bertino, 1999).

Decreased drug activation

Many anti-cancer agents are pro-drugs that require metabolic activation within cells before they can exert cytotoxic effects. A decrease in the activity of enzymes that have key functions in drug activation has been seen in cell lines resistant to several drugs. For example, decreased activity of deoxycytidine kinase confers resistance to cytosine arabinoside, and 6-mercaptopurine resistance is conferred by a loss of hypoxanthine guanine phosphoribosyl transferase activity. Cyclophosphamide and ifosfamide are activated by cytochrome P450-dependent mono-oxygenases; resistant experimental tumours show reduced expression of these enzymes.

Methotrexate requires intracellular metabolism by polyglutamation to increase its ability to inhibit its target enzyme, dihydrofolate reductase, and decrease the rate at which it is excreted from the cell. Polyglutamation is decreased in resistant human tumour cell lines. In clinical studies, polyglutamation has been found to be lower in acute myeloid leukaemia blast cells which are intrinsically resistant to methotexate than in acute lymphocytic leukaemia blasts which are sensitive to the drug (Goker et al., 1998).

Increased drug metabolism and detoxification

Rapid drug metabolism and detoxification within the cytoplasm of a tumour cell can decrease the level of active drug. One key pathway in the detoxification of the highly reactive chemical groups generated by anthracyclines and cisplatin is the glutathione system. Glutathione binds to highly reactive molecules, preventing them binding to DNA. The level of glutathione in tumour cell lines correlates with the degree of resistance to cisplatin. The extent to which glutathione mediates clinical resistance to cisplatin is not known, but buthionine sulphoxide, a compound which depletes glutathione from cells, is undergoing clinical evaluation. Phase I studies of buthionine sulphoxide have been completed, but randomized trials of platinum-based chemotherapy with and without buthionine sulphoxide will be needed to show if this approach will be of clinical benefit (Perez, 1998).

Altered expression of target proteins

Some drugs act to inhibit the function of key cellular proteins. Increased expression or mutation of the target protein can confer resistance. For example, dihydrofolate reductase (DHFR) is the target enzyme of methotrexate; when DHFR is inhibited the cell is unable to synthesize purines or thymidylate de novo. Amplification of the DHFR gene, resulting in increased DHFR protein expression, is commonly found in methotrexate-resistant cell lines and has also been seen in leukaemic blast cells from relapsed patients with acute lymphoblastic leukaemia who have clinical methotrexate resistance (Goker et al., 1998).

An example of a mutation in a target gene that confers resistance occurs with the taxane, paclitaxel. Taxanes are thought to act by disrupting the function of the microtubules that form the cytoskeleton of the cell. Microtubules consist of a polymerized form of a protein called tubulin. In order to undergo mitosis, cells have to restructure the microtubular network. This is achieved by depolymerizing microtubules to form tubulin monomers, followed by reassembly of the microtubules. The taxanes block this process by binding to tubulin within microtubules and blocking depolymerization. As a result, the cell undergoes metaphase arrest and apoptosis is triggered.

Cell lines that are resistant to taxanes express mutant forms of β-tubulin that form less stable microtubules than the normal protein, and therefore are presumably able to depolymerize in spite of the stabilizing effect of paclitaxel (Gonzalez-Garay et al., 1999). There is recent evidence to suggest that this mechanism of resistance may be important clinically. In a study that involved sequencing β-tubulin genes in non-small cell lung cancer patients treated with single-agent paclitaxel, the presence of β-tubulin mutations was found to be able to predict paclitaxel resistance (Monzo et al., 1999). None of the

16 patients with β-tubulin mutations had an objective response, whereas 13 of 33 patients without a β-tubulin mutation had complete or partial responses.

Multiple drug resistance

The exposure of tumour cells to one drug is capable of inducing resistance to multiple other drugs in the surviving cells. This induced resistance affects drugs that may be structurally unrelated to the drug used for the first treatment and/or have different mechanisms of action. Thus a typical cell with multiple drug resistance (MDR) is resistant to anthracyclines, vinca alkaloids, actinomycin D and paclitaxel. The common feature of agents affected by MDR is that they are hydrophobic compounds that enter cells by passive diffusion. Several mechanisms have been proposed to account for the MDR effect. Although these clearly operate in experimental models, the extent to which they are responsible for clinical MDR remains unclear.

P-GLYCOPROTEIN

Several proteins that function to transport drugs and other molecules out of cells can give rise to MDR in cell culture and experimental tumours in animals. The first protein to be described in humans was P-glycoprotein (P-gp), encoded by the *MDR-1* gene. P-gp is a cell-membrane protein pump expressed at high levels in several normal tissues, including haemopoietic stem cells, endothelial cells in the brain (the blood–brain barrier), renal tubular cells, pancreatic ducts and intestinal epithelium (Goldstein, 1996). The role of the protein has been clarified in a P-gp 'knockout' mouse. Animals lacking P-gp have a less effective blood–brain barrier and are more sensitive to chemotherapy, as cytotoxic drug elimination is decreased and tissue levels of drugs are increased (Schinkel *et al.*, 1994). P-gp expression alone converts previously chemosensitive cancer cell lines into MDR-type cells. P-gp pumps cytotoxic drugs rapidly out of the cell, keeping the amount of drug in the cytoplasm below the toxic level. Adding P-gp inhibitors to cell lines that have P-gp-mediated transport can cause the cells to lose MDR.

The extent to which P-gp is responsible for MDR in human tumours is not known. The study of P-gp in some solid tumours is complicated by expression of the protein in surrounding normal tissues. The clearest results have come from studying leukaemia cells taken directly from the blood of patients. Pure populations of cancer cells can be analysed rapidly using flow cytometry for expression of P-gp. Another test that can be done is to load cells with rhodamine 123, a fluorescent dye that is pumped out by P-gp. By determining the rate at which the dye is pumped out of the cells, the level of P-gp activity can be estimated. In a study of 352 patients with acute myeloid leukaemia, one-third of the patients had leukaemic blast cells that expressed P-gp and rapidly pumped out rhodamine 123. The patients with P-gp activity at presentation were significantly more likely to have chemotherapy-resistant disease (Leith *et al.*, 1999). In childhood acute lymphoblastic leukaemia, P-gp expression was found in only 13 per cent of patients at presentation and in 34 per cent of patients who relapsed; patients who relapsed with P-gp-positive cells had poorer survival (Dhooge *et al.*, 1999). These results imply that P-gp-positive cells are more likely to survive primary chemotherapy, consistent with P-gp conferring a survival advantage to leukaemic cells by MDR.

Studies in the more heterogeneous solid tumours are more difficult to interpret. Different methods to analyse PGP, such as Northern blotting, Western blotting and immunohistochemistry, have been used to analyse small numbers of samples (Goldstein, 1996). Some tumours frequently express high levels of P-gp at diagnosis, including renal cell carcinoma, colonic carcinoma and pancreatic tumours. This reflects the fact that the normal tissues from which these tumours derive express P-gp. It is tempting to speculate that high P-gp levels contribute to the intrinsic resistance of these tumours to chemotherapy, but there is no direct evidence to support this hypothesis. P-gp expression has also been studied in chemotherapy-responsive tumours. The majority of untreated breast cancers do not express P-gp (Trock *et al.*, 1997). However, the proportion of P-gp-positive tumours rises substantially after hormonal treatment or chemotherapy. Patients whose tumours express P-gp at presentation are three times more likely to fail to respond to chemotherapy than those whose tumours are P-gp negative. Patients with P-gp-positive tumours after therapy do even worse, having a fourfold increase in the rate of treatment failure. This suggests P-gp is a predictive marker for treatment failure in breast cancer, although it does not prove a role for P-gp in breast cancer MDR. Several clinical trials of agents that inhibit P-gp have been undertaken, based on this correlative evidence, and these are discussed below.

OTHER PROTEINS ASSOCIATED WITH MDR

MDR has also been described in cells that are P-gp negative but express another cell membrane protein pump, called multidrug-resistance-associated protein or MRP. In acute myeloid leukaemia patients there was no relationship between MRP expression and clinical outcome (Leith *et al.*, 1999). By contrast, in a study of patients with neuroblastoma, high levels of MRP were associated with poor clinical outcome in a multivariate analysis (Norris *et al.*, 1996). There was no relationship between P-gp expression and survival in this study. A second protein, called lung resistance-related protein (LRP) is also associated with non-P-gp-mediated MDR in cell lines. LRP expression is not associated with differences in clinical outcome in leukaemia (Leith *et al.*, 1999), but is correlated with outcome in ovarian cancer (Scheffer *et al.*, 1995). Whether either MRP or LRP expression accounts directly for the poorer outcome in neuroblastoma or ovarian cancer, or whether these proteins are just markers for other factors that determine outcome, is not clear.

OVERCOMING MDR

Several agents have been found which inhibit the function of P-gp in preclinical models. These include calcium-channel blockers such as verapamil, immunosuppressants such as cyclosporin, and several other drugs used for the treatment of non-malignant disease (Dalton, 1998). Several clinical trials have been undertaken with both verapamil and cyclosporin. High-dose infusional verapamil has been shown to reverse MDR when given in combination with vincristine, doxorubicin and dexamethazone (VAD), to myeloma patients who had become resistant to VAD alone (Dalton, 1998). However, the benefits were short lived and the cardiac toxicity from verapamil was high. Using oral verapamil in addition to VAD in myeloma patients has been tried as a less toxic alternative to infusional treatment, but this shows no advantage over VAD alone in a randomized trial (Dalton *et al.*, 1995). Cyclosporin A has been added to chemotherapy in trials in myeloma and acute myeloid leukaemia (AML), apparently overcoming MDR. However, this was at the price of increased chemotherapy-related toxicity, possibly due to the decreased clearance of drug caused by cyclosporin rather than inhibition of P-gp (Bartlett *et al.*, 1994).

Further P-gp-inhibiting agents have now been developed in an attempt to overcome the problems of toxicity seen with verapamil and cyclosporin. Dex-verapamil is a less cardiotoxic stereoisomer of verapamil, currently under investigation in clinical trials.

Similarly PSC-833, a derivative of cyclosporin, has been evaluated in a phase II study in leukaemia (Advani *et al.*, 1999). Like cyclosporin, it decreases drug clearance so cytotoxic doses need to be reduced. PSC-833 is now undergoing evaluation in randomized phase III studies in AML.

Several other established drugs have shown the ability to inhibit P-gp function, but none has shown convincing activity in a randomized study. Further new agents have been developed and are entering clinical trials, but it remains to be seen if P-gp inhibitors that are well tolerated can be developed, and whether these have any role in overcoming clinical drug resistance. Other proteins that are implicated in MDR, such as MRP, are also targets for future drug development.

Chemotherapy-induced apoptosis

One of the major advances in recent years has been the understanding that many, though not all, chemotherapeutic agents act by inducing apoptosis or programmed cell death, rather than simply poisoning the cell so that it dies by necrosis. Apoptosis is an active, energy-dependent process in which a cascade of enzymes destroys the organelles of the cell, including the nucleus, in a characteristic way. Apoptosis is a part of normal development and in the adult acts to delete cells with damaged DNA. For example, cells in the epidermis which have DNA damage following ultraviolet light exposure undergo apoptotic cell death. An early stage in the development of most tumours is disruption of the controls that regulate apoptosis. Once apoptosis following DNA damage is blocked, the cell can survive and acquire the further mutations required for malignant transformation.

The details of how apoptosis is regulated have still to be determined, but it is clear that two protein families are involved, Bax and BCL2. Bax proteins promote apoptosis while BCL2 proteins inhibit death. Both proteins can form dimers with themselves and with each other. Bax–Bax dimers trigger apoptosis, Bax–BCL2 dimers and BCL2–BCL2 dimers do not (Fig. 8.2). Hence the relative amounts of the two proteins determine whether apoptosis can be triggered (Korsmeyer, 1999).

Three p53 family members, p53, p73 and p63, have been shown to have a key role in regulating apoptotic cell

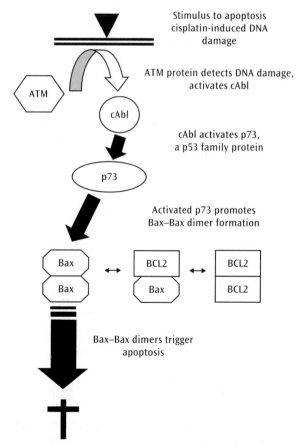

Figure 8.2 *Apoptotic cell death. The probable mechanism of cell death following cisplatin exposure is illustrated. How activated p73 triggers apoptosis is not clear, but this is likely to involve alteration of the Bax : BCL2 ratio, see text for details.*

death. These proteins also have a key role in triggering apoptosis following DNA damage. In part this is achieved by regulating the levels of Bax protein. Proteins that detect DNA damage activate p53, which in turn increases the level of Bax protein, promoting apoptosis (Schmitt and Lowe, 1999).

Cytotoxic drugs that damage DNA appear to activate apoptosis by a process that involves members of the p53 protein family. For example, cisplatin binds covalently to DNA. The damaged DNA is recognized by enzymes, probably including the enzyme ATM (ataxia telangiectasia mutant), which is mutated in ataxia telangiectasia (Gong et al., 1999; Pratesi et al., 1999). Activation of ATM in turn activates the nuclear enzyme cAbl, resulting in activation of p73. p73 then triggers the apoptotic cascade, resulting in the death of the cell (see Fig. 8.2). Drugs that do not damage DNA directly are also able to trigger apoptosis. For example the taxanes, which disrupt microtubule formation, induce apoptosis by a mechanism independent of p53. Taxanes induce phosphorylation of BCL2, which prevents BCL2 binding to Bax, increasing the number of Bax–Bax dimers and triggering apoptosis (Schmitt and Lowe, 1999).

Studies in 'knockout' mice lacking apoptosis-activating genes provide strong evidence that loss of p53 or Bax results in decreased apoptotic cell death following chemotherapy (Schmitt and Lowe, 1999). When chemotherapy-resistant cells lacking p53 are repaired by expression of p53, chemosensitivity is restored. Over expression of BCL2 also blocks apoptosis induced by a wide range of cytotoxic drugs in mouse and human cancer cell lines.

Mutations in apoptosis-regulating genes are common in human tumours. The most common gene to be mutated in human tumours is *p53*; over 50 per cent of tumours carry a *p53* mutation (Hickman, 1998). Mutations that lead to a loss of Bax protein have been found in haematological malignancy and colon cancer, and a chromosome translocation resulting in overexpression of BCL2 occurs in 85 per cent of follicular lymphoma (Korsmeyer, 1999). High levels of BCL2 are also found in over 80 per cent of one of the most chemotherapy-resistant tumours, malignant melanoma (Jansen et al., 1998). These observations suggest that mutation of genes related to apoptosis plays some part in clinical drug resistance.

OVERCOMING APOPTOSIS-RELATED DRUG RESISTANCE

Attempting to repair the effects of mutations in apoptosis-regulating genes has been a major focus of gene therapy programmes in cancer. Adenovirus vectors designed to express normal p53 protein in tumour cells have been developed and are undergoing clinical evaluation in non-small cell lung cancer and head and neck cancer. The virus is delivered by direct injection into the tumour. In a small phase I/II study in lung cancer, 28 patients had their tumours injected up to six times. Virally delivered p53 was detected in just under half the tumours. There was little toxicity and 2 of 25 evaluable patients had partial responses (Swisher et al., 1999). Clearly, this mode of treatment is not suitable for patients with metastatic disease. If the considerable problems of administering gene therapy systemically with a high efficiency of infection of tumour cells can be solved, repair of p53 and possible restoration of drug sensitivity may be achievable.

An alternative way to manipulate apoptosis is to reduce the levels of BCL2 in overexpressing tumours. Antisense oligonucleotides are short pieces of DNA that disrupt the production of RNA from the specific gene to which they are targeted, by hybridizing to the DNA encoding the gene in a way that blocks RNA transcription. A phase I study has been carried out using antisense oligonucleotide therapy to attempt to reduce BCL2 expression in refractory follicular lymphoma (Webb et al., 1997). Nine patients were treated with only minimal toxicity. A fall in BCL2 levels was seen in 2 of 5 patients in whom BCL2 was measured. There was one minor and one complete response; the complete response being maintained for over 2 years. This study suggests that BCL2 antisense therapy may have activity in follicular lymphoma. If this technology can be refined and improved, it may help to overcome the drug resistance of solid tumours as well as haematological toxicities. The chemosensitivity of human melanoma grafted into mice is improved by administration of antisense BCL2 oligonucleotides (Jansen et al., 1998).

Enhanced DNA repair

Most chemotherapy agents act by directly or indirectly damaging DNA. The degree of DNA damage caused by the drug depends on the balance of the rate of DNA damage and the rate of DNA repair. As described above, there are certain nuclear proteins that recognize DNA damage. Damaged DNA can be repaired by a series of enzymatic steps. The two major mechanisms of DNA repair are excision repair and direct enzymatic removal of alkyl groups from DNA.

DNA excision repair is used to repair damage caused by drugs such as alkylating agents, platinum compounds, mitomycin C and bleomycin. The damaged base is recognized and excised and the resulting gap in the DNA repaired using the other DNA strand as a template. Repair-deficient cell lines are highly sensitive to drugs such as mitomycin C and cisplatin, while resistant lines have increased efficiency of DNA repair (Zamble and Lippard, 1995; Gornati et al., 1997). One way in which excision repair may be able to be overcome is by combining drugs such as cisplatin with antimetabolites that can block DNA synthesis, which is required to complete the process of excision repair.

The other method of DNA repair is specific to drugs that cause O^6-alkylguanine adducts on DNA, such as dacarbazine (DTIC) and nitrosoureas. The enzyme O^6-alkylguanine transferase (AGT) removes these adducts directly from the DNA, becoming inactivated as it does so. Studies of human cell lines in culture have demonstrated a correlation between AGT activity and resistance to a DTIC metabolite and nitrosoureas. There is also a correlation between AGT levels in blood lymphocytes and cellular resistance to nitrosoureas in patients with chronic myeloid leukaemia. One way to target resistance based on DNA repair by AGT is by using agents that block the enzyme, such as O^6-benzylguanine. In a phase I study in cancer patients, O^6-benzylguanine was well tolerated and was able to deplete peripheral blood lymphocytes of AGT activity (Dolan et al., 1998). Further clinical trials of this agent are awaited.

FUTURE PROSPECTS

Defining the molecular basis of drug resistance

Studies of drug resistance to date have relied on detecting differences in protein expression between resistant and sensitive cancer cell lines. The protein being measured may have a function in drug resistance, but may simply be a marker that is co-expressed with the protein(s) responsible for resistance. It is necessary to identify all the genes that are differentially expressed in sensitive and resistant cells. This is now becoming a possibility using DNA microarrays, in which DNA sequences complementary to RNA derived from thousands of genes are immobilized on a glass slide. Microarrays enable a snapshot of many of the genes being transcribed in a cell to be obtained with relative ease, by hybridizing labelled RNA from the cell with the microarray.

It has also become clear that mouse or human cell lines may not be the best way of studying certain resistance mechanisms. Processes such as DNA repair can be studied much more rapidly and precisely in model organisms such as yeast. Once the candidate resistance gene has been identified from microarray analysis of yeast strains, the mouse or human homologue can be characterized in cell lines and animal models. It is to be hoped that this approach will speed up the elimination of spurious genes that do not mediate resistance much more rapidly than is possible at present (Marton et al., 1998). Once proteins conferring resistance to particular drugs have been defined by microarray technology, they can be used to guide drug design. Microarrays can allow rapid screening of tumour biopsies to predict resistance to a specific drug (Certa et al., 2001). This technology needs to become more cost effective before clinical trials can be carried out, but offers the hope of sparing patients unnecessary treatment with drugs to which their tumour is resistant, while selecting the combination of agents most likely to yield a response.

Improvements in imaging

The direct demonstration of drug resistance in human tumours would be a major advance in research and treatment of cancer patients. A recent study using positron emission tomography (PET) scanning suggests that by following the rate that a tracer is lost from tumour tissue, it is possible to identify lung cancer patients who will be resistant to subsequent chemotherapy with a high degree of accuracy (Fukumoto et al., 1999). If this result is borne out in future studies, it offers the prospect of reliable prospective prediction of chemotherapy resistance.

New drugs to block resistance

The formidable challenges that remain to giving efficient systemic gene therapy make it seem more likely that the development of new drugs, such as well-tolerated P-glycoprotein inhibitors or hypoxically activated agents, will occur before gene therapy becomes a reality. Improvements in drug scheduling and administration also offer the hope of small but significant steps in overcoming drug resistance, which remains the biggest challenge in modern chemotherapy practice.

SIGNIFICANT POINTS

- Drug resistance is the most important reason for cancer treatment failure.
- Genetic instability and the multi-clonal nature of tumours enables them to adapt to environmental changes.
- The use of combinations of drugs increases tumour cell killing, as predicted by the Goldie–Coldman hypothesis.
- Cell killing by drugs only active in certain phases of the cell cycle can be improved by altering schedules of drug administration.
- Hypoxia reduces the sensitivity of tumour cells to many drugs.
- The MDR-1 gene product, P-glycoprotein is able to confer resistance to multiple drugs by pumping them out of the tumour cell cytoplasm.

- Tumours often have mutations that make them resistant to chemotherapy-induced programmed cell death.
- DNA damage repair is important in resistance to many alkylating agents.
- Understanding the biological mechanisms of drug resistance allows the design of strategies to overcome drug resistance, with potential to improve the efficacy of cytotoxic drugs.

KEY REFERENCES

Brown, J.M. and Giaccia, A.J. (1998) The unique physiology of solid tumors: opportunities (and problems) for cancer therapy. *Cancer Res.* **58**, 1408–16.

Cahill, D.P., Kinzler, K.W., Vogelstein, B. and Lengauer, C. (1999) Genetic instability and Darwinian selection in tumours. *Trends Biol. Sci.* **24**, M57–M60.

Pinedo, H. and Giaccone, G. (eds) (1997) *Drug resistance in the treatment of cancer.* Cambridge: Cambridge University Press, 223–44.

Schmitt, C.A. and Lowe, S.W. (1999) Apoptosis and therapy. *J. Pathol.* **187**, 127–37.

REFERENCES

Advani, R., Saba, H.I., Tallman, M.S. *et al.* (1999) Treatment of refractory and relapsed acute myelogenous leukemia with combination chemotherapy plus the multidrug resistance modulator PSC 833 (Valspodar). *Blood* **93**, 787–95.

Antman, K. (1999) Critique of the high-dose chemotherapy studies in breast cancer: a positive look at the data. *J. Clin. Oncol.* **17**, 30s–35s.

Bartlett, N.L., Lum, B.L., Fisher, G.A. *et al.* (1994) Phase I trial of doxorubicin with cyclosporine as a modulator of multidrug resistance. *J. Clin. Oncol.* **12**, 835–42.

Brown, J.M. and Giaccia, A.J. (1998) The unique physiology of solid tumors: opportunities (and problems) for cancer therapy. *Cancer Res.* **58**, 1408–16.

Cahill, D.P., Lengauer, C., Yu, J. *et al.* (1998) Mutations of mitotic checkpoint genes in human cancers. *Nature* **392**, 300–3. [See comments.]

Cahill, D.P., Kinzler, K.W., Vogelstein, B. and Lengauer, C. (1999) Genetic instability and Darwinian selection in tumours. *Trends Biol. Sci.* **24**, M57–M60.

Certa, U., Seiler, M., Padovan, E and Spagnoli, G.C. (2001) High density oligonucleotide array analysis of interferon-alpha 2a sensitivity and transcriptional response in melanoma cells. *Br. J. Cancer* **85**, 107–14.

Dalton, W.S. (1998) The reversal of multidrug resistance. In Pinedo, H. and Giaccone, G. (eds), *Drug resistance in the treatment of cancer.* Cambridge: Cambridge University Press, 223–44.

Dalton, W.S., Crowley, J.J., Salmon, S.S. *et al.* (1995) A phase III randomized study of oral verapamil as a chemosensitizer to reverse drug resistance in patients with refractory myeloma. A Southwest Oncology Group study. *Cancer* **75**, 815–20.

de Gramont, A., Bosset, J., Milan, C. *et al.* (1997) Randomized trial comparing monthly low-dose leucovorin and fluorouracil bolus with bimonthly high-dose leucovorin and fluorouracil bolus plus continuous infusion for advanced colorectal cancer: a French intergroup study. *J. Clin. Oncol.* **15**, 808–15.

Dhooge, C., De Moerloose, B., Laureys, G. *et al.* (1999) P-glycoprotein is an independent prognostic factor predicting relapse in childhood acute lymphoblastic leukaemia: results of a 6-year prospective study. *Br. J. Haematol.* **105**, 676–83.

Dolan, M.E., Roy, S.K., Fasanmade, A.A. *et al.* (1998) O^6-benzylguanine in humans: metabolic, pharmacokinetic, and pharmacodynamic findings. *J. Clin. Oncol.* **16**, 1803–10.

Fennelly, D., Raptis, R., Crown, J.A.P. and Norton, L. (1998) Resistance to tumour alkylating agents and cisplatin. In Pinedo, H. and Giaccone, G. (eds), *Drug resistance in the treatment of cancer.* Cambridge: Cambridge University Press, 245–79.

Fukumoto, M., Yoshida, D., Hayase, N. *et al.* (1999) Scintigraphic prediction of resistance to radiation and chemotherapy in patients with lung carcinoma: technetium 99m-tetrofosmin and thallium-201 dual single photon emission computed tomography study. *Cancer* **86**, 1470–9.

Gatzemeier, U., Rodriguez, G., Treat, J. *et al.* (1998) Tirapazamine-cisplatin: the synergy. *Br. J. Cancer* **77**(suppl. 4), 15–17.

Goker, E., Gorlick, R. and Bertino, J.R. (1998) Resistance mechanisms to antimetabolites. In Pinedo, H.M. and Giaccone, G. (eds), *Drug resistance in the treatment of cancer.* Cambridge: Cambridge University Press, 1–13.

Goldie, C.H. and Coldman, A.J. (1984) The genetic origin of drug resistance in neoplasms: implications for systemic therapy. *Cancer Res.* **44**, 3643–53.

Goldie, J.H. and Coldman, A.J. (1986) Application of theoretical models to chemotherapy protocol design. *Cancer Treat. Rep.* **70**, 127–31.

Goldstein, L.J. (1996) MDR-1 expression in solid tumours. *Eur. J. Cancer* **32A**, 1039–50.

Gong, J.G., Costanzo, A., Yang, H.Q. *et al.* (1999) The tyrosine kinase c-Abl regulates p73 in apoptotic response to cisplatin-induced DNA damage. *Nature* **399**, 806–9. [See comments.]

Gonzalez-Garay, M.L., Chang, L., Blade, K. *et al.* (1999) A beta-tubulin leucine cluster involved in microtubule assembly and paclitaxel resistance. *J. Biol. Chem.* **274**, 23875–82.

Gore, M.E., Fryatt, I., Wiltshaw, E. and Dawson, T. (1990) Treatment of relapsed carcinoma of the ovary with cisplatin or carboplatin following initial treatment with these compounds. *Gynecol. Oncol.* **36**, 207–11.

Gorlick, R. and Bertino, J.R. (1999) Clinical pharmacology and resistance to dihydrofolate reductase inhibitors. In Jackman, A.L. (ed.), *Antifolate drugs in cancer therapy*. New Jersey: Humana Press.

Gorlick, R., Goker, E., Trippett, T. *et al.* (1997) Defective transport is a common mechanism of acquired methotrexate resistance in acute lymphocytic leukemia and is associated with decreased reduced folate carrier expression. *Blood* **89**, 1013–18.

Gornati, D., Zaffaroni, N., Villa, R. *et al.* (1997) Modulation of melphalan and cisplatin cytotoxicity in human ovarian cancer cells resistant to alkylating drugs. *Anticancer Drugs* **8**, 509–16.

Herrin, V.E. and Thigpen, J.T. (1999) High-dose chemotherapy in ovarian carcinoma. *Semin. Oncol.* **26**, 99–105.

Hickman, J.A. (1998) Genes that regulate apoptosis; major determinants of drug resistance. In Pinedo, H. and Giaccone, G. (eds) *Drug resistance in the treatment of cancer*. Cambridge: Cambridge University Press, 178–98.

Hortobagyi, G.N. (1999) High-dose chemotherapy for primary breast cancer: facts versus anecdotes. *J. Clin. Oncol.* **17**, 25–9.

Jansen, B., Schlagbauer-Wadl, H., Brown, B.D. *et al.* (1998) bcl-2 antisense therapy chemosensitizes human melanoma in SCID mice. *Nat. Med.* **4**, 232–4.

Korsmeyer, S.J. (1999) BCL-2 gene family and the regulation of programmed cell death. *Cancer Res.* **59**, 1693s–1700s.

Leith, C.P., Kopecky, K.J., Chen, I.M. *et al.* (1999) Frequency and clinical significance of the expression of the multidrug resistance proteins MDR1/P-glycoprotein, MRP1, and LRP in acute myeloid leukemia: a Southwest Oncology Group Study. *Blood* **94**, 1086–99.

Lilenbaum, R.C., Langenberg, P. and Dickersin, K. (1998) Single agent versus combination chemotherapy in patients with advanced nonsmall cell lung carcinoma: a meta-analysis of response, toxicity, and survival. *Cancer* **82**, 116–26.

Livingston, R. and Crawley, J. (1999) Commentary on the PBT-1 study of high dose consolidation versus standard therapy in metastatic breast cancer. *J. Clin. Oncol.* **17**, 22–4.

Marton, M.J., DeRisi, J.L., Bennett, H.A. *et al.* (1998) Drug target validation and identification of secondary drug target effects using DNA microarrays. *Nat. Med.* **4**, 1293–301. [See comments.]

Meta-analysis group in cancer. (1998) Efficacy of intravenous infusion of fluorouracil compared with bolus administration in advanced colorectal cancer. *J. Clin. Oncol.* **16**, 301–8.

Monzo, M., Rosell, R., Sanchez, J.J. *et al.* (1999) Paclitaxel resistance in non-small-cell lung cancer associated with beta-tubulin gene mutations. *J. Clin. Oncol.* **17**, 1786.

Morrison, V.A. and Peterson, B.A. (1999) High-dose therapy and transplantation in non-Hodgkin's Lymphoma. *Semin. Oncol.* **26**, 84–98.

Norris, M.D., Bordow, S.B., Marshall, G.M. *et al.* (1996) Expression of the gene for multidrug-resistance-associated protein and outcome in patients with neuroblastoma. *N. Engl. J. Med.* **334**, 231–8.

Overgaard, J., Hansen, H.S., Overgaard, M. *et al.* (1998) A randomized double-blind phase III study of nimorazole as a hypoxic radiosensitizer of primary radiotherapy in supraglottic larynx and pharynx carcinoma. Results of the Danish Head and Neck Cancer. Study (DAHANCA) Protocol 5-85. *Radiother. Oncol.* **46**, 135–46.

Perez, R.P. (1998) Cellular and molecular determinants of cisplatin resistance. *Eur. J. Cancer* **34**, 1535–42.

Pratesi, G., Perego, P., Polizzi, D. *et al.* (1999) A novel charged trinuclear platinum complex effective against cisplatin-resistant tumours: hypersensitivity of p53-mutant human tumour xenografts. *Br. J. Cancer* **80**, 1912–19.

Scheffer, G.L., Wijngaard, P.L., Flens, M.J. *et al.* (1995) The drug resistance-related protein LRP is the human major vault protein. *Nat. Med.* **1**, 578–82.

Schinkel, A.H., Smit, J.J., van Tellingen, O. *et al.* (1994) Disruption of the mouse mdr1a P-glycoprotein gene leads to a deficiency in the blood–brain barrier and to increased sensitivity to drugs. *Cell* **77**, 491–502.

Schmitt, C.A. and Lowe, S.W. (1999) Apoptosis and therapy. *J. Pathol.* **187**, 127–37.

Sethi, T., Rintoul, R.C., Moore, S.M. *et al.* (1999) Extracellular matrix proteins protect small cell lung cancer cells against apoptosis: a mechanism for small cell lung cancer growth and drug resistance *in vivo*. *Nat. Med.* **5**, 662–8.

Slevin, M.L., Clark P., Joel, S. *et al.* (1989) A randomised trial to evaluate the effect of schedule on the activity of etoposide in small cell lung cancer. *J. Clin. Oncol.* **7**, 1333–40.

Sobecks, R.M. and Vogelzang, N.J. (1999) High-dose therapy with autologous stem-cell support for germ cell tumours, a critical review. *J. Clin. Oncol.* **26**, 106–18.

Swisher, S.G., Roth, J.A., Nemunaitis, J. *et al.* (1999) Adenovirus-mediated p53 gene transfer in advanced non-small-cell lung cancer. *J. Natl Cancer Inst.* **91**, 763–71.

Tannock, I.F. (1968) The relation between cell proliferation and the vascular system in a transplanted mouse tumour. *Br. J. Cancer* **22**, 258–73.

Tannock, I.F. (1978) Cell kinetics and chemotherapy: A critical review. *Cancer Treat. Rep.* **62**, 1117–33.

Teicher, B.A. and Frei, E. (1998) Resistance to tumour alkylating agents and cisplatin. In Pinedo, H. and Giaccone, G. (eds), *Drug resistance in the treatment of cancer*. Cambridge: Cambridge University Press, 14–99.

Trock, B.J., Leonessa, F. and Clarke, R. (1997) Multidrug resistance in breast cancer: a meta-analysis of MDR1/gp170 expression and its possible functional significance. *J. Natl Cancer Inst.* **89**, 917–31.

Valagussa, P., Tancini, G. and Bonadonna, G. (1986) Salvage treatment of patients suffering relapse after adjuvant CMF chemotherapy. *Cancer* **58**, 1411–17.

Von Pawel, J., von Roemeling, R., Gatzemeier, U. *et al.* (2000) Tirapazine plus cisplatin versus cisplatin in advanced non-small-cell lung cancer: a report of the international CATAPULT I study group. Cisplatin and Tirapazamine in Subjects with Advanced Previously Untreated Non-Small-Cell Lung Tumors. *J. Clin. Oncol.* **18**, 1351–9.

Webb, A., Cunningham, D., Cotter, F. *et al.* (1997) BCL-2 antisense therapy in patients with non-Hodgkin lymphoma. *Lancet* **349**, 1137–41.

Zamble, D.B. and Lippard, S.J. (1995) Cisplatin and DNA repair in cancer chemotherapy. *Trends Biochem. Sci.* **20**, 435–9.

9

The endocrinology of malignancy

ROSHAN AGARWAL AND JONATHAN WAXMAN

Approximately 25 per cent of all malignant tumours in men and 40 per cent in women have a hormonal basis. Hormonal treatment results in dramatic responses without the toxicity associated with cytotoxic chemotherapy. Recent developments within the field of molecular biology have led to an understanding of the mechanisms of hormone action and the concept of autocrine and paracrine regulation of malignant cells. This increase in our knowledge of the endocrine control of tumour growth has led, in the past three decades, to a proliferation of new endocrine treatments for cancer with greater efficacy and lower toxicity. This chapter reviews normal endocrine physiology, the association between hormones and cancer and currently available hormonal therapies in cancer.

STEROID HORMONE REGULATION

The pituitary–gonadal axis

The anterior pituitary gonadotroph synthesizes and secretes luteinizing hormone (LH) and follicle stimulating hormone (FSH). The synthesis and secretion of these hormones is under the aegis of gonadotrophin releasing hormone (GnRH). It was suggested at the beginning of this century by Heape that fertility control related to changes in the constitution of the blood effected by a secretion termed gonadin. Harris, in 1937, demonstrated by electrophysiological techniques that ovulation could be induced by stimulation of the hypothalamus. In 1947, Green and Harris postulated that neurohumoral factors originating in the median eminence of the tuber cinereum might regulate pituitary function. McCann, in 1960, showed that a hypothalamic extract could release LH from the pituitary. This hormone was purified in 1967 by Schally and Bowers. Schally et al. described the amino acid composition of porcine LH releasing hormone in 1971, identifying its structure by thin layer chromatography and countercurrent electrophoresis. In dosages of less than 1 mg, porcine LH released both LH and FSH in men and women and therefore it was renamed GnRH.

GnRH is released from the median eminence of the hypothalamus in short pulses occurring approximately every 1–3 hours. The frequency and amplitude of these pulses vary, differing between childhood, puberty and sexual maturity, and varying with menstrual phase. Within the pituitary, GnRH has a short half-life and is metabolized by pituitary arylamidases. It is to the pulsatile release of this decapeptide that the pituitary gonadotroph responds. The synthesis and secretion of GnRH is itself under the control of several hormones, including oestrogen, progesterone, testosterone and prolactin.

The GnRH receptor of the pituitary gonadotroph is a member of the G-protein-linked heptahelical transmembrane receptor family, and is sited on the cell surface (Kakar et al., 1992). Binding of GnRH to its receptor results in the activation of the phospholipase C β pathway and the generation of inositol phosphate (IP_3) and diacylglycerol (Limor et al., 1989). These, in turn, result in the mobilization of intracellular calcium and activation of protein kinase C, respectively (Shangold et al., 1988). These processes cause the activation of MAP kinase, synthesis of LH and FSH and exocytosis of secretory granules. In addition, the process of exocytosis is mediated by an increase in intracellular calcium related to the opening of L-type voltage-gated calcium channels due to the activation of the GnRH receptor.

In women, LH and FSH stimulate the secretion of oestradiol and progesterone by ovarian theca externa and granulosa cells. In men LH is responsible for the synthesis and secretion of testosterone and, to a lesser degree, oestradiol by testicular Leydig cells. The feedback loop is completed by the secretion of a polypeptide known as inhibin, synthesized by ovarian granulosa cells and testicular Sertoli cells, which inhibits FSH release by pituitary gonadotrophs.

The adrenal glands are also involved in the synthesis of steroid hormones, which is regulated by adrenocorticotrophic hormone (ACTH). Although the total amount of sex hormone produced by the adrenals in young adults is small, it is of significance in postmenopausal women and castrated men.

Hypothalamic–pituitary–adrenal axis

Corticotrophin releasing factor (CRF) was identified in 1981 as a 41-amino-acid peptide by Vale and others at the Salk Institute (Vale *et al.*, 1981). The release of CRF depends upon noradrenergic and cholinergic signals originating in the brainstem, cortex and limbic systems acting on the parvular portion of the hypothalamic paraventricular nucleus. Hypothalamic release of CRF stimulates the CRH-1 receptor of adenohypophysial corticotrophic cells. This stimulates the activity of adenyl cyclase, and the synthesis and release of ACTH.

ACTH is a 39-amino-acid peptide formed from the cleavage of a large precursor molecule, proopiomelanocortin (POMC). POMC contains within its structure β- and γ-lipotropin, pro-gamma melanocyte stimulating hormone and β-endorphin (Fig. 9.1). All of these peptides are released with ACTH. There is a circadian rhythm for ACTH release, with the highest levels occurring just prior to waking and the lowest levels at midnight. ACTH release is inhibited by a negative feedback loop, with circulating cortisol acting at both the pitu-itary and hypothalamus to decrease ACTH synthesis and release.

In the adrenal cortex, ACTH controls both glucocorticoid and steroid synthesis. The action of ACTH is mediated via its receptor melanocortin receptor type 2

(MC2-R), which is a G-protein-coupled heptahelical membrane receptor, and by modulation of the desmolase enzyme system.

Desmolase converts cholesterol to pregnenolone, which is then acted upon by hydroxylase enzymes. As a result of the activity of these enzymes within the delta 4 and delta 5 pathways, the adrenal cortex synthesizes aldosterone, cortisol, androstenedione and oestradiol (Fig. 9.2).

Peripheral oestrogen synthesis and the effects of age on gonadal function

In postmenopausal women there is maintained production of small amounts of oestrogenic steroids by the ovary, but the main source of circulating oestrogenic steroids is the peripheral aromatase system. This system, which is sited in fat, muscle and liver, metabolizes androstenedione, the main adrenal androgen, converting it to oestrone and oestrone sulphate via the sulphatase system (Fig. 9.3).

In men, spermatogenesis continues throughout life and the testis remains the principal source of androgens in noncastrate men. There is, however, a gradual reduction in absolute levels of circulating testosterone, and an increase in concentration of sex hormone binding globulin, which results in a net fall in free circulating testosterone with age.

Sex hormone mediated cellular signalling

Oestradiol- and testosterone-mediated cell signalling occurs via specific receptors which belong to the nuclear

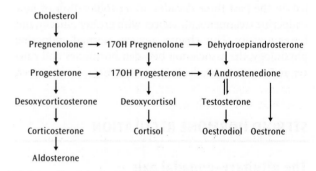

Figure 9.2 *Adrenal steroidogenesis.*

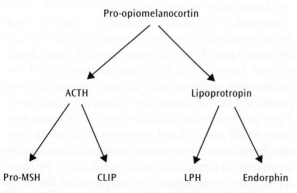

Figure 9.1 *Pro-opiocortin and its cleavage products.*

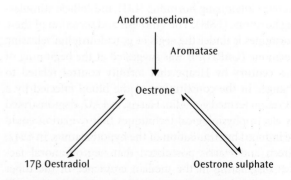

Figure 9.3 *Peripheral synthesis of oestrogenic steroids.*

steroid receptor superfamily, which also includes the gluco-corticoid, thyroxine, vitamin D and retinoic acid receptors.

Testosterone acts via the androgen receptor (AR), which was first described in 1969 by Fang *et al.* The gene for the receptor is localized on the long arm of the X-chromosome and is 90 kb in size (Chang *et al.*, 1988). The AR itself comprises 918 amino acids, molecular weight 100–110 kDa. It is subdivided into five domains, A–E. The N-terminal domains A and B are responsible for mediating transcriptional activation, and contain two homopolymeric stretches of glutamine and glycine repeats. Variations in length of the repeats correlate with transcriptional activation by ligand-bound receptor (Janne *et al.*, 1993). Domain C consists of two DNA-binding zinc fingers which are responsible for localizing the ligand-bound receptor to androgen response elements (AREs) of androgen-regulated genes. Domain D acts as a hinge and ligand-dependent nuclear localizing signal, while domain E corresponds to the ligand-binding domain which is activated by both testosterone and dihydrotestosterone (DHT).

DHT is derived from testosterone by its conversion in target tissues by the enzyme 5-alpha reductase. DHT has a tenfold greater affinity for the AR relative to testosterone and is therefore the principal ligand for the AR.

Unliganded ARs are localized in the cell nucleus and bound to heat-shock proteins. Binding of the androgen to AR results in dimerization. The AR–androgen complex diffuses passively into the nucleus and binds to AREs within DNA. This activates transcription through interactions with the pre-initiation complex in the promoter region and accessory activation factors such as SRC-120 and ARA70 (Janne *et al.*, 1993).

The effects of oestrogen are similarly mediated by the oestrogen receptors (ER). Two distinct subtypes, α and β, have been identified (Dickson and Stancel, 2000). ER-α is a 67-kDa protein encoded by a gene on chromosome 6, while ER-β weighs approximately 54 kDa and is encoded at chromosome 14. Overall the two receptors have a similar structure but share only 47 per cent amino-acid homology. The receptor DNA and ligand-binding domains are located at the centre of the protein and flanked at N- and C-termini by activation function-1 (AF-1) and activation function-2 (AF-2) domains.

Unliganded ERs are usually found in the cell nucleus and, like the AR, on binding oestradiol undergo conformational changes and dimerization, phosphorylation, dissociation from heat-shock proteins and binding to oestrogen response elements (EREs). The transcriptional activity of genes containing EREs is then modulated by AF-1 and/or AF-2.

Although the ligand-binding affinity for oestradiol is identical for the two ER subtypes, they differ significantly in their expression profiles and response to other ligands, such as tamoxifen. This is an area of active research and several tissue-selective oestrogen receptor modulators (SERMs) have been developed to exploit this phenomenon in clinical practice.

Membrane-bound oestrogen receptors are also known to exist, which may be responsible for mediating rapid non-genomic effects of oestrogens. However, these receptors have yet to be characterized.

HORMONAL FACTORS IN THE AETIOLOGY OF CANCERS

The incidence of a number of cancers, notably breast, prostate, ovary and endometrium, are recognized as being, in part, related to the patient's previous hormonal exposure. In each of these organs, epithelial proliferation is stimulated by sex steroids which, over time, may lead, with repeated cycles of DNA replication, to the accumulation of mutations in oncogenes, tumour suppressor genes and, ultimately, transformation into a malignant clone.

The proliferation of glandular breast tissue is stimulated by both oestrogen and progesterone, and the risk of breast cancer is proportional to the lifetime exposure to these hormones and the duration of cyclical proliferation of breast tissue during the menstrual cycle. This has been demonstrated in a number of studies which show an increased risk of breast cancers in patients with a late menopause, obesity and in those patients who have received prolonged oestrogen replacement therapy. However, pregnancy and lactation exert a protective effect, which is in excess of the reduction in the lifetime experience of menstrual cycles as a consequence of pregnancy.

The cyclical proliferation of ovarian tissue during the menstrual cycle under the influence of the gonadotrophins and oestrogen has also been shown to increase the risk of ovarian cancer. This is supported by the higher risk of ovarian cancer in nulliparous women and the duration-dependent reduction in risk related to oral contraceptive use (Hankinson *et al.*, 1992). In comparison, cyclical proliferation of endometrial tissue is stimulated by oestrogen and inhibited by progesterone. In endometrial cancer, oestrogen replacement therapy without concurrent progesterone or the use of sequential oral contraception is associated with an increased risk of malignancy, but the use of the combined oral contraceptive pill, which contains both oestrogen and progesterone, is associated with a reduction in cancer risk.

Prostate cancer shows a significant geographical variation in incidence, with lowest levels in Japan and highest levels in North America and Europe (Akazakis and Stennerman, 1973). Some studies have shown that this is related to differences in base levels of circulating testosterone and these may be higher in patients developing testicular cancer compared to controls. This hypothesis, however, has been challenged and other studies have shown no association between testosterone levels and prostate cancer incidence. Instead, a number of polymorphisms of the 5-alpha reductase gene and also the androgen receptor have recently been identified, some of which are more frequent in certain ethnic groups (Coetzee and Ross, 1994). As these polymorphisms result in differences in the conversion of testosterone to dihydrotestosterone and the binding and activation of the androgen receptor by testosterone or DHT, they can result in markedly different rates of proliferation of prostatic tissue despite similar plasma testosterone levels. Patient groups with higher net activity of testosterone may therefore be at higher risk of prostate cancer.

BIOCHEMICAL BASIS FOR HORMONAL TREATMENTS

Hormonal therapies for cancer are commonly regarded as cytostatic. They are not, and their application leads to cell death. Although the biochemical effects of most hormone therapies of cancer can be explained, the exact mechanisms by which responses are mediated are not fully understood. It is conventional to consider hormonal treatments limiting tumour growth via deprivation of the hormonal growth stimulus. The four main approaches are: downregulation of the hypothalamal pituitary gonadal axis; blockade of hormone receptors; inhibition of adrenal steroidogenesis; and inhibition of peripheral conversion of testosterone to oestrogen within tumour cells. In clinical practice, these approaches are utilized either in combination or sequentially, as these tumours only show a period of response following which relapse occurs due to the proliferation of resistant clones of cells. In this section we describe how each of the main groups of endocrine therapies function to regulate tumour cell proliferation.

Ovarian ablation

In premenopausal women ovarian ablation results in a significant fall in circulating oestrogen to menopausal levels. In 1896 Beatson first demonstrated the efficacy of oophorectomy in the treatment of premenopausal patients with metastatic disease. Since then techniques for ovarian ablation using radiotherapy and GnRH analogues have been developed. All three techniques are essentially equivalent and produce regression rates of 25–30 per cent in metastatic disease, with a duration of response of between 9 and 12 months (Litherland and Jackson, 1988). However, surgical oophorectomy is associated with the risk and complications of general anaesthesia and laparotomy, while radiation to the ovaries may require several weeks to be effective and may result in only incomplete destruction of the follicles. The development of GnRH analogues has therefore been a significant advantage as patients can be reliably treated using monthly or 3-monthly depot injections of leuprorelin or goserelin to achieve postmenopausal plasma-oestrogen levels. Medical ovarian ablation is potentially reversible. Ovarian ablation has also been shown to produce a survival benefit equal to that of adjuvant chemotherapy in premenopausal women, and the value of combined adjuvant chemo-hormonal therapy is currently under evaluation.

Castration

Reduction in plasma testosterone by either medical or surgical castration has been shown to be highly effective in the treatment of patients with prostate cancer. Surgical castration is a simple procedure with a good safety profile. However, it may be associated with significant psychological morbidity and, in analysis, has been found to be equivalent in cost. It has been shown that when given a choice patients prefer medical castration with GnRH analogues to orchiectomy. Leuprorelin and goserelin are the two most commonly used GnRH analogues and can be administered either as 1- or 3-monthly depot preparations subcutaneously.

In addition, medical castration can also be achieved using diethylstilboestrol in doses of either 3 or 1 mg/day (Byar, 1973). Although diethystilboestrol is extremely effective in suppressing testosterone to castrate levels and inducing responses in prostate cancer equivalent to that of orchiectomy and GnRH analogues, it is associated with a significant cardiovascular toxicity and increased incidence of thromboembolic events. This toxicity remains when low-dose oestrogens are prescribed.

Overall medical or surgical castration in metastatic prostate cancer results in a response rate of approximately 80 per cent and a median duration of response of 12–15 months.

GnRH analogues

The elucidation of the structure of GnRH in 1971 led to the development of a number of substituted analogues. Analogues which were nonapeptides or decapeptides with substitutions at the sixth or tenth amino-acid residues were found to be superagonists, i.e. a single injection produced supraphysiological release of both LH and FSH. In addition, these analogues had prolonged pituitary half-lives and so after initial stimulation of pituitary gonadotrophs the absence of pulsatile stimulation renders the pituitary unresponsive.

These compounds have become of value in those patients where gonadal downregulation is an advantage. They have been applied in endocrinology to the management of patients with precocious puberty and are also used to treat endometriosis. The greatest application of these compounds, however, is in the management of patients with sex-hormone-dependent malignant diseases, where they will provide a medical alternative to oophorectomy in breast cancer and orchiectomy in prostatic cancer.

Leuprorelin and goserelin are the two most commonly used GnRH analogues, although a number of others are available. These compounds may be administered as monthly subcutaneous depot preparations. Three-monthly depot preparations are also available and annual formulations are in development.

Due to the initial surge in LH and FSH with the use of GnRH agonists, tumour growth may be enhanced at the initiation of therapy and is termed 'tumour flare'. This is generally more common in patients with prostate cancer than breast carcinoma, and in the former can be prevented by the use of an anti-androgen prior to, and continued for several weeks beyond, the initiation of GnRH agonist therapy. GnRH antagonists should overcome the problem of tumour flare and are currently about to be launched into the market.

Anti-oestrogens

The most widely used 'anti-oestrogen' is tamoxifen. Tamoxifen is metabolized to 4-hydroxy tamoxifen and N-desmethyl tamoxifen (Adam et al., 1980). The most active metabolite is 4-hydroxytamoxifen. Peak plasma levels of tamoxifen are seen 3–7 hours after oral administration and the terminal half-life of tamoxifen is reported to be in the range between 4 and 11 days, enabling once-daily dosing. There is no evidence to suggest that increasing the dose of tamoxifen to greater than 40 mg/day increases therapeutic efficacy. The standard dose of tamoxifen is therefore 20 mg once a day. Tamoxifen acts by blocking the oestrogenic stimulation of breast cancer cells by inhibiting both the dimerization and translocation of the oestrogen receptor. This is thought to be its main mode of action. In vitro tamoxifen-induced inhibition of protein kinase C and reversal of multidrug resistance has also been demonstrated.

However, tamoxifen is a partial oestrogen receptor antagonist and therefore in some patients treatment may be associated with an initial period of tumour flare (Dickson and Stancel, 2000). The beneficial aspects of this oestrogenic activity, however, are a reduction in total cholesterol and a tend towards decreased cardiovascular morbidity. In postmenopausal women tamoxifen use is associated with an increase in bone mineral density. In premenopausal women tamoxifen-related oestrogen receptor antagonism causes osteoporosis.

Tamoxifen is active in the treatment of breast cancer in both premenopausal and postmenopausal women and its activity increases with the patient's age. This correlates with the increased likelihood of oestrogen-receptor-positive tumours in older patients. In women with metastatic breast cancer, tamoxifen induces a therapeutic response in about a third of patients. The selection of patients in whom response is likely has become possible with the development of monoclonal antibodies for the detection of oestrogen receptors in tumours by immuno-histochemistry. Patients whose tumours are both oestrogen- and progesterone-receptor positive have a response rate of 80 per cent, compared with 5 per cent in patients who are both oestrogen- and progesterone-receptor negative (Clark and McGuire, 1983).

Tamoxifen has also been used in the treatment of metastatic ovarian cancer, and response rates of 5–10 per cent have been reported.

The most common side-effect of tamoxifen is hot flushes, experienced by approximately 50 per cent of postmenopausal women on tamoxifen, which can be treated in some patients with low doses of progestogens. Tamoxifen also increases the risk of endometrial cancer and thromboembolic events (Early Breast Cancer Trialists' Collaborative Group, 1998). Recent evidence suggests that tamoxifen is hepatotoxic, causing a steatohepatitis which may progress to cirrhosis. In animal models tamoxifen forms DNA adducts and can induce hepatomas. For these reasons there is significant interest in the development of the SERMs, which are currently undergoing clinical trials in breast cancer.

Progestogens

In Europe medroxyprogesterone acetate is the progestogen most commonly used to treat cancers, while in the United States megestrol acetate is used. These compounds are thought to act via progesterone receptors (PGRs). PGRs are most frequently present in breast cancer and expressed in up to 60 per cent of tumours (Clark and McGuire, 1983). However, response to progestogens occurs in only a third of patients.

The biochemical effects of progestogens are complex and not necessarily confined to direct activity at the level of the tumour cell. Progestogens decrease circulating levels of the gonadotrophins, interfere with steroid hormone synthesis and have glucocorticoid activity. This can lead to steroidal side-effects and adrenocorticotrophic hormone suppression.

The optimal dose of these progestogens that should be used to treat hormone-dependent malignancies is controversial. In one study of parenteral medroxyprogesterone acetate, the highest response rate in breast cancer was seen at a dose of 1 g/day. Subsequent studies of medroxyprogesterone acetate given orally at a dose of 200 mg three times a day and 500 mg twice daily suggest equivalent efficacy (Gallagher et al., 1987). In practice, doses of 200–400 mg/day of medroxyprogesterone and 80–160 mg of megestrol acetate are used.

Standard oral dosing of medroxyprogesterone results in a delay of several weeks in achieving therapeutic tissue levels. This is in contrast to megestrol acetate which achieves steady-state levels by the third treatment day. Megestrol also has a sufficiently long half-life to enable once-daily dosing.

In the treatment of prostate cancer the progestogen, cyproterone acetate, has been used as both as a single agent for metastatic disease and also in combination to achieve total androgen blockade. However, prolonged use of cyproterone acetate is associated with a significant risk of progression to fulminant hepatic failure. Indeed, cyproterone acetate is no longer licensed for long-term use in prostate cancer, and has been replaced by the pure anti-androgens instead.

Progestogens are also active in endometrial cancer, with a response in 10–20 per cent of patients (Reifinstein, 1971). In renal carcinoma a response is seen in approximately 5 per cent of patients.

New anti-progestational agents, such as RU486, are currently being investigated in breast cancer. In one study a response rate of 18 per cent was noted with a dose of 200 mg/day orally of RU486 in patients with metastatic breast cancer.

Anti-androgens

A number of anti-androgens, androgen receptor antagonists, have been used in the treatment of prostate cancer over the past three decades. By binding to the androgen receptor these molecules deprive malignant cells of androgen-dependent proliferation signals.

Cyproterone acetate was the first drug to be used in this class for the treatment of prostate carcinoma. Although it inhibits the androgen receptor, its primary activity is progesterogenic. Although cyproterone acetate appears in clinical trials to be equivalent to diethylstilboestrol in response rate and overall survival, like the latter, it may be associated with an increased cardiovascular and thromboembolic risk.

The first pure anti-androgen to enter clinical practice was flutamide, followed by nilutamide and, most recently, bicalutamide. All three agents are effective in the prevention of tumour flare associated with GnRH analogues. In addition, they provide a significant but small survival advantage when used in combination with medical or surgical castration in the initial treatment of patients with metastatic prostate cancer (Prostate Cancer Triallist's Collaborative Group, 2000). Bicalutamide monotherapy has the advantage of maintaining potency in about 40 per cent of patients, and is an effective treatment of prostate cancer (Boccardo et al., 1999). Flutamide monotherapy is relatively ineffective and has been clearly shown to be inferior to medical or surgical castration alone.

The principal side-effects of flutamide are gynaecomastia, fatigue, diarrhoea and hepatotoxicity. The incidence of hot flushes and impotence are significantly less than with castration. In addition, nilutamide is associated with the development of interstitial pneumonitis and night blindness and therefore is no longer widely used in clinical practice.

Anti-androgens can be as second-line therapy in prostate cancer following the failure of medical or surgical castration. Addition of an anti-androgen to castration produces a response in 5–15 per cent of patients (Oh and Kantoff, 1998). While in patients initially treated with combined androgen blockade, 10–40 per cent respond to flutamide withdrawal, with a median duration of response of 3–4 months. This phenomenon is due to mutation of the androgen receptor with progressive disease which results in a paradoxical activation of the receptor by the anti-androgen. Anti-androgen withdrawal therefore results in deprivation of this mitogenic stimulus.

Inhibitors of adrenal steroidogenesis

Following castration in men and oophorectomy in women, the adrenals are the primary source of androgens, and these are converted by the aromatase system peripherally in the skin fat and muscle to oestrone and oestradiol. Historically, surgical adrenalectomy and hypophysectomy have both been used in an attempt to treat patients with progressive disease following castration or ovarian ablation in breast and prostate cancer. In both cases, significant responses are achieved and this has led to the development of inhibitors of adrenal steroidogenesis. Aminoglutethimide, ketoconazole, trilostane and metyrapone all inhibit various enzymes involved in the conversion of cholesterol to androstenedione (AS) and dihydroxyepiandrostene (DHEA).

Aminoglutethimide inhibits the action of adrenal P450 and has been used in the clinical setting in combination with hydrocortisone to prevent adrenal insufficiency. Pharmacological studies suggest that the action of aminoglutethimide on the adrenal P450 system is only transient and the production of androgens returns to baseline after several weeks of aminoglutethimide therapy. Indeed, in the treatment of prostate cancer long-term adrenal suppression and clinical response using hydrocortisone alone is equivalent to the combination of aminoglutethimide and hydrocortisone. Aminoglutethimide is also associated with a number of side-effects, including skin rashes and gastrointestinal toxicity, which also limit its use. The use of ketoconazole and trilostane in clinical practice is also limited by their toxicity.

Currently, hydrocortisone or prednisolone is used alone to inhibit adrenal steroidogenesis in patients with breast or prostate cancer. In breast cancer further suppression of oestrogens derived from adrenal steroidogenesis can be achieved with aromatase inhibitors, which are discussed below.

Aromatase inhibitors

Androstenedione and DHEA are converted to oestradiol and oestrone by the aromatase enzyme which is found in adipose tissue and skeletal muscle. Over the past two decades several inhibitors of aromatase have been developed for treating patients with breast cancer. These can be grouped into the steroidal (formestane and exemestane) and non-steroidal (letrozole and anastrozole and vorazole) inhibitors (Hamilton and Piccart, 1999). The non-steroidal aromatase inhibitors act by binding to the enzyme reversibly at a site distant from the hormone binding site.

Formestane is administered as a fortnightly intramuscular injection, while exemestane has good oral bioavailability and a long half-life, enabling once-daily oral dosing. Direct comparisons in terms of efficacy between formestane and exemestane are lacking. However, the ease of administration of exemestane has led to its greater acceptance in clinical practice. In patients with metastatic breast carcinoma with relapse following tamoxifen, exemestane at a dose of 25 mg/day has been shown to be equivalent to megestrol acetate 160 mg/day in terms of objective response. However, in these patients, treatment with exemestane results in a delay in the median time to tumour progression (20.3 weeks versus 16.6 weeks) and improved survival (Hamilton and Piccart, 1999).

Letrozole and anastrozole, of the non-steroidal inhibitors, are currently licensed for the treatment of patients with metastatic breast cancer who have relapsed following tamoxifen. Anastrozole, 1 mg/day, compared to megestrol acetate, 160 mg/day results in equivalent response rates (Buzdar et al., 1996). However, overall survival is improved with the aromatase inhibitor (27 versus 23 months). In comparisons of letrozole, 2.5 mg/day, and megestrol acetate, letrozole is associated with a higher response rate (24 versus 16 per cent) but overall survival is not significantly different (25 versus 22 months). Vorazole has not demonstrated any additional efficacy over megestrol acetate or aminoglutethimide in the treatment of these patients. However, all three agents show improved tolerability compared to megestrol acetate or aminoglutethimide in these patients.

Current data are insufficient to compare drugs within classes, or steroidal with non-steroidal aromatase inhibitors. In view of the improved tolerability and efficacy of these drugs compared to the traditional adrenal steroidogenesis inhibitors and progestagens, trials have been established to explore their use as first-line therapy in patients with metastatic disease and in the adjuvant treatment of patients with breast cancer.

CHEMOPREVENTION OF HORMONE-RESPONSIVE TUMOURS

The role of hormones in the development of breast and prostate cancer and the efficacy of hormonal therapy in the treatment of these diseases has led to the development of chemopreventive strategies aimed at inhibiting the hormone-mediated mitogenic stimulus to these organs.

In breast cancer trials on the use of adjuvant tamoxifen has consistently been shown to reduce by 30 per cent the risk of contralateral breast cancer (Early Breast Cancer Trialists' Collaborative Group, 1998). Based on these data, trials in both Europe and America have been conducted on the use of tamoxifen in primary prevention in high-risk patients. Although the European trial continues currently, the American trial conducted by the NSABP was terminated early as it showed a significant benefit from tamoxifen in postmenopausal women at high risk of breast cancer (approximately equal to that of a 60-year-old). However, an increased risk of endometrial cancer and thromboembolic events was also noted.

In prostate cancer, finasteride is being tested as a chemopreventive agent (Thompson et al., 1997). Finasteride is a specific inhibitor of 5-alpha reductase, which is responsible for the conversion of testosterone to the highly active dihydrotestosterone. Under physiological conditions, dihydrotestosterone is the principal androgenic stimulus in the prostate and its activity is thought to be related to the development of cancer. Finasteride is extremely well tolerated and does not cause impotence or other side-effects associated with androgen ablation. It is therefore being used in a 7-year trial of prostate cancer chemoprevention, being conducted by the National Cancer Institute in the United States, in which 18 000 healthy men aged 55 years or older have been randomized to receive either finasteride 5 mg/day or placebo.

In endometrial and ovarian cancer the use of non-sequential oral contraception is associated with a reduction in the risk of malignancy. Their use for primary prevention, however, has not been tested in a trial setting.

CONCLUSIONS

The past two decades have seen advances in both our understanding of the molecular biology of hormone-responsive cancers, and in the development of new agents for the treatment of these tumours. Patient with metastatic breast and prostatic cancer, however, ultimately become refractory to hormonal therapy. Elucidation of the mechanism by which hormonal resistance develops remains one of the greatest challenges in this field. It is hoped, with current advances in molecular biology, that this key to the mystery of hormonal regulation of tumour growth will be turned within the next decade.

SIGNIFICANT POINTS

- Therapeutic levels of tamoxifen take up to 6 weeks to be achieved.
- There is no evidence that doses of tamoxifen greater than 20 mg/day increase therapeutic efficacy.
- Tamoxifen is a partial oestrogen agonist and has stimulatory as well as inhibitory effects.

- Tumour flare may be seen with tamoxifen, especially in patients with hypercalcaemia and bone metastases.
- There is a small but definite increase in the incidence of uterine cancer in patients on long-term tamoxifen.
- In Europe medroxyprogesterone acetate is the most commonly used progestogen for malignancy, whereas in North America megestrol acetate is more frequently used.
- Sixty per cent of breast tumours contain progesterone receptors but only 30 per cent respond to progestogen therapy.
- The optimal progestogen dosage is controversial and various doses are used in practice.
- Peptide hormones have been used clinically in ovarian, breast and prostatic cancer as well as endometriosis and precocious puberty.
- Depot preparations of several types of peptide hormones are now widely used.

KEY REFERENCES

Grossman, A. (ed.) (1993) *Clinical endocrinology*. Oxford: Blackwell.

Lynn, J. and Bloom, S. (eds) (1993) *Surgical endocrinology*. Oxford: Butterworth–Heinemann.

Waxman, J. (ed.) (1995) *The molecular endocrinology of cancer*. Cambridge: Cambridge University Press.

REFERENCES

Adam, H.K., Patterson, J.S. and Kemp, J.V. (1980) Studies on the metabolism and pharmacokinetics of tamoxifen in healthy volunteers. *Cancer Treat. Rep.* **64**, 761.

Akazakis, K. and Stennerman, G.N. (1973) Comparitive study of latent carcinoma of the prostate among Japanese in Japan and Hawai. *J. Natl Cancer Inst.* **50**, 1137–44.

Boccardo, F., Rubagotti, A., Barichello, M. *et al.* (1999) Bicalutamide monotherapy versus flutamide plus goserelin in prostate cancer patients: results of an Italian Prostate Cancer Project Study. *J. Clin. Oncol.* **17**, 2027–38.

Buzdar, A., Jonat, W., Howell, A. *et al.* (1996) Anastrozole, a potent and selective aromatase inhibitor, versus megestrol acetate in postmenopausal women with advanced breast cancer. *J. Clin. Oncol.* **14**, 2000–11.

Byar, D.P. (1973) The Veterans Administration Cooperative Urological Research Group's studies of the cancer of the prostate. *Cancer* **32**, 1126–30.

Chang, C., Kokontis, J. and Liao, S. (1988) Structural analysis of complementary DNA and amino acid sequences of human and rat androgen receptors. *Proc. Natl Acad. Sci.* **85**, 7211–15.

Clark, G.M. and McGuire, W.L. (1983) Progesterone receptors and human breast cancer. *Breast Cancer Res.* **3**, 157–63.

Coetzee, G.A. and Ross, R.K. (1994) Prostate cancer and the androgen receptor. *J. Natl Cancer Inst.* **86**, 872.

Dickson, R.B. and Stancel, G.M. (2000) Estrogen receptor-mediated processes in normal and cancer cells. *J. Natl Cancer Inst.* **27**, 135–47.

Early Breast Cancer Trialists' Collaborative Group (1998) Tamoxifen for early breast cancer: an overview of the randomised trials. *Lancet* **351**, 1451–67.

Fang *et al.* (1969) Receptor proteins for androgens. On the role of specific proteins in selective retention of 17-β-hydroxy-5-α-androstan-3-one by rat ventral prostate *in vivo* and *in vitro*. *J. Biol. Chem.* **244**(24), 6584–95.

Gallagher, C.J., Cairnduff, F. and Smith E. (1987) High dose versus low dose medroxyprogesterone acetate. A randomized trial in advanced breast cancer. *Eur. J. Cancer Clin. Onc.* **23**, 1895–900.

Hamilton, A. and Piccart, M. (1999) The third-generation non-steroidal aromatase inhibitors: a review of their clinical benefits in the second-line hormonal treatment of advanced breast cancer. *Ann. Oncol.* **10**, 377–84.

Hankinson, S.E., Colditz, G.A., Hunter, D.J. *et al.* (1992) A quantitative assessment of oral contraceptive use and the risk of ovarian cancer. *Obstet. Gynecol.* **80**, 708.

Janne, O.A., Pavlimo, J.J., Kallio, P. *et al.* (1993) Androgen receptor and mechanism of action. *Ann. Med.* **25**, 83–9.

Kakar, S.S., Musgrove, L.C., Devor, D.C. *et al.* (1992) Cloning sequencing and expression of the human GnRH receptor. *Biochem. Biophys. Res. Comm.* **189**, 289–95.

Limor, R., Scharvtz, I., Hazum, E. *et al.* (1989) Effect of guanine nucleotides on stimulus secretion coupling mechanism in permealised pituitary cells: relationship to gonadotrophin releasing hormone action. *Biochem. Biophys. Res. Comm.* **159**, 51–8.

Litherland, S. and Jackson, I.M. (1988) Antioestrogens in the management of hormone-dependent cancer. *Cancer Treat. Rev.* **15**, 183–94.

Oh, W.K. and Kantoff, P.W. (1998) Management of hormone refractory prostate cancer: current standards and future prospects. *J. Urol.* **160**, 1220–9.

Prostate Cancer Triallist's Collaborative Group (2000) Maximum androgen blockade in advanced prostate cancer: an overview of the randomised trials. *Lancet* **355**, 1491–8.

Reifinstein, E.C. Jr (1971) Hydroxyprogesterone caproate therapy in advanced endometrial cancer. *Cancer* **27**, 485–502.

Shangold, G.A., Murphy, S.N. and Miller, R.J. (1988) Gonadotrophin-releasing hormone-induced calcium in single identified gonadotrophs. *Physiol. Sci.* **85**, 6566–70.

Thompson, I.M., Coltman, C.A. and Crowley, J. (1997) Chemo-prevention of prostate cancer: the Prostate Cancer Prevention Trial. *Prostate* **33**, 217–21.

Vale, W., Spess, J., Rivier, C. and Rivier, J. (1981) Characterisation of a 41 residue ovine hypothalamic peptide that stimulates secretion of corticotrophin and B endorphin. *Science* **231**, 1394–7.

References 151

10

Tumour imaging in oncology

RONALD BEANEY AND JOHN BINGHAM

The past 20 years have seen a rapid increase in imaging techniques. Most clinicians involved in the care of cancer patients now enjoy the luxury of having access to a wide variety of investigative techniques. X-ray procedures, ultrasound and radio-isotope techniques along with computed X-ray tomography (CT) and magnetic resonance imaging (MRI), provide us with most of the imaging data on which we make our clinical decisions. To this we must add the newer techniques which demonstrate functional change, such as positron emission tomography (PET), and immunogenic status, such as radio-isotope immunoscintigraphy (RIA). The ability to image in three dimensions has led to more accurate staging and diagnosis. This, in turn, has led to more appropriate and specifically tailored treatments. In addition, with the more elaborate imaging techniques it is becoming possible to monitor closely the morphological or physiological response to treatment. Tumour marker assays, together with improvements in imaging, have increased our ability to detect relapse sooner than previously possible. It is difficult to evaluate the actual contribution that imaging has made to the overall outlook of the cancer patient, since most of the improvement in survival figures over the past 10 years has come from advances in treatment rather than advances in imaging. However, the technical improvements have brought about increased sophistication, accuracy and specificity, improving staging and the determination of the most appropriate treatment. In this chapter a brief account of the basic principles of each investigative technique will be given, along with details of instrumentation and clinical usefulness. In making a comparison between different imaging techniques it is worth stressing that

one is not comparing like with like. In an article such as this it is impossible to be exhaustively comprehensive.

GENERAL PRINCIPLES

A wide range of physical principles is embodied in various imaging techniques. In general, the ability to see lesions depends upon the contrast between the lesion and the surrounding normal tissue. In two-dimensional imaging all the structures from the front to the back of the body are superimposed on a single film, reducing the contrast between the various structures. In addition there is the problem of interpreting three-dimensional information in a two-dimensional image. Tomography assists in two ways:

1 by displaying a cross-section of the body, thus 'separating' the structures and aiding anatomical interpretation;
2 by improving the contrast between organs or tumours and surrounding tissues. This reduced the minimum size of lesion detectable when compared with plain two-dimensional imaging. This is illustrated diagrammatically in Figure 10.1.

X-RAYS

Radiographs are created by passing a beam of X-rays through the subject and recording them on a sensitive medium. The beam is differentially absorbed according to the electron density of the tissues through which it

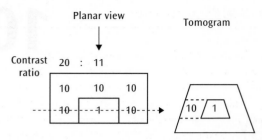

Figure 10.1 *Principle of tomography. When the three-dimensional structure is seen in two dimensions (left) the ratio of contrast between the normal and abnormal areas is 20:11. When a cross-section is taken through the lesion there is no superimposition of normal over abnormal areas and the contrast has increased 10:1.*

passes. The recording was initially made on silver oxide coated film but more recently digital techniques have been developed to allow the manipulation of the images in terms of both magnification and contrast resolution. The radiograph obtained is a two-dimensional representation of a three-dimensional structure and suffers the major disadvantage that all the structures along the path of the X-ray beam are superimposed. A density difference of approximately 5 per cent is required before organs can be visually separated from each other. This is amply sufficient in the chest, where the density of the lungs is very different from the mediastinal structures and the chest wall, but in the abdomen, where the organs are of very similar density, unless outlined by fat, they are inseparable. However, if there is calcification present, this may provide some information about the position and constitution of the organ of interest. Gas in the bowel aids its recognition, but is of little use for assessing tumours except when there is gross displacement by a mass or there is intestinal obstruction. Bony structures, because of their high calcium content, are easily separated from the adjacent soft tissues. To increase contrast resolution, two techniques were developed. First, tomography, literally 'slice writing', where a thin section of the structure of interest is obtained in a longitudinal plane by moving the X-ray tube and film in synchrony in opposite directions while exposing the film to the X-ray beam. By varying the degree of travel, the thickness of the slice could be varied, and this was very effective for detecting small nodules in the lungs. Second, a contrast medium can be introduced to increase the differential between the organ of interest and the surroundings. Iodinated contrast media have been used extensively for the opacification of arteries, veins and lymphatics and, with subsequent excretion, the urinary tract. Barium sulphate is used for examining the gastrointestinal tract from the mouth to the anus, while water-soluble contrast agents, again iodine containing, have been used for outlining structures such as the bronchus, as well as cavities, for example, the bladder.

Varying the voltage of the X-ray beam (kVp) can change the contrast discrimination, so that high-voltage X-rays are used for the lungs whereas low-voltage beams are used for discrimination of soft tissues, such as the breast in mammography.

COMPUTED TOMOGRAPHY

Computed tomography (CT) was developed in the 1970s and was first directed towards the brain, an organ that had proved to be difficult to investigate because of the surrounding skull. Invasive techniques such as angiography and air encephalography were required to show displacement of structures and abnormal blood flow associated with tumours. CT enabled direct visualization of the ventricular system and of parenchymal abnormalities and gained wide acceptance within a short time from introduction. The technique utilizes a source of X-rays with a bank of detectors which rotate around the patient in a 180° or 360° arc to obtain absorption data which are then reconstructed into a transverse section. Sectional thickness can be from 1 to 20 mm but is usually in the range 2–10 mm. The early generation machines passed the patient through the CT gantry in steps equal to the slice thickness, but technical developments have allowed the power source for the X-ray generator to be separated so that the tube and detectors can be rotated continuously as the patient is passed through the gantry. This is spiral or helical CT, which generates a continuous volume of data from which axial, coronal and sagittal images can be reconstructed with little loss in resolution. The development has resulted in shortening of the time of the examination so that the whole chest can be imaged in a breathhold. This reduces the chance of mis-registration of images and increases the quality of the non-axial reconstructed data. A further advantage has been the ability to image the patient during the peak of contrast opacification of the vessels, so that optimal enhancement of organs can be obtained as well as angiographic data. A further recent improvement has been made to provide multiple rows of detectors (multi-slice CT) so that the time of acquisition is reduced even further (Berland and Smith, 1998). Although improved collimation of the X-ray beam and the sensitivity of the detectors have increased, this has not resulted in a great deal of reduction in radiation dose associated with CT examination. However, low-dose techniques are now being developed which make CT as a screening test more feasible. This will be discussed later. The CT image being stored in digital form permits a variety of image manipulation techniques. The most valuable processing facility is that of windowing, where the desired range of attenuations can be spread over the dynamic range of the viewing screen. This enchances the contrast between the tissues of interest.

As in other types of X-ray diagnosis, contrast media can be introduced into the vascular system or body cavities to enhance contrast and assist the differentiation of the various structures. This is especially valuable in the mediastinum, where the diagnosis of lymphadenopathy can be difficult due to the proximity of the mediastinal vascular structures. Contrast is also used to outline the gut and vagina to assist in diagnosis of pelvic structures.

The identification of a lesion depends on the difference in density between the lesion and its surroundings: smaller lesions can be detected with CT than with conventional radiography. Small metastatic deposits only a few millimetres in diameter may be readily visible in the lung, whereas similar-sized metastases in the liver (because of the minor differences in density) would have to be two or three times larger before being identified. The administration of contrast agents can improve the contrast between tumours and the surrounding normal tissue. As in conventional radiography, tissue specificity is poor: CT cannot readily distinguish between benign lesions and malignant tumours; however, with the clinical history and a series of images it is normally possible to provide a diagnosis. CT images in three dimensions can be used to provide the basic data for radiotherapy treatment planning.

Advantages of CT scanning

CT scanning is ideal for looking at the body in a series of sections. Without the necessity for contrast media, it can demonstrate lesions in areas invisible to ultrasound. It produces better delineation of organs in obese subjects whereas, in ultrasound, fat often reduces the quality of the images. Unlike ultrasound, gas in the gut or lungs actually improves the image. CT scanning is also particularly useful in assessing sarcomas, where both bone and soft-tissue disease need visualization. Unlike lymphography, it can demonstrate enlarged nodes in virtually any region in the body. However, lymphography, unlike CT, can demonstrate the abnormal internal architecture of a pathological but normal-sized node. Despite this shortcoming of CT, enlarged intra-abdominal and mediastinal nodes greater than 1.5 cm in diameter are readily visualized. In addition, the technique of CT-guided percutaneous biopsy is now well established with a high success rate (Husband and Golding, 1983).

Some sites are particularly suited to investigation by CT, e.g. head and neck tumours, renal and adrenal tumours and retroperitoneal tumours, including nodal disease. The use of CT in different regions of the body is discussed later in this chapter.

CT and radiotherapy planning

CT, with its ability to accurately delineate a tumour volume in three dimensions, lends itself to radiotherapy planning. There are several commercially available packages where CT-integrated planning can be conducted directly on the CT image. Newer programmes allow off-axis data to be calculated and displayed. With the introduction of conformational radiotherapeutic techniques, CT imaging is essential.

ULTRASOUND IMAGING

High-frequency sound is transmitted through soft tissues and water, the absorption of the beam being determined by the nature of the tissue being traversed and the number of interfaces between tissues of different densities. Increased frequency enables higher resolution images to be obtained, although there is decreased penetration of the sound due to higher absorption. Ultrasound is not transmitted through an air/tissue interface to any significant extent, so it is essential for a coupling medium such as jelly or paraffin oil to be used between the transducer and interrogated tissue. Likewise, ultrasound cannot be used when air is present within the body, such as in the lungs or in the gastrointestinal tract.

As ultrasound traverses a series of tissues some of the ultrasound energy is scattered backwards towards the transducer each time a tissue interface is encountered (Fig. 10.2). The loss of energy and signal is compensated by appropriate amplification. With the use of a monitor it is possible to demonstrate the internal structures by modulating the brightness of the electron beam according to the strength of the returning ultrasound signal. Uniform solid tissues show up as a series of regular echoes, interfaces show as solid lines between organs or tissues; fluid-containing areas show relatively little echo pattern with distal enhancement of the beam while calcium-containing areas are seen as bright areas with no signal distal to them.

It is usual to use an electronic amplifier to compensate for the ultrasound absorption in the tissues. With cysts, for example, there is little absorption while the sound traverses the cyst, and so the signals behind the cysts are overamplified and shown up as a bright area (Fig. 10.3). The limitation of bone and air to the transmission of ultrasound means that acoustic windows have to be used, always ensuring that there is either soft tissue or fluid between the ultrasound transducer and the area of interest.

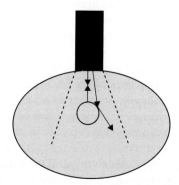

Figure 10.2 *The beam from the ultrasound transducer sweeps in an arc electronically or mechanically. When any part of the beam meets a tissue interface 'normally' the beam is reflected back and received by the same transducer. A time gain amplifier compensates for the absorption and scattering as the beam passes through the tissue.*

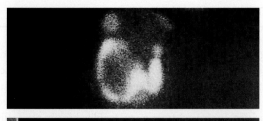

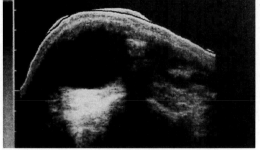

Figure 10.3 *Tc^{99m} pertechnetate scintigram of an enlarged right lobe of the thyroid (upper image). The ultrasound B-scan shows a large, circular abnormality without an echo pattern and enhancement of the echoes behind the lesion. The features are typical of a cyst (lower image).*

The transducers used for ultrasound imaging may be linear or sector. In sector scanning an electronic system sweeps the ultrasound beam in an arc; thus, although the transducer may be small, the area scanned at depth can be quite large. Electronic focusing ensures that each part of the arc is in focus. Since this is all done in real time, the ability to view the images dynamically greatly aids the diagnostic process, enabling the operator to build up a three-dimensional image in his mind.

Specialized transducers are available for transvaginal scanning of the pelvic structures. The static pictures which are taken for a permanent record often convey little of the information to be derived from real-time imaging. The small arc or rectangle displayed on the hard copy conveys only a fraction of the information visible to the ultrasound operator. In addition, the necessity to use an acoustic window restricts the value of the technique, since experience and skill are required to use ultrasound imaging effectively.

Doppler ultrasound employs the fact that moving structures alter the frequency of the returning sound waves. Moving red blood cells within vessels act as reflectors and the resulting changes in frequency can be displayed in colour on the monitor. The signals can be analysed to demonstrate the spectrum of velocities, and the results displayed as a graph or used to calculate the blood flow in a vessel. Doppler ultrasound is valuable for showing the flow in vessels for identification or to demonstrate obstruction to them or clotting within them. The vascularity of lesions can also be useful in differentiating between benign and malignant disease, for example, in the breast.

The organs immediately accessible to ultrasound include the thyroid, heart, liver, spleen, usually the pancreas and the pelvic structures, provided the bladder is well filled to provide an acoustic window. The degree of success will vary from patient to patient, depending on the preparation or gaseous state of the gastrointestinal tract.

Ultrasound uses a tomographic technique which improves the contrast and enables very small lesions to be visualized in certain circumstances. In the axial direction, the resolution at 5 MHz can be of the order of 1 mm, enabling the demonstration of very small blood vessels. The ability to see tumours depends upon the alteration in impedance between, for example, normal tissue of the liver and the tumour itself. This varies from tumour to tumour; for example, gut lesions show up clearly when the echo pattern is increased relative to the surrounding tissue, while in other cases there may be little difference in echo intensity. Thus, a negative examination may reflect the skill of the operator as well as the technical limitations of lack of contrast between a tumour and surrounding tissue.

The advantages of ultrasound are the lack of radiation hazard, its economy and ability to carry out many examinations with minimum discomfort to the patient. The disadvantages are the requirements of experience and skill and the problems associated with achieving a good acoustic window in the presence of variable amounts of gas in the abdomen.

RADIO-ISOTOPE STUDIES

Radionuclide imaging has played an important role in the investigation of cancer patients. The final image represents the degree of uptake of the labelled substance and depends on a combination of regional blood flow and biological function of the tissue being studied. The uptake of a radiopharmaceutical is thus related to function and is therefore able to complement the more detailed anatomical information provided by ultrasound, CT and MRI.

Each element has a series of isotopes, some of which are radioactive. Since the radioactive isotope of an element behaves in an identical fashion chemically to the nonradioactive isotope, the radioactive version can be used to trace biological processes inside the body (Belcher and Veall, 1971).

All radioactive isotopes decay in an exponential fashion, the half-life being the expression that represents the time taken for the radioactivity to decay to half its initial value. The half-life is particularly important since it must be long enough to enable the measurement process to be completed and yet short enough to keep the radiation dose to the patient to a minimum. For imaging purposes the ideal half-life is around 2–3 hours. The most commonly used radionuclide is the generator-produced technetium-99m (half-life = 6 hours). Long-lived isotopes such as gallium-67 (half-life = 78 hours) are used where the radiopharmaceutical takes days rather than hours to accumulate in the area of interest.

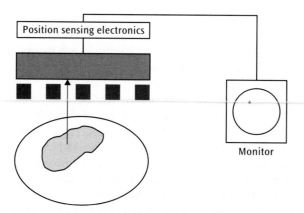

Figure 10.4 *The gamma camera consists of a sodium iodide crystal lead collimator and an electron detector to display the position of the interaction of the gamma rays from the radio-isotope on a monitor. In emission tomography, the gamma camera rotates around the patient.*

Radio-isotopes produce gamma, beta or alpha rays as they decay. For measurement purposes, the ideal radionuclide should decay with a pure gamma emission with an energy high enough to be detected outside the body yet low enough to be detected with maximum efficiency in the most commonly used detector, i.e. the sodium iodide containing gamma camera. Radionuclides with beta emissions are used for therapeutic purposes. The beta emission is stopped by the tissues in a small volume, all the energy being given up over a short distance. Alpha-particle emitters are not used for diagnosis since their high radiation dose can be carcinogenic. Imaging is performed with a gamma camera, the principle of which is illustrated in Figure 10.4.

A series of generators is also available for the production of short-lived radionuclides. This ensures that labelled compounds can be readily available at any time. Technetium-99m can be used to label compounds for imaging the brain, thyroid, lung perfusion and ventilation, the liver, kidneys, skeleton and some tumours. The choice of a particular labelled compound and its radiolabel depends upon the physiology or chemistry involved, the time required for adequate uptake in the lesion or tissue, and the equipment to be used for imaging. In most situations Tc^{99m} is used as the radionuclide for convenience and economy and because it has nearly the ideal characteristics for use with the gamma camera (160 keV pure gamma emission). In the case of the kidney, it can be used with dimercaptosuccinic acid (DMSA) for determining the anatomy and relative tubular function. Alternatively, diethylenetriaminepentaacetate (DTPA) can be used to demonstrate renal function and the outflow tract, for example, in suspected renal ureteric obstruction.

Most imaging is performed on gamma cameras. This device reproduces the photon interaction in the crystal detector on a cathode ray tube. With a computer the resulting image can be analysed to show time/activity changes in graphical form or a series of images synthesized into a whole-body image.

Tomography is also used in radio-isotope studies. The principle is similar to that used in CT scanning. A series of projections are taken around the body and sections reconstructed in the sagittal, coronal and transaxial planes. Although emission radio-isotope tomography can help to distinguish abnormalities more clearly than with planar imaging, it is more valuable for quantitation studies. The region of interest in each section is identified and the counts within it summed and corrected for attenuation by the overlying tissues. The series of regions of interest in each slice is summed to give the radioactivity within the volume of interest. A phantom with a known activity is used to calibrate the system. Sequential measurements give the activity in the lesion over a period of time and this, with the mass/volume of the lesion, can be used, for example, to calculate the radiation dose delivered to a tumour. Tomography can be carried out with either single photon emitters such as Tc^{99m} or with positron emitters where two gamma rays are emitted simultaneously at 180 degrees. For single photon emission tomography (SPECT) the detector is rotated around the patient. In positron emission tomography (PET) the detectors are usually in a ring around the patient and the photons detected in opposing crystals using a series of coincidence circuits. PET has the advantage of having improved resolution in most situations compared with SPECT. It usually also has higher sensitivity, the combination giving improved accuracy of quantitation of radioactivity in volumes of interest.

Radiopharmaceuticals used for radionuclide studies can be tailored to study any specific aspect of human physiology or metabolism. For example, blood flow to the brain can be studied using hexa-methyl propylene amine oxime (HMPAO). This compound, labelled with Tc^{99m}, is extracted with high efficiency during its first pass through tissues. The same compound can also be used to study tumour perfusion, to provide some indication of the availability of chemotherapeutic agents to the neoplastic tissue. On the other hand, the demonstration of lung perfusion to show up pulmonary emboli uses small particles of human albumin labelled with Tc^{99m}. Smaller particles can be used to study the lymphatic system or the reticuloendothelial system of the liver, spleen and bone marrow.

A series of radiolabelled compounds is available to study various aspects of metabolism. Metaiodobenzylguanidine traces the metabolic pathway in tumours of neuroectodermal origin. It can be labelled with ^{123}I for diagnostic purposes or ^{131}I for therapeutic applications. Both approaches have been used in phaeochromocytoma and neuroblastoma. The therapeutic application has had variable success. On the other hand, the diagnostic test has a high sensitivity for phaeochromocytoma.

Of the tests that show abnormalities as areas of increased radioactivity, perhaps bone imaging is the

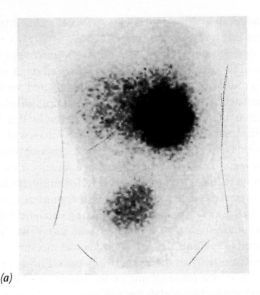

(a)

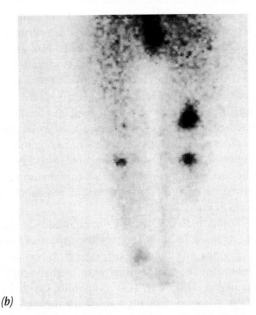

(b)

Figure 10.5 *(a) ^{131}I-labelled meta-iodobenzylguanidine uptake in carcinoid lesions involving the left lobe of the liver and the mesentery in the right iliac fossa. (b) ^{123}I-labelled meta-iodobenzylguanidine uptake in a child with secondaries in the femora and tibia from neuroblastoma. These lesions were not visible on plain X-rays or bone scintigrams.*

most successful. This test uses a labelled phosphate to demonstrate locally increased metabolism in the skeleton. The result is an image which predates changes seen on X-rays by several months. Unfortunately, altered metabolism is not confined to cancer, and therefore other abnormalities, which can be seen eventually on plain X-rays, are also detected by radio-isotope bone imaging, although the lack of resolution means that a specific diagnosis cannot be made at the early stage of the disease. Another situation where abnormalities are seen as areas of increased radioactivity is in the follow-up of

differentiated carcinoma of the thyroid gland. Differentiated primary or secondary thyroid cancer concentrates radio-iodine and can show up lesions in soft tissues of the neck, lung and skeleton before visible changes are found on the appropriate X-ray.

As stated above, compounds have been developed which can be used to trace neoplasms of the endocrine system other than the thyroid gland. These include ^{131}I-meta-iodobenzylguanidine (^{131}I-MIBG) which can be successfully used to demonstrate tumours arising from the neuroectodermal system, including phaeochromocytoma (Shapiro *et al.*, 1985), neuroblastoma and carcinoid (Fig. 10.5). Labelled octreotide may be used to image medullary carcinoma of thyroid.

Tumour-localizing agents

Edwards and Hayes (1969) discovered incidentally during a study of bone seekers that gallium-67 citrate localized in Hodgkin's disease. Since then it has been used in many different tumours, with variable success, for detection and staging purposes. ^{67}Ga produces three major photon peaks (91–93, 184 and 296 keV). For successful imaging it is important to utilize all three peaks to acquire as many counts as possible since the activities normally injected are low in comparison to other radio-imaging techniques. In addition, the use of emission tomography has also improved imaging. Gallium appears to be taken up by the lysosomal fraction of the tumour cell (Berry *et al.*, 1983) but the actual mechanism of uptake is still not completely understood. Intravenously administered ^{67}Ga citrate binds to serum transferrin and the gallium–transferrin complex, having traversed the abnormal tumour blood vessel endothelium, then binds to transferrin receptors on the cell surface (Larson *et al.*, 1979). Most ^{67}Ga scans are performed 48–72 hours after the administration of the radionuclide. Gallium-67 is normally taken up into liver, spleen, bone and bone marrow. Activity may also be seen in the female breast, salivary glands, lacrimal glands, external genitalia and thymus. Approximately 25 per cent of the administered dose is excreted in the urine. If the abdomen is to be imaged, then a bowel preparation is thought to be advisable since about 3 per cent per day is excreted into the bowel. Increased uptake is seen with tumour infiltration, infections and diseases such as sarcoidosis. The uptake in infections is lower than is usually seen in malignant neoplasms but the uptake in active sarcoidosis can be very high. In fact, the level of uptake can be used to monitor the course of the disease. The use of ^{67}Ga has fallen with the advent of PET scanning.

Clinical uses of gallium imaging

The most common use of radio gallium is in the detection of lymphoproliferative disorders (Beckerman *et al.*, 1984). The sensitivity of ^{67}Ga scans is dependent upon the histology, size of the lesion and anatomical location. The detection rate is greatest with Hodgkin's disease and histiocytic lymphoma (approximately 70 per cent) and falls to around 50 per cent for other types of lymphoma. Lesions less than 2 cm in diameter and greater than 5 cm are less reliably detected (the later presumably due to poorly perfused necrotic regions). Gallium-67 scans have a sensitivity in the region of 96 per cent and specificity of around 80 per cent for the detection of mediastinal disease. The sensitivity of detection of infradiaphragmatic disease is around 60 per cent. With the greater availability of CT scanning, the role of ^{67}Ga imaging in the diagnosis and staging of lymphoproliferative disease has diminished over the past few years.

Positron emission tomography

Positron-emitting radionuclides decay by ejecting positively charged electrons that travel a few millimetres in soft tissue before combining with negative electrons; both particles then undergo a transmutation process and are replaced by two photons of (0.51 MeV) given off at 180 degrees to each other (the so-called annihilation radiation). It is the coincident detection of these paired photons on either side of the body that forms the basis of PET (Fig. 10.6). Only the resolution of the detectors limit the resolution achievable inside the body, unlike single photon studies which are susceptible to the problems of scattering. The ability to correct for distortion of signal by tissue attenuation (by employing an external positron emitting ring source and performing a transmission scan or applying a geometric correction) allows the regional tissue concentration of the tracer to be measured in absolute units. Today's machines have multiple rings of

detectors providing transaxial resolutions of between 4 and 8 mm. Figure 10.7 shows a scanner which can collect data from eight rings of detectors simultaneously and compute and display 15 image planes. A detailed description of PET and second-generation scanner technology has been given by Phelps *et al.* (1978) and the latest scanner capabilities by Fahey (2001) and Turkington (2001).

The radionuclides most commonly used in cancer studies, along with their physical half-life and form of administration are given in Table 10.1. A heavy-particle accelerator, usually a cyclotron, is required for the production of most of these radionuclides, although some may be obtained from generators, e.g. ^{81}Rb and ^{68}Ga. With the short half-life of some of the tracers, an on-site cyclotron becomes essential but it is possible to carry out quite a variety of tests using positron emitters, provided that generators are available and the centre is within about 2 hours travelling time from a cyclotron.

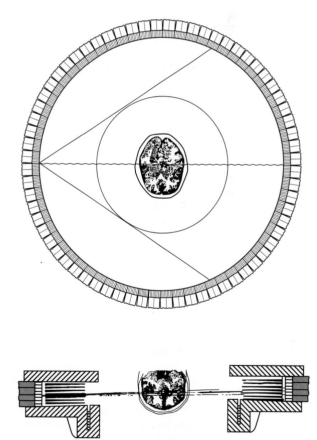

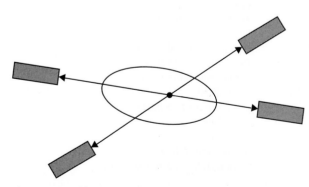

Figure 10.6 *Principle of positron emission tomography. When a positron is emitted it meets an electron, resulting in two simultaneous photons at 180°. The coincidence detecting system records these photons, which arrive simultaneously at each detector. The detectors record the events that occur in a line between the detectors, the width of the line depending upon the size of the detectors. By recording the positron emissions from all angles, the location of the radioactivity can be calculated.*

Figure 10.7 *The physical arrangement of the modern PET scanner, which comprises some 4096 individual detected elements. These are arranged in eight continuous rings of coincident detectors, which can record and reconstruct tomograph data of the distribution of positron-emitting isotopes within the human body. The upper part of the image shows the emission of the paired photons of annihilation radiation.*

Tracer kinetic models and tracer equations

Tracer kinetic models that accurately describe the fate of administered tracers are a necessary prerequisite for the measurement of regional tissue function using PET. The models provide a basis for the derivation of tracer kinetic equations. To solve these equations, both the blood activity and the tissue activity of the tracer must be known as a function of time. In practice, this means knowledge of the tissue concentration of the tracer (using PET) and either whole-blood or plasma concentration of the tracer in arterial blood (withdrawn during the scan) and measured in a cross-calibrated well counter. With the aid of a computer these equations can be solved pixel by pixel (voxel by voxel) and the initial cross-sectional display of regional tissue concentration of the tracer is replaced by a tomographic display of regional tissue function in absolute units. The complexities of the models will not be covered here. In practice, PET studies can be divided into two main categories: first, those studies where valid tracer models exist and the process under investigation can be measured in absolute units; and, secondly, studies in which the tracer models are thought to be less than complete (e.g. due to insufficient biological data) and the study is only semi-quantitative or qualitative. The images that are produced are really maps of regional tissue activity, for example, the metabolism of oxygen or glucose or regional blood flow. Table 10.2 lists some of the biological processes that have been studied using positron emission tomography.

Clinical positron emission tomography

Over the past 10 years where a semi-quantitative or qualitative approach has been taken to tumour imaging, PET has found its place in several clinical situations. The tracer most commonly used is [^{18}F] fluorodeoxyglucose (^{18}FDG). It exploits the aberrant glucose metabolism in cancer tissue. Lienhard *et al.* (1992) describe the uptake of glucose in terms of glucose transporters and its subsequent incorporation into the glycolytic pathway.

Table 10.1 *Useful positron-emitting radionuclides with their physical half-life, tracer form and clinical applications*

Radionuclide	Half-life (min)	Application
Oxygen-15	2.07	
$C^{15}O_2$		Blood flow
$H^{15}O$		Blood flow
$N^{15}O$		Blood flow
$^{15}O_2$		Oxygen utilization
$C^{15}O$		Blood volume
Carbon-11	20.4	
^{11}CO		Blood volume
^{11}C-alcohols		Cerebral blood flow
^{11}C-2 deoxyglucose		Glucose utilization
^{11}C-glucose		Glucose utilization
^{11}C-methylglucose		Glucose transport
^{11}C-amino acids		Amino acid uptake
$^{11}CO_2$		Cerebral pH
^{11}C-putrescine		Polyamine metabolism
^{11}C-drugs		Drug uptake and tissue pharmacokinetics, e.g. ^{11}C-BCNU
^{11}C-raclopride		Dopaminergic receptor studies
Nitrogen-13	10.0	
$^{13}NH_3$		Uptake/blood flow
^{13}N-labelled drugs		Drug uptake/pharmacokinetics
Rubidium-82	1.25	
$^{82}RbCl$		Blood–brain barrier integrity
Rubidium-81	274.8	
$^{81}RbCl$		Blood–brain barrier integrity
Fluorine-18	110.0	
^{18}F-FDG		Glucose utilization
^{18}F-labelled pyrimidines		Pyrimidine uptake in tumours
Gallium-68	68.3	
^{68}Ga EDTA		Blood volume, blood–brain barrier integrity

FDG-PET is used primarily in the staging of disease, but has been useful in confirming recurrence and, with some tumours, predicting response to treatment. The European Organization for Research and Treatment of Cancer (EORTC) PET study group have addressed the problem of assessing tumour response and have drawn up recommendations (Young *et al.*, 1999). In some studies a whole-body scan can be performed. FDG is actively taken up by any metabolically active tissue, and the brain and myocardium are easily visualized (Fig. 10.8). The tracer is excreted through the kidney and accumulates in the bladder. Maisey *et al.* (1999), in their atlas, illustrate some of the pitfalls of PET scanning.

Some studies refer to the standardized uptake value (SUV). This is a semi-quantitative approach which at least gives a number to any increase in FDG uptake. The SUV is defined as:

$$\frac{\text{tracer uptake (MBq ml}^{-1})}{\text{administered activity (MBq)/(patient weight in kg)} \times 1000}.$$

The tracer uptake is determined from a small region of interest placed over a region of the tumour in an attenuation-corrected image. A scanner calibration factor is required to convert this measured value into $MBq\,ml^{-1}$. There are several assumptions made in the application of this formula and there are some limitations. An SUV greater than 2.5 is thought to be indicative of cancer, although there is a wide range in tumours (2–15). Having an SUV allows serial monitoring of the patient's tumour and is extremely useful in those studies looking at the response to therapeutic intervention.

In many clinical situations the PET data alone may not provide enough information and the PET scan will be used along with MRI or CT images. A PET versus CT and MRI atlas has been produced where comparisons of these different techniques are provided (Bender *et al.*, 2000). There has been a great effort to co-register images accurately from different techniques, for example, CT and PET or MRI and PET, or even all three together. Never scanners have been produced with the capability of producing both CT and PET scans.

BRAIN TUMOURS

The present-day use of PET in neuro-oncology is really based on the findings in the early 1980s of increased glycolysis in brain tumours. Several workers, including

Table 10.2 *Some biological processes that have been studied with PET (those that can be measured quantitatively have the units provided)*

Biological process	Units
Blood flow	ml/100 ml tissue/min
Blood volume	ml/100 ml tissue
Oxygen utilization	ml O_2/100 ml tissue/min
Glucose utilization	mg of glucose/100 ml tissue/min
Uptake of amino acids	mmol/100 g/min
Uptake of pyrimidines	
Uptake of polyamines	
Blood–brain barrier permeability	
Drug uptake studies	
Receptor studies – ligands, antibodies	

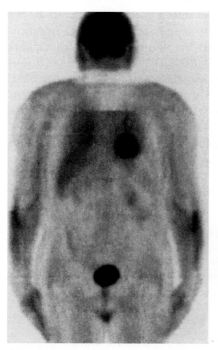

(a)

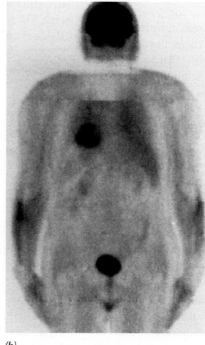

(b)

Figure 10.8 *Whole-body scan of a normal volunteer, showing high ^{18}FDG uptake in the brain and myocardium. In addition, because the tracer is excreted via the kidneys, activity is seen in the ureters and bladder.*

Di Chiro *et al.* (1982), found a correlation between [18]FDG uptake and the grade of the primary tumour. These workers characterized a tumour's metabolic rate for glucose by the peak value found within a region of the tumour. This was thought to be a valid approach as high-grade tumours were heterogeneous, with the highest-grade region being one of the main prognostic factors. [18]FDG uptake in high-grade tumours (grades 3 and 4) was significantly greater than in low-grade tumours (grade 2). Patronas *et al.* (1982) used [18]FDG in the evaluation of radiation-induced cerebral damage. These workers were able to differentiate between radiation-induced cerebral necrosis and recurrent tumour. The rate of [18]FDG uptake in the necrotic lesions was significantly lower than that of the surrounding normal brain. The recurrent tumours, on the other hand, had regions of [18]FDG uptake higher than that of normal brain.

The main indications for a PET scan in neuro-oncology include:

1 To obtain an idea of grade of tumour in patients with symptoms, signs and radiological evidence of a brain tumour but no pathological diagnosis. In other words, patients who either refused biopsy or biopsy was judged too risky by the neurosurgeons, or the biopsy was inconclusive.
2 To confirm recurrence in a previously treated high-grade glioma or differentiate between tumour recurrence and the late effects of radiation treatment.
3 To confirm transformation from a low-grade to a high-grade glioma.
4 To identify the site of the primary tumour in a patient with a cerebral metastasis from an unknown site. In other words, when all the simple staging investigations have been negative.

The natural history of a high-grade glioma is well known. For most patients, despite radical treatment with surgery, radiotherapy and possibly chemotherapy the disease returns. It is in this clinical setting that we have tried to establish the role, if any, of PET scanning. These studies fall into two groups. The first is where the technique is used simply to confirm the clinical diagnosis, and the second is where the technique provides unique data that may alter the clinical management. There are several clinical situations in which additional PET data may provide useful information to alter treatment. The management of low-grade brain tumours includes surveillance or post-operative monitoring until the patient develops symptoms or signs of progressive disease. This may be associated with transformation from a low grade to a higher-grade tumour. PET may allow this transformation to be detected sooner than simple clinical observation or from data available from MRI/CT scanning alone. This may allow more timely therapeutic intervention. In recent years there has been an increase in the interest shown in both stereotactic radiotherapy or radiosurgery and conformal radiotherapy. These techniques, which require the

accurate delineation of the tumour, which is not always easily obtained by MRI and CT, allow dose escalation and possibly better local control. Work is under way using co-registration techniques where data from CT, MRI and PET are integrated to give the most accurate delineation of the gross tumour volume (GTV).

[18]FDG SCANNING IN NON-CEREBRAL TUMOURS

Over the past 5 years most of the clinical PET studies have been on non-cerebral tumours. Again, the basis for these studies is the aberrant metabolism of glucose within cancerous tissue. The main indications for its use include the detection and staging of disease, the detection of recurrence and its differentiation from post-treatment sequelae and, in some studies, a tum-our's response to therapy. Some studies are performed through a restricted region of the body and some studies include whole-body PET scans. Figure 10.9 shows an [18]FDG scan image of a patient with a bronchogenic tumour with mediastinal node involvement. Figure 10.10 shows the first-ever images (CT and [18]FDG-PET) of a patient with a carcinoma of the left breast (Beaney, 1984). Whole-body imaging is commonly used in the study of Hodgkin's disease (HD) and non-Hodgkin's lymphoma, and other cancers where there is a high probability of metastatic disease. The whole-body scanning technique consists of a series of overlapping (interlaced) transaxial image sets from which two-dimensional projection (non-tomographic) images are generated (*see* Fig. 10.8). Ho *et al.* (1993) demonstrated the feasibility and potential of this technique for detecting primary and metastatic deposits. In most studies that include breast, colon, melanoma lymphoma and urothelial tumours (Rege *et al.*, 1993; Newman *et al.*, 1994) the sensitivity of detecting malignant disease was in the region of 87 per cent. The ability to examine the nature of post-treatment residual masses was first examined in germ-cell tumours (Beaney and Wong, 1994). Figure 10.11a shows a CT scan of the abdomen of a young man with a non-seminomatous germ cell tumour of the left testicle. Clinically this was judged stage 1 and the CT scan reported to be within the normal range. The patient's tumour markers did not return to normal after orchidectomy. An [18]FDG-PET scan

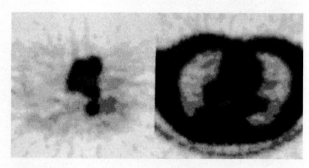

Figure 10.9 *Typical images of a patient with a bronchogenic carcinoma.*

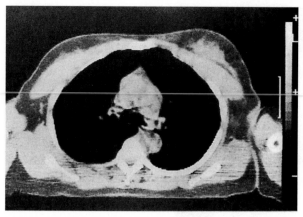

(a)

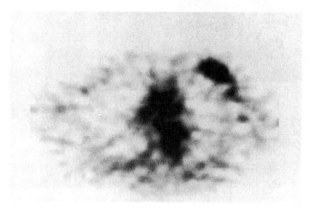

(b)

Figure 10.10 *(a) CT scan of a patient with a carcinoma of the left breast (on the reader's right). (b) PET ^{18}FDG uptake image after 45 min, showing increased uptake in the tumour.*

clearly demonstrated the abnormal node (Fig. 10.11b). After chemotherapy the tumour markers returned to normal and the repeat PET scan showed no increased uptake in the region of the node.

HODGKIN'S DISEASE AND NON-HODGKIN'S LYMPHOMA

The prognosis for patients with Hodgkin's disease (HD) and non-Hodgkin's lymphoma (NHL) depends partly on the histological subtype and partly on the stage of disease. CT is widely used in staging, but cannot reliably evaluate normal-sized lymph nodes and some extranodal sites, for example, liver, spleen and bone marrow. ^{18}FDG has been shown to preferentially accumulate in sites of lymphoma, both nodal and extranodal. Partridge *et al.* (2000) showed that significantly more sites were identified by PET than by CT. This resulted in the stage of disease being changed and the treatment modified in about 25 per cent of patients. ^{18}FDG-PET has been used as a prognostic indicator in the treatment of aggressive NHL. They found that PET is more accurate than CT in assessing remission and prediction of relapse-free survival.

An interim PET scan after 2–3 cycles of chemotherapy predicted the long-term outcome early in the course of treatment and had a high negative predictive value (100 per cent). The authors thought that this would be useful in separating, at an early stage, good-prognosis patients who are likely to be cured with standard chemotherapy from those patients with poorer prognosis who may require alternative treatment.

LUNG CANCER

PET scanning has an established role in patients with non-small cell lung cancer (NSLC). ^{18}FDG-PET imaging is a very powerful tool in the initial diagnosis and staging of the disease. It is also useful in the follow-up surveillance for recurrent tumour. Many groups would not subject a patient to a thoracotomy unless a PET scan has been performed. The use of ^{18}FDG-PET for staging lung cancer has now been included in the guidelines issued by the British Thoracic Society. A meta-analysis using pooled data from 14 PET studies (514 patients) and 29 CT studies (2226 patients) showed the superiority of PET in visualizing mediastinal disease (Dwamena *et al.*, 1999). One of the main indications for ^{18}FDG-PET is the investigation of the solitary pulmonary nodule. In a comparison with transthoracic fine-needle aspiration biopsy, ^{18}FDG-PET was found to be superior, with an overall accuracy of 94 versus 86 per cent (Dewan *et al.*, 1995).

HEAD AND NECK CANCER

Wong *et al.* (1997) evaluated the use of PET in the assessment of patients with head and neck cancer and found that it was extremely useful in not only detecting the primary tumour but also the presence of metastatic nodal disease. In this study the sensitivity and specificity of PET for detecting nodal disease was 67 and 100 per cent, respectively, compared with clinical assessment of 58 and 75 per cent. The co-registration of CT, MRI and PET data sets in head and neck cancer was covered by Wong *et al.* (1996).

MALIGNANT MELANOMA

^{18}FDG-PET is becoming part of an established staging procedure in patients with malignant melanoma. It is useful in detecting lymph-node metastases during staging and also in follow-up (Macfarlane *et al.*, 1998; Rinne *et al.*, 1998).

COLORECTAL CANCER

Increasing interest is being shown in PET scanning in patients with colorectal cancer. CT is used both in the staging of the disease prior to surgery and monitoring the patient at the time of recurrence. Unfortunately, CT has a low sensitivity. FDG-PET for initial diagnosis and staging and for preoperative assessment of recurrence

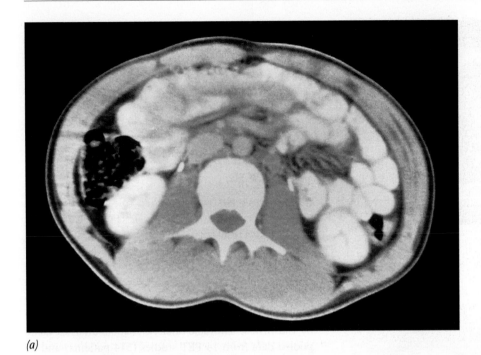

(a)

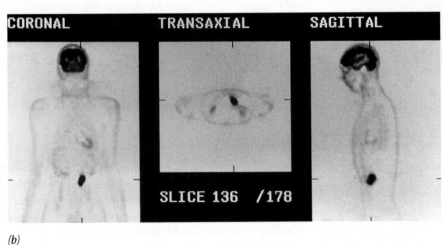

(b)

Figure 10.11 *(a) CT scan of a young patient with a stage 2 teratoma of the left testicle. The node on the left was about 1 cm in diameter and, by CT criteria, within the normal range. (b) PET [18]FDG scan in the same patient with a stage 2 teratoma of the left testicle. The node on the left is clearly abnormal, with markedly increased uptake. The patient's tumour markers remained elevated, indicating residual disease.*

has demonstrated a higher sensitivity than CT. Four studies comparing PET and CT in over 300 patients showed overall sensitivity for all sites of recurrence of 95 per cent for PET and 66 per cent for CT. Valk *et al.* (1999) also compared sensitivity and specificity of PET and CT by site of recurrence and determined the 95 per cent confidence interval for the difference between the two modalities for each site. PET was significantly more sensitive than CT overall. A review article gives one group's view on the role of PET in patients with colorectal cancer, indicating that it has a proven cost-effective role in the management of recurrent cancer and the monitoring of therapy (Arulampalam *et al.*, 2001).

OTHER TUMOURS

PET has now been used in the evaluation of most cancers, these include thyroid cancer, pancreatic cancer, oesophageal cancer and gynaecological neoplasms.

UNKNOWN PRIMARY

Patients with a solitary metastasis from an undetectable primary must undergo a battery of investigations including blood test, chest X-ray, CT, ultrasound scans and possibly MRI scans in a bid to find the source of the malignant cells. Even after these tests the primary may not be found. PET has been shown to be useful in detecting the primary.

Recently diagnostic imaging using more than one technique has been possible with a system that combines CT and PET data from one single non-invasive procedure. Co-registration of images capitalises on the spatial resolution of CT or MRI and the functional data provided by PET.

AMINO ACID METABOLISM IN TUMOURS

Several amino acids have been labelled with positron-emitting radionuclides and used successfully for studying

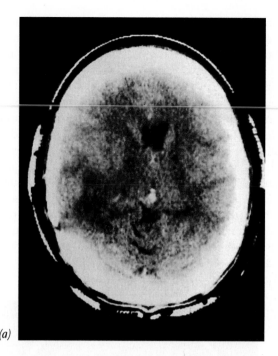

(a)

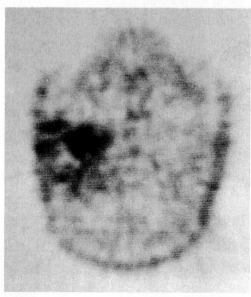

(b)

Figure 10.12 *(a) CT scan of a patient with low-grade astrocytoma in the left temporoparietal region. (b) PET [^{11}C]methionine scan, showing markedly elevated uptake of [^{11}C]methionine in the region of the tumour.*

tumour metabolism. Both natural and synthetic amino acids have been labelled with carbon-11. Kubota *et al.* (1984) conducted a comparative study with 10 ^{11}C-labelled amino acids and found that [^{11}C]L-methionine and [^{11}C]aminocyclopentane carboxylic acid (ACPC) showed the highest uptake in their animal tumour model and suggested that these amino acids may be useful for the detection of cancer in man. Several workers have used ^{11}C-labelled methionine and have successfully demonstrated tumour uptake in gliomas (Ericson *et al.*, 1985). They found this tracer particularly useful in delineating

the extent of the tumour into adjacent brain that was judged normal by conventional CT and PET ^{18}FDG studies. Bustany *et al.* (1985), using a three-compartment model, developed a method to quantify the regional cerebral uptake of [^{11}C]methionine and its rate of incorporation into protein. Recent data have highlighted some deficiencies in the model dealing with the protein incorporation of labelled amino acid when applied to neoplastic tissue. Nevertheless, the consensus of opinion is that [^{11}C]methionine uptake scans may be the best method of delineating low-grade gliomas, especially those that are poorly visible on conventional CT scanning or MRI. Figure 10.12 shows a typical [^{11}C]methionine scan of a patient with a low-grade glioma. Lung tumours have also been visualized using ^{11}C-labelled methionine. Quantitative evaluation of methionine uptake in tumour tissue suggested a positive correlation with tumour viability.

PET has also been used to 'map out' the cerebral tissue pharmacokinetics of ^{11}C-labelled BCNU (Yamamoto and Diksic, 1985), to study dopaminergic receptor status in pituitary tumours (Muhr *et al.*, 1986) and to monitor the physiological effects of treatment with steroids, surgery and radiotherapy (Beaney, 1986). Perhaps one of the most important uses of the PET technique in the future will be the study of tumour uptake and metabolism of labelled drugs used in the treatment of cancer.

MAGNETIC RESONANCE IMAGING

Interest in the use of magnetic resonance imaging (MRI) for the diagnosis of tumours was aroused in the early 1970s. *In vitro* studies on rat tumours revealed the abnormal magnetic resonance properties of neoplastic tissue (Damadian, 1971). This was quickly followed by the demonstration that nuclear magnetic resonance signals could be rendered spatially dependent (Lauterbur, 1973) and the first description of the appearance of a tumour (Hawkes *et al.*, 1980). Recent improvements in machine design and coil design provide a spatial resolution of less than 1 mm.

MRI is based on the ability to induce and record resonance of the magnetic moment of nuclei in the presence of magnetic fields. Nuclei with an odd number of protons and neutrons act like tiny magnets. In the presence of a strong magnetic field they have a net alignment with the field. If a pulse of radiofrequency (RF) energy of the appropriate resonant frequency is then applied, some of the nuclei will flip and align themselves against the field. After the pulse the nuclei will flip back to their original alignment, producing an RF signal of the same frequency as the one applied. It is possible to define both the location and concentration of resonant nuclei and then generate images that reflect their distribution in tissue. Hydrogen, since it is the most sensitive of the stable nuclei to NMR and because it is also the most abundant nucleus in the body, is ideally suited for MRI studies.

Instrumentation

All MRI scanners contain a large magnet which provides a uniform static magnetic field. When placed in this field the hydrogen nuclei align with this static magnetic field, producing a net proton magnetization in the long axis of the patient. Radiofrequency (RF) pulses are used to rotate the net magnetization. Thereafter, the magnetization recovers or relaxes back to its original position. In the longitudinal direction, the magnetization returns exponentially to its original state with a time constant T_1, the spin-lattice relaxation time. The magnetization in the transverse place returns to zero with a time constant T_2. The signal is induced in a receiver coil which surrounds the patient. The electrical signal detected by the coil is known as free induction decay and it is this signal that is used to reconstruct the image. The data can be manipulated to provide images taken in all the conventional body planes. NMR images are therefore obtained using short RF pulses to perturb the patient's nuclear magnetization, after which the electrical signal is detected; these pulse sequences are derived from classical spectroscopy and produce images which in part depend upon proton density (ρ), T_1 and T_2. The images do not simply depict the distribution of ρ modified by T_1 and T_2 but are also dependent on the particular radiofrequency pulse sequence and spatial encoding techniques used. The signal intensity is critically dependent on the imaging sequence (Pykett et al., 1982). The latter has resulted in rather complicated-sounding jargon that describes the sequences used to generate the images and should accompany each MRI scan (Figs 10.13 and 10.14).

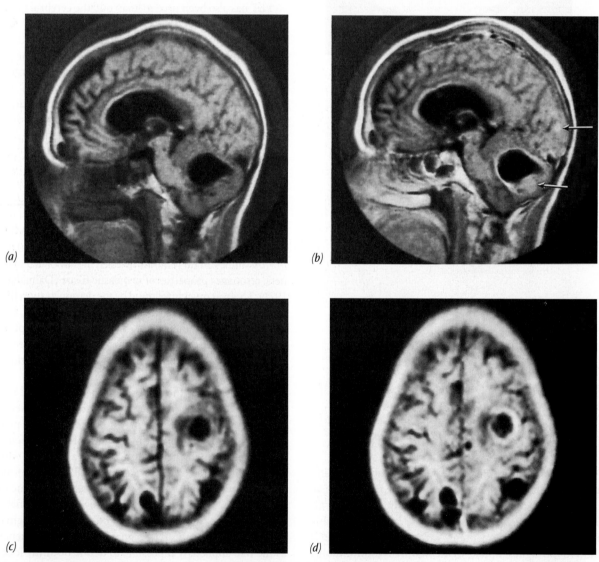

(a)   *(b)*   *(c)*   *(d)*

Figure 10.13 *MRI scan of a patient with cerebral metastases from a bronchogenic carcinoma: sagittal inversion recovery images (a) before and (b) after intravenous gadolinium-DTPA. The contrast-enhanced scan shows an area of enhancement around the cystic lesion in the occipital lobe (arrows). Images (c) and (d) are from another patient with cerebral metastases from breast carcinoma: IR1500/500/44 scans (c) before and (d) after intravenous Gd-DTPA. Ring enhancement is seen around the lesion in (d).*

As in CT scanning, the reconstructed images have all the advantages of tomography, i.e. separation of organs and improvement in contrast. Unlike CT, where images represent the regional attenuation coefficients and energy of the incident X-rays, MRI has a whole series of factors that finally contribute to the appearance of the final image. Longitudinal relaxation T_1 (Fig. 10.15) depends on the interaction of protons with surrounding nuclei and molecules (the 'lattice') and in practice shows up anatomy delineating fat from other tissues particularly well. The T_2 or transverse relaxation time (Fig. 10.16) depends on the interaction of protons with each other, and is often increased in tumours.

The spatial and contrast resolution of the final image depends largely upon the regional proton density and the relaxation times. The variation in proton density in soft tissue is relatively small (± 20 per cent) but the variation in relaxation times is much greater (about 200 per cent):

the latter therefore have the dominant influence on image contrast. The greater the concentration of protons, the stronger the signal, so soft tissue will appear white or grey and air and bone black. The differences in relaxation times are relatively large and it is mainly this phenomenon which gives MR images the improved soft-tissue contrast over CT. Altering the pulse sequences produces images with varying dependence on ρ, T_1 and T_2. Saturation-recovery (SR) pulse sequences produce images where contrast is mostly dependent upon proton density and T_1. An increase in ρ produces a light appearance and an increase in T_1 a dark appearance on the grey scale. Inversion-recovery (IR) sequences are similar, but the final images are more dependent on T_1; again an increase in T_1 produces a dark appearance. Spin-echo (SE) pulse sequences are more T_2 dependent. Lesions with a long T_2 appear lighter than the surrounding tissue.

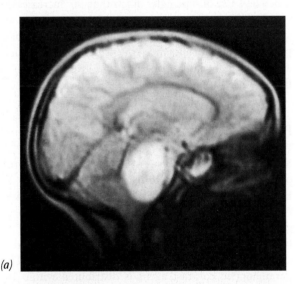
(a)

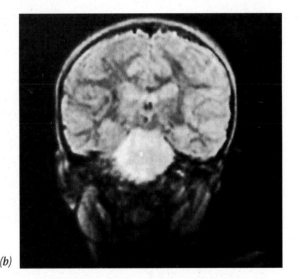
(b)

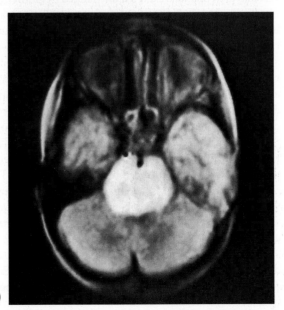
(c)

Figure 10.14 *MRI images of a patient with a brainstem glioma: SE 1500/80 scan in the (a) sagittal, (b) coronal and (c) transverse planes. The tumour has a high signal intensity and is encasing the basilar artery.*

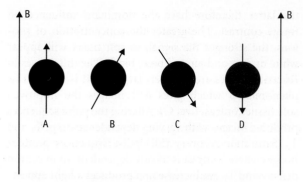

Figure 10.15 *In a strong magnetic field (B) nuclei line up with the field. When irradiated with the appropriate frequency (which depends upon the magnetic field strength) some of the nuclei absorb the energy and line up in the direction opposite to the field. They return (relax) to their original orientation with a half-time (T_1) which depends upon the surrounding molecules. This process is called longitudinal or spin-lattice relaxation.*

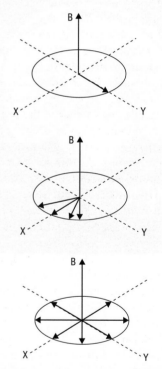

Figure 10.16 *If RF energy is supplied so that the nuclei rotate through 90°, they initially rotate in phase in the transverse orientation. They gradually become dephased and the magnetic moment in the transverse plane decays with a time constant, T_2.*

To describe the pulse sequences in detail the following information is necessary: the interval between successive pulse sequences (TR), the interval between the measuring pulse and point of sampling (TE), and the time between the initial inverting pulse and the measuring pulse (T_1). An example of an inversion recovery sequence would be

IR 1500/44/500 where TR = 1500 ms, TE = 44 ms and T_1 = 500 ms. Many sequences have been established to try and characterize pathological tissue in terms of T_1 and T_2.

Increases in T_1 and T_2 are seen in a variety of pathological conditions where there is an increase in the water content of a lesion, such as inflammation, oedema and most tumours. On the other hand, a relative decrease in T_1 is seen in subacute haemorrhage, fatty lesions and some forms of fibrosis. Changes in T_1 and T_2, even of great magnitude, are relatively non-specific. Not all tumours have an increase in T_1 and T_2. Specificity is usually derived from the clinical context and location of the lesion.

The parameters set up in advance skew the major component of each image so that it predominates, therefore they are referred to as T_1-weighted, T_2-weighted, etc. The characteristics of fluid show the greatest degree of change between T_1 and T_2 weighting, altering from low to high signal. Other soft tissues, such as muscle and fat, change much less. Use of flip angles of less than 90° increases the speed of the examination and results in images that are similar to T_1- and T_2-weighted sequences. Further radio pulses introduced into the sequence can result in negation of signal from fat or water, and give fat (STIR) or fluid (FLAIR) suppressed sequences.

Paramagnetic contrast agents

Most of the contrast apparent in MR images is a result of differences in the tissue relaxation times T_1 and T_2. Paramagnetic agents which usually contain unpaired electrons, for example, the metallic ions, manganese, gadolinium or iron, can regionally change the T_1 and T_2 of tissue (Runge, 1991). The first compound to be used in clinical practice was gadolinium-DTPA (Gd-DTPA). This paramagnetic contrast agent is distributed within the vascular system and is excreted unchanged by glomerular filtration with a half-life of approximately 90 minutes in humans. After intravenous injection, Gd-DTPA diffuses rapidly into the interstitial space, enhancing tissues with a high proportion of interstitial fluid. If it crosses the disrupted blood–brain barrier it produces a decrease in T_1 and T_2 in the brain. Its initial application has been in defining the abnormal blood–brain barrier in order to delineate the margin between tumour and peritumoral oedema (Carr *et al.*, 1984). Before the use of Gd-DTPA the lack of differentiation between tumour and oedema was a severe limitation in cerebral tumour studies. The results using this contrast agent are similar to that found with iodinated contrast agents in X-ray CT. Figure 10.13 shows MRI scan images from two patients with intracerebral metastases, before and after contrast.

Paramagnetic contrast agents are also of value for demonstrating tumours in the abdomen and limbs. Carr *et al.* (1986) clearly demonstrated the presence of both primary and metastatic liver tumours and studied the uptake of Gd-DTPA. However, few additional lesions were seen on contrast-enhanced MRI scans compared to contrast-enhanced CT scans.

New contrast media are being introduced for specific indications, and there is now a range of agents available for imaging the liver, with specific uptake in both the hepatocytes and the reticulo-endothelial cells so that different aspects of hepatic function can be investigated. There is now a contrast agent that is taken up in lymph nodes which has the potential for determining the morphology of the gland, so that enlargement due to metastatic replacement can be separated from reactive hyperplasia.

One of the limitations of MR has been the length of the sequences. Unlike CT, where the sections are generated one at a time in about 1 second, the data for MR are acquired over 2 or 3 minutes and then displayed as sections. This means that movement during the acquisition period results in considerable degradation of the image quality. This is particularly so in the chest, where respiratory and cardiac motion considerably affects the quality of the images. In the abdomen the main problem is peristaltic and respiratory motion artefact and, for these reasons, MR has been at its most useful in structures where there is very little movement, such as the brain, the spine, joints and soft tissues. Technical advance in the past few years has resulted in a considerable shortening of acquisition times so that breath-hold imaging is now available. This has resulted in a considerable improvement in resolution, particularly of the liver and the other upper abdominal organs. It is now becoming practical to substitute MR for CT for a number of organs, with the resultant abolition of radiation hazard.

Advantages of MRI

Magnetic resonance imaging has been shown to demonstrate the presence of tumours effectively. It does this without using ionizing radiation. It seems to be harmless (National Radiological Protection Board, 1991), and is relatively well tolerated by patients. In addition, one of the widely recognized benefits of MRI is the ability to acquire images directly from any viewing angle – axial, sagittal, coronal and even oblique (multi-angle MRI). The important question is whether MRI is of greater diagnostic value than that of established non-invasive techniques such as X-ray, CT, ultrasonography and isotope imaging.

Magnetic resonance imaging is of particular value in the central nervous system. Lesions such as tumours have high contrast and therefore small abnormalities can be seen clearly. The technique does not suffer from artefacts due to surrounding bone in the way that X-ray computed tomography does. Elsewhere in the body respiratory,

vascular and bowel movements produce artefacts. In the limbs and pelvis, however, the quality of images produced by MRI is at least equal, if not superior, to CT or ultrasonography (Fischer *et al.*, 1985; Poon *et al.*, 1985). Tumour spread into soft tissue or within bone, particularly bone marrow, is better demonstrated by MRI than by other techniques (Zimmer *et al.*, 1985; Petasnik *et al.*, 1986). When the quality of body images reaches that of the brain then it is likely that MRI will be used to replace some of the existing techniques.

The main hazard associated with magnetic resonance relates to the very strong magnetic field. The majority of metallic implants now utilized in the body are of predominantly non-ferromagnetic material and there is no significant displacement of the implants within the magnetic field. However, electrical currents generated within the conducting material of implants will result in a magnetic field which creates a void in the image and therefore the area around the implant cannot be adequately imaged. This is particularly important in the examination of the postoperative spine where the presence of supporting metalwork may preclude adequate visualization of the spinal canal and of the cord. Shrapnel tends to be more ferromagnetic than implanted materials and, although there is no significant displacement of the metal in the magnet as it is usually firmly bound down by fibrous tissue, considerable artefact can be generated. Care must be taken to exclude metal injury to the eye as this has a potential for displacement in the magnetic field and can give rise to damage to the eyes. The majority of cerebral aneurysm clips are now non-ferromagnetic as they are made of titanium, but the older clips did have a significant content of ferromagnetic material, and it is generally considered prudent to exclude patients with aneurysm clips from the magnetic environment. Cardiac pacemakers and cochlea implants are also affected by the magnetic field and may not function following MRI; therefore they are considered a contraindication to imaging. Although the intravenous contrast media are extremely safe in clinical practice, little information is available about their effects on the fetus and therefore they should not be administered during pregnancy. It is generally considered wise to exclude patients from the magnetic environment during the first trimester of pregnancy as the potential long-term effects of a magnetic field on the developing child are unknown. None the less, if there is an overwhelming need for MRI in these circumstances, then imaging is possible as long as appropriate precautions are taken.

A further consideration must be cost effectiveness (Evens and Evens, 1988). The expensive high-field machines of 1.5–2.0 Tesla are likely to have a more restricted distribution, but for imaging alone low-field systems of 0.08–0.5 Tesla provide satisfactory results (Kean *et al.*, 1986). The cost of low-field systems may come down, and rapid imaging should improve the time taken to image each patient, and improve cost effectiveness. This type of system can provide a routine clinical service for imaging the central nervous system. For those readers seeking a comprehensive text on MRI or the use of MRI specifically in imaging the CNS, Stark and Bradley (1992) and Atlas (1991), respectively, are recommended.

INTERVENTIONAL RADIOLOGY

Image-guided interventional techniques have vastly increased the therapeutic scope of radiology in the management of patients with cancer. These range from very simple procedures, such as the drainage of pleural effusions and ascites under ultrasound control, to the insertion of stents into stenotic structures, such as the oesophagus to relieve dysphagia and the biliary tree to treat obstructive jaundice. Obtaining samples for histological and cytological examination is now routinely employed as an alternative to surgical biopsy. This is normally performed with ultrasonic or CT control. The choice of guidance is made according to the visibility, size and accessibility of the lesion. The disadvantage of CT from this point of view is that the operator only finds out where the tip of the biopsy needle is after it has been moved, whereas real-time ultrasound allows the position of the needle to be viewed throughout the procedure and is much quicker. However, intervening bowel loops are more difficult to appreciate with ultrasound. The development of non-ferromagnetic biopsy needles and open configuration is opening MR to similar application. Laser thermal ablation of metastases in the liver can be guided with all three cross-sectional techniques, but MR can also be used to assess the extent of the surrounding thermal damage. Intra-arterial introduction of materials into vessels following selective catheterization can allow localized therapy or reduction of blood flow to tumours using embolic particles.

CLINICAL APPLICATIONS OF DIAGNOSTIC TECHNIQUES

Brain

For the detection of suspected space-occupying lesions, most clinicians prefer X-ray CT scanning as the first line of investigation (Baker *et al.*, 1980). It gives a high level of anatomical detail, showing the relationship of the tumour to the surrounding tissues and its relation to the ventricular system. For radiation treatment planning purposes, it can be difficult to distinguish the outline of the tumour from the surrounding oedema. Intravenous contrast media can help a little in outlining that part of the tumour where there is disruption of the blood–brain barrier.

Magnetic resonance imaging is especially valuable in the central nervous system, clearly demonstrating tumours of the brain and spinal cord (Bydder *et al.*, 1982, 1984; Brant-Zawadski *et al.*, 1984).

CT is a very practical and rapid diagnostic technique for the brain, particularly above the tentorium cerebelli. However, in the posterior fossa, the presence of artefact generated by the very dense bone of the base of the skull considerably degrades the quality of the images, with a reduction in sensitivity for detection of tumours. MR is totally unaffected by the presence of the skull vault as bone generates very little signal. The contrast resolution is also superior to CT even without the use of intravenous contrast medium and, when this is included as well, MR has a much higher detection rate for cerebral tumours particularly when they are small. The safety of the gadolinium-based contrast agents and the lack of ionizing radiation now makes MR the technique of choice for the imaging of all brain tumours. The added advantage of multi-directional display means that both a surgical approach to tumours and radiotherapy can be planned accurately. The ability of MRI to provide sagittal and coronal reconstructions makes this the imaging modality of choice for brainstem and spinal-cord lesions. Acute haemorrhage may be difficult to visualize with MR, as it may be hypo- or iso-intense with surrounding structures. Within 1–2 days, blood becomes bright on T_1-weighted images and is more conspicuous than on CT, particularly beyond about 10 days after the occurrence. When equivalent scans are compared, MR takes little longer than CT but may be limited by the patient's condition if he or she cannot lie still within the magnetic environment. Tissue characterization remains a problem and measurements of T_1 and T_2 values have not resulted in accurate discrimination between tumour types. Factors such as the age of the patient, the length of the history and the precise site of involvement are much more crucial in determining what is the most likely tumour type. Most tumours are slightly hyper-intense in T_2-weighted images and hypo-intense compared with the brain in T_1-weighted images. They are frequently surrounded by vasogenic oedema, which is of higher signal than the tumour in T_2-weighted sequences. Injection of intravenous contrast medium results in enhancement of the tumour mass and allows accurate delineation from the surrounding oedema.

MR is particularly effective for the detection of small metastatic deposits when the patient is symptomatic but has had a normal CT. Meningeal disease can be seen in T_1-weighted images but its detection is considerably aided by intravenous contrast medium, when it enhances intensely. It should be remembered that there are other causes of meningeal thickening and enhancement, including infection, previous surgery, chemotherapy and radiotherapy as well as repeated lumbar puncture. Subtle meningeal disease may be difficult to detect by all imaging techniques and cytological examination of the CSF may be necessary if imaging techniques are negative.

Grading intra-cerebral tumours by CT and MR is difficult although, as a general principle, the more vascular the tumour, the more likely it is to be of higher grade. PET imaging with both FDG and methionine can be used to assess the grade of primary tumours, and may also confirm the presence of malignancy when this has been in doubt from the previous imaging studies. PET is also useful for following treatment in patients when there is difficulty in distinguishing between enhancement due to radiation necrosis and that due to recurrent tumour, as there is normally no FDG or methionine uptake in radiation necrosis.

In the spinal cord the advantage of not requiring intra-thecal contrast media makes magnetic resonance imaging the modality of choice. The advantages of MRI are: the high degrees of contrast between grey and white matter, the absence of bone artefact in the posterior fossa, cranio-cervical junction or neural canal and the ability to image in the sagittal and coronal planes. Figure 10.14 shows a brainstem tumour. Most tumours show the pattern of increased proton density (probably in part due to increase in water content) and increased relaxation times, T_1 and T_2. There are exceptions, however: malignant melanoma metastases may produce a decrease in T_1 relative to normal tissue (Fig. 10.17). A number of benign tumours, including meningiomas and acoustic neuromas, may also have T_1 and T_2 values within the normal range.

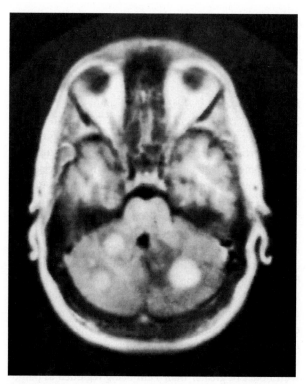

Figure 10.17 *MIR image of a patient with metastases from a malignant melanoma: IR1500/44/500 scan. The lesions in the cerebellar hemispheres have a high signal intensity.*

Spinal cord

Although CT is effective for showing the destruction of bone in metastatic disease and soft-tissue infiltration into the spinal canal, MR has a greater sensitivity for both the bony disease and for the depiction of the associated soft-tissue mass. The cord, in particular, is difficult to identify on CT in the absence of intrathecal contrast medium and therefore intramedullary tumours are difficult to identify. As a consequence, MR is now the investigation of choice for all disease of the spine unless there is a contraindication to examination. The most common intramedullary spinal tumour is the glioma and this results in expansion of the cord, often with an associated syrinx. The tumour usually enhances with intravenous contrast medium and there is surrounding oedema. It is unusual for tumours to present until the expansion of the cord reaches the capacity of the spinal canal, and tumour may extend over many vertebral segments. Intradural but extramedullary tumours are frequently benign and the two most common lesions are the meningioma and neurofibroma. It may be difficult to distinguish these two tumours from drop metastases and it is therefore important to examine the whole of the neuro-axis when this is a problem as many derive from a tumour arising in the brain. Meningeal spread of tumour may be vizualized as nodules along the nerve roots of the cauda equina, but intravenous contrast medium may be required to show meningeal enhancement with certainty. Extradural disease usually arises from secondary involvement of bone and is visible in T_1-weighted images because of the replacement of the fat of the bone marrow by tumour. There may be extension through the cortex with compression of the theca and a surrounding soft-tissue mass. Both osteoclastic and osteoblastic disease result in bone-marrow replacement, but it is more apparent with the former. It may be difficult to distinguish acute osteoporotic collapse from metastatic disease as both replace the bone marrow and there may be enhancement after intravenous contrast medium. However, benign collapse is rarely associated with a soft-tissue mass. Infection may mimic tumour involvement and therefore an image-guided biopsy may be necessary.

The orbit

Direct vision is usually used for assessment of tumours in the back of the eye but ultrasound can be utilized when a cataract impairs direct visualization of the retina. For retro-orbital tumours both CT and MR are effective, but the lack of radiation hazard to the lens means that MR is slightly preferred. Intra-ocular melanoma may be distinguished from other tumours by the unusually high signal in the T_1-weighted image, which is due to a combination of the haemorrhagic content and the paramagnetic effects of melanin.

Recent technical developments in MRI using surface coil data acquisition have provided a spatial resolution of less than a millimetre. Contrast discrimination is such that the cortex and nucleus of the lens can be distinguished. Although CT shows important information about the surrounding bone, MRI provides a similar diagnostic capability. The short T_1 and T_2 values of intra-ocular melanomas may allow distinction from other intra-ocular tumours (Worthington *et al.*, 1986).

Thyroid

In the diagnosis of primary thyroid disease the clinical examination is all important. Thyroid carcinomas usually present as hard masses which are relatively easily palpable. A radio-isotope image using either pertechnetate or radio-iodine can help in the differential diagnosis by detecting lesions with an increased metabolism by an increase in uptake. Although carcinoma cannot be completely excluded, the incidence of carcinoma in hot lesions is less than 3 per cent. Non-radioactive lesions, on the other hand, can pose a problem, 25 per cent of non-radioactive lesions are found to be malignant. The ultrasound examination is valuable in making the diagnosis of a thyroid cyst. However, experience to date has shown that ultrasound cannot confidently differentiate between benign and malignant neoplasms of the thyroid (Ikekubo *et al.*, 1986). Ultrasound is valuable for directing needle aspirations or defining the area for a trucut biopsy. With an incidence of between 10 and 25 per cent of carcinoma in patients presenting with what are thought to be single nodules of the thyroid, usually the lump has to be removed since current non-surgical diagnostic methods cannot exclude malignancy. In patients with proven follicular and some mixed thyroid carcinoma radio-iodine-131 is used to ablate residual normal thyroid and to trace the metabolism of differentiated thyroid tumours (Rosler, 1986). Scans following the administration of ablation and therapy doses are valuable in demonstrating the spread of metastases, if present. In patients without normal thyroid tissue, the *in vitro* thyroglobulin measurement is valuable for determining residual thyroid tissue which, of course, must then be carcinomatous. It may be that in future this test will replace routine scanning in the follow-up of patients thought to be free of thyroid carcinoma following therapy.

Medullary carcinoma of the thyroid does not concentrate radio-iodine and thus it cannot be used for diagnostic or therapeutic purposes. The diagnosis is often clinical with the assistance of calcitonin measurements. Patients suspected of having medullary carcinoma of the thyroid can be studied with Tc^{99m} V dimercaptosuccinic acid (DMSA). This compound has demonstrated proven metastases with a sensitivity of 85 per cent whereas radio-iodine-labelled meta-iodobenzylguanidine has a sensitivity of approximately 11 per cent (Clarke *et al.*,

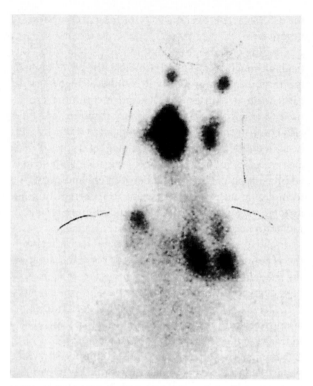

Figure 10.18 *Tc^{99m} (V) DMSA scan in a patient with medullary carcinoma of the thyroid with rising calcitonin levels, whose only clinical signs were enlarged cervical lymph nodes. CT scanning confirmed tumour in the left lobe of the thyroid, but did not show the lesions in the mediastinum.*

1988) (Fig. 10.18). A somatostatin analogue, octreotide, labelled with ^{111}In or ^{131}I has been used successfully to image medullary carcinoma of the thyroid and many other tumours.

Lung tumours

The high contrast denoted by the air in the lungs enables most soft-tissue abnormalities in the peripheral lung fields to be diagnosed by plain radiography with a high degree of confidence. However, much of the lung field is obscured by the bony rib cage and lesions can be missed when small. None the less, CT provides better contrast resolution and, with spiral CT, the chance of missing small lesions in the lungs because of mis-registration during respiration has been considerably reduced. Mediastinal adenopathy may be very difficult to visualize on a chest radiograph, particularly in the subcarinal region and, for staging, CT is essential. Intravenous iodinated contrast media are usually employed so that nodes can be distinguished from the normal mediastinal vascular structures. Various criteria are usually used for determination of involvement by tumour, with nodes of greater than 1 cm being regarded as pathological. However, metastases may be present in nodes smaller than this, and in this situation PET imaging with FDG may be extremely useful in the preoperative staging of carcinoma of the lung. Lesions close to the chest wall and chest wall invasion are conveniently studied with CT, but bone involvement may, on occasion, be better demonstrated with radionuclide imaging. MR has contributed little in the evaluation of the chest because of motion artefact, but increasingly with breath-hold techniques MR can be used for the mediastinum, chest wall invasion and particularly for apical tumours, where infiltration of the brachial plexus can be very elegantly demonstrated in the coronal plane. Unfortunately, small nodules are difficult to visualize with MR and it is not yet a suitable screening test for metastatic disease. Low-dose spiral techniques have recently been used for screening high-risk populations of smokers for early lung tumours so that they can be detected and excised before they metastasize. Early studies have shown that this is a viable approach for screening suitable populations for carcinoma of the lung (Kaneko *et al.*, 1996; Sone *et al.*, 1998). Although the hazard from iodinated contrast media has been reduced by the introduction of isosmolar contrast agents, there remains a small risk of both non-fatal and fatal idiosyncratic reactions to the contrast medium. The blood vessels in MR are predominantly visualized as 'flow voids' and mediastinal adenopathy may be demonstrated reliably without recourse to contrast media.

Liver

Ultrasound is the cheapest and quickest method of evaluating the liver for both primary and secondary tumours. For most centres ultrasound remains the easiest and most atraumatic examination (Cosgrove and McCready, 1982). Radio-isotope imaging of the liver has virtually been abandoned. Echo patterns in the various tumours do vary, ranging from hypo-echoic areas to well-defined areas of increased echogenicity (Fig. 10.19). Plain CT has a poor sensitivity for space-occupying lesions in the liver, but when intravenous contrast medium is administered the sensitivity exceeds that for ultrasound, particularly when a biphasic examination is used with imaging during the arterial phase of enhancement of the liver and the portal phase. Characterization of very small lesions in the liver may be extremely difficult as partial volume averaging of the adjacent liver tissue may prevent the water density of small cysts being recognized. In this situation, directed ultrasound may be extremely helpful for confirming the true nature of these small lesions. Failing that, core biopsy using ultrasound guidance can achieve a very high diagnostic specificity. In longitudinal studies of tumour response to chemotherapy, CT is more reproducible than ultrasound as it is much less operator dependent, particularly if identical protocols are used on each occasion. The highest sensitivity is achieved with CT portography, where a catheter is positioned in the hepatic artery and CT scans obtained during optimal contrast enhancement. MR techniques with liver-specific contrast agents are now approaching a similar sensitivity and specificity and may

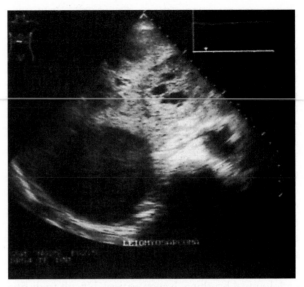

Figure 10.19 *A transverse ultrasound section through the liver, showing a variety of appearances of secondary deposits from a leiomyosarcoma. The large echo-poor (dark lesion) secondary is easily visible, while the more medial lesion is less obvious as the echo pattern is of the same intensity as the surrounding normal liver. The echo-poor ring around the lesion is often seen in metastases. In the centre are several fluid-containing, irregular, echo-free regions, presumably due to necrosis.*

well completely replace CT portography (Bluemke *et al.*, 2000; Semelka and Helmberger, 2001). Primary liver tumours may be difficult to identify with both ultrasound and CT as they may be very similar in appearance to the surrounding hepatic parenchyma. MR with specific liver agents is extremely useful for identifying the tumour and recognizing multi-focal involvement of the hepatic parenchyma. The most common benign tumour in the liver, the haemangioma, may be difficult to distinguish from a solitary metastatic deposit. The ultrasound features are of a small echogenic lesion, usually lying close to the dome of the diaphragm, and on CT these lesions enhance after contrast and attain equilibrium about 5–10 minutes after injection of contrast. Some metastatic deposits may show the same enhancement characteristics but the features of the haemangioma on MR are very typical, with a very high-intensity lesion visible in strongly T_2-weighted images. Intravenous contrast medium administration may confirm their enhancement characteristics with a similar time course to CT. It is generally considered unwise to biopsy these small lesions for confirmation but provided a biopsy path through the liver is chosen for access, these can be biopsied with a low incidence of bleeding.

The biliary system

Ultrasound is usually the first investigation of gallbladder disease and has completely replaced oral cholecystography. Although tumours of the gall-bladder wall may be detected with ultrasonic imaging, cholangiocarcinoma involving the bile ducts may be difficult to recognize and may be appreciated only because of dilatation of the biliary tree secondary to the tumour mass, or invasion into the surrounding liver parenchyma. Cholangiocarcinoma frequently lacks characteristic features on CT and will appear either as a hypo- or isodense lesion with liver parenchyma and may have either ill- or well-defined margins. Occasionally the lesions enhance with contrast, and there may also be delayed contrast accumulation thought to be due to the fibrous content of these tumours. MR imaging is also relatively non-specific and contrast administration contributes little to the diagnosis. Involvement of the biliary tree by tumour may be demonstrated at ERCP and this provides an opportunity to obtain cytological confirmation by endoluminal brushing. It may be very difficult to distinguish strictures of the bile duct due to a malignant cause from sclerosing cholangitis, which may be a predisposing cause for cholangiocarcinoma.

Spleen

The easiest technique for visualizing the spleen is ultrasound (Cosgrove and McCready, 1982). By this technique the size of the spleen and the echo pattern within it can be quickly and easily estimated. Tumours of the spleen, cysts and infarcts can all be demonstrated and the size of the splenic vessels, together with any abnormalities at the splenic hilum can be seen. Primary tumours of the spleen are unusual and metastatic disease, including lymphomatous involvement, is less common than that of the liver. Both ultrasound and CT can be used to detect tumours and, if necessary, to direct biopsy. Since the spleen is such a vascular organ, fine-needle aspiration is preferred to core biopsy, which may necessitate plugging of the biopsy track to reduce the possibility of bleeding. As with other areas of the body, malignant infiltration of the spleen can be detected with FDG-PET imaging.

Pancreas

Tumours in the pancreas can be demonstrated with ultrasound, particularly in slim subjects, and their recognition can be aided by the presence of dilatation of the common bile duct and of the pancreatic duct. However, the sensitivity for the identification of pancreatic tumours is impaired in those patients with an unsuitable body habitus for ultrasound imaging and where gastric or colonic gas overlies the pancreatic bed. Imaging can be improved in the latter situation by filling the stomach with water to act as an acoustic window and then giving intravenous Buscopan® or glucagon to reduce gastric emptying. However, CT using intravenous contrast medium, to firstshow the vascular phase of enhancement and to identify

encasement of the adjacent arteries and, secondly, to show a parenchymal phase to identify tumour involvement of the pancreas, is preferred. Identification of the pancreatic duct is greatly improved by optimization of the contrast enhancement of the pancreas with the use of multislice technique and curved reconstruction. Unfortunately, mass lesions in the pancreas due to tumour are very difficult to separate from focal pancreatitis, and it is usually necessary to confirm the diagnosis of tumour by percutaneous biopsy, which can be either ultrasound- or CT-guided. MRI using conventional spin-echo sequences has been limited for the evaluation of pancreatic disease, due to the long times of acquisition and the presence of both technical and movement artefact. Breath-hold imaging with fat suppression and dynamic acquisition after admin-istration of intravenous contrast agents has considerably improved the ability of the technique to recognize pancreatic neoplasms. None the less, specificity is limited and, as with CT, there is considerable overlap between focal pancreatitis and tumour.

Endoscopic ultrasound has a much higher resolution for pancreatic lesions than transabdominal examination and is more sensitive for the detection of small tumours, vascular encasement and local lymph-node involvement (Zerbey *et al.*, 1996).

Urinary tract and prostate

The basic investigations of renal-tract pathology include a plain film of the abdomen for the evaluation of stones and an intravenous urogram (IVU), which involves injection of iodinated contrast medium which is excreted through the upper tracts and accumulates in the bladder. Ultrasound is particularly simple and quick in demonstrating hydronephrosis (Fig. 10.20). Space-occupying lesions in the kidney will be shown on the IVU by displacement of the adjacent structures, but simple cysts may be totally indistinguish-able from tumours and ultrasound is invaluable for the differentiation between a solid mass and

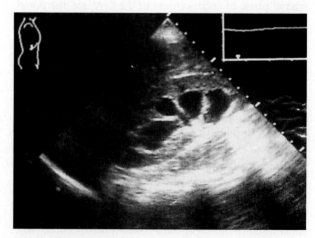

Figure 10.20 *An ultrasound scan of a hydronephrotic kidney, showing a very obvious dilatation of the calyces.*

a cyst. CT is reserved for evaluation of indeterminate cysts. Ultrasound may also be used for staging of renal tumours. Direct invasion into the peri-renal fat can be detected, as well as tumour thrombus in the renal vein and inferior vena cava, local lymph-node spread and pulmonary metastatic disease. MR has been limited by movement artefact, but breath-hold fat suppression techniques with contrast can be used to confirm the presence of tumours, and are particularly useful when there are multiple lesions present and long-term screening is required, as in conditions such as von Hippel–Lindau disease. The ureters are more difficult to visualize with cross-sectional techniques, and if the IVU does not show an intrinsic lesion then insertion of a catheter into the ureter via the bladder with retrograde instillation of iodinated contrast medium may be necessary to show small urothelial tumours. Although small bladder tumours may be shown by trans-abdominal ultrasound of the filled bladder, as a general principle, cystoscopy with direct visualization of the bladder mucosa is more accurate. At the same time as visualization of the tumour directly, biopsy can be performed. When bladder tumours are larger and staging is required, both CT and MR can be utilized to show perivesical involvement and spread to local lymph nodes. MR, particularly with gadolinium-DTPA enhancement and T_1-weighted images, appears slightly superior to CT for detection and staging of tumours and has the added advantage of multiplanar imaging, which is invaluable for the dome of the bladder (Barentsz *et al.*, 1993).

PROSTATE

Prostate cancer is now the most common cancer in men. The introduction of screening by serum prostate-specific antigen (PSA) has increased awareness of this disease, and more tumours are detected at an earlier stage. Screening can be effective for the improvement of prognosis and can permit radical surgery in patients with early disease. The aim of imaging is to improve preoperative staging so that appropriate therapy is carried out. Digital examination can detect primary lesions, which can be confirmed by endorectal ultrasound. The majority of tumours are in the peripheral zone, which is easily accessible to both the examining finger and the ultrasound probe. The presence of a hypo-echoic mass on ultrasound can confirm the presence of the cancer, but since focal prostatitis may give rise to very similar findings, biopsy is necessary for confirmation. Sensitivity for the detection of lesions in the prostate may be increased by intravenous contrast agents, although the specificity does not appear to be changed (Halpern *et al.*, 2001). The biopsy needle can be guided along the ultrasound probe and representative samples obtained. In patients with a raised PSA, representative biopsies from both sides of the prostate are recommended if a focal abnormality is not identified. From these, histological grading of the tumour can be determined. Spread outside the prostate is much more difficult to assess with ultrasound and for this both CT and MR have been used. Although CT is effective for detection of nodal involvement both within the pelvis and in the abdomen, MR is more effective for local staging of disease and to detect invasion of the neurovascular bundle which lies postero-lateral to a prostate and is an early site of invasion. Accuracy of diagnosis is improved by utilization of an endorectal coil but may be poorly tolerated by patients and needs to be supplemented by images obtained with a pelvic array coil for the determination of spread to local nodes. T_2-weighted images are used for imaging the prostate and intravenous contrast medium is rarely of any value. The bones of the pelvis and lower lumbar spine should be examined carefully for bone-marrow replacement by tumour, since these are a common site for bony metastatic disease.

Skeleton and soft tissues

While X-ray techniques provide the detail required in imaging the skeleton, radio-isotope techniques provide early warning of developing abnormalities. It is relatively easy and quick to survey the whole skeleton with the radio-isotope technique.

The precise mechanism by which the Tc^{99m} phosphate or diphosphonate localizes in the skeleton is not known. Most pathological processes which produce bone turnover in the skeleton result in a positive bone scan, whether the end result is an osteolytic or an osteoblastic area on the X-ray. It is thought that up to 50 per cent of the mineral content of a bone must be lost before small lesions become apparent on the X-ray, and this accounts for the delay between the positive bone scan and the positive X-ray. Table 10.3 lists some of the benign causes of positive bone scans. Prostate cancer usually produces lesions in the skeleton which have very intense uptake. Lung and breast cancer lesions are not usually so dramatic. Multiple myeloma is one of the more difficult diseases to diagnose by bone imaging. Opinions differ on the sensitivity of the test in this condition, particularly in the ribs where there is movement, lack of osteoblastic reaction and the lesions are small (Leonard *et al.*, 1981). In the spine, most of the positive lesions are due to collapsed

Table 10.3 *Some benign disorders that may produce a positive bone scan*

Osteoarthritis
Rheumatoid arthritis and other arthritides
Ankylosing spondylitis
Postfracture or postbiopsy repair
Osteomalacia
Localized osteoporosis
Paget's disease of bone
Osteomyelitis
Hyperostosis frontalis interna
Aseptic bone necrosis

vertebrae. Occasionally cold lesions are seen on bone scans: the causes include radiation damage (Hattner *et al.*, 1982) and quickly growing tumours. An added bonus of bone imaging is the ability to monitor renal function by evaluating the excretion of the radiopharmaceutical through the kidneys.

The usual reason for requesting a bone scan is to confirm metastatic disease in patients with bone pain. Often a plain X-ray is required to exclude trauma in areas of increased activity. Areas which may be difficult to interpret on X-ray, including the ribs, scapula and sternum, can be more easily evaluated on bone scans.

The consensus of opinion is that it is rarely justified to perform routine bone scanning in early carcinoma where there are no symptoms. The exception would be where accurate staging is required as part of a clinical trial. The value of bone scanning in carcinoma of the lung has been discussed by Merrick and Merrick (1986), the breast by Kunkler and Merrick (1986), the bladder by Davey *et al.* (1984) and the prostate by Constable and Cranage (1981). A typical bone scintigram in a patient with prostatic cancer is seen in Figure 10.21.

CT is used increasingly for localized areas of uptake, particularly when radiographs do not provide a cause. Increasingly, MR is being used in symptomatic patients with possible metastatic disease, particularly in the spine where the additional information about cord, cauda equina and root compression is so important in the management of the patient. Recent developments in faster sequences with fat suppression, as well as the utilization of moving-table technology, means that MR has the potential to replace isotope bone scanning for screening in metastatic disease without the requirement for radiation and the 3-hour wait between the injection of isotope and localization in the skeleton. As a general principle, osteoblastic lesions from primary neoplasms such as the prostate are better visualized by isotope bone scanning. Lytic lesions, particularly from breast carcinoma and myeloma may be relatively inapparent on bone scans but, because of the marked marrow replacement, are easy to visualize with MR and CT. Solitary vertebral abnormalities due to vertebral body collapse may be very difficult to evaluate. If the bone marrow signal is maintained in the MR images, then a benign cause such as osteoporosis is likely. Unfortunately, with acute collapse, bone marrow oedema may simulate replacement by tumour and the dilemma may only be resolved by waiting for the marrow signal to return to normal or to resort to biopsy or PET imaging to determine whether malignant infiltration is the cause. Rib lesions may be difficult to evaluate with plain films; CT and MR and isotope bone scans can be very sensitive for small lesions.

SOFT TISSUES

The most common soft-tissue tumour is the benign lipoma, which is usualy superficial within the subcutaneous fat and easily demonstrated by ultrasound. The more malignant tumours, such as sarcomas, can also be visualized with ultrasound but are usually evaluated with CT or MR so that their full extent can be determined and characteristics such as vascular encasement and bony invasion determined. As a general principle, MR and CT are poor at tissue characterization and biopsy is normally required (Kransdorf and Murphey, 2000). Although this can be directed by imaging, a large surgical biopsy, preferably performed by the person doing the definitive surgery, is recommended to ensure that a representative sample is obtained and the true malignant potential identified. The most suitable site to biopsy can usually be estimated from the solid component as shown by MR, but PET imaging may be more suitable for recognizing the most active part of the tumour to produce a representative biopsy.

Female pelvis

Ultrasound, both trans-abdominal and, particularly, transvaginal is utilized extensively for screening for both ovarian and uterine abnormalities. It is effective in separating simple cysts of the ovary from solid lesions, but care has to be taken as cystic tumours of the ovary are relatively common. These usually have a slightly thicker wall than a simple cyst and the contents are more echogenic than simple water. Bleeding into a simple cyst may result in what appears to be a solid lesion of the ovary. CT is predominantly used for staging of ovarian carcinoma and although peritoneal disease can be visualized, it is insensitive for

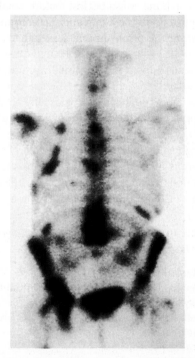

Figure 10.21 *A typical Tc^{99m}-methylene diphosphonate scintigram in a patient with prostatic carcinoma. The very intense focal lesions are typical of prostatic skeletal secondaries.*

early disease of the peritoneum. When spread extends into the upper abdomen the typical pattern is of subcapsular involvement of the liver rather than parenchymal. MR is less effective for peritoneal disease because motion artefact from peristalsis degrades the images, but it can be useful for characterization of ovarian tumours. All imaging investigations are insensitive for early uterine cervical disease, the diagnosis of which is usually made by direct inspection and biopsy. Spread into the parametrium is better demonstrated by MR than CT but nodal involvement can be recognized with both techniques. Fibroid change within the uterus is conveniently shown by MR, where heavily T_2-weighted images show the fibroids as low-signal masses within the uterine muscle. The ability to view the pelvis in trans-axial, sagittal and coronal sections is useful in patients with cervical cancer and may become the imaging technique of choice.

Lymphatic system

A variety of techniques are required to image the several parts of the lymphatic system. In the chest, a plain chest X-ray is often the only examination required. CT scanning yields more information but there are indications that [18]FDG-PET scanning will assist in the differential diagnosis and in determining areas of active disease spread. Gallium-67 scanning is rarely used now but Figure 10.22 demonstrates uptake in a patient with Hodgkin's disease.

Several radioactive techniques for imaging the lymphatic system are available. These involve the injection of labelled colloids subcutaneously or into the lymphatic ducts (Thornton and Pickering, 1985). Perhaps the most successful area for this technique has been in the evaluation of retrosternal lymph nodes in patients with breast cancer (Ege and Clark, 1985). Elsewhere the technique is not really competitive with CT imaging. A figure of

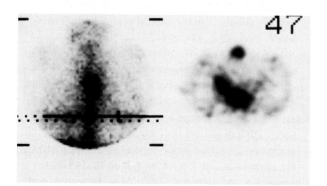

Figure 10.22 *Gallium-67 scan in a patient with Hodgkin's lymphoma. Increased activity is seen at the right hilum in lymphadenopathy not detectable on a CT scan. The planar view is seen on the left. The transaxial view on the right demonstrates the benefit of emission computerized tomography. A normal concentration of gallium is seen in the sternum anteriorly and spine posteriorly.*

about 80 per cent in overall accuracy is often quoted (Husband *et al.*, 1981). The accuracy of pelvic CT in detecting metastatic nodal disease from pelvic cancer is much lower (Walsh and Gopelrud, 1981).

Breast

Mammography using a low kV technique is used for radiological evaluation of the breast for tumours, both as a screening investigation and for symptomatic patients. Lesions may be seen as spiculated masses with or without coarse calcification. There may be evidence of skin thickening and axillary adenopathy. Mammography is particularly effective in older patients where there is reduction in the glandular tissue and fat replacement, whereas the density of the breast tissue may mask lesions in younger patients. Ultrasound is mainly used to clarify palpable masses, examine mammographically dense breasts or lesions visible in mammograms, particularly to distinguish cystic from solid. Unfortunately, US is not effective for screening, or for distinguishing benign from malignant with certainty, and biopsy is normally required. This can be US guided and involve either a fine-needle aspiration with cytology or a core biopsy with histological examination of the specimen. The use of colour flow imaging may add specificity to the identification of solid masses, as malignant tumours have an increased blood flow. MR tends to be reserved for problem patients, particularly the postoperative breast where mammography has difficulty in distinguishing fibrous scarring from surgery and radiotherapy from recurrence. It is also useful to detect multifocal tumour involvement in patients with a known carcinoma and to assess the contralateral breast.

CONCLUSIONS

This chapter has outlined the principles and applications of a wide variety of techniques used in the diagnosis and follow-up of tumours. The choice has widened greatly over the last few years. It is important to understand the principles involved in each test so that a correct choice can be made until such time that a patient is referred to the diagnostic department, leaving the choice to the diagnostician. It is also important to understand and know the limitations of each technique so that a level of confidence can be put on the diagnosis made on the image. For example, in an ultrasound examination a normal report means that the parts of the liver that were visible through an acoustic window were normal while other parts could be abnormal. It would be impossible for the radiologist to qualify each diagnosis with the limitations of the technique. It is usually the case that when there is a difficulty with one technique the answer is available with another. It is best to start with the simplest technique that is likely to give an answer. With the advent of computer-assisted diagnosis it will be possible to give an estimate of the probability of a correct diagnosis from a given set of features on a particular image. In the meantime, there should be close co-operation between the diagnostician and the oncologist in determining the best way of investigating a lesion so that the correct diagnosis and staging can be made before prescribing the appropriate treatment (with its side effects and impact on the quality of life of the patient). Each technique has both advantages and disadvantages, but the drive away from using methods that involve ionizing radiation has meant that ultrasound and MR have become used increasingly. It is important to remember that unless breath-hold techniques are used, CT is probably the most effective investigation, particularly in the chest and upper abdomen. No technique will give a definitive histological diagnosis and, in many cases, biopsy is required to confirm primary tumour histology, the presence of recurrence and to distinguish tumour from the effects and complications of treatment, including superadded infection. However, PET scanning with FDG shows great potential in the distinction of benign from malignant disease and for detecting recurrent disease on a background of postsurgical or radiation-induced change.

In this chapter the newer techniques have been dealt with in more detail than the older more established techniques. The latter are described in many general textbooks, including Vanel and Stark (1993).

SIGNIFICANT POINTS

- In making a comparison between different imaging techniques it is important to remember that one is not always comparing exactly the same parameters.
- MRI is particularly useful in that it provides improved definition of differing soft tissues and allows image reconstruction in multiple planes.
- Positron emission tomography examines tissue function and complements the information obtained by CT or MRI.
- In the future co-registration of images from different techniques will become more freely available.

KEY REFERENCES

Atlas, S.W. (ed.) (1991) *Magnetic resonance imaging of the brain and spine.* New York: Raven Press.
Bender, H., Palmedo, H., Biersack, H.-J. and Valk, P.E. (2000) *Atlas of clinical PET in oncology.* Berlin: Springer.

Bragg, D.G., Rubin, P. and Youker, J.E. (eds) (1985) *Oncological imaging.* Oxford: Pergamon Press.
Husband, J.E.S. and Resnek, R.H. (eds) (1998) *Imaging in oncology.* Oxford: Isis Medical Media.
Lee, J.K.T., Sagel, S.S., Stanley, R.J. and Heiken, J.P. (eds) (1998) *Computed body tomography with MRI correlation.* Philadelphia: Lippincott-Raven.
Vanel, V. and Stark, D. (1993) *Imaging strategies in oncology.* London: Martin Dunitz.

REFERENCES

Arulampalam, T.H.A., Costa, D.C., Loizidou, M. *et al.* (2001) Positron emission tomography and colorectal cancer. *Br. J. Surg.* **88**, 176–89.
Atlas, S.W. (ed.) (1991) *Magnetic resonance imaging of the brain and spine.* New York: Raven Press.
Baker, H.L., Houser, O.W. and Campbell, J.K. (1980) National Cancer Institute Study: evaluation of computed tomography in the diagnosis of intra-cranial neoplasms. I. Overall results. *Radiology* **136**, 91–6.
Barentsz, J.O., Ruijs, J.H.J. and Strijk, S.P. (1993) The role of MR imaging in carcinoma of the urinary bladder. *AJR* **160**, 939–47.
Beaney, R.P. (1984) Positron emission tomography in the study of human tumours. *Semin. Nucl. Med.* **XIV**, 324–41.
Beaney, R.P. (1986) Functional aspects of human brain tumours as studied by positron emission tomography. In Bleehen, N.M. (ed.), *Tumours of the brain.* Berlin: Springer-Verlag, 63–82.
Beaney, R.P. and Wong, W.L. (1994) The role of positron emission tomography in the assessment of germ cell tumours. In Jones, W. *et al.* (eds), *Advances in biosciences,* vol. 91. *Germ cell tumours III.* Elsevier Science, pp. 169–75.
Beckerman, C., Hoffer, P.B. and Bitran, J.D. (1984) The role of gallium-67 in the clinical evaluation of cancer. *Semin. Nucl. Med.,* **XIV**, 296–23.
Belcher, E.H. and Veall, H. (1971) *Radioisotopes in medical diagnosis.* London: Butterworths.
Bender, H., Palmedo, H., Biersack, H.-J. and Valk, P.E. (2000) *Atlas of clinical PET in oncology.* Berlin: Springer.
Berry, J.P., Escaig, F., Poupon, M.F. and Galle, P. (1983) Localisation of gallium in tumour cells. Electron microscopy, electron probe microanalysis and analytical ion microscopy. *Int. J. Nucl. Med. Biol.* **10**, 199–204.
Bluemke, D.A., Paulson, E.K., Choti, M.A., DeSena, S. and Clavien, P.A. (2000) Detection of hepatic lesions in candidates for surgery: comparison of ferumoxides-enhanced MR imaging and dual-phase helical CT. *AJR* **175**, 1653–8.
Brant-Zawadzki, M. *et al.* (1984) Primary intracranial tumour imaging: a comparison of magnetic resonance and CT. *Radiology* **150**, 435–40.

Bustany, P., Henry, J.F., De Rotrou, J. *et al.* (1985) Correlations between clinical state and positron emission tomography, measurement of local protein synthesis in Alzheimer's dementia, Parkinson's disease, schizophrenia and gliomas. In Greitz, T. *et al.* (eds), *The metabolism of the human brain studied with positron emission tomography*. New York: Raven Press, pp. 241–9.

Bydder, G.M., Steiner, R.E., Young, I.R. *et al.* (1982) Clinical NMR imaging of the brain: 140 cases. *AJR* **139**, 215–36.

Bydder, G.M., Kingsley, D.P., Gadian, D.G. *et al.* (1984) The NMR diagnosis of cerebral tumours. *J. Mag. Res. Med.* **1**, 5–29.

Carr, D.H., Brown, J., Bydder, G.M. *et al.* (1984) Intravenous chelated gadolinium as a contrast agent in NMR imaging of cerebral tumours. *Lancet* **i**, 484–6.

Carr, D.H., Graif, M., Niendorf, H.P. *et al.* (1986) Gadolinium DTPA in the assessment of liver tumours by magnetic resonance imaging. *Clin. Radiol.* **37**, 347–53.

Clarke, S.E.M., Lazarus, C.R., Wraight, P. *et al.* (1988) Pentavalent technetium ^{99m}DMSA, ^{131}I MIBG, and ^{99m}Tc MPD – an evaluation of 3 imaging techniques of patients with medullary carcinoma of the thyroid. *J. Nucl. Med.* **29**, 33–8.

Constable, A.R. and Cranage R.W. (1981) Recognition of the superscan in prostatic bone scinitigraphy. *Br. J. Radiol.* **54**, 122–5.

Cosgrove, D.O. and McCready, V.R. (1982) *Ultrasound imaging: liver, spleen and pancreas.* Chichester: Wiley.

Damadian, R. (1971) Tumour detection by nuclear magnetic resonance. *Science* **171**, 1151–3.

Davey, P., Merrick, D.V., Duncan, W. and Redpath, A.T. (1984) Bladder cancer: the value of routine bone scintigraphy. *Clin. Radiol.* **36**, 77–9.

Dewan, N.A., Reeb, S.D., Gupta, N.C. *et al.* (1995) PET-FDG imaging and transthoracic needle lung aspiration biopsy in evaluation of pulmonary lesions: a comparative risk-benefit analysis. *Chest* **108**, 441–6.

Di Chiro, G., DelaPaz, R.L., Brooks, R.A. *et al.* (1982) Glucose utilisation of cerebral gliomas measured by [^{18}F] fluorodeoxyglucose and positron emission tomography. *Neurology* **32**, 1323–9.

Dwamena, B.A., Sonnad, S.S., Angobaldo, J.O. and Wahl, R.L. (1999) Metastases from non-small cell lung cancer: mediastinal staging in the 1990s – meta-analytic comparison of PET and CT. *Radiology* **213**, 530–6.

Edwards, C.L. and Hayes, R.L. (1969) Tumour scanning with gallium citrate. *J. Nucl. Med.* **10**, 103–5.

Ege, G.N. and Clark, R.M. (1985) Internal mammary lymphoscintigraphy in the conservative management of breast carcinoma: an update and recommendations for a new TNM staging. *Clin. Radiol.* **36**, 469–72.

Ericson, K., Lilja, A., Bergstrom, M. *et al.* (1985) Positron emission tomography (PET) using ^{11}C-methionine, ^{11}C-glucose and 68-Ga-EDTA in the examination of supratentorial tumours. *J. Comput. Assist. Tomogr.* **9**, 683–9.

Evens, R.G. and Evens, R.G. (1988) Economic and utilization analysis of magnetic resonance imaging units in the United States in 1987. *Radiology* **166**, 27–30.

Fahey, F.H. (2001) Positron emission tomography instrumentation. *Radiol. Clin. North Am.* **39**(5), 919–29.

Fischer, M.R., Hricak, H. and Crooks, L.E. (1985) Urinary bladder MR imaging. Parts A and B. *Radiology* **157**, 467–77.

Halpern, E.J., Rosenberg, M. and Gomella, L.G. (2001) Prostate cancer: contrast-enhanced US for detection. *AJR* **219**, 219–25.

Hattner, R.S., Hartmeyer, J. and Wara, W.M. (1982) Characterization of radiation-induced photopenic abnormalities on bone scans. *Radiology* **145**, 161–3.

Hawkes, R.C., Holland, G.N., Moore, W.S. and Worthington, B.S. (1980) Nuclear magnetic resonance (NMR) tomography of the brain: a preliminary clinical assessment with demonstration of pathology. *J. Comput. Assist. Tomogr.* **4**, 577–86.

Ho, C.K., Hawkins, R.A., Glasby, J.A. *et al.* (1993) Cancer detection with whole body PET using 2-[^{18}F]fluoro-2-deoxy-D-glucose. *J. Comp. Ass. Tomog.* **17**, 582–9.

Husband, J.E. and Golding, S.J. (1983) The role of computed tomography-guided needle biopsy in an oncology service. *Clin. Radiol.* **34**, 255–60.

Husband, J.E., Barrett, A. and Peckham, M.J. (1981) Evaluation of computed tomography in the management of testicular teratoma. *Br. J. Urol.* **53**, 179–83.

Ikekubo, K., Higa, T., Hirasa, M. *et al.* (1986) Evaluation of radionuclide imaging and echography in the diagnosis of thyroid nodules. *Clin. Nucl. Med.* **11**, 145–9.

Kaneko, M., Eguchi, K., Ohmatsu, H. *et al.* (1996) Peripheral lung cancer: screening and detection with low-dose spiral CT versus radiography. *Radiology* **201**, 798–802.

Kean, D.M., Smith, M.A., Douglas, R.H. and Best, J.J. (1986) A description of a low field resistive magnetic resonance imaging system and its application in imaging midline central nervous system pathology. *Clin. Radiol.* **37**, 211–17.

Kransdorf, M.J. and Murphey, M.D. (2000) Radiologic evaluation of soft-tissue masses: a current perspective. *AJR* **175**, 575–87.

Kubota, K., Yamada, K., Fukada, H. *et al.* (1984) Tumour detection with carbon-11 labelled amino acids. *Eur. J. Nucl. Med.* **9**, 136–40.

Kunkler, I.A. and Merrick M.V. (1986) The value of non-staging skeletal scintigraphy in breast cancer. *Clin. Radiol.* **37**, 561–2.

Larson, S.M., Rasey, J.S., Allen, D.R. and Nelson, N.J. (1979) A transferrin-mediated uptake of gallium-67 by EMT-6 sarcoma. I. Studies in tissue culture. *J. Nucl. Med.* **20**, 837–42.

Lauterbur, P.C. (1973) Image formation by induced local interactions: examples employing nuclear magnetic resonance. *Nature* **242**, 190–1.

Leinhard, G.E., Slot, J.W., James, D.E. and Muecler, M.M. (1992) How cells absorb glucose. *Sci. Am.* **266**, 34–9.

Leonard, R.C.F., Owen, J.P., Proctor, S.J. and Hamilton, P.J. (1981) Multiple myeloma: radiology or bone scanning? *Clin. Radiol.* **32**, 291–5.

Macfarlane, D.J., Sondak, V., Johnson, T. *et al.* (1998) Prospective evaluation of 2-[18F]-2-deoxy-D-glucose positron emission tomography in staging of regional lymph nodes in patients with cutaneous malignant melanoma. *J. Clin. Oncol.* **16**, 1770–6.

Maisey, M., Wahl, R.L. and Barrington, S.F. (eds) (1999) *Atlas of clinical positron emission tomography.* London: Arnold.

Merrick, M.V. and Merrick, J.M. (1986) Bone scintigraphy in lung cancer: a reappraisal. *Br. J. Radiol.* **59**, 1185–94.

Muhr, C., Bergstrom, M., Lundberg, P.O. *et al.* (1986) Dopamine receptors in pituitary adenomas: PET visualisation with 11C-N-methyl spiperone. *J. Comput. Assist. Tomogr.* **10**, 175–80.

National Radiological Protection Board (1991) *Documents of the WKPB NRPB.* Didcot Oxon: Chilton, 1–29.

Newman, J.S., Francis, I.R., Kaminski, M.S. *et al.* (1994) Imaging of lymphoma with PET with 2-[F18]-fluoro-2-deoxy-o-glucose: correlation with CT. *Radiology* **190**, 111–16.

Partridge, S., Timothy, A., O'Doherty, M.J. *et al.* (2000) 2-Fluorine-18-fluoro-2-deoxy-D-glucose positron emission tomography in the pre-treatment staging of Hodgkin's disease: influence on patient management in a single institution. *Ann. Oncol.* **11**, 1273–9.

Patronas, N.J., Di Chiro, G., Brooks, R.A. *et al.* (1982) Work in progress: [18F] fluorodeoxyglucose and positron emission tomography in the evaluation of radiation necrosis of the brain. *Radiology* **144**, 885–9.

Petasnick, J.P., Turner, D.A., Charten, J.R. *et al.* (1986) Soft tissue masses of the locomotor system: comparison of MR imaging with CT. *Radiology* **160**, 125–33.

Phelps, M.E., Hoffman, E.J., Huang, S.C. and Kuhl, D.E. (1978) ECAT: a new computerised tomographic imaging system for positron-emitting radiopharmaceuticals. *J. Nucl. Med.* **19**, 635–47.

Poon, P.Y., McCallum, R.W., Herkelman, M.M. *et al.* (1985) Magnetic resonance imaging of the prostate. *Radiology* **154**, 143–9.

Pykett, I.L., Newhouse, J.H., Buonarro, F.S. *et al.* (1982) Principles of nuclear magnetic resonance imaging. *Radiology* **143**, 157–68.

Rege, S.D., Hoh, C.K., Glaspy, J.A. *et al.* (1993) Imaging of pulmonary mass lesions with whole-body positron emission tomography and fluorodeoxyglucose. *Cancer* **72**, 82–90.

Rinne, D., Baum, R.P., Hor, G. *et al.* (1998) Primary staging and follow-up of high risk melanoma patients with whole-body 18F-fluorodeoxyglucose positron emission tomography: results of a prospective study of 100 patients. **82**, 1664–71.

Rosler, I. (1986) Radioiodine treatment of thyroid carcinomas. In Cunowinkler, K. (ed.), *Nuclear medicine in clinical oncology.* Berlin: Springer-Verlag, 309–20.

Runge, V.M. (1991) *Contrast media in magnetic resonance imaging.* Philadelphia: J.B. Lippincott.

Semelka, R.C. and Helmberger, T.K.G. (2001) Contrast agents for MR imaging of the liver. *AJR* **218**, 27–38.

Shapiro, B., Copp, I.E., Sisson, J.C. *et al.* (1985) Iodine-131 metaiodobenzylguanidine for the locating of suspected pheochromocytoma: experience in 400 cases. *J. Nucl. Med.* **26**, 576–85.

Sone, S. Takashima, S., Li, F. *et al.* (1998) Mass screening for lung cancer with mobile spiral computed tomography scanner. *Lancet* **351**, 1242–5.

Stark, D.D. and Bradley, W.G. (1992) *Magnetic resonance imaging*, (2nd edn). St Louis: C.V. Mosby.

Thornton, A. and Pickering, D. (1985) Abdominal lymphoscintigraphy: an effective substitute for lymphography? *Br. J. Radiol.* **58**, 603–10.

Turkington, T.G. (2001) Introduction to PET instrumentation. *J. Nucl. Med. Technol.* **9**(1), 4–11.

Valk, P.E., Abella-Columna, E., Haseman, M.K. *et al.* (1999) Whole-body PET imaging with [18F] fluorodeoxyglucose in management of recurrent colorectal cancer. *Arch. Surg.* **134**, 503–11.

Vanel, V. and Stark, D. (1993) *Imaging strategies in oncology.* London: Martin Dunitz.

Walsh, J.W. and Gopelrud, D.R. (1981) Prospective comparison between clinical and CT staging in primary cervical carcinoma. *AJR* **137**, 997–1003.

Wong, W.-L., Hussain, K., Chevretton, E. *et al.* (1996) Validation and clinical application of computer-combined computed tomography and positron emission tomography with 2-[18F] fluoro-2-deoxy-D-glucose head and neck images. *Am. J. Surg.* **172**, 628–32.

Wong, W.-L., Chevretton, E.B., McGurk, M. *et al.* (1997) A prospective study of PET imaging for the assessment of head and neck squamous cell carcinoma. *Clin. Otolaryngol.* **22**(3), 209–14.

Worthington, B.S., Wright, J.E., Curati, W.L. *et al.* (1986) The role of magnetic resonance imaging techniques in the evaluation of orbital and ocular disease. *Clin. Radiol.* **37**, 219–26.

Yamamoto, Y.L. and Diksic, M. (1985) Positron emission tomography studies of pharmacokinetics. In Revich, M. and Alavi, A. (eds), *Positron emission tomography.* New York: Alan Liss, 413–23.

Young, H., Baum, R., Cremerius, U. *et al.* (1999) Measurement of clinical and sub-clinical response using [18F]-fluorodeoxyglucose and positron emission tomograph; review and EORTC recommendations. *Eur. J. Cancer* **13**, 1773–82.

Zerbey, A.L., Lee, M.J., Brugge, W.R. and Mueller, P.R. (1996) Endoscopic sonography of the upper gastrointestinal tract and pancreas. *AJR* **166**, 45–50.

Zimmer, W.D., Berquist, T.H., McLeod, R.A. *et al.* (1985) Bone tumours: magnetic resonance imaging versus computed tomography. *Radiology* **155**, 709–18.

11

Interventional radiology

TARUN SABHARWAL, ANNE P. HEMINGWAY AND ANDREW ADAM

Over the past three decades, a variety of invasive diagnostic and therapeutic procedures have been developed by radiologists. The term 'interventional radiology'(Adam, 1998) most appropriately refers to therapeutic procedures performed under imaging guidance. However, diagnostic invasive techniques are usually carried out by interventional radiologists and will be included in this chapter. The emergence of interventional radiology as a specialty has been made possible by the enormous technological advances in relation to catheter and instrument design and manufacture, imaging systems and radiological expertise. Some of these procedures have largely replaced more invasive and hazardous surgical alternatives; for example, tunnelled central venous catheters are now usually inserted using imaging-guided percutaneous techniques under local anaesthesia, rather than open surgery under general anaesthesia. The major techniques are listed in Table 11.1 and have been subdivided into diagnostic and interventional categories, although these are frequently combined in any one patient.

The term 'invasive' is relative; most of the procedures described in this chapter are considerably less invasive than their surgical alternative. However, they all carry some risk, which is interdependent on the underlying condition, the nature of the procedure and the experience of the radiologist. It is important that the clinicians who request a procedure are aware of its risks as well as its benefits, and that informed consent is obtained.

Emphasis is placed on the indications, contraindications and results rather than detailed technical descriptions.

Table 11.1 *Invasive radiological procedures*

Diagnostic procedures
  Biopsy
    percutaneous
    transluminal
      endoscopic
      fluoroscopic
  Venous sampling
    systemic
    portal
  Percutaneous puncture techniques
Interventional procedures
  Drainage
  Dilatation
  Extraction/retrieval
  Infusion
  Embolization
  Filters
  Shunts
  Neurolysis
  Thermal and chemical tumour ablation
  Gene therapy

DIAGNOSTIC MANOEUVRES

Biopsy procedures

The development of fine needles (Chiba needles) and small-gauge cutting instruments (automated biopsy devices such as the Quick-core, Temno and Biopty gun), which can be accurately directed to virtually any site within the body, under imaging control and local anaesthesia, has dramatically reduced the number of patients requiring open surgical biopsy to obtain tissue for a histological diagnosis. It is possible to perform most of these procedures on an outpatient basis. Needle placement for obtaining a cytological or histological specimen may be carried out under fluoroscopic, ultrasonic (US), computed tomographic (CT) or magnetic resonance imaging (MRI) guidance (Haubeck *et al.*, 1982; Husband and Golding, 1983; Mueller *et al.*, 1986). An efficient and accurate biopsy service is dependent upon the co-operation and expertise of the local departments of cytology and histology. Ideally, a cytologist should be present at the time of biopsy to determine if the specimen is adequate for examination. An initial cytological report should be available within hours; when larger specimens are sent for histological examination (as may be required with lymphoreticular malignancies), processing, sectioning and staining take longer.

It is possible to perform image-guided biopsy either percutaneously (transthoracic, abdominal, musculoskeletal, lymph nodes, etc.) or transluminally.

PERCUTANEOUS TRANSTHORACIC BIOPSY

Percutaneous transthoracic biopsy (Allison and Hemingway, 1981; Greene, 1981) is a rapid, safe and effective means of establishing a diagnosis in a patient with an opacity visible on a chest radiograph. The procedure is performed under local anaesthesia using either biplane fluoroscopy, ultrasound or computed tomography for guidance (Fig. 11.1).

US guidance is useful for pleural biopsy, rib lesions, subcutaneous deposits and peripheral lung lesions reaching a pleural surface. For other more central or difficult access lesions either fluoroscopy or CT guidance is recommended (van Sonnenberg *et al.*, 1988).

In general it is easier, quicker and less expensive to carry out a biopsy under fluoroscopic guidance than to

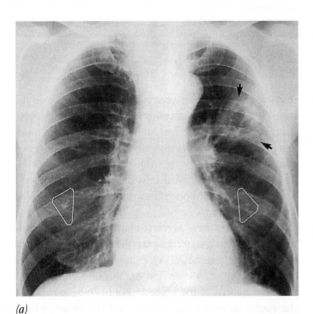

(a)

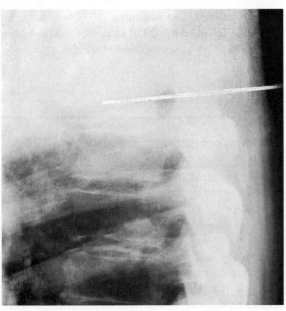

(c)

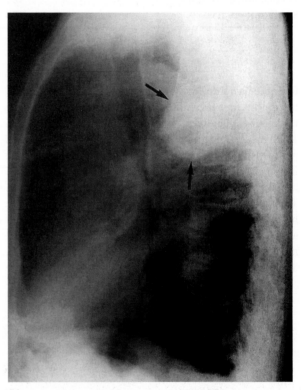

(b)

Figure 11.1 *(a) Percutaneous lung biopsy. An opacity is noted in the left upper zone (a) posteriorly (b) (The triangular metallic opacities are nipple markers). The biopsy needle has been inserted under biplane fluoroscopic control (c) Reproduced with permission from Allison (1987).*

use CT scanning for the procedure. However, CT has several advantages over fluoroscopy:

- It is easier to visualize small lesions on CT, especially when they are located in such a position as to be projected over the mediastinum or the spine on lateral fluoroscopy.
- Biopsies from partially necrotic lesions should be taken from the viable parts of the wall of the mass rather than the necrotic areas. It is easier to ensure that this is done under CT guidance.
- When multiple lesions are present, it is difficult to be certain that one is looking at the same lesion in both the anteroposterior and lateral projections on fluoroscopy, but much easier on CT.
- When a mass is close to a large vascular structure it is better to use CT for the biopsy as the vessel is easier to avoid because of the greater precision of the procedure.

CT guidance is also particularly useful in the performance of mediastinal biopsies. It is easier to distinguish abnormal masses from vascular structures by CT than by fluoroscopy. In addition, it is possible to avoid puncturing the lung, especially when a posterior approach is used, thus minimizing the risk of pneumothorax (Adam *et al.*, 1989). The major drawback with CT is the lack of real time imaging and slow image display time. To overcome this limitation, CT fluoroscopy (continuous imaging CT or real-time reconstruction CT) has recently been developed (Katada *et al.*, 1996). This combines the real-time advantage of ultrasound and fluoroscopy with the wide field of view and better soft-tissue contrast provided by standard CT, to allow for rapid and more confident imaging-guided biopsies (Fig. 11.2) and drainages (Meyer *et al.*, 1998).

The success rate of imaging-guided biopsy is approximately 80–90 per cent. The most serious complications are pneumothorax and bleeding. On most occasions these can be managed in the interventional suite, e.g. lung aspiration or chest drain insertion for pneumothorax, and embolization for haemoptysis. Although a small pneumothorax is seen on CT images in the majority of patients after lung biopsy, it is present on plain radiograph only in 15–20 per cent of patients; less than 2 per cent require insertion of a chest drain (cf. open lung biopsy, when all patients require a drain). Needle lung biopsy is contraindicated in patients with a bleeding diathesis, emphysema, contralateral pneumonectomy, hydatid disease or suspected arteriovenous malformation, i.e. any patients who could not withstand a pneumothorax or who might bleed uncontrollably. The procedure is of value not only in pulmonary parenchymal lesions but also in the investigation of pleural and mediastinal abnormalities. If the lesion to be biopsied shows evidence of cavitation, it is useful to obtain material from both the centre and periphery of the lesion; this may require multiple passes of the biopsy needle, increasing the risk of pneumothorax. It is important to realize that with percutaneous lung biopsy, as with any other form of biopsy, a single negative result cannot be taken as proof that malignancy is not present. It is generally accepted that three consecutive negative biopsies constitute a 'true' negative result.

PERCUTANEOUS ABDOMINAL BIOPSY

Fine-needle aspiration biopsy (FNAB) employing a 19–22 gauge needle inserted under image guidance has significantly reduced the need for exploratory laparotomy to determine the nature of abdominal, pelvic or retroperitoneal masses. For example, an ultrasound examination of a patient with haematuria may reveal a cystic or solid lesion. FNAB can be performed (often on an outpatient basis) and a cytological diagnosis made within a matter of hours. The success rate of FNAB in obtaining positive cytology exceeds 80 per cent (Mueller *et al.*, 1981) and complications are uncommon. In most cases a percutaneous abdominal biopsy is performed under ultrasound

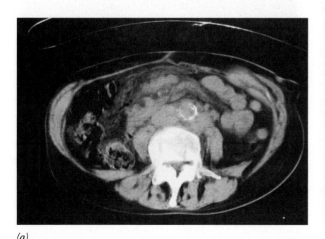

(a)

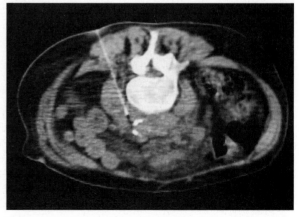

(b)

Figure 11.2 *Percutaneous CT fluoroscopy-guided biopsy of retroperitoneal mass: (a) CT scan, showing soft-tissue mass surrounding the aorta and inferior vena cava; (b) with the patient in the prone position, biopsy needle positioned from left approach (photon starvation artefact confirming position of needle tip). Reproduced with permission from Dr M. Roddie.*

or CT guidance. Both of these methods allow the radiologist to visualize not only the lesion to be targeted for biopsy but also the intervening organs, thus increasing the accuracy and safety of the procedure. The choice between the two techniques depends on the experience and preference of the radiologist and on the precise location of the lesion to be biopsied. For example, retroperitoneal masses are usually easier to visualize on CT scans, whereas lesions in the superior part of the right lobe of the liver immediately below the diaphragm are best biopsied under ultrasound guidance because this modality allows an oblique approach which avoids the lung. US is usually quicker to perform, does not involve ionizing radiation and is available as a portable technique.

In patients with a bleeding diathesis or massive ascites, percutaneous liver biopsy carries an increased risk of major, uncontrollable intraperitoneal haemorrhage. In such patients it is possible to obtain a liver biopsy via a transvascular route (Gilmore *et al.*, 1978; Gamble *et al.*, 1985). Specially designed biopsy instruments can be passed via the right internal jugular vein into the hepatic veins. Bleeding arising from a biopsy taken from this position passes directly back into the patient's circulation and is not therefore of haemodynamic significance. Although successful, this technique is technically demanding and not applicable to focal lesions.

An alternative method of percutaneous liver biopsy, which can be used in patients with abnormal blood coagulation, is plugged liver biopsy. The needle is introduced into the liver within a guiding sheath. The biopsy is performed and the needle is withdrawn, leaving the sheath in place. The biopsy track is then embolized with Sterispon or steel coils as the sheath is withdrawn (Allison and Adam, 1988).

More recently sheaths have become available for use with automated biopsy devices. As these devices allow biopsies to be carried out using relatively small-calibre needles, the tracks are smaller and easier to embolize, thus increasing the safety of the procedure (Dawson *et al.*, 1992).

MUSCULOSKELETAL BIOPSY

The presence of an abnormality within bone on either an isotopic bone scan and/or plain radiography in a patient with known malignancy does not necessarily herald dissemination of the tumour, and it may prove necessary to obtain material for cytology (Armstrong and Chalmers, 1978; Laredo *et al.*, 1994). Solitary bony abnormalities discovered incidentally in a patient who is otherwise well also pose a difficult diagnostic problem. Lytic lesions are relatively straightforward to biopsy (Fig. 11.3), whereas sclerotic lesions give rise to more difficulties and the

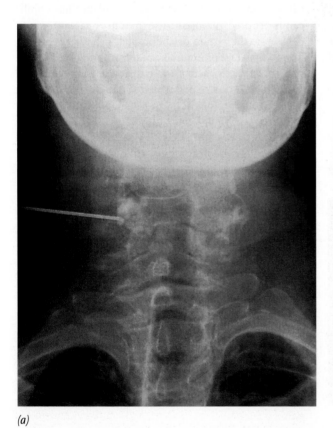

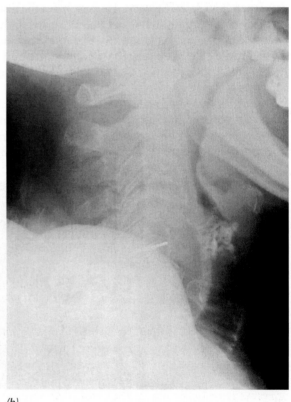

(a)   *(b)*

Figure 11.3 *A musculoskeletal biopsy. A fine-gauge needle has been inserted into a lytic lesion at the level of C5 using biplane fluoroscopic control: (a) = AP; (b) = lateral. The biopsy was performed under local anaesthesia and a diagnosis of osteoclastoma was made. Reproduced with permission from Allison (1987).*

procedure may need to be performed under very heavy sedation or general anaesthesia. CT is extremely useful during the performance of musculoskeletal biopsy because it allows the needle to be guided precisely to the abnormal area. Quite frequently a soft-tissue mass may be associated with lytic bone lesions and CT allows this to be visualized and biopsied. In addition, CT demonstrates areas where the cortex is thinnest and thus easiest to penetrate with a biopsy needle. Another advantage of CT, especially when biopsying lesions in thoracic vertebrae, is that the needle can be guided extrapleurally, thus avoiding the danger of pneumothorax. In a few cases, ultrasound guidance is sufficient. The great benefit of percutaneous biopsy is that the recorded incidence of complications is exceptionally low, the overall success rate is high (70–80 per cent) and the procedure is readily repeatable if the initial result is inconclusive.

MISCELLANEOUS BIOPSY TECHNIQUES

When a mass extends into the superior or inferior vena cava, the transvascular route provides a safe and convenient way of obtaining a biopsy. The femoral vein is punctured at the groin, and a long sheath is introduced into the inferior vena cava and advanced to lie adjacent to the mass to be biopsied. A modified cardiac bioptome is then inserted via the sheath and the biopsy taken (Jackson and Adam, 1991).

Developments in endoluminal ultrasound have allowed lesions deep in the pelvis to be biopsied transrectally (prostate biopsies) or transvaginally (ovarian cysts). The advent of endoscopic and intra-operative ultrasound probes has further extended the versatility of this imaging modality (Machi *et al.*, 1990; Ziegler *et al.*, 1993).

In the management of breast cancer, non-palpable lesions are biopsied or localized using either sterotactic mammography or ultrasound for guidance.

Venous sampling

The diagnosis of a hormone-secreting neoplasm is made on the basis of the clinical history and characteristic biochemical abnormalities. The localization of these tumours may, however, be quite difficult. Ultrasound and CT scanning of the common sites for tumours (e.g. adrenal glands for phaeochromocytomas, pancreas for insulinomas, etc.) will reveal the majority of tumours. However, a few are either too small to be detected by these means or are found in ectopic sites. In these instances, venous sampling techniques can prove invaluable (Allison, 1980). Both systemic and portal blood specimens are obtained from various sites in the venous system and the areas sampled recorded on a map (Fig. 11.4). The specimens are numbered accordingly and taken immediately for appropriate analysis. Areas of high hormone concentration can then be charted on the map and then searched by ultrasound, CT, angiography, MRI or surgery. While

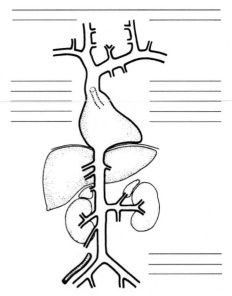

Figure 11.4 *Systemic venous sampling map. A diagram of a systemic venous system indicates the main venous tributaries. Each of these vessels can be selectively catheterized and a sample of blood obtained for hormone analysis.*

systemic venous sampling is relatively safe and has a high success rate, localization of pancreatic or gastrointestinal hormone-producing tumours is a more hazardous technique, as it requires the percutaneous transhepatic cannulation of the portal veins. The reader is referred to more specialized texts for detailed descriptions of these techniques.

THERAPEUTIC PROCEDURES

These are shown in Table 11.1.

Percutaneous puncture and drainage procedures

With the use of fluoroscopy, ultrasound or CT it is possible to image and drain obstructed renal and biliary systems, cysts, abscesses and effusions.

RENAL TRACT

Antegrade pyelography and percutaneous nephrostomy are useful in the management of benign and malignant obstruction of the urinary tract (Papanicolaou, 1996). The technique is also of value in a variety of other situations, e.g. in patients with malignancy undergoing chemotherapy resulting in haemorrhagic cystitis, in whom it is desirable to divert the urine to 'rest' the bladder. In patients with pelvic malignancy, either the disease or the treatment may result in the development of fistulas between the bladder and rectum or vagina, leading to incontinence. Diversion of urinary flow may assist in healing of the fistulas, ease nursing problems and allow patients to become 'dry'.

The procedure, usually performed under local anaesthetic and US guidance, involves an initial puncture of the pelvicalyceal system with a fine needle, followed by the instillation of radiographic contrast medium to demonstrate the anatomy and determine the level of obstruction. Urine can be aspirated for microbiological and cytological examination. Percutaneous nephrostomy entails the insertion of a pigtail catheter with multiple large side ports into the collecting system (Fig. 11.5). The catheter is introduced employing a needle, guide-wire and catheter exchange technique. If drainage is to be of short duration, it is satisfactory to allow the urine to drain externally into a bag. When long-term drainage is required, a J-J stent is inserted with the proximal pigtail coiled in the renal pelvis and the distal end in the bladder (Lu *et al.*, 1994), thus allowing the patient to be free of 'bags'.

In patients with pelvic malignancy and fistulas to the perineum, percutaneous nephrostomy is often insufficient

to achieve complete diversion of the urine. It is frequently necessary to combine nephrostomy with ureteric embolization using steel coils and fragments of gelatin sponge, in order to ensure that no urine reaches the skin of the perineum (Dick *et al.*, 1997).

BILIARY TRACT

Patients with obstructive jaundice due to irresectable malignant biliary strictures can be palliated by the insertion of endoprostheses. For surgical candidates, preoperative biliary drainage may be performed to correct metabolic disturbances and stabilize the patient.

Most patients with malignant obstructive jaundice undergo endoscopic retrograde cholangiopancreaticography (ERCP) as part of the diagnostic work-up. If ERCP confirms a malignant stricture, an endoprosthesis can be inserted immediately after cholangiography. Endoscopic drainage is less invasive than percutaneous biliary drainage (PBD), is associated with fewer complications and avoids the discomfort of a percutaneous biliary catheter. The majority of strictures of the mid and lower common bile ducts, which are mainly due to carcinoma of the head of the pancreas, can be drained effectively by the endoscopic approach, the percutaneous approach being reserved for patients in whom endoscopic drainage attempts have failed. Patients with obstructive jaundice due to malignant tumours at the hilum of the liver are best palliated by percutaneous drainage methods, as the endoscopic approach in such patients often fails and is associated with a high rate of complications. In most cases unilateral drainage is sufficient for relieving jaundice and pruritus.

The procedure is usually carried out under fluoroscopic and US guidance. First a percutaneous transhepatic cholangiogram (PTC) is performed, using a 22-gauge needle. It is important to visualize the entire biliary system prior to selecting the most suitable duct for insertion of a drainage catheter. Self-expandable metallic stents are now widely available and generally preferable to the conventional plastic endoprostheses. Such stents can be inserted using a relatively small introducing catheter and yet achieve a large internal diameter when released across the lesion (Fig. 11.6). The large calibre of these devices ensures that the rate of occlusion is lower than that of plastic endoprostheses. In our experience, the rate of haemorrhage and cholangitis is approximately three times lower with metallic endoprostheses than plastic stents. Most importantly, the rate of re-intervention for the purpose of replacement of occluded stents has also been found to be three times lower with metallic stents (Adam *et al.*, 1991). A randomized comparison of endoscopically inserted self-expanding metal stents and plastic stents has confirmed the longer patency of metallic endoprostheses and has shown that, although these stents are more expensive than the conventional plastic devices, the cost per patient is lower because of the lower rate of re-intervention (Davids *et al.*, 1992).

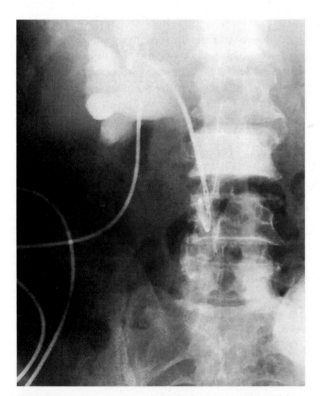

Figure 11.5 *Percutaneous renal drainage. A patient with obstruction of the renal tract secondary to prostatic malignancy (note the sclerotic vertebral body due to metastatic infiltration). A pigtail catheter has been introduced under local anaesthetic into the dilated pelvicalyceal system and ureter. Urine is able to drain via the side ports in the catheter into a drainage bag on the skin surface. Reproduced with permission from Allison (1987).*

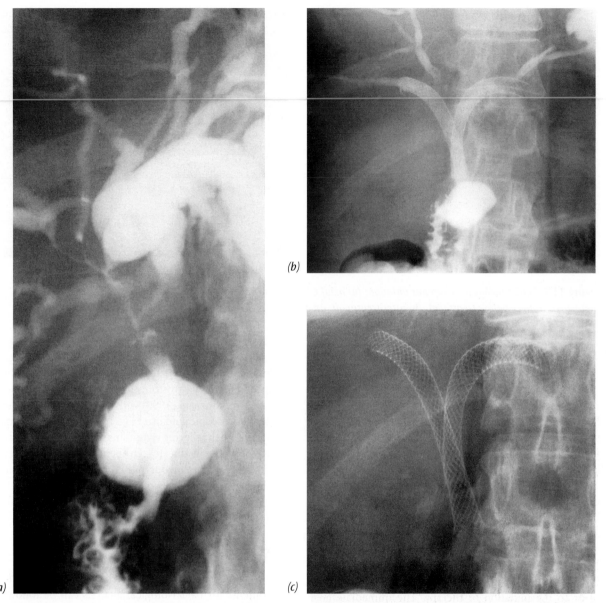

(a) *(b)* *(c)*

Figure 11.6 *(a) Percutaneous transhepatic cholangiogram in a patient with hilar cholangiocarcinoma involving the left and right hepatic ducts and the upper common hepatic duct. (b) Self-expandable metallic endoprostheses have been inserted into both hepatic ducts using separate punctures. Drainage of contrast medium is taking place into the duodenum. (c) The stents are shown in position following complete drainage of the contrast medium.*

Percutaneous treatment of liver metastases

Hepatic resection is the mainstay in the curative management of primary and secondary hepatic malignancies. Surgical resection significantly improves survival, but only a minority of patients are surgical candidates because of the size or location of the lesions, extrahepatic disease or, in the case of hepatoma, limited hepatic functional reserve secondary to associated cirrhosis.

Percutaneous liver tumour ablation Percutaneous techniques of local tumour ablation may be categorized into three major groups: injectables (ethanol, acetic acid, hot saline), heating (radiofrequency, electrocautery, interstitial laser therapy, microwave coagulation therapy and high

intensity focus ultrasound) and freezing (cryotherapy). Of these the most widely used are percutaneous ethanol injection for hepatocellular carcinoma and thermal ablation methods for hepatic metastases.

Percutaneous ethanol injection therapy (PEIT) was first described in 1983 (Sugiura *et al.*, 1983) and since that time has been used extensively for treatment of unresectable hepatocellular carcinoma (Livraghi and Solbiati, 1993). There is no absolute limitation to the size or number of lesions treated.

Lesional heating techniques such as radiofrequency (RF) ablation and interstitial laser photocoagulation (ILP) achieve tumour necrosis by hyperthermia. RF electrodes

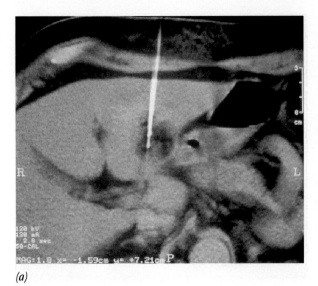
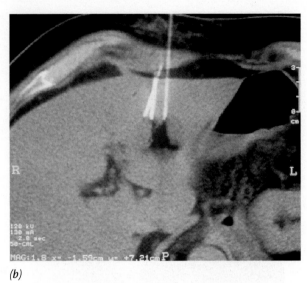

(a)   *(b)*

Figure 11.7 *Percutaneous liver tumour ablation: (a) axial CT scan showing radiofrequency electrode positioned within metastasis in liver before treatment; (b) after treatment, an area of necrosis is seen, indicating successful ablation.*

or laser fibres are inserted into the tumour under ultrasound, CT or MRI guidance (Fig. 11.7). Intralesional hyperthermia causes almost immediate coagulation necrosis.

Radiofrequency waves induce ionic agitation, which results in frictional heat production within the tissue. Serious complications are rare and consist mainly of intraperitoneal haemorrhage and liver abscess formation. Interstitial laser photocoagulation produces thermal coagulation by conversion of absorbed light energy into heat.

The follow-up of patients after all forms of percutaneous tumour ablation includes a combination of imaging, tumour marker assay and selected use of fine-needle aspiration biopsy. It is useful to follow serial levels of α-fetoprotein or carcinoembryonic antigen, in cases of hepatocellular carcinoma or metastatic disease respectively, when the serum levels of these markers are elevated prior to the initiation of therapy. The immediate goal of imaging is to assess whether complete necrosis has been achieved. Ultrasound does not usually provide useful information, as the echogenicity of fibrosis and neoplastic tissue overlap. Contrast-enhanced MRI and contrast-enhanced CT are capable of demonstrating remaining viable tumour requiring treatment. However, in difficult cases, PET scanning may provide additional information.

Better methods of imaging guidance and more sophisticated equipment are likely to increase the importance of percutaneous tumour ablation in the future.

GASTROINTESTINAL TRACT

In the management of patients with malignant disease, nutritional support is essential, particularly in those who are severely debilitated or unable to swallow. Parenteral nutrition can be provided using central venous catheters, but this is associated with significant morbidity and considerable expense. Enteric feeding is more desirable and can be provided by the insertion of gastrostomy tubes.

Gastrojejenostomy tubes are preferable when there is gastric outlet obstruction or in cases of gastro-oesophageal reflux. Several different techniques have been described for percutaneous gastrostomy insertions (van Sonnenberg *et al.*, 1986; Saini *et al.*, 1990) with and without gastropexy under fluoroscopic guidance (Fig. 11.8). Gastrostomy may also be useful in relieving symptoms in patients with gastric outlet obstruction due to retroperitoneal or mesenteric malignancy. Percutaneous puncture for decompression of the caecum (in cases of distal obstruction) and for afferent loop obstruction have been described (Casola *et al.*, 1986; Lee *et al.*, 1987).

ABSCESS DRAINAGE

Percutaneous puncture of an abscess cavity and aspiration of contents for bacteriological analysis can be followed by insertion of a drainage catheter (Gerzof *et al.*, 1981). It is possible to instil antibiotics into the cavity, and percutaneous drainage may be effective either as the definitive treatment or as a temporary measure until the appropriate surgery can be contemplated.

Ultrasound, CT or MRI guidance may be used for abscess drainage. CT is particularly useful for retroperitoneal or mediastinal abscesses where visualization by ultrasound scanning may be inadequate. Transvaginal or transrectal drainage under ultrasound guidance is very useful for certain abscesses in the pelvis.

PERCUTANEOUS VERTEBROPLASTY

Metastases to the vertebrae are common. Radiation therapy is not always effective in relieving the pain. Percutaneous vertebroplasty provides immediate and sustained pain relief, and contributes to spinal stabilization (Weill *et al.*, 1996). The procedure consists of percutaneous injection of acrylic surgical cement into a vertebra under

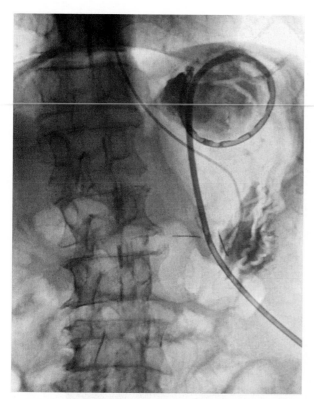

Figure 11.8 *Fluoroscopic insertion of gastrostomy feeding tube. Gastrostomy catheter is locked with pigtail in fundus of stomach. Nasogastric tube and the two 'stay' sutures used for the safe insertion of gastrostomy tube are then removed.*

radiological guidance (fluoroscopy and/or CT). This technique can also be used for treated bone metastases at other sites.

Dilatation techniques

Dilatation procedures (Allison *et al.*, 1997) are most widely employed for non-malignant conditions in the vascular tree. These techniques can also be applied to stenoses and occlusions in other systems, such as the gastrointestinal tract, renal, biliary and respiratory systems.

Fluoroscopically guided oesophageal dilatation has proved to be a particularly useful technique. A guide-wire is manipulated through the narrowed area and a balloon catheter of suitable dimensions is then passed over the wire. Intravenous analgesia should be given immediately prior to balloon inflation, as this can cause moderate discomfort. Dilatation alone is unlikely to be effective in malignant oesophageal strictures and should be followed by some form of stenting. Rigid plastic tubes inserted endoscopically or under fluoroscopic guidance have been used for several years. However, recently, self-expandable metallic endoprostheses have become available (Neuhaus, 1991; Song *et al.*, 1994). With recent advances and increased experience in the use of metallic stents, over 95 per cent of patients with inoperable

oesophageal strictures can be palliated successfully with these devices (Fig. 11.9). Strictures at other sites in the gastrointestinal tract can also be treated successfully by radiological dilatation techniques. The relief of obstruction at anastomotic strictures (gastroenterostomies, antral–pyloric strictures, enteroenterostomies and colorectal strictures) is particularly useful (Grundy, 1992). In cases of acute malignant obstruction of the large bowel, the insertion of self-expanding stents can provide immediate relief (Fig. 11.10). This may be a temporizing measure allowing stabilization of the patient prior to definitive surgery, or alternatively, in patients who are not surgical candidates, the stent may provide adequate palliation (De Gregori *et al.*, 1998).

Malignant airways obstruction can cause considerable distress to patients. When surgical resection is not possible, self-expanding metallic stents can provide good palliation (Tan *et al.*, 1996) (Fig. 11.11). Plastic covered stents are very effective in managing tracheo-oesophageal fistulas unsuitable for treatment with covered oesophageal stents (Morgan *et al.*, 1997). The stents are inserted under general anaesthesia using combined fluoroscopic and bronchoscopic guidance, following balloon dilatation of the strictures.

VENOUS DILATATION AND STENTING

The superior vena caval syndrome is most commonly related to mediastinal neoplasia, particularly primary and secondary lung tumours and lymphoma. The obstruction, which can be partial or complete, may be caused by caval compression or invasion by the tumour, and is sometimes complicated by venous thrombosis.

Cavography delineates the site and extent of the obstruction. Percutaneous transfemoral dilatation of the narrowed cava, combined with thrombolysis where necessary, followed by the insertion of self-expandable metallic endoprostheses, restores flow and provides excellent palliation of symptoms (Irving *et al.*, 1992) (Fig. 11.12).

Malignant involvement of the inferior vena cava can be managed in a similar fashion. Percutaneous insertion of an inferior vena cava filter is indicated in patients with recurrent pulmonary embolism refactory to, or unsuitable for, treatment with medical therapy. In patients with iliac or iliofemoral venous thrombosis due to pelvic malignancy, a temporary filter inserted prior to surgical resection of the tumour may protect from pulmonary embolism.

Extraction techniques

Developments in intravenous feeding therapy and monitoring techniques have led to a vast increase in the number of indwelling venous cannulas and catheters. Unfortunately, these occasionally break or become disconnected, resulting in loss of part or all of the catheter within the venous system (Gibson *et al.*, 1985). It is

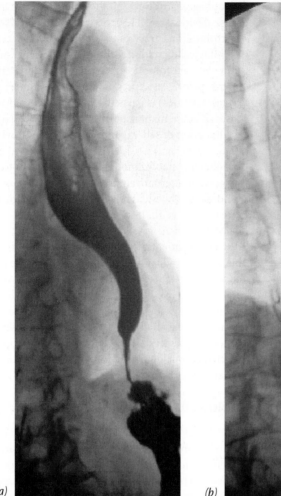
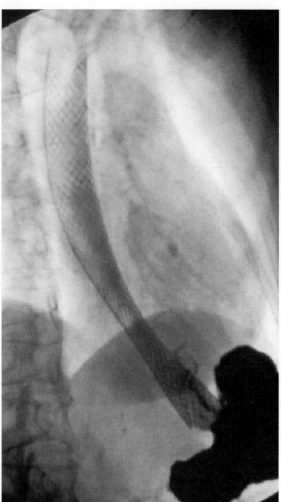

(a)

(b)

Figure 11.9 *Oesophageal stenting: (a) contrast swallow showing lower oesophageal carcinoma stricture; (b) Flamingo Wallstent (self-expanding metallic endoprosthesis) has been placed fluoroscopically across the stricture. Contrast is now flowing freely into the stomach.*

important to retrieve these intravascular foreign bodies as they can perforate vascular structures and cause dysrhythmias, and can be a source of infection, particularly in immunosuppressed patients. Surgical retrieval of catheter fragments necessitates a thoracotomy and carries significant risk. It is almost invariably possible to retrieve these catheter fragments percutaneously under fluoroscopic guidance (Rossi, 1982; Allison *et al.*, 1997) (Fig. 11.13). They usually lodge within the right side of the heart or the pulmonary arteries. A wide variety of instruments has been found to be useful in 'catching' these foreign bodies, including wire-loop snares, grasping forceps, steering catheters and Dormia baskets.

It is usually possible to retrieve the foreign body under local anaesthesia via a percutaneous femoral venous puncture. Detailed descriptions of all the techniques available are beyond the scope of this chapter but any interventional radiologist offering a comprehensive vascular service is well advised to acquaint himself or herself with the various methods and have the necessary equipment available (Belli and Hemingway, 1994).

The ability to snare or 'catch' the end of a catheter can also be of value in patients receiving intravenous cytotoxic chemotherapy in whom the tip of an indwelling central venous catheter has become displaced and lodged in the jugular vein instead of the superior vena cava. It is usually possible to 'pull' such a catheter back to the appropriate position using a percutaneous vascular approach under local anaesthesia.

Infusion techniques

The ability of the radiologist accurately to site a catheter into virtually any blood vessel within the body has brought into play the concepts of regional infusion of chemotherapeutic agents, monoclonal antibodies and isotopes. The principle underlying these techniques is that a high dose of the therapeutic agent is delivered to the tumour(s) with minimal systemic side-effects. Recent advances include the addition of embolic materials (*see* embolization section, below) and the microencapsulation of cytotoxic agents to achieve gradual and sustained

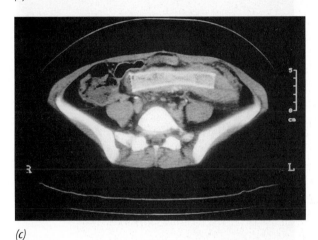
(a)

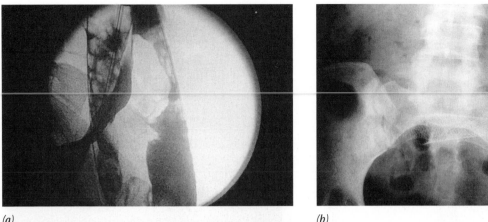
(b)

(c)

Figure 11.10 *Colonic stenting. (a) Contrast study of the sigmoid colon; lateral view of the pelvis, showing carcinoma stricture of the sigmoid colon. A guide-wire and catheter have been placed across the stricture. (b) A self-expanding metallic endoprostheses has been deployed across the stricture. (c) CT scan, showing the expanded stent within the sigmoid tumour. The patient's obstructive symptoms were successfully palliated.*

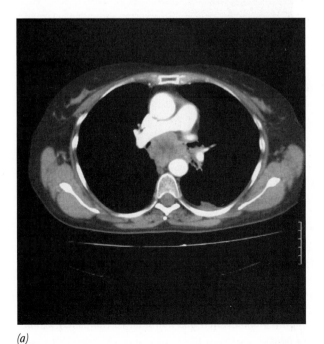
(a)

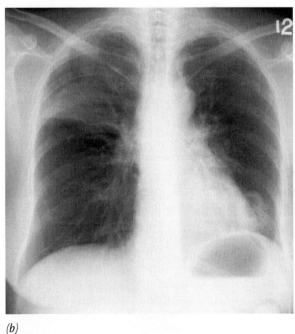
(b)

Figure 11.11 *Tracheal stenting. (a) Axial CT scan of a section through the chest, showing tumour and nodal mass encasing and compressing both main bronchi. (b) Chest X-ray after deployment of two self-expanding metal endoprostheses situated in the trachea and extending into both main bronchi.*

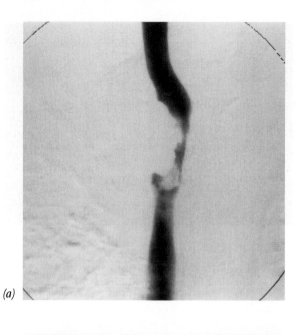

(a)

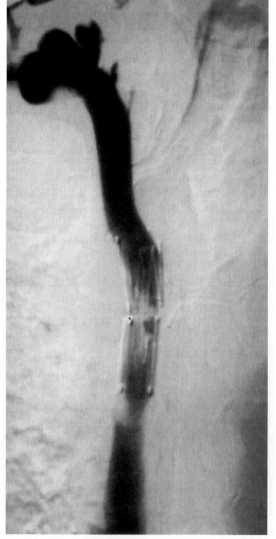

(c)

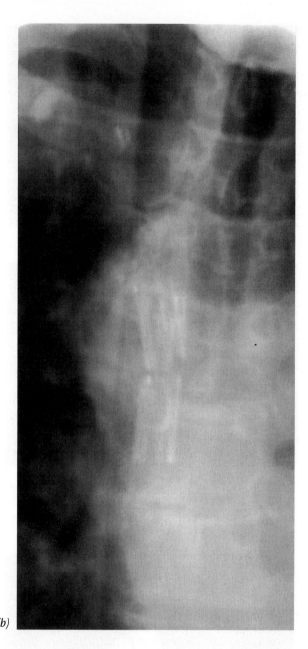

(b)

Figure 11.12 *Superior vena caval stenting. (a) Superior vena cavogram reveals severe narrowing of the superior vena cava (SVC) by tumour in the mediastinum. (b) Metal stents have been placed across the compressed area, which was initially dilated with a balloon. (c) A repeat venogram confirms patency of the SVC. The patient's symptoms improved immediately and had resolved completely within 24 hours.*

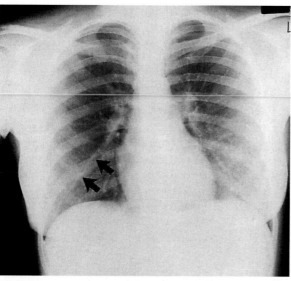

(a)

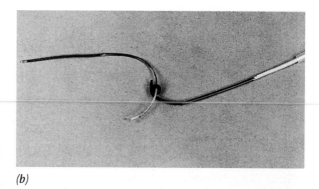

(b)

Figure 11.13 *(a) A chest radiograph in a young girl undergoing cytotoxic therapy in whom part of a central venous catheter became detached and migrated into a right lower lobe pulmonary artery (arrows). (b) The catheter fragment after extraction via the femoral vein, grasped in the catheter used for retrieval.*

release. Lipiodol is now also used in combination with cytotoxic drugs for the treatment of certain hepatic tumours; it is retained in tumour vessels and also acts as a contrast agent, thus allowing monitoring of tumour response to treatment using CT guidance.

These techniques have been used with varying degrees of success to treat primary and metastatic liver tumours (Balch and Levin, 1987), bone neoplasms, cerebral neoplasms, sarcomas, melanomas and pelvic neoplasms. It is possible to insert fine catheters that can be left in place for weeks at a time (Chuang and Wallace, 1987a).

A variety of long-term venous access lines (tunnelled central venous catheters, peripherally inserted central catheters (PICC) and Portacaths), have been developed for insertion under fluoroscopic and ultrasound guidance (Robertson *et al.*, 1989). Radiological techniques are best suited for their insertion (Adam, 1995). Tunnelled external catheters are most frequently used. The preferred access sites are the internal jugular and subclavian veins, but other veins can be used in cases of difficulty, including the common femoral, translumbar, inferior vena cava and hepatic veins. PICC lines are more usually inserted for shorter duration of therapy, with the basilic vein being the preferred site of puncture.

Vascular embolization

This technique (Allison *et al.*, 1997) involves the deliberate occlusion of arteries and/or veins by the injection of embolic agents through selectively placed catheters. It is one of the major applications of interventional radiology in patients with neoplastic disease and has been employed in the management of a wide variety of tumours.

Embolization, usually performed by a percutaneous approach under local anaesthesia, offers an attractive alternative to surgery and, in some situations, it is the only therapeutic option available. A wide variety of embolic agents is available (Hemingway, 1986) and a detailed description is beyond the scope of this chapter. The broad categories of substances used include particulate emboli (sterile sponge (Spongostan), polyvinyl alcohol (Ivalon)), mechanical emboli (balloons, steel coils) and liquids (50 per cent dextrose, absolute alcohol, lipiodol). The appropriate agent or combination of agents depends on the lesion to be treated and its site, with particular attention paid to adjacent vulnerable vascular structures.

There are three ways in which embolization can assist in the management of neoplasms: definitive, preoperative or palliative. Definitive treatment can only be offered in benign lesions.

PREOPERATIVE EMBOLIZATION

This has been widely employed in the management of renal carcinomas, although not all urologists find the technique useful. The tumour is embolized and surgery undertaken within 24–48 hours, while there is maximum devascularization and minimal oedema. Preoperative embolization reduces blood loss, and may minimize dissemination of malignant cells during tumour mobilization. Preoperative tumour embolization has proven to be of value in other situations, including nasopharyngeal tumours, paragangliomas, meningiomas and bone tumours (Fig. 11.14) (Allison *et al.*, 1997). In the latter example, the inclusion of a cytotoxic agent within the embolization 'cocktail' may further reduce the risk of tumour dissemination during surgery.

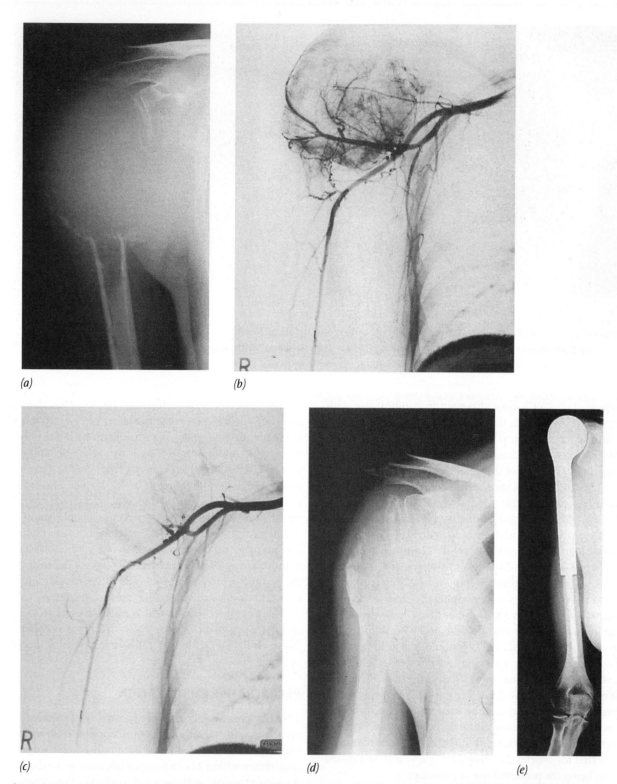

(a)

(b)

(c)

(d)

(e)

Figure 11.14 *Preoperative embolization of a bone neoplasm (osteoclastoma) in a 17-year-old girl which had proved resistant to radiotherapy. A plain radiograph (a) reveals a large soft-tissue mass with extensive bone destruction. Axillary arteriography shows the lesion to be highly vascular. (b) The feeding vessels selectively catheterized and embolized. The postembolization angiogram (c) shows the lesion to be completely devascularized. A plain radiograph 3 months later (d) shows considerable reduction in the size of the mass and bone regrowth. This improvement allowed reconstructive surgery to be performed. A humeral replacement (e) was successfully carried out. Reproduced with permission from Allison (1987).*

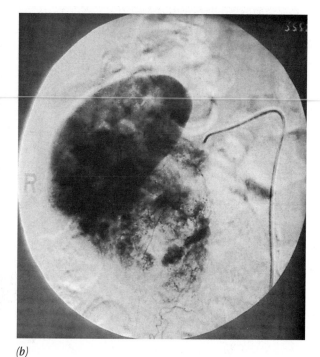

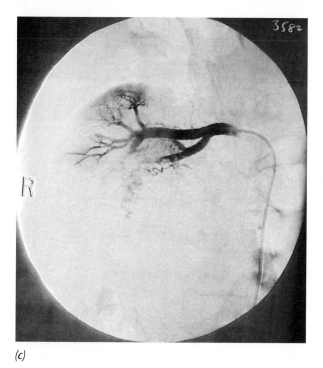

Figure 11.15 *Selective right renal arteriography, (a) arterial and (b) and (c) venous phases, reveals a highly vascular renal tumour in the lower pole of the kidney. The vessels supplying the tumour were selectively catheterized and embolized with particulate material, depriving it of its blood supply and relieving the patient of pain and haematuria. Reproduced with permission from Allison (1987).*

PALLIATIVE EMBOLIZATION

This technique is employed to control pain, haemorrhage and hormone production, as well as to reduce tumour bulk. It may be used as the primary mode of treatment in inoperable malignancy. Embolization of metastatic deposits has, in some situations, been shown to extend survival times in advanced disease (Chuang and Wallace, 1987b). Tumours in many organs have been treated in this fashion (liver, kidney (Fig. 11.15), bone,

lung, soft tissues, nervous system and gastrointestinal tract). Hormone-secreting neoplasms (e.g. metastatic carcinoid and APUD cell tumours) (Fig. 11.16) show the greatest therapeutic response to arterial embolization. Appropriate pharmacological blockade is necessary during the embolization to avoid the effects of a massive outpouring of hormone as the tumour is deprived of its blood supply. The beneficial effects of embolization may become apparent within a matter of hours.

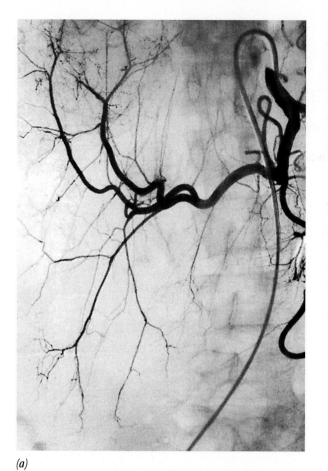

(a)

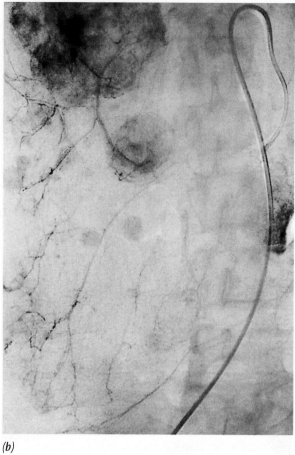

(b)

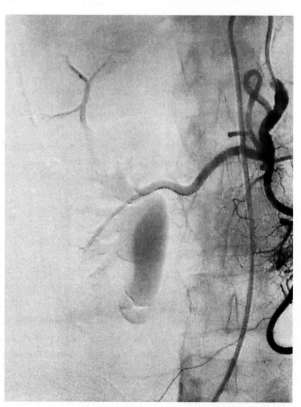

(c)

Figure 11.16 *Hepatic embolization for metastatic carcinoid tumour. (a) The early arterial phase shows hepatic enlargement. (b) The parenchymal phase reveals multiple tumour deposits. (c) Post-embolization arteriogram shows that the arterial supply has been obliterated. The patient's symptoms (flushing and diarrhoea) were dramatically alleviated by this procedure. Reproduced with permission from Allison (1987).*

In embolization procedures it is important that adequate premedication is given prior to the procedure, including broad-spectrum antibiotics. In many situations, e.g. liver and bone, it is advisable to continue antibiotics for 10 days after the procedure to prevent sepsis developing in the devascularized tissue.

After embolization, patients commonly experience some discomfort and pain. They may have a pyrexia for a few days, accompanied by a feeling of malaise and an elevated white cell count. This combination of signs and symptoms is known as the post-embolization syndrome (PES), an indicator of the presence of necrotic tissue. Any sustained pyrexia should alert the clinician to the possibility of abscess formation, and blood cultures and regional ultrasound should be performed. Serum C-reactive protein (CRP) estimations can also provide a useful indication that infection may be present. Following embolization, CRP reaches a peak at about 4 days, falling off thereafter to reach normal levels at 10 days. A continued CRP rise, or failure to fall, indicates infection. (Hemingway and Allison, 1988).

Neurolysis

Alcohol injection is useful in the palliation of intractable pain which occasionally accompanies retroperitoneal malignancy. For example, certain patients with carcinoma of the pancreas experience severe pain due to infiltration of the coeliac ganglion by the tumour. In these patients the ganglion may be ablated by injecting alcohol in its immediate vicinity under CT guidance (Fig. 11.17).

CHEMOEMBOLIZATION

Embolic agents in combination with chemotherapeutic drugs are being used in the treatment of certain malignancies. In this technique, known as chemoembolization (Kato *et al.*, 1981), the emboli cause ischaemia of the tumour cells and, by increasing the transit time through the tumour vascular bed, the contact time between the cytotoxic agent and the neoplastic cells is prolonged, resulting in a greater therapeutic effect.

Gene therapy

The most rapidly evolving area in medicine is gene therapy. The underlying principle is to identify and clone a gene, and then to insert it into a vector capable of directing expression in mammalian tissues (Voss and Kruskal, 1998). The main aim at present is to treat genetic deficiencies and malignant diseases refractory to conventional therapies. The delivery systems involved include retroviral vectors (RNA viruses), adenoviral vectors (DNA viruses) and cationic liposomes, along with strategies that involve ultrasound-directed gene transfer, CT-guided gene transfer and transcatheter gene delivery, in particular via the hepatic artery. Examples of genes being evaluated in trial include oncogenes, tumour suppressor genes, suicide genes and antiangiogenesis factors. The liver is an ideal therapeutic target for gene therapy. Hepatic malignancies being considered for treatment include metastatic colorectal carcinoma, hepatoma, cholangiocarcinoma, lymphoma, metastatic melanoma and haemangioma. Gene therapy strategies for managing occluded biliary stents (resulting from tumour ingrowth) and vascular transjugular intrahepatic portosystemic stents (resulting from neoendothelialization) are also under consideration. In gene delivery, angiographic guidance will be of use in localizing tumour blood supply and directing the targeted intra-arterial delivery of genes of interest, so that vector–DNA complexes can be delivered with accuracy and specificity. Embolization techniques may also be of benefit, by prolonging vector contact with the target cells, thus delaying washout and further enhancing target cell uptake. Radiological monitoring will be

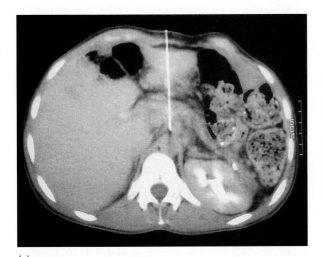

(a)

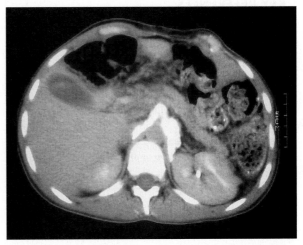

(b)

Figure 11.17 *Coeliax axis block for intractable pain in a patient with pancreatic carcinoma. (a) Axial CT scan with a 22-gauge needle positioned with its tip at level of the coeliac ganglion. (b) Bilateral spill seen following injection of alcohol.*

of considerable importance during gene delivery, e.g. the process of liposomal vector delivery can be monitored accurately with ultrasound because lipid vesicles are echogenic. Guided biopsy of transduced tissues for histopathologic analysis after gene delivery should also improve confidence in the evaluation of gene expression.

SIGNIFICANT POINTS

- An interventional procedure should only be contemplated if it is likely to benefit the patient's quality of life.
- Some interventional procedures are replacing surgical alternatives; others are totally new forms of treatment.
- Diagnostic invasive procedures, e.g. biopsy, are significantly less traumatic than their surgical alternatives.
- All interventional procedures require a team approach to ensure the best possible outcome for the patient.
- Advances in imaging technology and instrumentation are constantly occurring, leading to the emergence of new interventional techniques.
- Many interventional procedures, e.g. tunnelled central venous catheter insertion, SVC stenting, percutaneous drainage, are carried out in conjunction with, and enable the more effective use of, conventional forms of cancer therapy.

KEY REFERENCES

Allison, D.J., Wallace, S. and Machan, L. (1997) Interventional radiology. In Grainger, R.G. and Allison, D.J. (eds), *Diagnostic radiology: an Anglo-American textbook of organ imaging*, (3rd edn). Edinburgh: Churchill Livingstone, 2483–550.

Watkinson, A. and Adam, A. (eds) (1996) *Interventional radiology, a practical guide.* Oxford: Radcliffe Medical Press, 88–118.

REFERENCES

Adam, A. (1995) Insertion of long term central venous catheter: time for a new look. *BMJ* **311**, 341–2.

Adam, A. (1998) The definition of interventional radiology (or, 'When is a barium enema an interventional procedure?'). *Eur. Radiol.* **8**, 1014–15.

Adam, A., McSweeney, J.E., Whyte, M.K.B. *et al.* (1989) CT-guided extra-pleural drainage of bronchogenic cyst. *J. Comput. Assist. Tomogr.* **13**, 1065–8.

Adam, A., Chetty, N., Roddie, M. *et al.* (1991) Self-expandable stainless steel endoprostheses for treatment of malignant bile duct obstruction. *AJR* **156**, 321–5.

Allison, D.J. (1980) Therapeutic embolization and venous sampling. In Taylor, S. (ed.), *Recent advances in surgery*, vol. 10. Edinburgh: Churchill Livingstone, 27–64.

Allison, D.J. and Adam, A. (1988) Percutaneous liver biopsy followed by embolization of the track with steel coils. *Radiology* **169**, 261–3.

Allison, D.J. and Hemingway, A.P. (1981) Percutaneous needle biopsy of the lung. *BMJ* **282**, 875–8.

Allison, D.J., Wallace, S. and Machan, L.S. (1997) Interventional radiology: In Grainger, R.G. and Allison, D.J. (eds), *Diagnostic radiology: an Anglo-American textbook of organ imaging*, (3rd edn). Edinburgh: Churchill Livingstone, 2483–550.

Armstrong, P. and Calmers, A.H. (1978) Needle aspiration of the spine in suspected disc space infection, *Br. J. Radiol.* **51**, 333–7.

Athanasoulis, C.A., Pfister, R.C., Greene, R.E. and Roberson, G.H. (1981) *Interventional Radiology.* Philadelphia: WB Saunders.

Balch, C.M. and Levin, B. (1987) Regional and systemic chemotherapy for colorectal metastases to the liver. *World J. Surg.* **11**, 521–6.

Belli, A.M. and Hemingway, A.P. (1994) Retrieval of intravascular foreign bodies. In Belli, A.M. (ed.), *Interventional radiology in the peripheral vascular system.* London: Edward Arnold, 81–92.

Casola, J., Withers, C., van Sonnenberg, E. *et al.* (1986) Percutaneous cecostomy for decompression of the massively distended cecum. *Radiology* **158**, 793–4.

Chuang, V.P. and Wallace, S. (1987a) Arterial infusion and occlusion in cancer patients. *Semin. Roentgenol.* **16**, 13–25.

Chuang, V.P. and Wallace, S. (1987b) Hepatic artery embolization in the treatment of hepatic neoplasms. *Radiology* **140**, 51–8.

Davids, P.H.P., Groen, A.K., Rauws, E.A.J. *et al.* (1992). Randomized trial of self-expanding metal stents verses polyethylene stents for distal malignant biliary obstruction. *Lancet* **340**, 1488–92.

Dawson, P., Adam, A. and Edwards, R. (1992) Technique for steel coil-embolization of liver biopsy track for use with the 'Biopty' needle. *Br. J. Radiol.* **65**, 538–40.

De Gregorio, M.A., Mainar, A., Tejero, E. *et al.* (1998) Acute colorectal obstruction: stent placement for palliative treatment-results of a multicenter study. *Radiology* **209**, 117–20.

Dick, R., Adam, A. and Allison, D.J. (1997) Interventional techniques in the hepatobiliary system. In Grainger, R. and Allison, D.J. (eds), *Diagnostic radiology: an Anglo-American textbook of organ imaging*, (3rd edn). Edinburgh: Churchill-Livingstone, 1235–58.

Gamble, P.M., Colapinto, R.F., Stronell, R.G. *et al.* (1985) Transjugular liver biopsy: a review of 461 biopsies. *Radiology* **157**, 589–93.

Gerzof, S.G., Spira, R. and Robins, A.H. (1981) Percutaneous abscess drainage. *Semin. Roentgenol.* **16**, 62–71.

Gibson, R.N., Hennessy, O.F., Collier, N. and Hemingway, A.P. (1985) Major complications of central venous catheterization. A report of five cases and brief review of the literature. *Clin. Radiol.* **36**, 204–8.

Gilmore, I.T., Bradley, R.D. and Thompson, R.P.H. (1978) Improved method of transvenous liver biopsy. *BMJ* **ii**, 249.

Greene, R.E. (1981) Transthoracic needle aspiration biopsy. In Athanasoulis, C.A., Pfister, R.C., Greene, R.E. and Robertson, G.H. (eds), *Interventional radiology*. Philadelphia: WB Saunders, 587–637.

Grundy, A. (1992) The radiological management of gastrointestinal strictures and other obstructive lesions. In Adam. A. and Allison, D.J. (eds), *Clinical gastroenterology. Interventional radiology of the abdomen*. London: Bailliere Tindall, vol. 6 No. 2, 319–40.

Haubeck, A., Gammelgaard, G., Gronvall, S. and Holm, H.H. (1982) Ultrasonically-guided percutaneous puncture and biopsy technique. In Wilkins, R.A. and Viamonte, M.J.R. (eds), *Interventional radiology*. Oxford: Blackwell Scientific Publications, 373–408.

Hemingway, A.P. (1986) Materials for embolization. *Radiology Now* **3**, 63–4.

Hemingway, A.P. and Allison, D.J. (1988) Complications of embolization: analysis of 410 procedures. *Radiology* **166**, 669–72.

Husband, J.E. and Golding, S.J. (1983) Recent developments in whole body computed tomography. In Steiner, R.E. (ed.), *Recent advances in radiology*. Edinburgh: Churchill Livingstone, vol. 7, 88–106.

Irving, J.D., Dondelinger, R.F., Reidy, J.F. *et al.* (1992) Gianturco self-expanding stents: clinical experience in the vena cava and large veins. *Cardiovasc. Intervent. Radiol.* **15**, 351–5.

Jackson, J. and Adam, A. (1991) Percutaneous transcaval tumour biopsy using a 'road map' technique. *Clin. Radiol.* **44**, 195–6.

Katada, K., Kato, R., Anno, H. *et al.* (1996) Guidance with real-time CT fluoroscopy: early clinical experience. *Radiology* **200**, 851–6.

Kato, L., Nemeto, R., Mori, H. *et al.* (1981) Arterial chemoembolization with microencapsulated anticancer drug. *JAMA* **245**, 1123–7.

Laredo, J.D., Bellaiche, L., Hamze, B. *et al.* (1994) Current status of musculoskeletal interventional radiology. *Radiol. Clin. North Am.* **32**, 377–98.

Lee, L.I., Teplick, S.K., Haskin, P.N. *et al.* (1987) Refactory afferent loop problems: percutaneous transhepatic management of two cases. *Radiology* **165**, 49–50.

Livraghi, T. and Solbiati, L. (1993) Percutaneous ethanol injection in liver cancer: methods and results. *Semin. Intervent. Radiol.* **10**(2), 69–77.

Lu, D.S.K., Papanicolaou, N., Girard, M. *et al.* (1994) Percutaneous internal ureteral stent placement: review of technical issues and solutions in 50 consecutive cases. *Clin. Radiol.* **49**, 256–61.

Machi, J., Sigel, B., Kurohisi, T. *et al.* (1990) Operative ultrasound guidance for various surgical procedures. *Ultrasound Med. Biol.* **16**, 37–42.

Meyer, C.A., White, C., Wu, J. *et al.* (1998) Real-time CT fluoroscopy: usefulness in thoracic drainage. *AJR* **171**, 1097–101.

Morgan, R., Ellul, J., Denton, E. *et al.* (1997) Malignant esophageal fistulas and perforations: management with plastic-covered metallic endoprostheses. *Radiology* **204**, 527–32.

Mueller, P.R., Wittenberg, J. and Ferrucci. J.T. Jr (1981) Fine needle aspiration biopsy of abdominal masses. *Semin. Roentgenol.* **16**, 52–61.

Mueller, P.R., Stark, D.D., Simeone, J.F. *et al.* (1986) MR-guided aspiration biopsy: needle design and clinical trials. *Radiology* **161**, 605–9.

Neuhaus, H. (1991) Metal oesophageal stents. *Semin. Intervent. Radiol.* **8**, 305–10.

Papanicolaou, N. (1996) Uroradiological intervention. In Watkinson, A. and Adam, A. (eds), *Interventional radiology, a practical guide*. Oxford: Radcliffe Medical Press, 88–118.

Robertson, L.J., Mauro, M.A. and Jacques, P.F. (1989) Radiologic placement of Hickman catheters. *Radiology* **170**, 1007–9.

Rossi, P. (1982) Percutaneous removal of intravascular foreign bodies. In Wilkins, R.A. and Viamonte, M. (eds), *Interventional radiology*. Oxford: Blackwell Scientific Publications, 359–69.

Saini, S.J., Mueller, P.R., Gaa, J. *et al.* (1990) Percutaneous gastrostomy with gastropexy: experience in 125 patients. *AJR* **154**, 1003–6.

Song, H.-Y., Do, Y.S., Han, Y.M. *et al.* (1994) Covered, expandable oesophageal metallic stent tubes: experiences in 119 patients. *Radiology* **193**, 689–95.

Sugiura, N., Takara, K., Ohto, M. *et al.* (1983) Percutaneous intratumoral injection of ethanol under ultrasound imaging for treatment of small hepatocellular carcinoma. *Acta Hepatol. Jpn* **24**, 920–3.

Tan, B.S., Watkinson, A.F., Dussek, J.E. and Adam, A. (1996) Metallic endoprosthesis for malignant tracheo-bronchial obstruction: initial experience. *Cardiovasc. Intervent. Radiol.* **19**, 91–6.

van Sonnenberg, E., Wittich, G.R., Cabrera, O.A. *et al.* (1986) Percutaneous gastrostomy and gastroenterostomy: 2. Clinical experience. *AJR* **146**, 581–6.

van Sonnenberg, E., Casola, G., Ho, M. *et al.* (1988) Difficult thoracic lesions: CT guided biopsy experience in 150 cases. *Radiology* **167**, 457–61.

Voss, S.D. and Kruskal, J.B. (1998) Gene therapy: a primer for radiologists. *Radiographics* **18**, 1343–72.

Weill, A., Chiras, J., Simon, J.M. *et al.* (1996) Spinal metastases: indications for and results of percutaneous injection of acrylic surgical cement. *Radiology* **199**, 241–7.

Ziegler, K., Sanft, C., Zimmer, T. *et al.* (1993) Comparison of computed tomography, endosonography and intraoperative assessment in TN staging of gastric carcinoma. *Gut* **34**, 604–10.

12

Bio-immunotherapy approaches to cancer treatment

ANTHONY MARAVEYAS, HARDEV PANDHA AND ANGUS DALGLEISH

INTRODUCTION

Immunotherapy is undergoing a resurgence of interest following several decades of relative neglect. The turn of the twentieth century saw much interest in immunotherapy-type of approaches, e.g. toxin treatment. The advent of radiotherapy and chemotherapy, with their ability to induce visible tumour kill, deflected any further development in this field. This led to the development of 'objective response criteria' to help assess the relative merit of these treatments in the clinical situation. It has slowly become apparent that these criteria do not relate to some of the therapeutic effects often expected or sought from immuno/biotherapeutic strategies. This has been a recurrent and important issue of contention. Only over the past few years it is becoming more accepted that conventional criteria (e.g. WHO response criteria) used for the assessment of cytotoxic responses are inadequate and possibly misapplied when one tries to assess immunobiotherapy outcomes, specifically vaccine-based treatments. Quantification of criteria that assess cytotoxic treatment efficacy, such as dose-limiting toxicity, response rate, response duration, tumour-free survival or time to progression, in phase I/II studies allows the researcher to assess whether the agent in question has comparable activity/toxicity to existing compounds and whether further assessment in a randomized phase III trial is warranted. Although, for some biotreatments (cf. mono-clonal antibodies, below), these criteria may be legitimate end points, dose response is certainly not evident.

Furthermore, in other settings response criteria can be too crude to assess biological treatments which could be functioning by transforming the cancer process into a chronic illness (e.g. anti-angiogenesis targeting, cancer vaccines, etc.). The only outcome, therefore, that one can reasonably measure at present is overall survival. The development of surrogate end points for these treatments is a crucial field of research.

Before the advent of cytotoxics, biotherapies, although largely unsuccessful, were the mainstay of non-radiotherapy cancer therapeutics. It is not difficult to see how these approaches, where the inability to reproduce results or formulas and the complete lack of any scientific principles underpinning the expected efficacy, were eclipsed by the advent of cytotoxics. The current renaissance does not mean that bio-immunotherapies are even close to becoming as effective as some of the mainstream modalities in what they do, and they are unlikely to supplant these in the foreseeable future, if ever. Nevertheless, years of persevering, changes in expectations and a more rational positioning of these treatments as adjuncts to the mainstays are starting to bear fruit. This chapter will focus on the potential and impact of immune-based biotreatment approaches to cancer.

TUMOUR IMMUNOLOGY

The activation of the immune system is an attractive concept because it inherently implies specificity and amplification of the anti-tumour response once achieved. A comprehensive review of tumour immunology is beyond the scope of this chapter (Maraveyas *et al.*, 1998), nevertheless a basic outline of the mechanisms presumed to explain the potential of cancer to escape from the intact immune system is necessary.

Despite some indirect evidence, the existence of cancer immunosurveillance in the normal host is an unproven axiom, which is, however, central to cancer immunotherapeutics. It is postulated that a breach in this system allows the development of a tumour *de novo*. Of interest is that even micrometastases in the bone marrow of patients with early breast cancer, or even ductal carcinoma *in situ* (DCIS), exhibit genetic heterogeneity consistent with metastatogenic potential; nevertheless, many years may elapse before macrometastases actually develop. This state, currently known as tumour dormancy, can be interpreted as a general host characteristic (state of immune competence versus immune dysfunction of the host), or conversely a tumour characteristic (e.g. inability to induce neovasculature). A different possibility, however, arises from the assumption that all hosts are immunocompetent at the outset. This would indicate that the cancer cell harbours, at a specific point in its evolution, a feature or features that 'holds it hostage' to the immune response without this being a specific property of immunocompetence.

While, as mentioned above, the concept of immunosurveillance remains speculative, there is ample evidence that the presence of advanced cancer perpetuates a situation of immune dysfunction. It is probably inappropriate to term this state 'immunosuppression' as it bears little, if any, resemblance to immunosuppression in the classical sense, e.g. drug (cyclosporin) or virus (HIV) induced immunosuppression.

A number of theories to explain this immune dysfunction have been proposed, and experimental evidence exists which points to various possible mechanisms, operating either in isolation or in combination:

1 Cell heterogeneity enables subsets of the tumour cell population to evade the host's immune response as well as to evolve to resist chemical, physical and biological therapies (Heppner, 1984; Nowell, 1986). The melanoma ganglioside profile, for example, has been shown to change in parallel to the increase in the radial dimension of the tumour (Ravindranath *et al.*, 1989). This is consistent with the possibility that antigenic variants are being selected, under a constant backdrop of immunosurveillance evolutionary pressures, for their ability to escape from this defence mechanism.

2 Functional deficits to T cells through dysfunction of the T-cell receptor ζ-chain (TCR$_\zeta$) and to natural killer (NK) cells through inactivation of NF-κB p65, although seeming to start at the site of the tumour infiltrating monocyte population, eventually become detectable in the peripheral blood. TCR$_\zeta$ undergoes an ordered series of phosphorylations in response to receptor engagement, the level of phosphorylation being dependent on the nature of the ligand. Modulation of these phosphorylations may induce qualitative changes in the T-cell reaction (Kersh *et al.*, 1998). However, there also seems to be a reduction in the levels of TCR$_\zeta$. It is likely that loss of TCR$_\zeta$ is due to proteolysis, as no change has been found at the mRNA level (Reichert *et al.*, 1998). This suggests that the tumour microenvironment (tumour cells, stroma or other host cells infiltrating the area) induces signalling deficiencies, which are not antigen specific. Of interest is that either removal of tumour-infiltrating lymphocytes (TILs) from the tumour environment and culture in the presence of interleukin-2 (IL-2), or extirpation of the tumour, restores TIL function. In a study in renal cell carcinoma (RCC) patients treated with IL-2-based therapies, restoration of TCR$_\zeta$ was seen only in complete responders (Gratama *et al.*, 1999), and similar findings, although to a lesser extent, were reported in patients with malignant melanoma (Rabinowich *et al.*, 1996; Kersh *et al.*, 1999).

3 The density of the antigen on a cell may be lower than a threshold level required for recognition by the immune system (Welt *et al.*, 1987). The pattern of a surface distribution of the antigen may differ between normal and tumour cells. Sialylated tumour-associated antigens (TAAs) are only weakly immunogenic. Removal of sialic acid with neuraminidase can enhance immune recognition and tumour cell destruction (Takita *et al.*, 1976).

4 The host immune system may be overwhelmed by an overload of continuously shed TAAs, with a net result of induction of tolerance. This would be proportionate to the tumour's size, offering one explanation of the progressive deterioration of the immune status of the host with progression of the cancer (Herlyn *et al.*, 1985). Removing the growing neoplasm may reverse such suppression. It has also been shown that circulating TAA–antibody complexes may reduce the ability of circulating antibodies to mediate complement-dependent ADCC (antibody-dependent cell-mediated cytotoxicity) (Gupta *et al.*, 1979), or may even induce apoptosis of activated T cells by shedding HLA class I antigens.

5 T cells can be stimulated only if they encounter the relevant antigen presented by APCs (antigen-presenting cells). Activated T cells can home-in on cancer cells only if expression of MHC class I is present on the tumour cells. Furthermore, the expression of co-stimulatory molecules, such as B7, is mandatory for T-cell activation (Townsend and Allison, 1993). Many tumour cells evolve into states where these molecules are either deficient or non-existent (Freeman *et al.*, 1993). Also of great interest is the observation that if antigen is presented without the co-stimulatory

molecules, a state of anergy can be induced (reviewed by Dalgleish, 1996). Events at different levels in the HLA expression pathway can lead to loss or down-regulation of MHC class I, for example:

(a) mutations in HLA and related genes (β2m gene and heavy chain gene) or the promoter regions;
(b) defects in the transcription and translation pathways due to abnormal methylation of the DNA;
(c) deficient peptide transport into the endoplasmic reticulum (ER) due to transporter associated with antigen processing (TAP) gene downregulation or mutation; and
(d) defective glycosylation of the class I molecule.

However, recent evidence is emerging that even this mechanism of evasion needs to be finely balanced. Total loss of HLA, which is a frequent finding (9–52 per cent), through interference, for example, with β-microglobulin synthesis or transport, may not be the most effective method of evasion of the immune system. This may expose these tumour variants to NK cell attack since these cells lyse HLA class I-deficient targets. The experimental evidence tends to favour a modulatory function of HLA through KIRs (killer-cell inhibitory receptors) on NK cells. Some of these receptors belong to the immunoglobulin superfamily (Ig-SF, e.g. HLA-A [p140] and HLA-B [p70]) while others bear a C-type lectin domain (e.g. CD94). From the above one can postulate that the maximum loss of HLA that will not induce NK attack is the tumour phenotype that will be selected by the environmental pressures of the immune system (Ljunggren and Karre, 1990; Ward et al., 1990).

6 Humoral effects of tumour milieu on the T-cell population; tumour infiltrating lymphocytes proliferate less readily in response to IL-2 or mitogens, yet CD4 T cells are more abundant in TIL subpopulations, possibly furthering immunosuppression through propagation of local Th2 response cytokines. Cell suspensions from melanomas derived from patients have been shown to manufacture immunosuppressant cytokine, e.g. IL-10 (Sato et al., 1996). Even more interestingly, vascular endothelial growth factor (VEGF), a growth factor expressed ubiquitously by cancer cells, has been shown to have a profound immunosuppressant effect on APCs, perturbing adequate antigen presentation (Gabrilovich et al., 1996). The observation that most cancers are in areas of chronic inflammation that induces angiogenesis and suppression of cell-mediated immunity strongly suggests that immunoregulatory escape by cancer cells is necessary for further oncogenesis to develop. For instance, oncogene mutations would be detected by CTLs in a normal environment but could be immune silent in a suppressed cell-mediated environment (see O'Byrne et al., 2000). More recently IL-8, manufactured by stroma or other infiltrating cells within the tumour microenvironment, has been shown to act as a growth factor for melanoma cells.

7 The ability of tumours to induce apoptosis of activated T cells through a FasL–Fas-mediated pathway was recently postulated in metastatic melanoma (Hahne et al., 1996) and other cancers. The interesting finding was that the melanoma cells had lost expression of the receptor and consequently were protected from apoptosis through this mechanism. However, this is a controversial field, as some of the early results may have been reagent-induced false-positives (Chappell et al., 1999), while recent studies have indicated that, depending on the experimental model studied, both enhanced tumour growth but also tumour rejection may be mediated by CD95L upregulation. There is intense interest in apoptosis pathways at present. It is possible that apoptosis is involved in tolerogenic pathways, but it is also possible that prevention of the premature deletion of activated T-cell subpopulations may have a therapeutic potential (see later, anti-CD137 Mabs).

In conclusion, there does not seem to be a 'master mechanism' solely responsible for tumour-induced immune dysfunction. Ongoing characterization of the immune-dysfunction-inducing properties of tumours is taking place, the evidence pointing to a multitude of mechanisms, many of which are still to be clarified. These could be model-dependent, working both at the level of the tumour milieu and at the level of the host's immune system. These processes are not mutually exclusive and could feature either in isolation or in combination at one time or another as the tumour progresses through the different stages of growth and propagation.

CYTOKINES AND CANCER THERAPY

Introduction

The 1998 edition of the cytokine/chemokine periodic table features 116 molecules and is already out of date. It is clearly outside the scope of this chapter to delve into the complicated alphabet of the immunological language. Table 12.1, for example, where the molecules (ligands and receptors) which make up the tumour necrosis factor (TNF) superfamily are shown, gives an idea of the complexity, expansion and gaps in knowledge in this field. We now recognize that there are five major cytokine families:

- the type I cytokines (interleukins);
- the type II cytokines (interferons);
- the tumour necrosis factor family;
- the immunoglobulin supergene family; and
- the chemokines.

The focus of this chapter can only be on the cytokines in clinical use, reviewing track record and clinical potential

Table 12.1 *Molecules that are classified within the TNF superfamily (most of these were identified in the late 1990s)*

Ligand	Receptor
TNF-α	a) TNFRII/p75/CD120b
	b) TNFRI/p55/CD120a
NGF	LNGFR/p75
CD40L	CD40
CD137L/4-1BBL	CD137/4-1BB/ILA
LT-β	LT-β R
CD134L/0X40L	CD134/0X40/ACT35
CD27L/CD70	CD27
TRAIL	a) DR4
	b) DR5
	c) Dc/TRID
FASL	Fas/CD95/APO-1
CD30L	CD30/Ki-1
TNF-β/LT-α	LT-β R
Unknown	DR3/TRAMP/APO-3/LARD/WSL-1
Unknown	TR2
Unknown	GITR
Unknown	Osteoprotegerin/OPG

in greater detail. Tables 12.2 and 12.3 represent a short exposition of the currently known molecules classified as type I and type II cytokines. No list is comprehensive, and any such list is usually out of date at publication. For a continually up-to-date source of information and state-of-the-art reviews on these molecules, we would recommend the interested reader to visit http://www.rndsystems.com/ and, for an up-to-date textbook review of the field, *The cytokine network and immune functions* by Jacques Thèze (1999).

Interferons

INF-α

First discovered in 1957 by Isaacs and Lindemann, interferon-α (IFN-α) is currently available in recombinant formulations and licensed for the treatment of malignant diseases. It is now a regular therapeutic choice for a number of haematological malignancies (e.g. hairy-cell leukaemia, multiple myeloma and chronic myeloid leukaemia).

The major areas of contention remain the solid malignancies. Despite initially promising results in colon cancer, it is now clear from a number of randomized trials that no benefit can be demonstrated either in the adjuvant setting or in the metastatic setting in combination with 5-fluorouracil/folinic acid (5-FU/FA) compared to 5-FU/FA alone. On the other hand, a recently completed study from the Medical Research Council (MRC collaborators, 1999) into metastatic renal-cell cancer, using a relatively low dose (10 MU subcutaneously (s.c.) three times a week for 12 weeks) showed a survival advantage. The administration of INF-α in metastatic RCC conferred

a 28 per cent reduction in risk of death (HR 0.72 [95% confidence interval (CI) 0.55–0.94] $P < 0.02$) when compared to medroxyprogesterone acetate. This also seems to be the interpretation of a further study (Purhönen *et al.*, 1999) where INF-α (18 MU three times a week s.c.) and vinblastine (0.1 mg/kg every 3 weeks) were compared to vinblastine alone. The median survival was in favour of the interferon-containing arm (68 versus 38 weeks; $P < 0.005$) and the response rate was also in favour of the INF-α treatment (16.5 versus 2.5 per cent; $P < 0.005$). Unfortunately, by not including an interferon-α-only arm, this trial has failed to provide data on an ongoing debate as to whether the combination of a biological response modifier and a cytotoxic are synergistic. For example, a further randomized trial of INF-α (18 MU three times a week s.c. for 23 weeks) versus intravenous IL-2 (18×10^6 U/m^2 daily continuous i.v. for 5 days, repeated every 3 weeks for a maximum of six cycles) versus INF-α with IL-2 has indicated greater efficacy for the combination. Interestingly, the response rate for single-agent INF-α was only 6.5 per cent, compared to the 16.5 per cent seen for INF-α and vinblastine, and compared to the 18.6 per cent seen for INF-α and IL-2. While interferon and vinblastine are well tolerated, the doses of INF-α and IL-2 in the quoted trial induce marked toxicity. Currently a randomized trial of INF-α and retinoid, compared to INF-α, in the metastatic setting is still accruing (EORTC). The combination of INF-α and subcutaneous IL-2 with i.v. 5-FU has been advanced in Europe (Atzpodien *et al.*, 2001) as an active regimen in renal-cell cancer. It is currently being tested in a randomized EORTC/CRC trial as an adjuvant but also in metastatic renal cancer (MRC trial RE04). Further results from a larger randomized trial from the Hanover group are also expected. It is hoped that the administration of IL-2 in this manner will avoid the cardiovascular toxicity associated with the i.v. administration, making it a more acceptable regimen, especially since it is proposed as an adjuvant treatment.

The greatest controversy at present is that raging in stage III and stage II malignant melanoma. While a randomized WHO trial failed to demonstrate any advantage for low-dose interferon in stage III disease (lymph-node (LN) metastases) (Cascinelli *et al.*, 1994), in 1996 a trial (EST 1684) was published showing that high-dose INF-α (20 MU/m^2 i.v. five times a week for 4 weeks, followed by maintenance with 10 MU/m^2 s.c. three times a week for a further 11 months) initially improved time to relapse and overall survival in patients with stage III malignant melanoma (Kirkwood *et al.*, 1996). This was at the expense of quite severe toxicity and some mortality. As the use of this regime became more widespread, the toxicity profile reported or seen in the above study expanded, but better management also improved on the toxic death profile (liver failure). This was the first randomized trial of an adjuvant treatment in melanoma indicating improvement in disease free and overall survival.

Table 12.2 *Type I cytokines (interleukins). The molecular weight, amino-acid number, chromosomal location, main in vitro function in human cell systems and possible clinical therapeutic potential are shown*

Interleukin	Molecular weight, amino-acid (aa) number, chromosomal (Chr) location	Biological effects	Clinical therapeutic potential
IL-1 system (α, β)	14–17 kDa. IL-1α precursor, 271aa; IL-1β precursor, 269aa. Chr 2q13	(*Similar to TNF*). Co-stimulates T-cell proliferation. Favours development of Th1 response. Colony-stimulating-factor activation in bone marrow stroma. Activation of vascular endothelial cells. Induction/release of other cytokines. Inhibits thrombus dissolution. Induces colony-stimulating factor (CSF) production by accessory cells. Haemopoietin 1 activity. Activates macrophages. Induces acute-phase responses. Pyrogen. Mediates catabolic processes and inflammation. Affects the HPAA (hypothalamus–pituitary axis) directly ($\uparrow$ ACTH). Co-stimulates proliferation and differentiation of B cells. Induces maturation of pre-B cells	Platelet recovery and direct anti-tumour activity. Co-stimulatory molecule radioprotection (severe clinical toxicity [circulatory collapse] reached at doses of 100 ng/ml before clinical activity noted). Interest in therapeutic strategies blocking IL-1 receptor in septic shock and graft-versus-host disease (GVHD)
IL-1γ (or IL-18)	24 kDa. Some homology with IL-1 but does not interact with IL-1 receptors. 1995: Potent inducer of interferon-γ (IFN-γ) production by T cells. 1996: Human IL-18/IGIF cloned	(*Parallel activities with IL-12*). Induces IFN-γ production by T cells and NK cells. Rapid activation of monocyte/macrophage system. Apoptosis induction through the FasL pathway. Induction of FasL expression on CD4+ Th1 cells and NK cells	Undetermined (possibly in conjunction with IL-2 as vaccine adjuvants)
IL-2	15.5 kDa. 153aa precursor; 133aa mature. Chr 4q. 1965: 'soluble mitogenic factor'. 1976: soluble factor from stimulated mononuclear cells. 1979: cDNA cloned. Human IL-2, IL-4, IL-7, IL-9, IL-13, IL-15 close in structure and function	Co-stimulates T cells. Activates cytotoxic responses in T cells. Stimulates monocytes to become tumoricidal. Chemotactic for T cells. Cofactor for growth and differentiation of B cells; induction/release of cytokines. Induces non-MHC-restricted cytotoxic T lymphocyte (CTL) killing. Co-stimulates proliferation and differentiation of B cells	(*see text*) Co-stimulatory. Immunoadjuvant for immunotherapy schedules (antibody 17-1A, adoptive immunotherapy and vaccines). IL-2/antibody constructs. Indirect gene therapy (vaccines). Direct tumour cytotoxicity (renal cell carcinoma [RCC] and melanoma) in combination with chemotherapy or single agent. Some level III evidence, currently IV. Regimens thought to be very toxic but tested in the USA together with DVC in a randomized phase II trial. High-dose subcutaneous + INF-α + 5-fluorouracil (5-FU) in randomized phase III for RCC. IL-2 immunotoxin Food and Drug Administration (FDA) approved for cutaneous T-cell lymphoma (CTL)

Table 12.2 (continued)

Interleukin	Molecular weight, amino-acid (aa) number, chromosomal (Chr) location	Biological effects	Clinical therapeutic potential
IL-3	28 kDa. Chr 5. 'Haemopoetic cytokine' in same group as granulocyte/macrophage colony-stimulating factor (GM-CSF), IL-5, granulocyte colony-stimulating factor (G-CSF), erythropoietin, thrombopoietin and macrophage colony-stimulating factor (M-CSF)	Major haemopoietic factor in the vicinity of IL-3-secreting T cells. Supports mast-cell growth. Stimulates early progenitor cell growth (erythrocyte, monocyte, granulocyte, megakaryocyte). Supports growth of pre-B-cell lines	Acceleration of platelet recovery (clinical studies inconclusive). General clinical use of the haemopoetic factors in bone-marrow support for dose intensification of chemotherapy, bone-marrow stimulation for harvesting stem cells prior to stem-cell transplants and patient support/prophylaxis of chemotherapy induced myelosuppression. IL-3 may be useful specifically in rare bone-marrow disorders
IL-4	15–20 kDa (≥60 hyperglycosylated). 152aa precursor. Chr 5. 1982: 'T-cell derived factor with B-cell stimulatory effects'. 1986: cDNA cloned human IL-4. (See IL-2 family)	Co-stimulates (in proliferation of normal resting T cells). Stimulates thymocyte proliferation and differentiation to CTLs (in presence of lectin or phorbol myristate acetate). Helper factor for CTL generation in primary mixed lymphocyte culture (MLC), and induces/amplifies in vitro primed MLC memory cells. Promotes growth of tumour-infiltrating lymphocytes (TILs) cytotoxic for autologous human melanoma. Generates lymphokine-activated killer (LAK) activity and augments IL-2-induced LAK activity (in mouse). Supports mast-cell growth. Synergizes with other growth factors to promote colony growth. Induces monocyte cytotoxicity (in mouse). Induces MHC class II antigens on B cells and monocytes. Growth factor for activated B cells. Increases expression of Fcε receptors. Increases IgG1 and IgE secretion by B cells. Decreases IgG2a, IgG2b, IgM, and IgG3 secretion by B cells	Indirect gene therapy strategies (tumour cell transfection ex vivo and vaccination of patient with transfected cells). IL-4 immunotoxins. Co-stimulatory immunoadjuvant. Ineffective as a direct anti-cancer drug in phase I trials
IL-5	12–18 kDa (45–60, hyperglycosylated). Chr 5. (See also IL-3)	Induces proliferation and differentiation of eosinophil and basophil precursors. Function most closely associated with inflammatory and allergic reactions. Eosinophil chemotactic agent promoting degranulation	Treatment of nematode-induced eosinophilia by anti-IL-5 injections
IL-6	25–30 kDa. 222aa; 184aa, mature. Chr 7p21. Based on sharing the gp-130 chain as a receptor classed in the same family as IL-11, leukaemia inhibitory factor (LIF), OSM, CNTF and CT-1	Induces B-cell differentiation and terminal maturation. Enhances Ig secretion by B cells. Stimulates thymocyte growth and neuronal differentiation. Co-stimulates T cells. IL-2 production. CTL differentiation factor. Augments human and mouse antibody-dependent cell-mediated cytotoxicity (ADCC). Enhances MHC class I expression. Induces acute-phase responses. Synergizes with other growth factors to promote colony growth. Stimulates hepatocyte growth	Central role in pathogenesis of myeloma, acting as a growth and survival factor of myeloma cells (cf. recent success of thalidomide in malignant myeloma). Potent IL-6 inhibitors waiting to be tested

Table 12.2 *(continued)*

Interleukin	Molecular weight, amino-acid (aa) number, chromosomal (Chr) location	Biological effects	Clinical therapeutic potential
IL-7	17.4 kDa (unglycosylated). 177aa precursor; 152aa mature. Chr 5	*(T-cell stimulation profile similar to that of IL-2)* Factor in B-cell ontogenesis; Growth and differentiation factor for precursor B-cells of the pro-B/pre-B phenotype. Growth factor for thymocytes. Mostly effective on mature and immature double-negative T cells (CD4-/CD8-) subsets. Augments IL-1 and TNFα production by monocytes. Trophic factor for embryonic neurons	Possibly similar applications in indirect gene therapy as IL-2 but very few data as yet
IL-8	11 kDa (un-glycosylated). 99aa precursor; 77aa mature. Chr 4q. Classified within the CXC chemokine; other members: NAP2, GROα, GROβ, GROγ ENA-78, PF-4, GCP-2, SDF-1, Mig, and IP-10	Strongly chemotactic for neutrophils, T and B cells, NK cells and monocytes. Mitogen for endothelial cells, keratinocytes and smooth muscle cells, and enhances or inhibits growth of haematopoietic progenitors (depending on cofactor). Produced by almost all cell varieties including tumour cells	Prognostic indicator (melanoma). Increased IL-8 associated with poor prognosis and aggressive disease. Probable target for anti-angiogenesis strategies
IL-9	32–39 kDa (glycosylated). 144aa precursor; 126aa mature. Chr 8q	Major function is the promotion of mast-cell growth and differentiation; potentiates effects of IL-4 on IgE, IgM and IgG synthesis by B cells	IL-9 inhibition may have a therapeutic effect in haematological malignancies, where this factor sustains autocrine growth loops (T-cell non Hodgkin's lymphoma and acute myeloid leukaemia)
IL-10	17–21 kDa. Precursor, 160aa; mature, 157aa. Chr 1	Cytokine synthesis inhibitory factor for T-helper 1 (Th1) cells. Inhibits macrophage activity and monocyte-dependent stimulation of NK cell production of IFN-γ. Prevents IL-2, IL-5 and IL-6 generation from CD4+ T lymphocytes. Induces the proliferation of activated Tr1 (T regulatory) T-cell subset, which may be responsible for peripheral immune tolerance. Stimulates NK-cell activation. Increases MHC class II molecules on unstimulated B cells. Increases viability of resting B cells. Co-stimulates (with IL-3 or IL-4) enhanced growth of mast-cell lines and progenitors	Downregulation of IL-10 may enhance anti-tumour activity of the immune system, e.g. AS101. May be developed as an anti-allergic agent. Potent IL-10 blocking agents may prove beneficial in systemic lupus erythematosus
IL-11	*(See also* IL-6) 23 kDa. 199aa. Chr 19q13.3	(Many activities similar to IL-6 or through IL-6 stimulation). Stimulates T-cell-dependent development of Ig-producing B cells. Synergizes with IL-3 in supporting megakaryopoiesis. Stimulates erythropoiesis. Supports the proliferation of committed macrophage progenitors. Promotes osteoclastogenesis. Inhibits lipoprotein lipase in adipocytes. Stimulates acute-phase protein synthesis from hepatocytes. Regulates neuronal differentiation	Nil postulated or defined

Table 12.2 *(continued)*

Interleukin	Molecular weight, amino-acid (aa) number, chromosomal (Chr) location	Biological effects	Clinical therapeutic potential
IL-12	75 kDa [heterodimer of heavy chain (40 kDa) and light chain (35 kDa)]. Chr (40 kDa), 5q31–q33; Chr (35 kDa), 3p12–q13.2	Potent inducer of Th1 responses. Stimulates antigen-activated CD4+ and CD8+ T cells (independent of IL-2). Synergizes with IL-2 in induction of CTL and additive with IL-2 and CTL proliferation. Enhances NK activity. Stimulates IFN-γ secretion by resting and activated human peripheral blood lymphocytes (PBLs)	Possible role similar to IL-2 as a Th1-inducing molecule (vaccine adjuvant). Promising single-agent activity in preclinical tumour models and some phase I trials
IL-13	12.1 kDa (unglycosylated). 132aa precursor; 112aa mature. Chr 5. (*See also* IL-2)	Marker of Th2-cell production (similar to IL-4). Induces proliferation and differentiation of human B cells activated by CD40 ligand. Induces IgE synthesis. May cause STAT-6 activation on T lymphocytes	No role in cancer therapeutics at present
IL-14	468aa. Initially known as HMW-BCGF (high molecular weight B-cell growth factor)	Induces B-cell proliferation. Inhibits immunoglobulin secretion. Selectively expands certain B cells	No role in cancer therapeutics defined
IL-15	14–15 kDa (glycosylated). 162aa precursor; 114aa mature. Chr 4q. (*See also* IL-2)	Stimulates proliferation of activated T cells. Induces generation of cytolytic cells and LAK cells *in vitro*	Similar activation profile to IL-2 indicates that a similar therapeutic potential may exist; however, no clinical work has been published to date
IL-16	56 kDa (tetramer). Pro-IL-16 (67 kDa), 130aa. Chr 15	Inhibits IL-2 production by CD4+ cells. Also inhibits IL2r signalling. Chemotactic factor for lymphocytes; induces IL-2 receptor and HLA-DR expression. Growth factor for CD4+ T cells	By virtue of mRNA expression, almost exclusively limited to lymphatic tissue. Indicates immunomodulating potential. May be useful for selective CD4+ T-cell reconstitution following chemotherapy (fludarabine)
IL-17	20–30 kDa; homodimeric. 155aa. 1993: rat IL-17 cloned; initially erroneously assumed to be a mouse cytotoxic T lymphocyte-associated protein (CTLA) factor. 1995: human IL-17 cloned	Communication vehicle for T cells with the haemopoietic system. Induces haemopoiesis regulator in conjunction with other cytokines (IL-3, IL-4, IL-5, GM-CSF); induces IL-6, IL-8, G-CSF and prostaglandin E_2 (PGE_2) production by fibroblasts, endothelium, marrow stroma cells and RCC cells. Role in early Th2 type of responses	May have important role in pathophysiology of herpes simplex virus (HSV) infection
IL-18 (*see* IL-1γ)			

Table 12.3 *Class II cytokines (the interferons). The molecular weight, amino-acid number, chromosomal location, main in vitro function in human cell systems and possible clinical therapeutic potential are shown*

Cytokine	Molecular weight, amino-acid (aa) number, chromosomal (Chr) location	Biological effects	Clinical therapeutic potential
Type I interferons			
INF-α	16–27 kDa (mature). 165–166aa. Chr 9. INF-α is the collective names for 21 different type I interferons made by leucocytes	Signal transduction alterations through STAT pathways. Promotes partial reversal of the malignant phenotype. Enhances the expression of surface molecules, including β₂-microglobulin, Fc receptors, tumour-associated antigens, and MHC class I antigens. Augments natural killer (NK) activity. Modulates B-cell function. Inhibits suppressor T-cell activity. Activates monocytes/macrophages. Exerts antiviral activity. Interacts (enhance, inhibit) with growth factors, oncogenes and other cytokines. Activates cytotoxic T lymphocytes (CTL). Inhibits angiogenesis through IL-8, fibroblast growth factor (FGF) and monokine induced by γ interferon (MIG) pathways	(*See text.*) Intensively studied in renal cell carcinoma and melanoma. Has clinical status in haematological malignancies, Kaposi's sarcoma and carcinoid. No proven clinical efficacy in adenocarcinomas despite trials in colorectal and pancreatic cancer
IFN-β	20–26 kDa. 166aa. Chr 9. INF-β is a single type I interferon made by fibroblasts or epithelial cells		
Type II interferon			
IFN-γ	34–50 kDa. 143aa. Chr 12	Exerts antiviral activity. Augments NK activity. Induces expression of MHC class I and II molecules. Activates macrophages. Interacts (enhance, inhibit) with other cytokines. Induces IL-2 receptors. Mediates antimicrobial activity. Regulates lipid metabolism. Induces B-cell Ig production. Suppresses IL-4 activities on B-cells. Activates CTL. Enhances tumour-associated antigen expression. Regulates differentiation	Not active in any clinical model studied. Remains in use experimentally in ILP (isolated limb perfusion) combinations but efficacy not proven compared to TNF and melphalan

However, a confirmatory study (EST 1690), concluded and published in abstract form in 1999, failed to verify the increase in overall survival, although an increase in time to relapse was again substantiated. Kirkwood and associates published analyses of the possible causes of this disparity (Kirkwood *et al.*, 1999). The explanation favoured has been that high-dose INF-α was an effective salvage treatment in the control arm, having improved the survival of control patients who relapsed and subsequently received it. Although the researchers state that the handling of regional lymph nodes was not dramatically different between trials, it is also clear from the entry criteria of these trials that patients entering EST 1684 were not stratified according to lymph-node status (number of LNs positive). An imbalance in the randomization arms of ECOG 1684, due to lack of stratification according to positive LN number status, may have influenced the result. On the other hand, EST 1690, stratified for LN status, had a greater survival in the control arm compared to the control arm of EST 1684. This could have been due to administration of high-dose INF-α salvage in the metastatic setting, as favoured by Kirkwood and associates, but could also have been due to a stage migration effect from the randomization differences. Our own unpublished experience of high-dose INF-α in stage IV malignant myeloma (MM) demonstrated a <10 per cent response (7 per cent; 1/14) rate, with the one responder demonstrating a delayed response despite documenting progressive disease (PD) by computed tomography (CT) restaging after a month of high-dose INF-α. The results of the intergroup study, where high-dose INF-α was compared to a vaccine, GM-2KLH/QS-21 were not expected for a few years but were actually rushed out recently after the trial was stopped by the monitoring committee due to the significantly better survival in the standard treatment arm (high-dose interferon) compared to the experimental arm (Kirkwood *et al.*, 2001).

Despite this result there is still scepticism given that the effect of the vaccine was not controlled against a non-treatment arm and the possibility of a detrimental effect cannot be ruled out. A large recent meta-analysis of the interferons which included 3700 patients from 10 trials (Wheatley *et al.*, 2001) seems to indicate that a clear disease-free survival benefit can be seen across the dose range but an overall survival advantage is much more difficult to substantiate. Neither do the data point towards a dose effect. The high cost, increased toxicity and small benefit make the widespread adoption of high-dose interferon-α problematic.

As far as stage II (high-risk) melanoma is concerned, there have been two recent randomized trials of low-dose IFN-α, administered for a duration ranging from 12 to 18 months. In both studies, disease-free survival was prolonged ($P < 0.04$) without, however, a clear impact on overall survival. Based on these results, subcutaneous INF-α has been licensed for the adjuvant treatment of

high-risk malignant melanoma in Europe. However, this agent has not been licensed in the US. There are concerns about the end point of time to relapse being subject to observer bias after the 3 years follow-up that the protocol stipulated (Grob *et al.*, 1998). Furthermore, the analysis was not on an intention-to-treat basis, as nine patients on the treatment arm and one on the control arm were excluded from analysis. At present, since the overall survival benefit is probably very small (of the order of 4 per cent), the recommendation would be that patients should continue to enter trials as the issues are far from resolved.

Although HIV-related Kaposi's sarcoma has shown a good response to INF-α (50 per cent) this is becoming a rarer occurrence in the Western world. Treatment of these patients can be more difficult, especially if they have low CD counts and poor general health, but the existence of more effective treatments with very little toxicity (e.g. liposomal doxorubicin) have relegated the role of interferon in this setting.

As far as efficacy in other cancers are concerned, the evidence is anecdotal. Some efficacy has been seen in carcinoid tumours, but the lack of randomized data makes any recommendations difficult. The use of intravesical INF-α for the treatment of transitional carcinoma *in-situ* of the bladder may be a promising new niche. A 43 per cent complete response (CR) has been reported, with a better side-effect profile than BCG.

INF-γ AND INF-β

These cytokines have been used as single agents or in combination with other cytokines, e.g. INF-α or interleukin-2. There has been no real evidence of efficacy and, other than increased toxicity, they have not enhanced the therapeutic effect of the other cytokine used in combination. The use of INF-γ in combination with TNF-α and melphalan for the treatment, by isolated-limb perfusion (ILP), of in-transit metastases from melanoma remains controversial. Of interest is the use of an INF-γ retroviral vector for indirect (homologous cell transfection) and direct (intra-tumoral) gene therapy (*see* Chapter 14).

Interleukins

IL-2

Interleukin-2 (IL-2) is also known as T-cell growth factor (TCGF). It is able to expand activated T cells by providing the second-helper signal. In animal studies, it was noted that activated lymphocytes expanded *in vitro* with IL-2 could kill tumour cells when subsequently returned to the host, with additional IL-2 given intravenously. These cells were not MHC restricted and were labelled lymphokine-activated killer (LAK) cells. This approach was tried in the clinic, with 11 out of 25 advanced cancers responding to *ex-vivo* expanded LAK cells and high-dose

IL-2. Unfortunately, this treatment was not only very expensive in terms of infrastructure and man-hours, but also extremely toxic, resulting in intensive care for many of the patients. Subsequent studies showed that the response rate was considerably less than the 44 per cent originally reported, and ranged from 5 to 20 per cent (Rosenberg *et al.*, 1988). Several subsequent studies have shown similar response rates between IL-2 and LAK and IL-2 alone, although the original group maintains that more long-term remissions are seen with the IL-2 and LAK patients. IL-2 was given intravenously in high dose initially over a month, and led to severe toxicity involving flu-like symptoms, rashes, vascular leak syndrome and psychotic behaviour. As the main purpose of IL-2 is to expand activated T cells, both specific and non-specific, the need for such doses is dubious. Hence many subsequent studies have used lower subcutaneous doses in addition to combining IL-2 with IFN and chemotherapy (Philip and Flaherty, 1997). Although higher-dose IL-2 appears to be more beneficial than low dose in raising CD4 counts in HIV-positive patients, the effects observed in cancer patients support the use of lower doses, and this is now being pursued in several studies (cf. renal-cell carcinoma).

Cytokines such as IL-2 have a very small range of action and a short half-life, hence it is probably more important that they are delivered to relevant nodes, such as lymph nodes, than given intravenously (Dalgleish *et al.*, 1991). Very low-dose IL-2 administered into tumour-draining lymph nodes and/or tumour-affected lymph nodes has produced marked softening of the node/tumour and the occasional response. However, responses have been sporadic and have not influenced survival in studies undertaken in head and neck cancer; therefore none of these studies have been taken further (Mattijssen *et al.*, 1994).

TNF-α

The first suggestion that a molecule able to induce tumour necrosis existed was based on the observation that some patients with serious pyogenic infections would experience spontaneous regressions. In the 1960s it became apparent that the host, as a reaction to the infection, probably manufactured such a molecule. In 1975 it was shown that a circulating factor induced by bacterial infection had strong anti-tumour activity against subcutaneously implanted tumours in mice. This molecule was subsequently isolated and cloned in 1984. Known now as TNF-α, it has become clear that this molecule and its receptor are just the prototype of a family of molecules (the TNF superfamily) involved in the regulation of immune responses and inflammation (Table 12.1) (*see also* http://www.rndsystems.com/ for continually updated information). An insight into the therapeutic potential that these molecules offer is given in the monoclonal antibody section of this chapter. The current clinical

status of TNF-α, the major representative of this family of cytokines, is reviewed here.

With a maximum tolerated dose (MTD) of 300 mg/m² being well below that expected for a tumour response, it is now clear that this agent is too toxic for systemic administration, whether given alone or in combination (Old, 1985). However, this cytokine has shown some impressive results when used in isolated-limb perfusion for stage IIIAB and IIIB (in-transit metastases) malignant melanoma. From a total of 261 patients treated with 10 times the MTD and mild hyperthermia on a number of phase II multi-centre EORTC protocols (with or without melphalan or INF-γ) a CR of 70 per cent was demonstrated. From a total of 208 patients with soft-tissue sarcomas, where the only surgical procedure would have been limb amputation, a 25 per cent CR rate was noted. Ninety per cent of these patients had a limb-salvage procedure. For patients undergoing TIM-ILP (TNF-α + INF-γ + melphalan) the respective CR rates were 80 and 36 per cent. It has to remain clear that, for melanoma at least, these remain palliative procedures, as the overall survival rate of these patients does not seem to be affected (Lejeune *et al.*, 1998). Many other issues remain unresolved, such as the need for INF-γ, given no evidence of efficacy in any human trials, and the actual dosing of TNF-α. Randomized trials are in progress but, overall, the response rates and palliation from quite distressing disease is impressive in these relatively infrequent disease-settings.

ANTIBODY-BASED THERAPEUTICS

It has taken 22 years (since the Nobel prize winning discovery by Kohler and Milstein) for the first monoclonal antibody to be approved for the treatment of cancer. Antibodies had already been proposed towards the end of the nineteenth century (Hericourt and Richet, 1895) as the ultimate targeting device, to be conceptualized later, by Ehrlich, as the magic bullet (Himmelweit, 1957). The development of pharmaceuticals within this field has been one of the most rigorous and has established the need for better methods to evaluate these treatments. Monoclonal antibodies have undergone numerous modifications (fragmentation, humanization, effector function conjugation, etc.) to improve transport, access and anti-tumour efficacy. Critically, the amount of antibody targeting a solid tumour nodule is typically less than 0.01 per cent per injected dose per gram; furthermore, it is also clear that great heterogeneity exists throughout the targeted tumour volume. This is attributed to antibody characteristics (e.g. size, affinity) but also to tumour physiological properties (e.g. vascularization, necrosis and interstitial pressure). Table 12.4 lists some of the physiological and pharmacological hurdles that tumour-targeting molecules have to overcome. Rationalizing the initially

Table 12.4 *Factors that limit the use of monoclonal antibodies for tumour targeting*

Antibody catabolism by liver and reticuloendothelial system

Few tumour specific antigens (mostly tumour-associated antigens, TAAs)

Cross-reaction with normal, critical tissues

Interstitial pressure of tumours high

Ischaemic underperfused areas in tumours

Poor penetration of solid tumours by whole antibodies

Passive diffusion of antibody into tumour (law of mass action)

Poor stability of complex molecules (immunoconjugates) *in vivo*

Loss of radioactive isotope from antibody *in vivo* (RIT)

Development of neutralizing human antibodies (against toxin or antibody)

Reduced immunoreactivity after *in vitro* manipulations

high expectations has led to significant therapeutic gains. Approaching tumours (e.g. chronic lymphatic lymphoma (CLL)) or tumour states (minimal residual disease) which do not have such high physiological barriers, and using antibodies at earlier stages, is yielding significant efficacy with very low toxicity. In this setting the most crucial determinant of efficacy seems to be the growth regulatory function of the type of tumour antigen targeted (anti-idiotypic, CD20, Her 2-neu). Most of the licensed available agents at present stand out for this one property. This has highlighted the importance of understanding the cell signalling pathways, and the fact that we do not know how all antigens that have been identified to date either as 'tumour specific' or 'tumour associated' work. It seems that the majority of antigen/antibody combinations at present result in relatively 'neutral' targeting effects, necessitating 'arming' of the antibody. This may be due to the function of the antigen (inert protein on the cell surface), but it may also be a function of an antibody. For example, for a growth factor receptor one can develop antibodies that either transmit a positive signal, a negative signal, have an intermediate partial agonist effect, just block the binding site or have no effect whatsoever. Other antibodies can induce receptor complex internalization while others abrogate it. A further problem is that functionality seen in *in vitro* or *in vivo* preclinical models may have no bearing on the actual clinical efficacy. Many antibodies have gone on to clinical trials without this having been elucidated. Some of these issues will be highlighted later.

Unconjugated antibody immunotherapy

IMMUNE-ACTIVATING ANTIBODIES (ADCC/CDC)

Two mechanisms were thought to be essential in explaining the efficacy of the lone antibody in killing cancer cells – complement-mediated cytotoxicity (CDC) and antibody-dependent cellular cytotoxicity (ADCC) mediated through the Fc receptor of effector cells. Although single IgM molecules can activate and fixate complement, no substantial evidence has ever been generated to establish that CDC is actually one of the mechanisms of tumour cell death mediated by monoclonal antibodies. However, for ADCC, at least as it is tested *in vitro* and based on correlation with *in vivo* therapeutic efficacy, a substantial body of evidence has accrued indicating that this is a likely mechanism of action, at least in part (Herlyn and Koprowski, 1982). It has been shown, for example, that among the features that influence the amount of killing in ADCC are:

- the species origin of the antibody;
- IgG subclass;
- the number if antibody molecules bound per target cell;
- the ratio of effector cells to targets; and
- the activation state of effectors.

The species origin appears to have a significant influence on the ability of an antibody to recruit human effectors to kill human tumours. While human and rat antibodies mediate ADCC with human effectors, murine antibodies are often less potent in this role. The match of antibody to effector cell FcR is a significant feature of ADCC and there is clear experimental evidence that, at least *in vitro*, one can see a significant modulation of cytotoxic T-cell recruitment and activation for different Fc chimeras of the same antibody (e.g. 17-1A).

All IgG subclasses are, in principle, capable of ADCC. However, the IgG1 subclass of humans, IgG2a and IgG3 of the mouse, and IgG2b and IgG3 of the rat have been found to be the most active with human cells (Seto *et al.*, 1983; Hale *et al.*, 1985). This does not always parallel the order of FcR binding affinity, and other factors of Fc–FcR binding probably influence induction of cytolysis. Great efforts have been made to engineer on to antibodies characteristics that confer the capability to induce ADCC, for example changing the antibody isotype to IgG2b, which induced the most potent cytotoxicity with human effector cells (Shaw *et al.*, 1988). CAMPATH 1H, a humanized anti-CD52 antibody, is an example of this process, where the murine component has been grafted on to a human IgG1 Fc 'frame'.

Selection of a target antigen that is highly expressed will have a direct impact on the likelihood of the antibody being able to kill the cell with ADCC. There is very nearly a linear relationship with cytolysis. This therefore indicates that both the density of antigen and the amount of antibody reaching the target would be limiting factors for *in vivo* efficacy (Velders *et al.*, 1998). It follows that higher effector/target ratios yield increased killing. While a plateau in killing efficacy can be achieved *in vitro*, in the clinical setting the ratio of effector cells to targets is not so readily controlled. However, it is logical to believe that the greatest likelihood of achieving optimal ratios would be in minimal disease, for example in adjuvant settings (Riethmuller *et al.*, 1998).

The activation state of effector cells has been shown in several systems, *in vitro* and *in vivo*, to play an important role in the lysis of targets. The immune dysfunction of a host bearing a large tumour would clearly compromise efficacy of ADCC. This is exactly the thrust of adoptive immunotherapy (*see* below), where tumour-infiltrating lymphocytes are primed *in vitro* and then re-infused in the host. IL-2 continues to be given to maintain activation of the reinfused population of T cells. It is this principle that is now pursued in clinical studies of ADCC-mediating antibodies in conjunction with IL-2 or granulocyte/macrophage colony stimulating factor (GM-CSF). Clearly, from our current understanding of tumour-mediated immune dysfunction, such strategies are more likely to succeed in the setting of minimal disease.

The classical concept of the recruitment of effector cells to the tumour site/cells is linked with:

1 the destruction of the target cell through activation of cytotoxic mechanisms (e.g. perforin and granzyme release) which induce apoptosis; and
2 the phagocytosis of the cell-suicide products.

Of interest, however, is the recently proposed notion that the recruitment of effector cells may have a more subtle contribution to cell death. Namely, the multiple Fc receptors on the effector cell surface deliver multivalency to the cross-linking of the Fc regions of the antibody bound to the tumour, which, in turn, induces increased receptor cross-linking (hyper-crosslinking) and transduces a more potent cytostatic/cytotoxic signal (Shan *et al.*, 1998). Of similar potential may be the development of homo-dimeric antibodies. Whichever mechanism is functional, the main message from this work is that the choice of the antibody target-antigen is of vital importance.

Two antibodies with significant clinical activity, which are thought to mediate their clinical result at least in part through the ADCC mechanism, are the murine antibody 17-1A (Edrecolomab® (formerly known as Panorex®) and the 'humanized' anti-CD20 antibody rituximab (Rituxan®).

Colon cancer

Antibody 17-1A Murine antibody 17-1A (Edrecolomab®) is a mouse IgG2a that reacts with a 37–40 kDa glycoprotein, thought to be an adhesion molecule and found on some carcinomas and normal tissues. It is a first-generation antibody with low affinity. Very few responses were seen in phase I/II trials in metastatic colorectal cancer. Remarkably, however, when this antibody was given by Riethmuller and co-workers to patients with colorectal cancer Dukes' C in an adjuvant setting it conferred a similar survival advantage to adjuvant 5-FU-based chemotherapy. Side-effects were mild and treatment was a monthly injection for 4 months. The initial study was updated recently, showing the long-term efficacy of

this treatment. A recently completed large multi-centre phase III European trial of this antibody (Edrecolomab®) compared to 5-FU/FA or a combination of Edrecolomab® and 5-FU/FA has been reported (Punt *et al.*, 2001). Unfortunately, it was evident that the monoclonal antibody Edrecolomab® is inferior to regular treatment (5-FU/FA) and adds nothing to the treatment as a combination. Efforts at refining this antibody's functionality by increasing affinity, and increasing ADCC by simultaneous treatment with a variety of cytokines, are continuing. From the existing evidence it is clear that newer-generation antibodies are both better as far as affinity and induction of ADCC *in vitro* are concerned, but whether this will translate to superior clinical results is not known.

Lymphoma

Anti-CD20 antibody Rituximab (Rituxan®) received approval from the Food and Drug Administration (FDA) for clinical use in low-grade non-Hodgkin's lymphoma (NHL) in November 1997. Rituximab is a chimeric antibody with murine variable regions grafted on to a human IgG1 framework. It binds to epitopes on the CD20 molecule found on normal (95 per cent) and malignant (90 per cent) B cells with minimal normal tissue cross-reactivity. There are data that seem to indicate that cytotoxicity is mediated through ADCC; however, both the fact that CD20 may actually be a calcium-receptor channel and evidence showing that cross-linking of CD20 may deliver a cytotoxic/apoptotic signal to the cell, has lent support to the possibility that this antibody may also act through a signalling mechanism (*see* below).

The initial clinical testing of rituximab has indicated that, given CD20 positivity (most common in follicular lymphoma), patients have a very good chance of responding, irrespective of age, performance status, tumour bulk, lactate dehydrogenase (LDH) levels, previous treatment schedules (including transplant failures) or even previous exposure to rituximab (Davis *et al.*, 2000). Some degree of mild anaphylactoid reactions, especially after the first treatment, is very common. Severe anaphylaxis is a possibility, but is rare. This seems to be associated with the number of circulating CD20 cells, the higher the number, the greater the toxicity, reaching the extreme in CLL; therefore, a slower infusion rate is recommended in these patients.

The breakthrough trial was a phase II investigation of this agent in patients with relapsed follicular and low-grade lymphoma following one or more courses of chemotherapy, demonstrating a 60 per cent response rate for follicular lymphoma, with a median duration of 13.2 months (Moloney *et al.*, 1997). However, the greatest potential seems to be in the treatment of early disease in combination with chemotherapy, both for low-grade and also intermediate to high-grade lymphomas. Overall objective response rates approaching 100 per cent have been reported (Czuczman *et al.*, 1996). These results need to be confirmed and time to relapse and overall survival data are necessary, but the future for follicular lymphoma patients does look to have come a long way from single-agent chlorambucil.

Anti-CD52 antibody This is a chimeric humanized IgG1 anti-CD52 monoclonal antibody called CAMPATH-1H, which binds to the majority of B-cell and T-cell lymphomas. Although this antibody was designed specifically to enhance ADCC, recently evidence has emerged that cross-linking of the CD52 receptor mediates growth inhibition in the target cell. Despite going into pharmaceutical development earlier than Rituxan®, it has had more modest activity than the anti-CD20 antibodies. In a recent multi-centre phase II trial, 50 patients were treated. Clinical efficacy was mostly seen against circulating lymphoma cells, which were cleared from the circulation in over 90 per cent of patients. In over 30 per cent of patients, the bone marrow was also found to be completely clear. Nevertheless, actual objective responses in lymph nodes and spleen were rare (5 and 15 per cent, respectively). A total response rate (RR) of 14 per cent was reported, of which 8 per cent (four patients) was in skin. These patients had mucosis fungoides. Moreover, a significant number of patients had opportunistic infections (14 per cent) and bacterial septicaemia (18 per cent). Fourteen patients (28 per cent) had grade IV neutropenia (Lundin et al., 1998).

SIGNAL-TRANSDUCING ANTIBODIES

At least three clinically effective antibodies can be classified in this category. The realization that antibodies that are not delivering a classical cytotoxic agent can be effective by delivering a cytostatic *message* is one of the most interesting developments in our understanding of how antibodies may work. Furthermore, this message can be either positive (inducing) or negative (inhibitory). Inhibition may be achievable by simply blocking or disrupting the ligation of a receptor complex or by actually transducing a negative signal. The qualitative and quantitative complexities of signalling through these receptors could be likened to the adjustment capabilities (volume and tuning) of a radio (receptor), the listener's brain being the cell. Unravelling these complicated processes will lead to the identification of functional anti-tumour targets.

Lymphoma

There are two classes of effective antibodies in this group for the treatment of NHL. The first class of antibody, called rituximab (Rituxan®), which we have already discussed in greater detail, targets the CD20 receptor. This antibody has a very strong *in vitro* ADCC induction profile and, until recently, this was the proposed mechanism of action (*see* above). However, evidence is accruing that, at least in part, similarly to the anti-idiotypic antibodies, activation of a signalling pathway may explain efficacy, especially in view of the clinical observation of

prolonged tumour stabilization or prolonged time to response. Cross-linking of CD20 induces a number of signalling messages. These include an increase in protein tyrosine phosphorylation activation of phospholipase Cγ and upregulation of c-*myc* (Deans *et al.*, 1993). It also seems to be the case that CD20 is functionally linked to a number of membrane receptors, and *in vitro* experiments have shown that induction of apoptosis and growth inhibition is dependent on antibody cross-linking (Leveille *et al.*, 1999).

The second class is that of the anti-idiotypic antibodies. Although unlikely to become a widespread therapeutic modality, given the difficulties and costs of developing custom-made antibodies from each patient's tumour, they have demonstrated encouraging clinical efficacy in the treatment of non-Hodgkin's lymphoma (Davis *et al.*, 1998). This antibody targets the B-cell receptor complex, initiating cross-linking and internalization. This, in turn, activates a downstream signalling cascade that leads to cell cycle arrest, which can have, as a consequence, the induction of apoptosis but also the entry of the cell into a state of dormancy (Tutt *et al.*, 1998). What actually will happen to the B cell, assuming an intact signalling pathway, depends on the extent of B-cell receptor cross-linking, the level of co-stimulation, the duration of the signal, the stage of cell differentiation and the position of the cell in the cell cycle. This 'fine-tuning' of signalling receptors is a recurring theme (*see also* KIR and T-cell receptors, above). Although anti-idiotypic antibodies can induce dormancy, it is still unknown how this state is maintained over time.

Breast cancer

The licensing of herceptin, a chimeric IgG1 anti-HER2/neu antibody (Trastuzumab®), for the treatment of breast cancer is probably the most significant development in monoclonal antibody therapeutics for solid malignancies. HER2/neu is a 185 kDa transmembrane receptor and a member of the epidermal growth factor (EGF) tyrosine kinase receptor family. About 25–30 per cent of patients with metastatic breast cancer have tumours that overexpress this receptor. Initial work clearly indicated that antibodies against the HER2 receptor could reverse the malignant phenotype of cancer cells *in vitro*. Treatment of HER2-overexpressing breast cancer cell lines with herceptin results in induction of p27KIP1 and the Rb-related protein, p130, which in turn reduces the cells undergoing S-phase. Other phenotypic changes noted are the down-regulation of HER2, restored E-cadherin expression levels and reduced VEGF production. Other signalling phenomena have also been noticed, such as increased levels of protein tyrosine phosphorylation and activation of the MAP kinase pathway, which regulates p21WAF1, a key cell-cycle regulator. How this complicated signalling relates to the actual activity *in vivo* in the human host is still not clear. Whether this activity is a result of interfering with the pathway simply by blocking ihe receptor, or whether the signalling alterations are much more subtle, is also unknown (Mendelsohn, 1997). Although signalling, or disruption of signalling, is felt to be the major mechanism through which herceptin may work, there is significant experimental evidence suggesting that recruitment of effector cells may also be significant (Cooley et al., 1999).

The first large multi-centre open-label trial included 222 patients who were HER2/neu positive, who were treated with single-agent herceptin. Sixty-six per cent of patients had received adjuvant chemotherapy, the majority of patients had received at least two chemotherapy combinations for metastatic disease and 25 per cent had also received high-dose chemotherapy with stem-cell support. An objective response rate of 16 per cent, which included a 2 per cent CR rate, was documented. A further randomized trial of herceptin in combination with chemotherapy versus chemotherapy alone involved 469 patients. Anthracyclin-naïve patients received anthra-cyclin plus herceptin while patients who had been treated with anthracyclins in the past received herceptin and paclitaxel. The response rate was significantly increased in the chemotherapy plus antibody arms, and correlated with HER2/neu positivity (Dillman, 1999). Many trials are in progress to clarify the therapeutic potential of this new agent. It seems likely that a combination of antibody with chemotherapy will be the treatment of choice in the adjuvant setting, especially for patients whose tumour is HER2/neu positive.

Other developments

Although yet to reach the clinic, a class of antibodies targeting molecules from the TNF superfamily have given intriguing pre-clinical results through what are thought to be entirely novel mechanisms. In a study of anti-CD40 in a murine syngeneic lymphoma model, activation of a T-cell cytotoxic response was achieved which eradicated the tumour independent of T-helper cells (French et al., 1999). Mice, in which eradication of the tumour was achieved, were resistant to tumour re-challenge. A slightly different approach was seen with an anti-CD137 (4-1BB) antibody. Ligation of this receptor prevents clonal deletion of activated T cells, providing long-term survival (Takahashi et al., 1999) and, similarly, tumour eradication (Molero et al., 1997). Although these developments in the signalling antibody field are still early, they give an indication of the potential of this field.

Conjugated antibody treatment (targeted therapy)

Antibodies used in this setting are usually of the inert type (this may not be strictly true, as will be seen later). They are designed to have maximum tumour specificity (i.e. targeting a tumour specific/associated antigen) and, depending on the 'arming' process, to have either the capability to internalize (immunotoxins) or, conversely,

to remain bound to the cell surface (antibody-directed enzyme prodrug therapy, ADEPT). The use of recombinant molecular biology technology has allowed a bewildering array of modifications of these antibodies, designed to improve pharmacokinetics, affinity/avidity, tumour penetration and immunogenicity (human and mouse antibody (HAMA)). Initially monovalent fragments were in vogue. These had fast clearance kinetics and seemed to give higher tumour to normal tissue ratios than the parent compounds. Radio-antibody imaging seemed improved, but it quickly became clear that the absolute amounts of these reagents reaching the tumour were too low for therapy; they were even lower than those of the intact antibody. Increase in affinity of these monovalent fragments by using in vitro maturation techniques did not enhance efficacy. It became clear that the uptake of antibody by the tumour was a passive process, governed by the laws of mass action and receptor/target affinity variables. Mathematical modelling indicated that the ideal size of the targeting molecule should be above the renal clearing threshold of 60 kDa and not much larger than 100–120 kDa. Although very high affinity/ avidity of the antibody has been felt to be a desired property, it is not very clear whether this enhances or encumbers the targeting process. There is, for example, evidence that a very high affinity antibody administered intravenously in suboptimal amounts may suffer from an 'antigen-barrier' effect. In other words, it would be sequestered in the first few microns of its journey into the tumour, the high affinity defeating convection. There are many theoretical arguments of this sort that cannot be dealt with in detail in this chapter. Details for the interested reader can be found in Epenetos (1991) and Goldenberg (1995) and references therein.

At present a number of these constructs are available. They range from multivalent 'minibodies' (bivalent bi-bodies, trivalent tri-bodies, etc.) through engineered multi-specific antibodies and engineered antibody-toxin constructs. A few of these products are at an advanced pharmaceutical stage but, given the fact that the effective molecules now reaching the clinic are first- (mouse monoclonals) or second-generation reagents (chimeras), it is conceivable that these technologies will refine tumour response and reduce toxicity substantially.

IMMUNOTOXINS/MONOCLONAL ANTIBODY–DRUG CONJUGATES

Although called 'immunotoxins' the targeting moiety of these complex molecules is not always an antibody. Some of the most advanced in pharmaceutical development products target IL-2 receptors or even growth factor receptors such as cERBb2. The necessary prerequisite is cell internalization translocaton to the cytosol and, if possible, localization to the protein synthesis machinery. These are complicated pathways and internalization does not necessarily mean that the molecule will enter appropriate intracellular trafficking pathways needed for efficacy. It may be compartmentalized and metabolized painlessly. Refinements of these molecules may include the engineering of specific localization sequences on to the toxin. For example, the peptide sequence KDEL (Kreitman and Pastan, 1995) would localise a molecule bearing it to the cell nucleus. Theoretically, these toxins are extremely potent molecules, therefore even small amounts escaping into the cytosol may be enough to kill the target cell (Kreitman, 1999).

Toxins originate from plants or bacteria and are, by nature's design, equipped with their own binding specificity. These binding domains are essential for the toxin to internalize into the cell. It is necessary for these domains to be neutralized to avoid widespread toxicity. The binding specificity is then 'redirected' to a tumour antigen by either conjugating or engineering the toxin on to an antibody or ligand of the appropriate anti-tumour specificity. Great pains are taken in purification steps to avoid 'free' toxin within the injectate, or constructs containing other ratios than a strictly 1:1 toxin:ligand conjugate. The most common toxins used have been derivatives of ricin, diphtheria toxin and pseudomonas exotoxin.

Pharmaceutical products exist in relatively advanced stages of development for haematological malignancies (phase I/II/III trials). The main toxicity has been profound fatigue, hypoalbuminaemia and a capillary leak syndrome, while immunogenicity of these xenogeneic proteins has also been found to be high and reduces the number of possible administrations substantially. Objective response rates have been documented in lymphomas, ranging from 5 to 10 per cent of patients, with some patients achieving complete responses (CR). The most interesting results have been obtained in the rare cutaneous T-cell lymphoma (CTCL) group, where initially a small phase II study of 35 patients with CTCL documented five CRs and eight partial responses (PRs), using an IL-2 and truncated diphtheria toxin construct (DAB389-IL-2). This was verified in a phase III trial, where 71 patients had seven CRs and 14 PRs were documented, giving an overall response rate (ORR) of 30 per cent (LeMaistre et al., 1998). This led to approval of DAB389-IL-2 for treatment of CTCL by the FDA.

Although early clinical trials are in progress for solid malignancies, the results have been less encouraging. Systemic administration of a pseudomonas exotoxin targeting Le^y expressing cancers showed a ORR of 5 per cent (2/38) (Pai et al., 1996). There are ongoing trials of intravesical administration for bladder cancer and intratumoral administration for high-grade gliomas.

BISPECIFIC ANTIBODIES

Bispecific antibodies are single molecules that have been produced either by chemical conjugation, biological processes (hybridoma technology) or, more recently, by recombinant molecular genetic techniques. These molecules contain antigen-binding specificity for two different epitopes. The hypothesis is that one of the binding sites binds the tumour target while the other redirects either an effector function (e.g. T-cell cytotoxicity or NK cells) or a toxic agent, injected at a later point, to the tumour site. It is postulated that for this technology to work the antibody has to target a 'triggering' receptor on the effector cell.

The production of these molecules has been a stumbling block. The use of 'quadroma' technology, for example, suffers from low yields of functionally bispecific antibodies of the required immunoglobulin species. Chemical conjugation is laborious and expensive. This field is set to benefit from the great strides in recombinant molecular biology techniques, but at present there is no product at advanced pharmaceutical development stages.

An interesting approach to antibody-directed adoptive immunotherapy was evaluated in patients with glioma (Nitta et al., 1990). A bispecific antibody, with one arm recognizing CD3 and the other anti-glioma, was added in vitro to autologous lymphokine-activated killer (LAK) cells, after which the antibody-coated cells were reinfused intra-tumorally. The results suggest that bispecific antibody-treated LAK cells can lyse tumour cells. The intra-tumour application of bispecific antibodies continues, but remains at a very early developmental stage.

Some promising preclinical work with an anti-leukaemia/anti-saporin bispecific antibody indicated that the delivery of saporin to a tumour cell line could be increased by about 10^5 times (Glennie et al., 1988). This work subsequently progressed into the clinic, where a patient with non-Hodgkin's lymphoma was treated with an anti-CD22/anti-saporin bispecific antibody with documentation of an objective response. However, no further clinical work followed this initial trial.

The use of a bispecific antibody intraperitoneally in patients with ovarian cancer seemed to have a beneficial local effect, but did not hinder progression outside the peritoneal cavity. This antibody, having an anti-CD3 monospecific arm, was designed to 'redirect' a relatively broad T-cell specificity to tumour cells bearing a folate-binding tumour-associated protein. Being a mouse antibody produced by 'quadroma' technology, it induced human anti-mouse antibody responses in all of the patients.

Overall progress in this field has been slow and difficulties have been identified in a number of early clinical trials. There has been no clear therapeutic pattern to the results seen, which have been modest at best.

Pretargeting strategies

One of the finer modifications of targeted cancer therapy has been the concept of splitting the treatment into two or more phases. The first step constitutes the antibody or targeting molecule step. This antibody carries a moiety either chemically conjugated to it or genetically engineered into the antibody framework. Time is given for excess antibody to be cleared. Often an antibody-clearing step is incorporated to accelerate this event. This could be a further antibody (ADEPT) or it could even involve extracorporeal immunoadsorption. Subsequently the second step is administered. In the case of ADEPT, the first antibody has an enzyme conjugated to it while the second step is a prodrug catalysed by the enzyme to an active cytotoxic metabolite. Another application is the *in vivo* administration of streptavidin-conjugated antibodies, followed, after an appropriate period, by radioactive biotin (Hnatowich *et al.*, 1987), or injection of a biotinylated Ma followed by radioactive streptavidin (Paganelli *et al.*, 1990). Biotin has an extremely high affinity for streptavidin ($K_d = 10^{-15}$ M) and, at the same time, is small enough to diffuse rapidly through most tissues in the body. A pilot radio-immunolocalization study in patients with non-small cell lung carcinomas was conducted, with encouraging results (Kalofonos *et al.*, 1990). This has been taken further by other groups, and recently a pharmaceutical product (Pretarget®, by NeoRx) has become available, which is currently in phase I radio-immunotherapy trials for lymphoma, using Rituxan® as the first-step antibody (Breitz *et al.*, 1999).

Another strategy, similar in basic concept, is that of using high-affinity complementary oligonucleotides which could anneal to each other *in vivo*. Using monoclonal antibodies (Mabs) that localize to, and remain at, the cell surface, conjugated to an oligonucleotide, Kuijpers *et al.* (1993) effectively coated a target cell with an oligonucleotide that can be reached, in a two-step strategy, by a subsequently administered radiolabelled complementary oligonucleotide.

The most celebrated strategy put forward to ameliorate the limited amount of antibody that reaches target tissue (solid malignancies) was to use the enzymatic process to catalyse a large number of non-toxic pro-drug molecules into toxic drug at the tumour site (Bagshawe, 1993). Conjugating an enzyme on to the antibody and administering it as a non-toxic first step allows initial localization. This is then followed by a second infusion of an anti-enzyme antibody to selectively clear the circulation from excess circulating conjugated antibody. This would then allow, in theory, the infusion of a non-toxic pro-drug that would be converted to a cytotoxic in the targeted tumour tissue. A bystander effect from diffusion of the drug molecules is to be expected. Since the first pilot studies with carboxypeptidase anti-carcinoembryonic antigen (anti-CEA) antibody followed by an anti-carboxypeptidase antibody and then by benzoic mustard glutamate, which was catalysed to benzoic mustard, a number of limitations have been noted (Martin *et al.*, 1997). Although some responses were seen in these pilot studies, systemic chemotherapy side-effects were noted, the problem likely being residual enzymatic activity in normal tissues or very long drug half-lives.

A series of enzyme pro-drug systems have been reported for ADEPT. Most involve activation of pro-drugs for anthracyclines, methotrexate, etoposide and 5-FU. A pro-drug system called AGENT has also been developed, which is based on the enzyme β-glucosidase catalysing the production of cyanide *in situ* from a targeted anti-PLAP-amygdalin conjugate (Rowlinson-Busza *et al.*, 1991). However, this is still in a preclinical stage of development. Pro-drug systems do not, at present, exist for some of the more effective anti-cancer agents (e.g. platinums and taxanes). Despite many modifications to the early concept, there is still some way to go before these strategies reach the clinic.

Radiolabelled antibodies

General concepts There are two important factors related to the efficacy of this approach:

1 a sufficient amount of the radio-isotope must reach the tumour, which means that the antibody uptake by the tumour should reach a certain level; moreover
2 the injected dose needed to eradicate the tumour mass should not exceed maximal tolerable toxicity in the normal organs.

Radio-immunotherapy, i.e. the use of monoclonal antibodies to target radiation specifically to lesions, is not the sole form of targeted isotopic therapy. Broadly, it could be defined as a radiation treatment directed against a tissue by using a carrier molecule, biological or not, that exhibits a high propensity of accumulating in the target tissue. In some cases no carrier compound is needed as the isotope encompasses both functions. It is this selectivity that is so appealing. Theoretically, deposition of a high radiation dose to the target tissue should be achieved with only minor radiation exposure of normal structures, unlike external-beam radiotherapy where the dose is achieved at great expense to adjacent tissues.

Following the first physiological clinical studies, in which the blood velocity in normal subjects and patients with heart disease was compared using a radium solution injected in the one arm and detection of activity in the other (Blumgart and Yens, 1927), the use of ^{32}P as a treatment for leukaemia and ^{131}I for the diagnosis and treatment of thyroid conditions was soon proposed (Chievitz and Hevesy, 1937). However, the construction of the first nuclear reactors, after the Second World War, was the impetus for wider application, as radiopharmaceuticals could now keep pace with ideas.

The development of protein-labelling techniques was soon followed by the first radioactive polyclonal antibody preparations receiving clinical testing (Mach *et al.*, 1974; Goldenberg *et al.*, 1978). The further development of monoclonal antibodies (Kohler and Milstein, 1975), and the analogous enthusiasm that followed, led to greater expansion of the field of targeted radiation treatment.

Dosimetry considerations The problem of dose specification of radiobiological treatments, and how to

Table 12.5 *Promising β-emitting isotopes for radio-immunotherapy*

Radio-isotope	Emission	Energy (keV)	Abundance	$T_{1/2}$ (h)	Tumour size (mm)[a]
Iodine-131	beta	606	89	193	2.4–3.8
	beta	334	7.4		
	gamma	364	81		
Yttrium-90	beta	2284	100	64	23–34
Rhenium-186	beta	1077	71	91	6–10
	beta	939	21		
	gamma	137	10		
Rhenium-188	beta	2120	71	17	17–28
	beta	1965	25		
	gamma	155	15		
Copper-67	beta	390	57	61	1.2–1.6
	beta	482	22		
	beta	575	20		
	gamma	185	49		
Samarium-153	beta	632	34	47	2.6–4.0
	beta	702	44		
	beta	805	21		
	gamma	103	28		
Luthetium-177	beta	497	79	161	1.3–1.8
	beta	176	12		
	gamma	208	11		
Phosphorus-32	beta	1710	100	343	14–21

[a] Optimal tumour size treated by the respective isotope (adapted from O'Donoghue, 1993).

relate this to an observed or expected response, is being approached from a variety of directions.

Despite obvious misgivings about the ability of simplistic mathematical or computer simulation models to explain the complicated *in vivo* events, the usefulness of this form of modelling is exemplified by the hypotheses put forward based on a simple compartmental biodistribution model, relating to the efficacy of radio-immunotherapy and the possible dose-limiting toxicity that would hinder the treatment's applicability (Dykes *et al.*, 1987; Vaughan *et al.*, 1987). The predictions have withstood the experimental/clinical test remarkably.

Similarly, as for interstitial brachytherapy, a 'continuous hyperfractionation' scheme with an infinite number of small doses being delivered can be invoked for biologically targeted radiotherapy. There are, however, fundamental differences. The radiation distribution of biologically targeted radiotherapy (BTR) is completely unpredictable, as a variety of unquantifiable tumour-related physiological and pathological factors come into play. Tumour vascularity and vascular permeability, binding sites per tumour cell, the composition of the extracellular matrix and cell–cell interactions, the rate of antigen shedding and possibly other microenvironmental factors, such as pH, interstitial pressure and P_{O_2} are all ill-defined parameters of the target *milieu* that may exert an influence on the final result (Jain, 1988, 1991; Jain and Baxter, 1988; Cobb, 1989).

Until reproducible and suitable methodologies are developed to measure *in vivo* the multiple variables that may influence efficacy at both the micro- and macro-levels, dosimetry at the required level of accuracy will be impracticable. At this point, the dosimetry for internally administered radiobiological agents in the clinical situation is still calculated by use of the medical internal radiation dose (MIRD) formalisms (Loevinger and Berman, 1968; Snyder *et al.*, 1978; Watson *et al.*, 1993). The relatively crude pharmacokinetic models, such as the ones mentioned above, improve our understanding of the requirements for successful treatment; moreover, there is still a continuing need for better modelling of the dose distribution of an internally or regionally administered isotope at the macroscopic level.

Isotopes for biologically targeted radiotherapy A number of β-emitting isotopes have been advocated as targeting agents (Table 12.5). Coupling methods have been developed for most of these isotopes; however, difficulties stemming from availability, carrier contamination, low specific activity of eluate and cost are still substantial problems for the majority of these (Goldenberg, 1993; Mausner and Srivastava, 1993).

Radio-immunotherapy in practice The numerous successful examples of radio-immunotherapy in the preclinical nude mouse model have not been accompanied by an analogous success in the human situation (Epenetos *et al.*, 1986; Wessels, 1990). Studies using radiolabelled antibodies for tumour therapy have demonstrated substantial tumour responses in animal models; however, in humans the infrequent responses of epithelial cancers have usually been short-lived or incomplete. Hodgkin's disease and B-cell lymphoma have responded fairly well, probably because of the radiosensitivity of these tumours. Reasons cited for failure include the heterogeneity of antigen expression by the tumour, inadequate tumour: tissue ratios, low absolute amount of antibody uptake by the tumour, dehalogenation at the tumour site in the case of ^{131}I-labelled antibody or leaching of the isotope from the chelator, e.g. for ^{90}Y, and limitations due to normal tissue toxicity (Maraveyas and Epenetos, 1991). Dose will also depend on the radionuclide used. High-energy radionuclides, such as ^{90}Y, may produce overlapping dose distributions from radionuclide deposited in adjacent areas, leading to bystander killing of antigen-negative cells. The dose distribution of lower-energy radionuclides, such as ^{131}I, will overlap to a lesser extent.

Even before monoclonal antibodies became available, polyclonal antibodies were used for isotopic therapy. One of the first trials indicated that antibodies as a multimodality treatment may have a role to play. It is interesting that, despite this opinion having being put forward as a clinical observation at the initial stages of radio-immunotherapy, it remained little investigated. As various antibodies became available, each research unit interested in a specific neoplastic process pursued its own objectives. It has taken more than 10 years for the therapists hesitantly to recognize the practical inefficiency of antibody-mediated radio-immunotherapy for the treatment of solid epithelial cancers. The infrequently voiced theoretical opinion for their use as a multimodality treatment has not received the required attention to date (Wheldon *et al.*, 1991; Stewart *et al.*, 1993). In line with the theoretical dosimetry, results from radio-immunotherapy (RIT) of colorectal cancer (Welt *et al.*, 1994), gastrointestinal cancer (Sharkey *et al.*, 1994), ovarian cancer (Stewart *et al.*, 1990), glioma (Kalofonos *et al.*, 1989) and adenocarcinomas (Breitz *et al.*, 1993) have been generally disappointing. Two studies investigating regional treatments (Lashford *et al.*, 1988; Hird *et al.*, 1993), where neoplastic cells/minimal deposits in the meninges or in the peritoneum have been the object of treatment, have indicated possible efficacy.

In contrast to solid tumours, treating classically radiosensitive haematological malignances has led to reproducible and often gratifying results. It was well known that chemoresistant low-grade lymphomas could go into complete remission with a 100–250 cGy total-body irradiation (TBI) dose (Hellman *et al.*, 1977; Siegel *et al*, 1993). TBI of 1000–1575 cGy with bone-marrow transplantation (BMT) has led to complete remission and long-term survival in 40 per cent of patients (Appelbaum

et al., 1987). These doses are notable for the fact that they are practically achievable by radio-immunotherapy. In addition, the promise of selective tumour targeting may decrease toxicity of the above treatment.

Over 500 patients with NHL have now been treated with RIT with a variety of antibodies and have shown remarkable clinical responses (DeNardo *et al.*, 1999): 184 patients of a total of 260 (70 per cent) with relapsed NHL have demonstrated objective responses (CR + PR) when treated with an anti-CD20 antibody coupled either to ^{131}I or ^{90}Y in a series of phase I/II studies. There are now at least three randomized studies in progress. Rituxan® (humanized anti-CD20) is one of these antibodies in clinical trials. A further anti-CD20 antibody (anti-B1) recognizing a different epitope (Bexxar®) has also shown intriguing results and is currently in randomized trials. The approach of using myeloablative doses of radio-active antibody with stem-cell support has also been studied, with impressive results, in relapsed refractory NHL patients. Twenty-five of 29 patients thus treated had objective responses (Press *et al.*, 1993).

What is striking about the anti-CD20 antibodies is that they have clinical efficacy even without the radiolabel. Given the dosimetry considerations developed earlier in this chapter, the actual clinical effect of the radioconjugate is clearly synergistic. It is becoming apparent that the serendipitous combination of a signalling molecule that may be affecting apoptosis pathways is sensitizing cells to the relatively low dose of irradiation delivered by the radiolabel. This has led to a strong synergistic result through radio-sensitizing mechanisms still relatively poorly understood. Some recent preclinical evidence supports this line of thinking. A possible mechanism, postulated to explain increased cell death in irradiated cells treated with anti-Her-2 antibodies, is the activation of the mitotic cycle by this antibody, which reduces time for DNA repair during cell-cycle arrest induced by the irradiation. Cells forced to divide with critical damage to DNA trigger apoptotic mechanisms (Pietras *et al.*, 1999).

Compared to the excellent results in haematological malignancies, progress with radiolabelled antibody treatments for solid tumours has been slower. Breast cancer, colon cancer and ovarian cancer have been some of the solid malignancies where continuing efforts have shown some clinical results, albeit rarely and mostly transiently in advanced malignancies. Combinations with chemotherapy agents are being studied, but are in early development. Myeloablative doses and fractionated doses using humanized antibodies are also being studied, but it is too early yet for objective assessment of results. The pharmaceutical product in the most advanced stage of development is an anti-mucin antibody called HMFG-1 coupled to ^{90}Y (Theragyn®). Following prolonged phase I/II trials a survival benefit was found in patients treated with this antibody intraperitoneally, with no evidence of disease on second-look laparoscopy (Nicholson *et al.*, 1998). This has subsequently been put to the test in a randomized phase III trial that is ongoing.

VACCINE-BASED IMMUNOTHERAPY

The recognition that the immune system could be stimulated into rejecting established tumour came from the work of Coley (1893/1894) who refined earlier observations of a number of workers, such as Fehleisen (1882) and Bruns (1887–1888), that infectious empyemas occasionally led to the resolution of an established tumour. This led him to develop a heat-killed pool of bacteria that came to be known as Coley's toxins. Therapy with tumour cell vaccines *per se* was first described in 1902 by von Leyden and Blumenthal. From the start, however, similar procedures were to yield conflicting results at the hands of different researchers; for example, Coca and colleagues reported tumour regression in some patients while Risley found no response in his cancer patients using Coca's 'vaccine emulsion' (Coca and Gilman, 1909; Risley, 1911; Coca *et al.*, 1912). Both researchers administered autologous or allogeneic tumour cell extracts at 14-day intervals. Experimentation continued, for example, with intraperitoneal administration of tumour extracts by Vaughan (1914) or the investigation of combination treatments with radiotherapy by Graham and Graham (1962), who reported that the administration of a tumour cell vaccine to patients from whom tumour had been removed appeared to radiosensitize the residual disease. These therapeutic 'blends', with or without live bacteria, fell into disuse/disrepute as alternative treatments to radiotherapy, following the rediscovery of the effects of mustard-based chemicals after the Second World War. Cause and effect in the form of dose response were easier concepts to transfer to the clinic, ability to study pharmacokinetic and pharmacodynamic variables and correlate these to response end points transformed the treatment of cancer to a less empirical and more scientific field. Nevertheless, the work of these early pioneers helped establish the basic principles of immunotherapy, such as the need for minimal residual disease and the need for an immune response from the host.

Several observations support the potential value of active specific immunotherapy for the treatment of cancer, including:

1 vaccine-induced immunity against cancer in animal models;
2 the regression and eradication of tumours injected directly with immunostimulants;
3 occasional regression of non-injected tumours after the intralesional injection of bacillus Calmette–Guérin (BCG), mostly noted in melanoma, a tumour

where spontaneous regression is a well-described phenomenon (Morton *et al.*, 1974); and
4 the development of anti-tumour antibodies by the host.

Recently our increasing ability to dissect the immune response both *in vitro* and *in vivo* in the clinic is now generating a new interest in the concept of using immunotherapy to achieve surrogate end points, i.e. a Th1 or a CTL response, and then correlating this with a clinical response. At the present time the setting of minimal residual disease is, and should remain, the primary target for these treatments.

Prior to the development of what now is coined active specific immunotherapy, a large number of molecules, including BCG, have been used as non-specific immunostimulants which, despite early promise, have now mostly been abandoned as single agents (Table 12.6). They do, however, appear as adjuvants in composite 'specific' vaccines.

The recognized goals of active immunotherapy with cancer vaccines are:

1 to overcome the immunosuppression produced by tumour-derived factors/milieu;
2 to stimulate specific/selective immunological processes (e.g. T-cell, antibody response or NK-cell response) that will destroy tumour cells; and
3 to focus the immune response against antigens borne by the host's tumour by enhancing the immunogenicity/presentation of relevant tumour-associated antigens.

Adjuvants/carrier molecules

Although currently a number of therapeutic vaccines have been developed, and it is clearly not possible to discuss the rationale of each and every one, the majority contain an immunostimulatory/immunopotentiating component (adjuvant) combined with an antigen, in the hope of inducing an immune response against the host's tumour.

IMMUNOSTIMULATION – ADJUVANTS/IMMUNOPOTENTIATORS

Repeated efforts have been made to increase the immunogenicity of tumour vaccines by adding an adjuvant. Adjuvants used in clinical trials have included live vaccinia virus, salmonella extracts, viable BCG and BCG derivatives such as cell wall cytoskeleton, trehalose dimycolate, muramyl dipeptide and glycolipids (Table 12.6). Data obtained in clinical trials and in animal models (Hanna *et al.*, 1989) underline the importance of the ratio of tumour cells to adjuvant, as well as the sequence and site of administration of the tumour cell preparation and the adjuvant.

Table 12.6 *Non-specific host immune system stimulants (adjuvants)*

Category	Example	Notes
Intact micro-organisms	Viable: BCG Viable inactivated: OK-432 (Picibanil) Non-viable: C. *parvum*	
Microbial cell wall	BCG cell-wall skeleton *Nocardia* cell-wall skeleton Methanol extraction residue of BCG	
Glucans	Glucan (yeast) and fungal derivatives	Reported as effective in Japan. Not pursued by others
Protein-bound polysaccharide	PSK (Krestin) (fungal)	
Microbial glycoproteins	*Klebsiella* glycoprotein (Biostim)	
Purified or synthetic components	Peptidoglycans Muramyl dipeptide (MDP) MDP derivatives of BCG Trehalose dimycolate (P_3) Endotoxins (lipopolysaccharide) to reduce systemic modified endotoxins (detoxified) toxicity	Active component Used in liposomes
Interferon inducers, polynucleotides	Poly IC, poly IC-LC, poly AU	Early promise
Pyran copolymers	Ampligen, MVE-2	Not confirmed
Low molecular weight inducers	Prymidinones (ABPP, AIPP)	

PROTEIN ADJUVANTS

Addition of a highly antigenic carrier protein to an otherwise non-antigenic substance can often evoke an immune response. The antibodies formed against the complex are specifically directed against the previously non-antigenic substance as well as against the foreign protein in the complex. Early reports using rabbit gammaglobulin attached to proteins of autologous tumour cells reported some therapeutic benefit (Czajkowski *et al.*, 1967; Cunningham *et al.*, 1969) but the efficacy of this type of treatment has not been confirmed.

VIRAL ADJUVANTS

There is convincing evidence in animal models that infection of tumour cells with viruses augments the immunogenicity of tumour antigens (Cassel *et al.*, 1983; Wallack and Michaelides, 1984). Based on animal models, randomized clinical trials have been undertaken with viral oncolysates, allogeneic or autologous tumour cells infected with Newcastle disease virus, vesicular stomatitis virus (Livingston *et al.*, 1985) and vaccinia virus in patients with melanoma and osteosarcoma.

BACTERIAL ADJUVANTS

Immunological adjuvants such as BCG (Morton *et al.*, 1992), extract from salmonella Minnesota (Livingston *et al.*, 1987), C. *parvum* (Livingston *et al.*, 1985), methanol-extractable residue of the tubercle bacillus (Mitchell *et al.*, 1988) and Freund's complete adjuvant (Hollinshead *et al.*,

1982) are potent immunostimulants in animal systems, capable of enhancing the humoral and cellular immune response to a variety of antigens. We have recently completed two phase I/II studies of a novel bacterial immunoadjuvant called SRL-172 in patients with metastatic prostate cancer and metastatic melanoma (Maraveyas *et al.*, 1999). These patients were monitored with an intracellular cytokine assay for IL-2 and INFγ and IL-4. In both studies roughly 30 per cent of patients seemed to make a Th1 response. This was correlated with a drop in prostate-specific antigen (PSA) in prostate cancer patients and an increased survival in the melanoma patients. A comparison with historical controls seemed to indicate a significant increase in survival; furthermore, the subgroup with Th1 responses faired much better than those without such responses. However, pending a randomized trial to test these intriguing data, it was not clear whether the assays were identifying a subpopulation of patients with a less dysfunctional immune system who were capable of mounting Th1 responses, rather than a therapeutic effect of the vaccine itself.

CHEMICAL ADJUVANTS

Tumour-associated differentiating antigens (TAA) in human tumour cells can also be modified in a variety of ways by chemicals such as iodoacetate and cholesteryl hemisuccinate, which increase the immunogenicity of tumour cells (Seigler *et al.*, 1972). Certain enzymes, such as neuraminidase, enhance the immune response to neoplasms by chemically altering the surface glycoconjugates

(Simmons and Rios, 1971). Repeated intradermal immunization with neuraminidase-treated allogeneic acute myeloid leukaemic cells prolonged disease-free survival in patients treated with chemotherapy.

Tumour antigens

The main problem in designing tumour antigen vaccines is to identify tumour antigens that are truly tumour specific and also immunogenic. Although tumour cells do express potentially immunogenic molecules, these are often found in normal tissues at much lower concentrations, therefore they are commonly referred to as tumour-associated antigens (TAAs). TAAs can be broadly grouped into four categories. The first includes oncofetal antigens that are not expressed by any normal tissues but may be expressed on fetal tissues at some point of embryonic development (Carney, 1988), a classical example of which is α-fetoprotein. A second group of TAAs include neoantigens that are usually not expressed by the normal cells from which the cancer cells are derived, but that can be found in other normal tissues, e.g. the human melanoma associated ganglioside GD2, which is expressed on the surface of human melanomas but not normal melanocytes, can be found in human brain and spinal cord (Volk, 1975). The third group consists of cell-surface molecules that are commonly abundant but have antigenic epitopes 'unmasked' due to aberrant metabolism of the tumour cell, e.g. core protein of regular mucins (Gendler et al., 1988; Burchell et al., 1989). Finally, a small group of antigens appear to be tumour-specific antigens in that they are not found in normal adult or fetal tissues; an example of which is the truncated c-erb-b3 receptor on glioblastomas (Hills et al., 1995). Under appropriate conditions, antigens of all three groups can serve as targets for active immunotherapy with cancer vaccines. If one assumes sequential steps in tumorigenesis, it is very likely that during the cell's life-events, leading to the completely transformed immortal cell with malignant potential, novel mutated proteins/products of mutated genes will be expressed (Vogelstein et al., 1988).

CELL-BASED VACCINES

Autologous cell vaccines

Autologous cells can be used in two ways: a cell line raised from either excised tissue or a cell suspension can be reintroduced into the host with the appropriate adjuvant. Since autologous tumour cells express the same blood group and histocompatibility antigens as the host, they are considered ideal for tumour cell vaccines. However, the availability of autologous tumour tissue is limited and hence the amount of vaccine, and thus the number of immunizations possible, is restricted. Moreover, antigen expression may vary from site to site and a vaccine prepared from autologous cells isolated

from any particular nodules may not have the same TAA profile as tumour at another metastatic site. Cell-line production is also fraught with problems, e.g. infection of cultures, failure of cultures, lengthy procedure and culturing a dominant clone that is not representative of the actual initial tumour

Several uncontrolled trials or series using unmodified or modified autologous melanoma cells have been reported. Adjuvants were variably used and in some cases pre-sensitization of the host's immune system was undertaken (Oettgen and Old, 1991). Although some efficacy has been claimed, recently the final results of a randomized phase III vaccine of autologous tumour cells in patients with colorectal cancer treated in an adjuvant setting was reported (Harris et al., 2000). In this trial, 412 patients with either stage II or III disease were randomized either to receive the vaccine commencing 4 weeks after surgery or to observation only. Vaccination consisted of three doses given weekly, consisting of 10^7 irradiated cancer cells. BCG was co-administered with the first two injections (10^7 cfu). The main analysis showed no effect of the vaccine on survival or time to relapse.

Hapten-attached cell vaccines

Based on the understanding that a strong T-cell response to adjuvant/hapten-modified antigen may be accompanied by a response to unmodified antigen which otherwise would not have arisen, researchers have attached hapten (dinitrophenyl, DNP) to autologous melanoma cells (Berd and Mastrangelo, 1987, 1988a, b; Berd et al., 1986, 1990). An ingenious treatment protocol, involving cutaneous priming of the host with the hapten to ensure a delayed-type hypersensitivity (DTH) and administering low-dose cyclophosphamide designed to suppress a Th2 response, was followed by 4-weekly administration of the modified irradiated melanoma cells mixed with BCG in 64 patients with advanced-stage malignant melanoma. Eight cycles were given and DTH responses, CD8+ infiltrate of tumour nodules, was documented. Response of tumour nodules was reported and increased survival of disease-free patients was claimed. However, the number of patients was small and the comparison was made to a historical control group treated with the non-hapten modified vaccine; a phase III randomized trial is definitely required.

Cell lysate vaccines

Although a number of oncolysates have been introduced into clinical trials (Savage et al., 1986), the principal examples in this field are the viral melanoma oncolysate (VMO) using vaccinia virus and the DETOX-melanoma cell lysate, known as Theracine, where DETOX is an adjuvant mixture of cell-wall skeletons of Mycobacterium phlei in squalene oil and Tween-80 and lipid A from salmonella Minnesota. Melanoma cells are procured from allogeneic melanoma cell lines in culture and they are rendered nucleus-free. Ongoing work since the late seventies (Wallack et al., 1977) demonstrated antibody and CTL responses in melanoma patients, correlating with therapeutic efficacy (Wallack and Michaelides, 1984; Wallack et al., 1986; Kan-Mitchell et al., 1993; Mitchell et al., 1993; Wallack and Sivanandham, 1993) in limited phase I/II studies. Phase III double-blind randomized trials (Wallack et al., 1995) have been initiated but have failed to verify the optimistic preliminary results for both preparations (Wallack et al., 1986; Hersey et al., 1987; Dore et al., 1990; Mitchell et al., 1993; Wallack and Sivanandham, 1993). Marginal, if any, efficacy of the VMO-vaccinia preparation has been found (Wallack et al., 1995), while no activity of DETOX is anticipated, although the final trial analysis has not been published to date.

Allogeneic polyvalent cell vaccines

Allogeneic tumour cell cultures can provide a sufficient number of cells for multiple injections. Mixtures of cells from different tumours can provide a spectrum of TAAs. Similarly, however, passage of tumour cells in culture may introduce contaminants and favour the growth of subpopulations that diverge from the antigenic phenotype of the original cancer. Tumour cells grown in culture may also undergo antigenic alterations similar to those documented for ganglioside profiles of human melanoma and glioma. In some cases, these alterations have been used to advantage by mixing different cell lines with increased TAA expression to prepare allogeneic tumour cell vaccines.

This vaccine strategy employs allogeneic melanoma cells harvested from cell lines established and maintained for their immunogenicity (Jones et al., 1981). A number of trials have been undertaken where patients with melanoma are treated with these cell lines administered intradermally with contemporaneous priming with BCG. Over a period of 15 years survival and immunological data have been compiled on numerous patients receiving this treatment with or without other immunomodulatory treatment, e.g. cimetidine, cyclophosphamide, indomethacine or low-dose interferon/IL-2. The main observation, apart from establishing the minimal toxicity of these procedures, was that efficacy is associated with a reaction by the host. This concurs with data from other contemporary trials but, other than qualifying the response, does not offer an advance on the primary observation made 83 years by Vaughan (1914), who thought that minimal disease and a leucocyte reaction to the administration of the vaccine equated to a more hopeful outcome. Indicators of efficacy are: a positive DTH (Morton et al., 1992, 1993), increase in IgM antiganglioside antibodies (Ravindranath et al., 1989), a positive mixed lymphocyte tumour reaction (Morton et al., 1992, 1993) and ability to minimize tumour load even by extensive surgical intervention. A twofold increase in survival for stage IIIA and a threefold increase in survival for stage IV patients has been claimed (Morton et al., 1992). However, this has only recently

been put to the test. An international multi-centre randomized phase III trial sponsored by the National Institutes of Health (NIH) has now commenced for both stage III and stage IV American Joint Committee on Cancer (AJCC) patients following total resection of disease.

PROTEIN/POLYPEPTIDE VACCINES

Advocates of the use of specific soluble antigen as a vaccine, whether it is a peptide, supernatant or cloned protein, believe that patients can, and should, be matched to the immunogen. As our capability to do so improves, so should this method of vaccination become more effective. Eligibility criteria should include HLA typing and analysis of expression by the tumour of the genes encoding the available antigens for treatment (Radrizzani et al., 1991). The purified HLA-depleted vaccines include recombinant proteins/peptides, gangliosides, anti-idiotypic antibodies and polyvalent shed antigen vaccines.

The category carrying a great deal of pharmaceutical potential is that of the recombinant peptides, as they can be easily characterized, produced, purified and standardized, they are free of viral, DNA or other contaminants and study of responses in vivo are not confounded by allo- or xeno-responses. Many promising melanoma antigens have been cloned, all carrying the potential of being tumour immunogens (Farzaneh et al., 1991; Wollina et al., 1991; Demetrick et al., 1992). The best characterised is MAGE1, expressed in 40 per cent of melanomas, presented by HLA-A1 and located on the X chromosome (Xq27-qter) (Van Der Bruggen, 1991; Carrel and Johnson, 1993; Oaks et al., 1994). Clinical trials with these reagents, with or without adjuvants, are in very early stages, and encouraging clinical responses have been reported (Rosenberg et al., 1998; Marchand et al., 1999), although correlation with CTL responses was not demonstrated where these were monitored (Marchand et al., 1999).

Highlighting the difficulties in developing an effective peptide-based cancer vaccine is the cervical cancer paradigm. This disease can be viewed as a sexually transmitted virus-induced disease with the pathogen (HPV, human pappilomavirus) extremely well characterized. Intuitively, the development of a vaccine in this setting both as a preventative measure (third world burden from this disease is large) but also with a therapeutic potential (targeting immune responses to 'viral early proteins' E6 and E7) should be relatively straightforward. This, however, has not proved to be the case. Despite the fact that HPV have not developed any immunoregulatory mechanisms that would allow immune subversion of the host immune system, they seem to have been evolutionarily selected for their 'minimal exposure' to the immune system (Tindle, 2001).

CARBOHYDRATE VACCINES

In initial serological studies in melanoma patients immunized with whole-cell vaccines, the only clearly defined response was an occasional antibody response to the carbohydrate (polyglycosylated) antigens GD2 and/or GM2 (gangliosides). Based on this finding, purified GM2 ganglioside was promoted for clinical studies (Livingston 1993; Livingston et al., 1985). The results of a phase III randomized trial in melanoma patients, where patients were randomized to receive GM2 with BCG or GM2 alone or BCG alone, showed no statistically significant advantage for GM2 on an intention-to-treat analysis (Livingston et al., 1994). However, subset analysis showed significant survival benefit to patients responding serologically with high IgM anti-GM2 titres. The results from the randomised trial of GM2-KLH/QS-21 vs high dose interferon (Kirkwood et al., 2001) have, however, dealt a blow to this approach (see interferons). Despite some subset analyses indicating improved results in the patient subgroup that mounted an actual antibody response there is no avoiding the fact that the intention to treat analysis reveals, at the very least, that the vaccine had no effect either on overall survival or on disease-free survival. An EORTC trial of this vaccine in earlier stage melanoma (Stage II) is underway, but mustering enthusiasm for this approach may be difficult.

Recently a carbohydrate vaccine [Sialyl Tn (Stn) + KLH + Detox™-B] called Theratope® from Biomira Inc. has advanced to a randomized phase III trial following some intriguing early clinical results in two small phase III trials assessing the usefulness of co-administered cyclophosphamide (Maclean et al., 1996a; Miles et al., 1996). It was found that a single low-dose (l.d.) intravenous cyclophosphamide injection given prior to vaccination seemed to convey a survival advantage to patients with metastatic breast cancer. Patients receiving Theratope® + l.d. cyclophosphamide (25 patients) had a median survival of 26.5 months compared to controls (12.3–14.4 months). Encouragingly, those patients with a good immune response to Theratope® were the ones with an increased survival (Maclean et al., 1996b). Further trial results are awaited.

DNA-BASED VACCINES

The first demonstration of DNA vaccine efficacy in an animal model was accomplished using the influenza virus. Cytotoxic T cells were generated against epitopes from influenza virus nucleoprotein, and these effector cells provided cross-strain protection in a mouse model, even at very low doses (10 μg) of plasmid DNA injection (Ulmer et al., 1993). In its simplest form, a DNA vaccine contains the gene or genes encoding a cancer-specific antigen or an antigenic portion of a virus, such as the core protein or envelope protein. Direct injection of naked plasmid DNA induces strong and long-lived immune responses to the antigen encoded by the gene vaccine. DNA plasmids have two immunogenic components: the transcriptional unit, driven by a powerful viral promoter able to direct synthesis of tumour antigen

protein, and the plasmid backbone. The latter contains immunostimulatory sequences containing specific unmethylated CpG dinucleotide repeats, which stimulate an innate immune response. The mediators released include IFNγ, IL-12 and IL-18 from macrophages and monocytes, and IFNγ from natural killer cells. This particular cytokine profile directs the differentiation of naïve T cells to T helper 1 (Th1) cells.

Muscle cells express only low levels of MHC class I molecules and virtually no co-stimulatory molecules, so are unlikely to play a major role in the initial priming of T cells. It is probable that vaccine efficacy is by professional antigen-presenting cells, such as dendritic cells, being attracted to sites of muscle 'injury' from inoculation, capturing antigen released by myocytes and presenting peptides and priming T cells in draining lymph nodes. All routes of DNA introduction lead to efficient production of antibody and the activation of both CD8+ and CD4+ T lymphocytes. DNA immunization has a number of advantages over traditional peptide vaccines due to purity, ease of production, prolonged antigen expression, strong CTL and Th1 responses elicited and the resistance of the antigen source to antibody-mediated clearance. The endogenous tumour antigen gene expression achieved in APCs by naked DNA immunization may optimize the desirable MHC class I responses to the tumour bearing the same antigen. Alternatively, induction of CTL responses may occur by 'cross-priming' – a process by which antigen may be delivered to APCs either in membrane form or by heat-shock proteins. Gene transfer efficiency by DNA injection is relatively inefficient, with low frequency of integration into host chromosomes and therefore reduced risk of insertional mutagenesis. Some of the deficiencies may be viewed as strengths: inefficient expression of a target molecule may spare normal healthy cells while fostering an immune response. Similarly, for transient episomal (non-integrated) expression of potentially toxic agents, such as cytokines, it would be desirable to limit gene expression. Potential candidates for T-cell mediated immunity stimulated by DNA vaccination are shown in Table 12.7.

DNA vaccines against idiotypic determinants of B-cell lymphoma

The idiotypic (Id) determinants expressed by immunoglobulins (Ig) at the surface of a neoplastic B cell represent ideal tumour-associated targets for the immune response. Component idiotypic (variable) region genes can be identified in a patient's tumour biopsies and rapidly assembled as ScFv (single-chain) sequences. These can be used to produce recombinant ScFv protein in bacteria, or as naked DNA vaccines. Although these immunostimulant proteins would be unique to each patient, there would be obvious problems in individual vaccine production in economic terms. Injection of expression vectors encoding antibody fragments such as the variable (V)

Table 12.7 *Targets for DNA vaccination strategies*

Target	Class of antigen	Associated cancer(s)
EGFR	Growth factor receptor	Breast, ovary, stomach
ERBB3	Growth factor receptor	Breast, bladder, colon
p53	Mutated tumour suppressor	>50% all human cancers
RAS	Mutated oncogene product	>10% all human cancers
		>80% pancreatic, colorectal
Ig idiotypes	Idiotypic epitope	B-cell lymphoma
T-cell receptor idiotypes	Idiotypic epitope	T-cell lymphoma
Human papillomavirus E6 E7	Viral gene products	Cervical cancer
p210$^{BCR/ABL}$	Mutated oncogene product	Chronic myeloid leukaemia
MAGE-1	Embryonic gene product	Melanoma, breast
Tyrosinase	Normal differentiation antigen	>50% melanomas

EGFR, epidermal growth factor receptor.

genes of immunoglobulins into mouse models has resulted in the elicitation of anti-idiotypic antibodies. Similar results may be obtained using known T-cell receptor idiotypes. Immunization with DNA constructs encoding the idiotype of a murine B-cell lymphoma has recently been shown to induce specific anti-idiotypic antibody responses and protect mice against tumour challenge. Vaccine efficacy was improved subsequently by the use of DNA encoding an idiotype/GM-CSF fusion protein, or by simply co-injection of plasmids encoding murine GM-CSF or murine IL-2 (Stevenson *et al.*, 1995). Alternatively, the use of DNA encoding fusion genes of immunotoxins, such as tetanus toxin fragment (FrC), and the 3′ end of the ScFv sequence resulted in amplification of Id-specific antibody response, compared to injection of plasmid DNA encoding these genes separately. Immunization of lymphoma patients with ScFv DNA has now entered clinical trials. This approach has been extended to phase I trials in patients with malignancies expressing CEA (carcinoembryonic antigen) and tumour associated mucin (MUC-1). These anti-idiotypic responses may break immunological tolerance to self-antigen by providing an alternative source of epitope (a surrogate antigen) that serves as an autoimmunogen for the production of antibodies to CEA/MUC-1. Circulating populations of CTL may be detected in melanoma patients, which demonstrate lytic activity against autologous melanoma cells *in vitro*. A number of potential antigens have been identified in human melanoma as targets for CTL, as discussed earlier in this chapter. Several epitopes for these groups of antigens have been identified as targets for CTLs in the context of HLA-A2.1 and other MHC molecules. Such antigens could be used as DNA vaccines in patients with tumours that are known to express the antigen and who have the correct MHC haplotype to enable the antigen to be correctly presented to the immune system.

Cervical carcinoma is strongly associated with human papillomavirus (HPV) infection, with over 90 per cent of tumours containing DNA of HPV types 16 or 18. Two HPV genes encoding the E6 and E7 proteins are consistently retained and expressed: they can immortalize cells in tissue culture and induce transformation in co-operation with activated oncogenes (Vousden, 1994). Thus E6 and E7 proteins in tumour cells provide a truly tumour-specific target for immunotherapy. There is considerable evidence of beneficial immunotherapy directed against HPV antigens from observations that natural and experimental papillomavirus-associated tumours can be attenuated by immunization with E6 and E7. A phase I/II immunization strategy for treatment of eight patients with advanced cervical carcinoma using a recombinant vaccinia virus encoding modified forms of the HPV16 and 18 E6 and E7 protein sequences has been completed (Borysiewicz *et al.*, 1996). Vaccination was via the intradermal route using dermal scarification. Each of the eight patients mounted an anti-vaccinia antibody response and three of the eight patents developed an HPV-specific antibody response that could be ascribed to vaccination. Only one patient exhibited HPV-specific CTL, the effector mechanism thought to be most likely of benefit therapeutically.

DNA vaccination has great potential as an anticancer agent, particularly with rapid development of methods of detecting tumour-associated antigens, such as microarrays. The obvious advantages in terms of ease of preparation, purification and storage, plus the delivery of encoded antigens to processing sites capable of activating humoral and cellular immune responses, mean that the evaluation of these vaccines in clinical trials should be prompt. The recent development of oral vectors, such as attenuated strains of *Salmonella* sp., for DNA vaccine delivery provides further optimism for this growing field.

DENDRITIC CELL-BASED VACCINES

A relatively recent development to enhance presentation, whether it be protein peptide or DNA, is the *ex vivo* expansion and maturation of the most effective 'professional' antigen-presenting cell (APC) – the dendritic cell (DC). These cells, which can be claimed from either lymphoid or myeloid lineage and which are selected by negative selection due to the lack of absolute specific markers, are remarkably effective at inducing an immune response and even breaking tolerance. They express the necessary co-stimulatory receptors and other signals. DCs can be prepared from peripheral blood samples by expansion with GM-CSF and IL-4 or TNFα. They can then be pulsed with a variety of antigens, which they process and mature into an active APC, which can be reinfused or reinjected into patients. In the case of patients with renal cell carcinoma and melanoma, responses have been seen using DCs pulsed with cell lysates and peptides. In a recent study, objective responses were seen in 5 of 16 evaluable patients with malignant melanoma (Nestle *et al.*, 1998). With the ability to pulse DCs with tumour DNA and RNA, or even fuse them to whole tumour cells, this is going to be an intensely studied field in the next decade.

ANTI-IDIOTYPIC VACCINES

Finally, anti-idiotypic antibodies, the binding sites of which resemble epitopes on tumour antigen, have been used as immunogens. Two such antibodies (MF11-30 and MK2-23) resembling epitopes on high molecular weight melanoma associated antigen (HMW-MAA) have been used in the clinic in phase I trials in advanced stage IV melanoma (Mittelman *et al.*, 1992). Minimal toxicity and some activity in 57 patients have been documented, but the overall procedure has to be optimized and the results are not encouraging enough at this stage for a phase III trial to be undertaken. Similarly, a murine anti-idiotypic antibody which mimics ganglioside GD3, called BEC-2, has shown promising results in early trials in melanoma (McCaffery *et al.*, 1996), where it has been given with either BCG or QS-21 or KLH (Yao *et al.*, 1999). The data are still too immature to assess, but a randomized trial is in progress in small cell lung carcinoma (SCLC) (Grant *et al.*, 1999).

ADOPTIVE IMMUNOTHERAPY: LAKs, TILs AND CTLs

Adoptive immunotherapy involves sensitization or activation of autologous or allogeneic cells *in vitro* followed by re-infusion of cells into the patient. Host immunity is thus stimulated in an attempt to overcome the natural tolerance to the established tumour. The basic principle was developed by Borberg and co-workers in 1972, who showed intravenous injection of lymph-node cells from mice and sheep immunized with a methylcholanthrene-induced sarcoma induced regression or inhibition of established grafts of the same tumour in syngeneic mice. Since then a number of effector cells have been shown to be involved in the anti-tumour response and therefore

have subsequently been used in adoptive strategies. Natural killer (NK) cells are lymphocytes possessing cytotoxic activity against tumours, and possibly a role in anti-tumour 'surveillance'. This toxicity is not antigen-specific and is not MHC-restricted, unlike cytotoxic T cells (CTLs). There is evidence of functional interaction between CD4+ T cells and NK cells. Cytokines released from CD4+ cells in response to tumour challenge stimulated NK cells to act as effector cells to cause their destruction. Most NK cells express a cell-surface receptor for the Fc portion of IgG (CD16) and are associated with antibody-dependent cellular cytotoxicity. A subpopulation for cells lacking the CD16 phenotype can be activated *in vitro* by IL-2. The lymphokine-activated killer (LAK) cells display a wider spectrum of cytotoxicity. LAK cells have been used clinically by adoptive transfer in conjunction with high-dose infusional IL-2 (Rosenberg *et al.*, 1993) and associated with a higher response rate than IL-2 alone (22 per cent versus 13 per cent overall response rate) without evidence of a survival benefit. The small gain in response rate was at the expense of unacceptably severe systemic toxicity that was attributed to the IL-2 therapy. A number of further studies failed to capitalize on the initial advances in this field and the emphasis has since shifted to targeting specific tumour antigens and defining effector cell populations more accurately.

Compelling evidence of the existence of specific T-cell-mediated reactivity to tumour antigens came from the recovery of MHC-restricted CD8+ cells that had infiltrated the tumour. These tumour-infiltrating lymphocytes (TILs) were grown *in vitro* and were capable of lysis of autologous tumour cells from the same patient. There have been a number of attempts to apply this form of adoptive immunotherapy, predominantly for patients with malignant melanoma (Rosenberg *et al.*, 1988; Lotze *et al.*, 1992). TILs are expanded *in vitro* in the presence of high levels of IL-2 and returned to the patient in the hope that they traffic to sites of tumour which express the same antigens as those to which the TILs were raised. In a melanoma patient treated with TIL infusions, tumour regression was associated with a clonal expansion of T cells expressing a specific $V(\beta)16+$ gene segment of the T-cell receptor. These T cells demonstrated specific cytolytic activity against the patient's melanoma cells *in vitro* (Mackensen *et al.*, 1994). Although evidence of responses in individual patients have been recorded, trafficking of cells to liver and spleen have limited their efficacy. Since the early studies involving TILs, it is now a common finding that T lymphocytes from cancer patients can be stimulated *in vitro* to produce cytotoxic T cells (CTLs) specific for antigens expressed by autologous tumour cells. CTLs derived from autologous mixed lymphocyte–tumour cell cultures have been propagated using IL-2, and their lytic activity evaluated against a range of tumour and control targets. Resulting CTL populations are mostly CD8+ that recognize antigens presented by MHC class I molecules, and can be re-stimulated to produce CTL clones that can be maintained almost indefinitely. These clones can select antigen-loss variants of the tumour cells by several rounds of selection with different CTL clones. It is important to note that merely isolating antigens that T cells recognize *in vitro* may be insufficient for anti-tumour immune responses *in vivo*. CTLs for melanoma and other human cancers are known frequently not to be expanded, i.e. CTL precursors are not necessarily increased in numbers compared with humans infected with, for example, influenza virus, who frequently show expansions in virus-specific CTL precursors which may remain stable for years.

'MINI'-ALLOTRANSPLANTS

Patients with leukaemia who undergo an allogeneic bone-marrow transplant often develop graft-versus-host disease (GVHD). It is clear that the efficacy of this treatment rests on a graft-versus-leukaemia (GVL) effect (Porter and Antin, 1998). The extraordinary success in manipulating this reaction, by the use of donor mononuclear cell infusions given to patients who relapse after their allograft, has opened the possibility of new strategies to combat solid tumours. The reassessment of the therapeutic effect of bone-marrow transplantation has led to the realization that a graft-versus-tumour effect may be the main therapeutic benefit of this procedure. The development of non-myeloablative allogeneic peripheral-blood stem-cell transplants, which result in a chimeric marrow but have significantly lower morbidity, is an exciting development. Early work has led to a recent case report of a complete response in a patient with stage III renal cell cancer (Childs *et al.*, 1999a) and reasonably good responses in two of four very advanced malignant melanoma patients (Childs *et al.*, 1999b). It is expected that this approach will be the object of intensive investigations.

FUTURE DIRECTION

The success of some of these treatments in the hands of some and failure in the hands of others requires that positive results be viewed with caution. Several factors may have influenced the outcome of different trials, including the type of immunological approach, the adjuvant, method of preparation and schedule of administration, as well as patient-associated parameters (selection, tumour burden-distribution, etc.) prior to therapy. Unfortunately, none of these parameters are rigorously controlled in early often promising trials.

The only appropriate method of discrimination is the randomized, controlled trial with simple but well-defined end points. To date, the majority of randomized trials that have been undertaken investigating initially promising biotherapy treatments have failed to impress. In some trials, positive results have been gleaned from subset analyses looking at immunological end points that researchers happen to monitor. This has the pitfall of selecting patients out with more intact immune systems, who are able to make immune responses to the vaccines only as a surrogate marker to their innate ability to keep the tumour at bay longer than other patients who do not make immune-responses to the vaccine.

The problems of experimental design and performance of clinical trials for immunotherapy/biotherapy are not fundamentally different from those encountered more generally in cancer clinical trials. However, the yardstick of follow-up decision making, i.e. complete or partial response, is different. The clinician will often have to persevere even in the face of progressive disease before abandoning a line of treatment. The mounting of a successful immune response, especially in studies involving advanced-stage cancer, may be prolonged, and support by frequent surgical cytoreductive procedures may be warranted. Furthermore, it is likely that biotherapeutic approaches would have to be viewed as complementary treatments to other mainstream modalities.

SIGNIFICANT POINTS

- Immune surveillance by competent hosts is an unproven axiom that underpins the thinking of 'immune evasion' of the tumour.
- Established malignancy induces a state of 'immune dysfunction' which should be viewed as a different entity to that of classical immunosuppression. A state of host tolerance towards the tumour is established through a multitude of mechanisms which are not mutually exclusive.
- The field of bio-immunotherapy is finally finding justification through the production of agents that have got clear therapeutic benefits i.e. monoclonal antibodies for lymphoma and breast cancer interferons for haematological malignancies.
- Cytokines in cancer therapy have a significant role in haematological malignancies and probably in the adjuvant treatment of melanoma and the treatment of metastatic renal cell cancer. The developed 'effective' treatments are all characterized by high dose delivery and high levels of toxicity. High-cost high toxicity with small advantage treatments that are difficult to recommend.

- Monoclonal antibody technology has now delivered at least two low-toxicity high efficacy treatments: Rhituximab for CD20 positive lymphomas and Herceptin for her2 neu positive breast cancer. High-cost low morbidity and moderate benefit treatments that are easy to deliver and espouse.
- The efficacy of the antibody technology is clearly dependent on the target antigen. Both antibodies in clinical practice target signalling pathways of the cell.
- Vaccine-based immunotherapy has no representative agents in general usage. There are promising early results from trials of HLA-matched peptide vaccines, dendritic cell vaccines and allogeneic cell vaccines. However, to date all sufficiently powered and well conducted randomized trials have been negative.

ACKNOWLEDGEMENT

We would like to acknowledge the particular help of Nicola Dale in the typing and preparation of this manuscript.

KEY REFERENCES

Colombo, M.P. and Forni, G. (1994) Cytokine gene transfer in tumour inhibition and tumour therapy: where are we now? *Immunol. Today* **15**, 48.

Gong, J., Chen, D., Kashiwaba, M. and Kufe, D. (1997) Induction of antitumour activity by immunization with fusions of dendritic and carcinoma cells. *Nat Med.* **3**, 558–61.

Johnson, P.W. and Glennie, M.J. (2001) Rituximab: mechanisms and applications. *Br. J. Cancer* **85**, 1619–23.

Nestle, F.O., Burg, G. and Dummer, R. (1999) New perspectives on immunobiology and immunotherapy of melanoma. *Immunol. Today* **20**(1), 5–7.

Taylor-Papadimitriou, J. and Finn, O.J. (1997) Biology, biochemistry and immunology of carcinoma-associated mucins. *Immunol. Today* **18**, 105–7.

REFERENCES

Appelbaum, F.R., Sullivan, K., Buckner, C.D. *et al.* (1987) Treatment of malignant lymphoma in 100 patients with chemotherapy, total body irradiation and marrow transplantation. *J. Clin. Oncol.* **5**, 1340–7.

Atzpodien, J., Kirchner, H., Illiger, H.J. *et al.* (2001) IL-2 in combination with IFN-alpha and 5-FU versus tamoxifen in metastatic renal cell carcinoma: long-term results of a controlled randomized clinical trial. *Br. J. Cancer* **85**, 1130–6.

Bagshawe, K.D. (1993) Antibody-directed enzyme prodrug therapy (ADEPT). *Adv. Pharmacol.* **24**, 99–121.

Berd, D. and Mastrangelo, M.J. (1987) Effect of low dose cyclophosphamide on the immune system of cancer patients: reduction of T suppressor function without depletion of the CD8+ subset. *Cancer Res.* **47**, 3317.

Berd, D. and Mastrangelo, M.J. (1988a) Active immunotherapy of human melanoma exploiting the immunopotentiating effects of cyclophosphamide. *Cancer Invest.* **6**, 335.

Berd, D. and Mastrangelo, M.J. (1988b) Effect of low dose cyclophosphamide on the immune system of cancer patients: depletion of CD4+ 2H4+ suppressor-inducer T-cells. *Cancer Res.* **48**, 1671.

Berd, D., Maguire, H.C. Jr and Mastrangelo, M.J. (1986) Induction of cell-mediated immunity to autologous melanoma cells and regression of metastases after treatment with a melanoma cell vaccine preceded by cyclophosphamide. *Cancer Res.* **46**, 2572.

Berd, D., Maguire, H.C. Jr, McCue, P. and Mastrangelo, M.J. (1990) Treatment of metastatic melanoma with an autologous tumor-cell vaccine: clinical and immunological results in 64 patients. *J. Clin. Oncol.* **8**, 1858.

Blumgart, H.L. and Yens, O.C. (1927) Studies on velocity of blood flow: the method utilised. *J. Clin. Invest.* **4**, 1–13.

Borberg, H., Oettgen, H.F., Choudry, K. and Beattie, E.J. (1972) Inhibition of established transplants of chemically induced sarcomas in syngeneic mice by lymphocytes from immunised donors. *Int. J. Cancer* **10**, 539–43.

Borysiewicz, L.K., Fiander, A., Nimako, M., Man, S. and Inglis, S.C. (1996) A recombinant vaccinia virus encoding human papillomavirus types 16 and 18, E6 and E7 proteins as immunotherapy for cervical cancer. *Lancet* **347**, 1523–7.

Breitz, H.B., Fisher, D.R., Weiden, P.L. *et al.* (1993) Dosimetry of rhenium-186-labelled monoclonal-antibodies: methods, prediction from technetium-99m-labelled antibodies and results of phase I trials. *J. Nucl. Med.* **34**(6), 908–17.

Breitz, H.B., Weiden, P.L., Appelbaum, J.W. *et al.* (1999) Pretargeted radioimmunotherapy (PRIT) for the treatment of non-Hodgkin's lymphoma: preliminary results. *J. Nucl. Med.* **40**, 19.

Bruns, P. (1887–1888) Die Heilwirking des Erysipelas of Geschwulste. *Beitr. Klin. Chir.* **3**, 443.

Burchell, J., Taylor-Papadimitriou, J., Boshell, M., Gendler, S. and Duhig, T. (1989) A short sequence, within the amino acid tandem repeat of a cancer-associated mucin, contains immunodominant epitopes. *Int. J. Cancer* **44**, 691–6.

Carney, W. (1988) Human tumor antigens and specific tumor therapy. *Immunol. Today* **9**, 363.

Carrel, S. and Johnson, J. (1993) Immunologic recognition of malignant melanoma by autologous lymphocytes. *Curr. Opin. Oncol.* **5**, 383–9.

Cascinelli, N., Bufalino, R., Morabito, A. and Mackie (1994) Results of adjuvant interferon study in WHO melanoma programme. *Lancet* **343**, 913–14.

Cassel, W.A., Murray, D.R. and Phillips, H.S. (1983) A phase II study on the post-surgical management of stage II malignant melanoma with a Newcastle disease virus oncolysate. *Cancer* **52**, 856.

Chappell, D.B., Zaks, T.Z., Rosenberg, S.A. and Restifo, N.P. (1999) Human melanoma cells do not express Fas (Apo-1/CD95) ligand. *Cancer Res.* **59**, 59–62.

Chievitz, O. and Hevesy, G. (1937) Studies on the metabolism of phosphorus in animals. *KGL Danske Videnskabernes. Selskab. Biol. Meddelelser.* **13**, 9–33.

Childs, R.W., Clave, E., Tisdale, J. *et al.* (1999a) Successful treatment of metastatic renal cell carcinoma with non-myeloablative allogeneic peripheral-blood progenitor cell transplant: evidence for a graft-versus-tumour effect. *J. Clin. Oncol.* **17**, 2044–9.

Childs, R.W., Clave, E., Bahceci, D. *et al.* (1999b) Non-myeloablative peripheral stem cell transplantation (N-PBSCT) as adoptive allogeneic immunotherapy for metastatic melanoma (MM) and renal cell carcinoma (RCC). *Proc. Am. Soc. Clin. Oncol.* **18**, 52a.

Cobb, L.M. (1989) Intratumour factors influencing the access of antibody to tumour cells. *Cancer Immunol. Immunother.* **28**, 235–40.

Coca, A.F. and Gilman, G. (1909) The specific treatment of carcinoma. *Phil. J. Sci. Med.* **4**, 381.

Coca, A.F., Dorrance, G.M. and Lebredo, M.G. (1912) Vaccination in cancer: a report of the results of vaccination therapy as applied to seventy-nine cases of human cancer. *Z. Immun. Exp. Ther.* **13**, 543.

Coley, W.B. (1894) Treatment of inoperable malignant tumours with the toxins of erysipelas and the Bacillus prodigosus. *Trans. Am. Surg. Assoc.* **12**, 183.

Cooley, S., Burns, L.J., Repka, T. and Miller, J.S. (1999) Natural killer cell cytotoxicity of breast cancer targets is enhanced by two distinct mechanisms of antibody-dependant cellular cytotoxicity against LFA-3 and HER2/neu. *Exp. Hematol.* **27**, 1533–41.

Cunningham, T.J., Olson, K.B., Laffin, R., Horton, J. and Sullivan, J. (1969) Treatment of advanced cancer with active immunization. *Cancer* **24**, 932.

Czajkowski, N.P., Rosenblatt, M., Wolf, P.L. and Vasquez, J. (1967) A new method of active immunization to autologous human tumour tissue. *Lancet* **2**, 905.

Czuczman, M., Grillo-Lopez, A.J., White, C.A. *et al.* (1996) IDEC-C2B8/CHOP chemoimmunotherapy in patients with low-grade lymphoma: clinical and Bcl-2 (PCR) results. *Blood* **88**, 453a.

Dalgleish, A.G. (1996) Co-stimulatory molecules and their role in tumour immunity. *Tumor immunology: immunotherapy and cancer vaccines.* Cambridge: Cambridge University Press.

Dalgleish, A.G., Sauven, P., Fermont, D. *et al.* (1991) Local IL-2 in locally advanced breast cancer. *J. Exp. Clin. Cancer Res.* **9**, 4–5.

Davis, T.A., Maloney, D.G., Czerwinski, D.K. *et al.* (1998) Anti-idiotype antibodies can induce long-term complete remissions in non-Hodgkin's lymphoma without eradicating the malignant clone. *Blood* **92**, 1184–90.

Davis, T.A., Grillo-Lopez, A.J., White, C.A. *et al.* (2000) Rituximab anti-CD20 monoclonal antibody therapy in non-Hodgkin's lymphoma: safety and efficacy of re-treatment. *J. Clin. Oncol.* **18**, 3135–43.

Deans, J.P., Schieven, G.L., Shu, G.L. *et al.* (1993) Association of tyrosine and serine kinase with the B cell surface antigen CD20: induction via CD20 of tyrosine phosphorylation and activation of phospholipase C-γ-I and phospholipase C-γ-II. *J. Immunol.* **151**, 4494–504.

Demetrick, D.J., Herlyn, D., Tretiak, M. *et al.* (1992) ME491 melanoma-associated glycoprotein family: antigenic identity of ME491, NKI/C-3, neuroglandular antigen (NGA) and CD63 proteins. *J. Natl Cancer Inst.* **84**(6), 422–9.

DeNardo, S.J., Kroger, L.A. and DeNardo, G.L. (1999) A new era for radiolabelled antibodies in cancer? *Curr. Opin. Immunol.* **11**, 563–9.

Dillman, O. (1999) Unconjugated monoclonal antibodies for the treatment of hematological and solid malignancies. ASCO Educational Book, 461–8.

Dore, J.F., Portoukalian, J., Berthier-Vergnes, O. *et al.* (1990) Response in patients with melanoma to immunization using oncolysates of vaccine virus. *Bull. Cancer* **77**, 881–91.

Dykes, P.W., Bradwell, A.R., Chapman, C.E. *et al.* (1987) Radioimmunotherapy of cancer: clinical studies and limiting factors. *Cancer Treat. Rev.* **14**, 87–106.

Epenetos, A.A. (ed.) (1991) *Monoclonal antibodies; applications in clinical oncology*, vols 1 and 2. London: Chapman and Hall.

Epenetos, A.A., Snook, D., Durbin, H. *et al.* (1986) Limitations of radiolabelled monoclonal antibodies for localization of human neoplasms. *Cancer Res.* **46**, 3183–91.

Farzaneh, N.K., Walden, T.L., Hearing, V.J. and Gersten, D.M. (1991) B700, an albumin-like melanoma-specific antigen, is a vitamin D binding protein. *Eur. J. Cancer* **27**(9), 1158–62.

Fehleisen, F. (1882) Uber die Zuchtung der Erysipel-Kokken auf kuntschlichen Nahrboden und die Ubertragbarkeit auf den Menschen. *Deutsche Med. Wschr.* **8**, 533.

Freeman, G.J., Gribben, J.G., Boussiotis, V.A. et al. (1993) Cloning of B7-2: a CTLA-4 counter receptor in B7-deficient mice. Science 262(5135), 909–11.

French, R.R., Chan, H.T., Tutt, A.L. and Glennie, M.J. (1999) CD40 antibody evokes a cytotoxic T-cell response that eradicates lymphoma and bypasses T-cell help. Nat. Med. 5, 548–53.

Gabrilovich, D.I., Chen, H.L., Girgis, K.R. et al. (1996) Production of vascular endothelial growth factor by human tumors inhibits the functional maturation of dendritic cells. Nat. Med. 2, 1096–103.

Gendler, S., Taylor-Papadimitriou, J., Duhig, T., Rothbard, J. and Burchell, J. (1988) A highly immunogenic region of a human polymorphic epithelial mucin expressed by carcinomas is made up of tandem repeats. J. Biol. Chem. 263, 12280–3.

Glennie, M.J., Brennand, M.J., Bryden, F. et al. (1988) Bispecific F(ab'-γ)$_2$ antibody for the delivery of saporin in the treatment of lymphoma. J. Immunol. 141, 3662–70.

Goldenberg, D.M. (1993) Monoclonal antibodies in cancer detection and therapy. Am. J. Med. 94, 297–312.

Goldenberg, D.M. (ed.) (1995) Cancer therapy with radiolabeled antibodies. Boca Raton: CRC Press.

Goldenberg, D., Deland, F. et al. (1978) Use of radiolabelled antibodies to carcinoembryonic antigen for the detection and localisation of diverse cancers by external photoscanning. N. Engl. J. Med. 298, 1384–8.

Graham, J.B. and Graham, R.M. (1962) Autologous vaccine in cancer patients. Surg. Gynec. Obstet. 109, 121.

Grant, S.C., Kris, M.G., Houghton, A.N. and Chapman, P.B. (1999) Long survival of patients with small cell lung cancer after adjuvant treatment with the anti-idiotypic antibody BEC2 plus bacillus Calmette–Guérin. Clin. Cancer Res. 5, 1319–23.

Gratama, J.W., Zea, A.H., Bolhuis, R.L. and Ochoa, A.C. (1999) Restoration of expression of signal-transduction molecules in lymphocytes from patients with metastatic renal cell cancer after combination immunotherapy. Cancer Immunol. Immunother. 48, 263–9.

Grob, J.J., Dreno, B., de la Salmonière, P. et al. (1998) Randomised trial of interferon α-2a as adjuvant therapy in resected primary melanoma thicker than 1.5 mm without clinically detectable node metastases. Lancet 351, 1905–10.

Gupta, R.K., Golub, S.H. and Morton, D.L. (1979) Correlation between tumor burden and anticomplementary activity in sera from patients. Cancer Immunol. Immunother. 6, 63.

Hahne, M., Rimoldi, D., Schröter, M. et al. (1996) Melanoma cell expression of Fas (Apo-1/CD95) ligand: implications for tumour immune escape. Science 274, 1363–6.

Hale, G., Clark, M. and Waldmann, H. (1985) Therapeutic potential of rat monoclonal antibodies: isotype specificity of antibody-dependant cell-mediated cytotoxicity with human lymphocytes. J. Immunol. 134, 3056–61.

Hanna, M.G. Jr, Peters, L.C., Hoover, H.C. Jr (1989) Fundamentals of active specific immunotherapy of cancer using BCG-tumor cell vaccines. Prog. Clin. Biol. Res. 310, 51–65.

Harris, J.E., Ryan, L., Hoover, H.C. et al. (2000) Adjuvant active specific immunotherapy for stage II and III colon cancer with an autologous tumour cell vaccine: eastern co-operative oncology group study E5283. J. Clin. Oncol. 18, 148–53.

Hellman, S., Chaffey, J.T., Rosenthal, D.S. et al. (1977) The place of radiation therapy in the treatment of non-Hodgkin's lymphomas. Cancer 39, 843–51.

Heppner, G.H. (1984) Tumor heterogeneity. Cancer Res. 44, 2259.

Hericourt, J. and Richet, C. (1895) Traitment d'un cas de sarcome par la serotherapie. Compte Rendu Hebdomadaire des Sceances de l'Academie des Sciences 120, 948–52.

Herlyn, D. and Koprowski, H. (1982) IgG2a monoclonal antibodies inhibit human tumor growth through interaction with effector cells. Proc. Natl Acad. Sci. USA 79, 4761–5.

Herlyn, M., Thurin, J., Balaban, G. et al. (1985) Characteristics of human melanocytes isolated from different stages of tumor progression. Cancer Res. 45, 5670.

Hersey, P., Edwards, A., Coates, A. et al. (1987) Evidence that treatment with vaccinia melanoma cell lysates (VMCL) may improve survival of patients with stage II melanoma. Cancer Immunol. Immunother. 25, 257–63.

Hills, D., Rowlinson-Busza, G. and Gullick, W.J. (1995) Specific targeting of a mutant, activated EGF receptor found in glioblastoma using a monoclonal antibody. Int. J. Cancer 63, 537–43.

Himmelweit, F. (1957) The collected papers of Paul Ehrlich. Immunology and Cancer Research. London: Persimmon Press.

Hird, V., Maraveyas, A., Snook, D. et al. (1993) Adjuvant therapy of ovarian cancer with radioactive monoclonal antibody. Br. J. Cancer 68, 403–6.

Hnatowich, D.J., Virzi, F. and Rusckowski, M. (1987) Investigations of avidin and biotin for imaging purposes. J. Nucl. Med. 28, 1294–302.

Hollinshead, A., Arlen, M., Yonemoto, R. et al. (1982) Pilot studies using melanoma tumor-associated antigens (TAA) in specific active immunotherapy of malignant melanoma. Cancer 49, 1387.

Jain, R.K. (1988) Determinants of tumour blood flow: a review. Cancer Res. 48, 2641–58.

Jain, R.K. (1991) Haemodynamic and transport barriers to the treatment of solid tumours. Int. J. Radiat. Oncol. Biol. Phys. 60, 85–100.

Jain, R.K. and Baxter, L.T. (1988) Mechanisms of heterogeneous distribution of monoclonal antibodies and other macromolecules in tumours: significance of elevated interstitial pressure. *Cancer Res.* **48**, 7022–32.

Jones, P.C., Sze, L.L., Liu, P.Y., Morton, D.L. and Irie, R.F. (1981) Prolonged survival for melanoma patients with elevated IgM antibody to oncofetal antigen. *J. Natl Cancer Inst.* **66**(2), 249–54.

Kalofonos, H.P., Pawlikowska, T.R., Hemingway, A. *et al.* (1989) Antibody guided diagnosis and therapy of brain gliomas using radiolabelled monoclonal antibodies against epidermal growth factor receptor and placental alkaline phosphatase. *J. Nucl. Med.* **30**, 1636–45.

Kalofonos, H.P., Ruscowski, M., Siebecker, D.A. *et al.* (1990) Imaging of tumor in patients with indium-111 labelled biotin and streptavidin-conjugated antibodies: preliminary communication. *J. Nucl. Med.* **31**, 1791–6.

Kan-Mitchell, J., Huang, X.Q., Steinman, L. *et al.* (1993) Clonal analysis of *in vivo* activated CD8+ cytotoxic T lymphocytes from a melanoma patient responsive to active specific immunotherapy. *Cancer Immunol. Immunother.* **37**, 15–25.

Kersh, E.N., Shaw, A.S. and Allen, P.M. (1998) Fidelity of T-cell activation through multistep T cell receptor zeta phosphorylation. *Science* **281**, 572–5.

Kersh, E.N., Kersh, G.J. and Allen, P.M. (1999) Partially phosphorylated T cell receptor zeta molecules can inhibit T-cell activation. *J. Exp. Med.* **190**, 1627–36.

Kirkwood, J.M., Strawderman, M.H., Ernstof, M.S. *et al.* (1996) Interferon alfa-2b adjuvant therapy of high risk resected cutaneous melanoma: the eastern co-operative oncology group trial EST 1684. *J. Clin. Oncol.* **14**, 7–17.

Kirkwood, J.M., Ibrahim, J., Sondak, K. *et al.* (1999) Preliminary analysis of the E1690/S9111/C9190 intergroup postoperative adjuvant trial of high- and low-dose IFNa2b (HDI and LDI) in high-risk primary or lymph node metastatic melanoma. *Proc. Am. Soc. Clin. Oncol.* **18**, 537a.

Kirkwood, J.M., Ibrahim, J.G., Sosman, J.A. *et al.* (2001) High-dose interferon alfa-2b significantly prolongs relapse-free and overall survival compared with the GM2-KLH/QS-21 vaccine in patients with resected stage IIB-III melanoma: results of intergroup trial E1694/S9512/C509801. *J. Clin. Oncol.* **19**, 2370–80.

Kohler, G. and Milstein, C. (1975) Continuous culture of fused cells secreting antibody of predefined specificity. *Nature* **256**, 1197–203.

Kreitman, R.J. (1999) Immunotoxins in cancer therapy. *Curr. Opin. Immunol.* **11**, 570–8.

Kreitman, R.J. and Pastan, I. (1995) Importance of the glutamate residue of KDEL in increasing the cytotoxicity of pseudomonas exotoxin derivatives and for increasing binding to the KDEL receptor. *Biochem. J.* **307**, 29–37.

Kuijpers, W.H.A., Bos, E.S., Kasparsen, F.M. *et al.* (1993) Specific recognition of antibody oligonucleotide conjugate by radiolabelled antisense nucleotide: a novel approach to two-step radioimmunotherapy of cancer. *Bioconjugate Chem.* **4**, 94–102.

Lashford, L.S., Davies, A.G., Richardson, R.B. *et al.* (1988) A pilot study of ^{131}I monoclonal antibodies in the therapy of leptomeningeal tumours. *Cancer* **61**, 857–68.

Lejeune, F.L., Uegg, C. and Lienard, D. (1998) Clinical applications of TNF-α in cancer. *Curr. Opin. Immunol.* **10**, 573–80.

LeMaistre, C.F., Saleh, M.N., Kuzel, T.M. *et al.* (1998) Phase I trial of a ligand fusion-protein (DAB389IL-2) in lymphomas expressing the receptor for IL-2. *Blood* **91**, 399–405.

Leveille, C., Aldacca, K.R. and Mourad, W. (1999) CD20 is physically and functionally coupled to MHC class II and CD40 on human B cell lines. *Eur. J. Immunol.* **29**, 65–74.

Livingston, P.O. (1993) Approaches to augmenting the IgG antibody response to melanoma ganglioside vaccines. *Ann. N.Y. Acad. Sci.* **690**, 204–13.

Livingston, P.O., Kaelin, K., Pinsky, C.M. *et al.* (1985) The serological response of patients with stage II melanoma to allogeneic melanoma cell vaccines. *Cancer* **56**, 713–18.

Livingston, P.O., Calves, M.J. and Natoli, E.J. (1987) Approaches to augmenting the immunogenicity of the ganglioside GM2 is superior to whole cells. *J. Immunol.* **138**, 1524–31.

Livingston, P.O., Wong, G.Y., Adluri, S. *et al.* (1994) Improved survival in stage III melanoma patients with GM2 antibodies: a randomized trial of adjuvant vaccination with GM2 ganglioside. *J. Clin. Oncol.* **12**, 1036–44.

Ljunggren, H.G. and Karre, K. (1990) In search of the 'missing self': MHC molecules and NK recognition. *Immunol. Today* **11**, 237–44.

Loevinger, R. and Berman, M.A. (1968) *A schema for absorbed-dose calculations for biologically-distributed radionuclides.* New York.

Lotze, M.T., Rubin, J.T., Edington, H.D. *et al.* (1992) The treatment of patients with melanoma using interleukin-2, interleukin-4 and tumour infiltrating lymphocytes. *Hum. Gene Ther.* **3**, 167–77.

Lundin, J., Osterborg, A., Brittinger, G. *et al.* (1998) CAMPATH-1H monoclonal antibody in therapy for previously treated low-grade non-Hodgkin's lymphomas: a phase II multicenter study. European study group of CAMPATH-1H treatment in low-grade non-Hodgkin's lymphoma. *J. Clin. Oncol.* **16**, 3257–63.

Mach, J.P., Carrel, S., Merenda, C. *et al.* (1974) *In vivo* localisation of radiolabelled antibodies to carcinoembryonic antigen in human colon carcinoma grafted into nude mice. *Nature* **248**, 704–6.

Mackensen, A., Carcelain, G., Viel, S. et al. (1994) Direct evidence to support the immuno-surveillance concept in a human regressive melanoma. *J. Clin. Invest.* **93**, 1397–402.

Maclean, G.D., Miles, D.W., Rubens, R.D., Reddish, M.A., and Longenecker, B.M. (1996a) Enhancing the effect of theratope STn-KLH cancer vaccine in patients with metastatic breast cancer by pretreatment with low-dose intravenous cyclophosphamide. *J. Immunother. Emphasis Tumor Immunol.* **19**, 309–16.

Maclean, G.D., Reddish, M.A., Koganty, R.R. and Longenecker, B.M. (1996b) Antibodies against mucin-associated sialyl-Tn epitopes correlate with survival of metastatic adenocarcinoma patients undergoing specific immunotherapy with synthetic STn vaccine. *J. Immunother. Emphasis Tumor Immunol.* **19**, 59–68.

Maraveyas, A. and Epenetos, A.A. (1991) An overview of radioimmunotherapy. *Cancer Immunol. Immunother.* **34**, 71–3.

Maraveyas, A., Hrouda, D. and Dalgleish, A.G. (1998) Tumour immunology. In Mackiewicz, A. and Sehgal, P.B. (eds), *Molecular aspects of cancer and its therapy*. Basel/Switzerland: Birkhäuser Verlag, 73–87.

Maraveyas, A., Baban, B., Kennard, D. et al. (1999) Possible improved survival of patients with stage IV AJCC melanoma receiving SRL 172 immunotherapy: correlation with induction of increased levels of intracellular interleukin-2 in peripheral blood lymphocytes. *Ann. Oncol.* **10**(7), 817–24.

Marchand, M., van Baven, N., Weynants, P. et al. (1999) Tumour regressions observed in patients with metastatic melanoma treated with an antigenic peptide encoded by gene MAGE-3 and presented by HLA-A1. *Int. J. Cancer* **80**(2), 219–30.

Martin, J., Stribbling, S.M., Poon, G.K. et al. (1997) Antibody-directed enzyme prodrug therapy: pharmacokinetics and plasma levels of prodrug and drug in a phase I clinical trial. *Cancer Chemother. Pharmacol.* **40**, 189–201.

Mattijssen, V., De Mulder, P.H., De Graeff, A. et al. (1994) Intratumoural PEG-interleukin-2 therapy in patients with locoregionally recurrent head and neck squamous-cell carcinoma. *Ann. Oncol.* **5**, 957–60.

Mausner, L.F. and Srivastava, S.C. (1993) Selection of radionuclides for radioimmunotherapy. *Med. Phys.* **20**(2), 503–9.

McCaffery, M., Yao, T.J., Williams, L. et al. (1996) Immunization of melanoma patients with BEC2 anti-idiotypic monoclonal antibody that mimics GD3 ganglioside: enhanced immunogenicity when combined with adjuvant. *Clin. Cancer Res.* **2**, 679–86.

Mendelsohn, J. (1997) Epidermal growth factor receptor inhibition by a monoclonal antibody as anticancer therapy. *Clin. Cancer Res.* **3**, 2703–7.

Miles, D.W., Towlson, K.E., Graham, R.D. et al. (1996) A randomised phase II study of sialyl-Tn and DETOX-B adjuvant with or without cyclophosphamide pretreatment for the active specific immunotherapy of breast cancer. *Br. J. Cancer* **74**, 1292–6.

Mitchell, M.S., Kan-Mitchell, J., Kempf, R.A., Harel, W., Shau, H. and Lind, S. (1988) Active specific immunotherapy for melanoma: phase I trial of allogeneic lysates and a novel adjuvant. *Cancer Res.* **48**, 5883.

Mitchell, M.S., Harel, W., Kan-Mitchell, J. et al. (1993) Active specific immunotherapy of melanoma with allogeneic cell lysates. Rationale, results and possible mechanisms of action. *Ann. N.Y. Acad. Sci.* **690**, 153–66.

Mittelman, A., Chen, Z.J., Yang, H. et al. (1992) Human high molecular weight melanoma associated antigen (HMW-MAA) mimicry by mouse anti-idiotypic monoclonal antibody MK2-23: induction of humoral anti-HMW-MAA immunity and prolongation of survival in patients with stage IV melanoma. *Proc. Natl Acad. Sci. USA* **89**(2), 466–70.

Molero, I., Shuford, W.W., Newby, S.A. et al. (1997) Monoclonal antibodies against the 4-1BB T-cell activation molecule eradicate established tumors. *Nat. Med.* **3**, 682–5.

Moloney, D.G., Grillo-Lopez, A.J., Bodkin, D.J. et al. (1997) IDEC-CD2B8: results of a phase I multiple dose trial in patients with relapsed non-Hodgkin's lymphoma. *J. Clin. Oncol.* **15**, 3266–74.

Morton, D.L., Eilber, F.R., Holmes, E.C. et al. (1974) BCG immunotherapy of malignant melanoma: summary of a seven year experience. *Ann. Surg.* **180**, 635.

Morton, D.L., Foshag, L.J., Hoon, D.S. et al. (1992) Prolongation of survival in metastatic melanoma after specific immunotherapy with a new polyvalent melanoma vaccine. *Ann. Surg.* **216**(4), 463–82.

Morton, D.L., Hoon, D.S., Nizze, J.A. et al. (1993) Polyvalent melanoma vaccine improves survival of patients with metastatic melanoma. *Ann. N.Y. Acad. Sci.* **690**, 120–34.

MRC collaborators (1999) Interferon-α and survival in metastatic renal carcinoma: early results of a randomised controlled trial. Medical Research Council Renal Cancer Collaborators. *Lancet* **353**, 14–17.

Nestle, F.O., Alijagic, S., Gilliet, M. et al. (1998) Vaccination of melanoma patients with peptide- or tumor lysate-pulsed dendritic cells. *Nat. Med.* **4**, 328–32.

Nicholson, S., Gooden, C.S.R., Hird, V. et al. (1998) Radioimmunotherapy after chemotherapy compared to chemotherapy alone in the treatment of advanced ovarian cancer: a matched analysis. *Oncol. Rep.* **5**, 22–6.

Nitta, T., Sako, K., Yagita, H. et al. (1990) Preliminary trial of specific targeting therapy against malignant glioma. *Lancet* **335**, 368–71.

Nowell, P.C. (1986) Mechanisms of tumor progression. *Cancer Res.* **46**, 2203.

Oaks, M.K., Hanson, J.P. Jr and O'Malley, D.P. (1994) Molecular cytogenetic mapping of the human melanoma antigen (MAGE) family to chromosome region Xq27-qter: implications for MAGE immunotherapy. *Cancer Res.* **54**, 1627–9.

O'Byrne, K.J. and Dalgleish, A.G. (2000) Evolution, immune response and cancer. *Lancet* **356**, 242–4.

O'Donoghue, J.A. (1993) Optimal therapeutic strategies for RIT. *Strahlenther. Onkol.* **169**, 372.

Oettgen, H.F. and Old, L.J. (1991) The history of cancer immunotherapy. In Devita, V. (ed.), *Biologic therapy of cancer*. Philadelphia: Lippincott, 216–20.

Old, L.J. (1985) Tumour necrosis factor (TNF). *Science* **230**, 630–2.

Paganelli, G., Pervez, S., Siccardi, A. *et al.* (1990) Intra-peritoneal radio-localizaton of tumours pre-targeted by biotinylated monoclonal antibodies. *Int. J. Cancer* **45**, 1184–9.

Pai, L.H., Wittes, R., Setser, A. *et al.* (1996) Treatment of advanced solid tumors with immunotoxin LMB-1 an antibody linked to pseudomonas exotoxin. *Nat. Med.* **2**, 350–3.

Philip, P.A. and Flaherty, L. (1997) Treatment of malignant melanoma with interleukin-2. *Semin. Oncol.* **24**, S32–38.

Pietras, R.J., Poen, J.C., Gallardo, D. *et al.* (1999) Monoclonal antibody to HER2-neu receptor modulates repair of radiation induced DNA damage and enhances radiosensitivity of human breast cancer cells over-expressing this oncogene. *Cancer Res.* **59**, 1347–55.

Porter, D.L. and Antin, J.H. (1998) Infusion of donor peripheral blood mononuclear cells to treat relapse after transplantation for chronic myelogenous leukemia. *Hematol. Oncol. Clin. North Am.* **12**, 123–50.

Press, O.W., Eary, J.F., Appelbaum, F.R. *et al.* (1993) Radiolabelled-antibody therapy of B-cell lymphoma with autologous bone-marrow support. *N. Engl. J. Med.* **329**(17): 1219–24.

Punt, C.J., Nagy, A., Douillard, J. *et al.* (2001) Edrecolomab (17-1A antibody) alone or in combination with 5-fluorouracil based chemotherapy in the adjuvant treatment of stage III colon cancer: results of a phase III study. *Proc. Am. Soc. Clin. Onc.* **20**, 123a.

Purhönen, S., Salminen, E., Ruutu, M. *et al.* (1999) Prospective randomized trial of interferon alfa-2a plus vinblastine versus vinblastine alone in patients with advanced renal cell cancer. *J. Clin. Oncol.* **17**, 2859–61.

Rabinowich, H., Banks, M., Reichert, T.E. *et al.* (1996) Expression and activity of signalling molecules in T lymphocytes obtained from patients with metastatic melanoma before and after interleukin 2 therapy. *Clin. Cancer Res.* **2**, 1263–74.

Radrizzani, M., Benedetti, B., Castelli, C. *et al.* (1991) Human allogeneic melanoma-reactive T helper lymphocyte clones: functional analysis of lymphocyte-melanoma interactions. *Int. J. Cancer* **49**(6), 823–30.

Ravindranath, M.H., Morton, D.L. and Irie, R.F. (1989) An epitope common to gangliosides O-acetyl-GD3 and GD3 recognized by antibodies in melanoma patients after active specific immunotherapy. *Cancer Res.* **49**, 3891–9.

Reichert, T.E., Rabinowich, H., Johnson, J.T. and Whiteside, T.L. (1998) Mechanisms responsible for signalling and functional defects. *J. Immunother.* **21**, 295–306.

Riethmuller, G., Holz, E., Schlimok, G. *et al.* (1998) Monoclonal antibody therapy for resected Dukes' C colorectal cancer: seven year outcome of a multi-center randomised trial. *J. Clin. Oncol.* **16**, 1788–94.

Risley, E.H. (1911) The Gilman–Coca vaccine emulsion treatment of cancer. *Boston Med. Surg. J.* **165**, 784.

Rosenberg, S.A., Packard, B.S., Aebersold, P.M. *et al.* (1988) Use of tumour-infiltrating lymphocytes and interleukin-2 in the immunotherapy of patients with metastatic melanoma. *N. Engl. J. Med.* **319**, 1676–80.

Rosenberg, S.A., Lotze, M.T., Yang, J.C. *et al.* (1993) Prospective randomised trial of high dose interleukin-2 alone or in conjunction with lymphokine activated killer cells for the treatment of patients with advanced cancer. *J. Natl Cancer Inst.* **85**, 622–6.

Rosenberg, S.A., Yang, J.C., Schwartzentruber, D.J. *et al.* (1998) Immunological and therapeutic evaluation of a synthetic peptide vaccine for the treatment of patients with metastatic melanoma. *Nat. Med.* **4**, 321–7.

Rowlinson-Busza, G., Bamias, A., Kraus, T. *et al.* (1991) Cytotoxicity following specific activation of amygdalin. In Epenetos, A.A. (ed.), *Monoclonal antibodies: applications in clinical oncology*. London: Chapman and Hall, 179–83.

Sato, T., McCue, P., Masuoka, K. *et al.* (1996) Interleukin 10 production by human melanoma. *Clin. Cancer Res.* **2**, 1383–90.

Savage, H.E., Rossen, R.D., Hersh, E.M., Freedman, R.S., Bowen, J.M. and Plager, C. (1986) Antibody development to viral and allogeneic tumor cell-associated antigens in patients with malignant melanoma and ovarian carcinoma treated with lysates of virus infected cells. *Cancer Res.* **46**, 2127–33.

Seigler, H.F., Shingleton, W.W., Metzgar, R.S. *et al.* (1972) Non-specific and specific immunotherapy in patients with melanoma. *Surgery* **72**, 162–74.

Seto, M., Takahashi, T., Nakamura, S. *et al.* (1983) *In vivo* antitumor effects of monoclonal antibodies with different immunoglobulin classes. *Cancer Res.* **43**, 4768–73.

Shan, D., Ledbetter, J.A. and Press, O.W. (1998) Apoptosis of malignant human B cells by ligation of CD20 with monoclonal antibodies. *Blood* **91**, 1644–52.

Sharkey, R.M., Goldenberg, D.M., Badger, C.C. *et al.* (1994) Phase-I clinical evaluation of a new murine monoclonal antibody (mu-9) against colon-specific antigen-p for targeting gastrointestinal carcinomas. *Cancer* **73**(3), 864–77.

Shaw, D.R., Khazaeli, M.B. and Lobuglio, A.F. (1988) Mouse/human chimeric antibodies to a tumor-associated antigen; biologic activity of the four human IgG subclasses. *J. Natl Cancer Inst.* **80**, 1553–9.

Siegel, J.A., Goldenberg, D.M. and Badger, C.C. (1993) Radioimmunotherapy dose estimation in patients with B-cell lymphoma. *Med. Phys.* **20**, 579–82.

Simmons, R.L. and Rios, A. (1971) Combined use of BCG and neuraminidase in experimental tumor immunotherapy. *Surg. Forum* **22**, 99.

Snyder, W.S., Ford, M.R., Watson, S.B. *et al.* (1978) Estimates of specific absorbed dose fractions for photon sources uniformly absorbed in various organs of a heterogenous phantom. Medical Internal Radiation Dose (MIRD). Ed. S. N. Med. New York, 5–67.

Stevenson, F., Zhu, D., King, C., Ashworth, L., Kumar, S. and Hawkins, R. (1995) Idiotypic DNA vaccines against B-cell lymphoma. *Immunol. Rev.* **145**, 211–28.

Stewart, J.S.W., Hird, V., Snook, D. *et al.* (1990) Intraperitoneal Yttrium-90-labelled monoclonal antibody in ovarian cancer. *J. Clin. Oncol.* **8**, 1941–50.

Stewart, S., Maraveyas, A., Stafford, N. *et al.* (1993) Combined antibody targeted radiotherapy with external beam irradiation for loco-regional tumour control. *Br. J. Radiol.* **66**, 145.

Takahashi, C., Mittler, R.S. and Vella, A.T. (1999) Cutting edge: 4-1BB is a bona fide CD8 T cell survival signal. *J. Immunol.* **162**, 5037–40.

Takita, H., Minowada, J., Han, T. *et al.* (1976) Adjuvant immunotherapy in bronchogenic carcinoma. *Ann. N.Y. Acad. Sci.* **277**, 345–54.

Thèze, J. (1999) *The cytokine and immune functions.* Oxford: Oxford University Press.

Tindle, R.W. (2001) Immune evasion in human papillomavirus-associated cervical cancer. *Nat. Rev.* **2**, 59–65.

Townsend, S.E. and Allison, J.P. (1993) Tumour rejection after direct costimulation by B7-transfected melanoma cells. *Science* **259**(5093), 368–70.

Tutt, A.L., French, R.R., Illidge, T.M. *et al.* (1998) Monoclonal antibody therapy of B-cell lymphoma: signalling activity on tumour cells appears more important than recruitment of effectors. *J. Immunol.* **161**, 3176–85.

Ulmer, J.B., Donnelly, J.J., Parker, S.E. *et al.* (1993) Heterologous protection against influenza by injection of DNA encoding a viral protein. *Science* **259**, 1745–9.

Van Der Bruggen, P. (1991) A gene encoding an antigen recognised by cytolytic T lymphocytes on a human melanoma. *Science* **254**, 1643.

Vaughan, A.T.M., Anderson, P., Dykes, P.W. *et al.* (1987) Limitations to the killing of tumours using radiolabelled antibodies. *Br. J. Radiol.* **60**, 567–78.

Vaughan, J.W. (1914) Cancer vaccine and anti-cancer globulin as an aid in the surgical treatment of malignancy. *JAMA* **63**, 1258.

Velders, M.P., van Rhijn, C.M., Oskam, E. *et al.* (1998) The impact of antigen density and antibody affinity on antibody-dependent cellular cytotoxicity: relevance for immunotherapy of carcinomas. *Br. J. Cancer* **78**, 478–83.

Vogelstein, B., Fearon, E.R., Hamilton, S.R. *et al.* (1988) Genetic alterations during colorectal tumor development. *N. Engl. J. Med.* **319**(9), 525–32.

Volk, B.W. (1975) The gangliosidoses. *Hum. Pathol.* **6**, 555.

von Leyden, V.E. and Blumenthal, F. (1902) Vorlautige Mitteilungen ubber einige Ergebnisse der Krebsforschung auf der 1. medizinischen klinik. *Dt. Med. Wschr.* **28**, 637.

Vousden, K. (1994) Mechanisms of transformation by human papillomavirus. In Stern, P. and Stanley, M. (eds), *Human papillomavirus and cervical cancer – biology and immunology.* Oxford: Oxford Medical Publications, 92–115.

Wallack, M.K. and Michaelides, M. (1984) Serologic response to human melanoma lines from patients with melanoma undergoing treatment with vaccinia melanoma oncolysates. *Surgery* **96**, 791–9.

Wallack, M.K. and Sivanandham, M. (1993) Clinical trials with VMO for melanoma. *Ann. N.Y. Acad. Sci.* **690**, 178–89.

Wallack, M.K., Steplewski, Z., Koprowski, H. *et al.* (1977) A new approach in specific, active immunotherapy. *Cancer* **39**(2), 560–4.

Wallack, M.K., McNally, K.R., Leftheriotis, E. *et al.* (1986) A south-eastern cancer study group phase I/II trial with vaccinia melanoma oncolysates. *Cancer* **57**(3), 649–55.

Wallack, M.K., Sivanandham, M., Balch, C.M. *et al.* (1995) A phase III randomised, double blind, multi-institutional trial of vaccinia melanoma oncolysate-active specific immunotherapy for patients with stage II melanoma. *Cancer* **75**(1), 34–42.

Ward, P.L., Koeppen, H.K., Hurteau, T., Rowley, D.A. and Schreiber, H. (1990) Major histocompatibility complex class I and unique antigen expression by tumors that escaped from CD8+ T cell dependent surveillance. *Cancer Res.* **50**, 3851–8.

Watson, E.E., Stabin, M.G., Siegel, J.A. *et al.* (1993) MIRD formulation. *Med. Phys.* **20**, 511–13.

Welt, S., Carswell, E.A., Vogel, C.W. *et al.* (1987) Immune and non-immune effector functions of IgG3 mouse monoclonal antibody R24 detecting the disialganglioside GD3 on the surface of melanoma cells. *Clin. Immunol. Immunopathol.* **45**, 214.

Welt, S., Divgi, C.R., Kemeny, N. *et al.* (1994) Phase I/II study of iodine 131-labeled monoclonal antibody A33 in patients with advanced colon cancer. *J. Clin. Oncol.* **12**, 1561–71.

Wessels, B.W. (1990) Current status of animal radioimmunotherapy. *Cancer Res.* **50**, 3.

Wheatley, K., Hancock, B., Gore, M. *et al.* (2001) Interferon-α as adjuvant therapy for melanoma: a meta-analysis of the randomised trials. *Proc. Am. Soc. Clin. Onc.* **20**, 349a.

Wheldon, T.E., O'Donoghue, J.A., Barrett, A. *et al.* (1991) The curability of tumours of differing size by targeted radiotherapy using ^{131}I or ^{90}Y. *Radiother. Oncol.* **21**, 91–9.

Wollina, U., Kilian, U., Henkel, U., Schaarschmidt, H. and Knopf, B. (1991) The initial steps of tumour progression in melanocytic lineage: a histochemical approach. *Anticancer Res.* **11**(4), 1405–14.

Yao, T.J., Meyers, M., Livingston, P.O. *et al.* (1999) Immunization of melanoma patients with BEC2-keyhole limpet hemocyanin plus BCG intradermally followed by intravenous booster immunizations with BEC2 to induce anti-GD3 ganglioside antibodies. *Clin. Cancer Res.* **5**, 77–81.

13

Angiogenesis and the treatment of cancer

GUY F. NASH, AJAY K. KAKKAR AND ROBIN C.N. WILLIAMSON

BACKGROUND

Angiogenesis is the ability of pre-existing vasculature to form new microvessels. The term was first used to describe the formation of new blood vessels in the placenta (Hertig, 1935). In the early 1970s the potential relevance of tumour angiogenesis for tumour growth and metastasis was originally proposed (Folkman, 1971). Whereas small tumours could be nurtured with oxygen and energy simply by diffusion, growth would require newly formed blood vessels. It was therefore postulated that, in future, a more specific treatment of tumours might be developed by inhibition of angiogenesis (Folkman, 1971). Thus, investigations into tumour angiogenesis have concentrated on suppression of the neovascularity rather than direct tumour cell inhibition.

ANGIOGENESIS, TUMOUR GROWTH AND METASTASES

Direct evidence that tumour growth depends upon angiogenesis can be shown by suppressing tumour growth with monoclonal antibody against human basic fibroblast growth factor (bFGF) (Hori et al., 1991). It is now accepted that both progression of the primary tumours and the establishment of metastases is dependent on angiogenesis (Folkman, 1990). Previously, the increased vascularity noted in tumours was assumed to be a consequence of elevated metabolite excretion. Angiogenesis does not always correlate with the malignancy of a tumour; for example, highly vascularized benign tumours do not have the potential to spread.

There are several well-defined stages in the process of tumour cell detachment to form metastases; degradation of extracellular matrix (ECM), escape from apoptosis, locomotion in the ECM, immunologic escape in the circulation, adhesion to vascular endothelial cells and extravasation from the circulation at the target site of metastasis. Subsequently, the metastatic cells must undergo neovascularization within the target organ to reach a clinically detectable size. Potential metastatic cells cannot shed from the primary tumour until it becomes neovascularized (Liotta et al., 1974). Metastasis is therefore dependent upon angiogenesis at two steps of the cascade (Zetter, 1990).

The rate of division of tumour cells has been shown to decrease according to the distance from the nearest capillary providing nutrients (Tannock, 1968). The overall rate of tumour growth is dictated not by proliferation of the tumour cells themselves but by the lower rate of proliferation of endothelial cells. Thus the supply of oxygen and nutrients appears to be the dominant factor in limiting tumour growth (Tannock, 1968).

The stages of neovascularization are endothelial cell proliferation, migration, organization into functional vessels and subsequent remodelling of this vessel network. Vascular cell integrins assist in the formation of these immature vessels (Varner and Cheresh, 1996). The newly formed capillaries are composed of endothelial cells and pericytes. Pericytes facilitate the invasion of new vessels by degradation of the ECM (Nehls et al., 1994); this process being essential for angiogenesis and metastasis.

Matrix metalloproteinases (MMPs) are a family of zinc-dependent endoproteinases that are capable of breaking down the ECM. Tissue inhibitors of metalloproteinases (TIMPs) play an important role in the homeostasis of the ECM by controlling the activity of MMPs, and have been shown to inhibit angiogenesis in an animal model (Takigawa *et al.*, 1990).

Tumour cells are generally less adhesive than normal cells and deposit less ECM. The loosened matrix adhesion that results facilitates the escape of tumour cells from the tissue architecture. When detached, normal cells stop growing and undergo apoptosis caused by loss of adhesion. Integrin-activated pathways seem to be important in this anchorage dependence (Ruoslahti, 1999), although oncoproteins are capable of shunting these pathways. Malignant cells can evade anchorage dependence with the help of these oncoproteins.

MECHANISMS OF ANGIOGENESIS

Under physiological conditions, localized and tightly controlled angiogenesis occurs during embryonic development, in the female reproductive cycle and in wound repair. By contrast, many pathological conditions, including atherosclerosis, diabetic retinopathy and cancer, are characterized by persisting uncontrolled angiogenesis. Angiogenesis is regulated by pro-angiogenic and anti-angiogenic factors, and their balance in the healthy adult results in minimal net blood vessel growth. These molecules are collectively known as TAFs (tumour angiogenesis factors). The equilibrium between proliferation and apoptosis is important in the dormancy of tumours and the control of metastatic spread.

TAFs derive from the tumour cell themselves, platelet–endothelial interactions and infiltrating cells, such as macrophages, which are found in high concentrations in pathological angiogenic states.

Tumour cells often exhibit increased expression of growth factor mRNA (Berse *et al.*, 1992), or increased secretion of angiogenic factors (Dvorak *et al.*, 1991). The expression of angiogenic factors reflects the 'malignancy' of the tumour. The malignant phenotype occurs as a result of genetic changes that activate oncogenes and inactivate tumour suppressor genes. Angiogenesis can be influenced *in vitro* by tumour suppressor genes such as *p53* (Bouck, 1996).

Platelets release several positive regulators of angiogenesis, primarily from α-granules: hepatocyte growth factor (Nakamura *et al.*, 1986), epidermal growth factor (Ben-Ezra *et al.*, 1990) and basic fibroblast growth factor (Brunner *et al.*, 1993). Platelets also contain inhibitory factors, such as platelet factor 4 (PF4) and thrombospondin, which are contained abundantly and participate in efficient platelet aggregation (Jaffe *et al.*, 1982).

Endothelial cells may change from the resting state to the angiogenic phenotype; endothelial cell receptors are upregulated in tumour neovascularization (Plate *et al.*, 1992). They produce both proteolytic enzymes, such as urokinase-type plasminogen activator, and protease inhibitors, such as plasminogen activator inhibitor. Pro-angiogenic factors can upset this equilibrium, by stimulating proteolysis in the ECM.

Macrophages play an important role in regulating new vessels during tumour growth. Tumour necrosis factor-α (TNF-α) is a secretory product of activated macrophages and is believed to mediate cytotoxicity; it is a potent inducer of angiogenesis (Leibovich *et al.*, 1987). Macrophages may also inhibit angiogenesis by secretion of granulocyte–macrophage colony stimulating factor, which stimulates the production of plasminogen activator inhibitor type 2 (Joeseph and Isaacs, 1998).

PRO-ANGIOGENIC FACTORS

Vascular endothelial growth factors

Vascular endothelial growth factors (VEGFs) are a group of powerful angiogenic mitogens (Leung *et al.*, 1989). VEGFs are regulators of both physiological and pathological angiogenesis; they have overlapping but specific roles in controlling the growth of new blood vessels. The first member of the VEGF family (VEGF A) is the most specific and potent inducer of endothelial cell growth (Claffey *et al.*, 1996). VEGF is likely to contribute to tumour growth directly by promoting angiogenesis and stroma creation through neovascularization activity, but also indirectly by increasing vascular permeability. In addition, VEGF assists

Table 13.1 *Pro-angiogenic factors*

Pro-angiogenic factors	Year described
Vascular endothelial growth factors (VEGF)	1983
Angiogenin	1985
Hepatocyte growth factor	1986
Transforming growth factor-β (TGF-β)	1986
Tumour necrosis factor-α (TNF-α)	1987
Basic fibroblast growth factors (bFGF)	1989
Epidermal growth factor	1990
Interleukin-1, -4, -6, -8, -15	1993–7
Nitric oxide	1994
Platelet-activating factor	1995
Urokinase plasminogen activator	1995
Prostaglandin E_1 and E_2	1995
Acidic fibroblast growth factors (aFGF)	1995
Matrix metalloproteinases (MMPs)	1995
Vascular integrins	1996
Platelet-derived endothelial cell growth factor	1996

tumour dispersion by enhancing metastatic spread of cancer cells. VEGF receptors transduce signals mediating the basic stages of angiogenesis (Veikkola and Alitalo, 1999).

Most tumour angiogenesis factors function by producing either endothelial proliferation or migration, or both. VEGF derived from tumour has a paracrine effect in increasing angiogenesis, but seems also to have a stimulating autocrine effect (Liu et al., 1995). Tumour cell lines that over express VEGF result in angiogenesis stimulation followed by accelerated tumour growth.

Interestingly, the genetic mutations in von Hippel–Lindau syndrome cause increased VEGF production, resulting in familial renal carcinomas (Iliopoulos et al., 1996). VEGF is structurally related to platelet-derived growth factor (PDGF), which is another endothelial cell mitogen and is also released from platelets activated by the clotting cascade (Miyazono et al., 1987).

Fibroblast growth factors

Fibroblast growth factors (FGF) are a family of mitogenic (Schweigerer et al., 1987) and angiogenic compounds found in normal and abnormal cells. Acidic FGF (aFGF) binds heparin and aids wound healing and angiogenesis (Klagsbrun, 1989). Basic FGF (bFGF) has an autocrine effect, being promoted by heparin (Folkman and Shing, 1992) to act as an endothelial cell mitogen. bFGF, stored in both cells and extracellular matrix, may be released secondary to tumour ischaemia, thus stimulating angiogenesis (D'Amore and Thompson, 1987).

Angiogenin

Angiogenin was first found in adenocarcinoma cells (Fett et al., 1985), but subsequently was identified in normal tissues and serum (Weiner et al., 1987). It has RNAase activity that is essential for its angiogenic effect, but this is also dependent upon a second site on the angiogenin molecule (Hallahan et al., 1990).

Interleukins

Several interleukins display angiogenic effects. For example, interleukin-8 has angiogenic activity after rat cornea implantation, also inducing chemotaxis and proliferation of human endothelial cells (Koch et al., 1992). Interleukin-12 has been found to inhibit angiogenesis in vivo (Voest et al., 1995).

Nitric oxide and prostaglandins

Nitric oxide synthase (NOS) is an enzyme produced by vascular endothelium that catalyses the formation of nitric oxide (NO). NO is short lived and a major regulator of vascular permeability. NO production is induced by vasoactive agents, and one of its functions is to regulate the microvascular events necessary for neovascularization; in addition it mediates angiogenesis (Ziche et al., 1994). Cyclo-oxygenases (COXs) are important in the formation of eicosanoids from arachidonic acid. COX has two isoforms, COX-1 and COX-2 (Chiarugi et al., 1998); NOS also has two forms, one of which is inducible by COX-2. COX is important in the production of tumour-related angiogenesis in colon cancer (Tsujii et al., 1998), an effect that is inhibited by non-steroidal anti-inflammatory drugs (NSAIDS). NSAIDS may therefore have a role in prophylaxis of patients at high risk of colorectal cancers.

Prostaglandin E_2 (PGE_2), an eicosanoid, is an inducer of several regulators of angiogenesis, including VEGF, bFGF, PDGF and endothelin-1 (ET1). ET1 is a vasoconstrictor peptide (Rubanyi and Polokoff, 1994) that belongs to a family of endothelins, comprising ET1, 2 and 3. ET1 has been found in high concentration in prostate, breast and colon cancer tissue. It has two receptor types, ETA and ETB. An ETA antagonist has been shown to reduce cell turnover in a human colorectal cell line (Ali et al., 1988).

The role of hypoxia

Oncosuppressor gene p53 inhibits the angiogenic process at various stages. Mutations in p53 may enhance tumour cell survival through influencing their response to hypoxia (Graeber et al., 1996), and they facilitate the release of pro-angiogenic factors such as VEGF (Mukhopadhyay et al., 1995). Hypoxia may possibly enhance the survival of more malignant clones with p53 mutations. The growth of many solid tumours depends on a delicate balance of vascular perfusion: a relatively small insult may precipitate hypoxia then necrosis.

Hypoxia can be found in several areas of malignant tumours and is likely to be due to independent tumour angiogenesis. The presence and extent of these hypoxic tumour microenvironments have been shown to influence tumour progression by regulating tumour cell survival. VEGF probably functions as a hypoxia-induced angiogenic factor (Shweiki et al., 1992), and it may be the link between hypoxia and increased vascular permeability. The neovasculature formed in tumours is leaky, as it has an incomplete basement membrane, and this property facilitates tumour invasion (Nagy et al., 1989). Increased vascular permeability in tumour capillaries can manifest itself clinically as a malignant effusion or ascites (Senger et al., 1983). The combination of leaky vessels and paucity of lymphatics leads to an increase in intra-tumoral interstitial pressure. The resulting central hypoxia reduces delivery of traditional chemotherapeutic drugs to the tumour, an effect that can be reversed by administration of anti-angiogenic agents (Teicher et al., 1994).

Angiogenic balance, 'switch' and dormancy

Tumour angiogenesis, controlled by a balance of stimulators and inhibitors of angiogenesis, 'switches' on when the stimulants are upregulated, combined with down-regulation of the inhibitors of angiogenesis. The exact mechanism of the 'switch' is unclear in physiological or pathological angiogenesis. A study involving mouse fibroblasts containing transfected cDNA for human bFGF showed that bFGF may be a sole mediator of angiogenesis involved in the human angiogenic switch (Hori *et al.*, 1991). The influx of inflammatory cells such as macrophages may also contribute to the switch mechanism by increasing angiogenic activity (Koch *et al.*, 1986). In addition, the regulation of angiogenesis may involve changes at a genetic level (Hanahan and Folkman, 1996). Angiogenic activity in hamsters results from inactivation of a suppressor gene during carcinogenesis (Bouck *et al.*, 1986).

The 'angiogenic switch' enables tumour angiogenesis to play a critical role in the growth of solid tumours and their metastases, which may be dormant. Dormancy is distinct from premalignancy in that dormant cells are malignant but under growth control. Without neovascularization, most solid tumours stop growing when they reach 2–3 mm in size, and then enter a dormant phase that may last for many years. This process may explain the recurrence seen in some cancers even decades after the primary tumour is diagnosed. A superficial melanoma (less than 0.76 mm thick) is a visible example of a tumour before the angiogenic switch (prevascular state), as it grows slowly when confined to the epidermis, superficial to the intact capillary basement membrane. Deeper melanomas undergo angiogenesis and accelerated growth when they penetrate into the dermis (Smolle *et al.*, 1989).

Dormant micrometastases may undergo a decrease in apoptosis and subsequently proliferation (Uhr *et al.*, 1997). Whether the primary tumour or its metastases predominate, the clinical presentation at diagnosis depends upon the degree of suppression the tumour exerts upon its metastases. Once these metastases are detected, they seem to grow at a comparable rate to those metastases that appear only a few months after removal of the primary tumour (Crowley and Siegler, 1992).

Specific tissue affinities may explain the tendency of some tumours to preferentially establish distal metastases in certain organs. Most metastases develop in the first capillary bed encountered after escape from the primary tumour. However, tumours also metastasize to distant locations that cannot be predicted on the basis of blood flow patterns. The high proportion of bony metastases in breast, prostate and lung cancers are examples of selective 'homing' of tumour cells to a specific organ. Three major types of homing mechanisms have been proposed (Woodhouse *et al.*, 1997).

Interestingly, physiological and pathological angiogenesis is seen to vary with the age of the host (Pili *et al.*, 1994). Despite their low turnover, adult endothelial cells do retain the potential to form new blood vessels; consequently, pro-angiogenic drugs have the potential to 'revascularize' ischaemic organs.

The role of thrombosis, platelets and heparin

As knowledge of each process improves, the dose relationship between haemostasis and angiogenesis is emerging more clearly (Browder *et al.*, 1999). Both angiostatin (a plasminogen fragment) and endostatin (a collagen XVIII fragment) are potent inhibitors of angiogenesis and both are cleaved fragments from factors implicated in the clotting cascade. Blood coagulation tests are deranged in most patients with cancer (Sun *et al.*, 1979); in fact, thrombocytosis has been used as a prognostic indicator for cancer patients (Montreal *et al.*, 1998).

In mice, tissue factor (TF) has been shown to control the angiogenic and antiangiogenic properties of tumour cells (Zhang *et al.*, 1994). TF and several other tumour procoagulants seem likely primary stimuli for the generation of thrombin and mature fibrin in the tumour microenvironment. Activated thrombin induces release of VEGF from platelets (Mohle *et al.*, 1997). TF is also implicated in VEGF synthesis by tumour cells. Thrombin can be generated by some tumours, and it can stimulate tumour–platelet adhesion *in vitro* and metastases *in vivo* (Nierodzik *et al.*, 1991). Thrombin can also promote angiogenesis by a mechanism independent of fibrin formation (Tsopanoglou *et al.*, 1993).

Heparin prevents the formation of thrombin and inhibits its activity by binding to antithrombin III. The role of TF in metastasis appears to involve the coagulation pathway, as thrombin may be generated by TF on tumour cells and on the endothelium of tumour-induced microvessels (Contrino *et al.*, 1996). Distinct tumour production methods of thrombin generation versus plasminogen activators have resulted in a classification of tumour types (Zacharski *et al.*, 1992). Heparin minimizes angiogenesis via the inhibition of VEGF, TF and platelet activating factor. Heparin decreases tumour cell adherence by competitive inhibition (Engelberg, 1999). Therefore, besides preventing the venous thromboembolism associated with cancer, antithrombotic therapy (Kakkar and Williamson, 1999) and aspirin (Kort *et al.*, 1986) may have a beneficial role via a direct effect on the tumour.

Thrombin-catalysed, cross-linked fibrin formation is a characteristic histopathological finding in healing wounds and tumour stroma. In fact, there are many similarities between these two processes. Tumour stroma generation and wound healing (Dvorak, 1986) both entail plasma entering the extravascular space to initiate the clotting cascade. Proteins generated by the haemostatic system help to co-ordinate the localization and timing of clot/endothelial cell stabilization, followed by endothelial cell growth and repair of the damaged blood vessels. Activated platelets release platelet-derived growth factors and this is followed by an influx of inflammatory cells. Synthesis of fibronectin and interstitial collagen matures to produce a relatively hypoxic area that induces angiogenesis in the tumour (or the healing wound). It has therefore been suggested

Table 13.2 *Anti-angiogenic factors*

Anti-angiogenic factors	Year described
Platelet factor 4	1982
Corticosteroid and heparin	1985
Thrombospondin (TSP)	1988
Metalloproteinase inhibitors	1990
Cyclosporin A	1992
Retinoids	1993
Interferon-α, -β, -γ	1993–5
Angiostatin	1994
Linomide	1995
Interleukin-12	1995
Dexamethasone	1996
Fumagillin analogues	1997
Tamoxifen	1997
Diclofenac	1997
Endostatin	1997
Prostate-specific antigen	1999

that a tumour may appear to the host as a 'never-healing wound'.

ANTI-ANGIOGENIC FACTORS

Anti-angiogenic factors may be classified according to the stage of the angiogenesis process that they inhibit. For example, endothelial locomotion is inhibited by platelet factor 4 (PF4), whereas endothelial proliferation is inhibited by angiostatin, endostatin, thrombospondin 1 and inhibitors of FGF/VEGF. Fumagillin analogues and interferon-α/β inhibit both stages.

Anti-angiogenic factors may also be divided into direct and indirect inhibitors. Indirectly acting inhibitors of angiogenesis influence the microenvironment of the tumour, which in turn is influenced by the specific type of tumour and organ affected. Since a given tumour may secrete several angiogenic factors, it seems unlikely that a single indirect factor will prevent tumour proliferation and growth. The quantitative inhibitory power of these factors may now be compared (Chen *et al.*, 1995). Inhibiting a common angiogenic factor to most tumours (e.g. VEGF or bFGF) may have wider use than inhibiting more tumour-specific factors. Therefore, both the use of VEGF neutralizing antibody and interference with the function of one of its two angiogenic growth factor receptors (VEGFR 2) could be promising strategies for treating various types of tumour.

Platelet factor 4

Platelet factor 4 (PF4) was the first haemostatic protein shown to be anti-angiogenic *in vivo* (Taylor and Folkman, 1982). By linking to and blocking glycosaminoglycans receptors on the endothelial cell surface, PF4 will suppress endothelial growth factors (Maione *et al.*, 1990) as one of its many inhibitory effects on the angiogenic process.

Angiostatin and endostatin

Angiostatin and endostatin, both isolated from tumours (O'Reilly *et al.*, 1997), directly reduce endothelial cell mitogenesis. Angiostatin accumulates in the circulation in the presence of a growing primary tumour, and will induce and sustain dormancy of human primary tumours in mice (O'Reilly *et al.*, 1996). It is not clear whether angiostatin is produced directly or indirectly by the primary tumour, but it disappears within 5 days of removal of the primary (O'Reilly *et al.*, 1994). Accelerated angiogenesis then follows in metastases. Angiostatin is derived from kringles 1–4 of plasminogen (Hill *et al.*, 1996). Portions of all five kringle domains of plasminogen have anti-angiogenic properties (Cao *et al.*, 1996). Recombinant murine angiostatin has been synthesized and appears to be more potent than human angiostatin (Wu *et al.*, 1997).

Thrombospondin

Thrombospondin is a heparin-binding protein. It is a natural inhibitor of angiogenesis and may downregulate VEGF (Mantovani, 1994). Thrombospondin was identified as anti-angiogenic after the resemblance of its amino acid sequence to that predicted from an anti-angiogenic tumour suppressor gene was established (Good *et al.*, 1990). The anti-angiogenic effect is demonstrated by the presence of thrombospondin around mature vessels, in contrast to its absence from growing capillaries (O'Shea and Dixit, 1988).

Steroids and heparin

Steroids, such as hydrocortisone or cortisone, are inhibitors of angiogenesis, but this action is only seen in the presence of heparin (Crum *et al.*, 1985). A possible mechanism for this effect is the breakdown of the capillary basement membrane (Ingber *et al.*, 1986), via induction of plasminogen activator inhibitor (Blei *et al.*, 1993). The steroid–heparin combination can strongly inhibit angiogenesis in some tumours but others are refractory (Folkman *et al.*, 1983). This discrepancy suggests that some angiogenesis inhibitors are limited to specific capillary beds.

The immunosuppressant cyclosporin A is chronically administered to transplant patients, who demonstrate an increased incidence of many tumours. Cyclosporin A has angiostatic properties in the rat (Norrby, 1992). Linomide, which has a low toxicity profile (like many angiogenesis inhibitors) will decrease tumour growth and metastasis of murine B16 melanoma cells (Kallard, 1986); its long-term effects are under investigation.

ANTI-ANGIOGENIC TRIAL EXPERIENCE

The inhibition of angiogenesis is considered one of the most promising strategies for the development of novel antineoplastic therapies. Approximately 30 angiostatic agents are currently undergoing clinical trials, and almost twice this number are in preclinical testing. It is possible that an endothelial mitogen *in vitro* may not be angiogenic *in vivo*. Therefore, reliable *in vivo* bioassays are necessary if more sophisticated *in vitro* models cannot be developed to parallel the clinical situation. Unfortunately, any test substance causing inflammation or cell damage may induce a false-positive angiogenesis effect.

Animal studies have shown that angiogenesis inhibitors can prevent metastasis and shrink established experimental tumours to small dormant microtumours. For example, interleukin-12 causes tumour regression and reduces metastasis in animal models (Hiscox and Jiang, 1997), both by promoting anti-tumour immunity and by inhibiting angiogenesis and upregulating E-cadherin, a metastasis suppressor.

Several MMP inhibitors are already being used in clinical trials for malignant tumours, including the prototype MMP inhibitor, marimastat (and its analogue, batimastat), which is effective in patients with malignant ascites, and causes no major toxicity, even at high dose (Wojtowicz-Praga *et al.*, 1996). In another pilot study, patients with advanced inoperable gastric or gastro-oesophageal tumours given a 4-week course of marimastat are assessed macroscopically by endoscopy (Tierney *et al.*, 1999). A multicentre American trial of marimastat versus placebo is currently enlisting patients. The end point is survival of patients with stage III non-small cell lung cancer who have minimal residual disease following chemotherapy, radiotherapy and/or surgical resection.

In addition to these angiogenesis inhibitors, several compounds derived from natural sources, such as flavonoids, sulphated carbohydrates and cartilage, are undergoing evaluation. Cartilage-derived factors have collagenase inhibition properties as well as inhibiting angiogenesis (Brem and Folkman, 1975). This fact may explain why cartilage is rarely invaded by tumour and is one of the few avascular tissues in the body. In a phase I trial, shark cartilage was given to 60 patients with a variety of advanced cancers that were refractory to treatment; no improvement was seen in quantity or quality of life among those that completed the trial (Miller *et al.*, 1998). Another phase I trial with disappointing results involved nine patients with metastatic colorectal cancer who had failed conventional 5-fluorouracil treatment. They received recombinant PF4 at doses ranging from 0.3 to 3.0 mg/kg via 30-minute intravenous infusion. In 11 evaluable patients, who were treated with the 3 mg/kg dose over a longer infusion period, there were no clinical responses (Belman *et al.*, 1996).

Specific inhibitors of particular steps of the metastatic process are in various stages of investigation. TNP-470 (Takeda Neoplastic Product-470) is currently being tested in phase I and II clinical trials. One such fumagillin analogue reduced growth factor-mediated endothelial proliferation *in vivo*. TNP-470 (a non-specific angiogenic factor inhibitor) significantly inhibited subcutaneously implanted primary colonic tumours and their liver metastases in mice (Konno *et al.*, 1996). It was the first angiogenesis inhibitor to be given to humans. The effect of TNP-470 was to induce tumour dormancy and improved mouse survival.

Many different advanced cancers have responded in clinical trials after prolonged intravenous administration of TNP-470. Eighteen patients with advanced squamous cell carcinoma of the cervix, received an alternate-day infusion of TNP-470 (Levy *et al.*, 1996). After the 18-week course, there was one complete response, albeit at the cost of central nervous system toxicity. Histologically proven lung metastases vanished in this patient, who continued with the same therapy without subsequent toxicity or drug resistance.

Thirty-eight patients with AIDS-related Kaposi's sarcoma received TNP-470 by weekly intravenous infusion as part of a trial. The drug was well tolerated at doses up to and including the highest dose tested. Seven patients only (18 per cent) achieved a partial response. The median time to partial response was 4 weeks, and the median duration of response was 11 weeks (Dezube *et al.*, 1998). IM862 is a naturally occurring, small peptide, shown to inhibit angiogenesis. After an encouraging pilot study, a phase III randomized, double-blind, placebo-controlled study of intranasal IM862 has been set up in patients with mucocutaneous AIDS-related Kaposi's sarcoma to assess safety and responses to therapy.

Another anti-angiogenic clinical trial involved the treatment of haemangiomas that threatened life or sight. Haemangiomas are the most common tumours of infancy, but only one-third respond to the traditional corticosteroid therapy. On average, anti-angiogenic treatment lasted 8 months (range of 2–13 months) and was administered by daily subcutaneous injection. Interferon-α 2a, which is less toxic in children than in adults, induced regression by at least 50 per cent in 18 of 20 patients (Ezekowitz *et al.*, 1995).

Phase I trials of human recombinant endostatin are currently under way for advanced solid tumours at the MD Anderson cancer centre, Texas, USA. The treatment is on an outpatient basis, and serial biopsies after every two cycles will be analysed to gauge response to therapy.

DIAGNOSTIC APPLICATIONS

The onset of neovascularization may be heralded by the appearance of sinister symptoms, such as the discharge or excretion of sanguinous fluid, for example, haematuria with underlying bladder tumour.

Basic growth factor concentrations in the serum or urine may provide sensitive diagnostic markers for early tumours. Used as a diagnostic tool, prostate-specific antigen (PSA) was thought to be specific for prostate cancer but, interestingly, PSA levels also correlate with a good prognosis in breast tumours. PSA has subsequently been shown to inhibit endothelial proliferation, migration and invasion in mice (Fortier et al., 1999). Rather than being a marker of tumour progression, it may therefore represent an endogenous anti-angiogenic response. The distinct patterns of angiogenesis VEGFR-2 expression already allow differentiation between benign and malignant tumours (Skobe et al., 1997).

Prognostic indicators

The inhibition of angiogenesis can limit tumour growth, for example, by increasing the rate of apoptosis. Several clinical studies have shown that apoptosis and angiogenesis are prognostic indicators for patient survival. Apoptosis and angiogenesis may be valuable as response markers for patients having primary or adjuvant chemotherapy for cancer. Angiogenesis is an independent prognostic variable in several cancers: colonic carcinoma (Takahashi et al., 1995), prostate carcinoma (Weidner et al., 1993), non-small cell lung cancer (Macchiarini et al., 1992) and node-negative breast cancer (Heimann et al., 1996). Those lesions with high angiogenesis scores or microvessel densities are associated with a higher risk of metastases, recurrence and early patient death (Weidner, 1995).

Although the ability to exploit tumour angiogenesis as a prognostic marker is limited by the methods currently available for capillary identification and quantification, the potential clinical applications of these angiogenic markers lie in both prognosis and subsequent patient treatment. Identification of 'high-risk' tumours may allow more selective use of cytotoxic adjuvant therapy, and will assume increasing importance in the investigation of new therapies directed at inhibiting angiogenesis and targeting tumour vasculature.

Measuring anti-angiogenic effect

The intended effect of anti-angiogenic agents is to reduce tumours and their metastases to resting states. When compared with the cytotoxic effect of more traditional chemotherapy, this cytostatic effect requires new methods of measurement. Trials are needed to focus on appropriate end points and relevant biological markers. The techniques used for assessing tumour angiogenesis in tissue specimens include histopathological methods and the use of computer image analysis. Angiogenic factors assays, proteolytic enzymes and cell adhesion molecules may also act as surrogate end points for quantifying tumour

response to treatment. Since current clinical trials involve patients with advanced tumours intractable to conventional therapy, their effect is measured in terms of delay in tumour progression.

The assessment of intra-tumoral microvessel density and quantification of angiogenic factors or tumour markers in tissue, urine (Nguyen et al., 1994) or plasma may be of prognostic value in many cancers, but the two parameters do not necessarily correlate. Their use in clinical practice remains controversial due to the lack of prospective studies in humans, and the difficulties in the scoring and standardization of immunohistochemical methods. For measures of angiogenesis to be a reliable prognostic factor, they must have low inter and intraobserver variability. Standardized angiogenesis quantification would then allow comparison between institutes. An 'International Consensus on the Methodology and Criteria of Evaluation' has proposed a standard method for intra-tumoral microvessel density assessment that should allow such multicentre collaboration and meta-analysis (Vermeulen et al., 1996). These techniques are producing a new independent marker of prognosis and may be helpful in selecting patients for anti-angiogenic therapy.

Stabilization of tumour proliferation by inhibiting new vessel growth would seek reduction in vascularity by imaging techniques such as contrast-enhanced CT, MRI (also MR spectroscopy), duplex (Doppler-ultrasound) and PET scans. Serial imaging, which should be complementary to histological assays, could measure response to treatment and assess follow-up. These investigations have the advantage over serial biopsies in that they are non-invasive. At least 10^9 tumour cells must generally be present for clinical detection of a metastasis, but these newer tests could allow earlier detection and treatment.

Gradient-recalled echo MRI (GRE-MRI) offers a dynamic non-invasive method for monitoring tumour response to a change in vascularity (Robinson et al., 1998). The mature blood vessel wall contains smooth muscle cells that can cause vasodilatation in response to elevated CO_2 levels. GRE-MRI has shown that the non-dilating neovasculature of certain tumours can be affected differentially by VEGF withdrawal (Abramovitch et al., 1999). For contrast-enhanced MRI, increased capillary permeability emerges as the factor that best differentiates malignant from benign tissue (Delorme and Knopp, 1998). Another MRI-dependent technique for identifying angiogenic vasculature is the use of a paramagnetic contrast agent targeted to an angiogenesis marker, such as endothelial integrin $\alpha V \beta 3$ (Sipkins et al., 1998). Magnetic resonance spectroscopy (MRS) has shown encouraging early results in assessing response to anti-angiogenic therapy (Hoffer et al., 1988). MRS ^{31}P resonance is increased in untreated breast tumours and decreases before other evidence of regression in treated tumours (Glaholm et al., 1989).

PREVENTION OF TUMOUR GROWTH AND SPREAD

Screening tests, for those at 'high risk', may be developed in future to identify a premalignant state in certain tumours or predict the risk of future malignant transformation. Angiogenic assays can distinguish lesions undergoing neoplastic transformation before atypia or invasion are detected histologically (Brem et al., 1978). The growth of both carcinoma in-situ and dormant metastases may be controlled by long-term therapy with anti-angiogenic medication that prevents the 'angiogenic switch'. Although angiogenesis is unlikely to play a role in early dissemination of single or small group of cells, it does precede the formation of malignant tumours (Weidner, 1995). Angiostatin, endostatin and a fumagillin analogue have all been shown to prevent the angiogenic switch in some premalignant lesions (Bergers et al., 1999), and could therefore have some future preventative role.

Anti-angiogenic therapies

It is interesting to note that some traditional cancer therapies work by impairing angiogenesis; for example, tamoxifen is known to have anti-angiogenic effects (Donovan et al., 1997). The recent advent of pharmacological inhibitors of angiogenesis might best be used initially to prevent, treat or maintain those neoplasms not effectively treatable by other therapies.

Following recognition of the importance of the vascular bed for growth and metastasis of solid tumours, many researchers have attempted to attack the tumour vascular bed instead of the tumour cells themselves in anti-cancer therapy. 'Vascular targeting' aims to destroy the existing vasculature, while the theory of anti-angiogenesis specifically involves therapy against targets on the neovasculature. Such approaches have become possible with the expanding knowledge of the angiogenic process and the factors that regulate it. Possible biochemical targets of antiangiogenic therapy are the intercommunication between angiogenic factors and their receptors, the interaction of endothelial cells with the ECM and intracellular signalling pathways.

Endothelial damage is one method by which conventional treatments cause tumour shrinkage. The use of TNF in isolated limb perfusion for melanoma is one example of chemotherapy using vascular targeting. Unfortunately, TNF is too toxic for effective systemic use, whereas angiostatin, a specific inhibitor of endothelial cell proliferation, has no such toxicity. At present the doses of angiostatin used successfully against various experimental tumours seem to be too high for clinical use (Cao, 1999).

Potential therapy problems

Inactivation of VEGF or its receptors can lead to a marked negative effect on the development of experimental tumours. However, despite the encouraging results obtained in animal studies, it remains to be established whether human tumours are as sensitive to anti-VEGF treatment as the fast-growing tumours that have been used in the mouse.

As with any novel treatment, caution is required with regard to side-effects, especially one that may continue daily for months or even years. Some agents can worsen angina, peripheral vascular disease or fertility, and others may be teratogenic. The effect of thalidomide as an inhibitor of angiogenesis (D'Amato et al., 1994) may explain its infamous teratogenicity, and the same may be true of retinoids. As anti-angiogenic therapy is directed at endothelial cells, it is unlikely to cause bone-marrow suppression or hair loss. Conversely, the use of pro-angiogenic agents to improve vascular disease by encouraging revascularization has excluded those patients with recent cancers, for fear of waking dormant micrometastases.

It is likely that both pro-angiogenic and anti-angiogenic factors influence the growth of a particular tumour, and that a single anti-angiogenic agent may prove ineffective. Therefore, combination treatments may need to be developed that act on different aspects of angiogenesis, perhaps specific for that tumour type. Acquired drug resistance, which is a major problem with conventional chemotherapy, does not seem to develop in those tumours treated with angiogenesis inhibitors (Boehm et al., 1997).

Effect of surgical operations

Surgery is recognized as the best first-line treatment for the majority of solid tumours. However, a substantial proportion of patients eventually develop metastases despite an apparent curative excision. Both the operative insult and the subsequent process of wound healing are thought to induce angiogenesis (Uhr et al., 1997). This healing after surgical trauma seems to provide dormant tumour cells a permissive environment in which to grow. Excision of the primary tumour may cause proliferation of its dormant micrometastases (Folkman, 1995). The loss of the inhibitory angiogenesis factors, angiostatin and endostatin, from the primary tumour may explain this finding.

The healing wound is a pro-angiogenic site that favours local recurrence. This situation is seen to occur in clinical practice when colorectal anastomotic recurrences occur locally after resection. The timing of postoperative anti-angiogenic treatment may be important to allow wound healing but inhibit the pro-angiogenic climate that permits growth of metastases.

Combination therapy

Anti-VEGF treatment may represent a powerful tool in many human anti-cancer therapies, either alone or in combination with other inhibitors of angiogenesis.

Combined anti-angiogenic therapy can cure some tumours, whereas single agents may only be inhibitory (Teicher *et al.*, 1994). A promising early use of anti-angiogenic factors in anti-cancer therapy seems to lie in their combination with traditional chemotherapy or radiotherapy. The effect is found to be potentiated in tumour-bearing animals, partly because it reduces tumour hypoxia (Teicher *et al.*, 1994). More recently it has been found that ionizing radiation can increase VEGF mRNA, which may, in turn, confer protection against further radiation (Gorski *et al.*, 1999). This effect, which is inhibited by anti-VEGF antibody, could be exploited clinically by its administration prior to radiotherapy.

Immunotherapy

Tumour dormancy may also depend upon a functioning immune system. The future use of passive administration of humanized antibody and vaccination against tumour-associated antigens to induce cellular immunity would use the maximal immune response to perhaps maintain dormancy.

Gene therapies

Tumour suppressor genes may function as modulators of angiogenesis (Sager, 1986). Oncogenes and tumour suppressor genes are appealing targets for therapy since they are thought to be responsible for several different cancers. The clinical development of selective inhibitors of the Ras-processing enzyme to uncouple Ras activity is a promising area which is supported by the dramatic results of gene inactivation experiments in mice, which have identified several vascular endothelial related molecules as rate limiting for embryonic angiogenesis (Augustin, 1998).

Intra-tumoral injection of PF4 can reduce tumour growth, but for maximal effect this exposure should be sustained and uninterrupted; gene transfer may provide for such sustained administration (Tanaka *et al.*, 1997). Maintaining a prolonged systemic state of tumour dormancy may be difficult and costly, as many proteins are cleared rapidly from the circulation. Gene transfer potentially provides a localized area of angiogenesis inhibition by transduction of genes that code for anti-angiogenic proteins. Unfortunately, transduction of a large proportion of target cells is required for efficient tumour growth inhibition; current gene delivery vectors may find this difficult to achieve. Nevertheless, gene therapy offers great promise, as demonstrated by the transfection of thrombospondin 1 cDNA into a human breast carcinoma cell line with recurrent reduction in tumour angiogenesis, growth and metastatic potential (Weinstat-Saslow *et al.*, 1994).

Recent reports using local administration of IL-12 to the tumour site by retroviral vectors have suggested reduced tumour mass, with complete response occurring in cases (Hiscox and Jiang, 1997). Adenovirus-mediated regional anti-VEGF therapy using a gene encoding a soluble form of flt-1 (a VEGF receptor) can also be used for regional control of tumour growth (Crystal, 1999). The critical dependence of many tumours on VEGF for neovascularization and subsequent metastases implies that future methods of inhibiting VEGF may be applicable to many different tumour types.

CONCLUSIONS

Angiogenesis is a physiological process subject to autocrine and paracrine regulation, which has the potential to become aberrant and which is integral in several pathological states, including cancer. Each step in the angiogenic process represents a potential target for therapeutic anti-cancer strategies. Many endogenous angiogenic factors have been described, including VEGF, FGF and PDGF, but also a number of angiogenesis inhibitors, including thrombospondin, endostatin and angiostatin. These agents exhibit reduced toxicity and a decreased likelihood for the development of drug resistance when compared to conventional chemotherapies. Angiogenesis suppression should not be considered 'a cure for cancer'; it is more likely that it will be effective for certain stages of certain cancers. Preclinical data coupled with animal and early clinical studies indicate that combining anti-angiogenic therapy (probably as part of long-term regimes) with conventional treatment modalities has the potential to control cancer growth and improve survival.

SIGNIFICANT POINTS

- Angiogenesis must precede tumour growth beyond more than a few thousand cells.
- Multiple endogenous stimulators and inhibitors help to control angiogenesis.
- Tumour dormancy results from an equilibrium between proliferation and apoptosis.
- Tumour growth stability is the treatment aim, response measurement should reflect this parameter.
- Anti-angiogenic therapy may need to be delivered as prolonged and uninterrupted, but toxicity may be low and resistance has not yet been shown.
- Combination treatment with other anti-angiogenic agents, chemotherapy or radiotherapy may enhance therapeutic effect.

KEY REFERENCES

Folkman, J. (1971) Tumor angiogenesis: therapeutic implications. *N. Engl. J. Med.* **285**, 1182–6.

Harris, A.L. (1997) Antiangiogenesis for cancer therapy. *Lancet* **349**, S13–15 [review].

McNamara, D.A., Harmey, J.H., Walsh, T.N., Redmond, H.P. and Bouchier-Hayes, D.J. (1998) Significance of angiogenesis in cancer therapy. *Br. J. Surg.* **85**, 1044–55 [review].

REFERENCES

Abramovitch, R., Dafni, H., Smouha, E., Benjamin, L.E. and Neeman, M. (1999) *In vivo* prediction of vascular susceptibility to endothelial growth factor withdrawal: magnetic resonance imaging of C6 rat glioma in nude mice. *Cancer Res.* **59**(19), 5012–66.

Ali, H., Dashwood, M., Loizidou, M. *et al.* (1988) Endothelin A receptor antagonist affects growth of colorectal cancer cells. *Eur. J. Surg. Oncol.* **24**, 622–3.

Augustin, H.G. (1998) Antiangiogenic tumour therapy: will it work? *Trends Pharmacol. Sci.* **19**(6), 216–22.

Belman, N., Bonnem, E.M., Harvey, H.A. and Lipton, A. (1996) Phase I trial of recombinant platelet factor 4 (rPF4) in patients with advanced colorectal carcinoma. *Invest. New Drugs* **14**(4), 387–9.

Ben-Ezra, J., Sheibani, K., Hwabg, D.L. and Lev-Ran, A. (1990) Megakaryocyte synthesis is the source of epidermal growth factor in human platelets. *Am. J. Pathol.* **137**, 755–9.

Bergers, G., Javaherian, K., Kin-Ming, L., Folkman, J. and Hanahan, D. (1999) Effects of angiogenesis inhibitors on multistage carcinogenesis in mice. *Science* **284**, 808–11.

Berse, B., Brown, L.F., Van de Water, L., Dvorak, H.F. and Senger, D.R. (1992) Vascular permeability factor (vascular endothelial growth factor) gene is expressed differentially in normal tissues, macrophages and tumors. *Mol. Biol. Cell* **3**, 211–20.

Blei, F., Wilson, E.L., Mignatti, P. and Rifkin, D.B. (1993) Mechanism of action of angiogenic steroids: suppression of plasminogen activator activity via stimulation of plasminogen activator inhibitor synthesis. *J. Cell Physiol.* **155**, 568–78.

Boehm, T., Folkman, J., Browder, T. and O'Reilly, M.S. (1997) Antiangiogenic therapy of experimental cancer does not induce acquired drug resistance. *Nature* **390**, 404–7.

Bouck, N. (1996) p53 and angiogenesis. *Biochim. Biophys. Acta* **1287**, 63–6.

Bouck, N., Stoler, A. and Polverini, P.J. (1986) Coordinate control of anchorage independence, actin cytoskeleton and angiogenesis by human chromosome 1 in hamster-human hybrids. *Cancer Res.* **46**, 5101.

Brem, H. and Folkman, J. (1975) Inhibition of tumor angiogenesis mediated by cartilage. *J. Exp. Med.* **141**, 427–39.

Brem, S.S., Jensen, H.M. and Gullino, P.M. (1978) Angiogenesis as a marker of preneoplastic lesions of the human breast. *Cancer* **41**, 239–44.

Browder, T., Folkman, J. and Pirie-Shepherd, S. (1999) The hemostatic system as a regulator of angiogenesis *J. Biol. Chem.* **275**, 1521–4.

Brunner, G., Nguyen, H., Gabrilove, J., Rifkin, D.B. and Wilson, E.L. (1993) Basic fibroblast growth factor expression in human bone marrow and peripheral blood cells. *Blood* **81**, 631–8.

Cao, Y. (1999) Therapeutic potentials of angiostatin in the treatment of cancer. *Haematologica* **84**(7), 643–50.

Cao, Y., Ji, R.W., Davidson, D. *et al.* (1996) Kringle domains of angiostatin: characterization of the anti-proliferative activity on endothelial cells. *J. Biol. Chem.* **271**, 29461–7.

Chen, C., Parangi, S., Tolentino, M.J. and Folkman, J. (1995) A strategy to discover circulating angiogenesis inhibitors generated by human tumors. *Cancer Res.* **55**, 4230.

Chiarugi, V., Magnelli, L. and Gallo, O. (1998) Cox-2, iNOS and p53 as play-makers of tumor angiogenesis. *Int. J. Mol. Med.* **2**(6), 715–19.

Claffey, K.P., Brown, L.F., del Aguila, L.F. *et al.* (1996) Expression of vascular permeability factor/vascular endothelial growth factor by melanoma cells increases tumor growth, angiogenesis and experimental metastasis. *Cancer Res.* **56**, 172–81.

Contrino, J., Hair, G., Kreutzer, D. and Rickles, F.R. (1996) *In situ* detection of tissue factor in vascular endothelial cells: correlation with the malignant phenotype of human breast disease. *Nat. Med.* **2**, 209–15.

Crowley, N.J. and Siegler, H.F. (1992) Relationship between disease-free interval and survival in patients with recurrent melanoma. *Arch. Surg.* **127**, 1303–8.

Crum, R., Szabo, S. and Folkman, J. (1985) A new class of steroids inhibits angiogenesis in the presence of heparin or a heparin fragment. *Science* **230**, 1375.

Crystal, R.G. (1999) *In vivo* and *ex vivo* gene therapy strategies to treat tumors using adenovirus gene transfer vectors. *Cancer Chemother. Pharmacol.* **43**(Suppl.), S90–9.

D'Amato, R.J., Loughnan, M.S., Flynn, E. and Folkman, J. (1994) Thalidomide is an inhibitor of angiogenesis. *Proc. Natl Acad. Sci. USA* **91**, 4082–5.

D'Amore, P.A. and Thompson, R.W. (1987) Mechanisms of angiogenesis. *Ann. Rev. Physiol.* **49**, 453–64.

Delorme, S. and Knopp, M.V. (1998) Non-invasive vascular imaging: assessing tumour vascularity. *Eur. Radiol.* **8**(4), 517–27.

Dezube, B.J., Von Roenn, J.H., Holden-Wiltse, J. *et al.* (1998) Fumagillin analogue in the treatment of Kaposi's sarcoma: a phase I AIDS Clinical Trial Group study. AIDS Clinical Trial Group No. 215 Team. *J. Clin. Oncol.* **16**(4), 1444–9.

Donovan, D., Harmey, J.H., Redmond, H.P. and Bouchier-Hayes, D. (1997) Ascites revisited: a novel role for tamoxifen. *Eur. J. Surg. Oncol.* **23**, 570.

Dvorak, H.F. (1986) Tumors: wounds that do not heal. Similarities between tumor stroma generation and wound healing. *N. Engl. J. Med.* **315**, 1650–9.

Dvorak, H.F., Sioussat, T.M. and Brown, L.F. (1991) Distribution of vascular permeability factor (vascular endothelial growth factor) in tumors: concentration in tumor blood vessels. *J. Exp. Med.* **174**, 1275–8.

Engelberg, H. (1999) Actions of heparin that may affect the malignant process. *Cancer* **85**(2), 257–72.

Ezekowitz, R.A., Mulliken, J.B. and Folkman, J. (1995) Interferon alfa-2a therapy for life threatening hemangiomas of infancy. *N. Engl. J. Med.* **333**, 595.

Fett, J.W., Strydom, D.L., Lobb, R.R. *et al.* (1985) Isolation and characterization of angiogenin, and angiogenic protein from human carcinoma cells. *Biochemistry* **24**, 5480–6.

Folkman, J. (1971) Tumor angiogenesis: therapeutic implications. *N. Engl. J. Med.* **285**, 1182–6.

Folkman, J. (1990) What is the evidence that tumours are angiogenesis dependent? *J. Natl Cancer Inst.* **82**, 4–6.

Folkman, J. (1995) Angiogenesis in cancer, vascular, rheumatoid and other diseases. *Nat. Med.* **1**, 27–31.

Folkman, J. and Shing, Y. (1992) Angiogenesis. *J. Biol. Chem.* **267**, 10931–4.

Folkman, J., Langer, R., Linhardt, R., Haudenschild, C. and Taylor, S. (1983) Angiogenesis inhibition and tumor regression caused by heparin or a heparin fragment in the presence of cortisone. *Science* **221**, 719.

Fortier, A.H., Nelson, B.J., Grella, D.K. and Holaday, J.W. (1999) Antiangiogenic activity of prostate-specific antigen. *J. Natl Cancer Inst.* **91**, 1635–40.

Glaholm, J., Leach, M.O., Collins, D.J. *et al.* (1989) *In vivo* [31]P magnetic resonance spectroscopy for monitoring treatment response in breast cancer. *Lancet* **1**, 1326–7.

Good, D.J., Polverini, R.J., Rastinejad, F. *et al.* (1990) A tumor suppressor dependent inhibitor of angiogenesis is immunologically and functionally indistinguishable from a fragment of thrombospondin. *Proc. Natl Acad. Sci. USA* **87**, 6624–8.

Gorski, D.H., Beckett, M.A., Jaskowiak, N.T. *et al.* (1999) Blockade of the vascular endothelial growth factor stress response increases the antitumor effects of ionising radiation. *Cancer Res.* **59**, 3374–8.

Graeber, T.G., Osmanian, C., Jacks, T. *et al.* (1996) Hypoxia-mediated selection of cells with diminished apoptotic potential in solid tumours. *Nature* **379**, 88–91.

Hallahan, T.W., Shapiro, R. and Vallee, B.L. (1990) Dual site mode for the organogenic activity of angiogenin. *Proc. Natl Acad. Sci. USA* **88**, 2222–6.

Hanahan, D. and Folkman, J. (1996) Patterns and emerging mechanisms of the angiogenic switch during tumorigenesis. *Cell* **86**, 353–64.

Heimann, R., Ferguson, D., Powers, C., Recant, W.M., Weichselbaum, R.R. and Hellman, S. (1996) Angiogenesis as a predictor of long-term survival for patients with node-negative breast cancer. *J. Natl Cancer Inst.* **88**, 1764–9.

Hertig, A.T. (1935) Angiogenesis in the early human chorion and in the primary placenta of the Macaque monkey. *Contrib. Embryol.* **25**, 37–81.

Hill, S.A., Shaughnessy, S.G., Joshua, P., Ribau, J., Austin, R.C. and Podor, T.J. (1996) Differential mechanisms targeting type I plasminogen activator inhibitor and vitronectin into the storage granules of a human megakaryocytic cell line. *Blood* **87**, 5061–73.

Hiscox, S. and Jiang, W.G. (1997) Interleukin-12, an emerging anti-tumour cytokine. *In Vivo* **11**(2), 125–32.

Hoffer, F.A., Taylor, G.A., Spevak, M., Ingber, D. and Fenton, T. (1988) Metabolism of tumor regression from angiogenesis inhibition [31]P Magnetic Resonance Spectroscopy. *Magn. Reson. Med.* **11**, 202–8.

Hori, A., Sasada, R., Matsutani, E. *et al.* (1991) Suppression of solid tumor growth by immunoneutralizing monoclonal antibody against human basic fibroblast growth factor. *Cancer Res.* **51**, 6180.

Iliopoulos, O., Levy, A.P., Jiang, C., Kaelin, W.G. and Goldberg, M.A. (1996) Negative regulation of hypoxia-inducible genes by the von Hippel–Lindau protein. *Proc. Natl Acad. Sci. USA* **93**, 10595–9.

Ingber, D.E., Madri, J.A. and Folkman, J. (1986) A possible mechanism for inhibition of angiogenesis by angiostatic steroids: induction of capillary basement membrane dissolution. *Endocrinology* **119**, 1768.

Jaffe, E., Leung, L.L.K., Nachman, R.L., Levin, R.L. and Mosher, D.F. (1982) Thrombospondin is the endogenous lectin of human platelets. *Nature* **295**, 246–8.

Joeseph, I.B. and Isaacs, J.T. (1998) Macrophage role in the anti-prostate cancer response to one class of antiangiogenic agents. *J. Natl Cancer Inst.* **90**(21), 1648–53.

Kakkar, A.K. and Williamson, R.C. (1999) Prevention of venous thromboembolism in cancer patients. *Semin. Thromb. Hemost.* **25**(2), 239–43.

Kallard, T. (1986) Effect of immunomodulators LS-2616 on growth and metastasis of the murine B16-F10 melanoma. *Cancer Res.* **46**, 3018–22.

Klagsbrun, M. (1989) The fibroblast growth factor family: structure and biological properties. *Prog. Growth Factor Res.* **1**, 207–35.

Koch, A.E., Polverini, P.J. and Leibovich, S.J. (1986) Induction of neovascularization by activated human monocytes. *J. Leukoc. Biol.* **39**, 233.

Koch, A.E., Ploverini, P.J., Kunkel, S.L. *et al.* (1992) Interleukin-8 as a macrophage-derived mediator of angiogenesis. *Science* **258**, 1798–800.

Konno, H., Tanaka, T., Kanai, T., Maruyama, K., Nakamura, S. and Baba, S. (1996) Efficacy of an angiogenesis inhibitor, TNP-470, in xenotransplanted human colorectal cancer with high metastatic potential. *Cancer* **77**(Suppl. 8), 1736–40.

Kort, W.J., Hulsman, L.O., van Schalkwijk, W.P., Weijma, I.M., Zondervan, P.E. and Westbroek, D.L. (1986) Reductive effect of aspirin treatment on primary tumor growth and metastasis of implanted fibrosarcoma in rats. *J. Natl Cancer Inst.* **76**(4), 711–20.

Leibovich, S.J., Polverini, P.J., Shepard, H.M., Wiseman, D.M., Shively, V. and Nuseir, N. (1987) Macrophage-induced angiogenesis is mediated by tumour necrosis factor-alpha. *Nature* **329**, 630–2.

Leung, D.W., Cachaines, G., Kwang, W.-J., Goeddel, D.V. and Ferrera, N. (1989) Vascular endothelial growth factor is a secreted angiogenic mitogen. *Science* **246**, 1306–9.

Levy, T., Kudelka, A., Verschraegen, C.F. *et al.* (1996) A phase 1 study of TNP-470 administered to patients with advanced squamous cell cancer of the cervix. (Abstract 1140). *Proc. Am. Assoc. Cancer Res.* **37**, 166.

Liotta, L., Kleinerman, J. and Saidel, F. (1974) Quantitative relationships of intravascular tumor cells, tumor vessels and pulmonary metastases following tumor implantation. *Cancer Res.* **34**, 997–1004.

Liu, B., Earl, H.M., Baban, D. *et al.* (1995) Melanoma cell lines express VEGF receptor KDR and respond to exogenously added VEGF. *Biochem. Biophys. Res. Commun.* **217**, 721–7.

Macchiarini, P., Fontanini, G., Hardin, M.J., Squartini, F. and Angelletti, C.A. (1992) Relation of neovascularisation to metastasis of non-small cell lung cancer. *Lancet* **340**, 145–6.

Maione, T.E., Gray, G.S., Petro, J. *et al.* (1990) Inhibition of angiogenesis by recombinant human platelets factor-4 and related peptides. *Science* **247**, 77–9.

Mantovani, A. (1994) Tumor-associated macrophages in neoplastic progression: a paradigm for the *in vivo* function of chemokines. *Lab. Invest.* **71**, 5–16.

Miller, D.R., Anderson, G.T., Stark, J.J., Granick, J.L. and Richardson, D. (1998) Phase I/II trial of the safety and efficacy of shark cartilage in the treatment of advanced cancer. *J. Clin. Oncol.* **16**(11), 3649–55.

Miyazono, K., Okabe, T., Urabe, A., Takaku, F. and Heldin, C.H. (1987) Purification and properties of an endothelial cell growth factor from human platelets. *J. Biol. Chem.* **262**, 4098–103.

Mohle, R., Green, D., Moore, M.A. *et al.* (1997) Constitutive production and thrombin-induced release of vascular endothelial growth factor by human megakaryocytes and platelets. *Proc. Natl Acad. Sci. USA* **94**, 663–8.

Montreal, M., Fernandez-Llamazares, J., Pinol, M. *et al.* (1998) Platelet count and survival in patients with colorectal cancer – a preliminary study. *Thromb. Haemost.* **79**, 916–18.

Mukhopadhyay, D., Tsiokas, L. and Sukhatme, V.P. (1995) Wild type p53 and v-src exert opposing influences on human vascular endothelial growth-factor gene-expression. *Cancer Res.* **55**, 6161–5.

Nagy, J.A., Brown, L.F., Senger, D.R. *et al.* (1989) Pathogenesis of tumor stroma generation: a critical role for leaky blood vessels and fibrin deposition. *Biochim. Biophys. Acta* **948**, 305–26.

Nakamura, T., Teramoto, H. and Ichihara, A. (1986) Purification and characterization of a growth factor from rat platelets for mature parenchymal hepatocytes in primary culture. *Proc. Natl Acad. Sci. USA* **83**, 6489–93.

Nehls, V., Schuchardt, E. and Drenckhahn, D. (1994) The effect of fibroblasts, vascular smooth muscle cells, and pericytes on sprout formation of endothelial cells in a fibrin gel angiogenesis system. *Microvasc. Res.* **48**, 349–63.

Nguyen, M., Watanabe, H., Budson, A.E., Richie, J.P., Hayes, D.F. and Folkman, J.F. (1994) Elevated levels of an angiogenic peptide, basic fibroblast growth factor, in the urine of patients with a wide spectrum of cancers. *J. Natl Cancer Inst.* **86**, 356–61.

Nierodzik, M.L., Plotkin, A., Kojumo, F. and Karpatkin, S. (1991) Thrombin stimulates tumor-platelet adhesion *in vitro* and metastasis *in vivo*. *J. Clin. Invest.* **87**, 229–36.

Norrby, K. (1992) Cyclosporin is angiostatic. *Experientia* **48**, 1135–8.

O'Reilly, M.S., Holmgren, L., Shing, Y. *et al.* (1994) Angiostatin: a novel angiogenesis inhibitor that mediates suppression of metastases by a Lewis lung carcinoma. *Cell* **79**, 315–28.

O'Reilly, M.S., Holmgren, L., Chen, C. and Folkman, J. (1996) Angiostatin induces and sustains dormancy of human primary tumors in mice. *Nat. Med.* **2**, 689–92.

O'Reilly, M.S., Boehm, T., Shing, Y. *et al.* (1997) Endostatin: an endogenous inhibitor of angiogenesis and tumor growth. *Cell* **88**, 277–85.

O'Shea, K.S. and Dixit, V. (1988) Unique distribution of extracellular matrix component thrombospondin in the developing mouse embryo. *J. Cell Biol.* **107**, 2737–48.

Pili, R., Guo, Y., Chang, J. *et al.* (1994) Altered angiogenesis underlying age-dependent changes in tumor growth. *J. Natl Cancer Inst.* **86**, 1303–14.

Plate, K.H., Breier, G., Weich, H.A. *et al.* (1992) Vascular endothelial growth factor is a potential tumour angiogenesis factor in human gliomas *in vivo*. *Nature* **359**, 845–8.

Robinson, S.P., Howe, F.A., Rodrigues, L.M., Stubbs, M. and Griffiths, J.R. (1998) Magnetic resonance imaging techniques for monitoring changes in tumor oxygenation and blood flow. *Semin. Radiat. Oncol.* **8**(3), 197–207.

Rubanyi, G.M. and Polokoff, M.A. (1994) Endothelins: molecular biology, biochemistry, pharmacology, physiology and pathophysiology. *Pharmacol. Rev.* **46**, 325–415.

Ruoslahti, E. (1999) Fibronectin and its integrin receptors in cancer. *Adv. Cancer Res.* **76**, 1–20.

Sager, R. (1986) Genetic suppression of tumour formation: a new frontier in cancer research. *Cancer Res.* **46**, 1573–80.

Schweigerer, L., Neufield, G., Friedman, J., Abraham, J.A., Fiddes, J.C. and Gospodarowicz, D. (1987) Capillary endothelial cells express basic fibroblast growth factor, a mitogen that promotes their own growth. *Nature* **325**, 257–9.

Senger, D.R., Galli, S.J., Dvorak, A.M., Perruzzi, C.A., Harvey, V.S. and Dvorak, H.S. (1983) Tumor cells secrete a vascular permeability factor that promotes the accumulation of ascites fluid. *Science* **219**, 983–5.

Shweiki, D., Itin, A., Soffer, D. and Keshet, E. (1992) Vascular endothelial cell growth factor induced by hypoxia may mediate hypoxia-initiated angiogenesis. *Nature* **359**, 843–5.

Sipkins, D.A., Cheresh, D.A., Kazemi, M.R., Nevin, L.M., Bednarski, M.D. and Li, K.C. (1998) Detection of tumor angiogenesis *in vivo* by αVβ3-targeted magnetic resonance imaging. *Nat. Med.* **4**(5), 623–6.

Skobe, M., Rockwell, P., Goldstein, N., Vosseler, S. and Fusenig, N.E. (1997) Halting angiogenesis suppresses carcinoma cell invasion. *Nat. Med.* **3**, 1222–7.

Smolle, J., Soyer, H.P., Hofmann-Wellenhof, R., Smolle-Juettner, F.M. and Keri, H. (1989) Vascular architecture of melanocytic skin tumors. *Path. Res. Pract.* **185**, 740.

Sun, N.C.J., McAfee, M., Hunt, G.J. and Weiner, J.M. (1979) Hemostatic abnormalities in malignancy, a prospective study of one hundred and eight patients. *Am. J. Clin. Pathol.* **71**, 10–16.

Takahashi, Y., Kitadai, Y., Bucana, C.D., Cleary, K.R. and Ellis, L.M. (1995) Expression of vascular endothelial growth factor and its receptor, KDR, correlates with vascularity, metastasis and proliferation of human colon cancer. *Cancer Res.* **55**, 3964–8.

Takigawa, M., Nishida, Y., Suzuki, F., Kishi, J., Yamashita, K. and Hayakawa, T. (1990) Induction of angiogenesis in chick yolk-sac membrane by polyamines and its inhibition by tissue inhibitors of metalloproteinases (TIMP and TIMP-2). *Biochem. Biophys. Res. Commun.* **171**, 1264–71.

Tanaka, T., Manome, Y., Wen, P., Kufe, D.W. and Fine, H.A. (1997) Viral vector-mediated transduction of a modified platelet factor 4 cDNA inhibits angiogenesis and tumor growth. *Nat. Med.* **3**, 437–42.

Tannock, I.F. (1968) The relationship between cell proliferation and the vascular system in a transplanted mouse mammary tumour. *Br. J. Cancer* **22**, 258–73.

Taylor, S. and Folkman, J. (1982) Protamine is an inhibitor of angiogenesis. *Nature* **297**, 307.

Teicher, B.A., Holden, S.A., Ara, G. *et al.* (1994) Potentiation of cytotoxic cancer therapies by TNP-470 alone and with other anti-angiogenic agents. *Int. J. Cancer* **57**, 920–5.

Tierney, G.M., Griffin, N.R., Stuart, R.C. *et al.* (1999) A pilot study of the safety and effects of the matrix metalloproteinase inhibitor marimastat in gastric cancer. *Eur. J. Cancer* **35**(4), 563–8.

Tsopanoglou, N.E., Pipili-Synetos, E. and Maragoudakis, M.E. (1993) Thrombin promotes angiogenesis by a mechanism independent of fibrin formation. *Am. J. Physiol.* **264**, 1302–7.

Tsujii, M., Kawano, S., Tsujii, S., Sawaoka, H., Hori, M. and DuBois, R.N. (1998) Cyclooxygenase regulates angiogenesis by colon cancer cells. *Cell* **93**, 705–16.

Uhr, J.W., Scheuermann, R.H., Street, N.E. and Vietta, E.S. (1997) Cancer dormancy: opportunities for new therapeutic approaches. *Nat. Med.* **3**, 505–9.

Varner, J. and Cheresh, D.A. (1996) Tumour angiogenesis and the role of vascular cell integrin αVβ3. In DeVita, V.T., Hellman, S. and Rosenberg, S.A. (eds), *Important advances in oncology*. Philadelphia, Pennsylvania: Lippincott, 69–87.

Veikkola, T. and Alitalo, K. (1999) VEGFs, receptors and angiogenesis. *Semin. Cancer Biol.* **9**(3), 211–20.

Vermeulen, P.B., Gasparini, G., Fox, S.B. *et al.* (1996) Quantification of angiogenesis in solid human tumours: an international consensus on the methodology and criteria of evaluation. *Eur. J. Cancer* **14**, 2474–84.

Voest, E.E., Kenyon, B.M., O'Reilly, M.S., Truitt, G., D'Amato, R.J. and Folkman, J. (1995) Inhibition of angiogenesis in vivo by interleukin 12. *J. Natl Cancer Inst.* **87**, 581–6.

Weidner, N. (1995) Intratumor microvessel density as a prognostic factor in cancer. *Am. J. Pathol.* **147**, 9–15.

Weidner, N., Carroll, P.R., Flax, J., Blumenfeld, W. and Folkman, J. (1993) Tumor angiogenesis correlates with metastasis in invasive prostate carcinoma. *Am. J. Pathol.* **143**, 401–9.

Weiner, H.L., Weiner, L.H. and Swain, J.L. (1987) Tissue distribution and developmental expression of the messenger RNA encoding angiogenin. *Science* **237**, 280–-2.

Weinstat-Saslow, D.L., Zabrentzky, V.S., Frazier, W.A., Roberts, D.D. and Steeg, P.S. (1994) Transfection of thrombospondin 1 complementary DNA into a human breast carcinoma cell line reduces primary tumor growth, metastatic potential and angiogenesis. *Cancer Res.* **54**, 6504–11.

Wojtowicz-Praga, S., Low, J., Marshall, J. *et al.* (1996) Phase I trial of a novel matrix metalloproteinase inhibitor batimastat (BB-94) in patients with advanced cancer. *Invest. New Drugs* **14**(2), 193–202.

Woodhouse, E.C., Chuaqui, R.F. and Liotta, L.A. (1997) General mechanism of metastasis. *Cancer* **80**(Suppl.), 1520–37.

Wu, Z., O'Reilly, M.S., Folkman, J. and Yuen, S. (1997) Suppression of tumor growth with recombinant murine angiostatin. *Biochem. Biophys. Res. Commun.* **236**, 651–4.

Zacharski, L.R., Wojtukiewicz, M.Z., Costantini, V., Ornstein, D.L. and Memoli, V.A. (1992) Pathways of coagulation/fibrinolysis activation in malignancy. *Semin. Thromb. Hemostasis* **18**(1), 104–16.

Zetter, B. (1990) The cellular basis of site-specific tumor metastases. *N. Engl. J. Med.* **322**, 605–12.

Zhang, Y., Deng, Y., Luther, T. *et al.* (1994) Tissue factor controls the balance of angiogenic and antiangiogenic properties of tumor cells in mice. *J. Clin. Invest.* **94**, 1320–7.

Ziche, M., Morbidelli, L., Masini, E. *et al.* (1994) Nitric oxide mediates angiogenesis *in vivo* and endothelial cell growth and migration *in vitro* promoted by substance P. *J. Clin. Invest.* **94**, 2036–44.

14

Gene therapy

HARDEV S. PANDHA AND KAROL SIKORA

INTRODUCTION

The key problem in the effective treatment of patients with solid tumours is the similarity between tumour and normal cells. Local therapies such as surgery and radiotherapy can succeed, but only if the malignant cells are confined to the area treated. This is so in around one-third of cancer patients. For the majority some form of systemic selective therapy is required. While many cytotoxic drugs are available, only a small proportion of patients are actually cured by their use. The success stories of Hodgkin's disease, non-Hodgkin's lymphoma, childhood leukaemia, choriocarcinoma and germ-cell tumours have just not materialized for the common cancers such as those of the lung, breast or colon. Despite enormous efforts in new drug development, clinical trials of novel drug combinations, the addition of cytokines, high-dose regimens and even partial or fully myeloblative transplants and stem cell rescue procedures, the gains have been marginal.

Against this disappointing clinical backdrop we have seen an explosion of information on the molecular biology of cancer. Although our knowledge of growth control is still rudimentary, we have at last had the first glimpse of its complexity. This has brought a new vision with which to develop novel selective mechanisms to destroy tumours. There are many potential avenues to follow in devising future therapies (Table 14.1). The first task is to learn how the growth signalling apparatus works in detail and to develop drugs that can target specific components within it. Examples being actively pursued include the construction of growth factor analogues which can competitively bind receptors (Woll and Rozengurt, 1990) and dimerization inhibitors to block cell surface receptor activity by preventing the aggregation of receptors – an essential process in their activation (Lofts *et al.*, 1993). Other targets lie within the cell and include key signalling enzymes such as tyrosine kinase and protein kinase C. In the nucleus, specific transcription factors that control gene expression are interrupted (Hickman, 1992). Another approach is to use molecular genetics to specifically manipulate tumour cells, resulting in their destruction.

Gene therapy can be described as the transfer and expression of genetic material into human cells for a therapeutic purpose. The main problem facing the gene therapist is how to get new genes into every tumour cell. If this

Table 14.1 *Molecular strategies for cancer treatment*

Receptor blockade	Ligand analogues
	Antibodies
Oncoprotein inhibitors	Dimerization blockers
	Protein kinase inhibitors
	Nucleoside analogues
	Transcription factor blockade
Gene expression inhibition	Antisense oligonucleotides
	Ribozymes
	Triplex DNA formation
Gene insertion	Mutant oncogene replacement
	Tumour suppressor gene replacement
Selective drug activation	Oncogene promoters
	Tumour marker promoters

cannot be achieved, then any malignant cells that remain unaffected will emerge as a resistant clone. Presently we do not have ideal gene transfer vehicles (vectors). Despite this drawback, there are already over 300 protocols accepted for clinical trial in cancer patients worldwide – the majority in the USA. The ethical issues are fairly straightforward, with oncology providing some of the highest possible benefit–risk ratios. The following strategies are currently under investigation.

GENE DELIVERY

The addition, substitution or ablation of DNA sequences may be achieved by any of the following:

1 Injection of naked DNA into skeletal muscle by simple needle and syringe.
2 DNA transfer by liposomes (delivered by the intravascular, intratracheal, intraperitoneal or intracolonic routes).
3 DNA coated on the surface of gold pellets which are air-propelled into the epidermis (the 'gene gun').
4 Biological vectors such as viruses and bacteria. Viruses are genetically engineered not to replicate once inside the host. They are currently the most efficient means of gene transfer.

Other techniques involve fusion of whole cells or viral envelopes, electroporation, microinjection or chemical precipitation of DNA into cells (Wu and Wu, 1991).

The efficiency of transfer of the required therapeutic DNA (dictated by the nature of the genetic defect) influences the choice of vector; e.g. for gene replacement, high-efficiency viral vectors are desirable, whereas short-term gene expression to prime an immune response or sensitize cells to radiotherapy may be achieved by liposomal delivery. The poor efficiency of gene transfer by the currently available vectors has been identified as one of the most important factors that may limit gene therapy as a realistic treatment strategy for common cancers. Some of the above strategies can be achieved *ex vivo* by transfer of a therapeutic gene into isolated cancer or non-cancer cells which are then re-implanted into the host. Others require delivery and expression of genes to target cancer cells *in vivo* (at much lower efficiency than *ex vivo* transfer) by exploiting transcriptional differences of specific genes between cancer and normal cells. The efficiency of gene transfer also varies greatly according to cell type targeted (low in neural and haemopoietic cells, high in myocytes, fibroblasts, hepatocytes and variable among different tumours).

GENETIC TAGGING

There are several situations where the use of a genetic marker to tag tumour cells may help in making decisions on the optimal treatment for an individual patient. The insertion of a foreign marker gene into cells from a tumour biopsy and replacing the marked cells into the patient prior to treatment can provide a sensitive new indicator of minimal residual disease after chemotherapy. The most common marker is the gene for neomycin phosphotransferase, the *neor* gene, an enzyme that metabolizes the aminoglycoside antibiotic G418. This gene, when inserted into an appropriate retroviral vector, can be stably incorporated into the host cell's genome. Originally detected by antibiotic resistance, it can now be picked up more sensitively by the polymerase chain reaction. In this way as few as one tumour cell amongst 1 million normal cells can be identified. This procedure can help in the design of aggressive chemotherapy protocols.

A particularly elegant use of this strategy has been the analysis of the reasons for failure of autologous bone-marrow transplantation in childhood acute mycloblastic leukaemia (AML). Failure can be due to inadequate chemotherapy or to reinfusion of viable tumour cells in the stored marrow. Reinfused marrow was labelled with *neo* and recurrent tumour analysed for the presence of this gene. In the majority of cases, tumour cells contained the marker, indicating a failure of the purging process (Brenner *et al.*, 1993). Similar studies are now in progress for neuroblastoma as well as chronic myeloid and acute lymphoid leukaemia.

ENHANCING TUMOUR IMMUNOGENICITY

The presence of an immune response to cancer has been recognized for many years. The problem is that human tumours seem to be predominantly weakly immunogenic. If ways could be found to elicit a more powerful immune stimulus, then effective immunotherapy could become a reality. Several observations from murine tumours indicate that one reason for weak immunogenicity of certain tumours is the failure to elicit a T-helper cell response (James and Sikora, 1993) which releases the necessary cytokines to stimulate the production of cytolytic T-cells which can destroy tumours. The expression of cytokine genes such as interleukin-2 (IL-2), tumour necrosis factor (TNF) and interferon in tumour cells has been shown to bypass the need for T-helper cells in mice (Fearon *et al.*, 1991). Similar clinical experiments are now in progress. Melanoma cells have been prepared from biopsies and infected with retrovirus containing the IL-2 gene. These cells are being used as a vaccine to elicit a more powerful immune response.

Many tumours express small amounts of the products of the major histocompatibility complex (MHC). These molecules are necessary for antigen presentation and their absence may help tumours to evade immune scrutiny. There are now several examples of mouse model systems where tumour cells transfected with MHC class I genes can be used, not only to prevent tumour spread when given as a prophylactic vaccine, but also to induce remission of established leukaemias, lymphomas, carcinomas and sarcomas. Clinical experiments involving the direct intra-tumoral injection of foreign HLA genes are currently in progress for several tumour types.

VECTORING CYTOKINES TO TUMOURS

Cytokines, such as the interferons and interleukins, have been actively explored for their tumoricidal properties (Thomas and Sikora, 1991). Although there is evidence of cytotoxicity, their side-effects are profound, so limiting the dose that can be administered safely. It is possible to insert cytokine genes into cells that can potentially home in on tumours, so releasing a high concentration of their protein product locally. TNF genes have been inserted into tumour-infiltrating lymphocytes from patients with melanoma, and given systemically (Rosenberg, 1992). These experiments are controversial for two reasons. First, it appears from *in vitro* studies that the amount of TNF expressed from such cells is unlikely to be sufficient to cause a significant cytotoxic effect and, secondly, the inser-tion of a foreign gene limits the ability of the lymphocyte to target into tumour masses (Anderson, 1992). Over 15 patients have so far been treated at the US National Cancer Institute and formal publication of the results is eagerly awaited.

GENETIC PRODRUG ACTIVATION THERAPY

The fundamental problem with current chemotherapy is its lack of selectivity. If drug-activating genes could be inserted which would be expressed only in cancer cells, then giving an appropriate prodrug could be highly selective. There are many examples of genes preferentially expressed in tumours. In some cases their promoters have been isolated and coupled to drug-activating enzymes or suicide genes (Martin and Lemoine, 1996). Genetic pro-drug activation therapy (GPAT, also known as GDEPT or VDEPT – virally dependent enzyme prodrug therapy) exploits differences in gene expression between cancer cells in this way to increase the specificity of cell destruction.

Two targeting strategies may be used independently or in combination to keep suicide gene expression limited to malignant tissue:

1 Transcriptional targeting exploits regulatory sequences of genes overexpressed in cancer cells to drive the expres-sion of a suicide gene selectively within tumour cells, e.g. ERBB2 in breast cancer, tyrosinase in melanoma (Pandha *et al.*, 1999).
2 Transduction targeting relies on preferential delivery of vectors constitutively expressing a suicide gene into

actively dividing cells only, e.g. glioma cells and not into normal neighbouring central nervous system cells.

Improvements in the efficacy of GPAT have resulted from successfully modifying both retroviral and adeno-viral tropism, and the use of chimeric transcriptional ele-ments combining strong tissue-specific promoters with tissue-specific enhancers to improve targeting further, e.g. combining the ERBB2/MUC-1 transcriptional elem-ents to drive the *HSV-tk* gene in breast cancer cells increases their sensitivity to prodrug activation compared to using single elements to drive the same suicide gene expression (Ring *et al.*, 1997).

An important additional feature of GPAT systems is the 'bystander effect'. This is the process whereby non-transduced cells in a mixed population die in the presence of a given prodrug, due to diffusion, active transport or recruitment of a local immune response (Freeman *et al.*, 1993). This effect varies in magnitude with the GPAT sys-tem and tumour cell line studied, but as little as 2 per cent transduction of a colorectal tumour cell line resulted in almost complete cell kill upon exposure to prodrug (Huber and Lazo, 1994). This may indicate that sustained high-efficiency gene transfer may not necessarily be required. Current clinical trials consist of transductional targeting of glioma and mesothelioma, and transcriptional target-ing of ovarian and breast carcinomas and melanoma, using adenoviral or retroviral transduction, or direct intralesional injection of plasmid DNA.

SUPPRESSING ONCOGENE EXPRESSION

The downregulation of abnormal oncogene expression has been shown to revert the malignant phenotype in a variety of *in vitro* tumour lines (Shirasawa *et al.*, 1993). It is possible to develop *in vivo* systems such as the insertion of genes encoding complementary (antisense) mRNA to that produced by the oncogene. Antisense oligodeoxynu-cleotides are short (10–50 base) synthetic nucleotide sequences formulated to be complementary to specific DNA or RNA sequences. They are able to enter all cells relatively easily and have the potential specificity to target individual oncogenes. If that gene is responsible for a dis-ease process, then its downregulation could result in a reversal of the clinical abnormalities. By the binding of these nucleotides to their targets, the transcription or translation of a single gene can be selectively inhibited. The mutant form of the *RAS* oncogene is an obvious tar-get for this approach. Up to 75 per cent of human pan-creatic cancers contain a mutation in the twelfth amino acid of this protein, and reversion of this change in cell lines will lead to the restoration of normal growth control. Clearly the major problem is to ensure that every single tumour cell becomes infected. Any cell that escapes will have a survival advantage and will produce a clone of resist-ant tumour cells. For this reason it may be that future treatment schedules will require the repetitive administration of vectors in a similar way to fractionated radiotherapy or chemotherapy. This approach has not lived up to initial expectations, due to poor specificity and observations of opposite and undesirable effects, such as the downregulation of gene expression resulting, paradoxically, in increased cell invasiveness. Recent pilot clinical trials in lymphoma and AML patients have provided encouraging results with no evidence of adverse effects.

GENETIC IMMUNOTHERAPY

Attempts at enhancing the naturally weak immunogenicity to tumours have resulted from a clearer understanding of antigen recognition, processing and presentation at the molecular level, and in particular, the nature of effector (T-cell) responses to antigenic stimulation.

A number of approaches are currently being evaluated:

1 Systemic immunotherapy for cancer with recombinant cytokine therapy is associated with low response rates at the expense of high systemic toxicity. Small doses of cytokines can be delivered at the tumour site by inserting cytokine genes into cultured tumour-infiltrating lymphocytes (TILs) *ex vivo*, then re-infusing the cells. Anti-tumour efficacy of this subset of T cells has been shown to improve with the transfer of the genes for tumour necrosis factor and interleukin-2 (Rosenberg, 1991).
2 Transducing tumour cells *ex vivo* with the same cytokine, allogeneic HLA (human leucocyte antigen) or genes encoding co-stimulatory molecules, such as the B7 family of genes, prior to re-infusion (after irradiation to eliminate malignant activity) so that T-cell recognition of tumour antigens is enhanced. Cytotoxic T lymphocytes (CTLs) recognize tumour-specific antigens presented on the surface of these cells. They are induced by the local secretion of the transferred cytokine gene product to expand, target and destroy cancer cells.
3 Polynucleotide (naked DNA) vaccinations (as opposed to vaccines consisting of peptides, whole tumour cells or tumour cell lysates) have great therapeutic potential, in that delivery of genes that express unique oncoproteins, such as K-RAS or lymphoma idiotypic protein, endogenously within a cell may then result in an MHC class I CD8+ response and proliferative activation of CTLs, rather than a less effective class II CD4+ response induced by exogenous peptides. This may be a further means of breaking down immunotolerance to tumours and may lead to the generation of tumour-specific responses. The limitation of this approach is the paucity of truly tumour-specific antigens which may be exploited as molecular targets. However, most target antigens are tumour-associated and tumour-specific, i.e. normal cellular genes inappropriately expressed in cancer, and lack epitopes to activate T cells. Delivery of genes encoding the E6 and E7 proteins of HPV 16 and 18 in patients with advanced cervical cancer has resulted in antibody and human papillomavirus (HPV)-specific T-cell responses (Borysiewicz *et al.*, 1996).
4 Dendritic cells (DCs) are potent professional antigen-processing and antigen-presenting cells, which are critical to the development of primary MHC-restricted T-cell immunity to infectious agents, in autoimmune diseases and anti-tumour immunity. Recent technological advances have allowed their expansion *in vitro* from CD34+ peripheral blood precursors or monocytes, using cytokines (Banchereau and Steinman, 1998). Cultured DCs are able to take up exogenous antigen (as tumour protein, peptide or RNA), or may be transduced with genes encoding tumour antigen using physical or viral methods of gene transfer, and then present it to T cells to induce a measurable anti-tumour effect. However, a number of basic issues in the design of a dendritic cell vaccine still need to be addressed. These include route of administration (intradermal injection avoids sequestration effects observed in the lung after intravenous injection), number of cells in each vaccine, and timing and number of vaccines. It is clear from murine DC studies using model antigens that co-injection of biological adjuvants, such as keyhole limpet haemocyanin (KLH), are required to provide an additional CD4+-mediated signal to augment the anti-tumour response. There are numerous clinical trials currently in progress after early pilot trials of peptide-pulsed DCs for relapsed B-cell lymphoma (Hsu *et al.*, 1996) and malignant melanoma (Nestle *et al.*, 1998).

INTRODUCING TUMOUR-SUPPRESSOR AND DRUG-RESISTANCE GENES

The inactivation of tumour-suppressor genes, such as those for retinoblastoma (Rb1), p53, Nm23, p16 or E-cadherin, may result in the initiation or the progression of a cancer. Replacement with normal copies of these genes using viral vectors has resulted in suppression and/or reversal of the malignant phenotype in *in vitro* tumour models. Furthermore, combining successful restoration of genes such as wild-type p53 and sequential administration of chemotherapy (such as cisplatin) appears to be synergistic in reducing the malignant expression in these cell lines. The clinical efficacy of intratumoural adenoviral delivery of wild-type p53 into p53-mutant squamous cell head and neck tumours and non-small cell lung cancers is currently being evaluated.

The *MDR1* multiple drug resistance gene has been transduced *ex vivo* into normal marrow or blood-derived stem cells to produce a selectable population of cells resistant to high doses of chemotherapy, which would then be re-infused into the patient. This has allowed higher doses of Taxol® to be administered in breast and ovarian cancer patients.

RISKS

The potential risks of gene therapy include:

1 insertional mutagenesis, leading to cancer;
2 recombination of disabled vector, resulting in environmental pollution by infectious recombinant virus;
3 toxic shock caused by viraemia;
4 transfer of non-viral exogenous genetic material;
5 contamination with other deleterious viruses or organisms.

Perhaps the biggest risk is the possibility of insertional mutagenesis and the activation of oncogenes, leading to neoplasia. Such risks are clearly important factors in the consideration of the ethical basis for gene therapy for disorders such as cystic fibrosis, haemophilia and the haemoglobinopathies. For patients with metastatic cancer, the risks are low. Such patients are often desperate for some form of treatment and are already searching for the gene therapy programmes described in the media. Therapies with even minimal potential benefit will be avidly considered (Slevin *et al.*, 1990). In this situation the biggest problem is offering false hope. It is unrealistic to expect such new strategies to be effective immediately. The first patients entering clinical trials are providing much information for little personal benefit. This must be recognized by both the investigator and patient to reduce the 'breakthrough' mentality that surrounds novel cancer treatments.

CONCLUSIONS

There have been remarkable advances in our understanding of the molecular biology of cancer. Interventional genetics is now poised to provide new selective tumour destruction mechanisms for patients with widespread cancer. There are many hurdles still to overcome: how to transfer genes efficiently and stably into tumour cells *in vivo*; how to ensure safety for both patient and staff; and how best to place genetic approaches alongside more familiar therapies. We are witnessing the beginnings of molecular therapy. Fifty years ago the first alkylating agents were discovered and were about to enter clinical trial as systemic chemotherapy. None of our predecessors could have predicted the successes and disappointments that have led to the practice of modern medical oncology. We are now leaving an era of empiricism and entering an age where our knowledge of genetics and logical molecular design is likely to change radically the future face of cancer treatment.

SIGNIFICANT POINTS – GENE THERAPY APPROACHES

- Genetic marking.
- Evaluating kinetics of adoptive immunotherapy – TIL and LAK cells.
- Genes inserted for immunomodulation, e.g. HLA B7, B7, IL-2, IL-4, IL-7, TNF, granulocyte/macrophage colony stimulating factor (GM-CSF).
- DNA vaccines for tumour antigens.
- Protection of normal cells from drug or radiation injury.
- Genetic prodrug activation vectoring biological products to tumours.
- Inhibition of oncogene expression.
- Expression of tumour suppressor genes.

REFERENCES

Anderson, C. (1992) Gene therapy researcher under fire for controversial cancer trials. *Nature* **360**, 399–400.

Austin, E.A. and Huber, B.E. (1993) A first step in the development of gene therapy for colorectal carcinoma – cloning, sequencing and expression of *E. coli* cytosine deaminase. *Mol. Pharmacol.* **43**, 380–7.

Banchereau, J. and Steinman, R.M. (1998) Dendritic cells and the control of immunity. *Nature* **392**, 245–52.

Borysiewicz, L.K., Fiander, A., Nimako, M. *et al.* (1996) A recombinant vaccinia virus encoding human papillomavirus types 16 and 18, E6 and E7 proteins as immunotherapy for cervical cancer. *Lancet* **347**, 1523–7.

Brenner, M.K., Rill, D.R., Moen, R.C. *et al.* (1993) Gene marking to trace origin of relapse after autologous bone marrow transplantation. *Lancet* **341**, 85–6.

Fearon, E.R., Pardoll, D.M., Itaya, T. *et al.* (1991) Interleukin 2 production by tumour cells bypasses the T helper cell function in the generation of an antitumour response. *Science* **254**, 713–16.

Freeman, S.M., Abboud, C.N., Whartenby, K.A. *et al.* (1993) The 'bystander effect': tumor regression when a fraction of the tumor mass is genetically modified. *Cancer Res.* **53**, 5274–83.

Harris, J. and Sikora, K. (1994) Human genetic therapy. *Mol. Asp. Med.* **14**, 453–546.

Hickman, J.A. (1992) Membrane and signal transduction targets. In Workman, P. (ed.), *New approaches in cancer pharmacology: drug design and development*. ESO Monographs. London: Springer-Verlag, 33–46.

Hsu, F.J., Benike, C., Fagnoni, F. *et al.* (1996) Vaccination of patients with B-cell lymphoma using autologous antigen-pulsed dendritic cells. *Nat. Med.* **2**, 52–8.

Huber, B.E. (ed.) (1995) *Genetic approaches to cancer therapy*. Cambridge: Cambridge University Press.

Huber, B.E. and Lazo, J.S. (eds) (1994) Gene therapy for neoplastic diseases. *Ann. NY Acad. Sci.* **716**.

James, N. and Sikora, K. (1993) Tumour-associated antigens. In Lachmann, P., Peters, K. and Walport, M. (eds), *Clinical immunology* (4th edn). Oxford: Blackwells, 1773–84.

Latchman, D.S. (ed.) (1994) *From genetics to gene therapy*. Oxford: BIOS.

Lofts, F.J., Hurst, H.C., Sternberg, M.J.E. and Guilick, W.J. (1993) Specific short transmembrane sequences can inhibit transformation by the mutant neu growth factor receptor *in vitro* and *in vivo. Oncogene* **8**, 2813–26.

Martin, L. and Lemoine, N. (1996) Direct killing by suicide genes. *Cancer Metastasis Rev.* **15**, 301–16.

Mercer, W.E., Shields, M.T., Lin, D., Apella, E. and Ulrich, S.J. (1991) Growth suppression induced by wild type p53 protein is accompanied by selective down regulation of proliferating-cell nuclear antigen in colon carcinoma cell lines that express c*myb. Cancer Res.* **51**, 2897–901.

Nestle, F.O., Alijagic, S., Gilliet, M. *et al.* (1998) Vaccination of melanoma patients with peptide- or tumor lysate-pulsed dentritic cells. *Nat. Med.* **4**, 328–32.

Pandha, H.S., Martin, L.A., Rigg, A. *et al.* (1999) Genetic prodrug activation therapy for breast cancer: A phase I clinical trial of erbB-2-directed suicide gene expression. *J. Clin. Oncol.* **17**, 2180–9.

Ring, C.J., Blouin, P., Martin, L.A., Hurst, H.C. and Lemoine, N.R. (1997) Use of transcriptional regulatory elements of the MUC1 and ERBB2 genes to drive tumour-selective expression of a prodrug activating enzyme. *Gene Ther.* **4**, 1045–52.

Rosenberg, S.A. (1991) Immunotherapy and gene therapy of cancer. *Cancer Res.* **51**, 5074s–9s.

Rosenberg, S.A. (1992) Gene therapy for cancer. *JAMA* **268**, 2416–19.

Shirasawa, S., Furuse, M., Yokoyama, N. and Sasazuki, T. (1993) Altered growth of human colon cancer cell lines disrupted at activated K-ras. *Science* **260**, 85–8.

Sikora, K. (1994) Genes, dreams and cancer. *BMJ* **308**, 1217–20.

Slevin, M.L., Stubbs, L., Plant, H.J. *et al.* (1990) Attitudes to chemotherapy: comparing view of patients with cancer with those of doctors, nurses, and general public. *BMJ* **300** (6737), 1458–60.

Thomas, H. and Sikora, K. (1991) New therapeutic modalities for cancer. *Acta Oncol.* **30**, 107–20.

Woll, P.J. and Rozengurt, E. (1990) A neuropeptide antagonist that inhibits the growth of small cell lung cancer *in vitro. Cancer Res.* **50**, 1968–73.

Wu, G.Y. and Wu, C.H. (1991) Delivery systems for gene therapy. *Biotherapy* **3**, 87–95.

Practice

Practice

15

Central nervous system

ROY RAMPLING

The central nervous system (CNS) is host to a remarkable variety of primary tumours that demonstrate an equal diversity of clinical behaviour, response to treatment and prognosis. While most malignant tumours still carry a bleak prognosis, useful extension of life can be achieved in many patients. Those with more responsive tumours can enjoy prolonged survival or cure if adequately managed. Hence an accurate diagnosis is required in almost all cases and this has been facilitated in recent years by advances in neuroimaging, neurosurgical technique and neuropathology. The practising neuro-oncologist needs a detailed knowledge of a modern classification system and how this relates to tumour management.

PATHOLOGY

Incidence

The overall incidence of primary malignant brain tumours in the UK is around 7 per 100 000 person years at risk (Parkin et al., 1997). Incidence estimates are dogged by methodological problems but geographical and racial variations do seem to occur (Giles and Gonzales, 1995). High rates are reported in Israeli Jews, whether born in Israel or elsewhere. Whites in Los Angeles have a higher incidence than those in England and Wales. The incidence in Japan is low but is doubled in Japanese living in Los Angeles.

Brain tumours account for approximately 1.6 per cent of all primary tumours (Parkin et al., 1997) but nearly 7 per cent of the number of years of life lost from cancer before age 70. There is some evidence that the overall incidence of brain tumours is increasing, particularly in the elderly (Fleury et al., 1997).

The distribution of histological types is fairly uniform worldwide (Table 15.1). Exceptions to this include high rates of pineal germ cell tumours in Asia, medulloblastomas in New Zealand Maoris and primary CNS lymphomas in regions with a high incidence of acquired immunodeficiency syndrome (AIDS).

Age

Brain tumours occur at any age from neonates to great old age. The age-specific incidence shows a small peak in early childhood, a poorly defined minimum in teenage years, rising at an increasing rate to a second major peak at around 65 (Harris et al., 1999) (Fig. 15.1). After age 70 most series report a rapid decline into old age.

Table 15.1 *Approximate incidence rates (worldwide) for brain tumour types (per 100 000/year)*

Tumour type	Incidence
Astrocytoma	1.5
Anaplastic astrocytoma	1.0
Glioblastoma	3
Meningioma	3
Primary CNS lymphoma	
Immune competent	0.3
Overall	0.8–6.8
Medulloblastoma	0.5
Germ cell tumours	0.2
Pinealoma/pineoblastoma	0.1
Metastases	8

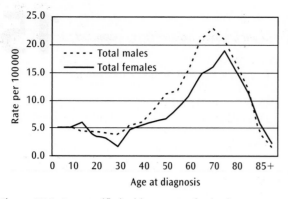

Figure 15.1 *Age-specific incidence rates for brain tumours in Scotland 1986–1995.*

This decline is possibly an artefact of data collection, and a Swedish series, based on high routine autopsy rates, shows the high incidence continuing into old age (Muir *et al.*, 1987). The brain is the most common site for solid tumours in childhood.

The tumour spectrum also varies with age. The majority of brain tumours in children (70–80 per cent) arise infratentorially (glial tumours, medulloblastoma) or in the midline (germ-cell tumours, craniopharyngioma). Low-grade glial tumours are common, particularly pilocytic astrocytoma. In adults most brain tumours are supratentorial. Gliomas, particularly glioblastomas, and meningiomas predominate.

Sex

Most brain tumours occur more commonly in males than in females, particularly medulloblastomas, germ-cell tumours, astrocytomas and oligodendrogliomas. Some, such as ependymomas and nerve-sheath tumours, are equally distributed and meningiomas are more common in females.

Aetiology

Ionizing radiation is the only environmental factor that is clearly associated with an increased risk of developing a brain tumour. This has been shown in adults and children receiving radiation for therapeutic purposes and following occupational exposure. Radiation-induced tumours include astrocytomas of all grades, benign and malignant meningiomas, sarcomas and nerve-sheath tumours. Although brain tumours may be induced in animals by a variety of viruses, none is known conclusively to do so in man although it is suspected in some, e.g. CNS lymphoma. Likewise, chemical agents can reliably induce tumours in some animal species (e.g. nitrosourea in rats) but neither industrial nor agricultural exposure in man has been definitely associated with an increased risk. Other putative agents have included

bacteria, head injury, diet, exposure to non-ionizing radiation (power lines, mobile phones) and tobacco. None has a proven relationship, although appropriate epidemiological studies are ongoing.

A number of genetic syndromes are associated with an increased risk of brain tumour (Kleihues and Cavenee, 2000). These are described in Table 15.2. A few other host-related factors are associated with an increased risk of acquiring a brain tumour. Immunosuppression, both environmental (e.g. AIDS) and iatrogenic, as in transplant recipients, predisposes to CNS lymphoma. The EBV genome is present in 95 per cent of these tumours and probably plays a major role in their development. Breast cancer may be associated with a higher incidence of meningioma (Markopoulos *et al.*, 1998).

Tumour types

The value of a pathological classification system to a clinician is that it can be used to direct management and predict behaviour. The most widely used classification for brain tumours is the World Health Organization system (Kleihues *et al.*, 1993; Kleihues and Cavenee, 2000). It has well over 100 entries. An abridged version is shown in Table 15.3. The scheme is based on a separation of tumour types according to their (presumed) tissue of origin (neuroepithelium, meninges, etc.) and then according to the derivative cell type (astrocyte, oligodendrocyte, etc.). Further classification recognizes features of the tumour cells and the associated microenvironment which grade the tumour according to its degree of malignancy. These features (for example cellular pleomorphism and necrosis in glioblastoma) relate to the clinical behaviour of the tumour. The WHO and other modern classification schemes such as St. Anne/Mayo (Daumas-Duport *et al.*, 1988) have now replaced older systems (Kernohan *et al.*, 1949) which placed undue emphasis on tumour cytology alone. Great care must be taken when comparing clinical series that use different classification schemes.

Although conventional light microscopy still provides the backbone of pathological analysis, it is often insufficient to produce a complete diagnosis. Immunohistochemistry is frequently an indispensable discriminant and electron microscopy can also provide useful information. In particular, glial fibrillary acidic protein (GFAP) is valuable in identifying normal astrocytes and cells from all astrocytic tumours. However, non-astrocytic and even some non-glial tumours may be positive. S-100 may also be useful but is not specific to the nervous system. Lymphomas, germ-cell tumours, sarcomas and metastases immunostain, as do their systemic counterparts (*see* under relevant sections elsewhere in this book). Molecular biology reveals differences between tumours already separated on the WHO scheme and also between tumours thought previously to be similar, e.g. glioblastomas types I and II. This is discussed below under their separate sections.

Table 15.2 *Genetic syndromes associated with an increased risk of brain tumour*

Syndrome	Brain tumour	Other associations	Genetics
Neurofibromatosis 1	Neurofibromas Gliomas Sarcomas	Pigmentation Peripheral neurofibromas Osseous and vascular lesions	*NF1* on 17q12 Autosomal dominant
Neurofibromatosis 2	Schwannomas (acoustic neuromas) Meningiomas Gliomas (especially spinal)	Cerebral calcification Lens opacities	*NF2* on 22q12 Autosomal dominant
Von Hippel–Lindau	Haemangioblastoma	Retinal haemangioblastoma Renal carcinoma Phaeochromocytoma Visceral cysts	*VHL* on 3p25–26 Autosomal dominant
Cowden	Dysplastic gangliocytoma of cerebellum	Peripheral hamartomas Breast cancer Thyroid neoplasia	*PTEN/MMAC1* on 10q23 Autosomal dominant
Turcot	Glioblastomas Medulloblastomas	Colorectal tumours	5q21 Autosomal dominant
Tuberous sclerosis	Subependymal giant cell astrocytoma Hamartomas	Angiofibromas Hypomelanotic patches	*TSC1* on 9q *TSC2* on16p
Li Fraumeni	Gliomas PNETs	Sarcomas Breast cancer	*TP53* on 17p13 Autosomal dominant
Basal naevus	Medulloblastomas	Basal cell carcinomas Bone abnormalities Palmer pits	*PTCH* on 9q31 Autosomal dominant

PNETs, primitive neuroectodermal tumours.

The molecular biology of brain tumours

The molecular pathogenesis of brain tumours is becoming increasingly clear (Rasheed *et al.*, 1999). Early changes comprise loss of tumour suppressor function, while gene amplification is almost exclusively seen in high-grade tumours and represents late change.

GENETIC ALTERATIONS IN BRAIN TUMOURS

Loss of heterozygosity (LOH) is common (Table 15.4). LOH 17p is usually associated with *p53* mutations and is associated with loss of tumour suppressor function. This is not the case in medulloblastoma where LOH 17p is not associated with *p53* mutation. LOH 9p (homozygous deletion) is associated with inactivation of *CDKN2A* (and B). LOH 13q (Rb inactivation) inhibits the same pathway. The two abnormalities are almost never seen together. LOH 10q is particularly common in all types of high-grade glioma but the specific LOH 10q 23 (the phosphatase and tensin (*PTEN*) gene) is largely confined to the subgroup of primary glioblastoma. Oncogene amplification is a late event. *EGFR* amplification in glioblastoma is most common but is restricted to the primary subtype and is frequently aberrant. *PDGFR*, *CDK4*, *MDM2* and a novel gene *GAS41* are amplified less frequently in gliomas.

LOW-GRADE GLIOMAS

LOH for 17p occurs commonly (>30 per cent), the majority associated with mutations of *p53* (*p53* mutations do not occur in pilocytic astrocytomas but are very common (>80 per cent) in gemistocytic astrocytomas).

GLIOBLASTOMA

There appear to be at least two types of glioblastoma based on their molecular abnormalities (Table 15.4). The *de novo*, or primary, glioblastoma tends to occur in older patients, with no prior history of tumour and have a particularly poor prognosis. They are characterized by oncogene amplification (typically epidermal growth factor receptor, *EGFR*, *CDKN2A* deletions and *PTEN* mutations). Secondary or progressive glioblastomas arise in younger patients, frequently with preceding astrocytoma, and have a slightly better prognosis. Common abnormalities are *p53* mutations and platelet-derived growth factor receptor (*PDGFR*) amplification. LOH 10 is common in both types of glioblastoma. Overexpression of *Mdm2*, without gene amplification, occurs in the majority of glioblastomas. Its role is unclear.

OLIGODENDROGLIOMA

Both oligodendroglioma and anaplastic oligodendroglioma exhibit LOH 1p and 19q (>80 per cent of patients). LOH 4, 6 and 11 occur much less frequently. There is a mutually exclusive pattern of LOH 1p, LOH 19q and *p53* gene mutation in oligoastrocytomas, suggesting that the former are of oligodendrocyte origin and the latter are astrocytic. LOH for 1p is associated with a good response to chemotherapy (Cairncross *et al.*, 1998). The minority

Table 15.3 *World Health Organization brain tumour classification system (abridged and adapted) (Kleihues and Cavenee, 2000)*

Tumours of neuroepithelial tissue	**Tumours of cranial and spinal nerves**

Tumours of neuroepithelial tissue

A. *Astrocytic tumours*
1. Astrocytoma (variants: fibrillary, protoplasmic, gemistocytic, mixed)
2. Anaplastic (malignant) astrocytoma
3. Glioblastoma (variants: giant cell, gliosarcoma)
4. Pilocytic astrocytoma
5. Pleomorphic xanthoastrocytoma
6. Subependymal giant cell astrocytoma

B. *Oligodendroglial tumours*
1. Oligodendroglioma
2. Anaplastic oligodendroglioma

C. *Ependymal tumours*
1. Ependymoma
2. Anaplastic ependymoma
3. Myxopapillary ependymoma
4. Subependymoma

D. *Mixed gliomas*

E. *Choroid plexus tumours*
1. Choroid plexus papilloma
2. Choroid plexus carcinoma

F. *Neuroepithelial tumours of uncertain origin*
1. Astroblastoma
2. Polar spongioblastoma
3. Gliomatosis cerebri

G. *Neuronal and mixed neuronal–glial tumours*
1. Gangliocytoma
2. Ganglioglioma
3. Anaplastic ganglioglioma
4. Dysembryoplastic neuroepithelial tumour (of childhood)

H. *Pineal tumours*
1. Pineocytoma
2. Pineoblastoma

I. *Embryonal tumours*
1. Medulloepithelioma
2. Neuroblastoma
3. Primitive neuroectodermal tumours (PNET)
4. Medulloblastoma

Tumours of cranial and spinal nerves

A. *Schwannoma (neurilemmoma, neurinoma)*

B. *Neurofibroma*

C. *Malignant peripheral nerve-sheath tumour*
1. Malignant schwannoma
2. Neurogenic sarcoma (and others)

Tumours of the meninges

A. *Tumours of meningothelial cells*
1. Meningioma (and variants)
2. Atypical meningioma
3. Anaplastic (malignant) meningioma

B. *Mesenchymal, non-meningothelial tumours*
1. Lipoma
2. Fibrous histiocytoma (etc.)

C. *Malignant neoplasms*
1. Haemangiopericytoma
2. Chondrosarcoma

D. *Primary melanocytic lesions*

E. *Tumours of uncertain histiogenesis*
1. Haemangioblastoma

Haematopoeitic neoplasms
1. Primary malignant lymphomas
2. Plasmacytoma

Germ-cell tumours
Germinoma
Teratoma (immature, mature)
Choriocarcinoma
Mixed

Cysts and tumour-like lesions
1. Rathkes cleft cyst
2. Dermoid cyst (and others)

Tumours of the anterior pituitary
1. Pituitary adenoma
2. Pituitary carcinoma

Local extensions from regional tumours
Craniopharyngioma
Paraganglioma
Chordoma
Chondrosarcoma

Metastatic tumours

---

of oligodendrogliomas, without LOH 1p, appear to be chemoresistant.

MEDULLOBLASTOMAS

LOH 17p occurs in 30–40 per cent of medulloblastomas but is associated with mutated *p53* in only 5–10 per cent. It is not considered the target of 17p loss.

MENINGIOMAS

Deletions on chromosome 22 occur in the majority of meningiomas. Half of these incur loss at 22q12. Atypical meningiomas show further loss on 1p, 9q and 10q, suggesting that progression may be associated with genes at these loci.

Local environment

The tumour extracellular matrix (ECM) comprises proteoglycans, glycoproteins and collagens. Fibronectin and laminin are present and may assist invasion. Gliomas modify the ECM by enzymatic digestion of the ECM proteins. There are changes in cell–cell and cell–matrix interactions and abnormalities in water and electrolyte

Table 15.4 *Molecular abnormalities in brain tumours*

Tumour type	High frequency	Low frequency
Astrocytoma (low-grade)	p53 mutations, PDGFR amplifications	
Primary glioblastoma	LOH 10q, EGFR amplification, PTEN alterations, CDKN2A deletions, p16 deletion	p53 mutations
Secondary glioblastoma	LOH 10q, p53 mutations, PDGFR amplifications	PTEN alterations, EGFR amplifications
Oligodendroglioma	LOH 1p, LOH 19q	LOH 10q, PTEN alterations
Anaplastic oligodendroglioma	LOH 1p, LOH 19q, CDKN2A deletions	LOH 10q, PTEN alterations
Medulloblastoma	LOH 17p, PAX overexpression	
Meningioma	Deletions of Chr 22 (especially 22q12). LOH 10q (atypical only)	

EGFR, epidermal growth factor receptor; PDGFR, platelet-derived growth factor receptor; PTEN, phosphatase and tensin; PAX, Paired Box containing (genes).

composition. A characteristic of many tumours, particularly glioblastomas, is heterogeneity. The intracellular and extracellular pH varies from a borderline alkalosis in regions of high perfusion to acidosis in regions of insufficiency. Likewise the pO_2 varies both in and around the tumour. It is clear, however, that large regions of the tumour are markedly hypoxic (Rampling *et al.*, 1994). The region adjacent to many tumours is characterized by oedema and inflammatory cell infiltrate.

Immunology

The brain does not have a lymphatic system. However, there are phagocytic, microglial cells, which probably derive from monocytes in the developing brain. They express macrophage markers and act in the same way as macrophages elsewhere in the body. Abnormal vessels in and around tumours allow the transfer of proteins and cells that would normally be prevented by an intact blood–brain barrier (BBB).

Brain tumour cells exhibit a number of tumour-associated antigens, such as Mel-14 and tenacsin, which may also be found on other neuroectodermal tumours and fetal cells. Astrocytic tumours overexpress CD10 and EGFR. *In vitro*, human glioma cells secrete a number of inhibitory factors, such as transforming growth factor-β2 (TGF-β2), prostaglandin E_2 (PGE$_2$) and interleukin-10 (IL-10), which act to reduce the local immune response to the tumour. Other cytokines are secreted, including interleukin-2, -6 and -8 and granulocyte/macrophage colony stimulating factor (GM-CSF). A variable, but often marked, cellular immune response occurs at the site of a brain tumour. The infiltrate is predominantly of CD8+ T lymphocytes and macrophages, with a minor component of B cells and natural killer (NK) cells. The systemic cellular immune response in patients with malignant brain tumours is often markedly impaired.

Tumour spread

By definition, benign tumours in the brain are non-invasive and non-metastatic. Their clinical effects arise

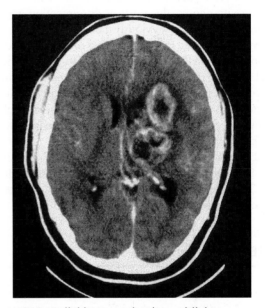

Figure 15.2 *A glioblastoma, showing multilobar involvement, transcallosal spread and oedema extending along the white-matter tracts.*

from compression of adjacent structures and the associated functional detriment. Primary malignant tumours, on the other hand, are usually highly infiltrative. Cellular motility occurs early in their development. These cells typically disseminate along white-matter tracts, following the pattern set by the tumorigenic oedema, and may be found many centimetres from the apparent 'edge' of the tumour (Kelly *et al.*, 1987). Spread in this way does not respect boundaries between the lobes of the brain or opposing hemispheres. Spread across the corpus callosum is common. This pattern is followed by many malignant tumours but is characteristic for malignant gliomas (Fig. 15.2). The term 'butterfly tumour' is frequently used to describe a lesion that involves both frontal lobes. Local spread will also occur along the meningeal surface in superficially placed tumours. Spread via the cerebrospinal fluid (CSF) is common in a few tumour types – medulloblastoma, pineoblastoma, germ-cell tumours and lymphoma – but is clinically less apparent in gliomas.

Table 15.5 *Categorization of the influences of brain tumours*

Site	Effect	Symptom	Outcome following treatment
Local	Infiltration Haemorrhage	Local syndromes	Usually irreversible
	Electrical	Seizure	Sometimes reversible
	Pressure/distortion Metabolic	Local syndromes	Usually reversible
Global	Pressure due to space occupation or obstructive hydrocephalus	Headache, nausea, tiredness, cognitive change, brainstem syndrome	Often reversible
	Electrical	Seizure	Sometimes reversible

However, if a post-mortem search is made in late survivors with glioma, this route of dissemination appears more common than previously thought.

Systemic spread for primary CNS tumours is uncommon. Exceptions to this are medulloblastoma, mesenchymal lesions (e.g. haemangiopericytoma and meningeal sarcoma) and, possibly, lymphomas and germ-cell tumours. In these latter, however, it may be difficult to know whether the brain lesion was part of a systemic process from the outset.

The pattern of spread of brain tumours is quite different from that of the more common cancer sites. Hence the TNM staging system, which works well for systemic cancer, has little relevance in brain tumours.

PRESENTATION

The functions of the brain are so numerous and diverse that it is not surprising that brain tumour presentation is also highly varied. A detailed description of the many syndromes is beyond the scope of this chapter and the reader is referred to a standard neurology text (Bannister, 1992). Some general principles can be applied.

The effects of brain tumours can be divided into local and global categories (Table 15.5). Symptoms due to pressure may be completely or partially reversed following tumour decompression, shunting or treatment with steroids. Damage to brain tissue due to infiltration or haemorrhage is frequently irreversible, although delayed recovery or compensation can occur after successful treatment.

The brain's inflammatory response to a tumour, particularly the development of oedema, may contribute to symptoms. Clinical response to steroids in these circumstances is often dramatic but may not be associated with corresponding changes on brain imaging. The mechanism of steroid action is far from clear. Likewise, the cause of seizure in patients with brain tumours is not understood. Seizures frequently persist, even after anti-tumour treatment and appropriate treatment with anticonvulsants.

Table 15.6 shows the first presenting symptom in 120 consecutive patients with glioblastoma. However, the

Table 15.6 *Initial symptom in 120 consecutive patients with newly diagnosed glioblastoma presenting to the neuro-oncology unit at Institute of Neurological Sciences in Glasgow*

Symptom	%	Symptom	%
Headache	34	Altered consciousness	4
Seizure	23	Incoordination	4
Limb weakness	12	Sensory disturbance	3
Cognitive change	8	Speech disturbance	3
Visual disturbance	5	Other	4

individual symptom prevalence is much higher, with headache a feature in over 70 per cent at presentation. While both headache and seizure are common symptoms in patients with brain tumours, in the community as a whole, brain tumours are a rare cause of these symptoms. A general practitioner will, on average, see five new patients with primary brain tumours in their career but thousands with headache. Suspicion should be aroused when the headache fits the pattern for raised intracranial pressure, is unremitting, arises in unexpected circumstances or is accompanied by vomiting or neurological deficit.

The great majority of patients presenting with seizure require a brain scan, but this is not feasible in all patients with headache. Evidence of recent neurological, psychological or behavioural change should be actively sought and examination of the fundi performed. If an abnormality is found, or if the headache intensifies in the face of conservative management, referral for examination is indicated.

Less usual presentations include the effects of hormonal disturbance, intellectual decline, developmental failure, disturbance of special senses and psychological disturbance.

IMAGING

The mainstay of brain tumour diagnosis is structural imaging, using either computed tomography (CT) or magnetic resonance imaging (MRI). The use of contrast enhancement in both techniques is indispensable. CT is quick, has scalar integrity, is relatively easy to interpret

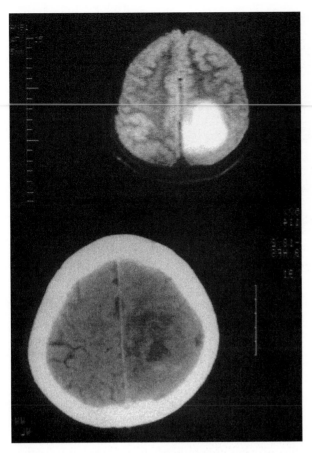

Figure 15.3 *A low-grade astrocytoma that is difficult to see on CT scan but which is clearly identified on MRI.*

and is inexpensive. Tumours less than 0.5 cm and those adjacent to bone may be missed. The basis of CT is differential absorption of X-rays. Since this is related to electron density, the derived Hounsfield numbers can be used as input to CT planning systems for radiotherapy. MRI relies on radiofrequency emission from perturbed atoms in a strong magnetic field. It is more expensive, prone to distortions and is more difficult to interpret. However, it is the more sensitive investigation and does not suffer from bone artefact. It is the diagnostic modality of choice for brain tumours in most circumstances (Fig. 15.3; *see also* Fig. 15.7).

A few patients with potentially magnetizable metal in their bodies, either from previous surgery or accidents, may not be eligible for MRI scan.

Brain tumour images appear as infiltrative or space-occupying lesions. The position and distribution of the tumour, together with the density variation, particularly after contrast injection, provides important diagnostic information. Tumours enhance with contrast (on CT and MRI) if they are hypervascular or if the vessels are abnormal and leak excessive contrast material. Areas of enhancement often indicate actively growing tumour. High-grade gliomas enhance in their actively growing rim (Fig. 15.2) but not in their necrotic centres or in the

associated oedema. Lymphomas (*see* Fig. 15.14), meningiomas (*see* Fig. 15.13) and many metastases (*see* Fig. 15.17) are usually uniformly enhancing. Slowly growing tumours, such as low-grade gliomas, often fail to enhance at all (Fig. 15.3). Some tumours may show calcification. While this is particularly frequent in oligodendrogliomas (*see* Fig. 15.11) and craniopharyngiomas, it may be seen in almost any slowly growing tumour.

It is important to realize that whereas imaging appearances can give a good indication of the nature of a tumour, they are not totally diagnostic. For example a solitary, mixed-density, enhancing, space-occupying lesion may suggest an intrinsic malignant tumour. However, these appearances are also common in metastases, and can be seen less commonly in meningioma, lymphoma or non-malignant lesions such as abscess or radiation necrosis. Histological examination is the only sure way to categorize a tumour.

Prior surgical intervention can also produce diagnostic problems. Postoperative imaging for residual tumour assessment should be done within 72 hours of the operation. After this time appearances can be misleading, particularly due to the presence of altered blood.

So-called functional imaging provides complementary information. Positron emission tomography (PET) scanning relies on the use of positron-emitting isotopes integrated into metabolically active molecules (e.g. [18F]fluorodeoxyglucose, 18FDG). The oppositely directed, colinear γ-rays can be detected by scintillation counters and turned into a three-dimensional image which represents the metabolic activity associated with the imaging agent. For example 18FDG uptake into glioma recurrence may distinguish it from radionecrosis in a patient treated with radiation. Single photon emission computed tomography (SPECT) similarly uses a radiolabelled, metabolically active molecule. In this technique, single γ-ray photons are imaged by a rotating gamma camera and three-dimensional images created using standard tomography algorithms. An example is thallium-201 (chloride) which is an analogue of potassium and is taken up preferentially into rapidly proliferating tumours. It may differentiate low- and high-grade tumours (Fig. 15.4). Other uses of functional imaging include assessing tumour response to treatment and measuring blood flow.

TREATMENT MODALITIES

Surgery

Surgery has three roles in brain tumour management: to obtain a diagnosis, to contribute to survival and to relieve symptoms.

Biopsy alone may be attempted either as an open procedure or using stereotactic techniques. The technique of burr-hole and 'blind' biopsy is uncertain in outcome

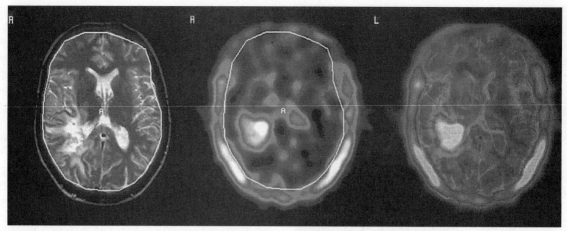

Figure 15.4 *A thallium SPECT scan of a glioblastoma (centre), showing dramatic uptake in the right deep parietal region. The corresponding T_2 MRI is shown on the left and the overlaid images on the right.*

and has a high morbidity/mortality. It should have little place in modern neurosurgical practice. Stereotactic biopsy relies on relating a CT (or MRI) acquired brain image to an external coordinate set. The image can then be used to direct a biopsy needle to the point of interest with an accuracy of 1–2 mm through a burr-hole. The diagnostic yield is very high (>90 per cent) and the morbidity/mortality correspondingly low (Krieger *et al.*, 1997). There are situations where even stereotaxy may be considered hazardous. In these circumstances biopsy under direct vision may be required using craniotomy or ventriculoscopy to visualize the tumour. Biopsies (multiple where possible) should be taken from the most active-looking part of the tumour. Functional imaging (e.g. SPECT) may be helpful in achieving this.

When interpreting the biopsy, it is important to provide the pathologist with full clinical information, such as the patient's demography, presentation, previous treatment and any previous insult to that area of brain (e.g. prior irradiation). Full radiological information is also invaluable. It is important to remember that sampling error may lead to underdiagnosis in a heterogeneous tumour. Hence adequate weight must be given to the clinical situation and the imaging appearances in making treatment decisions and prognostic forecasts. It is best practice for the managing clinician to review every biopsy with the pathologist and the radiologist.

The morbidity associated with neurosurgery for tumour has been greatly reduced by the routine use of corticosteroids. These are prescribed before operating and for some days thereafter. In many cases they can be reduced steadily in the days following surgery as the reaction settles, provided the source of pressure has been removed. Drugs that modify platelet function, and other potential anticoagulating agents, should be stopped preoperatively. Anticonvulsants are prescribed routinely in some countries, but in the UK may be given only to patients who are known to suffer from seizures or are at high risk because of the site of the intended operation.

For the resection of a tumour, access is gained by craniotomy. A scalp incision is made and a flap of skin and pericranial tissue turned. The siting of the craniotomy will depend on the position of the tumour. Most surgeons prefer a free bone flap, which is created first by making burr-holes, freeing the dura and then cutting the flap using a high-speed craniotome. The dura is then opened only by an amount that will give adequate exposure of the tumour-bearing brain. The operating microscope is used routinely to give good visualization. Minimal retraction of the brain is performed to permit access to the tumour. It is common practice to confirm the diagnosis with an intra-operative frozen section or cytological smear, prior to performing the full resection. The resection itself is normally performed by internal decompression, using a mixture of bipolar coagulation, sharp dissection, cautery, ultrasonic aspiration and, if appropriate, laser vaporization. The aim is always to remove as much of the tumour as is safely possible.

The operation is completed with dural closure, replacement of the bone flap and skin closure. The devitalized free bone flap is a potential site for infection that will be resistant to antibiotics. Infection in the flap following surgery will necessitate its removal.

The possibility of tumour removal has recently been improved by image-guided surgery. In this technique, a CT image of the tumour is displayed into the operating field via the operating microscope, allowing the surgeon to visualize the tumour more clearly. This technique has been enhanced by the ability to fuse multi-modality images (CT, MRI, SPECT) prior to projection. In this way the advantages of each imaging modality can be used to improve the accuracy of localization and completeness of resection. Most recently it has become possible to perform surgery within the magnetic field of a magnetic resonance imaging system. This allows the intraoperative generation of MR images which can be projected onto the patient to improve the completeness and safety of resection.

The technique of awake craniotomy involves 'cortical mapping' of neurological function. When performed during the operative procedure and it can be used to avoid resection of eloquent brain tissue.

Radiotherapy

The value of radiotherapy in the treatment of brain tumours depends largely on their intrinsic radiosensitivity. In some it may be curative (medulloblastomas, germ-cell tumours), whereas in others it will only contribute to a modest prolongation of survival. Most radiotherapy is delivered using postoperative external-beam X-rays. However, a variety of other techniques is possible, including intra-operative radiotherapy, particle radiotherapy and brachytherapy. In all situations the ambition is to deliver a maximal (or curative) dose to the entire tumour, while minimizing the normal tissue dose and volume. The particular applications are discussed under the individual tumour types.

RADIOTHERAPY TECHNIQUE

Partial brain irradiation
In the majority of patients, the head should be immobilized in preparation for treatment planning. Mouldable plastics, such as Aquaplast or Orfit, have the advantage of speed and simplicity but are perforated and less rigid and do not carry marking information well (Fig. 15.5b). Beam-direction shells (BDSs) can reproduce a set-up position to an accuracy of 3–5 mm. They are rigid and easy to mark (Fig. 15.5a). However, they are cumbersome and time consuming to prepare. Patients are most commonly positioned supine (Fig. 15.5b) but it may be necessary to plan the patient in the prone position (Fig. 15.5a) or even lying on their side, in order to facilitate beam placement.

It is standard practice to incorporate good-quality CT images into the planning of brain tumours. This can be done by simple screening at the simulator or by using a manual method of image transfer on to orthogonal radiographs of the skull (Fig. 15.6). MR images can be used in a similar way, but care must be taken to avoid errors due to distortion. If a patient has had surgery for a malignant brain tumour, it is conventional to use the preoperative scans as the basis for radiotherapy planning. The logic of this is not entirely clear, but the use of postoperative scans may be complicated by the difficulty of differentiating residual tumour from postoperative change.

Patients can also be planned using a CT planning system. This is the method of choice for unresected tumours, but in the postoperative patient the problem of image interpretation arises. This dilemma may be solved by fusing pre- and postoperative images. The possibility of fusing CT, MRI and functional images in the planning system further enhances target definition (Figs 15.4 and 15.7).

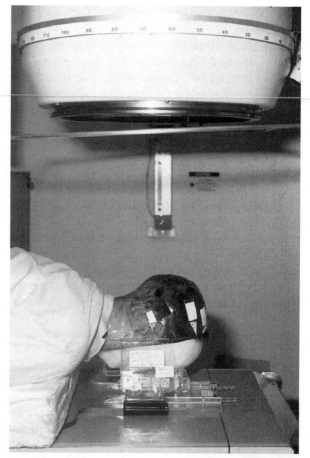

(a)

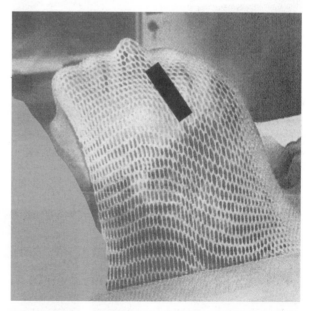

(b)

Figure 15.5 *Immobilization devices for brain tumour therapy. (a) Thermolabile beam-direction shell (BDS). Notice the 'cut out' region to preserve skin sparing. (b) An Orfit shell.*

It is now best practice to use multiple fields to deliver the radiation and minimize dose to non-tumour-bearing brain. Whole-brain radiotherapy is rarely used for gliomas. Limited opposed pair arrangements can be used for tumours affecting both sides of the brain or in very palliative set-ups. Otherwise the choice is usually three fields with appropriate wedging (Fig. 15.8). CT planning facilitates the use of non-coplanar beams to optimize radiation delivery, and the use of conformal shaping can further reduce the dose to normal brain.

It is usual to treat patients with brain tumours using a 4–6 MV linear accelerator. It has good depth–dose characteristics over the required depth range, typically 2–12 cm. The build-up depth of around 1 cm gives good skin sparing. High dose rates lead to short treatment times and the high energy means that bone doses are not excessive. Cobalt-60 can also be used but does not match these characteristics and also the penumbra is greater. Orthovoltage should not be used except in the most palliative of situations.

In radical treatments for brain tumours, fractionation is generally kept below 2 Gy per fraction (*see* below). Treatments are given daily, 5 days per week. No radiobiological advantage has been shown for accelerated or hyperfractionated treatments. It is customary to maintain patients on corticosteroids during their radiotherapy. However, the need for high doses is probably overemphasized, particularly if a good decompression has been performed. Decompressed patients may require only low doses of dexamethasone (2–4 mg/day) or none at all.

Hair loss is universal in the irradiated site but re-growth may occur if the dose at the hair follicle is kept below about 35 Gy. Other side-effects from radiotherapy include tiredness, which is common and may persist for weeks after completion of treatment, and skin erythema. By using megavoltage radiation and cutting out the BDS (Fig. 15.5), skin sparing and the possibility of hair re-growth may be maximized. Nausea is rare with modern radiotherapy and vomiting exceptional if the correct dose of steroids is used. Other possible causes of gastrointestinal upset must be actively excluded.

Whole-neuraxis radiotherapy

This technique is used in situations where the entire meningeal content is at risk from tumour dissemination in the CSF, e.g. medulloblastoma. The problem is one of irradiating, in continuity, the brain, which is best approached with an opposed pair of photon beams, and the spine, which requires a direct posterior field of photons or electrons.

The standard technique uses a 4–6 MV linear accelerator. The patient is immobilized in a prone cast extended over the shoulders to reduce movements of the trunk. A pair of lateral fields is used to irradiate the head. These are shaped using individually cast blocks to include the entire meningeal surface (Fig. 15.9). Particular attention must be paid to the region of the cribriform plate and the temporal lobes, which may extend lower than often appreciated. Centring the field on the outer canthus reduces divergence dose to the opposite lens. Compensators may be used to account for varying head width. In children care must be taken to irradiate the whole of the growing vertebra. The spine is irradiated using a direct posterior field (Fig. 15.9).

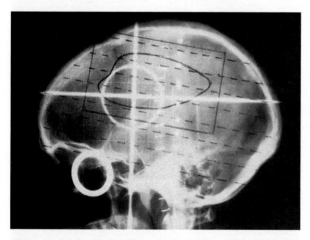

Figure 15.6 *Hand planning a brain tumour by transferring CT information on to orthogonal radiographs.*

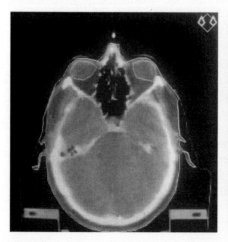
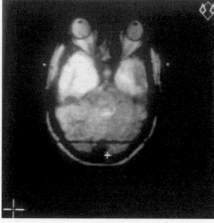

Figure 15.7 *A treatment planning system capable of inter-relating CT and MRI images.*

A collimator rotation on the head fields matches the divergence of the spine field (typically 7°). Two spinal fields, also matched, may be needed in adults. A compensator is used to produce a uniform dose to the cord (prescribed at the anterior cord surface). The spinal field extends at least to the bottom of S2. There is no evidence that a sacral 'spade' width extension to cover the sacral roots is required. Because of the uncertainties involved in

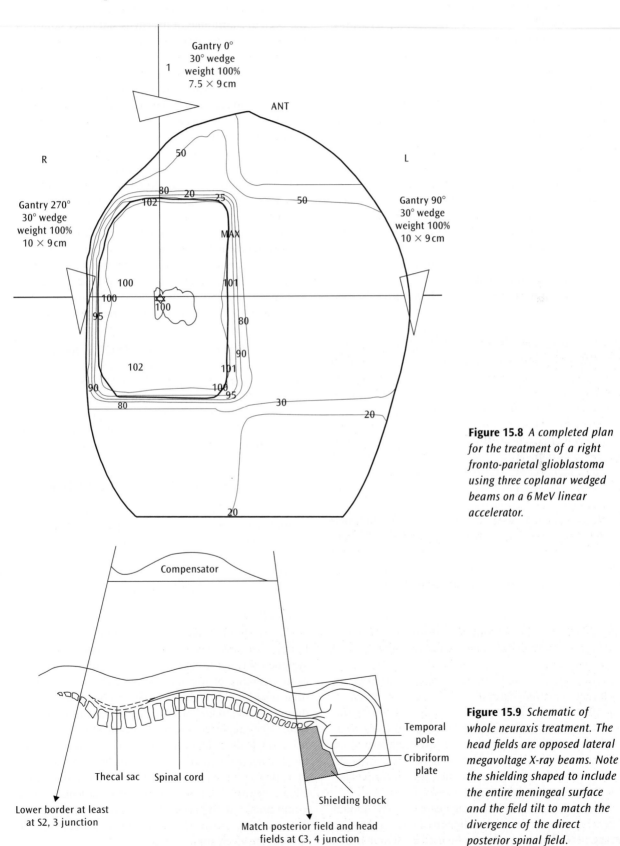

Figure 15.8 *A completed plan for the treatment of a right fronto-parietal glioblastoma using three coplanar wedged beams on a 6 MeV linear accelerator.*

Figure 15.9 *Schematic of whole neuraxis treatment. The head fields are opposed lateral megavoltage X-ray beams. Note the shielding shaped to include the entire meningeal surface and the field tilt to match the divergence of the direct posterior spinal field.*

establishing the junctions at each treatment, it is conventional in many departments to move them by 1 cm every seven treatments. Similar treatments to the spine have been described using electrons. The entire nueraxis irradiation technique is amenable to treatment planning with CT. This allows automated block cutting and spinal compensator production.

Special techniques

Conformal therapy implies shaping the radiation planning target volume to fit an irregularly shaped tumour. Modern imaging techniques produce better delineation of tumours in the brain, which can be turned into three-dimensional volumes in treatment planning systems. Technical advances in linear accelerator design allow the delivery of radiation to these volumes using either fixed cast blocks or a micro multileaf collimator, conformed to the tumour shape in 'beam's eye view'. In principle this should lead to a reduction in toxicity by reducing the volume of irradiated normal brain and offer the possibility of dose escalation. Clinical studies to confirm the value of this approach are awaited.

Stereotaxy simply relates to a method of localization in which the target is defined by an external coordinate system. This has the potential for great accuracy and implies the need for rigid fixation. This fixation may be 'one off' using pins screwed into the skull or may use a relocatable system based on a dental mouth bite or accurate BDS (Gill *et al.*, 1991). Accuracies of 1–2 mm are standard. Treatment is delivered using multiple sources, collimated to the same spherical volume (gamma knife) or using multiple coplanar arc therapy on a linac. Although the isodose volumes will be spherical in these cases, more complex shapes can be constructed from multiple, superimposed spheres. Multiple fixed conformed beams can also be delivered stereotactically.

Stereotactic radiosurgery delivers a single high (often necrotizing) dose treatment. It has an established role in the treatment of arteriovenous malformations (AVM) and small metastases. Fractionated stereotactic radiotherapy, using a relocatable frame, is being explored as a means of dose escalation in primary brain tumours. Its role has yet to be established. It is important to note that the radiobiology of radiosurgical treatments and those employing fractionated stereotactic radiotherapy are quite different.

Beam Intensity Modulated Radiotherapy (IMRT). This technique uses moving multi-leaf collimators to create complex dose distributions across multiple fields. In this way 3-D dose distributions are constructed to fit complex tumour shapes with the aim of complete tumour coverage but with improved sparing of normal tissues. This technique could prove extremely useful, particularly for tumours around the base of the skull.

Protons travelling in a medium deposit a large amount of energy into the final few millimetres of their path – the Bragg peak. This property can be used to deliver highly localized three-dimensional conformed dose distributions, even to volumes with concavities. This has led to the use of protons in the treatment of tumours requiring high doses but which lie immediately adjacent to vital structures. The most common application in the CNS has been to chordomas of the clivus, but other skull-base tumours would be appropriate targets. The production of high-energy proton beams is expensive and the technique is available in very few centres.

Brachytherapy, usually using temporary, high-energy ^{125}I seed implants, has been used to treat high-grade gliomas at relapse or as a boost at first presentation (Gutin *et al.*, 1991). The early results of randomized trials appeared encouraging, but mature results are still awaited. In Europe low-energy implants have been used to treat low-grade gliomas (Kreth *et al.*, 1995) and iridium wire afterloading has been used for palliation in glioblastoma.

Boron neutron capture therapy (BNCT) relies on the capture interaction of very low-energy (thermal) or low-energy (epithermal) neutrons with the stable isotope boron-10 ([10]B). Capture causes the [10]B to split, releasing an α and a lithium particle:

$$N + {}^{10}B \rightarrow {}^{4}He + {}^{7}Li$$

The requirement for successful BNCT is for selective accumulation of [10]B into brain tumours using boron-labelled compounds, such as [10]B-labelled bovine serum albumin (BSA). Irradiation with low-energy neutrons causes the release of short-range, high linear energy transfer (LET) particles in the vicinity of the tumour. The technique is under study in a few centres worldwide.

NORMAL TISSUE REACTIONS TO RADIOTHERAPY

As in other sites, radiation injury in the CNS depends on a number of factors which may be patient related (age, vasculopathy, infection) or treatment related (total dose, dose per fraction, volume irradiated). In general, the CNS is a late-responding tissue; however, both early and intermediate effects can also occur.

Acute effects

Acute effects of radiation begin within days or even hours and are probably an oedematous response, although this has never been clearly demonstrated. The acute tolerance of the brain is higher, both in terms of total dose (up to 80 Gy in 2-Gy fractions) and single doses (6–8 Gy), than is acceptable for late effects. Sheline *et al.* (1980) reported 4 acute deaths in 54 patients when using single doses of 10 Gy. The symptoms are generally those of acute raised intracranial pressure or a worsening of neurological symptoms caused by the lesion itself. Hence they are more commonly seen in patients who are symptomatic at the start of treatment. Using conventional dosing, acute effects are rarely troublesome if steroids are given appropriately.

Early delayed effects

An intermediate radiation reaction can begin within weeks of completing radiation therapy to the brain and may continue for 6–10 weeks thereafter. It comprises somnolence, lethargy and, frequently, recurrence of the original presenting symptoms and signs. It is usually self-limiting, but will respond to steroids. Recovery is the rule. The condition was originally described in children as 'somnolence syndrome' and later in adults treated to moderate brain doses (55 Gy in 27 fractions) (Rider, 1963). The pathogenesis is not known but is believed to correlate with interruption of myelin synthesis secondary to damage to the oligodendroglial cells. In the rare cases that fail to recover, autopsy has shown extensive demyelination, central necrosis, diminished numbers of oligodendroglial cells and gliosis, but without evidence of vascular, neuronal or axonal injury. A corresponding condition occurs after spinal irradiation and presents with Lhermitte's sign. This, too, is self-limiting.

DELAYED RADIATION DAMAGE

This is the most sinister form of radiation damage and is uniformly irreversible. The onset may be from around 3–4 months up to many years after the exposure. Injury is predominantly to the white matter and is dose and volume dependent. The clinical manifestations are diverse and may vary from subtle deterioration in higher cognitive function and behavioural changes, to gross neurological deficit associated with a space-occupying lesion. Pathologically the lesion may also vary in severity. Milder forms demonstrate gliosis, demyelination, vascular proliferation and thickening and neuron fallout.

Radiation necrosis is the most severe form of damage. It appears as an expansive lesion within the gyrus, which, on section, typically comprises haemorrhagic coagulation necrosis, restricted largely to the white matter. A fibrinous exudate typically accumulates in a lamina of hypocellularity along the grey–white junction. Fibrinoid necrosis is very common. Vascular proliferation can occur in the early phase of late damage and can resemble tumour. A further characteristic of irradiated brain is a large, bizarre, widely disseminated cell, the nature of which is not clear. In the more chronic phase some of the necrotic foci are resorbed and can evolve into multiple cysts. Calcification is characteristic of the later stages along with encephalomalacia, telangiectasia and vascular thickening. The underlying cause of radiation necrosis is not known, but there is accumulating evidence that fibrinolytic inhibitors are involved.

Late radiation damage can be difficult to differentiate clinically and radiologically from tumour recurrence. Furthermore, they can coexist. Functional rather than structural imaging has played an increasing role in differentiating the processes. Both FDG-PET and thallium SPECT can show good differentiation.

The rate of onset and the severity of the late radiation response in the brain depend strongly on the fraction size and total dose. However, the dependence on overall treatment time is weak for treatments more than 12 hours apart. Accepted levels of tolerance vary according to the situation. The dose commonly given to high-grade tumours – 60 Gy in 30 fractions – may cause around 5 per cent symptomatic late damage. In less demanding situations, 50–54 Gy in 2-Gy fractions is considered the upper limit. To minimize late damage, fraction sizes for radical brain treatments should not exceed 2 Gy.

Other late consequences of brain irradiation include hormone (pituitary) failure and second malignancy.

Late radiation damage in the cord may be sudden or insidious in onset, with sensory and motor abnormalities (paraplegia or quadriplegia), bowel and bladder sphincter disturbance and diaphragm dysfunction in high lesions. The most serious consequence is complete transection of the cord at the irradiated level. The pathology is similar to that in the brain. A combination of vascular lesions with demyelination and malacia is characteristic of radiation myelopathy. The pathogenesis remains obscure, with both the vasculature and oligodendrocytes identified as principle targets (Schultheiss et al., 1995).

Imaging may aid diagnosis. A myelogram should be negative but cord swelling can sometimes occur. MRI performed within 8 months of the onset of symptoms shows low signal intensity on the T_1-weighted image and high signal intensity on T_2-weighted images, often with cord swelling. Gadolinium enhancement is common. Late scans show an atrophic cord with normal signal intensity.

There is no evidence that either the volume irradiated or the anatomical level of irradiation materially affects the incidence of myelitis in patients receiving standard doses of radiotherapy. Accepted wisdom has been that spinal-cord tolerance at conventional fractionation was between 45 and 50 Gy, depending on the clinical situation. Others have argued that the spinal-cord tolerance should be revised upwards to 50 Gy or even higher (Marcus and Million, 1990; Rampling and Symonds, 1998) according to the clinical circumstance. A dose of 57–60 Gy carries a 5 per cent risk of myelitis (Schultheiss et al., 1995). Furthermore, there is evidence that re-irradiation of CNS tissue is possible. Some tolerance develops with increasing time from the initial radiation and is virtually complete (50–70 per cent) by 2 years. However, full tolerance is never regained.

Some chemotherapeutic drugs can enhance radiation damage. These include methotrexate, cytosine arabinoside and the nitrosoureas. These are all drugs that have good CNS penetration and can produce toxic damage in their own right. Others, such as Adriamycin®, become toxic when given following disruption of the BBB. The toxic pathological changes are similar to those produced by radiation, with both fibrinoid and coagulation necrosis, but with much greater involvement of the grey matter and much more generalized brain changes.

Chemotherapy

For a chemotherapeutic drug to be effective it must be active against the tumour and have access to it. In the brain the intact BBB generally inhibits the passage of molecules with molecular weights greater than 200 Da. Drugs with a high partition coefficient (e.g. nitrosoureas) or which are small (temozolomide) can circumvent this barrier. Although in the vicinity of tumour the barrier is partially defective, as is demonstrated by the penetration of contrast scanning agents, large hydrophilic molecules remain largely excluded from the brain/tumour structures and are not useful for therapy. However, some agents thought to be only modestly penetrating can be very effective, for example platinum compounds in germ-cell tumours and medulloblastoma.

THE ROLE OF CHEMOTHERAPY IN BRAIN TUMOURS

Chemotherapy can be given in a neo-adjuvant, adjuvant, consolidation or palliative setting. For astrocytoma of any grade the role is very limited, but another glial tumour, oligodendroglioma, has genetic subtypes which are much more sensitive. For the rare chemosensitive tumours (teratoma and lymphoma), neo-adjuvant treatment is well established, whereas in others, such as medulloblastoma, the role of adjuvant or neo-adjuvant remains unclear despite good response rates. This is discussed in more detail in the relevant sections.

ACTIVE AGENTS

Nitrosoureas

The chloroethyl nitrosoureas are held to be the most effective group of drugs for the treatment of brain tumours, although very few comparative studies against other agents have been reported. They are highly lipid soluble, non-ionized drugs which rapidly cross the BBB. They degrade rapidly into two reactive compounds, one with a carbamylation activity and the other an alkylating agent. Carmustine (BCNU), lomustine (CCNU), semustine (MeCCNU), tauromustine (TCNU), and streptozotocin have different pharmacokinetic properties while retaining

the same basic chemical activity and toxicity problems. None has proved more effective than any other, although BCNU is regarded as the benchmark drug. Given intravenously, the single-agent response rate for glioma is 20–40 per cent. CCNU is reported to have a similar response rate and is administered orally. Adverse effects include delayed myelosuppression and lung fibrosis (Rampling, 1997).

Procarbazine

Procarbazine is activated in the liver to an alkylating agent. The single-agent response rate for glioma is believed to be around 20 per cent. It causes nausea, vomiting and myelosuppression and it interacts adversely with alcohol and some smoked and preserved foods.

Temozolomide

Temozolomide is a small molecule which acts as an alkylating agent. It penetrates readily into brain tumours. It is active against glioblastoma and anaplastic astrocytoma and has a predictable and modest toxicity, principally myelosuppression.

Epidophyllotoxins and platinum compounds

Drugs such as VP-16, *cis*-platinum, and carboplatin, are valuable for treating non-glial brain tumours such as medulloblastoma and germ-cell tumours. They have only minor activity against gliomas.

COMBINATIONS

Few drugs are effective as single agents in glioma therapy and hence combinations have been little studied. PCV (*see* Table 15.7) is considered by many to be standard therapy as first-line treatment in relapsed glioma. However, the evidence that it is superior to single-agent nitrosourea is very sparse (Levin *et al.*, 1980) and it is equally acceptable to use single-agent nitrosourea in relapsed glioblastoma. Combinations may be more successful for some rarer tumours. Some relevant combinations are given in Table 15.7 and their use is discussed further in the relevant section.

NOVEL APPLICATIONS OF CHEMOTHERAPY

Because of the difficulty of access of many agents to the brain, alternative strategies have been considered to try to

Table 15.7 *Combination chemotherapy regimes used in CNS therapy*

Acronym	Regime	Reference
BEP	Bleo, etoposide, Cis plat (3-weekly)	Senan *et al.* (1991)
BEC	Bleo, etoposide, Carbo	Robertson *et al.* (1997)
CHOD-BVAM	Cyclo, DOX, VCR, Dex (one cycle) then BCNU 6-weekly and VCR, HDMTX and ARA-C 2-weekly	Bessell *et al.* (1996)
MACOP-B	HDMTX, DOX, Cyclo, VCR, Pred, Bleo	Brada *et al.* (1998)
PCV	Procarbazine, CCNU,VCR 6-weekly	Levin *et al.* (1980)
VCEP	VCR, Cyclo, alternating with etoposide, Carbo	Gaze *et al.* (1994)

ARA-C, cytosine arabinoside; Carbo, carboplatin; CCNU, lomustine; Cis plat, *cis*-platinum; Cyclo, cyclophosphamide; Bleo, bleomycin; Dex, dexamethasone; DOX, doxorubicin; HDMTX, high-dose methotrexate; MTX, methotrexate; VCR, vincristine; Pred, prednisolone.

increase the concentration of drug in the tumour. Arterial catheterization has been used to deliver agents, such as the nitrosoureas, to the tumour. Results have been disappointing and the complication rates high. This technique remains confined to a few centres. Global BBB disruption has been achieved with high-dose mannitol prior to infusion of hydrophilic drugs. Again this approach has proved unacceptably toxic since the BBB disruption is non-selective. Selective BBB breakdown can be achieved using the drug Ceroport® that affects blood vessels around the tumour. When agents such as carboplatin are given, higher tumour concentrations are achieved while the remainder of the brain is unaffected, increasing the therapeutic ratio. Perhaps the most successful innovation has been the biodegradable product Gliadel®. This polymer wafer is impregnated with BCNU and inserted into the cavity of a brain tumour immediately following its resection. The cytotoxic drug is released slowly into the neighbouring brain and residual tumour. This has been shown to produce a modest extension of remission in patients undergoing resection of glioma at first relapse (Brem *et al.*, 1995). Results in newly diagnosed patients are awaited.

New modalities

GENE THERAPY

As in other sites, there are two distinct aspects to this treatment approach. First, there must be a killing, or growth limiting, strategy. There are many possibilities, such as genes that sensitize the transfected cells to drugs that would otherwise be harmless, so-called suicide gene therapy (e.g. *HSV-tk* gene sensitizes to ganciclovir); or genes whose products can switch off activated oncogenes (e.g. antisense compounds). Such strategies often work well *in vitro*. However, a more formidable problem is delivery of the gene therapy. Vehicles that have been proposed include naked DNA and liposomes, but most work has looked at the potential role of viruses. Retroviruses, adenoviruses and Herpes virus have all been proposed and a randomized trial using retroviral producer cells and an *HSV-tk*/ganciclovir strategy has been performed. As yet there is no proven role for gene therapy in the treatment of brain tumours.

TARGETING ANGIOGENESIS

Abnormal angiogenesis is fundamental to the growth of most brain tumours. It is controlled by a variety of growth factors, particularly vascular endothelial growth factor (VEGF) and platelet-derived growth factor (PDGF). VEGF has been shown to be significantly upregulated in glioblastoma. Angiogenesis would seem to be a logical target in these tumours.

Thalidomide has been shown to block VEGF-induced angiogenesis in laboratory studies and to produce responses in a small proportion of tumours in the clinic. This and other approaches, e.g. with suramin, protamine and antisense strategies, are being examined.

IMMUNOTHERAPY

The immunobiology of brain tumours is still poorly understood. In spite of this, some clinical attempts at immunotherapy have been made. In an example of adoptive immunotherapy, lymphokine-activated killer (LAK) cells were injected concomitantly with IL-2 in patients with recurrent glioma. This met with little success and proved quite toxic. Other strategies have included radiolabelled antibodies directed, for example, at the EGFR but few results are yet available.

Adjunctive treatments

It has long been recognized that corticosteroids produce symptomatic benefit in patients with brain tumours. The physiological basis for this is not clear. The explanation that the steroid effect is by reversing cerebral oedema is not borne out fully by imaging studies and is almost certainly not wholly correct (Chumas *et al.*, 1997). Dexamethasone is most frequently used, in doses up to 64 mg daily. It is unusual for patients to be maintained on doses greater than 16 mg for more than a few days and any dose should be titrated down to the minimum needed to control symptoms. This will minimize the impact of severe side-effects, which in the elderly are particularly proximal myopathy, diabetes and osteoporosis, and in the young, acne and appetite stimulation. All patients may suffer weight gain, sleep disturbance and disorders of mood and perception.

Epilepsy is common in patients with brain tumours. Anticonvulsants should be given in doses determined by the efficacy and toxicity of a drug in a particular patient and not by the measured plasma level. The established agents, carbamazepine, phenytoin and sodium valproate, are still the drugs of first choice, with the newer agents lamotrigene, gabapentin, vigabatrin and topiramate giving greater scope for those not fully controlled. Probably half of all patients with tumour-associated epilepsy will not have their fits completely controlled, even with 'optimal' doses of anticonvulsants.

Although headache is a common presenting symptom, severe pain is fortunately unusual in patients with treated brain tumours, even following recurrence. When pain is a problem, the same analgesic ladder should be used as for other malignant conditions. The liberal use of morphine in the later stages of the disease is entirely justified.

Nausea can be a particularly troublesome symptom and may have a variety of causes. It may arise in posterior fossa syndrome and secondary to raised intracranial pressure, but it is also associated with seizure, drug toxicity (particularly anticonvulsants) and peptic pathology. Limited-field brain irradiation uncommonly causes nausea and this should be a diagnosis of exclusion. Clearly the cause of the toxicity should be sought and, where possible, treated. Where the usual anti-emetics fail to control nausea of intracranial origin, it may be useful to try continuous subcutaneous delivery of agents, such as the major tranquillizers or antihistamines.

Additional support

Brain tumours are rare but their effects are devastating. Cognitive decline and major physical disability often accompany the late stages. Because of their rarity, family doctors will have managed very few cases. Patients may require input from physiotherapists, speech therapists, social workers, palliative care workers, the GP and the district nurse. The specialist 'brain tumour clinical nurse specialist' who has knowledge of the patient's current condition, needs and likely prognosis, as well the facilities available in a particular area, can provide invaluable support to all workers involved in care, particularly the GP. Even if a brain tumour is incurable, the quality of the patient's life can be greatly enhanced by efforts to minimize the impact of his or her deficit. It is not sufficient to prolong the life of patients without maximizing its quality.

INDIVIDUAL TUMOURS

Astrocytomas

Diffuse astrocytomas are a group of tumours, more common in adults, which can arise anywhere in the CNS but are most frequent in the cerebral hemispheres. Irrespective of their histological grade, they infiltrate diffusely into adjacent and distant brain. Tumour grade is based on cell density, cytological features (nuclear atypia, nucleus: cytoplasmic ratio), mitotic activity and features of the microenvironment (vascular proliferation and necrosis). The grade allocated to the tumour is the highest grade seen in any part of the specimen. The prognosis is strongly dependent on the grade. Other important prognostic factors are the patient's age, performance status and presentation with seizure. These can be combined into a highly predictive prognostic index (MRC Brain Tumour Working Party, 1990) (*see* Fig. 15.10), which can be extended by including treatment variables (Scott *et al.*, 1998).

Lower grades of astrocytoma (except pilocytic) progress to a more malignant phenotype. The rate of progression is very variable. Transformation (to glioblastoma) may be complete within a year or may not begin for 10 or even 20 years. When transformation occurs, it is accompanied by a cumulative acquisition of genetic alterations.

The aetiology of the majority of astrocytomas is obscure. The only known associations are with some inherited conditions (Table 15.2) and exposure to ionizing radiation.

GRADE I: PILOCYTIC ASTROCYTOMA

Pilocytic astrocytoma is a tumour of children and young adults. It most commonly arises in the posterior fossa but is also found in the cerebral hemispheres, the optic nerve and chiasm, the thalamus and basal ganglia, the brainstem and the spinal cord. On imaging pilocytic astrocytomas appear as hyperdense, well-delineated, solid or solid/cystic tumours. They break the rule for low-grade tumours in that they frequently enhance with contrast. They are characterized by slow growth and may, without intervention, stop growing or even regress. Rarely, they may seed in the CNS. Unlike other low-grade astrocytomas they very rarely progress to a more malignant phenotype. However, a rare, intrinsically aggressive form exists (possibly more common in adults), which progresses relentlessly without change in the low-grade histology.

The histology is characterized by the presence of bipolar, GFAP-positive 'pilocytes' and eosinophilic

Definition of prognostic index

Prognostic factor	Category	Score
Age (years)	≤44	0
	45–59	6
	≥60	12
WHO performance status	0–1	0
	2	4
	3–4	8
Extent of neurosurgery	Complete resection	0
	Partial resection	4
	Biopsy	8
History of fits (months)	≥3	0
	<3	5
	None	10

Prognostic index = sum of scores for each factor, a low score indicating a better prognosis.

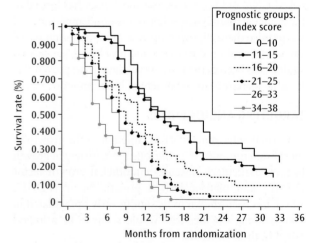

Figure 15.10 *Survival according to a prognostic index following treatment with radiotherapy in patients with glioblastoma. (Reprinted from* British Journal of Cancer, **64**, *Bleehan, N.M., Stenning, S.P. and Party, M.R.C.B.T.W, A Medical Research Council trial of two radiotherapy doses in the treatment of grades 3 and 4 astrocytoma, pp. 769–74, 1991, by permission of Churchill Livingstone.)*

hyaline masses, known as Rosenthal fibres. They are often highly vascularized and, in contrast to other low-grade astrocytomas, may show endothelial hyperplasia identical to glioblastoma. They do not demonstrate inactivation of *p53*.

The treatment of pilocytic astrocytoma is surgical. Maximal safe resection should be performed. Even if this is incomplete, further tumour progression may not occur. There is no evidence that postoperative radiation improves on surgery alone. If re-growth occurs, the treatment is again surgical. Should the second resection be incomplete, then adjuvant radiotherapy can be tried (45–50 Gy), but there is no clear documentation that this is beneficial.

Overall the prognosis for pilocytic astrocytoma is very good, with long-term control or cure rates of 80–90 per cent. The achievement of a complete resection is an important prognostic factor (Dirven *et al.*, 1997).

GRADE II: (DIFFUSE) ASTROCYTOMA

Low-grade diffuse astrocytomas (LGA) are well-differentiated, slow growing, diffuse tumours, more commonly seen in young adults but which can occur at any age. They usually arise in the cerebral hemispheres, but also occur in the brainstem and spinal cord. They are uncommon in the cerebellum. On imaging they typically appear as ill-defined, hypodense infiltrative lesions which may or may not displace other structures (Fig. 15.3). They are usually not contrast enhancing. They most commonly present with seizure.

Histologically they are recognized to contain abnormal numbers of astrocytes that show monotonous, minor degrees of anaplasia (nuclear pleomorphism and cytoplasmic changes). Mitoses are uncommon. The background may contain increased numbers of cellular processes and microcysts, which aid diagnosis. GFAP positivity is common. These tumours are sometimes subgrouped into fibrillary, protoplasmic and gemistocytic forms. This has prognostic significance only for the gemistocytic variant, which is generally regarded as more aggressive in nature and is treated in many departments as an anaplastic astrocytoma.

The management of low-grade astrocytoma is one of the most controversial areas in neuro-oncology. We know that these tumours will progress and that the majority will transform to higher-grade malignancy. However, patients presenting with controllable seizures as their only symptom and who have non-distorting, low-density lesions on scan may remain well for many years. There is no evidence that early treatment intervention improves the survival (Karim *et al.*, 2002). It is perfectly acceptable to observe these patients in the first instance until there is evidence of progression, sparing them the morbidity of treatment. This policy may, however, disadvantage a minority of patients whose tumours are misdiagnosed on scan (e.g. those having a more malignant lesion) and who may benefit from early intervention. Patients who find a policy of observation unacceptable after full consultation can be treated as outlined below.

Patients whose tumours are clearly progressing, as witnessed by demonstrable growth on scan or who develop neurological deficit or possibly loss of seizure control, require treatment. Maximal safe resection is usually recommended, although the data to support this concept are sparse. Likewise the role of radiotherapy is controversial, with neither the timing nor the intensity being clearly established. The balance of the retrospective literature appears to support early intervention at least to moderate dose (50 Gy) (Morantz, 1995). Two EORTC (European Organization for the Research and Treatment of Cancer) studies appear to show that neither the timing nor the dose of radiation is critical in improving overall survival, although the progression-free survival appears to be improved with early radiotherapy (Karim *et al.*, 2002).

Our recommendation is to offer radiotherapy within 4–8 weeks of surgery. The gross tumour volume (GTV) chosen is defined by the tumour margin identified on the CT/MRI scan and this is expanded by 1–2 cm to create the clinical target volume (CTV). In the absence of adequate postoperative imaging, the preoperative scans can be used. The additional margin required to create the planning target volume (PTV) is determined by local facilities and techniques. Two to four fields may be required to produce an adequate plan. These should be conformed to minimize the volume of non-tumour-bearing brain irradiated to high dose. Forty-five to 50 Gy are delivered in 1.8-Gy fractions, depending on the size of the irradiated volume.

The outcome after this form of management is variable. The majority of patients will relapse with ultimate tumour progression and death. Overall the median survival is about 5–8 years. However, some patients will continue well for many years showing no sign of progression even 20 years after treatment.

The role of chemotherapy is even less clear than that of surgery and radiotherapy. There is no good evidence that early intervention is of value. On relapse it is probably worth trying the same agents as used for high-grade tumours.

GRADE III: ANAPLASTIC ASTROCYTOMA

Anaplastic astrocytoma (AA) is also a diffusely infiltrating, astrocytic tumour but is typified by increasing cellularity, increasing nuclear size and variation, and the presence of mitoses (growth fraction around 5–10 per cent). In the WHO classification, tumour necrosis must not be present. (It is allowed in some other classifications, e.g. Mayo/St. Anne, and this can lead to confusion.) It is a tumour of middle age. It usually appears as a low-density lesion on CT/MRI and enhances with contrast, though not in the classical ring-enhanced way of glioblastoma. Unlike LGA, rapid growth is the rule in AA. It is treated as glioblastoma but the prognosis is considerably better, with a median survival of 2–4 years. There is also evidence of increased chemosensitivity as compared to glioblastoma and the two groups of patients should be distinguished in clinical trial work. The disease is almost uniformly fatal and transformation to glioblastoma usually occurs in the later stages.

GRADE IV: GLIOBLASTOMA

Glioblastoma is a poorly differentiated, extensively invasive, highly mitotic, astrocytic tumour. It is characterized by areas of necrosis and the presence of microvascular proliferation (previously known as capillary endothelial hyperplasia). It can arise at any age but is most common in the sixth and seventh decades. It occurs preferentially in the cerebral hemispheres, from where it extends into adjacent structures such as basal ganglia and across the corpus callosum to form the classical 'butterfly tumour'. It can arise rarely in the cerebellum, brainstem and spinal cord. It is universally fatal.

The tumour was previously called glioblastoma 'multi-forme' because of the marked intra- and inter-tumoral pathological heterogeneity. Macroscopically these tumours appear as grey masses with areas of haemorrhage, yellow necrosis and sometimes cysts. They may appear to have a capsule, but this is always an artefact of rapidly growing tumour and compressed brain. Adjacent brain is commonly swollen with peritumoral oedema. This tends to spread along the white matter tracts and can form a conduit for the migratory tumour cells, which can be found many centimetres from the main tumour mass. These migratory cells may form secondary masses. Hence, although glioblastomas may appear to be multifocal, this usually represents spread from a single tumour. The tumours are also highly heterogeneous at a cellular level, with almost any size and shape of cell being seen, including multinucleated giant cells, which are a hallmark of glioblastoma. Secondary glioblastoma is more likely to have areas comprising lower-grade astrocytoma. Heterogeneity also applies to immunohistochemical staining, with GFAP, S-100 and vimentin positivity variably present. An inflammatory infiltrate is usually seen. This comprises predominantly CD8+ T lymphocytes. CD4+ and B lymphocytes are much less frequent. Recognized glioblastoma variants are giant cell glioblastoma and gliosarcoma.

Microvascular proliferation and tumour necrosis are the histological hallmarks of glioblastoma. Angiogenic tyrosine receptors (e.g. VEGFR-1 and -2) are upregulated in proliferating tumour vessels and the ligands (e.g. VEGF) are found in the glioblastoma cells themselves, leading to paracrine stimulation of angiogenesis. There are two types of tumour necrosis: large-scale coagulation necrosis, which is usually visible on imaging studies, and microscopic serpiginous foci of necrosis, which form the pseudo-pallisading pattern typical of glioblastoma. The molecular biological changes have been discussed earlier in the chapter.

The typical imaging appearance of glioblastoma is a rim-enhancing, irregular tumour with a low-density (necrotic/cystic) centre and surrounding low-density oedematous brain. They tend to centre in the deep white matter. The brain is frequently distorted with evidence of raised intracranial pressure (Fig. 15.2). Metastases may produce a similar appearance but tend to lie preferentially at the grey/white junction, are often smaller, less heterogeneous and are commonly multiple. In the 1980s the Mayo Clinic group performed important studies. By taking serial stereotactic biopsies through glioblastomas and peritumoral brain they were able to correlate the pathology with the imaging appearances (Kelly et al., 1987). They showed that while the main growing tumour mass corresponded to the enhancing rim of tumour, isolated tumour cells could be found throughout the peritumoral oedema.

The overall strategy of management will depend on the likely prognosis. A diagnosis of glioblastoma will be suspected from the imaging in the majority of cases. The very elderly, or patients with severe, steroid-resistant symptoms may need only symptomatic care, since their outlook will be little changed by provision of the precise diagnosis and treatment. All other patients need a minimum of biopsy proof of diagnosis. It would appear to be good practice to resect as much of the tumour as is safely possible. The clinical ambitions are to relieve symptoms and to delay re-growth of tumour. However, no randomized study has ever shown that maximal resection improves quality of life or longevity when compared to lesser forms of surgery. While the surgical debate continues it is, nevertheless, a matter of common clinical experience that patients tolerate subsequent forms of treatment, particularly radiotherapy, much better when their tumours have been adequately decompressed. Surgery to provide adequate symptomatic relief is to be encouraged.

Between 1978 and 1981 four seminal studies showed beyond any doubt that treatment with radiation improves survival in patients with malignant glioma when compared to best supportive care alone (e.g. Walker et al., 1978). Surgery followed by limited-volume radiation therapy is now the standard treatment in this disease. Whole-brain radiotherapy has been abandoned. There are two approaches to choosing the radiotherapy target volume. In the first, we rely on the Mayo studies (Kelly et al., 1987), which show that tumour cells extend at least to the low-density oedema seen on CT (or the region of abnormality seen on T_2-weighted MRI). This region then defines the phase 1 volume to be irradiated (usually to two-thirds the dose). A second phase, to the full radical dose, is then applied to the region of the enhancing tumour (GTV) plus a modest margin of 1–2 cm.

The second approach is more pragmatic. It recognizes that when glioblastomas relapse they do so within 2 cm of the original enhancing rim in 85 per cent of cases (Wallner et al., 1989). If this problem is not solved, then what happens outside this region of relapse is of little consequence. In this one phase approach, the CTV is therefore defined throughout as the enhancing tumour rim (GTV) plus 2 cm.

Radiotherapy is usually delivered using a 4–6 MeV linear accelerator. The standard dose is 60 Gy in 30 fractions over 6 weeks to the enhancing tumour plus 1–2 cm. If an initial phase is used, this is usually restricted to 40 Gy. Alternative regimens are 45 Gy in 20 treatments (which can be delivered on a twice-daily basis) for patients in whom the more protracted regimen cannot be justified and 30 Gy in six fractions on alternate days as a very palliative approach (Thomas *et al.*, 1994).

The outcome following this approach remains poor. Figure 15.10 shows the survival in patients treated with radical radiotherapy according to the known prognostic factors (MRC Brain Tumour Working Party, 1990). Overall median survival is around 1 year, with less than 10 per cent surviving 2 years and almost no one alive at 5 years. Good prognostic indicators are youth and good performance status, with presentation with seizure and completeness of resection having a lesser impact.

Chemotherapy has a minor role in the management of glioblastoma. Although recent overviews have claimed a small statistical benefit to adjuvant treatment immediately after surgery (Fine *et al.*, 1993) this was not confirmed in the largest prospective randomized study ever performed (Thomas *et al.*, 2001). However the most recent overview (GMT group, 2002), which includes the Thomas study, shows a significant prolongation of survival associated with adjuvant chemotherapy, amounting to an absolute increase in 1-year survival of 6 per cent and a 2 month increase in median survival time. Whether this modest benefit is sufficient to justify routine treatment with adjuvant chemotherapy with its associated toxicity and morbidity is still a matter of contention. However, given the apparent benefit, it is now reasonable to offer the patient the choice. The most commonly used regimes contain a nitrosourea, classical PCV being the most common.

When patients relapse, around 30 per cent of those with good prognostic factors may enjoy a further brief improvement with chemotherapy. Single-agent CCNU (or other nitrosourea), PCV and temozolomide can all be given as outpatient treatment and produce about the same level of response with only modest acute toxicity. Temozolomide is probably better tolerated in the longer term for the few who respond well.

Oligodendrogliomas

Oligodendrogliomas are diffusely infiltrating glial tumours which are believed to arise from oligodendrocytes or their progenitor cells. They account for around 5–10 per cent of gliomas and have a peak age incidence between 30 and 50 years. They arise in white matter, with a predilection for the frontal and parietal lobes. They are

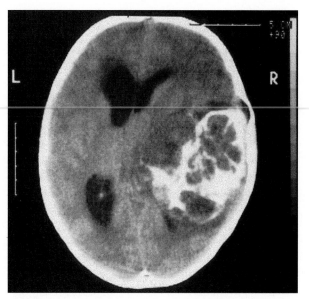

Figure 15.11 *A CT scan without contrast, showing a large, heavily calcified oligodendroglioma in a 24-year-old male whose only symptom was seizure.*

slow-growing tumours and the most common presentation is with seizure. The imaging characteristics are similar to those of low-grade astrocytoma, but calcification is very common ($\approx$50 per cent) (Fig. 15.11). Long-standing tumours in the frontal brain may extend across the corpus callosum to affect the contralateral lobe, even when the tumour is low grade.

Macroscopically the tumours usually appear as grey/pink masses, often well demarcated and with calcium frequently evident to the naked eye. Microscopically, the tumour comprises abundant uniform, small cells with round nuclei and a fine chromatin pattern. Although the majority of oligodendrogliomas are low grade, a substantial minority are more aggressive. Although the usual features of increased cellularity, mitotic activity, pleomorphism, vascular proliferation and necrosis are identified, it remains unclear just which features determine prognosis. Unlike glioblastomas, some patients with aggressive-appearing oligodendrogliomas can fare unaccountably well after treatment.

Grade for grade, the conventional management of these tumours is much as for astrocytomas. However, it has recently been shown that oligodendrogliomas have a better response to chemotherapy (Van den Bent *et al.*, 1998) and that LOH 1p acts as a marker for chemoresponsiveness in the great majority of cases (Cairncross *et al.*, 1998). PVC is currently the regime of choice, although few studies compare this with other regimens. A study is currently evaluating the role of chemotherapy along with surgery and radiotherapy in the initial management of these tumours. Overall the outcome for oligodendroglioma is better than for the equivalent grade of astrocytoma (Celli *et al.*, 1994; Olson *et al.*, 2000).

Ependymoma

Ependymoma is a glioma arising from the ependymal cells that normally line the cerebral ventricles and the central canal of the spinal cord. The incidence of intracranial tumours is greatest in young children and decreases steadily thereafter. They can arise at any site, usually in association with the ventricular system. They are most common in the posterior fossa, where they present with obstruction or with posterior fossa syndrome. Imaging usually shows a well-circumscribed tumour with variable contrast enhancement in the characteristic location. Differentiation from medulloblastoma may be difficult.

Ependymomas are soft, grey/pink tumours which often show their ependymal origin. Histologically, the monotonous cellular background is interrupted by perivascular pseudorosettes and ependymal rosettes. Anaplastic tumours may, in addition, show pleomorphism, disorganized cyto-architecture, increased mitosis and necrosis. Although ependymomas do spread via the CSF, the influence of spinal seeding on outcome has probably been overestimated. Whereas post-mortem series have shown up to 30 per cent spinal seeding, in life it is detected in around 10 per cent and is symptomatic in less than 5 per cent (Nazar *et al.*, 1990). Spread is more likely with infratentorial high-grade tumours.

All patients should be staged with neuraxis imaging as for medulloblastoma. Maximal tumour resection should be attempted regardless of site. The role of radiotherapy is more controversial and cannot be determined clearly from published studies. A reasonable policy is to deliver postoperative irradiation (50 Gy in 1.8-Gy fractions) to the tumour site for all low-grade tumours and to supratentorial high-grade tumours (54–60 Gy). Whole-neuraxis radiotherapy is then reserved for high-grade infratentorial tumours and those where seeding is already apparent. Adjuvant chemotherapy is of no proven value, although many clinicians add it to their treatment regimes for poorly differentiated tumours.

The 5-year survival for patients with low-grade tumours is between 30 and 50 per cent. It is worse for younger children. The 5-year survival for high-grade tumours is almost zero. Treatment failure is most commonly due to local recurrence.

The rare subependymoma is a very low-grade lesion which should be treated with surgery alone.

Rare neuroepithelial tumours

ASTROBLASTOMA

This unusual (probably astrocytic) tumour is regarded by some as a growth pattern rather than a separate pathological entity. The lesion comprises prominent elongated tumour cells which form pseudorosettes around the blood vessels. Tumours are often superficial, well circumscribed and amenable to surgical resection. The use of radiation and chemotherapy should follow the guidelines for astrocytomas.

PLEOMORPHIC XANTHOASTROCYTOMA

This is usually a cystic and peripherally located tumour of children and young adults. Histologically it is characterized by a mixture of spindle-like cells and mono- or multinucleated giant cells. There is often intracellular lipid accumulation and the marked presence of reticulin fibres. Although normally a low- to very low-grade tumour best treated with complete excision alone, radiation may be of value for the treatment of more aggressive tumours or those that recur after surgery.

SUBEPENDYMAL GIANT CELL ASTROCYTOMA

This very slow-growing tumour is (almost) always associated with tuberous sclerosis. Treatment is with surgery or observation only. There is no role for either radiotherapy or chemotherapy in this condition.

BRAINSTEM GLIOMA

Gliomas of all types may arise in the brainstem, most frequently in the pons. Biopsy can be very dangerous and it is acceptable in these cases to treat on the basis of the imaging appearances and clinical features alone. Treatment is usually with radiotherapy (54 Gy for high-grade and 45–50 Gy for low-grade tumours). Studies of hyperfractionation and adjuvant chemotherapy have not improved outcome. The majority of patients have high-grade tumours and their outlook is very poor. Patients with lower-grade gliomas may survive for years after treatment. As well as the familiar prognostic factors, patients with exophytic tumours appear to do better.

OPTIC NERVE GLIOMA

This tumour, which is most common in children and young adults, is usually low grade and very slow growing. Because of its position, it causes devastating symptoms of visual and hormonal disturbance. Management is controversial. Surgery (for unilateral disease), radiotherapy and sometimes chemotherapy have been advocated, but the timing is crucial and some tumours will spontaneously cease to progress and even sometimes regress. Simple guidelines to management cannot be offered and the reader is referred to more detailed text (Jenkin *et al.*, 1993).

GLIOMATOSIS CEREBRI

This is a diffuse glial tumour with varied histological appearances. It diffusely affects the brain, involving multiple lobes and sometimes extending infratentorially, even into the spine. It may affect any age. Imaging appearances, although abnormal, are frequently non-specific. Biopsy may often be non-diagnostic and the diagnosis is often only made at post-mortem. Surgery has almost no therapeutic role in this condition. Whole-brain radiotherapy may delay the disease process and is the treatment of choice. However, the outlook is dismal; most patients die within months of presentation.

DYSEMBRYOPLASTIC NEUROEPITHELIAL TUMOUR

This is a benign tumour which arises predominantly in the temporal lobes of children and young adults where typically it presents with seizure, often longstanding. Histopathologically this is characterized by a specific glioneuronal element, often with a nodular component and associated cortical dysplasia. Treatment is by surgical excision, there is no evidence for the value of either radiotherapy or chemotherapy.

GANGLIOCYTOMA AND GANGLIOGLIOMA

These tumours comprise neoplastic ganglion cells alone (gangliocytoma) or in association with neoplastic glial cells (ganglioglioma). Most patients are under 30 years of age and the great majority present with seizure. The primary treatment of both tumours is with surgery. In the event of incomplete resection postoperative radiotherapy (≈ 50 Gy) is often given to gangliogliomas (which are regarded as WHO grade II lesions). An anaplastic ganglioglioma may arise usually due to anaplastic change in the glial component.

CENTRAL NEUROCYTOMA

This is a rare tumour which arises within the ventricles of young adults. Histological features are of small, round cells with neuronal differentiation. Treatment is mainly surgical and the outcome, even after incomplete resection, can be good. However, troublesome recurrence can occur, at which time radiotherapy and even chemotherapy may be of value.

CHOROID PLEXUS TUMOURS

Choroid plexus papillomas are rare intraventricular tumours derived from the choroid plexus epithelium. They are found predominantly in children. The malignant choroid plexus carcinoma is even less common. Treatment is surgical and the outcome is highly dependent on the completeness of resection. Radiotherapy is reserved for incompletely removed tumours and malignant lesions. CSF spread can occur even in low-grade lesions.

Medulloblastoma and other primitive neuroectodermal tumours

Primitive neuroectodermal tumours (PNETs) are a group of highly malignant embryonal tumours that can differentiate along neuronal, astrocytic and ependymal (muscular and melanotic) pathways. PNETs, although arising at different sites in the CNS, have often been assumed to derive from a common progenitor cell in the subependymal matrix layer. This assumption is not proven and has recently been questioned (Pomeroy et al., 2002). They are undifferentiated, round-cell tumours, which include medulloblastoma, pineoblastoma and supratentorial PNET. They occur predominantly in children and young adults and have similar morphological and behavioural characteristics.

It has recently been shown that medulloblastomas are molecularly distinct from other brain tumours including primitive neuroectodermal tumours and atypical rhabdoid tumours (Pomeroy et al., 2002). Particularly, they show changes in genes that encode for transcription factors that are specific for cerebellar granule cells providing increasing molecular evidence that this is the cell of origin. Furthermore among the molecular changes in medulloblastomas, certain patterns are strongly predictive of outcomes.

Medulloblastoma has an annual incidence of 0.5 per 100 000. Seventy per cent of medulloblastomas occur in children under 16 (peak 7 years) and are rare after 40. The male preponderance is slightly less than 2 : 1. By definition, medulloblastomas arise in the posterior fossa, usually in the midline (vermis). They spread by local invasion into the cerebellar hemispheres and rostrally into the fourth ventricle and project into the brainstem. They readily spread via CSF to produce metastases on the leptomeninges of the brain and cord and to involve the ventricular surfaces.

Clinically they present with a cerebellar syndrome (Bannister, 1992) or with raised intracranial pressure due to CSF outflow obstruction. The characteristic imaging appearance is of a solid, often uniformly enhancing mass with a discrete edge (Fig. 15.12). Sometimes the tumour is more irregular, inhomogeneous and occasionally cystic.

The tumours may be soft or firm and are frequently haemorrhagic. The typical histological appearance comprises densely packed, small, hyperchromatic cells which have a high nuclear : cytoplasmic ratio and a high mitotic rate. Rosettes are seen in <50 per cent of cases. Apoptosis is more frequently seen than necrosis. Cellular differentiation, usually glial or neuronal, is often a feature. The prognostic significance of this is not established. Immunostaining with synaptophysin and vimentin is typical in medulloblastoma, and staining with GFAP and rhodopsin is also common. The desmoplastic variant is more common in older patients and is generally regarded as carrying a better prognosis.

The diagnosis will usually be suspected from the clinical presentation and the imaging appearances. If hydrocephalus is present, this may constitute an emergency and require prompt ventricular drainage and steroids prior to a definitive operative procedure, although some surgeons will undertake both the drainage and the tumour decompression simultaneously. Full neuraxis imaging (Gd-MRI) should be done preoperatively to look for metastatic spread before blood is introduced into the CSF at operation.

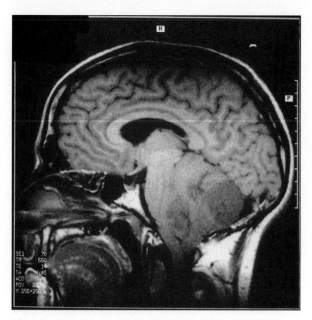

Figure 15.12 *A sagittal MRI of a medulloblastoma. The lesion appears as two masses with discrete edges, one encroaches the fourth ventricle, distorting the brainstem and causing obstruction.*

If this is not possible, then the investigation should be done within 48 hours of surgery. The tumour is removed through a posterior fossa craniectomy, using either suction or the ultrasound aspirator. Complete tumour removal is associated with a better prognosis. Whether this is due to the resection or to the property of resectability is not clear but, wherever possible, a complete removal should be attempted. In some situations the tumour involves the brainstem and total excision is not possible. A postoperative CT (or MRI) should be done within 48 hours of surgery to assess the amount of residual disease.

The prognosis for this disease improved dramatically in the late 1960s with the introduction of whole-neuraxis radiotherapy (Bloom *et al.*, 1969). Current practice involves the irradiation of the entire brain and spinal cord with the meningeal coverings to a dose of 35 Gy (in 20 fractions) with a boost of 19.8 Gy (in 11 fractions) being delivered to the posterior fossa. The technique is given on pp. 268–70. Attempts to reduce the dose, and hence toxicity, have led to lower rates of control.

Patients are treated daily. Adequacy of shielding should be checked with portal imaging and *in vivo* dose measurements to the eyes. Acute toxicity includes complete alopecia, and frequently nausea (and vomiting) which requires an anti-emetic. The exit dose from the spinal field may produce a radiation oesophagitis. Leucopenia and thrombocytopenia may occur, but rarely require support or interruption of treatment (even if prior chemotherapy has been used). Later consequences are ongoing nausea (especially in teenagers), loss of IQ, hormonal deficits, loss of height due to direct and indirect (growth hormone) effects on bone, and cataracts from scattered radiation dose.

There is no doubt that medulloblastoma is a chemosensitive tumour. However, in spite of large randomized controlled trials (Bailey *et al.*, 1995) the role of adjuvant chemotherapy has not been established for the totality of patients, although a subset with adverse prognostic factors at presentation appear to benefit and should be treated. However, despite the lack of evidence from randomized studies that adjuvant chemotherapy confers a survival benefit in non-high-risk patients there is widespread European and North American acceptance from non-randomized studies to justify its use (Kortmann *et al.*, 2000). In this difficult situation the entry of such patients into clinical trials to attempt to clarify the issue would seem sensible.

Overall 5-year survival is around 50–70 per cent, depending on the prognostic mix, although patients may still relapse many years after primary treatment. Good prognostic factors are age (infants fare worse), completeness of resection, lack of metastatic disease and desmoplastic histology.

Patients who relapse should be treated aggressively with a mixture of chemotherapy, further surgery, focal radiotherapy and high-dose therapy. Durable remissions can be induced using a variety of chemotherapy regimes, including VAC (vincristine, adriamycin/doxorubicin and cyclophosphamide) and platinum-based combinations e.g. VCEP (*see* Table 15.7) (Gaze *et al.*, 1994).

Meningiomas

A variety of tumours develop in the meninges but the most common by far are meningiomas, which arise from the meningothelial cells themselves. They are usually benign. They occur most commonly on the convexity or falcine brain regions but may arise anywhere that meninges are present, and cause particular difficulties in sites around the base of the skull. Spinal meningiomas are most common in the thoracic region.

Meningiomas arise most commonly in middle age and are more common in women (F : M = 3 : 2). They occur rarely in children, when they tend to be more aggressive. They can be induced by radiation in high or low doses when, again, they are aggressive in character. Some genetic syndromes, particularly neurofibromatosis type 2 (NF2), are associated with the development of meningiomas. A majority of tumours show the presence of the progesterone receptor and a minority are oestrogen-receptor positive. Whether this is important in the aetiology is not established. Loss of chromosome 22 is a consistent finding in meningioma and is particularly prominent in the atypical form.

Most meningiomas are round or lobulated, smooth, firm, well-delineated tumours, often indenting and compressing brain but rarely attached to, or invading it. More commonly they invade into or through the dura and induce hyperostosis in the overlying skull. In the

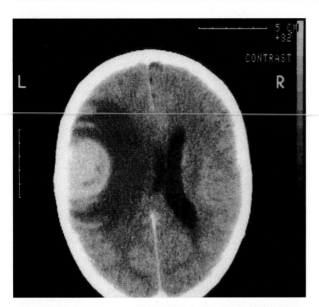

Figure 15.13 *Convexity meningioma arising in the left parietal region. Note the position adjacent to the dura, the strong, uniform enhancement and the sharp, marginal demarcation.*

base of skull they may grow as plaque-like tumours. Meningiomas derive their blood supply from the adjacent meningeal artery and are highly vascular. Identification and embolization of this artery can be therapeutic in its own right and can aid surgical removal.

A variety of histological variants is identified. These include the commonly recognized meningothelial, fibrous and transitional subtypes, as well as the rarer psammomatous, angiomatous, microcystic and choroid tumours. In spite of this variety, their clinical behaviour is similar. The great majority of these lesions are benign. However, aggressive behaviour may present in any of them. The WHO identifies an atypical meningioma, when areas are present that show increased cellularity with 'sheet-like' growth (loss of growth pattern), increasing numbers of mitoses, high nucleus : cytoplasm ratio and geographic necrosis. Malignant meningioma is said to be present when these features become increasingly prominent, and particularly if invasion of the brain or metastasis is identified. It is clear that these definitions are not precise and are subject to variation from pathologist to pathologist. The rare papillary variant is associated with a high rate of invasion and recurrence.

Presentation in patients with meningioma is diverse. Although headache is most common, seizure and functional deficit are also frequent. CT imaging usually reveals an iso- to hyperdense lesion, with a meningeal base, which enhances strongly with contrast (Fig. 15.13), although 15 per cent or more may have atypical appearances. Gd-MRI is the most sensitive detection method for meningioma. Angiography may add further diagnostic information and also provides the basis for embolization.

Surgery dominates the treatment of meningioma (DeMonte and Ossama, 1995). The aim is to remove the

entire tumour and any involved adjacent structure (dura, soft tissue and bone) to maximize the prospect for enduring local control. Preoperative embolization of the main feeder vessel is often performed as an aid to surgical removal. The site of the tumour determines the surgical procedure. Convexity meningiomas have the best chance of total removal. Removal of parasagittal tumours risks damage to the sagittal sinus and its draining veins. Tumours of the base of skull are particularly problematic because of the difficult access and the proximity of sensitive structures. A newly diagnosed meningioma is often separated from the brain by an intact layer of arachnoid, which can define a 'plane of safety' during the removal procedure.

The outcome following surgery depends largely on the extent of resection. Re-growth varies from less than 10 per cent for patients with a 'complete' excision to over 40 per cent for patients undergoing partial resection. It follows that patients with tumours in the most accessible regions (convexity) have better prospects than patients with tumours in difficult areas, such as the sphenoid ridge. Second operation for recurrence is possible in the majority of patients.

Radiotherapy is increasingly used in the management of meningioma, usually in the adjuvant setting following incomplete resection, or when the histology is unfavourable (Glaholm *et al.*, 1990). The GTV will include any imageable residual or recurrent tumour. The CTV will include a margin for spread into adjacent structures, particularly the dura. For malignant tumours, the brain and overlying bone must also be considered at risk. The dose for benign lesions is usually restricted to 50 Gy though up to 60 Gy should be used for atypical or frankly malignant lesions. Fractionation is 1.8–2.0 Gy per fraction. In base of skull tumours, proximity to sensitive structures may limit the dose. However, sophisticated immobilization, localization and blocking techniques can minimize the amount of irradiated normal tissue and improve the chance of delivering the desired high dose. Treated in this way, recurrence rates can be reduced (McCarthy *et al.*, 1998). Stereotactic radiosurgery has also been used to treat meningiomas but the tendency to dural spread and the damaging effect of large single doses may limit the success of this approach.

Chemotherapy is of no proven value in benign meningioma, although sarcoma regimes may be tried for palliation in the malignant form. The identification of hormone receptors in the majority of meningiomas has led to the use of anti-androgen hormone therapy, but with little success. The use of interferon has been advocated by some, but any benefit is minor and short lived. Meningiomas frequently show an excess of somatostatin receptors which can be imaged either with PET or SPECT. In principle these could form a therapeutic target (Cavalla and Schiffer, 2001) and studies on this are proposed.

Not all patients with meningioma require immediate surgery. Small lesions may be found serendipitously. Particularly in the elderly, these tumours may be so slow growing as to pose no threat during the patient's lifetime. They can be managed with follow-up and observation, intervening only if the clinical or imaging situation deteriorates.

Haemangiopericytoma

Previously thought of as a variant of meningioma, this tumour is now believed to be indistinguishable from haemangiopericytoma in other sites. It is probably derived from the meningeal capillary pericyte. In comparison to meningiomas, the tumours tend to arise in a younger age group and more frequently in men. They arise in the dura as highly vascular lobulated masses. They are densely cellular and often highly mitotic. Their behaviour is sarcomatous with a marked tendency to recur after surgery alone and to metastasize within and outside the CNS, particularly to bone. Surgery alone is rarely curative and they are best treated with radical excision followed by high-dose radiotherapy (55–60 Gy). Median survival is around 5 years.

Chordoma

Chordomas are malignant, embryonal tumours that arise from the notochordal remnant. They arise predominantly in the region of the clivus and at the sacrococcygeous. Rarely, other sites are affected. They normally arise in the extradural space but grow slowly and may invade the dura as they do. Histologically the identifying features are 'physaliferous' cells, which contain large mucus-filled vacuoles. They are arranged in lobules and are usually surrounded by extracellular mucus.

The management of these tumours is complex. The best possibility for cure probably results from aggressive surgical resection. However, even after apparent complete resection, local recurrence can be a problem. Conventional high-dose radiotherapy is often given in the postoperative setting, but the value of this is not proven. Dose escalation using highly conformed target volumes using proton-beam facilities appears to produce better results and, where possible, referral of these rare cases to these specialist centres is appropriate. The prospect of stereotactically localized, intensity-modulated radiotherapy offers the prospect of similar, linac-based dose escalation.

Primary CNS lymphoma

Primary CNS lymphoma (PCNSL) is defined as lymphoma arising in the CNS in the absence of obvious lymphoma elsewhere at the time of diagnosis. Previous names have included microglioma and reticulum cell sarcoma of the CNS. Its development is strongly related to immunosuppression due either to disease or therapy. Hence there is a high incidence in patients with AIDS, following organ transplantation and possibly in rheumatoid disease.

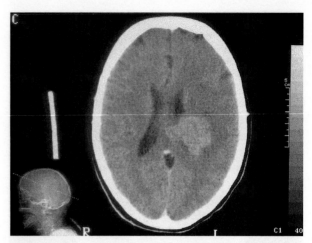

Figure 15.14 *A contrast-enhanced CT scan showing a primary CNS lymphoma. Note the periventricular location and the uniform enhancement. Although not shown here, these tumours are often multifocal.*

The incidence in both immune-competent and compromised patients appears to be rising. PCNSL may occur at any age but, in immune-competent patients, is most common in middle age. It is slightly more common in men.

Why PCNSL occurs at all is not clear, since the brain lacks a lymphatic system. It has been suggested that malignant lymphoma cells, which develop outside the brain, are imported and develop in this relatively immune-protected site. An alternative idea is that a polyclonal inflammatory lesion in the brain may expand clonally to a neoplastic state.

PCNSL arises preferentially in periventricular regions of the brain. On imaging it usually appears as iso- or hyperdense lesions which enhance uniformly (Fig. 15.14). They are frequently multiple at presentation (20–60 per cent). Characteristically they respond rapidly to treatment with steroids and may 'disappear' within 48 hours of starting treatment (the ghost tumour). Ocular disease is present in 15–20 per cent of cases. Clinically they usually present as mass lesions, much as high-grade gliomas. CSF cytology is positive in about 10 per cent. Primary spinal lymphoma is extremely rare.

The pathology is much as for systemic extranodal lymphomas. They can be firm or friable, well delineated or diffuse. They may be necrotic or haemorrhagic, yellow, grey or indistinguishable from adjacent brain. The great majority of PCNSLs are B-cell and express the usual pan B markers (e.g. CD20). Only 2 per cent are T-cell. The literature is confused over the incidences of the various subtypes, and the systemic classification schemes do not apply well. Large cell types (diffuse and immunoblastic) are more common than small cell (cleaved and non-cleaved) tumours. High-grade tumours are more common than low-grade. In most series a percentage of tumours cannot be classified. When primary Hodgkin's disease and plasmacytoma occur in the CNS, they are usually dural based. Both are extremely rare.

Although imaging may suggest PCNSL, histological proof is essential for adequate management. Response to non-surgical therapy, including steroids, is usually rapid and a (stereotactic) biopsy alone is needed. Once the diagnosis is established, the patient should be fully staged (*see* Chapter 45). This should also include ophthalmological examination, a lumbar puncture (where possible) and an immunological screen, including an human immunodeficiency virus (HIV) test.

In the past, patients with confirmed PCNSL were treated with radiotherapy alone. Survivals were dismal (median 18 months, 5 year disease-free survival 10–20 per cent) (Hayabuchi *et al.*, 1999). Modern management includes primary chemotherapy followed by radiotherapy for most patients, although no randomized trial has shown the supremacy of this approach and many questions concerning management remain unanswered (Maher and Fine, 1999).

Chemotherapy regimes that have been shown to be effective include CHOD-BVAM and MACOP-B (*see* Table 15.7). They have in common a reliance on agents, particularly high-dose methotrexate, which penetrate the BBB and deliver adequate drug concentrations to the brain. Response to these agents is high (complete response (CR) ≈ 60 per cent). Most regimes follow chemotherapy with radiation treatment. A typical regimen for single lesions delivers 40 Gy to the whole brain with a boost of 10–14 Gy to the primary site. For multiple lesions, where boost is not possible, 40–50 Gy of whole-brain radiotherapy is given. Where CSF cytology is positive, whole CNS treatment has been advocated, although the value has not been proven and it is not possible in older individuals. If the patient is not fit for chemotherapy, the radiotherapy regimes are used alone.

The outcome from this approach as yet is unclear. Median survival from methotrexate-containing regimens is claimed to be around 3 years (Maher and Fine, 1999). About 10 per cent relapse outside the CNS. Prognosis is related to age at presentation and performance status. The toxicity of this combined approach is high, with early onset dementia (in up to 30 per cent) a particular problem. There are important questions that remain unanswered. Does a combined approach truly increase survival and quality of survival? Is radiotherapy necessary after chemotherapy? Should it be high dose? Why does radiotherapy, at doses that control lymphoma in other sites, fail to do so in the brain?

The treatment of HIV-positive patients is even less well defined. If their condition allows it, an aggressive approach, as for the immune-competent patient, can be followed. For less well patients, radiotherapy alone can often be given. It is important to continue antiviral therapy.

Tumours of the pineal region

While pineal-cell and germ-cell tumours are particularly associated with this region of the brain, other tumour types, including gliomas, meningiomas, benign (cystic) tumours and metastases, also occur. Presentation is most commonly with hydrocephalus and is often accompanied by complete or partial Parinaud's syndrome.

TUMOURS OF THE PINEAL PARENCHYMA

These are uncommon tumours of the pineocytes. They always arise in the pineal gland but may disseminate in the CSF. They occur in childhood or, more commonly, in mid adult life and show no gender preference. On imaging they most frequently show as uniform iso- or hypodense lesions that enhance uniformly and often appear to have a well-defined margin. Cysts or calcifications may be present, but are not so prominent as in germ-cell tumours (GCTs).

Two types of pineal tumours are recognized; the well-differentiated pinealoma and the highly malignant pineoblastoma. Pinealomas comprise cells identical to normal pineocytes and contain few mitotic figures. Pineoblastomas contain undifferentiated cells with high mitotic activity and are often indistinguishable from other PNETs. These represent two ends of a continuum and, not infrequently, tumours may have features intermediate between these. Precise classification, then, is difficult.

The management of pineal tumours includes imaging of the entire neuraxis, immediate decompression of hydrocephalus and establishing a tissue diagnosis. Pineocytoma is a surgical disease and may be cured by total resection. Pineoblastoma is unlikely to be cured by surgery. It requires whole-neuraxis radiotherapy as for medulloblastoma but with the boost directed at the tumour (plus ventricular system if appropriate). The difficulty lies with 'intermediate' tumours. Our general attitude has been to treat these aggressively on the assumption of pineoblastoma.

The outcome in these rare tumours is difficult to estimate. Pineocytoma is likely to be cured by surgery. Pineoblastoma has a sinister reputation, although failure to recognize it and treat adequately has probably contributed to this. The outcome, if treated aggressively, is likely to be similar to that of medulloblastoma.

GERM-CELL TUMOURS

This comprises a group of tumours that present a spectrum of pathology indistinguishable histologically from their gonadal counterparts. It includes pure germinoma (seminoma), teratoma, choriocarcinoma, embryonal and yolk-sac tumours. They are tumours of the young, approximately 90 per cent occur before the age of 20. The male : female ratio is >2 : 1. They are predominantly midline tumours, most common around the pineal and third ventricle (80 per cent), though suprasellar presentation is not uncommon. Tumours arising elsewhere tend to be non-germinomatous. There is a marked geographical variation, with a higher incidence in the Far East, particularly Japan.

Typically, pure germinomas comprise sheets or lobules of large cells with abundant, glycogen-rich cytoplasm with round, centrally placed nuclei. They immunostain with placental alkaline phosphatase (PLAP), usually on the surface membrane. Human chorionic gonadotrophin (hCG)-positive syncytiotrophoblastic giant cells may be present and do not represent a major adverse prognostic factor. The presence of α-fetoprotein (AFP) staining in a specimen indicates the presence of non-germinomatous tumour and implies treatment as for immature teratoma.

Teratomas may be mature or immature. Mature teratomas contain only fully differentiated elements from any or all of the three germinal layers. The presence of incompletely differentiated elements automatically classifies the tumour as immature teratoma. Production of AFP is common. Teratoma with malignant transformation indicates a teratoma in which a malignancy of conventional somatic type (e.g. sarcoma, carcinoma) has arisen.

Yolk-sac tumours are characterized by primitive, AFP-positive, epithelial cells in a loose myxoid matrix. Embryonal carcinomas may appear similar to germinomas but are distinguished by staining for cytokeratin. Choriocarcinomas are characterized by the presence of cytotrophoblastic elements and syncytiotrophoblastic giant cells. Staining for hCG is a regular feature, PLAP is more variable.

Germ-cell tumours may grow locally, producing potentially reversible effects of pressure and obstruction. Local infiltration of adjacent brain with irreversible destruction may also occur. They tend to spread along the ventricular linings and have a marked tendency to disseminate via the CSF to affect other areas of the brain and spinal cord. The incidence of this is variably reported but is probably around 15 per cent. Systemic spread, either blood-borne or via ventriculo-peritoneal (V-P) shunts, can also occur. Presentation is as for other mass lesions in the pineal region (or other site).

The testicular tumour markers, hCG and AFP, can frequently be detected in the serum and CSF of these patients, and can be a useful guide to response to treatment. Decay of the marker may be delayed by the presence of cysts which act as reservoirs. The CSF to serum marker ratio is normally >1. If the ratio is reversed, systemic disease is likely. The detection of serum AFP is diagnostic of teratoma and may obviate the need for biopsy.

Gd-enhanced MRI is the imaging modality of choice and is essential for planning surgery. Germinomas tend to be homogeneous and enhance uniformly with contrast. Calcification is common and cystic areas may be present. Teratomas, benign and malignant, are notably heterogeneous, with variable signal characteristics and irregular contrast enhancement. The whole neuraxis should be imaged.

All patients presenting with a suspicion of a GCT require serum estimation for AFP and hCG. CSF levels should also be evaluated. This may be done following the placement of a shunt which is commonly required for the relief of hydrocephalus.

The management of GCT is complex and highly dependent on the precise histology of the lesion. Tissue (or marker) diagnosis is essential. However, the extent of surgery required is a matter of debate. The previous practice of 'test dose of radiation' as a surrogate for biopsy is now difficult to justify.

Biopsy of this region using stereotaxy may be possible but is frequently considered hazardous because of the localization of the tumour and the risk of bleeding. An open procedure may be considered safer, providing also the opportunity for therapeutic resection. The recently introduced technique of ventriculoscopy and biopsy can be valuable in otherwise difficult cases. Surgical excision is usually curative for differentiated teratoma but offers no advantage over biopsy alone in germinoma (Sawamura et al., 1997). Surgical resection of non-germinomatous GCT may be valuable (Bruce et al., 1995) but, because of the increasing success of non-surgical treatment, the risk of complications should be considered in each case.

The standard treatment for localized germinoma is whole-neuraxis radiotherapy with a tumour boost. The technique is as for medulloblastoma, but the doses required are lower: 30 Gy is delivered to the whole neuraxis. The primary lesion (including the adjacent ventricular system) is boosted to a total of 45–50 Gy (Dearnley et al., 1990). The toxicity from this treatment is similar to that for medulloblastoma. The use of chemotherapy with radiation confined to the tumour has only recently been explored. Early results suggest that comparable control can be obtained, possibly with less toxicity (Baranzelli et al., 1997). For patients with metastatic disease at the outset, a combined approach with chemotherapy and radiotherapy is required.

Patients with malignant non-germinomatous GCT require treatment with initial chemotherapy (2–4 cycles). Various platinum-based regimes have been used, e.g. BEP, BEC (see Table 15.7) (Senan et al., 1991; Robertson et al., 1997). This should be followed by radiotherapy as for germinoma but with doses of 35 Gy to the neuraxis and 50–54 Gy to the primary site. It is argued by some that following adequate chemotherapy the irradiated volume may be reduced or radiation omitted altogether. This proposal has not been adequately tested.

The outcome following these approaches is good. Five-year, disease-free survivals of 85–100 per cent can be expected in pure germinoma (Huh et al., 1996). Radiotherapy alone for non-germinomatous GCT produces only around 20 per cent long-term survivors, but the introduction of platinum-based chemotherapy has improved this to around 70 per cent or better (Senan et al., 1991; Robertson et al., 1997). As in gonadal GCT, it is not uncommon to image residual abnormality in the tumour site following treatment. In the absence of evidence of progression this needs observation only. However, if there is doubt concerning the completeness of treatment, surgery may be indicated.

The functional outcome following treatment is often good, although the same complications of treatment experienced by medulloblastoma survivors occur. Patients presenting with severe Parinaud's syndrome often suffer persistence of deficit and require the input of a neuro-ophthalmologist. Patients with suprasellar tumours may suffer long-term endocrine problems.

Craniopharyngioma

Craniopharyngioma is a benign epithelial tumour of the sellar region, thought to arise from a remnant of Rathke's pouch. It is most common in children and young adults. It grows slowly and presents with pressure symptoms, endocrine and visual disturbance. Hydrocephalus may be present. The typical imaging properties of an enhancing solid and cystic lesion, often with calcification in a sellar site, strongly suggest the diagnosis.

Two forms are recognized histologically: papillary and adamantinomatous. Both are slow growing, and excite intense gliosis in neighbouring brain tissue. Tongues of tumour also extend into adjacent brain tissue and may be very difficult to remove surgically. Single or multiple cysts are very common and contain a thick, cholesterol-rich fluid. The fluid in the adamantinomatous tumour is often oilier than the papillary type and calcification is much more common.

Optimal management of these tumours is controversial. A common approach in the UK is to attempt maximal surgical removal. If this is shown to be complete, then routine follow-up with interval imaging is sufficient. Because of the growth pattern, however, total excision is often not possible and the recurrence rate then is higher (Fahlbusch *et al.*, 1999). In these cases radiotherapy can be given. The volume should be minimized using accurate CT localization and conforming techniques as a dose of at least 50 Gy in 1.8-Gy fractions is needed. This treatment restores the level of tumour control to that of complete excision (Habrand *et al.*, 1999). In very young children, where radiotherapy might produce high levels of morbidity, observation may be appropriate, even after partial resection. Follow-up in all cases includes endocrine assessment, neuro-ophthalmology and neuropsychology as well as tumour surveillance.

Treatment of recurrence is difficult, as re-operation is hazardous. Radiotherapy naïve patients can be irradiated and cystic tumours may be treated with radioactive intracavitary yttrium-90, even after prior external-beam treatment.

Although the 10-year survival is around 90 per cent, fewer are free of disease. There is no clear difference in outcome between the histological subtypes.

Spinal tumours

A similar spectrum of tumours arises in the spine as in the brain, although the frequency of occurrence is different and some types are absent. Tumours may be grouped according to their site of occurrence into extradural (metastasis, chordoma, sarcoma), intradural–extramedullary (meningioma, neurofibroma) and intramedullary (astrocytomas, ependymomas, benign tumours).

For all sites the most common presentation is with pain and/or loss of function at and below the level of the lesion. The pain may be exacerbated by straining or coughing and may be felt in the spine itself or in the appropriate root distribution. Tumours cause functional loss by direct pressure, generation of spinal oedema, spinal infarction, invasion into spinal tissue and growth along nerve roots. Almost any pattern of motor deficit may occur. Combinations of complete and partial, upper and lower motor neuron lesions arise at and below the level of the lesion as the tumour develops. Likewise, sensory deficits may be complex. However, localization of the upper vertebral limit of the symptoms and signs can be a useful guide to identifying the position of the tumour within the spine. It is worth remembering that, in the adult, the spinal cord segmental level is approximately two above the bony vertebral level and that the cord ends in the conus at the level of L1–2. Lesions below this level can only produce lower motor neuron lesions.

Plain spinal X-rays still have an important role in the early evaluation of the patient suspected of having metastatic disease, but the widespread availability of MRI scanning has revolutionized the investigation of spinal tumours (Fig. 15.15). The clear identification of the tumour and its boundaries allows the surgeon to plan his operation accurately and the radiotherapist to make rational judgements on field size and placement.

Surgery is the mainstay of treatment for many low-grade spinal tumours. Good results can be expected from the complete excision of meningiomas, neurofibromas,

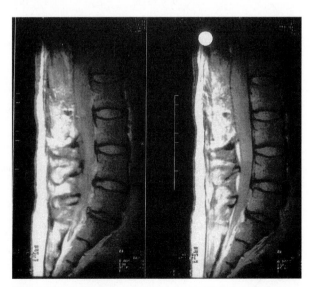

Figure 15.15 *A sagittal MRI of an ependymoma of the filum. Note the well-delineated lesion lying between lumbar vertebrae 3 and 4.*

pilocytic astrocytomas and ependymomas. However, surgical decompression of spinal metastases, fibrillary and anaplastic astrocytomas and high-grade ependymomas should usually be followed by treatment with postoperative radiotherapy. Spinal cord compression due to an intramedullary tumour nearly always requires urgent decompression. When loss of function develops rapidly (hours to days) the prospects for recovery of neurological function is likely to be worse than when cord compression develops slowly (weeks to months).

Radiotherapy may be given with palliative or radical intent. For palliation either direct posterior or opposed fields are used to deliver short courses of treatment. Doses of 30 Gy in 10 fractions or 20 Gy in 5 fractions are common in metastatic disease. Higher doses for radical treatments are often delivered using a technique based on a wedged pair of fields (Fig. 15.16). Optimal planning may involve the use of CT. For treatments to low-grade tumours doses of 45–50 Gy in 1.8-Gy fractions are usual, but for highly malignant tumours, doses up to 60 Gy may be appropriate. While the risk to the spinal cord from the radiation is increased at these doses, it may not be as high as previously thought, provided megavoltage X-rays are used and the dose per fraction is kept below 2 Gy (Rampling and Symonds, 1998). This risk must be balanced against the risk of undertreating the tumour and the consequences of early re-growth.

ASTROCYTOMAS

The majority of spinal astrocytomas are low grade but an important distinction exists here based on the precise histology. If the tumour is a pilocytic astrocytoma, the outcome following surgery is usually good. The value of adjuvant radiotherapy is not clear, though it is usually given. Diffuse astrocytoma, usually fibrillary, has a less good prospect. It is difficult for the surgeon to find any plane between tumour and normal tissue and there is less argument about the need for additional radiotherapy. Most patients are dead within 5 years (Minehan *et al.*, 1995). Anaplastic astrocytomas and glioblastomas rarely occur in the spine but, when they do, should be treated as their cerebral counterparts, with surgery and radiotherapy. The prognosis is very poor.

EPENDYMOMAS

Ependymomas may arise anywhere in the spine but have a predilection for the lower end, around the conus. Ectopic extraspinal tumours may develop in the pre-sacral region. Most are low grade. A clear operative plane is often found and it may be possible for the surgeon to excise the tumours completely. In this situation follow-up only is required. If complete excision is not obtained, then adjuvant-dose radiotherapy is often given, but clear evidence of its value is lacking. High-grade tumours can rarely be excised completely and postoperative whole-spine radiotherapy with a local tumour boost should be considered.

The variant myxopapillary ependymoma is found almost exclusively in the conus/cauda equina region. It is treated surgically and has a particularly favourable prognosis.

Metastases

The brain is a common site of metastasis for systemic malignancy, which may be found in up to 25 per cent of

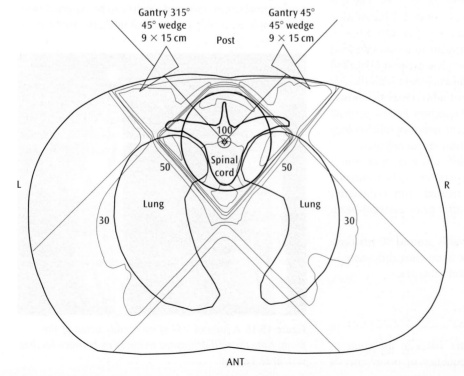

Figure 15.16 *A stylized diagram of a wedged pair treatment planned on CT for a spinal tumour. Treatments to intramedullary tumours would use smaller field widths (≈4 cm). If doses to vital structures (here lungs) are excessive, then the plan can be modified by using a posterior field together with the wedged pair.*

patients at autopsy (Posner and Chernick, 1978). However, the incidence varies with tumour type. Metastases from carcinomas of the bronchus, breast, bowel and from melanoma are very common, while spread from prostate cancer is almost never seen. They arise most commonly at the junction of cortex and white matter (Fig. 15.17) but cerebellar, dural and leptomeningeal metastases are also common. Less commonly metastases are found in sites such as the pituitary and choroid plexus. Patients with suspected intracranial metastases should undergo a minimum of a CT scan, with and without intravenous contrast. However, MRI will show additional metastases in around 15 per cent of cases and, where available, is the imaging modality of choice. Prognosis in this condition is very variable and depends on a number of factors (Priestman *et al.*, 1996) (Table 15.8), which in turn determine the management approach.

SOLITARY METASTASIS

Patients with one potentially resectable metastatic lesion diagnosed after adequate imaging (including MRI), and who have additional good prognostic factors, particularly controlled systemic disease, require an aggressive approach. Where possible, the lesion should be excised

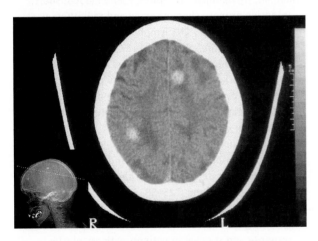

Figure 15.17 *A contrast-enhanced CT scan showing three metastases. Note their spherical shape, their position at the junction of grey and white matter and the uniform enhancement.*

completely. This goal is more easily achieved than for many intrinsic tumours as tumour growth is often less diffuse. The position of postoperative radiotherapy is not clear, although the limited randomized data available suggest that it is advantageous (Patchell *et al.*, 1998). Furthermore, the optimum volume, dose and fractionation are not known. Fractionated radiotherapy to the whole brain to at least 30 Gy in 10 fractions is advisable if longer survival is expected in the patient with good prognostic factors. It may also be appropriate, especially in older patients, to restrict the radiotherapy to the boost site only.

An alternative approach to the solitary metastasis is to treat the identified lesion with radiosurgery using either a modified linac or gamma knife. Again, the need for whole-brain treatment in addition is not known, although most clinicians will apply it. Tumour control rates appear to be as good as for surgery, although control of symptoms may be delayed and a good quality of life comparison of the techniques is not available.

MULTIPLE METASTASES

Patients with multiple metastases should be assessed carefully after treatment of their symptoms with steroids. Patients then who have better prognostic features should be offered radiotherapy. For these patients whole-brain radiotherapy is appropriate. Radiation Therapy Oncology Group (RTOG) studies have shown that the regimes 40 Gy in 20 fractions, 30 Gy in 10 fractions and 20 Gy in 5 fractions are equivalent in both efficacy and morbidity (Borgelt *et al.*, 1980). A Royal College of Radiologists (RCR) study has shown that 16 Gy in 2 fractions on consecutive days has much the same outcome as 30 Gy in 10 fractions, but may be associated with more side-effects (Priestman *et al.*, 1996). For patients who fall into the poor prognostic categories, the survival is brief irrespective of therapy (median 6–10 weeks) and it is doubtful that any radiotherapy is justified.

Chemotherapy may be used to treat cerebral metastases in those tumours known to be chemoresponsive. Hence this may be first-line treatment in patients with germ-cell tumours, small cell carcinoma and lymphoma. It can also be considered, usually second-line treatment, in less sensitive conditions such as breast cancer.

Table 15.8 *Factors affecting outcome in patients with brain metastases*

Factor	Good prognosis	Poor prognosis
Histology	Adenocarcinoma (especially slow-growing, breast, bowel, kidney)	Squamous carcinoma, poorly differentiated tumours
Age	Younger	Older
Performance status	Good	Poor
Disease-free interval	Long (or initial presentation)	Short
Number of metastases	Solitary	Multiple
Systemic disease	Controlled	Uncontrolled

The regimes used are those appropriate to the tumour concerned but, where a choice is possible, BBB-penetrating agents are selected.

SIGNIFICANT POINTS

- Tumours of the brain are characterized by their histological variety.
- Optimal structural and functional imaging can give good insight into the nature of the tumour and is essential for adequate management planning.
- Accurate histological diagnosis is essential for appropriate management.
- Modern histological classification schemes, particularly WHO (Kleihues and Cavenee, 2000), should be used exclusively to determine management.
- Molecular biology is defining further categories of tumour which correlate with variations in biological behaviour and response to treatment.
- Surgery and radiotherapy remain the mainstays of treatment for the majority of tumour types.
- Surgical and radiotherapeutic techniques should be tailored to the specific tumour.
- Chemotherapy can contribute both to tumour cure and palliation.
- Cure can be obtained for some patients with brain tumours (particularly children) and useful extension of life offered in many.

KEY REFERENCES

Davies, E.H. and Hopkins, A. (eds) (1997) *Improving care for patients with malignant glioma*. London: Royal College of Physicians.

Kay, A.H. and Laws, E.R. (eds) (1995) *Brain tumours: an encyclopedic approach*. Edinburgh: Churchill Livingstone.

Kleihues, P. and Cavenee, W.K. (eds) (2000) *Pathology and genetics of tumours of the nervous system*. Lyon: International Agency for Research on Cancer.

REFERENCES

Bailey, C., Gnekow, A., Wellek, S. *et al.* (1995) Prospective randomised trial of chemotherapy given before radiotherapy in childhood medulloblastoma. International Society of Paediatric Oncology (SIOP) and the German Society of Paediatric Oncology (GPO): SIOP II. *Med. Pediatr. Oncol.* **25**(3), 166–78.

Bannister, R. (1992) *Brain and Bannister's clinical neurology*. Oxford: Oxford University Press.

Baranzelli, M.C., Patte, C., Bouffet, E. *et al.* (1997) Nonmetastatic intracranial germinoma: the experience of the French Society of Pediatric Oncology. *Cancer* **80**(9), 1792–7.

Bessell, E., Graus, F., Punt, J. *et al.* (1996) Primary non Hodgkins lymphoma of the CNS treated with BVAM or CHOD/BVAM chemotherapy prior to radiotherapy. *J. Clin. Oncol.* **14**, 945–54.

Bloom, H.J., Wallace, E.N., Henk, J.M. *et al.* (1969) The treatment and prognosis of medulloblastoma in children. *AJR* **105**, 43–62.

Borgelt, B., Gelber, G., Kramer, S. *et al.* (1980) The palliation of brain metastases: final results of the first two studies by the Radiation Therapy Oncology Group. *Int. J. Radiat. Oncol. Biol. Phys.* **6**, 1–9.

Brada, M., Hjiyiannakis, D., Hines, F. *et al.* (1998) Short intensive primary chemotherapy and radiotherapy in sporadic primary CNS lymphoma (PCL). *Int. J. Radiat. Oncol. Biol. Phys.* **40**, 1157–62.

Brem, H., Piantadosi, S., Burger, P.C. *et al.* (1995) Placebo controlled trial of safety and efficacy of intraoperative controlled delivery by biodegradable polymers of chemotherapy for recurrent gliomas. *Lancet* **345**, 1008–12.

Bruce, J.N., Connolly, S. and Stein, B. (1995) Pineal and germ cell tumours. In Kaye, A.H. and Laws, E.R. (eds), *Brain tumours: an encyclopedic approach*. Edinburgh: Churchill Livingstone, 725–58.

Cairncross, J.G., Ueki, K., Zlatescu, M. *et al.* (1998) Specific genetic predictors of chemotherapeutic response and survival in patients with anaplastic oligodendrogliomas. *J. Natl Cancer Inst.* **90**(19), 1473–9.

Cavalla, P. and Schiffer, D. (2001). Neuroendocrine tumours of the brain. *Ann. Oncol.* **12**(2), 131–4.

Celli, P., Cervoni, L., Cantore, G. *et al.* (1994) Cerebral oligodendroglioma: prognostic factors and life history. *Neurosurgery* **35**, 1018–34.

Chumas, P., Condon, B., Olouch-Olunya, D. *et al.* (1997) Early changes in peritumorous oedema and contralateral white matter after dexamethasone: a study using proton magnetic resonance spectroscopy. *J. Neurol. Neurosurg. Psychiatry* **62**(6), 590–5.

Daumas Duport, C., Scheithauer, B., O'Fallon, J. *et al.* (1988) Grading of astrocytomas. A simple and reproducible method. *Cancer* **62**, 2152–65.

Dearnaley, D.P., A'Hearn, R.P., Whittaker, S. and Bloom, H.C.G. (1990) Pineal and CNS germ cell tumours: Royal Marsden Hospital experience 1962–87. *Int. J. Radiat. Oncol. Biol. Phys.* **18**, 773–81.

DeMonte, F. and Ossama A. (1995) Meningiomas. In Kay, A.H. and Laws, E.R. (eds), *Brain tumours: an encyclopedic approach.* Edinburgh: Churchill Livingstone, 675–704.

Dirven, C., Mooij, J. and Molenaar, W. (1997) Cerebellar pilocytic astrocytoma: a treatment protocol based on the analysis of 73 cases and a review of the literature. *Childs Nerv. Syst.* **13**(1), 17–23.

Fahlbusch, R., Honegger, J., Paulus, W. *et al.* (1999) Surgical treatment of craniopharyngioma: experience with 168 patients. *J. Neurosurg.* **90**(2), 237–50.

Fine, H.A., Dear, K.B., Loeffler, J.S. *et al.* (1993) Meta-analysis of radiation therapy with or without adjuvant chemotherapy for malignant gliomas in adults. *Cancer* **71**, 2585–97.

Fleury, A., Menegoz, F., Groscalaude, P. *et al.* (1997) Descriptive epidemiology of cerebral gliomas in France. *Cancer* **79**(6), 1195–202.

Gaze, M.N., Smith, D.B., Rampling, R.P. *et al.* (1994) Combination chemotherapy for primitive neuroectodermal and other malignant brain tumours. *Clin. Oncol.* **6**(2), 110–15.

Giles, G.G. and Gonzales, M.F. (1995) Epidemiology of brain tumours and factors in prognosis. In Kay, A.H. and Laws, E.R. (eds), *Brain tumours: an encyclopedic approach.* Edinburgh: Churchill Livingstone, 349–60.

Gill, S., Thomas, D.G., Warrington, A.P. *et al.* (1991) Relocatable frame for stereotactic external beam radiotherapy. *Int. J. Radiat. Oncol. Biol. Phys.* **20**, 599–603.

Glaholm, J., Bloom, H. and Crow, J. (1990) The role of radiotherapy in the management of intracranial meningiomas: the Royal Marsden Experience with 186 patients. *Int. J. Radiat. Oncol. Biol. Phys.* **18**, 755–61.

Glioma Meta-analysis Trialists (GMT) Group (2002) Chemotherapy in adult high grade glioma: a systematic review and meta-analysis of individual patient data from 12 randomised trials. *Lancet* **359**, 1011–18.

Gutin, P.H., Prados, M.D., Phillips, T.L. *et al.* (1991) External irradiation followed by an interstitial high activity iodine-125 implant 'boost' in the initial treatment of malignant gliomas: NCOG study 6G-82-2. *Int. J. Radiat. Oncol. Biol. Phys.* **21**, 601–6.

Habrand, J.-L., Ganry, O., Couanet, D. *et al.* (1999) The role of radiation therapy in the management of craniopharyngioma: a 25 year experience and review of the literature. *Int. J. Radiat. Oncol. Biol. Phys.* **44**(2), 255–63.

Harris, V., Sandridge, A., Black, R. *et al.* (1998) *Cancer registration statistics Scotland 1986–1995.* Edinburgh: ISD Scotland Publications.

Hayabuchi, N., Shibamoto, Y., Onizuka, Y. *et al.* (1999) Primary central nervous system lymphomas in Japan: a nationwide survey. *Int. J. Radiat. Oncol. Biol. Phys.* **44**(2), 265–72.

Huh, S.J., Shin, K.H., Kim, I.L. *et al.* (1996) Radiotherapy for intracranial germinomas. *Radiother. Oncol.* **38**(1), 19–23.

Jenkin, D., Angyalfi, S., Becker, L. *et al.* (1993) Optic glioma in children: surveillance, resection or irradiation? *Int. J. Radiat. Oncol. Biol. Phys.* **25**, 215–25.

Karim, A., Afra, D., Cornu, P. *et al.* (2002) Randomized trial on the efficacy of radiotherapy for cerebral low grade glioma in the adult: European Organisation for Research and Treatment of Cancer study 22845 with the Medical Research Council study BRO4: an interim analysis. *Int. J. Radiat. Oncol. Biol. Phys.* **52**, 316–24.

Kelly, P.J., Daumas Duport, C., Kispert, D.B. *et al.* (1987) Imaging based stereotaxic serial biopsies in untreated intracranial glial neoplasms. *J. Neurosurg.* **66**, 865–74.

Kernohan, J., Mabon, F., Svien, H.J. *et al.* (1949) Simplified classification of gliomas. *Proc. Staff Meeting Mayo Clinic* **24**, 71–5.

Kleihues, P. and Cavenee, W.K. (eds) (2000) *Pathology and genetics of tumours of the nervous system.* Lyon: International Agency for Research on Cancer.

Kleihues, P., Burger, P. and Scheithauer, B. (1993) The new WHO classification of brain tumours. *Brain Pathol.* **3**, 255–68.

Kortmann, R.D., Kuhl, J., Timmermann, B. *et al.* (2000) Postoperative neoadjuvant chemotherapy before radiotherapy as compared to immediate radiotherapy followed by maintenance chemotherapy in the treatment of medulloblastoma in childhood: results of the German prospective randomised trial HIT91. *Int. J. Radiat. Oncol. Biol. Phys.* **26**(2), 269–79.

Kreth, F.W., Faist, M., Warnke, P.C. *et al.* (1995) Interstitial radiosurgery of low grade gliomas. *J. Neurosurg.* **82**, 418–29.

Krieger, M.D., Chandrasoma, P.T., Zee, C.-S. *et al.* (1997) Role of stereotactic biopsy in the diagnosis and management of brain tumors. *Semin. Surg. Oncol.* **14**(1), 13–25.

Levin, V.A., Wilson, C.B., Rubenstein, L. *et al.* (1980) Adjuvant chemotherapy with BCNU or the combination of CCNU, procarbazine and vincristine following irradiation for glioblastoma multiforme. *Proc. Ann. Meet. Am. Assoc. Cancer Res.* **21**, 474.

Maher, E. and Fine, H. (1999) Primary CNS lymphoma. *Semin. Clin. Oncol.* **26**(3), 346–56.

Marcus, R.B. and Million, R.R. (1990) The incidence of myelitis after irradiation of the cervical spinal cord. *Int. J. Radiat. Oncol. Biol. Phys.* **19**, 3–8.

Markopoulos, C., Sampalis, F., Givalos, N. *et al.* (1998) Association of breast cancer with meningioma. *Eur. J. Surg. Oncol.* **24**(4), 332–4.

McCarthy, B., Davis, F., Freels, S. *et al.* (1998) Factors associated with survival in patients with meningioma. *J. Neurosurg.* **88**(5), 831–9.

Minehan, K.J., Shaw, E.G., Scheithauer, B.W. *et al.* (1995) Spinal cord astrocytoma: pathological and treatment considerations. *J. Neurosurg.* **83**(4), 590–5.

Morantz, R.A. (1995) Low grade astrocytomas. In Kay, A.H.and Laws, E.R. (eds), *Brain tumors: an encyclopedic approach.* Edinburgh: Churchill Livingstone, 433–48.

MRC Brain Tumour Working Party (1990) Prognostic factors for high grade malignant gliomas: development of a new prognostic index. *J. Neurooncol.* **9**, 47–55.

Muir, C., Waterhouse, J., Mack, T. *et al.* (1987) *Cancer incidence in five continents.* Lyon: International Agency for Research on Cancer, Scientific Publications.

Nazar, G.B., Hoffman, H.J., Becker, L.E. *et al.* (1990) Infratentorial ependymomas in childhood: prognostic factors and treatment. *J. Neurosurg.* **72**, 408–17.

Olson, J., Riedel, E. and De Angelis, L.M. (2000). Long-term outcome of low-grade oligodendroglioma and mixed glioma. *Neurology* **54**(7), 1442–8.

Parkin, D.M., Whelan, S.L., Ferlay, J. *et al.* (eds) (1997) *Cancer incidence in five continents.* Lyon: International Agency for Research on Cancer, Scientific Publications.

Patchell, R., Tibbs, P., Regine, W. *et al.* (1998) Postoperative radiotherapy in the treatment of single metastases to the brain: a randomised trial. *JAMA* **280**(17), 1485–9.

Pomeroy, S., Tamayo, P., Gaasenbeek, M. *et al.* (2002) Prediction of central nervous system embryonal tumour outcome based on gene expression. *Nature* **415**(6870), 436–42.

Posner, J.B. and Chernick, N.L. (1978) Intracranial metastases from systemic cancer. *Adv. Neurol.* **19**, 579–92.

Priestman, T., Dunn, J., Brada, M. *et al.* (1996) Final results of the Royal College of Radiologists' trial comparing two different radiotherapy schedules in the treatment of cerebral metastases. *Clin. Oncol.* **8**, 308–15.

Rampling, R. (1997) Chemotherapy: determining the appropriate treatment. In Davies, E.H. and Hopkins, A. (eds), *Improving care for patients with malignant glioma.* London: Royal College of Physicians, 63–74.

Rampling, R.P. and Symonds, R.P. (1998) Radiation myelopathy. *Curr. Opin. Neurol.* **11**, 627–32.

Rampling, R., Cruickshank, G., Lewis, A.D. *et al.* (1994) Direct measurement of pO_2 distribution and bioreductive enzymes in human malignant brain tumors. *Int. J. Radiat. Oncol. Biol. Phys.* **29**(3), 427–31.

Rasheed, B.A., Wiltshire, R.N., Bigner, S.H. and Bigner, D.D. (1999) Molecular pathogenesis of malignant gliomas. *Curr. Opin. Oncol.* **11**, 162–7.

Rider, W.D. (1963) Radiation damage to the brain: a new syndrome. *J. Can. Assoc. Radiol.* **14**, 67–9.

Robertson, P.L., DaRosso, R.C. and Allen, J.C. (1997) Improved prognosis for intracranial non germinoma germ cell tumors with multimodality therapy. *J. Neurooncol.* **32**(1), 71–80.

Sawamura, Y., De Tribolet, N., Ishii, N. and Abe, H. (1997) Management of primary intracranial germinomas: diagnostic surgery or radical resection? *J. Neurosurg.* **87**(2), 262–6.

Schultheiss, T.E., Kun, L.E., Ang, K.K. and Stephens, D.V. (1995) Radiation response of the central nervous system. *Int. J. Radiat. Oncol. Biol. Phys.* **31**(5), 1093–112.

Scott, C.B., Scarantino, C., Urtasun, R. *et al.* (1998) Validation and predictive power of Radiation Therapy Oncology Group (RTOG) recursive partitioning analysis classes for malignant glioma patients: a report using RTOG 90-06. *Int. J. Radiat. Oncol. Biol. Phys.* **40**(1), 51–5.

Senan, S., Rampling, R. and Kaye, S.B. (1991) Malignant pineal teratomas: a report on three patients and the case for craniospinal irradiation following chemotherapy. *Radiother. Oncol.* **22**(3), 209–12.

Sheline, G.E., Wara, W.M. and Smith, V. (1980) Therapeutic irradiation and brain injury. *Int. J. Radiat. Oncol. Biol. Phys.* **6**, 1215–28.

Thomas, R., James, N., Guerrero, D. *et al.* (1994) Hypofractionated radiotherapy as a palliative treatment in poor prognosis patients with high grade glioma. *Radiother. Oncol.* **33**(2), 113–16.

Thomas, D., Brada, M. *et al.* (2001) Randomised trial of procarbazine, lomustine, and vincristine in the adjuvant treatment of high-grade astrocytoma: a Medical Research Council trial. *J. Clin. Oncol.* **19**(2), 509–18.

Van den Bent, M., Kros, J., Heimans, P. *et al.* (1998) Response rate and prognostic factors of recurrent oligodendroglioma treated with procarbazine, CCNU, and vincristine chemotherapy. *Neurology* **51**(4), 1140–5.

Walker, M.D., Alexander, E., Hunt, W.E. *et al.* (1978) Evaluation of BCNU and/or radiotherapy in the treatment of anaplastic gliomas. *J. Neurosurg.* **49**, 333–43.

Wallner, K.E., Galicich, J.H., Krol, G. *et al.* (1989) Patterns of failure following treatment for glioblastoma multiforme and anaplastic astrocytoma. *Int. J. Radiat. Oncol. Biol. Phys.* **16**, 1405–509.

16

Ocular and adnexal tumours

JOHN L. HUNGERFORD AND P. NICHOLAS PLOWMAN

PAEDIATRIC TUMOURS

Although rare, malignant tumours arising in the eye and orbit in childhood are of great importance because of their curability. Benign tumours of the retina are of vascular or glial origin. Choroidal haemangiomas may occur as part of the Sturge–Weber syndrome and retinal haemangiomas as part of the von Hippel–Lindau syndrome. Uncomplicated angiomas require no treatment, but when larger lesions threaten vision, by producing a retinal detachment, circumscribed tumours benefit from radioactive plaque therapy, and diffuse haemangiomas require lens-sparing external-beam radiotherapy as described for retinoblastoma but at lower doses. In tuberous sclerosis and neurofibromatosis, benign astrocytic tumours may occur in the retina and optic nerve. The retinal lesions rarely require treatment, although large optic-nerve gliomas may require radiotherapy or resection to prevent proptosis or local invasion into the central nervous system. Very occasionally, juvenile xanthogranuloma involves ocular structures, especially the iris, producing hyphaema and secondary glaucoma. Where topical or systemic steroids fail to control these complications, external-beam radiotherapy to doses as low as 300 cGy may be very effective.

Retinoblastoma

Although a rare form of childhood cancer, retinoblastoma (RB) assumes a very important position in clinical oncology because of its high curability without significant loss of vision with modern treatment in early stage disease, its high lethality in late stage disease, its autosomal dominant inheritance and its tendency to affect both eyes (Hungerford *et al.*, 1992; Kingston and Hungerford,

1992). Whereas approximately one-third of all cases of RB are genetically determined and have multifocal or bilateral disease, only 10–20 per cent of affected children have a positive family history, implying a high new mutation rate. Survivors of genetically determined RB are at increased risk of developing second non-ocular cancers. Because of its familial tendency, the genetics of predisposition to RB and second tumours, genetic counselling and screening programmes have been the subject of much recent research.

Knudson (1971) proposed that at least two gene changes are required for the development of retinoblastoma. In genetically determined cases, one gene change is already present in the genotype and only one further change needs to occur in the somatic cell to produce RB. In non-genetic cases, two changes must occur in a single somatic cell for RB formation. It is implicit in the Knudson hypothesis that the normal genotype has a suppressive influence on RB induction. The RB gene has been localized to band 13q14. Cavenee *et al.* (1986) used recombinant DNA probes that recognize individual chromosome-specific markers, termed restriction fragment length polymorphisms (RFLPs), to probe this chromosomal region. Comparisons between the chromosome 13-associated RFLPs from RB cells and those from the leucocytes of patients revealed that loci that were heterozygous in the normal white cells were often homozygous in the tumour. Cavenee concluded that homozygosity for a mutant allele on chromosome 13 is a likely prerequisite for RB. Furthermore, Cavenee extended his studies to *in utero* prediction of RB risk, by the use of chromosome 13-specific RFLPs and esterase D isozymes – the esterase D gene being known to be close to the RB gene at 13q14. By comparing RFLP and isozyme patterns of individual family members over two or more generations, Cavenee and co-workers determined which haplotype pattern was associated with the maternally or paternally derived RB allele. They analysed amniotic fluid cells from second-trimester pregnancies and successfully predicted in four out of five cases whether a fetus at risk from RB would later develop the tumour (Cavenee *et al.*, 1986). These preliminary genetic studies are of much wider significance in the field of genetic oncology.

Friend *et al.* (1986) identified the gene that predisposes to retinoblastoma (*RB1*) and it was subsequently cloned by Lee *et al.* (1987). *RB1* was the first human recessive cancer gene ever cloned. It appears to occupy a key position in the cell cycle, possibly regulating the choice between proliferation and differentiation. The gene product, pRB, may exercise control on proliferation of cells by regulating the transcription of messenger RNA from the DNA of genes that promote growth (Nevins, 1991).

In London it is now possible to carry out prenatal or perinatal diagnosis of *RB1* carrier status through linkage analysis in over 95 per cent of RB families. It is planned to extend this service to sporadic bilateral cases with no previous family history, employing mutation analysis. Meanwhile, non-informative family members at risk of inheriting *RB1* are examined regularly under anaesthesia. The first examination takes place at age 2 weeks and the second 2 months later. Thereafter, examinations proceed 3-monthly during the remainder of the first year of life, 4-monthly during the second, and 6-monthly during the third and fourth years. Two further examinations are made, with the child awake, in the fifth year, before examinations can cease.

It has long been recognized that survivors of genetic retinoblastoma are at increased risk of developing second, non-ocular cancers. Estimates of the risk have ranged between 8.4 per cent at 18 years (Draper *et al.*, 1986) and 90 per cent at 30 years (Abramson *et al.*, 1984). It is now clear that inactivation of both copies of *RB1* may be responsible for many of these histologically distinct second neoplasms (Draper *et al.*, 1986).

The affected child usually presents under 3 years of age. The mean age of onset of the genetically determined, multifocal type is 1 year and that of the non-genetic, unifocal variant, 2 years. In developed countries, most children present with the tumour confined within the eye and with either a white pupil, a squint, or occasionally an expanded glaucomatous eye. In advanced cases the tumour may spread via the choroid to the bone marrow, or via the optic nerve to the central nervous system. In developing countries, RB tends to present late, with local extra-ocular extension leading to proptosis and spread to regional lymph nodes.

The initial assessment of the child with suspected RB should be carried out by an experienced ophthalmologist, employing binocular indirect ophthalmoscopy with scleral indentation, preferably under general anaesthesia. The diagnosis is a clinical one and RB must be distinguished from simulating lesions that include nematode endophthalmitis and various forms of retinal detachment.

Active RB lesions must be distinguished from non-progressive or spontaneously regressed tumours that are quite common and require no treatment. Intra-ocular procedures to sample a suspected tumour are contraindicated because of the very real risk of disseminating it locally within the orbit, but non-invasive ancillary tests, including ultrasound and computed tomography (CT) scanning, may be helpful by demonstrating a characteristic pattern of calcification (Arrigg *et al.*, 1983). The histogenesis of RB has been a matter of dispute (Hungerford, 1990) and the tumour has been variously considered to arise from glial cells and from photoreceptors. Recent immunohistochemical reactivity to a panel of monoclonal antibodies has suggested that RB may arise from an early multipotential cell, so that the resulting tumour cell population is heterogeneous (Tarlton and Easty, 1990). Whatever the cell of origin, there is clinical evidence that the progenitor cells lose the capability of malignant change as they mature and that this process occurs centrifugally in the retina. Thus, new tumours developing later during the risk period arise more peripherally than earlier lesions and the technique described is needed to see these neoplasms arising at the very edge of the retina.

Once the diagnosis has been made, systemic staging investigations are probably unnecessary in children with small intra-ocular tumours that can be managed without enucleation (Pratt *et al.*, 1989). CT prior to surgery is usually recommended when an eye is to be enucleated, mainly to confirm the intra-ocular diagnosis. CT cannot detect minor optic nerve invasion. Only very rarely seen on routine CT are ectopic intracranial retinoblastomas, which arise as a component of multifocal disease in cells within the pineal and suprasellar region, which have a similar embryonic origin to that of the eye (Kingston *et al.*, 1985). These tumours affect approximately 4 per cent of children with genetically determined RB and may be better seen in their early stages by magnetic resonance imaging (MRI) (Schulman *et al.*, 1986). They have a poor prognosis, probably due to late detection, but screening for them is impractical because the risk period during which they may develop after the diagnosis of RB extends for some 6 years.

Bone marrow and cerebrospinal fluid (CSF) cytology can be deferred until after enucleation, and is only required when there is histological evidence of extensive optic nerve or choroidal invasion. Technetium bone scans are needed only if there is clinical evidence of bony involvement. There is no satisfactory staging system for the overall management of retinoblastoma. The classification proposed by Reese and Ellsworth (1963) was designed to predict the prognosis for retaining an eye with RB irrespective of the visual outcome (Table 16.1). It has been used widely for 30 years to compare outcomes of treatments for intra-ocular RB. Pratt (1972) proposed a classification based on the clinical features at diagnosis and on histology, as a guide to treatment and prognosis.

Table 16.1 *Reese–Ellsworth classification of retinoblastoma*

Group I	Single or multiple tumours less than 4 disc diameters at or behind the equator (one optic disc diameter = 1.5 mm)
Group IIA	Solitary lesion 4–10 disc diameters at or behind the equator
Group IIB	Solitary lesion larger than 10 disc diameters
Group III	Lesions anterior to the equator
Group IVA	Multiple tumours, some larger than 10 disc diameters
Group IVB	Any lesion extending anteriorly beyond the limits of ophthalmoloscopy
Group VA	Massive tumours
Group VB	Vitreous seedlings

The aim of treatment of RB is to preserve vision where possible, with minimal morbidity and without compromising survival. The choice of treatment depends on whether or not retinoblastoma is confined to the eye, on the size, number and location of the intra-ocular tumours, and on whether one or both eyes are involved. Most children present with RB confined to the eye and there are now several conservative treatment options. External-beam radiotherapy has been used extensively for large and multifocal tumours, and for tumours of any size near the optic disc and macula, but has been largely supplanted by chemotherapy as the first-line management of such lesions.

The best outcomes in the treatment of retinoblastoma stem from combinations of treatments. Focal treatment is still preferable wherever possible for small tumours located away from the optic disc and macula. When choosing a focal treatment, methods such as cryotherapy and laser, which do not involve radiation, are to be preferred over plaque radiotherapy. Salvage treatment by cryotherapy or laser is unlikely to lead to loss of vision by potentiating the effects of earlier radiotherapy or chemotherapy. By contrast, salvage methods that involve radiation or chemotherapy must be planned very carefully to take account of earlier treatments by these methods if consequent visual loss is to be minimized. When focal treatment fails, many eyes can be salvaged by prompt use of chemotherapy or external-beam radiotherapy. Conversely, focal treatments are useful in salvaging eyes with new or persistent tumour activity after primary chemotherapy or external radiation.

The eye should be removed when retinoblastoma is too advanced for conservative treatment or when conservation fails. The decision to enucleate depends to some extent on the status of the contralateral eye. Eyes with extrascleral extension, glaucoma and tumour occupying more than half of the globe are best removed whatever the condition of the fellow eye. Eyes with tumour occupying half the volume of the globe are unlikely to be retained with useful vision and are best enucleated if the contralateral eye is healthy or has minor disease. It is justified, however, to attempt conservative treatment if the contralateral eye has been lost or has equally serious involvement. In infants, growth of the face is so retarded by whole-eye radiotherapy that it is rarely justified to employ this method when the other eye is reasonably healthy.

The survival prospects of these young patients can be maximized by subjecting the enucleated eye to a rigorous histopathological examination, on which is based a decision whether or not to give adjuvant chemotherapy. The histological risk factors predictive of metastatic death following enucleation have been well defined (Hungerford, 1993a). The presence of choroidal invasion significantly increases the risk of metastasis, but only when there is concurrent optic nerve invasion (Olver et al., 1991). In London, prior to 1985, 83 per cent of 74 children with concurrent major choroidal invasion and retrolaminar optic nerve invasion died from metastatic disease or direct intracranial extension. Subsequently, all children with these risk factors have received systemic adjuvant chemotherapy after enucleation, together with orbital radiotherapy when the optic nerve resection margin was involved. On this regimen there were no deaths in the first 11 children (Hungerford, 1993a) and only one death from CNS relapse subsequently.

Orbital recurrence may follow extra-ocular extension, optic nerve involvement to the resection margin, or an injudicious biopsy (Stevenson et al., 1989), although orbital relapse was occasionally seen in children with none of these features. Prompt orbital radiotherapy was formerly advised when there was an obvious risk factor, and usually prevented relapse in the orbit. Lately, adjuvant treatment for high-risk histology has dramatically reduced the incidence of orbital recurrence and radiotherapy is now recommended only for tumour extension to the optic nerve resection margin.

Most orbital recurrences occur within a year of enucleation, and were formerly associated with a poor survival rate even if local tumour control was established by orbital radiotherapy. Chemotherapy has greatly reduced the mortality rate in the few cases of orbital recurrence that still occur. In a prior series of 16 children not receiving chemotherapy, 15 died (Hungerford et al., 1987). The one long-term survivor had been treated with simple excision of the recurrent tumour, adjuvant chemotherapy and orbital radiotherapy. In a subsequent report from the same group, all five children with an isolated orbital recurrence were cured with a similar regimen (Goble et al., 1990).

With the advent of adjuvant chemotherapy where appropriate after enucleation, metastatic retinoblastoma has become a rarity in the UK. Metastases from retinoblastoma are usually apparent within a year of diagnosis of the ocular primary. Direct spread may take place through the sclera into the orbit or along the optic nerve into the central nervous system. Haematogenous dissemination may result in spread to bones, bone marrow and brain. Local extension into the lymphatic territory of the eyelids may lead to preauricular and submandibular lymph-node deposits and to subcutaneous deposits around the orbit and in the scalp (MacKay *et al.*, 1984). Initial responses to chemotherapy with vincristine, VM26 and platinum analogues for metastatic retinoblastoma are usually good but are rarely sustained, and early fatal relapse is common (Kingston *et al.*, 1987). Recently, however, reports have been appearing in the literature of long-term survival following intensive chemotherapy (Petersen *et al.*, 1987; Saleh *et al.*, 1988).

Ectopic intracranial retinoblastoma was formerly seen in around 1 in 20 children with the genetic form of the disease (Kingston *et al.*, 1985). Some children with genetic RB develop other midline primitive neuro-ectodermal tumours, for example in the region of the ethmoid sinuses, and these may be *forme fruste* of ectopic intracranial retinoblastoma. Like orbital recurrence, however, the incidence of ectopic intracranial retinoblastoma seems to have reduced significantly following the use of chemotherapy, either as a primary or as an adjuvant treatment. This entity presents with symptoms and signs of secondary hydrocephalus or, when arising in the suprasellar region, of diabetes insipidus. Treatment by radiotherapy alone or in combination with chemotherapy may prolong survival, but there have been very few durable remissions reported, with most children dying from spinal metastases.

CHEMOTHERAPY

The indications for chemotherapy currently in use at Saint Bartholomew's Hospital are summarized in Table 16.2.

The JOE regimen of vincristine, etoposide and carboplatin is the most widely used for primary and for adjuvant treatments, and is well tolerated. Six cycles are normally given for treatment of overt disease and four for adjuvant therapy. Second-line treatment with ifosphamide may be given for orbital and metastatic disease, but is rarely recommended for intra-ocular relapse, which is better managed by enucleation or radiotherapy. Intrathecal methotrexate should be considered for intracranial disease and should be combined with whole-neuraxis radiation. Local intra-ocular thiotepa and intra-orbital carboplatin have been tried for local intra-ocular relapse, but sustained local tumour control is unusual after this approach.

With the advent of primary chemotherapy for intra-ocular disease, the concept of 'chemoreduction' has been popularized. In this approach, chemotherapy is followed by a second treatment on the assumption that, by itself, it will be insufficient to destroy the tumour(s) in the eye. Chemotherapy is first given to reduce the size of the tumour. The aim is that a large lesion may then respond better to radiotherapy, or a smaller tumour may be treatable with a lower dose of external radiation, by focal radiation treatment with a radioactive plaque or, preferably, by a non-radiational focal treatment such as laser hyperthermia. This approach is severely limited by the poor visual outcome that results from the additive effects of chemotherapy and radiotherapy on the retina (Kingston *et al.*, 1996). It has been suggested that chemotherapy drug resistance in retinoblastoma may be due to a chemical pump in the tumour cell wall that can be blocked by the drug cyclosporin. This principal has been applied clinically by combining cyclosporin with chemotherapy. Early results have been encouraging (Chan *et al.*, 1996) but the method is not yet fully tested.

EXTERNAL-BEAM RADIOTHERAPY

This is indicated for retinoblastomas which are too large, too numerous or too close to the optic disc or macula for focal treatment, when vitreous seeding is present, and for tumours which have failed to respond to focal therapy. Any tumour larger than 13 mm in diameter is best treated by external-beam radiotherapy. Foote *et al.* (1989) analysed the dose–response rates and patterns of failure of external-beam radiotherapy for retinoblastoma. Using 4 or 6 MV photons they recommended a dose of 45 Gy in 1.8 Gy fractions and reported no eyes lost from radiation side-effects when treatment was given over 4 weeks in at least 20 fractions.

External-beam radiotherapy can be given using an anterior whole-eye field when one eye requires treatment, and by lateral whole-eye fields when both need radiotherapy. Using such techniques radiation-induced cataract is inevitable and the results of cataract surgery are limited by corneal opacification resulting from eyelid shrinkage, dryness and lagophthalmos, which also result from whole-eye radiotherapy and which are resistant to treatment. The result is usually a poorly sighted, photophobic, painful and unsightly eye.

A sophisticated and reproducible radiotherapy technique, developed by Schipper (1980) at Utrecht, has made it possible to treat the whole retina accurately up to, but not including, the lens. This technique has been

Table 16.2 *Indications for chemotherapy for retinoblastoma*

Extra-ocular disease
    Orbital relapse
    Metastatic disease
    Ectopic intracranial retinoblastoma
Adjuvant therapy following enucleation with adverse histology
    Retrolaminar invasion of optic nerve with or without extension to the resection margin
    Extensive choroidal invasion
    Scleral invasion
    Anterior chamber involvement
Intra-ocular disease
    Primary treatment of tumour(s) too large, too numerous or too close to the optic disc or macula for focal therapy
    Salvage therapy for recurrent disease bilaterally or in an only eye

developed for routine service at St Bartholomew's Hospital, London (Harnett *et al.*, 1987). A contact lens on the cornea of the anaesthetized infant provides a fixed reference point from which all measurements are made. This point is connected accurately to a linear accelerator, the beam of which has been split to minimize divergence and to create a very sharp cut-off point anteriorly. The distance from the front of the cornea to the back of the lens is determined before treatment by A-scan ultrasound, and the beam edge is placed at this depth with 0.5 mm accuracy. A lateral beam encompasses the retina up to the back of the lens, and may be angled at 40° to avoid the contralateral eye when only one globe is to be treated. The approach is recommended for posteriorly placed tumours without vitreous seeding and without retinal detachment extending to the ora serrata. Tumours not fulfilling these criteria and requiring external-beam radiotherapy are best treated by the whole-eye approach. Lens-sparing external-beam radiotherapy is particularly suited to smaller lesions located critically on the temporal side of the optic disc (Fig. 16.1). Small tumours located

very anteriorly at the edge of the beam may receive a suboptimal dose and are best pretreated by cryotherapy.

Response to external-beam radiotherapy is assessed by examination under anaesthesia 4–6 weeks after completion of treatment, whichever approach is utilized. Several patterns of regression are recognized and experience is necessary for correct interpretation of the results. Recently, the relationship of regression pattern after external-beam radiotherapy to recurrence has been analysed (Singh *et al.*, 1993). Complications of radiotherapy are now less than those that followed poorly fractionated whole-eye treatments (Fig. 16.2). Cataract and dry eye have been successfully eliminated by the lens-sparing technique, but some degree of growth retardation of the middle face is inevitable, though less marked than with the whole-eye method.

RADIOACTIVE SCLERAL PLAQUE THERAPY

This is particularly useful for tumours up to 10 mm in diameter located at least 5 mm away from the optic disc

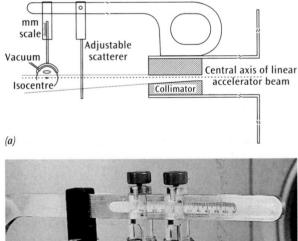

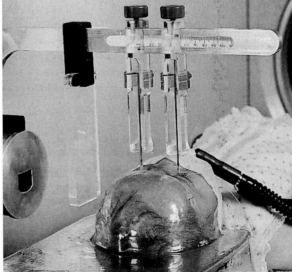

(a)

(b)

Figure 16.1 *(a) Schematic illustration of lateral beam technique used for lens-sparing external-beam radiotherapy. (b) Child in set-up position in treatment.*

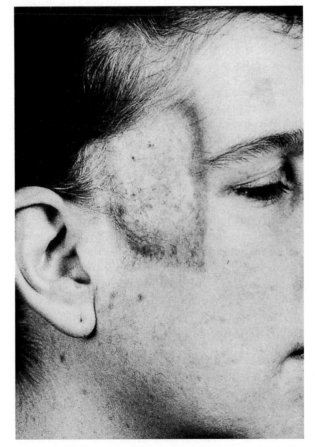

Figure 16.2 *Patient surviving from poorly fractionated radiotherapy for retinoblastoma. The punched-out square skin portal is most prominent. The other ocular complications (listed in text) are more serious than in the modern series of patients.*

and macula. The plaque is temporarily sutured to the sclera precisely over the base of the tumour and removed as soon as it has delivered 40 Gy to the apex of the lesion. Although most plaque therapy has been carried out with high-energy cobalt-60 applicators, these sources cannot be shielded on their external surface and have now been largely replaced by low-energy plaques employing either low-energy X-rays from iodine-125 (Harnett and Thomson, 1988) or β-rays from ruthenium-106 (Lommatzsch, 1977). Plaque therapy may be repeated at least once and two plaques may be applied for separate lesions. Radiation doses from plaques are cumulative and multiples of three or more tumours requiring radiation are best managed by an external-beam approach.

PHOTOCOAGULATION

Photocoagulation can destroy small retinoblastomas confined to the retina and at least 3 mm from the optic disc and macula. It is most applicable to postequatorial tumours. Most centres have employed the indirect technique described by Höpping (Höpping and Meyer-Schwickerath, 1964) to destroy the tumour by divorcing it from its blood supply (i.e. infarcting it). Shields et al. (1990) reported a local tumour control rate of 76 per cent in 45 photocoagulated eyes and best cure rates were achieved when treating tumours 1.5 mm in diameter or less.

HYPERTHERMIA

Photocoagulation has been substantially superseded by hyperthermia applied directly to the tumour using infrared radiation generated by a diode laser. Some clinics have employed argon green laser to achieve the same effect. This technique is now commonly applied as an adjunct to primary chemotherapy for intra-ocular disease under the term 'chemothermotherapy'. The method has not been fully evaluated. It is as yet uncertain whether it increases local tumour control rate compared with chemotherapy alone. Furthermore, it has not been investigated for adverse effects such as macular scarring and vitreous relapse due to direct treatment of the tumour. Both of these side-effects have been seen in the clinical application of this technique at St Bartholomew's Hospital.

CRYOTHERAPY

Cryotherapy is useful for the treatment of small tumours (Abramson and Ellsworth, 1982) anterior to the equator. The treatment is usually applied transconjunctivally, using a triple freeze–thaw technique, but posterior lesions may be treated through a small conjunctival incision provided that they are located at least 5 mm from the optic disc and macula. Abramson and Ellsworth (1982) and Shields et al. (1989) have reported local tumour control rates, respectively, of 70 and 79 per cent. Cryotherapy is not recommended for tumours more than 3.5 mm in diameter (Shields et al., 1989).

Orbital rhabdomyosarcoma

Rhabdomyosarcomas (RMS) are the most common soft-tissue sarcomas of childhood and are of unknown cause. Over one-third of all new cases present with head and neck primaries. Orbital RMS accounts for one-quarter of all head and neck primary sites (Sutow et al., 1982) and this particular primary RMS has long been recognized as having a later pattern of dissemination than tumours arising at other sites. Early surgical series demonstrated that, following orbital exenteration, up to 18 per cent of patients could remain long-term survivors. Similarly, Sagerman et al. (1972) found an excellent local control rate of 91 per cent following radical radiotherapy. However, in the late 1960s it was found that combination cytotoxic chemotherapy was extremely powerful against this condition. Following the success of adjunctive chemotherapy in Wilms' tumour, cytotoxic drugs quickly achieved a place in standard therapy of all patients with RMS. Furthermore, it became conventional practice to deliver one or two pulses of chemotherapy prior to radiotherapy to the orbit, to achieve cytoreduction and perhaps improve vascularity of the tumour at the time of irradiation. Together, chemotherapy and radiotherapy have improved the prognosis of RMS at all sites and, for patients with primary orbital RMS, orbital exenteration is now reserved as a salvage procedure.

Typically, the patient with an orbital RMS is a child aged between 1 and 15 years who presents with a painless orbital mass, a squint or proptosis. It is essential to confirm the diagnosis histopathologically by orbital biopsy. The histological subtype is usually embryonal RMS, although older children may be found to have alveolar RMS, which has an earlier pattern of dissemination. Staging of the disease includes a high-definition orbital CT scan to supplement plain skull X-rays, chest X-ray, bone scan and bone marrow examination. The majority of patients will have localized disease. Bad prognostic features at presentation include large tumour bulk, bone erosion, alveolar histology and metastases.

Conventional treatment might then comprise two cycles of VAC (vincristine 1.5 mg/m², actinomycin D 1.0 mg/m² and cyclophosphamide 600 mg/m²) to achieve initial tumour shrinkage, followed by external-beam radiotherapy to the entire orbit, only the vincristine and cyclophosphamide being continued during the radiotherapy. Thereafter, VAC chemotherapy is continued for one more year. Recently, ifosfamide has been used in preference to cyclophosphamide and such primary chemotherapy alone (without radiotherapy in scanning complete responders) is still championed by some workers for better histology (embryonal) tumours.

Radiotherapy is delivered by either megavoltage photons or an electron portal. Using a 60° wedge-pair technique (Fig. 16.3a) a dose distribution that well fits the orbit is achieved, but there is forward projection of the isodoses towards the pituitary and hypothalamus and late

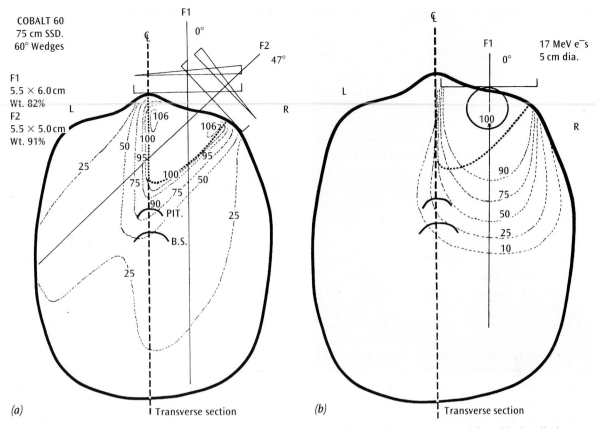

Figure 16.3 *(a) Wedge-pair photon technique for orbital radiotherapy. (b) Anterior electron portal for orbital radiotherapy.*

neuroendocrine sequelae may result. The alternative is a single anterior electron portal (Fig. 16.3b). At first this second technique is attractive because it is theoretically possible to choose the correct energy to draw up the beam at the apex of the orbit. However, the air spaces in the ethmoid region make dosimetry less certain in the midline. Thus, the large penumbra of an electron beam and the straight antero-posterior alignment of the nasal boundary of the orbit make it essential that the medial border of an anterior electron portal extends to the midline of the patient. Nevertheless, and particularly for anteriorly placed orbital RMS, the anterior electron portal is the favoured technique, whereas wedged photon portals are preferred for extensive orbital disease. If the photon technique is chosen, an 'eyes open' treatment position may reduce the keratoconjunctivitis risk by minimizing the bolus effect of the eyelids.

The radiation dose prescription varies with bulk of the tumour, age of the patient, histology and presence or absence of bone erosion. For younger children and small bulk disease, doses of the order of 40 Gy are prescribed in daily fractions of 1.75–1.8 Gy. For older children and large bulk disease, alveolar histology or bone erosion, a higher dose of 50 Gy or more is chosen, and given in similar daily dose fractions. Ophthalmic follow-up is advisable during and after irradiation, as radiation conjunctivitis and xerophthalmia are, respectively, acute and late

complications of high-dose treatments. Acute radiation conjunctivitis is usually inflammatory and treated by topical steroids. Secondary infection will require antibiotic drops. Dry eyes require long-term lubrication with artificial tears during the day and with ointment at night if there is significant nocturnal lagophthalmos.

Careful follow-up by CT scanning allows early detection of relapse. Almost without exception, relapse will be manifest within 2 years of treatment and radical orbital exenteration is the treatment of choice. Following exenteration we have successfully employed a brachytherapy technique where the margins of the resection were microscopically involved (Fig. 16.4).

Similarly, and particularly in patients relapsing off therapy, a very short period of some other chemotherapy, such as Doxorubicin, etoposide and cisplatin, may precede surgery in order to test the responsiveness of the tumour for postoperative chemotherapy. However, radical surgery must not be long delayed.

Following such a treatment scheme, 16 patients treated at St Bartholomew's Hospital and the Royal Marsden Hospital (Kingston *et al.*, 1984) have a 5-year survival of 94 per cent and the American intergroup RMS study reported 21 of 23 cases relapse-free at 2 years (Sutow *et al.*, 1982). With such excellent results, several groups have attempted to reduce the morbidity of therapy. The intergroup RMS studies have suggested that, in

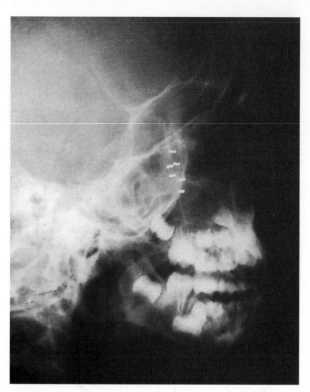

Figure 16.4 *Lateral skull X-ray to show the position of a six gold-grain implant technique performed by the authors. This girl relapsed locally following chemoradiotherapy for orbital rhabdomyosarcoma. The child underwent orbital exenteration but there was residual disease in the orbital apex despite orbital wall and ethmoid resection. She remains disease-free at 14 years.*

good-prognosis cases, two-drug chemotherapy with vincristine and actinomycin D is not significantly inferior to VAC, and the subtraction of cyclophosphamide may reduce the incidence of second tumours and infertility. Similarly, the trend downwards in total radiation dose below 50 Gy in selected cases is also expected to reduce late effects.

The late morbidity of patients with orbital RMS treated by chemoradiotherapy has been well studied by Heyn *et al.* (1986). The incidence of acute non-lymphocytic leukaemia following the alkylating agent containing VAC chemotherapy is approximately 4 per cent (Meyers and Ghavimi, 1983) and there will be a small incidence of other second tumours following chemoradiation. Following radiotherapy to the orbit there is always some retardation of growth, which is inversely related to age, cataract and a substantial incidence of dry-eye syndrome with photophobia and keratoconjunctivitis. Where the hypothalamus has received the majority of the radiation dose, clinically important deficits in growth hormone secretion have been demonstrated. Particularly in boys, the alkylating agent in VAC may lead to infertility.

There is continuing controversy as to whether, for good histology tumours, it is optimal to omit the alkylating agent (with its fertility and second cancer potential) or the radiation.

Other paediatric tumours

UVEAL MALIGNANT MELANOMA

Uveal malignant melanoma may occur in the choroid, ciliary body or iris. It is exceedingly uncommon in childhood, although benign naevi may arise in the choroid or iris and increase in size without malignant change. Continued growth and a raised lesion should arouse suspicion of malignancy and management is as for adult disease.

MEDULLOEPITHELIOMA

This is a rare tumour of the non-pigmented ciliary epithelium, presenting in children and young adults. The tumour is usually benign or of low-grade malignancy, with between one-quarter and two-thirds of medulloepitheliomas containing malignant cells (Anderson, 1962; Broughton and Zimmerman, 1978). Medulloepithelioma has been reported outside the uveal tract in the retina (Mullaney, 1974) and optic nerve (Green *et al.*, 1974), but usually arises in the iris and ciliary body. The clinical presentation is very variable. It usually presents as a grey mass arising from the ciliary body and displacing the lens to produce astigmatism, amblyopia and squint. There may be an associated pupillary abnormality, cataract or a painful glaucoma. Rare posterior lesions may produce a white pupil reflex similar to that seen in retinoblastoma. Extrascleral extension may lead to proptosis and ultimately a tumour may fungate between the eyelids (Fig. 16.5). Non-invasive investigations, including ultrasound and CT, cannot distinguish between medulloepithelioma and simulating lesions such as amelanotic melanoma, *Toxocara* granuloma, and leiomyoma. The diagnosis is best established by biopsy, but this approach is contraindicated for a posterior tumour in case it may prove to be a retinoblastoma. Medulloepitheliomas are friable lesions which are difficult to excise. Small iris tumours may be resectable (Morris and Garner, 1975), but most cannot be removed completely (Canning *et al.*, 1988). The eye should be removed when excision is incomplete and especially when malignant cells are seen. Primary enucleation is probably best for all except the most localized medulloepitheliomas (Canning *et al.*, 1988). Malignant medulloepitheliomas show a tendency to invade the orbit. The overall mortality rate is only 10 per cent, and the presence of extrascleral extension is the most important adverse prognostic indicator (Broughton and Zimmerman, 1978). In fatal cases, death commonly results from invasive local recurrence with intracranial extension. Metastases to regional lymph nodes and occasionally to distant sites may sometimes be seen late in the course of the disease in neglected cases.

OPTIC NERVE GLIOMA

Glioma of the optic nerve is a rare tumour, now classified as a juvenile pilocytic astrocytoma, which may occur anywhere in the optic nerve or chiasm. Most examples are histologically benign but inexorable growth of some

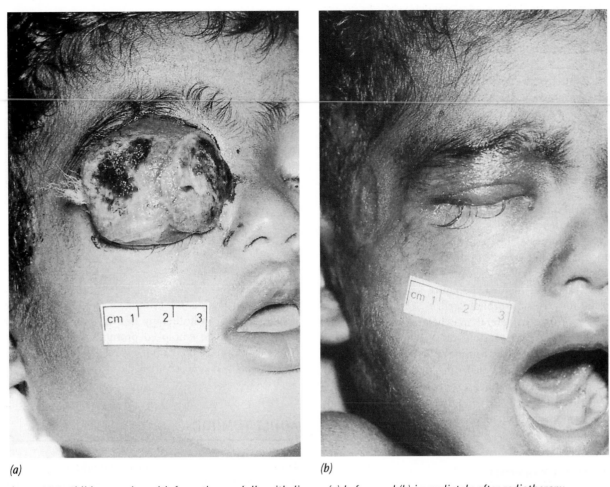

(a)   *(b)*

Figure 16.5 *Child presenting with fungating medulloepithelioma: (a) before and (b) immediately after radiotherapy.*

intracranial lesions may lead to death. Other astrocytomas grow episodically or cease to grow without treatment. Nine out of 10 of these tumours present in the first two decades (Chutorian *et al.*, 1964) and there is evidence of neurofibromatosis in nearly 40 per cent of affected individuals (Manschot, 1954). The clinical presentation depends on whether the tumour is mainly intra-orbital or intracranial (Crowe and Schull, 1953). The earliest sign is often loss of vision, called to attention by a squint, nystagmus or a dilated pupil. Involvement of the intra-orbital optic nerve results in painless axial proptosis and optic disc swelling or atrophy may be visible ophthalmoscopically. Chiasmal gliomas present with hydrocephalus, diabetes insipidus, somnolence, seizures, obesity or hypogonadism. The tumour is best seen on CT scanning, although intracranial extension may lead to enlargement of the optic foramen on plain X-ray and chiasmal involvement may be detected when visual field testing shows a quadrantic or hemianopic defect in the contralateral eye. Treatment is controversial. The tendency to slow or episodic growth and to spontaneous remission has made it difficult to assess the results of policies of no treatment, surgical excision or radiotherapy. Intra-orbital lesions with good vision and not involving the chiasm may be observed for evidence of growth before considering

excision, although gross proptosis in a blind eye is an indication for surgical removal of the tumour via a lateral orbitotomy. Some have advocated a combined orbital and neurosurgical approach if excision is incomplete or if the optic foramen is enlarged, and the weight of evidence from very long-term follow-up studies suggests that the death rate is high if an attempt is not made to remove these tumours surgically (Innes and Hoyt, 1986). Nevertheless, there is now a body of opinion that only tumours not involving the chiasm are resectable. Carefully fractionated external-beam radiotherapy to a dose of 40–50 Gy may be considered for progressive chiasmal lesions. Although some have claimed that improvement after radiotherapy is temporary (Reese, 1963), there is evidence (Taveras *et al.*, 1956; Lloyd, 1973) that good regression can be achieved and that treatment should be advised as soon as the chiasm is involved and not delayed until there are symptoms of this involvement. The overall mortality rate ranges up to 56 per cent for tumours with chiasmal involvement (Rush *et al.*, 1982).

HISTIOCYTOSIS X

Histiocytosis X usually has its onset in childhood and histiocytes accumulate throughout the body in soft tissues and bone. Bony involvement is seen more often in Hand–Schüller–Christian than in Letterer–Siwe disease. The membrane bones of the skull and sella turcica are preferentially affected. Orbital bone involvement is relatively infrequent (Moore *et al.*, 1985) and leads to non-axial proptosis, whereas a soft-tissue deposit within the optic nerve sheath may lead to axial forward displacement of the eye. Proptosis, bone deposits and diabetes insipidus constitute a triad of signs which suggest the diagnosis of histiocytosis X, which can be confirmed by radiological examination and biopsy. Before treatment is commenced the patient should be staged to assess the full extent of the disease. Multifocal involvement requires systemic therapy, which may begin with prednisolone alone. Cytotoxic drugs such as vincristine and vinblastine may be added and etoposide may be considered for resistant disease. Bony deposits respond well to intralesional injection of methyl sodium succinate, which is useful for accessible orbital deposits. The injection may need to be repeated several times before regression occurs (Moore *et al.*, 1985). Lesions resistant to this treatment and inaccessible deposits causing optic-nerve compression or severe proptosis may be treated with low-dose radiotherapy. Carefully planned external-beam radiotherapy to a dose of 12 Gy in eight fractions is followed by good regression with little morbidity (Harnett *et al.*, 1988).

SECONDARY DEPOSITS

Secondary deposits may be seen in the eye and orbit in children. Choroidal involvement is fairly common in uncontrolled acute lymphoblastic leukaemia (ALL) but, with the adequacy of modern systemic treatments and cranial radiation prophylaxis, the ocular relapse rate and pattern have both changed. We have encountered isolated anterior chamber relapses in children in bone marrow remission, usually soon after stopping maintenance chemotherapy, and it may be speculated that the radiation dose received by the back of the globe during cranial radiation prophylaxis is cytocidal and that chemotherapy is suppressive only with regard to the poor drug penetration to the anterior chamber sanctuary. Leukaemic infiltration of the bones and soft tissue of the orbit by green-coloured granulocytic tumour is seen in acute myeloblastic leukaemia (AML) and has led to the term 'chloroma'. Occasionally, intra-ocular relapse is seen in AML. Both orbital and ocular ALL and AML respond well to radiotherapy to a dose of 24 Gy given in 12 fractions over 15 days. Unlike adult non-Hodgkin's lymphoma, involvement of the orbit by lymphoma in childhood is usually associated with disseminated disease and the emphasis of management is on chemotherapy. The orbit is involved in 50 per cent of cases of the African form of Burkitt's lymphoma, usually by secondary extension from a maxillary primary. Neuroblastoma preferentially metastasizes to the orbits, often bilaterally (Fig. 16.6), and very occasionally

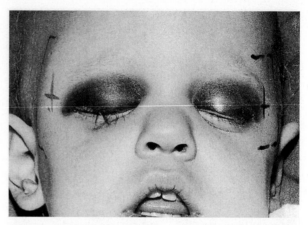

Figure 16.6 *The 'black eyes' of orbital involvement by metastatic neuroblastoma.*

a primary orbital neuroblastoma may arise in the ciliary ganglion. Local radiotherapy to a dose of 25 Gy in 13 fractions must be employed promptly if there is any threat to vision, as the tumour is reliably radiosensitive and unreliably chemosensitive.

ADULT TUMOURS

Tumours of the eye and of the ocular adnexa are much more common in adults than in children. Apart from choroidal naevi and benign papillomas of the eyelids, the most frequently encountered neoplasms are malignant. In contrast to those of children, many adult intra-ocular malignant neoplasms are metastatic, and for most affected individuals, treatment can only be palliative. For adult primary malignant intra-ocular tumours the overall cure rates remain relatively low, although a trend towards earlier detection during routine eye testing has produced some improvement in outlook.

Unlike intra-ocular malignancies, the majority of adult adnexal neoplasms are primary tumours. This contrasts once again with the situation in children where adnexal malignancies are commonly metastatic or related to a blood dyscrasia. Orbital malignant tumours now have relatively good cure rates in the adult because most are only locally invasive. Death from such a neoplasm usually results from direct local extension rather than from metastatic spread. The outlook is similarly good for most malignant tumours of the eyelids and conjunctiva, because they seem to have a lower propensity to regional and distant spread than their equivalents in other structures.

Benign tumours are common in the eye and its adnexa. The importance of these tumours is that many are associated with widespread diseases, some of which are heritable, and that, because of their location, complex treatment may be required to preserve vision or to reduce cosmetic deficit.

Benign tumours of the eye

The more common benign intra-ocular tumours in adults are of melanocytic, smooth muscle or vascular origin.

MELANOCYTIC TUMOURS

Melanocytic tumours are overwhelmingly the most numerous. Naevi arise from uveal melanocytes in the iris, ciliary body and choroid. There is no doubt that naevi may occasionally undergo malignant change and that most uveal-tract malignant melanomas arise in this way. Choroidal naevi are extremely common, but the chance of malignant change has been estimated to be less than 1 in 500 during a 5-year period (Ganley and Comstock, 1973). It is impractical to propose regular follow-up for all innocent, flat naevi. Nevertheless, repeated examinations are advised for all iris naevi and for raised choroidal lesions, those developing orange lipofuscin pigment, those with an associated serous retinal detachment or visual field defect, and multiple naevi. Patients with ocular or oculodermal melanocytosis also have an increased risk of uveal melanoma (Gonder et al., 1982) and should undergo regular examination of the ocular fundi.

SMOOTH MUSCLE TUMOURS

Smooth muscle tumours are represented by leiomyomas, which are slow-growing, pale, benign tumours. Leiomyomas are rare in the eye and have been described most frequently in the iris, with a few cases reported in the ciliary body (White et al., 1989). Re-evaluation of archival histological material suggests, however, that most so-called iris leiomyomas are really amelanotic benign melanocytic lesions (Foss et al., 1994). The only true ocular leiomyomas arise in the ciliary body, where they may grow quite large and be difficult to distinguish clinically from amelanotic melanomas. Ciliary-body leiomyomas are very circumscribed tumours which are easily excised from within the eye, the main indication for this procedure being exclusion of the alternative diagnosis of malignant melanoma.

VASCULAR TUMOURS

Vascular tumours may occur in the retina but are more common in the choroid. Most retinal lesions are capillary haemangiomas, which may be solitary or multiple. New retinal haemangiomas may arise throughout life in the von Hippel–Lindau syndrome. They tend to grow and may ultimately lead to bilateral blindness from retinal detachment. Large capillary haemangiomas may respond to cryotherapy (Annesley et al., 1977) but the best response rates are obtained by treating smaller lesions by cryotherapy or laser photocoagulation (Goldberg and Koenig, 1971). For this reason, a policy of annual ocular assessment of von Hippel–Lindau patients from infancy is wise, with early treatment of all new tumours. Cavernous haemangiomas are less common in the retina than tumours of the capillary type. The lesions are usually solitary, although the ocular tumour may be associated with skin or central nervous system vascular lesions as part of an inherited neuro-oculocutaneous syndrome, of which one bilateral case has been reported (Goldberg et al., 1979). The cavernous type of haemangioma rarely grows and is unlikely to lead to loss of vision unless it involves the macular area or unless it bleeds. Haemorrhage from one of these tumours may be treated by photocoagulation or by cryotherapy. Haemangiomas affecting the choroid are of cavernous type, though their histology and clinical behaviour are different from cavernous haemangiomas occurring at other sites. They are of two types. Most are circumscribed and first detected in adult life. Circumscribed choroidal haemangiomas are not associated with systemic abnormalities. A minority of haemangiomas are diffuse. Diffuse haemangiomas commonly present in children and young adults and are usually associated with vascular abnormalities of the skin and central nervous system, often as part of the Sturge–Weber syndrome. Choroidal haemangiomas grow slowly, if at all. Nevertheless, they may threaten vision by producing a localized or extensive serous retinal detachment. Serous exudation may be reduced by argon laser grid photocoagulation with retinal reattachment, but usually without destruction of the tumour. Should detachment persist or recur, sustained retinal reattachment and good tumour regression may be achieved by irradiating a circumscribed choroidal haemangioma to a dose of only 40 Gy to the apex of the lesion, using a radioactive scleral plaque. Diffuse choroidal haemangiomas commonly produce extensive, blinding serous retinal detachment. These tumours are usually too extensive to respond to photocoagulation or to focal radiotherapy using a scleral plaque. Sustained retinal reattachment has been achieved in diffuse haemangioma by using fractionated external-beam radiotherapy to a dose of 12 Gy, using the lens-sparing approach advocated for retinoblastoma (Plowman and Harnett, 1986), although usually without significant regression of the tumour.

Benign tumours of the eyelids, conjunctiva and orbit

Benign tumours of the ocular adnexa are common and are of epithelial, vascular, neurogenic, melanocytic or lacrimal gland origin. Benign orbital tumours must be distinguished from idiopathic inflammatory pseudotumour (Garner, 1973).

EPITHELIAL TUMOURS

Epithelial tumours mainly comprise benign papillomas of the eyelid margin, which are extremely common and of viral origin. They are easily treated by shaving and light cautery to the base, but tend to recur. Recurrent tumours may be managed by wedge excision. Seborrhoeic keratosis is particularly common in the elderly and may be treated by curettage. Cryotherapy may be performed for tumours of this type in pale-skinned individuals, but should be avoided in those with darker colouring because it is likely to be followed by noticeable depigmentation.

VASCULAR TUMOURS

Vascular tumours predominantly affect the orbit. In the adult, cavernous haemangioma is one of the most common primary orbital tumours. It usually presents in middle-aged women and is best managed by surgical resection via a lateral orbitotomy.

PERIPHERAL NERVE TUMOURS

Peripheral nerve tumours are mostly neurofibromas. Most orbital neurofibromas in adults are solitary and not associated with neurofibromatosis. Recurrence after surgical excision is unusual. Schwannomas are much less common and are encapsulated tumours which rarely recur after surgical excision.

MELANOCYTIC TUMOURS

Melanocytic tumours are mainly naevocellular naevi which are common in the skin of the eyelids and must be distinguished from pigmented basal cell and squamous cell lesions. Occasionally, a divided naevus is encountered which occupies the adjacent margins of both the upper and lower eyelid and which has arisen from a single naevus by separation of the eyelids in embryonic life (Hamming, 1983). Naevocellular naevi are best managed by infrequent observation. In oculodermal melanocytosis (naevus of Ota) there is widespread infiltration of the eyelid skin and of all ocular structures with plump melanocytes. The condition is most frequent in individuals of Asian and African extraction. Malignant change does not occur in the cutaneous element of naevus of Ota but, as well as being associated with an increased incidence of intra-ocular melanoma, it may very occasionally be linked with the development of a primary orbital melanoma. Benign conjunctival naevi are frequently cystic. They are easily excised and, bearing in mind that malignant change can occur, this option should be considered as an alternative to long-term follow-up.

LACRIMAL GLAND TUMOURS

These are usually of benign mixed-cell histology and are encapsulated. The whole affected lacrimal gland should be excised with the capsule intact via a lateral orbitotomy (Wright *et al.*, 1979). Incisional biopsy is contraindicated because recurrence is common if the capsule is ruptured and there is a significant chance of malignant change in the recurrent tumour.

Primary malignant tumours of the eye

By contrast with those of children, the vast majority of adult intra-ocular malignancies arise in the uveal tract and primary malignancies in the retina are very rare indeed.

MALIGNANT TUMOURS OF THE UVEAL TRACT

Malignant tumours of the uveal tract are mainly malignant melanomas. Uveal melanoma is the most common of all primary intra-ocular tumours. The neoplasm is most frequently encountered in the choroid but also arises in the ciliary body and occasionally in the iris. This tumour was formerly managed by enucleation of the eye. The survival rate following enucleation has been shown to be dependent on the size of the tumour, on the histological cell type, on its position within the eye, on the presence or absence of extrascleral extension and on the age of the patient. Large melanomas, ciliary-body melanomas and melanomas containing epithelioid cells or extending extrasclerally have a relatively bad prognosis, particularly in the elderly. For large tumours the overall mortality rate approaches 50 per cent (Shields, 1977) and the mean interval reported from treatment to the development of metastases is 43 months (Einhorn *et al.*, 1974). Metastases are rarely detectable at the time of diagnosis of the ocular primary, and it has been suggested that enucleation of the eye may in some way potentiate the development of widespread melanoma (Zimmerman *et al.*, 1978). This view is no longer widely held, but it has served to foster conservative management of ocular melanoma and the majority of eyes are no longer removed as the primary treatment of this tumour.

The treatment of choice depends mainly on the location of the tumour within the eye and on its size (Hungerford, 1993b, c). The diagnosis of an intra-ocular tumour is usually based entirely on clinical criteria, with an accuracy of almost 98 per cent (Char *et al.*, 1980) but fine-needle aspiration and cytology or formal biopsy through a scleral trapdoor incision may be considered in cases of doubt which cannot be resolved by a period of observation with serial photographs and ultrasound measurements of tumour size, looking for evidence of growth.

Iris melanomas are generally relatively benign spindle-cell lesions and overall mortality rates appear to be as low as 3 per cent. Most iris tumours can be managed by observation alone, with treatment reserved for those that are documented to grow or which are large at presentation. By contrast with their counterparts in the iris, melanomas of the choroid, and particularly those that develop in the ciliary body, are associated with particularly poor survival rates, of around 50 per cent at 5 years for larger lesions.

Three main methods of conservative treatment are available: photocoagulation, radiation and resection. Photocoagulation is applicable only to very small melanomas situated in the posterior choroid outside the macular arcades of vessels and not directly abutting the optic disc. Most of the reported experience has been obtained using xenon arc photocoagulation (François, 1982) but lately argon and krypton laser have been employed and the role of photosensitization with haematoporphyrin derivatives is being explored (Tse *et al.*, 1984). More recently still, hyperthermia using diode laser-generated infra-red radiation, so-called 'transpupillary thermotherapy', has been employed with good short-term results (Shields *et al.*, 1998). Photocoagulation and hyperthermia are not applicable to melanomas anteriorly located in the iris and ciliary body.

By contrast, local surgical resection is technically possible for some intra-ocular melanomas. Although easier to perform on small lesions arising anteriorly in the iris and ciliary body, the complication rate is higher than for tumours that develop posteriorly in the choroid and to which the method is most applicable (Foulds, 1983). The technique is limited to young, otherwise fit patients by the need for anaesthesia with profound hypotension while cutting the highly vascular choroid. Tumours up to 15 mm in diameter may be excised and overlying retinal detachment facilitates this operation. Local resection alone has a lower tumour control rate than plaque radiotherapy alone, so it is now advised that this operation should always be combined with adjuvant plaque therapy (Damato *et al.*, 1996). Radiotherapy has been by far the most widely used treatment modality for conservative therapy of intra-ocular melanomas and may be applicable to tumours in all locations within the uveal tract. Melanoma is a radioresistant neoplasm, whereas the lens of the eye and the choroid, retina and optic nerve are relatively radiosensitive structures. A radiation cataract can be safely removed but radiation choroidoretinopathy and optic neuropathy are not amenable to treatment. The risk of these side-effects increases at doses to the whole eye in excess of 50 Gy, whereas a tumour dose of between 80 and 120 Gy is required to regress uveal melanoma.

The treatment methods employed have depended on the difficulty of confining this high dose to the vicinity of the ocular tumour and of thereby limiting the dose to the adjacent retina, choroid and optic nerve. Until recently it has only been possible to preserve the healthy structures of the eye by brachytherapy techniques, employing radioactive applicators temporarily sutured to the surface of the sclera over the base of the tumour within the eye. After initial successes with radon (Stallard, 1949), the most widely used source was the cobalt-60 applicator, because the conveniently long half-life of this isotope allows the source to be reused many times and because it is simple to reactivate (Stallard, 1966; Bedford, 1973; MacFaul, 1977). The γ-rays emitted by cobalt-60 are of high energy and the external surface of the applicator cannot be effectively shielded. More recently, the low-energy β-ray-emitting ruthenium-106 and X-ray-emitting iodine-125 plaques used for retinoblastoma treatments (Fig. 16.7) have been

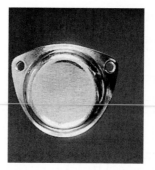
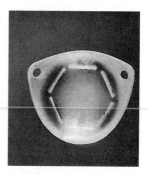

Figure 16.7 *Iodine-125 ophthalmic applicator currently in use at St Bartholomew's Hospital. Iodine-125 seeds are embedded in epoxy resin in a gold carrier.*

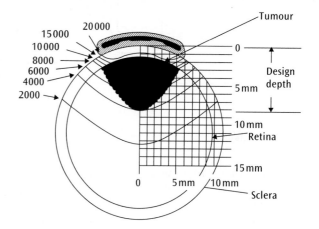

Dose distribution for CKA.3 (in cGy/6 days)

Figure 16.8 *Dose distribution plot of 10 mm cobalt-60 applicator.*

employed to treat ocular melanomas up to 5 or 8 mm thick, respectively (Lommatzsch, 1983; Packer, 1987). These plaques can be shielded, which allows them to be used to treat anterior melanomas without damage to the eyelids and lacrimal apparatus, as well as making them safer to handle. A dose of 80–120 Gy is prescribed at the apex of the tumour at a dose rate of at least 0.4 Gy per hour. Radiation-induced maculopathy and optic neuropathy limit the visual results of plaque therapy for tumours near the macula or optic disc. Because of the effects of the inverse square law, the dose received by the base of a neoplasm escalates substantially with increasing tumour thickness. Furthermore, the higher the dose at the base of the tumour, the larger is the area of surrounding choroid and retina which receives a dose in excess of the 50 Gy above which there is a significant risk of ischaemic damage to normal ocular structures (Fig. 16.8).

Over the last two decades, it has become possible to avoid this important limitation of radioactive scleral plaques. The special properties of positively charged particles give them an advantageous dose distribution. Not only is the dose uniform from base to apex of the tumour, but the Bragg peak effect means that the entry

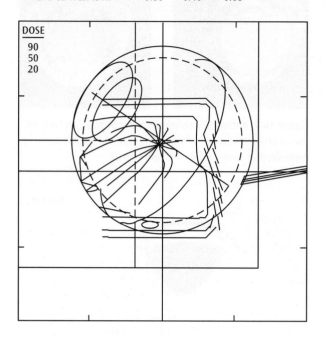

```
8411210          RIGHT EYE         8-SEP-84
PLANE WITHIN THE EYE
FIXATION LIGHT: POLAR 45 AZIMUTHAL 45 TWIST 0
EYE CENTER IS AT        0.50      0.40      0.00

DOSE
90
50
20
```

```
APERTURE IS: AP2
   RANGE: 1.60        RANGE MODULATION: 1.60
PLANE POSITION PARALLEL TO BEAM X- −0.7 Y-0.0 Z-0.0
```

Figure 16.9 *Computer-constructed plan for treatment by proton beam of an eye containing a malignant melanoma; 100%, 90% and 50% isodose plots are shown and demonstrate the Bragg peak effect.*

dose is reduced and that the beam is extinguished behind the treated volume (Fig. 16.9). Employing protons (Gragoudas *et al.*, 1977; Munzenrider *et al.*, 1988) or helium ions (Char and Castro, 1982) generated by a cyclotron, these properties have allowed a high dose prescription of 60–70 Gy in four or five fractions to be delivered to ocular melanomas over 4–5 days, with the 50 per cent isodose occurring within 2 mm of the tumour edge and with successful tumour regression. Survival rates have been comparable with those following enucleation (Seddon *et al.*, 1990). Although charged particles can be used to treat melanomas which are too close to the optic disc to apply a radioactive scleral plaque or too thick for plaque brachytherapy, the surface-sparing advantages of the Bragg peak are progressively lost with increasing modulation of beam to treat thicker and thicker tumours and with anterior location. Consequently, eyelid damage limits the benefits of charged particle therapy for larger and more anteriorly located melanomas. Moreover, treatment of larger tumours is not uncommonly followed by painful neovascular glaucoma, sometimes requiring enucleation (Foss *et al.*, 1997).

Gamma-knife stereotactic radiosurgery can also be used for the treatment of posterior uveal-tract melanomas (Zehetmayer *et al.*, 1995). The treatment is delivered in

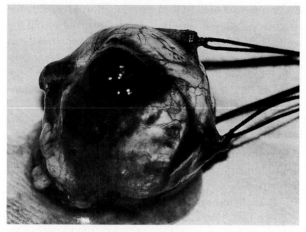

Figure 16.10 *Enucleated eye, showing an encapsulated nodular extrascleral extension of malignant melanoma.*

one or two fractions and this plainly contributes to the high rate of side-effects, which are not dissimilar to those of charged particle therapy. Nevertheless, easier access to this method compared with charged particles has lent it a certain popularity.

When appropriately selected for radiotherapy, more than 90 per cent of eyes can be retained (Wilson and Hungerford, 1999). The criteria of treatment success are shrinkage of the tumour or cessation of growth. Regression is slow and can continue episodically for 2 years or more. Melanomas less than 5 mm thick will often regress to a flat scar, but larger tumours will usually have some residual thickness when regression ceases.

Enucleation is advised for large melanomas measuring more than 1.5 cm³ in volume. Ciliary-body melanomas occupying more than one-third of the circumference of the globe are too large to manage by resection or plaque therapy and are also best treated by enucleation. Circumscribed nodular extrascleral extension may be managed by plaque therapy or by resection with a scleral graft, but extensive extrascleral spread is better treated by removal of the eye. The presence of extrascleral extension (Fig. 16.10) reduces the survival rate and significantly increases the risk of orbital recurrence (Starr and Zimmerman, 1962). Orbital exenteration following enucleation for extrascleral extension confers no survival advantage, and the risk of orbital recurrence can be substantially reduced without mutilation by postoperative orbital radiotherapy (Hykin *et al.*, 1990).

MALIGNANT TUMOURS OF THE RETINA

These are exceedingly uncommon. Cytologically malignant adenocarcinomas of the retinal pigment epithelium have been reported (Garner, 1973), although these lesions rarely, if ever, metastasize. They are pigmented and are usually a chance finding when an eye is removed for what is thought to be a malignant melanoma (Shields and Zimmerman, 1973). For this reason there are no data on whether or not they can be managed conservatively.

MALIGNANT LYMPHOMAS OF THE EYE

Malignant lymphomas are usually large-cell non-Hodgkin's tumours (Freeman *et al.*, 1987). They may present late in the course of a systemic lymphoma or they may be the initial manifestation of widespread lymphoma. They tend to affect elderly people, beginning in one eye and later affecting the other, and they have an insidious onset that is often confused with uveitis in the early stages. The more common variant affects predominantly the retina and vitreous. In this form of lymphoma the central nervous system may be involved. The rarer type affects the choroid and is associated with nodal and visceral lymphoma. The diagnosis is established by fine-needle biopsy and treatment is by chemotherapy (with high dose methotrexate and probably cytosine arabinoside) and then ocular radiotherapy.

SECONDARY DEPOSITS

Secondary deposits are usually seen in the uveal tract and only rarely in the retina, although choroidal metastases often present with a serous retinal detachment. The most common source of a choroidal metastasis is breast cancer. The ocular secondaries rarely present before the breast primary and the deposits are commonly multiple and bilateral. The second most common source is lung cancer. An ocular deposit is, more often than not, detected before the lung primary and is usually solitary and unilateral. The treatment of ocular metastases is palliative and mainly by radiotherapy, although it is legitimate to postpone irradiation and to watch for evidence of regression if the patient is to start chemotherapy, unless there is extensive retinal detachment.

Primary malignant tumours of the eyelids, conjunctiva and orbit

Like their benign counterparts, primary malignancies of the ocular adnexa are of epithelial, vascular, neurogenic, melanocytic or lacrimal gland origin.

MALIGNANT EPITHELIAL TUMOURS

These are relatively common. Basal cell carcinoma (BCC) is by far the most frequently encountered eyelid tumour, and the inner canthus is one of the most common sites for this neoplasm. The treatment of choice for eyelid BCCs depends on whether the tumour is of the nodular or morphoea type and on its size, location and the presence or absence of infiltration of underlying periosteum and bone. Small lesions may be treated effectively by liquid nitrogen cryotherapy. Cryotherapy or surgical excision is to be preferred for small BCCs on the upper eyelid, as radiotherapy may lead to keratinization of the eyelid margin and thereby to ocular discomfort from corneal epithelial abrasion. Very high cure rates can be obtained from surgical resection provided that complete excision is confirmed by frozen section at the time of surgery, especially for morphoea-type tumours. Extensive inner canthal lesions may be treated either by excision or by radiotherapy, although it is difficult to avoid epiphora with either approach. Radiotherapy is particularly suitable for tumours that have recurred after excision and for those tethered to the periosteum. Occasionally, orbital exenteration will be required for persistent or very extensive tumours.

Adenocarcinoma is the second most common primary eyelid malignancy and most examples are sebaceous carcinomas. The eyelid is copiously supplied with glandular structures and is a site of predilection for this neoplasm, which may also arise in sebaceous glands in the caruncle or eyebrow. The tumour tends to be multifocal, and pagetoid spread from the lid on to the bulbar conjunctiva is characteristic. Diagnosis is difficult and often delayed because the tumour is mistaken for a simple meibomian cyst or for chronic conjunctivitis or blepharitis. Persistent or recurrent meibomian cysts and chronic, indeterminate 'infections' of the conjunctiva and eyelid should therefore be subjected to biopsy. After melanoma it has the highest mortality rate of all eyelid cancers (Rao *et al.*, 1982) and is best managed by wide excision. Where the orbit is invaded, orbital exenteration is recommended and, although radiotherapy may be considered when an advanced sebaceous carcinoma involves the only good eye, this neoplasm is not very radiosensitive.

Invasive squamous carcinoma is rare in the eyelid (Aurora and Blodi, 1970), often arising in a focus of actinic keratosis. It may also arise in the conjunctiva, either *de novo* or in an area of pre-existing intraepithelial squamous carcinoma (Zimmerman, 1969). Surgical excision of eyelid lesions is to be preferred and block dissection may be added in the rare instances where regional lymph node spread occurs. Tethered lymph glands may be better treated by radiotherapy. Metastasis from an eyelid primary is uncommon and death very rare (Jakobiec *et al.*, 1979).

The mortality rate is similarly low for conjunctival primary epithelial tumours. Most are intra-epithelial, carcinoma *in situ* lesions that show a low propensity to develop into invasive carcinomas. The majority of these lesions are classified as 'conjunctival (or corneal) intra-epithelial neoplasia' or 'CIN' by ophthalmologists. They have indistinct margins and may be multifocal. Consequently, they show a strong tendency to recur after simple excision. The risk of recurrence may be reduced by adjuvant cryotherapy, although very persistent lesions are best managed by radiotherapy, particularly if there is any histopathological evidence of an invasive element. Radiotherapy for bulbar conjunctival lesions is best administered using a strontium-90 β-ray source. Recently, topical Mitomycin C therapy has been shown to be effective in the treatment of CIN that has recurred after surgery and for the primary treatment of some extensive, and therefore irresectable, *in situ* lesions. Mitomycin C therapy alone is not recommended for thick tumours or for invasive conjunctival carcinoma. Thick *in situ* lesions should first be debulked and Mitomycin C used in an adjuvant setting. Invasive tumours require wide excision.

MALIGNANT VASCULAR TUMOURS

Malignant vascular tumours may occur in the orbit but are uncommon. Haemangiopericytoma is a slow growing, encapsulated tumour (Jakobiec *et al.*, 1974). If the capsule is not breached during surgical removal, a total cure is usually effected. Postoperative radiotherapy may be indicated. Radiotherapy alone has not been shown to achieve sustained control of recurrent lesions (Jakobiec and Jones, 1979a) and recurrence should be managed by orbital exenteration. Malignant haemangioendothelioma is much less common. It is not encapsulated and local recurrence is likely after attempted surgical excision unless a wide margin of normal tissue is excised. Recurrence should be managed by orbital exenteration. There is a high mortality rate from distant spread (Stout, 1943).

MALIGNANT NEUROGENIC TUMOURS

Malignant neurogenic tumours of neural crest origin may arise *de novo* or may develop in a pre-existing benign tumour, particularly in association with neurofibromatosis. Malignant schwannoma (Grinberg and Levy, 1974) is an infiltrative tumour which tends to grow along neural channels and to present with pain. Local surgical excision is frequently followed by recurrence and orbital exenteration may be required. Persistent local recurrence may be managed by radiotherapy. Death may occur from direct intracranial extension or from distant metastases.

Most of the meningiomas seen in the orbit represent secondary orbital invasion by an intracranial tumour (Stern, 1973), but very occasionally a primary orbital meningioma may arise in the optic nerve sheath. Primary meningiomas of the orbit may be excised via a lateral orbitotomy and the local recurrence rate after this operation is much less than that following removal of an intracranial meningioma.

MALIGNANT MELANOCYTIC TUMOURS

Malignant melanocytic tumours are mostly melanomas. Their management is largely surgical (Hungerford, 1993b). Malignant melanoma of the eyelid skin is extremely rare and is best managed by wide surgical excision (Garner *et al.*, 1985; Collin *et al.*, 1986). Malignant melanoma is more common in the conjunctiva (Fig. 16.11), but nevertheless still rare. The majority of conjunctival melanomas arise in a pre-existing conjunctival lesion (Paridaens *et al.*, 1994a). Approximately 18 per cent of tumours arise in a pre-existing naevus and 57 per cent in primary acquired melanosis (PAM). Primary acquired melanosis was formerly termed precancerous melanosis and may be a manifestation of the atypical mole syndrome (Bataille *et al.*, 1993). Atypical melanocytes spread to involve much of

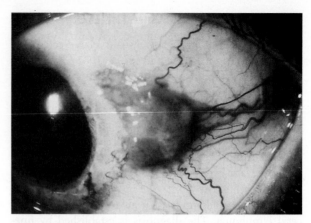

Figure 16.11 *Conjunctival malignant melanoma arising in primary acquired melanosis.*

the conjunctiva and on to the cornea (Paridaens *et al.*, 1992a) and eyelid (Robertson *et al.*, 1989a). Ultimately, melanoma develops in most cases of PAM in which atypia are found, as indicated by biopsy or by impression cytology (Paridaens *et al.*, 1992c), and in most cases multifocal tumours develop sequentially. Patients with PAM should have regular re-evaluation, looking for signs of a developing invasive melanoma. Cryotherapy is recommended to try to delay or prevent the onset of malignant change in PAM (Jakobiec *et al.*, 1988). This treatment should be directed towards the areas of acquired conjunctival pigmentation. Unfortunately the success of this approach is limited by the facts that most patients with PAM do not present until the first melanoma has developed and that in some instances the melanosis is not pigmented and is therefore invisible (Paridaens *et al.*, 1992b). Eyelid skin melanomas are also associated with PAM (Robertson *et al.*, 1989b) and the conjunctival involvement may not be apparent or may be unsuspected at the time the lid tumour is diagnosed (Hicks *et al.*, 1994).

Survival rates are excellent following surgical excision of solitary bulbar conjunctival tumours not associated with PAM. The local recurrence rate is low after simple excision of melanomas that do not involve the corneoscleral limbus and after en bloc lamellar corneoscleral dissection of those that do. Recurrence after incomplete excision may be reduced by adjuvant cryotherapy (Collin *et al.*, 1986) or by β-ray radiotherapy (Lederman *et al.*, 1984). It is more difficult to eradicate a melanoma arising in the palpebral conjunctiva, partly because adjunctive treatments are more difficult to apply in this location. Accordingly, survival rates are poorer for such tumours. Additionally, melanomas arising in this location are more often than not associated with PAM, and other interrelated prognostic factors apply (Paridaens *et al.*, 1994a). Tumours arising in unfavourable locations have 2.2 times the mortality of epibulbar melanomas. Unfavourable locations include the palpebral conjunctiva, the conjunctival fornices and the plica, caruncle and lid margin.

Histology is relevant and mixed-cell tumours have three times the mortality of spindle-cell lesions. Access to lymphatics may be the underlying reason why some locations are less favourable prognostically than others, and lymphatic invasion carries a fourfold increase in mortality rate. Multifocal and thick tumours attract a worse prognosis than solitary, thin ones. The various risk factors conspire to make conjunctival melanoma arising in PAM a much more serious disease than melanoma arising *de novo* or in a naevus.

Because of their poor outlook, melanomas arising in the eyelid, the conjunctival fornix and, particularly, in the caruncle have been managed by orbital exenteration. In a recent study the role of exenteration has been compared retrospectively in two groups of patients, one of which underwent the operation as the primary treatment of their disease while, in the other, conservative treatment was tried first, with exenteration reserved for palliative treatment (Paridaens *et al.*, 1994b). This second group of patients was not seen to be disadvantaged by prior conservative surgery in terms of survival. The key to survival appeared to be the thickness of the largest tumour rather than the treatment method, with overall melanoma-related mortality ranging between zero in tumours with a maximum thickness of 1 mm and 50 per cent in those in excess of 2 mm thick. A particularly poor outcome was noted for caruncular melanoma, with six out of seven patients dying despite primary exenteration. These results suggest that, where possible, a conservative approach should be tried first. Following exenteration, some patients have been documented to develop recurrences in the orbit, nasal passages and paranasal sinuses (Robertson *et al.*, 1989b; Paridaens *et al.*, 1992d).

Orbital recurrence is seen in large, neglected tumours and nasal recurrence in inner canthal lesions, probably because of implantation of tumour cells shed down the nasal passages. At St Bartholomew's Hospital, patients exenterated for large melanomas now receive adjunctive orbital radiotherapy, and those undergoing exenteration for inner canthal melanomas receive radiotherapy postoperatively to the ipsilateral nasal passages, in the hope of eliminating local recurrence.

MALIGNANT LACRIMAL GLAND TUMOURS

The most common malignant tumour of the lacrimal gland is adenocystic carcinoma. This tumour is not encapsulated and is locally invasive. There is a high mortality rate, with death usually resulting from direct intracranial extension. The tumour grows rapidly and the history of painful proptosis is short. The pain results from infiltration of neural channels. Radical resection may be performed if adenocystic carcinoma does not extend to the orbital apex and appears to be confined within the periosteum (Wright, 1985). Radiotherapy (and chemotherapy) may be considered for patients with primary or recurrent tumour that is locally extensive or metastatic.

MALIGNANT LYMPHOMAS OF THE ORBIT

The orbit may be the presenting site for generalized lymphoma or the primary site for subsequent dissemination (Wright, 1985; Jenkins *et al.*, 2000). The conjunctiva is commonly an extranodal primary site and, when this is so, these tumours are often of low grade and survival rates are good. Primary conjunctival lymphomas are now recognized as mucosal-associated lymphoid tissue (MALT) tumours, and this explains their frequent bilaterality (Hardman-Lea *et al.*, 1994). Almost all orbital lymphomas are of B-cell origin and Hodgkin's lymphoma is very rare in the orbit. Lymphocytic lymphoma is the most common tumour of the orbit, and well-differentiated variants may be very difficult to distinguish from benign reactive lymphoid hyperplasia, also common at this site (Morgan and Harry, 1978). Most patients presenting with poorly differentiated lymphocytic lymphoma in the orbit will have a short history and subsequently develop widespread disease. Biopsy is necessary and histologically malignant lymphocytic tumours are treated by fractionated radiotherapy (Foster *et al.*, 1971) (Fig. 16.12). Systemic staging investigations are mandatory except for elderly patients with a well-differentiated tumour. Chemotherapy is indicated for systemic involvement. Occasionally, orbital involvement is seen in association with systemic histiocytic lymphoma in middle-aged and elderly people (Jakobiec and Jones, 1979b).

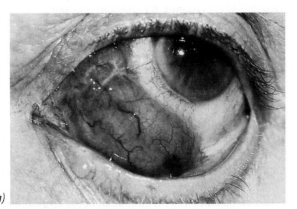
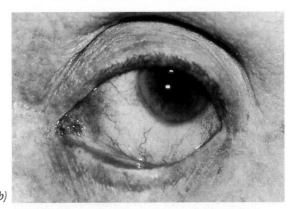

(a) *(b)*

Figure 16.12 *Subconjunctival deposit of lymphoma (a) before and (b) after treatment by fractionated radiotherapy.*

SECONDARY DEPOSITS

Secondary deposits are uncommon in the ocular adnexa in adults, although they may occasionally be seen in the orbit. Breast carcinoma is the most common primary source, although almost any tumour can spread to the orbit, including carcinoma of the lung, prostate, thyroid, gastrointestinal tract and bladder, and cutaneous or ocular. Most are treated by radiotherapy.

in which case the tumours are usually sequentially multifocal. Survival rates in conjunctival melanoma are generally better than those in the uveal tract variant of this tumour and can be maximized by a rigid policy of life long observation with a high index of suspicion and early treatment of potential new lesions.

SIGNIFICANT POINTS

- The modern treatment of tumours of the eye and ocular adnexa is still primarily surgical, but a multidisciplinary approach with radiotherapy or chemotherapy is increasingly employed, particularly for malignancies in childhood.
- Retinoblastoma has one of the highest survival rates of all childhood cancers, achieved mainly by adjuvant chemotherapy after enucleation for tumours with high risk histology. In the conservative treatment of retinoblastoma, focal methods and chemotherapy are currently preferred to external beam radiotherapy in order to reduce local morbidity and to minimize the chance of inducing other cancers in genetically susceptible children.
- Chemoreduction is still recommended for orbital rhabdomyosarcoma with high risk histology but it remains controversial whether it is permissible to eliminate either the alkylating agent or radiotherapy in tumours of favourable cell type.
- Both the choice of treatment and the life prognosis for uveal tract melanoma depend on the size and location of the tumour within the eye. Particularly if there is extensive retinal detachment or neovascular glaucoma, globes with large melanomas are still best enucleated, although mortality rates are relatively undiminished by aggressive treatment. Employing a variety of techniques, almost all eyes with smaller tumours, can be preserved with excellent cosmesis, often with good visual function, and with a fairly optimistic survival prospect.
- Most ocular adnexal melanomas arise in the conjunctiva. Almost all are associated with unilateral, premalignant, atypical melanosis

KEY REFERENCES

Hungerford, J.L. (1993) Uveal melanoma. *Eur. J. Cancer* **29**, 1365–8.

Hungerford, J.L. (1993) Surgical treatment of ocular melanoma. *Melanoma Res.* **3**, 305–12.

Hungerford, J.L., Plowman, P.N. and Kingston, J.E. (1992) Tumours of the eye and orbit. In Voute, P.A., Barrett, A. and Lemerie, J. (eds), *Cancer in children*. Berlin: Springer Verlag, 207–25.

Kingston, J.E. and Hungerford, J.L. (1992) Retinoblastoma. In Plowman, P.N. and Pinkerton, C.R. (eds), *Paediatric oncology. Clinical practice and controversies*. London: Chapman & Hall, 268–90.

REFERENCES

Abramson, D.H. and Ellsworth, R.M. (1982) Cryotherapy for retinoblastoma. *Arch. Ophthalmol.* **100**, 1253–6.

Abramson, D.H., Ellsworth, R.M., Kitchin, D. and Tung, G. (1984) Second monocular tumors in retinoblastoma survivors. Are they radiation induced? *Ophthalmology* **91**, 1351–5.

Anderson, S.R. (1962) Medulloepitheliomas of the retina. *Int. Ophthalmol. Clin.* **2**, 483–506.

Annesley, W.H., Leonard, B.C., Shields, J.A. and Tasman, W.S. (1977) Fifteen-year review of treated cases of retinal angiomatosis. *Trans. Am. Acad. Ophthalmol. Otolaryngol.* **83**, 446–53.

Arrigg, P.G., Hedges, T.R. and Char, D.H. (1983) Computed tomography in the diagnosis of retinoblastoma. *Br. J. Ophthalmol.* **67**, 588–91.

Aurora, A. and Blodi, F. (1970) Lesions of the eyelids: a clinicopathologic study. *Surv. Ophthalmol.* **15**, 94–104.

Bataille, V., Boyle, J., Hungerford, J.L. and Newton, J.A. (1993) Three cases of primary acquired melanosis of the conjunctiva as a manifestation of the atypical mole syndrome. *Br. J. Dermatol.* **128**, 86–90.

Bedford, M.A. (1973) The use and abuse of cobalt plaques in the treatment of choroidal malignant melanomata. *Trans. Ophthalmol. Soc. UK* **93**, 139–43.

Broughton, W.L. and Zimmerman, L.E. (1978) A clinicopathologic study of 56 cases of intraocular medulloepitheliomas. *Am. J. Ophthalmol.* **85**, 407–18.

Canning, C.R., McCartney, A.C.E. and Hungerford, J. (1988) Medulloepithelioma (Diktyoma). *Br. J. Ophthalmol.* **72**, 764–7.

Cavenee, W.K., Murphree, A.L., Shull, M.M. *et al.* (1986) Prediction of familial predisposition to retinoblastoma. *N. Engl. J. Med.* **314**, 1201–7.

Chan, H.S.L., DeBoer, G., Thiessen, J.J. *et al.* (1996) Combining cyclosporin with chemotherapy controls intraocular retinoblastoma without requiring radiation. *Clin. Cancer Res.* **2**,1499–508.

Char, D.H. and Castro, J.R. (1982) Helium ion therapy for choroidal melanoma. *Arch. Ophthalmol.* **100**, 935–8.

Char, D.H., Store, R.D., Irvine, I.R. *et al.* (1980) Diagnostic modalities in choroidal melanoma: sensitivity, specificity and reproducibility. *Am. J. Ophthalmol.* **89**, 223–30.

Chutorian, A.M., Schwartz, J.F., Evans, R.A. *et al.* (1964) Optic gliomas in children. *Neurology* **14**, 83–95.

Collin, J.R.O., Allen, L.H., Garner, A. and Hungerford, J.L. (1986) Malignant melanoma of the eyelid and conjunctiva. *Aust. N. Z. J. Ophthalmol.* **14**, 29–34.

Crowe, F.W. and Schull, W.J. (1953) The diagnostic importance of café au lait spot in neurofibromatosis. *Arch. Intern. Med.* **91**, 758–66.

Damato, B.E., Paul, J. and Foulds, W.S. (1996) Risk factors for residual and recurrent melanoma after trans-scleral local resection. *Br. J. Ophthalmol.* **80**, 102–8.

Draper, G.J., Sanders, B.M. and Kingston, J.E. (1986) Second primary neoplasms in patients with retinoblastoma. *Br. J. Cancer* **53**, 661–71.

Einhorn, L.H., Burgess, M.A. and Gottlieb, J.A. (1974) Metastatic patterns of choroidal melanoma. *Cancer* **34**, 1001–4.

Foote, R.L., Garretson, B.R., Schomberg, P.J. *et al.* (1989) External beam irradiation for retinoblastoma: patterns of failure and dose-response analysis. *Int. J. Radiat. Oncol. Biol. Phys.* **16**, 823–30.

Foss, A.J.E., Pecorella, I., Alexander, R.A. *et al.* (1994) Are most intraocular 'leiomyomas' really melanocytic lesions? *Ophthalmology* **101**, 919–24.

Foss, A.J., Whelahan, I., Hungerford, J.L. *et al.* (1997) Predictive factors for the development of rubeosis following proton beam radiotherapy for uveal melanoma. *Br. J. Ophthalmol.* **81**, 748–54.

Foster, S.C., Wilson, C.S. and Treffer, P.K. (1971) Radiotherapy of primary lymphomas of the orbit. *Am. J. Roentgen. Radiat. Ther. Nucl. Med.* **111**, 343–9.

Foulds, W.S. (1983) Current options in the management of choroidal melanoma. *Trans. Ophthalmol. Soc. UK* **103**, 28–34.

François, J. (1982) Treatment of malignant choroidal melanomas by photocoagulation. *Ophthalmologica* **184**, 121–30.

Freeman, L.N., Schachat, A.P., Knox, D.L. *et al.* (1987) Clinical features, laboratory investigations, and survival in ocular reticulum cell sarcoma. *Ophthalmology* **94**, 1631–9.

Friend, S.H., Bernard, R., Rogel, S. *et al.* (1986) A human DNA segment with properties of the gene that predisposes to retinoblastoma and osteosarcoma. *Nature* **323**, 643–6.

Ganley, J.P. and Comstock, G.W. (1973) Benign nevi and malignant melanomas of the choroid. *Am. J. Ophthalmol.* **76**, 19–25.

Garner, A. (1973) Pathology of 'pseudotumour' of the orbit: a review. *J. Clin. Pathol.* **26**, 639–48.

Garner, A., Koornneef, L., Levane, A. and Collin, J.R. (1985) Malignant melanoma of the eyelid skin: histopathology and behaviour. *Br. J. Ophthalmol.* **69**, 180–6.

Goble, R.R., McKenzie, J., Kingston, J.E. and Plowman, P.N. (1990) Orbital recurrence of retinoblastoma successfully treated by combined therapy. *Br. J. Ophthalmol.* **74**, 97–8.

Goldberg, M.F. and Koenig, S. (1971) Argon laser treatment of von Hippel–Lindau retinal angiomas. I. Clinical and angiographic findings. *Arch. Ophthalmol.* **92**, 12–15.

Goldberg, R.E., Pheasant, T.R. and Shields, J.A. (1979) Cavernous hemangioma of the retina: a four generation pedigree with neuro-oculocutaneous involvement and an example of bilateral retinal involvement. *Arch. Ophthalmol.* **97**, 2321–4.

Gonder, J.R., Shields, J.A., Albert, D.M. *et al.* (1982) Uveal malignant melanoma associated with ocular and oculodermal melanocytosis. *Ophthalmology* **89**, 953–60.

Gragoudas, E.S., Goitein, M., Koehler, A.M. *et al.* (1977) Proton irradiation of small choroidal malignant melanomas. *Am. J. Ophthalmol.* **83**, 665–73.

Green, W.R., Iliff, W.J. and Trotter, R.R. (1974) Malignant teratoid medulloepithelioma of the optic nerve. *Arch. Ophthalmol.* **91**, 451–4.

Grinberg, M. and Levy, N.S. (1974) Malignant neurilemmoma of the supraorbital nerve. *Am. J. Ophthalmol.* **78**, 489–92.

Hamming, N. (1983) Anatomy and embryology of the eyelid. Review with special reference to the development of divided nevi. *J. Pediatr. Dermatol.* **1**, 518.

Hardman-Lea, S., Kerr-Muir, M., Wotherspoon, A.C. *et al.* (1994) Mucosal-associated lymphoid tissue lymphoma of the conjunctiva. *Arch. Ophthalmol.* **112**, 1207–12.

Harnett, A.N. and Thomson, E. (1988) An iodine-125 plaque for radiotherapy of the eye: manufacture and dosimetric considerations. *Br. J. Radiol.* **61**, 835–8.

Harnett, A.N., Hungerford, J., Lambert, G. *et al.* (1987) Modern lateral external beam (lens sparing) radiotherapy for retinoblastoma. *Ophthal. Paediatr. Genet.* **8**, 53–61.

Harnett, A.N., Doughty, D., Hirst, A. *et al.* (1988) Radiotherapy in benign orbital disease, II. Ophthalmic Graves' disease and histiocytosis X. *Br. J. Ophthalmol.* **72**, 289–92.

Heyn, R., Ragab, A., Raney, R.B. Jr *et al.* (1986) Late effects of therapy in orbital rhabdomyosarcoma in children. *Cancer* **57**, 1738–43.

Hicks, C., Liu, C., Hiranandani, M. *et al.* (1994) Conjunctival melanoma after excision of a lentigo maligna melanoma in the ipsilateral eyelid skin. *Br. J. Ophthalmol.* **78**, 317–18.

Höpping, W. and Meyer-Schwickerath, G. (1964) Light coagulation treatment in retinoblastoma. In Boniuk, M. (ed.), *Ocular and adnexal tumors: new and controversial aspects.* St Louis: Mosby, 192–6.

Hungerford, J.L. (1990) Histogenesis of retinoblastoma. *Br. J. Ophthalmol.* **74**, 131–2.

Hungerford, J.L. (1993a) Factors influencing metastasis in retinoblastoma. *Br. J. Ophthalmol.* **77**, 541.

Hungerford, J.L. (1993b) Uveal melanoma. *Eur. J. Cancer* **29**, 1365–8.

Hungerford, J.L. (1993c) Surgical treatment of ocular melanoma. *Melanoma Res.* **3**, 305–12.

Hungerford, J.L., Kingston, J.E. and Plowman, P.N. (1987) Orbital recurrence of retinoblastoma. *Ophthal. Paediatr. Genet.* **8**, 63–8.

Hungerford, J.L., Plowman, P.N. and Kingston, J.E. (1992) Tumours of the eye and orbit. In Voute, P.A., Barrett, A. and Lemerle, J. (eds), *Cancer in children.* Berlin: Springer Verlag, 207–25.

Hykin, P.G., McCartney, A.C.E., Plowman, P.N. and Hungerford, J.L. (1990) Postenucleation orbital radiotherapy for the treatment of malignant melanoma of the choroid with extrascleral extension. *Br. J. Ophthalmol.* **74**, 36–9.

Innes, R.K. and Hoyt, W.F. (1986) Childhood chiasmal gliomas: update on the fate of the patients in the 1969 San Francisco study. *Br. J. Ophthalmol.* **70**, 179–82.

Jakobiec, F.A. and Jones, I.S. (1979a) Vascular tumors, malformations and degenerations. In Jones, I.S. and Jakobiec, F.A. (eds), *Diseases of the orbit.* Hagerstown: Harper and Row, 269–308.

Jakobiec, F.A. and Jones, I.S. (1979b) Lymphomatous, plasmacytic, histiocytic, and hematopoietic tumors. In Jones, I.S. and Jakobiec, F.A. (eds), *Diseases of the orbit.* Hagerstown: Harper and Row, 309–53.

Jakobiec, F.A., Howard, G.M., Jones, I.S. *et al.* (1974) Hemangiopericytoma of the orbit. *Am. J. Ophthalmol.* **78**, 816–34.

Jakobiec, F.A., Rootman, J. and Jones, I.S. (1979) Secondary and metastatic tumors of the orbit. In Jones, I.S. and Jakobiec, F.A. (eds), *Diseases of the orbit.* Hagerstown: Harper and Row, 503–6.

Jakobiec, F.A., Rini, F.J., Fraunfelder, F.T. and Brownstein, S. (1988) Cryotherapy for conjunctival primary acquired melanosis and malignant melanoma. *Ophthalmology* **95**, 1058–70.

Kingston, J.E. and Hungerford, J.L. (1992) Retinoblastoma. In Plowman, P.N. and Pinkerton, C.R. (eds), *Paediatric oncology. Clinical practice and controversies.* London: Chapman & Hall, 268–90.

Kingston, J.E., McElwain, T.J. and Malpas, J.S. (1984) Childhood rhabdomyosarcoma: experience of the Children's Solid Tumour Group. *Br. J. Cancer* **48**, 195–207.

Kingston, J.E., Plowman, P.N. and Hungerford, J.L. (1985) Ectopic intracranial retinoblastoma in childhood. *Br. J. Ophthalmol.* **69**, 742–8.

Kingston, J.E., Hungerford, J.L. and Plowman, P.N. (1987) Chemotherapy in metastatic retinoblastoma. *Ophthal. Paediatr. Genet.* **8**, 69–72.

Kingston, J.E., Hungerford, J.L., Madreperla, S.A. and Plowman, P.N. (1996) Results of combined chemotherapy and radiotherapy for advanced intraocular retinoblastoma. *Arch. Ophthalmol.* **114**, 1339–43.

Knudson, A.G. (1971) Mutation and cancer: statistical study of retinoblastoma. *Proc. Natl Acad. Sci.* **68**, 820–3.

Lederman, M., Wybar, K. and Busby, E. (1984) Malignant epibulbar melanoma: natural history and treatment by radiotherapy. *Br. J. Ophthalmol.* **68**, 605–17.

Lee, W.-H., Bookstein, R., Hong, F.D. *et al.* (1987) Human retinoblastoma susceptibility gene; cloning, identification and sequence. *Science* **235**, 1394–9.

Lloyd, L. (1973) Gliomas of the optic nerve and chiasm in childhood. *Trans. Am. Ophthalmol. Soc.* **72**, 488–535.

Lommatzsch, P. (1977) Beta-irradiation of retinoblastoma with 106Ru/106Rh applicators. *Mod. Probl. Ophthalmol.* **18**, 128–36.

Lommatzsch, P.K. (1983) P-irradiation of choroidal melanoma with 106Ru/106Rh applicators, 16 years' experience. *Arch. Ophthalmol.* **101**, 713–17.

MacFaul, P.A. (1977) Local radiotherapy in the treatment of malignant melanoma of the choroid. *Trans. Ophthalmol. Soc. UK* **97**, 421–7.

MacKay, C.J., Abramson, D.H. and Ellsworth, R.M. (1984) Metastatic patterns of retinoblastoma. *Arch. Ophthalmol.* **102**, 391–6.

Manschot, W.A. (1954) Primary tumours of the optic nerve in von Recklinghausen's disease. *Br. J. Ophthalmol.* **38**, 285–9.

Meyers, P.A. and Ghavimi, F. (1983) Secondary acute non-lymphocytic leukaemia (ANLL) following treatment of childhood rhabdomyosarcoma. *Abstracts of the Proceedings of the American Society of Clinical Oncology* **2**, 77.

Moore, A.T., Pritchard, J. and Taylor, D.S.I. (1985) Histiocytosis X: an ophthalmological review. *Br. J. Ophthalmol.* **69**, 7–14.

Morgan, G. and Harry, J. (1978) Lymphocytic tumours of indeterminate nature: a 5-year follow up of 98 conjunctival and orbital lesions. *Br. J. Ophthalmol.* **62**, 381–3.

Morris, A.T. and Garner, A. (1975) Medulloepithelioma involving the iris. *Br. J. Ophthalmol.* **59**, 276–8.

Mullaney, J. (1974) Primary malignant medulloepithelioma of the retinal stalk. *Am. J. Ophthalmol.* **77**, 499–504.

Munzenrider, J.E., Gragoudas, E.S., Seddon, J.M. *et al.* (1988) Conservative treatment of uveal melanoma: probability of eye retention after proton treatment. *Int. J. Radiat. Oncol. Biol. Phys.* **15**, 553–8.

Nevins, J.R. (1991) Transcriptional activation by viral regulatory proteins. *Trends Biol. Sci.* **16**, 435–9.

Olver, J.M., McCartney, A.C.E., Kingston, J. and Hungerford, J. (1991) Histological indicators of the prognosis for survival following enucleation for retinoblastoma. In Bornfeld, N., Gragoudas, E.S., Happing, W. *et al.* (eds), *Tumors of the eye.* Amsterdam: Kugler, 59–67.

Packer, S. (1987) Iodine-125 radiation of posterior uveal melanoma. *Ophthalmology* **94**, 1621–5.

Paridaens, A.D.A., Kirkness, C.M., Garner, A. and Hungerford, J.L. (1992a) Recurrent malignant melanoma of the corneal stroma: a case of 'black cornea'. *Br. J. Ophthalmol.* **76**, 444–6.

Paridaens, A.D.A., McCartney, A.C.E. and Hungerford, J.L. (1992b) Multifocal amelanotic conjunctival melanoma and acquired melanosis sine pigmento. *Br. J. Ophthalmol.* **76**, 163–5.

Paridaens, A.D.A., McCartney, A.C.E., Curling, O.M. *et al.* (1992c) Impression cytology of conjunctival melanosis and melanoma. *Br. J. Ophthalmol.* **76**, 198–201.

Paridaens, A.D.A., McCartney, A.C.E., Lavelle, R.J. and Hungerford, J.L. (1992d) Nasal and orbital recurrence of conjunctival melanoma 21 years after exenteration. *Br. J. Ophthalmol.* **76**, 369–71.

Paridaens, A.D.A., Minassian, D.C., McCartney, A.C.E. and Hungerford, J.L. (1994a) Prognostic factors in primary malignant melanoma of the conjunctiva: a clinicopathological study of 256 cases. *Br. J. Ophthalmol.* **78**, 252–9.

Paridaens, A.D.A., McCartney, A.C.E., Minassian, D.C. and Hungerford, J.L. (1994b) Orbital exenteration in 95 cases of conjunctival malignant melanoma. *Br. J. Ophthalmol.* **78**, 520–8.

Petersen, R.A., Friend, S.H. and Albert, D.M. (1987) Prolonged survival of a child with metastatic retinoblastoma. *J. Pediatr. Ophthalmol. Strabismus* **24**, 247–8.

Plowman, P.N. and Harnett, A.N. (1986) Radiotherapy in benign orbital disease, I. Complicated ocular and orbital angiomas. *Br. J. Ophthalmol.* **72**, 286–8.

Pratt, C.B. (1972) Management of malignant solid tumors in children. *Pediatr. Clin. North Am.* **19**, 1141–55.

Pratt, C.B., Meyer, D., Chenaille, P. and Crom, D.B. (1989) The use of bone marrow aspirations and lumbar punctures at the time of diagnosis of retinoblastoma. *J. Clin. Oncol.* **7**, 140–3.

Rao, N.A., Hidayat, A.A., McLean, I.W. and Zimmerman, L.E. (1982) Sebaceous carcinomas of the ocular adnexa: a clinicopathologic study of 104 cases with five-year follow-up data. *Hum. Pathol.* **13**, 113–22.

Reese, A.B. (1963) Glioma of the optic nerve, retina and orbit. In Reese, A.B. (ed.), *Tumors of the eye.* New York: Hoeber, 162–79.

Reese, A.B. and Ellsworth, R.M. (1963) The evaluation and current concept of retinoblastoma therapy. *Trans. Am. Acad. Ophthalmol. Otolaryngol.* **67**, 164–72.

Robertson, D.M., Hungerford, J.L. and McCartney, A.C.E. (1989a) Pigmentation of the eyelid margin accompanying conjunctival melanoma. *Am. J. Ophthalmol.* **108**, 435–9.

Robertson, D.M., Hungerford, J.L. and McCartney, A.C.E. (1989b) Malignant melanomas of the conjunctiva, nasal cavity, and paranasal sinuses. *Am. J. Ophthalmol.* **108**, 440–2.

Rush, J.A., Younge, B.R., Campbell, R.J. *et al.* (1982) Optic glioma: long term follow up of 85 histologically verified cases. *Ophthalmology* **89**, 1213–19.

Sagerman, R.H., Treffer, P. and Ellsworth, R.M. (1972) The treatment of orbital rhabdomyosarcoma of children with primary radiation therapy. *Am. J. Roentgen. Radiat. Ther. Nucl. Med.* **114**, 31–4.

Saleh, R.A., Gross, S., Cassano, W. and Gee, A. (1988) Metastatic retinoblastoma successfully treated with immunomagnetic purged autologous bone marrow transplantation. *Cancer* **62**, 2301–3.

Schipper, J. (1980) Retinoblastoma: a medical and experimental study. Thesis, University of Utrecht.

Schulman, J.A., Peyman, G.A., Mafee, M.F. *et al.* (1986) The use of magnetic resonance imaging in the evaluation of retinoblastoma. *J. Pediatr. Ophthalmol. Strabismus* **3**, 144–7.

Seddon, J.M., Gragoudas, E.S., Egan, K.M. *et al.* (1990) Relative survival rates after alternative therapies for uveal, melanoma. *Ophthalmology* **97**, 769–77.

Shields, J.A. (1977) Current approaches to the diagnosis and management of choroidal melanomas. *Surv. Ophthalmol.* **21**, 443–63.

Shields, J.A. and Zimmerman, L.E. (1973) Lesions simulating malignant melanoma of the posterior uvea. *Arch. Ophthalmol.* **89**, 466–71.

Shields, J.A., Parsons, H., Shields, C.L. and Giblin, M.E. (1989) The role of cryotherapy in the management of retinoblastoma. *Am. J. Ophthalmol.* **108**, 260–4.

Shields, J.A., Shields, C.L., Parsons, H. and Giblin, M.E. (1990) The role of photocoagulation in the management of retinoblastoma. *Arch. Ophthalmol.* **108**, 205–8.

Shields, C.L., Shields, J.A., Cater, J., Lois, N., Edelstein, C., Gündüz, K. and Mercado, G. (1998) Transpupillary thermotherapy for choroidal melanoma: tumour control and visual results in 100 consecutive cases. *Ophthalmology* **105**, 581–90.

Singh, A.D., Garway-Heath, D., Love, S. *et al.* (1993) Relationship of regression pattern to recurrence in retinoblastoma. *Br. J. Ophthalmol.* **77**, 12–16.

Stallard, H.B. (1949) A case of malignant melanoma of the choroid successfully treated by radon seeds. *Trans. Ophthalmol. Soc. UK* **69**, 293–7.

Stallard, H.B. (1966) Radiotherapy for malignant melanoma of the choroid. *Br. J. Ophthalmol.* **50**, 147–55.

Starr, H.J. and Zimmerman, L.E. (1962) Extrascleral extension and orbital recurrence of malignant melanoma of the choroid and ciliary body. *Int. Ophthalmol. Clin.* **2**, 369–84.

Stern, W.E. (1973) Meningiomas in the cranio-orbital junction. *J. Neurosurg.* **38**, 428–37.

Stevenson, K.E., Hungerford, J., Garner, A. (1989) Local extraocular extension of retinoblastoma following intraocular surgery. *Br. J. Ophthalmol.* **73**, 739–42.

Stout, A.P. (1943) Hemangio-endothelioma: a tumor of blood vessels featuring vascular endothelial cells. *Ann. Surg.* **118**, 445–64.

Sutow, W.W., Lindberg, R.D., Geban, E.A. *et al.* (1982) Three year relapse free survival rates in childhood rhabdomyosarcoma of the head and neck. *Cancer* **49**, 2217–21.

Tarlton, J.F. and Easty, D.L. (1990) The immunohistological characterisation of retinoblastoma related ocular tissue. *Br. J. Ophthalmol.* **74**, 144–9.

Taveras, J.M., Mount, L.A. and Wood, E.H. (1956) The value of radiation therapy in the management of glioma of the optic nerves and chiasm. *Radiology* **66**, 518–28.

Tse, D.T., Dutton, J.J., Weingeist, T.A. *et al.* (1984) Hematoporphyrin photoradiation therapy for intraocular and orbital malignant melanoma. *Arch. Ophthalmol.* **102**, 833–8.

White, V., Stevenson, K., Garner, A. and Hungerford, J. (1989) Mesectodermal leiomyoma of the ciliary body: case report. *Br. J. Ophthalmol.* **73**, 12–18.

Wilson, M.W. and Hungerford, J.L. (1999) Comparison of episcleral plaque and proton beam radiation therapy for the treatment of choroidal melanoma. *Ophthalmology* **106**, 1579–87.

Wright, J.E. (1985) Management of malignant orbital tumours. In Oosterhuis, J.A. (ed.), *Ophthalmic tumours*. Dordrecht: W. Junk, 229–39.

Wright, J.E., Stewart, W.B. and Krohel, G.B. (1979) Clinical presentation and management of lacrimal gland tumours. *Br. J. Ophthalmol.* **63**, 600–6.

Zehetmayer, M., Menapace, R., Kitz, K. and Ertl, A. (1995). Stereotatic radiosurgery for uveal melanoma. In Kogelnik, H.D. (ed.), *Progress in radio-oncology*. Bologna: Monduzzi, 451–4.

Zimmerman, L.E. (1969) The cancerous, precancerous, and pseudocancerous lesions of the cornea and conjunctiva. The Pocklington Memorial Lecture. In Ryeroft, P.V. (ed.), *Corneoplastic surgery*. New York: Pergamon Press, 547–55.

Zimmerman, L.E., McLean, I.W. and Foster, W.D. (1978) Does enucleation of the eye containing a malignant melanoma prevent or accelerate the dissemination of tumour cells? *Br. J. Ophthalmol.* **62**, 420–5.

17

Head and neck

ALASTAIR J. MUNRO, R. HUGH MACDOUGALL AND NICHOLAS D. STAFFORD

INTRODUCTION

The management of cancer of the head and neck has a reputation for being difficult. The factors contributing to the difficulties and problems involved in the management of head and neck cancer are summarized in Table 17.1. Many of the apparent difficulties can be resolved by realizing that the management of head and neck cancer follows the same basic principles that apply to the management of any tumour. Good communication between specialists is fundamental to the sound management of head and neck cancer. No individual specialist is omniscient: surgical and radiotherapeutic techniques are evolving rapidly, new drugs are being introduced for prevention and treatment of disease: the limitations of the past are no guide to the possibilities of the present. Decision making often involves careful appraisal of competing options: the welfare of the patient is the paramount concern. The defence of turf or the maintenance of reputation should be of no consequence. The key decision-maker should be the patient: it is, after all, the patients who, once they have been properly informed of the risks and advantages of the various options, are in the best position to make decisions that are right for them, as individuals. In order

Table 17.1 *Some of the factors contributing to complexity in the management of head and neck cancer*

The anatomy of the head and neck region is complicated. This is reflected in the number of primary tumour sites specified by the TNM system for staging head and neck cancer

There have been several revisions of the TNM system over the past 15 years

Tumours of apparently identical histological appearance may, according to their primary site of origin, behave very differently

The role of chemotherapy in head and neck cancer is poorly defined

For many tumours the decision between surgery and radiotherapy as definitive treatment is not clear cut

The close proximity of vulnerable normal structures to head and neck tumours means that both radiotherapy and surgery are technically demanding. A wide repertoire of techniques is required to treat these tumours effectively

The side-effects of the treatments available for head and neck cancer mean that effective palliative therapy is often difficult

Patients are often elderly, in poor physical condition, or have limited social support

Table 17.2 *Members of the multidisciplinary team required for the effective management of head and neck cancer*

Otorhinolaryngologist/head and neck surgeon
Oral and maxillofacial surgeon
Plastic and reconstructive surgeon
Oral surgeon
Clinical oncologist/radiotherapist
Diagnostic radiologist
Pathologist
Speech therapist
Prosthetist
Prosthodontist
Clinical nurse specialist (care of stoma, rehabilitation, supportive care)
Macmillan nurse (symptom control, palliative care)
Social worker/counsellor
Medical secretary/administrator

for patients to be adequately assessed and informed, it is essential that there be a multidisciplinary team characterized, not just by technical competence, but by open communication.

The easiest way to achieve the co-operation and the communication between various specialists involved in managing head and neck cancer is through combined clinics (Table 17.2). Such clinics require commitment and flexibility from those who participate – the surrender of autocracy involved in the process may not always suit the individual clinician but is undoubtedly in the patient's best interests. The recognition that the term 'clinician' embraces disciplines, such as nursing, radiography and speech therapy, other than surgery and medicine is an open acknowledgement of the importance of the team approach to managing cancer. The patient is always the most important member of the team.

ORGANIZATION OF SERVICES FOR PATIENTS WITH HEAD AND NECK CANCER

By their very nature and constitution, the multidisciplinary team and the combined clinic have to be based at a specialist centre. This immediately creates a problem: patients with head and neck cancer will not always present to large centres, they will present to local hospitals and they will not arrive neatly diagnosed and staged. In the UK each year otorhinolaryngologists see nearly 1 million patients, 50 000 of whom have change in their voice as a symptom. Fewer than 5 per cent of this 50 000 will have cancer: 48 000 patients with voice changes will not have cancer, they cannot all be referred to combined clinics for specialist assessment and opinion. Even a comparatively common head and neck cancer, laryngeal cancer, is rarely encountered in general practice. The average British GP will see one new patient with carcinoma of the larynx every 15 years or so.

The current model for delivering cancer care in the UK assumes that diagnosis will be made at a hospital near the patient's home but that patients will then need to travel to specialist centres for assessment and treatment. It is the ease which this transfer can take place which is crucial to the success of this model of care. One method is to have managed clinical networks, in which there are protocols and guidelines in place at district, regional and supra-regional levels. These are intended to ensure that, wherever possible, patients with a given problem are managed uniformly and that a high standard of care is not dependent upon a combination of serendipity and postcode.

Data on the interval between first symptom and specialist referral is, in the UK at least, encouraging: patients delayed a median of 4 weeks before consulting their family doctor and the majority of patients had been seen by a specialist within 12 weeks. This suggests that the initial phases of presentation and diagnosis are being managed effectively.

In spite of the theoretical advantages associated with management at a specialist centre, there is little actual proof that referral to a specialist centre influences outcome. Given the technical demands of surgery and radiotherapy for potentially curable patients with advanced disease, it would be surprising if experience and technical aptitude counted for naught. However, these patients are a small subset of all patients with head and neck cancer and so it would be difficult to design a study with sufficient statistical power to show an overall survival difference. Average improvements from specialist referral will be hard to prove and are largely irrelevant: it is failures at an individual level that are important (the 'if one sparrow falls' argument). When non-specialist services are examined, then some strange facts emerge. One-third of non-academically based oncologists in the United States used induction chemotherapy for head and neck cancer primarily in a desire to 'maintain spirit of multidisciplinary care'. This is a very suburban reason for prescribing toxic, and somewhat ineffective, treatment: an oncological version of keeping up with the neighbours.

INCIDENCE

Just over 800 patients are diagnosed with cancer of the head and neck in Scotland each year (data from Information and Statistics Division (ISD), NHS in Scotland). The majority are tumours of the larynx or tumours of the oral cavity. Males outnumber females by 2 to 1. Cancers of the head and neck are the sixth most common tumour in men, and the thirteenth most common in women. The lifetime risk for developing cancer of the head and neck before the age of 74 is 2.0 per cent for men and 0.6 per cent for women. Nearly 350 people die in Scotland each year from head and neck cancer. At any one time there are 4000 people who are living with head and neck cancer, or the consequences of its treatment. Extrapolating this figure to the UK as a whole produces a total of over 45 000 people – enough to fill a large football stadium.

Recent trends

There has been a steady increase in the incidence of head and neck cancer in Scotland between 1980 and 1995: from 650 registrations per annum in 1980 to the current figure of around 800. The standardized incidence rates (Fig. 17.1) suggest that the increase in numbers is mainly due to changes in the size and age structure of the population. The incidence of head and neck cancer is related to social deprivation (Fig. 17.2a) and there has been a rise in head and neck cancer in the most deprived sections of the community (Fig. 17.2b).

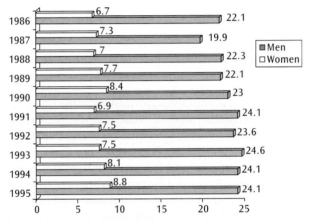

Figure 17.1 *Incidence per 100 000 population per annum of head and neck cancer in Scotland during the period 1986–95 (data from Information and Statistics Division, NHS in Scotland).*

These data clearly point to the social and environmental origins of head and neck cancer: as the rich become richer and the poor become poorer, then these social changes have a measurable impact upon those cancers where incidence is related to personal behaviours associated with social deprivation. This has important implications for any programmes aimed at cancer prevention. Someone whose existence is fairly miserable, whose quality of life is eroded by social deprivation, and with no prospect of improving their lot, is unlikely to be swayed by arguments involving the foreswearing of pleasures that are immediate, and actual, for gains that are both deferred and theoretical.

Head and neck cancer is a global problem

Head and neck cancer is an important problem in the developing world. As tobacco companies move into what is, for them, the lucrative market of the developing nations, then the harvest of their salesmanship will be an ever-increasing number of head and neck tumours in those nations who can least afford to treat them. A recent estimate suggests that a third of Chinese males currently under 29 years old will die from smoking-related illness: this corresponds to a total of 100 million premature deaths. The 1990 Globocan estimates provide a baseline assessment for head and neck cancer, a problem which, with time, will only get worse (Table 17.3).

It is a measure of the rapidity of world population growth and the impact of head and neck cancer in the developing world that the total of around 500 000 cases in 1990 is now surpassed by the estimate of 900 000 new cases in 1995. There are wide geographical variations in the standardized incidence rates for specific types of head and neck cancer. One of the poorest countries in the

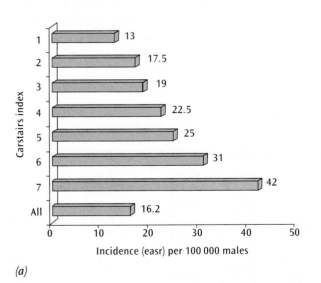

(a)

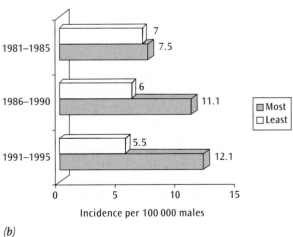

(b)

Figure 17.2 *(a) Incidence of head and neck cancer according to Carstairs category of social deprivation (7 is most deprived, 1 is least deprived). easr, European Age Standardized Rate. (b) Change in head and neck cancer according to social deprivation during the period 1981–95. (Data from Information and Statistics Division, NHS in Scotland.)*

world, Bangladesh, has some of the highest incidence rates for head and neck tumours. These wide differences provide important clues concerning the causes of head and neck cancer and the role of genetic susceptibility to the development of cancer (Table 17.4).

The distribution of nasopharyngeal cancer (NPC) is a case in point. The highest incidence occurs in Hong Kong and South-East Asia, with world age-standardized rates per 100 000 men of 25.2 (Hong Kong), 15.8 (Singapore) and 13.4 (Malaysia). The incidence is also high in parts of North Africa (10.9 in Tunisia) and this is, both clinically and epidemiologically, a distinct form of the disease. This, because of the colonial links with France, in turn affects the clinical features of NPC as it presents to some French hospitals. The practical point is that experience obtained in Hong Kong does not necessarily translate into appropriate guidelines for patients being treated in Paris. The reverse is also true.

Another feature of the global epidemiology of head and neck cancer is the emerging problem of laryngeal cancer in the countries of the former Eastern bloc.

Standardized rates per 100 000 men are approximately triple those observed in the UK (4.8): Ukraine (12.5); Russian federation (12.5); Croatia (13.2); Poland (12.1); Bosnia-Herzegovina (12.6). Worldwide, these rates are only exceeded by the figures for France (15.3), Spain (14.2) and Bangladesh (16.0).

Even within Europe and the developed world there are, on a regional basis, wide variations in the incidence of particular types of head and neck cancer. These differences are particularly marked for men: suggesting that many of the tumours in men might, potentially at least, be preventable.

The astonishingly high incidence in the Bas-Rhin region of France (Fig. 17.3) has usually been attributed to excessive consumption of the apple brandy (Calvados) that is the characteristic *digestif* of the region. The combination with heavy smoking appears to be a particularly potent carcinogenic stimulus to the hypopharynx and oesophagus.

OUTCOME

The statement is often made, particularly in the US literature, and particularly when defending the role of a new and expensive intervention, that survival has changed little over the past 30 years. The two Eurocare studies show that in Europe the 5-year survival for men with laryngeal cancer improved from 56 per cent for patients diagnosed between 1978 and 1985 to 63 per cent for men diagnosed between 1985 and 1989: an absolute improvement of 7 per cent, a relative improvement of 13 per cent. The corresponding survival figures for patients with tumours of the oral cavity and pharynx were 29 per cent (1978–85) and 34 per cent (1985–89): an absolute improvement of 5 per cent, a relative improvement of 16 per cent. Recent Scottish data are similarly encouraging: 5-year survival was 34.6 per cent for men and 42.5 per cent for women between 1978 and 1985; the corresponding figures for 1988–92 were 48.3 per cent (men) and 53.3 per cent (women).

Table 17.3 *Globocan data on absolute numbers (worldwide) of deaths from head and neck cancer by site (1990 estimates)*

Site	Deaths	ASR
Oral cavity, m	65939	3.14
Oral cavity, f	34096	1.42
Nasopharynx, m	24292	1.11
Nasopharynx, f	10788	0.44
Pharynx, m	49992	2.39
Pharynx, f	11565	0.48
Larynx, m	64598	3.12
Larynx, f	8934	0.37
Total head and neck cancers	270204	
Lung, m	692753	33.73
Lung, f	228441	9.23

Numbers and rates for lung cancer are included for comparative purposes. ASR, age-standardized rate; f, female; m, male.

Table 17.4 *Incidence of head and neck cancers according to economic development (worldwide data, Globocan, 1990)*

Site	World	Rate	Developed	Rate	Less developed	Rate
Oral cavity, m	140860	6.63	57456	8.42	83386	5.82
Oral cavity, f	70135	2.89	21162	2.25	48972	3.25
Nasopharynx, m	39701	1.77	4078	0.62	35628	2.28
Nasopharynx, f	17659	0.72	1638	0.2	16019	0.99
Pharynx, m	76645	3.64	30031	4.47	46601	3.34
Pharynx, f	17335	0.72	5270	0.59	12068	0.8
Larynx, m	118380	5.69	58079	8.48	60279	4.4
Larynx, f	17282	0.72	6556	0.72	10733	0.73
Total	497997		184270		313686	

f, female; m, male.

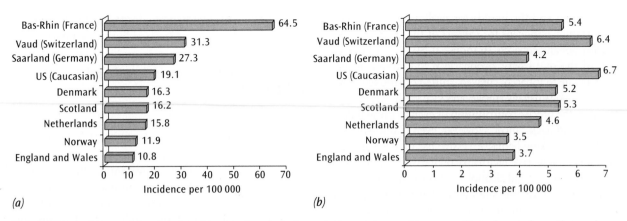

(a)   *(b)*

Figure 17.3 *Incidence of head and neck cancer in selected populations; (a) men; (b) women. (Data from Information and Statistics Division, NHS in Scotland.)*

Table 17.5 *Five-year survival (%) for patients with tumours of the oral cavity and pharynx diagnosed between 1985 and 1989 (data from Eurocare study)*

	Men	**Women**	**Ratio**
Europe	34	48	0.71
Poland	20	30	0.67
Italy	35	46	0.76
France	32	57	0.56
Estonia	17	15	1.13
Germany	37	45	0.82
Denmark	33	47	0.70
Scotland	35	44	0.80
England	37	46	0.80
Finland	35	54	0.65
Netherlands	47	46	1.02

Table 17.6 *Environmental factors implicated in the cause of head and neck cancer*

Alcohol	Oral cavity
	Pharynx
	Oesophagus
	Larynx
Tobacco	Oral cavity
	Pharynx
	Oesophagus
	Larynx
Betel nut/Pan masala (a complex mixture of areca nut, tobacco, lime, cardamom, etc.)	Oral cavity
Thorium dioxide	Paranasal sinuses
Radiotherapy for ringworm	Parotid
	Skin
Chromium dust/fumes	Nasal cavity and sinuses
Leather working	Nasal cavity and sinuses
Nickel dust/fumes	Nasal cavity and sinuses
Wood dust (e.g. beech)	Nasal cavity and sinuses
Iron deficiency	Post-cricoid carcinoma
Salt fish	Nasopharynx
HIV infection	Oral cavity
	Oropharynx

The data on survival for men compared with that for women are interesting (Table 17.5). Looking at the data for tumours of the oral cavity and pharynx, the men have, with two exceptions, survival rates about 70 per cent of those enjoyed by women. The two exceptions are the two countries at the extremes of the variation: which could be interpreted to mean that you can't get much worse than Estonia and you can't get much better than The Netherlands. In other words, there are potentially remediable factors in the other countries, the correction of which might bring survival for men closer to that observed for women.

These data also show considerable survival differences between countries. It is often assumed that countries with poorer survival provide a lower standard of care than countries with higher survival rates. This may occasionally be the case but, particularly for head and neck cancer, other factors will also be important. Social and behavioural factors will not only affect incidence, they will affect survival. These factors are often beyond the control of even the most technically efficient services providing care for patients with cancer. The solutions to many of these disparities in outcome will be economic and social rather than medical and technological.

AETIOLOGY

The current belief is that cancers arise as a result of the interaction between the outside world and an inherent, genetically based, susceptibility. The fact that genetic factors may be important is indicated by the finding that first-degree relatives of patients with head and neck cancer have a risk of head and neck cancer that is 3.5 times that of the general population. Environmental factors are, however, particularly important in the aetiology of cancers of the head and neck (Table 17.6). This is hardly surprising since our interactions with the environment largely occur by way of the structures within this region. Our noses sniff the air we breathe, our mouths taste the food we eat and the liquids we swallow. The two most important carcinogens for cancers of the head and neck are alcohol and tobacco. In India, 70–80 per cent of cancers of the oral cavity, oropharynx and larynx in men may be due to tobacco: chewed, sniffed or smoked. Since heavy drinkers usually smoke, and vice versa, it is difficult to assess the precise contribution of each to the aetiology of head and neck cancer. However, even if adjustment is made for smoking habits, excessive use of alcohol is still an independent risk factor, particularly for pharyngeal tumours. Tobacco and alcohol function as co-carcinogens, and so the effect of both smoking and drinking is approximately 2.5 times greater than simply adding the risks from each.

Tobacco and cancer of the head and neck

It has been estimated that, in the European Community (EC), between 33 and 44 per cent of deaths from cancer in men are due to smoking and/or alcohol. The higher figure is the UK estimate, the lower figure is the Danish estimate (IARC rep 107), the estimate for the EC as a whole is 39 per cent. Data from the Yorkshire Cancer Registry show that the absolute number of head and neck cancers which can be attributed to smoking is increasing: in men, from 190 per annum in the 1960s to 260 per annum in the 1990s; in women, from 65 per annum in the 1960s to 100 per annum in the 1990s. The current data suggest that 48 per cent of the tumours in men, and 35 per cent of the tumours in women are related to smoking. These figures are based on the Yorkshire population of 3.6 million. Extrapolating to the UK as a whole, these data suggest that, each year, approximately 5500 people develop cancers of the head and neck that can be attributed to smoking and that, since the 1960s, this figure has risen from 3900.

Dietary factors and cancer of the head and neck

The role of dietary factors in the causation of head and neck cancer is uncertain. There are reasonable theoretical grounds for thinking that vitamin A, retinoids and beta-carotene might be important in protecting against carcinogenesis in the epithelium of the upper aerodigestive tract. Dietary investigations in epidemiology, particularly those that are retrospective, are difficult: our eating habits change and recall is imperfect. There are nevertheless some data to suggest that people whose diets contain low levels of beta-carotene, vitamin A or vitamin C might be at increased risk of developing cancer of the head and neck. Other dietary factors that may help prevent cancers of the head and neck include genistein (from soya beans) and curcumin (in curry).

Dietary nitrosamines may also be important in the epidemiology of cancer of the head and neck. The consumption of smoked and salted fish, rich in carcinogenic nitrosamines, may be associated with a high incidence of head and neck cancers in parts of South-East Asia.

Occupational factors in head and neck cancer

Occupational exposure is an important aetiological factor in the development of cancer in the head and neck. The relationship between adenocarcinoma of the nose and para-nasal sinuses and employment in the furniture-making industry is well known. The associations between asbestos exposure and carcinoma of the larynx, between nickel refining and squamous carcinoma of the nose and para-nasal sinuses, and between work with vulcanization processes and carcinoma of the larynx are less well appreciated.

Viruses in head and neck cancer

Three main viruses have been associated with head and neck cancer: human papillomavirus (HPV), herpes simplex virus (HSV) and Epstein–Barr virus (EBV) (Table 17.7).

HPV may be associated with tumours of the oral cavity, tonsil and larynx. Using the polymerase chain reaction (PCR), between 15 and 35 per cent of squamous carcinomas of the head and neck can be shown to contain HPV sequences. The most common HPV is type 16 although other types (18, 33 and 31) are occasionally associated. A recent study of 248 tumours showed no relation between the presence of HPV sequences and T stage, tobacco use, race, gender, age or nodal status. There was, however, a relationship with tumour site: HPV was particularly frequent (56 per cent) in tumours of the oropharynx and less commonly found in tumours of the oral cavity (15 per cent) and larynx (17 per cent). The role of HPV in carcinogenesis is complex and is mediated by oncoproteins

Table 17.7 *Viruses associated with malignant and pre-malignant conditions involving the head and neck*

Epstein–Barr virus (EBV)
   Oral hairy leukoplakia
   Lymphomas
   Nasopharyngeal carcinoma

Human herpesvirus 8 (HHV8)
   Lymphoproliferative disorders
   Kaposi's sarcoma

Human herpesvirus 6 (HHV6)
   Squamous carcinoma
   Lymphomas

Human papilloma virus (HPV)
   Papillomas: larynx, oral cavity, etc.
   Epithelial dysplasia
   Squamous carcinomas

E6 and E7 which are produced by virally transformed cells within the epithelium. These oncoproteins, both of which possess a zinc-binding motif, inhibit the function of tumour-suppressor genes such as p53 and the Rb gene. The E7 protein may also have a more direct effect on the cell cycle by increasing the activity of cyclin A and E. The effect is to abolish the G_1–S transition checkpoint. These functional abnormalities correlate with histological evidence of premalignant change. Further abnormalities, loss of the viral regulatory proteins E1 and E2, together with acquired mutations (especially on chromosome 3), correlate with the appearance of invasive squamous carcinoma.

There is a clear association between EBV and nasopharyngeal carcinoma (NPC) but the mechanism, if any, whereby the virus causes the tumour is unclear. As with HPV, the infection may be associated with loss of function of tumour suppressor genes. The characteristic serological abnormalities can be used in screening for NPC. There are increases in antibodies to the viral capsid antigen (VCA), to the early antigen (EA) and to EBNA (Epstein–Barr nuclear antigen). There are also antibodies to the EBV transactivator (ZEBRA).

Herpes simplex virus, by increasing expression and activation of pre-existing oncogenes, may act as a cofactor in the development of squamous carcinomas.

THE PROBLEM OF SECOND PRIMARY TUMOURS IN HEAD AND NECK CANCER

There are defined criteria which need to be fulfilled before a cancer of the head and neck can be classified as a second primary, rather than simply a recurrence of the original tumour:

1 It must be more than 3 years since eradication of the original tumour, or the new tumour must be separated from the original tumour by at least 2 cm of normal epithelium.
2 If the second tumour is in the lung, then it should be solitary and, if less than 3 years from the time of diagnosis of the original tumour, the histological appearance should be different.

Field cancerization, a concept introduced by Slaughter in 1953, imposes a major constraint on the successful treatment of head and neck cancer. Slaughter's idea was that patients who developed head and neck cancer did so because the mucosal lining of the upper aerodigestive tract had become unstable. This instability represents the outcome, for that particular individual, of the interplay between environment and heredity. Comparison of *p53* mutations between the primary tumours and the second tumours suggests that the second tumours are genetically distinct from the original tumour. This supports the concept of environmental carcinogens, such as tobacco, acting

upon a vulnerable target – the mucosa of the aerodigestive tract in susceptible individuals.

Following successful treatment of a primary cancer of the head and neck, the risk of developing a second malignancy is relatively constant, at between 4 and 6 per cent per annum. Overall, 10–30 per cent of patients will develop second malignancy. The majority of these second tumours occur in the head and neck, lung or oesophagus, and, once a second tumour has developed, long-term survival is unlikely. Only 10 per cent of such patients survive for 5 years.

Screening routinely for new primary tumours at each follow-up visit may detect second primaries early but it will not prevent them. A policy of annual panendoscopy under general anaesthetic might detect second tumours at an even earlier stage, but compliance is likely to be poor. Annual chest X-ray may be worthwhile, but has not, in terms of its cost-effectiveness, been rigorously evaluated.

STRATEGIES FOR THE PREVENTION OF HEAD AND NECK CANCER

These can be divided into primary prevention, in which the aim is to prevent individuals developing head and neck cancer in the first place, and secondary prevention, in which the goal is to prevent further primary tumours in patients who have already had head and neck cancer.

Primary prevention

Given that, in the UK, almost half of the head and neck cancers in men, and over one-third of those in women, are caused by tobacco, there is one obvious strategy: encourage people not to smoke. However, as with many cancer-prevention programmes, the most vulnerable population is that which is hardest to reach: particularly if the persuasive strategies are based upon cosy middle-class values as opposed to any attempt to understand what it might actually feel like to be poor, unemployed and without any hope of socio-economic improvement.

There is an enormous literature on interventions designed to encourage people to give up smoking: there are several Cochrane reviews of the various methods that have been employed. The results of some of these interventions are summarized in Table 17.8. Even simply posting a self-help manual appears to be of some slight, but measurable, benefit. The Scottish telephone helpline (Smokeline), in its first year of operation helped an estimated 1.5 per cent of Scottish smokers to quit: a total of between 16 700 and 22 350 adults. Recidivism is an issue, how many of those not smoking at 6 months are still abstaining 2 years or more beyond the intervention?

Interventions designed to stop people smoking are amongst the most cost-effective measures in the whole of healthcare (Table 17.9). Simple advice at a routine clinic

Table 17.8 *Summary of some interventions intended to help patients stop smoking (data from Cochrane library, December 1999)*

General intervention	Specific type	Number of studies	Effect	Result
Nicotine replacement therapy (Silagy *et al.*)	All	91	Abstinence for ⩾6 m	OR 1.72 (1.60–1.84)
	Gum	49	Abstinence for ⩾6 m	OR 1.63
	Patches	32	Abstinence for ⩾6 m	OR 1.77
	Nasal spray	4	Abstinence for ⩾6 m	OR 2.27
	Inhaled	4	Abstinence for ⩾6 m	OR 2.08
	Sublingual	2	Abstinence for ⩾6 m	OR 1.73
	All		Rate difference	7% (17% Rx versus 10% controls)
			NNT	14
Physician advice (Silagy and Ketteridge)	Brief	16	Abstinence for ⩾6 m	OR 1.69 (1.45–1.98)
			Rate difference	2.5%
			NNT	40
Nursing interventions (Rice and Stead)	All	15	Abstinence for ⩾6 m	OR 1.43 (1.24–1.66)
	High intensity	10	Abstinence for ⩾6 m	OR 1.39 (1.19–1.64)
	Low intensity	5	Abstinence for ⩾6 m	OR 1.67 (1.14–2.45)
Self-help (Lancaster and Stead)	No personal contact	7	Abstinence for ⩾6 m	OR 1.23 (1.01–1.51)

OR, Odds ratio (with 95% confidence interval); NNT, number needed to treat; Rx, intervention.

Table 17.9 *Cost effectiveness of interventions intended to save lives*

Intervention	Cost per life year (1993 US$)
Nicotine gum plus smoking cessation advice, men aged 35–69	7 500
Nicotine gum plus smoking cessation advice, women aged 35–69	11 000
Smoking advice for pregnant women who smoke	0
Chemotherapy for adult non-ALL	27 000
Captopril for 35–64-year-olds with no cardiac disease, diastolic blood pressure >95 mmHg	93 000
Beta-blocker for 35–64-year-olds with no cardiac disease, diastolic blood pressure >95 mmHg	14 000
Haemoccult screening for colorectal cancer in asymptomatic 55-year-olds	1 300
Annual mammography plus breast exam, women 40–49	62 000
Postoperative adjuvant chemotherapy for premenopausal breast cancer	18 000
Compulsory annual motor vehicle inspection	20 000

ALL, acute lymphoblastic leukaemia.

or GP visit will persuade 2 per cent of smokers to give up for at least a year, at a cost of US$1500 per life year saved. This has to be set against the medical costs associated with smoking. In the USA it has been estimated that between 6 and 8 per cent of personal health expenditure, about $50 000 million in 1993 US dollars is spent on smoking-related illness.

Secondary prevention

Given the known carcinogenic effects of tobacco and alcohol, and given the concept of field cancerization, it would seem sensible to advise patients treated radically for early tumours of the head and neck to stop smoking and to cut down on their alcohol intake. Unfortunately there is no direct proof that these measures have any immediate beneficial effect.

Chemoprevention is a potentially useful strategy for preventing further tumours in patients with head and neck cancer. Chemopreventative agents are summarized in Table 17.10. Retinoids interact with specific nuclear retinoic acid receptors (RARs). The RARs function as ligand-dependent transcription factors. There are several subtypes of receptor, the most important being designated α, β and γ. The retinoid X-receptor (RXR), again with α, β and γ subtypes, is another crucial constituent of this system. Clinical and laboratory evidence suggests that it is the interaction with the β-receptor which is particularly important in growth inhibition. If insufficient

Table 17.10 *Agents used in the treatment of premalignant conditions and in the chemoprevention of squamous carcinoma of the head and neck*

Class	Action	Drugs	Acute toxicity	Chronic toxicity
Retinoids	Bind to nuclear receptors and, by transactivation, modulate gene expression; promote differentiation; anti-angiogenic	Vitamin A = retinol Tretinoin	Dry skin Desquamation	Liver damage Bone remodelling
		Etretinate (Tigason) 13-*cis*-retinoic acid (Roaccutane) 4-Fenretinide (HPR) 9-*cis*-retinoic acid: binds only to RXR All-*trans*-retinoic acid: binds to RAR and RXR	Dry eye Dry mucosa Hyper-triglyceridaemia Arthralgia Myalgia Bone tenderness Raised ICP	Skin erythema Teratogenic
Carotenoids	20% converted to vitamin A; ? independent protection via the remaining 80% through inactivation of free radicals	Beta-carotene		Yellow skin
Interferon	Anti-angiogenic; immune stimulation	Interferon-α	Flu-like syndrome Abnormal liver function tests Myalgia	
Tocopherols	Inactivation of nitrate carcinogens (e.g. nitrosodimethylamine); inactivation of free radicals (anti-oxidant effect)	Vitamin E		Antagonizes vitamin K, causing prolonged PT
N-Acetylcysteine	Scavenges free radicals (intracellular glutathione precursor); anti-oxidant: detoxifies carcinogens extracellularly and intracellularly; inhibits formation of DNA adducts by carcinogenic metabolites; lowers the rate of mutation – both acquired and spontaneous	*N*-Acetylcysteine	Non-toxic	

ICP, intracranial pressure; PT, prothrombin time; RAR, retinoic acid receptor; RXR, retinoid X-receptor.

levels of β-RAR are expressed, then retinoic acid is unlikely to have much preventative effect upon malignant change. Cultured squamous carcinoma cells expressing large amounts of the β-receptor will, when exposed to retinoic acid, undergo terminal differentiation. The retinoids that have been most widely used in clinical practice are 13-*cis*-retinoic acid and all-*trans*-retinoic acid. Since each RAR subtype may be associated with specific cellular effects, agents with selectivity for each type of receptor are now being developed and tested.

The use of a combined approach to chemoprevention is now being explored. Interferon and retinoids may act synergistically, possibly by inhibiting the neovascularization that is essential for tumours to grow and invade. The addition of *N*-acetylcysteine (NAC) is also logical, since its mechanisms of action are rather different from those of the retinoids. NAC acts primarily against the environmental stimuli causing malignant transformation, whereas the retinoids can affect the regulation of those intracellular processes controlling growth and differentiation.

Several randomized trials of chemoprevention have now been published. The practical results have not, by and large, fulfilled the theoretical promise. Compliance is a problem: only about 25 per cent of eligible patients are prepared to enter chemoprevention studies. In those patients persuaded to participate, the toxicity of the agents used poses another problem. The evidence from the randomized studies shows that time erodes any benefit that has been achieved. The risk ratio for second tumours (control to treated) is high at 1 year: 6.9 in the M.D. Anderson study, but by a median follow-up of 55 months the risk ratio had fallen to 2.0. The difference in the rate of second malignancy was still significant: 14 per cent in the treated group versus 31 per cent in the controls ($P = 0.04$). In spite of this impressive reduction in the rate of second tumours, there was no demonstrable increase in survival.

In interpreting chemoprevention trials the important denominator is not the number of patients completing the protocol as planned, nor even the number of patients entering the study: the truly important denominator is the total number of eligible patients.

GENERAL PRINCIPLES OF SURGERY IN HEAD AND NECK CANCER

Full discussion of the principles and practices of head and neck surgery is beyond the scope of this chapter and is covered in other specialist texts. For the general oncologist there are, however, a few principles and practical points to be considered. Surgery can be associated with significant long-term morbidity and should, therefore, only be undertaken in those patients who are fit enough to withstand its effects and who are aware of the likely functional outcome. Apart from diversions of the airway or digestive tract, aimed at relieving symptoms, there is little role for palliative surgery. Surgery should only be undertaken when there is a realistic chance of curing the patient.

Patients undergoing major oral cavity or oropharyngeal tumour resections are usually given a temporary tracheostomy to safeguard the airway. This should be undertaken at the start or end of the main procedure. Similarly, in patients undergoing major resections in whom the likelihood of an early return to normal swallowing is small, thought should be given to undertaking a percutaneous, or if needs be, open gastrostomy. This will safeguard the airway from overspill and allow good and safe nutritional support during the early postoperative period. Having decided on major surgery, the following issues need to be considered:

1 Accurate preoperative assessment of the size of the tumour and involvement of adjacent structures (e.g. mandible). This can usually be provided by competent endoscopy and the use of appropriate computed tomography (CT) and/or magnetic resonance imaging (MRI) scanning.
2 The extent of the excision that will be required to remove the tumour adequately. Standard texts talk of

allowing a 2 cm rim of macroscopically normal tissue around the tumour. However, such a margin is not always feasible in the head and neck, and recourse to frozen-section analysis of the excision margins is often necessary at the time of surgery. Not surprisingly, positive histological margins are associated with a worse prognosis.

3 The reliance on frozen section for histological diagnosis of the primary tumour. Although frozen-section analysis is reliable for squamous cell carcinoma, it is notoriously unreliable for salivary gland malignancies. Whenever possible, the histological diagnosis should be sought at the time of the initial endoscopy.
4 Management of nodal disease. Certain primary tumour sites in the head and neck are associated with a high incidence of metastatic nodal disease, which may be too early to be clinically palpable. Such sites include nasopharynx, tongue base, tonsil, supraglottis, pyriform fossa. It is therefore logical to consider a prophylactic ipsilateral neck dissection when undertaking excision of a primary tumour at one of these sites. The majority of surgeons dissect the neck if the primary tumour is stage T2 or above. In the absence of palpable disease, it would be appropriate to undertake a selective neck dissection and send off any suspicious-looking nodes for frozen section analysis. A full modified radical neck dissection for clinical N0 disease is only justified if intra-operative frozen section proves positive.
5 Reconstruction of the defect. Primary closure of a defect is sometimes possible where there is adequate mobile surrounding epithelium. However, this is not often the case in the head and neck region. Attempts to close a defect primarily can result in tethering of nearby structures (e.g. the tongue) or subsequent wound breakdown. If the defect cannot be closed primarily, then consideration must be given to the use of transposed tissue.

The types of flaps or grafts available along with situations where they are most commonly applied can be summarized as follows:

1 Free grafts:
   (a) Skin: split-skin grafts can be used on a well-vascularized bed, e.g. post hemiglossectomy or post buccal mucosa excision.
   (b) Bone: free bone has been employed to reconstruct a bony defect, e.g. after segmental mandibular resection. However, the bone graft is unlikely to become fully revascularised and free bone grafts are now rarely used.
2 Local mucosal or skin flaps. These can be:
   (a) Random: these flaps do not have a defined vessel supplying them. They are therefore relatively small and the length of the flap must never exceed the width of its base. They can be used for small defects in the oral cavity or on the facial skin.

(b) Axial: such flaps have a named blood supply. They can be cutaneous (e.g. the nasolabial flap, which is supplied by the superior labial branch of the facial artery and which can be used to reconstruct the anterior floor of the mouth) or mucosal (e.g. a tongue flap which is based on a branch of the lingual artery). Local axial flaps should be used with care in instances where the surgical field has previously been irradiated.

3 Distant axial flaps – these are distant in that the base of the flap is not immediately adjacent to the area of excision:

(a) Cutaneous: the best example of a distant cutaneous axial flap is the delto-pectoral flap. Although now rarely employed, this flap is still useful for providing neck skin cover. It is based on the perforating branches of the internal mammary artery.

(b) Myocutaneous: these flaps rely on the principle that the muscle involved carries with it a specific named blood supply which is preserved. Perforating branches can spread out into the skin overlying the muscle and allow a small paddle of skin to be preserved on the distal portion of the muscle. Such a muscle/skin flap can then be tunnelled up into the neck and the skin paddle on the muscle used to reline the mucosal surface appropriately. The two most popular myocutaneous flaps are:
   (i) the pectoralis major flap
   (ii) the latissimus dorsi flap.

(c) Osseomyocutaneous flaps are really a variation on (b) and incorporate a portion of rib to provide reconstruction of the jaw.

4 Free flaps. These are portions of tissue which carry an identifiable arterial supply and venous drainage, allowing the tissue to be raised, the vessels divided and the flap inset into the surgical defect with anastomosis of the vessels to appropriate vessels in the neck. Free flaps can be:

(a) Skin, e.g. radial forearm flap. This flap has the advantage that it can be harvested with a vascularized piece of radius which can be used to reconstruct a composite resection of the jaw and oral cavity. The groin flap provides a similar type of reconstruction to the radial forearm flap.

(b) Muscle – rectus abdominis. This flap can also be harvested with overlying skin. It provides a good bulky flap, e.g. for defects after glossectomy.

(c) Jejunum – a segment of jejunum can be harvested along with its vascular arcade and can be inset to provide a neo-pharynx, without disturbing the lumen of the small bowel. Alternatively, the jejunum can be opened along its anti-mesenteric border and used as a 'patch' type of reconstruction in the pharynx.

5 Pedicled viscera. Following a pharyngolaryngo-oesophagectomy (e.g. for a post-cricoid or cervical oesophageal carcinoma) the best way to reconstruct the upper digestive tract may be to mobilize and transpose the stomach into the neck. Colon can be used in a similar fashion but is often less reliable in view of its relatively poor vascular supply.

One of the major surgical developments over the past two decades has been post-laryngectomy speech restoration. There are a number of systems available, e.g. Blom Singer and Provox. Whichever device is used, the outlook for the patient after laryngectomy can be improved dramatically. The essence of speech restoration is to create a small fistula between the posterior wall of the trachea and the reconstructed pharynx. A catheter is kept in this tract to allow it to epithelialize and is then replaced by a one-way indwelling valve with flanges to keep it in place. By occluding the stoma and exhaling, the patient can divert air through the valve and into the pharynx. The slit type valve at the pharyngeal end of the prosthesis will set the air into vibration and the patient can then articulate in the normal way and produce excellent speech.

As with any medical treatment, head and neck surgery carries with it a host of potential complications. The most relevant of these are:

1 Fistula formation. The development of an oro- or pharyngo-cutaneous salivary fistula can occur after any major excision involving resection of digestive tract mucosa and synchronous dissection of the neck. It is more commonly seen in patients who have previously undergone radiotherapy. The management is initially conservative, and with modern antibiotics the risk of a subsequent carotid artery haemorrhage is very low. However, a persistent fistula should be treated with suspicion: not only is a carotid bleed possible but the presence of the fistula may indicate a recurrence of the original tumour. A chylous fistula is most likely to occur following a modified radical neck dissection. Although these fistulas usually settle spontaneously, re-exploration and surgical closure is occasionally necessary. Unlike a salivary fistula, they rarely prolong the patient's stay in hospital by many days.

2 Aspiration. After any major resection of the oral cavity or oropharynx a reconstructive flap will need to be employed. This flap will be anaesthetic and immobile and, not surprisingly, swallowing will suffer as a consequence. Depending on factors such as the site of the flap, the patient's age, previous surgery/radiotherapy, the patient may quickly learn to compensate. However, in certain instances long-term overspill becomes a serious problem. Management can be very difficult and the patient may benefit from a permanent tracheostomy to safeguard the airway. Following total glossectomy, a minority of patients will require salvage laryngectomy purely in order to prevent chronic aspiration.

3 Wound breakdown. This is rare unless there is an associated fistula.

4 Facial oedema. Significant facial oedema is unusual unless synchronous neck dissections are undertaken with removal of both internal jugular veins. Because of this and the associated problem of suddenly raised intracranial pressure, every attempt should be made to preserve at least one vein.

5 Frozen shoulder. Often seen following the conventional (Crile) radical neck dissection where the accessory nerve is divided. Postoperative radiotherapy makes the problem even more likely to occur. The 'solution' is to preserve the axillary nerve whenever possible, or to provide physiotherapy in the postoperative period.

GENERAL PRINCIPLES OF RADIOTHERAPY FOR HEAD AND NECK CANCER

Kinetics of squamous cell carcinoma of the head and neck

The volume doubling time of squamous cell carcinomas of the head and neck is between 40 and 80 days. The potential doubling time can be calculated from:

$$T_{pot} = \lambda \, (Ts/LI)$$

where LI is the labelling index, λ is a constant describing the age distribution of the population (values are typically in the range 0.75–1.0) and Ts is the duration of DNA synthesis. The results of a comprehensive review of kinetic parameters in 476 squamous carcinomas of the head and neck are summarized in Table 17.11. An important feature of these data, obtained from 11 separate centres, is that significant differences emerged when the results were stratified by centre. Only 2 of the 11 centres reported T_{pot} values of over 45 days, at five of the centres the maximum reported T_{pot} value was less than 20 days. This clearly demonstrates that, even in expert hands, there is considerable variation in the estimation of these parameters. There was no clear or consistent relationship between any of the three parameters and T-stage, site or histological grade. The median T_{pot} was 6.4 days for well-differentiated tumours and 7.8 days for undifferentiated tumours. These T_{pot} values are much shorter than the volume doubling times. The discrepancy between the two parameters can be explained by cell loss.

$$\phi = 1 - (T_{pot}/T_d)$$

where ϕ is the cell loss factor and T_d is the cell population doubling time, which will usually be longer than the volume doubling time.

Cell loss by desquamation is part of the repertoire of normal squamous epithelium. Cell loss factors of around 95 per cent are characteristic of squamous cell carcinomas of the head and neck. These high cell loss factors have important implications for the response to therapy. A 1-cm diameter tumour contains approximately 10^9 cells, without cell loss this size would be achieved within 30–35 generations. With cell loss, however, it could take up to 1000 generations or more to reach this size. A small tumour of the head and neck is therefore genetically old (Fig. 17.4a).

Mutations conferring resistance to radiation and/or drugs will occur randomly and may precede exposure to the toxic agent. The chance of such a mutation occurring depends on the number of cellular divisions that it has taken a tumour to reach a given size, rather than the absolute number of cells within the tumour. Cell loss thereby increases the probability of a mutation conferring resistance having occurred before diagnosis. Successful treatment may be jeopardized by events that have taken place during the preclinical phase of tumour development.

Cell loss will exaggerate the response to treatment observed clinically. Modest reductions in the number of clonogenic cells present will, through the amplificatory effect of cell loss, produce rapid shrinkage of tumour. The underlying problem is the presence of resistant cells and, imperceptibly at first, these will grow through treatment and ultimately dominate. The failure of chemotherapy, in spite of impressive initial responses, significantly to improve outcome in head and neck cancer may, in part, be related to the kinetic behaviour of squamous cell carcinomas (Fig. 17.4b).

Radiobiology of head and neck cancer

Clinical research in the radiotherapy of head and neck cancer has, historically, been dominated by the oxygen effect and it is only recently that the importance of other radiobiological factors has been rediscovered.

THE OXYGEN EFFECT

Hypoxic but viable cells may exist within tumours, these cells are relatively resistant to radiation-induced cell killing. Survival of such cells after a course of radiation treatment might limit cure. Three main methods have been used to attempt to overcome the potential problem of hypoxic cells limiting cure in head and neck cancer: hyperbaric oxygen, neutron therapy and hypoxic cell

Table 17.11 *Data on tumour kinetic parameters from 476 squamous carcinomas of the head and neck (from Begg et al., 1999)*

Parameter	Median	Range
Ts	10.7 hours	4.4–45.7 hours
LI	8.85%	0.6–47.7%
T_{pot}	5.1 days	0.8–72.9 days

LI, labelling index; Ts, duration of S phase; T_{pot}, potential doubling time.

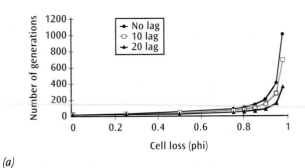

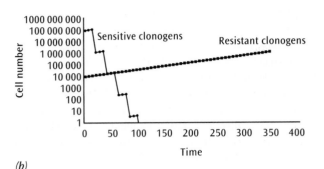

(a)

(b)

Figure 17.4 *(a) Number of generations to reach 10^9 clonogenic cells, corresponding to a diameter of 1 cm, plotted against cell loss factor under three separate assumptions: NO LAG, cell loss begins when tumour develops; 10 LAG, cell loss only kicks in after 10 generations; 20 LAG, cell loss only kicks in after 20 generations. For clinically relevant values for cell loss (between 0.8 and 0.99) it could take up to 1000 generations for a tumour to reach a size of 1 cm; ample time for mutations to accumulate. (b) This illustrates the eradication of sensitive clonogens by cytotoxic treatment, when cell loss is high ($\phi = 0.9$) followed by regrowth of resistant cells. Clinically, there will be rapid shrinkage of tumour followed by recurrence and death from resistant disease.*

sensitizers. There are other approaches to the problem, summarized in Table 17.12, and future research on the problems posed by the oxygen effect will be more broadly based than in the past.

Oxygen levels within tumours of the head and neck

Several studies have now reported on direct measurement, using polarographic electrodes, of oxygen levels in head and neck tumours. A significant proportion of the cells within squamous cancers of the head and neck are hypoxic. There is, as yet, no universally acceptable definition of hypoxia. Some authors have used a Po_2 threshold of 2.5 mmHg, others use 5 mmHg, others have used 10 mmHg.

Another approach is to measure the median Po_2 value: using a median Po_2 threshold of 10 mmHg, Brizel *et al.* (1997) found that the probability of disease-free survival was three times greater in the patients with well-oxygenated tumours. The distribution of median Po_2

Table 17.12 *Methods that could be used to circumvent the problems caused by the relative radioresistance of hypoxic cells within tumours*

Increase oxygen delivery to tumour
  Hyperbaric oxygen
  Normobaric oxygen
  Carbogen
  Nicotinamide
  Modify blood viscocity
  Increase haemoglobin
  Lower interstitial fluid pressure within tumour
Increase killing of hypoxic cells
  Hypoxic cell sensitizers (e.g. nimorazole)
  Bioreductive drugs (e.g. mitomycin C, tirapazamine)
  High LET radiation (e.g. neutrons)
Decrease oxygen demand within tumour
  Hypothermia
  Calcium channel blockers
  MIBG
Crabtree effect (acute hyperglycaemia)

LET, linear energy transfer; MIBG, [131I]meta-iodo benzyl guanadine.

values in tumours of the head and neck regions is completely different from that of the adjacent normal tissues: the median Po_2 in normal tissues follows a Gaussian (normal) distribution, with no values below 20 mmHg. The distribution of the median Po_2 values from tumours is skewed to the left, with the majority of patients having tumour median Po_2 values of less than 20 mmHg. It is probably the absolute number of hypoxic cells within a tumour, rather than the proportion, which is important. The concept of the 'hypoxic subvolume' has been introduced to describe this. The hypoxic subvolume is simply the product of the tumour volume × the hypoxic fraction (percentage of cells with Po_2 values below threshold, e.g. 5 mmHg). In a multivariate analysis in 59 patients with squamous cell carcinoma (SCC) of the head and neck, both hypoxic subvolume and pre-treatment haemoglobin level were of prognostic value in predicting survival.

A crucial question is whether or not, during a course of fractionated radiotherapy, hypoxic cells are able to re-oxygenate. Hypoxic cells will be relatively radioresistant and any such cells persisting after radiotherapy will compromise cure. If, however, fractionation permits all cells to regain normal oxygenation, then all cells, ultimately, will become vulnerable to radiation and it should be possible to eliminate every last clonogenic cell. Although some experimental evidence suggests that re-oxygenation may occur during fractionated radiotherapy, there is at least one clinical study showing the reverse. Stadler *et al.* (1999), using the Eppendorf electrode, studied sequential Po_2 measurements in patients with head and neck cancer. They showed a progressive fall in median Po_2 during treatment. This was partially reversed during the gap in their split course schedule, only to fall again once daily treatments were resumed.

Clinical studies on attempts to overcome the limitations to cure imposed by the presence of hypoxic cells within tumours

Pooling the results from 10 randomized trials of hyperbaric oxygen therapy in head and neck cancer shows an absolute difference in survival of 8.6 per cent (95 per cent confidence limits, 1.3–15.9 per cent) in favour of hyperbaric oxygen treatment. This difference is small, hyperbaric treatment is both cumbersome and potentially dangerous, and the technique is no longer used in the UK.

Fast neutrons kill hypoxic cells as efficiently as they kill well-oxygenated cells. Neutron therapy appeared to offer a logical means of circumventing the problems posed by the oxygen effect. The pooled results from seven randomized trials of neutron therapy in head and neck cancer show a statistically insignificant rate difference of 1 per cent in favour of neutron therapy (95 per cent confidence limits from −7 per cent to +9 per cent). The early promise of this form of treatment has not been fulfilled. Although local control of tumour may be slightly better, the late damage to normal tissues caused by neutrons is grossly excessive and abrogates the benefit from any increase in local control that might have been achieved.

Hypoxic cell sensitizers are still under active investigation in head and neck cancer. Initial studies used metronidazole and misonadazole, but cumulative neurotoxicity caused by the sensitizer proved limiting. These early studies showed no convincing benefit from the addition of the radiosensitizer. This failure to show benefit may, in part, have been due to the use of reduced doses of sensitizer dictated by the need to avoid excessive toxicity. One study, DAHANCA-5, using nimorazole as the radiosensitizer, initially showed a 13.9 per cent improvement in survival. Longer follow-up has shown a more modest, and statistically non-significant, benefit. The 10-year survival with radiotherapy alone was 16 per cent at 10 years compared with 26 per cent for patients treated with nimorazole plus radiation (Table 17.13). There was a statistically significant reduction in deaths attributed to cancer in the group treated with nimorazole, 41 per cent versus 52 per cent ($P = 0.002$).

Two large-scale randomized studies have assessed the effectiveness of etanidazole (SR 2508) as a radiosensitizer.

Although the sensitizer was well tolerated, it appeared ineffective in improving either local control or survival. For the moment at least, the most clinically useful radiosensitizer appears to be nimorazole.

Combined approaches have been used clinically in an attempt to circumvent the oxygen effect. The ARCON schedule uses accelerated radiotherapy (AR), carbogen (CO) and nicotinamide. Carbogen is a mixture comprising 95 per cent oxygen and 5 per cent carbon dioxide and is a means of increasing oxygen delivery to tissues while minimizing the vasoconstrictive effects of high concentrations of oxygen. Nicotinamide acts as a vasodilator and so the ARCON schedule aims to give a rapid course of radiotherapy to a tumour that has an excellent supply of oxygen-rich blood. Preliminary results in patients with head and neck cancer show that the approach is feasible, although toxicity from the nicotinamide causes problems with compliance. The acute reactions are no worse than with the equivalent radiotherapeutic schedule given alone. In a series of 62 patients with advanced laryngeal tumours the local control rate at 2 years was a somewhat astonishing – 92 per cent.

Haemoglobin and oxygenation There is some evidence that haemoglobin level before, and during, radiotherapy may influence therapeutic outcome in patients with head and neck cancer. There are over 16 studies that have looked at this question, and 11 of them suggest that patients with low haemoglobin levels fare less well than patients with higher levels. Six studies suggest that survival rates are lower in anaemic patients; two studies suggest that haemoglobin level has no influence on survival. Seven studies suggest a relationship between haemoglobin level and local control; four studies found no such relationship. The problem in interpreting these data is that the criteria used to distinguish 'low' from 'normal' or 'high' haemoglobin levels have varied. One general point does, however, emerge: haemoglobin levels at the lower end of the generally accepted 'normal range' may be suboptimal for patients undergoing radiotherapy for head and neck cancer. Current clinical trials are addressing the question of whether erythropoietin, used to maintain optimal haemoglobin levels, can improve the results

Table 17.13 *A summary of the results from recent large-scale trials of hypoxic cell sensitizers in head and neck cancer*

End point	Trial	Sensitizer (%)	Control (%)	*P* value
Survival at 2 years	RTOG etanidazole	43	41	0.65
Survival at 2 years	IGR etanidazole	54	54	0.99
Survival at 10 years	DAHANCA-5 nimorazole	26	16	0.32
Locoregional control at 2 years	RTOG etanidazole	40	40	NS
Locoregional control at 2 years	IGR etanidazole	53	53	0.93
Locoregional control at 5 years	DAHANCA-5 nimorazole	49	33	0.002

NS, not significant.

of radiotherapy for patients with cancer of the head and neck.

Bioreductive drugs Bioreductive drugs, unlike hypoxic cell sensitizers, are cytotoxic in their own right. They are, however, selectively toxic to poorly oxygenated cells. Mitomycin C is a bioreductive drug that has been used in cancer treatment, and particularly in combination with radiotherapy, for many years. Tirapazamine, porfiromycin, AQ4N and BMS-181174 are more recently introduced bioreductive agents. Tirapazamine has been used synchronously with radiotherapy for the treatment of head and neck cancer in two phase II studies. The rationale behind the use of bioreductive drugs synchronously with radiotherapy is that there may be true synergy between the two treatments: there may be a supra-additive effect. There are only four randomized trials, all using Mitomycin C, of bioreductive drugs in head and neck cancer. There are a further 16 phase II studies, 14 with Mitomycin C as well as the two studies using tirapazamine. Pooling the results of the randomized trials shows a modest survival benefit from the synchronous use of a bioreductive drug (Mitomycin C alone or in combination). The survival rate in the control group is 35 per cent versus 44 per cent in the group treated with synchronous chemotherapy containing Mitomycin C: the confidence interval on this absolute rate difference of 10 per cent extends from 1 to 19 per cent. The relative merits of porfiromycin and Mitomycin C are now being assessed in a randomized trial at Yale.

FRACTIONATION

Radiotherapists, and particularly head and neck radiotherapists, have recently been re-exploring fractionation as a means of improving the therapeutic ratio for radiation therapy. Much of the impetus has come from the realization that tumour kinetics may be perturbed by treatment and, in particular, that tumour cells may proliferate more rapidly as a response to treatment (Withers *et al.*, 1988). Whether this represents a true acceleration or simply the unmasking of the latent T_{pot} (of 5–10 days) is debated. There is no doubt that the phenomenon is clinically important. Even short unanticipated gaps in clinically effective schedules can significantly reduce local control and/or survival.

Various strategies have been devised to deal with the problem of accelerated repopulation. If accelerated repopulation is important, then either you must keep treatment as short as possible or you must, if using longer treatments, increase the total dose to compensate for proliferation during treatment. If you choose the latter approach, then you cannot simply increase the dose per fraction because the combination of increased dose per fraction and the increased total dose will produce unacceptably severe late effects. One solution to this dilemma is to use multiple daily fractions. An alternative approach is both to shorten treatment and to use multiple daily fractions. Three main strategies for unconventional fractionation have emerged over the past decade:

1 Pure hyperfractionation: overall treatment time is neither shortened nor prolonged and total dose is increased by using multiple fractions per day. The interval between fractions should be at least 6 hours to allow time for repair in damaged, but viable, cells of the normal tissues. If the interval between fractions is any shorter than this, then repair is incomplete and the damage to normal tissues may be unacceptable. Recent evidence suggests that repair half-times may be even longer than originally thought, and that some repair processes may take over 6 hours.

2 Pure acceleration: the overall treatment time is shortened, either by using multiple fractions per day or by treating at weekends. The size of each individual fraction is usually 1.8 Gy or greater.

3 Accelerated hyperfractionation: the overall time is shortened and multiple fractions per day are used. The fraction size is usually less than 1.8 Gy. The reduction in treatment time achieved with this approach may, at least in part, be offset by the need to introduce a gap in treatment to permit recovery of the normal mucosal cells. The use of the concomitant boost is a variation on this theme: a large tumour volume is treated with a conventional schedule but, during the latter phase of treatment, a supplementary treatment is given each day to a smaller, boost, volume. This boost is given at least 6 hours after the treatment to the large volume.

The schedules employed in those randomized trials of fractionation, for which data are currently available, are summarized in Table 17.14. The results of a meta-analysis of these trials are summarized in Table 17.15. Unconventional fractionation, particularly with regimens using pure hyperfractionation or pure acceleration, provides a modest benefit in survival and local control, but at the cost of an increase in acute side-effects. Regimens which combine hyperfractionation with acceleration appear to offer no gain in therapeutic ratio, in fact the reverse seems true: an increase in acute effects without any increase in locoregional control or survival. The overall conclusions are similar to those of a similar analysis of synchronous chemoradiotherapy in head and neck cancer: any gain in tumour control is offset by increased acute toxicity. There may, however, be some therapeutic gain in terms of late effects. The CHART study suggests that late effects may be less severe in the patients treated with the unconventional schedule. Interestingly, this does not appear to have measurable impact upon quality of life. Quality of life was significantly better in only two respects in the patients treated with CHART: sexual interest and sore muscles. It is difficult to attribute either of these observations to a biological effect of the radiation schedule. The CHART regimen has now evolved into CHARTWEL (Continuous Hyperfractionated Accelerated RadioTherapy WEekend

Table 17.14 *A summary of recent phase III trials of unconventional fractionation in head and neck cancer*

Study	Year	Type	Size	Conv. dose	Conv. dpf	Conv. time	BED 3	BED 10	Exp. dose	Exp. dpf	Exp. time	BED 3	BED 10
Sanchiz	1990	hf	559	60	2	42	100	72	70.4	1.1	42	96	78
RTOG 9003 hfx	1999	hf	556	70	2	49	117	84	81.6	1.2	49	114	91
TEO	1996	hf	100	60	2.5	30	110	75	71.2	1.6	30	115	84
EORTC 22791	1992	hf	325	70	2	49	117	84	80.5	1.15	49	111	90
PMH	1996	hf	336	51	2.55	26	94	64	58	1.45	26	86	66
Datta	1989	hf	176	66	2	45	110	79	79.2	1.2	45	111	89
Pinto	1991	hf	98	66	2	45	110	79	70.4	1.1	45	96	78
RTOG 9003 afx-s	1999	ha	556	70	2	49	117	84	67.2	1.6	42	103	78
RTOG 9003 afx-c	1999	ha	556	70	2	49	117	84	72	1.8	42	113	84
Awwad	1992	ha	56	50	2	35	83	60	42	1.4	11	62	48
Awwad	1998	ha	72	60	2	42	100	72	46.2	1.4	14	68	53
EORTC 22811	1995	ha	348	75	1.7	63	118	88	72	1.6	49	110	84
CHART	1997	ha	918	66	2	45	110	79	54	1.5	12	81	62
EORTC 22851	1997	ha	512	70	2	49	117	84	72	1.6	35	110	84
Dobrowsky	1998	ha	127	70	2	49	117	84	55.3	1.6	17	86	65
Gliwice	1996/8	a	100	72	2	55	120	86	72	2	36	120	86
Jackson	1997	a	82	66	2	48	110	79	66	2	25	110	79
DAHANCA 5 and 7	1998	a	540	68	2	45	113	82	68	2	39	113	82
Trans tasman	1999	a	191	70	2	47	117	84	59.4	1.8	24	95	70

afx-s, accelerated with split; afx-c, accelerated with concomitant boost; hf, pure hyperfractionation; ha, mixed acceleration and hyperfractionation; a, pure acceleration; Conv., conventional; Exp., exposure; dpf, dose per fraction; BED 3, biologically effective dose for α/β of 3 Gy (late effects); BED 10, biologically effective dose for α/β of 10 Gy tumours and acute effects.

Table 17.15 *Summary of overview of randomized trials of fractionation in head and neck cancer*

Type	Survival (%)	LRC (%)	Acute effects (%)	Late effects (%)
hf	13 (4–21)	15 (9–22)	18 (2–39)	4 (−1 to 9)
ha	2 (−3 to +7)	5 (−1 to +11)	32 (20–44)	0 (−6 to +7)
a	19 (9–30)	18 (7–28)	24 (15–33)	5 (−3 to +13)
All	9 (3–15)	12 (6–17)	26 (12–40)	2 (−2 to +7)

The method used for pooling results was that of DerSimonian and Laird (1986). Results are expressed as absolute rate difference (with 95% confidence limits), i.e. rate in experimental arm – rate in control arm. hf, Pure hyperfractionation; ha, accelerated and hyperfractionated; a, pure acceleration.

Less). The dose is 51 Gy in 34 fractions (1.5 Gy per fraction) given on 12 treatment days within an overall treatment time of 16 days. It is permissible to give a localized boost of 3 Gy in two fractions to a small volume (total dose 54 Gy in 36 fractions).

The definition of a 'conventional' fractionation schedule for treating cancers of the head and neck is by no means straightforward. The phase III trials, with only two exceptions, one of them a postoperative study, have adopted schedules lasting 6 weeks or more as the 'conventional' arm. However, this choice is not in accordance with the actual routine clinical practice of many radiotherapists in the UK. The Royal College of Radiologists Fractionation survey, published in 1989, showed that 52 per cent of UK radiotherapists would use a schedule lasting 5 weeks or less to treat an early cancer of the larynx;

37 per cent would use a schedule of 4 weeks or less. The available randomized studies have therefore failed to address questions of importance to most British radiotherapists. If accelerated proliferation of tumour clonogens does not begin until the third week of radiotherapy, then simply using a treatment schedule no longer than 4 weeks might be sufficient to prevent the problem of accelerated repopulation. It is perfectly feasible to treat in 4 weeks or less using single daily fractions; typical regimens use 50–55 Gy in 20 fractions over 4 weeks, at 2.5–2.75 Gy per fraction. Because there was concern that such short schedules might be associated, through the use of relatively high doses per fraction, with unacceptable late morbidity, the British Institute of Radiology performed a randomized comparison of short (≤4 weeks) versus long (>4 weeks) treatment times in cancer of the

laryngopharynx. The results of this large study show that tumour control was the same in the two arms, but the longer treatment schedules actually produced a higher incidence of late reactions (Wiernik *et al.*, 1991). For patients treated with five fractions per week, only 22 ± 6 per cent of patients treated on the longer schedules were free of late reaction for 10 years. The corresponding figure for the shorter schedules was 49 ± 4 per cent ($P = 0.008$).

This result is not so surprising as it at first seems. Total dose is just as important as dose per fraction in determining late effects. If, in order to counteract tumour proliferation during treatment, longer regimens require higher total doses, then keeping dose per fraction to 2 Gy or less will not necessarily protect against the development of late effects. The challenge for the future in fractionated radiotherapy is to make the punishment fit the crime: to identify before treatment those factors that influence kinetic behaviour during treatment and to treat with appropriately designed fractionation regimens.

Unfortunately the attempts to use kinetic parameters to predict response to radiotherapy have, so far, failed to deliver a clinically useful strategy. There is no relationship between T_{pot} and the ability of radiotherapy to control a tumour. There are clinical data to suggest that well-differentiated tumours may respond rather better than poorly differentiated tumours to the CHART regimen, and that patients with poorly differentiated tumours might benefit from longer overall treatment time. Experimental data from human squamous carcinomas growing in a xenograft system suggest precisely the opposite.

The intrinsic radiosensitivity of tumours in patients with cancers of the head and neck has been assessed using SF_2 (surviving fraction after 2 Gy). The technique takes about 4–5 weeks to produce a result and therefore, to use SF_2 as a guide to choosing treatment for an individual patient would involve delaying the start of treatment by a month or so. This is rarely acceptable, either to patients or to clinicians. Most of the investigation of this approach to choosing therapy has been confined to modelling, in which the theoretical benefits to a population of patients, were there feasible assays of intrinsic radiosensitivity for both tumours and normal tissues, are explored. Even the modellers disagree: some suggesting that there is no overall gain from predictive testing for individual patients, others believing that there are genuine gains to be made.

The proliferation of tumours and normal tissues follows circadian rhythms. This has already been exploited in the chrono-chemotherapy of cancer of the colon and, somewhat belatedly, is now being investigated in the radiotherapy of head and neck cancer. The National Cancer Institute of Canada is co-ordinating a trial (NCIC HN3) in which the randomization is simple: between single daily treatments given between 08.00 hours and 10.00 hours or between 16.00 hours and 18.00 hours. The rate of division of normal mucosal cells is maximal in the evening, cells are at their most radiosensitive at the G_2/M boundary. The proportion of normal mucosal cells at the G_2/M boundary is maximal between 18.00 hours and 20.00 hours. This suggests that mucositis may be less severe for patients treated in the morning. There is little evidence on circadian rhythms in squamous carcinomas of the head and neck. But such evidence as there is suggests that periodicity may be lost and that the time of day at which radiotherapy is given makes little difference to the killing of tumour cells. In theory, therefore, treatment in the morning might improve the therapeutic ratio for patients irradiated for cancers of the head and neck. Some of the increase in mucositis that is observed with schedules using multiple fractions per day may be explained on the basis of circadian variations in the radiosensitivity of the normal mucosa.

Whatever the merits, or otherwise, of shorter schedules, there is no doubt that unplanned interruptions of treatment significantly impair the effectiveness of radiotherapy in head and neck cancer. A series of 971 patients with supraglottic laryngeal tumours treated in Gliwice, Poland, using a standard 6–7-week schedule, showed that, if there were no unplanned interruptions to treatment, local control was 52 per cent. In patients with any gap, defined as an unplanned interruption of treatment, the local control rate was 40 per cent ($P = 0.014$). The longer the gap, the greater the decrease in local control: 3–7-day gap, local control 37.5 per cent; $\geqslant$15-day gap, local control 29.5 per cent. A comprehensive analysis, using pooled data from Manchester (3-week schedule) and Toronto (5-week schedule), on patients treated radically for T2 or T3 carcinomas of the larynx, again demonstrated the deleterious effect of unplanned gaps during treatment. Each extra day added to the overall treatment time corresponded to a decrease in effective dose of between 0.6 and 0.8 Gy (Hendry *et al.*, 1994). Similar data have been reported from Edinburgh and many other centres, for all sites and stages of squamous cancers of the head and neck.

It is possible to compensate for unplanned gaps in treatment by keeping the overall treatment time within the desired schedule, either by treating at weekends or by treating twice per day. If this is logistically impossible, then a less satisfactory alternative is to use a radiobiological model, such as the L–Q formula, as a guide to an upward adjustment of total dose.

Complications of radiotherapy

The acceptance of a degree of damage to normal tissues is implicit within the basic principles that underlie the use of radiotherapy to treat malignant disease. This problem is brought sharply into focus in the treatment of cancers of the head and neck. A painful, unpleasant, acute mucosal reaction almost invariably accompanies the use of radiation to treat these tumours. Because of the differing kinetics of the cells concerned, this mucosal reaction precedes any cutaneous reaction.

ACUTE REACTIONS AND THEIR MANAGEMENT

The sequential stages in the development of a mucosal reaction are: hyperaemia with erythema and oedema; the formation of an exudate (membrane) which is patchy at first but becomes confluent; with a severe reaction the mucosa may ulcerate and in extreme cases never heal. When treatment is fractionated over 4 weeks reaction usually starts during the third week, is at its peak during the fifth week and has abated by the sixth week. With longer courses of treatment the reaction arises later and lasts longer.

Patients should be warned of the acute mucosal reaction that they should expect, otherwise they might assume that the symptoms are due to the progression of their tumour. Patients should be seen and examined at least once a week during treatment. Careful supervision of oral hygiene is important, as is prompt identification and management of any secondary infection. The most common secondary infection is oral candidiasis.

Patients can take a considerable share of the responsibility for their own care during a course of radiotherapy, provided they are given adequate instruction. Simple measures will often reduce the duration and severity of the acute mucosal reaction; the most important steps are to stop smoking and to avoid alcohol. Advice is best given as a set of written instructions which are explained carefully to patients at the start of treatment and reinforced during treatment. The major points are summarized in Table 17.16. In addition to these general measures, several specific interventions are now being investigated.

Eliminating Gram-negative bacilli and yeasts from the oral cavity and oropharynx before treatment may lessen the acute mucosal reaction. The usual technique is to give lozenges containing polymyxin E, tobramycin and amphotericin B starting 2 days before the initiation of radiotherapy and continuing until 2 weeks after the completion of treatment. Randomized studies suggest that the incidence of confluent mucositis in the oral cavity is decreased but there is little effect on oropharyngeal reactions.

Haemopoietic growth factors may also affect mucosal reactions to radiotherapy. The use of granulocyte colony stimulating factor (G-CSF) is being investigated currently in controlled clinical trials. Haemopoietic growth factors presumably act by recruiting proliferation in normal mucosal stem cells.

Selective protection of normal cells against the adverse effects of radiation and chemotherapy is an alternative strategy for mitigating the acute side-effects of treatment. Most clinically available radioprotective agents act by increasing the supply of sulphydryl (thiol) groups. WR2721 (amifostine) has been used for many years as a radioprotector and has recently undergone a minor renaissance. It is a pro-drug, converted by alkaline phosphatase into the active compound WR1065. Randomized trials suggest that treatment with WR2721 will decrease

Table 17.16 *The prevention and management of mucosal reactions during radiotherapy to the head and neck*

Suggestions for self-care in patients undergoing radiotherapy to the head and neck:

Skin care	Avoid aftershave or astringent cosmetics
	Wash gently, pat the skin dry
	Avoid wet shaving
	Avoid collars or other clothes which chafe the treated area
	Try not to scratch the skin
Mucosal care	Stop smoking
	Do not drink alcohol
	Avoid hot or spicy foods
	Use regular mouthwashes
	Careful dental hygiene
	Chew sugar-free gum
	Drink plenty of clear fluids
Diet and nutrition	Bland high-protein diet
	Use dietary supplements
	Supplementary vitamins
	Put food through blender if necessary
	Avoid constipation
Care of the voice	Don't talk too much
	Rest voice as much as possible
	Don't try to force the voice
	Speak slowly and quietly
	Avoid dry or smoky atmospheres
	Reduce background noise
	Avoid excessive coughing and hawking

both the mucosal reactions and the xerostomia caused by radiotherapy. However, there are disconcerting reports of unexpectedly severe myelosuppression with chemoradiotherapy plus WR2721 and there is, as yet, no proven role for radioprotective agents in the treatment of head and neck cancer.

A wide variety of topical preparations is available for the treatment of the established mucosal reaction. Systemic analgesia, up to and including opiates, will be required for severe reactions.

Patients will normally lose some weight during treatment; if this becomes excessive (greater than 15 per cent of initial body weight) then admission to hospital and feeding via a fine-bore nasogastric tube may be necessary. When the larynx is within the treated area speech therapy, for expert advice on the care and preservation of the voice, is advisable.

The acute effects of radiation treatment, although unpleasant and distressing, are usually self-limiting. Only rarely are serious problems encountered. The dose that can be given to treat a tumour is limited by the late effects on normal tissues rather than by the acute reactions. The distinction between early and late effects of radiation is arbitrary but useful; arbitrary in that the temporal distinction cannot be universal for all tissues; useful that it draws attention to the possible differences in pathogenesis for the two types of response.

The shape of the initial portion of the cell-survival curves for acutely responding normal tissues differs from that for the cells of late-responding tissues. The difference in shape implies that increasing the number of fractions will selectively spare the late-responding tissues. Another implication is that the intensity of the acute reaction cannot be used to predict the severity of the late effects.

LATE EFFECTS OF RADIATION

The late effects of a course of radiotherapy will depend upon which vulnerable structures are within the radiated volume. The structures of relevance to the radiation treatment of carcinoma of the head and neck, the clinical consequences of radiation damage, and an indication of the limiting dose are summarized in Table 17.17. In general, the late complications of radiotherapy are more severe in patients who have had surgical procedures in addition to radical radiotherapy.

The effects of radiation on the salivary glands

The effects of radiation upon salivary glands are complex and straddle the conventional division between early and late effects. The incidence and severity of the effects of radiation upon the function of the salivary glands depend upon the amount of glandular tissue within the radiation field as well as upon time, dose and fractionation. Shielding even a proportion of one parotid gland may preserve a considerable proportion of salivary flow. Since a chronically dry mouth is unpleasant for the patient, and can be associated with rapidly progressive dental caries, it is important to exclude as much of the salivary glands as possible from the irradiated volume. Radiation-induced parotitis, manifest as acute swelling and inflammation of the salivary glands, can occur during the first few days of treatment. The syndrome itself is self-limiting. No specific management, other than reassurance is required. Serum amylase levels may rise as a response to this damage and, to some extent, provide a marker for the degree of damage to the salivary glands.

A decrease in the rate of flow of saliva occurs within 10–14 days of the start of treatment, a timing which suggests that cell death by apoptosis may be an important mechanism whereby radiation damages the salivary glands. The effects of radiation on salivary function are at their maximum 4–6 weeks after the start of treatment. The serous acini are more sensitive to radiation than are the mucinous acini, this means that the saliva changes and becomes thick and sticky. The return of salivary function is slow, it can take several years and is almost invariably incomplete. Chronic severe xerostomia can be one of the most distressing long-term side-effects of treatment for head and neck cancer. Recent randomized studies using pilocarpine have shown that it can, to some extent, alleviate radiation xerostomia. Pilocarpine can produce both an objective increase in salivary flow and a subjective improvement in symptoms.

Disturbances of taste

Radiation treatment to the mouth produces disturbances in the sensation of taste; these changes occur early in the course of treatment and persist for many months. Failure to appreciate the texture of food is a major feature. Many patients complain that food tastes like blotting paper or cotton wool. Cancer itself, or radiotherapy to regions of the body other than the head and neck, can also produce changes in the perception of taste. These disturbances are not easily managed and will interfere with eating in patients who are already having nutritional problems.

Radionecrosis

Necrosis of soft tissue is an uncommon late complication of radiotherapy. It is usually precipitated by trauma. Late

Table 17.17 *Structures in the head and neck which are vulnerable to the adverse late effects of radiotherapy: the doses given indicate a level at which approximately 5% of patients might be expected to experience the complication*

Tissue	BED ($\alpha/\beta = 3$ Gy)	Total dose at 2 Gy pf	Total dose at 2.75 Gy pf	Sequel
Lens	11	6	6	Cataract
Retina	88	52	46	Loss of vision
Optic nerve	99	59	52	Loss of vision
Anterior eye	117	70	61	Dry eye
VIIIth nerve	108	65	57	Hearing loss
Cranial nerves	108	65	57	CN palsy
Temporal lobe	92	55	48	Epilepsy, dementia
Brainstem	88	52	46	Dysarthria, nystagmus, ataxia, disturbed consciousness
Spinal cord	75	45	39	Myelopathy
Temporal bone	107	64	56	Osteonecrosis

BED, biologically effective dose; pf, per fraction.

effects of radiation, manifest as depletion of parenchymal stem cells and obliterative changes in blood vessels, will impair healing. Trivial trauma, for example injury by fish bones or excessively hot fluids, can occasionally produce extensive necrosis. Patients should be advised to chew their food carefully and to avoid very hot drinks. Cartilage necrosis is a rare complication of megavoltage radiotherapy for head and neck cancer: it was far more common in the days of orthovoltage treatment for carcinomas of the larynx.

The care of the teeth

The care of the teeth is one of the more contentious issues in the management of cancer of the head and neck. The issue hinges on the question of osteoradionecrosis of the mandible and its prevention. Routine dental clearance has been proposed for all patients with head and neck cancer. This view is too extreme and, given modern conservative dental technique, a less radical approach is justified. However, in patients who are unlikely to participate in programmes of dental care and surveillance, dental clearance may still be necessary. The ideal conservative dental programme is summarized in Table 17.18. With a conservative approach the majority of patients can keep their teeth, and the incidence of osteoradionecrosis can be kept acceptably low. When it does occur, it can usually be managed without surgery, using systemic antibiotics and vigorous oral hygiene. Small bony sequestra may be extruded spontaneously from time to time but this often causes only minor inconvenience. Less than 20 per cent of patients require surgery; this can vary from simple

Table 17.18 *Dental assessment and care for patients being treated with radiotherapy for head and neck cancer*

Oral assessments
   Plaque score
   Indexed record of pocket depth
   Vitality tests
   Restoration of carious teeth
   Panoramic X-ray
   Checking fit of dentures
   Inspection of oral mucosa
   Surveillance culture of oral flora
   Measurement of mouth opening
   Assessment of salivary flow rate
Prophylactic care
   Professional tooth cleansing
   Root planing and curettage
   Oral hygiene instructions
   Tooth brushing
   Interdental cleansing
   Use of disclosing agents
   Cleansing of mucosal surfaces
   Massage of oral mucosa
   Discouraging denture wearing during radiotherapy
   Instruction in fluoride usage
   Consultation with dietician

removal of sequestrum, to major procedures involving complete reconstruction of the mandible. The wearing of dentures after radiotherapy can produce problems. Ill-fitting dentures can damage the musoca and initiate necrosis of the underlying bone. Since some remodelling of the mouth will occur after radiotherapy, patients should be discouraged from wearing dentures for 3–6 months following treatment.

Muscles and soft tissue

The main effect of radiation on muscles and other soft tissues is to produce fibrosis. This develops slowly, usually several years after treatment. It may not be noticed by the patient but can confuse doctors. Diffuse fibrosis of the sternocleidomastoid muscle may be mistaken for cervical lymphadenopathy. Conversely, infiltrative nodal disease can mimic post-radiation fibrosis.

Severe fibrosis of the muscles and tissues around the mandible can produce trismus. This may be severe and can affect both eating and speaking. Regular jaw opening exercises, using rubber wedges of gradually increasing thickness, can prevent or ameliorate trismus. Such treatment must be started early. If trismus is allowed to become severe, then the patient's life becomes miserable.

Endocrine deficiency

When the pituitary is within the treatment volume, as it may well be for tumours of the nasopharynx or ethmoid sinuses, then pituitary failure may be a late complication of treatment. The onset is usually insidious, lethargy and lack of libido may go unnoticed. The diagnosis should be made as early as possible since hypopituitarism can so easily be treated by appropriate replacement therapy.

If the thyroid gland is within the radiation field, up to 50–60 per cent of patients irradiated for head and neck tumours may develop biochemical hypothyroidism, manifest as a raised thyroid stimulating hormone (TSH) level. Only about a third of these patients will develop clinical hypothyroidism. Risks of hypothyroidism developing are increased if there has been surgery to the neck – either laryngectomy or neck dissection. Incidence also depends upon total radiation dose and whether or not midline structures were shielded. Awareness of the potential problem of hypothyroidism after radiotherapy is the best aid to prompt diagnosis and treatment.

Spinal cord

The spinal cord is vulnerable to the late effects of radiotherapy for head and neck cancer. The spinal cord will often be within the treatment volume, particularly in patients with primary tumours of the nasopharynx, maxillary antrum or posterior pharyngeal wall, as well as in patients who have extensive nodal disease in the neck. L'hermitte's sign is a transitory complication of radiotherapy to the cord and its occurrence does not imply any increased risk of serious damage to the spinal cord. It typically occurs 3–15 months following the completion of treatment. It is self-limiting and requires no specific treatment.

Radiation-induced myelopathy is an avoidable catastrophe. Avoidable, in that limiting the dose to the cord will usually prevent its occurrence; catastrophic, in that, since the damage is inflicted to the cervical cord, quadriplegia is the usual consequence. The figures for cord tolerance given in Table 17.17 should be regarded as indicating the upper limit of cord tolerance: they are appropriate for patients with a low probability of cure, in whom a 10 per cent risk of cord damage might be considered worth taking, given that the likely alternative is death from uncontrolled tumour. For patients with a high probability of cure, a 10 per cent risk of severe late toxicity is unacceptable and the tolerance dose for the spinal cord should be revised downwards as follows: at 2 Gy per fraction, 42–44 Gy; at 2.75 Gy per fraction, 35–37 Gy. For experimental fractionation schemes, such as CHART, particular attention needs to be paid to cord doses – particularly because the phenomenon of slow repair may limit recovery in the spinal cord when multiple fractions per day are used. The cord dose for CHART should never exceed 44 Gy and, ideally, should be less than 40 Gy.

Temporal lobe necrosis

Temporal lobe necrosis is a potentially devastating consequence of radiotherapy for nasopharyngeal carcinoma. The necrosis is usually bilateral and this precludes surgical resection of the necrotic area. The only treatment is empirical use of steroids. The overall rate of temporal lobe necrosis following treatment for nasopharyngeal carcinoma is between 0 and 3 per cent. The latent interval is between 18 months and 13 years after treatment, with a median of 5 years. Once necrosis has developed, by a median of 3 years 30 per cent of patients are severely incapacitated.

Cranial nerves

Peripheral nerves are traditionally regarded as being relatively radioresistant. However, there is evidence from clinical studies that cranial nerves and sympathetic nerves in the head and neck are less radioresistant. This is particularly important in the management of tumours of the nasopharynx (*see* p. 373).

Sensorineural hearing loss after radiotherapy

The potential severity of the direct effects of radiation upon the eighth nerve is now well appreciated. The precise contribution of radiotherapy to sensorineural hearing loss is difficult to evaluate: hearing declines with age (presbyacusis) and, since there may be several years latency between the treatment and the demonstration of impaired eighth nerve function, which is to blame – time or radiation? Loss is minimal up to 50 Gy but doses of 60 Gy will cause approximately 10 dB loss. In a series of patients treated with short fractionation regimens for benign parotid tumours, 12 of 28 had significant sensorineural deafness 5 years or more after treatment. The deafness was predominately high tone: significant deafness was defined as more than 10 dB loss at 0.5, 1 and 2 kHz and more than 20 dB at 4, 6 and 8 kHz.

The late effects of radiation on the eye

The eye is vulnerable when radiotherapy is used to treat tumours of the sinuses or nasopharynx. The eye is a complex structure and several forms of late radiation damage may occur.

Lens Radiation-induced cataract is a classical example of a deterministic effect of radiation: the higher the dose, then the more severe the cataract. Cataracts arise as a result of radiation effects upon the germinative zone of the lens epithelium. This zone is located peripherally about 3–4 mm from the centre of the lens and about 1 mm in front of the equator of the lens. Changes in the lens are not usually detectable until 3 years or more after radiotherapy, and there is a lag of approximately 2 years between the first changes appearing and any detectable change in visual acuity. A single fraction of 5 Gy is sufficient to produce cataract whereas the same dose given in 10–20 fractions is unlikely to do so. The rate of cataract formation 8 years after 15 Gy in 15 fractions to the germinative zone of the lens is around 60 per cent and the probability of decreased visual acuity is approximately 40 per cent. Radiation-induced cataracts can be treated surgically and the radiosensitivity of the lens should not necessarily be the prime concern in planning radiotherapy to the head and neck: it is better to sacrifice the lens than the retina, and cure should not be put in jeopardy simply to avoid a later cataract extraction.

Anterior structures The lacrimal apparatus and cornea can be affected by radiation therapy. Severe damage will cause a painful dry eye and sometimes enucleation is required. Fortunately the tolerance dose of the anterior structures is high (BED = 110 Gy).

Retina Doses of radiation that exceed the tolerance of the retina will cause an exudative retinopathy. This will cause impaired vision and, although steroids and laser coagulation may buy time, vision may ultimately be lost.

Optic nerve The tolerance to radiation of the optic nerve is higher than that of the retina, but if damage does occur, blindness is inevitable and there is no effective treatment.

Radiotherapy: practical aspects of treatment

A detailed discussion of techniques and practices for the irradiation of head and neck tumours is beyond the scope of this chapter. There are several useful references on the subject (Dobbs *et al.*, 1999).

The principles involved are no different from those that apply elsewhere in the body: to devise a treatment technique that homogeneously irradiates the clinical target volume (CTV) while minimizing the dose to the adjacent normal structures. The definition of the CTV is a key issue in the radiotherapy of head and neck cancer. One approach is to keep the CTV as small as possible and irradiate with doses in the range of 2.75–3.5 Gy per fraction, using an overall treatment time of 4 weeks or less. Another approach is to use more generous fields and treat with lower doses per fraction (1.8–2 Gy) over a longer time, 6–7 weeks. Whichever approach is used, the CTV must be defined accurately and the patient must be positioned precisely each day for treatment. This is vital for treatment in the head and neck region because of the close proximity of vulnerable normal structures, such as the eye and spinal cord, to the CTV. An immobilization shell made individually for each patient and used throughout the processes of planning and treatment is the best way of achieving this positional accuracy.

The CTV should be defined using all available information: clinical examination, under anaesthesia if necessary, and imaging. If there is difficulty defining the tumour site, then marking the margins with radiopaque seeds can be useful. Computer-assisted treatment planning techniques should be standard. The CTV is marked on outlines taken at several levels through the intended treatment fields. The optimal combination of field sizes, beam arrangements, beam weights and wedges can be defined. The beam arrangements useful in treating cancers of the head and neck are similar to those used at other sites: parallel opposed; parallel opposed with unequal weighting; three fields with wedged lateral fields; orthogonal wedged pair; ipsilateral wedged pair. Electron fields can be used to boost the dose superficially while sparing structures at depth. There is no particular magic to radiotherapy planning for head and neck tumours, simply that the anatomy is more complicated and more compact than at other sites. Recent innovations in radiotherapeutic techniques are proving useful in the treatment of head and neck cancers. These include multileaf collimators, conformal therapy, stereotactic techniques, intensity modulated therapy and inverse planning algorithms.

The optimal energy for treating head and neck tumours with external-beam treatment is in the range 4–6 MV. The optimal source of radiation is a linear accelerator. Some advantage has, in the past, been claimed for treating certain tumours on ^{60}Co units: the argument being that too focused a beam might miss the tumour. Relying on the penumbra of a poorly collimated beam to treat a tumour is not, however, best practice.

INTERSTITIAL RADIATION THERAPY (BRACHYTHERAPY)

The use of flexible radioactive sources (such as ^{192}Ir wire) as an interstitial implant enables a high dose of radiation to be localized precisely to the site of a tumour. This can be used in the treatment of carcinomas of the lip, oral cavity, oropharynx and nasopharynx. Implantation can also be used in the treatment of lymph nodes. For tumours within the mouth and pharynx either looped implants or ^{192}Ir hairpins can be used. Simple planar implants can be used to treat the lip or nodes in the neck. Special applicators are used to treat tumours in the nasopharynx. Implants can either be used as part of the initial treatment, as a means of boosting the dose to the main bulk of the tumour, or they can be used as a palliative measure to treat symptomatic recurrences.

POSTOPERATIVE RADIOTHERAPY

The role of postoperative radiotherapy in the management of head and neck cancer has, in recent years, become more prominent. In part, it reflects the emergence of combined clinics and a multi-disciplinary approach to treatment. It also reflects the ability to exploit advances in both radiotherapy and surgery.

There is no evidence to suggest that routine postoperative treatment is of benefit to all patients. There are, however, several factors that aid in the selection of patients who might benefit from postoperative radiation. These include: positive resection margins; extracapsular involvement of lymph nodes; bulky nodes (>3 cm); perineural invasion; multifocal origin; multiple nodes positive, particularly if more than one group of nodes is involved; extensive carcinoma in-situ. The tolerance of the normal tissues is reduced following radical surgery and doses should be adjusted accordingly: 47.5–50 Gy in 20 fractions or 55–60 Gy in 30–35 fractions.

RE-TREATMENT WITH RADIOTHERAPY

This is a possible, but potentially hazardous approach, to the problem of recurrent disease, or a second primary tumour, within an area that has already been treated radically with radiotherapy. By definition, radical treatment is close to the tolerance of normal tissues and, therefore, a second course of treatment is likely to exceed tolerance. Nevertheless, the approach is feasible. The tolerance to re-treatment increases with lapsed time following initial treatment. The Institut Gustave Roussy (De Crevoisier et al., 1998) has reported on 169 patients given a second radical course of radiotherapy for head and neck cancer. The median survival was 10 months and nearly a quarter of the patients survived for 2 years. However, by 5 years, fewer than 10 per cent were still alive. As would be expected, the morbidity was high. Acute toxicity was only a little worse than would have been expected in naïve patients: the main problem was late damage (Table 17.19).

Table 17.19 Data from Institut Gustave Roussy on severe late complications following radical re-irradiation of patients with head and neck cancer (from De Crevoisier et al., 1998)

Complication	Rate (%)
Severe subcutaneous fibrosis	41
Mild to severe trismus	30
Osteoradionecrosis (ORN)	6.5
ORN requiring hemi-mandibulectomy	2
Mucosal necrosis	21
Fatal carotid blow-out	3

In highly selected patients, who have had the risks explained to them, and who accept those risks, radical re-treatment may offer useful prolongation of life. The issue of whether the symptoms from radiation effects are worse than those from the tumour itself has not been addressed.

REHABILITATION

The main issues in the rehabilitation of the patient with head and neck cancer are summarized in Table 17.20. Sensitive and careful counselling may be required for patients who have problems with body image following surgical resections. Many of these patients have difficulties with relationships and there is a surprising high incidence of sexual dysfunction. Communication between patients and their partners is often disrupted – each having a completely different understanding of what is going on. Prompt and sensitive intervention can prevent unnecessary psychological morbidity.

The most common physical problems after treatment for head and neck cancer involve mastication and swallowing. Close co-operation between surgeon, prosthodontist, speech therapist and dietician is required.

Table 17.20 *Summary of issues of concern in the rehabilitation of patients with cancers of the head and neck*

Prevention of second primary tumours
  Change in smoking and drinking habits
  Chemoprevention
  Regular ENT assessment
Physiotherapy
  After radical neck dissection or other major surgery
Speech therapy
  After laryngectomy
  Care of the voice during and after radiotherapy
  Swallowing and mastication problems
   (videofluoroscopy)
Prosthetics/prosthodontics
  After major head and neck surgery
Dental care
  After radiotherapy (xerostomia, caries)
Psychological support
  Accepting and dealing with diagnosis
  Specific issues related to perceived damage from
   treatment
  Relationships and sexuality
  Problems with body image
Social support
  Financial and social worries
   loss of earnings
   homelessness
   alcoholism

Videofluoroscopy can be extremely helpful in defining the functional anatomy of the problem and can indicate possible solutions.

The loss of muscle and sacrifice of the spinal accessory nerve during radical neck dissection can cause problems with movements of the shoulder and neck. Appropriate physiotherapy can minimize these difficulties.

Rehabilitation after laryngectomy is complex and has both physical and psychological aspects. Before consenting to laryngectomy, patients should have the opportunity to meet, and to converse with, a patient who has achieved reasonable speech following laryngectomy. Speech therapy is essential postoperatively. Many patients develop satisfactory oesophageal speech. Other options are also available: the electrolarynx, either as an external device or via an intraoral tube; the Blom–Singer valve, inserted into a surgically created fistula between the oesophagus and the trachea. The ability to use the telephone after treatment is a reasonable measure of functional rehabilitation – approximately 40 per cent of patients are able to communicate by telephone after laryngectomy.

THE ROLE OF CHEMOTHERAPY IN HEAD AND NECK CANCER

Chemotherapy can play several roles in the management of head and neck cancer, these are defined and summarized in Table 17.21.

Squamous carcinomas of the head and neck respond extremely well to chemotherapy, the problem is that these responses are short lived and contribute but little to the cure of the disease. The pooled data from over 500 phase II and phase III studies are summarized in Table 17.22. Data from controlled trials may more accurately reflect the real world: the complete response rate in phase III studies is significantly lower than that observed in phase II studies. The explanation for the disparity between response rates and survival benefit may lie in the kinetic behaviour of squamous carcinomas of the head and neck. The high cell loss factor allows ample opportunity for resistant

Table 17.21 *The potential roles played by chemotherapy in the management of head and neck cancer*

As sole treatment
  For cure
  For palliation
Given before definitive treatment (neo-adjuvant)
  To improve survival
To permit less radical ('organ conserving') surgery to be
  performed without compromising cure
Given synchronously with radiotherapy
An attempt to improve the therapeutic ratio: increased
  survival without increased toxicity
Given after definitive treatment (post-adjuvant)
  An attempt to lower the risks of recurrence

Table 17.22 *Data from phase II and phase III studies of chemotherapy for head and neck cancer*

Group	CR rate (%)	95% CI	Number of patients
Chemo alone	29	(28–30)	9 482
Chemo + xrt	61	(60–62)	5 330
Any chemo ± xrt	40	(39–40)	15 353
Platinum and 5-FU	37	(35–38)	4 439
Neither 5-FU nor platinum	22	(21–23)	4 180
Chemo only phase II	36	(34–37)	5 188
Chemo only phase III	20	(19–22)	4 294
Taxanes	49	(45–54)	421

CR, complete response; CI, confidence interval; chemo, chemotherapy; xrt, radiotherapy; 5-FU, 5-fluorouracil.

cells to evolve during the preclinical phases of tumour development. The rapid clinical response reflects high cell loss at a time of impaired production, the persistence and re-growth of the tumour reflects the presence of a small proportion of cells that are able to persist in spite of treatment and, ultimately, to dominate.

The most active combination of drugs for treating squamous carcinoma of the head and neck is cisplatin + 5-fluorouracil (5-FU). Radiotherapy is a potent addition to chemotherapy: the complete response rate to drugs alone is 29 per cent, when chemotherapy is given synchronously with radiotherapy this rate increases to 61 per cent. The taxanes are showing early promise in the treatment of head and neck cancer and, in the future, the most potent combination, on the basis of the early phase II data, may turn out to be a platinum compound plus 5-fluorouracil plus a taxane. These intensive and toxic schedules now need to be tested in prospective randomized trials.

Metastatic disease and palliative treatment

The response of metastatic head and neck cancer to chemotherapy is disappointing. The overall response rate is around 34 per cent (95 per cent CI 32–35 per cent) but only 8.2 per cent (95 per cent CI 7.4–9.0 per cent) of patients achieve a complete response.

There is very little evidence, other than the evanescent responses observed with chemotherapy for head and neck cancer, upon which to base recommendations for chemotherapy as a palliative treatment in this disease. Although over 15 000 patients have been included in published studies of chemotherapy in head and neck cancer, we have no idea whether or not the side-effects of treatment outweigh any reduction in tumour-related symptoms that might have been achieved. The question of quality of life is being belatedly addressed but there is, as yet, no information upon which to base an informed decision as to the palliative benefit, or lack of benefit, of chemotherapy for patients with head and neck cancer.

Chemotherapy in the curative treatment of locoregional disease

The conclusions of a systematic review of 73 randomized comparisons between standard treatment alone and similar treatment plus chemotherapy in the curative treatment of head and neck cancer can be summarized as:

1 neoadjuvant chemotherapy has minimal impact on survival;

2 the 'organ conserving' approach is feasible: it is possible to perform less radical surgery without sacrificing locoregional control;

3 when chemotherapy is given synchronously with radiotherapy then both the local control rates and the survival rates are higher than when radiotherapy is given alone. This benefit is achieved at the cost of increased acute toxicity – an effect that might possibly have been achieved with radiation alone, simply by increasing the dose of radiation.

The data on which these statements are based are summarized in Tables 17.23 to 17.26. A recently completed UK multi-centre randomized study of 971 patients has produced results which broadly confirm that synchronous chemotherapy is beneficial (J. Tobias, personal communication). Interestingly, this study, conceived in 1990, did not use platinum-based chemotherapy.

Although chemotherapy may contribute little to the cure of head and neck cancer, it is none the less useful. In the USA, the use of neo-adjuvant chemotherapy has proved helpful in convincing surgeons that T3 laryngeal carcinomas can be managed successfully without laryngectomy.

New drugs, and old drugs in new disguises, are constantly entering clinical practice. This is both a problem and a gift: a problem in that we do not yet know how best to use what we already have; a gift in that current chemotherapy is not particularly effective. Conventional drugs, such as *cis*-platinum and doxorubicin, can be encapsulated within liposomes and this can increase their specificity so that the effect on the tumour is maintained, but toxicity is less. This is yet another promising way forward.

In spite of over 30 years of clinical trials, we have not yet defined a role for chemotherapy in head and neck cancer. All too often, the assumption has been made that more must be better. We have limited data on the effectiveness of single agents and abundant data on the relative ineffectiveness of combinations of drugs. The present illustration of this is the addition of taxanes to existing regimens. Crucial information is missing, both from published studies, and, sadly, from studies that are currently being carried out. We know a great deal about blood counts and whether or not mucosal reactions were confluent. We know hardly anything about the pain, suffering, disruption and distress experienced by patients treated with chemotherapy for head and neck cancer. Until we do, bearing in mind that over 60 per cent of patients treated

Table 17.23 *Data on survival from a systematic review of randomized trials of chemotherapy in head and neck cancer. The rate difference (with 95% confidence interval) is simply rate in experimental arm − rate in control arm. Data were pooled using the random effects method of DerSimonian and Laird (1986)*

	Number of trials	Number of patients	Rate difference (%)
Survival all trials	73	11 355	8 (5–11)
Survival neo-adjuvant	43	6 205	4 (2–6)
Survival synchronous	28	3 910	16 (11–21)
Survival post-adjuvant	3	326	−9 (−22 to +4)

Table 17.24 *Data on locoregional control and the need for radical surgery from a systematic review of randomized trials of chemotherapy in head and neck cancer. The rate difference (with 95% confidence interval) is simply rate in experimental arm − rate in control arm. Data were pooled using the random effects method of DerSimonian and Laird (1986)*

	Number of trials	Number of patients	Rate difference (%)
Locoregional control (synchronous chemo–rt)	26	3353	16 (10–23)
Locoregional control (neo-adjuvant)	26	4726	−2 (−7 to 2)
Radical surgery required (neo-adjuvant)	19	2878	−15 (−27 to −3)

Chemo, chemotherapy; rt, radiotherapy.

Table 17.25 *Data on adverse consequences of treatment from a systematic review of randomized trials of chemotherapy in head and neck cancer. The rate difference (with 95% confidence interval) is simply rate in experimental arm − rate in control arm. Data were pooled using the random effects method of DerSimonian and Laird (1986)*

	Number of trials	Number of patients	Rate difference (%)	Control (%)	Chemo–rt (%)
Mucositis (synchronous)	24	3453	16 (10–21)	15	28
Rx related death (synchronous)	22	2963	0.06 (−4 to +5)	0.1	0.7
Rx related death (neo-adjuvant)	30	4902	0.9 (0.3–1.6)	1.3	3.5

Chemo, chemotherapy; rt, radiotherapy.

Table 17.26 *Per-patient meta-analysis of the role of chemotherapy added to locoregional therapy for head and neck cancer (data from Pignon et al., 2000)*

Type of chemo–rt	Absolute improvement in 5-year survival (%)
Adjuvant	1
Neo-adjuvant	2
Concomitant	8
All	4

Chemo, chemotherapy; rt, radiotherapy.

with curative intent are not actually cured, rational decision making will be impossible. There is little justification, outwith a clinical trial, for using chemotherapy to treat patients with head and neck cancer. The problem is to find a trial that asks a worthwhile question.

QUALITY OF LIFE

Quality of life is, like beauty, a concept that everyone understands but no-one can put adequately into words.

There are particular aspects of quality of life that are important to patients with head and neck cancer: appearance, eating and swallowing, speech and communication. These domains are not adequately covered by many of the generic instruments used to measure whatever happens to be called 'quality of life'. The largest single body of data on quality of life in patients with head and neck cancer comes from the CHART trial of accelerated hyperfractionation in the radical treatment of cancers of the head and neck. Patients were followed up for 2 years after treatment and, at each of 10 assessments, each patient completed a 33-item questionnaire based on the Rotterdam Symptom Check List. Over 200 000 data items were generated from the 615 patients in this part of the CHART trial. Somewhat surprisingly, the patients were not asked about many important issues and problems: difficulty swallowing, problems with communication, ability to eat in public, changes in taste, etc. The data on symptoms at presentation are summarized in Table 17.27.

There are now several quality of life instruments available specifically for patients with head and neck cancer. These include the University of Washington QOL (UWQOL), the Performance Status Scale–Head and Neck (PSS–HN) and the EORTC head and neck module

Table 17.27 *Symptoms assessed immediately before starting radiotherapy in patients with cancer of the head and neck: ranked in order by frequency and by distress (data from Griffiths et al., 1999; Munro and Potter, 1996)*

Ten most frequent (CHART)		Ten most distressing (CHART)	Ten most distressing (Bart's)
Tiredness	1	Hoarseness	Feeling anxious
Worrying	2	Difficulty sleeping	Hoarse
Anxious feelings	3	Tiredness	Worry about effects on family
Hoarseness	4	Lack of energy	Tired
Sore mouth/pain on swallowing	5	Sore mouth/pain on swallowing	Dry mouth
Lack of energy	6	Pain	Needing to be immobilized for treatment
Feeling tense	7	Decreased libido	Difficulty sleeping
Cough	8	Cough	Weight loss
Difficulty sleeping	9	Lack of appetite	Lack of appetite
Pain	10	Tense	Change in taste

Table 17.28 *Patients' priorities as assessed by Sharp et al. (1999)*

Rank	Effect of treatment
1	Being cured of my cancer
2	Living as long as possible
3	Having no pain
4	Keeping my natural voice
5	Having my speech understood easily
6	Being able to swallow all foods and drinks
7	Being able to chew normally
8	Keeping my normal sense of taste and smell
9	Having a comfortably moist mouth
10	Keeping my appearance unchanged
11	Having a normal amount of energy for me
12	Returning to my normal activities as soon as possible

These data were obtained from a small sample, $n = 20$, of patients with head and neck cancer.

(EORTC QLQ-H&N35). These tools will prove invaluable in future clinical studies in head and neck cancer and should help put decision making on to a more rational and less prejudiced basis.

Patients' expectations and desires regarding the treatment of head and neck cancer have been investigated recently in a small study from the University of Chicago (Table 17.28). As might be anticipated, patients rank cure as their highest priority. Keeping their natural voice is also important and, as was shown by Pauker and McNeil many years ago, some individuals are prepared to compromise their chances of cure in order to retain their natural voice.

There is a tendency to regard patients with head and neck cancer as non-sexual beings. This is totally inappropriate. The data from both the CHART trial and from the validation studies on the EORTC QLQ-H&N35 (Table 17.29) show that sexuality is important to patients with head and neck cancer and that worries and concerns about sexuality are a cause of considerable distress. The data from the CHART study show that over 20 per cent of patients rated their distress concerning loss of interest in sex as moderate or severe. These were patients who had not had major surgery. Imagine what it is like to kiss if you have had a tracheostomy, or to be kissed by someone who has had their larynx removed. These issues and concerns have to be addressed before, during and after treatment. There is more to treating cancer than extirpating a tumour, although, admittedly, that is an excellent start.

PALLIATIVE CARE

Tumours of the head and neck have the potential to destroy people in ways that do not apply to more deeply seated tumours. Head and neck cancers are often highly visible, and even small tumours can produce severe symptoms. Treatment often adds to the mutilation and deformity and exacerbates the stigma that patients already feel. Isolation, pain, cachexia and fear can all combine to produce a miserable existence: the challenge in the palliative management of head and neck cancer is to prevent such problems developing. The challenge is not trivial – 50 per cent of patients with head and neck cancer die from uncontrolled locoregional disease. Only about 10 per cent of patients will die from metastatic disease with the primary tumour controlled. A dignified, painless, death from liver metastases or renal failure is unusual in patients with head and neck cancer.

This raises an important question: is it justifiable to put a patient through a protracted, painful, debilitating and potentially mutilating sequence of treatments for what may turn out to be a very low chance of cure? The only sensible answer to such a question is that such a course of action may be justifiable provided that the individual patient, fully appraised of the benefits and harms associated with radical treatment, chooses to be so treated.

Given the heterogeneity that is intrinsic to cancers of the head and neck, and to the patients who are afflicted by them, there can be no stock solutions to clinical problems. Each patient, with their hopes, their fears, their own unique predicament, has to be managed and treated as an individual. Guidelines can provide advice but should

Table 17.29 *Problems before treatment in patients with head and neck cancer assessed using the EORTC QLQ-H&N35. Problems are ranked according to severity and grouped according to site of the primary tumour (Bjordal et al., 1999)*

Rank	Larynx	Oral	Pharynx
1	Speech	Pain	Sticky saliva
2	Cough	Dental problems	Pain
3	Sticky saliva	Sexuality	Sexuality
4	Dry mouth	Dry mouth	Cough
5	Sexuality	Sticky saliva	Feeling ill
6	Feeling ill	Social eating	Swallowing
7	Dental problems	Opening mouth	Dry mouth
8	Pain	Cough	Speech
9	Swallowing	Swallowing	Needing painkillers
10	Needing analgesics	Speech	Dental problems

not dictate management. There can be no useful protocol to dictate how the Goldberg Variations should be played, nor can the rigid implementation of protocols play a major role in the provision of care for patients with cancers of the head and neck.

The specific symptoms and problems associated with head and neck cancer are outlined in Table 17.30. Management depends first upon the recognition of the symptom then upon the appreciation of the mechanism by which it is occurring, and finally upon applying appropriate treatment. Psychological support, explanation and reassurance should be an integral part of this process.

The most logical approach is often to treat the tumour itself and combine treatment with whatever adjunctive treatments (analgesia, dietary supplements, etc.) are necessary. The problem is that treatment itself often produces symptoms and thus violates a basic principle of palliative treatment – first do no harm. The acute mucosal reaction caused by radiotherapy may prove more troublesome than the symptoms produced by the tumour. Split courses of treatment, by allowing time for repopulation of normal mucosal cells, offer a way round the problem: 14.8 Gy in 4 fractions over 2–4 days repeated 2–3 times at 3-week intervals is a useful schedule. Xerostomia may, however, still be troublesome.

Palliative surgical resections of tumour are not usually helpful but laser therapy, including photodynamic therapy, may provide usual palliation for lesions that are superficial and accessible. Cranial nerve sections may be useful for intractable pain.

Pain

Pain is a frequent and distressing symptom in patients with head and neck cancer. The causes and mechanisms are summarized in Table 17.31. Nearly 50 per cent of patients have pain at and around the time of diagnosis, 8 per cent of patients rated their pain as severe (Chaplin and Morton, 1999). Successful treatment of head and neck cancer provides effective pain control: by 2 years after successful treatment the proportion of patients complaining of pain was 26 per cent, and 4 per cent of patients had severe pain.

In order to manage pain rationally it is essential to discriminate between nociceptive pain caused by stimulation of free nerve endings and non-nociceptive, neuropathic pain related to abnormal excitability of nerve fibres. Nociceptive pain is managed primarily by prostaglandin antagonists and opiates whereas membrane stabilizers and nerve blocks are more appropriate for non-nociceptive pain.

The palliative treatment of head and neck cancer is not simply about attempting to shrink tumours. Broader existential issues have to be considered: fear (of pain, of disfigurement, of dying), emotional isolation, problems of body image (wasting, weakness), social function, nurture, nourishing and nutrition. If these, and many other, issues are to be properly dealt with, then there has to be adequate and open communication between the patient, the patient's family, the hospital-based services and the services based in the community. The Macmillan Nursing services and the district nurses can be an essential part of this liaison; however, the comparative rarity of these tumours means that individual nurses may have limited experience in dealing with the problems involved.

NOVEL APPROACHES TO THE MANAGEMENT OF HEAD AND NECK CANCER

Photodynamic therapy

Photodynamic therapy (PDT) is based on the principle that some tissues, including tumours, will specifically take up light-sensitizing chemicals. If light of a wavelength that will specifically excite the photochemical is shone upon the tumour and its immediate environment, then only the illuminated cells will be exposed to the toxic effects of singlet oxygen produced by the photochemical reaction. The biological effects of photodynamic therapy

Table 17.30 *Specific symptoms and problems which may require palliation in head and neck cancer*

Obstruction
  Upper airway
    dyspnoea
    fatigue
    stridor
  Pharynx
    dysphagia
  Nose
    anosmia
    headache
    sinusitis
    cacosmia
  Blood vessels
    facial congestion/swelling
    headache
    CNS symptoms (confusion, blurred vision)
  Eustachian tube
    otitis media
    deafness

Pain
  Nociceptive
    spread of tumour; infection
  Non-nociceptive
    nerve involvement
    neuropathy following radical neck dissection

Aspiration
  Destruction of upper airway sphincters by
    tumour
  Fibrosis following XRT
  Distorted anatomy following surgery

Bleeding
  From local tumour
    internally
    externally
  From eroded vein or artery

Dysphagia
  Obstruction by tumour
    intrinsic
    extrinsic

Dysphagia *(continued)*
  Fibrosis after surgery and/or XRT
  Reduced tongue mobility
  Secondary to involvement or destruction of lower
    cranial nerves
  Secondary to aspiration
  Secondary to dry mouth

Dry mouth
  Secondary to XRT

Special senses
  Diplopia
    invasion of orbit
    cranial nerve involvement
  Anosmia
    ethmoid tumours
    after craniofacial resection
    after XRT
  Deafness
    naso-pharyngeal carcinoma via VIIIth nerve
    rarely directly due to tumour
    post radiotherapy
  Balance
    usually secondary to other factors (anaemia, vascular
      insufficiency, hypotension)
  Communication
    receptive difficulties
    expressive difficulties
    psychological difficulties

Syncope
  IXth nerve syndrome (pain, hypotension, bradycardia)
  Carotid sinus hypersensitivity (bradycardia)

Weight loss
  Lack of appetite
  Inability to eat (tumour, side-effects of treatment)
  Cancer-induced cachexia

Foetor
  Infected tumour
  Mucositis
  Dental problems

XRT, radiotherapy.

Table 17.31 *Causes and mechanisms of pain in patients with cancer of the head and neck*

Related to tumour	Related to therapy
Infection	Mucositis (radiation, chemotherapy)
Inflammation	Nerve damage (spinal accessory)
Ulceration	Fibrosis
Bone invasion	Shoulder pain after radical neck dissection
Invasion of nerves	Trismus after radiotherapy
Lymphatic obstruction and raised pressure	Necrosis
within tissues	Surgery
	Radiotherapy

are complex. Cell death, by apoptosis or necrosis, occurs within 4 hours of treatment. Vascular effects are also important: obliterative changes cause ischaemia and impaired perfusion. Unlike ionizing radiation, for which the dependence upon oxygen is only relative, the biological effects of PDT have an absolute dependence upon oxygen: PDT has no effect when oxygen concentration falls below 0.5 per cent. Oxygen is rapidly depleted within tissues treated with PDT, this imposes a biological limitation upon the duration of effect.

The selectivity of uptake with currently available photosensitizers is not particularly impressive: the tumour to normal tissue ratios are typically around 2:3. For true therapeutic selectivity, ratios of at least 10, and preferably 100, would be required. Any benefits from PDT at present are more to do with the localization of light penetration, and subsequent sensitization, than any selectivity of the photochemical for tumour cells.

In practice, photodynamic therapy works as follows. Before exposing the tumour to light, the patient is treated with a photosensitizing chemical. Typical compounds are derived from porphyrins. The drug is concentrated within the tumour and eliminated from the normal tissues. The tumour is treated using a coherent source of laser light of appropriate wavelength. The approach is only feasible for tumours that are endoscopically accessible and relatively superficial. As technology develops, more tumours will be accessible using fibre optic sources and higher light energy will enable the light to penetrate more deeply into tumours. Currently the limit of penetration is between 5 and 10 mm. Systemically administered sensitizers will affect all tissues, this is only of practical importance for the skin. Those sensitizers with long total body clearance times will cause prolonged photosensitization of the skin. Patients should be warned to avoid exposure to sunlight, or fluorescent light, until the drug has been eliminated – for Photofrin this could take as long as 6–12 weeks.

A variety of photosensitizers is now available for clinical use. These are summarized in Table 17.32.

The main role of PDT in the management of head and neck cancer has been in the curative treatment of premalignant conditions, such as erythroplasia and leucoplakia in the oral cavity. It is establishing a niche in the palliative treatment of superficial recurrent disease. In the future, flexible light sources implanted into tumours may allow more homogeneous PDT for larger and deeper tumours. The integration of PDT with more conventional treatments as part of the primary management of head and neck cancer may be a promising area for future research.

Hyperthermia

As a means of specifically killing cancer cells, heat has many biological advantages over ionizing radiation. Unfortunately there are major physical disadvantages in terms of therapeutic equipment and dosimetry. Interstitial hyperthermia can be used, with or without radiation, in the palliative treatment of recurrent disease. There is, however, little indication that hyperthermia will have a major role to play in the primary management of head and neck cancer. It may have a useful contribution to make, in combination with radiotherapy, in the re-treatment of disease that has recurred locally following previous treatment with radiation.

Table 17.32 *A summary of clinically useful photosensitizers for photodynamic therapy (PDT)*

Haematoporphyrin derivative (HpD)
  The original photosensitizer
  Complex mixture of a variety of porphyrins
Photofrin
  A purified version of HpD containing a mixture of various porphyrins together with their ether and ester derivatives
  Several absorption peaks, maximal at 630 nm
  Skin sensitization lasts 6–12 weeks
5-Aminolaevulinic acid (5-ALA)
  A pro-drug which is metabolically converted to the active agent, protoporphyrin IX (PpIX)
  Can be used topically or systemically
meta-Tetrahydroxyphenychlorin (mTHPC, Foscan)
  A stronger absorption peak than Photofrin, peak is at 652 nm
  Skin toxicity lasts 3–6 weeks
Benzoporphyrin derivative (BPD)
  Strong peak at 690 nm, mono-acid form (BPD-MA) is more active
  Skin photosensitization lasts less than 5 days
Mono aspartyl chlorin e6 (Npe6)
  Peak is at 664 nm
  Short duration of action, skin photosensitization lasts less than a week
Lutetium texaphyrin (Lu-Tex)
  A third-generation sensitizer, preferential accumulation within tumours
  Transient skin toxicity, rapidly excreted
  Peak is at 732 nm
  Can be used for repeated treatments, a possible way round the problems of photobleaching and oxygen depletion

Biological therapies

The finding that many subtle abnormalities can be identified in squamous carcinomas has prompted the development of treatments aimed at specifically targeting those abnormalities which may be unique to the malignant cells.

Abnormal p53 is present in about 50 per cent of patients with head and neck cancer and thus presents an obvious target for therapeutic manipulation. Restoration of normal (wild-type) p53 has been attempted using a construct based on an adenovirus as vector. The construct (Ad–p53) uses the wild-type *p53* gene inserted into an adenoviral backbone. In a phase I study of 34 patients with advanced, recurrent or refractory head and neck cancer the Ad–p53 construct was administered by injection directly into the tumour. The data on expression of the *p53* transgene is scanty but persisting gene expression was observed in at least one patient. One patient obtained a pathological complete response, two patients achieved partial responses, six patients had stable disease, nine patients had progressive disease, 16 patients were not evaluated in terms of any disease response. There was little systemic toxicity. Interestingly, there is the suggestion that the treatment can be effective even in tumours which express wild-type *p53*. An alternative approach has been to use ONYX-015. This is an adenovirus which has had the E1B gene deleted and which will therefore selectively replicate within, and destroy, cells that lack wild-type *p53*. Phase I/II studies have shown that about 30 per cent of advanced cancers of the head and neck will respond to injection of ONYX-015 directly into the tumour. Even though the role of ONYX-015 as a single agent has not been clearly established it is already being combined, in further phase II trials, with chemotherapy.

Squamous cancers of the head and neck often express epidermal growth factor receptor (EGFR). There are two ways in which tumour cells can be targeted using this receptor. One is to use a monoclonal antibody, such as C225, directed against the receptor. Early clinical studies suggest that this approach has some biological effect. An alternative approach is to inhibit the tyrosine kinase that is responsible for the onward transmission of the signal generated when EGF binds to its receptor. Specific inhibitors of this kinase, such as the quinazolin compound CP-358, have been identified and are currently being assessed in phase I studies.

As our knowledge of the molecular biology of head and neck cancer increases then it is likely that many new therapeutic agents will be developed. It is equally likely that the initial clinical impact of molecular biology in head and neck cancer will be upon the assessment of prognosis and the definition of patients at particularly high risk of local recurrence or distant spread. Staining for p53 has already demonstrated that cancer cells may be present at resection margins defined as clear by conventional histology. The presence of such cells may be of independent prognostic significance.

STAGING AND PROGNOSIS

The factors that influence the prognosis of patients with head and neck cancer can be grouped into three main categories: factors related to the tumour, factors related to the host and factors related to treatment. The traditional clinical staging systems have concentrated primarily on those factors related to the tumour. Table 17.33 summarizes host- and tumour-related factors of potential relevance to prognosis.

The primary purpose of staging head and neck cancer is to classify tumours reproducibly so that valid comparisons can be made between groups of patients. Classification should also provide an indication of the prognosis for an individual patient. The UICC TNM system for cancer has undergone several revisions, most recently in 1997. The system has to cope with the heterogeneity of head and neck cancer, the wide variety of sites and subsites,

Table 17.33 *Prognostic factors in head and neck cancer*

Host related
Demographic/behavioural
  Gender (males worse)
  Age (under 40 worse)
  Ethnic group
  Tobacco use
    previous (worse)
    continuing (worse)
  Performance status (poorer performance worse)
  Nutritional status and diet (poorer worse)
  HIV status (positive worse)
Laboratory
  Haemoglobin (low worse)
  Albumin (low worse)
  Immune competence (impaired worse)

Treatment related
Surgery (adverse factors)
  Positive margins
  Wound infection
  Transfusion requirement
  Tracheostomy requirement
Radiotherapy
  Dose (lower worse)
  Overall treatment time (longer worse)

Tumour related
Primary
  Macroscopic
    Site
    Size
    T stage
    Appearance
      infiltrating (worse)
      exophytic (better)
    Local invasion
    Associated field change (worse)
  Microscopic
    Depth of invasion
    Differentiation (poor worse)
    Mitotic rate
    Pleomorphism
    Vascular invasion
  Molecular biology
    Ploidy (aneuploid worse)
    Tumour angiogenesis
      increased nodal metastases
      ?improved control of primary
    Syndecan-1, cell adhesion molecule
     (higher levels better)
    p53 mutations (?better ?worse)
    EGFR (high levels worse)
      p27 (low levels worse)
      c-*erb B-2* overexpression (worse)
      c-*myc* expression (worse)
      Loss of heterozygosity at 2q or 10q (worse)
Nodes
  Macroscopic
    Size
    N stage
    Fixation
    Density on CT scanning
  Microscopic
    Extracapsular spread
    Lymphocyte depletion
    Plasmacytic response

Table 17.34 *N staging (UICC, 1997) of head and neck cancer*

NX	Regional lymph nodes cannot be assessed
N0	No regional lymph-node metastasis
N1	Metastasis in a single ipsilateral lymph node, 3 cm or less in greatest dimension
N2	Metastasis in a single ipsilateral lymph node, more than 3 cm but not more than 6 cm in greatest dimension, or in multiple ipsilateral lymph nodes, none more than 6 cm in greatest dimension, or in bilateral or contralateral lymph nodes, none more than 6 cm in greatest dimension
	N2a Metastasis in a single ipsilateral lymph node more than 3 cm but not more than 6 cm in greatest dimension
	N2b Metastasis in multiple ipsilateral lymph nodes, none more than 6 cm in greatest dimension
	N2c Metastasis in bilateral or contralateral lymph nodes, none more than 6 cm in greatest dimension
N3	Metastasis in a lymph node more than 6 cm in greatest dimension

as well as the conflicting demands of surgeons and radio-therapists. It therefore represents a pragmatic compromise which is broadly useful, but is not entirely perfect.

There is a uniform N staging for nodal disease in the neck (Table 17.34), an exception is made for nasopharyngeal cancer. This has its own staging system, based primarily on the extensive experience of radiotherapists in the Far East.

The TNM system recognizes four degrees of histological differentiation for head and neck cancer:

- G1: well differentiated
- G2: moderately well differentiated
- G3: poorly differentiated
- G4: undifferentiated.

GX indicates that the degree of differentiation cannot be assessed.

There is also an R classification for indicating the presence and extent of residual tumour after primary therapy:

- R0 no residual tumour
- R1 microscopic residual tumour
- R2 macroscopic residual tumour
- RX residual tumour cannot be assessed.

The primary anatomical sites in the head and neck recognized by the TNM system are the lip, oral cavity, pharynx, larynx, maxilla, salivary glands and thyroid. The staging of thyroid and salivary tumours is considered in detail elsewhere (Chapters 19 and 18). The anatomical subsites and details of T staging for the other sites are considered in the appropriate later sections of this chapter. In general, Tis indicates carcinoma *in-situ*, Tx indicates that the primary tumour cannot be assessed and T0 indicates that there is no evidence of primary tumour.

Stage grouping

The recognition that the TNM system can produce a daunting array of permutations in head and neck cancer has led to the grouping of combinations of TNM categories into five larger groups, designated stage 0 to IV (Table 17.35). The main problem with stage grouping is that inherent to any process of aggregation: loss of fine

Table 17.35 *Stage groupings, based on TNM, for cancers of the head and neck*

Stage group	T	N	M
0	Tis	0	0
I	1	0	0
II	2	0	0
III	3	0	0
	1	1	0
	2	1	0
	3	1	0
IV			
A	4	0, 1	0
	Any T	2	0
B	Any	3	0
C	Any	Any	1

discrimination and the collapse of disparate entities into biologically implausible categories. This is particularly true of stage IV disease, which encompasses a spectrum extending from patients with locally advanced disease and minimal nodal involvement all the way through to patients with widespread metastatic disease. In recognition of this problem, the latest stage grouping subdivides stage IV into:

- IVA – advanced locoregional, non-metastatic: T4N0M0, T4N1M0, T(any)N2M0
- IVB – advanced nodal disease, non-metastatic: T(any) N3M0
- IVC – metastatic: T(any) N(any)M1.

Stage migration

Stage migration, that process whereby an artefactual improvement in stage-specific results can be produced simply by changing staging investigations or classification criteria, can cause problems in the interpretation of clinical results in head and neck cancer. It is obvious that patients with pathologically negative necks diagnosed as N0 by radical neck dissection are not directly comparable to patients staged clinically as N0. It is less immediately obvious that patients staged as II or III after CT and/or MRI will have a better prognosis than patients staged conventionally as stage II or III.

Table 17.36 *The consequences of persistent smoking for patients treated with radical radiotherapy for head and neck cancer*

End point	Continued to smoke (*n* = 53)	Non-smokers or quit (*n* = 62)	*P* by χ^2
Complete remission	45%	74%	0.003
2-year survival	40%	70%	0.003

Host-related prognostic factors

The most immediately relevant host-related factors are those that, unlike age, gender or previous social habits, are capable of favourable manipulation. Low pre-treatment haemoglobin is an adverse prognostic factor for survival in patients with tumours of the larynx and pharynx treated primarily with radiotherapy. The effect can be demonstrated even within a range that would be defined as physiologically normal. Transfusion would be beneficial if the low haemoglobin directly caused impaired survival, but it would not necessarily improve matters if the lower haemoglobin was simply a surrogate marker for some unidentified underlying factor in tumour or host – for example impaired nutritional status. The role of erythropoietin in increasing haemoglobin levels, and, perhaps, thereby improve the results of radiotherapy for head and neck cancer, is currently being investigated in randomized trials.

There is evidence that persistent smoking can adversely affect prognosis in patients treated with radiotherapy for head and neck cancer. The data from a Canadian study on 115 patients are summarized in Table 17.36. These data can be used to try to persuade patients to stop smoking.

ASSESSMENT OF THE PATIENT WITH HEAD AND NECK CANCER

A full clinical history and appropriate physical examination are essential. The history should pay particular attention to the duration of symptoms, possible aetiological factors and symptoms suggestive of metastatic disease, or a second (synchronous) primary tumour, should be actively sought. General physical examination should again be slanted towards the detection of systemic disease or second primary tumour. An adequate social history is also important, social and psychological problems should be anticipated and, wherever possible, dealt with.

The primary tumour should be assessed clinically. Site of origin, size, appearance and involvement of adjacent structures should all be formally recorded. Standardized diagrams are helpful both for initial assessment and subsequent follow-up. Wherever possible, patients should be assessed by more than one experienced clinician. The clinicians should make their assessments independently, record their findings, and only after so doing should they discuss and assign the TNM stage. The presence or absence of premalignant change should also be formally recorded.

Indirect endoscopy performed in the outpatient clinic can be supplemented by fibre-optic endoscopy but most patients will require formal assessment under anaesthesia. Adequate biopsy is mandatory: although the vast majority of head and neck tumours are squamous carcinomas, other histologies are encountered. It is a therapeutic disaster to mistake a lymphoma for a squamous carcinoma.

The following investigations should be performed in all patients: full blood count; liver function tests; urea and electrolytes; chest X-ray. CT scanning and MRI can provide important supplementary information, particularly concerning direct extension of tumour into bone or extent of nodal disease. CT is particularly useful in evaluating invasion of the laryngeal cartilage or spread into the pre-epiglottic or the paraglottic space. Although CT imaging enables very precise computation of tumour volume, this has not, for laryngeal cancer at least, proved to be of prognostic significance. CT imaging is not only useful diagnostically but can also facilitate radiotherapy planning – both for external-beam treatment and for brachytherapy. MRI scanning is particularly useful for assessing tongue tumours and in the assessment of the patient with amalgam-filled teeth.

Transcutaneous ultrasound in combination with flexible endosonography has proved useful in assessing bony involvement of the mandible in patients with oral tumours. Fine-needle aspiration cytology can be extremely useful, if there is a doubt about whether enlarged nodes are reactive or involved by tumour. There is no evidence that fine-needle aspirate performed before definitive treatment adversely affects prognosis. Although all these technological advances have improved the assessment of patients with head and neck cancer, there is still no substitute for careful clinical examination.

NECK NODES

There are three main areas of controversy concerning the management of cervical nodes in patients with head and neck cancer:

1 The management of the patient who presents with a malignant neck node in the absence of a clinically detectable primary tumour.
2 The role of prophylactic treatment to the neck in patients with primary tumours of the head and neck who have no evidence of cervical lymphadenopathy.

3 The management of potentially operable cervical lymphadenopathy in patients with primary tumours in the head and neck.

Presentation with malignant node in the neck

Between 5 and 10 per cent of patients with malignant disease seen in ENT departments have, as their presenting symptom, a lump in the neck. The majority of tumours are squamous cell carcinomas, the rest are adenocarcinomas, lymphomas or undifferentiated tumours. Prognosis depends critically upon histology: lymphomas have good prognosis, adenocarcinomas have an extremely poor prognosis – few patients survive for more than 3 years. The prognosis for patients with squamous carcinoma presenting in this fashion is intermediate (30–40 per cent 5-year survival).

The location of the lymphadenopathy, together with histology, may give an indication of whether the occult primary tumour lies above or below the clavicles. Nodes in the supra-clavicular fossa and/or adenocarcinoma usually indicate that the primary tumour is below the clavicles. The prognosis of adenocarcinoma presenting as a neck node is so poor that aggressive treatment cannot be justified for patients in whom a primary tumour cannot be found. Only treatable primary tumours should be sought. There is no point in performing extensive gastrointestinal endoscopies or barium studies. The potentially treatable primaries and the relevant investigations are outlined in Table 17.37.

SQUAMOUS CARCINOMA PRESENTING AS A CERVICAL LYMPH NODE

This subject has been reviewed by Jones *et al.* (1993): a total of 267 patients with squamous carcinoma presenting in this way were identified from the database of the Liverpool Head and Neck Unit. The findings are summarized in Table 17.38. Five-year survival for all the patients

presenting with squamous cell carcinoma in cervical nodes was 27 per cent. For those in whom a primary tumour in the head and neck could not be identified, survival was 31 per cent. The methods by which the primary site was identified are summarized in Table 17.39. All patients in whom a primary tumour was never found, or whose primary tumours were located below the clavicle, died within 5 years of diagnosis. Open biopsy of the neck nodes, as opposed to other ways of making the diagnosis, such as fine-needle aspiration, appeared adversely to affect survival.

The traditional approach to treatment when the primary site cannot be defined has been to use extended-field radiotherapy, with a treatment volume to include not just the neck nodes bilaterally but also the potential sites for the primary tumour. These would include the nasopharynx, the piriform fossa and the whole of the larynx. The Mayo Clinic reviewed, from their usual surgical perspective, their experience with neck nodes and unknown primary tumours (Coster *et al.*, 1992). Of 117 patients seen with this presentation between 1965 and 1987, 24 were treated by neck dissection without radiotherapy or any other treatment directed at possible primary sites. The 10-year survival in this highly selected group was 40 per cent. Experience from the radiotherapy department at the Middlesex Hospital, London also suggests that extended treatment may not always be necessary. The 5-year survival in 48 patients treated with radical radiotherapy to the neck only was 51 per cent – morbidity

Table 17.37 *Investigations, in addition to full history and examination, aimed at excluding treatable primary tumours as a cause of cervical lymphadenopathy*

Primary tumour	Investigations
Breast	Mammography
Ovary	CA 125
	Pelvic ultrasound
Prostate	Serum PSA
Germ cell tumour (gonadal or extragonadal)	Serum AFP and βhCG
	Pelvic ultrasound (female)
	Testicular ultrasound (male)
Thyroid	Serum thyroglobulin
	Thyroid ultrasound

AFP, α-fetoprotein; βhCG, human chorionic gonadotrophin; PSA, prostate-specific antigen.

Table 17.38 *Sites of primary tumour in the Liverpool series of patients presenting with nodes in the neck*

Site	%
Hypopharynx	17
Oropharynx	25
PNS	12
Mouth	7
Larynx	14
Bronchus	9
Cervix	2
Unknown	13

PNS, post-nasal space.

Table 17.39 *Method of diagnosis of primary site in patients presenting with nodes in the neck*

Method of identification	%
Outpatient history and examination	56
EUA	16
CXR	4
Follow-up or PM	11
Never	13

CXR, chest X-ray; EUA, examination under anaesthetic; PM, post mortem examination.

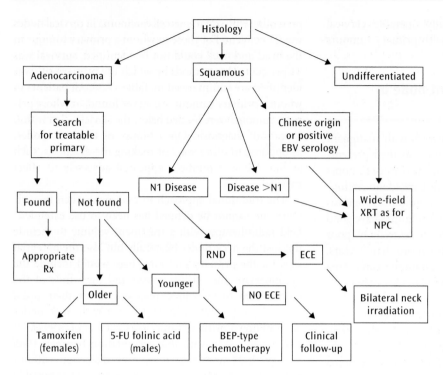

Figure 17.5 *A flow chart for the suggested management of a patient presenting with a node in the neck and no clinically obvious primary tumour. NPC, nasopharyngeal carcinoma; XRT, radiotherapy; BEP, bleomycin, etoposide, cis-platin; ECE, extracapsular extension; RND, radical neck dissection.*

was minimal, mainly because the bulk of both parotid glands could be spared (Glynne-Jones *et al.*, 1989).

Management

The flow chart (Fig. 17.5), based upon the available clinical evidence, illustrates an approach to the management of patients who present with neck nodes and an undetectable primary tumour. It assumes that all patients have been adequately investigated which, nowadays, should include a CT of thorax as well as CT of the head and neck.

For patients treated radically with radiotherapy for squamous or undifferentiated carcinomas the dose should be 47.5–52.5 Gy in 20 fractions. Palliative local radiotherapy may have a role in patients with adenocarcinomas in order to alleviate local discomfort or to prevent fungation of the nodes. It is reasonable to treat women presenting with adenocarcinomas with tamoxifen. Men presenting in this fashion, in whom prostate cancer has been excluded, and who seek active treatment, can be treated with systemic chemotherapy. For younger patients it is reasonable to use bleomycin, etoposide and carboplatin empirically, for older patients less toxic regimens such as 5-fluorouracil + folinic acid are preferable.

THE ROLE OF PROPHYLACTIC TREATMENT TO THE NECK IN PATIENTS WITH A CLINICALLY NEGATIVE NECK AND PRIMARY TUMOURS OF THE HEAD AND NECK

This question has generated controversy for many years and no randomized surgical trial has addressed the problem. In some clinical circumstances the argument is, in any event, superfluous. A tonsil 'commando' operation is

Table 17.40 *Advantages and disadvantages of elective radical neck dissection*

Advantages of elective neck dissection for N0 neck
  Provides definitive treatment
  Provides prognostic information:
    whether or not nodes are involved
    if so, how many
    presence or absence of extracapsular spread

Disadvantages of elective neck dissection
  Prolongs operating time with attendant
    anaesthetic risks
  Immediate surgical complications:
    haematoma
    lymphocoele
    wound dehiscence
    necrosis of flaps
    wound infection
    carotid rupture
    chylous fistula
    salivary fistula
  Later complications:
    facial oedema
    shoulder pain
    deafferentation pain
    XIth nerve damage

often combined with radical neck dissection since a pectoralis major flap can more easily repair the deficit if a block dissection has been performed. The advantages and disadvantages of elective block dissection are summarized in Table 17.40.

Prophylactic radiation of the entire neck requires large radiation fields and total doses of no more than 47.5–50 Gy can be given if treatment is given in 20 fractions over

4 weeks. These doses may be too low to control the primary tumour and boost doses to the primary may be required. Radiotherapists divide into two main schools – those who believe in high-dose, small-volume treatments and who therefore do not irradiate the neck prophylactically, and those who believe in using larger volumes, often encompassing all the potentially involved lymph nodes, but lower doses. The main side-effect of elective wide-field radiation to the upper cervical nodes is xerostomia, because much of the parotid gland is inevitably included within the fields. A randomized trial of prophylactic neck irradiation in patients with carcinomas of the oral cavity was performed at the Christie Hospital in the 1970s. This trial was briefly reported in an earlier edition of this textbook: no statistically significant benefit could be demonstrated, in terms of survival, for prophylactic radiotherapy to the ipsilateral neck when a dose of 50 Gy was given in 15 fractions over 21 days. Prophylactic radiotherapy to the neck did, however, significantly reduce the rate of recurrence in the neck: 79 per cent of 100 irradiated patients remained free of neck disease, compared with 64 per cent of 105 patients who received radiotherapy only to the primary tumour (P by $\chi^2 = 0.025$).

If isolated nodal relapse is to occur in patients not treated prophylactically, it usually does so within 2 years of first treatment. Careful follow-up, with patients being seen every 2–3 months, is obviously essential, so that if relapse does occur it can be diagnosed and treated promptly. Patients who are unlikely to co-operate with strict follow-up should have their necks treated prophylactically. Data from Liverpool show that unless follow-up is rigorous patients may relapse with unresectable nodal disease: 75 patients out of 155 patients irradiated radically for carcinoma of the oropharynx, relapsed in regional nodes. Of these 75 patients, only 19 had N1 disease, the rest had nodes >3 cm in diameter, 10/75 (13 per cent) of the patients were unsuitable for surgery.

THE MANAGEMENT OF POTENTIALLY OPERABLE CERVICAL LYMPHADENOPATHY

Traditionally, operable nodal disease was managed by block dissection in conjunction with removal of the primary tumour. Radiotherapy, as primary treatment to operable neck nodes, was used only in patients with inoperable primary tumours. Increasing unease with the morbidity associated with radical neck dissection, and an increased awareness of the effectiveness of radiotherapy in controlling both the primary tumour and nodal disease, has led to a reappraisal of the traditional position.

Bataini, at the Institute Curie, has clearly shown that even bulky nodal disease can be controlled by radiotherapy, provided the dose is sufficiently high (Bataini et al., 1988; Bataini, 1991). Factors which indicate that nodes are unlikely to be controlled by radiotherapy alone include nodes >3 cm, fixed nodes, primary T4 or T3 and prolonged overall treatment time. It is reasonable to recommend radiotherapy, with surgery held in reserve for failure, for patients with N1 disease (less than 3 cm). Patients with more advanced but operable neck disease and operable primary tumours should be considered for radical surgery. Patients with inoperable primary tumours and N2 or N3 disease will require high doses of radiation, preferably using concomitant boost techniques, if their neck disease is to be controlled adequately.

Radiotherapy need not routinely be given after adequate radical neck dissection. If, however, there is extensive evidence of extracapsular spread, or resection margins are positive, then postoperative radiotherapy can reduce the incidence of failure. There is some logic to using surgery for operable nodal disease in patients treated with radical radiotherapy (external beam plus implant) for tumours of the oral cavity and oropharynx. The morbidity from the radiotherapy will be increased if the whole ipsilateral neck has to be included within the radiation field. This can be avoided if the nodes are treated surgically. The functional and cosmetic advantages associated with the use of radiotherapy to treat the primary can be maintained without being jeopardized by the morbidity associated with wide-field irradiation.

TREATMENT OF INOPERABLE NODAL DISEASE AFTER PREVIOUS RADIOTHERAPY

Large, painful fungating nodes in the neck are extremely distressing to patients. This problem can occur with the primary tumour controlled in a patient who is otherwise generally well and is, therefore, condemned to a miserable existence with no immediate prospect of release. A combination of surgery and interstitial implantation can be used in an attempt to deal with this difficult problem. The bulk of the disease is removed surgically, in the full knowledge that disease is left behind at the base of the dissection. Afterloading tubes, for later ^{192}Ir interstitial implantation, are placed directly across the tumour bed at the time of the open operation. The tissue deficit is then closed using a myocutaneous flap. The radioactive sources are loaded several days later. This gives a high dose of radiation to the area, at depth, of residual disease. The skin and superficial tissues, having been brought in from elsewhere, have excellent tolerance to radiation. The surgical procedure deals directly with disease bulk and fungation and the radiation delays the regrowth of the tumour – thereby providing a significant period of relief from symptoms.

CARCINOMA OF THE LIP

Nearly all carcinomas of the lip are squamous carcinomas. Basal cell carcinomas can involve the lip but actually originate from the surrounding skin and cannot, by UICC criteria, be regarded as true tumours of the lip. Three sites are recognized – upper lip, lower lip and commisures.

Over 90 per cent of squamous carcinomas of the lip arise on the lower lip, presumably because the lower lip is more exposed to the most important aetiological factors: tobacco use, particularly pipe smoking, and sun exposure (Plate 1).

Tumours of the upper lip are uncommon and tend to be less well differentiated than tumours of the lower lip. Tumours of the upper lip and commisures, particularly those which are poorly differentiated, are more likely to spread to regional nodes than tumours of the lower lip. The classical description of lymph node spread is from the upper lip to the deep jugular chain, the centre of the lower lip to the submental nodes, the more lateral parts of the lower lip to the submandibular nodes. In practice, spread is variable. Overall, less than 10 per cent of well-differentiated tumours spread to nodes, whereas 30–40 per cent of poorly differentiated tumours are associated with nodal disease.

Clinically, carcinomas of the lip present as an indolent ulcer. A history of temporary regression followed by regrowth is characteristic. The ulcer often has a rolled margin and induration may be palpable well beyond the margins of the visible lesion. There may be evidence of associated leucoplakia. The differential diagnosis can be extensive, syphilis, chronic candidiasis and other infective causes must be excluded. Biopsy is essential.

The choice of treatment lies between surgery and radiotherapy. The final decision often rests on the local availability of specialist skills and techniques.

Radiotherapy

Radiotherapy can be administered either as external-beam treatment (electrons or orthovoltage) or as an interstitial implant. Electron-beam treatment has the advantage that the depth of penetration in tissue can be governed by the particular beam energy that is selected. The gums and teeth can easily be shielded using 3 mm or so of lead (backed with wax) as a gum shield. The technical set up is easy, the field size should be generous since electron isodoses constrict at depth.

Afterloaded iridium wire implants are straightforward and can easily be performed under local or general anaesthesia (Fig. 17.6). Two to three wires are placed in parallel 0.5–1.0 cm apart. There is a reciprocal relationship, governed by the size of the tumour, between the dose given via implant and the dose given by supplementary external-beam treatment (Table 17.41).

Surgery

The main indication for surgery for the treatment of carcinoma of the lip is the presence of leucoplakia adjacent to the invasive tumour. The tumour and the abnormal surrounding epithelium can be excised together. A W or V incision with primary closure is usually adequate when

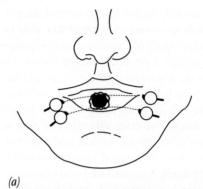

(a)

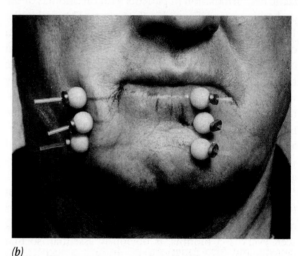

(b)

Figure 17.6 *Afterloaded implant to lower lip: (a) diagrammatic; (b) actual.*

Table 17.41 *Dose relationships between external-beam treatment and interstitial treatment for carcinoma of the lip*

Size of tumour	External-beam dose	Implant dose
≤1.5 cm	Nil	65–70 Gy
>1.5 cm <2.5 cm	25 Gy in 10 fractions	45 Gy
2.5–5 cm	45 Gy in 15 fractions	25 Gy
>5 cm	52.5 Gy in 20 fractions	Nil

the extent of the excision is less than one-third of the lower lip. For superficial lesions, lip shave and vermilion advancement will produce an excellent cosmetic result. Larger lesions will require excision and reconstruction using a flap.

There is no indication for routine treatment to the nodes in patients with carcinoma of the lip. However, patients with larger undifferentiated tumours or who are unlikely to attend for regular follow-up should be offered prophylactic treatment to the nodes, either block dissection or radiotherapy. Patients with clinically involved nodes should be managed along the line described previously (p. 346).

Prognosis

The overall prognosis for carcinoma of the lip is excellent. Radiotherapy will control 90 per cent of squamous carcinomas of the lip. The status of the neck nodes is important, less than 10 per cent of N0 patients fail, but radiotherapy fails to control disease in nearly 50 per cent of patients with clinically positive neck nodes.

TUMOURS OF THE ORAL CAVITY

Although relatively uncommon in Western societies, oral cavity tumours have a high incidence in the developing world – particularly India, where the incidence is 21/100 000 a year. This problem reflects social habits, the chewing of tobacco and betel nut. Snuff dipping (taking snuff orally: 'saffa' in the Sudan, 'nasswar' in Pakistan) and other forms of using smokeless tobacco are causally associated with oral cavity carcinomas. This is scarcely surprising since commercial snuff products contain extremely high levels of carcinogenic nitrosamines, over 2000 parts per billion. A worrying development is the increased use of smokeless tobacco products by socially disadvantaged young people in the developed world, including native people of Alaska and the North West territories of Canada, and Afro-Americans in the rural south of the USA. Other important aetiological factors in oral cavity cancer are cigarette smoking, alcohol and chronic sepsis and, mainly of historical interest nowadays, syphilis. Alcohol and cigarettes appear to have a 'catalytic' aetiological effect.

The T staging of tumours of the oral cavity is shown in Table 17.42.

Premalignant conditions of the oral cavity

LEUCOPLAKIA

Leucoplakia appears as a white patch on the mucous membrane. It cannot be removed by scraping and has a characteristic histological appearance – cellular atypia with acanthosis, hyperkeratosis and parakeratosis. Prevalence varies widely from country to country: 25/100 000 per year in the USA; in parts of rural India the rate is 40–50/1000. This represents a 200-fold difference in prevalence. The presence of leucoplakia indicates a high risk of developing carcinoma of the oral cavity, approximately 50 to 100 times compared to normal. The overall cumulative risk of developing invasive cancer for patients with leucoplakia is about 5 per cent at 20 years.

ORAL HAIRY LEUCOPLAKIA

Oral hairy leucoplakia (OHL) is increasingly recognized as one of the complications of infection with the HIV virus. Epstein–Barr virus is probably the direct cause.

Table 17.42 *T staging for primary tumours of lip and oral cavity (UICC, 1997)*

TX	Primary tumour cannot be assessed
T0	No evidence of primary tumour
Tis	Carcinoma *in-situ*
T1	Tumour 2 cm or less in greatest dimension
T2	Tumour more than 2 cm but not more than 4 cm in greatest dimension
T3	Tumour more than 4 cm in greatest dimension
T4	Lip: tumour invades adjacent structures (e.g. through cortical bone, inferior alveolar nerve, floor of mouth, skin of face)
	Oral cavity: tumour invades adjacent structures (e.g. through cortical bone, into deep (extrinsic) muscles of tongue, maxillary sinus, skin)
	Superficial erosion alone of bone/tooth socket by gingival primary is not sufficient to classify as T4

Characteristically there is an exuberant leucoplakia affecting the dorsum of the tongue. In a minority of patients with OHL and HIV infection there can be rapid progression to invasive cancer. Lesions in patients with positive tests for hepatitis B or syphilis are particularly likely to progress.

ERYTHROPLASIA

Erythroplasia appears as a velvety red patch on the mucous membrane, it is associated with a high rate of malignant transformation and histologically there is marked cellular atypia.

SUBMUCOUS FIBROSIS

Submucous fibrosis presents as oral discomfort, often exacerbated by spicy foods. The buccal mucosa is predominantly affected, the mucous membrane is thickened and pale. Histologically, the changes are those of chronic inflammation with accumulation of collagen at the dermo-epidermo junction. Submucous fibrosis is found predominantly in people from the Indian subcontinent, the incidence may be as high as 1 per cent in certain areas. There is an eightfold increase in the incidence of oral cancer in patients with submucous fibrosis.

Carcinoma of the mobile tongue

The mobile tongue (synonyms: oral tongue; anterior two-thirds of tongue) extends forwards from the circumvallate papilae. About 40 per cent of all oral cancers arise in the mobile tongue. There has recently been a change in the sex incidence of these tumours: formerly about 75 per cent of patients were male, the sex incidence is now approximately equal.

Most tumours of the oral tongue arise on the lateral borders (Plate 2), 15 per cent arise on the inferior surface and 10 per cent arise on the dorsum or the tip of the tongue. The presenting symptom is usually an ulcer, either painless or uncomfortable which does not heal. More advanced lesions will cause disturbances in speech; severe pain, often referred to the ear, is a late symptom. Secondary infection will produce foetor. Occasionally the primary lesion is unnoticed by the patient, who may present with a lump in the neck secondary to involved lymph nodes. The role of the general dental practitioner in early diagnosis is important.

The tip of the tongue drains to the submental lymph nodes, the rest of the mobile tongue drains to the submandibular, subdigastric and middle deep cervical nodes. Neck nodes are frequently involved – 30–40 per cent of patients have palpable lymphadenopathy at presentation and a further 30 per cent have occult disease. Contralateral nodal involvement may occur, even with well-lateralized lesions.

ASSESSMENT

Adequate biopsy, usually possible under local anaesthesia, and clinical examination of the primary and neck are routine. MRI scanning is superior to CT in the assessment of invasion and local spread (Fig. 17.7).

TREATMENT

There is little to choose, in terms of cure rate, between radiotherapy and surgery for early (stage I or stage II) tumours of the mobile tongue. In North America surgery is often preferred, whereas European centres have tended to treat with radiotherapy. Overall, the morbidity rate with surgery is less, but when it does occur after surgery, morbidity may be severe. Speech and swallowing are better preserved after radiotherapy, but often at the expense of xerostomia and long-term dental problems.

Surgery for larger lesions often has to be extensive, and it may be preferable to compromise surgical margins slightly and treat postoperatively with radiotherapy, rather than to create a tissue deficit that cannot be adequately reconstructed. Only 44 per cent of patients (12 of 27) in one series treated with near total glossectomy were able to swallow successfully. Certainly there is good evidence that postoperative radiotherapy can effectively prevent local recurrence in patients with a positive or 'close' (less than 0.5 cm) margin.

Surgery

Cryosurgery has been used successfully for superficial, less than 0.5 cm depth of invasion, tumours of the tongue. Simple wedge excision is equally effective for small superficial lesions. Larger tumours, but which do not extend across the midline, can be treated by hemiglossectomy. Primary closure may be sensible but excessive suturing should be avoided and granulation repair is rapid and preferable to avoid impaired function. Lesions which extend across the midline require a more

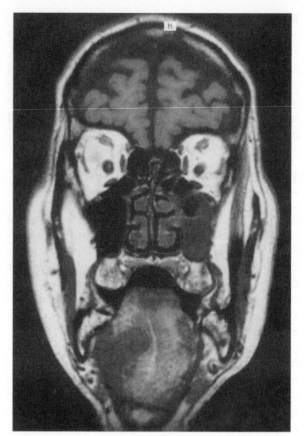

Figure 17.7 *Non-contrast-enhanced T_1 coronal MRI image of the tongue. There is a right-sided tongue cancer invading the normal fat planes, displacing but not breaching the midline fatty septum. The tumour abuts on to the mandible, but there is no invasion into the marrow cavity.*

aggressive approach. Exposure is best achieved by splitting the mandible anteriorly: the mandible and skin are then opened like the leaves of a book, providing excellent exposure. Sub-total excisions can be repaired using a radial forearm free flap. When the whole of the anterior two-thirds of the tongue has been removed, then bulkier flaps such as a pectoralis major, latissimus dorsi or rectus abdominis flap are required. The base of the tongue may then act as a piston and the flap is passively pushed forward during swallowing and speaking.

Radiotherapy

Small, less than 1 cm, lesions can be treated entirely by interstitial implant, either with ^{192}Ir wire or caesium needles. Alternatively, external-beam techniques using a ipsilateral wedged pair of fields may be employed. Such a field arrangement minimizes the volume of salivary tissue within the field and thereby may prevent troublesome xerostomia.

The results of radiotherapy for early tumours of the mobile tongue are summarized in Table 17.43. The careful studies at the Hôpital Henri Mondor in Creteil have provided a wealth of information on the technical and dosimetric factors of importance in interstitial

Table 17.43 *Local control and complications: series of patients with oral cavity tumours treated with radiotherapy*

Centre	Site	Stage	N	LC rate (%)	Complications (%)
Creteil	Tongue/FOM	T1	134	85	25
		T2	145	81	32
MGH	Oral tongue	T1,T2 N0	49 interstitial boost	54	12
	Oral tongue	T1,T2 N0	20 ioc	50	5
	Oral tongue	T1,T2 N0	73 electron boost	86	0
Lille	Tongue	Early	341	72	19
Curie	Tongue	T1	94	76	
		T2	288	69	
		T3	220	60	
RMH	Tongue/FOM	All	149	64	28
Tokyo	Tongue	T1	161	67	
		T2	Implants	74	
		All implants			10
	Tongue	T1	42	77	
		T2	ioe	50	
		All ioe			5
Charlottesville	Tongue	T1	Total	80	
		T2	49	56	
		T3		31	
		T4		0	
Creteil	FOM	T1	47	94	
		T2	72	71	
		All			51

FOM, floor of mouth; ioc, intra-oral cone; ioe, intra-oral electrons; LC, local control.

Table 17.44 *Technical and dosimetric considerations for ^{192}Ir implantation of tumours of the tongue and floor of mouth (derived from the experience of Hôpital Henri Modor, Creteil)*

Local control is significantly related to dose, independently of dose rate
Reducing the dose below 62.5 Gy leads to a rapid increase in failure rate
With dose rates less than 0.5 Gy/h, necrosis is significantly related to total dose
Necrosis is twice as common in floor of mouth implants compared to lateral tongue
Necrosis is related to dose rate, independently of dose
The optimal combination of dose and dose rate, when implant is used alone, is 65–70 Gy given at 0.3–0.5 Gy/h
The spacing between the sources does not significantly affect the necrosis rate
The spacing between sources may affect local control; <15 mm cf. ≥15 mm, relative risk = 0.51 ($P = 0.055$)
Tumour size >3 cm is associated with a significantly increased risk of necrosis

implantation. Their conclusions are summarized in Table 17.44 (Mazeron *et al.*, 1991).

The results from either surgery or radiotherapy alone for more advanced tumours (T3 and T4) are poor. The common approach is to combine surgery with postoperative radiotherapy, but the functional result may be poor. Treating the primary with radiotherapy and concomitant chemotherapy, and neck nodes surgically, is an alternative reasonable strategy.

Results of treatment, prognostic factors and causes of failure

According to one recent surgical series, the following histological features are independently associated with an increased risk of regional recurrence: perineural invasion, intralymphatic tumour emboli and T stage. Interestingly, the only adverse feature of independent significance for survival was tumour thickness. Patients with tumours greater than 3 mm thick had significantly reduced survival. Other series have shown that tumours more than 1–2 mm thick have a worse prognosis than the more superficial lesions. Palpable lymphadenopathy at presentation is an obvious adverse prognostic factor. Tongue carcinomas developing under the age of 40 appear to be biologically more aggressive than tumours developing in later years. However, patients over the age of 70 have a poorer prognosis compared with patients 10–20 years younger.

Between 20 and 30 per cent of patients with clinically negative necks, and who do not receive prophylactic radiotherapy to the neck, will relapse in cervical nodes. Five-year survival in such patients is approximately 30 per cent. There is, however, no clear evidence that routinely treating the neck in all patients improves overall survival. Patients with tumours more than 3 mm thick or with tumours $\geqslant 2$ cm in diameter are at sufficiently high risk of recurrence in the neck that routine treatment, at least to the first-echelon nodes, is justified.

Second malignancies and intercurrent deaths are a major problem in patients whose primary tumours are controlled. In the series from Creteil, 18.5 per cent of patients died from second tumours and 21 per cent of patients died from intercurrent causes. Only 20 per cent of patients actually died from tongue cancer. An autopsy series from Japan identified second malignancies in 19/83 patients with a cancer of the mobile tongue, 40/83 patients had control at the primary site, 28/83 patients died directly as a result of chest infections. These considerations dictate that the only fair way to compare treatments for early tumours of the tongue is in terms of actuarial local control or cause-specific survival.

Floor of the mouth

The boundaries of the floor of the mouth are the inner surface of the mandibular arch, the undersurface of the anterior part of the tongue and the anterior pillar of the tonsil. Tumours often arise adjacent to, and may spread along, Warthin's duct.

Comparison between series of patients treated for carcinoma of the floor of the mouth is not straightforward. Some authors include tumours of the floor of the mouth, tumours which involve the undersurface of the tongue, with tumours of the mobile tongue. Other authors simply recognize such tumours as a subgroup, with less favourable prognosis, of floor of the mouth tumours.

Cancer of the floor of the mouth is more common in males: 9 to 1 male to female ratio in the large series from Creteil. Tumours of the floor of the mouth may not be noticed by the patient. Eventually, difficulties with speech and excessive salivation may lead to the patient seeking medical advice. Pain usually indicates invasion of the mandible, involvement of the inferior dental nerve will cause anaesthesia of the lower lip on the affected side. *In-situ* carcinoma is not uncommon.

The management of carcinoma of the floor of the mouth is, in principle, very similar to that of carcinoma of the mobile tongue. For early lesions radiotherapy and surgery are equally effective. Where function is not compromised, surgery in experienced hands offers a rapid and straightforward approach. Invasion of mandible is a relative contraindication to radiotherapy. Larger lesions (T3, T4) may require a combined approach.

SURGERY

The tumour and the immediate lymphatic drainage should be removed *en bloc*. A neck dissection, either a radical or suprahyoid block dissection, should be performed in continuity with the primary procedure. If the tumour is large, or adherent to the mandible, then a marginal mandibulectomy is often required. If there is evidence of erosion of the mandible, then resection of the affected segment with suitable replacement is required. The radial forearm free flap is probably best for this purpose, although there are alternatives: groin flap with iliac bone, pectoralis major flap with rib, plating the mandible and packing the cavity with bone chips.

RADIOTHERAPY

In the report from Creteil, radiotherapy using implant alone controlled 93.5 per cent of 47 T1 tumours and 71 per cent of 72 T2 tumours, but for T2 node-positive tumours the local control rate was only 65 per cent. For T2N0 tumours with involvement of the undersurface of the tongue, the local control rate was only 68 per cent. For interstitial implant, a dose of at least 65 Gy at a dose rate of 0.3–0.6 Gy per hour is required. Tumours larger than 3 cm, or those that extend to the gum, are probably best treated surgically. External-beam radiotherapy can be given either using a parallel opposed pair, with or without unequal loading, or an ipsilateral wedged pair of fields (Fig. 17.8). A dose of 52–55 Gy in 20 fractions in 4 weeks, or its equivalent, is required.

There were 81 deaths in the series from Creteil. Of these, 33 were related to the original tumour and 48 to other causes. There were 26 deaths from second cancers, 10 intercurrent deaths and 12 deaths from unknown causes. The prognostic factors for tumours of the floor of the mouth are the same as for tumours of the mobile tongue. The results from other series are shown in Table 17.43.

Carcinoma of the buccal mucosa

The buccal mucosa forms the lining of the cheeks, the lymphatic drainage is to the submandibular and subdigastric nodes. Tumours often arise in relation to

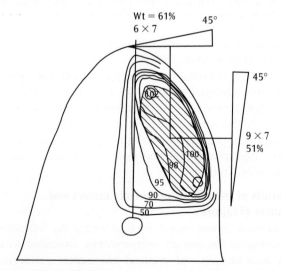

Figure 17.8 *Dose distribution for radiotherapy treatment for a tumour of the floor of the mouth, using a wedged pair of fields at right angles to each other.*

premalignant conditions such as submucous fibrosis or leucoplakia. The buccal mucosa is a common site of origin for verrucous carcinomas. The management of verrucous carcinomas of the oral cavity is controversial. Radiotherapy allegedly can cause these well-differentiated tumours to become less differentiated and thereby adversely affect prognosis. There is no evidence to support this contention and yet the view is often held that radiotherapy is contraindicated for verrucous carcinomas. These tumours should not be singled out for special treatment, their management should simply be as for any other squamous carcinoma.

Small tumours can be treated successfully either with surgery or radiotherapy. Larger tumours require a combined approach, but severe fibrosis may cause trismus and impair the functional and cosmetic results.

ASSESSMENT

Adequate biopsy, clinical examination and CT scanning of the primary and neck are routine.

SURGERY

Local excision for small lesions will leave a defect which can easily be closed, either with a locally rotated mucosal flap or by a split-thickness skin graft. More extensive resections will require major reconstruction: pectoralis major, latissimus dorsi flaps, cervico-facial flaps, or radial forearm free flap.

RADIOTHERAPY

Small tumours can be treated entirely by implant, larger lesions require external-beam treatment. The dose to the local tumour can be boosted either with implant or with electron beam. Electron-beam treatment can be administered externally or using an intra-oral cone. Fibrosis and trismus may cause problems after radiotherapy but can usually be minimized, provided careful attention is paid to technique and dose and to jaw opening exercises performed regularly after treatment.

Five-year survival for carcinoma of the buccal mucosa is poor: only 30–50 per cent. These figures reflect the poor general condition of many of these patients and the high incidence of second primaries.

Tumours of the gum

These tumours usually arise in relation to coexistent leucoplakia on the posterior part of the mandible. There is rich lymphatic drainage and 20–30 per cent of patients have positive nodes at presentation. The lingual surface of the mandible drains to subdigastric, upper deep cervical and retropharyngeal nodes. The buccal surface drains to the submandibular, submental and subdigastric nodes.

Invasion of bone is common and surgery is the treatment of choice. Only exuberant tumours with no evidence of bony erosion or involvement should be considered for radiotherapy. Overall 5-year survival is approximately 50 per cent.

Retromolar trigone

According to the UICC, tumours of the retromolar trigone are classified with tumours of the buccal mucosa. The retromolar trigone is that area of mucosa which overlies the ascending ramus of the mandible between and behind the lower third molar and the upper third molar (Plate 3). These tumours behave similarly to tumours of the anterior faucial pillar and should be managed similarly. There is a high risk of bone involvement and, as for gingival tumours, management should be primarily surgical in these cases. External-beam radiotherapy, using a wedged-pair technique, is adequate for the earlier tumours.

Tumours of the hard palate

The curious, and possibly apocryphal, habit of reverse smoking, apparently practised by Panamanian laundresses who smoke cigarettes with the lighted end in their mouths, presumably in order to stop the ash falling into the washing, is an interesting aetiological factor for these rare tumours.

SURGERY

When bone is involved, surgery is the preferred treatment. Lesions confined to the mucosa can be excised and the wound left to granulate. Attempts to repair the deficit are both unnecessary and futile. Resection of bone is often required and careful preoperative planning is necessary since some form of obturator will be required to close the defect. Teeth should be preserved if at all possible since they provide useful anchorage points for a wire-mounted prosthesis. Temporary obturators can be held in place by circumzygomatic wires.

RADIOTHERAPY

Small superficial tumours may be managed by radiotherapy. Electron-beam therapy, using an intra-oral cone, or gold grain implant can be used, either alone or in conjunction with external-beam treatment. The overall 5-year survival for primary tumours of the hard palate is between 30 and 50 per cent.

Carcinoma of the oropharynx

The oropharynx extends from the junction of the hard and soft palates to the level of the floor of the vallecula. The sites and subsites as defined by the UICC for carcinomas

Table 17.45 *UICC classification of sites and subsites in the pharynx*

Oropharynx
  Anterior wall
    tongue posterior to the vallate papillae
    vallecula
  Lateral wall
    tonsil
    tonsillar fossa and faucial pillars
    glossotonsillar sulci
  Posterior wall
  Superior wall
    inferior surface of soft palate
    uvula
Nasopharynx
  Posterosuperior wall
    from level of the junction of hard and soft palates to
      the base of the skull
  Lateral wall
    includes fossa of Rosenmuller
  Inferior wall
    superior surface of soft palate
Hypopharynx
  Post-cricoid area
    from the level of the arytenoids to the level of the
      inferior border of the cricoid cartilage
  Pyriform sinus
    from the pharyngo-epiglottic fold to the upper end
      of the oesophagus
    laterally: thyroid cartilage
    medially: ary-epiglottic fold and arytenoid and
      cricoid
  Posterior pharyngeal wall
    from the level of the floor of the vallecula to the
      level of the cricoarytenoid joints

of the pharynx are shown in Table 17.45, Figure 17.9 illustrates the oropharyngeal subsites.

When assessing the literature, it is important to remember that the epidemiology of oropharyngeal tumours in France may be very different from that elsewhere. For example, the ratio of male to female patients is typically between 2:1 and 3:1 in series from Denmark, Canada and the United States. In French series the ratio is between 12:1 and 15:1.

Most of these tumours are squamous carcinomas, although at this site non-Hodgkin's lymphoma is more common than elsewhere in the head and neck. Tumours characteristically present late – sometimes as a node in the neck from an occult primary. Difficulty swallowing or pain in the throat, or pain radiating to the ear are the usual symptoms from the primary itself. Spread to retropharyngeal nodes, which can occur late in the course of the disease, may cause cranial nerve palsies (IX, X, XI, XII). Infiltrating tonsillar tumours may produce trismus.

On examination, there is usually an ulcerating lesion at the primary site. Induration is caused by local infiltrative spread and is often more extensive than the visible lesion. Careful palpation, more kindly performed under general anaesthetic, is an essential part of the assessment of oropharyngeal tumours, together with adequate biopsy. CT scanning of the primary site and neck is essential.

Tumours of the posterior third of the tongue

About 70 per cent of patients with tumours of the posterior third of the tongue will have neck nodes at presentation.

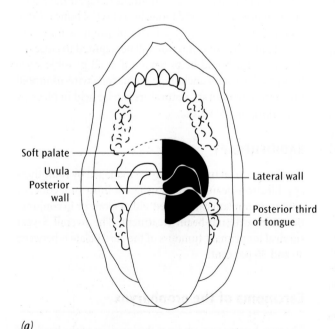

(a)

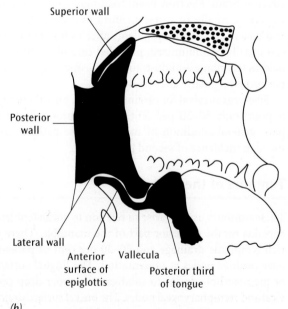

(b)

Figure 17.9 *The sites and subsites of the TNM classification for tumours of the oropharynx: (a) anterior view; (b) lateral view.*

The majority of patients, 59 per cent in the series from the Institut Curie, present with T3 or T4 tumours. In this large series, only 13 per cent of tumours were T1 and 28 per cent T2.

T1 and T2N0 tumours of the posterior tongue should be treated with radical radiotherapy to both the primary tumour and the neck nodes. The primary tumour and the first-echelon nodes can be treated by opposed lateral fields. The low neck can be treated by an anterior split cervical field. The dose to the primary should be 52–55 Gy in 20 fractions over 4 weeks (or its equivalent) the neck nodes should receive 50 Gy in 20 fractions in 4 weeks. This approach will produce 5-year disease-free survival rates of between 30 and 40 per cent.

For the majority of patients, those with a T3 or T4 tumour, the results of treatment are poorer, with 5-year survival rates of less than 30 per cent. Lymph-node spread is common. A series from the Institut Curie, using a primarily radiotherapeutic approach, reported 27 per cent overall survival at 5 years (Table 17.46). Of 166 patients in the series, 68 died because of failure in primary or nodes, 16 died from metastatic disease, 16 died from intercurrent causes and 8 died from second primaries.

Surgical options are limited. A total glossectomy and laryngectomy, with all that that implies in terms of loss of function and quality of life, is unacceptable to many patients. Less aggressive surgery, combined with post-operative radiotherapy, can, in carefully selected patients,

Table 17.46 *Local control and survival in selected series of patients with oropharyngeal cancer treated with radiotherapy*

Centre	Site	Stage	N	LC rate (%)	Survival (%)
Aarhus	OP	All	213	48	40
Rio de Janeiro	OP	III and IV	50 hyp	84	27
			48 conv	64	8
	BOT	III and IV	14 hyp		<20
			14 conv		<20
	Other OP	III and IV	36 hyp		31
			34 conv		15
MDA	Tonsil	T2–T4	28	71	
	BOT	T2,T3	17	81	
Curie	Tonsil <40 d	T1,T2	67	90–93	
	Tonsil <40 d	T3	68	75–83	
	Tonsil <40 d	T4	51	61–73	
	Tonsil 45 d	T1,T2	55	86	
	Tonsil 45 d	T3	91	60	
	Tonsil 45 d	T4	82	38	
	BOT	T1	22	96	49
		T2	47	57	29
		T3	64	45	23
		T4	33	23	16
Liverpool	OP	All	221	73	
Copenhagen	OP	All	222	41	45
	Tonsil	All	124	49	
	BOT	All	56	35	
	SP/uvula	All	28	40	
St Louis	Tonsil	T1,T2 N0	29	55	70
	Tonsil	T1,T2 N1	10	30	30
	Tonsil	T3 N0–2	21	52	58
	Tonsil	T4	12	25	20
Tours	OP	All	305	41	28
	OP	T1		82	
	OP	T2		56	
	OP	T3		31	
	OP	T4		4	
PMH	Tonsil	T1		87	
	Tonsil	T2		68	
	Tonsil	T3		50	
	Tonsil	All			54
EORTC	OP not BOT	T2,T3 N0,N1	166 hyp	60	40
	OP not BOT	T2,T3 N0,N1	159 conv	42	30

OP, oropharynx; BOT, base of tongue; SP, soft palate; hyp, hyperfractionated radiotherapy; conv, conventionally fractionated radiotherapy; LC, local control.

produce excellent results: 16/19 of T3 and T4 tumours were controlled in a recently published series. The ability to deliver effective brachytherapy to the posterior tongue may further improve results. Iridium-192 afterloaded wires can be placed either percutaneously or at open operation. Local control in 30/40 (75 per cent) of patients with T3 tumours and 8/12 (67 per cent) of T4 tumours, using external-beam radiotherapy and percutaneous iridium implants to both primary tumour and any involved cervical nodes, has been reported.

Treatment of the primary tumour with radiotherapy and lymph nodes by bilateral neck dissection is an acceptable combination, preserving function with reasonable local control. Concomitant chemotherapy with radiotherapy may improve local control rates by about 10 per cent at the expense of increased acute morbidity.

Tumours of the tonsillar area

The tonsillar area can be divided anatomically into the following sites: the tonsillar fossa, the anterior and posterior faucial pillars and the glosso-tonsillar sulcus. Since the anterior faucial pillar marks the point of embryological fusion between the oral cavity and the oropharynx, tumours arising from the anterior faucial pillar have more in common with oral cavity tumours than they do with carcinomas of the oropharynx.

The tonsil itself is a lymphatic organ and, together with lymphatic tissue in the posterior tongue, around the lower end of the Eustachian tube, in the nasopharynx and in the soft palate, forms Waldeyer's ring. Extranodal non-Hodgkin's lymphomas of the head and neck often arise from Waldeyer's ring. There is a clear association between non-Hodgkin's lymphoma arising extranodally in the head and neck and lymphomatous involvement of the stomach and small bowel. The investigation and treatment of non-Hodgkin's lymphoma is described in detail in Chapter 45.

Clinically, it is often possible to distinguish carcinomas of the tonsil from lymphomas. Patients with tonsillar lymphomas rarely complain of pain. Obstructive symptoms or the sensation of a foreign body in the throat predominate. The tumour itself is often smooth and purplish and ulceration of the overlying mucosa is uncommon. Cervical lymphadenopathy is often bilateral and bulky, the nodes have a characteristic elastic texture, in contrast to the hard, unyielding, nodes associated with squamous cell carcinomas.

Squamous carcinoma of the tonsil usually causes pain, often referred to the ear, and painful dysphagia. Typically there is an infiltrating ulcerated mucosal lesion, although occasionally tonsillar carcinoma can have an exophytic appearance with minimal ulceration or infiltration. Exophytic tumours may have a better prognosis than infiltrative tumours, this clinical impression is not, however, supported by evidence from formal multivariate analysis.

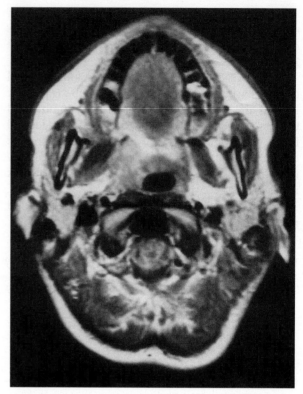

Figure 17.10 *MRI (T$_2$ proton density axial image) of a tonsillar tumour: there is a right-sided tumour invading laterally into the para-pharyngeal fat and into the medial pterygoid muscle. The pre-vertebral muscles have not been invaded.*

The lymphatic drainage of the tonsillar area is to the subdigastric and jugulo-digastric nodes initially and then to the middle deep cervical nodes. Between 60 and 75 per cent of patients will have palpable cervical nodes at presentation. In a large series of 466 patients from the Institut Curie, 27 per cent of patients were staged as T1 or T2, 37 per cent as T3 and 35 per cent as T4.

Assessment requires an examination under local or general anaesthesia with biopsy and a CT scan (Fig. 17.10).

Surgery alone or radiotherapy alone are probably equally effective for T1 or T2 tumours of the tonsillar area. Of the two, radiotherapy gives the better functional result, and therefore better quality of life. For T3 and T4 tumours, a combined approach is usually required. Radical surgery with postoperative radiotherapy is commonly used. A policy of radical radiotherapy with surgery reserved for operable failures is also reasonable and may give a better functional result. In one recent series, survival in patients operated upon for failure after primary radiotherapy was 24 per cent at 5 years. In a series from Liverpool, including all oropharyngeal sites, treated primarily with radiotherapy, 5-year survival after surgical treatment of recurrence at the primary site was 31 per cent. After nodal recurrence, survival was only 19 per cent at 5 years: 67 per cent of patients relapsing in nodes were clinically stage N2 or N3 when recurrence was detected.

This indicates the need for scrupulous follow-up and a low threshold of suspicion in patients with possible nodal recurrence. CT scanning of nodes at initial assessment makes comparison with such historical series difficult.

SURGERY

Radical surgery for tonsillar tumours was not really feasible until the development of the so called 'commando operation' in the 1940s: a neck dissection is performed initially and then the mandible is split behind or between the molar teeth. The tumour can then be visualized by rotating the posterior part of the mandible laterally and backwards. The tumour is then approached via the neck incision and the removal of the tumour and nodes can be carried out *en bloc*. Closure involves tissue replacement using, for example, a pectoralis major, latssimus dorsi flap, or free fibula or iliac crest when bone is resected. Overall 5-year survival after surgery for carcinoma of the tonsil is around 50 per cent.

RADIOTHERAPY

Early tumours of the tonsillar fossa, with no palpable cervical lymphadenopathy, can be treated using lateralized techniques: ipsilateral wedged pair or parallel opposed fields with unequal weighting (Fig. 17.11). These techniques will also treat the first-echelon nodes. Electron beams have appealing depth–dose characteristics but cannot be relied upon. The dose actually delivered to tissues behind the mandible may be less than expected because of the unpredictable absorption of electrons by bone.

For larger tumours, parallel opposed field arrangements, with treatment to the low neck using an anterior split cervical field, will be required. The primary tumour requires a dose of 50–55 Gy in 20 fractions in 4 weeks or its equivalant. A similar dose is required for palpable neck disease. The clinically negative neck can be effectively treated with 50 Gy in 20 fractions over 4 weeks or its equivalent. The results of external-beam radiotherapy for carcinoma of the tonsil are summarized in Table 17.46. Concomitant chemotherapy may offer a small but significant increase in local control.

The main cause of treatment failure in patients with carcinoma of the tonsil treated with radiotherapy is failure to control locoregional disease. Failure to control nodal disease is related to N stage: for N0 disease the failure rate with prophylactic radiotherapy to the neck is less than 5 per cent; for N3 disease the failure rate is 70 per cent.

It is possible to implant the tonsillar fossa with afterloaded ^{192}Ir wires. The results from series of patients treated with implants as part of their treatment are excellent. Possibly this has as much to do with careful selection of patients as it does to do with the effectiveness of the treatment. The data from Creteil report 100 per cent local control, a series from California reported control rate at the primary site of 84 per cent and 5-year actuarial survivals of 90 per cent (T1 and T2) and 60 per cent (T3 and T4).

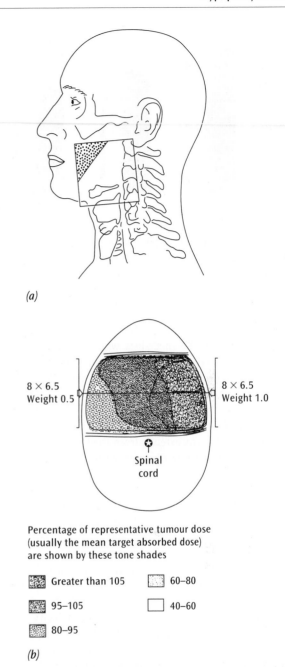

Percentage of representative tumour dose (usually the mean target absorbed dose) are shown by these tone shades

Greater than 105		60–80	
95–105		40–60	
80–95			

(b)

Figure 17.11 *Carcinoma of the tonsil: (a) radiation fields; (b) treatment plan for treating a well-lateralized tumour of the left tonsil using parallel opposed fields with 2 : 1 weighting.*

Overall treatment time is an important prognostic factor for local control in carcinoma of the tonsil treated by radiotherapy (Fig. 17.12 and Table 17.46). The main cause of treatment failure is recurrent or persistent locoregional disease.

HYPOPHARYNX

Tumours of the hypopharynx are relatively uncommon in the UK. A survey of ear, nose and throat specialists

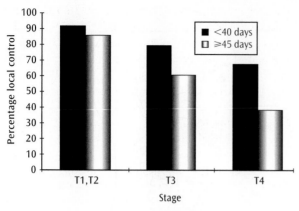

Figure 17.12 *Data from the literature on the effect of overall treatment time for the local control of carcinoma of the tonsil treated with radiotherapy. The adverse effect of prolonged treatment time is more marked with advanced T stage.*

reported that the 87 specialists who responded saw a total of only 213 new patients per annum with hypopharyngeal tumours. Half of the respondents (46/87) saw only one new patient per year, 21/87 (24 per cent) had seen no new cases of hypopharyngeal cancer during the previous 12 months.

The hypopharynx extends from the level of the tip of the epiglottis to the lower border of the thyroid cartilage. According to the UICC there are three main sites: the pyriform sinus, the posterior pharyngeal wall and the post-cricoid area. This classification of hypopharyngeal tumours can be criticized. Tumours arising on the pharyngeal surface of the ary-epiglottic folds might be more appropriately considered with tumours of the supraglottic larynx. Post-cricoid tumours are more closely related to tumours of the upper third of the oesophagus than they are to tumours of the pyriform sinus.

The lymphatic drainage of the hypopharynx is to retropharyngeal nodes and to the subdigastric, upper and middle deep cervical nodes. Post-cricoid tumours may spread to nodes in the upper mediastinum.

It is important to look at the distribution by site in series of hypopharyngeal tumours. For example, a series of 106 patients treated in Liverpool, with a policy of radical radiotherapy and possible salvage surgery for failure, reports 41 per cent 5-year survival (Jones, 1992). These results are better than several other surgical or radiotherapeutic series. It is relevant that only 30/106 patients in the Liverpool series had tumours of the pyriform sinus and that there was a relatively high proportion of post-cricoid tumours 53/106 (50 per cent). This distribution of sites is unusual and the results may reflect this.

Pyriform fossa

The pyriform (pear-shaped) fossae lie on each side of the laryngeal orifice; they are bounded, medially, by the ary-epiglottic fold, and laterally, by the thyroid cartilage and thyro-hyoid membrane. The apex usually extends inferiorally as far as the lower border of the thyroid cartilage.

Between 60 and 70 per cent of all hypopharyngeal tumours arise in the pyriform fossa. The vast majority (up to 80 per cent in one series) of patients are men. The primary tumour only rarely produces symptoms: the usual presentation is with a node in the neck. Eventually the primary tumour will produce pain, hoarseness and dysphagia. These tumours are usually advanced at presentation. In a series of 457 patients from Montpellier only 6.7 per cent had T1 tumours, 69.3 per cent had T3 or T4 tumours. Only 16.8 per cent of patients were N0 at presentation; 54.3 per cent were N3. Even small primary tumours may be associated with advanced neck disease; 18/31 patients with T1 tumours had N3 disease. The Memorial Hospital reported a series of 301 patients with hypopharyngeal tumours, 59 per cent of which arose in the pyriform fossa, and 35 per cent of which arose from the posterior pharyngeal wall: 15 per cent were T1; 61 per cent T2 and 24 per cent T3 (using the older TNM system). Clinically positive nodes were found in 66 per cent of patients and 18/46 patients with T1 tumours had nodal disease at presentation. It can be calculated that between 40 and 50 per cent of patients with clinically negative necks will have occult nodal disease at presentation. Prophylactic treatment of the neck is therefore indicated in all N0 patients accepted for radical treatment.

TREATMENT

Combined treatment is required for nearly all tumours of the pyriform fossa. The exception would be a small tumour arising from the hypopharyngeal surface of the ary-epiglottic fold, these tumours can often be adequately controlled by primary radiotherapy.

The basic surgical option for tumours of the pyriform sinus is pharyngo-laryngectomy, with all that implies in terms of functional loss. Postoperative radiotherapy will be required for the majority of patients.

Perhaps uniquely in the head and neck, neoadjuvant chemotherapy using *cis*-platinum and 5-fluorouracil may have a role to play in the management of these tumours – not because it improves survival, but because it may enable the larynx to be conserved. Response to chemotherapy may identify those patients who also respond well to radiotherapy. Responders to primary chemotherapy could be treated with radiotherapy (with salvage surgery for failure); non-responders could be treated with surgery and postoperative radiotherapy.

A study of 113 patients with hypopharyngeal tumours randomized one group of patients to total pharyngolaryngectomy plus radical neck dissection plus postoperative radiotherapy. The other group was treated with induction chemotherapy with radiotherapy for complete responders and surgery with postoperative radiotherapy for partial responders or patients who did not respond. The overall survival at 2 years was 67 per cent in the chemotherapy arm and 45 per cent in the control arm. This difference is not significant but suggests, at the very least, that neoadjuvant chemotherapy is not detrimental to survival. The important feature is that 23/57 (40 per cent) of the patients in the chemotherapy arm had complete responses and of these 13/23 were alive and well with larynx preserved. All patients in the control arm had laryngectomies.

A complementary study randomized patients to chemotherapy + radiotherapy or chemotherapy + surgery + postoperative radiotherapy. Results on the first 90 patients randomized show no significant survival difference: 75 per cent disease-free survival in the group treated without laryngectomy versus 89 per cent disease-free survival in the group treated with chemotherapy, surgery and postoperative radiotherapy.

These studies in advanced hypopharyngeal tumours have interesting parallels with similar studies in advanced laryngeal cancer. Longer-term follow-up is needed, the experience with primary chemotherapy and radiotherapy from Boston suggests that long-term local control with this approach is significantly worse for hypopharyngeal tumours than it is for laryngeal tumours.

The traditional treatment options (surgery alone, radiotherapy alone, surgery with pre- or postoperative radiotherapy) for carcinoma of the pyriform sinus have been formally modelled using decision analysis. This study concluded that radiotherapy alone was the least effective, and surgery and postoperative radiotherapy the most effective, option. The conclusion was sensitive to values chosen for operative mortality and survival increment to be gained by postoperative radiotherapy. Lack of information meant that it was difficult to incorporate factors relating to the quality of survival into this analysis, although these factors were undoubtedly important. Unfortunately, the recent data on neo-adjuvant chemotherapy may render this careful analysis obsolete.

Surgery

The choice of treatment for hypopharyngeal cancer in the UK may be heavily influenced by the individual surgeon's experience. Specialists seeing more than 10 new patients per annum with hypopharyngeal cancer, advocated primary surgery for 40 per cent of patients; specialists seeing fewer than five such patients per annum recommended primary radiotherapy for 93 per cent of patients.

The ablative surgical procedure required for patients with hypopharyngeal tumours is a pharyngolaryngectomy and block dissection of the ipsilateral neck. A permanent tracheostomy is inevitable. Several reconstructive methods have been used to restore continuity of the food passage. A recent non-randomized series from the MD Anderson Hospital showed that approximately 40 per cent of patients reconstructed with myo-cutaneous

flaps or colon transpositions failed to achieve normal swallowing and required long-term tube feeding. The failure rate with gastric transpositions or free jejunal grafts was 20 per cent or less. These results have been confirmed in the series from Pittsburgh. The hospital stay was shorter in those patients treated with jejunal graft than in those treated with gastric transposition. The long-term survival rates for patients treated with primary surgery for hypopharyngeal tumours are typically between 25 and 35 per cent: 25 per cent 5-year survival for 301 patients treated at Memorial Hospital (1950–70); 33 per cent in the more recent series from Montpellier.

Radiotherapy

The standard technique for treating these tumours is to use parallel opposed lateral fields to the primary tumour and the upper neck nodes, with an anterior split cervical field to treat the low neck. If there are concerns about the position of the junction between fields, then this can be moved halfway through treatment: for example, by adding 2 cm to the lower border of the lateral fields and subtracting 2 cm from the upper border of the anterior field. For patients with short necks, or where other technical or anatomical factors create problems, then more complex techniques, similar to those described for tumours of the supra-glottic larynx may be required.

The results of primary radiotherapy for cancer of the pyriform fossa are poor. Long-term survival is only 5–25 per cent. Inability to control locoregional disease is the usual cause of failure. Control of bulky nodal disease is particularly difficult. The macroscopic extent of the primary tumour may be misleading: skip lesions, occult cartilage involvement and clinically inapparent circumferential spread may all occur and will lead to underestimation of the extent of the tumour. Coping with this uncertainty by simply increasing field size may increase morbidity prohibitively. Calculations suggest that the serious morbidity rate, were all patients to survive long enough to develop problems, with current doses and techniques for T3 and T4 pyriform fossa tumours would be 13 per cent. This high rate reflects both field size and the local tissue destruction caused by these advanced tumours. If neo-adjuvant chemotherapy truly improves local control with radiotherapy, then this high morbidity rate might ultimately be expressed. A suggested scheme for the curative management of advanced T3 and T4 pyriform sinus tumour is shown in Figure 17.13.

The palliative management of patients with pyriform fossa tumours is difficult. Chemotherapy with carboplatin and 5-FU may produce rapid relief of symptoms but, since response is usually short, may only tantalize. Split-course radiotherapy – 14.8 Gy in 4 fractions over 1 week followed by a 3-week gap, followed by 14.8 Gy in 4 fractions over 1 week – may provide useful palliation without causing undue mucosal toxicity. For patients whose tumours and general condition improve with treatment, a third course of 4 fractions may be given after

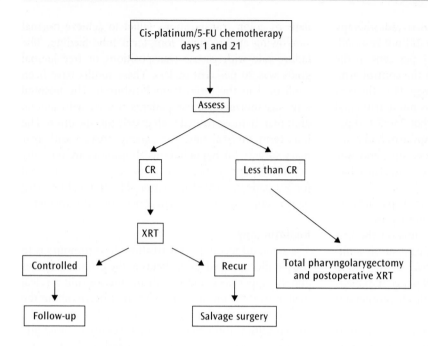

Figure 17.13 *A flow chart for the management of advanced tumours of the hypopharynx. CR, complete clinical response; 5-FU, 5-fluorouracil; XRT, radiotherapy.*

a further 3 weeks: total dose 44 Gy in 12 fractions over 12 weeks.

Second primary tumours are not a major cause of treatment failure for patients with hypopharyngeal carcinoma – perhaps because few patients survive long enough. Nevertheless, the rate of associated second malignancy is equivalent to other sites in the head and neck. The median prevalance of second malignancies in nine published studies is 13 per cent (range 7–37 per cent).

Post-cricoid tumours

These tumours are similar in their behaviour to tumours of the upper third of the oesophagus and should be treated as such (*see* Chapter 23).

Posterior pharyngeal wall

These tumours are uncommon and in most series account for 20 per cent or less of tumours of the hypopharynx. Clinically they present with dysphagia and the sensation of a foreign body at the back of the throat. As with carcinomas of the oesophagus, tumours commonly spread inferiorly and superiorly. Posterior spread of the tumour is limited by the prevertebral fascia. Surgical treatment for these tumours is extremely difficult and usually they are managed using radical radiotherapy. They can be treated using wedged lateral fields to a dose of 50–55 Gy in 20 fractions over 4 weeks. The spinal cord should be shielded at tolerance. Results of treatment are poor and only about 30 per cent of patients survive free of disease at 3 years. The usual cause of treatment failure is failure to control locoregional disease.

LARYNX

Approximately one-third of all cancers of the head and neck arise in the larynx. The majority of patients are middle-aged males (male : female ratio 8 : 1). Over 90 per cent of laryngeal tumours are invasive squamous carcinomas, between 2 and 10 per cent are *in-situ* carcinomas. Other tumours which may arise primarily in the larynx include oat cell carcinomas, lymphomas, tumours arising in ectopic salivary tissue and carcinoid tumours.

The UICC recognizes three anatomical subsites of the larynx: supra-glottis, glottis and sub-glottis. The supra-glottis is divided into five subsites: supra-hyoid epiglottis, laryngeal aspect of the ary-epiglottic fold, arytenoid, infrahyoid epiglottis and false cords (ventricular bands). There are three glottic subsites: cords, anterior commissure and posterior commissure. The T staging is shown in Table 17.47. Although the UICC recognizes five subsites for supra-glottic tumours, the most important distinction is between tumours of the epilarynx (supra-hyoid epiglottis, ary-epiglottic fold and arytenoid) and the rest. Tumours of the epilarynx tend to be more advanced than tumours of the lower supra-glottis, 52 per cent of patients in one series had T4 tumours. Nodal spread is also common.

The common defining feature of T3 laryngeal tumours is cord fixation. However, cord fixation can arise through a variety of mechanisms which may alter the prognosis. The sheer size of the tumour may physically trap the cord; the rotation of the arytenoid cartilage may be prevented by tumour involving the crico-arytenoid joint; the terminal branches of the recurrent laryngeal nerve may be affected by tumour, with consequent paralysis of the intrinsic muscles; the intrinsic laryngeal muscles may be

Table 17.47 *T staging (UICC, 1997) for laryngeal tumours*

TX	Primary tumour cannot be assessed
T0	No evidence of primary tumour
Tis	Carcinoma *in-situ*

Supraglottis

T1	Tumour limited to one subsite[a] of supraglottis with normal vocal cord mobility
T2	Tumour invades mucosa of more than one adjacent subsite[a] of supraglottis or glottis or region outside the supraglottis (e.g. mucosa of base of tongue, vallecula, medial wall of pyriform sinus) without fixation of the larynx
T3	Tumour limited to larynx with vocal cord fixation and/or invades any of the following: postcricoid area, pre-epiglottic tissues
T4	Tumour invades through the thyroid cartilage, and/or extends into soft tissues of the neck, thyroid and/or oesophagus

Glottis

T1	Tumour limited to vocal cord(s) (may involve anterior or posterior commissure) with normal mobility
T1a	Tumour limited to one vocal cord
T1b	Tumour involves both vocal cords
T2	Tumour extends to supraglottis and/or subglottis, and/or with impaired vocal cord mobility
T3	Tumour limited to the larynx with vocal cord fixation
T4	Tumour invades through the thyroid cartilage and/or to other tissues beyond the larynx (e.g. trachea, soft tissues of neck, including thyroid, pharynx)

Subglottis

T1	Tumour limited to the subglottis
T2	Tumour extends to vocal cord(s) with normal or impaired mobility
T3	Tumour limited to larynx with vocal cord fixation
T4	Tumour invades through cricoid or thyroid cartilage and/or extends to other tissues beyond the larynx (e.g. trachea, soft tissues of neck, including thyroid, oesophagus)

[a] Subsites include the following: ventricular bands (false cords) arytenoids suprahyoid epiglottis infrahyoid epiglottis aryepiglottic folds (laryngeal aspect).

directly infiltrated by tumour. Transglottic spread is an adverse prognostic factor within the T3 category of glottic tumours. The distinction is not made by the UICC but data from Liverpool show a 64 per cent 5-year relapse-free survival for T3 transglottic tumours compared with 80 per cent for T3 tumours where there is no transglottic spread.

The UICC TMN system also fails to discriminate between types of T2 glottic tumour. Impaired cord mobility may be an independently adverse prognostic factor. The supra-glottis has a rich lymphatic plexus draining to the subdigastric and mid cervical nodes. The sub-glottis drains to the lower cervical, para-tracheal and mediastinal nodes. The glottis itself is not well supplied with lymph vessels and tumours confined to the vocal cords rarely spread to nodes.

Clinical features

The cardinal symptom of laryngeal tumours is change in the quality of the voice. This can vary from mild hoarseness, often intermittent, to severe hoarseness with the voice reduced to the merest whisper. Hoarseness is a symptom that is usually taken seriously both by patients and their doctors and this, combined with the ease with which the larynx can be assessed by indirect laryngoscopy, means that patients with glottic tumours usually present with early disease. Hoarseness is a late symptom in patients with tumours of the epilarynx, mild dysphagia may be the only initial symptom from these tumours. This may go unnoticed, and patients with high supraglottic tumours may eventually present with a lump in the neck, from nodal disease. This delay in presentation may in part explain the poorer overall prognosis for tumours of the epilarynx.

Assessment

All patients with laryngeal cancer require direct laryngoscopy and biopsy as part of their initial assessment. This is usually best carried out under general anaesthesia, although fibreoptic nasendoscopy offers a possible alternative for patients in whom anaesthesia would be hazardous. Adequate biopsies are essential.

Cord mobility can usually be assessed on indirect laryngoscopy and cannot be adequately assessed in the anaesthetized paralysed patient. CT scanning is now routinely used in staging laryngeal tumours other than the obvious T1 tumour. Figure 17.14 shows CT images of invasive laryngeal tumours. By demonstrating early cartilage invasion, evidence of local spread beyond the larynx and nodal disease, the main effect of CT will be to classify as T4 tumours which, on clinical grounds alone, would have been staged as T1, 2 or 3. Stage migration should be remembered when comparing series in which CT has been used for staging and those using clinical staging only.

The patient who presents with stridor due to a laryngeal tumour usually has advanced disease but, if possible, careful assessment should take place. To avoid tracheostomy, endoscopic debulking may be possible to secure the airway. Although the adverse effect of tracheostomy followed by delayed primary treatment is known, emergency laryngectomy is rarely practicable.

Verrucous carcinomas of the larynx

The question of the radiosensitivity (or radioresistance) of verrucous carcinomas of the larynx is controversial.

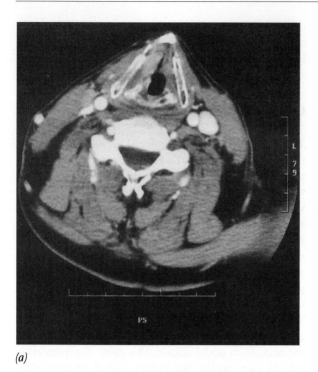

(a)

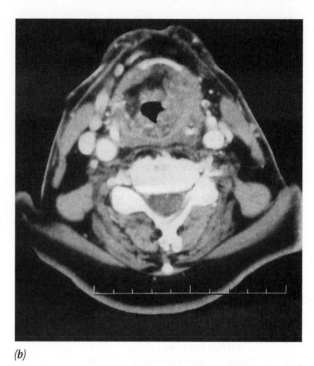

(b)

Figure 17.14 *(a) A CT image showing an enhancing tumour of the anterior two-thirds of the right vocal cord. There is no cartilage invasion but enhancing lymphadenopathy around the right carotid artery is demonstrated. (b) CT scan showing a large, left-sided supraglottic carcinoma with early breach of the thyrohyoid membrane.*

Table 17.48 *Radiotherapy versus surgery for verrucous carcinomas of the larynx*

	Radiotherapy ($n = 37$)	Surgery ($n = 144$)	P by χ^2
Local control	18 (49%)	133 (92%)	<0.0001
Death from laryngeal cancer	4 (11%)	5 (3%)	0.16

There is no evidence that radiotherapy in any way increases the aggressiveness of these tumours. On the other hand, there is evidence that radiotherapy is less effective for verrucous carcinomas than it is for other squamous carcinomas of the larynx (Table 17.48).

Supra-glottic tumours

Tumours of the supra-glottis account for 25–40 per cent of all laryngeal tumours in most series, although a much higher rate (>60 per cent) was reported from Finland. In a series of 325 patients from Leuven with supra-glottic tumours, 54 per cent had tumours arising in the lower supra-glottis and 46 per cent had tumours of the epilarynx. Nearly 50 per cent of patients with epilaryngeal tumours had palpable nodes at presentation, compared with only 23 per cent of patients with tumours of the lower supra-glottis. Tumours of the epilarynx behave more like pharyngeal tumours, tumours in the lower supra-glottis behave more like tumours of the larynx proper. The epiglottis has a pitted surface and is perforated by laryngeal nerves. This may facilitate direct extension of supra-glottic tumour into the pre-epiglottic space.

In a large series of patients from St. Louis with supra-glottic tumours, the main sites of origin of the primary tumour were: epiglottis, 24 per cent; false cords, 15 per cent; epiglottis and false cords, 28 per cent; epiglottis plus false cords, plus ventricle, plus arytenoids, 15 per cent. The distributions by T stage for these two series of supra-glottic carcinomas are shown in Figure 17.15.

The choice of treatment for early (T1, T2) supra-glottic tumours lies between voice-conserving surgery and radiotherapy. Supra-glottic laryngectomy will permit retention of the voice but is not always feasible. There may not be sufficient clearance between the lower end of the tumour and the vocal cords. Many patients are not fit for anaesthesia, involvement of both lingual arteries is also a contraindication to supra-glottic laryngectomy. In the series of 105 patients from Florida with T1 to T4 supraglottic carcinoma, 48 per cent were anatomically unsuitable for supra-glottic laryngectomy (SGL). Of the patients who were anatomically suitable for SGL, 40 per cent were inoperable on medical grounds. Overall, therefore, only 30 per cent of patients in this series could have been treated by supra-glottic laryngectomy and surgeons vary in their enthusiasm for the procedure.

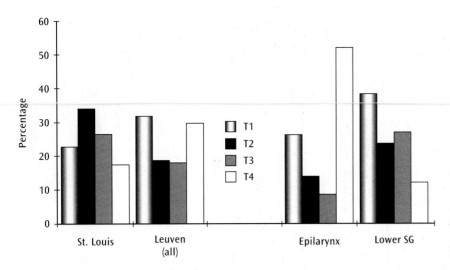

Figure 17.15 *The distribution of supra-glottic tumours by T stage. The majority of epilaryngeal tumours are staged as T4.*

For T3 tumours a policy of radical radiotherapy, with salvage laryngectomy reserved for failure, is appropriate for those tumours with favourable features: exophytic, limited local extension. Local control will be obtained with radiotherapy in 60–70 per cent of such patients. Infiltrating tumours, or those with extension or local invasion into the pyriform fossa or glottis, are best treated by laryngectomy. Postoperative radiotherapy should not be given routinely. Only patients with positive or minimal (less than 5 mm) surgical margins, or nodal disease with extracapsular spread, should be selected for postoperative radiotherapy.

RADIOTHERAPY TECHNIQUE

For early, T1,T2N0, supra-glottic tumours it is not necessary to treat the whole neck prophylactically, but fields need to take into account the high incidence of occult nodal disease. Parallel opposed fields extended up to cover potential lymph-node spread at the angle of the mandible with wedges to compensate for the contour of the neck can be used (Fig. 17.16). The dose should be 52–55 Gy in 20 fractions over 4 weeks, or its equivalent. The lower dose should be used for field sizes greater than 50 cm^2, otherwise late complications can be severe. More extended treatment schedules have been used, e.g. 66–74 Gy in 27–35 fractions at 2.2–2.4 Gy per fraction, but the late complication rate is, at 20 per cent, unacceptably high.

Patients with more advanced primary tumours, or who have nodal disease at presentation, will require treatment to the whole neck. This can, particularly in patients with short necks, pose a challenge. A variety of techniques have been used in order to avoid areas of underdosage within what is often an extensive treatment volume. The angled-down wedged pair offers the most elegant solution: the whole volume is treated en bloc and gaps are avoided. The downward angle is achieved by swinging the foot of the couch 10–15 degrees to the left for the right field and a similar amount to the right for the left

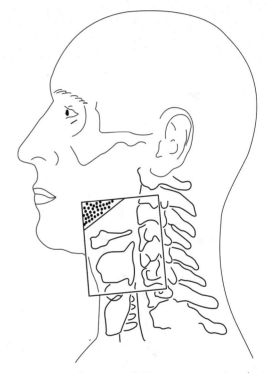

Figure 17.16 *Radiotherapy field arrangements for treating an early tumour of the supra-glottic larynx.*

field. The change in neck contour can be compensated by using wedges with the thick end anterior. The remaining problem is what to do about the cranio-caudal changes in separation, since this will produce inhomogeneities and there is a risk of overdosing the spinal cord. The best solution is probably to use a compensator, but, if this resource is unavailable, wedging in both directions may achieve a similar effect. The advent of three-dimensional conformal planning increases the potential accuracy of such treatments.

The results of radiotherapy alone for supra-glottic carcinoma depend critically upon stage (Fig. 17.17). The main cause of failure of radiotherapy for supra-glottic

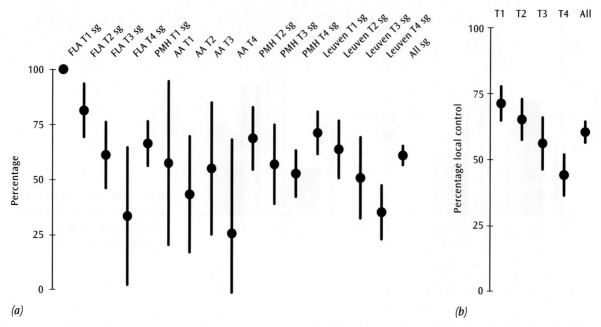

(a)

(b)

Figure 17.17 *(a) Local control for supra-glottic cancers treated with radiotherapy. FLA, Florida; PMH, Princess Margaret Hospital, Toronto; AA, Ann Arbor, Michigan; All sg, all supra-glottic tumours. (b) Data from (a) pooled by T stage.*

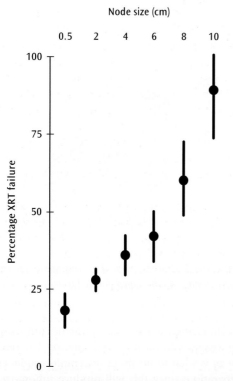

Figure 17.18 *Relationship between failure rate following radiotherapy and cervical node diameter in centimetres (pooled data from the literature).*

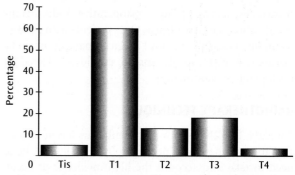

Figure 17.19 *Glottic cancers: distribution by T stage (pooled data from the literature).*

and neck in general. Other factors that decrease the probability of control of nodal disease by radiotherapy are fixation, smaller primary tumours and prolonged overall treatment time.

Glottic carcinoma

The majority (60–70 per cent) of laryngeal carcinomas arise from the vocal cords. The site distribution by T stage is shown in Figure 17.19. Nodal involvement at presentation is rare (less than 5 per cent), this reflects the poor lymphatic supply to the vocal cords.

CARCINOMA *IN-SITU*

This condition may be much more common than we suppose. In one autopsy series, 15 per cent of smokers had carcinoma *in-situ* of the larynx. This contrasts with

carcinoma is persistent or recurrence of the primary tumour, only about 10 per cent of patients fail solely in neck nodes. There is a clear relationship between the size of the neck nodes and failure rate. Figure 17.18 shows this relationship for squamous carcinomas of the head

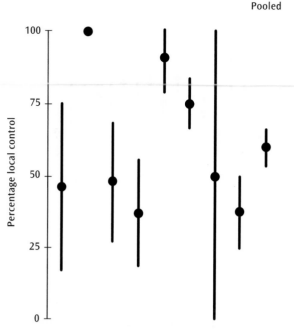

Figure 17.20 *Carcinoma* in-situ *of the larynx: local control after cord stripping (data from the literature).*

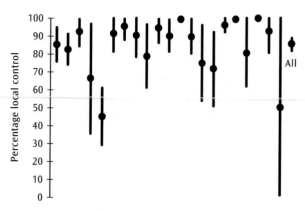

Figure 17.21 *Carcinoma* in-situ *of the larynx: local control after radiotherapy (data from the literature).*

the 2–10 per cent incidence of carcinoma *in-situ* observed in large series of patients with laryngeal carcinoma. For carcinoma *in-situ* of the vocal cords, simply stripping the cord can provide both material for diagnosis and, in the short term at least, effective treatment. The published data on cord stripping as primary management for carcinoma *in-situ* of the larynx are summarized in Figure 17.20. Laser excision is also now commonly used for *in-situ* carcinoma of the larynx. Experience is preliminary, but for selected patients it may provide a reasonably expedient alternative to radiotherapy. For more extensive lesions, the only surgical approach that is feasible may be cordectomy, which will invariably affect the quality of the voice.

Radiotherapy is undoubtedly effective in controlling *in-situ* carcinoma of the larynx, and there is no evidence whatsoever that irradiation of these lesions will cause them to become invasive. The results from radiotherapy for treating carcinoma *in-situ* of the larynx are summarized in Figure 17.21. The voice quality after radiotherapy is usually excellent, over 75 per cent of patients will have a normal voice after treatment. A radical dose is required, 50–52 Gy in 20 fractions over 4 weeks. Fields can be kept small, 4 × 4 cm or 5 × 5 cm, but care must be taken to include the whole of the anterior commissure in the high-dose volume.

EARLY, T1 OR T2, INVASIVE CARCINOMAS OF THE GLOTTIS

The results of radiotherapy for early glottic cancers are so good, Figure 17.22, that it is ethically difficult to introduce alternative treatments. Nevertheless, conservative surgical techniques may offer, for highly selected patients,

local control rates as good as those obtained by radiotherapy. The criteria for selecting patients for vertical hemilaryngectomy are summarized in Table 17.49. The main problem is that voice quality is not so reliable after conservative surgery as it is after radiotherapy. The Mayo clinic has recently reviewed their experience with conservative laryngeal surgery in patients with early (T1) glottic tumours. The median value for maximum tumour dimension was 8 mm – these were small tumours. Open operations were performed on 159 patients: frontolateral partial laryngectomy; laryngofissure with cordectomy; hemilaryngectomy; anterior commisure resection. There were 11 recurrences and 9 patients eventually required laryngectomy. The recurrence rate was 7 per cent (95 per cent CI, 3–11 per cent), the laryngectomy rate was 6 per cent (95 per cent CI, 3–10 per cent). The quality of voice after treatment was assessed in 123 patients: 14 per cent had poor voice, 49 per cent had 'fair' (hoarse) voice. The voice was normal, or nearly normal, in 37 per cent of patients. Uncorrected survival at 5 years was 84 per cent, the crude mortality rate was 44/159 (27 per cent; 95 per cent CI, 21–35 per cent), half of the deaths were due to intercurrent or unknown causes, a quarter were due to second primaries. Somewhat disconcertingly, 11 patients (25 per cent of the deaths) died from laryngeal cancer.

Laser excision of selected T1 tumours is being carried out by surgical enthusiasts. A randomized trial is being set up in the UK to compare laser with radiotherapy.

The vast majority of patients with T1 and T2 tumours of the glottis are treated with a policy of radical radiotherapy, with laryngectomy held in reserve for patients whose tumours persist or recur after primary radiotherapy. With this policy, about 90 per cent of patients with T1 tumours, and 70–75 per cent of patients with T2 tumours, will be cured without requiring laryngectomy. Long-term cause-specific survival is around 90 per cent for T1 tumours and 80–85 per cent for T2 tumours. Crude survival is much lower, typically around 50–60 per cent at 10 years. This difference reflects the high rate of intercurrent deaths and second malignancies in these

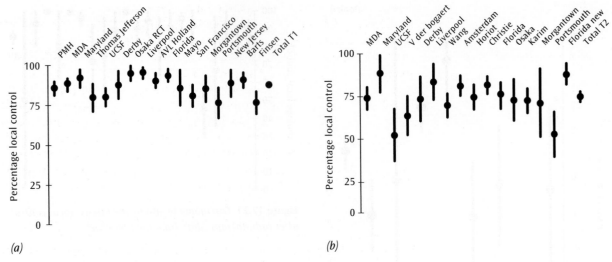

Figure 17.22 *Invasive tumours of the glottis: local control with radiotherapy. (a) T1 tumours; (b) T2 tumours. PMH, Princess Margaret Hospital, Toronto; MDA, M.D. Anderson Hospital, Houston.*

Table 17.49 *Criteria for performing vertical hemilaryngectomy*

No more than minimal extension to contralateral cord
No posterior extension beyond vocal process of arytenoid
<5 mm subglottic extension
Minimal supra-glottic extension
Vocal cords fully mobile
No involvement of cartilage

patients. Intercurrent deaths can cause difficulties with attribution in long-term follow-up of patients with tumours of the upper aerodigestive tracts. If treatment produces distortion and fibrosis of the structures around the epiglottis and larynx, then this may interfere directly with the protection of the airway during swallowing, and aspiration may occur. If significant aspiration goes unnoticed, and deaths are simply attributed to broncho-pneumonia, then this will underestimate the number of deaths occurring as a result of treatment-related complications. Any disparity in rates of death from intercurrent causes in comparisons of treatment for head and neck cancer should always be looked at carefully: this may be a clue to a significantly higher rate of complications in one treatment arm. This problem was particularly apparent in the Edinburgh neutron/photon trials in head and neck cancer, where there were many more intercurrent deaths in patients treated with neutrons.

T3 TUMOURS OF GLOTTIS

Less than 10 per cent of T3 glottic tumours are suitable for conservative surgery, and so for T3 glottic tumours the initial choice is almost always between total laryngectomy and radiotherapy. The choice is often difficult. Infiltrative ulcerative tumours are best treated surgically whereas the more exophytic tumours will often respond

well to radiotherapy. The general condition of the patient is also important since many of these patients are not medically fit for anaesthesia. The patient should be involved in the discussions and decision making from the start. Patients' attitudes to possible compromises between survival and voice preservation differ. Some patients value survival at all costs and will pay virtually any price to increase their certainty of cure. Other patients value their voices highly and would be prepared to compromise their chances of survival in order to retain normal speech. A recent detailed analysis of specialists' recommendations for the management of laryngeal cancer showed that the recommendations were heavily influenced by speciality (otolaryngologists as opposed to radiotherapists) and by geography (the USA and Australasia as opposed to Canada, the UK and Scandinavia). The specialists' recommendations for the management of a T3 glottic tumour are summarized in Figure 17.23 (O'Sullivan *et al.*, 1994). The surgical dominance of practice in the USA and Australia is well illustrated.

The results of primary radiotherapy for T3 glottic cancer are shown in Figure 17.24. Although local control rates vary widely, there is reasonable consistency between series in cause-specific survival. Case selection, with more unfavourable tumours being referred for surgery, invalidates any direct comparison of survival data between surgery and radiotherapy for T3 tumours of the vocal cord. No randomized trial has addressed this question. The influential Veterans Administration (VA) study on neo-adjuvant chemotherapy for laryngeal cancer has shed no real light on the issue. It has convinced many ENT surgeons that laryngectomy is not always necessary but, because there was no randomization to radiation alone, the relative contributions to tumour control of radiotherapy and chemotherapy in this study cannot be assessed. Careful review of the Veterans Administration data, and comparison with series using radiotherapy

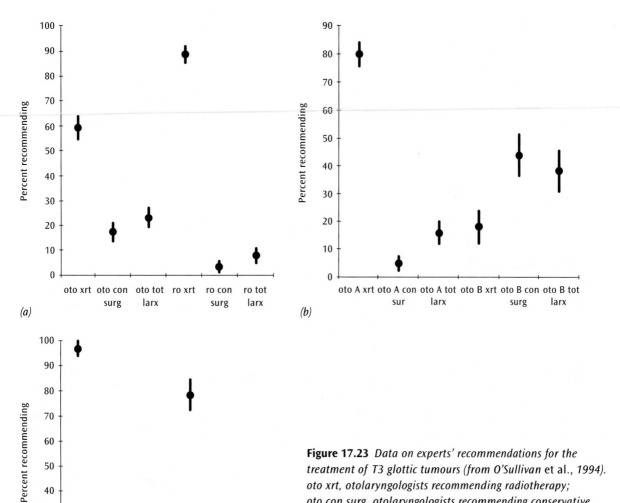

Figure 17.23 *Data on experts' recommendations for the treatment of T3 glottic tumours (from O'Sullivan et al., 1994). oto xrt, otolaryngologists recommending radiotherapy; oto con surg, otolaryngologists recommending conservative surgery; oto tot larx, otolaryngologists recommending total laryngectomy; ro xrt, radiation oncologists recommending radiotherapy; ro con surg, radiation oncologists recommending conservative surgery; ro tot larx, radiation oncologists recommending total laryngectomy. (a) Recommendations according to speciality; (b) otolaryngologists from Europe (A), USA and Australia (B); (c) radiation oncologists from Europe (A), USA and Australia (B).*

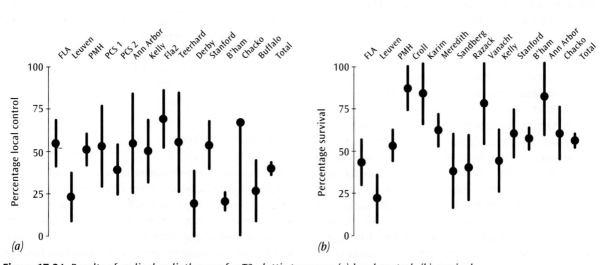

Figure 17.24 *Results of radical radiotherapy for T3 glottic tumours: (a) local control; (b) survival.*

alone, suggests that the chemotherapy in the Veterans Administration study may actually have contributed very little. There were 124 patients with glottic tumours in the VA study, the majority of which were presumably T3 tumours. Of the 61 patients randomized to chemotherapy 57 per cent achieved local control without requiring laryngectomy. Not all of the 43 per cent who required laryngectomy will have had a trial of radiotherapy, since failure of response to initial chemotherapy was one of the criteria for performing laryngectomy. The relative contributions of chemotherapy and radiotherapy to the conservative therapy of advanced laryngeal cancer are currently being addressed in an RTOG study and within the UKCCR head and neck study.

T4 TUMOURS OF GLOTTIS

The majority of patients with T4 glottic cancers who have operable disease and are fit for surgery should probably be treated by laryngectomy or pharyngolaryngectomy. This is particularly true for tumours involving the pyriform fossa, where the results from radiotherapy are particularly poor, less than 20 per cent local control at 5 years in the series from Princess Margaret Hospital (PMH). Early cartilage invasion is not, of itself, a contraindication to radical irradiation. In the series of patients from PMH, staged as T4N0M0 on the basis of cartilage involvement, the actuarial recurrence-free survival was 67 per cent at 5 years. Salvage laryngectomy is, however, rarely possible in patients with T4 glottic tumours who fail radiotherapy. This is a reflection of their poor general condition and the extensive local destruction that can be caused both by the primary tumour and post-irradiation perichondritis. Perichondritis of the thyroid cartilage is a potentially fatal complication of these tumours. Careful supervision after radiotherapy and prompt treatment with antibiotics is essential for its prevention. Surgical series on T4 glottic tumours report long-term local control rates of between 30 and 55 per cent.

RADIOTHERAPY TREATMENT TECHNIQUES FOR GLOTTIC CARCINOMAS

Most early glottic tumours can be treated using parallel opposed lateral fields with wedges used to compensate for the decreased separation of the neck anteriorly. In patients with short, fat necks it may be difficult physically to accommodate lateral fields, and oblique anterior fields with appropriate wedges may be used. Relatively small fields can be used for early tumours, provided that careful attention is paid to the anterior margin. The anterior commissure may lie as little as 2–3 mm below the skin surface, and the anterior field margin (defined at 50 per cent) should therefore extend beyond the skin surface. In patients with thin necks, bolus may be required to ensure adequate dose to the anterior commissure. All patients should be treated using an immobilization shell and a well-collimated beam from a 4–6 MV linear accelerator.

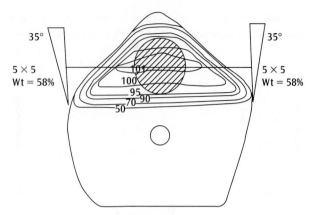

Figure 17.25 *Dose distribution for treatment of T1 carcinoma of the larynx, using 4 MV X-rays.*

All fields should be treated daily. It is no longer acceptable to use cobalt units for such treatment. Figure 17.25 shows a typical dose distribution achieved in the treatment of early laryngeal tumour.

The field should extend from the level of the hyoid to the lower border of the cricoid cartilage and the posterior border should overlie the vertebral bodies. A randomized study from Japan looked at the influence of field size upon local control and complications in patients with T1N0M0 glottic carcinoma. There was no difference in relapse-free survival between patients randomized to 6×6 cm fields compared with patients randomized to 5×5 cm fields. Patients treated with the larger fields had, however, a significantly higher incidence of chronic arytenoid oedema. It is important to remember that the physical size of the larynx varies on an individual basis and field sizes should be appropriate rather than standardized.

In patients with more advanced primary tumours larger fields may be necessary, but this will increase the risk of significant late morbidity. A dose of 52–55 Gy in 20 fractions over 4 weeks, or equivalent, is adequate for most glottic tumours. If field sizes exceed 50 cm^2 then it may be necessary, in order to avoid unacceptable late complications, to limit the dose to 52 Gy. There is a suggestion that, once the dose per fraction is less than 2 Gy, local control is impaired, even for very early glottic tumours. This effect is probably related to the prolonged overall treatment time and the consequent opportunity for repopulation of stem cells.

Subglottic tumours

These tumours are very uncommon, less than 5 per cent of all laryngeal tumours. Unlike glottic tumours they often spread to nodes; the nodal drainage is to the low neck, supraclavicular fossa and upper mediastinum. The clinical presentation is usually with wheeze or stridor, occasionally as a lump in the neck. The distinction between a true subglottic tumour and a glottic tumour with subglottic extension can sometimes only be made, since tumours will regress towards their site of origin, by observing the regression of tumour during treatment. For tumours arising at the level of the thyroid ring, surgery offers the best treatment. Tumours arising from the conus elasticus are more likely to respond to radiotherapy. Even advanced (T3, T4) subglottic tumours may be controlled with radiotherapy: overall local control rates for radiotherapy in subglottic tumours range from 30 to 70 per cent. Long-term survival is 30–50 per cent with radiotherapy and 40–50 per cent with surgery.

The radiation fields need to include the lymph nodes of the low neck, the upper mediastinum and supraclavicular fossa as well as the primary tumour. Cruciate anterior and posterior opposed fields are usually required, with a posterior cord block to keep the dose to the spinal cord within tolerable limits. The field size is usually such that a dose of 50 Gy in 20 fractions over 4 weeks, or its equivalent, cannot usually be exceeded.

Laryngectomy after radiotherapy

The indications for laryngectomy after radiation therapy provide interesting clues as to an institution's radiotherapeutic philosophy. Those centres with an aggressive approach will perform relatively more laryngectomies for necrosis and fewer for recurrence. The pattern will be reversed in centres with a less vigorous approach. In a series of 376 patients with laryngeal cancer reported from Edinburgh, 54/376 underwent laryngectomy. Of the 54 larynxes removed, 43 (77 per cent) contained tumour and 13 (23 per cent) showed no evidence of tumour. There was no difference in symptoms (pain, hoarseness, stridor) between patients with residual tumour and those with necrosis. In 7/56 patients, tumour was suspected clinically but the laryngectomy specimen contained no tumour. The overall rate, in this series, for laryngeal necrosis was 13/376 (3.5 per cent). The Edinburgh patients who required laryngectomy for necrosis enjoyed excellent survival, 92 per cent at 5 years. In a series of 250 patients from Liverpool with T1 or T2 glottic tumours, the proportion of patients requiring laryngectomy for necrosis was slightly lower, 2 per cent. This difference almost certainly reflects the lesser degree of tissue destruction caused by early glottic tumours rather than any difference in radiotherapeutic practice. The necrosis rate reported from the Christie is 4 per cent for patients treated with 55 Gy in 16 fractions over 24 days for patients with T2 glottic tumours. The data from Toronto, where radiation doses tend to be lower but fields larger, showed that only 3 per cent of laryngectomies performed after radiotherapy were for necrosis.

A depressing feature of the report from Liverpool is that 82 per cent of patients with recurrence had advance disease (pT3 pT4) on histological examination of the excised larynx. This is reflected in the poor survival figures: 40 per cent survival at 5 years in a series of patients with glottic tumours requiring laryngectomy for recurrence. This compares with 59 per cent 5-year survival in the Edinburgh series of laryngeal tumours requiring laryngectomy for recurrence. These data emphasize the importance of careful follow-up, a high degree of suspicion for recurrence, and a low threshold for performing microlaryngoscopy under anaesthetic in patients irradiated for laryngeal cancer. Follow-up should be every 4–8 weeks for the first year after treatment. In patients who are difficult to examine by indirect laryngoscopy, direct laryngoscopies should be performed at 3 and 6 months after treatment. Follow-up during the second year should be every 2 months. Thereafter the intensity of supervision can be decreased. Although occasional problems arise after 5 years, it is reasonable to discharge patients from routine follow-up at that time.

Data on the effectiveness of a policy of radical radiotherapy, with salvage surgery for failure, in advanced laryngeal cancer are shown in Figure 17.26. Using these data, it is possible to indicate outcome in an imaginary cohort of 100 patients with advanced laryngeal cancer treated with radical radiotherapy. Radiotherapy alone will produce long-term local control in between 50 and 56 patients. Salvage surgery will be attempted in 28 to 34 patients, and this will be successful in between 15 and 20 patients. There will be between 10 and 22 patients with persistent or recurrent disease who are, for one reason or another, unsuitable for salvage surgery. Ultimately, between 65 and 76 patients will obtain local control of their disease.

Previous radiotherapy undoubtedly increases the complication rate for laryngectomy. In the Edinburgh series of previously irradiated patients the complication rate was high: 30/56 (54 per cent) serious complications. Fistula was the most common complication, affecting 15/56 (27 per cent) patients. Other complications included infection, wound dehiscence and arterial rupture. In a series of 357 patients reported from Liverpool, 190 (of an original 796 radically irradiated patients) required laryngectomy for recurrence or residual tumour after radiotherapy: 167 patients had laryngectomy as primary treatment. The fistula rate was 39 per cent (74/190) in irradiated patients and 4 per cent (10/167) in unirradiated patients ($P < 0.001$). The median duration of the fistula in irradiated patients was 112 days, compared with 28 days in the unirradiated group ($P = 0.008$), six patients in the irradiated group died from fistula in the perioperative period. There were no such deaths in the unirradiated group.

The results of salvage laryngectomy for glottic tumours have been reported separately by the Liverpool group. The in-hospital mortality rate for 100 patients was 3 per cent. Fistulas occured in 32 per cent of patients. Over half the patients had no complications of their laryngectomy. The important features of all these different series is that they confirm the continuing viability of a long-standing

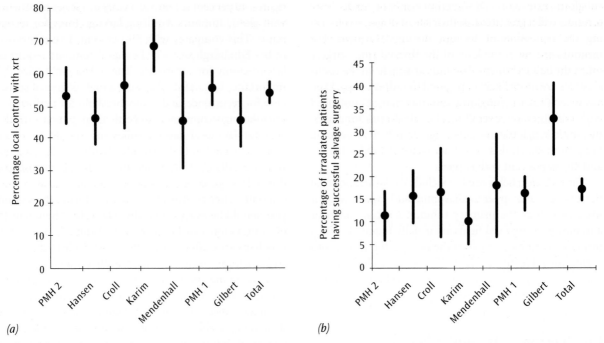

(a)   *(b)*

Figure 17.26 *(a) Local control rate with radiotherapy for advanced laryngeal cancer. (b) Successful salvage surgery, expressed as a percentage of all irradiated patients.*

policy of radical radiotherapy with salvage surgery for failure in the treatment of laryngeal cancer. The Liverpool data on 478 patients with T1 to T3 N0 glottic cancers treated with this policy shows that at 5 years 50 per cent of patients were alive with intact larynxes, 5 per cent were alive but had required laryngectomy, 13 per cent had died from their original cancer and 33 per cent had died from other causes. Most of these intercurrent deaths were due to smoking-related diseases – 50 per cent of the deaths in the Edinburgh series of patients requiring salvage laryngectomy. Encouraging patients, treated for laryngeal cancer, to stop smoking should improve their immediate prognosis (as shown in the Canadian data quoted previously in this section) but unfortunately can do little to prevent the long-term harmful effects of the cigarettes they have already smoked. Unless smoking habits change or strategies for secondary prevention prove effective, then long-term survival rates for patients with laryngeal cancer will always be eroded by a high rate of intercurrent death – despite curing the majority of patients.

NASOPHARYNX

Tumours of the nasopharynx are biologically distinct from other tumours of the head and neck. These tumours are common in the Far East and North Africa. Three main factors are important for the development of classical nasopharyngeal carcinoma: genetic susceptibility; Epstein–Barr virus infection; dietary factors. The importance of genetic factors in the origin of these tumours is

illustrated by their familial tendency. There is often serological evidence of EBV infection, with antibodies to the viral capsid antigen (VCA); in addition EBV-associated DNA sequences can sometimes be identified within the tumour itself. Recombinant DNA technology will increase the effectiveness of serological testing for the infection by providing large quantities of pure antigen for testing. The dietary factor that is particularly associated with nasopharyngeal carcinoma is the consumption of salted fish. Wistar rats fed powdered Chinese salt fish develop malignant tumours of the nasal cavity. Surveys in China have shown that fish from areas with a high incidence of nasopharyngeal carcinoma contained more carcinogenic nitrosamines than samples of fish from areas with a lower incidence of nasopharyngeal carcinoma. Thus it is not simply the consumption of salt fish in general that is important, the type of salt fish is also relevant.

It is difficult, from a Western perspective, to appreciate just how common nasopharyngeal carcinoma is in southern China, Hong Kong and Taiwan. In some areas of Guangdong province the incidence is as high as 40 per 100 000 per annum. This rate would, if applied to the UK, produce 21 000 patients per year with carcinoma of the nasopharynx. In Taiwan, 60–70 per cent of all patients treated with radiotherapy are treated for nasopharyngeal carcinoma.

Nasopharyngeal carcinoma in China and the Far East may be a somewhat different disease to that encountered in Western Europe. In Hong Kong less than 10 per cent of patients have metastatic disease at presentation. This contrasts with experience at the Institut Gustave Roussy

(IGR) in Paris, where 113/255 (44 per cent) of patients presented with metastatic disease. The IGR treats 100–150 new patients per annum for nasopharyngeal carcinoma – most of the patients are originally from North Africa or southern Italy. The age-incidence peak for nasopharyngeal carcinoma in China is between 40 and 60, males outnumber females by 3 : 1. In Caucasian patients there is a suggestion of a secondary peak in incidence around the age of 20. In the West there is also a significant incidence of nasopharyngeal carcinoma in childhood.

There are several pathological classifications for nasopharyngeal carcinoma. The WHO classification is the most widely used, three categories are recognized:

- Type 1: keratinizing squamous; found in 25 per cent of Caucasians with NPC; not related to EBV infections; behaves more like a typical SCC of the head and neck; has the worst prognosis.
- Type 2: transitional cell carcinoma.
- Type 3: undifferentiated tumours including lympho-epitheliomas (Schminke), anaplastic, spindle cell, clear cell. In Hong Kong 90–95 per cent of NPCs are type 3.

Anatomy

The roof of the nasopharynx is formed by the base of the skull, which slopes downwards and backwards to become continuous with the posterior pharyngeal wall. The anterior boundary is the posterior choanae and the free posterior edge of the nasal septum. Its lower limit is defined as the level of the uvula, opposite the second cervical vertebra. The lateral wall contains the fossa of Rosenmuller and the Eustachian tubes. The floor is the superior surface of the soft palate.

The nasopharynx is difficult to assess clinically. Surgery is rarely used in the management of NPC and so it is only comparatively recently, with the advent of CT scanning and MRI, that it has been possible to obtain accurate anatomical information about the origins and local spread of NPC (Figs 17.27 and 17.28). Most tumours originate in the fossa of Rosenmuller, and the earliest radiological sign is blunting of the angle at the Eustachian cushion. CT scanning has highlighted the importance of spread into the parapharyngeal space. This is defined as abnormal soft tissue lying in the space between the pharyngeal constrictors and the pterygoid plates. This was found in 120/403 (30 per cent) of patients in one recent series, and in 221/262 (84 per cent) in another. Another feature is the ability of the primary tumour to invade directly into the carotid sheath. Previously, involvement of the carotid sheath was assumed to be due to nodal spread. Retropharyngeal nodes are involved early in NPC.

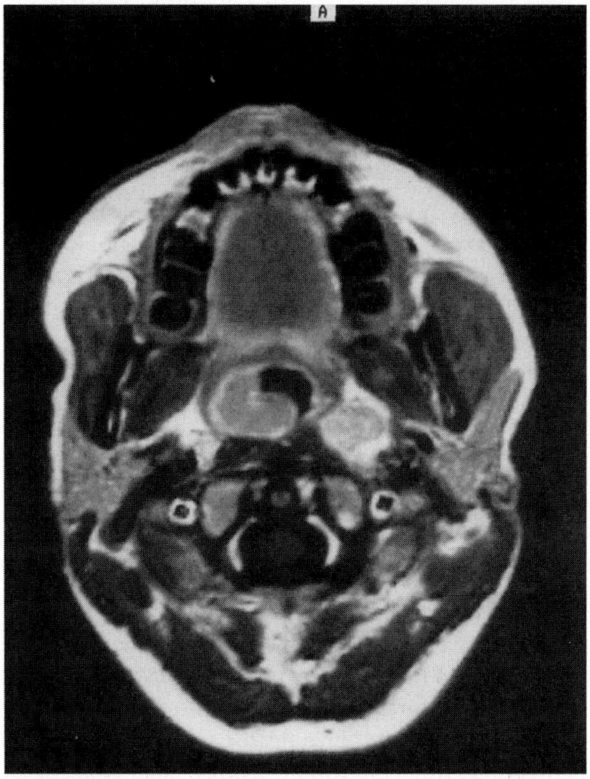

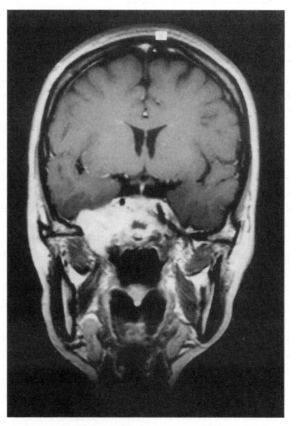

Figure 17.27 *Post-gadolinium T₁ coronal image of the nasopharynx. This shows a right-sided nasopharyngeal carcinoma with nodal metastases in the left parapharyngeal space.*

Figure 17.28 *Post-gadolinium T₁ coronal image of the nasopharynx. This shows a right-sided nasopharyngeal tumour invading the cavernous sinus in the middle cranial fossa.*

They cannot be detected by clinical examination but can readily be demonstrated by CT.

In a recent series of 119 patients with NPC who were staged both clinically and by CT scanning, 11/37 (30 per cent; 95 per cent CI, 15–44 per cent) of patients with clinically negative necks had nodal involvement detected by CT. In the series of 5037 patients from Queen Elizabeth Hospital, Hong Kong, mainly staged without CT, 1290 (26 per cent) were staged as N0. CT staging would possibly have reduced this to figure to between 700 and 1100 (14–21 per cent). CT scanning is also useful in the detection of base of skull involvement, which was found in 140/403 patients (35 per cent) in a CT-staged series. This compares with 633/5037 (13 per cent) when CT was not used routinely. Even if patients with cranial nerve palsies and/or evidence of skull base erosion are grouped together, the rate in this latter series rose only to 922/5037 (18 per cent).

Intracranial extension is also more common than was formerly supposed: 12 per cent of 262 patients in the series from Queen Elizabeth Hospital (QEH) had extension to the middle cranial fossa (Fig. 17.28). Extension beyond the nasopharynx can be demonstrated readily by CT: 27 per cent had sphenoid sinus involvement; 18 per cent had involvement of the ethmoid sinus and 22 per cent of the tumours invaded the nasal cavity, according to the data from the QEH series.

Clinical presentation

The nasopharynx, together with the pyriform sinus and the base of tongue, is a classic site for a silent primary tumour in the head and neck. About 75 per cent of patients have palpable neck nodes at presentation and the neck mass is the presenting symptom in from 40 to 50 per cent of patients. The remaining patients usually present with nasal symptoms: obstruction, epistaxis; or with symptoms from the ear: deafness, tinnitus. Headache, often severe, central and unresponsive to standard analgesics, usually indicates a locally advanced tumour. Between 20 and 25 per cent of patients have cranial nerve palsies at presentation. This indicates either erosion of the base of skull or spread via the various exit foramina of the cranial nerves. In a series of 109 patients with cranial nerve involvement, the frequency of individual nerve involvement was: VI, 70 per cent; V, 54 per cent; III, 39 per cent; VII, 34 per cent; XII, 28 per cent; IV, 28 per cent; X, 27 per cent; IX, 25 per cent; II, 18 per cent; IX, 4 per cent.

A syndrome of syncope has been described in NPC, and similar problems may occur in other patients with head and neck cancer. The mechanisms are complex but predominantly involve pressure on the carotid sinus, causing reflex bradycardia, and stimulation of the IXth nerve, again causing a fall in heart rate as well as hypotension due to direct vasodilatation.

A variety of paraneoplastic syndromes has been described in association with nasopharyngeal carcinoma: hypertrophic osteoarthropathy and the syndrome of inappropriate antidiuretic hormone (ADH) secretion occur rarely. A syndrome of NPC, leukaemoid changes in the peripheral blood and pyrexia of unknown origin has recently been described in 15/113 patients without metastatic disease from the Institut Gustave Roussy.

Clinical assessment

Examination under anaesthesia, with adequate visualization of the primary tumour and biopsy, is essential both for confirming the diagnosis and for clinical staging. CT scanning is essential and should include the skull base and lower parts of the anterior and middle cranial fossae and should extend down to the level of the suprasternal notch. Contrast enhancement allows discrimination between vascular structures and soft tissue. MRI is extremely useful in assessing NPC and has the potential to detect early evidence of spread beyond the primary tumour; for example, infiltration of the tensor veli palatini. Other routine investigations should include chest X-ray, routine haematology, liver function tests (including LDH) and EBV serology. The issue of routine bone scanning and liver ultrasound is contentious. The series from IGR has a remarkably high incidence of metastatic disease at presentation, 44 per cent. In this series 30 per cent of patients had liver metastases, 63 per cent had bone metastases and 20 per cent had lung metastases at presentation. Series from the Far East typically report much lower rates of metastatic disease (less than 20 per cent) and routine staging investigations have a much lower yield of positive results.

If there is any doubt about the histological diagnosis, then expert pathological review, with re-biopsy if necessary, is essential, particularly in non-endemic areas. The differential diagnosis of tumours at this site is extensive and includes lymphoma, rhabdomyosarcoma, extramedullary plasmacytoma, amelanotic melanoma, polymorphic reticulosis, Wegener's granulomatosis, sarcoidosis and pharyngeal tuberculosis.

Staging

The staging of NPC is a nightmare and the literature is extremely difficult to interpret (Teo *et al.*, 1991). There are at least six staging systems in use – the tendency has been for the Ho system to be used in the Far East and for the UICC system to be used in the West. Investigations influence stage, and investigative policies vary both between centres and within centres. The problem of stage shift therefore complicates the interpretation of clinical results and the only way to compare series is to use the overall data. Stage-specific comparisons are virtually impossible.

Table 17.50 *UICC (1997) T stage compared with Ho staging systems for nasopharyngeal cancer*

T staging	Original Ho (1978)	Modified Ho (1989)
T1	Tumour confined to nasopharynx	No change
T2	Extension to nasal fossa, oropharynx, or adjacent muscles or nerves below skull base	2n: Nasal fossa involvement, without parapharyngeal space involvement or T3 features
		2o: Oropharyngeal involvement, without parapharyngeal space involvement or T3 features
		2p: Parapharyngeal involvement without T3 features
T3	3a: Bone involvement below base of skull including floor of sphenoid sinus	3p: Parapharyngeal involvement with T3 features
	3b: Involvement of base of skull	3a,b,c,d as previously
	3c: Cranial nerve involvement	
	3d: Involvement of orbits, laryngopharynx or infratemporal fossa	

Table 17.51 *Ho N staging (no change between 1978 and 1989)*

N0	No cervical nodes palpable
N1	Nodes wholly above the skin crease extending laterally and backwards from just below the thyroid notch
N2	Nodes palpable between the skin crease and the supraclavicular fossa
N3	Nodes palpable in the supraclavicular fossa, of skin involvement

Table 17.52 *UICC (1997) staging for nasopharyngeal cancer*

TX	Primary tumour cannot be assessed
T0	No evidence of primary tumour
Tis	Carcinoma *in-situ*
T1	Tumour confined to the nasopharynx
T2	Tumour extends to soft tissues of oropharynx and/or nasal fossa
	T2a without parapharyngeal extension
	T2b with parapharyngeal extension
T3	Tumour invades bony structures and/or paranasal sinuses
T4	Tumour with intracranial extension and/or involvement of cranial nerves, infratemporal fossa, hypopharynx, or orbit

Regional lymph nodes (N)

NX	Regional lymph nodes cannot be assessed
N0	No regional lymph node metastasis
N1	Unilateral metastasis in lymph node(s), 6 cm or less in greatest dimension, above the supraclavicular fossa
N2	Bilateral metastasis in lymph node(s), 6 cm or less in greatest dimension, above the supraclavicular fossa
N3	Metastasis in a lymph node(s)
	N3a greater than 6 cm in dimension
	N3b extension to the supraclavicular fossa

There are major differences between the Ho systems (original and modified) and the UICC system (Tables 17.50–17.52). The N staging in the Ho system is entirely dependent upon the level of nodal involvement. Size, laterality and fixation are not considered. The UICC system uses size and bilaterality as its criteria. The Ho system T stage depends upon extent of the primary tumour, bone erosion and cranial nerve involvement. T stage, according to the UICC, depends initially upon involvement of subsites within the nasopharynx, a nebulous concept at best.

In spite of these problems, there is, for the Ho staging at least, remarkable uniformity in the distribution by stage for several large series of patients with NPC (Fig. 17.29). The original system has been modified recently in an attempt to produce a more even distribution by stage and improve discrimination in terms of survival. Although the original system produces an excess of patients with stage III disease, its ability to define prognostically useful categories is excellent (Fig. 17.30).

Management

Other than to provide tissue for diagnosis, there is little role for surgery in the initial management of the carcinoma of the nasopharynx. Radiotherapy is the mainstay of treatment. The role of chemotherapy is slowly being clarified. There are three major randomized studies specifically investigating adjuvant chemotherapy in patients irradiated for nasopharyngeal carcinomas. A multi-centre study in the USA (SWOG, RTOG, ECOG) randomized patients to radiotherapy alone, or to synchronous platinum and radiotherapy followed by cisplatin and 5-FU in stages III and IV NPC. The European study, organized by the IGR, randomized patients to neo-adjuvant chemotherapy with bleomycin, epirubicin and cisplatin plus radiotherapy versus radiotherapy alone. The American study showed a significant survival advantage to the chemotherapy treatment arm (78 versus 47 per cent). The European study shows an improvement in disease-free survival but not overall survival. In contrast, a randomized trial of chemotherapy plus radiotherapy versus radiotherapy alone for nasopharyngeal carcinoma randomized

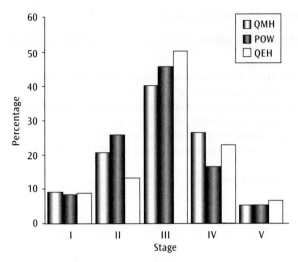

Figure 17.29 *Distribution of nasopharyngeal cancers by Ho stage in three major series from Hong Kong. QMH, Queen Mary Hospital; POW, Prince of Wales Hospital; QEH, Queen Elizabeth Hospital.*

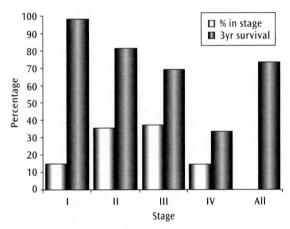

Figure 17.30 *Stage distribution and stage-related survival when patients with nasopharyngeal carcinoma are classified according to the latest version of the Ho staging system.*

patients to chemotherapy with cyclophosphamide, vincristine and Adriamycin or no further treatment after radical radiotherapy. Four-year survival was 66/113 (58 per cent) in the group given chemotherapy and 78/116 (67 per cent) in the group treated with radiotherapy alone.

For stage III and IV disease it appears that platinum and 5-FU with radiotherapy confers a survival advantage. The acute reactions to concomitant chemotherapy and radiotherapy are undoubtedly more severe and prolonged. The potential late complications of the combination have yet to be documented.

RADIOTHERAPY TECHNIQUE

A superb account of radiotherapeutic treatment techniques was given by Ho in the first edition of this textbook. The essential principle of his technique is to use small lateral fields and a supplementary anterior field to treat the nasopharynx. The neck is treated using an anterior field with a midline shield. An alternative technique is to use larger lateral fields to treat the nasopharynx, the nasal cavity and the upper neck, and to treat the low neck using an anterior split cervical field. A two-phase technique is required in order to shield the spinal cord at tolerance and also to change the level of the junction between the anterior and the lateral fields (Fig. 17.31).

The need to treat the whole neck in patients with early nasopharyngeal tumours has been questioned (Lee *et al.*, 1989). A series of 189 patients with stage I (Ho) NPC, treated at QEH Hong Kong with radiotherapy to the nasopharynx and first-echelon nodes only, had a 7-year survival of 85 per cent, but relapse-free survival was only 62 per cent. Neck relapse occurred in 30 per cent of patients, 81 per cent of whom were successfully re-treated. As might be expected, there was a significant difference in survival between patients with regional relapse (70 per cent) and those without (87 per cent). A randomized trial confirmed the effectiveness of nodal irradiation in preventing regional relapse, but there were no significant differences in survival or disease-free survival. The lower regional relapse rate in the patients whose necks were irradiated was offset by an increased rate of distant metastases (Table 17.53).

The dose required to treat carcinoma of the nasopharynx is 60–70 Gy in 30–35 fractions. Wang has used twice-daily fractionation to 64 Gy in 30 fractions with a further 7 Gy by intracavitary implant: overall 5-year survival is 85 per cent. Field size is an important consideration. A significant incidence of late complications is virtually inevitable in the treatment of nasopharyngeal carcinoma (Lee *et al.*, 1992a). In a series, from Queen Elizabeth Hospital, Hong Kong, of 4527 patients assessed for late complications, 1395 (31 per cent) had significant problems: 322/4527 (7 per cent) had severe late morbidity and 62/4527 (1.4 per cent) died as a result of treatment. Most of the fatalities were due to CNS damage, temporal lobe necrosis or damage to the brainstem. The most common form of severe late damage is hearing loss. This can arise from several treatment-related causes: serous otitis media, direct damage to the cochlea by radiation, damage to the auditory pathways in the mid brain. Soft-tissue fibrosis is the most common cause of minor morbidity; when the temporo-mandibular joint is involved, trismus results. Dry mouth and dental problems are frequent. The incidence of hypothalamo-pituitary dysfunction depends upon how hard it is looked for, clinical problems were recognized in only 4 per cent of patients in the retrospective review from Queen Elizabeth Hospital, but up to 60 per cent of patients followed prospectively have demonstrable endocrine dysfunction within 5 years of irradiation. The actuarial incidence of hormone deficiencies at 5 years in one series was: growth hormone,

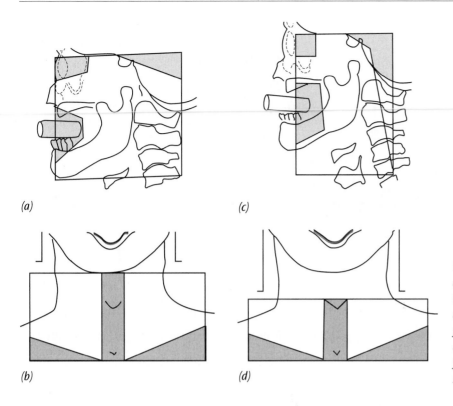

(a)

(c)

(b)

(d)

Figure 17.31 *Radiotherapy field arrangements suitable for the treatment of nasopharyngeal cancer: (a) phase I lateral facial fields; (b) phase I anterior split cervical field; (c) phase II lateral facial fields; (d) phase II anterior split cervical field.*

Table 17.53 *Randomized trial of elective neck irradiation in patients with nasopharyngeal carcinoma (data quoted in Lee et al., 1992a and b)*

	Elective neck XRT	No XRT to neck	P by χ^2
Survival	53/75 (71%)	59/77 (76%)	0.5
DFS	49/75 (65%)	55/77 (71%)	0.5
Local relapse	21/75 (28%)	19/77 (25%)	0.8
Regional relapse	4/75 (5%)	19/77 (25%)	0.002
Distant relapse	11/75 (15%)	4/77 (5%)	0.09

XRT, radiotherapy; DFS, disease-free survival.

63.5 per cent; gonadotrophins, 30.7 per cent; ACTH, 26.7 per cent; thyroid stimulating hormone (TSH), 15 per cent.

A significant proportion (10–20 per cent) of patients with nasopharyngeal carcinoma have clinically evident residual tumour in the nasopharynx at the completion of radiotherapy. A variety of techniques for boosting the dose to the primary tumour have been proposed: small external-beam fields, [198]Au grain implant, intracavitary therapy with ^{137}Cs or ^{192}Ir and ^{125}I seed implant. A non-randomized study from Beijing showed 54 per cent 5-year survival in 92 patients treated with a 20 Gy external boost after 70 Gy; the 5-year survival in 90 similar patients treated without a boost was 21 per cent. The local boost appeared to lower both the rate of local recurrence and distant metastases. The price paid was an unacceptable increase in brainstem damage, from 5 per cent in unboosted patients to 17 per cent when 90 Gy was given to the tumour. This contrasts with much lower complication rates reported from centres using intra-cavitary or interstitial boosts.

MANAGEMENT OF RECURRENCE

Patients in whom nodal disease is the sole site of recurrence or failure should be treated surgically. Re-irradiation of the neck nodes is of little benefit. Patients in whom local recurrence is the only problem can be treated by re-irradiation. The long natural history of nasopharyngeal carcinoma means that, although long-term survival after re-treatment may only be about 15 per cent, local control, and subsequent relief of symptoms, can be achieved in 30–35 per cent of re-irradiated patients. Late morbidity is a problem if re-irradiation is given solely by external beam. The best approach is probably to give 20–30 Gy by external beam and then 40–50 Gy by intracavitary treatment or implant.

Patients with metastatic disease should be considered for chemotherapy. The bleomycin, epirubicin and platinum

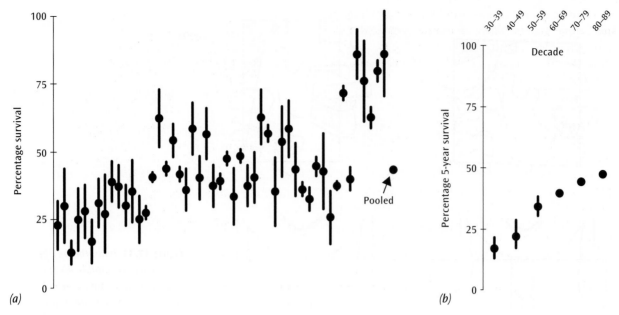

Figure 17.32 *Survival after radical radiotherapy for nasopharyngeal carcinoma: (a) series from the literature; (b) results pooled and grouped by decade.*

regimen used at the Institut Gustave Roussy has yielded the best results so far.

Prognostic factors

The main adverse prognostic factors for survival are: presence of metastatic disease; higher nodal stage, when the Ho system is used; cranial nerve paresis and base of skull involvement. Male patients and patients with parapharyngeal disease may also have a worse prognosis. The overall survival data from a variety of series, both Eastern and Western, are shown in Figure 17.32. It is a feature of most single-centre series that prognosis has improved steadily over the past 20 years. This reflects general improvements in radiotherapy technique and better pre-treatment evaluation, rather than any specific contribution from altered fractionation or the addition of chemotherapy. It also illustrates the danger of using historical controls when evaluating treatment for nasopharyngeal carcinoma. It is likely that this trend will continue as three-dimensional treatment planning and conformal therapy become more widely used. These techniques offer significant advantages over conventional treatment planning in the management of nasopharyngeal carcinoma.

Causes of treatment failure

The causes of failure in the series from Queen Elizabeth Hospital, Hong Kong, are summarized in Table 17.54. Half the patients died from nasopharyngeal carcinoma, 35 per cent survived, 7 per cent died from intercurrent or unknown causes, 1 per cent died from treatment-related

Table 17.54 *Causes of failure in management of nasopharyngeal carcinoma (data from Lee et al., 1992a and b)*

	N	(%)
Metastatic at presentation	292	6
Unfit for radical Rx	258	5
Metastases as first site of failure	924	19
LR failure then metastases	521	11
Regional failure alone	177	4
Failure of initial treatment to achieve LC	564	12
Local failure after initial LC	891	20

LR, locoregional; LC, local control; Rx, radiotherapy.

complications, 1 per cent died from second malignancies and 7 per cent were lost to follow-up.

TUMOURS OF THE NOSE AND PARA-NASAL SINUSES

Tumours of the nose and para-nasal sinuses are characterized by histological and anatomical heterogeneity. The diversity of the population of normal cells found in the lining of the sinuses is paralleled by the diversity of the histological types of tumour that are encountered in this region: squamous carcinoma, salivary gland tumours, adenocarcinoma, inverting papillomas, melanoma, esthesio-neuroblastoma, lymphomas and sarcoma. The nasal vestibule is lined with squamous epithelium but the nasal cavity and sinuses are lined with columnar ciliated epithelium. Goblet or mucous cells are interspersed amongst the columnar cells, and beneath the basement membrane there is a virtually continuous layer of mucous and serous glands. There is diffuse lymphoid tissue throughout the region. In the olfactory region, the lining comprises three types of cell: bipolar olfactory nerve cells, basal cells and sustentacular cells.

Anatomy

The nasal vestibule is defined as that small area of the nasal fossa just proximal to the nares. The nasal cavity begins at the squamo-columnar junction and extends backwards to the posterior choanae. The nasal septum divides it into left and right and laterally it is bounded by the ala nasi. The nasal septum ends inferiorly as the columella, that structure which separates the two nostrils. Tumours of the columella should be classified with tumours of the nasal vestibule. The olfactory portion of the nasal cavity comprises the roof, the superior concha and the adjacent upper part of the nasal septum.

The maxillary sinuses are pyramidal in shape. The lateral wall of the nasal cavity lies medially, the roof is formed by the orbital floor, the alveolar process forms the floor and the apex extends into the zygomatic process of the maxilla. The cheek lies anteriorly, the pterygoid plates and pterygo-palatine fossa lie posteriorly.

The maxillary sinus can be divided into a superior portion (the suprastructure) and an inferior portion (infrastructure) by an imaginary line, Ohngren's line, drawn between the medial canthus and the angle of the jaw. This division has prognostic significance. Tumours of the suprastructure have a worse prognosis, they present later and may invade locally into the orbit and adjacent structures.

The ethmoidal sinuses lie within the ethmoid bone between the medial plate of the ethmoid, part of the lateral wall of the nasal cavity, and the lateral plate of the ethmoid, part of the medial wall of the orbital cavity. The top of the ethmoid bone articulates with the frontal and splenoid bones, its floor articulates with the vomer and the septal cartilage of the nose. The frontal sinuses lie within the frontal bone, immediately above the orbits. Tumours of the frontal sinuses can easily spread into the orbits or to the anterior cranial fossa. The sphenoid sinuses lie within the body of the sphenoid bone. This sinus varies considerably in size and may extend into the occipital bone almost as far back as the foramen magnum. Tumours of the sphenoid sinus may extend directly into the middle cranial fossa.

The lymphatic drainage of the nasal cavity and para-nasal sinuses is poor. Tumours arising in this region rarely spread to lymph nodes. The main lymphatic drainage is to the submandibular, subdigastric and retro-pharyngeal nodes. Clinically enlarged nodes associated with these tumours should not be assumed to be metastatic. The nasal vestibule and columella drain to the submandibular and subdigastric nodes. Posterior parts of the ethmoid

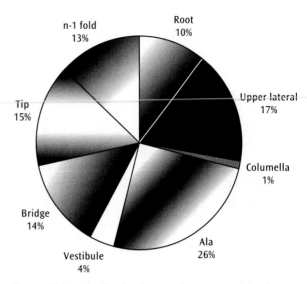

Figure 17.33 *Distribution by site of tumours arising from the skin of the nose.*

sinus and the whole of the sphenoid sinus drain to the retro-pharynygeal nodes.

The nose

The distribution by site of 1676 tumours of the skin of the nose treated with radiotherapy is shown in Figure 17.33. The majority were basal cell carcinomas but there was a high incidence of squamous carcinomas in the vestibule (75 per cent) and columella (48 per cent). There was no overall difference in control for squamous carcinomas compared with basal cell carcinomas. However, site was important. The control rate for carcinomas of the columella was 78 per cent (95 per cent CI, 60–95 per cent); the rate was 75 per cent (64–86 per cent) for tumours of the vestibule, and 95 per cent (93–96 per cent) for tumours at other sites. Given these differences, tumours of the nasal vestibule and columella should be considered separately from tumours at other sites on the nose. These latter tumours can be managed similarly to other tumours of the skin. The TNM staging system for skin tumours can also be used for staging carcinomas of the nasal vestibule and columella. The stage distribution for tumours of the nasal vestibule is shown in Figure 17.34. The absence of T3 tumours is unsurprising: it would be difficult to imagine a 5 cm tumour of the vestibule which had not invaded bone or cartilage. Tumours of the vestibule will invade bone, cartilage or the skin of the upper lip early, hence the high proportion of T4 tumours. This local invasion may occur surreptitiously, for example along the floor of the nasal fossa. This may, in part, explain the poorer prognosis of tumours at this site compared to other tumours of the nose.

Surgery has only a limited role to play in the primary management of tumours of the nasal vestibule or columella. An operation extensive enough to remove the tumour with adequate margins will be cosmetically

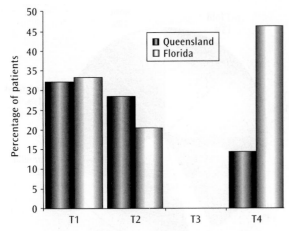

Figure 17.34 *Distribution by T-stage of tumours arising from the nasal vestibule.*

unacceptable. A cosmetically acceptable operation will almost certainly leave positive histological margins and the subsequent requirement for radiotherapy.

The appropriate radiotherapeutic technique for managing tumours of the nasal vestibule or columella is controversial. The debate concerns the relative roles of interstitial implantation and external-beam therapy. These tumours can be easily implanted using afterloaded ^{192}Ir wires. The procedure can be carried out under local anaesthetic: 60 Gy at 0.5 Gy/h produces excellent tumour control and good cosmetic results. External-beam treatment should either be with electrons or with an anterior wedged pair of fields using megavoltage X-rays. Orthovoltage is not to be recommended because of the uncertainties of dose at depth and because the skin will inevitably receive 100 per cent of the given dose. The vexed question of the relationship between cartilage necrosis and low-energy X-rays can be avoided entirely if orthovoltage therapy is not used. The dose for megavoltage therapy should be 50–55 Gy in 20 fractions, or its equivalent.

Only 5–15 per cent of patients have involvement of lymph nodes at presentation. Nodal relapse in the untreated neck is an uncommon course of treatment failure. Pooling data from the literature gives a nodal relapse rate of 31/288 (11 per cent; 95 per cent CI, 7–14 per cent). There is therefore little indication for treating the nodes prophylactically in patients with carcinoma of the nasal vestibule. Surgical salvage is sometimes possible after failure of radiotherapy. Overall actuarial 5-year survival is between 75 and 80 per cent; patients with T1 or T2 tumours have cause-specific survival of nearly 95 per cent at 5 years.

Nasal cavity and para-nasal sinuses

These tumours are uncommon and account for less than 10 per cent of all tumours of the head and neck.

A proportion of these tumours, particularly the adenocarcinomas, may be related to occupational factors: wood dust, chromium or nickel fumes and leather dust.

The distribution of histological types of tumour depends not only upon the site of origin of the tumour but also upon the centre reporting the results (Fig. 17.35a, b, c). The incidence of esthesio-neuroblastoma is high in the series of nasal cavity tumours from Florida; the high incidence of adenocarcinomas in the series of ethmoidal tumours reported from Bordeaux may reflect occupational factors. Selection criteria have a major influence, it is hard to believe that adenoid cystic carcinoma of the maxillary sinus only occurs in Houston and that lymphomas of this region are only found in Glasgow. Nevertheless, these differences in distribution of histological types will influence reported results.

Doubts about the precise site of origin of the tumour will provide another source of potential confusion. In the large series of sinus and nasal cavity tumours reported from the Christie Hospital it was possible to define a site of origin in only 48 per cent of patients (Logue and Slevin, 1991). The group of patients in whom the precise site of origin was undetermined had a much poorer survival than those for whom site could be defined. This uncertainty will produce an effect analogous to stage shift on site-specific prognosis.

NASAL CAVITY

Tumours of the nasal cavity characteristically present with nasal obstruction, discharge or epistaxis. Clinically, an ulcerating or infiltrating lesion is usually visible on nasoscopy. There is no UICC staging system but two staging systems for tumours of the nasal cavity have been suggested. The T staging proposed from St. Louis is as follows:

- T1: confined to the nasal cavity plus or minus vestibule.
- T2: extends to other sinuses or the nasopharynx.
- T3: extends beyond the nasal cavity and para-nasal sinuses.

The University of Florida system is somewhat different:

- Stage 1: limited to site of origin.
- Stage 2: local extension.
- Stage 3: extension to base of skull ± pterygoid plate destruction ± intracranial extension.

Nodal involvement at presentation is uncommon, between 10 and 15 per cent in most series.

Radiotherapy is the primary method of treatment. Anterior wedged oblique fields with 6 MV X-rays can be used. Alternatively a weighted anterior field plus wedged lateral fields can be used. [192]Ir implants may be particularly useful for treating tumours of the nasal septum. Overall survival after radiotherapy is between 50 and 75 per cent. Local recurrence is the predominant course of treatment failure. Isolated nodal relapse is uncommon

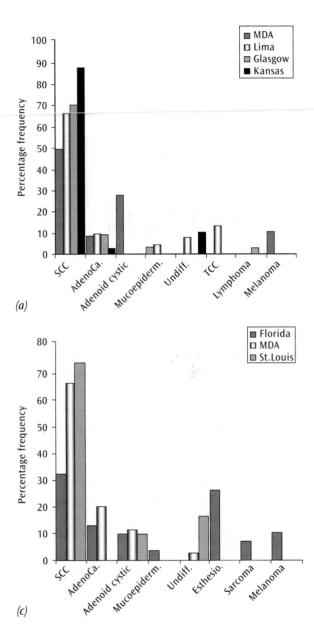

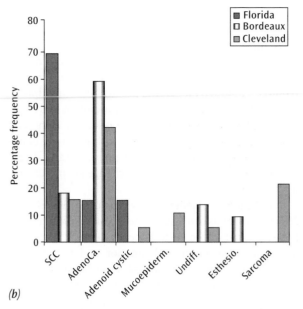

(a)

(b)

(c)

Figure 17.35 *Tumours of the nasal cavity and para-nasal sinuses: histology and site of origin. (a) Tumours of the maxillary antrum; (b) tumours of the ethmoid cavity; (c) tumours of the nasal cavity. SCC, squamous carcinoma; Mucoepiderm., mucoepidermoid carcinoma; Esthesio., esthesioneuroblastoma; Undiff., undifferentiated carcinoma; AdenoCa., adenocarcinoma; TCC, transitional cell carcinoma; MDA, M.D. Anderson Hospital, Houston.*

(less than 20 per cent of patients). Local control is a better yardstick than overall survival for assessing therapy, since approximately 50 per cent of deaths are unrelated to the original tumour. The local control by T stage in a series from St. Louis was: T1, 18/23 (78 per cent); T2, 6/11 (58 per cent); T3, 9/22 (42 per cent).

The most important complication after radiotherapy for nasal cavity tumours is blindness. When tumour extends into or close to the orbit then the ipsilateral eye will be within the high-dose volume. The incidence of visual loss in patients treated with radiotherapy for nasal cavity carcinoma is between 5 and 10 per cent and this must be accepted if tumour control is to be achieved.

INVERTING PAPILLOMA (RINGERTZ TUMOUR)

This is a rare tumour which arises primarily in the nasal cavity: the incidence is 0.6/100 000 per year. Although

histologically benign, it has a conspicuous tendency to recur after surgical resection. It can also, if left untreated, undergo malignant transformation either to squamous carcinoma or to adenocarcinoma. Radiotherapy has an important potential role in its management.

Histologically, these tumours are characterized by hyperplasia and metaplasia of the surface epithelium with infolding into the supporting stroma. Papillary projections are often prominent but, unless there has been malignant change, the basement membrane remains intact. Careful histological review suggests that the carcinomas arise directly from the inverting papilloma rather than as coincidental separate neoplasms. Analysis with *in-situ* hybridization and the polymerase chain reaction suggests an association between HPV and inverting papilloma. The pooled data from seven recent surgical series shows the overall rate of malignancy associated with inverting papilloma is 38/443 (8.5 per cent). Clinically, these tumours present as nasal obstruction and may be mistaken for polyps.

The initial treatment is surgical, lateral rhinotomy and medial maxilloectomy or cranio-facial resection may be required. Although the surgical procedures sound drastic, the cosmetic and functional results are often extremely good. For small tumours complete resection with good long-term control may be possible with per-nasal endoscopic resection. Recurrence after previous radical surgery or the presence of malignant change are indications for radiotherapy.

A radical dose of radiotherapy is required: 50–55 Gy in 20 fractions, or its equivalent. The ipsilateral eye may have to be included within the treatment volume. A three-field technique with a weighted anterior and two wedged lateral fields produces a reasonable dose distribution.

The largest series of patients irradiated for inverted papilloma published so far is of 25 patients treated in Boston: 18 of these patients had coexistent carcinoma. Local control was achieved in 6/7 patients with inverted papilloma alone, and 17/18 patients with malignant change. All 25 patients have survived, follow-up after radiotherapy is from 6 months to 12.9 years. The interval between initial diagnosis and referral for radiotherapy ranged from 6 weeks to 24 years. The serious late effects of radiation were mainly ocular: 2 of 25 patients had decreased visual acuity.

MAXILLARY SINUS

Sixty years ago Ohngren reported 38 per cent long-term survival for patients with maxillary sinus carcinoma treated by combined surgery and radiotherapy. Not a great deal has changed since. The results for several series, which include a variety of therapeutic approaches, are summarized in Figure 17.36.

Early tumours of the maxillary sinus cause few symptoms: epistaxis, nasal obstruction. Tumours of the infrastructure may present as a palatal or upper alveolar swelling and be mistaken for a primary tumour of the gum or palate. All patients with tumours of the gum or palate should have radiological investigation of the maxillary sinus to exclude the possibility that the tumour has arisen primarily at that site. Tumours that have spread beyond the sinus will cause swelling of the cheek, diplopia, proptosis, numbness and paraesthesia of the cheek or upper lip. Palpable lymphadenopathy at presentation is uncommon. The majority of tumours are squamous carcinomas (Fig. 17.35a). The UICC (1997) staging of maxillary sinus carcinoma is summarized in Table 17.55.

It is obvious from the criteria for T staging that clinical examination alone is insufficient for staging maxillary sinus carcinomas. CT scanning is an essential investigation in the assessment of these tumours. The images will indicate the extent of the tumour and aid in the evaluation of operability and the planning of radiotherapy (Fig. 17.37).

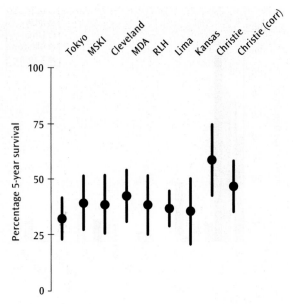

Figure 17.36 *Carcinoma of the maxillary antrum – 5-year survival data from the literature. MSKI, Memorial Sloan Kettering Institute, New York; MDA, M.D. Anderson Hospital, Houston; RLH, Royal London Hospital.*

Table 17.55 *UICC (1997) T-staging for tumours of the paranasal sinuses*

Maxillary sinus

TX	Primary tumour cannot be assessed
T0	No evidence of primary tumour
Tis	Carcinoma *in-situ*
T1	Tumour limited to the antral mucosa with no erosion or destruction of bone
T2	Tumour causing bone erosion or destruction, except for the posterior antral wall, including extension into the hard palate and/or the middle of the nasal meatus
T3	Tumour invades any of the following: bone of the posterior wall of maxillary sinus, subcutaneous tissues, skin of cheek, floor or medial wall of orbit, infratemportal fossa, pterygoid plates, ethmoid sinuses
T4	Tumour invades orbital contents beyond the floor or medial wall, including any of the following: the orbital apex, cribriform plate, base of skull, nasopharynx, sphenoid, frontal sinuses

Ethmoid sinus

T1	Tumour confined to the ethmoid with or without bone erosion
T2	Tumour extends into the nasal cavity
T3	Tumour extends to the anterior orbit, and/or maxillary sinus
T4	Tumour with intracranial extension, orbital extension including apex, involving sphenoid, and/or frontal sinus and/or skin of external nose

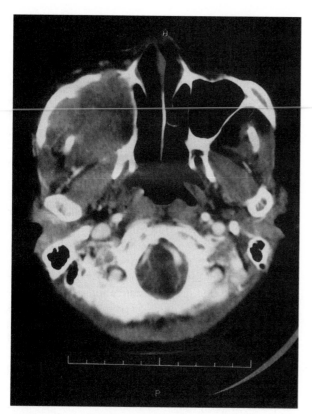

Figure 17.37 *CT image of a large right-sided antral carcinoma which has expanded the antrum and invaded through the anterior wall and into subcutaneous fat. The posterior wall has also been breached and there is extensive spread of tumour into the infra-temporal fossa.*

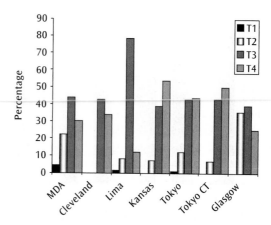

Figure 17.38 *Data from the literature showing the stage distribution of antral tumours at presentation. MDA, M.D. Anderson Hospital, Houston.*

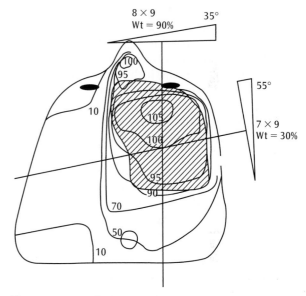

Figure 17.39 *Radiotherapy field arrangements which may be used for the treatment of a tumour of the maxillary antrum.*

The majority of tumours are advanced at presentation: 70–90 per cent are T3 or T4 (Fig. 17.38). Some early tumours can be treated successfully by surgery alone or by radiotherapy alone. Combined treatment is, however, required for the majority of patients. The optimal sequence for radiotherapy and surgery has, in the past, been controversial. Preoperative radiotherapy may facilitate the subsequent surgery but important prognostic information, from the surgical pathology, may be lost and post-surgical complications may be increased. Postoperative radiotherapy is now the preferred sequence in most centres, but extensive surgical procedures may be required for tumours of the maxillary sinus. A radical maxillectomy is usually the minimum procedure. If there has been orbital invasion, then more extended surgery, possibly including orbital exenteration, may be required. Reconstruction will usually involve a myocutaneous flap and, when the orbital contents have been removed, a suitable prosthesis. The removal of the hard palate provides good access to the sinus cavity and facilitates drainage during post-operative radiotherapy. In the longer term, an obturator will be required to permit eating and speaking. The management of these patients is complicated and involves many disciplines, rehabilitation is critical to successful functional results.

Radiotherapy can be given using an anterior and wedged lateral fields. The fields required for a well-lateralized tumour with no invasion of the orbit are shown in Figure 17.39. When the orbit has been invaded, the eye shielding on the anterior field cannot be used and the dose to the eye may well exceed radiation tolerance. When megavoltage beams are used to treat tumours invading the cheek, bolus will be required to eliminate skin sparing and bring the high dose volume anteriorly. Tumours that extend across midline will require both right and left wedged lateral fields. It is sometimes possible to spare some of the eye by angling these fields posteriorly; the problem with doing this is that the dose to the spinal cord will be increased. The dose required postoperatively is 50 Gy in 20 fractions, or its equivalent in 30 fractions. When radiotherapy is used alone then the doses need to be a little higher: 55 Gy or 65 Gy.

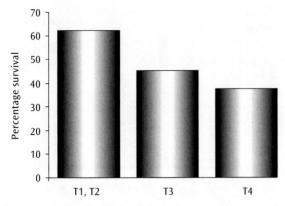

Figure 17.40 *Survival according to T stage for tumours of the maxillary antrum: 5-year survival estimates pooled from the literature.*

The 5-year survival data by T stage are shown in Figure 17.40. Data from the Christie show the best results: 58 per cent 5-year survival in 37 patients with tumours known to arise from the maxillary sinus. Unfortunately many tumours (48 per cent) in this series of 152 tumours of the para-nasal sinuses and nasal cavity could not have a site of origin assigned. If correction is made for this, the overall survival in the patients with maxillary sinus tumours treated at the Christie falls to 46 per cent of an estimated 74 patients. The majority of the patients in the series from the Christie were treated with radiotherapy alone whereas, in the other series shown in Figure 17.36, the majority of patients were treated with combined treatment. These data therefore call into question the absolute need for surgery in all patients with tumours of the maxillary sinus. Combined treatment is possibly unnecessary for T1 and T2 tumours and is often impossible for T4 tumours. It is probably only in the T3 tumours, therefore, that combined treatment will be required. The main cause of treatment failure is failure of local control: this accounted for over 80 per cent of failures in a large series from Tokyo. Only about 5–10 per cent of patients relapse in the regional nodes. About 5 per cent of patients develop distant metastases and less than 5 per cent develop second primaries.

The main late complications of radiotherapy are ocular and neurological. The temporal lobes lie closer to the antrum than is often appreciated and may, for advanced tumours, be within the high-dose volume. Temporal lobe necrosis, often manifest as temporal lobe epilepsy, may occur after radiotherapy. The brainstem and cord are also vulnerable and only careful treatment planning will avoid overdosage. If the eye is within the high-dose volume, then eventual blindness, either because of severe dry eye, cataract, or retinal damage, is virtually inevitable.

ETHMOID SINUS

Tumours of the ethmoid sinus present with headache, visual disturbances, nasal obstruction and, in the later stages, lateral displacement of the globe of the eye. Orbital involvement is frequent and the ipsilateral eye may have to be sacrificed; this applies whether treatment is by surgery or by radiotherapy.

These tumours are extremely rare and a variety of histological types may be encountered (Fig. 17.35b). This makes comparison of various approaches to treatment difficult. Of 41 tumours reported upon from Bordeaux, 22 were treated by a combination of surgery and radiotherapy. The local recurrence rate was 12/22 and the 5-year survival was 44 per cent. Patients with sarcomas, previous chemotherapy or treatment with radiotherapy alone were excluded from the published results. The 5-year survival rates reported from other, smaller, series range from 35 to 50 per cent. Local recurrence is the main cause of treatment failure, distant relapse is uncommon.

Radical surgery for these tumours may involve craniofacial resection and orbital exenteration. Radical radiotherapy requires a dose of 50–55 Gy in 20 fractions, or its equivalent. The optimal field arrangement is to use a heavily weighted anterior field, with bolus to the medial canthus if necessary, and wedged lateral fields. CT planning is essential to avoid overdosing the contralateral eye, and also to ensure that any intracranial extension is adequately encompassed.

SPHENOID SINUS

The main symptom of carcinoma of the sphenoid sinus is headache; persistent, severe and central. Cranial nerve palsies occur later. These tumours are usually advanced at presentation. Radical treatment with radiotherapy may be attempted, but the chance of cure is low. Surgery has little to offer, either as primary or as secondary therapy. For the majority of patients, palliative treatment is all that can be offered.

TUMOURS OF THE EAR

The ear can be divided anatomically into the pinna, the external auditory canal, the middle ear and the mastoid antrum.

Squamous carcinoma of the middle ear

These tumours are extremely rare, with an incidence in the UK of less than 1/1 000 000 per annum. There is an undoubted association with chronic suppurative ear disease: 65–70 per cent of patients with tumours of the middle ear have a history of chronic ear infection. The incidence of malignancy in patients with chronic ear disease has been estimated at between 1 in 4000 and 1 in 20 000. A crude calculation would suggest that chronic ear infection, of 10 years' duration, would be associated with a 5- to 25-fold risk of developing a carcinoma of the middle ear. Tumours of the middle ear can be classified by site of origin into petromastoid tumours and tympanotubal tumours. The petromastoid tumours present with pain and discharge and VIIth nerve palsy. The tympanotubal tumours can spread along the Eustachian tube and, with consequent multiple palsies of cranial nerves, imitate nasopharyngeal tumours. Nodal spread is uncommon in petromastoid tumours because the otic capsule provides a barrier to tumour spread.

Tumours of the middle ear are often diagnosed late, the symptoms of the associated ear infection mask those of the tumour. Only about 20 per cent of patients have T1 tumours at presentation according to the staging system proposed by Stell:

- T1: tumour limited to the site of origin, with no facial nerve paralysis and no bone destruction.
- T2: tumour extends beyond the site of origin, indicated by facial paralysis or radiological evidence of bone destruction, but no extension beyond the organ of origin.
- T3: clinical or radiological evidence of extension to surrounding structures, dura, base of skull, parotid gland, temporo-mandibular joint, etc.
- TX: patients with insufficient data for classification.

About 30 per cent of patients present with disease that is too far advanced to permit radical therapy.

Clinically, there is destruction of the middle ear and a visible tumour obscures any proper assessment of the extent of local invasion into the structures of the middle ear and adjacent bone. CT and MRI are therefore essential in the assessment of patients before treatment (Fig. 17.41).

These tumours are best managed by a combination of conservative surgery and postoperative radiotherapy (Birzgalis *et al.*, 1992). The advantages of using surgery first are that it removes the bulk of the tumour, any infection in bone is physically removed and the resulting cavity can be easily inspected and monitored during treatment. The surgical specimen also provides information which, taken in conjunction with the radiological investigations, enables the postoperative radiotherapy to be planned accurately and rationally.

Most tumours of the middle ear can be treated using an ipsilateral wedged pair of fields. Occasionally, for tumours extending deep into the temporal bone, a contralateral field may also be required. Additional fields using electrons may be useful when there is extensive involvement of the skin and subcutaneous tissues. The absorption of electrons by bone is unpredictable and it is unwise to rely on electrons to treat disease that is unquestionably invading bone.

The postoperative radiation dose should be 50 Gy in 20 fractions over 4 weeks. Some very early tumours may be satisfactorily treated solely by radiotherapy: the dose should be 52–55 Gy in 20 fractions. The main risk from radiotherapy to the temporal bone is osteoradionecrosis. Provided overdosage is avoided, and this will require careful attention to any hot spots seen on the treatment plan, and provided that any infection is treated aggressively, this complication is unlikely. The dose to the brainstem should be limited to 40 Gy in 20 fractions, or its equivalent.

The results of surgery and radiotherapy for carcinoma of the middle ear are summarized in Figure 17.42. The data

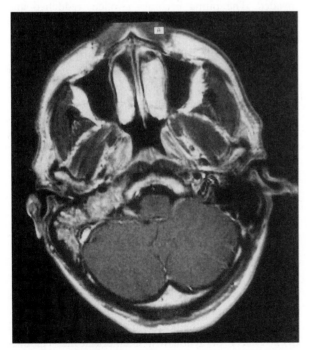

Figure 17.41 *MRI image (T1 axial scan with gadolinium), showing a tumour of the middle ear with involvement of the apex of the petrous temporal and mastoid.*

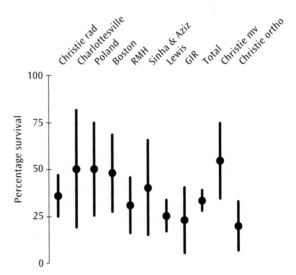

Figure 17.42 *Data from the literature on 5-year survival after surgery and radical radiotherapy for cancer of the middle ear. Christie rad, all patients treated radically at the Christie Hospital; Christie mv, patients treated with megavoltage X-rays at the Christie Hospital; Christie ortho, patients treated with orthovoltage radiotherapy at the Christie Hospital.*

from the Christie Hospital clearly show the advantages of megavoltage, as opposed to orthovoltage, radiotherapy. Overall the 5-year survival is around 33 per cent. Failure to control local disease is the usual cause of treatment failure, distant metastases or nodal relapse are uncommon.

Effective palliative treatment is extremely difficult for tumours of the middle ear. Extensive surgical resections produce morbidity that is often worse than the disease itself, and any relief of symptoms is often brief: 3 months in one series. Conventional radiotherapy is not very effective in controlling pain. In the series from Manchester, pain was effectively controlled with radiotherapy in only 50 per cent of patients. Unconventional palliative schedules such as 14.8 Gy in 4 fractions in 2 days, repeated 2–3 times at 3-weekly intervals, may provide some measure of control of the tumour with minimal morbidity or upset. Palliative chemotherapy using cisplatin and 5-fluorouracil may have a short-term benefit.

Tumours of the external auditory canal

The majority of malignant tumours of the external auditory canal are squamous carcinomas but other histologies may also be encountered: adenocarcinoma, adenoid cystic carcinoma and basal cell carcinoma.

Pain and discharge are the usual symptoms, although deafness and a mass around the ear may also occur. Mastoid tenderness may be present on physical examination, but the diagnosis is usually made on the presence of obvious tumour, often polypoidal, in the canal. Facial palsy is unusual (less than 20 per cent of patients).

The external auditory canal can be divided into two portions: the osseous and the cartilaginous. There are no defining differences in presentation between the two sites. Tumours of the bony canal may spread to the middle ear and it is sometimes difficult to decide whether a tumour has arisen primarily within the middle ear or has invaded secondarily from the osseous canal. CT and MRI are required to stage patients adequately. The staging system proposed by Stell can also be applied to tumours of the external auditory canal.

Conservative surgical excision and postoperative radiotherapy is the treatment of choice. Radiation dosage and technique is similar to that described for tumours of the middle ear. Prognosis for tumours of the external auditory canal is better than that for tumours of the middle ear, long-term survival is typically in the range of 30–50 per cent.

Tumours of the pinna

Tumours of the pinna usually arise from the skin. The majority are squamous carcinomas, a minority are basal cell carcinomas. Between 5 and 10 per cent of all skin tumours arise on the pinna, a disproportionately high incidence. Most of these tumours can be treated satisfactorily with radiotherapy. There are two sites, however, at which surgery may be the preferred treatment: tumours arising around the origin of the external auditory canal and tumours of the retroauricular sulcus.

The role of orthovoltage treatment in carcinoma of the pinna is controversial. The Z value for cartilage is unknown. If it is close to that of bone, the cartilage will be overdosed relative to the skin if orthovoltage is used: if it is closer to that of soft tissue, the problem of relative overdosage will not arise. Recent data from Liverpool suggest that, whatever the theoretical arguments might be, there is no practical disadvantage from treating carcinoma of the pinna with orthovoltage radiotherapy. Local control was achieved in 60/62 patients and the overall necrosis rate was 10 per cent. Only 1/62 patients required surgery for necrosis, the remaining five necroses healed with conservative therapy.

Electron-beam therapy produces excellent results for carcinoma of the pinna. The beam energy should be chosen according to the thickness of the tumour; build-up will be required for the lower energies. For tumours on the helix it is usually possible to shield the skin behind the ear using thin lead, backed with wax, to absorb any knock-on photons. It may be necessary to use a wax ear plug as a compensator for tumours arising around the concha. A dose of 45 Gy in 10 fractions in 2 weeks is adequate for small (less than 2 cm) tumours; for larger tumours a dose of 50–55 Gy in 20 fractions in 4 weeks may be required.

Perichondritis may complicate the treatment of these tumours, particularly when the cartilage has been directly invaded. The pinna becomes swollen, reddened and exquisitely tender. Fever may be present. The condition usually responds to prompt therapy with a broad-spectrum antibiotic. Late necrosis of cartilage is an accepted complication of treatment. It usually occurs after trauma, particularly from spectacles. Treatment with systemic antibiotics and topical steroids is usually effective.

The prognosis for carcinomas of the pinna is excellent. Local control with radiotherapy as sole treatment is over 90 per cent and survival is close to 100 per cent.

RARE AND UNUSUAL TUMOURS OF THE HEAD AND NECK

Paragangliomas

The nomenclature and classification of these rare tumours are complex, inconsistent and confusing. They can arise at a variety of sites in the head and neck, and are described by a variety of synonyms; chemodectomas, glomus tumours, etc. The literature is a poor guide – different authors applying different criteria for inclusion in ostensibly comprehensive series that often turn out to be fairly restricted. Management is controversial: extreme views are often taken with only slender, and highly selected, evidence to support them.

Paragangliomas are benign tumours arising from the APUD cells of the chemoreceptor bodies. Histologically they are highly vascular with cell nests (zellballen) separated by a dense capillary network. The cells are pale and uniform and, on electron microscopy, contain neurosecretory granules. Only 5–10 per cent of paragangliomas metastasize. They grow slowly, and respond slowly to non-surgical treatment. There is an association between chronic hypoxaemia, for example living at high altitude, and paragangliomas. Familial forms also occur, and there is some overlap with the multiple endocrine neoplasia (MEN) syndromes. A significant proportion, around 20 per cent, of patients will have multiple tumours. This is particularly true of familial cases. In keeping with their neuroendocrine origin, these tumours may secrete enzymes or amines into the bloodstream: neuron-specific enolase (NSE), vanillylmandelic acid (VMA) and 5-hydroxyindoleacetic acid (5-HIAA).

The simplest classification of paragangliomas is by site:

- middle ear = tympanicum;
- jugular bulb ± middle ear = jugulare;
- hypopharynx = vagale;
- carotid bifurcation = carotid body tumour.

The incidence is low, 2/100 000 per annum, and females outnumber males by approximately 3 to 1. The symptoms and clinical findings depend upon the site of origin. Tumours of the middle ear classically present with pulsatile tinnitus (75 per cent of patients), deafness (52 per cent), fullness in the ear (15 per cent) and dizziness or vertigo (10 per cent). Glomus vagale or carotid body tumours usually present as a mass in the neck; indentation of the pharyngeal wall is visible in approximately a third of patients with glomus vagale tumours, there is usually a corresponding external mass just behind the angle of the mandible.

A visible mass is usually present on examination of patients with tumours of the middle ear. About 30 per cent may have a visible polyp in the external auditory canal. Cranial nerve palsies are frequent: VIII, IX and X for tympanojugulare tumours; X and XII for vagale tumours. The investigation of patients with paragangliomas has been revolutionized by CT scanning and MRI. Assessment of operability and the planning of surgery or radiotherapy is now far more precise than when angiography was the only reliable investigation. Detection of multiple tumours is also important, and radioisotope imaging either with [131I]meta-iodobenzylguanidine (MIBG) or [111In]octreotide can be extremely useful.

The choice of treatment lies between surgical resection and radiotherapy. Data from the literature are shown in Figure 17.43a, b. These data are of very limited usefulness since many of the published series deal with highly selected groups of patients. Surgical techniques have improved considerably over the past 10–20 years and much of the older data on surgically treated patients is now only of historical interest. Microsurgical techniques and advances in anaesthesia, with hypothermia and cardiopulmonary bypass, have improved surgeons' ability to resect tympanicum and jugulare tumours while sparing blood vessels and nerves. Advances in diagnostic imaging mean that these tumours are now being diagnosed at an earlier, more easily resectable, stage. The relative roles of surgery and radiotherapy must be assessed on currently available techniques.

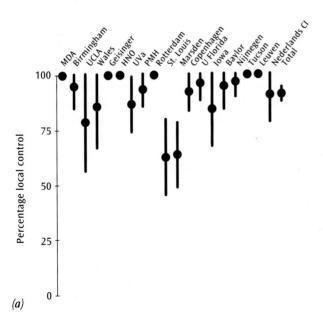

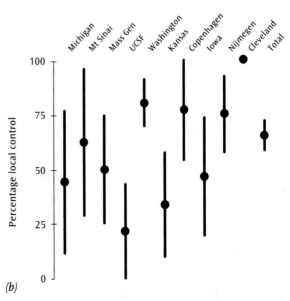

Figure 17.43 *Local control rates for paragangliomas: (a) patients treated with radiotherapy; (b) patients treated with surgery.*

For younger, fitter patients with resectable tumours, radical surgery is the treatment of choice. Older patients, or those in whom surgical resection would produce unacceptable morbidity, can be treated with radiotherapy.

CT planning is essential for tumours of the middle ear: an ipsilateral wedged pair of fields will usually produce a satisfactory dose distribution. Tumours extending deeply towards the midline may require a contralateral top-up field. The dose should be 50–55 Gy in 25 fractions over 5 weeks. This produces adequate control of disease without excessive morbidity. Response to treatment will depend upon how local control is defined. Para-gangliomas are, by virtue of their natural history, tumours in which stable disease is an acceptable and useful thera-peutic end point. Roughly speaking, about 15 per cent of tumours will regress completely after radiotherapy, 60 per cent will regress by ⩾50 per cent and 15 per cent will remain stable: 10 per cent of tumours will grow in spite of treatment (Powell *et al.*, 1992). Long follow-up is needed, since even an apparently well-controlled tumour may eventually regrow.

Esthesioneuroblastoma (olfactory neuroblastoma)

Esthesioneuroblastoma is a small, round-celled tumour which arises from the olfactory epithelium in the roof of the nasal cavity and which may spread into the ethmoid sinus. The age instance is bimodal, with peaks in the second and sixth decades. The histological appearance varies and the differential diagnosis from other small, round-celled tumours may be difficult. Two features are characteristic of olfactory neuroblastoma: an intracellu-lar fibrillary network and Homer Wright rosettes. These latter structures comprise a ring of cells around a central mass of eosinophilic fibrils. Hyams has devised a four-stage histological grading for olfactory neuroblastoma which may be of prognostic significance: grade is based upon an evaluation of architectural pattern, rosettes, necrosis, mitotic activity and nuclear pleomorphism.

Patients usually present with anosmia, nasal obstruc-tion, nasal discharge or epistaxis. Invasion of the orbit will produce proptosis and diplopia. The Kadish system has been used for clinical staging:

- A: confined to the nasal cavity;
- B: involvement of the para-nasal sinuses;
- C: spread beyond the nasal cavity or paranasal sinuses.

Treatment is primarily surgical, with cranio-facial resection the standard procedure. These tumours are radiosensitive and postoperative radiotherapy should be given to patients with high-grade tumours, or those in whom excision is incomplete. The dose should be 50 Gy in 20 fractions, or its equivalent. Inoperable tumours, or tumours in patients who are unfit for surgery, can be treated with radical radiotherapy. A dose of 55 Gy in

20 fractions, or its equivalent, is necessary. The radi-ation treatment technique is similar to that used for ethmoid tumours. CT planning is essential, MRI may demonstrate tumour extension beyond that which is visible on CT.

Experience with 49 cases of olfactory neuroblastomas accrued over 41 years at the Mayo Clinic has been reviewed recently. The overall 5-year survival was 70 per cent. Local control was achieved in nearly 90 per cent of the patients, but 20 per cent of the patients recurred locally. Late recurrence, beyond 10 years, was typical of this tumour. Distant metastases occurred in 18 per cent of patients. There is little experience with chemotherapy in these tumours: traditionally, regimens based upon Adriamycin, cyclophosphamide and vincristine have been used. Platinum-based regimens may also be effective.

Juvenile angiofibroma

This tumour, originally described by Hippocrates in the fourth century BC, characteristically occurs in adolescent males. The tumour is histologically benign but may behave in a malignant fashion, with local invasion and a tendency to recur after surgical resection. The tumour is nodular, bluish red, glistening and frequently ulcerated. It obtains its blood supply from the internal maxillary artery. The majority of tumours arise at the junction of the nasal cavity and the nasopharynx. The tumour will grow read-ily into soft tissues, and cavities and erosion of bone is frequent. Thirty of 38 cases from the Princess Margaret Hospital, Toronto had evidence of bone destruction.

Clinically, these tumours present with unilateral nasal obstruction, facial deformity and/or epistaxis. Careful evaluation is required with CT and MRI imaging and angiography. The latter may usefully be combined with preoperative embolization. Embolization alone, however, is not adequate treatment. Primary surgery has become the treatment of choice, although the results of radio-therapy are also satisfactory, with six recurrences in a series of 38 from Toronto. The hazards of surgery should not be underestimated but, in general, the principal of avoiding radiotherapy for benign disease, particularly in the young, should be adhered to. In cases that recur after surgery, or where there is residual tumour after surgery, radiotherapy is unquestionably of benefit. Low doses are sufficient: 30 Gy in 22 fractions over four and a half weeks produced local control, with minimal morbidity, in a series from Florida (Kasper *et al.*, 1993). In Toronto 30 Gy in 15 fractions is the norm. There is little to be gained from the use of higher doses. There are anecdotal accounts that these tumours respond to oestrogen ther-apy. Such an approach would be a therapy of last resort, because of unacceptable side-effects in the adolescent male. It is suggested that these tumours may regress spontaneously on maturation and observation is accept-able in some rare cases.

Merkel cell carcinoma

This neuroendocrine tumour of the skin was first described in 1972. It has, at varying times, also been called primary endocrine carcinoma of the skin or trabecular skin carcinoma. Cases presenting before 1972 were often classified as dermal adult neuroblastoma. Histologically, and in tissue culture, the tumour cells resemble small cell carcinoma of the lung. Merkel cell tumours may express NSE and/or calcitonin. Abnormalities of chromosomes 11 and 13, particularly translocations involving p36, have been described in up to 50 per cent of Merkel cell carcinomas. Over half the cases of Merkel cell carcinomas described in the literature have involved the skin of the head and neck.

Patients are typically elderly and present with a relatively short history. The lesions arise in the dermis and therefore rarely ulcerate; typically they appear as pinkish or greyish blebs. About 16 per cent of patients have nodal disease at presentation: survival is poor for patients with positive nodes, a median of 13 months in the series from the MD Anderson, compared with 40 months for patients with clinically negative nodes.

Local surgery alone was initially thought to be sufficient treatment for these tumours but 71/181 patients (39 per cent) treated in this way recurred locally and 83/181 (46 per cent) relapsed in regional nodes. The 5-year survival in patients treated with surgery alone at the MD Anderson was 30 per cent. Wide local excision and radical node dissection is now the recommended surgical approach and this should be combined with postoperative radiotherapy. The radiation dose should be 45–50 Gy in 20 fractions for prophylactic radiotherapy and 50–55 Gy in 20 fractions when microscopic disease is present. The recent data suggest that both local control and survival will be improved if radiotherapy is routinely used in the management of Merkel cell carcinoma. Approximately 25 per cent of patients will develop distant metastases. Chemotherapy, using regimens similar to those used for small cell lung cancer, has some logic, but the value is uncertain and the toxicity for the mostly elderly patients may be excessive.

Basaloid squamous carcinoma

This aggressive tumour was first recognized as a distinct pathological entity in 1986. Since then they have been reported more frequently. Histology characteristically shows a basaloid pattern with squamous differentiation. The tumours are cytokeratin positive and on electron microscopy there are no neurosecretory granules. This suggests that basaloid squamous carcinoma is an aggressive variant of squamous cell carcinoma rather than of any other cellular origin.

On fine-needle aspiration cytology these tumours can be confused with small cell undifferentiated carcinoma or adenoid cystic carcinoma. The tumours occur most commonly in the hypopharynx, larynx and floor of mouth, although other sites of involvement, such as the buccal mucosa and oesophagus, have been recognized recently.

The majority of patients have involved lymph nodes at presentation, extensive local invasion and distant metastases occur early in the course of the disease. The aggressiveness of the treatment should match that of the tumour. However, the value of chemotherapy remains to be defined.

Mucosal melanomas

Only about 0.5–4 per cent of melanomas occurring in the head and neck arise from the mucosa. The nose and paranasal sinuses are the most common sites and lymphatic spread is unusual. Since the structure of mucosa is different from that of skin, Clark's histological staging system is inappropriate for mucosal melanomas.

Historically, the management of mucosal melanoma has been surgical. However, there is increasing appreciation that mucosal melanomas may respond well to radiotherapy (Gilligan and Slevin, 1991). Tumours which are resectable should be treated surgically, and postoperative radiotherapy should be given to those patients in whom the tumours were large, thick or where there is doubt about the adequacy of the surgical margins. For patients whose tumours are inoperable, radiotherapy alone may be effective treatment. The dose required will be 50–55 Gy in 20 fractions, or its equivalent. Unconventional fractionation has also been used for melanomas, the 0, 7, 21 regimen (24 Gy in 3 fractions over 4 weeks) is simple and effective. Care must be taken with this regimen to the head and neck to ensure that vulnerable normal structures, such as brain, spinal cord or retina, are shielded after two fractions, as the full three fractions would exceed the tolerance of these organs. There is, however, no evidence that this is superior to conventional fractionation in head and neck melanomas.

Long-term survival for patients with mucosal melanomas is poor, with less than 25 per cent of patients in most series surviving for 5 years. Late relapses are typical, and so, given the limited data, it is unlikely that more than 20 per cent of patients with mucosal melanomas are cured by treatment.

The results for radiotherapy as primary treatment are shown in Figure 17.44. The 5-year survival in the Edinburgh series was 0 per cent, in the series from the Christie Hospital it was 5/28 (18 per cent; 95 per cent CI, 4–32 per cent).

Ameloblastoma

This rare tumour arises in the vicinity of the tooth socket, its precise histogenesis is uncertain. The classical site is in the mandible, close to the molar teeth. Patients

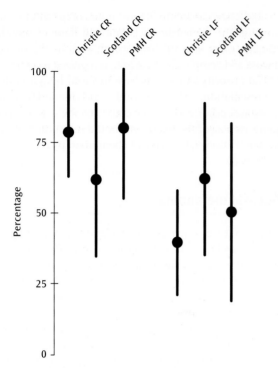

Figure 17.44 *Results of treating mucosal melanomas with radiotherapy. CR, complete response; LF, local failure; PMH, Princess Margaret Hospital, Toronto.*

The primary treatment of plasmacytoma of the head and neck is with radiotherapy. A dose of 40–45 Gy in 20 fractions is adequate. Supplementary chemotherapy may be used in patients with extensive tumours, although the role of adjuvant chemotherapy in this context is unproven. Patients who have been treated for plasmacytoma should be followed up carefully since many, if not all, may progress to develop systemic (multiple) myeloma.

SIGNIFICANT POINTS

- The optimal management of head and neck cancer requires the interplay of many medical specialities.
- Patients need to be involved in decisions affecting their care by understanding the risks and benefits of different interventions.
- Although there are certain broad principles, head and neck cancers have very different natural histories.
- To date chemotherapy has shown little benefit other than palliation.

are usually aged between 20 and 40 and give a history of a painless swelling often of several years' duration.

These tumours grow slowly and rarely metastasize. Plain X-rays show non-specific cystic changes, and bone involvement is much often more extensive than would be suspected radiologically. The standard treatment is surgical excision, islands of tumour may be found within the adjacent, apparently normal, bone and the excision may need to be fairly extensive. Curettage is not adequate therapy for ameloblastoma.

Plasmacytoma

Plasmacytomas can occur as apparently isolated tumours in the head and neck. The sites most often involved are the maxilla, the maxillary antrum and the mandible. Clinically the tumour presents as a tender swelling. In the extra-osseous form of the disease this is simply a reddish purple mass; in the intra-osseous form there is concomitant destruction of bone and pain may be severe.

The diagnosis of plasmacytoma should not be accepted without a search for evidence of multiple myeloma. All patients should have a skeletal survey, bone marrow aspirate, electrophoresis of serum proteins and urine tested for Bence Jones protein. The presence of a paraprotein does not necessarily imply that a patient has disseminated myeloma. The abnormal protein may be produced by the plasmacytoma itself and might prove useful in monitoring response to therapy.

KEY REFERENCES

Dimery, I.W. and Hong, W.K. (1993) Overview of combined modality therapies for head and neck cancer. *J. Natl Cancer Inst.* **85**, 95–111.

O'Sullivan, B., Mackillop, W.J., Gilbert, R. *et al.* (1994) Controversies in the management of laryngeal cancer: results of an international survey of patterns of care. *Radiother. Oncol.* **31**, 23–32.

Tannock, I.F. and Cummings, B.J. (1992) Neoadjuvant chemotherapy in head and neck cancer: no way to preserve a larynx. *J. Clin. Oncol.* **10**, 343–4.

Wiernik, G., Alcock, C.J., Bates, T.D. *et al.* (1991) Final report on the second British Institute of Radiology fractionation study: short versus long overall treatment times for radiotherapy of carcinoma of the laryngo-pharynx. *Br. J. Radiol.* **64**, 232–41.

REFERENCES

Bataini, J.-P. (1991) Head and neck cancer and the radiation oncologist. *Radiother. Oncol.* **21**, 1–10.

Bataini, J.-P., Bernier, J., Asselain, B. *et al.* (1988) Primary radiotherapy of squamous cell carcinoma of the oropharynx and pharyngolarynx: tentative multivariate modelling system to predict the radiocurability of neck nodes. *Int. J. Radiat. Oncol. Biol. Phys.* **14**, 635–642.

Begg, A.C., Haustermans, K., Hart, A.A. *et al.* (1999) The value of pre-treatment cell kinetic parameters as predictors for radiotherapy outcome in head and neck cancer: a multicenter analysis. *Radiother. Oncol.* **50**, 12–23.

Benner, S.E., Pajak, T.F., Lippman, S.M., Earley, C. and Hong, W.K. (1994) Prevention of second primary tumors with isotretinoin in patients with squamous cell carcinoma of the head and neck: long-term follow-up. *J. Natl Cancer Inst.* **86**, 140–1.

Birzgalis, A.R., Keith, A.O. and Farrington, W.T. (1992) Radiotherapy in the treatment of middle ear and mastoid carcinoma. *Clin. Otolaryngol.* **17**, 113–16.

Bjordal, K., Hammerlid, E., Ahlner-Elmqvist, M. *et al.* (1999) Quality of life in head and neck cancer patients: validation of the European Organization for Research and Treatment of Cancer Quality of Life Questionnaire-H&N35. *J. Clin. Oncol.* **17**, 1008–19.

Brizel, D., Sibley, G., Prosnitz, L., Sher, R. and Dewhirst, M. (1997) Tumor hypoxia adversely affects the prognosis of carcinoma of the head and neck. *Int. J. Radiat. Oncol. Biol. Phys.* **38**, 285–9.

Chaplin, J.M. and Morton, H.N. (1999) A prospective, longitudinal study of pain in head and neck cancer patients. *Head Neck* **21**, 531–7.

Coster, J.R., Foote, R.L., Olsen, K.D., Jack, S.M., Schaid, D.J. and deSanto, L.W. (1992) Cervical nodal metastasis of squamous cell carcinoma of unknown origin: indications for witholding radiotherapy. *Int. J. Radiat. Oncol. Biol. Phys.* **23**, 743–9.

De Crevoisier, R., Bourhis, J., Domenge, C. *et al.* (1998) Full-dose reirradiation for unresectable head and neck carcinoma: experience at the Gustave-Roussy Institute in a series of 169 patients. *J. Clin. Oncol.* **16**, 3556–62.

Department of Veterans Affairs laryngeal cancer study group (1991) Induction chemotherapy plus radiation compared with surgery plus radiation in patients with advanced laryngeal cancer. *N. Engl. J. Med.* **324**, 1685–90.

DerSimonian, R. and Laird, N. (1986) Meta-analysis in clinical trials. *Control Clin. Trials* **7**, 177–88.

Dobbs, J., Barret, A. and Ash, D. (1999) *Practical radiotherapy planning*. London: Arnold.

Dubray, B.M. and Thames, H.D. (1992) The influence of dose and time on the cure of larynx tumors. *Radiother. Oncol.* **23**, 199.

Gilligan, D. and Slevin, N.J. (1991) Radical radiotherapy for 28 cases of mucosal melanoma in the nasal cavity and sinuses. *Br. J. Radiol.* **64**, 1147–50.

Glynne-Jones, R.G.T., Anand, A.K., Young, T.E. and Berry, R.J. (1989) Metastatic adenocarcinoma in the cervical lymph nodes from an occult primary. *Clin. Oncol.* **1**, 19–21.

Griffiths, G.O., Parmar, M.K. and Bailey, A.J. (1999) Physical and psychological symptoms of quality of life in the CHART randomized trial in head and neck cancer: short-term and long-term patient reported symptoms. CHART Steering Committee. Continuous hyperfractionated accelerated radiotherapy. *Br. J. Cancer* **81**, 1196–205.

Hendry, J.H., Roberts, S.A., Slevin, N.J., Keane, T.J., Barton, M. and Agren-Cronqvist, A. (1994) Influence of radiotherapy treatment time on control of laryngeal cancer: comparisons between centres in Manchester, UK and Toronto, Canada. *Radiother. Oncol.* **31**, 14–22.

Jones, A.S. (1992) The management of early hypopharyngeal cancer: primary radiotherapy and salvage surgery. *Clin. Otolaryngol.* **17**, 545–9.

Jones, A.S., Cook, J.A., Phillips, D.E. and Roland, N.R. (1993) Squamous carcinoma presenting as an enlarged cervical lymph node. *Cancer* **72**, 1756–61.

Kasper, M.E., Parsons, J.T., Mancuso, A.A. *et al.* (1993) Radiation therapy for juvenile angiofibroma: evaluation by CT and MRI, analysis of tumor regression, and selection of patients. *Int. J. Radiat. Oncol. Biol. Phys.* **25**, 689–94.

Lee, A.W.M., Sham, J.S.T., Poon, Y.F. and Ho, J.H.C. (1989) Treatment of stage I nasopharyngeal carcinoma: analysis of patterns of relapse and the results of witholding elective neck irradiation. *Int. J. Radiat. Oncol. Biol. Phys.* **17**, 1183–90.

Lee, A.W.M., Law, S.C.K., Ng, S.H. *et al.* (1992a) Retrospective analysis of nasopharyngeal carcinoma treated during 1976–1985: late complications following megavoltage irradiation. *Br. J. Radiol.* **65**, 918–28.

Lee, A.W.M., Poon, Y.F., Foo, W. *et al.* (1992b) Retrospective analysis of 5037 patients with nasopharyngeal carcinoma treated during 1976–1985: overall survival and patterns of failure. *Int. J. Radiat. Oncol. Biol. Phys.* **23**, 261–70.

Logue, J.P. and Slevin, N.J. (1991) Carcinoma of the nasal cavity and paranasal sinuses: an analysis of radical radiotherapy. *Clin. Oncol.* **3**, 84–9.

Mazeron, J.J., Simon, J.M., Le Péchoux, C. *et al.* (1991) Effect of dose rate on local control and complications in definitive irradiation of T_{1-2} squamous cell carcinomas of mobile tongue and floor of mouth with interstitial iridium-192. *Radiother. Oncol.* **21**, 39–47.

Munro, A.J. and Potter, S. (1996) A quantitative approach to the distress caused by symptoms in patients treated with radical radiotherapy. *Br. J. Cancer* **74**, 640–7.

O'Sullivan, B., Mackillop, W.J., Gilbert, R. *et al.* (1994) Controversies in the management of laryngeal cancer: results of an international survey of patterns of care. *Radiother. Oncol.* **31**, 23–32.

Pignon, J.P., Bourhis, J., Domenge, C. and Designe, L. (2000) Chemotherapy added to locoregional treatment for head and neck squamous-cell carcinoma: three meta-analyses of updated individual data.

MACH-NC Collaborative Group. Meta-Analysis of Chemotherapy on Head and Neck Cancer. *Lancet* **335**, 949–55.

Powell, S., Peters, N. and Harmer, C. (1992) Chemodectoma of the head and neck: results of treatment in 84 patients. *Int. J. Radiat. Oncol. Biol. Phys.* **22**, 919–24.

Sharp, H.M., List, M., MacCracken, E., Stenson, K., Stocking, C. and Siegler, M. (1999) Patients' priorities among treatment effects in head and neck cancer: evaluation of a new assessment tool. *Head Neck* **21**, 538–46.

Stadler, P., Becker, A., Feldmann, H.J. *et al.* (1999) Influence of the hypoxic subvolume on the survival of patients with head and neck cancer. *Int. J. Radiat. Oncol. Biol. Phys.* **44**, 749–54.

Teo, P.M.L., Tsao, S.Y., Ho, J.H.C. and Yu, P. (1991) A proposed modification of the Ho stage-classification for nasopharyngeal carcinoma. *Radiother. Oncol.* **21**, 11–23.

UICC (1997) *TNM classification of malignant tumours.* Berlin: Springer Verlag.

Wiernik, G., Alcock, C.J., Bates, T.D. *et al.* (1991) Final report on the second British Institute of Radiology fractionation study: short versus long overall treatment times for radiotherapy of carcinoma of the laryngo-pharynx. *Br. J. Radiol.* **64**, 232–41.

Withers, H.R., Taylor, J.M.G. and Maciejewski, B. (1988) The hazard of accelerated tumor clonogen repopulation during radiotherapy. *Acta Oncol.* **27**, 131–46.

FURTHER READING

Calais, G., Reynaud-Bougnoux, A., Garand, G., Beutter, P. and Le Floch, O. (1990) Oropharynx carcinoma: irradiation alone versus induction chemotherapy plus irradiation – 5 year results. *Br. J. Radiol.* **63**, 340–5.

Davidson, J., Briant, D., Gullane, P., Keane, T. and Rawlinson, E. (1994) The role of surgery following radiotherapy failure for advanced laryngopharyngeal cancer. *Arch. Otolaryngol. Head Neck Surg.* **120**, 269–76.

Dimery, I.W. and Hong, W.K. (1993) Overview of combined modality therapies for head and neck cancer. *J. Natl Cancer Inst.* **85**, 95–111.

England, R.J. and Stafford, N.D. (1998) Conservative neck surgery in squamous cell carcinoma. *Surg. Oncol.* **7**(1–2), 91–4.

Grau, C. and Overgaard, J. (1998) Significance of hemoglobin concentration for treatment outcome. In Molls, M. and Vaupel, P. (eds), *Medical radiology – diagnostic imaging and radiation oncology. Blood perfusion and microenvironment of human tumors. Implications for clinical radiooncology.* Berlin: Springer, 101–12.

Hong, W.K., Lippman, S.M., Itri, L.M. *et al.* (1990) Prevention of second primary tumours with isotretinoin in squamous carcinoma of the head and neck. *N. Engl. J. Med.* **323**, 795–801.

Horiot, J.C., Le Fur, R., N'Guyen, T. *et al.* (1992) Hyperfractionation versus conventional fractionation in oropharyngeal carcinoma: final analysis of a randomized trial of the EORTC cooperative group of radiotherapy. *Radiother. Oncol.* **25**, 231–41.

Kaanders, J.H., Pop, L.A., Marres, H.A. *et al.* (2002) ARCON: experience in 215 patients with advanced head-and-neck cancer. *Int. J. Radiat. Oncol. Biol. Phys.* **52**, 769–78.

Liu, B.Q., Peto, R., Chen, Z.M. *et al.* (1998) Emerging tobacco hazards in China: 1. Retrospective proportional mortality study of one million deaths. *BMJ* **317**, 1411–22.

MacDougall, R.H., Munro, A.J. and Wilson, J.A. (1993) Palliation in head and neck cancer. In Doyle, D.V., Hanks, G.W.C. and Macdonald, N. (eds), *Oxford Textbook of Palliative Medicine.* Oxford: Oxford University Press, 422–33.

Million, R.R. (1992) The larynx … so to speak: everything I wanted to know about laryngeal cancer I learned in the last 32 years. *Int. J. Radiat. Oncol. Biol. Phys.* **23**, 691–704.

O'Sullivan, B. and Mackillop, W.J. (1986) An approach to the interpretation of the literature of head and neck cancer. *Clin. Oncol.* **5**, 411–33.

Parkin, D.M., Pisani, P. and Ferlay, J. (1993) Estimates of the worldwide incidence of eighteen major cancers in 1985. *Int. J. Cancer* **54**, 594–606.

Parkin, M., Whelan, S., Ferlay, J. *et al.* (1997) *Cancer incidence in five continents.* Lyon: IARC Scientific Publications.

Skladowski, K., Law, M.G., Maciejewski, B. and Steel, G.G. (1994) Planned and unplanned gaps in radiotherapy: the importance of gap position and duration. *Radiother. Oncol.* **30**, 109–20.

Stell, P.M. (1992) Adjuvant chemotherapy for head and neck cancer. *Semin. Radiat. Oncol.* **2**, 195–205.

Tannock, I.F. and Cummings, B.J. (1992) Neoadjuvant chemotherapy in head and neck cancer: no way to preserve a larynx. *J. Clin. Oncol.* **10**, 343–4.

Vokes, E.E., Weichselbaum, R.R., Lippman, S.M. and Hong, W.K. (1993) Head and neck cancer. *N. Engl. J. Med.* **328**, 184–94.

18

Salivary glands

HOWARD M. SMEDLEY AND ROBERT HEDDLE

Primary tumours arising in salivary gland tissue are uncommon; secondary tumours are generally only encountered in cases of widespread advanced disease and rarely need specific therapy.

The very scarcity of these tumours makes them hard to study. In all but specialized secondary referral centres, the number of cases encountered by an individual clinician each year will be only a handful. Most recorded series documenting the natural history and outcome for individual tumour types often extend over a 20-year period and may need cautious interpretation. For example, the total number of malignant tumours of salivary gland origin registered in a typical Regional Health Authority in England and Wales would be about 40 patients per year. This represents an incidence of approximately 0.75 patients per 100 000 population. There is no overall difference between male and female. The overall cancer incidence for the same region would be approximately 500 per 100 000 population (Kingsley-Pillers, personal communication 1987). These figures do not include the 'benign' tumours such as pleomorphic adenoma (mixed) tumours, which makes accurate epidemiological data even harder to obtain.

Salivary gland tumours also vary considerably in the site and manner of presentation. Although the majority arise in the major paired anatomically identifiable glands, such the parotid, submandibular and sublingual, salivary gland tissue is encountered widely in the body, but mostly in the head and neck. For this reason, patients may present to a general practitioner, dental surgeon, general surgeon, ophthalmic surgeon, ENT surgeon, oral surgeon or neurologist before a diagnosis is reached. There is a good case to be made for developing pathways of referral at a local level which allows a few individuals the opportunity to develop real expertise in the management of these rare tumours.

The other main feature of salivary gland tumours is the variability in behaviour, even amongst histologically similar groups. These tumours as a whole seem to exist with a spectrum of aggressive behaviour. The conventional concept of benign and malignant as two distinct entities has limited value. In a substantial proportion, the behavioural characteristics of a tumour for parameters such as likelihood of local recurrence and responsiveness to radiation will be poorly predicted by histological criteria. For this reason the treatment should be considered individually for each patient, and all relevant factors, such as age, general medical condition and extent of disease, evaluated before formulating any treatment plan (King and Fletcher, 1971).

ANATOMY

Salivary tissue can be divided into that which is concentrated in the so-called salivary glands – the parotid, submandibular and sublingual glands – and the remainder of the salivary tissue. This is scattered around the oral cavity, lying in the epithelium covering the hard and soft palates, the buccal mucosa and the surfaces of the lips. Pathology may arise in any of these areas but the principal areas for neoplasia are the parotid, submandibular, sublingual and extraglandular sites, in that order.

Parotid gland

The parotid gland is the largest of these glands and lies in the interval between the bones of the mastoid process and the vertical ramus of the mandible. It is wedge-shaped with the broad edge of the wedge lying subcutaneously and the apex of the wedge lying deep between two bony points. The gland is contained in an envelope of parotid fascia which is relatively unyielding. For descriptive purposes it is conveniently divided into a superficial and a deep lobe, these being separated from one another by the VIIth cranial nerve and its branches. Above, the gland extends as far as the zygomatic process and below it encroaches down on to the anterior border of the upper part of the sternomastoid muscle. Anteriorly it encroaches upon the masseter muscle. An accessory portion of the gland lies over the masseter muscle, along the line of the parotid duct which crosses the masseter to pierce the buccinator muscle, entering the mouth opposite the upper second molar tooth. At this point the duct is covered by a small valve. The apex of the wedge of parotid tissue lying deep in the notch between these bones lies close to the external carotid artery and internal jugular vein. Digastric muscle and the styloid apparatus are also close to the apex of the wedge.

The gland is traversed by the facial nerve which emerges from the stylomastoid foramen and is purely a motor nerve. The main trunk of the nerve descends almost vertically and just before entering the parotid gland divides into two major branches which subsequently subdivide within the parotid and then rejoin, producing a plexus or pes anserinus. The branches of the nerve emerge in five main groups from the parotid and spread over the face and neck to supply the muscles of facial expression.

The plane at which this nerve passes through the parotid gland is the plane used to remove the superficial proportion of the gland in a superficial parotidectomy. The gland receives its blood supply from the external carotid artery and the venous return is via small veins to the internal jugular. Parasympathetic secretomotor fibres arise from cell bodies in the otic ganglion travelling along the auriculotemporal nerve. Sensory fibres travel within the great auricular nerve.

Lying within the subcutaneous tissue, superficial to the parotid and within the parotid sheath, are a number of lymph nodes. These drain lymph from the parotid and also from the side of the face. Lymph from these lymph nodes is transmitted to the upper group of the deep cervical glands lying around the internal jugular and, when enlarged, they may be palpated anterior to the upper end of the sternomastoid muscle. The presence of nodes superficial to the parotid sometimes gives rise to diagnostic confusion since these glands may mimic parotid neoplasia.

Submandibular gland

The submandibular salivary gland is about 2.5 cm in diameter and is slightly flattened. It lies inferior to the horizontal ramus of the mandible, partly within the submandibular fossa and partly deep to the mandible, where its contact with the bone produces a concavity. The posterior aspect of the gland is narrower and follows the duct which curves from the gland around the posterior border of the myelohyoid. Part of the submandibular gland thus comes to lie along the submandibular duct and is therefore lying in the floor of the mouth. The duct passes anteriorly, emerging in the floor of the mouth just beneath the tongue, and the papilla is palpable. The submandibular duct at this point is surrounded by sublingual gland tissue and its ducts, and some of these ducts drain with the submandibular duct. The gland is closely related to the facial artery which may actually pass through it. It derives its blood supply from this artery. Lying on the surface of the submandibular salivary gland are some lymph nodes and it is into these submandibular lymph nodes that the submandibular lymph passes and then on to the deep cervical glands lying around the internal jugular vein.

CLASSIFICATION

All systems of classification vary slightly and none is universally acceptable. Table 18.1 contains a useful classification based not only on apparent histogenesis of the tumour but also on likely behaviour patterns. The apparent diversity of these tumours can be explained by the microscopic structure of the salivary gland (Fig. 18.1). This shows the basic structure common to all salivary glands. It can be seen that different types of cell are present. For example, there are two types of acinar cells, one producing mucus and the other producing watery secretions. Similarly, there are many types of epithelial cells lining the ducts of the glands. Particularly significant is the myoepithelial cell which is responsible for contractile mobility along the gland duct. This cell is of

Table 18.1 *A classification of salivary gland tumours (based on the American Forces Institute of Pathology System)*

Benign
  Mixed tumour (pleomorphic adenoma)
  Papillary cystadenoma lymphomatosum (Warthin's)
  Monomorphic adenoma, e.g. oncocytoma,
    myoepithelioma

Malignant
  Low grade: Adenoid cystic carcinoma
             Mucoepidermoid carcinoma
             Acinic cell carcinoma
             Myoepithelial (epidermoid) carcinoma
  High grade: Mucoepidermoid carcinoma
              Adenocarcinoma
              Undifferentiated carcinoma
              Squamous cell carcinoma
              Malignant mixed carcinoma

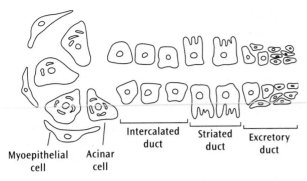

Figure 18.1 *Schematic representation of the basic structure of a salivary gland unit.*

Table 18.2 *Distribution in percentage terms of tumours of salivary gland origin by site*

Site of origin	Distribution (%)
Parotid	75–80 (of which 90% arise in the superficial lobe)
Submandibular	5–10
Sublingual	1–2
Minor glands (all sites)	10–20

ectodermal origin but has capacity for mesenchymal differentiation.

This spectrum of change accounts for the apparent appearance of tissue of both ectodermal and mesodermal origin in the so-called 'mixed' (pleomorphic) adenoma. The other cells present, together with associated lymphatic and connective tissue element, may also undergo malignant change.

AETIOLOGY

In most cases the aetiology of these tumours is unknown. There is an association in patients who have undergone previous radiation therapy which has directly involved salivary gland tissue. A similar weak link exists in patients who have a tendency to multi-centric cutaneous malignancy. This is thought to represent an unstable field change involving tissues of similar embryological origin. Squamous cell carcinomas arise in areas of squamous metaplasia associated with chronic irritation, such as chronic infection or long-standing calculi. Occasionally, some element in a 'mixed' pleomorphic tumour may undergo malignant change.

The distribution of tumours of the salivary gland by site of origin is shown in Table 18.2.

INDIVIDUAL TUMOUR TYPES

Despite their rarity, salivary gland tumours remain a favourite topic for discussion. Below is a list of various tumour types with some relevant features of clinical significance.

Pleomorphic adenoma

This is the commonest salivary gland tumour. Most commonly found in the superficial lobe of the parotid, it usually presents as an asymptomatic mass which has grown slowly over several years. The most common age of presentation is 30–50 years. Diagnosis is usually a clinical one. At surgery, there is frequently a pseudocapsule encompassing the tumour present. Enucleation may therefore appear to be technically easy but will lead to a high rate of local recurrence. This is because of a number of microscopic pseudopodia which will be left behind and will ultimately regrow.

For this reason wide local excision, usually amounting to superficial lobectomy, is preferred as the treatment of choice. If this is not technically possible, e.g. proximity of the facial nerve or poor condition of the patient, then postoperative radiotherapy to the parotid bed should be offered. This appears to be equally efficient at preventing local recurrence. Histologically these tumours show features of epithelial elements, together with mesenchymal features (so-called 'mixed' appearance). Sufficient sections should be examined to ensure no truly malignant focus is present. These tumours present a notoriously varied microscopic appearance.

Papillary cystadenoma lymphomatosum (adenolymphoma)

This is a benign, slow-growing tumour, almost exclusively confined to the parotid gland. It has the most characteristic pattern of all salivary tumours, presenting as a slow-growing mass in the inferior pole of the superficial lobe of the parotid. It is the tumour most likely to be bilateral (5 per cent).

Microscopically it appears to arise from salivary ductal cells trapped in intraparotid lymph nodes. It has a characteristic appearance of cystic spaces lined by two layers of epithelial cells. Complete wide excision is usually adequate treatment.

Oncocytoma (oxyphilic adenoma)

An uncommon tumour, usually arising in the parotid in patients over the age of 50. It is said to be more common in the minor glands of the upper lip. It is a well encapsulated tumour, with a lobulated appearance on cut section; wide local excision is the treatment of choice.

Acinic cell carcinoma

Acinic cell carcinoma is a slow-growing tumour, probably arising from serous fluid-secreting acinar cells. Mainly found in the parotid gland, their behaviour is hard to predict from histological appearances. They seem to have an increased potential for malignant behaviour with increased duration of history: the longer the mass has been present, the greater the risk of true malignant local infiltration and spread to adjacent lymph nodes in the neck and preparotid group. However, it is often very slowly progressive and associated with very good 5-year survival rates, even when suboptimal treatment is given.

Following excision, preferably through lobectomy, consideration is given to radiation. This should be offered if there is any reason to believe that there is a significant risk of local recurrence within the patient's lifetime. Factors to indicate this include incomplete excision, tumour breaching the parotid capsule, microscopically involved lymph nodes, or a high mitotic rate. Alternatively, these tumours usually grow so slowly that no survival disadvantage will accrue by waiting until there is evidence of frank recurrence in an elderly or frail patient.

Adenoid cystic carcinoma

This is the most common tumour of the submandibular glands. It can be fairly slow in onset with a long history, but can be differentiated from other tumours by the association of pain and nerve paralysis with the developing mass.

Microscopically the tumour has a poorly developed capsule and consists of two cell types, namely the duct-lining cells and myoepithelial cells. Histologically and clinically, an important feature of these tumours is a tendency to invade perineural spaces and so grow back directly along a nerve pathway, sometimes spreading directly back into the brain. This knowledge is important when planning surgical and radiation treatment.

Since the progression of the tumour is rather slow, the 5-year survival is good, although the 20-year survival is much worse. This is because of the notorious pattern of repeated local recurrence after apparently complete surgery. Various attempts at radical and supraradical surgery, together with surgery combined with radiation, have therefore been made. The series tend to be fairly small and collected over a number of years. Overall they suggest that radical surgery, even for apparently localized disease, gives a good chance of permanent local control (Stell *et al.*, 1985).

However, similar rates of local control can be achieved by conservative excision combined with radiotherapy. The effect of radiation appears to be dose-dependent, with significantly better control being achieved with tumour doses in excess of 6000 cGy. Other series have shown a significant local control rate achieved by radiotherapy in patients in whom only biopsy was possible (37 per cent). This suggests that radiotherapy is effective in providing useful growth restraint in these tumours, and should therefore be considered in all cases except those undergoing true radical surgery (Cowie and Pointon, 1984).

All series report a significant number of patients developing metastatic disease irrespective of the technique for treating the primary tumour. This is in the range of 35–50 per cent. Spread seems to be largely haematogenous to lungs and liver and only rarely to local lymph nodes. Even when present, metastases appear to grow only slowly. Radiation may have a palliative effect, but chemotherapy seems to have little part to play. The development of metastatic disease suggests that supraradical approaches to the primary disease have no part in routine management.

Mucoepidermoid carcinoma

This tumour arises from the ducts of major salivary glands. Mucin-secreting acinar cells are the major component. They exist as a spectrum of malignancy, ranging from very low-grade to a high-grade tumour with frequent mitoses and a capacity for local invasion and local lymph node metastases. Even at this end of the spectrum, truly aggressive local growth is uncommon. Approximately 65 per cent of mucoepidermoid tumours are histologically low grade. Occasionally it can arise in childhood, but usually presents in the 40–60 year age group.

Patients present with a mass, the duration of which varies from months to years. In 30 per cent pain or nerve paralysis is a feature. This tumour has the capacity for spread and, therefore, basic staging investigations to screen for distant disease seem appropriate before any radical local measure is undertaken. Approaches to treatment vary considerably. Given the varied nature of the disease, and the differences in the patient group affected, this seems inevitable. From published data the following general principles seem reasonable.

The best chance of cure will come from radical surgery used on tumours of limited extent. This will usually be superficial parotidectomy. In cases where the histology seems favourable, nothing further is necessary. In cases where histological features are unfavourable, e.g. vascular invasion, high mitotic rate, etc., further treatment is indicated at the local site. This may also be the case in patients with short clinical histories. The choice is between more radical surgery or radical radiotherapy. Although the best published results come from patients undergoing radical surgery, there may be an element of selection in this. Most clinicians in this country would be prepared to advocate radiotherapy for this group on the grounds that most deaths come from distant metastases and that these will occur whatever modality is used at the primary site. Overall, approximately 80 per cent of patients with high-grade tumours will be dead of disease at 5 years. Improvements in survival from this tumour therefore await the development of effective systemic chemotherapy.

Undifferentiated carcinoma

This is an uncommon salivary gland tumour. It occurs in the older age group, usually with a short history and early

VIIth nerve involvement. Microscopically it has few specific features and is said to resemble the small round cell appearances encountered in sarcomas. Its rarity and lack of identifying features mean that the possibility that this tumour is, in fact, the presenting metastasis from a primary tumour elsewhere, e.g. oat cell carcinoma of lung, must be excluded. The prognosis is poor and local spread rapid. Radical parotid removal may have a place, but it is first necessary to show that the tumour is not inoperable on technical grounds, e.g. medial growth to invade the base of the skull. This is best assessed by computed tomographic scanning. Radiotherapy may be used effectively to achieve palliation and postoperatively following complete excision.

Preoperative radiotherapy seems to be of little benefit.

Squamous cell carcinoma

This is also a very rare tumour and squamous metastases from other sites must be excluded. They are usually well to moderately differentiated tumours which can be associated with chronic infection or long-standing calculi. Diagnosis is made after biopsy. Depending on the extent of surgery undertaken, postoperative radiotherapy should be offered. This tumour shows the same responsiveness to radiotherapy as squamous cell carcinomas in other sites.

Adenocarcinoma

This is another rare tumour, found equally in the major and minor glands. Speed of growth and clinical appearance give some indication of the relative aggression shown by this tumour. Microscopically the tumour consists of single cell types which vary from well to poorly differentiated. It is important to distinguish this type from adenocarcinomatous transformation arising in a pleomorphic adenoma.

Malignant mixed carcinoma

Microscopically this shows histological features of malignancy in an otherwise pleomorphic adenoma. It occurs in 2–5 per cent of all mixed tumours. The malignant change is usually adenocarcinomatous, but can be sarcomatous or undifferentiated. Clinically, it is characterized by a sudden change in the shape and size of a long-standing pleomorphic adenoma. The distribution reflects that of benign mixed tumours. It can be distinguished from the rare event of distant metastases being found in a patient with an apparently benign pleomorphic adenoma. Treatment principles are the same as for other high-grade adenocarcinomas of salivary glands.

SYMPTOMS AND PRESENTATION

Parotid tumours normally present with a lump lying within the substance of the parotid gland. These lumps are commonly slow growing and may be present for some years. Signs of malignancy may supervene and rapid growth of a previously slowly growing parotid swelling is an indication of malignancy. Patients do not commonly complain of any other symptoms and clinical examination of a lump which is benign does not usually reveal any other physical signs. Malignancy should be suspected if there is any evidence of palsy of the facial nerve or its branches. Although facial nerve palsy is very obvious, a palsy of a single branch is more common and difficult to detect clinically.

Parotid malignancy may present with enlargement of the cervical or preauricular lymph node and occasionally the parotid swelling is so small that the patient may not notice it. This is partly due to the fact that malignant tumours of the parotid more commonly arise in the deep lobe and therefore do not bring themselves to attention as readily as the benign tumours lying in the more superficial and subcutaneous parts of the gland. Advanced parotid malignancy may present with skin ulceration or evidence of invasion of adjacent structures.

Tumours arising in the accessory portion of the parotid gland are often not initially recognized as being of parotid origin, since this structure lies anterior to the bulk of the parotid gland. Benign and malignant tumours do arise at this site and malignancy at this site often presents with a lump, together with palsy of the branches of the facial nerve supplying the upper lip. This palsy is not normally noticed unless specifically looked for.

There are few investigations of any value in the assessment of parotid swelling. If malignancy is suspected clinically, the regional cervical and preauricular lymph nodes should also be checked and it is possible that aspiration cytology may be helpful. Sialography has never been shown to be of any true value in the distinction between benign and malignant parotid tumours.

SURGERY

Parotid gland

Surgical exploration of the parotid should not be undertaken until complications of the operation, notably facial palsy, have been fully explained to the patient. Malignancy of the parotid is not commonly suspected until the operation of parotidectomy is under way and the operation plan has to be changed.

Exploration of the parotid involves operating on a patient who has not received neuromuscular blockade. A vertical incision in front of the ear, extending down on to the neck, parallel and below the mandible is used, and this skin flap is then elevated anteriorly at the level of the parotid fascia. The skin flap is lifted off as far as the anterior border of the masseter muscle. The parotid tissue is then displaced forwards and the VIIth cranial nerve sought in the depths of the wound. Many surgeons use a nerve stimulator to facilitate this detection but the location of the main trunk of the nerve does not normally present any great difficulties.

When the nerve has been found, the exact location of the tumour will become clear. Tumours of the superficial lobe are removed by dissecting the superficial part of the parotid off the VIIth cranial nerve branches and this part of the operation requires considerable care. If operative assessment of the parotid shows evidence of malignancy, it is still sometimes possible to remove the tumour plus most of the parotid gland and preserve the VIIth cranial nerve. On occasion, however, it is necessary to remove the whole gland plus the nerve within it, and this means that the main trunk of the facial nerve and its branches as far as the anterior border of the gland have to be divided.

Subsequent reconstruction involves VIIth nerve grafting, commonly involving the use of bridge graft of great auricular nerve (sensory) or a piece of sural nerve from the back of the calf. Such grafting involves delicate microvascular techniques and the results do not, by any means, provide perfect subsequent function of the muscles of the face. It may also be necessary, if the presence of malignant lymph nodes is detected at this operation, to proceed to an en bloc neck dissection and this can be of the radial variety, sacrificing sternomastoid muscle and the accessory nerve, or the functional variety where these structures are preserved.

Complications

Complications of this operation may be immediate or delayed. Immediate complications occur within the first week or two after surgery and may affect subsequent attempts to use radiotherapy in the treatment of the patient should the tumour prove to be malignant. Infection of the wound is rare but can occasionally occur. Haematoma formation under the flap of skin is an uncommon complication, requiring a return to theatre and evacuation of the clot. The apex of the skin flap, below the lobe of the ear, may undergo necrosis if it has been thinned excessively during the operation, and this may take a week or two to heal. A facial nerve palsy may occur and should be expected if the facial nerve has had to be resected during the operation. During the immediate postoperative phase an external parotid fistula occasionally may occur and these normally stop discharging saliva spontaneously within a short time. Local sensory nerves, such as the great auricular nerve and the auricular temporal nerve, may be damaged. These may give rise to sensory loss to the ear and cheek on the side of the operation.

Delayed complications include recurrence of the tumour, whether it was originally benign or malignant.

Recurrence of a benign tumour implies incomplete removal with rupture of the capsule during surgery and local recurrence of a malignant tumour may occur at any time after surgery.

A troublesome condition following parotidectomy is known as Frei's syndrome. This harmless condition is only evident when the patient eats, and involves the presence of gustatory perspiration in the skin in the preauricular area. It is thought to be due to damage to the auriculotemporal nerve. Persistent VIIth cranial nerve palsy may produce ocular damage and these patients may subsequently require a tarsorrhaphy to protect the cornea.

A rare long-term complication is factitious damage to the ear lobe produced by sensory denervation as a result of excision of the great auricular nerve. Patients suffering from this feel an irritation in the lobe of the ear on the side of the parotidectomy and eventually this irritation leads to persistent scratching and the ear lobe may be lost.

Submandibular tumours

Malignant or benign tumours of the submandibular salivary gland are rare and normally present with a lump in the region of the submandibular gland below the horizontal ramus of the mandible. When malignant and advanced, they may also present with the symptoms of palsy of the mandibular branch of the VIIth nerve, and an enlarging malignant tumour in this gland may affect the lingual and hypoglossal nerves. Treatment of tumours of the submandibular gland involves the total excision of the gland and this is performed through a horizontal incision below the ramus of the mandible and parallel to it. Complications include nerve damage, especially to the mandibular branch of the VIIth nerve, and haematoma formation. Delayed complications include infection.

Follow-up

Malignant and benign salivary tumours may recur at any time following an apparently successful treatment. Therefore, follow-up should be long term. Subsequent recurrence may be evident by a lump at the primary site or evidence of regional node enlargement.

RADIOTHERAPY

Parotid gland

Several techniques exist to irradiate the parotid gland. The first decision is the intention of treatment. By and large, palliative treatments are simple and fairly easy to plan. Radical treatments are demanding and require great care if long-term complications are to be avoided.

Palliative therapy is given for advanced, rapidly growing tumours to relieve pain or prevent fungation. It is also used when distant disease is present. A single direct field is usually sufficient. The patient is placed supine on the treatment couch with the neck well extended by a neck roll. A single lateral field is then marked. The boundary is determined by clinical examination. There is no need to take special care to shield the cord of the brain in this situation. Treatment may be given on a cobalt-60 machine using 1 cm wax build-up if there is evidence of skin infiltration. A dose in the order of 45–50 Gy, depending on field size, delivered over 20 daily fractions will provide good tumour control for the duration of the patient's lifetime. Alternatively, electrons are suitable for this technique. An energy of between 10 and 14 MeV is chosen, and the same dose and fractionation followed. There is little place for orthovoltage equipment in this situation.

Radical therapy means treatment is given with intent to cure, and therefore care must be taken to avoid long-term complications. An immobilization shell is essential. The most satisfactory technique employs a pair of anterior and posterior oblique wedged fields. This allows the definition of a volume of high dose which is triangular in cross-section (Fig. 18.2). The conventional dose is 60 Gy in 30 daily fractions over 6 weeks; other prefer 45 Gy in 20 daily fractions. The apex is adjacent to the brainstem and other dose-limiting structures, but can be adjusted to avoid long-term damage.

The other practical problem with this technique is caused by the exit beam from the posterior field. This usually passes through the contralateral eye. The dose to the lens can be reduced by angling this field inferiorly by 10–15° during set-up. It is important to take accurate dose measurement around the orbit during treatment to calculate the anticipated dose to the lens early on in treatment. Most clinicians accept an estimated lens dose of 8 Gy in 30 fractions over 6 weeks, a dose which causes a small increased risk of cataract formation. In some situations it may be impossible to avoid a higher dose. If so, the patient should be warned of the risk of cataract formation. It should be realized, however, that it may be better to treat a patient for cataract 5 years after radiation than to die of an uncontrolled tumour.

A final method of treating these tumours comes from a combination of cobalt photons and 8–12 MeV electrons. This is given as a split course – cobalt-60, 20 Gy in five fractions over 2 weeks followed by 8–12 MeV electrons, 20 Gy in five fractions over 2 weeks. This is particularly suitable for postoperative treatment of mixed pleomorphic adenomas, where a lower dose may be sufficient to control microscopic disease. It has the advantage of delivering a high dose over the whole parotid bed while keeping to a minimum the exit dose to the contralateral parotid gland (Tapley, 1977).

Early in the treatment of parotid glands, patients experience loss of taste and a dry mouth. This may be preceded by altered taste perception. Patients must be warned of this prior to treatment. As treatment progresses a mucositis will be seen; this can be valuable in delineating the treatment volume and to confirm that treatment is being given to the correct volume at the correct rate. Mucosal reaction is managed as for any other site, i.e. simple symptomatic measures initially are combined with scrupulous oral hygiene. Opportunistic fungal infections are common and should be treated by nystatin suspension or amphotericin lozenges. More severe reactions are soothed by topical steroids. Particularly helpful in this respect is aspirin and hydrocortisone mucilage which can be used every 2–3 hours.

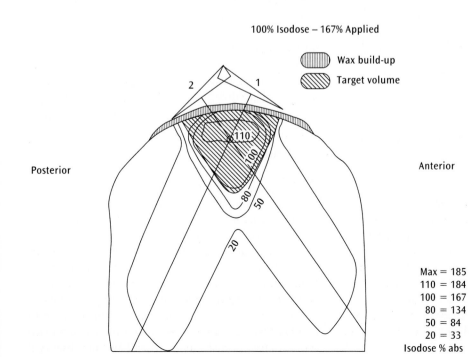

100% Isodose – 167% Applied

Wax build-up
Target volume

Posterior

Anterior

Max =	185
110 =	184
100 =	167
80 =	134
50 =	84
20 =	33
Isodose % abs	

Figure 18.2 *Anterior and posterior oblique wedged pair used to define a volume which is triangular in cross-section to treat a parotid gland tumour.*

Occasionally, painful reactions can interfere with swallowing. Viscous lignocaine gel can be used as a topical anaesthetic to help these symptoms. Taste can remain depressed for a considerable time after radiotherapy. Patients should be warned that 6 months is a common length of time to be affected. Moisture will return to the mouth after 4–8 weeks. At first the saliva tends to be thick and unpleasant. This can be helped by proprietary artificial saliva preparations.

Good oral hygiene is important. The same principles apply as when radiation is administered to other parts of the oral cavity. The ultimate aim is to prevent osteoradionecrosis. There is a chance of this if the gums and teeth present are unhealthy. Consultation with an oral surgeon is advisable. If there is much dental disease, then dental clearance and primary closure of gum flaps may save much trouble in the future. This can be done during the time a shell is being prepared. Even if oral hygiene is good, referral to an oral hygienist in the period following treatment is advisable. Appropriate treatment then, e.g. topical fluoride preparations, may slow down the increased rate of caries formation which follows radiotherapy. Heavily restored teeth are not usually a problem unless they shield the tumour volume from the radiation beam. The scatter they cause may increase the mucosal reaction.

Submandibular glands

Again, treatment must be divided into palliative and radical. Palliative treatment can be simple, using a single direct field to deliver a dose of 40–45 Gy in 15 daily fractions. Radical treatment will depend on the size and extent of tumour and the nature of any surgery. A small tumour volume not approaching the midline may be treated by an anterior and lateral wedged pair of fields. This keeps the high-dose area to a limited volume and may limit morbidity. Larger or more medially extending tumours are best treated by a parallel opposed pair of fields. Wedges may be used to ensure a homogeneous distribution over a changing skin profile. In both cases the prescribed dose is in the range of 50–55 Gy in 25 daily treatments.

Minor glands

Each site will present its own problems. The most common site for minor gland tumours is the hard palate. In this case a pair of parallel opposed wedged fields are used. Occasionally, for limited volume tumours in the elderly, a good result can be achieved by the use of an intra-oral applicator worked at 140 kV. The largest tube which can be used in this way is usually 4 cm in diameter. Large doses (e.g. 4 Gy) can be given up to three times per week in this way and give useful control of the tumour with minimal morbidity.

CHEMOTHERAPY

No chemotherapy regimen has been shown to be curative in these tumours. Reported series are small and reports of response to individual agents are anecdotal. Some salivary gland tumours have been included in series of miscellaneous head and neck tumours treated by combinations of chemotherapy and radiation. Regimens studied in these series include VBM (vincristine, bleomycin and methotrexate) and cyclophosphamide and platinum combinations. In general, these series show better local control rates together with increased disease-free intervals. The acute reactions are also more severe. There is little evidence of overall benefit in survival.

OTHER MODALITIES

Hyperthermia

Hyperthermia uses the principle of raising the temperature of tumour tissue to more than 42°C in order to produce cell death, which seems to be expressed more in tumour tissue than normal tissue. Limitation in technology at present restricts the depth at which tissue can be treated. There is also a physiological restriction in the volume of the body which can be heated to these potentially dangerous temperatures. Current research therefore tends to concentrate on relatively superficial tumours of limited volume. As such, parotid tumours are particularly suited for hyperthermia.

The mechanism of heat-induced cell damage is different from that caused by ionizing radiation. The two modalities can therefore be used with synergistic effect. Clinical trials are still at the experimental stage. However, early work suggests that local control of previously untreated disease may be better when hyperthermia and radiation are combined than by radiation alone. It is too early to know what impact this may have on overall survival. Hyperthermia seems to be of little value in previously heavily irradiated tissue, i.e. in local recurrence.

Neutrons

Fast neutrons are a form of high linear energy transfer (LET) radiation with a similarly high relative biological effect (RBE). On theoretical grounds, it might be possible to expect increased control rates in tumours where large anoxic primaries were a feature and control by conventional radiation was not good. Salivary gland tumours fall into that category. Catterall and Errington (1987) reported a series of 65 patients with salivary gland tumours treated with 7.5 MeV mean energy neutrons produced on the Hammersmith cyclotron. These patients had advanced disease (stages III and IV) and disease at various major and minor sites. A high proportion (93 per cent) achieved complete regression, with overall local control being achieved in 74 per cent. Control rates were better for patients who had not previously undergone surgery or radiotherapy. They also report preservation of facial nerve (VII) function in a greater proportion of patients receiving neutrons than those receiving surgery and conventional radiation.

The authors gave a tumour dose of 15.6 Gy in 12 fractions over a 4-week period. The series reports an acceptably low treatment morbidity. The authors conclude that the slow doubling time of many of these tumours relates to a high proportion of hypoxic cells and explains why neutrons may be superior. Further confirmation of these results is now under way. If neutrons prove to be a superior method of achieving local control, treatment of disseminated disease will become even more important.

PROGNOSIS

The prognosis of salivary gland tumours varies according to the grade and stage of the tumour. Within certain tumour types other independent variables for survival, such as age and sex, have been recorded, but generally histology and extent of disease have overriding importance. Table 18.3 shows an accumulated likely prognosis from several published series.

Table 18.3 *Median age at presentation and approximate 5-year survival rates according to tumour type*

Histological type	Median age at diagnosis (years)	5-year survival (%)
Adenoid cystic	49.5	50
Mucoepidermoid		
Low grade	53.5	80
High grade	53.5	20
Acinic cell	46.5	80
Squamous cell	62.3	20
Undifferentiated	60	20
Adenocarcinoma	57.7	25
Malignant mixed tumour	56.5	40

SIGNIFICANT POINTS

- Nearly all salivary gland tumours are primary; secondary tumours are rare.
- 75 per cent of all salivary gland tumours are pleomorphic adenomas.
- 65 per cent of all parotid tumours are pleomorphic adenomas.
- 80 per cent of pleomorphic adenomas occur in the parotid.
- 80 per cent of sublingual tumours are malignant.
- The palate is the most common site for minor gland involvement.
- 50 per cent of submandibular tumours are malignant.
- The most common tumour of submandibular glands is the adenoid cystic.
- Treatment for these uncommon tumours is best undertaken by joint planning by an oncologist and surgeon.
- Because of the indolent nature of some tumours, long-term follow-up is necessary.

REFERENCES

Catterall, M. and Errington, R.D. (1987) The implications of improved treatment of malignant salivary gland tumours by fast neutron radiotherapy. *Int. J. Radiat. Oncol. Biol. Phys.* **13**, 1313–18.

Cowie, V.J. and Pointon, R.C.S. (1984) Adenoid cystic carcinoma of the salivary gland. *Clin. Radiol.* **35**, 331–3.

King, J.J. and Fletcher, G.H. (1971) Malignant tumours of the major salivary glands. *Radiology* **100**, 381.

Stell, P.M., Cruikshank, A.H., Storey, P.J. *et al.* (1985) Adenoid cystic carcinoma, the results of radical surgery. *Clin. Otolaryngol.* **10**, 205–8.

Tapley, N.D. (1977) The place of irradiation in the treatment of malignant tumours of the salivary gland. *Ear Nose and Throat J.* **56**, 110.

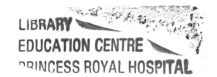

19

Thyroid

LOUIZA VINI AND CLIVE HARMER

INTRODUCTION

The thyroid follicular cell can give rise to a wide variety of neoplasms, ranging from indolent micropapillary carcinoma that has no effect on life expectancy despite minimal treatment, to lethal anaplastic cancer, invariably fatal despite aggressive treatment. Thyroid tumours most frequently develop in young adults; however, all age groups can be affected, including children and the elderly. Although the estimated incidence has increased by 14.6 per cent over the past four decades, the estimated death rate has decreased by 21 per cent. Mortality from thyroid cancer represents less than 1 per cent of all cancer deaths and only 9 per cent of patients with thyroid cancer will die from it. Because of these low rates, morbidity caused by treatment should not exceed that caused by the disease. Management of thyroid cancer demands multidisciplinary care, including consultation with pathologist, surgeon, oncologist, endocrinologist and nuclear physician.

EPIDEMIOLOGY

Thyroid cancer is rare, accounting for only 1 per cent of all malignancies. Incidence rates vary from 12 to 15 per 100 000 women in Iceland and Hawaii to only 1 per 100 000 in the British Isles; these geographical differences are probably caused by environmental or dietary factors rather than by race or heredity (Waterhouse, 1991). The incidence has been increasing, partly reflecting the past use of radiotherapy for benign childhood conditions, but also due to improvements in diagnostic techniques. In England and Wales a significant increase in incidence was seen between 1962 and 1984, especially in North and mid Wales where the highest levels of fallout radiation were documented (Dos Santos Silva and Swerdlow, 1993). Between 1973 and 1987, the estimated incidence increased worldwide by 14.6 per cent, whereas the estimated death rate decreased by 21 per cent (Coleman *et al.*, 1999).

Most cases occur in patients between 25 and 60 years of age, but thyroid cancer can occur in the very young and the elderly. The median age at diagnosis is earlier in females than in males, for both papillary and follicular tumours (Correa and Chen, 1995). For papillary carcinoma, the median age is 40 years for females and 44 years for males, while for follicular cancer median age at diagnosis is 48 years for females and 53 years for males. The incidence of both is higher in women, with a female to male ratio of between 1.5 : 1 and 4 : 1.

AETIOLOGY

Radiation exposure is the only risk factor known definitively to increase the incidence of well-differentiated cancer, although a large study from the Connecticut Tumour Registry showed that only 9 per cent of thyroid cancer could be related to radiation (Ron *et al.*, 1987). By contrast, in several American studies of the 1950s, between 32 per cent and almost 100 per cent of children with thyroid cancer had received prior irradiation for a variety of conditions, including enlarged thymus, tonsils, adenoids or acne. The recognition of the association between irradiation and thyroid cancer led to the elimination of the widespread use of radiotherapy for benign conditions in infants and children by 1960.

Large series of patients who had neck irradiation during childhood show that the latent period is at least 3–5 years, with most cases occurring between 20 and 40 years after exposure; there is no apparent drop-off in the increased risk even after 40 years following radiation exposure (Schneider et al., 1993). The age at exposure is inversely related to the risk. Analysis of the pooled individual data from seven studies showed that the probability of developing thyroid cancer is related to the radiation dose absorbed by the thyroid (Ron et al., 1995); this is strong indication that radiation is a cause of thyroid cancer. A radiation effect is seen at doses as small as 10 cGy. Over most of the dose range the data fit best to an excess relative risk model, although an absolute risk model cannot be excluded. At highest doses, cell killing was thought to overtake tumour formation; with increasing dose the slope (the excess relative risk) of the dose–response curve does not decline, indicating that the relative risk remains significant (Schneider et al., 1993). Data from the acute radiation exposure among the survivors of the atomic bombs in Hiroshima and Nagasaki are similar, showing an increased risk in the younger age population and in females in particular. The estimated dose to thyroid from these acute incidents also showed a proportional relationship to risk (Takeichi et al., 1991).

Improvements in multimodality therapy incorporating radiation for neoplastic conditions in infants, children and young adults, result in many patients cured of tumour who can then be followed up for long-term effects of the therapeutic radiation they received. A dramatically increased relative risk (between 132 and 310) of developing thyroid cancer among individuals who had been treated for neuroblastoma or Wilm's tumour indicates the significance of age at exposure (Tucker et al., 1991). Patients who had treatment for Hodgkin's disease or non-Hodgkin's lymphoma tend to be older and, although the radiation dose to thyroid is high, they more frequently develop hypothyroidism or thyroid nodules than thyroid cancer; the estimated relative risk of developing cancer is 16–80. In the adult population treated with therapeutic radiation the risk drops off. A relative risk of 2.3 was estimated among 150 000 women treated with radiotherapy for cervical cancer (Boice et al., 1988).

A second type of radiation exposure to the thyroid is from radio-isotopes which concentrate in the gland. Large, well-designed studies have shown no increase in thyroid cancer among individuals who had diagnostic nuclide scans or were treated with radioactive iodine for thyrotoxicosis (Holm et al., 1991). However, data regarding exposure to nuclear fallout in the Marshall Islands, Nevada, and

Chernobyl all show a significant increase in thyroid cancer. The importance of age at exposure is evident in recent studies showing a steady sequential increase in paediatric thyroid cancer as early as 3 years and increasing between 5 and 10 years after the later accident (Becker et al., 1996; Stiller, 2001).

Thyroid tumours can be produced in animals by iodine deficiency or drugs. A common factor in these experimental conditions is prolonged stimulation by thyroid-stimulating hormone (TSH). A sequence of reversible hyperplasia followed by irreversible hyperplasia and, in some cases, by the subsequent development of follicular carcinoma has been noted (Schaller and Stevenson, 1966). Evidence of primary TSH-related induction of thyroid tumours in humans is not convincing. However, papillary carcinoma is more frequent in iodine-rich areas, such as islands, while a number of case-controlled studies have strongly suggested that low dietary iodine content is responsible for the increased rates of follicular and anaplastic cancer in areas of endemic goitre (Franceschi et al., 1991). In addition, dietary iodine supplementation has been shown to increase the relative proportion of papillary cancer and to decrease the frequency of follicular cancer.

Because of the strong female predominance, the influence of sex hormone status has been investigated. Factors such as parity, early menopause, contraceptive use and late age of first birth have been associated with an increased risk of thyroid cancer, although these associations are weak and inconsistent. A pooled analysis of case-control studies also confirmed a weak association of menstrual and reproductive factors with thyroid cancer risk (Negri et al., 1999). The biological basis of these epidemiological observations could be that oestrogen acts as a growth promoter on thyrocytes. Some experimental evidence suggests that thyrocytes express oestrogen receptors and oestrogens may stimulate thyrocyte growth in cell-culture systems. It has been also shown recently that tamoxifen inhibits the growth of papillary cancer cells both in vitro and in vivo.

Genetic factors may play a role in a small group of patients with differentiated thyroid tumours. Familial syndromes associated with thyroid tumours of follicular cells include familial polyposis coli, Gardner's syndrome, Turcot's syndrome, Cowden's disease, Carney complex, and multiple endocrine neoplasia type I. Familial occurrence of differentiated thyroid cancer has been recently recognized, although it appears to be rare, occurring in only 2.5–4 per cent of cases (Hawkins et al., 1999).

PATHOGENESIS

Traditionally, thyroid adenoma and carcinoma have been considered as distinct entities. However, there is some evidence to suggest an adenoma to carcinoma multistep pathogenesis. Oncogene activation by a point mutation or translocation, particularly of the RAS oncogene, is common in both papillary and follicular tumours (approximately 40 per cent). Activation of this oncogene is found at all stages from benign through well-differentiated to undifferentiated carcinoma, suggesting that it represents an early event and that this defect is not by itself sufficient for carcinogenesis (Suarez *et al.*, 1988). There is also a spectrum of gradually increasing chromosome abnormalities in all benign and malignant thyroid tumours. Translocations involving chromosome band 19q13 are seen frequently in follicular tumours and are identical to those occurring in benign hyperplastic nodules, indicating that the events associated with translocation could be amongst the earliest steps in carcinogenesis. Recent studies suggest that loss of a tumour suppressor gene on chromosome 3p could be specific for follicular carcinoma and might be a key event in the progression from adenoma to carcinoma. A sequence of events, starting with 19q13 rearrangement in hyperplastic nodules, followed by *RAS* activation in some adenomas and finally tumour suppressor loss on 3p may be involved in the pathogenesis of some follicular cancers.

Histologically, there is no evidence that hyperplastic nodules or follicular adenomas ever undergo change to a malignant papillary tumour. Chromosomes 3 and 19 are rarely abnormal and *RAS* oncogene activation is uncommon. However, structural chromosomal abnormalities mainly involving chromosome 10, in particular 10q, occur in about 50 per cent of papillary carcinomas. Molecular genetic studies have revealed that these changes involve the intrachromosomal inversion of the *RET* proto-oncogene, leading to fusion with the *H4* gene and formation of an oncogene, designated as *RET/PTC1* (Bongarzone *et al.*, 1994). Two other rearrangements involving *RET* result in formation of the *RET/PTC2* and *RET/PTC3* oncogenes. *RET* rearrangements are seen in about 30 per cent of papillary cancers; they have been also documented in 4 out of 7 radiation-induced tumours from patients after the Chernobyl accident, suggesting that radiation exposure may be one mechanism for activation of *RET/PTC* oncogenes.

Whether either papillary or follicular tumours can progress to anaplastic carcinoma remains uncertain. The entity of poorly differentiated follicular carcinoma suggests that such an event may occasionally occur. Tumour progression and dedifferentiation are likely to be associated with further oncogene activation and tumour suppression loss. The tumour suppressor gene *p53* is only infrequently mutated in well-differentiated tumours, but point mutations inactivating the *p53* gene have been observed in almost 50 per cent of poorly differentiated and anaplastic tumours (Suarez *et al.*, 1988).

PATHOLOGY AND NATURAL HISTORY

Thyroid tumours can originate from the follicular epithelium, from parafollicular or C cells, or from non-epithelial stromal elements (LiVolsi and Merino, 1981). The World Health Organization classifies malignant epithelial thyroid tumours as: papillary carcinoma, follicular carcinoma, medullary carcinoma and undifferentiated (anaplastic) carcinoma. The pTNM classification is recommended to assist in management decisions and for uniformity of case-series reporting.

Papillary carcinoma

Papillary carcinoma is the most common type, comprising 80 per cent of all thyroid malignancies. These tumours are almost three times as common in women as in men, with a peak incidence in the third and fourth decades. The histological hallmarks are branching papillae arranged on a fibrovascular stalk. Tumour cells are cuboidal with homogeneous cytoplasm, characteristic hypochromatic nuclei with absent nucleoli (Orphan Annie eyes) and may contain laminated calcified psammoma bodies (Fig. 19.1a). The term 'mixed papillary and follicular carcinoma' is no longer used since the majority of papillary carcinomas do contain some follicular areas. Papillary cancer shows an infiltrating pattern of growth, multifocality (up to 75 per cent of cases) and spread to the regional lymph nodes. Obvious cervical adenopathy is seen in 50 per cent of patients at presentation but has been reported in as many as 90 per cent of those who underwent elective node dissection. Haematogenous metastases are uncommon and mainly involve the lungs; lung involvement at diagnosis is 5–10 per cent in adults but may be up to 25 per cent in children. Certain variants of papillary cancer, such as the tall cell, the columnar and the diffuse sclerosing variant, have been shown to be more aggressive.

Micropapillary or 'occult' carcinoma has the same histological features as papillary cancer but is less than 1 cm diameter (1.5 cm in some series). These tumours are a common incidental finding at autopsy, their incidence being dependent on overall age of the population, the ethnic group studied and the diligence with which the pathologist looks for these foci. Incidence ranges from 0.5 to 14 per cent, with a greater incidence in older age groups. The discrepancy between the incidence of occult and that of clinically detected thyroid cancer argues that these minimal lesions may have a different biology. Although they can metastasize to regional lymph nodes, they rarely cause significant morbidity or mortality (Bramley and Harrison, 1996).

Follicular carcinoma

Follicular carcinoma accounts for 5–20 per cent of thyroid tumours, is also three times more common in females than in males, but tends to present in middle life. It is a tumour of follicular origin but lacks the diagnostic features of papillary cancer. It may be extremely difficult to diagnose when well differentiated, as the appearance is

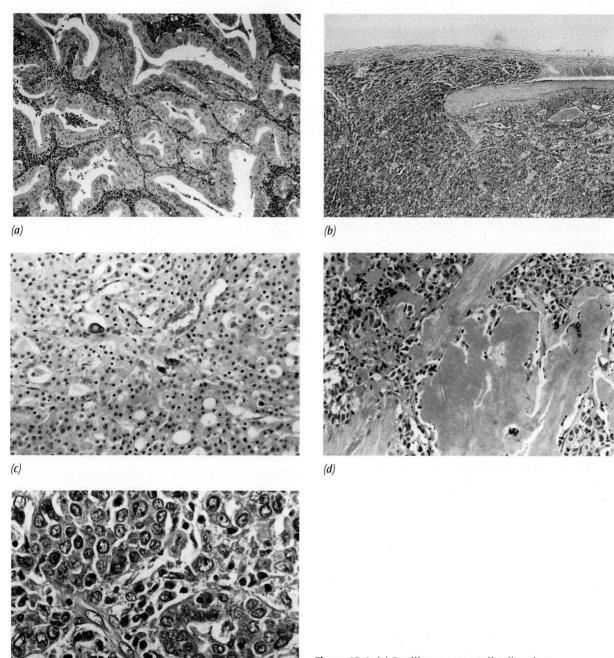

Figure 19.1 *(a) Papillary cancer, tall cell variant; (b) follicular cancer, showing capsular invasion; (c) Hürthle cell carcinoma; (d) medullary carcinoma with amyloid stroma; (e) non-Hodgkin's lymphoma of MALT type.*

similar to both normal thyroid and benign follicular adenoma. Invasion of either capsule or blood vessels is often the only feature to denote malignancy (Fig. 19.1b). It may be either minimally or widely invasive, reflecting good or poor prognosis, respectively. Lymph-node metastases are less frequent than in papillary tumours but haematogenous spread, mainly to bones and lungs, is present in 14 per cent of patients at diagnosis.

Hürthle cell carcinoma was previously considered a variant of follicular cancer and is composed of cells which exhibit oncocytic changes (Fig. 19.1c). However, it is now

recognized as a distinct entity because of its different oncogenic expression and may also be of papillary type. The majority of Hürthle cell tumours are benign, but malignancy is well documented in the form of local recurrence and distant metastases. Histopathological studies have shown that either capsular or vascular invasion is a reliable criterion of malignancy. Although they are usually well differentiated and produce thyroglobulin, these tumours do not take up iodine. This is probably a contributory factor to their less good prognosis than other follicular carcinomas (Vini *et al.*, 1998f). Insular carcinoma is a recently defined tumour of follicular origin which has a nested growth pattern and prominent vascularity. It invades both lymphatics and veins, resulting in nodal and distant metastases with a poor prognosis.

Anaplastic thyroid cancer

Anaplastic thyroid cancer is one of the most aggressive of all malignancies and one of the most lethal. Epidemiological studies indicate that the incidence has decreased to approximately 1–3 per cent of all thyroid tumours (Tan *et al.*, 1995). This decrease has been attributed partially to dietary iodine prophylaxis and an overall decrease in endemic iodine-deficient goitre. It is the predominant type of thyroid cancer in elderly people, with approximately 75 per cent of patients being over 60 years of age; in most series there are equal numbers of males and females. It may be associated with a long history of goitre but there is disagreement as to whether or not anaplastic transformation from differentiated carcinoma is involved in pathogenesis.

These tumours also arise from the follicular cell. However, the natural history, clinical presentation and outcome reflect their undifferentiated biology, with rapid growth and invasive characteristics. Histological variants include small cell, giant cell and spindle cell, although their behaviour does not differ significantly. Patients present with a rapidly enlarging collar of tumour and confluent lymphadenopathy, frequently invading trachea, larynx or oesophagus, resulting in stridor, hoarseness or dysphagia. The majority die within 6 months of the first symptom, from aggressive locoregional disease. At diagnosis 25–50 per cent of patients have pulmonary metastases and at death this figure approaches 100 per cent.

Medullary carcinoma

Medullary carcinoma of the thyroid (MTC) was first described by Hazard in 1959 as a solid neoplasm without follicular histology (Hazard *et al.*, 1959). It accounts for 8–12 per cent of thyroid tumours, the incidence increasing in recent years due to screening (Heshmati *et al.*, 1997). Sporadic or non-familial MTC accounts for 70–80 per cent of cases, with the remainder occurring as a hereditary entity. Hereditary MTC can occur alone (familial medullary thyroid carcinoma, FMTC) or as the thyroid manifestation of multiple endocrine neoplasia type II syndromes MEN IIA and MEN IIB, as shown in Table 19.1. These are autosomal dominant disorders due to germline mutations in the *RET* proto-oncogene, located on the long arm of chromosome 10, band q11.2, which codes for a receptor-like tyrosine kinase (Ponder, 1990).

MTC arises from the parafollicular or 'C' cells which are of neural crest origin and secrete calcitonin as well as other peptides: carcinoembryogenic antigen (CEA), adrenocorticotrophic hormone (ACTH), serotonin, bradykinin,

Table 19.1 *MTC syndromes*

Phenotype	Frequency (%)	Presentation
Sporadic MTC	80	MTC
MEN IIA	9	MTC, phaeochromocytoma, hyperparathyroidism
MEN IIB	3	MTC, phaeochromocytoma, ganglioneuromas, marfanoid habitus
FMTC	1	MTC (in at least 4 patients)
Other FMTC	7	MTC (in 2 or 3 patients)

MTC, medullary carcinoma of the thyroid; MEN, multiple endocrine neoplasia; FMTC, familial medullary thyroid cancer.

prostaglandin and vasoactive intestinal polypeptide (VIP). It is composed of small, round cells within an amyloid stroma, and immunohistochemical staining for calcitonin granules is the most accurate method to establish the diagnosis (Fig. 19.1d). Fewer than 20 per cent of sporadic tumours are bilateral but in the familial syndromes, medullary cancer is usually bilateral and multicentric. At presentation, involvement of cervical or mediastinal lymph nodes is seen in 11–75 per cent, and distant metastases (mainly to lung, bone and liver) in 12 per cent.

Lymphoma of the thyroid

Lymphoma of the thyroid is a rare disease, representing 5 per cent of thyroid malignancies and 2 per cent of extranodal lymphomas. Chronic autoimmune stimulation, as in Hashimoto's thyroiditis, is a predisposing factor. There is a strong female predominance, ranging from 3 : 1 to 8 : 1, while the median age at diagnosis is in the seventh decade, similar to that of anaplastic cancer from which it must be distinguished (Fig. 19.1e). Patients present with a rapidly enlarging painless neck mass, and compressive symptoms are experienced by one-third of patients, although B symptoms of fever, night sweats and weight loss are rare (Oertel and Heffess, 1987).

Almost all thyroid lymphomas are non-Hodgkin's of B-cell origin, intermediate or high grade. Biologically, many thyroid, breast, parotid, lung and gastrointestinal lymphomas are a distinct subset of extranodal lymphomas derived from mucosa-associated lymphoid tissue (MALT). These small-cell lymphomas are characterized by a low grade of malignancy, slow growth rate and a tendency for late relapse or second lymphomas in other MALT sites (Laing *et al.*, 1994).

DIAGNOSTIC EVALUATION

Palpable thyroid nodules are present in 4–7 per cent of all adults; age, gender, history of exposure to ionizing radiation and method by which the nodules are detected all influence significantly the findings of different retrospective studies. In one pathological study, up to 90 per cent of women over 70 years and 60 per cent of men over 80 years had nodular goitre. In most series a 5–15 per cent risk of cancer in all thyroid nodules for the total population is reported (Mazzaferri, 1992). Therefore, it is neither practical nor necessary to remove every nodule in order to exclude malignancy. Investigations should be directed to select those with an increased risk of malignancy. However, no single clinical feature, physical finding or laboratory test is pathognomonic for the detection of thyroid cancer, except for the serum calcitonin level in medullary carcinoma and fine-needle aspiration cytology (FNAC). A diagnostic algorithm is presented in Table 19.2.

Information from the history and physical examination may help in assessing the risk of malignancy. Exposure to ionizing radiation, extremes of age, family history of thyroid cancer or MEN syndromes and other inherited disorders, such as Gardner's syndrome and Cowden's disease, increase the suspicion of cancer. While not specific for malignancy, a history of rapid growth, pain, hoarseness and airway obstruction are of concern. On examination of the neck, attention should be paid to the size, consistency, mobility and number of nodules as well as to the presence of enlarged lymph nodes. The risk of malignancy is greater in a solitary nodule (5–20 per cent) than in multiple nodules; a dominant nodule or a nodule that changes size in a multinodular goitre requires further investigation. Cervical adenopathy is probably the most consistent feature of malignancy in a thyroid mass but lacks specificity.

High-resolution ultrasonography is a useful adjunct to clinical examination for assessment of nodule size,

Table 19.2 *Diagnostic evaluation for thyroid tumours*

Procedure	Finding	Significance
History	Radiotherapy to head and neck	Known aetiology of thyroid cancer
	Family history of MTC	Inherited in an autosomal dominant pattern
	Family or personal history of phaeochromocytoma or hyperparathyroidism	Suggestive of MEN IIA or IIB syndrome
	Diarrhoea, flushing	Common in MTC
	Hashimoto's thyroiditis	Known association with thyroid lymphoma
Physical examination	Solitary thyroid nodule	Higher incidence of cancer in solitary nodule (5–15%)
	Multiple nodules	Lower incidence of cancer; cancer may present in dominant nodule
	Thyroid fixation, hoarseness, Horner's syndrome	May indicate cancer
	Enlarged cervical lymph nodes	More consistent sign of malignancy
Fine-needle aspiration	Malignant, suspicious, benign, insufficient sample	70–97% accuracy
Ultrasonography	Differentiates solid from cystic nodules, assists in fine-needle biopsy	Solid nodules more often malignant
X-ray	Psammomatous calcification	Suggests thyroid nodule is malignant
Radionuclide imaging(^{131}I, ^{99m}Tc)	Cold, warm or hot nodule	15–25% of cold nodules are malignant; lower incidence of cancer in warm and hot nodules
^{131}I mIBG, ^{111}In octreotide	Imaging of medullary thyroid cancer	May detect residual, recurrent or metastatic cancer
CT scan, MRI	Extent of primary tumour, lymph nodes and metastases	Assist in treatment planning
Thyroglobulin	Preoperative elevated value	Does not distinguish between benign and malignant tumour
	Postoperative elevated value	Indicates residual, recurrent or metastatic thyroid cancer
	Normal value	Supportive evidence of lack of disease
Calcitonin	Preoperative elevated value	Indicates C-cell hyperplasia or MTC
	Postoperative elevated value	Indicates residual/recurrent/metastatic MTC
	Postoperative normal value	Indicates lack of disease

MEN, multiple endocrine neoplasia; MTC, medullary carcinoma of the thyroid; MIBG, *meta*-iodobenzylguanidine; CT, computed tomography; MRI, magnetic resonance imaging.

detection of multiple nodules and for assisting in FNAC. Despite advances allowing more sensitive detection of blood flow, differences in echogenicity or vascularity cannot distinguish benign from malignant lesions. Ultrasound can establish whether a lesion is solid or cystic. In a review of 16 series, 21 per cent of the solid lesions, 12 per cent of the mixed and 7 per cent of the cystic lesions were malignant (Shimamoto *et al.*, 1993). Therefore, a solid mass, although most often benign, has the highest chance of being malignant.

The single most important investigation for evaluating thyroid nodules is FNAC. It can often be undertaken in the clinic, without the need for ultrasound guidance. The impact this procedure has had on clinical practice is reflected by a reduction of the number of thyroid operations performed, a greater proportion of malignancies removed at surgery and an overall reduction in the cost of managing patients with nodules (Hamburger, 1994). Accuracy of cytological diagnosis ranges from 70 to 97 per cent, being dependent on the skills of the operator and the cytopathologist. Results typically comprise: benign (70 per cent), malignant (4 per cent), suspicious (9 per cent) and insufficient (17 per cent). The malignant potential of follicular neoplasms cannot be determined cytologically and surgical excision is mandatory. False-negative results are reported in 1–6 per cent and false-positive in 3–6 per cent. FNAC is adequate to diagnose anaplastic cancer but trucut biopsy is required to reliably distinguish the subtypes of primary thyroid lymphoma by immunohistochemistry and ascertain MALT status.

Radionuclide imaging with iodine-131 or sodium pertechnetate (^{99m}Tc) has been employed in evaluating thyroid nodules, although its use is limited and, since the advent of FNAC, it is no longer routine. Malignant thyroid tissue either does not incorporate iodine or incorporates less iodine than normal thyroid, so that a malignant lesion appears as a cold area on the scan (Sisson, 1997). Scanning cannot differentiate benign from malignant nodules and thus is used to assign only a probability of malignancy. A review of 22 studies in which all patients underwent operation regardless of the functional status of the nodule reported that 84 per cent were cold, 10.5 per cent were warm and 5.5 per cent were hot. Malignancy was documented in 16 per cent of cold nodules, 9 per cent of warm and 4 per cent of hot nodules (Ashcraft and van Herle, 1981). These results indicate that cold nodules are more likely to be malignant but warm and hot nodules can also be malignant.

The goals of scintigraphy in patients with established thyroid cancer are to locate metastases or residual neoplasm and to predict efficacy of therapy with ^{131}I. Following thyroidectomy and radio-iodine ablation of normal residual thyroid tissue, diagnostic whole-body ^{131}I scanning is highly sensitive; foci of uptake correspond to thyroid cancer metastases. While it is clear that higher scanning doses improve visualization of disease, even low doses of 75–111 MBq were found to diminish

uptake of the subsequent therapeutic ^{131}I. Proposals to avoid this tumour stunning by the scanning dose include use of smaller diagnostic doses or use of ^{123}I.

Less well-differentiated tumours and some that are well differentiated (especially in older patients) may concentrate so little ^{131}I that the diagnostic scan will prove false negative and the therapeutic dose will not treat effectively. Locating these tumours may be helpful in planning alternative treatment, such as surgical resection. Thallium-201 chloride accumulates in highly cellular, well-perfused lesions and has been found to concentrate in more than half of thyroid tumours not visualized by ^{131}I although an appreciable number of well-differentiated neoplasms concentrate iodine but not thallium (Ramana *et al.*, 1991). Fluorodeoxyglucose positron emission tomography (^{18}FDG PET) may also be useful in suspected recurrent well-differentiated tumour, but is of greater value for poorly differentiated carcinoma and MTC. ^{111}In octreotide and ^{131}I *meta*-iodobenzylguanidine (mIBG) are concentrated in 25–60 per cent of MTC and may be helpful in locating sites of disease, particularly in patients with an elevated calcitonin but no clinical or radiological evidence of tumour (Krenning *et al.*, 1993). Pentavalent dimercapto succinic acid (V-DMSA) whole-body scintigraphy is the best method for locating occult MTC, but has no therapeutic potential.

Computed tomography (CT) can define the morphology of the thyroid gland, tumour extension to structures such as trachea or vessels, and nodal involvement in the neck and mediastinum. Imaging of the chest may reveal micronodular disease in the lungs not shown on chest X-ray. In addition, CT is particularly valuable in radiotherapy treatment planning and in assessing the effectiveness of therapy. Magnetic resonance imaging (MRI) is preferred in order to avoid use of iodinated contrast medium which remains in the body for a considerable time, reducing uptake of subsequent radioiodine therapy. MRI is useful in depicting lesion margins, invasion of adjacent structures and cervical lymphadenopathy. The presence of a cystic node or a nodal diameter of ⩾15 mm suggests metastasis; using these two criteria, a specificity of 100 per cent with an 82 per cent accuracy but a sensitivity of only 60 per cent has been estimated (Takashima *et al.*, 1998). MR spectroscopy has yet to be evaluated.

MANAGEMENT OF DIFFERENTIATED THYROID CANCER

Differentiated thyroid cancer is one of the most controversial malignancies as regards treatment. Debate involves almost every stage of management decision: extent of initial surgery, need for lymph-node dissection, role of radioactive iodine ablation, value of dosimetry in radioiodine therapy and the role of adjuvant external-beam radiotherapy. The major reasons for these ongoing controversies are that thyroid cancer is rare and that its behaviour is indolent (although there are groups of tumours which behave more aggressively). Due to lack of prospective studies and well-structured guidelines, the potential for relapse may be either underestimated, resulting in patients receiving inadequate treatment, or, due to referral bias, it may be overstated and patients are overtreated. Evidence-based guidelines for the management of thyroid cancer in adults were published in 2002 by the British Thyroid Association in conjunction with the Royal College of Physicians of London.

Certain factors have been linked to the behaviour of well-differentiated carcinoma and are used to determine prognosis. Groups such as the Mayo Clinic, the Lahey Clinic and the European Thyroid Association have published data on factors identified through retrospective analyses which correlate with survival. Since all factors are closely interrelated, only multivariate analysis can identify their individual prognostic significance. In most studies age is found to be the most important predictor of outcome; a significant increase in mortality is seen over the age of 40 (Fig. 19.2). Males tend to fare worse compared with females, but gender is of much less prognostic importance. Tumour size, extent and grade are also related to the risks of recurrence and survival (Fig. 19.3). Patients with papillary cancer fare better than those with follicular well-differentiated carcinoma; less well-differentiated follicular tumours show a significantly higher relapse rate and

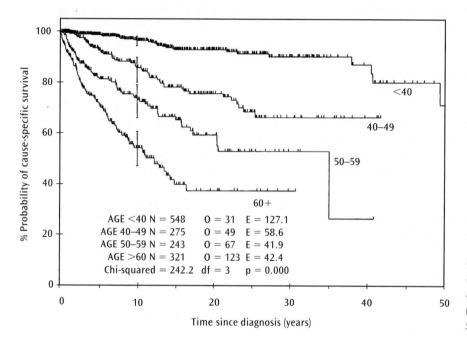

Figure 19.2 *Differentiated thyroid cancer: Royal Marsden Hospital experience 1929–99 (1390 patients). Cause-specific survival according to age.*

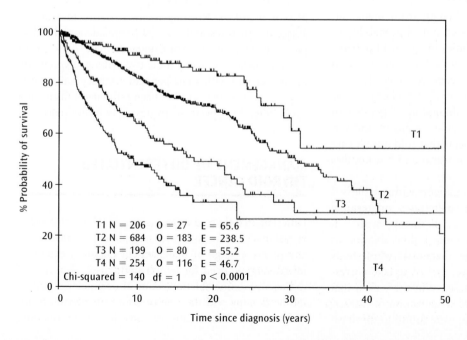

Figure 19.3 *Differentiated thyroid cancer: Royal Marsden Hospital experience 1929–99 (1390 patients). Survival according to tumour stage.*

shorter survival. The impact of nodal status is controversial. In some series, it is found to be associated with an increased risk of locoregional recurrence, although the effect on survival is less clear. The results of multivariate analysis for 1390 patients with differentiated thyroid cancer treated at the Royal Marsden Hospital between 1929 and 1999 are shown in Table 19.3 (Vini *et al.*, 1999).

Based on these prognostic factors, several scoring systems have been developed to help in assessing individual patient risk of dying from cancer and planning treatment (AGES, AMES, GAMES, MACIS). None of these systems is perfect, but all succeed in identifying at least high- and low-risk patients (Candy and Rossi, 1988; Loree, 1995). The low-risk group includes young patients with small ($\leqslant$1 cm) well-differentiated tumours confined to the gland and no evidence of nodal or distant spread. Prognosis in this group is excellent, with cancer-specific mortality of less

than 1 per cent at 30 years (Hay *et al.*, 1992). The recurrence and survival rates are strikingly different in the high-risk group, which includes older patients with locally advanced or metastatic disease at presentation or less well-differentiated tumours. Risk group analysis makes a selective approach to treatment possible and can spare many patients the morbidity of unnecessarily aggressive treatment, without compromising outcome.

Surgical treatment

Surgery remains the initial and potentially curative treatment for differentiated thyroid cancer. However, there is no universal agreement as to the extent of the surgical procedure, partly because many still regard thyroid cancer as a non-fatal disease. There have been no prospective

Table 19.3 *Prognostic factors for survival, local recurrence and distant recurrence for 1390 patients with differentiated thyroid cancer treated at RMH between 1929 and 1999 (Cox proportional hazards regression model for multivariate analysis)*

Factor	HR (95% CI) Survival	Local recurrence	Distant recurrence
Age (years)			
<40	1.0	1.0	1.0
40–49	2.5 (2.3–2.7)	1.4 (1.3–1.6)	1.8 (1.6–2.1)
50–59	6.2 (5.6–6.8)	2.1 (1.9–2.3)	3.3 (2.9–3.7)
$\geqslant$60	15.3 (13.9–16.8)	2.9 (2.7–3.2)	6.0 (5.3–6.8)
	$P < 0.001$	$P < 0.001$	$P < 0.001$
T stage			
T1	1.0	1.0	1.0
T2	1.9 (1.7–2.1)	1.7 (1.5–1.9)	1.8 (1.6–2.1)
T3	3.5 (3.1–3.9)	2.8 (2.5–3.2)	3.4 (2.9–3.9)
T4	6.5 (5.8–7.2)	4.8 (4.2–5.4)	6.2 (5.4–7.2)
	$P < 0.001$	$P < 0.001$	$P < 0.001$
M stage			
M0	1.0	1.0	1.0
M1	6.9 (5.4–8.7)	0.92 (0.51–1.6)	3.9 (2.6–6.0)
	$P < 0.001$	NS	$P < 0.001$
Surgery			
NT/TT	1.0	1.0	1.0
ST/HT/L	1.89 (1.49–2.4)	1.8 (1.38–2.36)	1.87 (1.3–2.5)
B/E	4.66 (3.56–6.1)	3.48 (2.49–4.85)	3.72 (2.5–5.5)
	$P < 0.001$	$P < 0.001$	$P < 0.001$
Iodine ablation			
No	1.0	1.0	1.0
Yes	0.67 (0.55–0.82)	0.39 (0.31–0.50)	0.4 (0.3–0.58)
	$P < 0.001$	$P < 0.001$	$P < 0.001$
Grade			
I	1.0	1.0	1.0
II	2.6 (2.3–2.9)	2.0 (1.7–2.3)	2.6 (2.1–3.1)
III	6.6 (5.9–7.5)	3.8 (3.3–4.5)	6.7 (5.6–8.0)
	$P < 0.001$	$P < 0.001$	$P < 0.001$

RMH, Royal Marsden Hospital; NS, not significant; NT, near total thyroidectomy; TT, total thyroidectomy; ST, sub-total thyroidectomy; HT, hemi-thyroidectomy; L, lobectomy; B, biopsy; E, enucleation.

randomized trials and in retrospective analyses there is always patient selection bias as well as the confounding effect of non-surgical adjuvant therapy. The minimum requirement is complete excision of all macroscopic disease, which usually includes ipsilateral lobectomy and isthmusectomy, avoiding damage to the parathyroid glands and recurrent laryngeal nerves.

A more radical initial approach is advocated by many surgeons in view of the high incidence of bilateral multi-focality (as high as 87 per cent), especially in papillary carcinoma. Most studies have showed a significant reduction in local recurrence rates following total or near-total thyroidectomy, with some also reporting improved overall survival (Hay et al., 1987; Mazzaferri and Jhiang, 1994). Even in the low-risk patients with tumours smaller than 1.5 cm diameter, the locoregional recurrence rate after lobectomy significantly exceeded that seen after total thyroidectomy: 20 per cent and 5 per cent, respectively, at 20 years, although overall survival was similar (Hay et al., 1992). Survival was improved with bilateral resection in patients with unfavourable prognostic factors (Hay et al., 1987). This is also true for locally advanced tumours invading the aerodigestive tract: following complete resection the 5-year survival is greater than 50 per cent but, without such intervention, 80 per cent of these patients are dead at 5 years (Ballantyne, 1994).

Other major advantages in favour of total thyroidectomy are that postoperative follow-up using serum thyroglobulin (Tg) and radio-iodine diagnostic scanning are facilitated, as well as subsequent ^{131}I therapy if this becomes necessary. Both serum Tg monitoring and iodine scanning may be difficult to interpret in the presence of a thyroid remnant of significant size. Remnant ablation in this situation is associated with a low success rate, of the order of only 30 per cent, with higher administered activities or repeat doses required to achieve complete ablation. The main argument against radical surgery, that is morbidity, is less important now that experienced surgeons are reporting reduced complication rates. Vocal cord paralysis occurs in only 1–3 per cent and permanent hypocalcaemia in 1–6 per cent in most specialist centres following total or near total thyroidectomy.

The role of elective level VI tracheo-oesophageal groove clearance of nodes down to the level of the thymus awaits clarification. Those in favour argue that this is the most common site of lymph-node metastases, that the potential morbidity associated with reoperating at a later date is much greater, and that there is an increased risk of subsequently finding inoperable disease. However, this procedure does carry a slightly increased risk of hypoparathyroidism and recurrent laryngeal nerve damage. Our policy is to perform an elective tracheo-oesophageal groove clearance on the ipsilateral side only, proceeding to therapeutic dissection if paratracheal disease is demonstrated clinically, radiologically or during the operation. If extensive superior mediastinal disease is detected, we favour a combined thoracocervical approach, using a sternal split to extend dissection down to the arch of the aorta (Ladas et al., 1999).

The surgical management of lymph-node metastases is also controversial. The presence of metastatic disease in nodes, especially in the lower-risk young patients, is not generally seen as an adverse prognostic factor (Mazzaferri and Jhiang, 1994). It does correlate with increased locoregional recurrence in most series, although the effect on survival is not clear. However, the largest single institution series of papillary carcinoma (2192 cases) confirmed a significant effect of clinical nodal status on survival (Noguchi et al., 1994). Papillary carcinoma can be found in the regional lymph nodes of 35–75 per cent of patients when dissections are performed and carefully examined. However, recurrence is not seen in 75 per cent of patients with clinically uninvolved nodes not undergoing routine neck dissection. This argues against the need for elective lateral deep cervical node dissection of the clinically uninvolved neck. If clinically apparent nodal disease is present, many surgeons recommend a modified neck dissection, preserving the sternomastoid, spinal accessory nerve and internal jugular vein (Shaha, 1998). However, some still perform simple node excision, previously known as 'berry picking'; although regional recurrence rates are high, a survival disadvantage has not been proven. If nodes are clinically involved, we favour a selective node dissection (levels II, III, IV and VI) since thyroid cancer rarely spreads to submandibular or posterior cervical lymph nodes (levels I and V).

Endocrine treatment

Thyroid stimulating hormone (TSH) is the main regulator of thyroid function, differentiation and proliferation. Binding of TSH to its receptor on thyroid cells primarily activates a cAMP cascade, leading to thyroid hormone synthesis and release, as well as expression of thyroid-specific genes including those encoding thyroglobulin and thyroperoxidase. Differentiated thyroid carcinomas retain some degree of thyroid-specific gene expression and function similar to normal thyroid cells; therefore they are responsive to stimulation by TSH. In thyroid cancer cell lines, TSH has been shown to stimulate vascular endothelial growth factor secretion and angiogenesis. Thus TSH may promote growth in some thyroid cancers (Soh et al., 1996).

The beneficial effect of TSH suppression has not been tested in prospective studies. However, available data suggest that thyroxine reduces the risk of recurrence, tumour progression and death from thyroid cancer (Mazzaferri, 1987). The degree of TSH suppression is controversial. Treatment with thyroxine in doses sufficient to lower the serum TSH to an undetectable level may cause subclinical thyrotoxicosis, while there is no evidence that undetectable

TSH levels offer any advantage over low but detectable levels. Monitoring the free thyroxine (T_4) level in the athyroid patient receiving exogenous thyroxine will give a false high value because of binding and can be confusing. We therefore favour total TSH suppression with monitoring of the free tri-iodothyronine (T_3) level, in order to avoid hyperthyroidism. Concern regarding permanently low TSH levels on bone metabolism has been resolved by a number of studies that have failed to show a detrimental effect on bone density, despite accelerated bone turnover (Giannini *et al.*, 1994).

Radioactive iodine ablation of residual thyroid tissue

The value of postoperative ^{131}I to ablate residual normal thyroid is still debated. Arguments in favour of remnant ablation are that it permits the subsequent identification by a whole-body scan of any residual or metastatic carcinoma and increases the sensitivity of Tg measurement for follow-up (Schlumberger *et al.*, 1981). Most importantly, several retrospective studies have documented that it decreases tumour recurrence and death (Mazzaferri and Jhiang, 1994; Vini and Harmer, 2000) (Fig. 19.4). However, the beneficial effect of ^{131}I ablation can be seen mainly in patients who are at high risk of recurrence, such as those with larger tumours, extrathyroid extension and involved lymph nodes, as well as those with residual disease (Taylor *et al.*, 1998). In low-risk patient groups, and especially in those with microcarcinoma (tumours up to 1.5 cm), prognosis is so favourable after surgery alone that little further improvement is possible with iodine ablation (Hay *et al.*, 1992).

The optimal activity of ^{131}I required to achieve successful ablation is controversial. In the literature, variable doses ranging from 0.85 to 9.5 GBq have been reported. Higher initial iodine doses were thought to be more effective in achieving complete ablation with a single administration. The philosophy of a large dose ablation was based on the possibility that it not only ablates remnants but also possible micrometastatic deposits (Beirwaltes *et al.*, 1984). The same authors also stressed the importance of delivering maximal radiation dose from the first iodine administration; due to mechanisms which are at present poorly understood, the biological half-life of subsequent administrations falls, therefore reducing the radiation dose delivered.

In 1976, McCowan *et al.* were the first to report that iodine doses of 3–3.7 GBq were no more effective than 1.1 GBq, findings which were confirmed by several retrospective analyses (Vermiglio *et al.*, 1999). The long-term tumour recurrence rate was 7 per cent following a low dose of 1.1–1.85 GBq, compared with 9 per cent following a high dose of 1.9–7.4 GBq (Mazzaferri, 1999). The advantages of administering the smallest effective dose of ^{131}I are patient convenience and lower cost, as well as a reduced risk of treatment-related complications from lower whole-body radiation exposure.

The only prospective randomized clinical trial to evaluate the optimal ^{131}I ablation dose (involving 149 patients) showed that increasing the administered activity beyond 1.85 GBq resulted in plateauing of the dose–response curve; a radiation absorbed dose to the thyroid remnant greater than 300 Gy did not result in a higher ablation rate (Bal *et al.*, 1996). Successful ablation, defined as absence of any detectable radio-iodine-concentrating tissue in a diagnostic 185 MBq ^{131}I scan with neck uptake of less than 0.2 per cent and Tg of less than 10 ng/mL, was achieved in 77 per cent of thyroid remnants with the lower dose of 1.85 GBq. Maxon *et al.* (1992) used dosimetry to individualize administered activity so as to

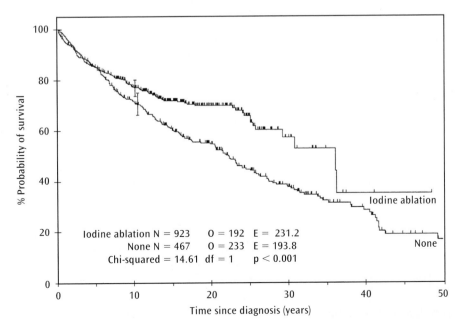

Figure 19.4 *Differentiated thyroid cancer: Royal Marsden Hospital experience 1929–99 (1390 patients). Survival in relation to radio-iodine ablation.*

deliver a radiation dose of 300 Gy to the thyroid remnants. They reported an 81 per cent ablation rate, with no apparent gain from using a dose greater than 300 Gy.

Four weeks after total thyroidectomy, by which time the level of TSH should be >33 mU/L (Harmer and McCready, 1996), we recommend an ablation dose of 3 GBq ^{131}I to all patients with differentiated thyroid cancer, except young women with tumours up to 1.5 cm in diameter, children over the age of 10 with small node negative tumours and patients in whom carcinoma is an incidental microscopic histological finding (Fig. 19.5). This dose ablates 75 per cent of remnants and delivers a mean radiation dose of 410 Gy (O'Connell *et al.*, 1993). Scans of the neck and whole body are obtained on the third day, when

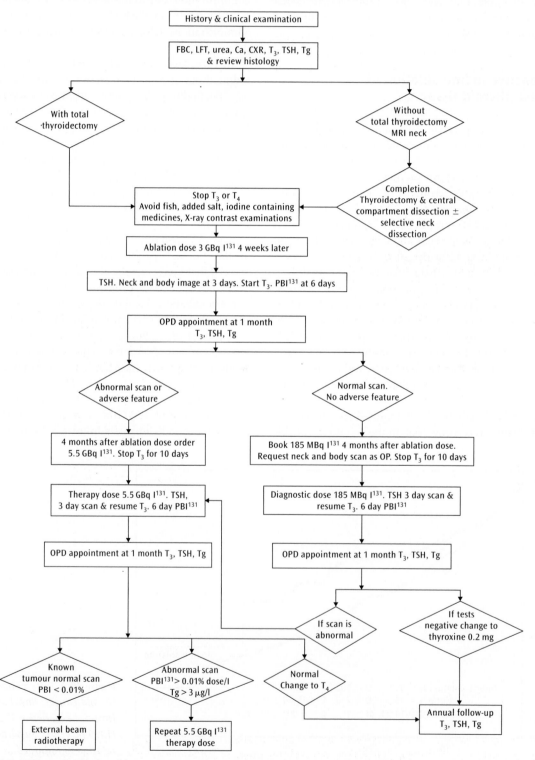

Figure 19.5 *Differentiated thyroid cancer: management protocol.*

the patient is usually discharged from the ward, subject to the total body radioactivity having fallen below the permitted level. Replacement thyroid hormone is then commenced in the form of tri-iodothyronine, 20 µg three times a day. Blood is also taken on day 6 to measure the protein-bound ^{131}I level (PBI). Four months later the neck and body scans are repeated following administration of 185 MBq [131]I. If scanning is negative and provided there are no adverse features, no further treatment is required (Fig. 19.6). The patient is switched to lifelong thyroxine at an average daily dose of 200 µg in order to suppress TSH to an undetectable level. Should the diagnostic scan reveal abnormal uptake in the neck or at any distant site, repeat therapeutic doses of radio-iodine are indicated until uptake disappears and the Tg level becomes negligible.

To optimize iodine uptake by both residual normal thyroid and cancer, TSH stimulation is necessary and therefore patients should be hypothyroid at the time of ^{131}I administration. Proper preparation is achieved by a low-iodine diet, avoidance of iodine-rich contrast media and discontinuation of tri-iodothyronine for 10 days. Clinical trials of recombinant human TSH (rh-TSH) as an alternative to thyroid hormone withdrawal and hypothyroidism are promising (Robbins *et al.*, 2001); rh-TSH is now available but has not been validated for ^{131}I therapy doses.

FOLLOW-UP

Annual follow-up, comprising clinical examination and estimation of free T_3, TSH and Tg, is essential to ensure normal thyroid function with TSH suppression and to detect recurrent tumour. Early discovery of recurrence is of paramount prognostic significance both for cure and survival (Schlumberger *et al.*, 1996a). Local or regional

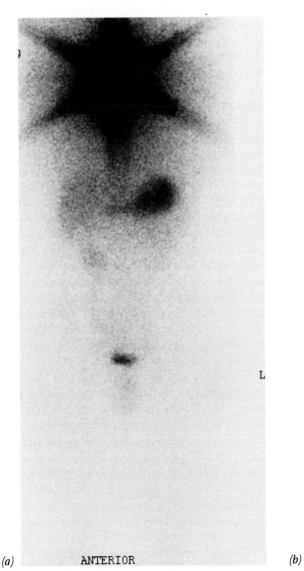

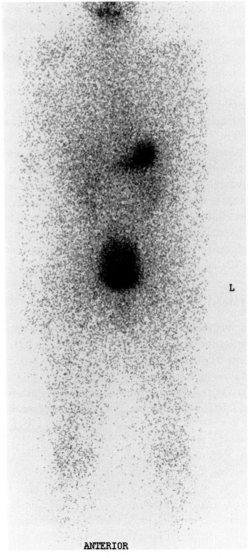

(a) ANTERIOR   *(b)* ANTERIOR

Figure 19.6 *(a) Whole-body scan following an ablation dose of 3 GBq ^{131}I, showing intense uptake in the thyroid bed. (b) Diagnostic whole-body ^{131}I scan (370 MBq) 4 months after ablation, confirming disappearance of iodine uptake (complete ablation).*

relapse develops in 5–20 per cent of patients with differentiated thyroid cancer. Most relapses occur during the early years of follow-up but may be detected even after 40 years; follow-up should therefore be lifelong. The risk of locoregional failure relates partly to tumour aggressiveness, being higher with certain histological subtypes (tall cell, columnar cell and diffuse sclerosing papillary variants), poorly differentiated carcinomas, large tumours and lymph-node involvement at presentation. The risk of recurrence is also closely related to the extent of initial treatment, with limited thyroidectomy resulting in higher recurrence rate than complete thyroidectomy (Mazzaferri, 1987).

Recurrence in the thyroid bed or cervical lymph nodes may be discovered by palpation. Ultrasonography or MRI are useful to delineate disease extent. Serum Tg is usually elevated although it may be undetectable in 20 per cent of patients on thyroxine who have isolated lymph-node metastasis (Schlumberger and Baudin, 1998). Whole-body scanning following administration of ^{131}I, especially high activities, will reveal uptake in 60–80 per cent of patients with lymph-node disease.

Surgery is the treatment for locoregional recurrence, and complete resection should be attempted in all patients who are fit. Even if disease cannot be removed completely, surgical debulking is beneficial and facilitates the subsequent use of radio-iodine. If surgical removal would result in unacceptable morbidity or has to be incomplete, both radio-iodine treatment and external-beam radiotherapy should be used to control local disease (Tubiana et al., 1985; O'Connell et al., 1994). Outcome of patients with locoregional recurrence is closely related to its site, initial prognostic factors and response to treatment. Mortality after local recurrence has been high in most series; a 10-year survival rate of only 60 per cent has been reported (Mazzaferri, 1999).

TREATMENT OF METASTATIC DISEASE

Distant metastases develop in 5–23 per cent of patients with differentiated thyroid carcinoma, mainly in lung and bone, less frequently in liver and brain. In any individual patient the long-term result of treatment is unpredictable; an interplay between patient and tumour characteristics seems to determine outcome. Both univariate and multivariate analyses have highlighted the adverse prognostic effect of older age at the time of discovery of metastases on survival (Schlumberger et al., 1996a). Treatment comprises repeated doses of radio-iodine. Activities ranging from 3.7 to 10.1 GBq at 3–9-month intervals have been employed; many centres use a dose of 5.5 GBq at 6-monthly intervals (Fig. 19.7). There is no maximum limit to the cumulative ^{131}I dose that can be given to patients with persistent disease, provided that individual doses do not exceed 2 Sv total body exposure, progressive improvement can be documented and each pretreatment blood count confirms absence of bone marrow damage.

A whole-body scan 3 days after iodine administration (by which time the blood background will be negligible) provides scintigraphic assessment of disease, and serial scanning will document response to treatment. Diagnostic scanning using a tracer dose of iodine is not necessary prior to therapy and may have an adverse effect since tumour stunning by the diagnostic dose may reduce uptake of therapeutic [131]I (Park et al., 1994). The value of ^{123}I as a scanning agent to prevent stunning has been confirmed (Siddiqi et al., 2001). In addition, a significant proportion of patients with residual tumour, as evidenced by an elevated Tg, demonstrate a negative diagnostic scan but uptake can be documented in the post-therapy scan (Pineda et al., 1995; Fatourechi et al., 2000).

The real benefit of iodine treatment has been questioned; however, at least one large study clearly demonstrated its independent prognostic benefit on survival. Younger patients with limited-volume disease, mainly in the lungs, who achieve a complete response to radio-iodine treatment, have been shown consistently to have the best prognosis, with a 15-year survival of 89 per cent (Schlumberger et al., 1996a). In contrast, older patients and those with large metastases or bone involvement are less likely to respond. Although distant metastases, particularly in the lung, may remain stable for years, there is evidence that early treatment may affect outcome. Microscopic foci are more radiosensitive; a complete response was reported in 82 per cent of patients with uptake in lung metastases not seen on chest radiography but in only 15 per cent of those with visible micro- or macronodules (Maxon et al., 1997). The radioresistance of large deposits may be due to poor vascularity, resulting in limited and inhomogeneous iodine distribution, or to the appearance of radioresistant clones. Bone lesions demonstrate a low response rate to radio-iodine; surgical excision, when possible, or external-beam radiotherapy, should be added (Niederle et al., 1986; Marcocci et al., 1989). Surgical resection with curative intent for patients with a solitary deposit not concentrating iodine and those with bulky disease resistant to iodine has achieved a 5-year post-metastasectomy survival of 46 per cent (Vini et al., 1998e).

Sometimes metastases persist despite administration of substantial ^{131}I therapy doses. This may be the consequence of rapid turnover of radio-iodine in the tumour (short effective half-life) with discharge before adequate energy has been deposited. The effective half-life in metastases responding to therapy has been shown to be more than twice as long as in those not responding: 5.5 days compared with 2.5 days (Maxon et al., 1983). Lithium carbonate slows the release of radio-iodine from normal thyroid as well as from thyroid tumours, and has been shown to prolong the biological half-life in 10 of 12 thyroid tumours without increasing the amount of radiation received by the whole body (Koong et al., 1999). Lithium therefore may be helpful in maximizing the radiation effect in cases with rapid discharge of iodine from tumour. However, blood levels need to be monitored closely to

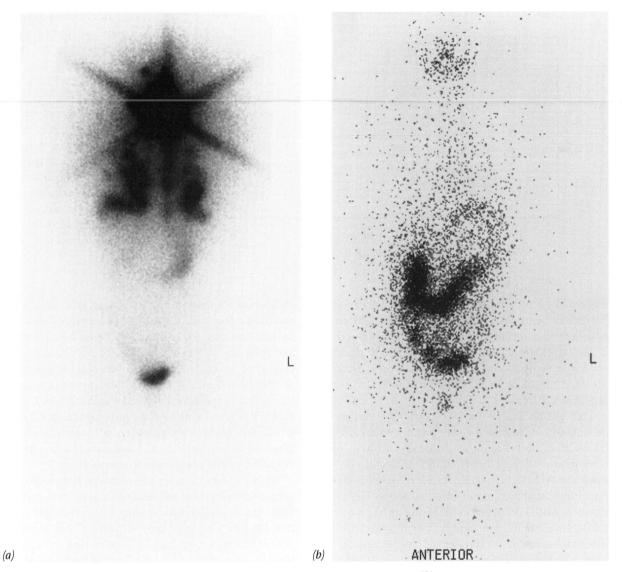

(a)   *(b)*   **ANTERIOR**

Figure 19.7 *(a) Whole-body gamma camera scan following administration of 5.5 GBq ^{131}I, showing intense uptake in thyroid bed, neck, mediastinum and both lung fields. (b) Diagnostic scan following administration of a cumulative activity of 14 GBq ^{131}I, showing complete response.*

avoid toxicity, and psychiatric expertise must be available; because of this its routine use is not a practical option.

DOSIMETRY OF ^{131}I THERAPY

Historically, use of radio-iodine has been empirical. Fixed activities of 1–3.7 GBq for remnant ablation and 3.7–7.5 GBq for therapy are still administered, based on experience and likely side-effects. However, measurement of the absorbed dose has several advantages. The first is that patients are not overtreated and their overall radiation exposure is kept as low as possible. Secondly, it is the only way to determine whether further ^{131}I therapy will be effective, so that alternative treatment can be considered in unsuccessful cases. But the most important reason for basing iodine therapy on lesion dosimetry is that optimizing the administered dose gives the highest

probability that the lesion will be eradicated. Because current information suggests that a stunning effect occurs with incomplete or inadequate therapy and may be permanent, the most effective strategy is to attempt to eradicate a tumour with either a single ^{131}I administration or as few treatments as possible.

Over the past decade attempts have been made to calculate the radiation absorbed dose by thyroid remnants and metastatic deposits (Maxon *et al.*, 1992; O'Connell *et al.*, 1993). In order to calculate the radiation dose (*D*) three parameters must be determined: the initial activity in the target tissue (A_0), the effective half-life of the radio-iodine (T_e) and the mass of tissue (*m*). We use single photon emission computerized tomography (SPECT) or positron emission tomography (PET) imaging to measure the volume of metabolically active thyroid tissue or tumour and, following iodine treatment, perform

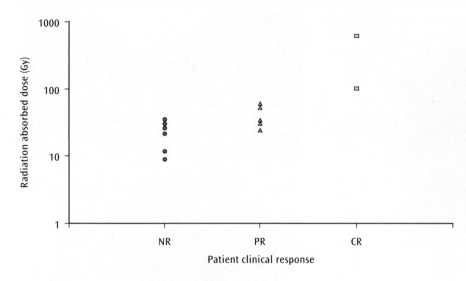

Figure 19.8 *Dose–response relationship in radio-iodine therapy for patients with metastatic thyroid cancer. NR, no response; PR, partial response; CR, complete response.*

sequential quantitative scans from which activity–time curves can be produced. By fitting the data and extrapolating to the time of administration, the initial activity in the target tissue and the effective half-life of iodine are determined. Calculations are then performed using the Medical Internal Radiation Dosimetry (MIRD) formula: $D = 0.16A_0T_e/m$.

Preliminary analysis of 25 dosimetry studies in patients with metastatic lesions showed a wide variation in radiation absorbed dose (5–621 Gy) from a fixed administered ^{131}I activity of 5.5 GBq (Vini *et al.*, 1998c). There was evidence of a dose–response relationship clearly explaining the spectrum of clinical response (Fig. 19.8). However, MIRD dosimetry calculations are based on two major assumptions: that radioactivity is uniformly distributed throughout the tumour and that washout of ^{131}I is governed by a single exponential function. If either of these assumptions is inaccurate, then errors will be introduced into the dosimetry estimates. In addition, errors on each parameter (percentage uptake, target activity, T_e and mass) will contribute to a combined error of absorbed dose (Flower and McCready, 1997). Given all the problems with dosimetry and the potential for large errors, it could be questioned whether trying to perform dose calculations is worthwhile. With current efforts to produce accurate sequential registered three-dimensional SPECT images and dose–volume histograms of therapy distributions, a greater level of accuracy may be achieved eventually, resulting in improved effectiveness of treatment.

COMPLICATIONS OF RADIO-IODINE TREATMENT

Radio-iodine therapy is well tolerated and usually lacks serious complications. Radiation thyroiditis may occur up to 4 days following ablation and is characterized by pain, swelling and localized tenderness in the neck. Symptoms may be severe if there is a large thyroid remnant, requiring steroid treatment. Acute sialadenitis affecting the parotid or submandibular glands occurs occasionally within 48 hours of administration and may last a few days. A liberal fluid intake and frequent use of lozenges containing sodium citrate should be routine to reduce salivary uptake and limit this reaction. Intravenous administration of amifostine has been reported to result in reduced salivary uptake (Bohuslaviski *et al.*, 1998). Sialadenitis may persist into a chronic phase with episodes recurring over years; about 70 per cent of patients showed a significant decrease in salivary function which can result in xerostomia and appeared to be dose related (Bohuslaviski *et al.*, 1996). Persistent painful masses may require excision.

Most patients demonstrate transient haematological depression, especially following administration of high doses, but myelodysplasia leading to aplastic anaemia is rare and likely to occur only in patients with extensive bone metastases who have received a high cumulative dose. In most of these cases the dose to the blood was in excess of 3 Gy (Benua *et al.*, 1962). Radiation pneumonitis and pulmonary fibrosis have been reported in patients with diffuse functioning lung metastases following repeated administrations (Rall *et al.*, 1957). A 6–12-month interval between iodine doses may reduce the risk of this complication; if serial lung-function tests indicate early damage, future iodine doses can be fractionated.

Because differentiated thyroid cancer occurs in women of childbearing age and young men, the possibility that iodine treatment may affect fertility has created concern. A temporary increase in follicular stimulating hormone (FSH) levels has been noted following ^{131}I treatment in both male and female patients, indicating temporary gonadal dysfunction. A positive correlation between FSH levels and the cumulative activity of iodine has been also reported (Pacini *et al.*, 1994). In a small prospective study using thermoluminescent dosimetry, we measured the radiation absorbed dose to the testes to be relatively low: 5.4–9.8 cGy and 12–19.2 cGy following administration of 3 and 5.5 GBq, respectively (Vini *et al.*, 1998f). Regarding female patients, no significant difference was observed in fertility rates, birth rates or prematurity among women treated with radio-iodine and those not treated (Dottorini *et al.*, 1995; Schlumberger *et al.*, 1996b). In 406 patients under the age of 40, temporary amenorrhoea and minor menstrual irregularities were seen in 20 per cent; 427 normal children were born to 276 women and only one patient was unable to conceive (Vini *et al.*, 1998b).

The carcinogenic hazard of ^{131}I in the treatment of both hyperthyroidism and thyroid cancer has been the subject of several large series. An excess risk of acute leukaemia was seen in the past, especially in patients receiving a cumulative activity over 40 GBq, although the numbers were small (Edmonds and Smith, 1986). In more recent series the incidence of leukaemia is much lower, probably due to efforts to limit the total body dose to 2 Gy and longer intervals of 6–12 months between doses. Among 802 patients in Sweden there were six leukaemias (SIR = 2.37; 95 per cent CI, 0.87–5.16); however, an increased risk was seen for chronic lymphocytic leukaemia (SIR = 4.49), a condition not normally related to irradiation (Hall *et al.*, 1992). With regard to solid tumours, there is a suggestion of an increased incidence of breast cancer as well as cancer in organs which concentrate ^{131}I, such as salivary glands, bladder, kidney and colon (de Vathaire *et al.*, 1997). The latter can be minimized by a liberal fluid intake plus routine use of a laxative.

External-beam radiotherapy and chemotherapy

The role of external-beam radiotherapy (RT) in the management of differentiated thyroid cancer remains controversial, the main reason being difficulty in interpreting published data. In most reports, results are presented without distinguishing between prophylactic (adjuvant) postoperative RT, RT following microscopically incomplete surgery and RT for macroscopic inoperable disease. In addition, in those series assessing prophylactic RT, there is no suitable control group. Furthermore, the slow growth rate requires long follow-up in order to evaluate results.

Radiotherapy is clearly not indicated in patients with good prognostic features, nor in young patients with residual disease and good iodine uptake. Data suggest that adjuvant RT should be restricted to patients older than 40 years with locally advanced tumours who do not show significant iodine uptake and demonstrate an elevated Tg postoperatively (Farahati *et al.*, 1995; Tsang *et al.*, 1998). Doses in excess of 50 Gy achieved local control in 90 per cent (Tubiana *et al.*, 1985). A fall in serum Tg levels following RT has also been documented. Irradiation of bulky inoperable tumours is less satisfactory; however, local control was obtained in half of the patients who received doses greater than 60 Gy. Radiotherapy is also effective for advanced and recurrent Hürthle cell carcinoma, having a relatively more important role here because this tumour does not take up iodine (Vini *et al.*, 1998d).

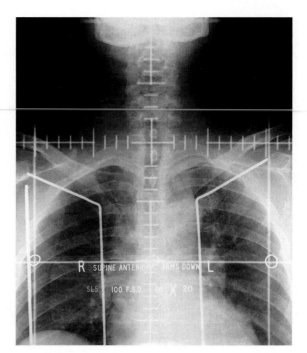

Figure 19.9 *Radiotherapy technique for thyroid cancer: phase I volume covering the thyroid bed, neck and superior mediastinum.*

Our policy is to use RT infrequently because high dose is required and side-effects, especially oesophagitis, are unavoidable. Indications include macroscopic unresectable residual tumour and suspected microscopic disease or involved excision margins, especially in older patients with less well-differentiated cancers unlikely to concentrate radio-iodine (O'Connell *et al.*, 1994). The treatment volume comprises the thyroid bed, bilateral deep cervical plus supraclavicular nodes, and superior mediastinum down to the level of the carina, using anterior and undercouched fields for phase I with lead protecting the mandible and subapical portions of the lungs, going to a maximum cord dose of 46 Gy in 2 Gy daily fractions (Fig. 19.9). A perspex shell is then fashioned for the phase II volume, which includes sites of micro- or macroscopic tumour (Fig. 19.10). We use three-dimensional planning and conformal beam shaping assisted by a multileaf collimator, to deliver a dose of at least 60 Gy with avoidance of adjacent normal tissues, as demonstrated in Figure 19.11 (Harmer *et al.*, 1998). Intensity-modulated RT improves the dose distribution and could allow dose escalation (Nutting *et al.*, 2001).

Experience with chemotherapy in differentiated thyroid cancer is limited by the rarity of tumours not controlled by surgery and radio-iodine. There is, however, a significant minority of patients who do not respond to conventional therapy and survive for many years with minimal symptoms. Because presently available drugs are of limited benefit and cause significant morbidity, chemotherapy is reserved for patients with progressive and symptomatic disease that fails to concentrate

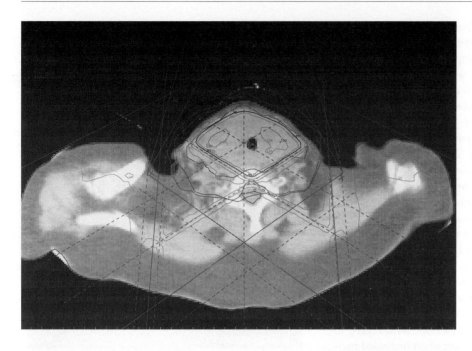

Figure 19.10 *Three-dimensional plan (anterior and pair of antero-oblique fields) for phase II volume covering microscopic disease in the thyroid bed.*

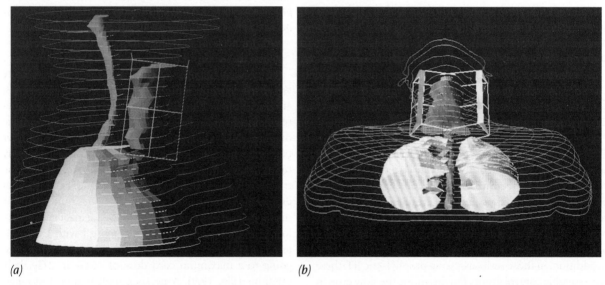

(a)   *(b)*

Figure 19.11 *Three-dimensional reconstruction showing field positions in relation to planning target volume and critical organs: (a) spinal cord; (b) lung apices.*

radio-iodine (Hoskin and Harmer, 1987). Of the several agents investigated, doxorubicin has been the most effective, with response rates of 30 to 40 per cent. The combination of doxorubicin and cisplatin has produced a similar response rate to that of doxorubicin alone, but with greater toxicity. Responses are usually partial and of short duration. However, worthwhile palliation in patients with advanced symptomatic disease has been reported (Ahuja and Ernst, 1987). Doxorubicin in combination with external-beam radiotherapy appeared to be effective in some patients with large inoperable tumours (Kim and Leeper, 1987). Chemotherapy may be beneficial in patients with advanced non-iodine-concentrating

thyroid cancer by inducing uptake and allowing subsequent radio-iodine therapy (Morris *et al.*, 1997).

MANAGEMENT OF ANAPLASTIC CARCINOMA

Patients with anaplastic carcinoma present with rapidly progressive local and regional nodal disease. Prognosis is dismal with a median survival of only 6 months from the original symptom. Local growth results in upper airway and oesophageal obstruction. For this reason, it was thought that maximal surgical debulking should be attempted, leaving residual tumour for treatment by radiation and/or chemotherapy (McIver et al., 2001).

Anaplastic cancer is the least radiosensitive of all thyroid tumours. Doses of less than 50 Gy given in conventional fractionation are associated with a very low probability of local control; evidence for control with higher doses is scant and subject to selection bias. Experience with 50–60 Gy administered in 5–6 weeks achieved local response in less than 45 per cent of patients, and 75 per cent still died from local progression (Levendag et al., 1993). There is little effect on survival and the majority of patients spend a significant period of their remaining life undergoing treatment and recovering from its toxicity.

In an attempt to improve local control, alternative approaches were investigated, including accelerated radiotherapy and chemotherapy. Clinical and some laboratory data on the proliferation rate of high-grade thyroid cancer suggest that the potential tumour doubling time is less than 5 days, making accelerated radiotherapy attractive. Several centres have shown an improvement in local tumour response. In our series of 17 patients treated twice daily, 5 days a week, to a dose of 60.8 Gy in 32 fractions over 20–24 days, significant response was achieved in 59 per cent (including three patients with a complete clinical response). Unfortunately, there was a corresponding increase in treatment toxicity which was unacceptable; grade 3–4 oesophagitis occurred in over 90 per cent of patients and persisted for several weeks following cessation of radiotherapy (Mitchell et al., 1999). Furthermore, despite success in achieving local control, survival remained poor, with almost all patients dying within 6 months of treatment.

Better response rates are reported with combined chemotherapy and radiotherapy, particularly if the latter is delivered in a hyperfractionated schedule, although at the cost of increased morbidity (Schlumberger et al., 1991b). Doxorubicin is the single most effective agent, and even low doses in combination with radiation appear to have a synergistic effect. There is a very small number of patients who demonstrate prolonged survival, having been rendered free of disease by subsequent surgery. In a study from Sweden, 33 patients were treated with hyperfractionated accelerated radiotherapy concurrently with small doses of doxorubicin followed by debulking surgery and postoperative chemoradiotherapy. Despite the patients' advanced age and locally extensive disease, such an aggressive treatment modality was feasible. Local control was achieved in 50 per cent and in only 24 per cent was death attributed to local failure; 10 per cent of patients survived with no evidence of disease for more than 2 years (Tennvall et al., 1994).

Control of local disease is important both for palliation and if there is to be any chance of prolonging survival. Improvements in radiotherapy fractionation schedules and conformal beam shaping could maximize the probability of local control while limiting toxicity. Finally, since almost all patients who achieve local control still die from metastatic disease, a more effective systemic treatment awaits discovery. Manumycin has enhanced the cytotoxic effect of paclitaxel on anaplastic thyroid carcinoma cell lines with no significant toxicity (Yeung et al., 2000); gemcitabine has also shown promising activity in cell lines (Voigt et al., 2000).

MANAGEMENT OF MEDULLARY CANCER

Total thyroidectomy with routine dissection of lymph nodes in the central compartment of the neck and sampling of lateral jugular nodes is the optimal surgical treatment for MTC. Total thyroidectomy is indicated since in over 90 per cent of familial and about 20 per cent of sporadic cases, disease is multicentric and bilateral. Furthermore, the incidence of local recurrence is lower in patients treated by radical surgery (Modigliani et al., 2000). Cervical lymph-node involvement at presentation ranges from 15 to 75 per cent. A modified neck dissection with preservation of the sternomastoid muscle, the spinal accessory nerve and the internal jugular vein is indicated if metastatic nodes are found during sampling (Dralle et al., 1995). Excision of mediastinal lymph nodes, if involved, should be attempted. Aggressive surgery is justified by the initial localized extent of disease in most cases. Ideally, the postoperative calcitonin will fall to an undetectable level. It should be repeated at annual follow-up, together with clinical evaluation.

Unfortunately elevated calcitonin levels often persist following initial operation and may be detected in up to 70 per cent of patients with node involvement (Block et al., 1978). The most frequent sites of disease are nodes in the neck and mediastinum, while distant metastases may involve the liver, lungs and bones. Non-invasive imaging methods for detecting occult disease include ultrasonography, CT scan or MRI, and radionuclide scanning (^{99m}Tc-pentavalent dimercaptosuccinic acid (DMSA), ^{123}I meta-iodobenzylguanidine (mIBG), ^{111}In octreotide, ^{201}Thallium), although none of the latter is very specific. We have previously reported a 30 per cent sensitivity of radionuclide imaging in MTC (Vini et al., 1998a). Other methods of investigating recurrent MTC include selective venous catheterization to assay calcitonin levels (Medina-Franco et al., 2001), radioimmunoscintigraphy with monoclonal antibodies such as ^{131}I anti-CEA (Juweid et al., 1997) and more recently positron emission tomography (Diehl et al., 2001).

Residual MCT is usually progressive, as reflected in a rise in calcitonin levels over time; a mean annual increase of 117 per cent of the initial value was calculated in 35 of 40 patients by Tisell, while in another study an exponential increase was detected in 19 of 23 patients (Tisell et al., 1996). This progressive increase can continue from the first postoperative measurement, but may not appear until after a long period of stability. The often indolent course of MCT despite the presence of regional metastatic disease has been emphasized by several authors. In a series from the Mayo Clinic, only 11 of 31 patients with raised calcitonin but negative imaging developed overt recurrent disease when followed for a mean period of 12 years. Reoperation for clinically documented local recurrence did not result in normalization in calcitonin level. However, overall survival at 5 and 10 years was 90 per cent and 86 per cent, respectively (van Heerden *et al.*, 1990).

A more aggressive approach towards localization of residual disease was adopted by Tisell, who performed meticulous 12-hour neck dissections, often removing 40–60 cervical lymph nodes (Tisell *et al.*, 1986). In a series of 11 patients, the calcitonin normalized in four (36 per cent) and dramatically improved in four. However, follow-up was short (2–4.5 years) and there is no evidence that these biochemical improvements translate into a survival advantage (Moley *et al.*, 1993). This policy is not without risk, with higher complication rates than conventional surgery. In view of this and the long-term survival seen with patients on observation, many advocate close follow-up, with surgery reserved for when clinical recurrence can be documented (Heshmati *et al.*, 1997).

The role of postoperative RT is controversial due to lack of prospective studies; retrospective series comparing surgery alone with surgery plus RT are subject to selection bias. Favourable responses in terms of tumour reduction and local control have been reported (Simpson, 1990; Fife *et al.*, 1996). At the Institut Gustave-Roussy, the survival of 68 patients treated with surgery alone was similar to that of 59 who received postoperative RT. However, in patients with involved lymph nodes, 5-year survival improved significantly with postoperative RT, from 36 per cent to 81 per cent (Schlumberger *et al.*, 1991a). In contrast, an adverse effect of RT was reported from the MD Anderson; survival was significantly worse for 24 patients given postoperative RT compared with 39 age- and disease-matched patients treated with surgery alone (Samaan *et al.*, 1988). We recommend the use of adjuvant RT in patients with locally advanced disease at presentation, and multiple involved lymph nodes in particular, who have persistently elevated calcitonin levels postoperatively, indicating microscopic residual disease (Fersht *et al.*, 1999). Radiotherapy should be also considered in patients with bulky inoperable tumours for whom significant palliation can be achieved with doses of 60 Gy in 6 weeks; occasionally subsequent surgery becomes possible. Palliative RT also has a role for inoperable mediastinal masses and painful bone metastases.

Many patients with metastatic medullary cancer survive for years having minimal symptoms and, apart from medication to control diarrhoea, may not require any other treatment. Chemotherapy should be considered for those with unresectable progressive and symptomatic disease. Doxorubicin produces symptomatic response in about 30 per cent of cases, but most are partial and of short duration (Hoskin and Harmer, 1987). In contrast, the combination of streptozocin, 5-fluorouracil and dacarbazine has been recommended, with response rate not improved by the addition of doxorubicin (Nocera *et al.*, 2000). The selective uptake of ^{131}I mIBG and ^{111}In octreotide by 30–50 per cent of medullary cancers has generated interest in their potential use for targeted radiotherapy, although early attempts have not been particularly successful (Wiseman and Kvols, 1995). Treatment with unlabelled somatostatin analogues may be helpful to control severe diarrhoea from metastatic disease, although side-effects can be troublesome. Finally, use of recombinant interferon-α-2a has been reported.

The clinical course of MTC varies widely, with overall 10-year survival rates ranging from 65 to 90 per cent (Heshmati *et al.*, 1997; Hyer *et al.*, 2000). Patients with multiple endocrine neoplasia (MEN) IIB have the most aggressive tumours, often with early development of metastases and death. Young age at diagnosis, male gender, lymph-node involvement and incompleteness of initial surgical resection have been identified as significant adverse prognostic factors (Schroder *et al.*, 1988). In some retrospective series, patients with familial cancer have a significantly longer survival compared to those with sporadic cancer (Samaan *et al.*, 1988); however, when patients were matched for age, gender, extent of disease and treatment, this difference disappeared.

MANAGEMENT OF FAMILIAL MEDULLARY THYROID CANCER

Since 1993 when *RET* proto-oncogene mutations were identified, considerable information has been accumulated on the clinical usefulness of genetic information. The goal of screening for MEN II is to identify gene carriers early, in an attempt to modify the outcome of the disease. The two manifestations that are life threatening are MTC and phaeochromocytoma. There is compelling evidence for both that early intervention will improve outcome (Wells *et al.*, 1994). Genetic testing is the most cost-effective approach to detect affected individuals (Ponder, 1993). All techniques currently use DNA fragments generated by polymerase chain reaction (PCR) amplification of genomic DNA. Several analytic techniques have been applied to detect specific mutations, including direct DNA sequencing, denaturing gradient gel electrophoresis, restriction analysis of amplified products and allele-specific hybridization. Each of these has proved reliable for detection of the most common mutations causing MEN II or familial medullary thyroid cancer (FMTC).

Genetic testing should be performed soon after birth. Family members found not to be gene carriers by *RET* mutation analysis do not require further genetic or biochemical testing and no tests need to be performed on their descendants. Adults who are gene carriers are at high risk of developing MTC; total thyroidectomy with central lymph-node dissection should be performed after exclusion of phaeochromocytoma. Two approaches have evolved for the management of children found to be gene carriers. The first is to use annual pentagastrin stimulation of calcitonin and defer total thyroidectomy until the test becomes abnormal (Brandi et al., 2001). This will identify affected children at an average age of 10–13 years. Concern related to pentagastrin testing is failure to identify C-cell abnormalities at the earliest stage, since approximately 50 per cent of children had microscopic MTC rather than C-cell hyperplasia (Gagel et al., 1988). The second approach is to perform total thyroidectomy based solely on the results of genetic testing at the age of 5–6 years. Surgery is well tolerated and the risks of recurrent laryngeal nerve damage or hypoparathyroidism are no greater than in older children (Wells et al., 1994). This approach is most cost-effective and eliminates the unpleasantness of annual pentagastrin testing.

Annual measurement of urinary catecholamines and metanephrines on a 24-hour specimen provides a straightforward outpatient screening approach to detect phaeochromocytoma. Elevated adrenaline or an elevated adrenaline/noradrenaline ratio are the most commonly observed patterns. Basal or exercise-stimulated plasma catecholamines provides an alternative method. MRI is used to confirm phaeochromocytoma or an enlarged medulla. In most cases abnormalities involve both adrenals and bilateral adrenalectomy is recommended (Heshmati et al., 1997). The procedure is well tolerated but must be preceded by α- and β-blockade for about 7–10 days.

Measurement of serum calcium should be performed annually in MEN IIA gene carriers to screen for hyperparathyroidism. Once hypercalcaemia is documented, serum intact parathormone (PTH) should be measured to confirm the diagnosis. The majority of patients with hyperparathyroidism will have diffuse but unequal multiglandular hyperplasia, with only a small proportion (10–15 per cent) having a single adenoma. There is controversy regarding total parathyroidectomy with immediate auto-transplantation versus subtotal parathyroidectomy.

The value of genetic screening is beyond doubt. However, it is important that family members be counselled regarding the impact of a positive genetic test. A long-term strategy of education and support is recommended.

MANAGEMENT OF THYROID LYMPHOMA

Most patients with primary thyroid lymphoma present with confluent cervical/mediastinal lymphadenopathy (stage IIE) but in about one-third tumour is confined to the thyroid gland (IE). Haematology and biochemistry, CT scan of the neck, thorax and abdomen, and bone marrow aspirate plus trephine are required for staging.

However, these patients are often elderly and may require urgent therapy to relieve airway obstruction, making full staging impracticable until later.

Aggressive surgery to debulk the tumour is neither feasible nor necessary. For localized disease, external-beam radiotherapy had been the standard practice for several decades, resulting in 5-year survival rates of approximately 35 per cent. Local bulky disease and gross mediastinal involvement were significantly associated with failure distant from the irradiated volume (Tupchong et al., 1986). Chemotherapy for high-grade lymphomas has demonstrated better local and distant disease control with overall long-term disease-free survival of about 50 per cent. The combination of radiotherapy preceded by chemotherapy has become the standard practice in most institutions and has resulted in 5-year survival rates of 65–90 per cent (Matsuzuka et al., 1993). Six cycles of cyclophosphamide, doxorubicin, vincristine and prednisolone (CHOP) given over 4 months is usually recommended.

Lymphomas showing mucosa-associated lymphoid tissue (MALT) characteristics usually present as localized extranodal tumour without adverse prognostic factors, and follow a more indolent course (Thieblemont et al., 2002). Radiotherapy as single-modality treatment resulted in a complete response rate of almost 100 per cent, a relapse rate of around 30 per cent, a salvage rate of over 50 per cent, and an overall cause-specific survival of almost 90 per cent at 5 and 10 years (Laing et al., 1994). Our policy is to treat stage IEA MALT-positive lymphomas with radiotherapy only, but to use combination treatment for all other tumours. The treatment volume includes the neck and superior mediastinum and is irradiated by a pair of anterior and undercouched fields to 40 Gy in 20 fractions over 4 weeks. If bulky disease remains in the neck, a reduced phase II volume is treated to total dose of 50 Gy. Primary Hodgkin's disease of the thyroid is excessively rare and is treated in a similar fashion to extranodal Hodgkin's at any other site.

FUTURE PROSPECTS

For treatment of differentiated thyroid carcinoma the exciting advance over the past decade has been the development of ^{131}I dosimetry to calculate the absorbed radiation dose in recurrent and metastatic disease. This has permitted construction of dose–response curves which explain the spectrum of clinical response from fixed activities of radio-iodine (Vini et al., 1998c). They allow for the tumoricidal dose to be calculated and thus enable precise prescription of further ^{131}I therapy, so as to maximize tumour kill while minimizing patient toxicity, staff exposure and unnecessary expense.

Effectiveness of treatment could also be improved by increasing radio-iodine uptake by tumour, altering tumour metabolism so that iodine is retained longer, and adding drugs that enhance the radiation effect. Administration of higher activities of ^{131}I is the simplest measure to increase iodine uptake. However, use of activities greater than the standard 5.5 GBq therapy dose is associated with an increased risk of marrow suppression, leukaemia, lung fibrosis (for patients with miliary lung metastases) and salivary gland damage (Carnell *et al.*, 1997). Chemical agents such as doxorubicin or cisplatin inhibit recovery from radiation damage and may be used to enhance the tumoricidal effect of ionizing radiation. Low-dose doxorubicin combined with ^{131}I therapy for patients with poor prognosis is under study.

Autoradiographs of thyroid tumours show a non-uniform distribution of ^{131}I, which may be a contributory factor to treatment failure in some cases. In an attempt to improve dose distribution and dose rate, alternative isotopes have been investigated. Astatine-211 (^{211}At), a member of the same chemical family as iodine, emits high-energy α particles, resulting in a more uniform distribution of dose delivered within thyroid cancer cells. Unfortunately, in animal experiments it has been associated with significant toxicity.

An alternative approach is the administration of the radio-isotope as a conjugate with monoclonal antibodies. Tg and TSH receptors are logical target antigens for antibody-directed therapy. Tg is present in both cells and colloid in most differentiated thyroid tumours. However, it is heterogeneously distributed and, in less-differentiated tumours, is present in lower concentrations. The initial results of immunoscintigraphy studies using ^{131}I-labelled antithyroglobulin antibodies were encouraging, but no clinical studies have been reported (Shepherd *et al.*, 1985). Radiolabelled antireceptor monoclonal antibodies or recombinant-produced human TSH may possibly be used to locate, or even treat, tumours possessing these receptors.

There is some evidence that immunological factors may play a role in the course of thyroid cancer. The sudden development of widespread metastases after years of an indolent course of disease suggests a change in tumour or host factors. Patients with large-volume metastases have been found to have suppressed T-cell function and patients with lymphocytic thyroiditis have been reported to have a better overall prognosis. Attempts to induce autoimmune thyroiditis in patients with advance thyroid carcinoma by immunizing them with a chemically altered Tg showed only minimal clinical response. Interleukin-1 and TNF-α have shown some promising results, although *in vivo* studies have not yet been conducted. Finally, for tumours that have reduced ability to concentrate iodine or have become dedifferentiated, retinoic acids have been shown to decrease tumour growth rate and increase the expression of sodium-iodine symporter (Schmutzler and Kohrle, 2000). Their clinical relevance in redifferentiation therapy-induced radio-iodine uptake is promising but not confirmed.

SIGNIFICANT POINTS

- The incidence of thyroid cancer has increased significantly over the past decades. However, cause-specific mortality rates during the same period have dropped significantly, possibly due to earlier diagnosis.
- Fine-needle aspiration cytology is the single most accurate method for evaluating thyroid nodules and has resulted in a significant reduction in the number of operations, a greater proportion of malignancies removed during surgery, and an overall reduction in the cost of managing patients with thyroid nodules.
- Multivariate analyses of large retrospective studies have identified patient and tumour characteristics that are related to prognosis; age is the most important independent predicting factor, while tumour size, grade, extension and presence of metastases also have a significant effect on tumour recurrence and survival. Based on these prognostic factors, any individual patient's risk of dying of cancer can be assessed, making a selective approach to treatment possible.
- Surgery remains the initial and potentially curative treatment for differentiated carcinomas. Following total thyroidectomy, ablation of thyroid remnants with radioactive iodine reduces the risk of locoregional recurrence and cancer-specific mortality for patients with poor prognostic factors.
- Radio-iodine therapy is the mainstay of treatment for disseminated thyroid cancer; a significant proportion of patients can be cured and, in others, durable palliation can be achieved.

KEY REFERENCES

Becker, D.V., Robbins, J., Beebe, G. *et al.* (1996) Childhood thyroid cancer following the Chernobyl accident: a status report. *Endocrinol. Metab. Clin. North Am.* **25**, 197–211.

Candy, B. and Rossi, R. (1988) An expanded view of risk-group definition in differentiated thyroid cancer. *Surgery* **104**, 947–53.

Dos Santos Silva, I. and Swerdlow, A.J. (1993) Thyroid cancer epidemiology in England and Wales: time trends and geographic distribution. *Br. J. Cancer* **67**, 330–40.

Harmer, C., Bidmead, M., Shepherd, S. *et al.* (1998) Radiotherapy planning techniques for thyroid cancer. *Br. J. Radiol.* **71**, 1069–75.

Heshmati, H.M., Gharib, H., van Heerden, J.A. and Sizemore, G.W. (1997) Advances and controversies in the diagnosis and management of medullary thyroid carcinoma. *Am. J. Med.* **103**, 60–9.

Mazzaferri, E.L. and Jhiang, S. (1994) Long-term impact of initial surgical and medical therapy on papillary and follicular thyroid cancer. *Am. J. Med.* **97**, 418–28.

Schlumberger, M., Challeton, C., De Vathaire, F. *et al.* (1996a) Radioactive iodine treatment and external radiotherapy for lung and bone metastases from thyroid carcinoma. *J. Nucl. Med.* **37**, 598–605.

REFERENCES

Ahuja, S. and Ernst, H. (1987) Chemotherapy of thyroid cancer. *J. Endocrin. Invest.* **10**, 303–10.

Ashcraft, M.W. and van Herle, A.J. (1981) Management of thyroid nodules. Scanning techniques, suppressive therapy and fine needle aspiration. *Head Neck Surg.* **3**, 216–30.

Bal, C., Padhy, A.K., Jana, S. *et al.* (1996) Prospective randomised clinical trial to evaluate the optimal dose of ^{131}I for remnant ablation in patients with differentiated thyroid carcinoma. *Cancer* **77**, 2574–80.

Ballantyne, A.J. (1994) Resections of the upper aerodigestive tract for locally invasive thyroid cancer. *Am. J. Surg.* **168**, 636–9.

Becker, D.V., Robbins, J., Beebe, G. *et al.* (1996) Childhood thyroid cancer following the Chernobyl accident: a status report. *Endocrinol. Metab. Clin. North Am.* **25**, 197–211.

Beirwaltes, W.H., Rabbani, R., Dmuchowski, C. *et al.* (1984) An analysis of ablation of thyroid remnants with ^{131}I in 511 patients from 1947 to 1984: experience at University of Michigan. *J. Nucl. Med.* **25**, 1287–93.

Benua, R.S., Cicale, N.R., Sonenberg, M. and Rawson, R.W. (1962) The relation of radioiodine dosimetry to results and complications in the treatment of metastatic thyroid cancer. *Am. J. Radiol.* **87**, 171–82.

Block, M.A., Jackson, C.E. and Tashjian, A.H. (1978) Management of occult medullary thyroid carcinoma evidenced only by serum calcitonin level elevations after apparently adequate neck operations. *Arch. Surg.* **113**, 368–72.

Bohuslaviski, K.H., Brenner, W., Lassmann, S. *et al.* (1996) Quantitative salivary gland scintigraphy in the diagnosis of parenchymal damage after treatment with radioiodine. *Nucl. Med. Commun.* **17**, 681–6.

Bohuslaviski, K.H., Klutmann, S., Brenner, W. *et al.* (1998) Salivary gland protection by amifostine in high-dose radioiodine treatment: results of a double-blind placebo controlled study. *J. Clin. Oncol.* **16**, 3542–9.

Boice, J.D., Engholm, G., Lkeinerman, R.A. *et al.* (1988) Radiation and second cancer risk in patients treated for cancer of the cervix. *Radiat. Res.* **116**, 3–55.

Bongarzone, I., Butti, M.G., Coronelli, S. *et al.* (1994) Frequent activation of ret protooncogene by fusion with a new activating gene in papillary thyroid carcinomas. *Cancer Res.* **54**, 2979–85.

Bramley, M.D. and Harrison, B.J. (1996) Papillary microcarcinoma of the thyroid gland. *Br. J. Surg.* **83**, 1674–83.

Brandi, M.L., Gagel, R.F., Angeli, A. *et al.* (2001) Guidelines for diagnosis and therapy of MEN type I and type II. *J. Clin. Endocrinol. Metab.* **86**(12), 658–71.

Candy, B. and Rossi, R. (1988) An expanded view of risk-group definition in differentiated thyroid cancer. *Surgery* **104**, 947–53.

Carnell, D., McCready, R.V., Vini, L. and Harmer, C. (1997) High activity radioiodine therapy for advanced differentiated thyroid carcinoma: efficacy and morbidity. In Bergmann, H., Kohn, H. and Sininger, H. (eds), *Radioactive isotopes in clinical medicine and research.* Basle: Birkhauser-Verlag, 443–9.

Coleman, P., Babb, P., Damiecki, P. *et al.* (1999) *Cancer survival trends in England and Wales 1975–1995: deprivation and NHS region.* London: Stationery Office, Series SMPS no. 61, 471–8.

Correa, P. and Chen, V.W. (1995) Endocrine gland cancer. *Cancer* **75**, 338–52.

de Vathaire, F., Schlumberger, M., Delisle, M.J. *et al.* (1997) Leukemias and cancers following iodine-131 administration for thyroid cancer. *Br. J. Cancer* **75**, 734–9.

Diehl, M., Risse, J.H., Brandt-Mainz, K., *et al.* (2001) Fluorine-18 fluorodeoxyglucose positron emission tomography in medullary thyroid cancer: results of a multicentre study. *Eur. J. Nucl. Med.* **28**(1), 1671–6.

Dos Santos Silva, I. and Swerdlow, A.J. (1993) Thyroid cancer epidemiology in England and Wales: time trends and geographic distribution. *Br. J. Cancer* **67**, 330–40.

Dottorini, M.E., Lomuscio, G., Mazzucchelli, L. *et al.* (1995) Assessment of female fertility and carcinogenesis after iodine-131 therapy for differentiated thyroid carcinoma. *J. Nucl. Med.* **36**, 21–7.

Dralle, H., Scheumann, G.F.W., Proye, C. *et al.* (1995) The value of lymph node dissection in hereditary medullary thyroid carcinoma: a retrospective European multicentre study. *J. Intern. Med.* **238**, 357–61.

Edmonds, C.J. and Smith, T. (1986) The long-term hazards of the treatment of thyroid cancer with radioiodine. *Br. J. Radiol.* **59**, 45–51.

Farahati, J., Reiners, C., Stuschke, M. *et al.* (1996) Differentiated thyroid cancer. Impact of adjuvant external radiotherapy in patients with perithyroidal tumour infiltration (stage pT4). *Cancer* **77**, 172–80.

Fatourechi, V., Hay, I., Mullan, B.I. (2000) Are post-therapy radioiodine scans informative and do they influence subsequent therapy of patients with differentiated thyroid cancer? *Thyroid* **10**(7), 573–7.

Fersht, N., Vini, L., A'Hern, R. and Harmer, C. (1999) Management of patients with elevated calcitonin following initial surgery for medullary thyroid cancer. *Br. J. Cancer* **8**(suppl. 2), 61 (P132).

Fife, K.M., Bower, M. and Harmer, C. (1996) Medullary thyroid cancer: the role of radiotherapy in local control. *Eur. J. Surg. Oncol.* **22**, 588–91.

Flower, M.A. and McCready, V.R. (1997) Radionuclide therapy dose calculations: what accuracy can be achieved? *Eur. J. Nucl. Med.* **24**, 1462–4.

Franceschi, S., Levi, F., Negri, E. *et al.* (1991) Diet and thyroid cancer: a pooled analysis of four European case-control studies. *Int. J. Cancer* **48**, 395–8.

Gagel, R.F., Tashjian, A.H., Cummings, T. *et al.* (1988) The clinical outcome of prospective screening for multiple endocrine neoplasia type 2a: an 18-year experience. *N. Engl. J. Med.* **318**, 478–84.

Giannini, S., Nobile, M., Sartori, L. *et al.* (1994) Bone density and mineral metabolism in thyroidectomised patients treated with long-term L-thyroxine. *Clin. Sci.* **87**, 593–7.

Hall, P., Boice, J.D., Berg, G. *et al.* (1992) Leukemia incidence after iodine-131 exposure. *Lancet* **340**, 1–4.

Hamburger, J.I. (1994) Diagnosis of thyroid nodules by fine needle biopsy. Use and abuse. *J. Clin. Endocrinol. Metab.* **79**, 335–9.

Harmer, C.L. and McCready, R.V. (1996) Thyroid cancer: differentiated carcinoma. *Cancer Treat. Review* **96**, 161–77.

Harmer, C., Bidmead, M., Shepherd, S. *et al.* (1998) Radiotherapy planning techniques for thyroid cancer. *Br. J. Radiol.* **71**, 1069–75.

Hawkins, M., Vini, L., Houlston, R. and Harmer, C. (1999) Familial differentiated thyroid cancer. *Br. J. Cancer* **8**(suppl. 2), 112 (P334).

Hay, I.D., Grant, C.S., Taylor, W.F. *et al.* (1987) Ipsilateral lobectomy versus bilateral lobar resection in papillary thyroid carcinoma: a retrospective analysis of surgical outcome using a novel prognostic scoring system. *Surgery* **102**, 1088–94.

Hay, I.D., Grant, C.S., van Heerden, J.A. *et al.* (1992) Papillary thyroid microcarcinoma: a study of 535 cases in a 50-year period. *Surgery* **112**, 1139–47.

Hazard, J.B., Hawk, W.A. and Crile, G. (1959) Medullary (solid) carcinoma of the thyroid: a clinicopathologic entity. *J. Clin. Endocrinol. Metab.* **19**, 152–6.

Heshmati, H.M., Gharib, H., van Heerden, J.A. and Sizemore, G.W. (1997) Advances and controversies in the diagnosis and management of medullary thyroid carcinoma. *Am. J. Med.* **103**, 60–9.

Holm, L.E., Hall, P., Wiklund, K. *et al.* (1991) Cancer risk after iodine-131 therapy for hyperthyroidism. *J. Natl Cancer Inst.* **83**, 1072–7.

Hoskin, P.J. and Harmer, C. (1987) Chemotherapy for thyroid cancer. *Radioth. Oncol.* **10**, 187–94.

Hyer, S., Vini, L., A'Hern, R. *et al.* (2000) Medullary thyroid cancer: multivariate analysis of prognostic factors influencing survival. *Eur. J. Surg. Oncol.* **26**, 686–90.

Juweid, M., Sharkey, R.M., Swayne, L.C. *et al.* (1997) Improved selection of patients for reoperation for medullary thyroid cancer by imaging with radiolabelled anticarcinoembryonic antigen antibodies. *Surgery* **122**, 1156–65.

Kim, J.H. and Leeper, R.D. (1987) Treatment of locally advanced thyroid carcinoma with combination doxorubicin and radiation therapy. *Cancer* **60**, 2372–5.

Koong, S.S., Reynolds, J.C., Movius, E.G. *et al.* (1999) Lithium as a potential adjuvant to ^{131}I therapy of metastatic well-differentiated thyroid carcinoma. *J. Clin. Endocrinol. Metab.* **84**, 912–16.

Krenning, E.P., Kwekkeboom, D.J., Baker, W.H. *et al.* (1993) Somatostatin receptor scintigraphy with [^{111}In]DTPA and [^{123}I-Tyr]-octreotide; the Rotterdam experience with more than 1000 patients. *Eur. J. Nucl. Med.* **20**, 716–31.

Ladas, G., Rhys-Evans, P.H. and Goldstraw, P. (1999) Anterior cervical transternal approach for the resection of neural tumours of the thoracic inlet. *Ann. Thorac. Surg.* **67**, 785–9.

Laing, R.W., Hoskin, P., Vaughan Hudson, G. *et al.* (1994) The significance of MALT histology in thyroid lymphoma: a review of patients from BNLI and Royal Marsden Hospital. *Clin. Oncol.* **6**, 300–6.

Levendag, P.C., De Porre, P.M. and van Putten, W.L. (1993) Anaplastic carcinoma of the thyroid gland treated by radiation therapy. *Int. J. Radiat. Oncol. Biol. Phys.* **26**, 125–8.

LiVolsi, V.A. and Merino, M.J. (1981) Histopathologic differential diagnosis of the thyroid. *Pathol. Annu.* **16**, 357–406.

Loree, T.R. (1995) Therapeutic implications of prognostic factors in differentiated carcinoma of the thyroid gland. *Semin. Surg. Oncol.* **11**, 246–55.

Marcocci, C., Pacini, F., Elisei, R. *et al.* (1989) Clinical and biological behaviour of bone metastases from differentiated thyroid carcinoma. *Surgery* **106**, 960–6.

Matsuzuka, F., Miyauchi, A., Katayama, S. *et al.* (1993) Clinical aspects of primary thyroid lymphoma: diagnosis and treatment based on our experience of 119 cases. *Thyroid* **3**, 93–9.

Maxon, H.R., Thomas, S.R., Hertzberg, V.S. *et al.* (1983) Relation between effective radiation dose and outcome of radioiodine therapy for thyroid cancer. *N. Engl. J. Med.* **309**, 937–41.

Maxon, H.R., Englaro, E.E., Thomas, S.R. *et al.* (1992) Radioiodine-131 therapy for well differentiated thyroid cancer. A quantitative radiation dosimetric approach: outcome and validation in 85 patients. *J. Nucl. Med.* **92**, 1132–6.

Maxon, H.R., Thomas, S.R. and Samaratunga, R.C. (1997) Dosimetric considerations in the radioiodine treatment of macrometastases and micrometastases from differentiated thyroid cancer. *Thyroid* **7**, 183–7.

Mazzaferri, E.L. (1987) Papillary thyroid carcinoma, factors influencing prognosis and current therapy. *Semin. Oncol.* **14**, 315–32.

Mazzaferri, E.L. (1992) Thyroid cancer in thyroid nodules: finding a needle in a haystack. *Am. J. Med.* **93**, 359–62.

Mazzaferri, E.L. (1999) An overview of the management of papillary and follicular thyroid carcinoma. *Thyroid* **9**, 421–7.

Mazzaferri, E.L. and Jhiang, S. (1994) Long-term impact of initial surgical and medical therapy on papillary and follicular thyroid cancer. *Am. J. Med.* **97**, 418–28.

McCowen, K.D., Adler, R.A., Ghaed, N. *et al.* (1976) Low dose radioiodine thyroid ablation in post surgical patients with thyroid cancer. *Am. J. Med.* **61**, 52–8.

McIver, B., Hay, I.D., Guiffrida, D.F. *et al.* (2001) Anaplastic thyroid carcinoma: a 50 year experience at a single institution. *Surgery* **130**(b), 1028–34.

Medina-Franco, H., Herrera, M.F. and Lopez, G. (2001) Persistent hypercalcitoninemia in patients with medullary thyroid cancer: a therapeutic approach based on selective venous sampling for calcitonin. *Rev. Invest. Clin.* **53**(3), 212–17.

Mitchell, G., Huddart, R. and Harmer, C. (1999) Phase II evaluation of high dose accelerated radiotherapy for anaplastic thyroid carcinoma. *Radioth. Oncol.* **50**, 33–8.

Modigliani, E., Franc, B. and Niccoli-siri, P. (2000) Diagnosis and treatment of medullary thyroid cancer. *Baillieres Best Pract. Res. Clin. Endocrinol. Metab.* **14**(4), 631–49.

Moley, J.F., Wells, S.A., Dilley, W.G. and Tisell, L.E. (1993) Reoperation for recurrent or persistent medullary thyroid cancer. *Surgery* **114**, 1090–6.

Morris, J.C., Kim, C.K., Padilla, M.L. and Mechanick, J.I. (1997) Conversion of non-iodine concentrating thyroid carcinoma metastases into iodine-concentrating foci after anticancer chemotherapy. *Thyroid* **7**, 63–6.

Negri, E., Dal Maso, L., Ron, E. *et al.* (1999) A pooled analysis of case-control studies of thyroid cancer. Menstrual and reproductive factors. *Cancer Causes Control* **10**, 143–55.

Niederle, B., Roka, R., Schemper, M. *et al.* (1986) Surgical treatment of distant metastases in differentiated thyroid cancer: indications and results. *Surgery* **100**, 1088–97.

Nocera, M., Baudin, E., Pellegriti, G. *et al.* (2000) Treatment of advanced medullary thyroid cancer with an alternating combination of doxorubicin-streptozocin and 5-FU-dacarbazine. *Br. J. Cancer* **83**(6), 715–18.

Noguchi, S., Murakami, N. and Kawamoto, H. (1994) Classification of papillary cancer of the thyroid based on prognosis. *World J. Surg.* **18**, 552–7.

Nutting, C.M., Convery, D.J., Cosgrove, V.P. *et al.* (2001) Improvements in target coverage and reduced spinal cord irradiation using intensity-modulated radiotherapy (IMRT) in patients with carcinoma of the thyroid. *Radiother. Oncol.* **60**, 173–80.

O'Connell, M.E.A., Flower, M.A., Hinton, P.J. *et al.* (1993) Radiation dose assessment in radioiodine therapy. Dose–response relationships in differentiated thyroid carcinoma using quantitative scanning and PET. *Radioth. Oncol.* **28**, 16–26.

O'Connell, M.E.A., A'Hern, R.P. and Harmer, C. (1994) Results of external beam radiotherapy in differentiated thyroid carcinoma: a retrospective study from the Royal Marsden Hospital. *Eur. J. Cancer* **30A**, 733–9.

Oertel, J.E. and Heffess, C.S. (1987) Lymphoma of the thyroid and related disorders. *Semin. Oncol.* **14**, 333–42.

Pacini, F., Gasperi, M., Fugazzola, L. *et al.* (1994) Testicular function in patients with differentiated thyroid carcinoma treated with radioiodine. *J. Nucl. Med.* **35**, 1418–22.

Park, H.M., Perkins, O.W., Edmondson, J.W. *et al.* (1994) Influence of diagnostic radioiodine on the uptake of ablative dose of iodine-131. *Thyroid* **4**, 49–54.

Pineda, J.D., Lee, T., Ain, K.B. *et al.* (1995) Iodine-131 therapy for thyroid cancer patients with elevated thyroglobulin and negative diagnostic scans. *J. Clin. Endocrinol. Metab.* **80**, 1488–92.

Ponder, B.A. (1990) Multiple endocrine neoplasia type 2: the search for the gene. *BMJ* **300**, 484–5.

Ponder, B.A. (1993) Genetic screening for multiple endocrine neoplasia type 2. *Exp. Clin. Endocrinol.* **101**, 53–6.

Rall, J.E., Alpers, J.B., Lewallen, C.G. *et al.* (1957) Radiation pneumonitis and fibrosis: a complication of radioiodine treatment of pulmonary metastases from cancer of the thyroid. *J. Clin. Endocrinol. Metab.* **17**, 1263–76.

Ramana, L., Waxman, A. and Braunstein, G. (1991) Thallium-201 scintigraphy in differentiated thyroid cancer: comparison with radioiodine scintigraphy and serum thyroglobulin determinations. *J. Nucl. Med.* **32**, 441–6.

Robbins, R.J., Tuttle, R.M., Sharaf, R.N. *et al.* (2001) Preparation by recombinant human thyrotrophin or thyroid hormone withdrawal are comparable for the detection of residual differentiated thyroid carcinoma. *J. Clin. Endocrinol. Metab.* **86**, 619–25.

Ron, E., Kleinerman, R.A., Boice, J.D. *et al.* (1987) A population based case-control study of thyroid cancer. *J. Natl Cancer Inst.* **79**, 1–12.

Ron, E., Lubin, J.H., Shore, R.E. *et al.* (1995) Thyroid cancer after exposure to external radiation: a pooled analysis of seven studies. *Radiat. Res.* **141**, 259–77.

Samaan, N.A., Schultz, P. and Hickey, R. (1988) Medullary thyroid carcinoma: prognosis of familial versus sporadic disease and the role of radiotherapy. *J. Clin. Endocrinol. Metab.* **67**, 801–5.

Schaller, R.T. and Stevenson, J.K. (1966) Development of carcinoma of the thyroid in iodine deficient mice. *Cancer* **19**, 1063–7.

Schlumberger, M. and Baudin, E. (1998) Serum thyroglobulin determination in the follow-up of patients with differentiated thyroid carcinoma. *Eur. J. Endocrinol.* **138**, 249–52.

Schlumberger, M., Fragu, P., Parmentrier, C. and Tubiana, M. (1981) Thyroglobulin assay in the follow-up of patients with differentiated thyroid carcinomas: comparison of its value in patients with or without normal residual tissue. *Acta Endocrinol.* **98**, 215–21.

Schlumberger, M., Gardet, P., de Vathaire, F. *et al.* (1991a) External radiotherapy and chemotherapy in MTC patients. In Calmettes, C. and Guliana, J.M. (eds), *Medullary thyroid carcinoma* Colloque INSERM/John Libbey. Eurotext Ltd, 211, 213–20.

Schlumberger, M., Parmentrier, C., Delisle, M.J. *et al.* (1991b) Combination therapy for anaplastic giant cell thyroid carcinoma. *Cancer* **67**, 564–6.

Schlumberger, M., Challeton, C., De Vathaire, F. *et al.* (1996a) Radioactive iodine treatment and external radiotherapy for lung and bone metastases from thyroid carcinoma. *J. Nucl. Med.* **37**, 598–605.

Schlumberger, M., De Vathaire, F., Ceccarelli, C. *et al.* (1996b) Exposure to radioactive iodine-131 for scintigraphy or therapy does not preclude pregnancy in thyroid cancer patients. *J. Nucl. Med.* **37**, 606–12.

Schmutzler, C. and Kohrle, J. (2000) Retinoic acid redifferentiation therapy for thyroid cancer. *Thyroid* **10**(5), 393–406.

Schneider, A.B., Ron, E., Lubin, J. *et al.* (1993) Dose–response relationships for radiation induced thyroid cancer and thyroid nodules: evidence of prolonged effects of radiation on the thyroid. *J. Clin. Endocrinol. Metab.* **77**, 362–9.

Schroder, S., Bocker, W., Baisch, H. *et al.* (1988) Prognostic factors in medullary thyroid carcinomas: survival in relation to age, sex, stage, history, immunohistochemistry and DNA content. *Cancer* **61**, 806–16.

Shaha, A.R. (1998) Management of the neck in thyroid cancer. *Otolaryngol. Clin. North Am.* **31**, 823–31.

Shepherd, P.S., Lazarus, C.R., Mistry, R.D. and Maisey, M.N. (1985) Detection of thyroid tumour using a monoclonal ^{123}I antihuman thyroglobulin antibody. *Eur. J. Nucl. Med.* **10**, 291–5.

Shimamoto, K., Endo, T., Ishigaki, T. *et al.* (1993) Thyroid nodules: evaluation with color Doppler ultrasonography. *J. Ultrasound Med.* **12**, 673–8.

Siddiqi, A., Foley, R., Britton, K. *et al.* (2001) The role of ^{123}I-diagnostic imaging in the follow-up of patients with differentiated carcinoma as compared to ^{131}I-scanning. Avoidance of negative therapeutic uptake due to stunning. *Clin. Endocrinol.* **55,** 515–21.

Simpson, W. (1990) Radioiodine and radiotherapy in the management of thyroid cancers. *Otolaryngol. Clin. North Am.* **23**, 509–21.

Sisson, J. (1997) Selection of the optimal agent for thyroid cancer. *Thyroid* **7**(2), 295–302.

Soh, E.Y., Sobhi, S.A., Wong, M.G. *et al.* (1996) Thyroid stimulating hormone promotes secretion of vascular endothelial factor in thyroid cancer cell lines. *Surgery* **120**, 944–7.

Stiller, C.A. (2001) Thyroid cancer following Chernobyl. *Eur. J. Cancer* **37**, 945–7.

Suarez, H.G., Du Villard, J.A., Caillou, B. *et al.* (1988) Detection of activated ras oncogenes in human thyroid carcinoma. *Oncogene* **5**, 403–6.

Takashima, S., Sone, S., Takayama, F. *et al.* (1998) Papillary thyroid carcinoma: MR diagnosis of lymph node metastasis. *Am. J. Neuroradiol.* **19**, 509–13.

Takeichi, N., Ezaki, H. and Dohi, K. (1991) A review of forty-five years study of Hiroshima and Nagasaki atomic bomb survivors. Thyroid cancer: reports up to date and a review. *J. Rad. Res. (Tokyo)* **32**(suppl.), 180–8.

Tan, R.K., Finley, R.K., Driscoll, D. *et al.* (1995) Anaplastic carcinoma of the thyroid: a 24 year experience. *Head Neck* **17**, 41–7.

Taylor, T., Specker, B., Robbins, J. *et al.* (1998) Outcome after treatment of high-risk papillary and non-Hurthle cell follicular thyroid carcinoma. *Ann. Intern. Med.* **129**, 622–7.

Tennvall, J., Lundell, G., Hallsquist, A. *et al.* (1994) Combined doxorubicin, hyperfractionated radiotherapy and surgery in anaplastic thyroid carcinoma. Report on two protocols. The Swedish Anaplastic Thyroid Cancer Group. *Cancer* **15**, 1348–54.

Thieblemont, C., Mayer, A., Dumontet, C. *et al.* (2002) Primary thyroid lymphoma is a heterogeneous disease. *J. Clin. Endocrinol. Metab.* **87**(1), 105–11.

Tisell, L.E., Hansson, G., Jansson, S. and Salander, H. (1986) Reoperation in the treatment of medullary thyroid carcinoma. *Surgery* **99**, 60–6.

Tisell, L.E., Dilley, W.G. and Wells, S.A. (1996) Progression of postoperative residual medullary thyroid carcinoma as monitored by plasma calcitonin levels. *Surgery* **119**, 34–9.

Tsang, R.W., Brierley, J.D., Simpson, W.J. *et al.* (1998) The effects of surgery, radioiodine and external radiation therapy on the clinical outcome of patients with differentiated thyroid carcinoma. *Cancer* **82**, 375–88.

Tubiana, M., Haddad, E., Schlumberger, M. *et al.* (1985) External radiotherapy in thyroid cancers. *Cancer* **55**, 2062–71.

Tucker, M.A., Jones, P.H.M., Boice, J.D. *et al.* (1991) Therapeutic radiation at a young age is linked to secondary thyroid cancer. The Late Effects Study Group. *Cancer Res.* **51**, 2885–8.

Tupchong, L., Hughes, F. and Harmer, C. (1986) Primary lymphoma of the thyroid: clinical features, prognostic factors and results of treatment. *Int. J. Radiat. Oncol. Biol. Phys.* **12**, 1813–21.

van Heerden, J.A., Grant, C.S., Grarib, H. *et al.* (1990) Long-term course of patients with persistent hypercalcitoninaemia after apparent curative primary surgery for medullary thyroid carcinoma. *Ann. Surg.* **212**, 395–401.

Vermiglio, F., Violi, M.A., Finocchiaro, M.D. *et al.* (1999) Short term effectiveness of low-dose radioiodine ablative treatment of thyroid remnants after thyroidectomy for differentiated thyroid cancer. *Thyroid* **9**, 387–91.

Vini, L. and Harmer, C. (2000) Radioiodine treatment for differentiated thyroid cancer. *Clin. Oncol.* **12**, 365–72.

Vini, L., Al-Saadi, A., Pratt, B. *et al.* (1998a) The role of radionuclide imaging (V-DMSA, ^{131}I-MIBG, ^{111}In-Octreotide) in medullary thyroid cancer. *Nucl. Med. Commun.* **19**, 384.

Vini, L., Al-Saadi, A., Pratt, B. *et al.* (1998b) Fertility after iodine therapy for thyroid cancer. *Br. J. Cancer* **78**(suppl.), 16.

Vini, L., Chittenden, S., Pratt, B. *et al.* (1998c) *In vivo* dosimetry of radioiodine in patients with metastatic differentiated thyroid cancer. *Eur. J. Nucl. Med.* **25**, 904 (OS-272).

Vini, L., Fisher, C., A'Hern, R. and Harmer, C. (1998d) Hurthle cell cancer of the thyroid: the Royal Marsden experience. *Thyroid* **8**(12), 1228.

Vini, L., Harmer, C. and Goldstraw, P. (1998e) The role of metastasectomy in differentiated thyroid cancer. *Eur. J. Surg. Oncol.* **24**, 348.

Vini, L., Pratt, B., Al-Saadi, A. *et al.* (1998f) Testicular dose from iodine-131 treatment for thyroid cancer and male fertility. *Eur. J. Nucl. Med.* **25**, 1058 (PS 300).

Vini, L., A'Hern, R., Fisher, C. *et al.* (1999) Differentiated thyroid cancer: the Royal Marsden experience. *Br. J. Cancer* **8**(suppl. 2), 112 (P336).

Voigt, W., Bulankin, A., Muller, T. *et al.* (2000) Schedule-dependent antagonism of gemcitabine and cisplatin in human anaplastic thyroid cancer cell lines. *Clin. Cancer Res.* **6**(5), 2087–93.

Waterhouse, J.A. (1991) Epidemiology of thyroid cancer. In Preece, P.E., Rosen, R.D. and Maran, A.G.D. (eds), *Head and neck oncology for the general surgeon* London: Saunders W.B., 1–10.

Wells, S.A., Chi, D.D., Toshima, K. *et al.* (1994) Predictive DNA testing and prophylactic thyroidectomy in patients at risk for multiple endocrine neoplasia type 2a. *Ann. Surg.* **220**, 237–50.

Wiseman, G.A. and Kvols, L.K. (1995) Therapy of neuroendocrine tumours with radiolabelled MIBG and somatostatin analogues. *Semin. Nucl. Med.* **25**, 272–8.

Yeung, S., Xu, G., Pan, J. *et al.* (2000) Manumycin enhances cytotoxic effect of paclitaxel on anaplastic thyroid carcinoma cell lines. *Cancer Res.* **60**(3), 650–6.

20

Endocrine system

ASHLEY B. GROSSMAN AND P. NICHOLAS PLOWMAN

THE 'APUD' CONCEPT AND APUDOMAS

In 1966 Pearse first described cytochemical and ultrastructural properties which were shared by several apparently disparate cell series in the body – initially adrenomedullary chromaffin cells, enterochromaffin cells, the corticotroph, the melanotroph, the pancreatic islet B cell and the thyroid C cell. Pearse later proposed the generic name APUD for these cells from the initial letters of their common cytochemical characteristics, which include Amine Precursor Uptake and Decarboxylase activity within the cells (Pearse, 1968). Since that time the list of APUD cells has expanded enormously. The structural and chemical similarity of APUD cells to neurons suggests a neural crest origin. Indeed, APUD cells of the adrenal medulla, melanocytes, thyroid, gastrointestinal tract and carotid body are of principally neuroectodermal lineage, and the ultrastructural similarity is true for all APUD cells. Pearse considered these cells as 'neuroendocrine' programmed cells derived from determined precursors arising in the embryonic epiblast, or in one of its principal early descendants. They are conceived as constituting a diffuse neuro-endocrine system (DNES) which may be regarded as a third division of the nervous system, products of which suppress, amplify or modulate the activities of the other two divisions (Pearse, 1979).

The DNES is divided into central and peripheral divisions, the first of which contains the cells of the hypothalamo-pituitary axis and the pineal gland, while the cells of the second division are primarily located in the gastrointestinal tract and pancreas, where they comprise the gastro-entero-pancreatic (GEP) endocrine cells. However, APUD cells are actually distributed throughout the body, where they are all prone to both hyperplasia and neoplasia, and more recent concepts have tended to decrease the emphasis on a truly discrete and distinct neuroendocrine 'network'.

This chapter will deal with many APUDomas, although pineal tumours and medullary carcinoma of the thyroid are covered in more detail in Chapters 15 and 19, respectively. The management of pituitary tumours will be discussed first, followed by some of the more important neoplastic conditions in other organs. Finally, the topic of adrenal cortical tumours is covered.

PITUITARY TUMOURS

Tumours of the pituitary gland are not uncommon and represent approximately 10 per cent of all intracranial tumours. However, this figure is usually based on mass lesions of the pituitary which present with visual field defects or local destructive changes, and it is now realized that small, hormonally active pituitary tumours are considerably less rare. These smaller tumours present due to the consequent endocrinopathy, most commonly sexual or reproductive dysfunction. The management of such tumours differs greatly from conventional oncological treatment programmes. Nevertheless, tumours of the pituitary form a continuum from the relatively insignificant minor aberration requiring no treatment, to the lethal massive tumour resistant to all modalities of therapy.

Classification

Pituitary tumours were originally classified in terms of their staining characteristics with conventional histological techniques and have been principally divided into eosinophilic, basophilic and chromophobe adenomas. In such a classification the majority of tumours are either eosinophilic or chromophobe, with 10–15 per cent being basophilic. However, the staining characteristics are principally a reflection of the nature of the secretory product of the cell, and these can now be visualized directly using immunohistochemistry or immunofluorescence in most instances. The hormone product of the cell is also more closely related to the function of the tumour, its clinical presentation and its biological behaviour, and is thus a more logical way to classify histological types. On this basis, pituitary tumours may be classified as either secretory or non-secretory, and the former may be subdivided on the basis of their principal hormone product.

The majority of secretory pituitary tumours are undoubtedly prolactin-secreting or prolactinomas. Prolactin-containing vesicles are usually seen throughout the cytoplasm, and may be released aberrantly from non-apical surfaces of the adenomatous lactotroph. Occasionally, tumours of the somatotrophs (growth hormone (GH)-secreting cells) have lactotrophs (prolactin-secreting cells) scattered throughout their substance, appearing as though such cells had become isolated in the tumour matrix during its growth. However, there are true mixed tumours consisting of adenomatous elements of both lactotrophs and somatotrophs, while certain tumours appear to secrete both prolactin and GH from the same cytoplasmic granules. It has been speculated that the latter tumours have arisen from a common prolactin–GH cell, the 'somato-mammotroph', which may be present in normal pituitary tissue or might represent a progenitor of both lactotrophs and somatotrophs.

Basophil tumours contain one of the glycoprotein hormones and most often consist of adenomatous corticotrophs. Adrenocorticotrophin (ACTH) is not itself glycosylated, but originates from a 31 kDa precursor, pro-opiomelanocortin, which has sugar moieties attached at several sites upstream and downstream to ACTH. Approximately 10–15 per cent of all pituitary tumours are classified conventionally as ACTH-secreting basophil adenomas. Tumours of the thyrotroph, secreting thyroid-stimulating hormone (TSH), are rare. However, approximately 30 per cent of all large pituitary tumours are said to be non-secretory or functionless, and are usually chromophobe adenomas. Many of these may be shown to contain secretory vesicles by electron microscopy. It appears increasingly likely that these tumours are related to, or originate from, gonadotrophin-secreting cells. They often secrete α-subunit, the common subunit of luteinizing hormone (LH), follicle stimulating hormone (FSH) and TSH, both *in vivo* and *in vitro*; in addition, secretion of LH and FSH may frequently be demonstrated *in vitro*.

However, they rarely present with clinical symptoms and signs of gonadotrophin excess: true gonadotrophinomas are extremely rare.

Tumours of the posterior pituitary are occasionally seen, but generally arise from the glial or non-endocrine elements of the gland. Secretory tumours of the neurohypophysis have not been described.

Treatment objectives

It is particularly important in the management of pituitary disorders that the objectives of treatment are clarified. In the case of pituitary tumours, the principal problems are due to the local mass effects of the lesion, especially visual impairment, partial or complete hypopituitarism, and the distant (target tissue) effects of any hormonal hypersecretion. Treatment thus needs to be directed towards reversing the neurological impairment and avoiding its recurrence, replacing any endocrine deficits and normalizing the levels of any elevated hormones. The disruption of the patient's lifestyle should be minimized; this implies careful consideration of the necessity for long-term medication, with its side-effects, and the frequency of outpatient visits and inpatient reassessments. It is difficult to optimize all these objectives, as it is usually the case that the more radical therapy with the highest probability of tumour sterilization will be most likely to induce long-term endocrine sequelae. Furthermore, individual patients may differ in their requirements for a normalization of their endocrine status and their desire to avoid medication. Not all neuroendocrine changes defined by subtle alterations during complex test procedures necessitate therapeutic intervention. It is, therefore, evident that often a range of treatment options can be made available, and a therapeutic plan optimized according to the needs and wishes of the individual patient.

Prolactinomas

Although there appears to be a gradation in size of pituitary tumours, the biological behaviour and clinical features of small and large tumours are so different that they are usually classified quite separately. This is particularly true in the case of prolactinomas. Microadenomas (also called microprolactinomas or small prolactinomas) are less than 1 cm in maximum diameter and are entirely contained within the pituitary fossa. Prolactin-secreting macroadenomas (also called macroprolactinomas or large prolactinomas) are greater than 1 cm in diameter and are likely to have expanded beyond the pituitary fossa to compress and distort adjacent structures.

MACROPROLACTINOMAS

Pituitary tumours associated with marked hyperprolactinaemia are usually prolactinomas, although mild hyperprolactinaemia may be seen in patients with hypothalamic or pituitary lesions regardless of aetiology. Prolactin is under predominantly inhibitory control by hypothalamic dopamine, such that any disruption of the portal vasculature may decrease the delivery of dopamine to the lactotrophs and elevate circulating prolactin. This is rarely very significant, although serum prolactin levels up to 6000 mU/L (normal range less than 400 mU/L) have been seen in association with non-secretory tumours in this region (Ross et al., 1985). For true prolactinomas there is an approximate correlation between tumour size and prolactin level.

The conventional first-line treatment for macroprolactinomas was previously transfrontal craniotomy, but is now virtually always by either transethmoidal or transsphenoidal removal. The trans-sphenoidal approach, originally devised by Harvey Cushing but particularly popularized by Guiot and Hardy, is used in conjunction with an operating microscope and intra-operative screening. It is most appropriate for tumours with minimal or small suprasellar extensions, although midline suprasellar extensions up to 2–3 cm can be tackled by this approach if the tumour is soft, as is most often the case. Surgical complications such as cerebrospinal fluid (CSF), rhinorrhoea and meningitis are very uncommon in experienced hands, and surgically induced diabetes insipidus (probably secondary to damage to the inferior hypophyseal artery) is usually transient. The tumour is decompressed from below and the suprasellar extension collapses centrally. The procedure is not appropriate for tumours with large lateral extensions, although even these may be attempted with an intra-operative endoscope, but with suprasellar lesions marked field defects may be improved rapidly and relatively easily. Nevertheless, trans-sphenoidal surgery for macroprolactinomas is rarely curative as small nests of cells are invariably left behind. Pituitary tumours are not encapsulated as such, but they compress surrounding tissue into a dense band around the bulk of the tumour and may frequently evaginate small processes into surrounding normal tissue, including the dura. It is, thus, not surprising that serum prolactin is rarely normalized following surgery, and that these tumours have a high recurrence rate. In general, large pituitary tumours causing visual impairment will almost certainly recur unless postoperative radiotherapy is also given. Recent data suggest that such radiotherapy reduces the risk of recurrence from >50 per cent to 3 per cent or less at 10 years (Brada et al., 1993).

In 1972 the ergot alkaloid bromocriptine was introduced into clinical practice in the treatment of galactorrhoea, and it was subsequently found that bromocriptine could activate the dopamine receptors on lactotrophs and inhibit the release of prolactin in patients with pathological hyperprolactinaemia. It became established that, in patients with prolactinomas, bromocriptine could lower, and usually normalize, the elevated serum prolactin, and it was thus used in conjunction with surgery and

radiotherapy in the management of such patients. It now also appears that the majority of prolactinomas will show significant tumour shrinkage with bromocriptine or one of the newer dopamine agonists; sometimes a large tumour with a significant suprasellar extension is transformed to a partially empty fossa. Although it had been reported that all significant shrinkage will occur within 6 weeks (Bassetti et al., 1984), it has been the general experience that prolactinomas may continue to show progressive diminution in size even after many months of treatment. These dramatic changes are also seen with other dopamine agonists such as pergolide, cabergoline and the non-ergot quinagolide. Cabergoline is particularly useful as it has a remarkably long duration of action and freedom from adverse effects: daily dosing in the acute phase can be tapered down to treatment with 0.5 mg twice or even once a week in time (Webster et al., 1994; Verhelst et al., 1999).

The remarkable efficacy of dopamine agonists in the treatment of prolactinomas, with over 90 per cent showing suppression of serum prolactin and some 80 per cent significant shrinkage, determines that this is now the initial treatment of choice. However, there is controversy regarding the optimal long-term therapy. In many cases the agent is simply tumoristatic, and on cessation the tumour will expand, sometimes extremely rapidly (Thorner et al., 1981). For example, Figure 20.1 demonstrates the serial CT scans of one of our patients treated for 2 years with bromocriptine who demonstrated marked tumour shrinkage; on cessation of therapy (due to patient non-compliance) for 5 weeks there was marked and rapid regrowth of the tumour to its former size. However, there are also reports of patients in whom withdrawal of dopamine agonist after several years of therapy did not induce tumour regrowth, at least in the short term.

One approach is to use external-beam radiotherapy if the dopamine agonist has caused the tumour to diminish considerably in size and is clear of the optic chiasm. Following our usual prescription (see below), there is evidence that the prolactin will fall when off treatment over a period of several years to within or near the normal range and, in female patients, fertility is likely (and conception safe) (Tsagarakis et al., 1991). Hypopituitarism may occur but will usually only involve GH in the short term: gonadotrophin deficiency is probable at 5–10 years after radiotherapy, but ACTH and TSH deficiency appear to be rare up to 10 years after treatment. It has been appreciated that the hypopituitarism that is described after irradiation may actually be due to radiation-induced hypothalamic morbidity – this is best documented for the growth hormone releasing hormone (GHRH)–GH axis (Grossman et al., 1984; Blacklay et al., 1986; Lam et al., 1986). Although the mediobasal hypothalamus is more likely to be in the radiation portal for larger adenomas, it seems likely, nevertheless, that the hypothalamus receives near to full dose in all pituitary radiotherapy plans. Following radiotherapy, interim

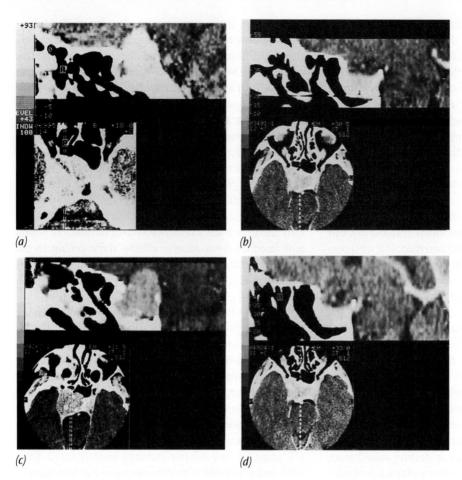

(a)

(b)

(c)

(d)

Figure 20.1 *CT scans of a patient with a large prolactinoma: (a) at presentation (prolactin = 206 000 mU/L) and (b) after 2 years bromocriptine treatment (prolactin = 170 mU/L); the patient then stopped bromocriptine treatment for 5 weeks and his tumour enlarged rapidly, as shown in (c) when his prolactin had risen to 50 000 mU/L. He was restarted on bromocriptine, and was rescanned 3 months later (d), by which time his serum prolactin had fallen to 400 mU/L.*

dopamine agonist therapy is used until serum prolactin is normalized.

As noted above, there is also a school of thought in favour of long-term use of dopamine agonist therapy alone, possibly with occasional withdrawal to assess drug and dose requirements. This is also increasingly our own practice. Where the serum prolactin or tumour mass are not sensitive to one or other of the dopamine agonists (and the use of the newer agents has greatly decreased drug intolerance as a reason for drug failure), then transsphenoidal surgery may be required.

In summary, dopamine agonist therapy has transformed the management of macroprolactinomas and surgery has been limited to those patients demonstrating residual chiasmal compression after attempted tumour shrinkage. Such surgery is rarely curative and may be complemented by radiotherapy. There remains uncertainty concerning the optimal long-term therapy; some centres advise tumour control with dopamine agonist therapy alone, while others would suggest that definitive treatment with radiotherapy will lead to gradual sterilization of the tumour with a low medium-term risk of hypopituitarism. However, the high incidence of GH deficiency, and the increasing acceptance of the morbidity associated with this state, has led to a decrease in enthusiasm for radiotherapy in this situation. With either approach, long-term close surveillance is necessary.

MICROPROLACTINOMAS

Autopsy series have revealed that some 10 per cent of adults harbour microprolactinomas within their pituitaries, although the secretory rate of these small tumours is sufficient to cause hyperprolactinaemia in only 0.1 per cent of female patients (Miyai *et al.*, 1986). The prevalence of prolactinomas is much less in men (around 0.005 per cent), presumably due to their different hormonal milieu; there is no evidence that oestrogen-containing oral contraceptives are oncogenic (Davis *et al.*, 1984). While many tests have been devised to differentiate patients with microprolactinomas from those with 'functional' or 'idiopathic' hyperprolactinaemia, there appears to be no clear dividing line between the two groups (Prescott *et al.*, 1985). High-resolution MRI scans reveal abnormalities of the pituitary fossa in the great majority of such patients, and thus most women with a serum prolactin persistently above 1000 mU/L are likely to harbour microprolactinomas. Most authorities would advise that primary treatment of secondary amenorrhoea in such patients should be with a dopamine agonist drug. The achievement of normoprolactinaemia is associated with the resolution of clinical symptoms and conception may be safely attempted. Previous estimates of pregnancy-induced tumour expansion were almost certainly exaggerated, and it seems unlikely that such problems will occur in more than 1 per cent of pregnancies, although authorities differ as to the exact incidence. When this does occur, it may be treated rapidly by the reinstitution of dopamine agonist therapy. However, treatment may need to be continued for many years as spontaneous resolution is only infrequently seen. Occasionally after treatment with a dopamine agonist serum prolactin may return to a level much lower than previously, such that therapy may be discontinued (Schlechte et al., 1989); this tends to occur particularly following a pregnancy (Rjosk et al., 1982). Very rarely there is progression from a microadenoma to a macroadenoma, with a gradual increase in tumour size and prolactin level and the onset of local compressive symptoms. In such a case the treatment should be adapted to that appropriate to a macroprolactinoma.

We now generally initiate treatment with cabergoline, starting with 0.25 mg once a week and increasing over 2–3 weeks to 0.5 mg once or twice a week. True resistance may occasionally be responsive to an alternative dopamine agonist such as bromocriptine or quinagolide, but this is rarely so in our experience. Most data on safety in inducing conception have been obtained with bromocriptine, with over 20 years evidence for a lack of teratogenicity or problems in pregnancy; to date, cabergoline and quinagolide appear to be equally safe, but the relative long-term experience is much more limited.

When the patient remains either intolerant or resistant to all available agents, surgical intervention may be considered. In large centres with an experienced surgeon, trans-sphenoidal microadenomectomy is immediately curative in 70–90 per cent of patients, the cure rate being inversely related to the serum prolactin level (Randall et al., 1983; Bevan et al., 1987). There is a risk of hypopituitarism but this is very low in the case of microadenomas. In our opinion trans-sphenoidal surgery is, on current evidence, an acceptable alternative to dopamine agonist therapy only for those patients unable or unwilling to take long-term medication: 10- and 15-year follow-up studies of these patients are awaited with interest.

If a patient's symptoms are minimal, it may be prudent in some cases to avoid treatment altogether. The natural history of the microprolactinoma is generally benign and many patients only require reassurance. There are, however, three provisos: first, since hyperprolactinaemia may cause subtle changes in sexual function and libido, every patient should at least be offered a trial of a dopamine agonist to assess their clinical response; secondly, hyperprolactinaemia is associated with oestrogen deficiency and long-term osteoporosis and therefore should necessarily be treated when it causes either complete amenorrhoea or low circulating oestradiol levels (Koppelman et al., 1984; Ciccarelli et al., 1988; Klibanski et al., 1988) (as a general rule we consider that menses should not be less frequent than every other month); finally, all patients should be followed up long-term to monitor the possible progression to a macroprolactinoma.

An alternative approach is simply to treat the patient with some form of oestrogen replacement therapy, to induce regular withdrawal bleeds and minimize the risk of osteoporosis. While such treatment has previously been contraindicated owing to the assumed risk of tumour growth stimulation, several recent studies have demonstrated that such a risk may be relatively small (Corenblum and Donovan, 1993).

Pregnancy in a patient with a microprolactinoma has a low but positive risk of oestrogen-induced tumour expansion. It is probably wise, therefore, to monitor such patients during pregnancy for clinical symptoms and visual-field defects. Postpartum, it is unlikely that the tumour will enlarge in size if it has not done so previously, and thus lactation should proceed normally.

Microprolactinomas appear to be extremely uncommon in men. It has been suggested that this is because the principal clinical symptom of impotence is not brought early to medical attention (Spark et al., 1982) and the patients are only seen if they progress to a macroprolactinoma some 10 years later. Whatever the case, the treatment of a male microprolactinoma follows the same guidelines as in the female. Finally, a number of patients with apparent hyperprolactinaemia and a relative absence of symptoms may have 'macroprolactinaemia', where biochemical assays show a spuriously elevated level due to prolactin's association with an immunoglobulin. This can be established by various techniques.

In summary, microprolactinomas generally have a benign natural history and therapy must take this into account. The mainstay of treatment is dopamine agonist therapy, supplemented where necessary by trans-sphenoidal surgery. Radiotherapy should only be considered where the tumour gives evidence of high growth characteristics such as local invasiveness or a very high serum prolactin, or there is resistance to dopamine agonist therapy.

Functionless tumours

The principal treatment modality for functionless tumours is surgical. A significant proportion (30–40 per cent) of large pituitary tumours are apparently functionless in so far as they are unassociated with a hypersecretory syndrome, although a proportion of these may be capable of secreting a hormonal product in very low quantities, so-called silent corticotroph adenomas or gonadotrophinomas. The rest are chromophobe adenomas, although sparse secretory granules and some endoplasmic reticulum may be evident ultrastructurally. These tumours usually present with visual defects and headache, but partial or complete hypopituitarism is often present on dynamic testing. Surgery is used to decompress the visual pathways, and nowadays this is almost always trans-sphenoidal in all but the most massive tumours (Harris et al., 1989). Early work suggested that pretreatment with dopamine agonists or somatostatin derivatives might cause tumour shrinkage, similar to that seen with prolactinomas, but prospective studies of patients carefully followed up for prolonged periods have shown that any shrinkage that does occur is relatively minor and does not obviate the need for surgery (Grossman *et al.*, 1985; Bevan *et al.*, 1992). It is conceivable that the slight but definite evidence of a decrease in apparent tumour size is due to a diminution in size of the normal lactotrophs or somatotrophs, but that once this has occurred, the inevitable tumour progression is seen. Whatever the mechanism, dopamine agonists or somatostain analogues only very rarely induce a clinically useful improvement in symptoms or signs in patients with functionless tumours, and we would advise urgent definitive treatment in patients with large pituitary tumours and a normal or minimally elevated serum prolactin (less than 1000 mU/L).

If the surgeon believes that he has achieved complete clearance, and if the tumour shows no obvious evidence of invasiveness, many centres would follow this by serial MRI scans (the first at 3–6 months) to assess recurrence. However, recent surveys have demonstrated significant recurrence rates even in those tumours thought to have been completely removed, of the order of 50 per cent at 10 years (Gittoes *et al.*, 1998; Turner *et al.*, 1999). It is therefore our own policy to mandate external-beam radiotherapy in the great majority of patients following surgery, accepting that there will be a gradual increase in hypopituitarism in those patients with postoperative preserved pituitary function. Of course, other factors need to be taken into account, such as the age of the patient and presence of pre-existing hormone defects, but, generally, adhering to this policy the rate of recurrence has been less than 5 per cent at 10 years. We have not seen clear evidence for second tumours or neurocognitive defects using our current prescription, although a second tumour rate of *c*. 3 per cent at 10 years has been reported.

However, there remains the group of patients whose serum prolactin varies between 1000 mU/L and 6000 mU/L, who may either have a prolactin-secreting tumour or a functionless tumour causing stalk compression hyperprolactinaemia. Both categories respond to dopamine agonists with a normalization of serum prolactin, but only the former are likely to show tumour regression. A short trial of cabergoline may be appropriate to test the response of the tumour, but this must be monitored extremely carefully by serial visual field testing and MRI scanning, as recourse to surgery is important in non-responders.

Silent corticotroph tumours, gonadotrophin-secreting and TSH-secreting tumours should be treated as functionless tumours. Some silent corticotroph tumours may progress to clinical Cushing's disease and should be treated particularly vigorously. TSH-secreting tumours may be sensitive to dopamine agonists or the somatostatin analogue octreotide, which may be given a therapeutic trial, while gonadotrophinomas may occasionally respond to gonadotrophin releasing hormone (GnRH) antagonists (and infrequently to GnRH agonists).

In summary, the primary approach to the functionless tumour is surgical, trans-sphenoidal in the great majority, followed either by radiotherapy or a policy of regular imaging and close monitoring.

Acromegaly and gigantism

Acromegaly is generally considered a rare condition with a prevalence in the UK of approximately 40 per million population. It is classically associated with a large pituitary tumour, the majority being macroadenomas. Very rarely, acromegaly due to somatotroph hyperplasia may be secondary to a carcinoid tumour secreting growth hormone releasing hormone (GHRH). However, as biochemical assays for GH have become more widespread, the spectrum of the disease has widened, with increasing numbers of patients having purely intrasellar tumours or microadenomas. This has, in turn, modified the balance of the principal therapeutic approaches. It is now clearly established that acromegaly is, when untreated, associated with an increased mortality, and definitive treatment aimed at lowering serum GH is indicated in almost all cases.

Trans-sphenoidal surgery is highly effective in substantially lowering mean GH levels in the majority of patients, although a surgical cure is rare. Older data often discussed a 'cure' of acromegaly as a mean serum GH, basally or after glucose, of less than 5, 10 or even 20 mU/L; however, it is now accepted that treatment should aim for a serum GH below a mean of 5 mU/L, as residual mean GH levels above 5 mU/L were still associated with elevated mortality (Bates *et al.*, 1993). There is also evidence that normalization of the insulin-like growth factor-I (IGF-I) level should be an additional goal of therapy (Swearingen *et al.*, 1998). Most series report a fall in mean serum GH to less than 5 mU/L in approximately 40–60 per cent of all acromegalic patients treated surgically, but this 'cure' rate rises to 65 per cent for microadenomas (Wass *et al.*, 1986; Nabarro, 1987); hypopituitarism occurs in approximately 25 per cent of such patients. External-beam radiotherapy has also been used extensively in the treatment of acromegaly and, although it induces a fall in mean serum GH, this may take several years to become fully effective (Fig. 20.2). In our own series of 80 patients treated with 45 Gy via a three-field technique, the 'cure' rate at 10 years was approximately 70–80 per cent, with levels below 10 mU/L in 90 per cent of patients at this time (Wass *et al.*, 1987). It has been argued that this fall is not paralleled by serum IGF-I levels (Barkan *et al.*, 1997), but most studies have confirmed its efficacy. In addition, normal pituitary function may be compromised. At 6 years we found that 25 per cent of patients who did not require replacement therapy beforehand now needed some form of therapy, including gonadal steroids (11 per cent), thyroxine (8 per cent) or hydrocortisone (16 per cent).

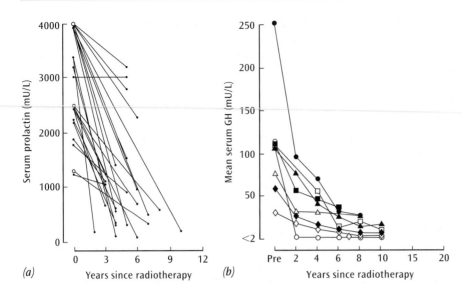

Figure 20.2 *Fall in serum prolactin (a) and serum GH (b) in patients with prolactinomas and acromegaly treated by our standard technique and prescription of external-beam radiotherapy (see text). In each case there was an initial rapid fall in the pathologically elevated hormone levels, followed by a more gradual decrease over succeeding years. Each data point was obtained with the patient at least 1 month off dopamine agonist therapy.*

Bromocriptine will lower GH levels in approximately 70 per cent of acromegalic patients, although in only 10 per cent of cases is this substantial. This is also seen more easily with cabergoline, although doses in the range 1–4 mg/week may be required. The long-acting analogue of somatostatin (octreotide, Sandostatin®) has also been used to lower elevated GH levels; most studies have demonstrated considerable falls in serum GH levels in the majority of patients (Lamberts *et al.*, 1985). The native drug must be given by regular subcutaneous injection, usually 100 μg three times a day, but new long-acting depot preparations may last from 1 to 6 weeks per dose. Inhibition of gut and pancreatic peptides may lead to mild diarrhoea/steatorrhoea and cholestasis, but this is rarely problematic. Inhibition of gastric acid output by octreotide has also been associated with chronic gastritis, but the clinical relevance of this has been disputed. More importantly, inhibition of gall bladder motility in conjunction with a change in bile composition, induced by octreotide, gives rise to a steady increase in the incidence of gallstones. Long-acting octreotide, Sandostatin LAR®, is given as a depot injection of 20–30 mg every 4–6 weeks, and after a gradual rise in drug level it produces a prolonged inhibition of GH release in more than 80 per cent of patients, often to within the 'safe' range (Lancranjan *et al.*, 1999). Long-acting lanreotide (Somatuline LA®) is more rapid in onset but only lasts for 1–2 weeks, although a longer-acting gel formulation can be given subcutaneously and lasts at least 4 weeks. Unfortunately, all of the long-acting preparations are extremely expensive, rendering their use as primary treatment for acromegaly inappropriate in all except a minority of patients. A growth hormone receptor, peguisamont, will normalize IGF-I levels in more than 90 per cent of patients when given as a daily subcutaneous injection, but is also likely to be expensive when it becomes available.

Dopamine agonists will occasionally cause marked tumour shrinkage in somatotroph tumours; this is more commonly seen with somatostatin analogues, but in this

case the degree of shrinkage is usually minor, *c.*10–30 per cent.

In summary, both surgery and radiotherapy can substantially lower GH levels in about 75 per cent of patients, but while the former is effective immediately the latter may take up to 10 years. Both are more efficacious with lower GH levels and may cause partial or complete hypopituitarism. For rapidity of results, therefore, primary therapy should usually be trans-sphenoidal adenomectomy, followed by external-beam radiotherapy for residual tumour (as revealed by elevated non-suppressible serum GH levels). The radiotherapy not only leads to a further fall in GH levels but also, as discussed above, greatly decreases the probability of regrowth or recurrence. Medical therapy is most useful as interim treatment, although it can occasionally be used as sole treatment in patients with very mild disease who are unenthusiastic about surgery, or in the very old. In all others, definitive treatment aimed at ablating the tumour and lowering serum GH and IGF-I levels into a 'safe' range is mandatory.

Cushing's disease

Cushing's disease, or pituitary-dependent Cushing's syndrome, is seen in 10–15 per cent of patients with pituitary tumours. Almost all cases are secondary to an ACTH-secreting basophil adenoma of the pituitary, although very occasionally patients with hyperplastic nests of basophilic cells have been reported. The tumours are usually small, and may often lie at or near the midline. Therapy is directed towards normalization of the excess secretion of corticosteroids and either removal of the tumour, or at least avoidance of its regrowth. In earlier years bilateral adrenalectomy was certainly able to treat the cortisol hypersecretion, but the pituitary tumour remained, and in most patients enlarged further in size, with a concomitant increase in circulating ACTH and hyperpigmentation – the development of Nelson's syndrome. In view of these data it is important that both the source of excess ACTH and the high levels of circulating corticosteroids are treated, which is most effectively obtained by trans-sphenoidal microadenomectomy. The tumours are usually small and in the best centres immediate 'cure' rates of 75–80 per cent are reported (Fahlbusch *et al.*, 1986; Swearingen *et al.*, 1999), although a true cure rate of around 50 per cent is produced when strict criteria are used. As the normal corticotrophs undergo long-term suppression (histologically demonstrable as Crooke's cell changes), serum cortisol postoperatively should be extremely low and patients will require long-term corticosteroid cover until their own pituitary–adrenal axis recovers. Recurrence appears to be uncommon (3–5 per cent) when patients are truly cured (i.e. many apparent recurrences simply reflect inadequate criteria for primary cure), but long-term follow-up is essential. Localization of these small tumours preoperatively may cause problems, although high-resolution MR scanning in conjunction with surgical expertise at the time of operation is certainly very helpful in demonstrating tumour tissue. Localization and lateralization within the fossa can also be greatly facilitated by means of the simultaneous measurement of plasma ACTH from bilateral catheters placed in the superior petrosal sinuses, following stimulation with corticotrophin releasing hormone (Kaltsas *et al.*, 1999). Where attempted microadenomectomy has not led to a cure, the alternatives are either to re-explore the fossa and perform a total hypophysectomy or to irradiate the pituitary tumour. Radiotherapy of ACTH-secreting tumours, as in the case of other hormonally active pituitary tumours, leads to a gradual fall in ACTH levels over several years and a decrease in requirements for medical therapy (Estrada *et al.*, 1997). In our series of 22 patients treated with radiotherapy and medical therapy alone, 60 per cent were cured 1–12 years after irradiation, in so far as they have been able to stop all medical treatment (Howlett *et al.*, 1989). It is particularly efficacious in childhood (Jennings *et al.*, 1977), where surgery may be hazardous or very difficult.

Metyrapone is an 11-hydroxylase steroid synthesis inhibitor that blocks the final stage in cortisol biosynthesis and which may be used to normalize cortisol levels while awaiting improvement following radiotherapy, or as preoperative preparation. The principal side-effects of metyrapone are associated with the increased shuttling of steroid precursors into adrenal androgen biosynthesis, causing menstrual problems and hirsutism in women; metyrapone may also be teratogenic. Mitotane (1,1-dichloro-2-(*o*-chlorophenyl)-1-(*p*-chlorophenyl)ethane; *o'p'*-DDD) is adrenolytic and causes a slow-onset fall in all adrenal products; impurities may render the drug toxic in high doses, but when pure it may be remarkably effective in lowering cortisol levels in the long term. Unfortunately, recent evidence suggests that *o'p'*-DDD causes severe hypercholesterolaemia; if essential, the drug may be combined with drugs that lower cholesterol such as lovastatin or simvastatin, but in general this finding has severely limited its long-term use. The antifungal agent ketoconazole is also adrenolytic and is finding increasing favour as first-line medical therapy of hypercortisolaemia, especially in young women. It should be used with care as it is potentially hepatotoxic. However, these drugs are only useful when the primary pituitary pathology has been tackled by other means. Intravenous etomidate is available to lower cortisol levels where oral therapy is not possible (Drake *et al.*, 1998a).

Bilateral adrenalectomy had been of mainly historical interest, but with the advent of laparoscopic adrenalectomy its place is again being recognized. Rather than persevere with long-term control with adrenostatic agents, both adrenals can be removed at a single procedure, or staged unilateral procedures. Indeed, it has been claimed recently that if control is achieved after pituitary radiotherapy and unilateral adrenalectomy, then the long-term results are equivalent to successful trans-sphenoidal surgery. Bilateral adrenalectomy may also be considered in the treatment of patients with the ectopic ACTH syndrome, where the source of ACTH has defied localization. It is uncertain as to whether pituitary irradiation following adrenalectomy for Cushing's disease will necessarily prevent the onset of Nelson's syndrome, but we consider that it is best given prophylactically. Our data suggest that the onset of Nelson's syndrome may be reduced, or at least delayed, by such treatment (Jenkins *et al.*, 1995). In Nelson's syndrome, or where the ACTH-secreting tumour presents as a macroadenoma, surgical cure is rare and radiotherapy usually essential. When the tumour recurs following conventional radiotherapy, 'radiosurgery' may still be applicable (*see* below). Such tumours may be extremely invasive and prone to recurrence, and often prove to be amongst the most difficult to treat in neuro-endocrinology. Certain drugs, such as bromocriptine, cyproheptadine, sodium valproate and octreotide, may be tumoristatic in some patients, and should certainly be tried in difficult cases. Unfortunately, these tumours may prove resistant to all modalities of treatment.

In summary, ACTH-secreting pituitary tumours are usually small and best-treated surgically, with radiotherapy reserved for postoperative residual tumour or recurrence. Of the drugs currently available for blocking cortisol production while definitive treatment is awaited, none is perfect but metyrapone, *o'p'*-DDD and ketoconazole may play a useful role. Drugs which may interact with central neurotransmitters are rarely necessary or effective, except where other therapeutic approaches have failed.

Pituitary radiation technique and dose prescription

The conventional external radiotherapy technique for pituitary tumours requires a head-fixation device – usually a plastic head-shell with the patient supine. Modern radiotherapy simulator facilities, together with modern-generation MRI scanning (in both transaxial and coronal planes), allow the field sizes to be minimized. The volume for irradiation comprises the boundaries of the tumour on the imaging procedures plus 0.5 cm in all planes. If a tumour has shrunk following medical therapy, then the post-drug imaging tumour size is used. If the tumour has been resected surgically, the preoperative tumour size is used for planning; we have documented evidence of suprasellar recurrences in such cases referred from other units where the postoperative radiation volume was confined to the fossa.

By such planning techniques, a day-to-day set-up reproducibility within 2 mm is achieved routinely, and a three-field technique using fixed portals has been adopted – two laterals and an antero-oblique or direct superior field (6–8 MeV X-rays are used at St Bartholomew's Hospital).

There have been differences in the dose prescriptions, but those publications employing 50 Gy or more have not produced superior control rates to those employing 44–45 Gy: our recommended prescription to the tumour volume is 45 Gy in 25 fractions over 35 days. The prescription utilizes daily dose fractions of 1.8 Gy and therefore respects the well-documented association between radiation damage to the nervous system and high fraction size. Utilizing this technique and dose prescription in the treatment of over 700 patients with pituitary adenoma presenting to St Bartholomew's Hospital, we have not encountered late optic chiasmal damage, but late defects in hypothalamo-anterior pituitary function may occur. Radiation-induced second tumours may also occur, but in our experience are extremely rare.

Newer forms of radiotherapy include stereotactically delivered, single high-dose radiation, or 'radiosurgery'. While there are initial attractions for using highly 'focused' radiation therapy methods in dealing with a benign tumour confined to the fossa, nevertheless, there are other considerations that should be taken into account: the optic chiasm lies just rostral to the pituitary fossa and is more sensitive to single high doses of radiation. Secondly, too highly focused radiation produces partial fossa radiation, and the initial results of gamma unit therapy for pituitary adenomas were not encouraging. However, recently, a good study by Landolt et al. (1998) (see review by Plowman, 1999) compared the endocrine results of treating acromegaly by gamma-unit radiosurgery or conventionally fractionated radiotherapy, and concluded that there is equivalence with regard to efficacy (albeit with considerably shorter follow-up in the radiosurgery-treated patients), with the extra bonus from radiosurgery being the faster normalization of the growth hormone levels following this high-dose, single-shot radiation therapy.

The question as to which radiation modality is appropriate for which patients will be much discussed in the next decade. The current authors remain of the persuasion that conventional radiotherapy should be the first choice for most macroadenoma therapy, but that there is a selective role for radiosurgery in the therapy of small, discrete and low-lying adenomas, and a very definite place in the therapy of recurring adenomas after conventional radiotherapy – particularly, in our experience, those recurring in the cavernous sinuses. We therefore espouse conventionally fractionated radiotherapy for the initial treatment of most pituitary tumours, and utilize single-treatment focused radiotherapy, radiosurgery, as salvage treatment.

Chemotherapy

Since the third edition of this text, there have been a number of anecdotal reports in the literature concerning the use of cytotoxic chemotherapy for patients with inoperable pituitary tumour recurrence after radiotherapy. However, in spite of a variety of treatment regimens, both single and multiple, with and without platinum-based drugs, there is little evidence that any is of substantial benefit. Pituitary tumours appear to be relatively chemoresistant (Kaltsas and Grossman, 1998; Kaltsas et al., 1998).

Replacement therapy

All patients with pituitary tumours require endocrine evaluation, often with dynamic function tests, to determine their requirements for replacement therapy. In steroid insufficiency, hydrocortisone should be given in a dose necessary to mimic the normal cireadian rhythm of cortisol. This is usually 10 mg on rising, 5 mg at around lunchtime and then a further 5 mg in the early evening; this should be doubled during any febrile illness. Parenteral hydrocortisone may be required during surgery and in the instance of vomiting or diarrhoea. Thyroid replacement consists of a dose of thyroxine, usually 0.1–0.2 mg once daily, to normalize circulating thyroxine levels. For gonadal replacement, women should be given cyclical oestrogen and progesterone, while men will require injectable depot testosterone every 3–4 weeks, testosterone undecanoate orally, testosterone implants (where available), or one of the newer testosterone patches. For fertility, regular injections of FSH and LH, or their analogues, are required, but this should be carried out in specialist units. The treatment of GH deficiency in adults remains highly controversial. There is good evidence that such deficiency is associated with decreased lean body mass and increased adipose tissue, and undoubted psychological dysfunction (Cuneo et al., 1992). This latter usually takes the form of increased lethargy and diminished vitality. There are also data suggesting that mortality, principally associated with premature atherosclerosis, is increased (Rosen and Bengtsson, 1990). We have generally found a marked improvement in general well-being and in the quality of life in patients with severe GH deficiency treated with replacement GH in a gradually incremental dose-titration regimen (Drake *et al.*, 1998b). GH deficiency should be treated vigorously with biosynthetic GH injections in children. Finally, diabetes insipidus responds to therapy with desmopressin (DDAVP®) subcutaneously (1–2 μg, once or twice daily), intranasally (10–20 μg daily), or orally (50–100 μg twice or three times daily).

PARATHYROID ADENOMA AND CARCINOMA

The normal adult parathyroid glands vary from 3 to 6 mm in diameter. The upper glands arise from the fourth pharyngeal pouch and are fairly constantly located by the upper poles of the thyroid. The lower glands arise, in conjunction with the thymus, from the third pharyngeal pouch, and this thymic association accounts for the, not infrequent, ectopic location of these glands in the mediastinum.

More than 95 per cent of parathyroid tumours are adenomas, the remainder being carcinomas. The tumours may present because of the complications of hypercalcaemia (primary hyperparathyroidism), such as nephrolithiasis, although asymptomatic hypercalcaemia revealed by routine screening is increasingly common. The tumours are more common in females (prevalence approximately 1 : 1000) and are equally frequently discovered in young adults as in the elderly. The discovery biochemically of a raised serum calcium, a lowered serum phosphate and an elevated plasma parathyroid hormone (PTH) level is diagnostic of the condition. Treatment is by surgical excision, but the critical question concerns which patients should be referred for surgery. Most authorities agree that a patient who has nephrolithiasis, renal dysfunction, nephrogenic diabetes insipidus or a serum calcium >3 mmol/L requires early surgery. Asymptomatic patients may be regularly observed, although recent data suggest that even these run a significant risk of osteoporosis, and some 10 per cent will require operation within 10 years (Silverberg *et al.*, 1999). Furthermore, many apparently 'asymptomatic' patients show improved mood and/or cognition following parathyroidectomy. It is therefore a matter of fine clinical judgement if, and when, to offer surgery to such patients.

Localization is not usually difficult in the hands of an experienced surgeon but may be aided by preoperative localization techniques such as subtractive isotope scanning (sestamibi), ultrasound, CT and/or MRI. Probably the optimal current modalities are ultrasound and sestamibi subtraction scanning. Sestamibi scanning is particularly helpful, and indeed should always be used before re-operation following failed surgical exploration (Johnston *et al.*, 1996).

Adenomas may consist of chief cells, oxyphil cells or water-clear cells. Carcinomas may also present as primary hyperparathyroidism, but are very rare: pathologically, they may be suspected if they show a trabecular pattern, while the presence of mitoses is diagnostic of carcinoma. Treatment comprises complete resection where possible; postoperative PTH levels will indicate the completeness of this operation. The operation may need to comprise a radical thyroidectomy and formal dissection of neck nodes, but this is not *de rigueur* and individual assessment is necessary as to the correct operative procedure. In a pooled series, Schantz and Castleman (1973) found a 30 per cent recurrence rate, with less than one-half of patients dying within 5 years of the disease, indicating the very slow growth pattern of this tumour. Refractory hypercalcaemia is often a considerable problem in these patients, but it may respond to oestrogen therapy. More recently, mithramycin and certain diphosphonate derivatives such as pamidronate (APD) have also been used to control persistent hypercalcaemia. While pamidronate is less effective in hyperparathyroidism than in malignant hypercalcaemia, either it, or one of its congeners (e.g. clodronate), should always be considered in such patients.

GASTRO-ENTERO-PANCREATIC ENDOCRINE TUMOURS

Another major group of apudomas are the gastro-enteropancreatic neuroendocrine tumours. Insulinoma is the most common (incidence: 1/1 000 000/year) and generally presents with 'Whipple's triad' of hypoglycaemic symptoms (headache, slurred speech, pallor, palpitations, sweating/fainting and impaired consciousness) associated with a demonstrable low blood glucose and alleviated by glucose administration; plasma insulin and/or C-peptide levels remain unsuppressed in the presence of the hypoglycaemia. Gastrinomas have an incidence of approximately 1/10 000 000/year, and present with intractable peptic ulceration (the Zollinger–Ellison syndrome); other functioning tumours include VIPomas (watery diarrhoea syndrome), glucagonomas (rash, weight loss, diabetes), somatostatinomas (diabetes, steatorrhoea, gall stones, weight loss, hypochlorhydria), GRFoma (acromegaly due to ectopic secretion of growth hormone-releasing factor) and ACTHoma (Cushing's syndrome). These are all relatively rare, and overlap with non-pancreatic gut-derived neuroendocrine tumours with and without the carcinoid syndrome. A significant proportion of these are associated with multiple endocrine neoplasia type I, and all have a capacity for metastatic spread, although this is rare for insulinomas and, even when present, may be compatible with long survival. Diagnosis is based on clinical suspicion, serum tests and imaging. Serum tests involve the gut hormone profile and other relevant endocrine testing.

Depending on location, CT and MRI have a 40–85 per cent detection rate for primary gastro-entero-pancreatic endocrine tumours, and as imaging techniques advance, the ability to locate tumours down to 5 mm or even less is possible. Selective angiography continues to play a (minor) role in localization, while simultaneous sampling of hepatic venous blood after arterial injections of calcium gluconate (a secretagogue for insulinoma; Doppman *et al.*, 1995) or secretin (a secretagogue for gastrinoma) during this procedure may 'regionalize' the tumour. Further 'non-functional' imaging is offered by endoscopic or peroperative ultrasound. A significant proportion of such tumours may also be localized by scanning with the radionuclide [^{123}I]*meta*-iodobenzylguanidine (MIBG): positive uptake allows for consideration of [^{131}I]MIBG as therapy. Recent data suggest that 6-monthly treatment with *c.* 200 mCi doses is safe and well-tolerated, and may improve survival, although bulk tumour regression is unusual (Mukherjee *et al.*, 2001). Scanning with somatostatin analogues such as ^{111}In-labelled octreotide or lanreotide is more frequently positive in these tumours (Kaltsas *et al.*, 2001), and early trials suggest that yttrium-99-labelled analogues, which are short range β-emitters, may be therapeutically beneficial. However, there is a family of at least five octreotide receptors: for example, octreotide binds only to subtype 2 receptors (expressed on 80 per cent of gastrinomas, VIPomas and glucagomas, but only 60 per cent of insulinomas), while a different analogue may have better potential as far as therapy is concerned. In the future, it may well be that a cocktail of different subtype-specific analogues specific for a particular patient's tumour will be prepared for therapy, all the molecules being tagged with yttrium-90 or a related β-emitter. Therefore we now have two radionuclide approaches in the treatment of such tumours, although the optimal sequencing of administration, possibly even simultaneously, has yet to be investigated fully.

However, the initial treatment for all these tumours should be the removal of all resectable disease, where possible. Gut neuroendocrine tumours frequently pursue an indolent course over many years, and where systemic therapy is ineffective or delayed in efficacy, surgical debulking or hepatic arterial embolization of large hepatic metastases may well be indicated. Chemotherapy with 5-fluorouracil and lomustine (CCNU), streptozotocin and/or doxorubicin is traditional chemotherapy, with a 30–50 per cent symptomatic and/or biochemical response rate, a 10–20 per cent tumour response rate; however, the treating physician must wait longer than for most other tumours to observe a tumour response, as these tumours regress very slowly and the oncologist should not expect any significant volume reduction or similar marker response in the first 3–6 cycles. We still employ this type of therapy for slow-growing tumours. For the faster-growing malignant neuroendocrine tumours, platinum/etoposide chemotherapy, as for small cell lung cancer, is currently our optimal therapy. However, we currently reserve intensive chemotherapy for tumours which are negative on radionuclide scanning, the latter modality of therapy currently being our first-line approach.

As noted above, many of these tumours are very slow growing, and symptomatic palliation of the sequelae of their endocrine products is an extremely important part of their management. In particular, diazoxide will often (but not invariably) inhibit neoplastic insulin secretion, while omeprazole (sometimes in high doses) may protect from the consequences of hypergastrinaemia. In addition, somatostatin derivatives such as octreotide or lanreotide can be very useful in inhibiting hormonal hypersecretion; both are available as long-acting formulations, with lanreotide having a more rapid onset of action.

CARCINOID TUMOURS

Carcinoid tumours most commonly occur in the gastrointestinal tract and arise from the argentaffin cells, essentially a pathological staining technique which identifies certain types of neuroendocrine cells. The most common sites are the appendix, the small bowel and the rectum. The overall incidence of appendiceal carcinoids is 1 in 150 to 1 in 1000, according to appendix histology reports. The histopathological reporting of appendiceal carcinoids is relatively more common in appendix specimens of young adults than in the elderly, which mirrors the incidence of argentaffin cells in the body, the total number of which rises and then falls in later life. This observation also implies an involution of some benign carcinoid tumours. Appendiceal carcinoid tumours are almost invariably benign; those rare examples that have metastasized have all been more than 2 cm diameter (itself a remarkable rarity for a carcinoid at this level).

In the Mayo Clinic experience, small bowel carcinoids occur with the following distribution: duodenum, 2 per cent; jejunum, 7 per cent; ileum, 89 per cent (with the distal ileum being much more commonly the site of origin than the proximal ileum); and 2 per cent occur in a Meckel's diverticulum: they are often multicentric. Most small bowel carcinoids are small and arise deep in the crypts. Tumours with metastatic potential are almost always more than 2 cm in diameter, but this malignant potential is otherwise difficult to assess by the morphology of the cells. Once the tumour reaches the bowel mesentery, it engenders a massive fibrous reaction. This contracts the mesentery and this 'encasement phenomenon' frequently leads to bowel obstruction, the most common presenting feature of extramural small bowel carcinoid tumours. Metastases almost invariably spread to the liver, to which they may be confined for long periods; metastatic carcinoids have one of the longest doubling times of any malignant human tumour. Despite enormous hepatomegaly, patients may remain well for long periods. Indeed, the mean natural history from operation on a malignant small bowel carcinoid to death is between 7 and 10 years.

The 'carcinoid syndrome' is a clinical syndrome due to the secretion by carcinoid tumour cells of vasoactive amines, particularly 5-HT (5-hydroxytryptamine), prostaglandins and tachykinins. The syndrome is virtually confined to patients with bulky liver metastases, ordinarily rarely seen in patients in whom the urine fails to contain abnormally high quantities of the 5-HT catabolite, 5-HIAA (5-hydroxyindole acetic acid). There is an approximate correlation between disease severity and the level of urinary 5-HIAA, although there is little doubt that many of the symptoms and signs are not a direct consequence of 5-HT excess. The dominant clinical features of the carcinoid syndrome are the flushing attacks, which may be precipitated by stress and alcohol, as well as calcium and pentagastrin infusions. It is difficult to demonstrate a rise in the blood 5-HT levels during a flushing attack, but recent studies have demonstrated a close association with circulating tachykinins. Diarrhoea, often with colic, is the second major clinical feature of the carcinoid syndrome, and this also does not seem to relate to 5-HT secretion. Other components to the carcinoid syndrome include bronchial asthma and congestive or right-sided cardiac failure due to tricuspid or pulmonary stenosis.

5-HT is not the only vasoactive substance or hormone secreted by gut carcinoids; motilin, substance P, prostaglandins, insulin and ACTH are other documented examples, some of which contribute to the syndrome. Nevertheless, serotonin (5-HT) antagonists may partially ameliorate the diarrhoea and colic and occasionally the flushing. By inhibiting tryptophan 5-hydroxylase, parachlorophenylalanine (PCPA) may have a role in particularly severe cases. However, in the great majority of patients the tumours are somatostatin-receptor positive, and both octreotide and lanreotide (see below) can be of major symptomatic benefit.

Operable disease is resected where possible, e.g. appendicectomy or right hemicolectomy if the appendiceal base nodes and mesentery are involved. Indeed, excision of discrete hepatic metastases of this very slowly growing tumour is also perceived to be advantageous. Nevertheless, the tumour seems to exhibit a strong desmoplastic response, whereby surrounding tissues readily become bound down to overlying gut, and surgical excision can be very difficult.

With regard to cytotoxic drug therapy, four conventional cytotoxic drugs have single-agent activity results of 20 per cent or more in the classic indolent carcinoid; these are Adriamycin (doxorubicin), 5-fluorouracil, streptozotocin and DTIC (dacarbazine). The combination of 5-fluorouracil plus Adriamycin or streptozotocin is active, and we still employ such therapy for slow-growing disease. However, for faster-growing disease, aggressive and atypical carcinoids, the combination of cis-platinum and etoposide is favoured, as for the more malignant islet cell tumours. Again, similar to other gastro-entero-pancreatic tumours noted above, radionuclide therapy is of increasing importance, and if the relevant tracer scanning is positive (Kaltsas et al., 2001), they have displaced

chemotherapy as far as initial systemic therapy is concerned (Mukherjee et al., 2001). As for the other tumours, the optimal radionuclide treatment stategies have yet to be defined.

In 1983 Oberg et al. reported that leucocyte interferon therapy ameliorated the carcinoid syndrome due to metastatic midgut carcinoids, and led to prompt decreases in urinary 5-HIAA levels, although these workers failed to demonstrate shrinkage of the tumour masses. The same Swedish group of workers later reported the treatment of 22 patients with advanced, malignant pancreatic apudomas with leucocyte interferon and demonstrated both endocrine and oncological remissions (Eriksson et al., 1986). These authors raise the fascinating, yet speculative, hypothesis that, for a carcinoid tumour to grow, tumour-derived hormones are required as autocrine growth factors; interferon may control cell growth via inhibition of such factors. Unfortunately, this method has not been substantiated in recent years and few are now employing interferon in the treatment of this disease.

In refractory cases with massive and painful hepatomegaly or carcinoid syndrome, hepatic artery embolization with gelatin sponge has satisfactorily palliated the disease for some time. Although there were some early reports that low-dose whole-liver radiotherapy similarly palliated the disease, this optimism may not be well founded.

Like appendiceal carcinoids, rectal carcinoids are usually benign. Rectal carcinoids occur above the dentate line and almost invariably on the anterior or lateral walls, almost never posteriorly. Above 13 cm, carcinoids are extremely rare in the sigmoid, descending, transverse and ascending colons, until the caecum and appendix are reached. When colonic carcinoids occur, they are usually malignant. Tumours more than 2 cm diameter should always be suspected of malignancy, and abdoperineal resections may well be appropriate for the rare, large, rectal carcinoid tumour.

Carcinoid tumours may arise at other sites – bronchial carcinoids are particularly well known and are the most common 'benign' bronchial tumour. Bronchial carcinoids arise endobronchially and frequently in the major bronchi, more commonly in the right lung. They usually present clinically due to haemoptysis or bronchial obstruction, and although resection (lobectomy, pneumonectomy) is usually curative, histopathologically these tumours usually show some evidence of local invasion. Indeed, approximately 5 per cent of bronchial carcinoids show node metastases and, in a considerably higher proportion, the histopathologist reports the primary tumour as containing 'cellular atypia'.

PHAEOCHROMOCYTOMA

Phaeochromocytomas are uncommon tumours with a prevalence of 1 in 10 000, and are also a rare finding in the hypertensive population (less than 1 per cent). These occur most commonly in adults (with a median presentation age of 35–55 years cited in the literature), with an equal sex incidence. There is a familial association in the multiple endocrine neoplasia type II syndrome (MEN II), von Hippel–Lindau syndrome, and (rarely) in neurofibromatosis (NF1). The majority of phaeochromocytomas are benign tumours, with some 10 per cent being malignant, although higher estimates of malignancy have been cited in association with MEN II. Approximately 90 per cent of phaeochromocytomas originate in the adrenal medulla and may be bilateral; other primary sites include the sympathetic chain, bladder, thorax and carotid arch. Histologically, the tumour cells are polygonal and contain cytoplasmic granules which contain the catecholamine stores.

Clinically, phaeochromocytomas may present due to their release of pressor amines into the vasculature; this release may occur in spontaneous bursts or be provoked by emotion, exertion, posture, foods or tumour handling. These episodes of catecholamine release may lead to the 'intermittent attacks' classically ascribed to this tumour. During such attacks a patient feels apprehension, usually with a headache and often pallor, sweating and palpitation; the blood pressure is usually very high during attacks, which may last from a few minutes to several hours. However, approximately half of all patients suffer sustained hypertension. Flushing is not an important clinical feature of phaeochromocytomas.

The diagnosis is suspected in any patient with attacks such as described and is remembered as a rare (but usually curable) cause of hypertension. The diagnosis is made biochemically by the demonstration of increased catecholamine formation, best quantified as total catecholamine excretion in the urine over a 24-hour period. Plasma levels of catecholamines are of lesser sensitivity than urinary catecholamines, but may be useful if measured during a suspect event. Urinary catecholamine metabolites such as vanillylmandelic acids (VMAs) and metanephrines do not have the sensitivity required of a screening test, and have now been replaced by direct catecholamine assay (by either high pressure liquid chromatography/electrochemical detection (HPLC/ECD) or gas chromatography–mass spectrometry (GCMS)) in most major centres. Suppression tests for differentiating high circulating catecholamines due to stress from phaeochromocytoma have been used (e.g. pentolinium, clonidine), although none has found universal favour. Even very small tumours secrete excess noradrenaline, and true 'adrenaline-secreting tumours' are exceptionally rare; dopamine excess is often associated with metastatic malignant tumours. Adrenal tumours are localized most commonly by CT/MRI scanning, but venous sampling at different levels in the inferior vena cava and elsewhere allows confirmation of tumour origin and detection of multiple tumours. It is particularly useful in the assessment of possible bilateral tumours in patients with one

of the genetic syndromes. Unlike arteriography, venous cannulation and sampling is unlikely to provoke a hypertensive crisis, but it would be wise to undertake full adrenoceptor blockade before this investigation. [123I]MIBG radionuclide scanning can be useful in confirming that a mass is catecholamine-secreting (more precisely, catecholamine-uptaking), and can also be extremely helpful in locating extra-adrenal or metastatic sites.

The treatment of phaeochromocytoma is surgical resection, which usually implies adrenalectomy. Most centres are now able to offer this via the laparoscopic approach. Preoperative preparation of the patient with several days of α_1- (e.g. phenoxybenzamine) and β_1-adrenergic blockade is very important. Without such preparation the relaxation of vascular tone following tumour removal may leave the patient acutely hypovolaemic. However, with several days' administration of particularly α-adrenergic blockade, vascular tone and normal blood volume can be largely and homeostatically restored before the operation, although great anaesthetic care is still vital during any phaeochromocytoma operation. Surgical resection of the primary may still have a role in the management of the patient with low bulk metastases. External-beam radiotherapy has little place in the management of phaeochromocytoma, and cytotoxic chemotherapy is as for the other malignant apudomas. In inoperable, metastatic cases, [131I]MIBG therapy may offer good long-term control (Mukherjee et al., 2001; Fig. 20.3); it is at least equally important to produce adequate adrenergic blockade to avoid pressor crises. Where phenoxybenzamine is poorly tolerated, newer α-blockers such as doxazosin may be tried.

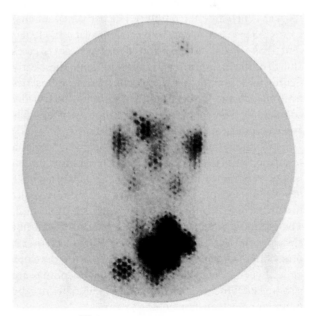

Figure 20.3 [123I]MIBG scan of a patient with a metastatic paraganglioma. Metastatic deposits are seen in the mediastinum and in the skull. Uptake in the nasopharynx and salivary glands is not pathological.

The adrenal medullary neuroblastomas are discussed in Chapter 41.

MULTIPLE ENDOCRINE NEOPLASIA

This title describes a group of syndromes, often familial, in which more than one endocrine gland in an individual undergoes hyperplasia or tumour formation. In 1954 Wermer described the association of tumours of the parathyroid, pituitary and pancreas within individuals and their families – noting an autosomal dominant inheritance. This syndrome is referred to as Wermer's syndrome or MEN I. In 1961 Sipple reported a patient with two phaeochromocytomas and a malignant thyroid tumour; Sipple's review of the literature demonstrated that there was, indeed, an association between phaeochromocytoma and thyroid cancer (now known to be medullary thyroid cancer). This association is now referred to as Sipple's syndrome or MEN IIA, and is also inherited as an autosomal dominant condition, often with parathyroid adenomas. A variant syndrome (MEN IIB) has been described where, in addition, the patient manifests mucosal neuromas and other phenotypic features, but without parathyroid disease. The genes for both MEN syndromes have now been identified, although their precise functions are still unclear.

MEN I (Wermer's syndrome)

Ballard et al. (1964) reviewed 85 patients with this syndrome. In order of frequency, the involved endocrine glands were: parathyroids (88 per cent), pancreatic islets (80 per cent), anterior pituitary (65 per cent), adrenal cortex (38 per cent) and thyroid parafollicular cells (19 per cent). Pairs of glands were involved in 60 per cent of cases and all of the first three glands in 40 per cent. These early figures have now been reviewed in several large series from the US and Europe, and they appear to be broadly compatible. There is also an association with lipomas and carcinoids, at least in certain families.

The parathyroid glands usually undergo hyperplasia or adenoma formation, and are usually the first abnormality to be noted; the islet cells of the pancreas either develop an adenoma or carcinoma or, more rarely, diffuse hyperplasia, and often the tumours are multifocal. The pituitary gland develops adenomas, usually but not always secretory; there is a particular predilection for prolactinoma formation. The adrenal cortex develops either hyperplasia or adenomas. Thyroid adenomas are also well documented. Adenomas in all these sites may be functioning or non-functioning.

The gene mutated has been identified as producing a peptide product, menin, which binds to and may repress the transcription factor JunD. Unfortunately, there is no common area of mutation throughout this large gene,

and little genotype–phenotype correlation. Genetic screening is therefore not usually possible outside of a research setting (Bassett et al., 1998).

MEN II (Sipple's syndrome)

Usually, but not invariably, this autosomal dominantly inherited condition presents in young adult life. In the most common form a medullary carcinoma of the thyroid is associated with a phaeochromocytoma. This association is common enough to warrant screening for the other tumours (by calcitonin or urinary catecholamines estimations) in any patient presenting with either one. Occasionally, patients present with parathyroid hyperplasia or adenoma. In other patients the medullary thyroid carcinoma and phaeochromocytoma occur with multiple small, subcutaneous and/or submucosal neuromas of the oral cavity and lips, plus autonomic ganglioneuromatosis and a Marfanoid habitus. These syndromes appear to result from a neural crest dysplasia during embryonic development. The gene involved is the ret oncogene, encoding a membrane-spanning peptide with multiple cysteines, which acts as the receptor for glial-cell derived neurotropic factor, GDNF. Mutations are clustered around a small number of 'hot spots', which renders screening relatively straightforward and which has greatly assisted in patient counselling (Chew and Eng, 1995; Marsh et al., 1997).

More recently it has been recognized that these syndromes are not mutually exclusive, and that occasional patients may be seen with features of both MEN I and MEN II syndromes – so-called 'overlap' MEN.

With regard to management, each endocrine disease should be treated on its own merits, but the clinician must remain wary to the possible development of other aspects of disease. Thus, it is reasonable to screen all phaeochromocytoma patients for the presence of a medullary thyroid carcinoma, and vice versa, while patients with pancreatic endocrine tumours, at the very least, require assessment of serum calcium and radiology of the pituitary fossa. Where the gene mutation has been identified, it is now common to offer total thyroidectomy to all affected individuals with MEN II at, or near, 5 years of age. The cloning of the genes for these conditions has considerably altered screening policies and follow-up plans for these families.

Other genetic disorders associated with phaeochromocytomas

The von Hippel–Lindau syndrome is an autosomal dominant condition in which tissues appear to sense hypoxia inappropriately due to mutations of the gene product elongin: this leads to a failure to break down vascular endothelial growth factor (VEGF), which in turn causes the development of vascular malformations in the eye (retinal angiomas) and central nervous system, especially cerebellar and spinal haemangioblastomas (Maxwell *et al.*, 1999). In addition, there is a high incidence of phaeochromocytomas, especially bilateral. However, for reasons which are unclear, there is also a very high incidence of renal cell carcinomas: these are prone to be multiple and recurrent, and patients may require sequential partial nephrectomies followed at some stage by bilateral nephrectomy and long-term dialysis. The optimal screening strategy is not well-defined, but any renal lesion on imaging screening must be treated as possibly malignant until proven otherwise. The gene is very large and there are no 'hot spots', so family screening is only possible if the index mutation has been identified.

In neurofibromatosis type 1, phaeochromocytomas occur with a frequency of around 1 per cent. They should be treated as for the sporadic disease.

ADRENAL CORTICAL TUMOURS

Although benign adrenal cortical adenomas are not infrequently found at autopsy, most are non-functioning and of no clinical importance. The majority of functioning cortical adenomas are found in female patients. Those occurring in prepubertal patients tend to present with virilization, while those in postpubertal patients present with Cushing's syndrome. An adrenal cortical adenoma producing aldosterone (Conn's syndrome) is a very rare cause of hypertension. Diagnostic tests include the endocrine demonstration of non-suppressible and excessive levels of circulating adrenal steroids, and the appropriate diagnostic imaging tests (e.g. MR/CT scanning). Treatment is by surgical excision (adrenalectomy).

Increasingly, small adrenal tumours are being detected on imaging of the abdomen by CT or MRI for an ostensibly unrelated reason – the so-called 'incidentaloma'. Various algorithms have been proposed to differentiate tumours that require surgical removal as opposed to those that can be simply monitored, most attempting to exclude a hypersecretory state biochemically, and assess the probability of adrenal malignancy on imaging criteria (Peppercorn *et al.*, 1998). In general, small (<3 cm) lesions with 'benign' imaging characteristics can be simply observed and rescanned at intervals, although the recent finding of 'subclinical Cushing's syndrome' in a significant minority, if not the majority, of such patients, renders the production of clear clinical guidelines extremely difficult.

Adrenal carcinoma is a rare malignancy afflicting women slightly more frequently than men (Didolkar *et al.*, 1981), and the mean age of presentation in women may be lower than in men (Nader *et al.*, 1983). Overall, the disease tends to afflict a younger age group than most carcinomas (median ages at presentation cited in the literature being in the range 37–55 years). The relative incidence of functioning to non-functioning carcinomas is equal; it seems to be unaffected by the age of presentation and may not be different between the sexes, although in the MD Anderson Hospital series more women had functioning tumours (Nader *et al.*, 1983). Interestingly, the left adrenal has been documented as the more common site of primary disease (Didolkar *et al.*, 1981; Nader *et al.*, 1983); rarely, the disease is bilateral.

The most common clinical presenting feature of this disease is abdominal symptomatology (fullness, indigestion, nausea, vomiting, pain or the patient finding an abdominal lump). However, other prominent symptoms include weight loss, weakness, fever, features of tumour function and symptoms due to metastases. Between one-quarter and one-third of patients with primary adrenal carcinoma have clinical evidence of endocrine dysfunction at presentation, most commonly Cushing's syndrome, often supplemented by virilism. A slightly higher fraction of the patients have chemical endocrine evidence of abnormal hormone secretion, i.e. subclinical dysfunction. Obviously, the weight gain of Cushing's syndrome may be absent from patients with an aggressive malignant tumour and the virilism may be more marked. As for suspected cortical adenomas, diagnostic tests include the demonstration of excessive and non-suppressible levels of adrenal steroids and relevant abdominal diagnostic imaging.

At least half of all patients presenting with adrenal cortical carcinoma will have metastatic disease at the time of diagnosis, the most common sites of spread being lung, liver, peritoneum and abdominal nodes. For patients with localized disease or disease apparently confined to this region, radical surgery is the recommended definitive treatment, with an appreciable cure rate for early disease 'completely' resected. Radiotherapy to the tumour bed is recommended if there is disease at resection margins or in regional nodes, and we use a parallel opposed pair of megavoltage portals to 40 Gy mid-plane in 20 fractions, considering the position of the adjacent kidney carefully.

For patients with more advanced adrenal carcinomas there is no curative treatment, and orthodox cytotoxic chemotherapy has yet to make any impact on this disease. Nevertheless, there is one specific therapy: *o'p'*-DDD (Hutter and Kayhoe, 1966). This drug causes necrosis and atrophy of normal adrenal tissue and also of differentiated adrenal carcinoma cells. In the original study a steroid response rate of 72 per cent was recorded, with an objective regression of tumour in 34 per cent. Other workers have subsequently confirmed this drug's usefulness in adrenal carcinoma, but responses may be slow (months) and there may be associated gastrointestinal (vomiting and diarrhoea) and neuromuscular side-effects (lethargy and weakness) in many patients so treated. However, recent data suggest that doses in the region of 1–3 g per day are as effective as much higher doses, and are better tolerated. The dose is slowly accumulative, and measurement of the drug level 2–4 months after treatment will allow precise control of therapeutic dosimetry. The drug is not myelosuppressive. Glucocorticoid cover is essential for patients receiving $o'p'$-DDD therapy. Alternative drugs are suramin and gossypol, but neither has been shown to have a major impact on disease progression. Cushing's syndrome due to adrenal carcinoma may also be palliated by metyrapone therapy (250 mg to 1 g four times daily, commencing at the lower dose). Metyrapone inhibits 11β-hydroxylase (the enzyme converting the metabolically inactive 11-deoxycortisol to cortisol), as previously discussed under Cushing's disease. When used as sole therapy, metyrapone may be highly effective, although the dose may require careful adjustment so as not to cause an Addisonian crisis. Some patients experience pronounced gastrointestinal upset on metyrapone and occasional allergic reactions have been documented. Metyrapone also shunts steroid precursors into androgen precursors and may cause marked virilism. The antifungal drug ketoconazole is also showing increasing promise. It should be noted that in any patient with Cushing's syndrome secondary to an adrenal tumour, removal or ablation of the tumour will need to be followed by long-term steroid-replacement therapy until the suppressed hypothalamo-pituitary-adrenal axis has recovered function: this may take several years. Similarly, removal of a Conn's tumour is often followed by transient hyperkalaemia. Phaeochromocytomas do not appear to inhibit adrenaline release from the normal adrenal gland, and there is, if anything, a tendency for patients with such tumours to remain mildly hypertensive postoperatively.

SIGNIFICANT POINTS

- Pituitary tumours represent around 10 per cent of intracranial tumours, and may cause problems due to local compression, hormone hypersecretion or hypopituitarism.
- For the majority of tumours, primary therapy is trans-sphenoidal surgery, followed where appropriate by external-beam radiotherapy to diminish the chance of recurrence.
- Prolactin-secreting tumours can frequently be shrunk with dopamine agonist therapy, thereby avoiding pituitary surgery.
- Growth hormone hypersecretion by growth hormone-secreting tumours may be well controlled medically with somatostatin analogues, while awaiting the effect of more definitive treatment.

- Parathyroid adenomas are common and best treated surgically.
- Modern chemotherapy regimens can often provide useful life extension in neuroendocrine tumours of the gut, while hormone oversecretion will usually respond to somatostatin analogue therapy. Radionuclide therapy with labelled MIBG or a somatostatin derivative should be considered in most cases.
- Phaeochromocytomas are an uncommon cause of hypertension: they are often not diagnosed in life and may be associated with a variety of genetic disorders.
- Adrenal 'incidentalomas' are being found increasingly: treatment protocols are designed to exclude hypersecretory states and adrenal carcinoma.
- Adrenal carcinomas are frequently highly malignant and refractory to therapy, but the adrenolytic drug mitotane is usually worth a therapeutic trial.

KEY REFERENCES

Bevan, J.S., Webster, J., Burke, C.W. and Scanlon, M.F. (1992) Dopamine agonists and pituitary tumor shrinkage. *Endocr. Rev.* **13**, 220–40.

Chew, S.L. and Eng, C. (1995) Multiple endocrine neoplasia type 2 and related genetic conditions. *Curr. Opin. Endocrinol. Dis.* **2**, 121–6.

Drake, W.M., Perry, L.A., Hinds, C.J., Lowe, D.G., Reznek, R.H. and Besser, G.M. (1998) Emergency and prolonged use of intravenous etomidate to control hypercortisolemia in a patient with Cushing's syndrome and peritonitis. *J. Clin. Endocrinol. Metab.* **83**, 3542–4.

Newell-Price, J., Trainer, P., Besser, M. and Grossman, A.B. (1998) The diagnosis and differential diagnosis of Cushing's syndrome and pseudo-Cushing's states. *Endocr. Rev.* **19**, 647–72.

Silverberg, S.J., Shane, E., Jacobs, T.P., Siris, E. and Bilezikian, J.P. (1999) A 10-year prospective study of hyperparathyroidism with or without parathyroid surgery. *N. Engl. J. Med.* **341**, 1249–55.

Turner, H.E., Stratton, I.M., Byrne, J.V., Adams, C.B.T. and Wass, J.A.H. (1999) Audit of selected patients with nonfunctioning pituitary adenomas treated without irradiation – a follow-up study. *Clin. Endocrinol.* **51**, 281–4.

REFERENCES

Ballard, H.S., Frame, B. and Hartsock, R.J. (1964) Familial multiple endocrine adenoma-peptic ulcer complex. *Medicine* **43**, 481–516.

Barkan, A.L., Halasz, I., Dornfield, K.J. *et al.* (1997) Pituitary irradiation is ineffective in normalizing plasma insulin-like growth factor-1 in patients with acromegaly. *J. Clin. Endocrinol. Metab.* **82**, 3187–91.

Bassett, J.H., Forbes, S.A., Pannett, A.A. *et al.* (1998) Characterization of mutations in patients with multiple endocrine neoplasia type 1. *Am. J. Hum. Genet.* **62**, 232–44.

Bassetti, M., Spada, A., Pezzo, G. and Giannattasio, G. (1984) Bromocriptine treatment reduces the cell size in human macroprolactinomas: a morphometric study. *J. Clin. Endocrinol. Metab.* **58**, 268–73.

Bates, A.S., Van't Hoff, W., Jones, J.M. and Clayton, R.N. (1993) An audit of outcome of treatment in acromegaly. *QJM* **86**, 293–300.

Bevan, J.S., Adams, C.B.T., Burke, C.N. *et al.* (1987) Factors in the outcome of transsphenoidal surgery for prolactinomas and non-functioning pituitary tumour, including pre-operative bromocriptine therapy. *Clin. Endocrinol.* **26**, 541–56.

Bevan, J.S., Webster, J., Burke, C.W. and Scanlon, M.F. (1992) Dopamine agonists and pituitary tumor shrinkage. *Endocr. Rev.* **13**, 220–40.

Blacklay, A., Grossman, A., Ross, R.J.M. *et al.* (1986) Cranial irradiation for cerebral and nasopharyngeal tumors in children – evidence for the production of a hypothalamic defect in growth hormone release. *J. Endocrinol.* **108**, 25–9.

Brada, M., Rajan, B., Traish, D. *et al.* (1993) The long-term efficacy of conservative surgery and radiotherapy in the control of pituitary adenomas. *Clin. Endocrinol.* **38**, 571–5.

Chew, S.L. and Eng, C. (1995) Multiple endocrine neoplasia type 2 and related genetic conditions. *Curr. Opin. Endocrinol. Dis.* **2**, 121–6.

Ciccarelli, E., Savino, L., Carlevatto, V. *et al.* (1988) Vertebral bone density in non-amenorrheic hyperprolactinaemic women. *Clin. Endocrinol.* **28**, 1–6.

Corenblum, B. and Donovan, L. (1993) The safety of physiological estrogen plus progestin replacement therapy and with oral contraceptive therapy in women with pathological hyperprolactinemia. *Fertil. Steril.* **59**, 671–3.

Cuneo, R.C., Salomon, F., MeGauley, G.A. and Sonksen, P.H. (1992) The growth hormone deficiency syndrome in adults. *Clin. Endocrinol.* **37**, 387–97.

Davis, J.R.E., Selby, C. and Jeffcoate, W.J. (1984) Oral contraceptive agents do not affect serum prolactin in normal women. *Clin. Endocrinol.* **20**, 427–34.

Didolkar, M.S., Bescher, A., Elias, E.G. and Moore, R.H. (1981) Natural history of adrenal cortical carcinoma. A clinicopathologic study of 42 patients. *Cancer* **47**, 2153–61.

Doppman, J.L., Chang, R., Fraker, D.L. *et al.* (1995) Localization of insulinomas to regions of the pancreas by intra-arterial stimulation with calcium. *Ann. Intern. Med.* **123**, 269–73.

Drake, W.M., Perry, L.A., Hinds, C.J., Lowe, D.G., Reznek, R.H. and Besser, G.M. (1998a) Emergency and prolonged use of intravenous etomidate to control hypercortisolemia in a patient with Cushing's syndrome and peritonitis. *J. Clin. Endocrinol. Metab.* **83**, 3542–4.

Drake, W.M., Coyte, D., Camacho-Hubner, C. *et al.* (1998b) Optimising growth hormone replacement therapy by dose titration in hypopituitary adults. *J. Clin. Endocrinol. Metab.* **83**, 3913–19.

Eriksson, B., Oberg, K., Alm, G. *et al.* (1986) Treatment of malignant endocrine pancreatic tumours with human leucocyte interferon. *Lancet* **ii**, 1307–9.

Estrada, J., Boronat, M., Mielgo, M. *et al.* (1997) The long-term outcome of pituitary irradiation after unsuccessful transsphenoidal surgery for Cushing's disease. *N. Engl. J. Med.* **336**, 172–7.

Fahlbusch, R., Buchfelder, M. and Muller, O.A. (1986) Transsphenoidal surgery for Cushing's disease. *J. R. Soc. Med.* **79**, 262–9.

Gittoes, N.J.L., Bates, A.S., Tse, W. *et al.* (1998) Radiotherapy for non-functioning pituitary tumours. *Clin. Endocrinol.* **48**, 331–7.

Grossman, A., Lytras, N., Savage, M.O. *et al.* (1984) Growth hormone-releasing factor: comparison of two analogues and demonstration of hypothalamic defect in growth hormone release after radiotherapy. *BMJ* **288**, 1785–7.

Grossman, A., Ross, R., Charlesworth, M. *et al.* (1985) The effect of dopamine-agonist therapy on large functionless pituitary tumours. *Clin. Endocrinol.* **22**, 679–86.

Harris, P.E., Afshar, F., Coates, P. *et al.* (1989) The effects of the transsphenoidal surgery on endocrine function and visual fields in patients with functionless pituitary tumours. *QJM* **265**, 417–27.

Howlett, T.A., Plowman, P.N., Wass, J.A. *et al.* (1989) Metyrapone and pituitary irradiation as primary treatment for Cushing's disease. Presented at 7th International Congress of Endocrinology, Quebec, July 1–7, Abstract 892.

Hutter, A.M. and Kayhoe, D.E. (1966) Adrenal cortical carcinoma. Results of treatment with o'p'DDD in 138 patients. *Am. J. Med.* **41**, 581–91.

Jenkins, P.J., Trainer, P.J., Plowman, P.N. *et al.* (1995) The long-term outcome after adrenalectomy and prophylactic radiotherapy in Cushing's syndrome. *J. Clin. Endocrinol. Metab.* **80**, 165–71.

Jennings, A.S., Liddle, G.W. and Orth, D.N. (1977) Results of treating childhood Cushing's disease with pituitary irradiation. *N. Engl. J. Med.* **297**, 957–62.

Johnston, L.B., Carroll, M.C., Britton, K.E., Lowe, D., Besser, G.M. and Grossman, A. (1996) The accuracy of parathyroid gland localisation in primary hyperparathyroidism using sestamibi radionuclide imaging. *J. Clin. Endocrinol. Metab.* **81**, 346–52.

Kaltsas, G.A. and Grossman, A.B. (1998) Pituitary carcinoma: a review. *Pituitary* **1**, 69–81.

Kaltsas, G.A., Mukherjee, J.J., Plowman, P.N., Monson, J.P., Grossman, A.B. and Besser, G.M. (1998) The role of cytotoxic chemotherapy in the management of aggressive and malignant pituitary tumors. *J. Clin. Endocrinol. Metab.* **83**, 4233–8.

Kaltsas, G.A., Giannulis, M.G., Newell-Price, J. *et al.* (1999) A critical analysis of the value of simultaneous inferior petrosal sinus sampling in Cushing's disease and the occult ectopic adrenocorticotropin syndrome. *J. Clin. Endocrinol. Metab.* **84**, 487–92.

Kaltsas, G., Korbonits, M., Heintz, E. *et al.* (2001) Comparison of somatostatin analog and metaiodobenzylguanidine (MIBG) radionuclides in the diagnosis and localisation of advanced neuroendocrine tumors. *J. Clin. Endocrinol. Metab.* **86**, 895–902.

Klibanski, A., Biller, B.M.K., Rosenthal, D.I. *et al.* (1988) Effects of prolactin and estrogen deficiency in amenorrheic bone loss. *J. Clin. Endocrinol. Metab.* **67**, 124–30.

Koppelman, M.C.S., Kurtz, D.W., Morrish, K.A. *et al.* (1984) Vertebral body bone mineral content in hyperprolactinemic women. *J. Clin. Endocrinol. Metab.* **59**, 1050–4.

Lam, K.S.L., Wang, C., Yeung, T.T. *et al.* (1986) Hypothalamic hypopituitarism following cranial irradiation for nasopharyngeal carcinoma. *Clin. Endocrinol.* **24**, 643–51.

Lamberts, S.W.J., Uitterlinder, P., Verschoor, L. *et al.* (1985) Long-term treatment of acromegaly with the somatostatin analogue, SMS 201–995. *N. Engl. J. Med.* **313**, 1576–80.

Lancranjan, I., Atkinson, A.B., and the sandostatin LAR group (1999) Results of a European multicenter study with sandostatin LAR in acromegalic patients. *Pituitary* **1**, 105–14.

Landolt, A.M., Haller, D., Lomax, N. *et al.* (1998) Stereotactic radiosurgery for recurrent surgically treated acromegaly: a comparison with fractionated radiotherapy. *J. Neurosurg.* **88**, 1002–8.

Marsh, D.J., Mulligan, L.M. and Eng, C. (1997) RET proto-oncogene mutations in multiple endocrine neoplasia type 2 and medullary thyroid carcinoma. *Horm. Res.* **47**, 168–78.

Maxwell, P.H., Wiesener, M.S., Chang, G.W. *et al.* (1999) The tumour suppressor protein VHL targets hypoxia-inducible factors for oxygen-dependent proteolysis. *Nature* **399**, 271–5.

Miyai, K., Ichihara, K., Kondo, K. and Mori, S. (1986) Asymptomatic hyperprolactinaemia and prolactinoma in the general population – mass screening by paired assays of serum prolactin. *Clin. Endocrinol.* **25**, 549–54.

Mukherjee, J.J., Kaltsas, G.A., Islam, N. *et al.* (2001) Treatment of metastatic carcinoids, pheochromocytomas, paragangliomas and medullary carcinoma of the thyroid with ^{131}I-metaiodobenzylguanidine. *Clin. Endocrinol.* **55**, 47–60.

Nabarro, J.D.N. (1987) Acromegaly. *Clin. Endocrinol.* **26**, 481–512.

Nader, S., Hickey, R.C., Sellin, R.V. and Samaan, N.A. (1983) Adrenal cortical carcinoma. A study of 77 cases. *Cancer* **52**, 707–11.

Oberg, K., Funa, K. and Alm, G. (1983) Effects of leucocyte interferon on clinical symptoms and hormone levels in patients with mid-gut carcinoid tumours and carcinoid syndrome. *N. Engl. J. Med.* **309**, 129–33.

Pearse, A.G.E. (1968) Common cytochemical and ultrastructural characteristics of cells producing polypeptide hormones (the APUD series) and their relevance to the thyroid and ultimobronchial C cells and calcitonin. *Proc. R. Soc. Lond.* **170**, 71–80.

Pearse, A.G.E. (1979) Embryology of the diffuse neuroendocrine system and its relationship to the common peptides. *Fed. Proc.* **38**, 2288–91.

Peppercorn, P.D., Reznek, R.H. and Grossman, A.B. (1998) Incidentally-discovered adrenal masses. *Clin. Endocrinol.* **48**, 379–88.

Plowman, P.N. (1999) Pituitary adenoma radiotherapy – when, who and how? *Clin. Endocrinol.* **51**, 265–71.

Prescott, R.W.G., Johnston, D.G., Taylor, P.K. *et al.* (1985) The inability of dynamic tests of prolactin and TSH secretion to differentiate between tumorous and non-tumorous hyperprolactinaemia. *J. Endocrinol. Invest.* **8**, 49–54.

Randall, R.V., Laws, E.R., Abboud, C.F. *et al.* (1983) Transsphenoidal microsurgical treatment of prolactin-secreting pituitary adenomas, results in 100 patients. *Mayo Clinic Proc.* **58**, 108–21.

Rjosk, H.-K., Fahlbusch, R. and von Werder, K. (1982) Spontaneous development of hyperprolactinaemia. *Acta Endocrinol.* **100**, 333–6.

Rosen, T. and Bengtsson, B.A. (1990) Premature mortality due to cardiovascular disease in hypopituitarism. *Lancet* **336**, 285–8.

Ross, R.J.M., Grossman, A., Bouloux, P., Rees, L.H., Doniach, I. and Besser, G.M. (1985) The relationship between serum prolactin and immunocytochemical staining for prolactin in patients with pituitary macroadenomas. *Clin. Endocrinol.* **22**, 227–36.

Schantz, A. and Castleman, B. (1973) Parathyroid carcinoma: a study of 70 cases. *Cancer* **31**, 600–5.

Schlechte, J.A., Dolan, K., Sherman, B. *et al.* (1989) The natural history of untreated hyperprolactinemia: a prospective analysis. *J. Clin. Endocrinol. Metab.* **68**, 412–18.

Silverberg, S.J., Shane, E., Jacobs, T.P., Siris, E. and Bilezikian, J.P. (1999) A 10-year prospective study of hyperparathyroidism with or without parathyroid surgery. *N. Engl. J. Med.* **341**, 1249–55.

Sipple, J.H. (1961) The association of phaeochromocytoma with carcinoma of the thyroid gland. *Am. J. Med.* **31**, 163–6.

Spark, R.F., Wills, C.A., O'Reilly, G. *et al.* (1982) Hyperprolactinaemia in males with and without pituitary macroadenomas. *Lancet* **ii**, 129–32.

Swearingen, B., Barker, F.G., Katznelson, L. *et al.* (1998) Long-term mortality after transsphenoidal surgery and adjunctive therapy for acromegaly. *J. Clin. Endocrinol. Metab.* **83**, 3419–26.

Swearingen, B., Biller, B.M.K., Barker, F.G. *et al.* (1999) Long-term mortality after transsphenoidal surgery for Cushing's disease. *Ann. Intern. Med.* **130**, 821–4.

Thorner, M.O., Perryman, R.L., Rogol, A.D. *et al.* (1981) Rapid changes of prolactinoma volume after withdrawal and reinstitution of bromocriptine. *J. Clin. Endocrinol. Metab.* **53**, 180–4.

Tsagarakis, S., Grossman, A., Plowman, P.N. *et al.* (1991) Megavoltage pituitary irradiation in the management of prolactinomas: long-term follow-up. *Clin. Endocrinol.* **34**, 399–40.

Turner, H.E., Stratton, I.M., Byrne, J.V., Adams, C.B.T. and Wass, J.A.H. (1999) Audit of selected patients with nonfunctioning pituitary adenomas treated without irradiation – a follow-up study. *Clin. Endocrinol.* **51**, 281–4.

Verhelst, J., Abs, R., Maiter, D. *et al.* (1999) Cabergoline in the treatment of hyperprolactinemia: a study of 455 patients. *J. Clin. Endocrinol. Metab.* **84**, 2518–22.

Wass, J.A.H., Laws, E.R., Randall, R.V. and Sheline, G.E. (1986) The treatment of acromegaly. *Clin. Endocrinol. Metab.* **15**, 683–707.

Wass, J.A.H., Plowman, P.N., Jones, A.E. and Besser, G.M. (1987) The treatment of acromegaly by external pituitary irradiation and drugs. In *Growth hormone, growth factors and acromegaly*. New York: Raven Press, 199–206.

Webster, J., Piscitelli, G., Polli, A., Ferrari, C.I., Ismail, I. and Scanlon, M.F. (1994) A comparison of cabergoline and bromocriptine in the treatment of hyperprolactinemic amennorea. *N. Engl. J. Med.* **331**, 904–9.

Wermer, P. (1954) Genetic aspects of adenomatosis and endocrine glands. *Am. J. Med.* **16**, 363–71.

21

Breast

JOHN YARNOLD

INCIDENCE AND MORTALITY

Approximately 24 000 women develop breast cancer every year in the UK. The age-specific incidence rate rises fourfold between the ages of 35 and 70 years, and the risk of developing breast cancer by the age of 80 years is 1 in 12. Fifteen thousand women die of the disease annually, representing 20 per cent of female cancer mortality. The age-standardized breast cancer mortality rate in England and Wales is among the highest in the world, the lowest being recorded in Japan. However, there has been a 15 per cent reduction in UK breast cancer mortality since 1990 (Peto, 1998). The explanation is probably more effective treatment, the fall in mortality appearing too early to credit the national mammographic screening programme.

CANCER GENETICS AND ENDOCRINOLOGY

Cancer genetics

Somatic mutation theory postulates the accumulation of mutations in somatic genes that progressively deregulate normal breast cell behaviour. The cell in question is believed to be the epithelial cell lining the terminal duct lobular unit. Several processes predispose to mutation, including exposure to mutagens, for example ionizing radiation, and mitogens such as oestrogen. The latter is thought to predispose to malignant transformation by increasing the risk of unrepaired DNA replication errors during stimulated cell division. However generated, somatic mutations activate or inactivate genes responsible for regulating genomic stability, cell growth, invasion and metastases (Osin et al., 1998; Invarsson, 1999). Genes which are activated and overexpressed in 20–30 per cent of breast cancers include the epidermal growth factor receptor (EGFR or c-erbB1), c-erbB2 (neu or HER2), bcl-2 and c-myc. Overexpression of c-erbB1, c-erbB2 or c-myc is associated with high nuclear grade, negative oestrogen receptor (ER) status and a poor prognosis (Hung and Lau, 1999). Overexpression of the bcl-2 gene is correlated with well-differentiated tumours and ER positivity. Overexpression of c-erbB2 is also reported in roughly 40 per cent of patients with solid, comedo-type duct carcinoma in-situ (DCIS), but not in invasive lobular carcinoma. Genes inactivated in a proportion of breast cancers include the Rb, p53 and NM23 tumour suppressor genes.

Inheritance of highly penetrant dominant mutations accounts for 5–10 per cent of breast cancer cases, and typically presents with a strong family history. The most important examples include the *BRCA1* and *BRCA2* genes, which account for about 2 per cent and 1 per cent, respectively, of breast cancer incidence (Yang and Lippman, 1999). Affected individuals are born heterozygous for the gene defect, but random loss of the normal allele in a breast duct epithelial cell leads to breast cancer in about 60 per cent of individuals, often at a young age. The biochemical basis of the cellular effect is a DNA repair defect, rendering the genome prone to mutation, a state referred to as genomic instability. Genomic instability is also introduced by an inherited defect in the *p53* gene, a rare cause of breast cancer predisposition (Li–Fraumeni syndrome). Ataxia telangiectasia (A-T) is a rare autosomal recessive disorder, that renders homozygous individuals more vulnerable to cancer via an elevated risk of mutation. A-T heterozygotes constitute 0.5–1 per cent of the general population and are probably breast-cancer prone (Lavin, 1998).

Low-penetrance mutations and genetic polymorphisms confer a lower increment of cancer risk than *BRCA1* and *BRCA2*, but may contribute a more important component of genetic predisposition than realized previously (Roberts *et al.*, 1999). Genetically determined differences in the expression or function of genes regulating steroid metabolism, for example, represent one of many possible mechanisms.

Molecular endocrinology

Oestrogen regulates the transcription of endocrine-responsive genes in tumours and normal tissues via oestrogen receptor (ER), a nuclear transcription factor. The ER has distinct amino-acid sequences (domains) determining oestrogen binding, ER dimerization, DNA binding and regulation of oestrogen-responsive genes. Activation of ER is initiated by the binding of one molecule of oestrogen (E_2) to one ER molecule, followed by pairing (dimerization) of two E_2/ER molecules (Jordan, 1998). The E_2/ER dimer binds specific DNA sequences (oestrogen response elements, EREs) in the vicinity of oestrogen-responsive genes. Gene transcription depends on specific E_2/ER domains responsible for the activating function (AF). There are two such domains, AF-1 and AF-2, the latter requiring bound oestrogen for gene activation. The progesterone receptor (PgR) is one of many oestrogen-regulated proteins, and its expression in a breast tumour indicates a functional oestrogen-response pathway.

Tamoxifen also induces dimerization of ER and specific DNA binding to ERE, but transcriptional activation does not occur in tumours. In some normal tissues, including endometrium, the tamoxifen–ER complex is able to activate transcription, thereby explaining its oestrogen agonist effect. Raloxifene also allows receptor dimerization

and DNA binding, but its oestrogen agonist properties appear to be confined to bone. The pure oestrogen antagonist ICI 182 780 also binds ER but blocks dimerization.

The pattern of oestrogen agonist and antagonist effects displayed by tamoxifen and more recent derivatives, such as raloxifene and draloxifene, is not fully understood, but may reflect the interplay of tissue-specific co-regulators (Jordan, 1998). The situation is likely to become much clearer following the cloning of a second ER gene (ERβ), which modulates the effects of the original ER (ERα). The different tissue distributions of ERα, ERβ and associated co-regulators are likely to underpin the functions of present and future selective oestrogen receptor modulators (SERMs) for the prevention of breast cancer, uterine cancer, osteoporosis, heart disease and hot flushes (Mitlak and Cohen, 1999).

Other medical strategies for depriving tumour cells of oestrogen include inhibition of aromatase enzyme, responsible for the peripheral conversion of androgens to oestrogen. Examples include anastrazole, exemestane, letrozole and vorozole. Recent research suggests that breast tumours are rich in aromatase enzyme, pointing to intra-tumoral as well as peripheral targets for conventional aromatase inhibitors.

IDENTIFICATION AND MANAGEMENT OF HIGH-RISK PATIENTS

Current epidemiological models of breast cancer causation emphasize the importance of increased exposure to the mitogenic effects of oestrogens, unopposed by normal levels of progestogens. These models incorporate both genetic and environmental factors, the latter including oral contraceptive use and hormone replacement therapy (CGHFBC, 1996, 1997). Family history is not a precisely defined term and does not necessarily indicate an inherited component, but is used to identify a minority of patients at increased lifetime risk of breast cancer. Definitions vary, but the average lifetime risk of 8 per cent is increased to 12–25 per cent if the family has just one or two first-degree relatives diagnosed with breast cancer before 50 years, or else two first- or second-degree relatives on the same side of the family with breast or ovarian cancer (these scenarios apply to 4 per cent of the female population). Women with three or more first- or second-degree relatives with breast or ovarian cancer on the same side of the family, a history of bilateral tumours, male breast cancer or sarcoma, or women aged <40 years at diagnosis, have a lifetime risk of breast cancer of 25–50 per cent (applies to 1 per cent of the female population). Women who inherit proven *BRCA1* or *BRCA2* mutations have a 60–80 per cent lifetime risk of breast cancer, plus a significant risk of ovarian cancer in the case of *BRCA1* (Ford *et al.*, 1998). Nevertheless, this leaves 95 per cent of the female population with a lifetime risk <12 per cent, including women with one first- or second-degree relative diagnosed with breast cancer at age 50 years or older, or women with one second-degree relative diagnosed with breast cancer at any age.

Genetic and epidemiological risk factors may be reflected in breast pathology. Women with atypical ductal hyperplasia also have a lifetime risk of breast cancer several times higher than average (Page, 1992). DCIS and lobular carcinoma *in-situ* (LCIS) confer a several-fold elevated risk of invasive carcinoma. In the former case, the invasive tumour is often close to the original site of DCIS in the same breast, whereas in the LCIS, the invasive cancer is less likely to develop at this site, and may appear in the opposite breast (Fisher *et al.*, 1996). The bilateral nature of the cancer risk in women with LCIS suggests an inherited component.

Women at intermediate or high risk according to the factors described above are increasingly offered referral to a specialist risk clinic, comprising a clinical geneticist, breast oncologist and nurse counsellor with close links to a molecular genetics laboratory dedicated to genetic testing (Vasen *et al.*, 1998). There is currently little evidence on which to base reliable guidelines. Women at moderately increased risk (up to 25 per cent) are advised to examine their breasts once a month, asked to attend for biannual or annual clinical breast examination and recommended annual mammography between ages 35 and 50 years. The frequency of screening is commonly reduced above this age and continued until age 69 years. Women considered or proven to have *BRCA1* mutations are referred for annual pelvic ultrasound in addition, in view of the elevated risk of ovarian cancer.

Women at high risk (>25 per cent) of breast cancer sometimes wish to consider further measures, including bilateral prophylactic mastectomies and reconstruction. These measures are taken only after careful consideration, including psychological counselling of the woman (Hopwood, 1998). Inclusion in a prevention trial may also be considered in the UK (*see* below).

BREAST CANCER PREVENTION

The 1995 overview by the Early Breast Cancer Trialists' Collaborative Group (EBCTCG) of all clinical trials testing adjuvant tamoxifen in women with early breast cancer reported an unexpected 47 per cent reduction (SD 9 per cent) in the risk of a contralateral tumour associated with 5 years of tamoxifen medication (EBCTCG, 1998a). The preliminary results of the American Breast Cancer Prevention Trial (NSABP P1) indicate a 45 per cent reduction in breast cancer incidence in a trial of 13 388 women comparing 5 years of tamoxifen and placebo (3.6 and 6.6 breast cancers in the tamoxifen and placebo groups, respectively, per 1000 woman-years) (Fisher *et al.*, 1998a). A web site news release by the National Institutes of Health (NIH) was followed by unblinding of the trial and the offer of tamoxifen to women in the placebo arm.

Preliminary analyses of two smaller European trials so far fail to confirm this effect. No effect was reported by a British study of 2471 high-risk women, nor by an Italian trial with 5408 average-risk women, with 2.1 and 2.3 breast cancers in the tamoxifen and placebo groups, respectively, per 1000 woman-years (Powles *et al.*, 1998b; Veronesi *et al.*, 1998). Lower statistical power fails to account for lack of a tamoxifen effect compared to NSABP P1. Poor compliance among Italian participants may be partly responsible for the negative result in the Italian study (26 per cent of women withdrew from the trial, most in the first year). Relatively young age and strong family history in the British study may signify a subset resistant to prophylactic tamoxifen by virtue of genetic risk.

Interpretation of the interim trial data is controversial. The early benefits seen in NASBP-P1 may be due to effects on occult invasive disease, rather than to a true preventive effect. In the UK, the International Breast Cancer Intervention (IBIS) Trial, testing 5 years of tamoxifen 20 mg daily against placebo, has closed, having achieved its target of 7000 women. Second-generation trials in the UK propose to evaluate the role of aromatase inhibitors, retaining the use of a placebo for the time being. In the USA, tamoxifen is now considered standard treatment for high-risk women. The successor to NASBP-P1 tests tamoxifen against raloxifene in 22 000 women at elevated risk (STAR trial). Raloxifene is a selective oestrogen receptor modulator with a proven role in reducing the risk of osteoporosis in postmenopausal women.

SCREENING

The ability of current mammographic techniques to identify small tumours does not guarantee that breast cancer mortality will fall. Some cancers may have spread despite earlier detection, while others may remain localized until symptomatic. Screening may also identify intraduct lesions that would not progress to invasive cancer within the woman's lifespan. Uncertainties about the benefits of screening are overcome by population-based randomized trials of mammographic screening in the USA and Sweden, which demonstrate significant mortality reductions in women between 50 and 69 years (Nystrom *et al.*, 1993). The results show a relative reduction in cancer mortality of approximately 30 per cent in this age group, depending on patient acceptance and frequency of screening. Controversy remains regarding the magnitude of benefit of the screening programme (Olsen and Gotzsche, 2001). Unresolved questions relate to the optimal screening interval and the benefits of screening patients under 50 years and over 70 years. When all trials in women under 50 years are submitted to meta-analysis, the mean odds ratio is consistent with a proportional reduction in the risk of death of about 10 per cent compared with controls, one-third of the benefit seen in women over 50 years (Harris, 1997). This works out as about one life saved for every 1000 women of this age group undergoing screening over a 10-year period. In the UK, routine population screening of women under 50 years is not currently recommended, although prospective randomized trials are under way.

The national target for breast cancer in the UK was to reduce the death rate in the 50–64 years age group by at least 25 per cent by the year 2000. These objectives could be met if at least 70 per cent of women in this age group accept two views (mediolateral and cranio-caudal) at the first screen and single mediolateral oblique views every 3 years thereafter, and attend for further assessment and treatment if necessary. During the initial prevalence screen 10 per cent of women are expected to be recalled because of some mammographic abnormality, and after additional mammographic views, clinical assessment and ultrasound, 1.5 per cent will require diagnostic biopsy and about 0.5 per cent will have a cancer. Overall, approximately 70 per cent of new cancers are expected to be screen-detected in a population attending for mammography at 3-yearly intervals, assuming 100 per cent compliance with the programme. Assuming 70 per cent uptake, these measures should save 1250 lives per year in the UK, representing about 25 000 woman-years of life saved.

PRESENTATION AND INVESTIGATION

Typical mammographic features of screen-detected cancer include spiculate densities, clusters of fine calcifications, retraction or thickening of the overlying skin or nipple, and enlarged axillary nodes. The investigation of a screen-detected impalpable abnormality requires localization for fine-needle aspiration cytology or core biopsy guided by stereotactic radiography or ultrasound. If negative, this is followed by wire-guided localization excision biopsy to establish a histological diagnosis. If positive, a therapeutic excision with wider margins is undertaken if the patient is suitable for breast-preserving surgery. Either way, specimen radiography is important to confirm that the radiological abnormality has been removed.

The management of a palpable lump is fairly straightforward. Cancer is always a possibility, but fibroadenomas are relatively common at around 30 years of age and cysts at around 40 years. Palpable fibroadenomas are usually removed, unless the woman is very young (e.g. <25 years), and cysts can be aspirated without further investigation or follow-up unless the fluid is bloodstained or a residual lump is felt. Any other discrete lump will have to be removed so fine-needle aspirate or Trucut biopsy can be performed before imaging, to complete the triple assessment. If the result is cancer, the first open surgery can be therapeutic, and the mammogram will influence the appropriate extent of surgery, based on the presence of multifocal disease (frozen section will be needed prior to mastectomy if only cytology is available). Simple staging investigations are adequate prior to surgery, namely haematology, biochemistry and chest radiograph, with further tests according to symptomatology or test results. If cytology or Trucut histology is negative, diagnostic excision biopsy is required before treatment decisions can be made. If the lump is clinically benign, mammography should be performed prior to fine-needle aspiration or core biopsy, since haematoma formation often prevents interpretation of the mammogram for up to 3 weeks.

PATHOLOGY

Structure of the breast

The breast is a modified sweat gland with 15–20 duct systems converging on the nipple. These are branching structures starting with 1 mm lobules in which the terminal branch divides into multiple blind-ending ductules called terminal duct lobular units. Several tens of thousand lobules in each breast are suspended in subcutaneous fat supported in a fibrous stroma and by elastic ligaments. Stereomicroscopy of whole-breast sections supports the origin of most breast carcinomas from the terminal duct lobular unit.

Histological classification

The large majority of breast carcinomas are adenocarcinomas, and most are classified on the basis of morphology as either ductal or lobular, despite their common origin from the terminal duct lobular unit. Invasive ductal carcinoma (IDC) with no special histological features accounts for 75 per cent of invasive breast cancers. It is referred to as ductal carcinoma not otherwise specified (NOS) or of no special type (NST). Invasive lobular carcinoma (ILC) accounts for 10 per cent and medullary carcinoma for 5 per cent of invasive breast cancers (Azzopardi et al., 1982). There are also three common special types of invasive breast cancer which have a significantly better prognosis than the others, including tubular or cribriform tumours, mucinous or colloid tumours and papillary carcinoma, which together account for 5 per cent of invasive disease.

Grading of carcinomas using the Bloom and Richardson system is based on the degree of tubule formation, nuclear pleomorphism and mitotic index, each scored on a three-point scale. Grading criteria have been difficult to standardize in the past, but progress in reducing observer variation has been made in recognition of its powerful prognostic significance. The proportion of tumours in different series is variable, roughly 1 : 2 : 2 for grades 1, 2 and 3, respectively. Histological grading is also applied to invasive lobular carcinoma, although tubule formation cannot be scored.

Duct carcinoma *in-situ*

DCIS comprises a spectrum of lesions characterized by proliferation of malignant cells within ducts without invasion of surrounding stromal tissue. It presents as a mass or nipple discharge, nowadays more commonly as a screen-detected mammographic abnormality. DCIS is commonly graded on morphological grounds, according to the Van Nuys system, into high (grade 3) and non-high grade lesions, the latter subdivided according to the presence of comedo-type necrosis (grade 2) or not (grade 1). Grade 3 DCIS is composed of cells with large pleomorphic nuclei, often with multiple mitotic figures, with or without comedo-type necrotic debris in the centre of the ducts. Calcification of necrotic debris produces characteristic microcalcifications on mammography, ranging in size from a single focus, measuring a few millimetres, to extensive involvement of a whole quadrant. DCIS is nearly always unilateral, in contrast to LCIS (*see* below). A classification that groups DCIS according to the risk of local recurrence after breast-preserving surgery has been proposed by Silverstein, combining the Van Nuys grade (1–3) with tumour size in millimetres (≤15, 16–40, ≥40) and excision margin in millimetres (≥10, 1–9, <1). With each predictor graded on a 3-point scale, a prognostic index scoring from a low of 3 to a high of 9 appears to identify subgroups with very different recurrence risks (Silverstein *et al.*, 1996). Margins appear to be particularly important in determining local recurrence risk (Silverstein *et al.*, 1999). The therapeutic implications of this are discussed later.

Lobular carcinoma *in-situ*

LCIS is not clinically palpable or detectable by mammography, but is identified incidentally in about 1 per cent of benign breast biopsies. Under the microscope, LCIS appears as a solid proliferation of small cells within breast lobules, with uniform small round/oval nuclei, rarely enlarging lobules to greater than 2–3 times their normal size. Mitoses are infrequent and necrosis is not seen. It is found predominantly in premenopausal women, always multicentric in the breast and often (35 per cent) bilateral. LCIS is regarded as an indicator of elevated cancer risk rather than as a premalignant condition in its own right, but recent data challenge this view (E. R. Fisher *et al.*, 1996). It is associated with approximately a 30 per cent lifetime risk of developing an invasive carcinoma. The invasive cancer is usually ductal and may present in the same or opposite breast.

PROGNOSTIC MARKERS AND PREDICTION OF THERAPEUTIC RESPONSE

Conventional pathological features of invasive carcinomas that correlate with prognosis include histological subtype, tumour size, grade, lymphovascular invasion and axillary node metastases. Pathological node status is the single most powerful prognostic indicator, node-positive patients having a 10-year survival of 40 per cent compared with 80 per cent for node-negative women. The 10-year survival for women with 1–3 nodes positive is approximately 55 per cent compared with 25 per cent for women with >3 nodes positive. Multivariate analyses have been used to generate algorithms based on pathological tumour size, grade and node status that separate patients into prognostic groups, the best-known being the Nottingham index (Todd *et al.*, 1987). The Nottingham index [NI = 0.2 × pathological tumour size (cm) + node stage (1–3) + grade (1–3)] is an empirical algorithm that identifies subgroups with very different prognoses. Just pathological tumour size and the number of positive axillary nodes discriminate pretty well (Carter *et al.*, 1989). Estimates of prognosis influence treatment recommendations, especially for adjuvant cytotoxic chemotherapy. They provide an indirect estimate of absolute gain from adjuvant systemic therapies, patients with a high risk of premature death usually having more to gain than those at low risk.

Morphological features such as histological subtype and grade reflect the interplay of hundreds of proteins, the identification and characterization of which are advancing rapidly via gene cloning. Some of the new prognostic markers that have been identified over the past decade include immunohistochemical analyses of cancer gene products, vascular growth factors, differentiation markers, proliferation indices and assays of the hormone-response pathway (Elston *et al.*, 1998). These may contribute to understanding the biology of cancer, but have not so far replaced conventional prognostic indices. One reason, beyond feasibility and cost considerations, may be that the influences of many gene products are expressed in the morphological phenotype scored by conventional pathology.

Reliable predictive markers of response to systemic therapies are needed more than new prognostic markers. Assays are needed that identify patients likely to benefit from endocrine therapy or chemotherapy, or a combination of both. The best-studied markers are the ER and PgRs, nuclear proteins detectable in about 70 per cent of tumours (Jordan, 1998; Harvey *et al.*, 1999). Receptor status can be established by immunohistochemistry, which correlates with tumour response to endocrine therapy in the adjuvant and metastatic settings. To be reliable, the surgical tissue must be fixed immediately to avoid degradation of labile receptor protein. Any nuclear staining is taken by some as evidence of ER positivity, although a semi-quantitative measure is provided by the 'H-score'. This parameter is the product of the nuclear staining intensity on a 4-point graded scale (0–3) and the percentage of cells showing nuclear staining. The maximum score is 300, and ER 'weak positive' is variably defined by an H-score between 1 and 20. About 20 per cent of patients are true ER− by these criteria, i.e. the H-score is zero. Note that about 20 per cent of ER− tumours are PgR+ (roughly 5 per cent of all tumours) and these are probably endocrine responsive.

Where benefit to adjuvant cytotoxic therapy is concerned, earlier reports that the 20 per cent of patients overexpressing *c-erbB2/neu/HER2* oncogene fail to benefit from adjuvant cyclophosphamide, methotrexate and 5-fluorouracil (CMF) are now much less secure (Gusterson *et al.*, 1992; Menard *et al.*, 1999). Recently, *c-erbB2* overexpression has been linked to tamoxifen resistance in the adjuvant setting, although the data are conflicting and should not influence routine treatment at the present time (Pegram *et al.*, 1998).

Selected retrospective studies suggest that resection during the period of unopposed oestrogen synthesis in the first half of the menstrual cycle is associated with a worse prognosis than surgery in the second half of the cycle. Meta-analysis of conflicting reports is consistent with a modest effect, although multiple subgroup analyses and publication bias could be potent causes of false-positive results (McGuire *et al.*, 1992). Prospective observational studies are under way to test the original observations. Finally, another therapeutic parameter reported to impact on prognosis is delay of more than 3 months in diagnosis and treatment (Richards *et al.*, 1999).

SURGERY FOR EARLY BREAST CANCER

After decades of uncertainty, the reduction in breast cancer mortality demonstrated by the systematic overview of radiotherapy effects proves the existence of patients with disease confined to the breast and lymphatic pathways (EBCTCG, 2000). The implications for surgery (and for radiotherapy, *see* p. 460) are that eradication of locoregional disease is necessary, and often sufficient, to ensure permanent cure of disease.

Primary surgery

Review of relevant randomized trials confirm that breast-conserving surgery plus radiotherapy are equivalent to mastectomy in terms of local control and overall survival (Margolese, 1998). Breast-conserving surgery can therefore be offered as an alternative to mastectomy to the majority of women with early stage disease. Clinical or radiological multicentricity is an indication for mastectomy, unless discrete multifocal lesions can be independently localized and completely excised. When the expected surgical defect is large or when the nipple needs to be removed, the patient may opt for mastectomy

(Sainsbury *et al.*, 1994). If the patient finds it difficult to lie in the radiotherapy treatment position, if she is pregnant or has a collagen vascular disease (systemic sclerosis, systemic lupus), there will also be a lower threshold for avoiding the need for radiotherapy.

With breast-conserving surgery, circumferential incisions that follow the contours of skin creases are less visible than radial incisions. A narrow (5 mm) slice of skin helps the pathologist to orientate the surgical specimen; a wider ellipse is unnecessary and worsens the cosmetic outcome. Breast and axillary incisions should be separate unless the primary tumour is located high up in the upper outer quadrant or axillary tail. The primary surgical specimen must be marked with surface sutures to allow orientation and the whole specimen Indian inked before fixation. The deep layers should not be sutured together and no suction drainage should be used. Local complications include seroma, haematoma and infection.

There is no consensus on the optimal margins of excision. A Milan trial testing tumorectomy (⩽1 cm margins of healthy tissue at surgery) against quadrantectomy, both followed by radiotherapy, reported superior local control with the latter at the expense of breast appearance (Mariani *et al.*, 1998). The absolute minimum requirement is a microscopic complete excision, and if this is not achieved, the patient must have a second operation (further excision or mastectomy). Complete microscopic clearance, based on pathological examination of multiple paraffin sections cut from blocks prepared at the narrowest macroscopic tumour margins, is possible in the large majority of cases. The depth of excision is variable, some operators aiming routinely to remove tissue down to the pectoral fascia, others not. If the resection extends to the deep fascia, microscopic evidence of disease at the deep margin is regarded by many surgeons as a complete resection unless the fascia is breached. Microscopic evidence of disease at the radial or superficial resection margins in women under 40 is a risk factor for local recurrence if there is associated extensive intraduct carcinoma (EIC). EIC is defined as DCIS occupying more than 25 per cent of the tumour cross-section at high-power microscopy plus extension of DCIS beyond the peripheral margins of the invasive component. The elevated recurrence risk seems to be accounted for by a higher probability of macroscopic residual disease in the tumour bed, which can often be dealt with by re-excision (Macmillan *et al.*, 1996). Even if there is no extensive intraduct carcinoma, microscopic evidence of disease at the resection margins is an absolute indication for re-excision.

Mastectomy or marked breast deficits and distortions can cause marked changes in body image and self-esteem, for which preoperative counselling and reconstruction should be offered (*see* p. 455). Patients may find it helpful to see photographs of patients who have had the operation or to meet patients who have been through the experience before. Postoperative complications include wound infections and seroma.

Breast reconstruction

Breast reconstruction can be performed as a one-stage procedure at the time of mastectomy, although some women defer a decision until other treatment is complete, including radiotherapy. It can be offered to a majority of women opting for mastectomy, and may be relevant to a minority of women after breast-preserving treatment (Evans and Kroll, 1998). Reconstruction of a breast mound can be achieved by placing an inflatable envelope (tissue expander) beneath the pectoralis major muscle, and inflating it with saline gradually over several weeks until moderately overfilled compared to the opposite breast. A few months later, the expander is replaced with a silicone implant. It is now common to use a Becker implant, a device that acts both as an expander and as an implant, having separate envelopes accessed via a single subcutaneous port that is removed at a later date. The alternative to tissue expansion is to transfer a musculocutaneous flap consisting of skin, fat and muscle, beneath which an implant is placed. The latissimus dorsi (LD) flap from the upper back or the transverse rectus abdominis myocutaneous-free (TRAM) flap from the abdominal wall may be combined with a reduction mammoplasty of the contralateral side. Complications include infection, seroma, necrosis and poor cosmesis. Breast reconstruction is consistent with subsequent local radiotherapy, although some, but not all, retrospective studies report higher rates of late adverse effects, including contraction and induration (Mark et al., 1996; Zimmerman et al., 1998).

Axillary surgery

A representative sample of lower axillary nodes may be removed as a diagnostic procedure to establish prognosis and to define the need for adjuvant sytemic therapy, especially chemotherapy. Another reason to sample the axilla is to define the node-positive patients (roughly one-third of the total) who require therapeutic complete axillary dissection or axillary radiotherapy.

Axillary sampling traditionally involves the surgeon identifying by palpation and inspection a minimum of four lymph nodes from the axillary fat pad, a diagnostic procedure defined and tested against axillary dissection in a well-designed randomized trial (Forrest et al., 1995). Sampling of the sentinel lymph node, defined as the nearest regional lymph node to take up a radiolabelled colloid injected subdermally superficial to the primary tumour, is now being widely adopted as a refinement of the sampling approach (Koops et al., 1999). A hand-held gamma-ray detector directs the surgeon to the precise location of the sentinel node, usually in the axilla but occasionally in the internal mammary chain. Methylene blue dye injected shortly before operation offers an additional visual guide. The routine role of sentinel-node biopsy is currently under evaluation in prospective trials.

A complete axillary dissection may be preferred as an alternative to axillary sampling, to avoid the need for a second axillary operation or axillary radiotherapy if the nodes are positive. Axillary surgery is preferable to radiotherapy in patients with palpably enlarged mobile nodes, of whom 70 per cent will have lymphatic metastases, sometimes bulky. Depending on the exent of surgery, a median of 10 nodes are recovered from below the lower border of pectoralis minor (level I), five nodes from beneath this muscle (level II) and a further five nodes above the upper border of pectoralis minor (level III). Axillary recurrence should be uncommon (1 or 2 per cent at 10 years) in node-positive women after a full dissection.

Numbness, shoulder stiffness and pain are common complications of complete axillary dissection (Ivens et al., 1992). The optimal timing of shoulder exercises is unclear, some surgeons introducing them gently on the first postoperative day and increasing in range once the drain and sutures are removed. The risk of arm oedema depends on the anatomical level of dissection, a 10 per cent risk being typical after a level II dissection. Arm oedema is managed with the early introduction of a well-fitting support stocking or sleeve. Breast oedema after axillary surgery is also common, and may last many months. Cording is a painful restriction of shoulder mobility after axillary surgery, of unknown aetiology, presenting with thickened strands in the subcutaneous tissues. The syndrome usually subsides on its own after several months, but physiotherapy with gentle stretching can help.

ENDOCRINE THERAPY FOR EARLY BREAST CANCER

The 5-yearly systematic overviews published by EBCTCG provide convincing evidence that adjuvant endocrine therapy and chemotherapy in women with early breast cancer each reduce annual mortality risk for at least 10 years. The benefits of each modality in women <50 years old add up to about 10 extra women alive at 10 years for every 100 women with stage II disease, and up to five extra women alive at 10 years for every 100 women with stage I disease. It is not formally possible to distinguish between cure of a small proportion of women or a modest extension of life in a large proportion (or a mixture of both). The benefits of adjuvant systemic therapies, including endocrine therapies, are summarized in Tables 21.1–21.3.

Adjuvant ovarian suppression

In women under 50 years, ovarian suppression as sole adjuvant treatment reduces the annual risk of death by almost 25 per cent for at least 15 years (EBCTCG, 1996). Although the greatest absolute benefit is seen in the first 5 years, ovarian suppression still prevents or delays deaths that would otherwise have occurred 10+ years after presentation.

Table 21.1 *Direct estimates of reduction in the annual odds of recurrence and death in trials of single-modality adjuvant therapy (EBCTCG, 1996, 1998b)*

Adjuvant therapy	Number	Reductions % (SD) in annual odds of:	
		Recurrence or prior death	Death
Chemotherapy only versus nil (age <50)	3900	37 (4)	28 (5)
Chemotherapy only versus nil (age 50–69)	4448	22 (4)	12 (4)
Ovarian suppression only versus nil (age <50)	1295	25 (7)	24 (7)
Tamoxifen only versus nil (all ages):			
1 year	3265	28 (4)	15 (4)
2 years	7381	34 (3)	17 (4)
5 years	6482	46 (4)	22 (5)

Table 21.2 *Proportional risk reductions achieved by adjuvant tamoxifen, subdivided by patient age and tamoxifen duration. Trials include those in which both arms received chemotherapy; analysis excludes oestrogen-receptor (ER) poor (Data from EBCTCG, 1998a, Figure 7)*

Adjuvant therapy	Number	Reductions % (SD) in annual odds of:	
		Recurrence or prior death	Death
Tamoxifen versus no tamoxifen (age <50):			
1 year	2248	2 (7)	−2 (8)
2 years	4173	14 (5)	10 (6)
5 years	1327	45 (8)	32 (10)
Tamoxifen versus no tamoxifen (age 50–59):			
1 year	2217	28 (6)	21 (6)
2 years	4382	32 (4)	19 (5)
5 years	2536	37 (6)	11 (8)
Tamoxifen versus no tamoxifen (age 60–69):			
1 year	2210	26 (6)	12 (6)
2 years	4466	33 (4)	12 (5)
5 years	3174	54 (5)	33 (6)
Tamoxifen versus no tamoxifen (age 70+):			
1 year	882	22 (9)	8 (8)
2 years	1476	42 (8)	36 (7)
5 years	390	54 (13)	34 (13)

Table 21.3 *Direct estimates of reductions in the annual odds of recurrence and death in trials testing combinations of chemotherapy (CT), ovarian suppression (OS) or tamoxifen (EBCTCG, 1996, 1998a, b)*

Type of systemic therapy	Number	Reductions % (SD) in annual odds of:	
		Recurrence or prior death	Death
Age <50:			
CT versus CT + OS	933	10 (9)	8 (10)
Tamoxifen versus tamoxifen + CT	640	21 (13)	25 (14)
Age 50–69:			
Tamoxifen versus tamoxifen + CT	9192	19 (3)	11 (4)
All ages:			
CT versus CT + tamoxifen			
1 year	4272	12 (5)	7 (5)
2 years	7096	22 (4)	16 (4)
5 years	945	52 (8)	47 (9)

For every 100 women with node-positive disease, the absolute survival benefit at 15 years is 13.4 per cent (SD 3.8), whereas for node-negative disease it is 8.9 per cent (SD 4.2). The benefits are less in the presence of chemotherapy, as expected in view of the chemical castration that occurs in a proportion of patients. It is not possible to say from the currently available data whether the benefits of ovarian suppression are confined to women with ER+ tumours, but this is an obvious hypothesis to test.

Ovarian suppression was at least as effective as classical CMF in terms of disease-free survival in ER+ pre/perimenopausal women in a trial of 1640 patients with stage II breast cancer (Kaufman, 2001). In ER− patients, CMF was superior to goserelin for disease-free survival. Patients treated with goserelin had superior quality of life scores during therapy. In a further study, 3-weekly i.v. CMF was equivalent to ovarian suppression in premenopausal women with node-positive ER+ disease, according to a Swedish trial of 732 patients (Ejlertsen et al., 1999). In a smaller Scottish trial of 332 premenopausal node-positive patients, there was a trend for ovarian suppression to be superior to 3-weekly i.v. CMF in ER+ patients, and inferior to the same chemotherapy in ER− patients (SCTBG, 1993). There are almost no data on the added benefits of chemotherapy and/or tamoxifen against a background of ovarian suppression. It may be unreliable to assume that the treatment benefits of chemotherapy and/or tamoxifen are identical to those reported for postmenopausal women >50 years.

Adjuvant tamoxifen

The 1998 overview by the EBCTCG confirms the benefits of adjuvant tamoxifen in women of all age groups with ER+ or ER-unknown tumours (excluding ER-poor patients because no benefit is reported for this subgroup in the overview; see Table 21.2) (EBCTCG, 1998a). However, it is likely that the ER− PgR+ subgroup do benefit from tamoxifen. It is also possible that the apparent failure of tamoxifen reported by the overview in the ER-poor subgroup is partly due to short tamoxifen duration in women <50 years receiving adjuvant chemotherapy. There is a strong tamoxifen duration effect in women of all ages, but particularly in women <50 years, who need a minimum of 5 years of therapy for any significant benefit. The benefits, and possible adverse effects, of longer-duration tamoxifen are being tested in the aTTom (adjuvant tamoxifen treatment, offer more) and other trials.

Very little is known about the combined effects of adjuvant tamoxifen and ovarian suppression. The benefit of ovarian suppression in addition to tamoxifen is currently being tested in several trials, including the Cancer Research Campaign (CRC) Zoladex trial and the Adjuvant Breast Cancer (ABC) trial. The effects of tamoxifen and chemotherapy in combination appear to be additive (see Table 21.3). In most trials testing tamoxifen and

chemotherapy in combination, both modalities were given concurrently, often with short tamoxifen duration (about 18 months on average in premenopausal women). Concerns about a negative interaction between the two modalities in young women are probably unfounded, being based on a combination of theoretical considerations, selected cell culture models and retrospective subgroup analyses of clinical trials. There is more justified concern that concurrent chemo-endocrine therapy may increase the risk of thromboembolism (Saphner et al., 1991; Ragaz and Coldman, 1998). If confirmed, this risk must be weighed against the potential dangers of delaying by several months the introduction of tamoxifen, a highly effective anti-cancer treatment.

Primary endocrine therapy

Primary endocrine therapy has been tested in two randomized clinical trials totalling 854 women over 70 years of age, comparing tamoxifen 20 mg alone to primary surgery plus tamoxifen. Both confirm higher rates of local disease progression, and greater need for salvage surgery, in the tamoxifen alone group, although no statistically significant differences in overall survival have yet been reported (Bates et al., 1991; Mustacchi et al., 1994). These trials do not establish tamoxifen as the treatment of choice for this group of women unless they are physically or mentally unfit for surgery. As an alternative to primary chemotherapy in women <70 years with ER+ tumours, primary endocrine approaches are now an active research area (Howell et al., 1998).

Adverse effects of endocrine therapy

Most adverse effects are related to oestrogen deprivation, with the exception that tamoxifen and other selective oestrogen-response modulators act as a weak oestrogen agonist in some tissues. The endometrial cancer risk associated with tamoxifen (approximately two additional deaths per 10 000 woman-years) and the beneficial effects on postmenopausal bone density are related directly to this agonist effect. In advanced disease, the side-effects of tamoxifen cause patients considerable distress, with hot flushes reported in up to 80 per cent (Leonard et al., 1996). The safety and effectiveness of alternative medicines and hormone replacement therapy in the management of hot flushes remain poorly clarified, with several common remedies performing poorly in placebo-controlled studies. Venlafaxine is an antidepressant which has been tested and reported helpful to a proportion of women. It is preferable to consider hormone replacement therapy against hot flushes in order to maintain women with ER+ tumours on adjuvant tamoxifen than to withdraw this drug (Cobleigh et al., 1994). Ideally, as many patients as possible should be considered for the current

UK randomized clinical trial testing the safety and effectiveness of hormone replacement therapy.

CHEMOTHERAPY FOR EARLY BREAST CANCER

Adjuvant chemotherapy

The benefits of adjuvant systemic therapies, including chemotherapy, are summarized in Tables 21.1–21.3. There is no identifiable subgroup of women age <70 years who fail to gain a statistically significant extension of overall survival after adjuvant chemotherapy. All women <50 years with early invasive breast cancer are usually considered for adjuvant chemotherapy as part of standard treatment if they have any of the following: pathologically node positive, lymphovascular invasion positive, grade 3, oestrogen receptor negative, tumour larger than 2 cm (pN+, LV+, G3, ER −, >pT1). This corresponds to a group of women with <90 per cent survival prospects at 10 years, in whom the 25 per cent reduction in the annual odds of death after chemotherapy corresponds to a minimum absolute overall survival benefit of 2–3 per cent. This is more-or-less standard practice in the UK now, although there is also much interest in adjuvant tamoxifen or ovarian suppression as an equally, or more, effective first-choice adjuvant therapy in ER+ cases. Between ages 50 and 69, the threshold for recommending chemotherapy is raised, taking into account the reduced chemotherapy benefit. Nevertheless, even postmenopausal women with pN− ER+ tumours randomized to 4 cycles of adjuvant AC (doxorubicin, cyclophosphamide) chemotherapy plus tamoxifen in the NSABP B-20 trial gained a statistically significant overall survival benefit compared to those allocated tamoxifen alone (Fisher et al., 1997a). In Europe at least, it is not clear that survival gains in the range 1–3 per cent are justified in terms of quality of life and health economic considerations in postmenopausal women (Gelber et al., 1996).

The relative reductions in mortality rate are similar in axillary node-negative and -positive women, with the possible exception of postmenopausal women. In this subgroup, the 1998 overview data suggest a larger absolute benefit in node-negative (6.4 per cent, SD 2.3) compared to node-positive women (2.3 per cent, SD 1.3). The authors consider this likely to be a false-positive result, estimating the absolute survival advantages for node-negative and node-positive women, aged 50–69, to be 2.4 per cent and 3.2 per cent, respectively (EBCTCG, 1998b). Until this uncertainty is clarified, it is reasonable to consider that the reduction in the annual odds of death achieved by any adjuvant systemic therapy is independent of node status.

The most common adjuvant schedule used in the UK is classical CMF (cyclophosphamide, $100\,mg/m^2$ p.o. days 1–14; methotrexate, $40\,mg/m^2$ i.v. days 1 and 8; fluorouracil (5-FU), $600\,mg/m^2$ i.v. days 1 and 8; repeated on a 28-day cycle). Several prospective randomized trials have failed to demonstrate any advantage to giving more than 6 months of classical CMF (EBCTCG, 1998b). Where dose intensity (mg/m^2 per week) of CMF and other common chemotherapy schedules is concerned, the relationship between dose intensity and clinical response appears linear over the standard range of dose intensity (Hryniuk and Levine, 1986; Hryniuk et al., 1998). The 3-weekly i.v. CMF (cyclophosphamide, $600\,mg/m^2$ i.v. day 1; methotrexate, $40\,mg/m^2$ i.v. day 1; 5-FU, $600\,mg/m^2$ i.v. day 1) corresponds to a summation dose intensity (SDI) of 1.27 compared to 1.98 for classical CMF, a difference in SDI of >0.65 appearing to identify schedules that differ significantly in terms of overall survival benefit. The only direct test of 6 cycles of classical CMF against 6 cycles of 3-weekly i.v. CMF demonstrated a clear benefit for the former in terms of reponse rate (48 per cent versus 29 per cent) and median survival (17 versus 12 months) in 254 patients with metastatic disease (Engelsman et al., 1991).

Reliable dose–response data for anthracyclines come from a Cancer and Leukaemia Group B (CALGB) trial randomizing 1550 patients with stage II breast cancer to a high-dose arm (cyclophosphamide $600\,mg/m^2$, doxorubicin $60\,mg/m^2$ and 5-FU $600\,mg/m^2$ every 28 days for 4 cycles) versus a low-dose arm (cyclophosphamide $300\,mg/m^2$, doxorubicin $30\,mg/m^2$ and 5-FU, $300\,mg/m^2$ every 28 days for 4 cycles) and a moderate-dose arm (cyclophosphamide $400\,mg/m^2$, doxorubicin $40\,mg/m^2$ and 5-FU $400\,mg/m^2$ every 28 days for 6 cycles) (Budman et al., 1998). At median follow-up of 9 years, there was no difference in survival between high- and moderate-dose arms, but statistically significant worse survival for the low-dose arm, corresponding to roughly 10 per cent fewer patients alive at 10 years. Where the dose intensity of cyclophosphamide is concerned, the NSABP B-22 trial testing $600\,mg/m^2$ versus $1200\,mg/m^2$ i.v. doses of cyclophosphamide in conjunction with i.v. doxorubicin $60\,mg/m^2$ found no benefit for the higher-dose arm (Fisher et al., 1997b).

The 1998 EBCTCG overview revealed a statistically significant absolute gain of 2.7 per cent (SD 1.4 per cent) in overall survival at 10 years for adjuvant schedules containing an anthracycline (EBCTCG, 1998b). This small benefit is considered clinically significant in many countries, where anthracycline schedules have all but replaced CMF. The potential for a lethal interaction between anthracyclines, radiotherapy and the heart in patients with left-sided tumours highlights the importance of cardiac shielding. The UK National Epirubicin Adjuvant trial (NEAT) has tested the added benefits of 4 cycles of epirubicin ($100\,mg/m^2$) i.v. every 3 weeks prior to classical CMF in a test of the earlier reports from Milan on the superiority of sequential anthraclines and CMF (Bonadonna et al., 1995). The results are awaited.

Taxanes are the latest group of drugs to be tested in the adjuvant setting, with several thousand patients randomized to date. On the basis of a very early analysis of the CALGB 9344 trial, which reported a statistically significant increase in disease-free (90 per cent versus 86 per cent) and overall survival (97 per cent versus 95 per cent) in favour of paclitaxol in 3170 women randomized to this drug after 4 cycles of AC, paclitaxel is now licensed for adjuvant use in the USA (Henderson *et al.*, 1998). However, longer follow-up of CALGB, and the results of a National Cancer Institute (NCI) trial testing paclitaxel, have cast doubt on the reliability of the early analysis. The latest NIH consensus statement in November 2000 agreed that considerable uncertainty remains, and imminent UK licensing is not expected. In the UK, the Taxotere as Adjuvant Chemo-therapy (TACT) trial is testing docetaxel and FEC (fluorouracil, epirubicin and cyclophosphamide) against FEC alone in the adjuvant setting.

Neoadjuvant, preoperative or primary medical therapy

Cytoreductive chemotherapy, endocrine therapy and/or radiotherapy have long been used to downstage inoperable tumours in an attempt to render them resectable by mastectomy (Bonadonna *et al.*, 1990). In the past decade, there has been a logical progression to test preoperative chemotherapy for patients with operable tumours, particularly those considered too large for breast-conservation surgery. This hypothesis has been tested most comprehensively by the NSABP B-18 trial, which randomized 1523 women with tumours (T1,3N0,1M0) of invasive breast carcinoma to 4 cycles of AC chemotherapy before or after primary surgery (Fisher *et al.*, 1997c). The study showed that women with tumours >5 cm given preoperative chemotherapy were much more likely to be treated with breast-conservation surgery as opposed to mastectomy – a consequence of tumour shrinkage. However, no differences in disease-free and overall survival were seen between the preoperative and postoperative chemotherapy arms of the trial. The conclusion is that there is currently no proven survival advantage to be gained from primary medical therapy compared to the adjuvant setting. The great appeal of primary medical therapy is that it allows biological studies to be undertaken, allowing not just research into cellular and molecular mechanisms of drug action, but also the identification of early markers of therapeutic benefit.

Dose intensification with marrow or peripheral stem-cell support

Several small, non-randomized phase I/II trials in patients with metastatic disease in the early 1990s reported encouraging responses and overall survival rates compared to historical controls. Only one relatively large randomized trial has evaluated this approach in patients with metastatic disease (Stadtmauer *et al.*, 1999). The study tested high-dose chemotherapy with the STAMP V regimen (cyclophosphamide 6000 mg/m², thiotepa 500 mg/m² and carboplatin, 800 mg/m²) plus stem-cell support against maintenance classical CMF in 184 randomized and evaluable patients who had already achieved complete or partial response to 4–6 cycles of induction CAF (cyclophosphamide, doxorubicin and fluorouracil) or CMF. The trial reported no differences in overall survival or serious toxicities between the two groups.

In the adjuvant setting, five relatively large randomized trials have tested high-dose regimens in patients with poor prognosis, non-metastatic disease, typically stage II patients with heavy node involvement. Four of the five trials reported negative results, including a small Dutch trial of 97 women (Rodenhuis *et al.*, 1998). The US Intergroup Trial, tested a single autologous marrow transplant regimen comprising cyclophosphamide (5635 mg/m²), cisplatin (165 mg/m²) and BCNU (600 mg/m²) against the same drugs without transplant at 900, 90 and 90 mg/m², respectively, following 4 cycles of CAF (cyclophosphamide 1200 mg/m², doxorubicin 60 mg/m² and 5-FU 600 mg/m² every 28 days) in 785 randomized patients (Peters *et al.*, 1999). No difference in overall survival was reported at 5 years (71 per cent versus 68 per cent for the transplant and control arms). No difference in overall survival was noted at a median of 24 months in a Scandinavian trial of 274 patients randomized to 3 cycles of standard FEC (5-FU 600 mg/m², epirubicin 60 mg/m² and cyclophosphamide 600 mg/m² every 21 days) followed by a single STAMP V regimen (*see* above) and stem-cell transplant against a control arm comprising 9 cycles of dose-intensive FEC (SBCSG, 1999).

The only positive trial was reported from South Africa (Bezwoda, 1999). It compared up-front tandem stem-cell transplants against 6 cycles of standard CAF (cyclophosphamide 600 mg/m², doxorubicin 50 mg/m² and 5-FU 600 mg/m²). Each stem-cell transplant was preceded by cyclophosphamide 4400 mg/m², mitoxantrone 45 mg/m² and etoposide 1500 mg/m². In 154 randomized patients at more than 5 years follow-up, 25 per cent patients had relapsed in the high-dose arm compared with 66 per cent in the control arm ($P < 0.01$). Mortality rates were 17 per cent (8/75) and 35 per cent (28/79), respectively. These dramatic benefits have been the subject of a fraud investigation by the NCI, which concluded that fraud had been committed.

Combined endocrine therapy and chemotherapy

Accumulating evidence, both indirect and direct, from randomized clinical trials supports the hypothesis that the benefits of adjuvant endocrine therapy and chemotherapy are additive. This is best reviewed in the systematic overviews of the Early Breast Cancer Trialists Collaborative Group summarized in Table 21.3 (EBCTCG, 1996, 1998a, b).

This does not imply that the different modalities interact in the same patients; they may benefit different subgroups in ways that are still poorly established. The example of ER− status as a possible indicator of endocrine resistance is an obvious instance. Many randomized clinical trials are testing various modalities in combination, including a CRC/Swedish trial testing goserelin versus no goserelin against a background of tamoxifen and/or chemotherapy. The ABC trial is another example of a pragmatic trial testing ovarian suppression (in premenopausal women) and/or chemotherapy against a background of tamoxifen in early breast cancer.

Adverse effects of chemotherapy

Dose-limiting complications relate most commonly to self-renewal tissues such as the marrow and intestinal mucosa, with the attendant risks of neutropenic sepsis, bleeding, anaemia and mucositis. Increased risk of thromboembolism is also a common feature of many common schedules. Virtually any organ system is vulnerable to adverse effects, depending on drugs and dose schedules, including gastrointestinal tract, liver, kidney, nervous system, heart, lungs, gonads, immune system and skin. Most acute toxicities are reversible if diagnosed early and managed appropriately, but fatal complications occur even under optimal conditions.

BISPHOSPHONATES IN EARLY BREAST CANCER

Although bisphosphonates were first introduced for the management of skeletal metastases (*see* below), recent trials have tested the benefits of these inhibitors of osteoclast function in the adjuvant setting. In two randomized trials of oral clodronate in 1079 and 284 women respectively, a statistically significant reduction in the incidence of bone metastases was reported (Diel *et al.*, 1998; Powles *et al.*, 1998a). In the smaller study from Germany, a reduced incidence of non-osseous metastases was also reported. These exciting findings are in contrast to a statistically increased incidence of metastases in a recent Finnish study testing adjuvant bisphosphonates. These agents are currently only appropriately prescribed in the context of a well-conducted randomized clinical trial.

RADIOTHERAPY IN EARLY BREAST CANCER

Impact on breast cancer mortality and cardiac deaths

The latest world overview of radiotherapy trials by the EBCTCG confirms a statistically significant reduction in the annual odds of death from breast cancer in patients randomized to radiotherapy after primary surgery, whatever the extent of surgery (EBCTCG, 2000). The relative reduction in risk is independent of node status, and is statistically significant in axillary node-positive and negative patients. It amounts to 8 per cent absolute reduction in breast cancer mortality at 20 years in node-positive and 3–4 per cent in node-negative patients. Meta-analysis of over 6000 patients shows the beneficial effects of radiotherapy to be additive with those of adjuvant chemotherapy. Roughly speaking, for every 20 isolated locoregional recurrences avoided by radiotherapy, 5 breast cancer deaths are prevented, a remarkably favourable 4 : 1 ratio. These substantial reductions in breast cancer mortality are offset by an increased risk of cardiac and vascular mortality, even in trials conducted in the megavoltage era, although less marked in trials started since 1975. Most recently, two Danish national trials comprising >3000 node-positive women tested radiotherapy to the chest wall (direct electron field), internal mammary chain, axilla and supraclavicular fossa after mastectomy and level I/II axillary dissection. They reported 10 per cent absolute overall survival with no excess cardiac mortality in high-risk pre- and postmenopausal women, respectively (Overgaard *et al.*, 1997; Overgaard, 1999).

There is every reason to expect that the same survival benefits are gained in women treated with breast-preserving surgery. In conclusion, there is overwhelming evidence for a major curative role for radiotherapy in women with early breast cancer provided cardiac shielding is implemented effectively, and exposure of major vessels is minimized. On the basis of a 2–3 per cent absolute reduction in breast cancer mortality in node-negative women, it can be argued that chest wall radiotherapy should be discussed with all patients opting for mastectomy, regardless of node status.

Indications for locoregional radiotherapy

The relative contributions to cure of radiotherapy to different target volumes (breast, chest wall, axilla, supraclavicular fossa, internal mammary chain) are currently unclear, since most trials have tested radiotherapy to all areas. Both local and lymphatic areas are likely to contribute, depending on the extent of primary surgery. Control of axillary disease is essential, but axillary radiotherapy is unlikely to contribute significantly after a complete axillary dissection. The contribution of radiotherapy to the supraclavicular fossa and internal mammary chain (IMC) is currently being tested in the EORTC 22922 protocol. It is quite possible that IMC irradiation will be shown to have an important role in reducing breast cancer mortality, since at least 30 per cent of axillary node-positive patients have involved IMC nodes (Handley, 1975). Until these uncertainties are resolved, it is important to achieve maximum locoregional control in at least

Table 21.4 *Trials comparing breast-conserving surgery with or without breast radiotherapy*

| Trial | Number | pT | Randomization | Actuarial rate % of breast recurrence: | | |
				RT	No RT	FU (years)
NSABP-B06 (Fisher *et al.*, 1989)	1265	<4 cm	LE ± RT	10.0	39.0	8
Uppsala (Liljegren *et al.*, 1994)	381	PT1pN-	WLE ± RT	2.3	18.4	5
Ontario (Clark *et al.*, 1996)	837	T1-2pN-	LE ± RT	11.3	35.7	10
Milan (Veronesi *et al.*, 1993)	567	T1-2	QU ± RT	0.3	9.0	3

LE, local excision; WLE, wide local excision; QU, quadrantectomy; RT, breast radiotherapy; FU, fluorouracil.

the breast/chest wall, axilla and supraclavicular fossa. The task is to identify women with, say, ≥10 per cent risk of recurrence at any local or regional site after taking into account tumour factors (tumour size, grade, lymphovascular invasion, node status) and treatment (extent of local and axillary surgery and impact of systemic therapy). For example, the reduction in breast cancer mortality expected in a population of patients at 10 per cent risk of locoregional recurrence cannot be estimated reliably at present; a benefit in the range of 2 per cent is likely, the threshold of effect commonly applied in discussions of adjuvant systemic therapy.

If a 10 per cent chest wall recurrence risk is adopted as a threshold for recommending adjuvant radiotherapy with curative intent, a high proportion of women qualify after mastectomy. So far, an international consensus has not been reached to recommend post-mastectomy radiotherapy in women with 1–3 positive axillary nodes (Recht *et al.*, 2001). The controversy focuses on the true rate of locoregional recurrence in these patients following optimal surgery and adjuvant systemic therapy, something that is best established by local audit. Traditional indicators identifying women at >30 per cent risk of chest wall recurrence (any tumour >5 cm, node positivity, lymphovascular invasion or microscopic evidence of tumour at the deep resection margins) will need to be revised to include any pT2 (pathological tumour diameter 2.1–5.0 cm) or G3 disease. Where axillary radiotherapy is concerned, the overview suggests that this is an effective alternative to axillary dissection. After a level I dissection (removing an average of 10 nodes) it may be preferable to refer node-positive patients back for level II/III clearance (Aitken *et al.*, 1989). The reported morbidity of axillary radiotherapy is very variable in the literature, but 10–40 per cent of patients suffer some degree of lymphoedema, depending on the dose and level of prior axillary surgery (Larson *et al.*, 1986). Node-positive patients have a 10–20 per cent lifetime risk of supraclavicular fossa relapse, depending on the number of affected axillary nodes, justifying radiotherapy to the supraclavicular fossa in view of the difficulty of relieving malignant lymphoedema and brachial plexopathy (McKinna *et al.*, 1999). It is rare for UK patients to be prescribed radiotherapy to the internal mammary chain, even in patients with central or axillary node-positive tumours, and it reflects poorly on UK practice that so few patients are entered into the European Organization for the Research and Treatment of Cancer (EORTC) 22922 trial.

After breast-preserving surgery for invasive carcinoma, radiotherapy to the whole breast is standard practice, although regional audits show that a significant proportion of patients >70 years are not offered treatment. In addition to reducing breast cancer mortality, radiotherapy achieves a fourfold reduction in the risk of breast relapse, even in patients with small tumours (Table 21.4). It is not yet possible to identify patients with such a low risk of breast cancer recurrence after tumour excision that subsequent radiotherapy is considered unnecessary. This question has been addressed in the UK by the British Association of Surgical Oncologists (BASO) II trial in patients with completely excised unifocal pT1G1LV-pN-M0 breast adenocarcinoma. So far, observational data from several sources suggest that even the most favourable tumours, in terms of size, grade and node status, have breast recurrence risks of >10 per cent by 10 years (Schnitt *et al.*, 1996).

The importance of a radiotherapy boost after tumour excision and whole-breast radiotherapy is now much clearer, having been tested in a large randomized trial of 5318 patients (90 per cent node-negative) by the EORTC (Bartelink *et al.*, 2001). A boost dose of 16 Gy in eight fractions after complete local excision and whole-breast radiotherapy to 50 Gy in 25 fractions reduced local recurrence risk by an average of 40 per cent (more in young women; less in older women). The biggest absolute effect was seen in women under 40 years of age, who suffered a 30 per cent local recurrence risk at 8 years without boost, reduced to just under 10 per cent with a boost. The added protection in women <50 years appears amply justified in relation to the added treatment morbidity in terms of altered breast appearance, pain and tenderness (Vrieling *et al.*, 1999). In node-negative women >50 years, the data suggest that a boost is not worthwhile, provided excision is microscopically complete.

Radiotherapy delivery

The patient lies supine and the position must remain unchanged for planning, simulation and treatment.

An adjustable inclined plane and stabilization devices are important components of a stable treatment position, requiring verification using orthogonal laser beams on reliable fiducial marks, such as surface point tattoos.

It is still too common for breast cancer patients to be planned by marking fields (50 per cent isodoses) on the skin, rather than by defining and planning a target volume. After breast-preserving surgery, the clinical target volume includes the soft tissues of the palpable breast down to the deep fascia, but excluding underlying muscle, rib-cage and overlying skin and scar. The shape and size of the clinical target volume after breast-preserving surgery corresponds to the edges of the palpable breast, although this is often difficult to define superiorly (the axillary tail defines the upper extent). After mastectomy, scar, skin and residual subcutaneous tissue are target tissues. The opposite breast can be used as a guide to defining clinical target volume, which ideally includes the whole mastectomy scar. The planning target volume includes the entire clinical target volume plus a 1 cm margin on all borders. After mastectomy, medial and lateral edges of the scar are sometimes excluded in order to minimize exposure of underlying heart and lung by tangential photon fields.

Transverse cross-sections through the target volume are taken with the patient in the treatment position, using a CT simulator or an external contouring device. The breast/chest wall is encompassed with 6 MeV X-rays (10 MeV for wide separations). The maximum thickness of lung should be 3 cm (preferably 2 cm) and cardiac shielding should be considered if any myocardium is included in the treatment volume, even at the cost of shielding target tissues (this can be a very difficult trade-off in the absence of precise risk:benefit data). If lymphatic fields are used, divergence of the superior border of tangential fields must be eliminated by the use of asymmetric collimators or couch rotation. Posterior divergence of tangential fields into heart and lung is overcome by widening the angle between the central axes by a few degrees, until the 50 per cent isodoses run parallel to each other at the back of the volume. Depending on the location of the primary tumour in the preserved breast, the medial and/or lateral field borders can be adjusted to minimize the amount of lung in the tangential fields. Heart shielding is easily implemented using a multileaf collimator or a manually placed shielding block, unless this involves shielding the tumour bed.

The breast-boost target allows a margin of several centimetres around the periphery of the tumour bed. The diameter of an electron field is influenced by the size of the original tumour, the amount of surrounding normal tissue removed by the surgeon and the accuracy of localization. A preoperative Polaroid photograph taken of the patient lying in the treatment position at the time of initial presentation is a useful way to localize the boost, but surgical clips are a guide if their exact relationship to the tumour is defined. The optimal target volume is not properly established but usually involves a 7–10-cm diameter 10–14 MeV electron field, treating down to the deep fascia without build-up to the skin or scar. Alternatively, an interstitial implant may be used.

The dose should be prescribed to the reference point at or near the centre of the target volume, typically halfway between the anterior skin surface and the lung/chest wall interface (ICRU, 1993). Radiotherapy dosimetry in the intact breast is inhomogeneous in the UK because it is often based on a single transverse contour of the patient, ignoring the dramatic changes in external contour above and below the central plane. In addition, reduced lung attenuation may be ignored, leading to added inhomogeneity. Under these conditions, 10–20 per cent dose variation through the breast is common, a potential determinant of increased complications and poor cosmesis.

The clinical target volume of lymphatic fields comprises the axillary lymph-node chain and the supraclavicular fossa, the latter depending on axillary lymph-node status. The volume is defined according to fixed anatomical landmarks, including soft tissue and bony structures. Some of these landmarks are defined at imaging, in which case clinical examination must ensure that palpable disease falls within the target volume. The field arrangement includes an anterior field with the reference points at the build-up depth, i.e. 100 per cent. A daily posterior axillary contribution may be added in order to ensure that the midline axilla dose does not fall below 80 or 85 per cent; this involves a posterior contribution of approximately 10 per cent in the current UK Standardization of Radiotherapy (START) trial. Improved lymphatic localization and dosimetry are current priorities for the UK.

The reproducibility of field localization should be monitored by machine check films or electronic portal imaging, the latter increasingly purchased as standard accessories with new treatment machines. Radiotherapy dose and fractionation for the whole breast is in the range 46–50 Gy to the ICRU reference point in 2.0 Gy fractions. The boost dose is usually 10 Gy to the reference point (100 per cent if electrons are used) in 2.0 Gy fractions. A variety of alternative fractionation schedules are in common use that aim to improve treatment outcome by reducing the number of fractions. The UK START trial compares 25 fractions of 2.0 Gy (50 Gy) over 5 weeks against 15 fractions of 2.67 Gy over 3 weeks. The initiative also tests 25 fractions of 2.0 Gy (50 Gy) against 13 fractions of 3.2 Gy (41.6 Gy) or 13 fractions of 3.0 Gy (39 Gy) over 5 weeks.

Risk factors for locoregional recurrence

The single most potent risk factor for chest wall recurrence after mastectomy is positive axillary node status, suggesting a pathogenesis linked to metastasis. After breast-conserving surgery, residual primary or multifocal disease appears to be more important than node status

(Kurtz, 1992). Clinical tumour size, lymphovascular invasion and pathological axillary node status are each reported as significant risk factors for breast recurrence after local excision in some studies, but not in all. Microscopic disease may be present several centimetres beyond the edge of macroscopic tumour (Holland *et al.*, 1985). The elevated risk of breast relapse with EIC is explained by a higher chance of bulky foci of residual invasive and intraduct disease in the tumour bed after local excision with narrow margins (Holland *et al.*, 1990b). EIC is more likely to affect young women and it appears to be partly responsible for the strongly elevated risk of breast relapse in women <40 years treated with breast-conserving surgery and radiotherapy, reported most vividly in the EORTC 'boost' trial (Bartelink *et al.*, 2001).

Tumours of different histological subtype have not been studied in sufficient numbers to allow a definitive statement to be made, but it is possible that favourable subtypes, e.g. tubular, medullary and mucinous, are less likely to recur locally after breast-conserving treatment. Where tumour grade is concerned, the small size of most clinico-pathological studies, tumour-sampling error, and wide inter-observer variation are cited as limiting the ability to interpret data. These, nevertheless, suggest a significant trend for high-grade tumours to carry a higher than average risk of breast relapse, as is the case for chest wall relapse after mastectomy.

The traditional view that breast relapse after breast-conserving surgery has a relatively favourable outcome is powerfully challenged by a combined analysis of two EORTC and Danish trials which randomized to breast-preserving therapy or mastectomy (van Tienhoven *et al.*, 1999). This shows the prognosis of patients relapsing in the breast to be no different and equally poor compared to patients relapsing on the chest wall after mastectomy.

Where lymphatic relapse is concerned, this is closely related to pathological node status, the presence of extracapsular extension and the extent and completeness of surgical resection (Yarnold, 1984). Extranodal extension is a risk factor for axillary (7 per cent) and supraclavicular (12 per cent) recurrence after therapeutic axillary dissection (Fisher *et al.*, 1997d). Axillary radiotherapy is justified in this context, provided the patient understands the possible cost in terms of iatrogenic morbidity.

SCHEDULING OF RADIOTHERAPY AND CHEMOTHERAPY

Adjuvant systemic therapies should be instituted within 2–4 weeks of primary surgery. The only randomized trial to have addressed the impact of treatment delay, tested adjuvant chemotherapy before radiotherapy against the reverse sequence in 244 women after primary surgery for early breast cancer (Recht *et al.*, 1996). Small sample size prevented firm conclusions being drawn, but delayed chemotherapy was associated with a marked, but non-significant, tendency for a higher rate of metastatic relapse, whereas delayed radiotherapy was associated with a marked, but non-significant, tendency for a higher rate of local relapse. Delays in starting breast radiotherapy after local excision have also been reported to predispose to breast recurrence in recent retrospective studies. In common with all retrospective data, they are extremely difficult to interpret because the timing of treatment may be clearly influenced by factors known to predispose to recurrence (McCormick *et al.*, 1993). The problem is that concurrent chemo-radiotherapy, especially with anthracycline combinations but to a lesser extent with CMF as well, increases the risk and severity of early and late normal tissue injury (Hji Yiannakis and Yarnold, 1996). The UK Sequencing of Chemotherapy and Radiotherapy in Early Breast Cancer (SECRAB) trial is currently testing the safety and effectiveness of intercalated versus sequential chemo-radiotherapy. Until reliable evidence is available on how to optimize the balance of risks and benefits, clinical practices will vary in a more or less arbitrary fashion. Doxorubicin and epirubicin must not be given concurrently with radiotherapy.

Adverse effects of radiotherapy

Fatigue is the most common side-effect of breast radiotherapy. Skin reactions during and after breast radiotherapy include erythema and dry and moist desquamation. Data from a randomized trial confirm that gentle washing is effective in reducing the intensity of acute skin reactions (Campbell and Illingworth, 1992). Loose cotton clothes are preferable to tight-fitting garments. Baby powder helps to absorb excess skin moisture and pruritus is relieved with 1 per cent hydrocortisone. Local areas of moist desquamation requiring Geliperm®, or similar dressing, can develop in the inframammary fold and axillary tail.

The breast becomes inflamed several months after radiotherapy in a minority of patients. If this is caused by a cellulitis, it improves with antibiotics. Occasionally it represents diffuse recurrence. Otherwise, breast swelling, erythema, pain and tenderness may be a radiotherapy reaction, which subsides over several months. The pathogenesis is unclear and non-steroidal anti-inflammatory agents occasionally help symptoms.

Breast atrophy and induration are the most obvious late effects of breast radiotherapy, causing variable degrees of shrinkage and distortion. Poor dosimetry is probably a major contributory factor to the worst results, although intrinsic radiation sensitivity may play a role in some patients. Matchline fibrosis can cause obvious changes in the subcutaneous tissues. Telangiectasia is seen most frequently when a build-up has been used for the boost, where skin surfaces are in apposition or where matchline problems have occurred. Other late effects include breast oedema, rib fracture and soft-tissue pain and tenderness.

Clinical or radiological pneumonitis seldom arises from tangential fields to the breast, unless attempts are made to include the internal mammary chain in the fields. Inclusion of heart muscle in tangential or internal mammary fields is responsible for a significantly raised risk of cardiac death in the second and subsequent decades of follow-up. If axillary/supraclavicular fossa fields are prescribed, pneumonitis may be symptomatic, especially if adjuvant chemotherapy is concurrent. Axillary dissection is associated with a 10 per cent risk of arm lymphoedema, double if radiotherapy is added (Swedborg and Wallgren, 1981; Werner et al., 1991). With proper attention to technical factors and dose prescription, radiation-induced brachial plexopathy is a rare occurrence.

The most important preventable complication of radiotherapy in women with left-sided tumours, is radiation-induced heart disease (Gyenes et al., 1997; Paszat et al., 1998). The 1999 world overview of radiotherapy trials indicate that this is responsible for 2–3 fatalities for every 100 women treated over a 20-year period. The elevated risk is not confined to the orthovoltage era. It is therefore not possible to say that partial volume exposure confined to the cardiac apex, which includes part of the anterior descending coronary artery, is free of risk. The risk of stroke and other vascular death is not yet fully quantified, but these complications need to be considered in relation to lymphatic techniques.

The increased risk of non-breast second malignancies is another important complication of treatment to consider, including sarcomas and carcinomas. Where cancer of the opposite breast is concerned, randomized trials of radiotherapy versus no radiotherapy in the treatment of early breast cancer show no suggestion of an increased risk of a contralateral primary in the irradiated patients, but the overall numbers of patients and events are relatively small. Several large, case-matched controlled cancer registry studies are consistent with a statistically significant increased risk associated with the use of radiation (Boice et al., 1992). The relative risk is about 1.3 but the absolute risk remains low at <1 per cent per year.

SPECIAL PRESENTATIONS OF EARLY BREAST CANCER

Duct carcinoma in-situ

Since mammographic screening programmes were introduced, the proportion of breast cancer patients presenting with pure DCIS has risen from a few per cent to approximately 20 per cent. The traditional management of patients with a palpable mass is mastectomy. DCIS is typically unifocal but local excision alone is associated with a significant risk of local recurrence, since the tumour often extends much more widely than clinical or mammographic examinations suggest (Holland et al., 1990a). The control arms of randomized trials testing the effects of radiotherapy by the NSABP and EORTC confirm this (Fisher et al., 1998b; Julien et al., 2000). In the NSABP B-17 trial, 818 patients with microscopically complete excision of localized pure DCIS were randomized to lumpectomy with or without whole-breast radiotherapy (50 Gy in 25 fractions over 5 weeks, with no planned boost). The outcome data at 8 years show a significant reduction in ipsilateral invasive breast recurrence from 13.4 per cent to 3.9 per cent and of all ipsilateral recurrence from 26.8 per cent to 12.1 per cent after radiotherapy. The EORTC 10853 trial addressed the same question in 1010 patients. The addition of whole-breast radiotherapy (50 Gy in 25 fractions over 5 weeks with no boost) significantly reduced the incidence of invasive breast recurrences from 8 to 4 per cent, and all recurrences from 16 to 9 per cent at 4 years. A peculiarity of this trial was that there were 16 contralateral tumours in the irradiated group and 5 in the non-irradiated. This is unlikely to be radiation-induced, and is more likely a chance finding. These two trials demonstrate that radiotherapy significantly reduces the risk of ipsilateral invasive recurrence, but do not have the power to test for a reduction in distant metastasis or breast cancer mortality. Neither were the trials set up to identify prognostic subgroups that would be better treated by mastectomy, on the one hand, or those who may not need radiotherapy after complete excision, on the other – issues that need to be addressed by the next generation of trials.

Even mastectomy is not always curative, with metastasis and death reported in 1–2 per cent of cases. Risk factors for ipsilateral recurrence retrospectively reported by the NSABP B-17 included degree of necrosis but not excision margin width. The EORTC identified age <40 years, symptomatic presentation, involved margins and solid/cribriform growth pattern as risk factors for ipsilateral recurrence after breast-conservation surgery. The Van Nuys index proposed by Silverstein offers a provisional measure of how different subgroups may vary in local recurrence risk, but this has not been independently or prospectively validated (Silverstein et al., 1999).

With regard to adjuvant tamoxifen, the NSABP B-24 trial reported a significant reduction in the recurrence of invasive and non-invasive disease in the ipsilateral breast from 14 per cent to 8 per cent at 5 years in 1804 women randomized to 5 years tamoxifen after local excision and whole-breast radiotherapy (Fisher et al., 1999). The United Kingdom Co-ordinating Committee for Cancer Research (UKCCCR) DCIS Trial (in press) used a 2 × 2 factorial design to compare the effectiveness of complete local excision alone, or followed by radiotherapy and/or tamoxifen, in 1694 patients. It is reported to show similar results to the NSABP B-17 and EORTC 10853 studies for the addition of radiotherapy (roughly a 50 per cent reduction in the risk of local recurrence). However, no difference in local progression is reported for the addition of tamoxifen to radiotherapy. This contrasts with the results of NSABP B-24, the most obvious difference between the study populations being age; the UK patients were mainly >50 years, whereas in the US trial a high proportion of women were <50 years. Neither trial offers any information on the influence of ER status on treatment benefit. The full results of the UKCCCR trial and a similar Radiation Therapy Oncology Group (RTOG) 9804 trial are awaited.

Elderly

Women over 70 years have an average life expectancy of 15 years and account for one-third of breast cancer presentations (Silliman *et al.*, 1993). Tamoxifen as sole treatment has been evaluated in this age group. In UK trials, half the patients required a change in local management within 2 years of presentation (Bates *et al.*, 1991). On the basis of these data, local excision or mastectomy should be offered to elderly women with early breast cancer unless co-morbidity prevents effective primary surgery. Adjuvant tamoxifen should be added in patients with oestrogen-positive tumours, in view of its beneficial effects on disease-free and overall survival. Women in their seventies and eighties are usually fit enough to cope with radiotherapy. There is no evidence that late normal tissue reactions are more likely with increasing age.

Bilateral breast cancer

The incidence of bilateral primary tumours at presentation is about 1 per cent. In patients presenting with unilateral disease, the annual incidence of a contralateral primary is about 0.75 per cent. Risk factors include known or suspected genetic predisposition, young age at first presentation, a positive family history, multicentric disease in the ipsilateral breast and lobular histological subtype. Some of these risk factors may reflect a genetic predisposition in a minority of patients. Where the management of bilateral or contralateral tumours is concerned, each cancer is treated on its own merits.

Pregnancy

Breast cancer arising during pregnancy presents a particularly difficult set of clinical problems to resolve, where the interests of the fetus and mother may not coincide (Clark and Chua, 1989; Doll *et al.*, 1989). Breast cancer during pregnancy or lactation is associated with a less favourable stage distribution, and about two-thirds of patients are node positive. Investigations are kept to a minimum. Haematology and a biochemical screen, including liver function tests and alkaline phosphatase, are needed to supplement the clinical assessment. Breast ultrasound

should be used in preference to mammography. A chest radiograph should not be performed routinely, especially in the first trimester.

In the first trimester the fetus is at its most vulnerable to developmental abnormalities as a result of exposure to general anaesthesia, radiation or cytotoxic agents. The patient should be asked to consider termination. If the patient decides against abortion, mastectomy or breast-conserving surgery should be considered. In the second and third trimesters adjuvant chemotherapy has not been associated with an increased risk of congenital abnormalities, although the literature is small. Methotrexate should be avoided. Endocrine therapy and radiotherapy should be postponed until after delivery. In node-positive women, it will often be necessary to introduce chemotherapy in the second or third trimester. If so, folate antagonists are often avoided, although fluorouracil has been used safely in 24 pregnant women (Berry *et al.*, 1999). Otherwise, 4 cycles of AC are usually given (Stevenson *et al.*, 1997).

Case-matched control studies show no reduction in life expectancy in women who become pregnant 6 months or more after treatment for early breast cancer. Patients are advised to wait at least several months after the end of radiotherapy, adjuvant systemic therapy and tamoxifen before trying to have a child. Depending on the intensity of chemotherapy, a majority of women under 40 years and a minority of premenopausal patients over 40 years resume ovulatory cycles.

Paget's disease

Paget's disease is a form of breast cancer presenting with eczematous changes of the nipple, which may extend onto the adjacent areola and skin. It may be associated with nipple discharge, inversion or erosion, and clinical or mammographic evidence of an underlying primary tumour mass. Malignant cells in the epidermis are diagnostic and have a characteristic appearance, with large, pale-staining cells with clear cytoplasm staining positively for mucin. The cells represent intra-epidermal spread from an underlying intraduct or invasive adenocarcinoma. The most common treatment is mastectomy but there are now several reports of successful breast conservation with radiotherapy following removal of the nipple and underlying tumour with clear surgical margins (Bulens *et al.*, 1990).

Male breast cancer

Breast cancer in men represents less than 1 per cent of breast cancer. Risk factors include a history of unopposed oestrogens resulting from primary or secondary testicular failure, including Klinefelter's syndrome and exogenous oestrogens. Patients present with a lump, with or without nipple retraction, bleeding, ulceration, deep fixation and axillary adenopathy. The main differential diagnosis is gynaecomastia. Staging procedures are the same as for female patients and the treatment of choice for operable disease is mastectomy. The principles of axillary surgery are the same as for women, with axillary clearance reducing the risk of regional recurrence.

There are no clear guidelines for the use of postmastectomy radiotherapy because of small patient numbers and data confined to retrospective studies. Some reports indicate a reduction in locoregional relapse after mastectomy, but not all. In the absence of good data it is reasonable to apply the same criteria as in women. There are indications from case-matched control studies that adjuvant tamoxifen and adjuvant chemotherapy are each effective in early male breast cancer (Ribeiro and Swindell, 1992). Given the modest toxicity of tamoxifen, it is reasonable to prescribe it to all patients. It is difficult to recommend a policy for adjuvant chemotherapy, given the retrospective nature of the data and the relative side-effects of treatment. It seems reasonable to make young node-positive patients aware of the possibilities of gain, and to administer it to those keen to have the treatment despite its uncertain benefit. It is not clear that men fare any worse than women after stratification for known factors such as TNM stage, oestrogen-receptor status and grade.

Axillary adenopathy

A presentation with enlarged axillary nodes accounts for less than 0.5 per cent of breast cancer. The differential diagnosis includes non-malignant causes such as infection and autoimmune disorders, and malignancies of the lung, gastrointestinal tract, melanoma and lymphoma. By far the likeliest primary site if the lymph node contains metastatic adenocarcinoma is the breast, and patients should be investigated accordingly with clinical assessment, mammography and, increasingly, magnetic resonance imaging (MRI).

In the absence of symptoms or signs of a primary tumour or distant metastases, the options for operable disease are axillary clearance and mastectomy or breast radiotherapy. An occult breast primary is found in more than half the mastectomy specimens in the larger series. Any mammographic abnormality should be resected first if breast preservation is being considered. It is reasonable to apply the same criteria for adjuvant systemic therapy as in patients with a palpable primary breast cancer. The prognosis is comparable to that of patients presenting with a breast lump and positive axillary nodes.

TREATMENT OF PATIENTS WITH LOCALLY ADVANCED DISEASE

About 20 per cent of patients present with locally advanced disease without evidence of metastases. Locally advanced disease refers to tumours over 5 cm in diameter (T3), and tumours of any size with overlying oedema, chest-wall fixation, skin infiltration or inflammatory features (T4). In terms of management, the locoregional disease is classified as operable (stage IIIA) or inoperable (stage IIIB). Several randomized trials have compared different local and systemic treatment strategies, either alone or in combination (Dorr et al., 1989). The general conclusions are that two modalities of treatment are better than one, and that three modalities (systemic therapy, surgery and radiotherapy) are more effective than two (Yarnold, 2001).

Primary surgery for patients with operable disease

Mastectomy with axillary dissection is associated with locoregional recurrence in at least 30 per cent of patients. Five-year survival rates for patients with positive nodes are in the range 40–50 per cent. A small subgroup of patients with large primary tumours and negative axillary histology have a more favourable outcome. On the basis of its proven effect in early stage disease, it is assumed that postmastectomy radiotherapy in patients with advanced local disease will also be useful in reducing the risk of locoregional relapse. Retrospective studies of mastectomy with radiotherapy report locoregional relapse rates in the range 10–20 per cent. An Eastern Co-operative Oncology Group (ECOG) randomized trial of 332 patients with stage IIIA disease tested combined chemo-endocrine therapy with and without locoregional radiotherapy after modified or standard radical mastectomy. A modest reduction in locoregional progression from 20 to 11 per cent was seen in patients randomized to radiotherapy, and, unexpectedly, an increased metastasis rate (Olson et al., 1997). This interpretation of this result is controversial, and is not considered sufficient to overturn the recommendation for radiotherapy in this group of patients (Fowble, 1997).

Primary medical therapy

The practice of introducing intensive chemo-endocrine therapy as primary treatment in women with locally advanced breast cancer is becoming common, as it is becoming clear that the majority of patients gain at least a partial response, and approximately 10 per cent of patients gain a complete pathological response (Kuerer et al., 1999). These response data lead to encouraging expectations that this approach will offer real benefits to patients in terms of locoregional control, relapse-free survival and, possibly, overall survival in the future. Radiotherapy alone, or as a prelude to surgery in patients with tumours of borderline operability, is increasingly reserved for patients who are too unfit for, or refuse, chemo-endocrine therapy.

Chemotherapy is also the mainstay of treatment for inflammatory carcinoma, with or without endocrine therapy (Jaiyesimi *et al.*, 1992). Retrospective studies suggest that optimal locoregional control is gained with mastectomy and postoperative radiotherapy after several months of chemotherapy, with approximately two-thirds of patients remaining locally disease-free for the remainder of their lives. Unfortunately, the prognosis is worse than for non-inflammatory cancer, and it is impossible to say whether the natural history of the metastatic disease is significantly affected by the systemic therapy. The contribution of radiotherapy has not been tested directly in randomized trials.

MANAGEMENT OF LOCOREGIONAL RECURRENCE

Recurrence in the breast after breast-conserving surgery and radiotherapy for ductal carcinoma usually develops close to the primary site (Kurtz *et al.*, 1990). The majority of local recurrences are discrete tumours in the breast parenchyma, which are operable by mastectomy or further wide excision. If staging investigations are negative and the disease operable, the prognosis of this selected subgroup is relatively good, with 70 per cent alive at 5 years. In patients entered into two randomized breast-conservation trials, 5-year survival rates of 58 per cent have been reported after ipsilateral breast relapse, no better than in patients relapsing on the chest wall after randomization to mastectomy (van Tienhoven *et al.*, 1999).

Locoregional relapse after mastectomy alone is associated with distant metastases on routine restaging in approximately 50 per cent patients. In these women, appropriate systemic measures constitute the treatment of first choice. Patients with isolated locoregional recurrence should be considered for surgery and high-dose radiotherapy. Roughly half the patients will be alive 5 years later and approximately half will achieve long-term locoregional control (Schwaibold *et al.*, 1991).

TREATMENT OF PATIENTS WITH METASTATIC DISEASE

Presentation and evaluation

Chest-wall or regional recurrence is associated with distant metastases in about 50 per cent of patients. Common sites of metastatic relapse include the skeleton, lung, pleura, liver, spinal cord and brain. Clinical assessment is used to guide staging investigations. Prognostic factors include relapse-free interval and the pattern of organ involvement. If the skeleton or pleura is the dominant site, the median survival is more than 2 years. Disease in the liver or central nervous system is associated with a median survival of less than 1 year.

Principles of management

Clinical trials have not demonstrated that conventional therapies prolong overall survival, although trials of new therapies are promising (*see* below). The principle of management is to select treatments that forestall or palliate cancer complications in exchange for the minimum iatrogenic toxicity. Beyond the management of co-morbid conditions, the first choice of systemic treatment is often endocrine therapy supplemented by other measures, including radiotherapy, to palliate specific symptoms. A durable symptomatic remission may be associated with less than a partial response, i.e. stable disease. Patients who relapse within 2 years of presentation, have multiple organ involvement, especially liver, or who have progressive symptoms of visceral disease are usually considered for cytotoxic therapy as first-line palliative treatment.

Endocrine therapy

Endocrine therapy is the first choice for a significant proportion of patients (Fossati *et al.*, 1998). The probability of a clinical response increases with a disease-free interval over 2 years, a pattern of relapse in bone, skin, lymph nodes and pleura, and positive ER status. Symptomatic responses tend to take longer to materialize than with chemotherapy, but this may reflect selection bias based on tumour type rather than the treatment.

The ER protein is an important component of the oestrogen-response pathway, and its concentration in tumour correlates with the chances of an endocrine response. Even so, response to ovarian suppression has been reported in about 20 per cent of premenopausal patients with metastatic ER− tumours, compared with 40 per cent of those with ER+ disease (Blamey *et al.*, 1992). Oestrogen blockade with tamoxifen (20 mg daily) is a reasonable first choice in premenopausal women (Crump *et al.*, 1997). Transient hypercalcaemia is a favourable therapeutic sign, referred to as a 'tamoxifen flare'. In premenopausal women tamoxifen increases pituitary gonadotrophins and total plasma oestradiol levels, and does not necessarily stop ovulation. The response rate to a second endocrine agent following response to tamoxifen is about 30 per cent. Ovarian suppression by laparoscopic oophorectomy, radiotherapy (e.g. 16 Gy in four fractions) or luteinizing hormone releasing hormone (LHRH) agonists in premenopausal women is an alternative to first-line tamoxifen in ER+ women, and is needed before a trial of an aromatase inhibitor. Third-generation aromatase inhibitors, such as anastrazole or letrozole, are currently used as second-line endocrine agents after failure of tamoxifen in postmenopausal women, causing fewer side-effects than their predecessors, formestane, fadrozole and aminoglutethimide. They are also less toxic than progestogens. After response to a third-generation aromatase inhibitor, the progestogen megestrol acetate (160 mg daily) may be introduced, depending on symptom progression and medical fitness. Side-effects of progestogens include troublesome weight gain and fluid retention, especially in the elderly. Sequential endocrine therapy appears to be superior to combined concurrent therapy.

Recent trials suggest that third-generation aromatase inhibitors are at least equivalent, and perhaps superior, to tamoxifen as first-line agents in postmenopausal women with advanced breast cancer (Goss and Strasser, 2001). In practice, the majority of ER+ patients will already have been exposed to tamoxifen in the adjuvant setting, so that aromatase inhibitors may be the first choice anyway. Aromatase inhibitors and inactivators are associated with hot flushes and sweats, but are not associated with thromboembolism and other oestrogen-agonist effects.

Chemotherapy

Failure of endocrine therapy and other measures to control progressive symptoms is a common context in which chemotherapy is introduced. Symptoms of visceral relapse are commonly an indication for introducing chemotherapy without a prior trial of endocrine therapy. The severity of symptoms and speed of progression at relapse are also factors that affect choice of first modality, serious or life-threatening symptoms or signs justifying chemotherapy because of the higher chances of symptomatic improvement (up to 70 per cent).

The trade-off between symptoms of disease and treatment toxicity can only be judged by patient self-assessments, testing their impact on physical and psychological function. These assessments are rarely performed in the routine setting, and therapeutic response is judged in terms of the change in parameters related directly to tumour bulk, combined with a broad measure of physical performance. Most routine clinical assessments are hence crude measures of patient benefit.

It is common to start with one of a number of schedules applied in the adjuvant setting, including classical CMF, although AC or one of several other commonly used, and more or less equivalent, anthracycline combinations are now more common starting points. Overall, tumour-response rates are in the range 50–70 per cent, with about 10 per cent of patients achieving a complete clinical remission. The median duration of response is in the range 6–9 months. After progression on anthracyclines, it is increasingly common to consider taxanes, which are clearly active in this disease. The clinical benefit of taxanes in the palliative setting is currently being tested in the UK ABO1 randomized trial, which is comparing epirubicin and paclitaxel against epirubicin and cyclophosphamide in terms of progression-free survival, treatment toxicities, quality of life and health-economic consequences. The two schedules appear to be equivalent in terms of progression-free survival. Taxanes are licensed for this application in the UK and have been approved by

the National Insitute of Clinical excellence (NICE) for use after failure of anthracyclines. Other agents under evaluation include vinorelbine and gemcitabine.

The importance of dose intensity in the palliative setting is difficult to address because most trials have failed to incorporate end points related to impact of therapy on life quality. In addition, many trials have tested standard schedules of polychemotherapy against lower doses of the same drugs. These and other points, including the likely importance of patient selection, are well reviewed in a meta-analysis of metastatic breast cancer treatment (Fossati et al., 1998). In 14 randomized clinical trials involving 2765 patients, higher (often standard) dose chemotherapy schedules conferred a modest reduction in the odds of death, equivalent to absolute survival gains of 6 per cent at 1 year and 3 per cent at 3 years, at the expense of a higher burden of toxicity. One well-conducted trial addressing dose intensity in the palliative setting suggested a dose response for better life quality as well as tumour response with standard- versus low-dose CMF (Tannock et al., 1988). There are fewer uncertainties concerning the relative benefits of intermittent versus continuous treatment regimens. The largest trial, which randomized 308 patients to 6 cycles of polychemotherapy versus 3 cycles plus a further 3 cycles at symptom progression, reported significantly superior objective response duration and life quality with the continuous-therapy approach (Coates et al., 1987). The effects of continuing CAF beyond 6 cycles has been tested in 145 stable or responding patients, randomized to continue CAF or resume at the onset of symptoms (Ejlertsen et al., 1993). The symptom-free survival was longer in the continuously treated group at the expense of greater treatment toxicity, but the lack of life-quality assessments make it impossible to evaluate the benefit to the patient. In routine practice, it is common to combine informal assessments of patient tolerance with formal evaluation of tumour response after two courses. Patients with progressive symptoms or signs do not proceed with that schedule.

Experimental approaches aimed at improving the quality of life and overall survival of women with metastatic disease include the evaluation of high-dose chemotherapy with marrow transplantation. In the only phase III trial of this type, cyclophosphamide $6000\,mg/m^2$, thiotepa $500\,mg/m^2$ and carboplatin $800\,mg/m^2$ plus transplant was tested against maintenance CMF in women induced with either CAF or CMF. Only 199/513 (39 per cent) women entered into the trial were randomized, with no gains in complete response (CR), time to progression or overall survival (Stadtmauer et al., 1999). Where trastuzumab (Herceptin®) against the c-erbB2/HER2 oncoprotein is concerned, a randomized clinical trial involving 469 patients with metastatic disease, overexpressing this plasma-membrane growth factor receptor, tested the addition of simultaneous trastuzumab to AC or paclitaxel (Slamon et al., 2001). At a median follow-up of 25 months, a statistically significant survival gain of several months was reported in favour of AC or paclitaxel combined with trastuzumab. The most significant toxicity was cardiac dysfunction in 27 per cent of patients given an anthracycline, cyclophosphamide and trastuzumab, in 13 per cent of patients given paclitaxel and trastuzumab, in 8 per cent of patients given anthracycline and cyclophosphamide, and in 1 per cent of patients given paclitaxel alone.

COMPLICATIONS OF METASTATIC DISEASE

Skeletal secondaries

Skeletal metastases occur in up to 70 per cent of patients with metastatic breast cancer, and are responsible for major morbidity, including pain, fracture and spinal-cord compression. The pathogenesis of bone pain is not well understood, but chemical mediators of pain are believed to play a role. Pressure on the periosteum, bone fracture, nerve-root compression and associated muscle spasm are other causes of pain associated with bone secondaries. Confirming the clinical diagnosis is seldom difficult with the help of radiographs and isotopic bone-scan evidence. The medical management of skeletal pain involves the use of non-narcotic analgesics, narcotics and non-steroidal anti-inflammatory agents. Antidepressants, steroids, anticonvulsants and muscle relaxants also have a role, depending on specific clinical features. Other approaches to pain management include bisphosphonates, radiotherapy and chemo-endocrine therapies.

Bisphosphonates interfere with tumour-mediated lysis by inhibiting osteoclast recruitment and function. Pamidronate (90 mg i.v. every 4 weeks) or clodronate (1500 mg i.v. every 2 weeks) reduce pain severity in about 50 per cent of patients, and is routinely considered for patients with multiple pain sites. Oral therapy has not, so far, been shown to be effective against skeletal pain (Robertson et al., 1995). If pain does not improve after 3 cycles of i.v. bisphosphonate therapy, it should be stopped; otherwise, it is often continued for 6 months in the absence of data on optimal duration. The role of bisphosphonates in managing skeletal metastases uncomplicated by pain or fracture is at an advanced stage of evaluation. Six randomized trials of oral clodronate or i.v. pamidronate confirm lower rates of pathological fractures of long bones and vertebrae, spinal-cord compression, analgesia, orthopaedic surgery and radiotherapy (Paterson et al., 1993; Conte et al., 1996).

Radiotherapy is a very effective treatment for breast cancer patients with painful skeletal metastases. Patients have at least a 65 per cent chance of worthwhile pain relief, with complete response in about 20 per cent, as judged by self-assessment questionnaires. No clear evidence for a dose response has emerged for the short-term relief of bone pain. The long-term effectiveness of a single fraction of 8 Gy compared to multifraction schedules has been established using patient self-assessments for 12 months in 761 patients with uncomplicated metastatic bone pain, more than half with breast cancer (BPTWP, 1999).

Pathological fracture of a long bone is a complication that should be prevented as often as possible by periodic review of femoral radiographs in patients with known skeletal disease. It is difficult to predict pathological fracture, but erosion of more than half the cortical thickness is an indication for an orthopaedic opinion concerning prophylactic surgical fixation or pinning. There is no randomized evidence relating to the contribution of post-surgical radiotherapy, or the optimal dose, but 20 Gy in five fractions is commonly prescribed.

Brain secondaries

Patients present with symptoms and signs of raised intracranial pressure, with or without focal neurological signs. The clinical diagnosis is confirmed by computed tomography (CT) or MRI scanning. There is a role for surgical resection followed by whole-brain radiotherapy for solitary lesions on MRI. Standard treatment for multiple symptomatic secondaries is palliative radiotherapy to the whole brain. No survival advantage has been demonstrated for high-dose palliation, and 20 Gy in five fractions is a commonly used schedule. A UK trial comparing 30 Gy in 10 fractions with 12 Gy in two fractions delivered 1 week apart reported no difference in functional status or overall survival, although it is not clear to what extent this trial has influenced routine practice (Priestman et al., 1996). Chemotherapy can offer effective palliation of intracerebral disease and should be considered for patients with symptomatic multisystem disease, especially those needing palliative chemotherapy for other symptoms (Boogerd et al., 1992).

Compression of the spinal cord and cauda equina

Diagnostic suspicion of cord compression constitutes an oncological emergency. Spinal-cord compression associated with bone secondaries occurs when a tumour in a vertebral body or neural arch extends beyond the bone into the spinal canal, or when a vertebral collapse narrows the spinal canal. MRI studies suggest that soft-tissue epidural deposits are a more common source of spinal-cord compression than previously realized. This diagnosis should be considered with the onset of back pain in a patient without plain radiological evidence of a local bony lesion. Local and radicular pains, sensory changes, motor deficits and bladder/bowel dysfunction are all common presenting features. Cauda equina lesions present with lower motor neuron weakness affecting the bladder and bowel, associated lax anal sphincter tone and sacral anaesthesia. The chance of preventing permanent paraplegia depends on urgent investigation and treatment in the earliest stages of development.

MRI of the whole spine is the investigation of choice, and needs to be performed on the same day if possible. Immediate surgical referral and decompression must be achieved within 24–48 hours of symptoms for the maximum chances of functional recovery. Dexamethasone 16 mg daily in divided doses should be introduced as soon as a clinical diagnosis is made, to reduce inflammation and ease pain. In non-surgical cases, urgent radiotherapy is the mainstay of palliative treatment. There are no data on the optimal dose prescription in this situation. It is common to give a tumour dose of 20 Gy in five fractions at 5 cm depth. Chemotherapy does not have a defined role in the management of this complication. The success of treatment and rehabilitation depends strongly on the neurological deficit at presentation. Patients who can still walk have good chances of full functional recovery, whereas paraplegic patients are unlikely to be helped to a useful degree.

Carcinomatous meningitis

Metastases to the meninges are usually established via the arachnoid vessels and affect the meninges along the whole cranio-spinal axis. Presenting features include headache, altered mental state, cranial nerve palsies, lower motor neuron signs and positive Babinski's sign. The diagnosis can be difficult and rests on noting a variety of symptoms and signs at more than one level in the central nervous system. Positive cytology in the cerebrospinal fluid is achieved in about half the patients after the first lumbar puncture, which may need to be repeated to confirm a clinical diagnosis.

Unfortunately, intrathecal or intraventricular chemotherapy seldom offers little more than transient improvement in symptoms and signs, and local palliative radiotherapy may be a more appropriate way of relieving local symptoms and signs in many patients. The prognosis is very poor, usually a few weeks, although some long-term responders to intrathecal methotrexate have been reported.

Malignant effusions

Malignant pleural effusions tend to develop ipsilaterally and affected patients have a more favourable prognosis than patients with other metastatic sites of relapse. Patients usually complain of dyspnoea, and a chest radiograph is usually sufficient to confirm a diagnosis. Cytology or pleural biopsy help to distinguish cancer from non-malignant causes of effusion. Heparinized pleural fluid is sent for cytology, which is positive in about 75 per cent of malignant effusions. If subsequent aspirations fail to confirm the diagnosis, pleural biopsy is justified. Management includes thoracocentesis of 1 litre prior to commencing endocrine or chemotherapy in a patient with multiple symptomatic sites of metastasis. If the pleura is the sole or main site of relapse, thoracoscopy plus talc pleurodesis is the treatment of choice.

Malignant pericardial effusions are far less common than pleural effusions, occasionally presenting as tamponade with dyspnoea, chest pain and cough. Cardiac ultrasound is the most sensitive way to confirm a clinical diagnosis of pericardial effusion. If the patient is mildy symptomatic, endocrine or chemotherapy can be considered as first options if the malignant nature of the effusion is not in doubt. In the presence of more marked symptoms or tamponade, a pericardial window will need to be considered urgently.

Hypercalcaemia

Hypercalcaemia is one of the most common complications in patients with advanced breast cancer and is nearly always associated with skeletal metastases. Parathyroid hormone-like factors appear to be less important than in some other cancers. Endocrine therapy is sometimes a cause of transient hypercalcaemia within a few weeks of instituting treatment. Symptoms of hypercalcaemia are highly variable and reflect alterations in neurological, gastrointestinal, renal, musculoskeletal and cardiac functions. The basis of management includes intravenous rehydration with correction of electrolyte imbalances, the use of bisphosphonates and a review of systemic therapy options.

PSYCHOSOCIAL SUPPORT

Shock, fear and disbelief are common initial reactions met by the clinician who imparts the diagnosis (Fallowfield, 1990). Speed in reaching the diagnosis is important. The ability of patients to cope with the uncertainty improves with counselling and good professional and social support (McArdle et al., 1996). Trained nurse counsellors are of great value in this respect, and breast care nurses are one of the most valuable components of a multidisciplinary breast clinic. Anxiety is common in the initial stages and is best managed by counselling in the first instance. Short-term anxiolytics may be needed to overcome severe anxiety or panic attacks. Clinical depression persists beyond the first few weeks in a proportion of patients, and antidepressants should be considered.

Women find it increasingly helpful to be informed and involved in decision making despite the additional responsibility this places upon them at a most stressful time in their lives. Many patients have clear ideas about the level of information that they find helpful. Others appear not to expect a lot of information. The approach needs to be modified to the patient's level of specialized knowledge and understanding.

HORMONE REPLACEMENT THERAPY

A history of breast cancer is considered a contraindication for hormone replacement therapy (HRT). A proportion of women with breast cancer develop natural or iatrogenic menopausal symptoms, especially hot flushes and sweats. If symptoms interfere significantly with life quality, it is reasonable to recommend HRT for at least a few months in the first instance after other remedies, including a trial of venlafaxine, have failed, especially if this helps compliance with adjuvant tamoxifen. Combined low-oestrogen/progestogen preparations are advised, although the progestogen can be omitted in patients who have had a hysterectomy. Oestrogen/progestogen skin patches allow greater flexibility in adjusting the minimum dose of hormone replacement to suppress symptoms. Historical data are scanty (DiSaia, 1993). A randomized trial has recently been started in the UK to resolve the issue, especially as there are proven benefits relating to protection from osteoporosis and heart disease.

FOLLOW-UP

Evidence-based guidelines based on randomized clinical trials are scarce, but alternatives to regular and endless hospital outpatient attendances are being explored, including the role of nurse-led clinics. Apart from breast examination, no routine investigations are required except for annual mammography (after mastectomy this is biennial for the opposite breast) for the first 5 years and every other year thereafter, at least up to the age of 70 years (Maher, 1995).

FUTURE DEVELOPMENTS

The number of new drugs under clinical testing has never been higher, and the pace is likely to quicken in the years ahead. These include fluorouracil analogues, such as capecitabine and vinorelbine, a vinca alkaloid that interferes with tubulin assembly. Current interest focuses on trastuzumab, a humanized monoclonal murine antibody to the Neu/c-erb B2/HER-2 plasma membrane receptor, the first successful clinical targeting of a tumour-specific defect in breast cancer. This drug is currently under test in phase III adjuvant trials. Angiogenesis and tumour telomerase are other targets under investigation. Restoration of depleted tumour-suppressor gene products, and targeting intracellular signalling molecules, including tyrosine kinase inhibitors, are also in clinical development and testing.

Virtually complete oestrogen suppression is already achievable with current oestrogen antagonists. Selective blockade of oestrogen action in tumour cells is a goal of research into selective oestrogen receptor modulators, based on recognition of the different roles of the different oestrogen receptors and the added level of tissue specificity conferred via cofactors that regulate transcription from oestrogen-responsive genes. Targeting intra-tumoral metabolism of oestrogen conjugates by sulphatase enzymes is one such approach.

Technical radiotherapy research will focus on improving treatment to the breast and lymphatic pathways. Techniques of beam intensity modulation for eliminating heart and lung exposure and reducing dose variation in the breast, which should greatly improve cosmetic outcome and reduce complications, are being developed. Where dose-fractionation is concerned, the START trial will clarify the relevance of fraction size, and will generate reliable dose–response data for tumour control and normal tissue injury. These data will help adjust the total dose more carefully to recurrence risk, thereby optimizing the trade-off between tumour complication and treatment complication risks. Genetic factors that predispose to radiotherapy-induced normal tissue complications are also likely to be identified within the next 5–10 years.

SIGNIFICANT POINTS

- Population-based mammography of the 50–64-year age group should save 1250 lives per year in the UK, assuming 70 per cent uptake by women in that age group.
- Breast cancer diagnosis relies on a triple assessment, namely clinical examination, mammography ($\pm$ultrasound) and aspiration cytology.
- Before cutting into an excised breast lump, the specimen must be tagged with sutures to enable orientation of the specimen, dipped into Indian ink and air dried before sending to the pathology laboratory.
- The pathological description of an excised tumour should include the dimensions and weight of the surgical specimen, the maximum microscopic diameter of invasive disease, the macroscopic and microscopic margins (and locations) of excision, tumour grade, oestrogen-receptor status, the presence of vascular invasion and the extent of an *in-situ* component.
- The doctor must know exactly what his/her breast surgeon means by a diagnostic/therapeutic axillary dissection

- in terms of anatomical level and number of nodes removed.
- For every 100 women with early breast cancer having single-modality adjuvant systemic therapy (chemotherapy, tamoxifen, or ovarian suppression if <50), there will be an extra 5–10 women alive at 10 years compared with women who have no form of adjuvant systemic therapy.
- The majority of ER+ women of all ages with early breast cancer should take tamoxifen 20 mg daily for 5 years, unless entered into a trial testing a longer duration. Randomized controlled trials are needed to identify women with the most to gain from chemotherapy and/or ovarian suppression in addition to tamoxifen.
- Locoregional radiotherapy reduces breast cancer mortality (approximately 5–10 per cent absolute benefit at 10 years). The prevention of four isolated local recurrences prevents one breast cancer death. The relative contribution to cure of treating the axilla, supraclavicular fossa and IMC is unclear.
- Tangential fields to the left breast must be localized carefully, and cardiac shielding employed. Junctions between tangential breast/chest wall portals and anterior axillary fields must be planned and monitored carefully to ensure that no field overlaps occur.
- Primary medical therapy and dose intensification in patients with non-metastatic breast cancer should be confined to research protocols, preferably randomized clinical trials.
- Most patients with metastatic breast cancer are suitable for a trial of endocrine therapy as first-line systemic treatment. Patients with ER− tumours, who relapse after a short disease-free interval or present with liver involvement, are unlikely to benefit from this approach, and should be considered for chemotherapy in the first instance.
- Taxanes should be considered for patients with metastatic disease only after a trial of anthracyclines.
- Women with breast cancer are well informed and must be given every opportunity to express their own preferences for/against treatment.

ACKNOWLEDGEMENT

I thank Dr Rubin Soomal, Dr Duncan Wheately and Dr Stephen Morris for their valuable contributions to this manuscript.

KEY REFERENCES

Bartelink, H., Horiot, J.-C., Poortmans, P. et al. (2001) European Organisation for Research and Treatment of Cancer Radiotherapy and Breast Cancer Groups. Recurrence rates after treatment of breast cancer with standard radiotherapy with or without additional radiation. N. Engl. J. Med. **345**(19), 1378–87.

Delmas, P.D., Bjarnason, N.H., Mitlak, B.H. et al. (1997) Effects of raloxifene on bone mineral density, serum cholesterol concentrations, and uterine endometrium in postmenopausal women. N. Engl. J. Med. **337**, 1641–7.

Diel, I.J., Solomayer, E.F., Costa, S.D. et al. (1998) Reduction in new metastases in breast cancer with adjuvant clodronate treatment. N. Engl. J. Med. **339**, 357–63.

EBCTCG (Early Breast Cancer Trialists' Collaborative Group) (1998a) Tamoxifen for early breast cancer: an overview of the randomised trials. Lancet **351**, 1451–67.

EBCTCG (1998b) Polychemotherapy for early breast cancer: an overview of the randomised trials. Lancet **352**, 930–42.

EBCTCG (2000) Favourable and unfavourable effects on long-term survival of radiotherapy for early breast cancer: an overview of the randomised trials. Lancet **355**, 1757–70.

Fisher, B., Costantino, J.P., Wickerham, D.L. et al. (1998) Tamoxifen for prevention of breast cancer: report of the National Surgical Adjuvant Breast and Bowel Project P-1 Study. J. Natl Cancer Inst. **90**, 1371–88.

Fisher, E.R., Dignam, J., Tan-Chui, E. et al. (1999) Pathological findings from the National Surgical Adjuvant Breast Project (NSABP) eight-year update of protocol B-17. Am. Cancer Soc. **86**(3), 429–38.

Hortobagyi, G.N., Theriault, R.L. and Lipton, A. (1998) Long-term prevention of skeletal complications of metastatic breast cancer with pamidronate. Protocol 19 Aredia Breast Cancer Study Group. J. Clin. Oncol. **16**, 2038–44.

Slamon, D.J., Leyland-Jones, B., Shak, S. et al. (2001) Use of chemotherapy plus a monoclonal antibody against HER2 for metastatic breast cancer that overexpresses HER2. N. Engl. J. Med. **344**(11), 783–42.

REFERENCES

Aitken, R.J., Gaze, M.N., Rodger, A., Chetty, U. and Forrest, A.P. (1989) Arm morbidity within a trial of mastectomy and either nodal sample with selective radiotherapy or axillary clearance. *Br. J. Surg.* **76**, 568–71.

Azzopardi, J.G., Chepick, O.H. and Harman, W.H. (1982) The World Health Organisation histological typing of breast tumours (2nd edn). *Am. J. Clin. Pathol.* **78**, 806.

Bartelink, H., Horiot, J.-C., Poortmans, P. *et al.* (2001) European Organisation for Research and Treatment of Cancer Radiotherapy and Breast Cancer Groups. Recurrence rates after treatment of breast cancer with standard radiotherapy with or without additional radiation. *N. Engl. J. Med.* **345**, 1378–87.

Bates, T., Riley, D.L., Houghton, J., Fallowfield, L. and Baum, M. (1991) Breast cancer in elderly women: A Cancer Research Campaign trial comparing treatment with tamoxifen and optimal surgery with tamoxifen alone. *Br. J. Surg.* **78**, 591–4.

Berry, D.L., Theriault, R.L., Holmes, F.A. *et al.* (1999) Management of breast cancer during pregnancy using a standardized protocol. *J. Clin. Oncol.* **17**, 855–61.

Bezwoda, W. (1999) Randomised, controlled trial of high dose chemotherapy (HD-CNVp) versus standard dose (CAF) chemotherapy for high risk surgically treated, primary breast cancer. *35th Annual ASCO Meeting, Atlanta, GA*, abstract 4.

Blamey, R.W., Jonat, W., Kaufmann, M., Bianco, A.R. and Namer, M. (1992) Goserelin depot in the treatment of premenopausal advanced breast cancer. *Eur. J. Cancer* **28A**, 810–14.

Bloom, H.J.G. and Richardson, W.W. (1957) Histological grading and prognosis and breast cancer. *Br. J. Cancer* **11**, 359–77.

Boice, J.D., Jr, Harvey, E.B., Blettner, M., Stovall, M. and Flannery, J.T. (1992) Cancer in the contralateral breast after radiotherapy for breast cancer. *N. Engl. J. Med.* **326**, 781–5.

Bonadonna, G., Veronesi, U., Brambilla, C. *et al.* (1990) Primary chemotherapy to avoid mastectomy in tumors with diameters of three centimeters or more. *J. Natl Cancer Inst.* **82**, 1539–45.

Bonadonna, G., Zambetti, M. and Valagussa, P. (1995) Sequential or alternating doxorubicin and CMF regimens in breast cancer with more than three positive nodes. Ten-year results. *JAMA* **273**, 542–7.

Boogerd, W., Dalesio, O., Bais, E.M. and van der Sande, J.J. (1992) Response of brain metastases from breast cancer to systemic chemotherapy. *Cancer* **69**, 972–80.

BPTWP (Bone Pain Trial Working Party, Chair J.R. Yarnold) (1999) 8 Gy single fraction radiotherapy for the treatment of metastatic skeletal pain: randomised comparison with a multifraction schedule over 12 months of patient follow-up. *Radiother. Oncol.* **52**, 111–21.

Budman, D.R., Berry, D.A., Cirrincione, C.T. *et al.* (1998) Dose and dose intensity as determinants of outcome in the adjuvant treatment of breast cancer. The Cancer and Leukemia Group B. *J. Natl Cancer Inst.* **90**, 1205–11.

Bulens, P., Vanuytsel, L., Rijnders, A. and van der Schueren, E. (1990) Breast conserving treatment of Paget's disease. *Radiother. Oncol.* **17**, 305–9.

Campbell, I.R. and Illingworth, M.H. (1992) Can patients wash during radiotherapy to the breast or chest wall? A randomized controlled trial. *Clin. Oncol. R. Coll. Radiol.* **4**, 78–82.

Carter, C.L., Allen, C. and Henson, D.E. (1989) Relation of tumor size, lymph node status, and survival in 24,740 breast cancer cases. *Cancer* **63**, 181–7.

CGHFBC (Collaborative Group on Hormonal Factors in Breast Cancer) (1996) Breast cancer and hormonal contraceptives: collaborative reanalysis of individual data on 53,297 women with breast cancer and 100,239 women without breast cancer from 54 epidemiological studies. *Lancet* **347**, 1713–27.

CGHFBC (1997) Breast cancer and hormone replacement therapy: collaborative reanalysis of data from 51 epidemiological studies of 52,705 women with breast cancer and 108,411 women without breast cancer. *Lancet* **350**, 1047–59.

Clark, R.M. and Chua, T. (1989) Breast cancer and pregnancy: the ultimate challenge. *Clin. Oncol. R. Coll. Radiol.* **1**, 11–18.

Clark, R.M., Whelan, T., Levine, M. *et al.* (1996) Randomized clinical trial of breast irradiation following lumpectomy and axillary dissection for node-negative breast cancer: an update. Ontario Clinical Oncology Group. *J. Natl Cancer Inst.* **88**, 1659–64.

Coates, A., Gebski, V., Bishop, J.F. *et al.* (1987) Improving the quality of life during chemotherapy for advanced breast cancer. A comparison of intermittent and continuous treatment strategies. *N. Engl. J. Med.* **317**, 1490–5.

Cobleigh, M.A., Berris, R.F., Bush, T. *et al.* (1994) Estrogen replacement therapy in breast cancer survivors: a time for change. *JAMA* **272**, 540–5.

Conte, P.F., Latreille, J., Mauriac, L. *et al.* (1996) Delay in progression of bone metastases in breast cancer patients treated with intravenous pamidronate: results from a multinational randomized controlled trial. *J. Clin. Oncol.* **14**, 2552–9.

Crump, M., Sawka, C.A., DeBoer, G. *et al.* (1997) An individual patient-based meta-analysis of tamoxifen versus ovarian ablation as first line endocrine therapy for premenopausal women with metastatic breast cancer. *Breast Cancer Res. Treat.* **44**, 201–10.

Diel, I.J., Solomayer, E.F., Costa, S.D. *et al.* (1998) Reduction in new metastases in breast cancer with adjuvant clodronate treatment. *N. Engl. J. Med.* **339**, 357–63.

DiSaia, P.J. (1993) Hormone-replacement therapy in patients with breast cancer: a reappraisal. *Cancer* **71**, 1490–500.

Doll, D.C., Ringenberg, Q.S. and Yarbro, J.W. (1989) Antineoplastic agents and pregnancy. *Semin. Oncol.* **16**, 337–46.

Dorr, F.A., Bader, J. and Friedman, M.A. (1989) Locally advanced breast cancer current status and future directions. *Int. J. Radiat. Oncol. Biol. Phys.* **16**, 775–84.

EBCTCG (Early Breast Cancer Trialists' Collaborative Group) (1996) Ovarian ablation in early breast cancer: overview of the randomised trials. Early Breast Cancer Trialists' Collaborative Group. *Lancet* **348**, 1189–96.

EBCTCG (1998a) Tamoxifen for early breast cancer: an overview of the randomised trials. Early Breast Cancer Trialists' Collaborative Group. *Lancet* **351**, 1451–67.

EBCTCG (1998b) Polychemotherapy for early breast cancer: an overview of the randomised trials. Early Breast Cancer Trialists' Collaborative Group. *Lancet* **352**, 930–42.

EBCTCG (2000) Favourable and unfavourable effects on long-term survival of radiotherapy for early breast cancer: an overview of the randomised trials. *Lancet* **355**, 1757–70.

Ejlertsen, B., Pfeiffer, P., Pedersen, D. *et al.* (1993) Decreased efficacy of cyclophosphamide, epirubicin and 5-fluorouracil in metastatic breast cancer when reducing treatment duration from 18 to 6 months. *Eur. J. Cancer* **4**, 527–31.

Ejlertsen, B., Dombernowsky, P., Mouridsen, H.T. *et al.* (1999) Comparable effect of ovarian ablation (OA) and CMF chemotherapy in premenopausal hormone receptor positive breast cancer patients (PRP). *ASCO 1999 Annual Meeting*, abstract No 248.

Elston, C.W., Ellis, I.O. and Pinder, S.E. (1998) Prognostic factors in invasive carcinoma of the breast. *Clin. Oncol. R. Coll. Radiol.* **10**, 14–17.

Engelsman, E., Klijn, J.C., Rubens, R.D. *et al.* (1991) 'Classical' CMF versus a 3-weekly intravenous CMF schedule in postmenopausal patients with advanced breast cancer. An EORTC Breast Cancer Co-operative Group Phase III Trial (10808). *Eur. J. Cancer* **27**, 966–70.

Evans, G.R. and Kroll, S.S. (1998) Choice of technique for reconstruction. *Clin. Plast. Surg.* **25**, 311–16.

Fallowfield, L.J. (1990) Psychosocial adjustment after treatment for early breast cancer. *Oncology (Huntingt)* **4**, 89–97; discussion 97–8, 100.

Fisher, B., Dignam, J., Wolmark, N. *et al.* (1997a) Tamoxifen and chemotherapy for lymph node-negative, estrogen receptor-positive breast cancer. *J. Natl Cancer Inst.* **89**, 1673–82.

Fisher, B., Anderson, S., Wickerham, D.L. *et al.* (1997b) Increased intensification and total dose of cyclophosphamide in a doxorubicin–cyclophosphamide regimen for the treatment of primary breast cancer:

findings from National Surgical Adjuvant Breast and Bowel Project B-22. *J. Clin. Oncol.* **15**, 1858–69.

Fisher, B., Brown, A., Mamounas, E. *et al.* (1997c) Effect of preoperative chemotherapy on local-regional disease in women with operable breast cancer: findings from National Surgical Adjuvant Breast and Bowel Project B-18. *J. Clin. Oncol.* **15**, 2483–93.

Fisher, B.J., Perera, F.E., Cooke, A.L. *et al.* (1997d) Extracapsular axillary node extension in patients receiving adjuvant systemic therapy: an indication for radiotherapy? *Int. J. Radiat. Oncol. Biol. Phys.* **38**, 551–9.

Fisher B., Costantino J.P., Wickerham D.L. *et al.* (1998a) Tamoxifen for prevention of breast cancer: report of the National Surgical Adjuvant Breast and Bowel Project P-1 Study. *J. Natl Cancer Inst.* **90**, 1371–88.

Fisher, B., Dignam, J., Wolmark, N. *et al.* (1998b) Lumpectomy and radiation therapy for the treatment of intraductal breast cancer findings from National Surgical Adjuvant Breast and Bowel Project B-17. *J. Clin. Oncol.* **16**, 441–52.

Fisher, B., Dignam, J., Wolmark, N. *et al.* (1999) Tamoxifen in treatment of intraductal breast cancer: National Surgical Adjuvant Breast and Bowel Project B-24 randomised controlled trial. *Lancet* **353**, 1993–2000.

Fisher, E.R., Costantino, J., Fisher, B. *et al.* (1996) Pathologic findings from the National Surgical Adjuvant Breast Project (NSABP) Protocol B-17. Five-year observations concerning lobular carcinoma *in-situ*. *Cancer* **78**, 1403–16.

Ford, D., Easton, D.F., Stratton, M. *et al.* (1998) Genetic heterogeneity and penetrance analysis of the *BRCA1* and *BRCA2* genes in breast cancer families. The Breast Cancer Linkage Consortium. *Am. J. Hum. Genet.* **62**, 676–89.

Forrest, A.P., Everington, D., McDonald, C.C., Steele, R.J., Chetty, U. and Stewart, H.J. (1995) The Edinburgh randomized trial of axillary sampling or clearance after mastectomy. *Br. J. Surg.* **82**, 1504–8.

Fossati, R., Confalonieri, C., Torri, V. *et al.* (1998) Cytotoxic and hormonal treatment for metastatic breast cancer: a systematic review of published randomized trials involving 31,510 women. *J. Clin. Oncol.* **16**, 3439–60.

Fowble, B. (1997) Postmastectomy radiation: a modest benefit prevails for high risk patients. *Cancer* **79**, 1061–8.

Gelber, R.D., Cole, B.F., Goldhirsch, A. *et al.* (1996) Adjuvant chemotherapy plus tamoxifen compared with tamoxifen alone for postmenopausal breast cancer: meta-analysis of quality-adjusted survival. *Lancet* **347**, 1066–71.

Goss, P.E. and Strasser, K. (2001) Aromatase inhibitors in the treatment and prevention of breast cancer. *J. Clin. Oncol.* **19**, 881–94.

Gusterson, B.A., Gelber, R.D., Goldhirsch, A. *et al.* (1992) Prognostic importance of c-erbB-2 expression in breast cancer. International (Ludwig) Breast Cancer Study Group. *J. Clin. Oncol.* **10**, 1049–56.

Gyenes, G., Gagliardi, G., Lax, I., Fornander, T. and Rutqvist, L.E. (1997) Evaluation of irradiated heart volumes in stage I breast cancer patients treated with postoperative adjuvant radiotherapy. *J. Clin. Oncol.* **15**, 1348–53.

Handley, R.S. (1975) Carcinoma of the breast. *Ann. R. Coll. Surg. Engl.* **57**, 59–66.

Harris, R. (1997) Variation of benefits and harms of breast cancer screening with age. *J. Natl Cancer Inst. Monogr.* **22**, 139–43.

Harvey, J.M., Clark, G.M., Osborne, C.K. and Allred, D.C. (1999) Estrogen receptor status by immunohistochemistry is superior to the ligand-binding assay for predicting response to adjuvant endocrine therapy in breast cancer. *J. Clin. Oncol.* **17**, 1474–81.

Henderson, I.C., Berry, D., Demetri, G. *et al.* (1998) Improved disease-free (DFS) and overall survival (OS) from the addition of sequential paclitaxel (T) but not from the escalation of doxorubicin (A) dose level in the adjuvant chemotherapy of patients (PTS) with node-positive primary breast cancer (BC). *ASCO 1998 Annual Meeting,* abstract No. 390A.

Hji Yiannakis, P. and Yarnold, J.R. (1996) Mixing anthracyclines and radiotherapy in early breast cancer: how safe is it? *Eur. J. Cancer* **32a**, 2374–7 [corrected and republished article, originally printed in *Eur. J. Cancer* (1996) Oct.; **32A**(11), 1845–8].

Holland, R., Veling, S.H., Mravunac, M. and Hendriks, J.H. (1985) Histologic multifocality of Tis, T1-2 breast carcinomas. Implications for clinical trials of breast-conserving surgery. *Cancer* **56**, 979–90.

Holland, R., Connolly, J.L., Gelman, R. *et al.* (1990a) The presence of an extensive intraductal component following a limited excision correlates with prominent residual disease in the remainder of the breast. *J. Clin. Oncol.* **8**, 113–18.

Holland, R., Hendriks, J., Verbeek, A.L.M., Mravunac, M. and Schuurmans Stekhoven, J.H. (1990b) Extent, distribution, and mammographic/histological correlations of breast ductal carcinoma in-situ. *Lancet* **335**, 519–22.

Hopwood, P. (1998) Genetic risk counselling for breast cancer families: Editorial. *Eur. J. Cancer* **34**, 1477–9.

Howell, A., Anderson, E., Blamey, R. *et al.* (1998) The primary use of endocrine therapies. *Recent Results Cancer Res.* **152**, 227–44.

Hryniuk, W. and Levine, M.N. (1986) Analysis of dose intensity for adjuvant chemotherapy trials in stage II breast cancer. *J. Clin. Oncol.* **4**, 1162–70.

Hryniuk, W., Frei, E., 3rd and Wright, F.A. (1998) A single scale for comparing dose-intensity of all chemotherapy regimens in breast cancer: summation dose-intensity. *J. Clin. Oncol.* **16**, 3137–47.

Hung, M.C. and Lau, Y.K. (1999) Basic science of HER-2/neu: a review. *Semin. Oncol.* **26**, 51–9.

ICRU (1993) *Prescribing, recording, and reporting photon beam therapy.* ICRU Report 50.

Invarsson, S. (1999) Molecular genetics of breast cancer progression. *Semin. Cancer Biol.* **9**, 277–88.

Ivens, D., Hoe, A.L., Podd, T.J., Hamilton, C.R., Taylor, I. and Royle, G.T. (1992) Assessment of morbidity from complete axillary dissection. *Br. J. Cancer* **66**, 136–8.

Jaiyesimi, I.A., Buzdar, A.U. and Hortobagyi, G. (1992) Inflammatory breast cancer: a review. *J. Clin. Oncol.* **10**, 1014–24.

Jordan, V.C. (1998) Molecular biology of the estrogen receptor aids in the understanding of tamoxifen resistance and breast cancer prevention with raloxifene. *Recent Results Cancer Res.* **152**, 265–76.

Julien, J.P., Bijker, N., Fentiman, I.S. *et al.* (2000) Radiotherapy in breast-conserving treatment for ductal carcinoma *in situ*: first results of the EORTC randomised phase III trial 10853. EORTC Breast Cancer Cooperative Group and EORTC Radiotherapy Group. *Lancet* **355**, 528–33.

Kaufman, M. (2001) 'Zoladex' (goserelin) versus CMF as adjuvant therapy in pre-/peri- menopausal node positive early breast cancer. Preliminary efficacy results from ZEBRA study. *Breast* **10**, 53.

Koops, H.S., Doting, M.H., de Vries, J. *et al.* (1999) Sentinel node biopsy as a surgical staging method for solid cancers. *Radiother. Oncol.* **51**, 1–7.

Kuerer, H.M., Newman, L.A., Smith, T.L. *et al.* (1999) Clinical course of breast cancer patients with complete pathologic primary tumor and axillary lymph node response to doxorubicin-based neoadjuvant chemotherapy. *J. Clin. Oncol.* **17**, 460–9.

Kurtz, J.M. (1992) Factors influencing the risk of local recurrence in the breast. *Eur. J. Cancer* **28**, 660–6.

Kurtz, J.M., Spitalier, J.M., Amalric, R. *et al.* (1990) The prognostic significance of late local recurrence after breast-conserving therapy. *Int. J. Radiat. Oncol. Biol. Phys.* **18**, 87–93.

Larson, D., Weinstein, M., Goldberg, I. *et al.* (1986) Edema of the arm as a function of the extent of axillary surgery in patients with stage I–II carcinoma of the breast treated with primary radiotherapy. *Int. J. Radiat. Oncol. Biol. Phys.* **12**, 1575–82.

Lavin, M. (1998) Role of the ataxia-telangiectasia gene (ATM) in breast cancer. A-T heterozygotes seem to have an increased risk but its size is unknown [editorial]. *BMJ* **317**, 486–7.

Leonard, R.C.F., Lee, L. and Harrison, M.E. (1996) Impact of side-effects associated with endocrine treatments for advanced breast cancer: Clinicians' and patients' perceptions. *Breast* **5**, 259–64.

Liljegren, G., Holmberg, L., Adami, H.O., Westman, G., Graffman, S. and Bergh, J. (1994) Sector resection with or without postoperative radiotherapy for stage I breast cancer: five-year results of a randomized trial. Uppsala-Orebro Breast Cancer Study Group. *J. Natl Cancer Inst.* **86**, 717–22.

Macmillan, R.D., Purushotham, A.D. and George, W.D. (1996) Local recurrence after breast-conserving surgery for breast cancer. *Br. J. Surg.* **83**, 149–55.

Maher, E.J. (1995) Non-surgical management of early breast cancer in the United Kingdom: follow-up. Clinical Audit Sub-committee of the Faculty of Clinical Oncology, Royal College of Radiologists, and the Joint Council for Clinical Oncology. *Clin. Oncol. R. Coll. Radiol.* **7**, 227–31.

Margolese, R.G. (1998) Mastectomy or lumpectomy? The choice of operation for clinical stages I and II breast cancer. *Can. Med. Assoc. J.* **158**, S15–S21.

Mariani, L., Salvadori, B., Marubini, E. *et al.* (1998) Ten year results of a randomised trial comparing two conservative treatment strategies for small size breast cancer. *Eur. J. Cancer* **34**, 1156–62.

Mark, R.J., Zimmerman, R.P. and Greif, J.M. (1996) Capsular contracture after lumpectomy and radiation therapy in patients who have undergone uncomplicated bilateral augmentation mammoplasty. *Radiology* **200**, 621–5.

McArdle, J.M.C., George, W.D., McArdle, C.S. *et al.* (1996) Psychological support for patients undergoing breast cancer surgery: a randomised study. *BMJ* **312**, 813–16.

McCormick, B., Begg, C.B., Norton, L., Yao, T.J. and Kinne, D. (1993) Timing of radiotherapy in the treatment of early-stage breast cancer [letter; comment]. *J. Clin. Oncol.* **11**, 191–3.

McGuire, W.L., Hilsenbeck, S. and Clark, G.M. (1992) Optimal mastectomy timing. *J. Natl Cancer Inst.* **84**, 346–8.

McKinna, F., Gothard, L., Ashley, S., Ebbs, S.R. and Yarnold, J.R. (1999) Lymphatic relapse in women with early breast cancer: a difficult management problem. *Eur. J. Cancer* **35**, 1065–9.

Menard, S., Valagussa, P., Pilotti, S. *et al.* (1999) Benefit of CMF treatment in lymph node-positive breast cancer overexpressing HER2. *ASCO 1999 Annual Meeting,* abstract no. 257.

Mitlak, B.H. and Cohen, F.J. (1999) Selective estrogen receptor modulators: a look ahead. *Drugs* **57**, 653–63.

Mustacchi, G., Milani, S., Pluchinotta, A., De Matteis, A., Rubagotti, A. and Perrota, A. (1994) Tamoxifen or surgery plus tamoxifen as primary treatment for elderly patients with operable breast cancer: The GRETA Trial. Group for Research on Endocrine Therapy in the Elderly. *Anticancer Res.* **14**, 2197–200.

Nystrom, L., Rutqvist, L.E., Wall, S. *et al.* (1993) Breast cancer screening with mammography: overview of Swedish randomised trials. *Lancet* **341**, 973–8 [published erratum appears in *Lancet* (1993) Nov. 27; **342**(8883), 1372].

Olsen, O. and Gotzsche, P.C. (2001) Screening for breast cancer with mammography (Cochrane Review). *Cochrane Database Syst. Rev.* 4.

Olson, J.E., Neuberg, D., Pandya, K.J. *et al.* (1997) The role of radiotherapy in the management of operable locally advanced breast carcinoma: results of a randomized trial by the Eastern Cooperative Oncology Group. *Cancer* **79**, 1138–49.

Osin, P., Shipley, J., Lu, Y.J., Crook, T. and Gusterson, B.A. (1998) Experimental pathology and breast cancer genetics: new technologies. *Recent Results Cancer Res.* **152**, 35–48.

Overgaard, M. (1999) Overview of randomised trials in high risk breast cancer patients treated with adjuvant systemic therapy with or without postmastectomy irradiation. *Semin. Rad. Oncol.* **9**, 292–9.

Overgaard, M., Hansen, P.S., Overgaard, J. *et al.* (1997) Postoperative radiotherapy in high-risk premenopausal women with breast cancer who receive adjuvant chemotherapy. Danish Breast Cancer Cooperative Group 82b Trial. *N. Engl. J. Med.* **337**, 949–55.

Page, D.L. (1992) The clinical significance of mammary epithelial hyperplasia. *The Breast* **1**, 3–7.

Paszat, L.F., Mackillop, W.J., Groome, P.A., Boyd, C., Schulze, K. and Holowaty, E. (1998) Mortality from myocardial infarction after adjuvant radiotherapy for breast cancer in the surveillance, epidemiology, and end-results cancer registries. *J. Clin. Oncol.* **16**, 2625–31.

Paterson, A.H., Powles, T.J., Kanis, J.A., McCloskey, E., Hanson, J. and Ashley, S. (1993) Double-blind controlled trial of oral clodronate in patients with bone metastases from breast cancer. *J. Clin. Oncol.* **11**, 59–65.

Pegram, M.D., Pauletti, G. and Slamon, D.J. (1998) HER-2/neu as a predictive marker of response to breast cancer therapy. *Breast Cancer Res. Treat.* **52**, 1–3.

Peters, W., O'Rosner, G., Vredenburg, J. *et al.* (1999) A prospective randomised comparison of two doses of combination alkylating agents as consolidation after CAF in high-risk primary breast cancer involving ten or more axillary lymph nodes: preliminary results of the CALGB9082/SWOG9114/NCIC MA-13. *35th Annual ASCO Meeting, Atlanta, GA,* abstract 2.

Peto, R. (1998) Mortality from breast cancer in UK has decreased suddenly [letter]. *BMJ* **317**, 476–7.

Powles, T.J., Paterson, A.H.G., Nevantaus, A. *et al.* (1998a) Adjuvant clodronate reduces the incidence of bone metastases in patients with primary operable breast cancer. *Prog. Proc. Am. Soc. Clin. Oncol.* **17**, 123a.

Powles, T., Eeles, R., Ashley, S. *et al.* (1998b) Interim analysis of the incidence of breast cancer in the Royal Marsden Hospital tamoxifen randomised chemoprevention trial. *Lancet* **352**, 98–101.

Priestman, T.J., Dunn, J., Brada, M., Rampling, R. and Baker, P.G. (1996) Final results of the Royal College of Radiologists' Trial comparing two different radiotherapy schedules in the treatment of cerebral metastases. *Clin. Oncol.* **8**, 308–15.

Ragaz, J. and Coldman, A. (1998) Survival impact of adjuvant tamoxifen on competing causes of mortality in breast cancer survivors, with analysis of mortality from contralateral breast cancer, cardiovascular events, endometrial cancer, and thromboembolic episodes. *J. Clin. Oncol.* **16**, 2018–24.

Recht, A., Come, S.E., Henderson, I.C. *et al.* (1996) The sequencing of chemotherapy and radiation therapy after conservative surgery for early-stage breast cancer. *N. Engl. J. Med.* **334**, 1356–61.

Recht, A., Edge, S.B., Solin, L.J. *et al.* (2001) Postmastectomy radiotherapy: clinical practice guidelines of the American Society of Clinical Oncology. *J. Clin. Oncol.* **19**, 1539–69.

Ribeiro, G. and Swindell, R. (1992) Adjuvant tamoxifen for male breast cancer (MBC). *Br. J. Cancer* **65**, 252–4.

Richards, M.A., Smith, P., Ramirez, A.J., Fentiman, I.S. and Rubens, R.D. (1999) The influence on survival of delay in the presentation and treatment of symptomatic breast cancer. *Br. J. Cancer* **79**, 858–64.

Roberts, S.A., Spreadborough, A.R., Bulman, B., Barber, J.B., Evans, D.G. and Scott, D. (1999) Heritability of cellular radiosensitivity: a marker of low-penetrance predisposition genes in breast cancer? *Am. J. Hum. Genet.* **65**, 784–94.

Robertson, A.G., Reed, N.S. and Ralston, S.H. (1995) Effect of oral clodronate on metastatic bone pain: a double-blind, placebo-controlled study. *J. Clin. Oncol.* **13**, 2427–30.

Rodenhuis, S., Richel, D.J., van der Wall, E. *et al.* (1998) Randomised trial of high-dose chemotherapy and haemopoietic progenitor-cell support in operable breast cancer with extensive axillary lymph-node involvement. *Lancet* **352**, 515–21.

Sainsbury, J.R., Anderson, T.J., Morgan, D.A. and Dixon, J.M. (1994) ABC of breast diseases. Breast cancer. *BMJ* **309**, 1150–3.

Saphner, T., Tormey, D.C. and Gray, R. (1991) Venous and arterial thrombosis in patients who received adjuvant therapy for breast cancer. *J. Clin. Oncol.* **9**, 286–94.

SBCSG (Scandinavian Breast Cancer Study Group) (1999) The Scandinavian Breast Cancer Study Group 9401. Results from a randomised adjuvant breast cancer study with high dose chemotherapy with CTCb supported by autologous bone marrow stem cells versus dose escalated and tailored FEC therapy. *35th Annual ASCO Meeting, Atlanta, GA*. abstract 3.

Schnitt, S.J., Hayman, J., Gelman, R. *et al.* (1996) A prospective study of conservative surgery alone in the treatment of selected patients with stage I breast cancer. *Cancer* **77**, 1094–100.

Schwaibold, F., Fowble, B.L., Solin, L.J., Schultz, D.J. and Goodman, R.L. (1991) The results of radiation therapy for isolated local regional recurrence after mastectomy. *Int. J. Radiat. Oncol. Biol. Phys.* **21**, 299–310.

SCTBG (Scottish Cancer Trials Breast Group) (1993) Adjuvant ovarian ablation versus CMF chemotherapy in premenopausal women with pathological stage II breast carcinoma: the Scottish trial. Scottish Cancer Trials Breast Group and ICRF Breast Unit, Guy's Hospital, London. *Lancet* **341**, 1293–8.

Silliman, R.A., Balducci, L., Goodwin, J.S., Holmes, F.F. and Leventhal, E.A. (1993) Breast cancer care in old age: what we know, don't know, and do. *J. Natl Cancer Inst.* **85**, 190–9.

Silverstein, M.J., Lagios, M.D., Craig, P.H. *et al.* (1996) A prognostic index for ductal carcinoma *in-situ* of the breast. *Cancer* **77**, 2267–74.

Silverstein, M.J., Lagios, M.D., Groshen, S. *et al.* (1999) The influence of margin width on local control of ductal carcinoma *in situ* of the breast. *N. Engl. J. Med.* **340**, 1455–61.

Slamon, D.J., Leyland-Jones, B., Shak, S. *et al.* (2001) Use of chemotherapy plus a monoclonal antibody against HER2 for metastatic breast cancer that overexpresses HER2. *N. Engl. J. Med.* **344**, 783–92.

Stadtmauer, E., O'Neil, A. and Goldstein, L. (1999) Phase III randomized trial of high-dose chemotherapy and stem cell support shows no difference in overall survival or severe toxicity compared to maintenance chemotherapy with cyclophosphamide, methotrexate and 5-fluorouracil for women with metastatic breast cancer who are responding to conventional induction chemotherapy: The 'Philadelphia' Intergroup Trial (PBT-1) *35th Annual ASCO Meeting, Atlanta, GA*, abstract 1.

Stevenson, J., Giantonio, B., Boyd, R.L. and Bruner, J.A. (1997) Adjuvant chemotherapy for breast cancer in pregnancy: can recommendations be made with confidence. *Semin. Oncol.* **24**, xxv–xxxvi; discussion xxxvi, xxxix.

Swedborg, I. and Wallgren, A. (1981) The effect of pre- and postmastectomy radiotherapy on the degree of edema, shoulder-joint mobility, and gripping force. *Cancer* **47**, 877–81.

Tannock, I.F., Boyd, N.F., DeBoer, G. *et al.* (1988) A randomized trial of two dose levels of cyclophosphamide, methotrexate, and fluorouracil chemotherapy for patients with metastatic breast cancer. *J. Clin. Oncol.* **6**, 1377–87.

Todd, J.H., Dowle, C., Williams, M.R. *et al.* (1987) Confirmation of a prognostic index in primary breast cancer. *Br. J. Cancer* **56**, 489–92.

van Tienhoven, G., Voogd, A.C., Peterse, J.L. *et al.* (1999) Prognosis after treatment for loco-regional recurrence after mastectomy or breast conserving therapy in two randomised trials (EORTC 10801 and DBCG-82TM). EORTC Breast Cancer Cooperative Group and the Danish Breast Cancer Cooperative Group. *Eur. J. Cancer* **35**, 32–8.

Vasen, H.F.A., Haites, N.E., Evans, D.G.R. *et al.* (1998) Current policies for surveillance and management in women at risk of breast and ovarian cancer: a survey among 16 European Family Cancer Clinics. *Eur. J. Cancer* **34**, 1922–6.

Veronesi, U., Luini, A., Del Vecchio, M. *et al.* (1993) Radiotherapy after breast-preserving surgery in women with localized cancer of the breast. *N. Engl. J. Med.* **328**, 1587–91.

Veronesi, U., Maisonneuve, P., Costa, A. *et al.* (1998) Prevention of breast cancer with tamoxifen: preliminary findings from the Italian randomised trial among hysterectomised women. Italian Tamoxifen Prevention Study. *Lancet* **352**, 93–7.

Vrieling, C., Collette, L., Fourquet, A. *et al.* (1999) The influence of the boost in breast-conserving therapy on cosmetic outcome in the EORTC 'boost versus no boost' trial. *Int. J. Radiat. Oncol. Biol. Phys.* **45**, 677–85.

Werner, R.S., McCormick, B., Petrek, J. *et al.* (1991) Arm edema in conservatively managed breast cancer: obesity is a major predictive factor. *Radiology* **180**, 177–84.

Yang, X. and Lippman, M.E. (1999) BRCA1 and BRCA2 in breast cancer. *Breast Cancer Res. Treat.* **54**, 1–10.

Yarnold, J.R. (1984) Selective avoidance of lymphatic irradiation in the conservative management of breast cancer. *Radiother. Oncol.* **2**, 79–92.

Yarnold, J. (2001) Radiation in the context of multidisciplinary approaches: radiotherapy and locally advanced breast cancer. *The Breast* **10**, 78–83.

Zimmerman, R.P., Mark, R.J., Kim, A.I. *et al.* (1998) Radiation tolerance of transverse rectus abdominis myocutaneous-free flaps used in immediate breast reconstruction. *Am. J. Clin. Oncol.* **21**, 381–5.

22

Bronchus

VANESSA A. POTTER, PENELLA J. WOLL AND NICHOLAS THATCHER

INCIDENCE AND AETIOLOGY

Lung cancer is the leading cause of cancer death in the developed world, with the majority of patients (80–90 per cent) dying within a year of diagnosis. Lung cancer accounts for 28 per cent of male cancer deaths in the UK, 33.2 per cent in the USA and 14.2 per cent in Japan. For women, lung cancer accounts for 17 per cent of cancer deaths in the UK, 14.2 per cent in the USA and 7.4 per cent in Japan. In 1996, 22760 men and 13000 women died from lung cancer in the UK. Mortality figures within England and Wales show significant regional differences in incidence, with the highest incidence in the North of England. The mortality in this region is the highest in Europe, in Tyneside the age-standardized mortality for men is 101.3 per 100000, compared to only 18.9 in Potenza, Italy, and 23.8 for women in Merseyside compared to 2.4 in Potenza.

The incidence of lung cancer has increased dramatically since the beginning of the twentieth century, although the number of deaths in men is now stable in the UK and has begun to fall in the USA (Fig. 22.1). However, in women the incidence of lung cancer continues to rise, and in Scotland and the USA has overtaken breast cancer as the most common cause of cancer death. The incidence of lung cancer increases with age. Less than 1 per cent of cases occur under 40, and 56 per cent of cases occur in the over-70 age group.

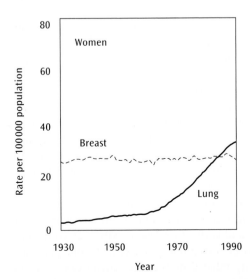
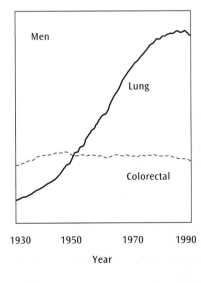

Figure 22.1 *Incidence of lung cancer in men and women in the UK during the twentieth century, compared with the incidence of breast cancer in women and colorectal cancer in men.*

Cigarette smoking is the main risk factor for lung cancer, accounting for up to 94 per cent of lung cancer deaths in men and 83 per cent in women. The relationship between cigarette smoking and lung cancer was established by the classic epidemiological studies of Doll and Hill (1964) but has been confirmed by numerous prospective and retrospective studies worldwide. The rapid rise in incidence of lung cancer in women over the past few decades is due to the fact that, for women, smoking was an uncommon habit until after the Second World War, while smoking had been socially acceptable for men several decades earlier. Although the overall consumption of cigarettes has decreased since the 1970s, it is particularly worrying that smoking is most common in the 20–24-year age group, and that the proportion of children who smoke has actually increased, with 30 per cent of 15-year-old girls in the UK being regular smokers (Cancer Research Campaign, 1996).

The risk of lung cancer is related directly to both the duration of exposure and the number of cigarettes smoked, and is 15-fold greater in smokers of 25 cigarettes per day than in non-smokers. The risk of developing lung cancer falls rapidly after stopping smoking, but even 15–20 years later the risk is still 1.5–4 times that of lifelong non-smokers (Mao et al., 1997). The risk of lung cancer is increased with the tar and nicotine content of the tobacco smoked, inhalation of smoke, taking more puffs from each cigarette, keeping the cigarette in the mouth between puffs and relighting half-smoked cigarettes. The lower risks of pipe and cigar smoking may be due to the social rituals associated with their use, including less inhalation.

The age of onset of smoking is an important factor in defining the risk from cigarette smoking. Therefore the increased prevalence of smoking in children is alarming as the resulting cancers will not be seen for several decades. The risk of lung cancer at the age of 60 is three times greater for those who started to smoke at age 15 than for those who started 10 years later. A recent study (Wiencke et al., 1999) has demonstrated significantly increased levels of tobacco-induced DNA damage in patients who began smoking before the age of 25 compared to those who began in later life.

In recent years there has been a slight reduction in male lung cancer deaths in Britain, possibly attributable to reductions in the tar content of cigarettes, as well as reduced consumption. However, since 1950 there has been a 500 per cent increase in lung cancer mortality in women. It has been proposed that women are more susceptible to tobacco carcinogens. Zang and Wynder (1996) examined the risk of women developing lung cancer compared to men, according to exposure (cumulative tar, pack-years and current number of cigarettes smoked), and found that for the same lifelong exposure to cigarette smoke, women were at a 1.5-fold higher risk of developing lung cancer than men. These clinical findings may be due to physiological differences that result in the slower detoxification of carcinogens in women.

Many non-smokers are exposed to tobacco smoke at home, during work and in public places. The health risks of such indirect (passive) smoking are difficult to quantify, but the incidence of lung cancer and ischaemic heart disease is increased. In the UK approximately 1 in 6 of the population are exposed passively to tobacco smoke at home. It is estimated that a non-smoker in a smoking household is exposed to the equivalent of 1 per cent of the cigarettes actively smoked. In this non-smoking population the risk of developing lung cancer is increased by 24 per cent (Hackshaw, 1998), the risk increasing with the number of cigarettes smoked and duration of cohabitation.

Additional factors associated with the development of lung cancer include atmospheric pollution, ionizing radiation and various occupational hazards. Atmospheric pollution appears to increase the risk of lung cancer, mainly in smokers. In some large industrial cities, there is considerable variation in lung cancer rates, which can be linked to material deprivation. Radiation exposure has been associated with increased rates of lung cancer in atomic bomb survivors and patients treated with radiotherapy for ankylosing spondylitis, breast cancer and Hodgkin's disease. The effects of natural radiation from radon are seen in the increased lung cancer risk of miners in these areas. There is concern that radon may accumulate in houses constructed with energy-saving features in areas of hard rock geology, causing a hazard to the inhabitants. Despite this, lung cancer incidence in Cornwall is well below the national average. Industrial carcinogens, such as asbestos, chromium, nickel, vinylchloride and arsenic, have been well documented. Workers engaged in the coal distillation and gas industry also have an increased risk of lung cancer. Interestingly, chloromethylether (unlike many other carcinogens) is particularly associated with a specific histological subtype, small cell lung cancer. In many of these cases, the effects of the carcinogens are seen mainly in smokers.

A number of broncho-pulmonary diseases may also predispose to the development of lung cancer, including tuberculosis, pulmonary scars from previous infection, and trauma. Fibrosing alveolitis is said to be usually associated with the development of non-small cell lung cancers.

Although most patients with lung cancer are smokers, only a minority of smokers develop lung cancer. This suggests that certain individuals are more susceptible to the effects of smoking than others, and has led to a search for heritable predisposing factors. In lung cancer patients aged less than 50, an autosomal recessive cancer-prone gene could contribute to the development of as many as 70 per cent of tumours. Genetic variations in metabolism, such as debrisoquine oxidation phenotype, glutathione transferase and arylhydroxylase activity, may contribute to lung cancer susceptibility. These metabolic pathways may detoxify inhaled or ingested carcinogens. Dietary factors such as vitamin A deficiency and exposure to nitrosoamines may also be important.

Genetic changes in the development of lung cancer

In order for normal cells to evade the normal regulatory processes and become malignant, it has been proposed that six or seven mutations are required. No clear hereditary component has yet been detected in lung cancer, although mutation of the p53 gene in the Li Fraumeni cancer syndrome and loss of heterozygosity of the Rb gene are associated with increased risk of developing lung cancer. A large number of mutations of both tumour suppressor genes and oncogenes have been described (Table 22.1). The loss of tumour suppressor activity requires the loss of heterozygosity to an inactive homozygous state. Each step of bronchial carcinogenesis is a result of accumulation of genetic damage involving several oncogenes and tumour suppressor genes (Fig. 22.2).

This process of carcinogenesis appears to be increased when exposed to cigarette smoke carcinogens. Mao *et al.* (1997) showed that loss of heterozygosity of 3p21–22, 17p13 and 9p21 was present in 82 per cent of smokers, but only 10 per cent of non-smokers. Clonal changes do persist in ex-smokers. It also appears that the presence of certain mutations (K-*ras* and c-*erb*-B2) may be associated with poor prognosis (Roland and Rudd, 1998).

PREVENTION AND SCREENING

Primary prevention

As the vast majority of lung cancer is caused by cigarette smoking, most prevention strategies are aimed at reducing tobacco consumption, and several approaches have been tried. Health education programmes aim to promote the image of smoking as an abnormal, unpleasant activity; to discourage non-smokers from taking up smoking and to help smokers to give up. However, while the advertising budget of the tobacco industry far outweighs that of health education, these will have limited effect. The ban on tobacco advertising and smoking in many public places should help further. It has also been clearly shown that increasing the price of cigarettes results in decreased consumption (by 0.5 per cent for every 1 per cent increase in real price; Cancer Research Campaign, 1996) and therefore governments should continue to increase taxation above inflation. Finally, new measures are being taken to prevent young children taking up the habit. The results from campaigns in Scandinavia in the 1970s have been favourable and can be attributed to integrated central government and local policies.

Chemoprevention has also been studied as a method for reducing the incidence of lung cancer. Many case-controlled and cohort studies have shown that the incidence of lung cancer is reduced in people who have

Table 22.1 *Genetic abnormalities detected in SCLC and NSCLC (from Roland and Rudd, 1998; Salgia and Skarvin, 1998)*

Site of mutation	Name and type	Frequency	Stage of carcinogenesis
Chromosome 3: 3p14, 3p21, 3p25	Fragile histidine triad (FHIT); tumour suppressor	SCLC *c.* 90%, NSCLC *c.* 50%	Early
Chromosome 9: 9p21	*p16*; oncogene	SCLC >80%, NSCLC >50%	Early
Chromosome 12: 12p	K-*ras*; oncogene	Adenocarcinoma *c.* 30%	Late
Chromosome 13: 13q	Retinoblastoma gene; tumour suppressor	SCLC *c.* 90%, NSCLC *c.* 30%	Intermediate
Chromosome 17: 17p13	*p53*; tumour suppressor	SCLC *c.* 80%, NSCLC *c.* 50%	Early
Chromosome 17: 17q	c-*erb*-B2; oncogene	NSCLC *c.* 25%	Late

SCLC, small cell lung carcinoma; NSCLC, non-small cell lung carcinoma.

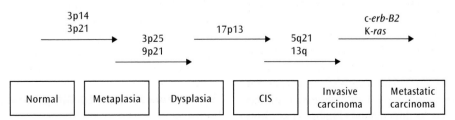

Figure 22.2 *Genetic changes that occur in the progression from normal epithelium to metastatic carcinoma in small cell lung cancer. CIS, carcinoma* in-situ. *From Thiberville* et al. *(1995), Petersen* et al. *(1998) and Salgia and Skarvin (1998).*

a high consumption of fruit and vegetables and, in particular, a high intake of β-carotene. In order to determine whether supplementation with β-carotene would reduce the risk of lung cancer in smokers, two large randomized studies have been performed. Surprisingly, both the Alpha-Tocopherol, Beta Carotene (ATBC) study, involving over 29 000 patients (Alpha-Tocopherol, Beta Carotene Cancer Prevention Study Group 1994) and the Beta Carotene and Retinol Efficacy Trial (CARET) (Omenn et al., 1996) demonstrated an increased incidence of lung cancer (16–28 per cent) in those receiving β-carotene. In addition, this group also had higher rates of overall mortality, particularly due to ischaemic heart disease. Studies in non-smokers show no significant benefit (Albanes, 1999). The current advice is that fruit and vegetable consumption should be increased, but that additional supplementation with β-carotene cannot be recommended.

Screening

The purpose of screening is to detect early stage tumours in the hope that treatment will lead to increased 5-year survival. Lung cancer should potentially be an ideal model, in that high-risk groups can easily be identified and methods for screening, such as sputum cytology and chest radiography, are widely available. Four large, randomized, controlled studies involving over 37 000 patients have shown that, using sputum cytology and/or plain chest X-rays, more early cases of lung cancer were detected, but all four failed to show any significant reduction in mortality (reviewed by Rizvi and Hayes, 1999; Smith, 1999).

Many new methods for early detection of the disease are currently under investigation. Conventional sputum cytology has a poor pick-up rate, but recent advances in molecular biology may allow the detection by polymerase chain reaction (PCR) techniques of chromosomal mutations found commonly in lung cancer; for example p53 and K-ras. Great interest has also been given to immunohistochemical techniques using an antibody staining the ribonucleoprotein (RNP)-binding protein, hnRNP A2/B1. Recent studies have shown that this may be one of the most powerful predictors of early disease, with a detection rate of 80 per cent (Tockman et al., 1997). Others have investigated automated methods of examining the nuclear changes in cells, such as those used in cervical screening. Payne et al. (1997) used this method both on lung biopsy specimens and sputum cytology from patients with cancer and demonstrated significant changes in over 75 per cent of normal-appearing specimens.

Other novel methods of early detection have used breath tests, this method relies on the fact that normal human breath contains volatile organic compounds. Several of these compounds have been identified as markers for lung cancer. Using this method (Phillips et al., 1999) predicted the diagnosis in 72 per cent of patients undergoing bronchoscopy.

RADIOLOGICAL SCREENING

Plain chest X-rays (CXR) are poor at detecting very early stage disease. In Japan, detection rates have been as low as 0.03–0.05 per cent. Therefore other radiological methods have been investigated. The use of low-dose spiral computed tomography (CT) scanning has been reported both in Japan and the USA. In the Japanese study (Sone et al., 1998), carried out in an area of low incidence, the rate of detection of lung cancer was 0.48 per cent, almost tenfold that using chest X-rays, and of these patients 84 per cent had stage I disease. The detection rate was considerably higher (2.7 per cent by CT versus 0.7 per cent by CXR) in the US study, which was performed in high-risk individuals (Henschke et al., 1999). However, in both of these studies a larger number of patients with benign non-calcified nodules were detected, who then underwent further investigation. While this method does seem to be particularly sensitive at detecting stage I disease in asymptomatic individuals, the survival benefits are unproven and the economic implications are enormous.

CLINICAL FEATURES

The vast majority of patients with lung cancer present with symptomatic disease. In a study of 678 patients only 7 per cent were asymptomatic, with over 60 per cent of patients presenting with systemic symptoms. Patients who present with a long history of symptoms related to the primary tumour have been found to have a better 5-year survival, suggesting that the growth of these tumours may be more indolent.

The presenting features of lung cancer depend on the location of the tumour, rapidity of growth and co-morbidity of the patient. The majority of patients (70 per cent or more) have regional or metastatic disease, making resection impossible. Small cell lung cancer (SCLC) has the most rapid growth rate of the four major types of lung cancer and metastasizes early. Symptoms from SCLC occur earlier and are more varied than those from non-small cell lung cancer (NSCLC). Non-metastatic syndromes affecting the nervous and endocrine systems are much more common with the small cell subtype.

The median interval between onset of symptoms and diagnosis is about 4 months. This delay occurs because symptoms are often of gradual onset and on a background of chronic obstructive airways disease in smokers. A summary of the initial symptoms of patients with lung carcinoma taken from a series of studies representing 8638 patients is given in Table 22.2 (Hyde and Hyde, 1974).

Symptoms related to the primary tumour

Cough is the most frequently reported symptom and is often disregarded by the patient and doctors for some

Table 22.2 *Initial symptoms of 8638 patients in seven studies (Hyde and Hyde, 1974)*

Initial symptoms	Percentage of patients
Cough	70
Weight loss	45
Chest pain	44
Dyspnoea	42
Haemoptysis	34
Lymphadenopathy	22
Hepatomegaly	22
Bone pain	18
Clubbing	17
Intracranial	9
Hoarse voice	7
SVCO	5

SVCO, superior vena cava obstruction.

time in smokers. The development of a new cough or change in its character is therefore important. In particular, the failure of a chest infection to resolve or the onset of haemoptysis should prompt further investigation. Dyspnoea may be secondary to intrinsic or extrinsic obstructive lesions or the development of pleural effusions. If tumour involves the major airways, very severe dyspnoea can develop rapidly and the presence of stridor must always be regarded as an emergency. Chest pain can arise from the primary tumour or superimposed infection, and does not necessarily imply metastatic disease. The pain is often described as heavy, is poorly localized and may be dismissed as unimportant. More severe pain can be caused by chest wall invasion.

Symptoms related to regional spread

Nerve involvement is often seen in the Pancoast syndrome, caused by superior sulcus tumours invading the brachial plexus and ribs. This is associated with severe shoulder pain radiating down the arm, classically in the T1 distribution, and weakness of hand grip. Horner's syndrome due to involvement of the sympathetic chain can also occur.

Superior vena caval obstruction (SVCO) is another dramatic and extremely unpleasant symptom complex occurring in about 4 per cent of patients at presentation. The syndrome results from local tumour extension or nodal metastases with compression of the superior vena cava (SVC). Venous engorgement of the face and neck is an early presenting feature but eventually a collateral circulation with dilatation of superficial chest wall veins develops. Other symptoms of SVCO may include headaches, drowsiness, vertigo, dyspnoea and dysphagia.

Symptoms of intra-thoracic spread of tumour include dysphagia from mediastinal lymphadenopathy or direct infiltration of the oesophagus. Pericardial infiltration can cause arrhythmias, effusions and occasionally tamponade.

Both the phrenic and left recurrent laryngeal nerves may be damaged by central tumours, resulting in paralysis of the diaphragm and hoarse voice, respectively. The use of Teflon injections behind the vocal cords can be helpful in improving the cough reflex to clear bronchial secretions and to strengthen the voice.

Extrathoracic metastases

Extrathoracic lymph-node metastases may be visible or palpable in the supraclavicular, cervical and axillary regions. The presence of upper abdominal lymphadenopathy, usually arising from SCLC, can cause poorly localized upper abdominal or back pain, jaundice, nausea, anorexia or vomiting. Other common sites of metastases include liver, bone and brain. Liver metastases are seen in over 35 per cent of patients at autopsy, and characteristic symptoms are pain and a feeling of fullness. Bone lesions occur in about 25 per cent of patients and are usually lytic and most commonly occur in the spine, pelvis and femur. Brain metastases are particularly common in small cell and adenocarcinoma, they are seen in up to 80 per cent of patients at autopsy. They can present with focal neurological deficits, with features of raised intracranial pressure such as headaches and vomiting, or impaired mental function or with personality changes. The adrenals and other endocrine organs are also prone to metastases in SCLC; the incidence may be as high as 30 per cent, although patients remain asymptomatic until 90 per cent of the gland has been replaced. Less common sites of metastases include choroidal metastases causing retinal detachment and skin metastases (less than 5 per cent).

Lung cancer is frequently associated with constitutional symptoms, including fatigue and weight loss which occur in over 50 per cent of patients at presentation. Pyrexia of uncertain origin and normochronic, normocytic anaemia are also features of lung cancer. Anaemia, particularly in the case of SCLC, may result from marrow infiltration.

A multitude of non-metastatic or paraneoplastic syndromes may occur, particularly in small cell lung cancer, some preceding the diagnosis of lung cancer by many months (Table 22.3).

PATHOLOGY

It is extremely important that an accurate pathological diagnosis is made. The current national guidelines state that the target for pathological verification should be at least 75 per cent. The initial diagnosis may be made by radiological means, for example CXR or CT scans. Confirmation may be performed by cytology or histology, using a variety of techniques. Sputum cytology is the least invasive method, but bronchoscopy with washings

Table 22.3 *Paraneoplastic syndromes associated with lung cancer, particularly small cell lung cancer*

System	Syndrome	Comments
Skeletal	Clubbing	*c.* 20% of patients, squamous cell carcinoma common
	Pulmonary hypertophic osteoarthropathy	*c.* 5% of patients, adenocarcinoma common, periostitis of long bones
Cutaneous	Dermatomyositis	Weakness of pelvic girdle muscles, heliotrope rash, 15–20% of patients will have underlying malignancy
	Acanthosis nigricans	Hyperkeratosis and pigmentation of axillae, neck and flexures
Neurological	Subacute cerebellar degeneration	Subacute, symmetrical cerebellar failure; anti-Purkinje and Yo antibodies detected
	Sensorimotor peripheral neuropathy	Distal motor and sensory loss; anti-Hu antibodies are a marker
	Polymyositis	Proximal muscle weakness
	Eaton–Lambert syndrome	Fatigue of proximal muscles, poor response to edrophonium test; 1–6% SCLC
	Autonomic neuropathy	Orthostatic hypotension, neurogenic bladder, GI dysmobility; SCLC
Endocrine	Ectopic parathyroid hormone	Squamous cell carcinoma; *c.* 15% of patients with hypercalcaemia
	Cushing's syndrome	Ectopic ACTH production, usually presents with hypokalaemia, SCLC
	Syndrome of inappropriate ADH secretion (SIADH)	Hyponatraemia, *c.* 30% patients with SCLC; may lead to seizures
	Hypercalcitonaemia	Hypocalcaemia, may present with paraesthesia, cramps and tetany
	Gynaecomastia	Due to ectopic gonadotropin production, common in large cell and adenocarcinomas
Renal	Nephrotic syndrome	Secondary to immune complexes, thrombus, amyloid
	Membranous glomerulonephritis	
GI	VIP secretion	Profuse diarrhoea, hypokalaemia

GI, gastrointestinal; ADH, antidiuretic hormone; VIP, vasoactive intestinal polypeptide.

or biopsy, transthoracic needle biopsy or biopsy of lymph nodes or metastatic deposits is often required.

Histologically, lung cancers are classified according to their light microscopic appearance rather than their histogenesis. They are divided pragmatically into two clinico-pathological groups, small cell and non-small cell. Non-small cell cancers include squamous cell, adenocarcinoma and large cell tumours as defined by WHO/IASLC in 1998 (Table 22.4).

In the UK and many European countries squamous cell carcinoma accounts for the majority of cases (40 per cent), with adenocarcinoma and small cell carcinoma 15–25 per cent each and large cell carcinomas and the other rarer forms accounting for 10–20 per cent. The incidence of the different forms of cancer varies considerably between countries, with adenocarcinoma being the most common in the USA. This range of incidence may reflect the source of tissue for diagnosis, for example as squamous cell carcinomas are more frequently resected these may be over-represented, while small cell carcinomas are prone to crushing, making interpretation difficult. Both intra and inter-observer disagreement can occur (Mooi, 1996), which obviously has implications for the management of patients. Therefore, in the context of clinical trials, appropriate review mechanisms should be available.

Squamous cell carcinomas occur more commonly in men than women and are most frequently related to smoking. The tumours typically occur in the major bronchi, and the surrounding epithelia commonly show areas of metaplasia or dysplasia. Macroscopically these tumours appear as firm lesions with a pale grey, gritty surface. Microscopically the hallmarks of squamous differentiation are apparent, with prominent intercellular bridges and keratinization. Immunohistochemical staining with antibodies against high molecular weight cytokeratins (>63 kDa) is helpful in the diagnosis, in particular cytokeratin 14. Other antibodies include those staining for involucrin and carcinoembryonic antigen (CEA).

Table 22.4 *Histological classification of lung tumours (WHO/IASLC, 1998)*

1. *Squamous cell carcinoma*
   Variants:
      Papillary
      Clear cell
      Small cell
      Basaloid

2. *Small cell carcinoma*
   Variant:
      Combined small cell carcinoma

3. *Adenocarcinoma*
   Acinar
   Papillary
   Bronchioloalveolar carcinoma
      Non-mucinous (Clara cell/type II pneumocyte type)
      Mucinous (goblet cell type)
      Mixed mucinous and non-mucinous (Clara cell/type II
         pneumocyte and goblet cell type) or indeterminate
   Solid carcinoma with mucin formation
   Mixed
   Variants:
      Well-differentiated fetal adenocarcinoma
      Mucinous ('colloid')
      Mucinous cystadenocarcinoma
      Signet ring
      Clear cell

4. *Large cell carcinoma*
   Variants:
      Large cell neuroendocrine carcinoma
         Combined large cell neuroendocrine carcinoma
      Basaloid carcinoma
      Lymphoepithelioma-like carcinoma
      Clear cell carcinoma
      Large cell carcinoma with rhabdoid phenotype

5. *Adenosquamous carcinoma*

6. *Carcinomas with pleomorphic, sarcomatoid or
   sarcomatous elements*
   Carcinomas with spindle and/or giant cells
      Pleomorphic carcinoma
      Spindle cell carcinoma
      Giant cell carcinoma
   Carcinosarcoma
   Blastoma (pulmonary blastoma)

7. *Carcinoid tumour*
   Typical carcinoid
   Atypical carcinoid

8. *Carcinomas of salivary gland type*
   Mucoepidemoid carcinoma
   Adenoid cystic carcinoma
   Others

9. *Unclassified carcinoma*

Adenocarcinomas occur with equal frequency in men and women and are less frequently associated with smoking. A precursor lesion, atypical alveolar hyperplasia, is now well recognized. These tumours are typically peripheral.

Macroscopically they form irregular, round masses, the cut surfaces of which often have a myxoid appearance. Microscopically, varying degrees of glandular differentiation are seen, and the nuclei often have prominent nucleoli. Immunohistochemistry and mucin histochemistry are often important to differentiate these tumours from mesotheliomas. Antibodies staining the surfactant apoprotein and CEA may be positive, while BerEP4 and the mesothelial markers CK5, thrombomodulin and calretinin are negative.

Carcinoid tumours account for only 2 per cent of all lung cancers and may behave in a benign fashion. They tend to arise in the major bronchi and contain large numbers of neurosecretory granules.

Small cell lung cancers are usually found in the major bronchi and are associated with smoking. The tumours are associated with the secretion of a number of hormones, including antidiuretic hormone (ADH), calcitonin and adrenocorticotrophic hormone (ACTH). Macroscopically the tumours are friable, with a pinky/tan cut surface. Microscopically they are characterized by the presence of small cells, approximately three times larger than a lymphocyte, with large pleomorphic nuclei and scanty cytoplasm. Crush artefacts following bronchoscopic biopsy are common. The use of antibodies such as Cam 5.2, chromogranin, synaptophysin, CD56 (neural cell adhesion molecule, NCAM) and NSE (neuron-specific enolase) are the most useful antibodies, but some NSCLCs may stain with these. Therefore morphology is very important and forms the principal means of diagnosis.

A problem that may arise for pathologists is that approximately 10 per cent of small cell tumours are of mixed cell type. Mixed small cell and large cell tumours are associated with a poorer prognosis and poor response to therapy. In addition, changes in cell type may occur following treatment: in one study 11 of 40 cases revealed NSCLC histology at relapse (Abeloff *et al.*, 1979).

The presence of tumours of mixed cell type implies either separate primary tumours or a common stem cell undergoing different differentiation processes. The proposition of a common stem cell is supported by the observation that neuroectodermal markers such as L-dopa decarboxylase and neuron-specific enolase, which were formerly associated exclusively with SCLC, can also be found in some NSCLCs. Indeed, the presence of these markers is associated with a more aggressive clinical course and greater sensitivity to chemotherapy.

The development of techniques for culturing lung cancer cell lines has led to improved understanding of the biology of lung cancer. SCLCs are characterized by the presence of dense core granules on electron microscopy. These are associated with the ability to secrete a variety of ectopic peptides and hormones. It is now increasingly evident that many of these can act as growth factors. They may act on the secreting cell (autocrine) or nearby cells (paracrine) to stimulate tumour growth.

The development of antagonists to these growth factors is being explored as a potential therapeutic intervention. Many researchers have established antibodies to lung cancer cells. These have been tested against each other on panels of different tissues to characterize the antigenic epitopes they recognize. Five such antigen clusters are now recognized for SCLC, and the most commonly expressed, cluster 1, has been identified as the neural cell adhesion molecule, NCAM. The development of monoclonal antibodies specific for SCLC will permit their use in diagnosis, imaging and treatment. Specific tumour markers would be useful in screening a high-risk population for early cancers and could also be useful in diagnosis, staging and monitoring the response to therapy. Unfortunately, none of the markers examined to date, including neuron-specific enolase, ACTH, calcitonin and neurophysin, have been sufficiently sensitive and specific to be useful clinically in this role.

STAGING AND OTHER PROGNOSTIC FACTORS

Staging

The extent or stage of the tumour should be established in pre-treatment investigations. Accurate staging is important; first, to give patients and carers accurate prognostic information; secondly, to help to decide the most effective treatment; and, finally, to allow comparison between different treatments and institutes. The international standard for staging in NSCLC is the TNM system, originally proposed by Denoix (Denoix, 1944). These TNM subgroups can then be amalgamated into a smaller number of disease stages (Table 22.6). The original TNM system adopted by the American Joint Committee on Cancer Staging was based on data from over 2000 patients with proven lung cancer assessed using 28 variables, and was shown to have a consistency of over 90 per cent between physicians. In 1986 a new international staging system for lung cancer was developed from a database of 3753 patients. This system has been updated recently (Mountain, 1997), with new elements to meet the needs of modern treatment and for better estimation of prognosis by dividing stage I and II disease into A and B categories and modifying stage IIIA. The new international TNM staging classification is given in Table 22.5 and the new stage groupings in Table 22.6 (Mountain, 1997).

Patients with clinical stage I, II and IIIa NSCLC can be considered for surgical treatment; for patients with stage IIIb and IV disease radiotherapy, chemotherapy or combined modality treatment might be appropriate. Detailed preoperative staging is required for NSCLC in order to avoid unnecessary surgery. The use of CT scanning of the mediastinum and mediastinoscopy has greatly improved the accuracy of staging. Additional investigations are required to assess the suitability of patients for surgery, including cardiovascular evaluation and pulmonary function tests, to assess postoperative reserve. The prognostic significance of various stages and TNM subsets are discussed later in the treatment section, but the overall influence of stage is shown in Figure 22.3.

Small cell lung cancer requires a different staging system, as no difference in survival is found in resected patients with TNM stages I, II and III. Small cell lung cancer has therefore been divided into two stages: limited and extensive. Limited disease describes about 30 per cent of patients and is defined as disease confined to one hemithorax with regional metastases, including hilar, ipsilateral and contralateral mediastinal, and ipsilateral and contralateral supraclavicular nodes and ipsilateral pleural effusions, whether or not the cytology is positive. Extensive-stage disease is defined as disease beyond this, including distant lymph nodes, brain, liver, bone, bone marrow and intra-abdominal soft-tissue metastases. The importance of stage for survival is discussed below.

Further restaging investigations are necessary to monitor the progress of the disease and the response to treatment. In SCLC if there is no reduction in tumour mass with the first few cycles of therapy, there is a significantly shorter survival time than in patients with a response detectable on chest X-ray. The definition of remission of the tumour requires full restaging to determine whether previous abnormalities have resolved and to what extent. It is recommended that patients be followed up regularly to identify progressive disease, complications of treatment, such as pulmonary fibrosis, or second malignancies. Patients who continue to smoke after resection of a lung cancer are at particularly high risk of developing a second tumour.

Other prognostic factors

Additional features at presentation can be useful in assessing prognosis, particularly in SCLC. Performance status is one of the most important prognostic indicators. As expected, patients who are fully mobile with few or no symptoms respond better to treatment and have better survival than those who are bed-bound. The various scales in common use (WHO, Karnofsky, ECOG and Zubrod) all predict for survival. In addition to assessing prognosis, performance status is also valuable in monitoring the effects of treatment. More complex measures of quality of life are now being incorporated in clinical studies to assess the benefit of different treatment strategies which have a similar survival. It is important to note that age has not been shown to be an independent prognostic factor affecting survival for either SCLC or NSCLC.

A number of multivariate analyses of adverse prognostic factors have been performed in SCLC. The

Table 22.5 *International TNM staging for lung cancer (from Mountain, 1997 with permission)*

Primary tumour (T)

TX   Primary tumour can not be assessed, or tumour proven by the presence of malignant cells in sputum or bronchial washings; not visualized by imaging or bronchoscopy

T0   No evidence of primary tumour

Tis   Carcinoma *in-situ*

T1   Tumour 3 cm or less in greatest dimension, surrounded by lung or visceral pleura, without bronchoscopic evidence of invasion more proximal than the lobar bronchus

T2   Tumour with any of the following features of size or extent:
- \>3 cm in greatest dimension
- involves main bronchus, at least 2 cm distal to the carina
- invades the visceral pleura
- associated with atelectasis or obstructive pneumonitis that extends to the hilar region but does not involve the entire lung

T3   Tumour of any size that directly invades any of the following: chest wall (including superior sulcus tumours), diaphragm, mediastinal pleura, parietal pleura; or tumour in the main bronchus less than 2 cm from the carina, but without involvement of the carina; or associated atelectasis or obstructive pneumonitis of the entire lung

T4   Tumour of any size that invades any of the following: mediastinum, great vessels, trachea, oesophagus, vertebral body, carina; or tumour with malignant pleural or pericardial effusion; or with satellite tumour nodule(s) within the ipsilateral primary-tumour lobe of the lung

Regional lymph nodes (N)

NX   Regional lymph nodes cannot be assessed

N0   No regional lymph node metastases

N1   Metastases to ipsilateral peribronchial and/or ipsilateral hilar lymph nodes, and intrapulmonary nodes involved by direct extension of the primary tumour

N2   Metastases to ipsilateral mediastinal and/or subcarinal lymph nodes

N3   Metastases to contralateral mediastinal, contralateral hilar, ipsilateral or contralateral scalene or supraclavicular lymph nodes

Distant metastases (M)

MX   Presence of distant metastases cannot be assessed

M0   No distant metastases

M1   Distant metastases present

Notes

T1   The uncommon superficial tumour of any size with its invasive component limited to the bronchial wall, which may extend proximal to the main bronchus is also classified as T1

T4   Most pleural effusions associated with lung cancer are due to the tumour. However, there are a few patients in whom multiple cytopathological examinations of pleural fluid show no tumour. In these cases, the fluid is non-bloody and is not an exudate. When these elements and clinical judgement dictate that the effusion is not related to the tumour, the effusion should be excluded as a staging element and the patient should be staged T1, T2 or T3. Pericardial effusion is classified according to the same rules

M1   Separate metastatic tumour nodules in the ipsilateral non-primary-tumour lobe(s) of the lung are also classified M1

---

parameters identified have included low performance status, low serum albumin, low sodium, high alkaline phosphatase, extensive disease, elevated lactate dehydrogenase (LDH), high aspartate aminotransferase and low bicarbonate. In an overview of eight UK study databases including almost 4000 patients, the most important independent prognostic factors were low performance status, high alkaline phosphatase and extensive-stage disease (Rawson and Peto, 1990). Placing patients into a defined prognostic group with, for example, no adverse features, allows treatment to be tailored. Thus, intensive treatment can be given to those patients in the better prognostic groups, while patients identified as having a poor prognosis can be offered a more palliative approach to therapy.

An analysis of prognostic factors for NSCLC examined features identifying patients who survived for more than 12 months following chemotherapy. Favourable characteristics were good performance status, female, no bone, liver or subcutaneous metastases, non-large cell histology, little weight loss and no shoulder or arm pain. Other groups reported a favourable prognosis for patients with a single site of extrathoracic metastases. The use of cisplatin-based therapy and a normal LDH have also been shown to be powerful independent predictors in multivariate analyses (Albain *et al.*, 1991).

Table 22.6 *Stage of lung cancer as defined by the TNM classification; 5-year survival is given according to clinical estimates of the extent of the disease (from Mountain, 1997 with permission)*

Stage	TNM subset	5-year survival (%)
0	Carcinoma *in-situ*	
IA	T1 N0 M0	61
IB	T2 N0 M0	38
IIA	T1 N1 M0	34
IIB	T2 N1 M0	24
	T3 N0 M0	
IIIA	T3 N1 M0	13
	T1 N2 M0	
	T2 N2 M0	
	T3 N2 M0	
IIIB	T4 N0 M0	5
	T4 N1 M0	
	T4 N2 M0	
	T1 N3 M0	
	T2 N3 M0	
	T3 N3 M0	
	T4 N3 M0	
IV	Any T Any N M1	1

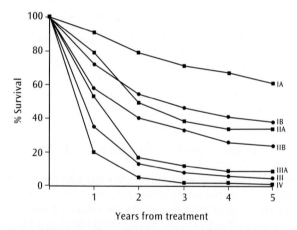

Figure 22.3 *Overall survival in patients with NSCLC according to stage at diagnosis.*

TREATMENT OF NON-SMALL CELL LUNG CANCER

Surgery for non-small cell lung cancer

While there is little evidence in terms of randomized controlled studies evaluating the benefits of surgery, many observational studies clearly show a survival advantage. Therefore surgical resection continues to be the prime modality of curative treatment for NSCLC. Resectability depends upon the tumour stage and the patient's ability to tolerate the procedure. Patients with stage I and stage II tumours should be considered for resection if preoperative assessment suggests that such a procedure would be safe. Patients with stage IIIA tumours also have potentially resectable disease. Survival is dependent on the extent of the disease, with patients with T3 N1 tumours doing better than those with N2 disease. N2 disease has a particularly poor prognosis if associated with T3 tumours, multiple nodal station involvement and adenocarcinoma histology. Patients with stage IIIB or IV disease are considered unresectable.

The most suitable type of resection is determined by tumour size, stage and other criteria. Pneumonectomy is only performed in approximately 20 per cent of patients and is required if the tumour or lymph nodes are involving proximal structures. Lobectomy is the most common procedure performed for N0 and N1 disease and results in similar survival to more extensive procedures when undertaken in patients with equivalent tumour size. As second primary tumours occur in 5–10 per cent of previously resected patients, conservation of lung tissue can allow further resection later. Very limited resections, such as wedge resections and segmentectomy, may be useful in patients with low pulmonary reserve, but the rate of local recurrence is increased threefold (Ginsberg and Rubenstein, 1995). Thoracoscopy and video-assisted thoracoscopy (VATS) have been developed to allow access to the chest cavity with minimally invasive surgical techniques. VATS has primarily been used for diagnostic purposes, being particularly useful in the evaluation of mediastinal pathology. Mediastinoscopy has therefore changed to some extent from confirming unresectable disease to identifying patients with minimal N2, stage IIIB disease who may be suitable for resection or multimodality treatment. Resections have been performed in selected centres with VATS and may allow resection in patients who are otherwise borderline for standard thoracotomy. However, the use of VATS in surgical resection needs to be evaluated very carefully as limited resection is associated with higher local recurrence rates. Nevertheless, these newer surgical approaches, together with improvements in anaesthesia, management of chronic obstructive airways disease and ischaemic heart disease have extended the surgical options for patients with lung cancer.

RESULTS OF SURGICAL TREATMENT FOR NON-SMALL CELL LUNG CANCER

Advances in anaesthetic and surgical techniques have reduced postoperative mortality. The risk of postoperative death is higher in patients over 70 years old, in those with co-morbid conditions and following more extensive resections. Current rates following pneumonectomy are 6–7 per cent, whereas after lobectomy this is only 3 per cent. Morbidity is high, with about 20 per cent of patients having minor complications, the most common being supraventricular tachycardia, and 10 per cent suffering from major problems such as embolus and pulmonary insufficiency. Studies examining quality of life post-resection have

Table 22.7 *Survival following surgical resection according to stage at diagnosis (from Mountain, 1997 with permission)*

Stage	TNM	5-year survival (%)
IA	T1 N0 M0	67
IB	T2 N0 M0	57
IIA	T1 N1 M0	55
IIB	T2 N1 M0	39
	T3 N0 M0	38
IIIA	T3 N1 M0	25
	T1–3 N2 M0	23

shown that preoperative levels are not achieved until at least 6 months after surgery (Dales *et al.*, 1994).

In Britain about 65 per cent of patients are inoperable at presentation and at exploratory thoracotomy a further 15 per cent are unresectable. Of the remaining 20 per cent who undergo 'curative' resection, only about 30–40 per cent are alive at 5 years and 16–18 per cent at 10 years or more. Survival is dependent on both the stage of tumour (Table 22.7) and histology, with squamous cell carcinomas having a better survival than adenocarcinomas. However, it is thought that approximately 15–20 per cent of the reported deaths are likely to be non-cancer related and therefore 5-year survival for stage IA disease is in the region of 85 per cent. T3 tumours that are difficult to resect, such as those in the superior sulcus and invading the chest wall, have been shown to have 5-year survival rates of 26–40 per cent.

Treatment failure results from lack of control of local disease in about a third of patients and from metastatic spread in the remainder, with up to 10 per cent of patients developing brain metastases. The majority of local relapses occur within the first 2 years following surgery, therefore close follow-up is required during this period. In addition to recurrent disease, a proportion of patients will develop second primary lung cancer. Resection of new primary lung cancers should be performed if possible, even in the unusual circumstance of synchronous lung cancer, although survival is poor (*c.* 25 per cent) even for low-stage disease.

It is clear that surgery can cure some patients; however, the problem remains that the majority of tumours are unresectable at presentation. There is increasing interest in the use of neo-adjuvant chemotherapy, to render the tumour resectable, especially in patients with N2 disease. This will be discussed below.

Radiotherapy for non-small cell lung cancer

Radiotherapy may be used with curative intent in patients with disease that is potentially operable but who are not suitable for surgery. These patients represent the minority of those who receive radiotherapy, with the majority receiving palliative treatment.

RADICAL RADIOTHERAPY

Radical radiotherapy given with curative intent should be considered as an alternative to surgery in patients with stage I and II tumours who decline operation and in patients whose co-morbid conditions would make surgery unsafe. It may be also considered in patients with stage III disease. Poor lung function may also preclude radical radiotherapy because radiation pneumonitis and fibrosis occur in almost all irradiated patients within 1 year.

In order to deliver appropriate doses of radiation to the tumour, careful planning is required, with CT playing an important role. The recommended fields include a 2 cm margin around the tumour. The maximum dose, however, is highly dependent on the total volume to be irradiated and the tolerance of the normal lung and spinal cord. Radical treatment is contraindicated in patients with distant metastases, malignant pleural effusions and poor performance status. Treatment schedules have varied widely, but it is now clear that survival is dependent on the radiation dose achieved. It is now recommended that patients should receive the biological equivalent of 60 Gy in 30 fractions to the primary tumour and that 45–55 Gy should be given to the mediastinum. For stage I, the recommendation is that the target volume encompasses the tumour only, while the ipsilateral hilum should be included in patients with stage II disease.

A study comparing surgery and radical radiotherapy, published in 1963, reported that the 4-year survival following radiotherapy was only 7 per cent compared to 23 per cent in patients who underwent surgery (Morrison *et al.*, 1963). More recent studies have shown 1-year survival after radiotherapy to be over 40 per cent, falling at 5 years to 10–15 per cent (Table 22.8). It is difficult to compare these findings directly with surgery as patients have rarely been as fully staged and may have other medical conditions contraindicating surgery. Independent prognostic indicators of survival include tumour size, radiation dose and performance status.

These results remain disappointing and therefore novel radiotherapy techniques have been investigated. The median doubling time for NSCLC cell lines is approximately 7 days, although it can be considerably faster. The use of hyperfractionation was therefore considered as a means to overcome rapid repopulation. The results of a randomized controlled study involving 563 patients were published in 1997 (Saunders *et al.*, 1997). Patients were randomized to receive either conventional radiotherapy (60 Gy in daily 2 Gy fractions over 6 weeks) or continuous hyperfractionated acclerated radiotherapy (CHART). For this, patients received 1.5 Gy three times a day (at least 6 hours apart) for 12 consecutive days. Patients who received CHART had significant improvements in both the incidence of local recurrence and in survival at 1 (63 per cent versus 55 per cent) and 2 years (29 per cent versus 20 per cent). Dysphagia occurred earlier and was of greater severity in patients receiving CHART, and later

Table 22.8 *Examples of recent studies demonstrating survival following radical radiotherapy for NSCLC*

Study	Number of patients	Tumour stage	Radiotherapy	Median survival (months)	1 year (%)	2 year (%)	5 year (%)
Talton *et al.* (1990)	77	T1–3 N0	60 Gy in 30 F	18	57	36	17
Rosenthal *et al.* (1992)	40	T1–2 N0	18–65 Gy	15	72	35	N R
		T1–2 N1		18	70	33	12
Dosoretz *et al.* (1992)	152	T1–3 N0	45–65 Gy in 1.8–2 Gy F	17	N R	40	10
Graham *et al.* (1995)	103	T1–2 N0–1	Median 60 Gy in 30 F	16	N R	35	13
Morita *et al.* (1997)	149	T1–2 N0	55–74 Gy in 2 Gy F	27	78	N R	22

F, fractions of radiotherapy; NR, not recorded.

complications such as myelitis and pulmonary fibrosis were increased. Although the results of this study were exciting, they have not been replicated elsewhere. The use of continuous hyperfractionated radiotherapy would be problematic in the majority of radiotherapy centres and many oncologists believe that similar results could be obtained with chemoradiotherapy. Modified hyperfractionated regimens have been investigated (Mehta *et al.*, 1998; Saunders *et al.*, 1998) and appear to produce similar results. The effect of these new regimens on quality of life has been shown to be similar to that of conventional therapy, with the exception of breathlessness, which was considerably worse in the CHART arm at 2 years.

NEO-ADJUVANT/ADJUVANT RADIOTHERAPY

The use of neo-adjuvant radiotherapy has shown no benefit in survival. In an attempt to reduce the risk of local recurrence following surgery, a number of studies have investigated the role of postoperative radiotherapy. A meta-analysis of the data from nine randomized controlled studies has shown that postoperative radiotherapy was detrimental to survival, resulting in a 7 per cent reduction in overall survival at 2 years (Stewart *et al.*, 1998). This effect appeared to be greatest in patients with stage I and II disease. A number of these studies have been criticized, one included some patients with SCLC and in others staging was not fully assessed.

PALLIATIVE RADIOTHERAPY

The aims of palliative treatment are symptom relief and symptom prevention rather than life extension. The vast majority (80 per cent) of patients referred for consideration of radiotherapy for lung cancer are only suitable for palliative treatment, and in about 10 per cent radiation is not considered to be worthwhile. For patients with inoperable tumours in whom there is a negligible chance of long-term survival, there is a difference of opinion as to whether patients who are relatively asymptomatic should receive immediate radiotherapy or whether treatment

should be deferred. The Medical Research Council study, LU17, has addressed this issue. Two hundred and thirty patients with untreated NSCLC whose disease was locally too advanced for resection or radical radiotherapy and with minimal symptoms were randomized to receive supportive care plus immediate thoracic radiotherapy, or supportive care plus delayed radiotherapy to treat symptoms. The study concluded that immediate palliative radiotherapy resulted in no improvement in symptom control or survival (Girling *et al.*, 2000).

The doses of thoracic radiotherapy used are lower than in radical treatments, duration of treatment is shorter and an important objective is to minimize side-effects. A number of randomized controlled studies have addressed the effect of radiation dose on palliation and survival. It has been demonstrated that shorter courses of treatment (10 Gy in a single fraction or 17 Gy in two fractions) are as good, if not better, at palliating symptoms as longer courses, with fewer adverse effects (Table 22.9). In a recently published MRC study (Medical Research Council, 1996a) the use of higher doses did produce a survival advantage and therefore many oncologists argue that high-dose palliation should be considered in patients with good performance status.

Symptoms which respond best to palliative radiotherapy include SVC obstruction and haemoptysis, which are relieved in 80 per cent or more of patients, while cough, chest pain and breathlessness are relieved in about 60 per cent of patients. There is evidence that radiotherapy may also improve non-specific symptoms such as tiredness.

The use of endobronchial radiotherapy has been shown to be effective in controlling cough, breathlessness and haemoptysis in selected tumours causing intrinsic or extrinsic bronchial compression, with improvement in symptoms in 75 per cent. The most serious complication of this treatment is major haemoptysis. There is no clear evidence that this method of delivery is better than external beam, but it may be useful in retreating patients who have received maximum doses to the spinal cord, although

Table 22.9 *Examples of recent trials investigating the effect of dose in palliative radiotherapy on symptom control in NSCLC*

Study	Radiotherapy	Number of patients	Comment
MRC Lung Cancer Working Party (1991)	30 Gy in 10 F vs 17 Gy in 2 F	369	Results for survival and palliation equivalent
MRC Lung Cancer Working Party (1992)	17 Gy in 2 F vs 10 Gy in 1 F	233	1F group better for control of haemoptysis; no difference in survival
MRC Lung Cancer Working Party (1996a)	39 Gy in 13 F or 36 Gy in 12 F vs 17 Gy in 2 F	509	Survival advantage in 13 F group, 9 vs 7 months median survival; palliation at 2–3 months better with 2 F and fewer side-effects
Rees *et al.* (1997)	22.5 Gy in 5 F vs 17 Gy in 2 F	216	Tendency towards better palliation in 2 F group

F, fractions of radiotherapy.

this needs evaluation in clinical trials. Laser therapy can also be used to destroy endobronchial tumours via the bronchoscope. Unfortunately, current laser delivery systems can only treat small endobronchial lesions and therefore multiple treatments are often needed.

Radiotherapy is also of benefit in the treatment of metastatic disease, with bone pain being relieved in more than 50 per cent of patients, frequently with a single fraction of irradiation. Large field, e.g. hemi-body, irradiation can be considered for widespread bony metastases. Palliative brain irradiation for metastatic disease can result in symptomatic improvement in 80 per cent or more of patients, particularly those who have fits and headaches. However, in patients with focal neurological signs from brain metastases and spinal cord compression the results of radiotherapy are much less impressive. A neurosurgical opinion should be sought in otherwise fit patients with spinal cord compression or solitary brain metastases and no evidence of metastatic disease elsewhere. Anorexia, weight loss, hoarseness, pleural effusion and non-metastatic features of lung cancer rarely respond to palliative radiotherapy. In the early Oxford studies of 1975–77 there was no clear benefit from radiotherapy when compared with observation, except for control of specific symptoms such as pain, haemoptysis and SVC obstruction. This has lent support to the policy of deferred radiotherapy in the absence of symptoms in patients with poor prognosis. Other methods of palliation, including chemotherapy, steroids, appropriate analgesia, nursing care and psychological support, should also be considered for patients with lung cancer.

ADVERSE EFFECTS OF RADIOTHERAPY

Side-effects can be divided into short, intermediate and long-term effects. The most common short-term toxicity is dysphagia secondary to oesophagitis. This can occur in up to 50 per cent of patients and typically lasts for 2 weeks after completion of therapy, although in a minority of patients (5 per cent) this may be prolonged. Radiation pneumonitis is evident in up to 100 per cent of

chest X-rays but is only clinically apparent in 5–10 per cent of patients, occurring 6–12 weeks following treatment. Long-term effects include radiation fibrosis, which again is more common radiologically than clinically significant, but these changes may make detection of recurrent tumour difficult. Transient radiation-induced myelitis may also occur and give rise to Lhermitte's sign. However, there is usually complete recovery and only a small minority of patients (<1 per cent) develop progressive limb weakness and paraparesis. Again this unusual side-effect (due to vascular impairment) may be difficult to distinguish from tumour involvement, although the latter often causes pain.

Chemotherapy for NSCLC

EARLY STAGE DISEASE

There has been increasing interest in the role of chemotherapy in stage I, II and IIIA NSCLC in combination with other treatment modalities. Studies have shown that the response to chemotherapy in locally advanced disease is approximately twice that seen in advanced disease.

Neoadjuvant chemotherapy prior to surgery

The rationale for using chemotherapy prior to surgery includes downstaging the tumour, eradication of micrometastases and reduction in growth factors produced by the primary tumour, so decreasing the stimulus to any residual cancer. It is clear that response rates to therapy are greater in early stage disease than in advanced disease. The majority of studies have been performed in patients with stage IIIA tumours, with the results suggesting a survival benefit. Two randomized studies comparing surgery alone to chemotherapy followed by surgery (Table 22.10) were closed prematurely, so only 120 patients were included in total. Although they both demonstrated a survival benefit for patients receiving neoadjuvant chemotherapy, a number of criticisms have been made of these studies. The numbers of patients were small and the survival for patients undergoing surgery alone in the

Table 22.10 *Examples of preoperative chemotherapy studies in NSCLC*

Study	Number of patients/stage	Randomization	Median survival
Rosell *et al.* (1994)	60/Stage IIIA	Surgery vs 3 $\times$ MIC + surgery	8 months vs 26 months[a]
Roth *et al.* (1994)	60/Stage IIIA	Surgery vs 3 $\times$ CEP + surgery + 3 $\times$ CEP	11 months vs 64 months[a]

[a]$P < 0.05$.

study of Rosell *et al.* (1994) was poor. In the Rosell study, 60 per cent of patients had an objective response to chemotherapy, with only one patient having progressive disease. In the Roth *et al.* (1994) study, 35 per cent of patients had an objective response, while four patients had progressive disease. The surgical resection rates did not differ significantly between the treatment groups in either study, and postoperative complications were not increased in the patients receiving preoperative chemotherapy. The median survivals have been revised with longer follow-up and are not as dramatic (Roth *et al.*, 1998; Rosell *et al.*, 1999). A recent study of 355 patients with stage I, II and IIIA disease randomized to receive neoadjuvant chemotherapy or surgery alone demonstrated that although disease-free survival was prolonged by chemotherapy (27 versus 13 months), improvements in median survival and three-year survival were not significant (Depierre *et al.*, 2002). At present, neoadjuvant chemotherapy cannot be recommended for routine use in stage IIIA patients. However, its role is being addressed further in randomized trials in a variety of stage settings, including the MRC study LU22.

Adjuvant chemotherapy following surgery

A meta-analysis of eight trials in which patients with resectable disease received cisplatin-containing combination chemotherapy following definitive surgery, demonstrated a survival benefit of 5 per cent at 5 years (Non-small cell lung cancer collaborative group, 1995), although the confidence intervals were large. The absolute benefit therefore remains unclear. In addition it has been found to be difficult to treat patients early postoperatively, because of the lengthy recovery time following thoracotomy.

Combination chemotherapy and radiotherapy

The results of a meta-analysis showed that addition of cisplatin-containing chemotherapy to radical radiotherapy improved survival at 5 years by 2 per cent (Non-small cell lung cancer collaborative group, 1995). The CALGB study has recently published data showing that those patients receiving combined modality therapy had improved survival (17 versus 6 per cent at 5 years) (Dillman *et al.*, 1996). ASCO guidelines (1997) state that chemotherapy in association with definitive dose radiotherapy prolongs survival in patients with locally advanced unresectable stage III

NSCLC but that the optimum sequence remains unclear. The sequential use of chemotherapy and radiotherapy has been the most studied and appears to have less toxicity than when given concurrently (Table 22.11). A phase III study in which 320 patients were randomized to receive concurrent or sequential thoracic radiotherapy with chemotherapy (mitomycin, vindesine and cisplatin) demonstrated that median survival was significantly improved (16.5 versus 13.3 months) in the concurrent group but that this was offset by significantly greater myelotoxicity (Furuse *et al.*, 1999). Further studies are required to determine the magnitude of benefit and the impact on quality of life.

CHEMOTHERAPY FOR ADVANCED DISEASE

For many years there was a great deal of pessimism concerning the role of chemotherapy in advanced NSCLC. However, a meta-analysis has confirmed that this modality does play an important role in the treatment of patients with advanced disease. Data from 11 trials comparing chemotherapy plus best supportive care (BSC) with BSC alone were evaluated, two studies used long-term alkylating agents, one used etoposide and eight used cisplatin-containing regimens. The analysis demonstrated that while alkylating agents had an adverse effect on prognosis (hazard ratio 1.26), the use of platinum-containing compounds resulted in improved survival (hazard ratio 0.73) equivalent to an increase in 1-year survival of 10 per cent from 15 to 25 per cent (Non-small cell lung cancer collaborative group, 1995). The response rates seen with single-agent chemotherapy, as reported in phase I and II studies in NSCLC, are shown in Table 22.12.

A number of new agents have been identified that are active against NSCLC as single agents. Of these new agents, vinorelbine and gemcitabine have been found to be particularly well tolerated. Indeed, in a meta-analysis comparing single-agent and combination therapies, vinorelbine alone was shown to have equivalent response rate and less toxicity than cisplatin-containing combinations (Lillenbaum *et al.*, 1998). Vinorelbine is a semisynthetic vinca alkaloid, normally given on a weekly schedule. Phase II and III studies have shown 1-year survival figures similar to those of cisplatin combinations. Of particular interest, single-agent vinorelbine has been shown to be well tolerated in patients over the age of 70.

Table 22.11 *Examples of recent randomized studies investigating the use of chemo-radiotherapy in NSCLC compared with radiotherapy alone*

Study	Number of patients	Sequence	Chemotherapy/ radiotherapy	Rx	Median survival (months)	2-year survival (%)
Dillman et al. (1990)	155	Sequential	Cis, vinblastine/60 Gy in 30 F	CT + RT	13.8	26
				RT	9.7	13
Schaake-Koning et al. (1992)	331	Concurrent	Cis 30 mg/m^2 weekly or 6 mg/m^2 daily/30 Gy in 10 F + 25 Gy in 10 F	CT30 + RT	NR	19
				CT6 + RT		26
				RT		13
Sause et al. (1995)	904	Sequential	Cis, vinblastine/60 Gy in 30 F	CT + RT	13.8	32
				RT	11.4	19
Jeremic et al. (1996)	131	Concurrent	Carbo + etoposide/69.6 Gy in 1.2 Gy F twice daily	CT + RT	22[a]	23[a]
				RT	14	9[b]
Cullen et al. (1999)	446	Sequential	MIC/>40 Gy in 15 F	CT + RT	11.7	20
				RT	9.7	16
Sause et al. (2000)	490	Sequential	Cisplatin + vinblastine/ 60 Gy in 30 F or 69.6 Gy in 1.2 F twice daily	CT + RT	13.2	32
				RT	11.4	21
				HFX RT	12.0	24

F, fractions; Cis, cisplatin; NR, not reported; CT, chemotherapy; RT, radiotherapy.
[a]$P < 0.05$; [b]4-year rather than 2-year survival.

Table 22.12 *Mean overall response rates using single agents in NSCLC*

Drug	Mean overall response (%)
Irinotecan	27
Ifosfamide	26
Paclitaxel	26
Docetaxel	26
Gemcitabine	21
Cisplatin	20
Mitomycin C	20
Vinorelbine	20
Vindesine	17
Doxorubicin	13
Topotecan	13
Etoposide	11
Methotrexate	10
Cyclophosphamide	8

In a randomized controlled trial of 161 patients aged over 70, an objective response rate of 19.7 per cent was seen and, more importantly, there was an improvement in quality of life, cancer-related symptoms and median survival in those patients receiving vinorelbine (Gridelli et al., 1999).

Gemcitabine is a pyrimidine antimetabolite, which has been shown to have impressive rates for response and symptom control. Up to 60 per cent of patients have reported symptomatic benefit, with low toxicity (Malayeri et al., 1997). Randomized studies have shown single-agent gemcitabine to be equivalent to cisplatin plus etoposide in terms of response rates and median survival, with a dramatic reduction in the number of patients developing neutropenia and nausea (Manegold et al., 1997; Perng et al., 1997).

The responses seen using single-agent therapy led to the investigation of combinations of these new agents with platinum agents. In general, these studies have shown that response rates and survival are increased, but at the cost of increased toxicity. Table 22.13 shows the results of some phase III studies investigating the addition of cisplatin.

In addition to those drugs shown, phase II data are available from trials investigating the addition of cisplatin to docetaxel and have shown increased response rates. Irinotecan is a topoisomerase I inhibitor and has also been shown to be effective in combination with cisplatin (Masuda et al., 1998). The results from phase III studies are awaited with interest. Tirapazamine has preferential activity towards hypoxic cells and acts in synergy with cisplatin. Phase II studies using a combination of cisplatin (80 mg/m^2) and tirapazamine (260–390 mg/m^2) have reported response rates of 21–30 per cent, higher than expected from single-agent cisplatin. In addition, toxicities were no greater than those seen with single-agent cisplatin, with fatigue and nausea predominating (Gatzemeier et al., 1998b; Treat et al., 1998).

These new agents appear to offer promise in improving survival in patients with advanced disease, and the low toxicity seen using single-agent therapy may allow older patients, or those with poor performance status, to be treated. In order to reduce the toxicity of cisplatin-containing combinations, phase II studies with its analogue carboplatin have been instigated and toxicity

Table 22.13 *Examples of phase III trials of new chemotherapy agents in the treatment of NSCLC*

New agent	Study	Chemotherapy regimens	Response rates (%)	Median survival	1-year survival (%)
Vinorelbine	Le Chevalier *et al.* (1994);	NVB	14	31 weeks	30
	n = 612	NVB + Cis	30[a]	40 weeks[a]	33[a]
		Vin + Cis	19	32 weeks	27
	Wozniak *et al.* (1998);	Cis (100)	12	6 months	20
	n = 432	NVB + Cis	26[a]	8 months[a]	36[a]
Gemcitabine	Crino *et al.* (1999);	Gem + Cis	38[a]	8.6 months	NR
	n = 307	MIC	28	9.6 months	
	Cardenal *et al.* (1999);	Gem + Cis	40.6[a]	8.7 months[a]	32[a]
	n = 135	Cis + Etop	21.9	7.2 months	26
Paclitaxel	Bonomi *et al.* (2000);	Tax (250/24) + Cis (75 + G)	27.7[a]	10 months	40.3
	n = 599	Tax (135/24) + Cis (75)	25.3[a]	9.5 months	37.4
	Giaccone *et al.* (1998);	Cis 75 + Etop	12.4	7.6 months	31.8
	n = 332	Tax (175/3) + Cis (80)	41[a]	9.7 months	48
		Cis + Tenip	28	9.9 months	41
	Gatzemeier *et al.* (1998a);	HD-Cis (100)	17	8.6 months	NR
	n = 414	Tax (175/3) + Cis 80	26[a]	8.1 months	
Tirapazamine	von Pawel *et al.* (2000);	Cis (75)	13.7	27.7 weeks	21
	n = 446	Cis (75) + Tir (390)	27.5[a]	34.6 weeks[a]	33[a]

NVB, vinorelbine; Cis, cisplatin; Vin, Vindesine; Gem, gemcitabine; MIC, Mitomycin C, ifosfamide, cisplatin; Etop, etoposide; Tax, paclitaxel; +G, +G-CSF; Tenip, teniposide; HD, high dose; Tir, tirapazamine; NR, not reported.
[a]$P < 0.05$.

Table 22.14 *The effect of combination chemotherapy compared to single-agent chemotherapy in the treatment of NSCLC on response rate, survival and toxicity, from a meta-analysis of 4642 patients (from Lillenbaum* et al., *1998)*

End-point	Relative risks of combination chemotherapy compared to single-agent therapy
Objective response rate	1.93 (95% CI = 1.54 − 2.42)
6-month survival	1.10 (95% CI = 1.02 − 1.19)
12-month survival	1.22 (95% CI = 1.03 − 1.45)
Toxic deaths	3.70 (95% CI = 2.2 − 6.4)

appears to be reduced. The National Institute of Clinical Excellence guidelines produced in 2001 state that of these new agents, gemcitabine, paclitaxel and vinorelbine should be considered as part of first-line therapy in patients with advanced NSCLC in combination with a platinum agent, while docetaxel should be considered for use as second-line therapy.

The efficacy of single-agent chemotherapy and combination chemotherapy has been compared in a number of randomized controlled studies, and meta-analyses of these studies have clearly shown that response rates increase with the use of combination therapy (Marino *et al.*, 1995; Lillenbaum *et al.*, 1998). Lillenbaum *et al.* (1998) demonstrated a twofold increase in response rates and increased 6- and 12-month survival in patients treated with combination chemotherapy (Table 22.14), although

this was associated with a higher incidence of toxicity and risk of treatment-related death.

Unfortunately, few studies have formally examined the effect of chemotherapy on quality of life (QL). In those that have, however, it is clear that the effect is beneficial (Cullen *et al.*, 1999) and is not limited to young, fit patients (Hickish *et al.*, 1998). In terms of specific symptom relief, Ellis *et al.* (1995) found that following a single cycle of Mitomycin C, vinblastine and cisplatin (MVP) chemotherapy 61 per cent of patients had a symptomatic response and that this increased to 96 per cent after two cycles. Symptoms that were best controlled included pain (60 per cent), cough (66 per cent), dyspnoea (59 per cent) and general malaise (53 per cent). Newer agents have also been shown to be beneficial, a randomized trial where QL was the primary end point demonstrated that gemcitabine plus BSC provided better symptom relief and quality of life with reduced need for palliative radiotherapy than BSC alone (Anderson *et al.*, 2000). In the light of these studies, both the American Society for Clinical Oncology (1998) and the Royal College of Radiologists (1999) have issued guidelines stating that chemotherapy should normally be discussed with patients with advanced NSCLC.

Cisplatin-containing regimens are currently the standard, with Mitomycin C, ifosfamide and cisplatin (MIC) or Mitomycin C, vinblastine and cisplatin (MVP) being the most widely used regimens in the UK. Both these regimens have objective response rates of approximately 50 per cent. In the other European Union countries gemcitabine/cisplatin and platinum/vinorelbine regimens are widely used. Carboplatin/paclitaxel has also been adopted widely in the USA following the Bonomi trial in 1996 (Bonomi *et al.*, 2000), although other studies have not shown significant benefit over standard treatments. In a randomized study, Schiller *et al.* (2002) demonstrated equivalence with respect to response rate and survival between the following regimens: cisplatin/paclitaxel, cisplatin/gemcitabine, cisplatin/docetaxel or carboplatin/paclitaxel. Further, direct comparisons are currently being tested in multicentre randomized trials. It remains unclear as to the best timing of chemotherapy in these patients. However, recent studies have shown that a good pretreatment performance status correlates with high response rates and less toxicity, therefore early treatment is likely to be more beneficial.

TREATMENT OF SMALL CELL LUNG CANCER

Chemotherapy

Without treatment the median survival from diagnosis of SCLC is 2 months and there have been no documented survivors at 2 years from diagnosis. Until the 1970s radiotherapy was the standard treatment for SCLC, but this had little effect on median survival (Table 22.15).

The introduction of chemotherapy has significantly improved survival and is now considered to be first-line therapy.

The beneficial effect of chemotherapy was first reported by Green *et al.* (1969), in patients with advanced SCLC. Those who received single-agent cyclophosphamide compared to an inert compound had significantly improved survival. Several active agents have been identified, including cyclophosphamide, ifosfamide, doxorubicin, epirubicin, vincristine, cisplatin, carboplatin, etoposide, topotecan, irinotecan and paclitaxel. Objective responses in the order of 15–45 per cent have been reported for single agents, but the impact on survival was minimal. This may reflect the inclusion of relapsed patients in phase II studies. These poor results led to the investigation of combination chemotherapy, which resulted in a dramatic improvement in median survival. As previously discussed (p. 486), the TNM classification is rarely used in SCLC, instead the use of prognostic indicators and extent of disease are used to determine prognosis and potential response to treatment.

It is clear that only patients with limited-stage disease and good performance status are likely to achieve long-term survival. Standard combination chemotherapy regimens result in response rates of 85–95 per cent in patients with limited-stage disease, with complete responses in about 50 per cent. The overall response rate in patients with extensive disease falls to 65–85 per cent, with complete responses in only 25 per cent. Few patients have disease progression on initial chemotherapy, so the vast majority achieve some symptomatic benefit. The use of prognostic factors allows prediction of patients who are likely to have a good outcome from treatment, and the choice of chemotherapy regimen can be selected to match potential gain and current performance status. The newer drug combinations, such as VICE and ICE (in which ifosfamide (I) is substituted for cyclophosphamide with vincristine, carboplatin and etoposide), have substantial response rates and, in some studies, a 5-year survival of 15–17 per cent, but are associated with greater toxicity. These combinations may be an appropriate choice for fit patients with limited or extensive disease and no other

Table 22.15 *Impact of treatment on survival in SCLC according to extent of disease (modified from Minna et al., 1989)*

Therapy	Median survival (months)		2-year survival (%)	
	LS	ES	LS	ES
Supportive care	3	1.5	–	–
Thoracic radiotherapy	3–9	–	2–7	–
Single-agent chemotherapy	6	4	–	–
Combination chemotherapy	10–14	7–11	5–15	1–3
Combination chemotherapy + thoracic radiotherapy	12–16	7–11	10–35	1–2

LS, limited stage; ES, extensive stage.

adverse prognostic features. In contrast, the aim of treatment in patients with poorer prognostic features is palliation to control the disease and improve symptoms with minimal chemotherapy.

Drugs are chosen for combination therapy because they are active as single agents, have different mechanisms of action and differing toxicities. Two important studies have compared single-agent with combination chemotherapy in patients of poor prognosis (Medical Research Council Lung Cancer Working Party 1996b; Souhami et al., 1997). Both studies compared oral etoposide (50 or 100 mg twice daily for 10 or 5 days, respectively) with intravenous chemotherapy (etoposide and vincristine (EV) or cyclophosphamide, doxorubicin and vincristine (CAV), or alternating cisplatin and etoposide (PE) and CAV, respectively). The response rates and 1-year survival were significantly better with intravenous combination chemotherapy (Table 22.16), whereas haematological toxicity and quality of life were worse with oral etoposide.

Combination chemotherapy is now generally accepted as being superior to single-agent treatment. There is little evidence to suggest that using more than three myelosuppressive drugs concurrently improves the overall outcome, as dosage is compromised by increasing myelosuppression with additional agents. The standard combination chemotherapy regimens, such as PE, CAV, and cyclophosphamide, doxorubicin and etoposide (ACE or CDE) all produce response rates of 85–95 per cent in patients with limited disease, with this being reduced to 65–85 per cent in extensive disease. Few direct comparisons between these combinations have been made. Studies comparing PE with CAV have shown that while overall response rates were higher in the PE arm, there was little effect on overall survival (Fukuoka et al., 1991; Roth et al., 1992). In the USA the PE regimen is favoured due to reduced toxicity, particularly when combined treatment with radiotherapy is given. The PE combination appears to be of benefit in patients who relapse after primary treatment with CAV, with response rates of 50 per cent, whereas second-line therapy with CAV has less benefit. In the UK, CAV is often preferred, as it is easier to administer in an outpatient setting and can be used in patients with cardiorespiratory and renal co-morbidity, for whom cisplatin would be problematic.

Although chemotherapy improves survival in patients with SCLC, the optimal duration has been unclear. Randomized studies have not shown an improved survival with prolonged treatment (Table 22.17). In a large Cancer Research Campaign (CRC) study (Spiro et al., 1989) 616 patients were randomized to receive either four or eight cycles of induction treatment with cyclophosphamide,

Table 22.16 *Outcome of the use of single-agent oral etoposide (E) compared to intravenous (IV) chemotherapy for poor-prognosis SCLC*

	Etoposide (E)	Intravenous (IV) chemotherapy	Overall response rate		1-year survival		Comments
			E	IV	E	IV	
MRC Lung Cancer Working Party (1996b); $n = 339$	50 mg twice daily for 10 days	EV or CAV	45%	51%	11%	13%; $P = 0.03$	Increased haematological toxicity in E arm
Souhami et al. (1997); $n = 155$	100 mg twice daily for 5 days	PE/CAV	32.9%	45.3%; $P < 0.01$	9.8%	19.3%; $P < 0.05$	Decreased QL in E arm

EV, etoposide/vincristine; CAV, cyclophosphamide/doxorubicin/vincristine; PE, cisplatin/etoposide; QL, quality of life.

Table 22.17 *The effect of extended courses of chemotherapy on survival in patients with SCLC*

Study	Chemotherapy	Median survival		2-year survival (%)	
		Long	Short	Long	Short
Bleehen et al. (1989); $n = 497$	EMCV 12 vs 6	35 weeks; NS	29 weeks	6	6
Spiro et al. (1989); $n = 616$	CVE 8 vs 4	39 weeks; $P = 0.007$	32 weeks	NR	NR
Bleehen et al. (1993); $n = 458$	EMCV 6 vs 3	8.6 months; NS	7.4 months	7	8

EMCV, etoposide/cyclophosphamide/methotrexate/vincristine; CVE, cyclophosphamide/vincristine/etoposide; NR, not reported; NS, not significant.

vincristine and etoposide (CVE). On progression, patients were randomized to receive either second-line chemotherapy or symptomatic treatment. The results showed that the response rate after four cycles was 61 per cent compared to 63 per cent after eight cycles. While patients who received only four cycles of induction chemotherapy and no second-line chemotherapy had the poorest survival, the length of induction therapy had no effect on survival in the patients who received further treatment on relapse. Two MRC studies, however, showed no survival advantage in patients who received extended courses of chemotherapy, indeed quality of life was worse in patients receiving 12 cycles of treatment (Bleehen et al., 1989).

The optimal timing of chemotherapy has also been investigated and it is now felt that it should be given as soon as possible after diagnosis. Two randomized studies have shown improvement in survival and quality of life if chemotherapy is given as soon as possible after diagnosis rather than being used to treat symptoms. The Medical Research Council Lung Cancer Working Party (1989) compared immediate treatment with six cycles of etoposide, cyclophosphamide, methotrexate and vincristine (ECMV) with the use of single-agent chemotherapy and radiotherapy for symptom control. The median survival was 32 weeks in patients receiving immediate therapy compared to only 16 weeks in those treated symptomatically. Earl et al. (1991) treated 300 patients either immediately with eight cycles of cyclophosphamide, etoposide and vincristine (CEV) or delayed treatment with the same regimen until onset of symptoms. While no difference in survival was shown, quality of life was higher in patients receiving immediate treatment.

NEW AGENTS

A number of new agents have been investigated in phase II studies in the treatment of relapsed or extensive SCLC (Table 22.18). Other agents, such as docetaxel and vinorelbine, have also been demonstrated to produce impressive response rates either as single agents or in combination with platinum agents. A phase III study comparing cisplatin and etoposide with cisplatin and irinotecan was closed early (154 patients) because interim analysis demonstrated significantly improved survival in the irinotecan and cisplatin arm (12.8 versus 9.4 months). Two-year survival was 19.5 per cent in the irinotecan arm compared to only 5.2 per cent in the control arm (Noda et al., 2002). These new agents may play an important role both in first-line therapy and also in the treatment of recurrent disease, which is resistant to standard agents.

CHEMOTHERAPY FOLLOWING RELAPSE

Despite dramatic responses to first-line therapy, the majority of SCLC patients will relapse with chemoresistant disease. A proportion of patients will benefit from second-line chemotherapy on relapse. The use of drugs that have not previously been used results in improved responses. The use of the PE regimen following CAV has been shown to produce response rates of 50 per cent. The response rates seen using other regimens have not been so impressive, Spiro et al. (1989) demonstrated rates of 18–25 per cent using methotrexate and doxorubicin after first-line treatment with CVE. Topotecan has been shown to produce response rates of 24 per cent and to be

Table 22.18 *Phase II trials of a number of new agents in the treatment of SCLC*

Study	Drug (dose mg/m^2)	Patient group	ORR	Median survival
Smit et al. (1998); n = 24	Paclitaxel 175	Resistant	29%	100 days
Groen et al. (1999); n = 35	Paclitaxel 175; carboplatin AUC7	Resistant	73.5 %	31 weeks
Deppermann et al. (1999); n = 75	Paclitaxel 200; carboplatin AUC 6	Chemonaïve extensive disease	61%	359 days
Lyss et al. (1999); n = 34	Paclitaxel 230; Cisplatin 75; G-CSF	Chemonaïve extensive disease	71%	7.6 months
Ardizzoni et al. (1997); n = 101	Topotecan	Resistant Sensitive	6.4% 37.8%	4.7 months 6.9 months
Kudoh et al. (1998); n = 75	Irinotecan + cisplatin	Chemonaïve Limited Extensive	Overall = 84%	14.3 months 13 months
Nakamura et al. (1999); n = 51	Irinotecan + etoposide	Chemonaïve extensive disease	66%	12 months
De Vore et al. (1998); n = 44	Irinotecan	Sensitive Resistant	35.3% 3.7%	5.9 months 2.8 months

ORR, overall response rate. Sensitive disease = relapse >3 months following first-line chemotherapy; resistant disease = progression within 3 months of first-line chemotherapy.

superior to CAV in terms of symptom control when used as second-line therapy (von Pawel *et al.*, 1999).

ATTEMPTS AT IMPROVING RESPONSE RATES AND SURVIVAL

Maintenance chemotherapy

As discussed above, there appears to be little benefit in increasing the number of cycles of chemotherapy given, indeed prolonged treatment has been shown to impair quality of life. Maintenance therapy with recombinant interferon following response to induction chemotherapy has been investigated by several groups, without clear evidence of benefit (Table 22.19). In some of these studies, the compliance with interferon treatment was limited by toxicity (Jett *et al.*, 1994). The use of low-dose interferon-α has been compared to maintenance chemotherapy and observation only (Mattson *et al.*, 1997). While no difference in median survival was seen between the groups, patients with limited disease who received interferon had a significant improvement in 5-year survival compared to the other two arms (10 per cent versus 2 per cent versus 2 per cent).

Alternating regimens

The rationale for the use of alternating regimens is to reduce the development of resistant clones within the tumour. There does appear to be at least some lack of cross-resistance between platinum/etoposide (PE) and

CAV, with an objective response rate of about 50 per cent compared with only 10 per cent for CAV following failure with PE. Benefit in survival has been reported using this regimen, particularly in patients with limited-stage disease (Fukuoka *et al.*, 1991), but these findings were not confirmed in a later study in patients with extensive disease (Roth *et al.*, 1992) (Table 22.20).

Dose intensification

Dose escalation can overcome cytotoxic drug resistance and increase cures in preclinical cancer models. A variety of methods have been used to increase cytotoxic dose intensity, including the use of increased doses, shorter treatment intervals, haemopoietic growth factor support and high-dose therapy with haemopoietic progenitor cell transplantation.

Suboptimal chemotherapy doses result in inferior survival, but it is uncertain how much survival in SCLC can be improved by increasing cytotoxic dose intensity. An early study in SCLC (Cohen *et al.*, 1977) showed significantly higher response rates, median survival and long-term survival when the cyclophosphamide dose was increased from 0.5 to $1 \, g/m^2$, lomustine from 50 to $100 \, mg/m^2$ and methotrexate increased from 10 to $15 \, mg/m^2$. Many would now consider the standard arm of this study to have been under-dosed. Five other studies have been reported testing increased dosage of drugs used in the same combination, including one study of standard-dose CAV, which was compared to high-dose

Table 22.19 *Results of maintenance therapy using recombinant interferon (IFN) compared to observation only following response to induction chemotherapy for SCLC*

Study	Number of patients	Interferon dose	Median survival
Mattson *et al.* (1992)	237 with OR	IFN-2α 3×10^6 units	IFN: 11 months Obs: 10 months
Jett *et al.* (1994)	100 with CR	IFN-γ 4×10^6 units per day for 6 months	IFN: 13.3 months Obs: 18.8 months
Kelly *et al.* (1995)	171 with OR	IFN-2α 3×10^6 units $3 \times$ week for 2 years	IFN: 13 months Obs: 16 months
van Zandwijk *et al.* (1997)	117 in CR or good PR	IFN-γ 4×10^6 units alternate days for 4 months or observation	IFN: 8.9 months Obs: 9.9 months

There was no significant difference between the IFN and observation arms in any of the above studies.
Obs, observation; CR, complete response; OR, objective response; PR, partial response.

Table 22.20 *Examples of the effect of alternating chemotherapy regimens on response rate and survival in SCLC*

	Overall response rate (%)			Median survival (months)			Number of patients	Extent of disease
	CAV	PE	CAV/PE	CAV	PE	CAV/PE		
Fukuoka *et al.* (1991)	55	78	76	9.9	9.9	11.8	300	LS + ES
Roth *et al.* (1992)	51	61	59	8.3	8.6	8.1	437	ES

LS, limited stage; ES, extensive stage.

CAV in extensive-stage patients and another comparing standard-dose etoposide and cisplatin versus higher doses of these agents. In none of these studies was survival significantly improved (Klastersky and Sculier, 1989; Johnson, 1993; Ihde et al., 1994). However, a French study of 105 SCLC patients with limited-stage disease, reported a significant survival benefit (2-year survival 43 per cent versus 26 per cent, $P = 0.02$) for those randomized to receive higher doses of cisplatin and cyclophosphamide for the first dose only (Arriagada et al., 1993).

Accelerated chemotherapy

Shortening the interval between cycles of chemotherapy might reduce the opportunity for tumour cells to regrow and mutate to drug-resistant clones. Typically, myelosuppressive drugs are alternated weekly with non-myelosuppressive agents. A summary of seven phase II studies, incorporating 285 patients, reported 40 per cent complete and 85 per cent overall responses with median survivals of 12 months or more. Furthermore, these intensive weekly regimens were generally well tolerated (Klastersky and Sculier, 1989).

Randomized trials using weekly cisplatin and dose reduction if there was toxicity have shown no advantage over standard treatment at 3-week intervals. A randomized trial alternated cisplatin and etoposide with ifosfamide and doxorubicin for 12 consecutive weeks, and compared this to the standard 3-weekly regimen of alternating CAV/PE in good performance status, limited- and extensive-stage patients. Response rates and median and 2-year survivals were not significantly different (Souhami et al., 1994). A similar study conducted by the European Lung Cancer Working Party has shown no survival advantage in

patients treated with weekly multiple-drug chemotherapy as against standard combination treatment with cyclophosphamide, doxorubicin and etoposide (ACE) (Sculier et al., 1993). The Canadian weekly regimen, CODE (cisplatin, vincristine, doxorubicin and etoposide) was compared with CAV/PE in a randomized study in 220 patients with extensive-stage SCLC (Murray et al., 1999). CODE increased twofold the dose intensity of the same drugs in the CAV/PE regimen and led to higher response rates (87 per cent versus 70 per cent) but was associated with more toxic deaths. There was no significant difference in progression-free or overall survival. Weekly chemotherapy is therefore not recommended for SCLC.

Haemopoietic growth factors

Granulocyte colony-stimulating factor (G-CSF, filgrastim, lenograstim) has been shown to reduce the depth and duration of neutropenia during standard chemotherapy for SCLC, leading to fewer infections and a higher proportion of patients receiving the planned dose on time (Crawford et al., 1991; Trillet-Lenoir et al., 1993). In contrast, granulocyte/macrophage colony stimulating factor (GM-CSF) was associated with more thrombocytopenia, toxic deaths, days in hospital and use of blood products and intravenous antibiotics in a South West Oncology Group (SWOG) study of concurrent chemotherapy and radiotherapy (Bunn et al., 1995). Several groups have tested the use of haemopoietic growth factors to increase cytotoxic dose intensity in SCLC. Modest increases have been achieved, and two recent studies have reported significantly improved survival in the dose-intensified arm and a policy of dose delay rather than dose reduction to allow recovery (Table 22.21).

Table 22.21 *Effect of dose intensification with or without haemopoietic growth factors in the treatment of SCLC*

Study	Regimen	RDI	Response rate (%)	Median survival	2-year survival (%)
Arriagada et al. (1993)	PCAE; n = 105	P = 100 vs 80 mg/m^2; C = 300 vs 225 mg/m^2	87 vs 70	–	43 vs 26
Woll et al. (1995)	VICE; n = 65	1.34 vs 1.17	93.5 vs 94.1	69 vs 65 weeks	32 vs 15
Trillet-Lenoir et al. (1996)	AVI; n = 54	1.76 × higher than 3 weekly	77	8 months	22
Wolf et al. (1996)	AIO/PE; n = 330	–	–	17.1 vs 15.1 months	34 both groups
Woll et al. (2001)	ICE 2 vs 4 weeks; n = 50	1.8 vs 0.99	80 vs 76	–	–
Steward et al. (1998)	VICE 3 vs 4 weeks; n = 301	26% higher	83 vs 84	443 vs 351 days	33 vs 18[a]
Thatcher et al. (2000)	ACE 2 vs 4 weeks; n = 403	–	89 vs 86	350 vs 330 days	25 vs 18[a]

RDI, relative dose intensity; P, cisplatin; C, cyclophosphamide; ACE, cyclophosphamide/doxorubicin/etoposide; AIO, doxorubicin/ifosfamide/vincristine; AVI, doxorubicin/etoposide/ifosfamide; ICE, ifosfamide/carboplatin/etoposide; PCAE, cisplatin/cyclophosphamide/doxorubicin/etoposide; PE, cisplatin/etoposide; VICE, vincristine/ifosfamide/carboplatin/etoposide.
[a]$P < 0.05$.

New approaches to dose intensification

The success of high-dose therapy with haemopoietic progenitor cell support in leukaemia and lymphoma gave impetus to using a similar approach in chemoresponsive solid tumours such as SCLC. High-dose chemotherapy has been administered as primary treatment or following tumour remission with conventional induction treatment. This requires hospitalization and reinfusion of previously stored autologous bone marrow or peripheral blood progenitor cells to abrogate the severe and potentially lethal bone marrow suppression. The most popular agents for late intensification have been cyclophosphamide and etoposide because myelosuppression is their dose-limiting toxicity. Most studies have been of very small patient numbers. Although the complete response rates have been high, in general no survival improvement has been noted. In 178 patients from seven studies, 37 per cent had a complete response after the procedure but only 9.5 per cent were alive 1 year after therapy and 7.8 per cent died during treatment (Klastersky and Sculier, 1989). In only one study did high-dose treatment result in better relapse-free survival (but not overall survival) (Humblet et al., 1987). The use of chemoradiotherapy and the introduction of peripheral blood progenitor cells led to renewed interest in high-dose therapy for SCLC during the 1990s. In selected patients of favourable prognosis, high response rates and encouraging survival rates were obtained (Humblet et al., 1996; Fetscher et al., 1997; Elias et al., 1999). Demonstrating the benefits of late intensification in a randomized study would be very difficult given the large numbers of patients required. Only about 30 per cent of patients in late intensification programmes are actually suitable for the procedure because of toxicity from the induction regimen, lack of initial response or inability to withstand the late intensification chemotherapy with its severe toxicity. An alternative approach is to use haemopoietic progenitor cells and G-CSF to support accelerated multicyclic chemotherapy (Pettengell et al., 1995).

Combined modality treatment for small cell lung cancer

THORACIC RADIOTHERAPY AND CHEMOTHERAPY

Despite the improvement in survival with the widespread use of chemotherapy for SCLC, 30–80 per cent of patients will develop local recurrence of their disease. The use of radiotherapy in addition to chemotherapy has therefore been investigated. A meta-analysis of 13 randomized trials comparing chemotherapy with chemotherapy plus radiotherapy, including 2103 patients with limited disease (Pignon et al., 1992), clearly demonstrated a significant survival advantage. Patients receiving combined modality therapy had a 14 per cent reduction in risk of death, with overall survival at 3 years being 14.3 per cent for combined

Table 22.22 *Three-year survival figures following single- or combined-modality treatment for SCLC (from Pignon et al., 1992)*

	3-year survival (%)	
	CT	**CT + thoracic RT**
<55 years	9.2	17.4
>70 years	10.2	8.7

CT, chemotherapy; RT, radiotherapy.

modality versus 8.9 per cent with chemotherapy alone. The greatest benefits were seen in patients under the age of 55 (Table 22.22).

Combined modality treatment improves local control of SCLC tumours by 10–50 per cent, but the optimal timing for the radiotherapy remains unclear. The meta-analysis and a number of other randomized trials have failed to show a consistent effect of the timing of radiotherapy on survival. However, two randomized studies (Murray et al., 1993; Takada et al., 1996) have shown a survival benefit with early radiotherapy, and this is now being tested in large multicentre trials. In the Canadian study, patients who received radiotherapy with the second cycle of platinum-based chemotherapy had a median survival of 21.2 months, compared to 16 months in those who received radiotherapy with cycle 6. Five-year survival was also significantly enhanced, being 21.5 per cent compared with 11 per cent (Murray et al., 1993). However, haematological, oesophageal and pulmonary toxicity is greater when radiotherapy is given concurrently (Takada et al., 1996). This risk of toxicity is increased with the use of doxorubicin. It is currently recommended in the UK that patients with limited disease and good performance status, who have achieved a good response to induction chemotherapy, should be offered consolidation thoracic radiotherapy.

The optimal dose of radiotherapy is also uncertain. A single randomized study has shown that higher doses (37.5 Gy versus 25 Gy) resulted in better control (Coy et al., 1988), and the majority of recent studies have used 45–50 Gy in 2 Gy fractions. The use of hyperfractionated radiotherapy given concurrently with cisplatin and etoposide has also been investigated (Turrisi et al., 1999). Patients were randomized to receive 45 Gy given twice daily over 3 weeks, or daily over 5 weeks, with chemotherapy. Twice-daily radiotherapy significantly improved survival. The median survival was 23 and 19 months, respectively, and 5-year survival 26 per cent and 16 per cent, respectively. Severe oesophagitis was more common in patients receiving the hyperfractionated radiotherapy.

PROPHYLACTIC CRANIAL IRRADIATION

Up to 50 per cent of SCLC patients achieving remission will develop brain metastases within 2 years. While palliative

Table 22.23 *Three-year survival and incidence of brain metastases in SCLC patients in complete remission treated with or without prophylactic cranial irradiation (PCI) (adapted from Auperin* et al., *1999)*

	PCI	No PCI	Significance
Overall 3-year survival (%)	20.7	15.3	$P = 0.01$
Incidence of brain metastases at 3 years (%)	33.3	58.6	$P < 0.001$

radiotherapy may improve symptoms in a proportion of patients, the effect of metastases can be devastating for both the patient and their carers. A number of early clinical trials investigating the effect of prophylactic cranial irradiation (PCI) demonstrated reduction in the incidence of metastases but no benefit in survival. A meta-analysis of 987 patients in seven randomized controlled trials comparing PCI with no PCI in patients with complete response following induction chemotherapy has recently been published (Auperin *et al.*, 1999). Overall survival was significantly increased in the patients receiving PCI, with a 16 per cent reduction in risk of death and a 5.4 per cent increase in survival at 3 years (Table 22.23). The risk of brain metastases was reduced by 54 per cent. There was no significant difference between doses of radiation received, although there was a trend towards better survival in patients receiving higher radiation doses.

One of the major concerns about the use of PCI is the possibility of long-term neurotoxicity. This includes memory loss, tremors, somnolence, ataxia and cortical atrophy. Evaluation of the impact of therapy on 64 patients who were in remission for at least 2 years showed that the majority of patients had a significant degree of cognitive dysfunction, demonstrated by neuropsychometric testing, although no pre-treatment assessment was available for comparison (Cull *et al.*, 1994). A randomized controlled study run by the European Organization for Research and Treatment of Cancer (EORTC) and the United Kingdom Co-ordinating Committee for Cancer Research (UKCCCR) (Gregor *et al.*, 1997), included cognitive function and quality of life as end points. This study showed that there was cognitive impairment even before treatment and increased impairment at both 6 and 12 months after treatment, although there was no consistent difference between those who received PCI and those who did not.

SURGICAL ADJUVANT THERAPY

Surgical resection is generally contraindicated in SCLC as most patients have bulky central and metastatic disease, either evident or occult at the time of presentation. Early studies comparing surgery and radiotherapy showed no survival advantage in patients undergoing surgical resection. However, the value of surgery in SCLC has recently been re-evaluated. In one of the largest reviews

(from the University of Toronto Lung Oncology Group), 79 SCLC patients underwent surgery as their first treatment, most then received CAV-based postoperative chemotherapy. Overall, the median survival for the entire group was 26 months, with a 5-year survival of 39 per cent. Five-year survival in a small group of these patients with stage I and II disease was 51 per cent (Shepherd *et al.*, 1991). The investigators still felt that surgery should not be employed initially other than in the rare situation of a small, peripherally located pulmonary lesion, or in patients in whom SCLC was found unexpectedly at thoracotomy and a complete excision was possible. In a recent prospective randomized phase III study, in which patients who achieved an objective response following induction chemotherapy with CAV were randomized to undergo surgical resection or observation only (Lad *et al.*, 1994), similar survival rates were demonstrated in both arms. All patients had received thoracic and cranial radiotherapy.

Salvage surgery may rarely be beneficial to patients with mixed SCLC and NSCLC histology who relapse within the chest, or in patients who at relapse are found to have purely NSCLC histology following chemotherapy for SCLC.

SIGNIFICANT POINTS

- Lung cancer accounts for 28 per cent of male and 17 per cent of female deaths in the UK.
- Cigarette smoking accounts for 94 per cent of male and 83 per cent of female lung cancer deaths.
- The major pathological types in the UK are squamous cell carcinoma (40 per cent), adenocarcinoma (20 per cent) and small cell lung cancer (20 per cent).
- The most common presenting symptoms are cough, weight loss, chest pain, dyspnoea and haemoptysis.
- Surgery is the treatment of choice for stages I and II NSCLC.
- Only 35 per cent of NSCLC are operable and only 20 per cent are resectable. Among these, the 5-year survival rate is 30–40 per cent.
- Curative radiotherapy is possible in less than 5 per cent of patients with NSCLC, but palliative radiotherapy is frequently beneficial.
- Chemotherapy in stage IIIB and IV NSCLC, using platinum agents, has been shown to increase 1-year survival by 10 per cent and can improve quality of life.

- Chemotherapy is the treatment of choice for SCLC. There is a high response rate and chemotherapy extends the median survival from 2 to 18 months.
- In limited-stage SCLC the use of consolidation thoracic radiotherapy and prophylactic cranial irradiation following a response to chemotherapy is beneficial.

KEY REFERENCES

Auperin, A., Arrigada, R., Pignon, J.P. *et al.* (1999) Prophylactic cranial irradiation for patients with small cell lung cancer in complete remission. *N. Engl. J. Med.* **341**, 476–84.

Mountain, C.F. (1997) Revisions in the International system for staging lung cancer. *Chest* **111**, 1710–17.

Non-small cell lung cancer collaborative group (1995) Chemotherapy in non-small cell lung cancer: a meta-analysis using updated data on individual patients from 52 randomised trials. *BMJ* **311**, 899–909.

Royal College of Radiologists (1999) Guidelines for the non-surgical management of lung cancer. *Clin. Oncol.* **11**, S14–S49.

Saunders, M., Dische, S., Barrett, A. *et al.* (1997) Continuous hyperfractionated accelerated radiotherapy (CHART) versus conventional radiotherapy in non-small cell lung cancer: a randomised multicentre trial. *Lancet* **350**, 161–5.

REFERENCES

Abeloff, M.B., Eggleston, J.C., Mendelsohn, G. *et al.* (1979) Changes in morphological and biochemical characteristics of SCLC: a clinicopathological study. *Am. J. Med.* **66**, 757–64.

Albain, K.S., Crowley, J.J., LeBlanc, M. and Livingston, R.B. (1991) Survival determinants in extensive-stage non-small cell lung cancer: the Southwest Oncology Group Experience. *J. Clin. Oncol.* **9**, 1618–26.

Albanes, D. (1999) Beta-carotene and lung cancer: a case study. *Am. J. Clin. Nutr.* **69**(suppl.), S1345–S1350.

Alpha-Tocopherol, Beta Carotene Cancer Prevention Study Group (1994) The effect of vitamin E and beta carotene on the incidence of lung cancer and other cancers in male smokers. *N. Engl. J. Med.* **330**, 1029–35.

American Society for Clinical Oncology (1998) Clinical practice guidelines for the treatment of unresectable non-small cell lung cancer. *J. Clin. Oncol.* **15**, 2996–3018.

Anderson, H., Hopwood, P., Stephens, R.J. *et al.* (2000) Gemcitabine plus best supportive care (BSC) versus BSC in inoperable non-small cell lung cancer – a randomized trial with quality of life as the primary outcome. *Br. J. Cancer* **83**, 447–53.

Ardizzoni, A., Hansen, H., Dombernowsky, P. *et al.* (1997) Topetecan, a new active drug in the second line treatment of small cell lung cancer: a phase II study in patients with refractory and sensitive disease. *J. Clin. Oncol.* **15**, 2090–6.

Arriagada, R., Le Chevalier, Y., Pignon, J.P. *et al.* (1993) Initial chemotherapeutic doses and survival in patients with limited small cell lung cancer. *N. Engl. J. Med.* **329**, 1848–52.

Auperin, A., Arriagada, R., Pignon, J.P. *et al.* (1999) Prophylactic cranial irradiation for patients with small cell lung cancer in complete remission. *N. Engl. J. Med.* **341**, 476–84.

Bleehen, N.M., Fayers, P.M., Girling, D.J. and Stephens, R.J. (1989) Controlled trial of twelve versus six courses of chemotherapy in the treatment of SCLC. *Br. J. Cancer* **59**, 584–90.

Bleehen, N.M., Girling, D.J., Machin, D. and Stephens, R.J. (1993) A randomised trial of three or six courses of etoposide, cyclophosphamide, methotrexate and vincristine or six courses of etoposide and ifosfamide in small cell lung cancer. I: survival and prognostic factors. Medical Research Council Lung Cancer Working Party. *Br. J. Cancer* **68**, 1150–6.

Bonomi, P., Kim, K., Fairclough, D. *et al.* (2000) Comparison of survival and quality of life in advanced non-small cell lung cancer patients treated with two dose levels of paclitaxel combined with cisplatin versus etoposide with cisplatin: results of an Eastern Co-operative Oncology Group trial. *J. Clin. Oncol.* **18**, 623–31.

Bunn, P.A., Crowley, J., Kelly, K. *et al.* (1995) Chemoradiotherapy with or without GM-CSF in the treatment of limited stage small cell lung cancer. *J. Clin. Oncol.* **13**, 1632–41.

Cancer Research Campaign (1996) *Lung cancer and smoking.* Factsheet 11.1–11.7.

Cardenal, F., Lopez-Cabrerizo, M., Anton, A. *et al.* (1999) Randomised phase III study of gemcitabine–cisplatin versus etoposide–cisplatin in the treatment of locally advanced or metastatic non-small cell lung cancer. *J. Clin. Oncol.* **17**, 12–18.

Cohen, M.H., Creavan, P.J., Fossieck, B.E. *et al.* (1977) Intensive treatment of small cell bronchogenic cancer. *Cancer Treat. Rep.* **61**, 349–354.

Coy, P., Hodson, I. and Payne, D.G. (1988) The effects of dose of thoracic irradiation on recurrence in patients with limited stage small cell lung cancer: initial results of a Canadian multicenter randomised trial. *Int. J. Radiat. Oncol. Biol. Phys.* **14**, 219–26.

Crawford, J., Ozer, H., Stoller, R. *et al.* (1991) Reduction by granulocyte colony-stimulating factor of fever and neutropenia induced by chemotherapy in patients with small cell lung cancer. *N. Engl. J. Med.* **325**, 164–70.

Crino, L., Scagliotti, G.V., Ricci, S. *et al.* (1999) Gemcitabine and cisplatin versus mitomycin, ifosfamide and cisplatin in advanced non-small cell lung cancer: a randomized phase III study of the Italian lung cancer project. *J. Clin. Oncol.* **17**, 3522–30.

Cull, A., Gregor, A., Hopwood, P. *et al.* (1994) Neurological and cognitive impairment in long-term survivors of small cell lung cancer. *Eur. J. Cancer* **30A**, 1067–74.

Cullen, M.H., Billingham, L.J., Woodroffe, C.M. *et al.* (1999) Mitomycin, ifosfamide and cisplatin in unresectable non-small cell lung cancer: effects on survival and quality of life. *J. Clin. Oncol.* **17**, 3188–94.

Dales, R.E., Belanger, R., Shamji, F.M. *et al.* (1994) Quality of life following thoractomy for lung cancer. *J. Clin. Epidemiol.* **47**, 1443–9.

Denoix, P.F. (1944) *Bull. Inst. Nat. Hyg. (Paris)* **1**, 1–69.

Depierre, A., Milleron, B., Moro-Sibilot, D. *et al.* (2002) Preoperative chemotherapy followed by surgery compared with primary surgery in resectable stage I (except T1N0), II, and IIIa non-small-cell lung cancer. *J. Clin. Oncol.* **20**, 247–53.

Deppermann, K.M., Serke, M., Oehm, C. *et al.* (1999) Paclitaxel and carboplatin in advanced SCLC: a phase II study. *Proc. Am. Soc. Clin. Oncol.* **18**, 482a.

De Vore, R.F., Blanke, C.D. and Denham, C.A. (1998) Phase II study of irinotecan in patients with previously treated small cell lung cancer. *Proc. Am. Soc. Clin. Oncol.* **17**, 451a.

Dillman, R.O., Seagren, S.L., Propert, K.L. *et al.* (1990) A randomised trial of induction chemotherapy plus high-dose radiation versus radiation alone in stage III non-small cell lung cancer. *N. Engl. J. Med.* **323**, 940–5.

Dillman, R.O., Herndon, J., Seagren, S.L. *et al.* (1996) Improved survival in stage III NSCLC: seven year follow-up of cancer and leukaemia group B (CALGB) 8433 trial. *J. Natl Cancer Inst.* **88**, 1210–15.

Doll, R. and Hill, A.B. (1964) Mortality in relation to smoking: ten years' observations of British doctors. *BMJ* **1**, 1399–450.

Dosoretz, D.E., Katin, M.J. and Blitzer, P.H. (1992) Radiation therapy in the management of medically inoperable carcinoma of the lung: results and implications for future treatment strategies. *Int. J. Radiat. Oncol. Biol. Phys.* **24**, 3–9.

Earl, H.M., Rudd, R.M., Spiro, S.G. *et al.* (1991) A randomised trial of planned versus as required chemotherapy in small cell lung cancer: a Cancer Research Campaign trial. *Br. J. Cancer* **64**, 566–72.

Elias, A., Ibrahim, J., Skarin, A.T. *et al.* (1999) Dose-intense therapy for limited-stage small cell lung cancer: long term outcome. *J. Clin. Oncol.* **17**, 1175–84.

Ellis, P.A., Smith, I.E., Hardy, J.R. *et al.* (1995) Symptom relief with MVP (mitomycin C, vinblastine and cisplatin) chemotherapy in advanced NSCLC. *Br. J. Cancer* **71**, 366–70.

Fetscher, S., Brugger, W., Engelhardt, R. *et al.* (1997) Dose-intense therapy with etoposide, ifosfamide, cisplatin and epirubicin (VIP-E) in 100 consecutive patients with limited and extensive disease small cell lung cancer. *Ann. Oncol.* **8**, 49–56.

Fukuoka, M., Furose, K., Saijo, N. *et al.* (1991) Randomized trial of cyclophosphamide, doxorubicin and vincristine versus cisplatin and etoposide versus alternation of these regimens in small cell lung cancer. *J. Natl Cancer Inst.* **83**, 855–61.

Furuse, K., Fukuoka, M., Kawahara, M. *et al.* (1999) Phase III study of concurrent versus sequential thoracic radiotherapy in combination with mitomycin, vindesine and cisplatin in unresectable stage III non-small cell lung cancer. *J. Clin. Oncol.* **17**, 2692–9.

Gatzemeier, U., von Pawel, J., Gottfried, M. *et al.* (1998a) Phase III comparative study of high dose cisplatin versus a combination of paclitaxel and cisplatin in patients with advanced non-small cell lung cancer. *Proc. Am. Soc. Clin. Oncol.* **17**, 454a.

Gatzemeier, U., Rodriguez, G., Treat, J. *et al.* (1998b) Tirapazamine–cisplatin: the synergy. *Br. J. Cancer* **77**, 15–17.

Giaccone, G., Splinter, T.A., Debruyne, C. *et al.* (1998) Randomized study of paclitaxel-cisplatin versus cisplatin-teniposide in patients with advanced non-small cell lung cancer – the European Organisation for Research and Treatment of Cancer Lung Cancer Cooperative Group. *J. Clin. Oncol.* **16**, 2133–41.

Ginsberg, R.J. and Rubenstein, L.V. (1995) Randomised trial of lobectomy versus limited resection for T1 N0 NSCLC. *Ann. Thorac. Surg.* **60**, 615–23.

Girling, D.J., Falk, S., White, R. *et al.* (2000) Immediate versus delayed thoracic radiotherapy (TRT) in patients with unresectable, locally advanced non-small cell lung cancer (NSCLC) and minimal symptoms: results of an MRC/BTS randomised trial. *Lung Cancer* **29**(suppl. 1), 164.

Graham, P.H., Gebski, V.J. and Langlands, A.O. (1995) Radical radiotherapy for early non-small cell lung cancer. *Int. J. Radiat. Oncol. Biol. Phys.* **31**, 261–6.

Green, R.A., Humphrey, E., Close, H. and Patino, M.E. (1969) Alkylating agents in bronchogenic carcinoma. *Am. J. Med.* **46**, 516–25.

Gregor, A., Cull, A., Stephens, R.J. *et al.* (1997) Prophylactic cranial irradiation is indicated following complete response to induction therapy in small cell lung cancer: results of a multicentre randomised trial. *Eur. J. Cancer* **33**, 1752–8.

Gridelli, C., Perrone, F. and Gallo, C. (1999) Effects of vinorelbine on quality of life and survival of elderly patients with advanced non-small cell lung cancer. *J. Natl Cancer Inst.* **91**, 66–72.

Groen, H.J.M., Fokkema, E., Biesma, B. *et al.* (1999) Paclitaxel and carboplatin in the treatment of small cell lung cancer patients resistant to cyclophosphamide, doxorubicin and etoposide: a non-cross resistant schedule. *J. Clin. Oncol.* **17**, 927–32.

Hackshaw, A.K. (1998) Lung cancer and passive smoking. *Stat. Methods Med. Res.* **7**, 119–36.

Henschke, C.I., McCauley, D.I., Yankelevitz, D.F. *et al.* (1999) Early Lung Cancer Project: overall design and findings from baseline screening. *Lancet* **354**, 99–105.

Hickish, T., Smith, I., O'Brien, M. *et al.* (1998) Clinical benefit from palliative chemotherapy in non-small cell lung cancer extends to the elderly and those with poor prognostic factors. *Br. J. Cancer* **78**, 28–33.

Humblet, Y., Symann, M., Bosly, A. *et al.* (1987) Late intensification chemotherapy with autologous bone-marrow transplantation in selected small cell carcinoma of the lung: a randomised study. *J. Clin. Oncol.* **5**, 1864–73.

Humblet, Y., Bosquee, L., Weynants, P. *et al.* (1996) High dose chemo-radiotherapy cycles for limited stage small cell lung cancer patients using G-CSF and blood stem cells. *Bone Marrow Transplant.* **18** (S1), S36–S39.

Hyde, L. and Hyde, C.I. (1974) Clinical manifestations of lung cancer. *Chest* **65**, 299–306.

Ihde, D.C., Mulshine, J.L., Kramer, B.S. *et al.* (1994) Prospective randomized comparison of high-dose and standard dose etoposide and cisplatin chemotherapy in patients with extensive-stage small-cell lung cancer. *J. Clin. Oncol.* **12**, 2022–34.

Jeremic, B., Shibamoto, Y., Acimovic, L. and Djuric, L. (1995) Randomised trial of hyperfractionated radiation therapy with or without concurrent chemotherapy for stage III non-small cell lung cancer. *J. Clin. Oncol.* **13**, 452–8.

Jeremic, B., Shibamoto, Y., Acimovic, L. and Milisavljevic, S. (1996) Hyperfractionated radiation therapy with or without concurrent low dose daily carboplatin/etoposide for stage III non-small cell lung cancer: a randomized study. *J. Clin. Oncol.* **14**, 1065–70.

Jett, J.R., Maksymiuk, A.W., Su, J.Q. *et al.* (1994) Phase III trial of recombinant interferon gamma in complete responders with small cell lung cancer. *J. Clin. Oncol.* **12**, 2321–6.

Johnson, D.H. (1993) Recent developments in chemotherapy treatment of small cell lung cancer. *Semin. Oncol.* **20**, 315–25.

Kelly, K., Crowley, J.J., Bunn, P.A. *et al.* (1995) Role of recombinant interferon alfa-2a maintenance in patients with limited stage small cell lung cancer responding to concurrent chemoradiation – A Southwest Oncology Group Study. *J. Clin. Oncol.* **13**, 2924–30.

Klastersky, J.A. and Sculier, J.P. (1989) Intensive chemotherapy of small cell lung cancer. *Lung Cancer* **5**, 196–206.

Kudoh, S., Fujiwara, Y., Takada, Y. *et al.* (1998) Phase II study of irinotecan combined with cisplatin in patients

with previously untreated SCLC. *J. Clin. Oncol.* **16**, 1068–74.

Lad, T., Piantadosi, S., Thomas, P. *et al.* (1994) A prospective randomized trial to determine the benefit of surgical resection of residual disease following response of small cell lung cancer to combination chemotherapy. *Chest* **106**, S320–S323.

Le Chevalier, T., Brisgand, D. and Douillard, J.Y. (1994) Randomised study of vinorelbine and cisplatin versus vindesine and cisplatin versus vinorelbine alone in advanced non-small cell lung cancer: results of a European multicentre trial including 612 patients. *J. Clin. Oncol.* **12**, 360–7.

Lillenbaum, R.C., Langenberg, P. and Dickersin, K. (1998) Single agent versus combination chemotherapy in patients with advanced non-small cell lung cancer. *Cancer* **82**, 116–26.

Lyss, A.P., Herndon, J.E., Lynch, T.C. *et al.* (1999) Paclitaxel cisplatin + G-CSF in patients with previously untreated extensive stage small cell lung cancer: preliminary analysis of Cancer and Leukemia Group B (CALGB) 9430. *Proc. Am. Soc. Clin. Oncol.* **18**, 468a.

Malayeri, R., Ulsperger, E., Baumgartner, G. *et al.* (1997) Gemcitabine in the treatment of advanced non-small cell lung cancer: a phase II trial. *Lung Cancer* **56**(Suppl. 1), 52.

Manegold, C., Stahel, R., Mattson, K. *et al.* (1997) Randomized phase II study of gemcitabine monotherapy versus cisplatin plus etoposide in patients with locally advanced or metastatic non-small cell lung cancer. *Proc. Am. Soc. Clin. Oncol.* **16**, 1651.

Mao, L., Lee, J.S., Kurie, J.M. *et al.* (1997) Clonal genetic alterations in the lungs of current and former smokers. *J. Natl Cancer Inst.* **89**, 857–62.

Marino, P., Preatoni, A., Cantoni, A. and Buccheri, G. (1995) Single-agent chemotherapy versus combination chemotherapy in advanced non-small cell lung cancer: a quality and meta-analysis study. *Lung Cancer* **13**, 1–12.

Masuda, N., Fukuoka, M., Fujita, A. *et al.* (1998) A phase II study of combination CPT-11 and cisplatin for advanced non-small cell lung cancer. *Br. J. Cancer* **78**, 251–6.

Mattson, K., Niiranen, A., Pyrhonen, S. *et al.* (1992) Natural interferon alfa as maintenance therapy for small-cell lung cancer. *Eur. J. Cancer* **28A**, 1387–91.

Mattson, K., Niiranen, A., Ruotsalainen, T. *et al.* (1997) Interferon maintenance therapy for small cell lung cancer: improvement in long-term survival. *J. Interferon Cytokine Res.* **17**, 103–5.

Medical Research Council Lung Cancer Working Party (1989) Survival, adverse reactions and quality of life during chemotherapy compared with selective palliative treatment for small cell lung cancer. *Respir. Med.* **83**, 51–8.

Medical Research Council Lung Cancer Working Party (1991) Inoperable non-small cell lung cancer (NSCLC): a Medical Research Council randomised trial of palliative radiotherapy with two fractions or ten fractions. *Br. J. Cancer* **63**, 265–70.

Medical Research Council Lung Cancer Working Party (1992) A Medical Research Council randomised trial of palliative radiotherapy with two fractions or a single fraction in patients with inoperable non-small cell lung cancer and poor performance status. *Br. J. Cancer* **65**, 934–41.

Medical Research Council Lung Cancer Working Party (1996a) Randomised trial of palliative two fraction versus more intensive 13-fraction radiotherapy for patients with inoperable non-small cell lung cancer. *Clin. Oncol.* **8**, 167–75.

Medical Research Council Lung Cancer Working Party (1996b) Comparison of oral etoposide and standard intravenous multidrug chemotherapy for small cell lung cancer: a stopped multicentre randomised trial. *Lancet* **348**, 563–6.

Mehta, M.P., Tannehill, S.P., Adak, S. *et al.* (1998) Phase II trial of hyperfractionated accelerated radiation therapy for non-resectable NSCLC: results of Eastern Cooperative Oncology Group 4593. *J. Clin. Oncol.* **16**, 351–23.

Minna, J., Pass, H., Glatstein, E. and Ihde, D.C. (1989) Cancer of the lung. In De Vita, V., Hellman, S. and Rosenberg, S.A. (eds), *Principle and practice of oncology.* Philadelphia: JB Lippincott, 591–705.

Mooi, W.J. (1996) Common lung cancers. In Hasleton P.S. (ed.), *Spencer's pathology of the lung.* New York: McGraw-Hill, 1009–64.

Morita, K., Fuwa, N., Suzuki, Y. *et al.* (1997) Radical radiotherapy for medically inoperable non-small cell lung cancer in clinical stage I: a retrospective analysis of 149 patients. *Radiother. Oncol.* **42**, 31–6.

Morrison, R., Deeley, T.J. and Cleland, W.P. (1963) The treatment of carcinoma of the bronchus: a clinical trial to compare surgery and supervoltage radiotherapy. *Lancet* **1**, 683–4.

Mountain, C.F. (1997) Revisions in the International system for staging lung cancer. *Chest* **111**, 1710–17.

Murray, N., Coy, P., Pater, J.L. *et al.* (1993) Importance of timing for thoracic irradiation in the combined modality treatment of limited stage lung cancer *J. Clin. Oncol.* **11**, 336–44.

Murray, N., Livingston, R.B., Shepherd, F.A. *et al.* (1999) Randomized study of CODE versus alternating CAV/EP for extensive stage small cell lung cancer: an intergroup study of the National Cancer Institute of Canada Clinical Trials Group and the Southwest Oncology Group. *J. Clin. Oncol.* **17**, 2300–8.

Nakamura, S., Kudoh, S., Komuta, K. *et al.* (1999) Phase II study of irinotecan (CPT-11) combined with etoposide for previously untreated extensive-disease small cell lung cancer: a study of the West Japan Lung Cancer Group. *Proc. Am. Soc. Clin. Oncol.* **18**, 470a.

Noda, K., Nishiwaki, Y., Kawahara, M. *et al.* (2002) Irinotecan plus cisplatin compared with etoposide plus cisplatin for extensive small-cell lung cancer. *N. Engl. J. Med.* **346**, 85–91.

Non-small cell lung cancer collaborative group (1995) Chemotherapy in non-small cell lung cancer: a meta-analysis using updated data on individual patients from 52 randomised trials. *BMJ* **311**, 899–909.

Omenn, G.S., Goodman, G.E. and Thornquist, M.D. (1996) Effects of a combination of beta carotene and vitamin A on lung cancer and cardiovascular disease. *N. Engl. J. Med.* **334**, 1150–5.

Payne, P.W., Sebo, T.J., Doudkine, A. *et al.* (1997) Sputum screening by quantitative microscopy: a reexamination of a portion of the National Cancer Institute Cooperative Early Lung Cancer Study. *Mayo Clin. Proc.* **72**, 697–704.

Perng, R.-P., Chen, Y.-M., Ming Liu, J. *et al.* (1997) Gemcitabine versus the combination of cisplatin and etoposide in patients with inoperable non-small cell lung cancer in a phase II randomized study. *J. Clin. Oncol.* **15**, 2097–102.

Petersen, S., Wolf, G., Bockmuhl, U. *et al.* (1998) Allelic loss on chromosome 10q in human lung cancer: association with tumour progression and metastatic phenotype. *Br. J. Cancer* **77**, 270–6.

Pettengell, R., Woll, P.J., Thatcher, N. *et al.* (1995) Multicyclic dose-intensive chemotherapy supported by sequential reinfusion of haemopoietic progenitors in whole-blood. *J. Clin. Oncol.* **13**, 148–56.

Phillips, M., Gleeson, K., Hughes, J.M.B. *et al.* (1999) Volatile organic compounds in breath as markers of lung cancer: a cross-sectional study. *Lancet* **353**, 1930–3.

Pignon, J.-P., Arriagada, R., Ihde, D.C. *et al.* (1992) A meta-analysis of thoracic radiotherapy for small cell lung cancer. *N. Engl. J. Med.* **327**, 1618–24.

Rawson, N.S.B. and Peto, J. (1990) An overview of prognostic factors in small cell lung cancer. A report from the subcommittee for the management of lung cancer of the United Kingdom Co-ordinating Committee on Cancer Research. *Br. J. Cancer* **61**, 597–604.

Rees, G.J.G., Devrell, C.E., Barley, V.I. and Newman, H.F.V. (1997) Palliative radiotherapy for lung cancer: two versus five fractions. *Clin. Oncol.* **9**, 90–5.

Rizvi, N. and Hayes, D.F. (1999) A breathalyser for lung cancer. *Lancet* **353**, 1897–8.

Roland, M. and Rudd, R.M. (1998) Somatic mutations in the development of lung cancer. *Thorax* **53**, 979–83.

Rosell, R., Gomez-Codina, J., Camps, C. *et al.* (1994) A randomized trial comparing pre-operative chemotherapy plus surgery with surgery alone in patients with NSCLC. *N. Engl. J. Med.* **330**, 153–8.

Rosell, R., Gomez-Codina, J., Camps, C. *et al.* (1999) Pre-resectional chemotherapy in stage IIIA non-small-cell lung cancer: a 7-year assessment of a randomized controlled trial. *Lung Cancer* **47**, 7–14.

Rosenthal, S.A., Curran, W.J., Herbert, S.H. *et al.* (1992) Clinical stage II non-small cell lung cancer treated with radiation therapy alone. *Chest* **70**, 2410–17.

Roth, B.J., Johnson, D.H., Einhorn, L.H. *et al.* (1992) Randomized study of cyclophosphamide, doxorubicin and vincristine versus etoposide and cisplatin versus alternation of these two regimens in extensive small cell lung cancer: a phase III trial of the Southeastern Cancer Study Group. *J. Clin. Oncol.* **10**, 282–91.

Roth, J.A., Fossella, F., Komaki, R. *et al.* (1994) A randomized trial comparing perioperative chemotherapy and surgery with surgery alone in resectable stage IIIA NSCLC. *J. Natl Cancer Inst.* **86**, 673–80.

Roth, J.A., Atkinson, E.N., Fossella, F. *et al.* (1998) Long-term follow-up of patients enrolled in a randomized trial comparing perioperative chemotherapy and surgery with surgery alone in resectable stage IIIA non-small-cell lung cancer. *Lung Cancer* **21**, 1–6.

Royal College of Radiologists (1999) Guidelines for the non-surgical management of lung cancer. *Clin. Oncol.* **11**, S14–S49.

Salgia, R. and Skarvin, A.T. (1998) Molecular abnormalities in lung cancer. *J. Clin. Oncol.* **16**, 1207–17.

Saunders, M., Dische, S., Barrett, A. *et al.* (1997) Continuous hyperfractionated accelerated radiotherapy (CHART) versus conventional radiotherapy in non-small cell lung cancer: a randomised multicentre trial. *Lancet* **350**, 161–5.

Saunders, M., Rojas, A., Lynn, B.E. *et al.* (1998) Experience with dose escalation using CHARTWEL continuous hyperfractionated accelerated radiotherapy (weekend less) in NSCLC. *Br. J. Cancer* **78**, 1323–8.

Sause, W.T., Scott, C., Taylor, S. *et al.* (1995) Radiation Therapy Oncology Group (RTOG) 8808 and Eastern Co-operative Oncology Group (ECOG) 4588: preliminary results of a phase III trial in regionally advanced unresectable non-small cell lung cancer. *J. Natl Cancer Inst.* **87**, 198–205.

Sause, W., Kolesar, P., Taylor, S. *et al.* (2000) Final results of a phase III trial in regionally advanced unresectable non-small cell lung cancer: Radiation Therapy Oncology Group, Eastern Cooperative Oncology Group, and Southwest Oncology Group. *Chest* **117**, 358–64.

Schaake-Koning, C., van den Bogaert, W., Dalesio, O. *et al.* (1992) Effects of concomitant cisplatin and radiotherapy on inoperable non-small cell lung cancer. *N. Engl. J. Med.* **326**, 524–30.

Schiller, J.H., Harrington, D., Belani, C.P. *et al.* (2002) Comparison of four chemotherapy regimens for advanced non-small cell lung cancer. *N. Engl. J. Med.* **346**, 92–8.

Sculier, J.P., Paesmans, M., Bureau, G. *et al.* (1993) Multiple-drug weekly chemotherapy versus standard combination regimen in small cell lung cancer: a phase III randomized study conducted by the European Lung Cancer Working Party. *J. Clin. Oncol.* **11**, 1858–65.

Shepherd, F.A., Ginsberg, R.J., Feld, R., Evans, W.K. and Johnasen, E. (1991) Surgical treatment for limited stage small cell lung cancer: the University of Toronto Lung Oncology Group experience. *J. Thorac. Cardiovasc. Surg.* **101**, 385–93.

Smit, E.F., Fokkema, E., Biesma, B., Snoek, W. and Postmus, P.E. (1998) A phase II study of paclitaxel in heavily pretreated patients with SCLC. *Br. J. Cancer* **77**, 347–51.

Smith, I.E. (1999) Screening for lung cancer: time to think positive. *Lancet* **354**, 86–7.

Sone, S., Takashima, S., Li, F. *et al.* (1998) Mass screening for lung cancer with mobile spiral computed tomography scanner. *Lancet* **351**, 1242–5.

Souhami, R.L., Rudd, R., Ruiz de Elvira, M.-C. *et al.* (1994) Randomized trial comparing weekly versus 3-week chemotherapy in small cell lung cancer: a Cancer Research Campaign trial. *J. Clin. Oncol.* **12**, 1806–13.

Souhami, R.L., Spiro, S.G., Rudd, R.M. *et al.* (1997) Five day etoposide for advanced small cell lung cancer: randomized comparison with intravenous chemotherapy. *J. Natl Cancer Inst.* **89**, 577–80.

Spiro, S.G., Souhami, R.L., Geddes, D.M. *et al.* (1989) Duration of chemotherapy in SCLC: a Cancer Research Campaign trial. *Br. J. Cancer* **59**, 578–83.

Steward, W.P., von Pawel, J., Gatzemeier, U. *et al.* (1998) Effects of granulocyte–macrophage colony-stimulating factor and dose intensification of VICE chemotherapy in small cell lung cancer: a prospective randomised study of 300 patients. *J. Clin. Oncol.* **16**, 642–50.

Stewart, L.A., Burdett, S. and Souhami, R.L. (1998) Post operative radiotherapy in NSCLC: a meta-analysis using individual patient data from randomised clinical trials. *Proc. Am. Soc. Clin. Oncol.* **17**, 457a.

Takada, M., Fukuoka, M., Furuse, K. *et al.* (1996) Phase III study of concurrent versus sequential thoracic radiotherapy in combination with cisplatin and etoposide for limited stage small cell lung cancer: preliminary results of the Japan Clinical Oncology Group. *Proc. Am. Soc. Clin. Oncol.* **15**, 372.

Talton, B.M., Constable, W.C. and Kersch, C.R. (1990) Curative radiotherapy in non-small cell carcinoma of the lung. *Int. J. Radiat. Oncol. Biol. Phys.* **19**, 15–21.

Thatcher, N., Girling, D.J., Hopwood, P., Sambrooke, R.J., Qian, W. and Stephens, R.J. (2000) Improving survival without reducing quality of life in small cell lung cancer patients by increasing the dose-intensity of chemotherapy with granulocyte colony stimulating factor support: results of a British Council Lung Cancer Working Party. *J. Clin. Oncol.* **18**, 396–404.

Thiberville, L., Payne, P., Vielkinds, J. *et al.* (1995) Evidence of cumulative gene losses with progression of premalignant epithelial lesions to carcinoma of the bronchus. *Cancer Res.* **55**, 5133–9.

Tockman, M.S., Mulshine, J.L., Piantadosi, S. *et al.* (1997) Prospective detection of preclinical lung cancer: results from two studies of hnRNP overexpression. *Clin. Cancer Res.* **3**, 2237–46.

Treat, J., Johnson, E., Langer, C. *et al.* (1998) Tirapazamine with cisplatin in patients with advanced non-small cell lung cancer: a phase II study. *J. Clin. Oncol.* **16**, 3524–7.

Trillet-Lenoir, V., Green, J., Manegold, C. *et al.* (1993) Recombinant granulocyte colony stimulating factor reduces the infectious complications of cytotoxic chemotherapy. *Eur. J. Cancer* **29A**, 319–24.

Trillet-Lenoir, V., Soler, P., Arpin, D. *et al.* (1996) The limits of chemotherapy dose intensification using granulocyte colony stimulating factor alone in extensive small cell lung cancer. *Lung Cancer* **14**, 331–41.

Turrisi, A.T., Kim, K., Blum, R. *et al.* (1999) Twice daily compared with once daily thoracic radiotherapy in limited stage small-cell lung cancer treated concurrently with cisplatin and etoposide. *N. Engl. J. Med.* **340**, 265–71.

van Zandwijk, N., Greon, H.J.M., Postmus, P.E. *et al.* (1997) Role of recombinant interferon-gamma maintenance in responding patients with small cell lung cancer. A randomised phase III study of the EORTC lung cancer cooperative group. *Eur. J. Cancer* **33**, 1759–66.

von Pawel, J., Schiller, J.H., Shepherd, F.A. *et al.* (1999) Topotecan versus cyclophosphamide, doxorubicin and vincristine for the treatment of recurrent small cell lung cancer. *J. Clin. Oncol.* **17**, 658–67.

von Pawel, J., von Roemling, R., Gatzemeier, U. *et al.* (2000) Tirapazamine plus cisplatin versus cisplatin in advanced non-small cell lung cancer: a report of the international CATAPULT I study group. *J. Clin. Oncol.* **18**, 1351–9.

Wiencke, J.K., Thurston, S.W., Kelsey, K.T. *et al.* (1999) Early age at smoking initiation and tobacco carcinogen DNA damage in the lung. *J. Natl Cancer Inst.* **91**, 614–19.

Wolf, M., Hans, K., Drings, P. *et al.* (1996) Treatment intensification with GM-CSF in patients with non-metastatic SCLC. Results of a multicenter trial including 330 patients. *Proc. Am. Soc. Clin. Oncol.* **15**, 270.

Woll, P.J., Hodgetts, J., Lomax, L. *et al.* (1995) Can cytotoxic dose intensity be increased by using granulocyte colony-stimulating factor? A randomised controlled trial of lenograstim in small cell lung cancer. *J. Clin. Oncol.* **13**, 652–9.

Woll, P.J., Thatcher, N., Lomax, L. *et al.* (2001) Use of hematopoietic progenitors in whole blood to support dose-dense chemotherapy: a randomized phase II trial in small cell lung cancer. *J. Clin. Oncol.* **19**, 712–19.

Wozniak, A.J., Crowley, J.J., Balcerzak, S.P. *et al.* (1998) Randomized trial comparing cisplatin with cisplatin plus vinorelbine in the treatment of advanced non-small-cell lung cancer: a Southwest Oncology Group Study. *J. Clin. Oncol.* **16**, 2459–65.

Zang, E.A. and Wynder, E.L. (1996) Differences in lung cancer risk between men and women: examination of the evidence. *J. Natl Cancer Inst.* **88**, 183–92.

23

Oesophagus

HUGO R. BAILLIE-JOHNSON

Despite much therapeutic effort and ingenuity, the results of treatment for this terrible disease remain very poor. Only a small proportion of patients have sufficiently limited disease to allow a realistic attempt at curative treatment. Around 10 per cent of patients are suitable for radical surgical resection, with a treatment-related mortality of 8–16 per cent. The majority of patients have locally extensive or metastatic disease at presentation. These patients have a median survival of 9–10 months. The difficult anatomy and anatomical relations of the oesophagus mean that attempts at radical surgical treatment are attended by a significant morbidity and mortality. Results of radical treatment, either by surgery or by radiotherapy, remain disappointing and it seems unlikely that they will be much improved using currently available treatment modalities. Chemotherapy has definite, but limited, value and is being integrated with surgery and radiation therapy through continuing clinical trials. Major effects on mortality rates continue to elude us, and in many patients, treatment is directed at palliation rather than cure. Even so, palliation is in itself a worthwhile therapeutic endeavour and one about which there remains much to be learned. New techniques are being developed to allow rapid and safe palliation and these will be described.

INCIDENCE, EPIDEMIOLOGY AND AETIOLOGY

Cancer of the oesophagus has an incidence in the UK of approximately 8 per 100 000 population, accounting for about 4000 deaths per annum. The male-to-female ratio for carcinoma of the thoracic oesophagus is about 2.5 : 1. For carcinoma of the cervical oesophagus, it is reversed, especially for post-cricoid carcinoma, which predominantly affects women. There has been a marked increase in the disease over recent decades and a striking increase in adenocarcinomas, especially of the lower third and cardia. The death rate increases sharply with age (Gardner et al., 1983), there being an eightfold increase between the age bands 45–54 years and 65–74 years. In this country, oesophageal cancer accounts for 0.7 per cent of all cancer deaths (DHSS, 1983) and broadly comparable figures apply to the USA and Western Europe. Pockets of abnormally high incidence occur in regions loosely grouped into a broad band which extends from the Eastern Mediterranean through the South Caspian and Iran, to the Lin Xiang and Honan provinces of China, which have an annual incidence amounting to 100 per 100 000 (Yang, 1980). In the Chinese population clusters, there has been an interesting circumstantial correlation with a similar condition in chickens, suggesting a possible dietary or environmental carcinogen. Closely adjacent populations (both human and fowl) have no such increased incidence. Food contaminants, such as mycotoxins and nitrosamines, have been proposed, but the reason for regions of increased incidence is probably multifactorial. Alcohol and tobacco consumption also correlate with risk of developing oesophageal cancer and a direct dose–effect relationship has been described (Wynder and Bross, 1961; Schottenfeld, 1984). In some predisposed populations, notably black

South Africans in the Transkei, poor black populations in the USA, and in Brittany, it is possible that contamination of homemade alcohol is a contributory factor.

With annual incidences such as those seen in high-risk regions of China, screening of the population at risk becomes an economically viable measure. Using endoscopy and abrasion cytology, results of treating screened populations have been encouraging (Crespi *et al.*, 1979; Munoz *et al.*, 1982). Early lesions, amounting to *in-situ* change, have been identified and successfully treated and the importance of reflux and chronic oesophagitis as a possible precursor in such patients has been stressed (Guanrei *et al.*, 1982). Screening programmes of this sort are unfortunately only practicable in high-risk, highly selected populations, but data suggest that early T1 tumours in Western populations, though rare, are also highly treatable (Skinner, 1984).

Molecular biology

The basic molecular defects which result in development of the malignant phenotype have not yet been comprehensively identified. A number of defects at gene level have now been characterized, but there appears to be considerable variation in the molecular genetics of these tumours. Studies of oesophageal tumour tissue, and tissue from premalignant epithelium including Barrett's epithelium, have identified mutations in *p53* (a tumour suppressor gene) in a high proportion of cases (Fléjou *et al.*, 1993). These mutations may result also in overexpression of the protein product of *p53*, and monoclonal antibody staining techniques have localized the overexpression to malignant and high-grade dysplastic epithelium. Low-grade dysplasia and non-dysplastic epithelium tend not to demonstrate *p53* protein overexpression. Similar findings were reported by Bennett *et al.* (1992) who identified *p53* mutations in some (but not all) cases of invasive carcinoma. One patient who had invasive carcinoma coexisting with pre-invasive lesions had two different mutations in different codons. The genetic alterations found are therefore far from constant. Although *p53* mutation is certainly not the sole cause of oesophageal cancer, stepwise mutation and accumulation of the mutant gene product appear to be associated with tumour formation in a substantial proportion of cases. The clinical relevance of such studies will develop as such work is carried further, but already it appears that molecular aberrations such as *p53* mutation and amplification, c-*myc* amplification, and *Rb* deletion may be of value as clinical markers of malignancy, allowing the early identification of lesions which are of high metastatic potential. (Montesano *et al.*, 1996). Chromosome studies have revealed a range of deletions, with allelic loss (variously) at 3p, 5q, 9p, 9q, 13q, 17p, 17q and 18q.

It is likely therefore that the genetic defect resulting in the malignant phenotype is complex, with several gene mutations co-operating functionally to produce malignant transformation. While there is good evidence that a single mutation is capable of malignant transformation under some circumstances, 'single-hit' carcinogenesis is probably the exception rather than the rule.

Several other oncogene proteins have been identified in human oesophageal tumours (Jankowski *et al.*, 1992), notably c-*erb-B2* *(neu)* and c-*erb-B2* *(CB11)*. Jankowski reported that 11 of 15 specimens stained strongly for these membrane-associated proteins and seven specimens stained strongly for *p53*; c-*erb-B2* overexpression was found also in nine specimens from Barrett's epithelium.

In addition to the histological morphology of the malignant phenotype, an aggressive metastatic behaviour is also a characteristic feature of these tumours. Features such as production and activation of metalloproteinases, scatter factor, and angiogenic factors may all participate in the development of aggressive metastatic behaviour.

Because the genetic alterations in oesophageal cancer are multiple and variable, potential molecular targets for therapeutic intervention are at present rather hard to define. Molecular testing may be of value in identifying premalignant cases with greater malignant potential, allowing their selection for early and aggressive treatment.

Predisposing conditions and risk factors

REFLUX STATES

Oesophageal reflux has long been suspected as a causative factor in oesophageal carcinoma but this is now beyond doubt. A variety of states known to predispose to malignancy are also associated with reflux. These include hiatus hernia, achalasia, and oesophageal ulceration with dysphagia. A concern that use of H2 blockers might predispose to malignancy has been substantially allayed by careful case-control study (Chow *et al.*, 1995) Barrett's oesophagus is also closely linked to, and probably caused by, chronic acid reflux. Refluxing gastric contents may also expose inflamed oesophageal epithelium to ingested carcinogen-containing tobacco residues. Oesophageal motility disorders impair the ability of the distal oesophagus to clear refluxed stomach contents, and it has been shown that exposure to even modest doses of alcohol produces surprisingly long episodes of reflux with drastic changes in oesophageal pH (Vitale *et al.*, 1987). Thus, the two major factors seen in Western populations, tobacco and alcohol, conspire together to derange oesophageal motility and set up chronic inflammation due to reflux, which may culminate in malignant transformation.

Certain other conditions predispose to the development of oesophageal cancer.

Tylosis palmaris

This is a rare inherited genetic disorder characterized by a gross waxy, hyperkeratotic scaling of palms and soles. It is known to exist in two forms. Type A has its onset in early adolescence, and carries a progressive risk of oesophageal malignancy with a 50 per cent incidence by the age of 45 and a 95 per cent incidence by the age of 65. The second form, designated type B, presents in infancy, and carries no excess risk of oesophageal carcinoma. Both variants of the condition have an autosomal dominant pattern of inheritance (Clarke and McConnell, 1954; Harper *et al.*, 1970).

Malnutrition states

Conditions of malnutrition, especially chronic iron deficiency states and the Paterson–Kelly syndrome, have been identified as risk factors. The prevalence of subsequent malignancy appears to be in the region of 10 per cent. Malnutrition states may be associated with high-risk lifestyles such as excess alcohol consumption and smoking which appear as independent factors to predispose to this malignancy. An increased incidence has also been reported in chronic malabsorption states (Halvorsen and Thompson, 1984). In addition to iron deficiency, micronutrient deficiency states also contribute to risk of malignancy.

Achalasia of the oesophagus

This carries a significant risk of subsequent development of carcinoma of around 7 per cent, probably as a result of oesophageal stasis and chronic irritation. Medical treatment consists of therapy with calcium channel blockers, such as nifedipine, or by injection of botulinum toxin, but success is rather limited. Surgical treatment consists of dilatation or myotomy, using Heller's technique or a modification thereof. A long-term follow-up study of 146 evaluable patients treated by myotomy revealed that 23 subsequently died of cancer, 10 of whom had carcinoma of the oesophagus. Whilst improving oesophageal function, surgery may not have a major effect on cancer risk.

Barrett's oesophagus and other reflux states

Reflux states are known to be significant risk factors, especially if associated with Barrett's epithelium. This is an acquired dysplastic condition of the oesophagus produced by chronic gastro-oesophageal reflux. Through the endoscope, Barrett's epithelium has a reddish velvet appearance reminiscent of small bowel mucosa. There is often an easily seen line of demarcation separating Barrett's from normal areas of mucosa (Fig. 23.1). Histologically it resembles a transitional or columnar epithelium with mucous glands and often a villiform surface. The histological pattern may be heterogeneous, with patches of small bowel or gastric epithelium. With high-grade dysplasia, carcinoma *in-situ* is a common and ominous finding. Areas of invasive carcinoma may coexist with dysplastic epithelium. Where true invasive carcinoma occurs it is commonly an adenocarcinoma, although squamous carcinomas are also frequently seen.

The risk of carcinoma developing in Barrett's epithelium appears to be greater than previously thought, perhaps up to 50 per cent where there is longitudinally extensive involvement with high-grade dysplasia. With lesser degrees of involvement, the risk of neoplasia is

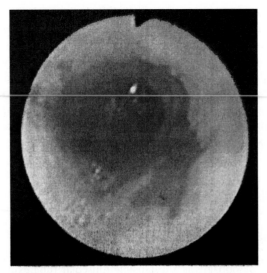

Figure 23.1 *Endoscopic view of Barrett's epithelium showing demarcation zone.*

around 0.8 per cent per annum, on an accumulating basis. This is about 40 times the risk for an unaffected population. Pera *et al.* (1992) described a series of 18 patients who underwent oesophagectomy for high-grade dysplastic Barrett's epithelium, nine of whom were found to have histological evidence of invasive carcinoma. These patients were all stage I or stage II, and had an overall 5-year survival of 37.5 per cent. Similar figures are confirmed by a larger series of 112 patients with adenocarcinoma in Barrett's oesophagus with survival at 5 years of 30 per cent for stages up to and including 2a. The fall-off of survival with increasing stage is seen when this figure is compared with comparable survival data for stage 0 + stage I patients, who achieved 63 per cent survival at 5 years (Menckepluymers *et al.*, 1992). A series of 55 patients reported by Collard contained 12 with high-grade dysplasia, 4 of whom had changes of invasive carcinoma in their surgical specimens (Collard *et al.*, 1997). There is evidence that the risk of dysplasia and carcinoma increases to significant levels when Barrett's epithelium is greater than 8 cm in length (Iftikhar *et al.*, 1992). Regression of Barrett's epithelium has been observed after antireflux surgery (Attwood *et al.*, 1992) and following treatment with omeprazole (Lundell, 1992). Dysplastic Barrett's epithelium is considered to be an indication for surgery, and resection should be considered at an early stage. Endoscopic surveillance may not be a safe option; patient compliance can prejudice the effectiveness of such a policy, and tumour progression may easily be missed (Collard *et al.*, 1997).

Oesophagectomy is a major undertaking, attended by significant risk, and alternative treatment techniques such as photodynamic therapy may have a part to play in conservative management of high-grade dysplasia. This technique depends on selective accumulation of protoporphyrin IX in dysplastic tissue, which is then activated by irradiation with 630 nm light. In a small series of patients, dysplasia was eradicated, but non-dysplastic Barrett's epithelium recurred in 2/5 (Barr *et al.*, 1996). An effective conservative alternative to surgery would be a very valuable development, since many of these patients are relatively asymptomatic and find it hard to accept the option of major surgical intervention. For the time being, however, surgical intervention remains the definitive treatment option for this potentially dangerous premalignant condition.

ANATOMY

Anatomical relations

The oesophagus is a distensible muscular tube extending some 25 cm from the level of C6 to traverse the diaphragm at the level T10. Arising just behind the lower border of the cricoid, it consists of an outer longitudinal and an inner circumferential muscle layer. In the cervical and upper thoracic oesophagus, the oesophageal muscle is of striated type, blending progressively and being replaced by non-striated muscle in the mid- and lower-thoracic oesophagus. The muscle layers are not invested with a serosa, allowing invasive tumours unimpeded access to the posterior mediastinum. The lumen of the oesophagus is lined with non-keratinizing stratified squamous epithelium, beneath which lies a rich plexus of blood and lymphatic vessels. Submucosal spread is an important feature of oesophageal cancer and is associated with early dissemination of metastases to regional lymph nodes, and to the systemic circulation.

The blood supply of the oesophagus is obtained by several routes. The upper third and cervical oesophagus are supplied by the inferior thyroid artery. The middle third is supplied by branches from the aorta and associated vessels and the lower third similarly, supplemented by branches from the left gastric artery.

Venous drainage relates to the arterial supply, the upper third draining into the inferior thyroid system, the middle third into the azygos and hemiazygos systems and the lower third partly into the azygos and partly into the left gastric vein. A portal systemic anastomosis exists around the lower third of the oesophagus and in circumstances of portal hypertension it may give rise to oesophageal varices.

The lymphatic drainage of the oesophagus is initially via the rich submucosal lymphatic plexus to a network of lymphatics, allowing cross-regional drainage and widespread nodal metastasis. The cervical oesophagus drains principally to deep cervical lymph nodes. The thoracic oesophagus drains to mediastinal nodes, paratracheal and pretracheal nodes and subcarinal and hilar nodes. The lower third of the oesophagus drains to the coeliac axis.

With such an extensive and intercommunicating lymphatic network, it is easy to see why the early spread of oesophageal tumours presents such formidable surgical problems. Longitudinal extension of oesophageal tumours allows lymphatic drainage by multiple routes and about 30 per cent of patients with upper oesophageal tumours will have transdiaphragmatic lymph node metastases at presentation. For tumours of the lower oesophagus, the figure is nearer 70 per cent (Halvorsen and Thompson, 1984).

The anatomical relations of the oesophagus contribute to the difficulties of both the surgeon and the radiation oncologist. Throughout its length it lies in close proximity to vital structures, especially in the upper oesophagus where radiation therapy is much more feasible than surgery. Conversely, the lower oesophagus is more surgically accessible and radiation therapy is limited by the anterior curvature of the spinal cord and by the limited radiation tolerance of the gastric cardia. For lower oesophageal tumours, a surgical approach, where possible, is generally preferred. Many tumours, however, are well beyond the possibility of surgery when they present. Computerized tomography displays the anatomical relationships which must be considered in planning treatment (Fig. 23.2).

In the upper oesophagus, the trachea and recurrent laryngeal nerves lie in close anterior relationship. The vertebral column and spinal cord lie posteriorly and the carotid sheaths laterally.

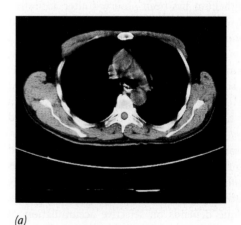

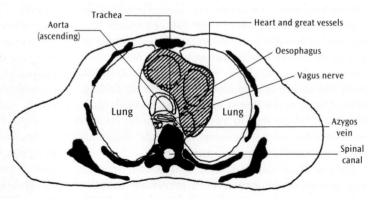

(a) *(b)*

Figure 23.2 *(a, b) CT anatomy of a carcinoma of the middle third of the oesophagus.*

The middle third of the oesophagus nestles adjacent to the trachea, the left main bronchus, the pulmonary artery, the pericardium and the heart. The azygos vein system and the vertebral column lie posteriorly. The lower third lies closely behind the heart and aorta and runs for about 2 cm below the diaphragm to the gastric cardia. The nerve supply to the oesophagus is via a plexus arising from the vagus and from the sympathetic chain.

It will be seen from the above that all the major intrathoracic structures are vulnerable to direct invasion by oesophageal tumours. Careful evaluation of the mediastinum by endoscopy and CT imaging is therefore needed in planning treatment.

Endoscopic anatomy

Seen through an endoscope, the oesophagus starts at 15 cm from the incisors, with the level of the aortic arch at 23 cm, that of the left main bronchus at 27 cm and the gastric cardia at 42 cm, subject to individual variation. The oesophagus curves in two planes as it traverses the thorax. The anterior curvature varies with the degree of spinal kyphosis and in elderly patients is often considerable. On occasions, it can be very difficult to treat upper or middle third lesions with a radiation field that entirely spares the spinal cord. The cervical oesophagus and middle third lie more or less in the midline, whilst the upper thoracic and, to a greater extent, the lower third, lie to the left of the midline. These deviations have to be considered in radiation treatment planning and may require individual shaping of treatment fields.

METASTASES AND NATURAL HISTORY

The natural history of this disease is one of more or less rapid progression to death following inexorable oesophageal obstruction. Malnutrition and dehydration, lack of resistance to infection and cardiopulmonary complications all play their part. Radical treatment, by surgery or radiation therapy, serves only to increase the survival of a small group of patients with limited disease, but even so, fewer than 8 per cent of patients survive for 5 years (Earlam and Cunha-Melo, 1980; Skinner, 1984; Giuli and Sancho-Garnier, 1986).

The biological behaviour of oesophageal cancer provides insurmountable therapeutic problems. The primary tumour has a tendency to spread locally, infiltrating the mediastinum and invading the vital structures within it. Longitudinal spread occurs early and extensively via the submucosal lymphatics and vascular network, and 'skip lesions', apparently discontinuous with the primary tumour, may occur several centimetres from its apparent limits (Fig. 23.3). Evidence of the high metastatic potential of this disease can be found in autopsy series such as that of Sons and Borchard (1986). In reviewing autopsies

of 171 cases of carcinoma of the distal oesophagus, 80.9 per cent had evidence of metastatic disease. In interpreting the study, it is important to recognize that these patients had end-stage disease and the greater proportion of them appear to have had carcinoma of the cardia, infiltrating the distal oesophagus. Forty-nine per cent of cases had mediastinal node involvement and 40 per cent had positive coeliac and perigastric nodes. Blood-borne metastases were found in 35 per cent of the series. Liver and lung involvement occurred in 23 per cent and 22 per cent of cases, respectively; 11 per cent had peritoneal metastases and 8 per cent had bone or kidney involvement.

A biological basis for this aggressive metastatic behaviour is suggested by the identification of metalloproteinase production by cells in oesophageal tumours (Shima *et al.*, 1992). Metalloproteinases are a class of zinc-motif-containing enzymes which are capable of breaking down a variety of extracellular matrix macromolecules. This ability allows the destruction of type 4 collagen, and enables tumour cells to breach basement membranes and invade beyond them, thus breaching vascular and other tissue boundaries. It is therefore likely that the ability to produce these classes of enzyme is a fundamental component in the mechanism of metastasis, and the inhibition of these enzymes is potentially of therapeutic importance. Other factors involving coagulation mechanisms, cell motility (scatter factors), and angiogenesis also have highly important roles in the metastatic process but it would be simplistic to conclude that controlling any one of these alone holds the key to the problem of metastatic disease. Their importance lies in the identification of possible new avenues for therapeutic intervention and several novel drugs are currently in trial.

Computed tomography (CT) scanning has recently provided information on the incidence of metastases in living patients. Halvorsen and Thompson (1984) emphasize the high incidence of subdiaphragmatic involvement.

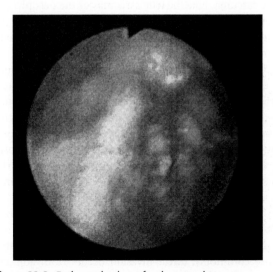

Figure 23.3 *Endoscopic view of submucosal tumour nodules.*

With middle third tumours, the figure was around 40 per cent and for tumours of the lower third, greater than 62 per cent. Comparable data were reported by Galandiuk *et al.* (1986). Reviewing 236 cases retrospectively, coeliac node involvement was found in 26 per cent of cases and 30 per cent of cases developed metastases before surgery, or were found to have metastatic disease at operation. Such data are adverse to the concept of radical treatment of local disease and it is perhaps unsurprising that treatment results are so poor.

PATHOLOGY

Eighty-five per cent of oesophageal tumours arise in the middle and lower two-thirds of the oesophagus and are distributed equally between these regions. Only 15 per cent arise in the upper third. The vast majority (90 per cent) of tumours are squamous carcinomas, but of lower third lesions, 30 per cent are adenocarcinomas (Giuli and Sancho-Garnier, 1986). The distinction between adenocarcinomas of the lower third of the oesophagus and adenocarcinomas of the gastric cardia involving the lower oesophagus has never been easy, or particularly meaingful, and they are best considered in clinical terms as essentially a single entity. In recent years, there has been a substantial increase in the numbers reported of adenocarcinomas of the lower third/cardia. Within these histological types, varying degrees of differentiation may occur, from well-differentiated keratinizing squamous carcinomas to undifferentiated tumours. Heterogeneity of histological pattern is well recognized, some tumours containing mixed histology (adenosquamous) or adenocarcinoma admixed with squamous epithelium (adenoacanthoma). Sarcoma-like tumours, designated pseudosarcoma and carcinosarcoma, rarely occur and may be squamous carcinoma variants, or contain elements of true sarcoma. Like the true sarcomas of the oesophagus, they are exceedingly rare. When these arise, they are generally leiomyosarcomas and may represent malignant transformation of a benign oesophageal leiomyoma.

Oat cell carcinoma of the oesophagus is analagous to the oat cell carcinoma of lung and behaves in a broadly similar way. It may exhibit neuroendocrine features such as dense cored vesicles on transmission electron microscopy and is sensitive to both radiation and cytotoxic drugs, though it carries a very poor long-term prognosis.

Mucous glands found in the oesophagus may give rise to tumours of adenoid cystic type, similar in appearance to adenoid cystic carcinomas of the salivary glands.

Melanomas occasionally occur as apparently localized entities, but are very rare.

Metastases from other sites are occasionally seen and, more commonly, direct invasion occurs from adjacent bronchial tumours or from involved mediastinal lymph nodes.

Premalignant conditions of the oesophagus have already been described.

SYMPTOMS AND PRESENTATION

Dysphagia

This is the presenting symptom in the vast majority of cases. The symptom has generally been experienced for some time prior to seeking advice and typically starts with discomfort on swallowing solids. At the onset of dysphagia, the tumour has obstructed about 50 per cent of the oesophageal lumen and has a minimum dimension of 2 cm. Some patients report symptomatic improvment with the use of some olive oil before eating, presumably for its lubricant properties. Difficulty with liquids follows when the obstruction has reached an advanced stage. The sensation of food sticking at the level of the sterno-manubrial joint signifies mechanical obstruction but does not necessarily correspond with the site of the obstruction. Pain frequently accompanies attempts at swallowing and total dysphagia may supervene as an acute and distressing event.

Conversely, a relatively small amount of tumour shrinkage produced by radiation therapy may be sufficient to allow considerable relief of obstructive symptoms. In simple obstruction, an attempt at swallowing is followed by forcible regurgitation after a short interval. If a tracheo-oesophageal fistula is present, an attempt at sipping even a very small quantity of water is followed by immediate explosive coughing and retching. The presence of a fistula can often be diagnosed by recognizing this sign. Total dysphagia due to complete obstruction may mean that patients are unable to swallow their own saliva and aspirate it into the bronchial tree. Historically, patients were maintained by feeding gastrostomy and had to endure this distressing state until they died of inanition and recurrent aspiration pneumonia. For this reason, many clinicians feel that feeding gastrostomies no longer have a place in management, but with the advent of the percutaneous gastrostomy (PEG) the question should probably be reopened. It is possible that PEG support may prolong survival through improvement in nutritional status, whilst providing a negative effect on quality of life by allowing the development of the distressing symptoms described above. This is a difficult situation where intervention, though possible, may not be in the best interests of the patient.

Pain

While this may be a prominent symptom in some patients, it is absent in others. When present, it typically accompanies attempts to swallow and occurs as the food bolus impacts at the site of obstruction. In locally advanced tumours infiltrating the mediastinum, pain may be severe and continuous. It is generally of an aching or boring character and may radiate to the back. Occasionally, pain from sites of metastatic disease in liver or bone may be a presenting problem.

Weight loss

This is an almost universal finding. It may be severe, of rapid onset, and out of proportion to the dietary limitations imposed by increasing dysphagia. Malnutrition, due to an inadequate dietary intake is a major cause, but patients with metastatic disease may also lose weight dramatically. The reasons for this cancer cachexia are obscure; undoubtedly, calorie deficiency is the predominant cause, but the wasting syndrome in cancer patients may be due to a poorly understood cytokine-mediated effect. When present, it is often a striking finding. These emaciated and dehydrated patients may exhibit signs of frank malnutrition and vitamin deficiency, and expert advice from a dietitian should be sought in order to make best use of the many dietary supplements which have become available.

Nutritional status is of particular relevance where radical treatment is contemplated. These patients are often exceedingly frail, hypoalbuminaemic, and quite unable to withstand the rigors of surgery or radiation therapy. Preparation of patients prior to surgery is undoubtedly of benefit and can often be accomplished by a relatively short period of rehydration with enteral nutritional support. There has been speculation about the value of intensive parenteral support in this situation, but a randomized trial (Vonmeyenfeldt *et al.*, 1992) has demonstrated benefit in terms of a reduction in major complications (mainly septic) in patients who had lost more than 10 per cent of their body weight. This study was not confined to patients with oesophageal cancer, but most oesophageal cancer patients would meet the trial criteria as 'depleted' patients, and would thus match the subgroup in which most benefit was seen. Short-term nutritional support appears to help severely depleted patients to withstand surgical treatment, but benefit for fitter patients has not clearly been demonstrated.

Symptoms from metastases

Occasionally, these are presenting symptoms but more commonly accompany advanced disease. Metastases to the liver and coeliac axis are very common. Where the liver capsule is distended, pain may occur and some relief may be obtained from the use of steroids in high doses (e.g. soluble prednisolone 60 mg/day). Metastases to bone may produce local pain, which responds to palliative radiation therapy: it is conveniently given as single fractions of 8–10 Gy applied dose.

Symptoms from locally extensive disease may produce mediastinal pain as described above. This can often be relieved by a course of fractionated palliative radiation therapy using 20 Gy in five daily fractions, or 27 Gy in six fractions, three fractions per week. Compression or encroachment on the trachea may give rise to an irritating cough. Invasion of adjacent great vessels may give rise to haematemesis or signs of upper gastrointestinal bleeding. Such small bleeds may precede massive haemorrhage.

Direct invasion of the pericardium may give rise to symptoms of cardiac irritation, mainly manifesting as rhythm disturbances.

Presentation as an incidental finding

Occasionally the diagnosis is made following endoscopy as part of the investigation of upper gastrointestinal symptoms. The advent of fibre-optic endoscopy has undoubtedly increased the number of lesions diagnosed in this way. Whether this will result in the identification of significantly greater numbers of early and treatable lesions remains to be seen. Evidence from endoscopic screening programmes in Japan suggests that aggressive treatment of very early lesions can be rewarding, and it is recommended that radical treatment should be considered on the rare occasions that a small tumour comes to light as an unexpected and incidental finding.

DIAGNOSIS

This is frequently suspected from the history, typically of progressive dysphagia worse for solids, often with pain and usually accompanied by weight loss. Recognition of symptoms of high gastrointestinal obstruction suggests a plan of investigation directed towards:

- establishing a tissue diagnosis;
- identifying the site, type and extent of obstruction; and
- assessing the suitability of tumour and patient for an attempt at radical treatment.

A contrast swallow (Fig. 23.4) gives a rapid assessment of the site and type of obstruction and can often differentiate between benign and malignant strictures. It may also demonstrate extrinsic compression by lymph nodes and may reveal the presence of a coexisting abnormality such as achalasia or an oesophageal web. Where there is evidence of obstruction, either clinical or radiographic, fibre-optic endoscopy and endoscopic biopsy should be carried out. Multiple biopsies are taken in order to maximize the chance of obtaining a tissue diagnosis. The endoscope should be negotiated past any visible tumour in order to determine the longitudinal extent of involvement. In many cases it is not immediately possible to do this, and a cautious dilatation should then be attempted. In most cases, this will allow successful completion of the endoscopy and the dilatation frequently helps the patient symptomatically. Where obstruction is such that complete

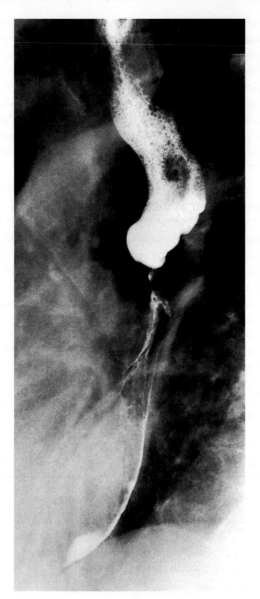

Figure 23.4 *Contrast swallow showing obstruction due to a carcinoma of the middle third of the oesophagus.*

endoscopy is not possible, it is sometimes worth repeating it after a short course of radiation therapy. It is most important to determine the full extent of the tumour and obtain a tissue diagnosis in every case.

FIBRE-OPTIC BRONCHOSCOPY

This is necessary to assess the integrity of the bronchial tree and to look for signs of encroachment by tumour or extrinsic compression by involved lymph nodes. High quality CT is a reasonably good predictor of tracheal involvement, with an accuracy exceeding 90 per cent.

MEDIASTINOSCOPY

This can give valuable information about involvement of first drainage lymph nodes and can provide histological proof of such involvement.

CHEST X-RAY

This may demonstrate involved lymph nodes in the mediastinum and is also useful as part of the cardiopulmonary assessment.

CT AND MAGNETIC RESONANCE (MR) SCANS

Scanning the chest and upper abdomen contributes information about the anatomy and extent of the intrathoracic tumour, which is often surprisingly extensive compared with the plain chest X-ray appearances. Upper abdominal scans allow a search for liver metastases and assessment of the coeliac axis lymph nodes. Local metastatic lymph node involvement is common, and is present in 70 per cent of patients at diagnosis. About 20 per cent of patients have detectable distant metastases at presentation, mainly in lymph nodes, liver and lung. Locally extensive tumours, which breach the oesophageal wall, have a 5 per cent survival at 5 years. CT scans are often used in assessing suitability for radical surgery. They are not entirely satisfactory for this purpose (Halvorsen and Thompson, 1984) especially in assessment of local invasion of the mediastinum. Compression of structures and obliteration of fat planes are helpful signs of involvement, but the lack of such signs is not a reliable indicator of operability. Thus, CT scans are relatively unreliable for detecting mediastinal invasion (unless gross), and may give false positives as well as false negatives. Infiltration of major airways, however, is detectable with an accuracy exceeding 90 per cent. Lymph nodes, unfortunately, are problematic for CT detection and diagnosis.

MR imaging gives similar results to CT, but may be less satisfactory for the detection of small lesions and lung metastases. MR technology continues to develop, however, and in making assessments of the extent of disease, it may be best to consider results from MR, CT and ultrasound together. The interpretation of imaging information is a guide, and only a guide, to the likely extent of disease, which at present is accurately revealed only when the patient comes to surgery.

ULTRASOUND

External ultrasound examination is of value in assessing for metastatic disease in the liver and coeliac axis lymph nodes. Internal ultrasound, carried out via a transducer placed endoscopically, is of value in assessing the primary tumour dimensions and local invasion. It can also demonstrate para-oesophageal nodes, and coeliac axis nodes. Endoscopic ultrasound is of considerable value in differentiating T4 disease from earlier T stages, and can usefully be deployed in selecting patients with apparently limited disease for resection. As with any endoscopic technique, there may be difficulties in negotiating the malignant stricture, even after dilatation, and it must not be forgotten that instrumentation of the oesophagus carries an appreciable risk and mortality, usually due to perforation of a malignant stricture. In many patients, perhaps 20 per cent, endoscopic ultrasound cannot be completed because of intractable obstruction.

MAGNETIC RESONANCE IMAGING (MRI)

MRI has been used extensively in the evaluation of oesophageal cancers. It is a developing art, but at present has no advantage over CT, and for some evaluations, it is inferior. It is at present as unreliable as CT in predicting lymph node involvement, but continues to develop, especially in terms of novel imaging contrast agents.

OTHER IMAGING TECHNIQUES

Positron emission tomography (PET) is currently an investigational technique. Fluorodeoxyglucose positron emission computed tomography (FDG-PET) allows imaging of regions of glucose metabolism, and tumours can be imaged by virtue of a local increase in such metabolism. The resolution tends to be rather poor, but the technique may in due course prove to be of value in detecting residual or recurrent disease following radical resection. At present there are physical and cost constraints on the availability of PET scanning but it has considerable promise and may well prove to be the best way of detecting low volume disease in locations which are difficult for CT/MR evaluation.

Clinical classification and staging

As in other tumours, clinical classification and staging is an attempt to ensure comparability in the evaluation of treatment results. With oesophageal cancers, non-invasive staging is of limited value, since surgical and autopsy series show that a high proportion of patients with locoregional tumours in fact have extensive disease. For practical purposes, the tumour node metastasis (TNM) system has the merits of being readily applied and, within the limitations of uncertainty, is as accurate as other staging systems. Modifications of the TNM system are frequently used:

Tumour
- T0: no evidence of tumour
- Tis: *in-situ* change only
- T1: invasion to, but not through, lamina propria
- T2: invasion of muscularis, but adventitia not breached
- T3: invasion of adventitia
- T4: invasion of adjacent anatomical structures

Node
- Nx: no node assessment data
- N0: node negative
- N1: node histologically positive

Metastasis
- Mx: no metastasis data
- M0: no metastases
- M1: metastases present

Stage grouping
- Stage I: TI N0 M0 or T1 Nx M0
- Stage IIa: T2 N0 M0 or T2 Nx M0 or T3 N0 M0
- Stage IIb: T1,2, N1 M0
- Stage III: T3 N1 M0 T4N0/1 M0
- Stage IV: any T any N + M1

Clinical staging has the limitation that in this anatomical site, autopsy data show that the extent of disease is consistently underestimated in life (Galandiuk *et al.*, 1986).

When full staging has been carried out, 75–80 per cent of patients are stage II or III. Uncertainty will make this figure something of an underestimate of the true state of affairs, and the proportion of patients with truly limited disease who are most suitable for radical treatment is indeed very small.

TREATMENT

Treatment of some sort is almost always indicated for oesophageal neoplasms. A small proportion of patients will be moribund on referral and therapeutic measures directed towards relieving distress may be required. In such patients, the use of subcutaneous infusion pumps to deliver opioid analgesic drugs is of great value.

For patients in whom more active management is possible, a decision must be made whether to attempt radical treatment with intent to cure. Only a very small proportion of patients will be suitable for such a treatment plan and the most careful selection is needed to obtain even a small proportion of long-term survivors. Radical treatment carries costs in terms of morbidity and a definite mortality, and inappropriate radical treatment carries no benefit for the patient, whose quality of life may be compromised needlessly by toxic effects of treatment.

Patients with limited lesions should be considered for surgical resection. Ideally, such patients will be in good general condition, with no coexisting medical conditions (especially cardiopulmonary conditions) which preclude surgery. They will have strictly limited tumours, with no evidence of local invasion or locoregional extension to adjacent organs. Evidence of metastatic disease at any site precludes radical surgery. Using the techniques of evaluation already described, inoperable criteria include vocal cord paralysis, fistula, cervical node enlargement, hepatic or other metastases, or evidence of encroachment upon trachea or great vessels.

All patients who are inoperable by any one or more of the above criteria may then be considered for radical radiation therapy or for palliative measures only. In general, radical radiation therapy is only applicable to patients who would be suitable for surgery were it not for coexisting medical conditions and patients with locoregional disease only. Palliative measures arc directed towards relieving pain and dysphagia and the measures selected should carry the best chance of rapid relief of symptoms, with the minimum of risk and hospitalization for the patient.

Surgery

In the rare early tumours, radical resection is justified with a prospect of long-term survival. These cases, it must again be stressed, are exceedingly uncommon. The chance of long-term survival in the vast majority of unselected cases lies around the 5 per cent mark. For the majority of patients, about 9 months of reasonable quality of life is the most that can be realistically expected from a very major and dangerous surgical procedure. Highly selected cases, where surgical staging corresponds with early-stage disease may have a survival at 5 years of 35 per cent. These cases account for about 5 per cent of all cases, so long-term survival is rare.

Surgical resection of oesophageal tumours is generally carried out with curative intent. Patients who survive surgery generally obtain palliative benefit and have a reduced requirement for subsequent dilatation and intubation. Many operations and variations in technique have been described but there is no doubt that the best results are obtained in units where such operations are performed frequently. Operative and postoperative mortality quoted in the literature varies around 10–15 per cent. Some centres quote much lower figures than this, no doubt as a result of a combination of management expertise and rigorous case selection. Operative and mortality is largely related to cardiopulmonary complications, including sepsis, and anastomotic leakage. Intensive and expert postoperative support, including ventilation where indicated, is an important factor in reducing surgical mortality.

MIDDLE THIRD LESIONS

The precise type of surgical procedure carried out varies according to surgeon and centre, but in the UK the two-stage technique of Ivor Lewis is favoured by many. In the first stage of the operation, the stomach is approached through an upper abdominal incision and is mobilized; in stage II, the oesophagus is approached through a right 5th interspace thoracotomy for dissection and resection of the tumour. A margin of approximately 8 cm on either side of the tumour is desirable. Continuity of the oesophageal remnant and the mobilized stomach is restored by anastomosis, which is carried out by hand, or with a staple gun, according to preference.

LOWER THIRD LESIONS

Surgery is the preferred approach for lesions of the lower third. A left thoracoabdominal incision allows access for mobilization of the stomach, resection of tumour and fashioning of the anastomosis.

Orringer's operation is carried out via a laparotomy and a cervical incision. The mobilized stomach is relocated by a pull-through procedure, and the anastomosis fashioned. The technique requires considerable expertise but is favoured by its exponents.

UPPER THIRD LESIONS

Surgical resection is not generally considered possible for the majority of cases. Palliation is best achieved with radiation therapy.

Where surgical resection is attempted, it involves pharyngolaryngectomy with total oesophagectomy and reconstruction. This is very major, arduous, and hazardous surgery and can be justified only for cases that have undergone the most careful selection, and where suitable surgical and supportive care expertise is available.

Radical surgical resection and reconstruction

This can be done by dissection and *en bloc* removal of the posterior mediastinum, with transposed stomach or colon being used to restore continuity of the alimentary tract. There is a serious danger of leakage from the colonic anastomoses or from sloughing of the transposed colon owing to ischaemia. The highest mortality from oesophageal surgery is encountered in association with this kind of resection but the operation does allow the possibility of achieving radical clearance of the tumour and associated lymph nodes. Lymphadenectomy forms part of the procedure, with two-field and three-field lymphadenectomy procedures, the latter providing superior results. It also allows the most definitive method of surgical staging. An alternative resection technique involves resection without thoracotomy. This operation has a lower postoperative mortality but is more likely to give inadequate resection margins. Unforeseen lateral tumour extension into great vessels can make this operation a disastrous undertaking and it is generally favoured more in the USA than in the UK.

Radical radiation therapy

This carries a lower mortality than surgery, but is, nevertheless, associated with significant morbidity. Tumours of the upper and middle oesophagus are most suited to this approach. Tumours of the lower third are best approached surgically. The limited tolerance of the upper portion of the stomach (about 40 Gy in 2-Gy fractions), together with the high probability of infradiaphragmatic spread, make a radical radiotherapeutic approach unrealistic. As with surgery, careful selection of patients for radical treatment is of great importance. Many patients are dehydrated and malnourished and will be able to withstand treatment better following palliative dilatation and pre-treatment preparation. Treatment planning must encompass all the tumour and draining lymph nodes if it is to stand a chance of being successful.

In order to determine an adequate treatment volume, all possible information about location and extent of the tumour must be obtained from endoscopy, plain and contrast X-rays (*see* Fig. 23.4) and CT scans, if available. Screening of a contrast swallow under direct vision often gives a truer appreciation of the extent of the tumour than hard copy films alone. Planning is carried out using a simulator with fluoroscopy, or with the help of a CT planning system. Calculation of isodose distribution is usually carried out by a dedicated radiation therapy planning computer. Current computerized planning systems and multileaf collimators allow conformal volumes to be planned where appropriate.

POSITIONING OF PATIENT

Patients are planned supine, with hands on or behind the head in order to keep the arms clear of posterior oblique treatment portals. Careful positioning with the spine as straight as possible will greatly help planning and treatment, by keeping the spinal cord out of the high-dose treatment volume throughout its length. Positioning is assisted by means of standard bolsters, which are carefully recorded so that an identical set-up can be achieved on the treatment machine.

A sip of thin contrast is given and the patient asked to retain it, swallowing under fluoroscopic control. The track of the contrast bolus will give an assessment of the location and functional extent of the tumour and will allow a centre corresponding with the centre of the obstructed oesophageal segment to be identified. If a CT scan is used for planning purposes, it is likewise important that the patient is scanned in the treatment position. It is often easier to obtain optimal bolstering by simulation before placing the patient on the scanner to ensure that the spinal cord remains parallel with the long axis of the treatment field.

Neither contrast swallow, CT scan, nor any other diagnostic technique will detect submucosal spread, which may extend well beyond the apparent tumour and which may be discontinuous with the main tumour bulk. The only way to attempt to treat submucosal spread is to use unusually large field margins and to treat at least 5 cm of apparently uninvolved oesophagus cranially and caudally (Fig. 23.5). It should be noted that recommended margins for radical surgery are somewhat greater, 8 cm in either direction.

In practical terms, this means that the treatment volume will never be less than 14 cm long, even for early lesions. Lateral margins must include mediastinal and hilar nodes, setting the lateral borders of the treatment volume about 8 cm apart. The AP diameter of the treatment volume is determined by lateral simulation and should allow for the changing position of the oesophagus relative to the spinal column as it progresses through the thorax. It is most important that the treatment volume does not encroach on the cord, since treatment must be to a dose in the region of 60 Gy – well beyond cord tolerance. Avoiding the cord can present considerable practical problems and meticulous positioning of the patient is

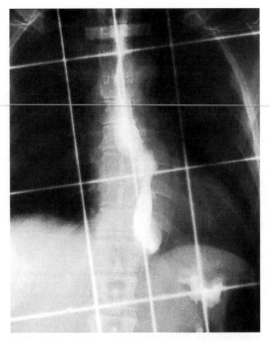

Figure 23.5 *Simulator film showing anterior field limits in the planning of radical treatment to a middle third oesophageal carcinoma.*

the best way of solving them. Angulation of the posterior oblique fields or judicious rotation of the treatment couch are other manoeuvres used to overcome problems of geometry. During simulation, magnification markers are placed so that the treatment volumes defined can be related to field dimensions and so that geometrical planning information, especially with reference to the spinal cord, can be derived. Because of the curvature of the oesophagus, it is necessary to consider the dosimetry throughout the length of the treatment volume. In order to do this, three plans are prepared: a central axis plan and two off-axis plans to provide transverse sectional dose distributions at the upper and lower limit of the treatment volume. These are absolutely essential to ensure that the cord tolerance is not locally exceeded.

Contours are therefore taken at these levels, either manually or with transverse axial tomography and the anatomical information from the planning films, corrected for magnification, is transposed to the contours. The treatment volume is drawn in on the planning films and the spinal cord is shaded throughout its length, using a wax pencil on the planning films. It is important on the planning contour to identify the tumour volume, the spinal cord and the lungs, so that the physicist may apply appropriate corrections for tissue inhomogeneity. A suggested arrangement of fields, typically a plain anterior and two posterior oblique wedged fields, will generally provide a satisfactory dose distribution (Fig. 23.6). The precise angulation and wedge angles are selected to provide the best possible treatment volume isodose distribution, with the minimum possible dose to the spinal cord throughout its length.

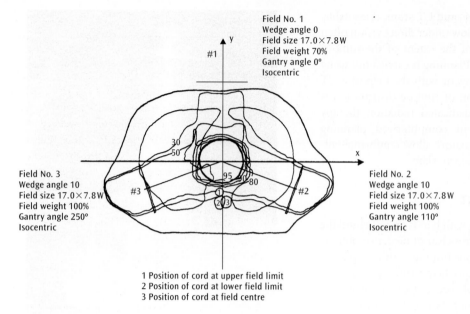

Field No. 1
Wedge angle 0
Field size 17.0×7.8W
Field weight 70%
Gantry angle 0°
Isocentric

Field No. 3
Wedge angle 10
Field size 17.0×7.8W
Field weight 100%
Gantry angle 250°
Isocentric

Field No. 2
Wedge angle 10
Field size 17.0×7.8W
Field weight 100%
Gantry angle 110°
Isocentric

1 Position of cord at upper field limit
2 Position of cord at lower field limit
3 Position of cord at field centre

Figure 23.6 *Classical three-field arrangement used for the second phase of radical treatment of a middle third oesophageal carcinoma. Note the proximity of the spinal cord to the high dose volume at the upper limit of the field (5 MeV Linac). Note the doses to lungs.*

Most centres will now use CT planning systems in preference to the procedure described above. They are rapid and convenient to use and give much better and more comprehensive dosimetry. In defining a treatment volume, the volume decided upon is entered into the planning computer using a light pen, by drawing round the contour to be treated on a CT section. Regions of interest, such as the spinal cord, can be defined for dose calculation. When planning from CT data, it is important to bear in mind that the true extent of the tumour cannot be seen on the CT image. Only limited diagnostic information is available on planning scan images. The volume to be treated should be defined by careful consideration of the extent of the tumour from a synthesis of pre-treatment staging investigations, and the temptation to use a small field with inadequate margins should be resisted. The existence of extensive submucosal spread and lateral extension should always be kept in mind.

Since the field is invariably a long one, care must also be taken to keep lung doses to a minimum. This is best achieved by a three-field plan. Four-field plans have been employed, sometimes with angulations and longitudinal compensation if the contour geometry is complex. A longitudinal contour will allow assessment of longitudinal inhomogeneity and, if there is a steeply sloping contour over the upper chest, it may sometimes be necessary to have a longitudinally wedged anterior field (thick end of wedge at the cranial end of the field) in order to compensate for this. Rotations are not satisfactory, since they irradiate an excessive lung volume and do not usually provide good longitudinal coverage of the treatment volume. Conformal therapy (Tate *et al.*, 1986) has been employed in some centres with suitable equipment which can be made to 'track' a complex volume. In addition to needing special equipment, the planning calculations required for such treatments are extremely specialized, with the advent of multileaf collimators and three-dimensional planning systems, conformal planning techniques are now widely available. Conformal therapy should allow much higher tumour doses to be achieved, with the aim of reducing local recurrence. Local control of tumours is a problem with conventional treatment techniques and dosages, with post-treatment local recurrence developing in around 70 per cent of radiation therapy patients.

A definitive and detailed account of the techniques of radiation therapy planning can be found in Dobbs *et al.* (1999). This is required reading for radiation oncologists treating these conditions.

DOSE AND COMPLICATIONS

Radical treatment of the oesophagus means delivering a dose of 60 Gy in 2-Gy fractions, or the equivalent dose with different fractionation regimens. Split courses are often better tolerated but may be less effective for radiobiological reasons. Continuous, hyperfractionated and accelerated radiotherapy (CHART) techniques are currently being evaluated. Palliative doses are typically 30 Gy in 10 fractions in 14 days, or 27 Gy in six fractions in 14 days (three times weekly). The main complications occur early.

HYBRID TECHNIQUES

These use external beam irradiation for initial treatment, with intracavitary brachytherapy using the Selectron to provide a local high-dose boost to the tumour volume. Careful selection of patients is necessary, since the limited transverse dimension of the high-dose volume means that locally extensive tumours will be irradiated inadequately at depth. Where high radical doses are delivered by such techniques, local control can be good, but at some cost in terms of radiation oesophagitis and stricture formation. The development of these techniques is still in progress, and assessment of their value is at present premature.

COMPLICATIONS OF RADIOTHERAPY

The common complications associated with radiation therapy are as follows.

Radiation oesophagitis

Radiation oesophagitis is common, and develops in the second and third weeks of treatment. It is often perceived by patients as a sensation of obstruction, and varies from a minor symptom to a severe problem. Aspirin and hydrocortisone mucilage, given orally, is usually helpful. Debilitated patients are also at risk of oesophageal candidiasis, which should be treated if oral candidiasis is present or suspected. Nystatin, amphotericin, and miconazole preparations are effective if used generously.

Radiation complications may be considerably exacerbated by concurrent chemotherapy, and caution is advised in circumstances of concurrent treatment, especially with drugs that are known to interact with radiation, such as methotrexate, cisplatin, and 5-fluorouracil (5-FU).

Patients who have diabetes or collagen diseases seem to tolerate radiation therapy relatively poorly. Radiation can sometimes exacerbate problems of nutrition and hydration in patients who are cachectic or debilitated.

Radiation pneumonitis

This may produce a dry cough, even some months after treatment has been completed. It may be precipitated by intercurrent infection. A hazy shadowing, corresponding to the boundaries of the radiation treatment fields, is sometimes seen. It responds promptly to soluble prednisolone (15 mg twice a day) and gradual tapering of the dose after symptoms have been controlled. Patients who experience such problems may have recurrences in response to subsequent infections, and should be advised to seek advice at an early stage if their symptoms recur.

Fistula formation

The most feared complication is that of bronchooesophageal fistula, the result of destruction of tumour which has invaded the tracheobronchial tree. It is not a necrosis of normal tissue due to radiation and is a complication of the disease itself. Tumours thought to be invading in this way should be irradiated with great caution. A fistula, when present, gives rise to the unmistakable symptom of explosive coughing and choking following a sip of water or other fluid. The bronchial tree may outline with thin contrast when this is swallowed and the site of the fistula can sometimes be seen. The formation of a fistula is an indication for intubation. In a similar manner, breakdown of tumour may occur where it is infiltrating large blood vessels with disastrous results and catastrophic haemorrhage.

Such catastrophic haemorrhage is often preceded by one or more minor haemoptyses.

Acute dysphagia

This may occasionally occur where the lumen of the oesophagus becomes further reduced by post-treatment radiation induced swelling. Such cases respond to steroids.

Late complications

Late complications of radical radiation therapy include mediastinal fibrosis and post-radiation stricture. The latter is treated by dilatation. Radiation damage to the spinal cord may occur where tolerance is locally exceeded, usually due to adverse patient geometry. It is very rare with modern planning and dosimetry. Patients treated palliatively with opposed portals may occasionally experience transient radiation myelopathy, with sensations like electric shocks in arms or legs following neck flexion (L'hermitte's sign). These symptoms are generally self-limiting without specific treatment.

Results of treatment

A direct prospective randomized comparison between radiation and surgery has not been carried out in spite of almost equally poor results with either treatment modality. The MRC Working Party on Oesophageal Cancer has proposed a study to address this question. Patients referred for radiation are almost always those who have extensive disease or who are otherwise unfit for surgery. Patients who are fit, and who have limited disease, are usually operated upon. In a review of nearly 84 000 patients culled from 49 papers, Earlam and Cunha-Melo (1980) found a 1-year survival of about 44 per cent, a 2-year survival of about 16 per cent and a 5-year survival of 6 per cent, 6 per cent and 20 per cent in three papers where patients were judged to be broadly comparable to surgical series. Overall survival figures, including large numbers of patients treated for palliation, were 18 per cent at 1 year, 8 per cent at 2 years and 6 per cent at 5 years.

Pearson's classic paper, describing a huge personal series of 1650 patients, quotes a 1-year survival in the region of 44 per cent and a 5-year survival of 22 per cent. These results remain amongst the best published, reflecting unusual expertise in case selection, the importance of which the author stresses. The dose used was in the region of 50 Gy in 27 days. Beatty et al. (1979) reported a substantial series and although they obtained a 2-year survival rate of 21 per cent, there were no 5-year survivors. Newaishy et al. (1982) reported a series of 444 patients in whom an 18 per cent 2-year survival was achieved, with only 9 per cent surviving to the fifth anniversary.

From the literature, it appears that radical radiation therapy can alter the natural history of this disease in a small number of patients and although a direct comparison has not yet been possible, results not unlike those from surgical series have been obtained in a motley population of patients. If new imaging techniques improve case selection, it is likely that future published results will show some improvement for patients treated radically, whilst the results of subradical treatment are likely to remain very poor.

COMBINED MODALITY TREATMENT

Adjuvant and neoadjuvant therapy

There have been many attempts improve the results of surgery by deploying other treatment modalities in an adjuvant or neoadjuvant setting. Although several studies have shown apparently encouraging results, these have not been confirmed by prospective randomized controlled trial. A recent review of the subject (Lehnert, 1999) examined more than 30 prospective randomized trials. No benefit in terms of improved survival was detected with adjuvant chemotherapy or radiotherapy, and in a neoadjuvant setting, no increase in resectability or survival was found, and indeed, postoperative mortality appeared to be increased in the treatment arms.

Preoperative radiation therapy

This has been now been examined by a number of randomized studies including a large EORTC trial in 1987. There was no evident benefit in terms of resectability or survival. All these studies used relatively low doses, however.

Current thinking does not support preoperative radiotherapy as a useful treatment option. The rationale underlying this approach is as follows. In certain circumstances, preoperative radiation therapy appears to improve operability and so it was logical to explore this in the treatment of oesophageal tumours. Various radiation schedules have been employed, but most authors have aimed for a dose in the region of 50 Gy. Much higher doses have been explored, with no apparent benefit, and indeed with a possible detrimental effect. As with other trial data, prospective randomized studies are lacking and many published studies use historical controls.

The Memorial Hospital reports a series of 89 patients (Goodner, 1969), of whom 59 underwent surgery; 47 out of 59 had technically resectable disease and 11.8 per cent died as a result of surgery. Only 3.5 per cent survived for 5 years.

Akakura et al. (1970) reported a series of 346 patients, of whom 229 underwent surgery and 117 had preoperative radiation therapy; 96 patients out of the 117 underwent resection. The group treated by surgery alone ($n = 229$) had a 40 per cent resection rate with an operative mortality of 13 per cent the study was non-randomized.

A paper from Stanford (Doggett et al., 1970) reported a series of 42 patients, of whom 29 underwent surgery. In 7 per cent of patients no tumour was found in the resected specimen. Eight out of 29 patients died postoperatively. Two out of 42 patients survived. Marks et al. (1976) reported 332 patients, of whom 137 underwent surgery: 101/137 were resected, with an operative mortality of 18 per cent; 13 per cent had either no detectable disease

or in-situ changes only. The 5-year survival was 6 per cent overall and 13 per cent for those patients successfully resected.

In a prospective randomized study, the EORTC compared 33 Gy in 12 days, with surgery alone. No significant differences were found in resection rate, operative mortality or survival.

Launois et al. (1981), in a prospective study of 124 patients, used intensive radiation therapy consisting of 40 Gy in 8–12 days and found a 5-year survival of 11.5 per cent in the surgical arm and 9.5 per cent in the group receiving preoperative radiation therapy. Berry et al. (1989) employed intracavitary irradiation with high- and low-dose external beam regimens 15 Gy (ICR) plus 40 Gy or 20–30 Gy. Histological examination of the surgical specimens showed residual tumour in only 1/11 high-dose patients, but in 8/10 low-dose patients. It appears from these and other data that high local doses can provide impressive local control. Survival, however, is usually related to metastasis status.

In summary, there is no doubt that radiation therapy has an effect upon oesophageal tumours in that several series contain a small number of cases in which either no tumour or in-situ change only was found. This effect is not substantially reflected in long-term survival, although some patients who are rendered resectable by preoperative radiation may have a marginally improved survival probability.

When subjected to randomized trial, however, good evidence of benefit is lacking.

Intraoperative and postoperative radiation therapy

The attractions of this approach are that surgical debulking has been carried out, leaving radiation to deal with subclinical disease and hopefully prevent local recurrence. Also, histological information regarding the extent of the disease is available from the resected specimen. In fact, relatively little work has been done on this aspect of treatment. Patients undergoing postoperative radiation therapy are necessarily self-selected since they are, by definition, resectable and have survived the substantial postoperative mortality. There is an understandable reluctance of surgeons to refer these patients (a group containing most of the few long-term survivors) for an additional and unproven treatment modality.

Kasai et al. (1978) reported full-dose postoperative radiation therapy in a small series of patients. Survival benefit was claimed in node-negative patients. Local recurrence was seen in 2/14 patients in the radiation therapy arm, compared with 14/18 in a group who received no such additional therapy. A randomized study by Fok et al. (1993) showed some improved local control without effect on survival. Another, reported by Teniere et al. (1991), showed a similar reduction in local recurrence, again without survival benefit. Lehnert's review, cited above, failed to reveal evidence of benefit, and suggests that postoperative radiation therapy can now be discounted.

A Japanese group has attempted intraoperative radiation therapy using single doses of 25 Gy. Serious complications due to tracheal damage were encountered in a substantial proportion of patients (Arimoto et al., 1993).

Combined modality including radiation, chemotherapy and surgery

Further progress in improving upon the results of surgery alone is now being reported by several groups in studies with substantial numbers of patients. The Duke University group (Wolfe et al., 1993) reported 229 patients in whom surgery was preceded by chemotherapy and radiation therapy. Of these patients 165 proceeded to surgery, and a 5-year survival of 25 per cent was reported. Forty per cent of patients with squamous carcinoma had a pathological complete response, with a 5-year survival for this subset of 40 per cent. Twenty per cent of patients with adenocarcinoma had a pathological complete response, but these patients had a 5-year survival of 60 per cent. It is also interesting to note that some patients who underwent chemotherapy and radiation therapy declined surgical intervention, but nevertheless had a 5-year survival of 18 per cent, a very respectable survival rate for this lethal disease. A Southwestern Oncology Group study (Izquierdo et al., 1993) treated 25 mainly T3 patients with cisplatin plus bleomycin daily for 21 days, followed, after three courses, by radiation therapy to a radical dose. The complete response rate was 16 per cent with 8 per cent surviving more than 4 years.

Matsuda et al. (1992) combined hyperthermia with chemotherapy and radiation therapy, but without surgery, in a small number of patients and reported an impressive complete response rate and long survival for some of their patients.

There is a tempting conclusion to be drawn from many studies of combined modality treatment that it may now be possible significantly to improve local control and long-term survival in some patients by the use of synchronous combined chemoradiotherapy, followed by surgery. Unfortunately, in most of these studies numbers are small and a large-scale randomized and properly controlled study is awaited to confirm or refute these impressions.

What is clear from even the smaller studies is that synchronous chemoradiotherapy has significant toxicity. The Intergroup study (Herskovic et al., 1992; al-Sarraf et al., 1997) demonstrated benefit from a combined chemoradiotherapy approach. However, there are several caveats attached to these conclusions, the improvements in the combined arm being offset by 20 per cent grade 4 toxicity, versus 3 per cent in the radiotherapy alone arm.

In the UK the Medical Research Council (MRC) have recently performed a randomized controlled trial of surgery with or without chemotherapy in potentially respectable patients. The MRC OEO2 study completed recruitment in June 1998 and was reported to participants in January 2001. This trial addressed the question of whether preoperative chemotherapy has a role in the management of respectable oesophageal carcinoma. A total of 802 patients were randomized to receive two preoperative chemotherapy cycles, 3 weeks apart, or alternatively to proceed to surgical resection without chemotherapy. Resection was considered complete in 84 per cent of patients receiving chemotherapy plus surgery, compared with 71 per cent in the surgery alone group. Postoperative complications and mortality were similar in the trial arms. Median survival, overall survival, and survival at 2 years were all superior for the chemotherapy plus surgery arm.

The median survival for the combined arm was 17.4 months versus 13.4 months for surgery alone. Two-year survival rates were 45 per cent and 35 per cent, respectively. Progression-free survival benefit was superior in the combined arm with $P < 0.001$.*

This important and rigorously designed trial confirms significant improvement of survival in respectable patients, without incurring additional serious adverse events, and preoperative chemotherapy should now be considered for all patients satisfying the clinical criteria of respectability. The chemotherapy regimen employed in this study was cisplatin 80 mg/m^2 by 4-hour infusion on day 1, 5-FU 1 g/m^2 per day continuous infusion for 4 days, cycle = 21 days, number of cycles = 2.

At least one study appears to show increased complication rates and decreased survival for the combined modality arm (Neuhaus et al., 1992). The chemotherapy regimen used in this study, while having an appreciable objective response rate, proved to be more toxic than anticipated. When considering combined treatment, the general condition of the patient and the ability to withstand the treatment regimen must be given the most careful consideration.

Brachytherapy as single agent and as a combined modality

Intraluminal brachytherapy is now a well established palliative treatment which can be given conveniently and safely. A dose of 12 Gy at 1 cm from the central axis is capable of producing useful and durable palliation of dysphagia. A logical step, especially with the advent of high dose-rate (HDR) equipment would be to use brachytherapy to boost the dose to the central axis of the tumour, and perhaps to combine this with concurrent

---

*The author is indebted to Dr D. Girling and the MRC for permission to publish these results as a personal communication.

chemotherapy. The latter approach was explored by RTOG in protocol 92-07 and was found to produce a very high incidence of serious and potentially life-threatening toxicity (Gaspar et al., 1997b).

Guidelines for the use of brachytherapy have been published by the Clinical Research Committee of the American Brachytherapy Society. These suggest the following conditions and regimens for optimal use of this modality. It should be borne in mind that trials to define optimal regimens continue, and there will undoubtedly be further developments in the field.

As part of radical or combined modality treatment with 5-FU, in unifocal lesions of 10 cm or less of the thoracic oesophagus, following 45–50 Gy external-beam treatment, brachytherapy may be given either as two fractions of 5 Gy each at weekly intervals (HDR) or a single fraction of 20 Gy (low dose rate; LDR). Brachytherapy should be given after external-beam therapy has been completed, and should not be given concurrently with chemotherapy.

As a single palliative modality, 15–20 Gy in two to four fractions (HDR) or 25–40 Gy (LDR) in two to four fractions may be given. In the UK, doses of 12–15 Gy in a single fraction have proved effective in palliating symptoms. Dosimetry conventions define the prescribed dose as that dose measured at 1 cm from the central axis at the mid-source point in a uniformly loaded source train. LDR defines dose rates at 1 cm from the source train as 0.4–1 Gy/h (Gaspar et al., 1997a).

A patient series reported by Hareyama et al. (1992) demonstrates that brachytherapy can boost local doses to provide encouraging results in patients with very localized disease. The problem is that these patients are rare in Western populations. As part of palliative treatment, suitable doses are 10–14 Gy in a single fraction (HDR) or 20–24 Gy (LDR) can be employed in conjunction with external-beam treatment of 30 Gy (fractionated).

Chemotherapy

Carcinoma of the oesophagus is undoubtedly chemosensitive, with appreciable response rates to several cytotoxic agents, notably cisplatin and 5-FU (Iizuka et al., 1992). Responses are seldom complete, however, and when they occur, are generally not durable, lasting only for an average of 8–10 weeks. While enthusiasm for chemotherapy as the sole treatment for this tumour is not great, early published data suggested that chemotherapy might be of significant value when combined with surgery and radiation therapy.

Several studies of combined modality treatment have shown histological absence of tumour in the surgical specimen, with possible survival benefit in these patients. Metastatic disease remains the major problem, and while local control is improved with survival benefit for a subset of patients with localized disease, the majority of patients with frank or occult metastatic disease at presentation are destined to have a much lower survival. When submitted to prospective randomized controlled trial, benefit appears to be illusory, and preoperative chemotherapy may be related to inferior therapeutic results. Although other studies give conflicting results, at this time a good case for neoadjuvant chemotherapy cannot be supported.

As may be seen above, the literature is extensive, and frequently conflicting. A thoughtful and conservative review of current opinion is found in Price et al. (1998), and a detailed review of trials in Lehnert (1999).

PALLIATIVE MEASURES

The easiest and safest palliative measure is simple dilatation of the oesophageal lumen. This is done with a variety of patterns of dilator, usually graduated metal olives or tapering mercury bougies. The procedure can be repeated many times but provides relatively short-lived palliation, usually for a matter of a few weeks.

Dilatation is often part of diagnostic endoscopy, which many patients subsequently regard as an effective therapeutic event. The technique is effective where only a short length of oesophagus is obstructed; obstruction of appreciable length is best treated by intubation.

Intubation has been used with good effect for many years, but has now been superseded by the use of self-expanding stents.

Intubation carries a significant mortality, of up to 20 per cent in some series, usually following oesophageal perforation during placement of the tube. Intubation is unsuitable for tumours of the upper thoracic and cervical oesophagus. Tubes are not well tolerated at these sites and are liable to become displaced. Stenting is now the preferred technique.

Oesophagectomy without thoracotomy has been practised as a palliative measure. Mortality from this operation runs in the region of 15 per cent, although in experienced hands it drops to 7 per cent (Sugimachi et al., 1986). Complications arise when the tumour is more locally extensive than anticipated and the dissection tears mediastinal great vessels or the tracheobronchial tree.

Radiation therapy may be employed to provide palliation of obstructing oesophageal tumours at all sites. It has the advantage of being non-invasive, safe and providing reasonably durable palliation of symptoms in a high proportion of patients. About 70 per cent of patients will achieve palliation lasting for more than 2 months and the average duration of palliation of symptoms is of the order of 6 months (Wara et al., 1976). This will, of course, carry many patients through the remaining course of their illness (Beatty et al., 1979). Palliation is often achieved with relatively low doses of 30 Gy in 10 fractions in 2 weeks but occasionally high doses requiring the use of planned

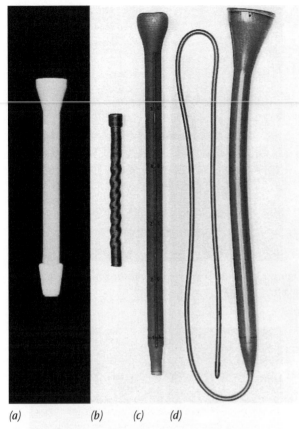

(a)   *(b)*   *(c)*   *(d)*

Figure 23.7 *Oesophageal tubes used for palliation of dysphagia. (a) Atkinson; (b) Souttar; (c) Celestin; (d) Mousseau-Barbin tubes.*

fields must be used. Where there is a threat of tumour necrosis leading to fistula, radiation is best avoided or used with protracted fractionation. This complication is unavoidable in a small number of cases, but awareness of the problem will minimize the likelihood of it developing.

Symptomatic recurrence of tumour following tolerance radiation therapy is best managed by dilatations or intubation. It may occasionally be necessary to exceed normal concepts of radiation tolerance in the hope of palliating intractable and distressing symptoms. Palliation of advanced disease also includes apparently mundane matters such as dietary advice, which can do much to enable patients to remain in the home environment for as long as possible. This should include emphasis on the importance of maintaining hydration and liquidizing foods. Various dietetic measures can be employed to give liquidized foods greater attractiveness and variety, this being of considerable practical importance to patients who may have to live on such a diet for many months.

Pain may occasionally be a problem, the basic principles of palliation as for other tumours being applicable. Locally painful metastases may be relieved with local radiation therapy. Incomplete control may be supplemented with analgesic drugs, which, of course, must be in a formulation which the dysphagic patient can cope with. Opioid mixtures are sometimes poorly tolerated.

In such instances, the drugs can usefully be given by small volume subcutaneous injection, or by continuous pump-driven infusion. Oxycodone (30 mg) suppositories or topical Fentanyl patches (25, 50, 75, 100 μg/h) are valuable for durable pain control the latter having the advantage of a 72-hour duration of action. Systemic steroids in high doses can be of great value in improving well-being and in the relief of pain from liver metastases. Doses of at least 20 mg soluble prednisolone twice daily, and often doses greater than this, are customarily employed.

Palliation of symptoms is always worth working on. Some patients can be restored sufficiently to return home for a considerable time, even though the eventual outcome of their disease is inevitable. In recent years, new techniques offering rapid and apparently safe palliation have been developed. These are discussed under 'Future trends', below.

Palliative radiation therapy

Radiation can provide effective palliation in all but the moribund. Since the aim of treatment is to relieve symptoms, there is by definition no indication for palliative radiation in the absence of symptoms. The simplest technique consistent with effective treatment is the use of opposed fields directed to irradiate the obstructed section of oesophagus. Good palliation can be achieved with a relatively low dose such as 30 Gy in 10 fractions in 2 weeks but it may sometimes be necessary to employ a higher dose to achieve results. Although it has been said in the past that lower third oesophageal tumours are resistant to radiation therapy, there is no good evidence that this is so, and palliative treatment can be very rewarding. The one major caveat regarding palliative radiotherapy is the suspected existence of a tracheo-oesophageal fistula. This was formerly considered a contraindication and if radiation therapy is carried out, caution is necessary. Such cases should be considered for palliative intubation or stenting with consideration of palliative radiotherapy after completion of such procedures.

Palliative surgery – intubation, stenting, and laser treatment

The principal palliative surgical procedures are dilatation and intubation. Various patterns of dilator and oesophageal tube are available. Dilatation with mercury bougies or graduated dilators can provide rapid palliation of symptoms. Though a definite morbidity is associated with all these procedures, they remain relatively safe in experienced hands. The major complications encountered are perforation and splitting of the stenosed segment.

Intubation is a long established procedure, now replaced by stenting, and involves the insertion of one of several patterns of tube designed to restore a usable lumen.

The original tubes were of natural materials, such as decalcified ivory, but have evolved with modern materials technology into different patterns, with devices to facilitate insertion and retention, and to avoid displacement. Intubation can only be used for lesions of the middle and lower oesophagus. The tubes are inserted by pulsion techniques, or by 'pull-through' techniques from below. There is a significant mortality associated with attempted intubation. Tube insertion often gives good palliation, although some patients will only be able to manage semi-solids. Patients with tubes need to be advised as to which foods should be avoided and how to prepare food in order to minimize the possibility of blockage. Where a fistula has developed, tube or stent insertion is more hazardous but is the only real way of reducing the tracheo-oesophageal leak. Although patients in whom a fistula has developed have very poor survival prospects, the symptoms they have are so distressing that a palliative measure is justifiable. The main complications encountered with tubes are as follows.

Dilatation and endoscopy may be associated with perforation and oesophageal splitting. Obstruction of the tube may occur and may require intervention. The most serious complications are displacement and perforation, and different designs have been contrived in an attempt to minimize these risks. Perforation requires the removal of the tube. In extreme cases, a short course of radiation treatment may allow subsequent dilatation and elective placement of a tube, which would otherwise have been impossible.

Stenting of obstructive neoplasms has proved to be a rapid and effective palliative measure and is now the preferred surgical palliative technique. Various types of stent have been devised, the commonest consisting of a coated wire mesh tube or an expanding helical spring. Stents can sometimes migrate, or give rise to pain and may need to be repositioned or revised to relieve these problems. Perhaps the commonest problem encountered is re-obstruction by tumour re-growth above, below, or sometimes through the stent. Plastic covered stents (Fig. 23.8) have a tendency to migrate, while uncovered stents are prone to obstruction by regrowth of tumour through the mesh. Tumour frequently grows over the entrance to oesophageal tubes, and sometimes a stent can successfully be inserted to relieve the obstruction (Fig. 23.9). Patients with stents need to be aware of the possibility of acute obstruction by food material, and should receive appropriate advice to minimize this possibility.

Laser photohistolysis with a YAG laser can rapidly relive obstruction, but unfortunately palliation is variable in degree, and usually of very short duration.

Alcohol injection into tumour masses can be carried out at endoscopy, and in appropriately skilled hands is a safe procedure, but palliation is typically of short duration, usually 3–4 weeks, and similar to laser treatment. It should be remembered that any instrumentation of the oesophagus carries significant risk, so short-duration treatments carry a cost in terms of morbidity and

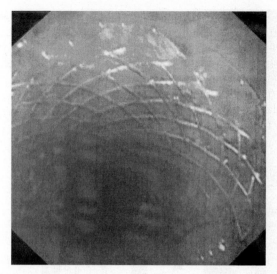

Figure 23.8 *Endoscopic view of plastic covered stent in-situ.*

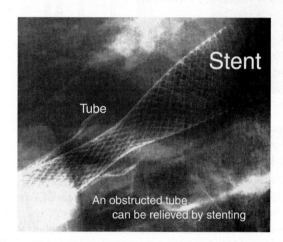

Figure 23.9 *Palliative stenting of obstructed Atkinson tube.*

mortality, which has to be set against the palliation obtained.

General palliation

Correction of nutritional deficiencies and anaemia makes patients feel better. Pain control is important and local radiation therapy to the mediastinum can provide good relief of pain due to mediastinal invasion. Painful bone metastases can be treated successfully with a single treatment of 8–10 Gy. Painful liver metastases are best treated with steroids and analgesics. Hepatic radiation has been used, with good palliation of pain, but at the cost of post-radiation nausea. It may occasionally merit consideration, and when given, is delivered in small fractions of 0.75–1 Gy, with steroid and chlorpromazine cover. A total dose of 6–8 Gy is generally used. The importance of regular analgesia must be stressed to the patient and alternative routes of administration, such as continuous subcutaneous infusion, are especially useful.

Steroids are often of great value in these patients and have the effect of improving well-being and allaying symptoms. Soluble prednisolone 15–20 mg twice daily is safe and effective. Many of these patients will benefit from continuing care in the later stages of the disease and there is much to be said for involving continuing care staff at a relatively early stage so that they are familiar to the patient by the time hospice admission becomes necessary.

COMPLICATIONS OF TREATMENT

Surgery

In addition to the hazards attendant upon major surgery in very sick and debilitated patients, the main surgical complications are as follows.

OESOPHAGEAL PERFORATION

This may occur following any attempt at instrumentation, even in the most experienced hands. It is best managed conservatively, with antibiotics and parenteral steroids, but is associated with a high mortality if frank mediastinitis supervenes. The risk of perforation is high, perhaps 15 per cent with every instrumentation procedure.

FISTULA FORMATION

Formation of a fistula may occur spontaneously, or following instrumentation or radiation therapy. It is a complication of the disease rather than the treatment. Management is generally by placement of a tube across the fistula in an attempt to seal the leak between oesophagus and airways. The procedure is not without hazard, most series carrying a very appreciable mortality following the procedure. Without a tube, however, the length of survival is very short, patients succumbing with very distressing symptoms. The pulsion technique is generally preferred if the procedure has to be undertaken.

ANASTOMOTIC LEAKAGE

Such leakage may occur following surgery and is managed conservatively.

CARDIOPULMONARY PROBLEMS

These are a major cause of death in surgical series, usually related to overwhelming infection. Patient preparation and careful case selection will reduce this factor as much as possible.

Radiation therapy

Early complications include radiation oesophagitis, generally seen after the second and third weeks of treatment and manifested as a recurrence of painful dysphagia. Topical analgesics such as mucaine may he helpful and can be used on a regular basis. Anti-inflammatory preparations such as aspirin and hydrocortisone mucilage are often very effective and should be used freely. Patients may need advice as to which foods to avoid in order to minimize symptoms until the radiation reaction subsides. Liquidized, bland, milk-based foods are preferred. Bread, meat and spicy or acidic foods are usually best avoided.

The extensive fields necessary to treat these tumours include an appreciable volume of lung and may produce a radiation pneumonitis; this may occur as an early or a delayed event following treatment.

The symptoms of radiation pneumonitis arc a dry, irritating, non-productive cough, sometimes associated with fever. A chest X-ray may demonstrate a paramediastinal haze corresponding to and bounded by the limits of the radiation fields. A rapid response to soluble prednisolone 10–20 mg twice daily is generally obtained. Following resolution, steroids should be reduced with caution. Interruption of radiation treatment may be necessary to allow symptoms to subside.

Nausea, sometimes with vomiting, is a problem during treatment. Minor symptoms may be controlled with anti-emetics such as metoclopramide or chlorpromazine. Treatment may also have to be suspended temporarily.

Fistula formation or erosion of a major blood vessel may develop catastrophically where a locally extensive tumour breaks down following treatment. The only steps that can be taken to minimize the likelihood of this are to attempt to identify patients at risk beforehand and, if radiation therapy has to be used, to proceed with caution and prolonged fractionation. Late complications following radiation therapy consist mainly of oesophageal strictures. These may, on rare occasions, develop surprisingly early, within the first 3 or 4 months following treatment, but most patients do not survive long enough to experience late complications. Where stricture does occur, it can be treated by dilatation, repeatedly if necessary.

Spinal cord damage is more a theoretical risk than a real one, partly because of the low survival time and mainly because radiation planning techniques keep the total dose delivered to the cord within accepted tolerance, i.e. 40 Gy in fractions not greater than 2 Gy each.

As with surgery, respiratory complications, including aspiration, are a major cause of morbidity and mortality. Most clinicians feel that complications are minimized in patients who are prepared prior to treatment by improving nutritional and pulmonary status as far as possible. Incidental conditions such as candidiasis should not be forgotten and are very commonly present in these patients. At post-mortem examination, evidence of *Candida* infection in the oesophageal mucosa is extremely common. Antifungal agents such as nystatin suspension, amphotericin B lozenges and miconazole gel should be offered if *Candida* infection is a possibility.

Follow-up visits should be scheduled to allow early identification of recurrent symptoms and allow further palliative measures to be introduced.

FUTURE TRENDS

The literature of oesophageal cancer is bedevilled by lack of data from prospectively randomized and numerically adequate series. Selection effects are hard to avoid and obscure interpretation of trial results. Full appraisal of the value of combined modality treatment cannot be made without such data, although it does appear unlikely that the results of radical treatment will change much using currently available techniques. Better imaging and patient selection will allow identification of patients at least risk from surgical intervention, though technical changes alone are unlikely to make much further impression on operative mortality. Improved palliation techniques, however, may have much to offer in optimizing quality of life with relatively little risk of morbidity. Two new techniques are currently under evaluation.

Intracavitary radiation therapy

Techniques of intracavitary therapy are certainly not new. Historically, radium bougies were described by Lederman and Clarkson in 1945. The dose administered was 12 000 röntgens (R) (3.12 C/kg), 200 R/h, 60 hours of treatment in 15 days. The bougie contained 75 mg radium-226 and, as can be imagined, staff were exposed to a degree which would now be unacceptable. Other radionuclides were used subsequently, such as gold-198, which was applied by wrapping it round a Souttar's tube. Lederman (1966), in a later paper, describes the use of this technique to deliver a dose of 3000–5500 R at 0.5 cm. Once again, staff exposure was a (largely unrecognized) problem. Tantalum and iridium wire have also been used, in specially designed applicators. More recently, remote after-loading systems have become available which are capable of delivering a locally high dose to oesophageal tumours. Rowland and Pagliero (1985) described a technique using a remote afterloading system (Selectron; Nucletron Trading, B.V., Holland) to deliver a source train of caesium spheres to a specially designed applicator, which is placed intraluminally spanning the oesophageal tumour. The technique is reasonably straightforward (Fig. 23.10). After dilatation, a guide-wire is passed under endoscopic control. The upper and lower extent of the tumour are defined and a Selectron applicator negotiated past the tumour. The intra-oesophageal catheter is fixed in position and the patient connected to the Selectron in the treatment suite. The Selectron can be made to assemble a source train of varying length and activity by selecting active caesium-137 spheres and spacing them with inert metal spheres. These are then driven pneumatically

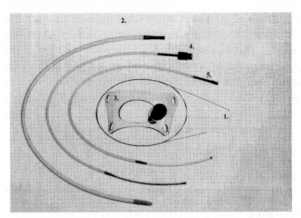

Figure 23.10 *Selectron oesophageal applicator set. In order of insertion: 1, guide-wire; 2, applicator (via guide-wire); 3, retainer mask; 4, dummy source train (X-ray to adjust position); 5, Selectron source carrier.*

down a flexible tube into the applicator. Since the procedure is carried out remotely, this afterloading technique involves no exposure of staff. If treatment is interrupted, the source train is immediately withdrawn into the Selectron safe until staff have reset the machine. Treatment times are typically in the region of 1.14 hours to deliver a dose of 15 Gy at 1 cm from the central axis (Rowland and Pagliero, 1985). A high degree of palliation has been reported using this technique. An obvious further application of this technique is in the treatment of successful resected patients and, hopefully, data from such studies will be forthcoming in due course.

Although the author prefers to carry out catheter placement under a light general anaesthetic, the technique can be used as an outpatient procedure under local anaesthesia or mild sedation. The dose distribution provided by the technique overcomes many practical problems encountered when delivering treatment to a radical dose by external beam techniques. An important limitation, however, is the transverse dimension of the high-dose volume, as many tumours will be found to have extended beyond the confines of a 2-cm diameter treatment envelope.

Flores *et al.* (1989) reported the results of combined intra-cavitary and external-beam treatment in 171 evaluable patients from a series of 211 patients, 131 of whom had T3 tumours. Complications reported by the group include radiation oesophagitis, which was moderate in 27 patients and severe in 25. Ninety-seven of the 171 patients (57 per cent) had complete restoration of swallowing for solids, 154 (90 per cent) had improved swallowing lasting for 3 or more months and 60 (35 per cent) required dilatations later. At 3-year follow-up, five of 26 evaluable patients survived, and at 2-year follow-up 14 of 55 evaluable patients survived. All patient with metastases succumbed within 8 months. A small number of this series subsequently underwent surgical resection of their tumours. Of these 26 patients, only four had macroscopic evidence of residual tumour. These data suggest that local control of limited tumours is an attainable goal with adequate primary treatment.

Hareyama *et al.* (1993) reported the results of treatment with a combination of external-beam radiation therapy and intra-cavitary irradiation in 161 patients, which resulted in a complete response rate of 53 per cent. At 5-year follow-up, local control was maintained in 32 per cent with 43 per cent in those patients who were stages I and II. Five patients developed radiation-related strictures and the authors suggest that radiation tolerance for their technique is close to their protocol dose of 55 Gy in 22 fractions plus two or three insertions totalling 15–2 0 Gy brachytherapy dose. By any standards these results are impressive, and there is now a real prospect of improving local control of early tumours.

Laser photohistolysis

Laser therapy has obvious advantages in this site. It is precise, haemostatic and can be performed non-invasively under direct endoscopic vision. As in obstructive bronchial lesions, laser debulking of oesophageal lesions has been reported to have immediate palliative value (Fleischer and Sivak, 1985). As further centres gain experience of the technique, it will be possible to assign it an appropriate place in palliative treatment strategies. Laser therapy can also be used to allow a more comprehensive clearance of tumour obstructing the oesophageal lumen.

Neodymium yttrium–aluminium–garnet (NdYAG) lasers (Pilkington Fibrelase 100) are capable of providing highly controllable pulses of laser energy. These are ideally suited for endoscopic use via specially designed optical fibres. Obstructing tumours are vaporized under direct vision, either in an antegrade or retrograde manner, using pulses of laser energy. At a power setting of 80–100 W, 2000–7000 J of energy is delivered per treatment session. The optical fibre also carries a low-power laser-aiming beam to enable precise resections to be carried out. Operators describe various technical problems, such as the need to keep the fibre tip clean in order to avoid damage. It is also possible to damage the endoscope if the laser is inexpertly applied, resulting in operator, rather than patient, morbidity.

Evaluation of these techniques has been carried out (Fleischer and Sivak, 1985) and the value of the technique has been established, although further data are required to define its place in the treatment of these tumours. In 60 patients with oesophagogastric cancer treated by Fleischer, 48/60 were rendered capable of eating most or all food after treatment. A further eight patients previously unable to eat solids were enabled to do so, although they could not manage every type of solid food. Poor results were obtained in four patients, three of whom developed perforations. The rapidity of treatment and advantages in reducing the hospitalization have a substantial cost–benefit attraction and it is likely that the technique will find a much wider application as the equipment becomes more generally available.

One drawback of laser treatment is that relief of symptoms appears to be of rather short duration, typically 2–3 months, after which it may be necessary to attempt to repeat the treatment. Laser treatment has been combined with radiation therapy in an effort to make responses more durable. In one such study, Sargeant (1992) combined laser treatment with high- and low-dose radiation therapy. The optimum dose regimen in this small series was the low-dose 30-Gy regimen, which allowed 14 of 16 patients to maintain dysphagia of grade 2 or less for the remainder of their lives. The results of a more extensive study by this group will help to determine whether this approach is, indeed, of value.

Photodynamic therapy (PDT)

This form of treatment is currently under evaluation but in entering clinical use for the treatment of Barrett's dysplasia. It is also applicable in cases of low bulk carcinoma as a palliative intervention. The procedure involves the administration of a drug that undergoes photochemical change to a cytotoxic species when irradiated with light of an appropriate wavelength. The photosensitizers most commonly used at the present time are Photophrin (Ipsen Ltd.) and Aminolaevulinic acid (ALA). These agents produce generalized sensitivity to light following administration, which is rather greater for Photophrin than for ALA, and of longer duration. It may be necessary to protect patients from exposure to strong light for from several days to a week following each injection. ALA is metabolized to Protoporphyrin IX, which is the active agent, and is felt to have milder systemic photosensitivity. However, there is some evidence that photosensitizers may also differ in their effectiveness (Tomaselli *et al.*, 2001).

The drug is given prior to the procedure (40 hrs for Photophrin, 4–6 hrs for ALA). The volume to be treated is identified endoscopically, and illuminated using a cylindrical applicator, with a suitable laser, delivering energy in the range of 100–300 J/cm at a wavelength (for Photophrin) of 630 nm. Other wavelengths are sometimes used with different photosensitizers. The drug then undergoes a photochemical change resulting in the liberation of highly reactive free singlet oxygen which has a cytotoxic effect on cells. Because the laser irradiation is local, and controlled, such treatment can be given with some precision, and dysplastic epithelium can, in many cases, be eliminated. What is less clear is whether such treatment can prevent the future development of malignant change in patients with high-grade dysplasia, and for the present it should only be considered an alternative to surgery in low-grade dysplastic lesions. Careful subsequent follow-up is extremely important. (Ackroyd *et al.*, 2000; Barr *et al.*, 2001).

This form of treatment is in active development, with new photosensitizers, lasers, and fractionation schedules under active evaluation. At this time it can be regarded as a safe procedure for the treatment of low-grade Barrett's dysplasia (Brown *et al.*, 2000) and for the palliation of selected patients with obstructing oesophageal cancer (Luketich *et al.*, 2000).

A variety of complications of photodynamic therapy have been reported including oesophagitis, strictures, abscess formation and sunburn. It may have a particular role in upper oesophageal tumours and other tumours which cannot satisfactorily be stented.

PDT may carry an increased risk of complications in patients who have previously been treated with radiation or chemotherapy (Sanfilippo *et al.*, 2001).

CONCLUSIONS

Poor results are still obtained from attempts at radical treatment of advanced oesophageal cancer. Therapeutic advances, albeit modest, are being made in terms of exploiting combined modality treatment to improve local control. The Selectron and the laser have now established themselves as practical and valuable local treatments, and larger prospective studies will more clearly define their place in combined modality radical treatment, as well as in palliation of symptoms. Early detection should improve results, but is unlikely to become practicable in Western populations. Increased awareness of reflux-associated risk factors, especially Barrett's epithelium, will allow early treatment of high-risk patients. Brush cytology combined with the techniques of molecular biology may develop to form diagnostic tests of predictive value in identifying patients before frankly invasive malignant transformation has occurred. Advances in imaging and non-invasive tumour staging will allow improved selection of treatments for patients. The greatest problem is still that of metastatic disease and for this there are, as yet, no satisfactory treatments available. Patients with advanced disease now have more rapid and effective palliative treatments, particularly endocavitary brachytherapy, intubation and laser debulking. The timing and deployment of these, together with medical symptom control and nutritional support, can greatly improve the quality of life for these unfortunate people.

SIGNIFICANT POINTS

- Very few patients are suitable for radical treatment.
- Non-invasive imaging tends to underestimate disease.

- Progress has been made in improving local control, but metastatic disease remains a major obstacle.
- The use of combined modality treatment is showing some promise, but patients should be entered into trials to resolve the place of this approach to treatment.
- The use of the Selectron and the laser should be considered in the management of selected patients. These modalities can provide rapid palliation of symptoms.
- The Selectron cannot effectively treat bulk disease which extends beyond the high-dose envelope. If the Selectron is to be employed as part of radical treatment, this should be borne in mind.

KEY REFERENCES

Berry, B., Miller, R.R., Luoma, A., Nelems, B., Hay, J. and Flores, A. (1989) Pathologic findings in total esophagectomy specimens after intracavitary and external beam radiotherapy. *Cancer* **64**, 1833–7.

Darnell, J., Lodish, H. and Baltimore, D. (1990) *Molecular biology of the cell*. Scientific American Books.

Dobbs, J., Barrett, A. and Ash, D. (1999) *Practical radiotherapy planning*, 3rd edn. London: Arnold.

Flores, A.D., Nelems, B., Evans, K., Hay, J.H., Stoller, J. and Jackson, S.M. (1989) Impact of new radiotherapy modalities on the surgical management of cancer of the oesophagus and cardia. *Int. J. Radiat. Oncol. Biol. Phys.* **17**, 937–44.

Watson, J.D., Hopkins, N.H., Roberts, J.W., Steitz, I.A. and Weiner, A.M. (1987) *Molecular biology of the gene*. Amsterdam: Benjamin Cummings.

REFERENCES

Ackroyd, R., Brown, N.J., Davis, M.F. *et al.* (2000) Photodynamic therapy for dysplastic Barrett's oesophagus: a prospective double blind, randomised, placebo controlled trial. *Gut* **47**, 612–17.

Akakura, I., Kakegawa, T. and Watanabe, H. (1970) Surgery of carcinoma of the oesophagus with preoperative radiation. *Chest* **57**, 47–57.

al-Sarraf, M., Martz, K., Herskovic, A. *et al.* (1997) Progress report of combined chemoradiotherapy versus radiotherapy alone in patients with esophageal cancer: an intergroup study. *J Clin Oncol* **15**, 277–84.

Arimoto, T., Takamura, A., Tomita, M., Suzuki, K., Hosokawa, M. and Kaneko, Y. (1993) Intraoperative radiotherapy for esophageal carcinoma – significance of IORT dose for the incidence of fatal tracheal complication. *Int. J. Radiat. Oncol. Biol. Phys.* **27**, 1063–7.

Attwood, S.E.A., Barlow, A.P., Norris, T.L. and Watson, A. (1992) Barrett's oesophagus – effect of antireflux surgery on symptom control and development of complications. *Br. J. Surg.* **79**, 1050–3.

Barr, H., Shepherd, N.A., Dix, A., Roberts, D.J., Tan, W.C. and Krasner, N. (1996) Eradication of high-grade dysplasia in columnar-lined (Barrett's) oesophagus by photodynamic therapy with endogenously generated protoporphyrin IX [*see* comments]. *Lancet* **348**, 584–5.

Barr, H., Dix, A.J., Kendall, C. and Stone, N. (2001) The potential role of photodynamic therapy in the management of upper gastrointestinal disease. *Aliment. Pharmacol. Ther.* **15**, 311–21.

Beatty, J.D., De Boer, G. and Rider, W.G. (1979) Carcinoma of the oesophagus. Pretreatment assessment, correlation of radiation treatment parameters with survival, and identification and management of radiation treatment failures. *Cancer* **43**, 2254–7.

Bennett, W.P., Hollstein, M.C., Metcalf, R.A. *et al.* (1992) p53 mutation and protein accumulation during multistage human esophageal carcinogenesis. *Cancer Res.* **52**, 6092–7.

Berry, B., Miller, R.R., Luoma, A., Nelems, B. and Flores, A. (1989) Pathologic findings in total esophagectomy specimens after intracavitary and external beam radiotherapy. *Cancer* **64**, 1833–7.

Chow, W.H., Finkle, W.D., McLaughlin, J.K. *et al.* (1995) The relation of gastroesophageal reflux disease and its treatment to adenocarcinomas of the esophagus and gastric cardia. *JAMA* **274**, 474–7.

Clarke, C.A. and McConnell, R.B. (1954) Six cases of carcinoma of the oesophagus occurring in one family. *Br. Med. J.* **2**, 1137–8.

Collard, J.M., Romagnoli, R., Hermans, B.P. and Malaise, J. (1997) Radical esophageal resection for adenocarcinoma arising in Barrett's esophagus. *Am. J. Surg.* **174**, 307–11.

Crespi, M., Bigotti, A., Casale, V. and Grasse, A. (1979) The value of blind abrasive cytology in cancer diagnosis. *Front. Gastrointest. Res.* **5**, 17–20.

DHSS (1983) *On the state of the public health.* London: HMSO.

Dobbs, J., Barrett, A. and Ash, D. (1999) *Practical radiotherapy planning*, 3rd edn. London: Arnold.

Doggett, R.L.S., Guernsey, J.M. and Bagshaw, M.A. (1970) Combined radiation and surgical treatment of carcinoma of the thoracic oesophagus. *Front. Radiat. Ther. Oncol.* **5**, 147–54.

Earlam, R. and Cunha-Melo, J.R. (1980) Oesophageal squamous carcinoma. 1. A critical review of surgery. 2. A critical review of radiotherapy. *Br. J. Surg.* **57**, 380–90; 157–61.

Fleischer, D. and Sivak, M.V., Jr (1985) Endoscopic Nd YAG laser therapy as palliation for oesophagogastric cancer. *Gastroenterology* **89**, 8227–31.

Fléjou, J.F., Potet, F., Muzeau, F. *et al.* (1993) Overexpression of p53 protein in Barrett's syndrome with malignant transformation. *J. Clin. Pathol.* **46**, 330–3.

Flores, A.D., Nelems, B., Evans, K., Hay, J.H., Stoller, J. and Jackson, S.M. (1989) Impact of new radiotherapy modalities on the surgical management of cancer of the oesophagus and cardia. *Int. J. Radiat. Oncol. Biol. Phys.* **17**, 937–44.

Fok, M., Law, S., Stipa, F., Cheng, S. and Wong, J. (1993) A comparison of transhiatal and transthoracic resection for oesophageal carcinoma. *Endoscopy* **25**, 660–3.

Galandiuk, S., Herman, R.E., Gassman, J.J. and Cosgrove, D.M. (1986) Cancer of the esophagus: the Cleveland Clinic experience. *Ann. Surg.* **203**, 101–8.

Gardner, M.J., Winter, P.D., Taylor, C.P. and Acheson, F.D. (1983) *An atlas of cancer mortality in England and Wales, 1968–1978.* Chichester: John Wiley & Sons.

Gaspar, L.E., Nag, S., Herskovic, A., Mantravadi, R. and Speiser, B. (1997a) American Brachytherapy Society (ABS) consensus guidelines for brachytherapy of esophageal cancer. Clinical Research Committee, American Brachytherapy Society, Philadelphia. *Int. J. Radiat. Oncol. Biol. Phys.* **38**, 127–32.

Gaspar, L.E., Qian, C., Kocha, W.I., Coia, L.R., Herskovic, A. and Graham, M. (1997b) A phase I/II study of external beam radiation, brachytherapy and concurrent chemotherapy in localized cancer of the esophagus (RTOG 92-07): preliminary toxicity report. *Int. J. Radiat. Oncol. Biol. Phys.* **37**, 593–9.

Giuli, R. and Sancho-Garnier, H. (1986) Diagnostic, therapeutic, and prognostic features of cancers of the esophagus: results of the international prospective study conducted by the OESO group (790 patients). *Surgery* **99**, 614–22.

Goodner, J.T. (1969) Surgical and radiation treatment of cancer of the thoracic oesophagus. *Am. J. Roentgenol.* **105**, 523–8.

Guanrei, Y., He, H., Sungliang, Q. and Yuming, C. (1982) Endoscopic diagnosis of 115 cases of early esophageal carcinoma. *Endoscopy* **114**, 157–61.

Halvorsen, R.A. and Thompson, W.M. (1984) Computed tomographic evaluation of oesophageal carcinoma. *Semin. Oncol.* **11**, 113–26.

Hareyama, M., Nishio, M., Kagami, Y. *et al.* (1992) Intracavitary brachytherapy combined with external-beam irradiation for squamous cell carcinoma of the thoracic esophagus. *Int. J. Radiat. Oncol. Biol. Phys.* **24**, 235–40.

Harper, P.S., Harper, R.M.J. and Howel-Evans, A.W. (1970) Carcinoma of the oesophagus with tylosis. *Q. J. Med.* **34**, 317–33.

Herskovic, A., Martz, K., al-Sarraf, M. *et al.* (1992) Combined chemotherapy and radiotherapy compared with radiotherapy alone in patients with cancer of the esophagus [*see* comments]. *N. Engl. J. Med.* **326**, 1593–8.

Iftikhar, S.Y., James, P.D., Steele, R.J.C., Hardcastle, J.D. and Akinson, M. (1992) Length of Barrett's oesophagus – an important factor in the development of dysplasia and adenocarcinoma. *Gut* **33**, 1155–8.

Iizuka, T., Kakegawa, T., Ide, H. *et al.* (1992) Phase II evaluation of cisplatin and 5-fluorouracil in advanced squamous cell carcinoma of the esophagus – a Japanese Esophageal Oncology Group Trial. *Jpn. J. Clin. Oncol.* **22**, 172–6.

Izquierdo, M.A., Marcuello, E., Desegura, G.G. *et al.* (1993) Unresectable nonmetastatic squamous cell carcinoma of the esophagus managed by sequential chemotherapy cisplatin and bleomycin and radiation therapy. *Cancer* **71**, 287–92.

Jankowski, J., Coghill, G., Hopwood, D. and Wommsley, K.G. (1992) Oncogenes and oncosuppressor gene in adenocarcinoma of the oesophagus. *Gut* **33**, 1033–8.

Kasai, M., Mon, S. and Watanabe, T. (1978) Follow-up results after resection of oesophageal cancer. *World J. Surg.* **2**, 543–51.

Launois, B., Delarue, D. and Campion, J.P. (1981) Preoperative radiotherapy for carcinoma of the oesophagus. *Surg. Gynecol. Obstet.* **153**, 690–2.

Lederman, M. (1966) Carcinoma of the oesophagus with special reference to the upper third. *Br. J. Radiol.* **39**, 193–701.

Lehnert, T. (1999) Multimodal therapy for squamous carcinoma of the oesophagus *Br. J. Surg.* **86**, 727–39.

Luketich, J.D., Christie, N.A., Buenaventura, P.O. *et al.* (2000) Endoscopic photodynamic therapy for obstructing esophageal cancer: 77 cases over a 2-year period. *Surg. Endosc.* **14**, 653–7.

Lundell, L. (1992) Acid suppression in the long-term treatment of peptic stricture and Barrett's oesophagus. *Digestion* **51**(Suppl 1), 49–58.

Marks, R.O., Jr, Scruggs, H.J. and Wallace, K.M. (1976) Pre-operative radiation therapy for carcinoma of the oesophagus. *Cancer* **38**, 84–9.

Matsuda, H., Tsutsui, S., Monita, M. *et al.* (1992) Hyperthermo-chemo-radiotherapy as a definitive treatment for patients with early esophageal carcinoma. *Am. J. Clin. Oncol. – Cancer Clinical Trials* **15**, 509–14.

Menkepluymers, M.B.E., Schoute, N.W., Mulder, A.H. *et al.* (1992) Outcome of surgical treatment of adenocarcinoma in Barrett's oesophagus. *Gut* **33**, 1454–8.

Montesano, R., Hollstein, M. and Hainaut, P. (1996) Genetic alterations in esophageal cancer and their relevance to etiology and pathogenesis: a review. *Int. J. Cancer* **69**, 225–35.

Munoz, N., Crespi, M., Grassi, A. *et al.* (1982) Precursor lesions of oesophageal cancer in high risk populations in Iran and China. *Lancet* **1**, 876–9.

Neuhaus, H., Hoffmann, W., Dittler, H.J., Niedermeyer, H.P. and Classen, M. (1992) Implantation of self-expanding esophageal metal stents for palliation of malignant dysphagia. *Endoscopy* **24**, 405–10.

Newaishy, G.A., Read, G.A., Duncan, W. and Kerr, G.R. (1982) Results of radical radiotherapy of squamous carcinoma of the oesophagus. *Clin. Radiol.* **33**, 347–52.

Pearson, J.G. (1966) The radiotherapy of carcinoma of the oesophagus and post-cricoid region in South East Scotland. *Clin. Radiol.* **17**, 242–57.

Pera, M., Trastek, V.F., Carpenter, H.A., Allen, M.S., Deschamps, C. and Pairolero, P.C. (1992) Barrett's esophagus with high-grade dysplasia: an indication for esophagectomy? *Ann. Thorac. Surg.* **54**, 199–204.

Price, P., Hoskin, P.J., Hutchinson, T. and Stenning, S. (1998) What is the role of radiation-chemotherapy in the radical non-surgical management of carcinoma of the oesophagus? Upper GI Cancer Working Party of the UK Medical Research Council. *Br. J. Cancer* **78**, 504–7.

Rowland, C.G. and Pagliero, K.M. (1985) Intracavitary irradiation in the palliation of carcinomas of the oesophagus and cardia. *Lancet* **2**, 981–3.

Sanfilippo, N.J., His, A., DeNittis, A.S. *et al.* (2001) Toxicity of photodynamic therapy after combined external beam radiotherapy and intraluminal brachytherapy for carcinoma of the upper aerodigestive tract. *Lasers Surg. Med.* **28**, 278–81.

Sargeant, I.R., Loizou, L.A., Tobias, J.S. *et al.* (1992) Radiation enhancement of laser palliation for malignant dysphagia – a pilot study. *Gut* **33**, 1597–601.

Schottenfeld, D. (1984) Epidemiology of cancer of the esophagus. *Semin. Oncol.* **11**, 92–100.

Shima, I., Sasaguri, Y., Kusukawa, J. *et al.* (1992) Production of matrix metalloproteinase-2 and metalloproteinase-3 related to malignant behavior of esophageal carcinoma – a clinicopathologic study. *Cancer* **70**, 2747–53.

Skinner, D. (1984) Surgical treatment for esophageal cancer. *Semin. Oncol.* **2**, 136–43.

Sons, H.U. and Borchard, F. (1986) Cancer of distal oesophagus and cardia. *Ann. Surg.* **203**, 188–95.

Sugimachi, K., Mackawa, S., Koga, Y. *et al.* (1986) The quality of life is sustained after operation for carcinoma of the oesophagus. *Surg. Gynecol. Obstet.* **162**, 544–6.

Tate, T., Brace, J.A., Morgan, H. and Skeggs, D.B.L. (1986) Conformation therapy in the treatment of carcinoma of the oesophagus. *Clin. Radiol.* **37**, 267–71.

Teniere, P., Hay, J.M., Fingerhut, A. and Fagniez, P.L. (1991) Postoperative radiation therapy does not increase survival after curative resection for squamous cell carcinoma of the middle and lower esophagus as shown by a multicenter controlled trial. French University Association for Surgical Research. *Surg. Gynecol. Obstet.* **173**, 123–30.

Unruh, H.W. and Pagliero, K. (1985) Pulsion intubation versus traction intubation for obstructive carcinomas of the oesophagus. *Ann. Thorac. Surg.* **40**, 337–42.

Vitale, G.C., Cheadle, W.G., Patel, B., Sadek, S.A., Michel, M.E. and Cuschieri, A. (1987) The effect of alcohol on nocturnal gastroesophageal reflux. *JAMA* **258**, 2077–9.

Vonmeyenfeldt, M.F., Meijerink, W.J.H.J., Rouflart, M.M.J., Builmaassen, M.T.H.J. and Soeters, P.B. (1992) Perioperative nutritional support – a randomised clinical trial. *Clin. Nutr.* **11**, 180–6.

Wara, W.M., Mauch, P.M., Thomas, A.N. and Phillips, T.L. (1976) Palliation for carcinoma of the oesophagus. *Radiology* **121**, 717–20.

Wolfe, W.G., Vaughn, A.L., Seigler, H.F., Hathorn, J.W., Leopold, K.A. and Duhaylongsod, F.G. (1993) Survival of patients with carcinoma of the esophagus treated with combined-modality therapy. *J. Thorac. Cardiovasc. Surg.* **105**, 749–55.

Wynder, E.L. and Bross, I.J. (1961) A study of etiological factors in cancer of the oesophagus. *Cancer* **14**, 389–413.

Yang, C.S. (1980) Research on oesophageal cancer in China. *Cancer Res.* **40**, 2633–44.

FURTHER READING

Adelstein, D.J., Forman, W.B. and Beavers, B. (1984) Esophageal carcinoma. A six-year review of the Cleveland Veterans Administration Hospital Experience. *Cancer* **54**, 918–23.

Andersen, A.P., Berdal, P., Edsmyr F. *et al.* (1984) Irradiation chemotherapy and surgery in oesophageal cancer: a randomized clinical study. The first Scandinavian trial in esophageal cancer. *Radiother. Oncol.* **2**, 179–88.

Aste, H., Munizzi, F., Martines, H. and Pugliese, V. (1985) Esophageal dilation in malignant dysphagia. *Cancer* **56**, 2713–15.

Attwood, S.E.A., Barlow, A.P., Norris, T.L. and Watson, A. (1992) Barrett's oesophagus – effect of antireflux surgery on symptom control and development of complications. *Br. J. Surg.* **79**, 1050–3.

Bader, M., Dittler, H.J., Ultsch, B. *et al.* (1986) Palliative treatment of malignant stenoses of the G1 tract using a combination of laser and afterloading therapy. *Endoscopy* **18**(suppl. 1), 27–31.

Bennett, W.P., Hollstein, M.C., Metcalf, R.A. *et al.* (1992) p53 mutation and protein accumulation during multistage human esophageal carcinogenesis. *Cancer Res.* **52**, 6092–7.

Birch, P.R. (1984) Esophageal cancer in relation to tobacco and cigarette consumption. *J. Chronic Dis.* **37**, 793–814.

Brace, J.A., Davy, T.J., Skeggs, D.B.L. and Williams, H.S. (1981) Conformation therapy at the Royal Free Hospital. *Br. J. Radiol.* **54**, 1068–74.

Brister, S.J., Chiu, R.C.J., Brown, R.A. and Mulder, D.S. (1984) Clinical impact of intravenous hyperalimentation on oesophageal carcinoma. *Ann. Thorac. Surg.* **38**, 617–21.

Campion, J.P., Bourdelat, D. and Launrois, B. (1983) Surgical treatment of malignant oesophagotracheal fistula. *Am. J. Surg.* **146**, 641–6.

Coonley, C.J., Bains, M., Hilaris, B., Chapman, R. and Kelsen, D.P. (1984) Cis-platinum and bleomycin in the treatment of esophageal cancer. A final report. *Cancer* **54**, 2351–5.

Coonley, C.J., Bains, M., Hilaris, B. *et al.* (1985) Therapeutic alternatives in patients with esophageal carcinoma. *Am. J. Surg.* **150**, 665–8.

Day, N.E. (1984) Geographic pathology of cancer of the oesophagus. *Br. Med. Bull.* **40**, 329–34.

Dinwoodie, W.R., Bartolucci, A.A., Lyman, G.H. *et al.* (1986) Phase II evaluation of cis-platinum, bleomycin and vindesine in advanced squamous carcinoma of the oesophagus: a South Eastern Cancer Study Group Trial. *Cancer Treat. Rep.* **70**, 67–70.

Doherty, M.A., McIntyre, M. and Arnett, S.J. *et al.* (1984) Oat cell carcinoma of the oesophagus. *Int. J. Radiat. Oncol. Biol. Phys.* **10**, 147–52.

Dubois, J.B., Balmes, J.L. and Pujol, H. (1984) Endoscopic irradiation technique using iridium-192. *Br. J. Radiol.* **57**, 351–2.

Ellis, F.H. (1984) Cancer of the oesophagus and cardia: role of surgery in palliation. *Postgrad. Med.* **75**, 139–43.

Ellis, F.H. Jr, Gibb, S.P. and Watkins, F. (1985) Overview of the current management of carcinoma of the oesophagus and cardia. *Can. J. Surg.* **128**, 493–6.

Fléjou, J.F., Potet, F., Muzeau, F. *et al.* (1993) Overexpression of p53 protein in Barrett's syndrome with malignant transformation. *J. Clin. Pathol.* **46**, 330–3.

Froehlicher, P. and Miller, G. (1986) The European experience with oesophageal cancer limited to mucosa and submucosa. *Gastrointest. Endosc.* **32**, 88–90.

Hishikawa, Y., Tanaka, S. and Miura, T. (1985) Early esophageal carcinoma treated with intracavitary irradiation. *Radiology* **156**, 519–22.

Hishikawa, Y., Kamikonya, N., Tanaka, S. and Miura, T. (1986) Esophageal stricture following high dose rate intracavitary irradiation for esophageal carcinoma. *Radiology* **159**, 715–16.

Hishikawa, Y., Tanaka, S. and Miura, T. (1986) Esophageal fistula after intracavitary irradiation. *Radiology* **159**, 548–51.

Izquierdo, M.A., Marcuello, E., Gomez de Segura, G. *et al.* (1993) Unresectable nonmetastatic squamous cell carcinoma of the esophagus managed by sequential chemotherapy (cisplatin and bleomycin) and radiation therapy. *Cancer* **71**, 287–92.

Keane, T.J., Harwood, A.R., Elhakim, T. *et al.* (1985) Radical radiation therapy with 5-FU infusion and mitomycin C for oesophageal squamous carcinoma. *Radiother. Oncol.* **4**, 205–10.

Kelsen, D. (1984) Chemotherapy of esophageal cancer. *Semin. Oncol.* **11**, 159–68.

Kelsen, D. (1985) Chemotherapy of esophageal cancer. *Eur. J. Cancer Clin. Oncol.* **21**, 5–7.

Li, M.X. and Cheng, S.J. (1984) Carcinogenesis of oesophageal cancer in Lin Xiang, China. *Chin. Med. J.* **97**, 311–16.

McKeown, J.C. (1985) The surgical treatment of carcinoma of the oesophagus. A review of the results in 478 cases. *J. R. Coll. Surg. Edin.* **30**, 1–14.

Matsuda, H., Tsutsui, S., Monita, M. *et al.* (1992) Hyperthermo-chemo-radiotherapy as a definitive treatment for patients with early esophageal carcinoma. *Am. J. Clin. Oncol.* **15**, 509–14.

Menkepluymers, M.B.E., Schoute, N.W., Mulder, A.H. *et al.* (1992) Outcome of surgical treatment of adenocarcinoma in Barrett's oesophagus. *Gut* **33**, 1454–8.

Nakayama, K. and Kinoshita, Y. (1974) Surgical treatment of carcinoma of the oesophagus combined with pre-operative irradiation. *JAMA* **227**, 178–81.

Panettiere, F.J., Leichman, L.P., Tilchen, E.J. and Chen, T.T. (1986) Chemotherapy for advanced epidermoid carcinoma of the oesophagus, with single agent cisplatin. *Cancer Treat. Rep.* **68**, 1023–4.

Paull, A., Trier, J.S., Dalton, M.D., Camp, R.C., Loeb, P. and Goyal, R.K. (1976) The histologic spectrum of Barrett's oesophagus. *N. Engl. J. Med.* **295**, 476–80.

Payne, W.S., Trastek, V.F., Pichler, J.M. *et al.* (1986) Current techniques for the surgical management of malignant lesions of the thoracic esophagus and cardia. *Mayo Clin. Proc.* **61**, 564–76.

Pizzi, G.B., Beorchia A., Contento G. *et al.* (1989) A new technique for endocavitary irradiation of the oesophagus. *Int. J. Radiat. Oncol. Biol. Phys.* **16**, 261–2.

Quint, L.E., Glazer, G.M. and Orringer, M.B. (1985) Esophageal imaging by MR and CT. Study of normal anatomy and neoplasms. *Radiology* **156**, 727–31.

Quint, L.E., Glazer, G.M., Orringer, M.B. and Gross, B.H. (1985) Esophageal carcinoma: CT findings. *Radiology* **155**, 171–5.

Roussel, A., Bleiberg H., Dalesio O. *et al.* (1989) Palliative therapy of inoperable oesophageal carcinoma with radiotherapy and methotrexate: final results of a controlled clinical trial. *Int. J. Radiat. Oncol. Biol. Phys.* **16**, 67–72.

Sargeant, I.R., Loizou, L.A., Tobias, J.S. *et al.* (1992) Radiation enhancement of laser palliation for malignant dysphagia – a pilot study. *Gut* **33**, 1597–601.

Schlag, P., Herman, R., Fritze, D. *et al.* (1985) Preoperative chemotherapy in localized cancer of the oesophagus with cis-platinum, vindesine and bleomycin. *Prog. Clin. Biol. Res.* **201**, 253–8.

Schottenfeld, D. (1979) Alcohol as a co-factor in the etiology of cancer. *Cancer* **43**, 1962–64.

Shima, I., Sasaguri, Y., Kusukawa, J. *et al.* (1992) Production of matrix metalloproteinase-2 and metalloproteinase-3 related to malignant behavior of esophageal carcinoma – a clinicopathologic study. *Cancer* **70**, 2747–53.

Skinner, D.B., Dowlatshahi, K.D. and DeMeester, T.R. (1982) Potentially curable cancer of the esophagus. *Cancer* **50**, 2571–5.

Sons, H.U. and Borchard, F. (1984) Oesophageal cancer. Autopsy findings in 171 cases. *Arch. Pathol. Lab. Med.* **108**, 983–5.

Steinberg, C., Kelsen, D., Dukeman, M. *et al.* (1985) Carboplatin; a new platinum analog in the treatment of epidermoid carcinoma of the esophagus. *Cancer Treat. Rep.* **69**, 1305–7.

Stoller, J.L. and Flores, A.D. (1985) Intracavitary irradiation for oesophageal cancer. *Lancet* **2**, 1365.

Sugimachi, K., Matsufuji, H., Kai, H. *et al.* (1986) Preoperative irradiation for carcinoma of the oesophagus. *Surg. Gynecol. Obstet.* **162**, 174–6.

Sun, De-Ren (1989) Ten year follow-up of esophageal cancer treated by radical radiation therapy: analysis of 869 patients. *Int. J. Radiat Oncol. Biol. Phys.* **16**, 329–34.

Thomson, W.M. (1983) Esophageal cancer. *Int. J. Radiat. Oncol. Biol. Phys.* **10**, 1533–65.

Van Andel, J.G., Dees, J., Eikenboom, W.M.H. *et al.* (1986) Therapy of oesophageal cancer: result from the Joint Group on Oesophageal Cancer in Rotterdam. *Acta Radiol. Oncol.* **25**, 115–20.

Wang, M., Gu, X.Z., Yin, W.B., Huang, G.J., Wang, L.J. and Zhang, D.W. (1989) Randomized clinical trial on the combination of preoperative irradiation and surgery in the treatment of esophageal cancer: report on 206 patients. *Int. J. Radiat. Oncol. Biol. Phys.* **16**, 325–7.

24

Liver

PHILIP J. JOHNSON

INTRODUCTION

In many parts of the world, particularly sub-Saharan Africa and the Far East, hepatocellular carcinoma (HCC) is a major public health problem. Although progress towards effective therapy has been slow, low-cost vaccines against the hepatitis B virus are now starting to reduce the incidence of this malignancy. Worldwide, the liver is the most common, and often the clinically predominant, site of metastatic cancer. After considering briefly the aetiological factors and the clinicopathological features of liver tumours, this chapter goes on to describe the possible modes of therapy. These have been grouped broadly into surgery, locoregional treatments and cytotoxic, and other systemic, chemotherapy. Within each section hepatocellular carcinoma will be considered first, then metastatic liver disease. Since management of hepatic metastases from primary carcinoid tumours may pose additional problems, because of the associated carcinoid syndrome, the possible therapeutic approaches are discussed separately.

INCIDENCE

Hepatocellular carcinoma is one of the most common malignant tumours in the world today. The highest annual incidence rates, of over 100 per 100 000 occur in parts of southern Africa and the Far East (Table 24.1). Some estimates suggest that male Chinese carriers of the hepatitis B virus (HBV), who may comprise up to 15 per cent of males in certain populations, carry a lifetime risk of developing the tumour of nearly 40 per cent. In contrast, HCC is much less common in northern Europe, the United States and Australia, although there is some evidence that the frequency may be increasing, perhaps in relation to the spread of hepatitis B and C viruses infection (El-Serag and Mason, 1999). In most series, between 10 and 20 per cent of primary liver tumours are accounted for by cholangiocarcinoma and about 1 per cent by primary hepatic sarcomas (Table 24.2).

Liver metastases are found at approximately 1 per cent of all autopsies. The liver is involved in up to 40 per cent of adult patients with primary extrahepatic malignancies who come to autopsy, and, as such, is the most common organ to be involved. Up to 75 per cent of primary tumours drained by the portal venous system will have spread to involve the liver before death occurs (Willis, 1973).

AETIOLOGY OF HEPATOCELLULAR CARCINOMA

In view of the limited therapeutic options that are available once HCC has developed, the identification of risk factors, which may, in turn, lead to interventional strategies that reduce its incidence, is of particular importance.

Table 24.1 *Typical age-adjusted incidence rates per 100 000 of population in various countries. Many registries do not distinguish between hepatocellular carcinoma and other primary liver tumours*

	Country	Male	Female
Low-incidence areas	UK	1.6	0.8
	USA (white)	2	1
	Australia	1.1	0.5
	Germany	4	1.2
	Denmark	3.6	2.3
Intermediate incidence areas	Italy	7.5	3.5
	Spain	7.5	4
	Roumania	11.8	7.9
	Argentina	8	5
High-incidence areas	Japan	20	5
	Hong Kong	32	7
	Zimbabwe	65	25
	Senegal	25	9
	Taiwan	85	–

Table 24.2 *Classification of the more common primary liver tumours*

Cell of origin	Benign tumour	Malignant tumour
Hepatocyte	Hepatocellular adenoma	Hepatoblastoma
		Hepatocellular carcinoma
Bile duct	Bile-duct adenoma	Cholangiocarcinoma
		intrahepatic
		extrahepatic
Blood vessels	Haemangioma	Angiosarcoma
		Epithelioid
		Haemangioendothelioma

Hepatoblastoma is confined to children.

The wide geographical variation in the incidence of HCC, as outlined above, has pointed to the likely importance of environmental factors. Prime among these have been the hepatitis B virus (HBV) and exposure to aflatoxin. Beasley (1988) followed up over 22 000 Chinese males, 15 per cent of whom were HBV carriers, for up to 9 years. The development of HCC was almost exclusively confined to those who had serum markers of HBV infection at presentation. There is now evidence that the annual incidence rate of HCC is starting to fall, at least among children, in countries such as Taiwan where universal vaccination against HBV is practised (Chang *et al.*, 1997) (Table 24.3). Preliminary evidence also suggests that antiviral therapy of chronic viral hepatitis may also decrease the incidence of subsequent HCC development. The epidemiological evidence linking chronic hepatitis C virus (HCV) infection and HCC is similar to that for HBV. Indeed, in Europe and Japan the attributable risk may be even higher (Okuda, 1997; Brechot *et al.*, 1998). However, since HCV has no reverse transcriptase activity and is not a retrovirus it should, in theory, have no direct oncogenic potential. Most authors have therefore

Table 24.3 *The effect of universal vaccination against hepatitis B virus on the incidence of hepatocellular carcinoma in Taiwan (from Chang* et al., *1997)*

	Average annual incidence
Children aged 6–14 years born	
1981–86	0.7
1990–94	0.36
Children aged 6–9 years born	
1974–84	0.52
1984–94	0.13

attributed the association with HCC to the chronic liver disease that chronic HCV infection may cause (*see* below). HCC usually arises in a cirrhotic liver although, particularly in high-incidence areas, the cirrhosis is not always symptomatic. Indeed, the development of HCC may be the first indication of the underlying cirrhosis. Males with cirrhosis are affected significantly more frequently than females. The relative importance of the

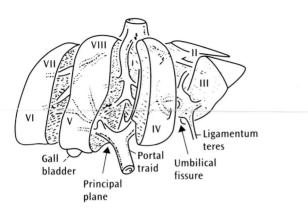

Figure 24.1 *Segmental anatomy of the liver.*

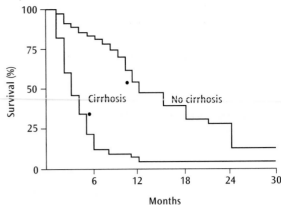

Figure 24.2 *Cumulative survival curves for patients with hepatocellular carcinoma with and without cirrhosis (reproduced with permission from Melia et al., 1984).*

chronic liver disease, as compared with HBV, HCV and aflatoxin exposure, may be different in different parts of the world (Johnson and Williams, 1987).

In the experimental animal, aflatoxin, formed by the fungus *Aspergillus fumigatus* which grows on cereals stored under damp conditions, is one of the most potent hepatic carcinogens known. In several high HCC incidence areas of the world a clear relation between intake and the incidence of HCC has been established, both by conventional dietary assessment (Linsell and Peers, 1977) and, more recently, by the use of biomarkers (Ross *et al.*, 1992). As well as the obvious approach of improving grain storage to overcome the problem of aflatoxin exposure, workers are currently exploring the possibility of chemoprevention with Oltipraz, a drug that can alter the metabolic pathway of aflatoxin to induce production of non-carcinogenic metabolites (Wang *et al.*, 1999).

NORMAL AND PATHOLOGICAL ANATOMY OF THE LIVER

Recognition of the segmental anatomy of the liver has been important in allowing more refined operative techniques for surgical resection. The portal vascular supply and bile ducts define two functional hepatic lobes, the line of demarcation running from the gall-bladder bed to the inferior vena cava. Each of these two lobes is split into four segments, none of which has any surface markings (Fig. 24.1). The standard surgical resections are based on this description. The left, and the right and the middle hepatic veins drain the conventional 'anatomical' left and right lobes, as defined by the falciform ligament, respectively. It has been recognized for more than half a century (Segall, 1923), that, whereas the normal liver receives about 70 per cent of its blood supply from the portal vein, the dominant blood supply to liver tumours is from the hepatic artery. This forms the rationale for several therapeutic approaches, including hepatic artery occlusion and regional chemotherapy.

NATURAL HISTORY AND PATTERNS OF METASTASIS

Hepatocellular carcinoma is usually rapidly fatal and most untreated patients die within 12 months of the onset of symptoms. In Africa and the Far East, the tumour appears to behave in a particularly aggressive manner. Geddes and Falkson (1970) reported a mean duration of symptoms of 5 months before death in South African Bantu mineworkers; in China the mean survival time from diagnosis is less than 3 months. In the West, patients without underlying cirrhosis survive longer (Melia *et al.*, 1984) (Fig. 24.2). The prognosis of patients with other primary liver tumours is equally poor. The only exceptions are the recently described, but very rare, 'epithelioid haemangioendothelioma' and the equally rare variant of HCC, 'fibrolamellar carcinoma' (*see* below). Both have a rather better prognosis, with a median survival of around 5 years.

The lung is the most common site of metastases from HCC (40 per cent of cases coming to autopsy), but in more than half of these cases the tumour is only detectable microscopically (Willis, 1973). As local treatment becomes more effective, symptomatic lung metastases are becoming more frequently detected. Retrograde spread to invade the portal vein is the next most common mode of dissemination; hepatic artery and bile-duct involvement are also common.

Secondary liver tumours

Untreated, the overall median survival is in the range of 6–9 months, with less than 1 per cent of patients surviving for more than 5 years. Metastases from primary carcinoid tumours are the only secondary tumours to exhibit a significantly better prognosis, survival periods of up to 10 years not being uncommon. With the wide use of more sophisticated radiological techniques, the diagnosis of liver metastases is being established earlier, often while the patient is asymptomatic, and this makes for an apparent increase in survival. As a rule, the major factor influencing survival is the percentage of liver involved by the tumour.

SYMPTOMS AND PRESENTATION

The most common mode of presentation for primary and secondary liver tumours is the triad of abdominal pain, weight loss and the presence of an hepatic mass (Johnson, 1999). In addition, patients with HCC often present with signs of hepatic decompensation, such as ascites, or variceal haemorrhage and cutaneous stigmata of chronic liver disease (Melia et al., 1984). A particularly dramatic presentation is spontaneous rupture of the tumour. There is a sudden onset of severe pain with shock, and paracentesis reveals blood-stained ascitic fluid. Rarer presentations of HCC include hypoglycaemia, hypercalcaemia and polycythemia. Spread to involve the portal or hepatic venous system may cause portal hypertension. Intrahepatic ('peripheral type') cholangiocarcinomas have no specific clinical features that distinguish them from HCC, but those arising at the bifurcation ('hilar type'), and below, present with obstructive jaundice, weight loss and abdominal pain (Altaee et al., 1991). Malignant liver tumours are increasingly diagnosed presymptomatically. In the case of HCC this follows screening patients with cirrhosis by serial estimations of α-fetoprotein (AFP) and ultrasound examination. Not surprisingly, such patients survive longer (up to 3 years) (Ebara et al., 1986).

Hepatomegaly, often massive, is an invariable feature of symptomatic malignant liver tumours. In the case of HCC, other clinical features usually relate to the underlying chronic liver disease. Certain metastatic tumours, particularly carcinoids, involve the liver with relatively little disruption of hepatic function. Indeed, patients with large tumours may have normal liver function tests and are often surprisingly well despite extensive tumour deposits.

IMAGING

In experienced hands, an ultrasound (USS) examination provides invaluable information. HCC is shown as hypoechoic when small, becoming progressively hyperechoic with ill-defined margins as it enlarges. Ultrasound scanning can also assess the patency of the portal and hepatic veins, particularly when Doppler flow studies are undertaken. It permits differentiation between solid and cystic space-occupying lesions, and can allow accurate measurement of the main tumour size and daughter nodules, if present. USS is particularly appropriate for regular screening of cirrhotic patients for the development of HCC, since lesions as small as 1 cm can be detected. Tumour and cirrhotic nodules can often be differentiated, but the entire examination is very operator dependent. The quoted sensitivity has been between 70 and 80 per cent and the specificity between 90 and 95 per cent (Kanematsu et al., 1985). However, such figures depend on the 'gold-standard' applied. When the gold standard is pathological examination of livers explanted after liver transplantation for end-stage liver disease, figures for sensitivity and specificity are considerably lower (Dodd et al., 1992).

Conventional contrast-enhanced CT scanning is at least sensitive but, in addition, a detailed search for primary or secondary lesions outside the abdomen is possible, although examination time and expense may limit applicability. HCC is seen as a hypodense lesion that does not enhance with contrast. Spiral CT is perhaps the most sensitive routinely applied technique (Oliver and Baron, 1996; Freeny, 1997). The lowly chest radiograph should not be forgotten as lung, or even bony, metastases may be seen at presentation, and this clearly has implications for further investigation. Also, HCC arising in the dome of the liver may be apparent on the plain chest radiograph as a 'bulge'. It is a common experience that a firm diagnosis of HCC cannot be made on the basis of the imaging evidence, and the physician is left with an area that is 'suspicious of HCC' rather than diagnostic. In such circumstances CT with lipiodol, hepatic angiography or combined CT and hepatic angiography may offer a more clear-cut diagnosis (Kanematsu et al., 1997). It should be noted that all imaging techniques are much less sensitive when the tumour is composed of numerous, small, multifocal lesions.

Haemangiomas, the most common of the solid hepatic tumours, arising in around 5 per cent of normal individuals, are a frequent source of confusion in assessing patients with suspected HCC. Although haemangiomas do not cause symptoms unless very large, they are frequently encountered when screening high-risk patients by ultrasound, a technique which cannot confidently distinguish them from HCC. There is no perfect test, but if the distinction is clinically important, then dynamic CT scanning is the most widely available technique and criteria for recognition of haemangiomas have been published (Ashida et al., 1987). There is progressive enhancement from the periphery until the lesion becomes isodense with the surrounding liver. An alternative approach is to use scanning with ^{99m}Tc-labelled red blood cells, but it is likely that in the future MRI will become the definitive investigation (Whitney et al., 1993).

SEROLOGICAL TUMOUR MARKERS

Serum AFP levels are elevated in 50–70 per cent of patients with HCC at the time of presentation, with a median value in the order of 3000 ng/ml (Tekata, 1990). The test is primarily of value in the diagnosis of HCC developing in patients with cirrhosis, where a level above 500 ng/ml is almost diagnostic. Levels between 10 and 500 ng/ml may occur in other, non-malignant, liver diseases, particularly severe untreated chronic active hepatitis and fulminant liver failure. However, a steadily rising value over a 1–2-month period is very strongly suggestive of HCC. The test is less useful in distinguishing between primary and secondary tumours in the non-cirrhotic normal liver – only 50 per cent of such cases of HCC have elevated levels, and up to 10 per cent of hepatic metastases will have elevated levels. AFP derived from HCC differs in respect of the structure of its carbohydrate side-chains from that arising in 'benign' liver disease (Johnson *et al.*, 1997). Carcinoembryonic antigen (CEA) is of value in monitoring the response of colonic metastases to therapy and disease recurrence after resection (Braunstein *et al.*, 1980).

TUMOUR BIOPSY

Ideally, histological confirmation should always be obtained, but at what stage of investigation biopsy should be undertaken remains contentious because of the small risk of tumour dissemination along the needle track. If the tumour is likely to be resectable, most surgeons prefer to avoid biopsy and rely on frozen section histology at the time of operation. Provided the prothrombin time is not prolonged by more than 3 seconds, or the patient is not deeply jaundiced, the conventional percutaneous approaches using Menghini, Trucut or fine-needle biopsy (depending on the availability of expert cytology) are safe. Most institutions will now use ultrasound or CT to guide the operator, or combine biopsy with laparoscopy to increase the frequency with which tumour tissue can be obtained.

PATHOLOGY

There is great variation in the degree of anaplasia and pleomorphism in HCC, both between different tumours and within the same liver, but most show some degree of hepatocellular differentiation. The presence of bile in the tumour cells or dilated canaliculi is diagnostic of HCC. The most typical histological growth pattern is microtrabecular, which may simulate normal liver except that there will be no portal tracts or bile ducts in evidence. Several other patterns are described, the most common being acinar, pseudoglandular or adenoid, but neither these, nor the cytological appearance, have any prognostic significance. The surrounding, non-tumorous liver appears compressed, and a Budd–Chiari-like picture of sinusoidal dilatation is seen when the tumour compresses the hepatic vein radicals.

Three histologically defined primary liver cancers deserve special consideration since they do have specific clinical correlates. The fibrolamellar variant of HCC, which accounts for about 5 per cent of cases in the West but less than 1 per cent in the East, is reported to have a better prognosis than the common form of HCC. It is defined histologically by its deep eosinophilic cytoplasm and pyknotic nuclei interspersed with acellular collagen. The patients are young (mean age 26 years), the male : female ratio is 1 : 1, the non-tumorous liver is not cirrhotic and α-fetoprotein (AFP) is not produced in excess (Craig *et al.*, 1980). Although resection rates are high, most patients will still die of their tumour, with a median overall survival of around 5 years. None the less, before attributing better survival to this particular historically defined subgroup we should note that being non-cirrhotic, young and AFP negative are all, in themselves, indicators of a relatively good prognosis in other types of HCC. For patients with non-resectable metastatic disease, median survival is 14 months, compared to 7 months in a group matched with the more common histological types (Epstein *et al.*, 1999). Another variant with which fibrolamellar carcinoma may be confused has marked sclerosis histologically but does not have a better prognosis. It is usually associated with hypercalcaemia (Peters, 1976). The recently described 'epithelioid' haemangioendothelioma can be shown to be of endothelial origin by staining for factor VIII-associated antigen, and some patients have survived several years (Ishak *et al.*, 1984).

When the primary tumour from which a hepatic metastasis has originated is not apparent, histological examination may provide a clue. Adenocarcinomas are usually of colorectal or pancreatic origin, but intrahepatic cholangiocarcinomas also have a similar appearance. Anaplastic tumours are usually of bronchial origin. Recently developed histological methods involving special stains, immunocytochemistry and electron microscopy often permit distinction of the origin of these highly anaplastic tumours. This means that the surgeon must collaborate very closely with the pathologist so that biopsy specimens can be placed in the appropriate medium. Detection of a lymphoma on the basis of positive B- or T-cell surface markers is particularly gratifying as relatively specific therapy is available.

STAGING AND PROGNOSIS

The simplest and most practical staging procedure for HCC is that described by Okuda *et al.* (1985a) on the basis of observations on 229 untreated patients. Tumour size, presence or absence of ascites and jaundice, and the serum albumin level are recorded and permit classification into stages 1 to 3 with clear prognostic discrimination (Table 24.4). The conventional TNM staging is used less widely for HCC than for other tumours, because the

Table 24.4 *Staging of hepatocellular carcinoma (adapted from Okuda et al., 1985a)*

Clinical feature		Points
Tumour size (on anterior	>50%	1
projection of liver scan)	<50%	0
Ascites	Present	1
	Absent	0
Serum albumin (g/l)	<30	1
	>30	0
Serum bilirubin (μmol/l)	>35	1
	<35	0

Total score	Stage	Median survival (months)
0	1	28
1,2	2	8
3,4	3	1

Table 24.5 *The TNM classification of HCC (Anonymous, 1998)*

Tumour T	
Tx	The primary tumour cannot be assessed
T0	No evidence of primary tumour
T1	Solitary, <2 cm tumour without vascular invasion
T2	Solitary, <2 cm tumour with vascular invasion
	Multiple, one lobe, <2 cm without vascular invasion
	Solitary, >2 cm without vascular invasion
T3	Solitary, >2 cm with vascular invasion
	Multiple, one lobe, <2 cm with vascular invasion
	Multiple, one lobe, >2 cm with or without vascular invasion
T4	Multiple, > one lobe
	Invasion of major branch of portal or hepatic veins
Nodes N	
Nx	Regional lymph nodes cannot be assessed
N0	No regional lymph node metastases
N1	Regional lymph node metastases
Metastases	
M0	Metastases absent
M1	Metastases present

state of the underlying liver function is at least as important in terms of management decisions and prognosis as are the 'tumour factors' that the TNM system uses (Anonymous, 1998) (Table 24.5).

Vascular invasion

The presence of vascular invasion is an important adverse prognostic factor. It is well recognized that some very large tumours can be resected with good long-term outcome if vascular invasion has not occurred. This observation has led to 'vascular invasion' being added to the most recent TNM classification. Presumably vascular invasion is an indication of the inherent malignancy of the lesion and a channel for intrahepatic and extrahepatic metastasis. Portal vein thrombosis is detected in about 10 per cent of cases at presentation and develops in up to 25 per cent during the course of the disease (Okuda *et al.*, 1985b). The diagnosis can usually be made accurately and non-invasively by ultrasound examination. In most instances the thrombosis is related to invasion of the portal system by tumour and, as such, presumably represents a further indication of vascular invasion. It is not surprising, therefore, that portal vein thrombosis has been consistently found to be an independent adverse prognostic factor (Calvet *et al.*, 1990; Stuart *et al.*, 1996; Groupe d'Etude et de Traitement du Carcinome Hepatocellulaire, 1999).

TREATMENT OF HEPATOCELLULAR CARCINOMA

The only hope of long-term survival for patients with HCC is surgical resection or liver transplantation. Although, for reasons detailed below, this proves feasible in less than 20 per cent of cases overall, the physician needs to consider this possibility in every patient in whom the diagnosis of HCC is established.

Surgical approaches

Liver tumours are unresectable if there is extrahepatic spread of the disease, extensive bilobar involvement or tumour invasion of the major vessels, including the inferior vena cava, main portal vein or common hepatic artery. A patient with a normal liver can tolerate resection of about three-quarters of the liver but in a cirrhotic liver a right lobectomy (55 per cent resection) is probably the upper limit of resectability. Liver resection is a major operation that carries an operative mortality of 1–5 per cent in non-cirrhotic and 10–15 per cent in cirrhotic patients. It should, therefore, not be undertaken lightly. The high operative mortality in cirrhotic patients needs to be balanced against the inevitably poor survival of patients with symptomatic HCC with cirrhosis. Child's Grade C cirrhosis is usually considered as a contraindication to surgery.

Intra-operative ultrasound gives much important information in addition to gross examination. It locates small tumours that may otherwise be undetected, it discovers small secondary lesions and it detects tumour thrombus in portal and hepatic veins. It also helps to determine the resection margins and the plane of liver transection in relation to the hepatic vasculature, thus helping to preserve as much functioning liver tissue as possible. This is especially important in patients with cirrhosis. Recent studies have shown that intra-operative ultrasound helps the

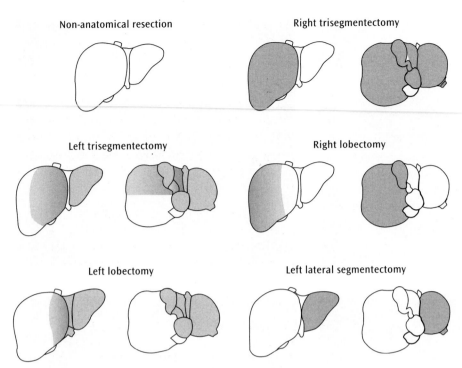

Non-anatomical resection

Right trisegmentectomy

Left trisegmentectomy

Right lobectomy

Left lobectomy

Left lateral segmentectomy

Figure 24.3 *Standard surgical resections.*

surgeons to make important surgical decisions during the operation in about one-quarter of cases (Lau *et al.*, 1993).

RESECTION

Couinaud (1957) divided the liver anatomically into eight segments, each receiving its hepatic arterial, portal venous and biliary duct branches (Fig. 24.1). The hepatic venous branches, however, are distributed differently since a number of their branches are between, rather than within, the individual segments. It is possible to resect individual segments. Accurate delineation of the segments to be excised has been facilitated by intra-operative ultrasound, and by the injection of dyes into the portal or arterial blood supply.

Apart from resection of individual liver segments, five lobar and/or segmental resections of the liver have commonly been used (Fig. 24.3). With right trisegmentectomy, the right lobe of the liver and medial segment of the left lobe are removed, except that the caudate lobe may be removed or retained, depending on the location of the tumour. With left trisegmentectomy, the left lobe of the liver and the anterior segment of the right lobe are removed, but the caudate lobe may be resected or retained. Non-anatomical resection refers to resection of the liver along non-anatomical planes. In general, this results in more bleeding and can leave behind parts of the liver remnants deprived of their blood supply.

TUMOUR RECURRENCE AND POSTOPERATIVE ADJUVANT THERAPY

About 15 per cent of HCC will come to operation and the 5-year survival rate is about one-third to one-half

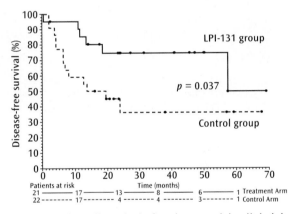

Figure 24.4 *Overall survival of patients receiving lipiodol ^{131}I after resection of HCC, compared to an untreated control group (from Lau et al., 1999).*

(Nagasue *et al.*, 1993; Fong *et al.*, 1999). A recently reported prospective randomized trial suggests that administration of a single dose of intrahepatic arterial lipiodol ^{131}I (1850 MBq) after complete resection significantly decreases the rate of recurrence from 59 to 28.5 per cent, and increases the overall survival rate (Fig. 24.4) (Lau *et al.*, 1999).

PREOPERATIVE NEOADJUVANT CHEMOTHERAPY

The combination of conventional cytotoxic drugs (*cis*-platinum, Adriamycin and 5-fluorouracil (5-FU)) and α-interferon, known as 'PIAF', has been reported to produce a partial response in about 25 per cent of cases. In itself, this is not a remarkable result. However, in 15–20 per cent of cases the tumour has become resectable.

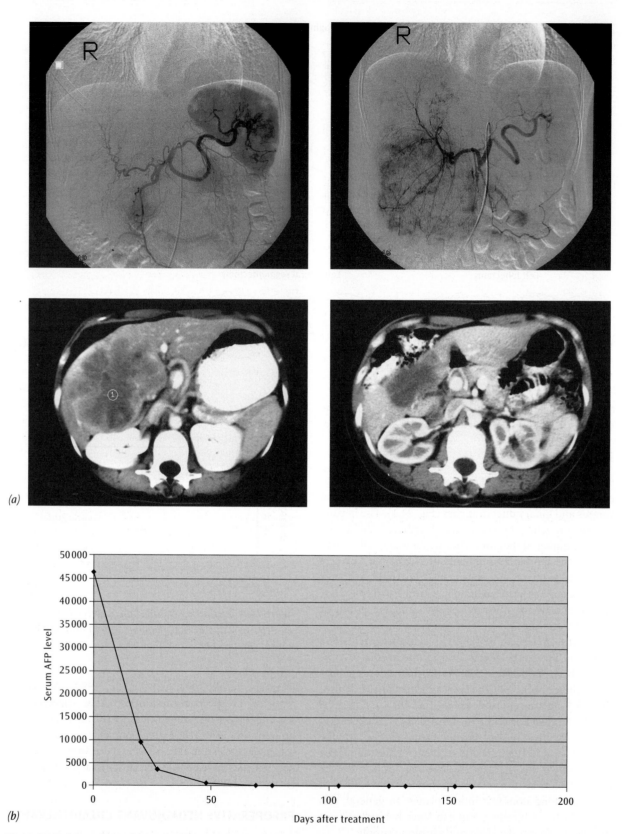

Figure 24.5 *(a) Angiographic and CT response to systemic chemotherapy. The left-hand figures show the situation before PIAF chemotherapy. After treatment (right-hand figures) the tumour became operable. Although the response was only partial on conventional CT criteria, histopathological examination of the resected tumour showed complete pathological remission, with no viable tumour cells detectable. (Courtesy of Dr Thomas Leung MD.) (b) Changes in serum α-fetoprotein (AFP) in the same patient as in (a). Note that the AFP fall to within the reference range reflects the true response as determined on histopathological grounds.*

Furthermore, the resected specimen has shown minimal or, in many cases, no residual disease (Leung *et al.*, 1999) (Fig. 24.5).

ORTHOTOPIC LIVER TRANSPLANTATION

Orthotopic liver transplantation overcomes the problems of diffuse tumour spread throughout the liver and the development of hepatic insufficiency after major liver resection, especially for cirrhotic patients. Many of the first recipients to achieve long-term survival after liver transplantation in the early 1970s had malignant liver disease. In general, they tolerated the operation well and recovered rapidly. However, despite careful preoperative assessment which attempted to exclude those with extrahepatic spread, tumour recurrence, presumably stemming from undetectable micrometastases, and perhaps favoured by the requisite immunosuppression, was frequent. This led many groups to abandon grafting for malignant disease, other than when the tumour was found incidentally in a patient undergoing transplantation for advanced cirrhosis. Indeed, the percentage of transplant operations for malignant disease fell from 25 per cent before 1988 to only 10 per cent between 1988 and 1997 (European Liver Transplant Registry, 1998).

Subsequently it became evident that the small group of patients in whom HCC was discovered incidentally in the explanted liver had an extremely good prognosis and recurrence in this group was less than 10 per cent. Recent figures suggest 5-year survival rates of around 80 per cent. Further, it is now evident that tumour size is a major factor influencing recurrence; small tumours may have a very good prognosis after transplantation, whereas recurrence is very frequent, but not inevitable, with tumours greater than 8 cm diameter or in those that are multifocal. Thus for patients with tumours of less than 5 cm in diameter, the expected 3- and 5-year survival rates are currently 72 and 68 per cent, respectively (McPeake *et al.*, 1993; Achkar *et al.*, 1998) (Table 24.6). Other groups have concentrated on the degree of vascular invasion as the indicator of whether or not recurrence is likely.

Locoregional therapies for hepatocellular carcinoma

Where surgical resection is not feasible, and no extrahepatic metastases are detected, some form of locoregional therapy is usually offered. This is usually based on hepatic arterial infusion of some form of therapy, or a direct attack on the tumour by injection of alcohol, radiofrequency ablation or cryo/laser therapy. It is emphasized that convincing improvement in survival has not been demonstrated for any of these approaches, and if they are to be used, it is with the intention of palliation. Under these circumstances, the procedure with the least morbidity and mortality should be used. Some of the more widely used methods are described below.

Table 24.6 *Recurrence rate and survival in relation to tumour size in patients undergoing liver transplantation (adapted from McPeake et al., with permission)*

Tumour dimensions (cm)	Recurrence number (%)	Survival		
		1 year	3 years	5 years
<4	0 (0)	83.9	69.9	69.9
4–8	5 (33)	73.3	73	59
>8	7 (78)	66	0	0
Multifocal	14 (78)	33	14	14

ARTERIAL EMBOLIZATION

As documented above, primary and secondary liver tumours derive the bulk of their blood supply from the hepatic artery, and embolization of the hepatic artery causes tumour necrosis. This is currently achieved by injecting emboli under fluoroscopic control, at the time of diagnostic hepatic arteriography, until blood flow ceases. This approach has largely superseded hepatic artery ligation at the time of laparotomy, not only because anaesthesia and laparotomy may be avoided but also because subsequent growth of a collateral circulation is less likely, or at least delayed, as occlusion is induced at the periphery. Effective embolization is often associated with fever, pain and vomiting for up to 5 days, after which it subsides spontaneously. Antibiotic prophylaxis is required for 1 week, starting on the day before the procedure, together with adequate analgesia. The procedure can be repeated on several occasions. The presence of Child's grade C cirrhosis is a relative contraindication. Only if the tumour is very small or can be catheterized very selectively should such patients be considered. The main indication is pain relief, which is effected in up to 65 per cent of cases. Although more than half the patients show evidence of tumour regression, clinical experience and a recent prospective randomized controlled trial suggest that there is no improvement in overall survival (Bruix *et al.*, 1998).

Direct infusion of cytotoxic agents may allow an increase in drug exposure (the time/concentration interval) of the tumour up to 400-fold so that dose-limiting toxicity becomes 'regional', i.e. hepatic and not systemic. There is no doubt that this route increases the response rate to chemotherapy but, again, convincing evidence of survival gain has not been forthcoming. The combination of these two approaches, together with the use of lipiodol has, until recently, been the most widely used locoregional therapy.

TRANSCATHETER OILY CHEMOEMBOLIZATION

When lipiodol, an oily contrast medium, is injected into the hepatic artery at the time of arteriography, subsequent CT scanning shows that it is cleared from normal hepatic tissues but accumulates in many HCCs (Okayasu *et al.*, 1988). It has been suggested, therefore, that lipiodol might be an ideal vehicle for targeting cytotoxic drugs. Typically, in transcatheter oily chemoembolization (TOCE) 60 mg of doxorubicin is mixed with 15 mL of lipiodol and injected into the tumour-feeding arteries. This is followed by embolization with 0.5–1 mm of gelatin cubes. Side-effects, other than those mentioned above, are uncommon, but include accidental embolization of other organs, including the gall bladder and spleen. Portal vein thrombosis is usually a contraindication to TOCE, since the cirrhotic liver is crucially dependent on the hepatic artery in this situation and any further interruption thereof may lead to liver failure.

The procedure has been supported enthusiastically, and by the late 1980s TOCE was widely regarded as standard treatment for inoperable disease. However, when agents such as doxorubicin are used it has become clear that systemic toxicity is, in fact, no different from that achieved with intravenous administration. Furthermore, although there is apparent tumour regression in over 50 per cent of cases, it has never been shown that this is any greater than that achieved by embolization alone. Recent prospective randomized trials have again confirmed the efficacy of the procedure in terms of achieving high response rates, but have failed to document any improvement in survival (Groupe d'Etude et de Traitement du Carcinome Hepatocellulaire, 1995; Pelletier et al., 1998).

PERCUTANEOUS ALCOHOL INJECTION

Percutaneous injection of absolute alcohol into liver tumours has been practised for more than 15 years now. Under real-time ultrasonic or CT guidance about 5 mL of sterile 95 per cent ethanol is injected through a 20-cm long, 21- or 22-gauge needle. The procedure is repeated, depending on the size of the tumour and extent of necrosis obtained. The most suitable patients are those with small solitary tumours with good underlying liver function (Child's grade A or B). The advantage of this approach is its simplicity, lack of side-effects and cheapness. On the other hand, while small tumours (<2 cm) only require 3–4 sessions, larger tumours require up to 20. Many workers have found it difficult to gain a homogeneous distribution of alcohol throughout the lesion. The patient often complains of mild pain and some fever. If the alcohol escapes into the peritoneal cavity, severe pain ensues. This can be avoided by very slow infiltration of the alcohol. Survival at 1, 3 and 5 years has been reported to be 96, 72 and 51 per cent for Child's A cirrhosis; 90, 72 and 48 per cent for Child's B cirrhosis and 94, 25 and 0 per cent for Child's C cirrhosis (Livraghi, 1998). Although prospective randomized trials have not been undertaken, using historical control groups, it appears that, at least over the first 3 years after treatment, results are not dissimilar to those obtained by surgical resection (Castells et al., 1993). Other injection agents, such as hot water and saline and acetic acid, are currently being assessed.

RADIOTHERAPY

The application of external-beam irradiation for the treatment of liver tumours has been severely limited by the radiosensitivity of normal hepatocytes. The maximum tolerance of normal liver to radiation is generally accepted to be between 2500 and 3000 cGy (Wharton et al., 1973) and above this the risk of radiation hepatitis, veno-occlusive disease with perivenular congestion and fibrosis increases rapidly. The Ann Arbor group used conformal radiotherapy and intrahepatic arterial 5-fluoro-2'-deoxyuridine (floxuridine; 5-FUDR) as a radiosensitizer. The hepatic tumour received between 4500 cGy and 6000 cGy without development of severe radiation hepatitis. The dose is potentially tumoricidal and produced durable responses of up to 8 months (Lawrence et al., 1991). In a subsequent study in which only primary hepatobiliary cancers were entered, the radiation dose to the tumour was between 4800 and 7260 cGy (Robertson et al., 1993). Objective responses were seen in all patients with focal tumours. Median survival for localized HCC was 11 months and there were only two cases, neither fatal, of radiation hepatitis.

INTERNAL IRRADIATION WITH INTRA-ARTERIAL RADIOISOTOPES

Therapeutic dose of radio-isotopes can be administered into the hepatic artery using yttrium-90 tagged to resin-based or glass microspheres or iodine-131 in conjunction with lipiodol. Yttrium-90, a pure β-emitter, is more powerful than iodine-131, with a physical half-life of 64.2 hours and with a mean energy 936.7 KeV (maximum 2270 KeV). The mean penetration in tissue is about 2.5 mm. With such an approach, tolerance of the liver to the effects of radiation by yttrium-90 microspheres is higher than expected from external radiation, and a therapeutic dose of radiation can be delivered without causing radiation hepatitis.

Of 71 patients treated with yttrium-90 tagged to resin-based microspheres, 27 per cent had a partial response by conventional imaging criteria (Lau et al., 1998). Of particular note, however, was the observation that AFP fell by more that 50 per cent in nearly all cases, and to within the normal range in 22 per cent. Furthermore, in four patients, the tumour could be resected after treatment, and in two of these, examination of the resected specimen showed there was complete pathological remission. Side-effects are usually confined to minor degrees of abdominal discomfort and, despite the presence of cirrhosis in all patients, there was no incidence of radiation hepatitis, even when the non-tumorous liver received up to 7000 cGy. Leakage of microspheres into the right gastric artery or gastroduodenal artery may occasionally cause radiation gastritis or duodenitis. Systemic leakage of the microsphere to involve the lungs, which are also sensitive to irradiation, may occur if there is extensive arteriovenous shunting within the tumour. For this reason, the degree of lung shunting must be determined before administration of the radio-isotope, by performing a technetium-99m macroaggregated albumin scan (Tc-MAA) with gamma camera scanning. This permits prediction of the percentage of lung shunting and the relative tumour to non-tumour uptake ratio (T/N ratio). Those with high lung shunting (>5 per cent) and poor T/N ratio are not suitable for yttrium-90 microsphere treatment (Leung *et al.*, 1994).

Systemic chemotherapy for hepatocellular carcinoma

A recent systematic review of randomized trials for HCC has concluded that current non-surgical treatments for HCC are non-effective or minimally and uncertainly effective (Simonetti *et al.*, 1997). Two of the three approaches considered minimally effective have since been shown to be ineffective in large prospective randomized trials.

Almost all the cytotoxic agents used in oncological practice have been evaluated and none has been shown, as a single agent or in combination with other agents, to improve survival or to achieve a consistent response rate of greater than 20 per cent. In a review of several published trials involving over 600 patients, Adriamycin (doxorubicin) was shown to have an objective response rate of 19 per cent with a median survival of 4 months (Nerenstone *et al.*, 1988). Combination therapy has not been shown to be superior to single-agent treatment, although, recently, encouraging results have been reported with a combination of cytotoxic agents (*cis*-platinum, Adriamycin, 5-fluorouracil and interferon), the so-called 'PIAF' regimen. With this combination, 10–15 per cent of initially unresectable tumours have been rendered resectable, and the resected specimens have, in some cases, shown complete pathological remission (Fig. 24.5a, b).

An alternative systemic approach has been endocrine manipulation, particularly with anti-oestrogenic and anti-androgenic agents. However, recent large-scale prospective controlled studies have largely refuted any role for anti-androgenic agents (Grimaldi *et al.*, 1998) or tamoxifen (CLIP Group, 1998). Early hopes that single-agent interferon may be effective have not been fulfilled (Llovet *et al.*, 2000). In a recent small, prospective, controlled study, octreotide led to a significant improvement in survival and appears worthy of larger-scale studies (Kouroumalis *et al.*, 1998).

An overall treatment strategy

Faced with such a wide range of options, what should the physician or surgeon offer? Surgical resection should be considered in every case. If the contraindication is poor underlying liver function, liver transplantation is the most effective treatment, but local factors frequently limit availability. If the tumour is not resectable but remains confined to the liver, some form of local palliative treatment is usually given. This depends again on local availability and expertise. Lack of side-effects should be a major criterion in choosing the most appropriate therapy. For those with metastatic disease, systemic chemotherapy can be tried, preferably within a clinical-trial setting. The most successful regimens appear to be those that contain interferon and 5-FU, but it should be noted that these regimens are toxic and randomized trials have not yet been reported.

TREATMENT OF SECONDARY LIVER TUMOURS

Metastases to the liver are present in 40 per cent of autopsy cases in which there is an extrahepatic primary tumour. This high figure has been attributed to the vascularity of the liver, its double arterial supply, and the characteristics of its endothelial membrane, which render the liver fertile ground for malignant cells. The most common sites of the primary lesion are the gastrointestinal tract, the lung, the breast and melanoma.

Surgical resection and neoadjuvant chemotherapy

The only large series of surgical resection for secondary liver cancer relate to patients with metastases from colorectal cancer, about 5–10 per cent of whom were suitable. Among those patients who appeared to have the disease confined to the liver, and in whom curative resection was attempted, survival at 1, 3 and 5 years was 85 per cent, 50 per cent and 33 per cent, respectively, with an operative mortality of less than 5 per cent (Gayowski *et al.*, 1994; Fong *et al.*, 1997; Scheele and Altendorf-Hofmann, 1999). Although no controlled trial has been undertaken, the cumulative evidence that surgical resection, when possible, is beneficial, is now overwhelming. The 5-year survival rate of patients not undergoing surgery, even with the most favourable prognostic factors, is less than 5 per cent. These figures are thus better than those achieved with any other form of therapy. After apparently successful resection, large or multiple tumours, positive resection margins or a disease-free interval of less than 12 months are adverse prognostic factors. In the light of these data, all patients without obvious evidence of extrahepatic disease should be actively assessed for possible surgical resection.

As initiated by those dealing with paediatric liver cancer (Ortega *et al.*, 1991), and increasingly with primary liver cancer, there is also a trend towards neoadjuvant therapy in patients with inoperable secondary liver cancer. In a recent publication, nearly all patients (78 per cent) with initially unresectable hepatic metastases were successfully resected after therapy with chronomodulated oxaliplatin, 5-FU and leukovorin (Borner, 1999; Giacchetti et al., 1999). The 5-year survival rate was almost 60 per cent. Although these data are very encouraging, it must be recognized that criteria for resectability are not clear-cut, and the results of ongoing controlled trials must be awaited before this approach becomes standard.

Systemic chemotherapy for secondary liver tumours

Generally, the response rates of metastatic tumours to chemotherapy are similar to the response rates of the primary lesion, or slightly less. It should be emphasized from the outset that most of the available data on systemic chemotherapy relate to patients with 'advanced', i.e. metastatic, colorectal carcinoma. Although liver metastases are common amongst such patients, other metastatic sites may affect survival. Data relating specifically to patients with isolated liver metastases is largely confined to studies on intra-arterial chemotherapy for which extrahepatic metastases are usually considered a contraindication.

SYSTEMIC CHEMOTHERAPY FOR HEPATIC METASTASES FROM COLORECTAL CANCER

5-Fluorouracil (5-FU) has been the standard chemotherapeutic agent for the treatment of advanced colorectal carcinoma for many years and remains the standard by which new treatments are judged. 5-FU alone offers a small but significant improvement in survival. Infusion-based regimens give better response rates but minimal improvement in survival, and are more labour intensive to administer. The role of modulation with folinic acid remains very controversial and the reader is referred a recent debate on the subject (Sobrero et al., 1999). None the less, most units now use a 5-FU and folinic acid regimen, while acknowledging that the definite improvement in response rate compared to single-agent 5-FU has not yet been shown convincingly to translate into survival benefit. There is a consistent response rate of 15–20 per cent, a complete response rate of 3–5 per cent, and an improvement in survival compared to 'best supportive treatment', in the order of 6–9 months. Responses are rare in elderly patients with extensive liver involvement or those in poor clinical condition. Such patients should usually be spared chemotherapy, as the risks of toxicity outweigh potential benefits. Enthusiasm for regimens involving the combination of 5-FU and interferon has waned following randomized trials suggesting no improvement over results obtained by 5-FU alone and at the expense of considerable haematological toxicity (Hill et al., 1995).

NEW AGENTS FOR ADVANCED COLORECTAL CARCINOMA

Several new agents are entering clinical trials. Amongst these, raltitrexed, oxaliplatin and irinotecan have received most attention. Raltitrexed is one of a new generation of specific and direct inhibitors of thymidylate synthase. After entry into the cell by the reduced folate carrier, the drug is polyglutaminated, thereby increasing time in the cells and allowing a cycle frequency of 3 weeks. Recent direct comparison with 5-FU and high-dose folinic acid has shown an almost identical response rate, a similar improvement in quality of life and overall survival in the two regimens, but with rather less toxic side-effects in those receiving raltitrexed (Cocconi et al., 1998). Oxaliplatin is a platinum analogue. Cisplatin itself is inactive in colorectal cancer, but oxaliplatin has a different spectrum of activity and toxicity. Cold-induced dysthesia is dose limiting, the compound showing little of cisplatin's effects of renal, auditory and myelosuppressive toxicity. The response rate is between 20 and 25 per cent in previously untreated patients and 10 per cent in those previously receiving 5-FU (de Gramont et al., 1997). When combined with 5-FU and folinic acid, response rates of over 50 per cent have been achieved. Recent studies have shown that irinotecan, an agent that inactivates topoisomerase I, when combined with fluorouracil and folinic acid improves survival in patients with colorectal cancer (Douillard et al., 2000). Of interest has been the application of chronotherapy, in which drugs are administered at specific times of the day in order to take into account circadian rhythms that affect the drug's toxicity and the tumour's responsiveness to chemotherapy. Chronotherapy has been shown to be significantly less toxic and to give higher response rates when compared to constant-rate infusion in patients with metastatic colorectal cancer (Levi et al., 1997).

Use of chemotherapy in an adjuvant setting

Although the majority of patients will have complete macroscopic clearance of disease, about 50 per cent will ultimately develop recurrence, usually within 4 years of operation. The recurrence presumably occurs because of pre-existing metastases, which are already present, but clinically undetectable, at the time of operation. Adjuvant therapy aims to eliminate these micrometastases before they become established and, indeed, there are good theoretical grounds for thinking that while small they are more amenable to cytotoxic chemotherapy.

On this basis, the role of adjuvant chemotherapy, particularly to the liver in patients with Dukes' stage B2 or C, has been investigated extensively. Several trials using 5-FU alone did not demonstrate any effect, nor did any of those involving combination chemotherapy, until two trials using the combination of 5-FU and levamisole both showed a significant survival advantage. The largest of these, the Intergroup trial involving 1296 patients (Moertel et al., 1990), showed that 1 year of treatment with the combination of systemic 5-FU plus levamisole in patients with Dukes' stage C disease gave a marked reduction in recurrence rate and death rate. The percentage of patients with recurrence at all sites, including the liver, was decreased. In this study, patients with rectal carcinoma were excluded, but equally good results have been reported recently for the combination of 5-FU and irradiation. The disease-free survival in those receiving adjuvant therapy at 3 years was 66 per cent, compared to 47 per cent in the control group – a very highly significant difference. Major prospective randomized trials have confirmed that there is an overall benefit in favour of adjuvant treatment that decreases the odds of dying from colon cancer by 25 per cent and gives an overall survival improvement of around 5 per cent. The optimal duration of therapy is currently considered to be 6 months (IMPACT investigators, 1995; O'Connell et al., 1997, 1998).

Intra-arterial infusion chemotherapy with 5-fluorouracil

The rationale for intra-arterial chemotherapy (hepatic arterial infusion, HAI) for liver metastases is similar to that described for HCC, namely that metastatic tumours derive most of their blood supply directly from the hepatic artery and the tumour is therefore to some extent 'targeted'. In addition, it has been suggested that the liver is the 'first stop' for metastatic cells from colorectal carcinomas, before they disseminate to other organs. If this first step can be interrupted, the subsequent dissemination may be avoided. These factors, combined with the observation that 5-FU and FUDR have favourable pharmacological properties (short plasma half-life and steep dose–response curve) make intra-arterial therapy an attractive approach for those patients with tumour confined to the liver. Successful arterial infusion therapy depends on adequate perfusion of the entire liver and a safe delivery system. Totally implantable pumps, much safer and more effective than percutaneous access, are now readily available and there are few of the original problems of clotting and infection.

There is no doubt that trials directly comparing systemic and intra-arterial therapies show that there is at least a doubling of response rate. However, as so often happens, there has been difficulty in establishing any effect on overall survival. This may reflect methodological problems in trial design rather than any inadequacy of the treatment itself. In the face of high response rates in the intra-arterial group it is ethically difficult to avoid crossover. None the less, the cumulative evidence now strongly suggests a significant benefit in overall survival, together with an improvement in patients' quality of life (Allen-Mersh et al., 1994; Kemeny and Atiq, 1999). Assuming that this treatment is confined to patients with hepatic involvement as the sole site of disease and who do not have resectable disease, then perhaps 3 per cent of patients with advanced colorectal cancer will be suitable candidates.

Portal vein infusion

Since, as noted above, it appears that micrometastases, in contradistinction to established metastases, gain their blood supply from the portal vein, cytotoxic drug infusion into the portal vein immediately after surgery (usually within 1 week) might decrease the recurrence rate. Efficacy of such an approach has been difficult to demonstrate, despite several studies, but recent reviews concluded that there was a small improvement in overall survival at 5 years despite no clear evidence of a decrease in the recurrence rate (Liver Infusion Meta-analysis Group, 1997; Rougier et al., 1998).

Side-effects of 5-fluorouracil

When the bolus approach is used, the predominant toxicity is myelosuppression; whereas with the infusion, the so-called 'hand–foot syndrome' (desquamation of the palms and soles) and diarrhoea are more common. With intra-arterial treatment, the toxicity is quite distinct from that seen with systemic administration of 5-FU. Nausea, vomiting, diarrhoea and myelosuppression are all uncommon. The toxicity relates to ulcer disease and hepatic toxicity. The former is presumed to be due to gastric and duodenal perfusion from small branches of the hepatic artery. The most common lesion is a chemical hepatitis, associated with, and progressing to, sclerosing cholangitis. This is probably due to primary damage of the blood vessels feeding the bile ducts that also derive their blood supply from the hepatic artery. Interruption of treatment is required in 50 per cent.

It seems likely that both intra-arterial therapy and the combination of 5-FU and folinic acid represent a significant advance for those with isolated liver metastases and advanced disease, respectively. They offer the prospect of palliation in terms of improvement in disease-related symptoms and improvement in overall well-being, together with the possibility of improved survival at an acceptable cost in terms of complications. However, it should be recognized that the benefits remain modest, not all investigators concur with these sentiments, and the extent to which response rate is influenced by performance status should not be underestimated.

What should patients with colorectal cancer metastatic to the liver be advised?

Whenever possible the tumour should be resected surgically. In a young patient, with good performance status and a small volume of liver disease that is inoperable, HAI is a reasonable recommendation, if not precluded by financial considerations. For the elderly patient with extensive disease replacing more than 50 per cent of liver and in poor physical condition, only supportive therapy should be offered. For those in between, the combination of 5-FU and folinic acid, based on either high or low folinic acid dose, is now standard therapy and should be started before symptoms develop, if possible. Newer agents, particularly irinotecan, are likely to enter routine practice shortly, and the possibility of resection in patients responding well to any form of chemotherapy should be kept in mind.

THE CARCINOID SYNDROME

The development of the carcinoid syndrome usually implies metastatic spread to involve the liver. The common primary sites are small bowel, appendix and rectum, but only those from the small bowel are commonly associated with hepatic metastases (Kulke and Mayer, 1999). Overall 5–10 per cent of patients with primary carcinoid will develop the syndrome. The syndrome comprises facial flushing and diarrhoea. Less common accompanying signs are wheezing, cardiac complications symptomatic in 10 per cent of cases (usually tricuspid regurgitation and/or stenosis), osteoarthropathy and pellagra. Abdominal pain may be due to obstruction by the primary small bowel tumour. Diagnosis is based on an elevated level of urinary 5-hydroxyindoleacetic acid (5HIAA) and the characteristic histological pattern of a neuroendocrine tumour involving the liver. It is characteristic of this tumour that the patient's clinical state, and liver function tests, appear remarkably good, even in the presence of extensive liver involvement.

In the absence of symptoms, there is little indication for active treatment of hepatic carcinoid metastases unless complete surgical resection is feasible. When the characteristic carcinoid syndrome does develop, the symptoms may be mitigated by reduction of tumour mass by surgery, arterial embolization (or cytotoxic chemotherapy), pharmacological interference with production or action of the tumour products, or by non-specific symptomatic control. It should be stressed that most of these approaches have unpleasant side-effects and should be only employed when symptoms are severe.

Measures to decrease tumour bulk

By the time the carcinoid syndrome has developed, the tumour is usually too widespread for curative resection to be attempted, but it may be successful in occasional patients and the approach to assessment is, as with other liver tumours, outlined above. Liver transplantation has been employed in carefully selected cases. Until recently, the usual approach was palliative resection, as symptom control could often be obtained by shelling out individual deposits. This approach has now been largely superseded by hepatic artery embolization (Fig. 24.6). Symptomatic control of hormone-producing tumours is now the best indication for this form of treatment, and it should be stressed that it is symptom control and pain relief which are being attempted and not prolongation of

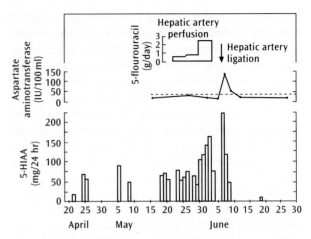

Figure 24.6 *Serial measurement of 24-hour urinary 5-HIAA levels before and after hepatic artery infusion of 5-FU followed by hepatic artery ligation.*

survival. About 80 per cent of patients achieve complete resolution of symptoms, and these remissions last from 1 month to 3 years. A major advantage of hepatic artery embolization over ligation of the hepatic artery is that the procedure can be repeated, and we have experience of one patient who had seven embolizations over a 10-year period (Melia *et al.*, 1982).

Streptozotocin is the most active cytotoxic agent to have been used, but it leads to a reduction in tumour mass in only 30 per cent of cases. The addition of other agents, such as Adriamycin and 5-FU, may give rather higher response rates but at the cost of considerably greater toxicity. Cytotoxic therapy is the last resort in the treatment of the carcinoid syndrome, and in the event that rapid symptomatic improvement does not occur, treatment should not be continued.

Pharmacological control

Previously, a wide variety of pharmacological agents have been used, but these have all now been superseded by the somatostatin analogues, such as octreotide, which are usually dramatically effective against diarrhoea and frequently against flushing too (Kvols *et al.*, 1986; Oberg *et al.*, 1991). The drug is also very effective in managing and preventing carcinoid crises that occur when there is massive release of vasoactive peptides from the tumour tissue after embolization or during surgery. When the disease symptoms are refractory to somatostatin analogues, the addition of interferon-α may induce a further remission. Interferon may be effective in its own right in about one-third of cases, but side-effects are often troublesome (Janson and Oberg, 1993). Octreotide needed to be given by injection three times per day, but long-acting preparations are now becoming available and preliminary evidence suggests that they are equally effective (Ruszniewski *et al.*, 1996). The aim of therapy is symptom control and early reports that there was tumour shrinkage have not been substantiated.

Control of diarrhoea with codeine phosphate or loperamide and careful avoidance of precipitating factors, such as alcohol and certain foods, may also be effective.

FUTURE PROSPECTS

Preoperative adjuvant therapy for unresectable primary and secondary liver tumours, with a view to rendering the tumours resectable, would seem an area worthy of further investigation. Similarly, postoperative adjuvant therapy after apparently successful resection may prove to have an important role in decreasing recurrence rates. Immunization against the hepatitis B virus, and increasingly effective antiviral treatments for chronic hepatitis B and C, may significantly decrease the incidence of HCC, but convincing proof that screening patients at high risk of HCC will significantly decrease mortality is a long way off.

SIGNIFICANT POINTS

Hepatocellular carcinoma (HCC)

- Hepatocellular carcinoma accounts for 5–10 per cent of all cancer worldwide. Major risk factors include chronic viral hepatitis (types B and C), any form of chronic liver disease, male gender, increasing age and exposure to aflatoxin.
- Universal vaccination against the hepatitis B virus is likely to lead to a major decrease in the incidence of HCC over the coming decades.
- Surgical resection or liver transplantation remains the best hope of long-term survival. Adjuvant therapies are showing promise of increasing operability rates and decreasing recurrence rates.
- Locoregional treatment for hepatocellular carcinoma offers good palliation but conclusive proof of survival benefit remains elusive.
- Systemic treatment of HCC has not yet been shown to prolong survival.

Colorectal liver metastases

- The liver is involved in up to 40 per cent of adult patients with primary extrahepatic malignancies; 7 per cent of primary tumours drained by the portal venous system will have spread to involve the liver.

- Surgical resection offers up to a 35 per cent 5-year survival rate and remains the best hope for long-term survival. Adjuvant therapies are showing promise of increasing operability.
- Intra-arterial therapy gives high response rates (<50 per cent) and there is also increasing evidence of improved survival.
- Where systemic treatment is indicated, 5-FU and leukovorin have become standard combination therapy. This combination gives response rates in the order of 20 per cent and modest increases in survival (6 months). Promising new agents are entering clinical practice.

Carcinoid syndrome

- Treatment should only be offered for symptomatic carcinoid tumours involving the liver unless curative resection is an option.
- Excellent palliation can be obtained with hepatic arterial embolization and somatostatin analogues.

KEY REFERENCES

Beasley, R.P. (1988) Hepatitis B virus. The major etiology of hepatocellular carcinoma. *Cancer* **61**(10), 1942–56.

Chang, M.H., Chang, M.H., Chen, C.J. *et al.* (1997) Universal hepatitis B vaccination in Taiwan and the incidence of hepatocellular carcinoma in children. *N. Engl. J. Med.* **336**,1855–9.

Fong, Y., Sun, R.L., Jarnagin, W. and Blumgart, L.H. (1999) An analysis of 412 cases of hepatocellular carcinoma at a Western center. *Ann. Surg.* **229**(6), 790–9; discussion 799–800.

Moertel, C.G., Fleming, T.R. and MacDonald, J.S. (1990) Levamisole and fluorouracil for adjuvant therapy of resected colon carcinoma. *N. Engl. J. Med.* **322**, 352–8.

Scheele, J. and Altendorf-Hofmann, A. (1999) Resection of colorectal liver metastases. *Langenbecks Arch. Surg.* **384**(4), 313–27.

Simonetti, R.G., Liberati, A., Angiolini, C. and Pagliaro, L. (1997) Treatment of hepatocellular carcinoma: a systematic review of randomized controlled trials. *Ann. Oncol.* **8**,117–36.

REFERENCES

Achkar, J.P., Araya, V., Baron, R.L. *et al.* (1998) Undetected hepatocellular carcinoma: clinical features and outcome after liver transplantation. *Liver Transplant. Surg.* **4**, 477–82.

Allen-Mersh, T.G., Earlam, S., Fordy, C., Abrams, K. and Houghton, J. (1994) Quality of life and survival with continuous hepatic-artery floxuridine infusion for colorectal liver metastases. *Lancet* **344**(8932), 1255–60.

Altaee, M.Y., Johnson, P.J., Farrant, J.M. and Williams, R. (1991) Etiological and clinical characteristics of peripheral and hilar cholangiocarcinomas. *Cancer* **68**, 2501–5.

Anonymous (1998) The new TNM classification in gastroenterology. *Endoscopy* **30**, 643–9.

Ashida, C., Fishman, E.K., Zerhouni, E.A., Herlong, F.H. and Siegelman, S.S. (1987) Computed tomography of hepatic cavernous hemangioma. *J. Comput. Assist. Tomogr.* **11**, 455–60.

Beasley, R.P. (1988) Hepatitis B virus. The major etiology of hepatocellular carcinoma. *Cancer* **61**(10), 1942–56.

Borner, M.M. (1999) Neoadjuvant chemotherapy for unresectable for liver metastases of colorectal cancer – too good to be true? *Ann. Oncol.* **10**, 623–6.

Braunstein, B.R., Steele, G.D. Jr, Ensminger, W. *et al.* (1980) The use and limitations of serial plasma carcinoembryonic antigen (CEA) levels as a monitor of changing metastatic liver tumour volume in patients receiving chemotherapy. *Cancer* **46**, 266–72.

Brechot, C., Jaffredo, F., Lagorce, D. *et al.* (1998) Impact of HBV, HCV and GBV-C/HGV on hepatocellular carcinomas in Europe: results of an European concerted action. *J. Hepatol.* **292**,173–83.

Bruix, J., Llovet, J.M., Castells, A. *et al.* (1998) Transarterial embolization versus symptomatic treatment in patients with advanced hepatocellular carcinoma: results of a randomized, controlled trial in a single institution. *Hepatology* **27**, 1578–83.

Calvet, X., Bruix, J., Gines, P. *et al.* (1990) Prognostic factors of hepatocellular carcinoma in the west: a multivariate analysis in 206 patients. *Hepatology* **12**, 753–60.

Castells, A., Bruix, J., Bru, C. *et al.* (1993) Treatment of small hepatocellular carcinoma in cirrhotic patients: a cohort study comparing surgical resection and percutaneous ethanol injections. *Hepatology* **18**, 1121–6.

Chang, M.H., Chang, M.H., Chen, C.J. *et al.* (1997) Universal hepatitis B vaccination in Taiwan and the incidence of hepatocellular carcinoma in children. *N. Engl. J. Med.* **336**, 1855–9.

CLIP Group (1998) Tamoxifen in treatment of hepatocellular carcinoma: a randomised controlled trial. CLIP Group. *Lancet* **352**,17–20.

Cocconi, G., Cunnningham, D., Van Cutsem, E. *et al.* (1998) Open, randomized, multicenter trial of raltitrexed versus fluorouracil plus high-dose leucovorin in patients with advanced colorectal cancer. *J. Clin. Oncol.* **16**, 2943–52.

Couinaud, C. (1957) *Le foie: etudes anatomiques et chirugicales.* Paris: Masson & Cie, 3–9.

Craig, J.R., Peters, R.L. and Omata, M. (1980) Fibrolamellar carcinoma of the liver – a tumour of adolescents and young adults with distinctive clinicopathologic features. *Cancer* **46**, 372–9.

de Gramont, A., Vignoud, J., Tournigand, C. *et al.* (1997) Oxaliplatin with high-dose leucovorin and 5-fluorouracil 48-hour continuous infusion in pretreated metastatic colorectal cancer. *Eur. J. Cancer* **33**, 214–19.

Dodd, G.D. III, Miller, W.J., Baron, R.L. *et al.* (1992) Detection of malignant tumors in end-stage cirrhotic livers: efficacy of sonography as a screening technique. *AJR* **159**, 727–33.

Douillard, J.Y., Cunningham, D., Roth, A.D. *et al.* (2000) Irinotecan combined with fluorouracil compared with fluorouracil alone as first-line treatment for metastatic colorectal cancer: a multicentre randomised trial. *Lancet* **355**, 1041–7.

Ebara, M., Ohto, M., Shinagawa, T. *et al.* (1986) Natural history of minute hepatocellular carcinoma smaller than three centimeters complicating cirrhosis. *Gastroenterology* **90**, 289–98.

El-Serag, H.B. and Mason, A.C. (1999) Rising incidence of hepatocellular carcinoma in the United States. *N. Engl. J. Med.* **340**, 745–50.

Epstein, B.E., Pajak, T.F., Haulk, T.L. *et al.* (1999) Metastatic nonresectable fibrolamellar hepatoma: prognostic features and natural history. *Am. J. Clin. Oncol.* **22**, 22–8.

European Liver Transplant Registry (1998) *European Liver Transplant Registry Data Analysis 05/1968–12/1997.* Villejuif, France: European Liver Transplant Association.

Fong, Y., Cohen, A.M., Fortner, J.G. *et al.* (1997) Liver resection for colorectal metastases. *J. Clin. Oncol.* **15**, 938–46.

Fong, Y., Jarnagin, W.R., Brennan, M.F. and Blumgart, L.H. (1999) Hepatocellular carcinoma: an analysis of 412 HCC at a Western center. *Ann. Surg.* **2296**, 790–9; discussion 799–800.

Freeny, P.C. (1997) Helical computed tomography of the liver: techniques, applications and pitfalls. *Endoscopy* **29**, 515–23.

Gayowski, T.J., Iwatsuki, S., Madariaga, J.R. *et al.* (1994) Experience in hepatic resection for metastatic colorectal cancer: analysis of clinical and pathologic risk factors. *Surgery* **116**(4), 703–10; discussion 710–11.

Geddes, E.W. and Falkson, G. (1970) Malignant hepatoma in the Bantu. *Cancer* **25**, 1275–8.

Giacchetti, S., Itzhaki, M. and Gruia, G. *et al.* (1999) Long term survival of patients with unresectable colorectal liver metastases following infusional chemotherapy with 5-Fluourouracil, Leucovorin, oxaliplatin and surgery. *Ann. Oncol.* **10**, 663–9.

Grimaldi, C., Bleiberg, H., Gay, F. *et al.* (1998) Evaluation of antiandrogen therapy in unresectable hepatocellular carcinoma: results of a European Organization for Research and Treatment of Cancer multicentric double-blind trial. *J. Clin. Oncol.* **16**(2), 411–17.

Groupe d'Etude et de Traitement du Carcinome Hepatocellulaire (1995) A comparison of lipiodol chemoembolization and conservative treatment for unresectable hepatocellular carcinoma. *N. Engl. J. Med.* **332**, 1256–61.

Groupe d'Etude et de Traitement du Carcinome Hepatocellulaire (1999) A new prognostic classification for predicting survival in patients with hepatocellular carcinoma. *J. Hepatol.* **311**, 133–41.

Hill, M., Norman, A. and Cunningham, D. (1995) Royal Marsden phase III trial of fluoruracil with or without interferon alpha 2b in advance colorectal cancer. *J. Clin. Oncol.* **1**, 1297–302.

IMPACT (International Multicentre Pooled Analysis of Colon Cancer Trials) Investigators (1995) Efficacy of adjuvant fluorouracil and folinic acid in colon cancer. *Lancet* **345**, 939–44.

Ishak, K., Sesterhenn, I.A., Goodman, M.Z.D. *et al.* (1984) Epithelioid haemangioendothelioma of the liver: a clinical pathologic and follow-up study of 32 cases. *Hum. Pathol.* **15**, 839–52.

Janson, E.T. and Oberg, K. (1993) Long-term management of the carcinoid synrome: treatment with octreotide alone and in combination with alpha-interferon. *Acta Oncol.* **32**, 225–9.

Johnson, P.J. (1999) Presentation and approach to diagnosis. In Leong, A.S.-Y., Liew, C.-T., Lau, J.W.Y. and Johnson, P.J. (eds), *Hepatocellular carcinoma. Contemporary diagnosis, investigation and management.* London: Arnold, 19–28.

Johnson, P.J. and Williams, R. (1987) Cirrhosis and the aetiology of hepatocellular carcinoma. *J. Hepatol.* **4**, 140.

Johnson, P.J., Leung, N., Cheng, P. *et al.* (1997) 'Hepatoma-specific' alphafetoprotein may permit preclinical diagnosis of malignant change in patients with chronic liver disease. *Br. J. Cancer* **75**, 236–40.

Kanematsu, M., Hoshi, H., Imaeda, T. *et al.* (1997) Detection and characterization of hepatic tumors: value of combined helical CT hepatic arteriography and CT during arterial portography. *AJR* **168**, 1193–6.

Kanematsu, T., Sonoda, T., Takenaka, K. *et al.* (1985) The value of ultrasound in the diagnosis and treatment of small hepatocellular carcinoma. *Br. J. Surg.* **72**, 23–5.

Kemeny, N.E. and Atiq, O.T. (1999) Non-surgical treatment for liver metastases. *Baillieres Best Practice Res. Clin. Gastroenterol.* **13**, 593–610.

Kouroumalis, E., Skordilis, P., Thermos, K. *et al.* (1998) Treatment of hepatocellular carcinoma with octreotide: a randomised controlled study. *Gut* **42**, 442–7.

Kulke, M.H. and Mayer, R.J. (1999) Carcinoid tumors. *N. Engl. J. Med.* **340**, 858–68.

Kvols, L.K., Moertel, C.G., O'Conneil, M.J. *et al.* (1986) Treatment of the malignant carcinoid syndrome: evaluation of a long-acting somatostatin analogue. *N. Engl. J. Med.* **315**, 663–6.

Lau, W.Y., Leung, K.L., Lee, T.W. *et al.* (1993) Ultrasonography during liver resection for hepatocellular carcinoma. *Br. J. Surg.* **80**, 493–4.

Lau, W.Y., Ho, S., Leung, W.T. *et al.* (1998) Selective internal radiation therapy for inoperable hepatocellular carcinoma with intraarterial infusion of yttrium[90] microspheres. *Int. J. Radiat. Oncol. Biol. Phys.* **40**, 583–92.

Lau, W.Y., Leung, T.W., Ho, S.K. *et al.* (1999) Adjuvant intra-arterial lipiodol–iodine-131-labelled lipiodol for resectable hepatocellular carcinoma – a prospective randomised trial. *Lancet* **353**, 797–801.

Lawrence, T.S., Dworzanin, L.M. and Walker-Andrews, S.C. (1991) Treatment of cancers involving the liver and porta hepatis with external beam irradiation and intraarterial hepatic fluorodeoxyuridine. *Int. J. Radiat. Oncol. Biol. Phys.* **20**, 555–61.

Leung, W.T., Lau, W.Y., Ho, S. *et al.* (1994) Intrahepatic-arterial technetium-99m macroaggregated albumin in measurerment of lung shunting in hepatocellular carcinoma. *J. Nucl. Med.* **35**, 70–3.

Leung, T.W.T., Patt, Y.Z., Lau, W.Y. *et al.* (1999) Complete pathological remission is possible with systemic combination chemotherapy for inoperable hepatocellular carcinoma. *Clin. Cancer Res.* **5**, 1676–81.

Levi, F., Zidani, R. and Misset, J.L. (1997) Randomised multicentre trial of chronotherapy with oxaliplatin, fluorouracil, and folinic acid in metastatic colorectal cancer. International Organization for Cancer Chronotherapy. *Lancet* **350**, 681–6.

Linsell, C.A. and Peers, F.G. (1977) Aflatoxin and liver-cell cancer. *Trans. R. Soc. Trop. Med. Hyg.* **71**, 471–3.

Liver Infusion Meta-analysis Group (1997) Portal vein chemotherapy for colorectal cancer: a meta-analysis of 4000 patients in 10 studies. *J. Natl Cancer Inst.* **89**, 497–505.

Livraghi, T. (1998) Percutaneous ethanol injection in hepatocellular carcinoma. *Digestion* **59**(Suppl. 2), 80–2.

Llovet, J.M., Sala, M., Castells, L. *et al.* (2000) Randomized controlled trial of interferon treatment for advanced hepatocellular carcinoma. *Hepatology* **31**, 54–8.

McPeake, J.R., O'Grady, J.G., Zaman, S. *et al.* (1993) Liver transplantation for primary hepatocellular carcinoma: tumour size and number determine outcome. *J. Hepatol.* **18**, 226–34.

Melia, W.M., Nunnerley, H.B., Johnson, P.J. and Williams, R. (1982) Use of arterial devascularization and cytotoxic drugs in 30 patients with the carcinoid syndrome. *Br. J. Cancer* **463**, 331–9.

Melia, W.M., Wilkinson, M.L., Portmann, B.C., Johnson, P.J. and Williams, R. (1984) Hepatocellular carcinoma in the non-cirrhotic liver: a comparison with that complicating cirrhosis. *QJM* (New Series LIII) **211**, 391–400.

Moertel, C.G., Fleming, T.R. and MacDonald, J.S. (1990) Levamisole and fluorouracil for adjuvant therapy of resected colon carcinoma. *N. Engl. J. Med.* **322**, 352–8.

Nagasue, N., Kohno, H., Chang, Y.C. *et al.* (1993) Liver resection for hepatocellular carcinoma. Results of 229 consecutive patients during 11 years. *Ann. Surg.* **217**, 375–84.

Nerenstone, S.R., Ihde, D.C. and Friedman, M.A. (1988) Clinical trials in primary hepatocellular carcinoma: current status and future directions. *Cancer Treat. Rep.* **15**, 1–31.

Oberg, K., Norheim, I. and Theodosson, E. (1991) Treatment of malignant carcinoid tumors with a long-acting somatostatin analogue octreotide. *Acta Oncol.* **30**, 503.

O'Connell, M., Maillard, J., Kahn, M.J. *et al.* (1997) Controlled trial of fluorouracil and low-dose leucovorin given for 6 months as post-operative adjuvant therapy for colon cancer. *J. Clin. Oncol.* **15**, 246–50.

O'Connell, M.J., Laurie, J.A., Kahn, M. *et al.* (1998) Prospectively randomized trial of postoperative adjuvant chemotherapy in patients with high-risk colon cancer. *J. Clin. Oncol.* **16**, 295–300.

Okayasu, I., Hatakeyama, S., Yoshida, T. *et al.* (1988) Selective and persistent deposition and gradual drainage of iodized oil, lipiodol in hepatocellular carcinoma after injection into the feeding hepatic artery. *Cancer* **90**, 536–44.

Okuda, K. (1997) Hepatitis C virus and hepatocellular carcinoma. In Okuda, K. (ed.), *Liver cancer*. New York: Churchill Livingstone, 39–49.

Okuda, K., Ohtsuki, T., Obata, H. *et al.* (1985a) Natural history of hepatocellular carcinoma and prognosis in relation to treatment. *Cancer* **56**, 918–28.

Okuda, K., Ohnishi, K., Kimura, J. *et al.* (1985b) Incidence of portal vein thrombosis in liver cirrhosis. An angiographic study in 708 patients. *Gastroenterology* **89**, 279–85.

Oliver, J. and Baron, R. (1996) Helical biphasic contrast-enhanced CT of the liver: technique, indications, interpretations, and pitfalls. *Radiology* **201**, 1–14.

Ortega, J.A., Krailo, M.D. and Haans, J.E. (1991) Effective treatment of unresectable or metastatic hepatoblastoma with cisplatin and continuous infusion of doxorubicin chemotherapy: a report from the Children's Cancer Study Group. *J. Clin. Oncol.* **9**, 2167–76.

Pelletier, G., Ducreux, M., Gay, F. *et al.* (1998) Treatment of unresectable hepatocellular carcinoma with lipiodol chemoembolization: a multicenter randomized trial. Groupe CHC. *J. Hepatol.* **29**, 129–34.

Peters, R.L. (1976) Pathology of hepatocellular carcinoma. In Okuda, K. and Peters, R.L. (eds), *Hepatocellular carcinoma*. New York: John Wiley.

Robertson, J.M., Lawrence, T.S., Dworzanin, L.M. *et al.* (1993) Treatment of primary hepatobiliary cancers with conformal radiation therapy and regional chemotherapy. *J. Clin. Oncol.* **77**, 1286–93.

Ross, R.K., Yuan, J.M., Yu, M.C. *et al.* (1992) Urinary aflatoxin biomarkers and risk of hepatocellular carcinoma. *Lancet* **339**, 9–11.

Rougier, P., Sahmoud, T., Nitti, D. *et al.* (1998) Adjuvant portal-vein infusion of fluorouracil and heparin in colorectal cancer: a randomised trial. European Organisation for Research and Treatment of Cancer Gastrointestinal Tract Cancer Cooperative Group, the Gruppo Interdisciplinare Valutazione Interventi in Oncologia, and the Japanese Foundation for Cancer Research. *Lancet* **351**,1677–8.

Ruszniewski, P., Ducreux, M., Chayvialle, J.A. *et al.* (1996) Treatment of the carcinoid syndrome with the long acting somatostatin analogue lanreotide: a prospective study in 39 patients. *Gut* **39**, 279–83.

Scheele, J. and Altendorf-Hofmann, A. (1999) Resection of colorectal liver metastases. *Langenbecks Arch. Surg.* **384**(4), 313–27.

Segall, H. (1923) An experimental anatomical investigation of the blood and bile channels of the liver. *Surg. Gynecol. Obstet.* **37**, 152–78.

Simonetti, R.G., Liberati, A., Angiolini, C. and Pagliaro, L. (1997) Treatment of hepatocellular carcinoma: a systematic review of randomized controlled trials. *Ann. Oncol.* **8**, 117–36.

Sobrero, A.F., Herrmann, R., Rischin, D. and Zalcberg, J. (1999) Current controversies in cancer. Does biomodulation of 5-fluorouracil improve results? *Eur. J. Cancer* **335**, 186–94.

Stuart, K.E., Anand, A.J. and Jenkins, R.L. (1996) Hepatocellular carcinoma in the United States. Prognostic features, treatment outcome, and survival. *Cancer* **7711**, 2217–22.

Tekata, K. (1990) Alpha-fetoprotein: re-evaluation in hepatology. *Hepatology* **12**, 1420–32.

Wang, J.S., Shen, X., He, X. *et al.* (1999) Protective alterations in phase 1 and 2 metabolism of aflatoxin B1 by oltipraz in residents of Qidong, People's Republic of China. *J. Natl Cancer Inst.* **91**, 347–54.

Wharton, J.T., Declos, L., Gallager, W. and Smith J.P. (1973) Radiation hepatitis induced by abdominal irradiation with cobalt-60 moving strip technique. *AJR* **117**, 73–80.

Whitney, W.S., Herfkens, R.J., Jeffrey, R.B. *et al.* (1993) Dynamic breath-hold multiplanar spoiled gradient-recalled MR imaging with gadolinium enhancement for differentiating hepatic hemangiomas from malignancies at 1.5 T. *Radiology* **189**, 863–7.

Willis, R.A. (1973) Secondary tumours of the liver. In *The spread of tumours in the human body*. London: Butterworths.

Pancreas

HEMANT M. KOCHER AND IRVING S. BENJAMIN

This is so common a major clinical problem throughout the world that patients in the later decades of life presenting with obstructive jaundice are regarded as having a tumour of the pancreas until proven otherwise.

INCIDENCE

From 1920 to 1970, the incidence had trebled in the United States but has started to level off now (Blumgart and Imrie, 1985; Gold and Goldin, 1998). In the same time period, it had doubled in England and Wales, but recent evidence from the West Midlands Cancer Registry data showed levelling off for pancreatic cancer for both sexes from 1970 onwards (Brahmall et al., 1995). The initial increase may now be considered as due to improved diagnostic modalities. Carcinoma of the exocrine pancreas is the fourth and fifth leading cause of death from malignant disease in men and women, respectively, in the USA (Carter, 1990; Boring et al., 1994). In Europe, there is preponderance in the northern European countries (Nordic countries and the UK), while the southern European countries have a lower incidence (Fernandez et al., 1994). In men, it is second as a site of gastrointestinal cancer only to the colon in the USA, and third to the colon and the stomach in the UK. It is twice as common in men as in women (McMahon, 1982) and in the USA almost twice as common in black as in white men (Gold and Goldin, 1998). There appears to be a higher incidence in Jews in the USA. The incidence is markedly age-dependent, with 80 per cent of cancers occurring between the ages of 60 and 80 (Maruchi et al., 1979). The incidence of pancreatic cancer in India is as low as 0.5–2.4 per 100 000 men and 0.2–1.8 per 100 000 for women (Dhir and Mohandas, 1999). In Japan, the incidence of pancreatic cancer is 12.5 and 6.8 per 100 000 males and females, respectively, with a rapid rise in early years (1950–85) which has plateaued since 1988 (Lin et al., 1998).

AETIOLOGY

This remains mostly unknown, with the only conclusive links being to tobacco smoking and dietary factors (Gold and Goldin, 1998). While several chemical agents, including benzidine and nitrosureas, produce pancreatic cancer in animal models (such as the Syrian hamster), careful studies have been conflicting about the higher incidence in persons subject to industrial exposure to these or other chemical substances (Selenskas et al., 1995; Tolbert, 1997; Calvert et al., 1998; Schwartz et al., 1998; Ji et al., 1999). There appears to be a doubling of the incidence in cigarette smokers (Doll and Peto, 1976). The risk increases with the amount smoked, and ex-smokers have a risk less than that of current smokers (Fontham and Correr, 1989). The incidence is increasing disproportionately in women and this may be due to changes in smoking habits amongst women (Rattner, 1992). Initial UK studies had shown a positive association between the frequency of coffee consumption and risk of pancreatic cancer, but corresponding Finnish and Norwegian studies have shown no such causal effect (McMahon 1982;

Stensvold and Jacobsen, 1994; Partanen et al., 1995). It seems unlikely that alcohol is related to pancreatic cancer. Human studies have suggested positive associations with meat consumption and carbohydrate intake and a protective effect of dietary fibre and consumption of fruits and vegetables (Howe and Burch, 1996; Gold and Goldin, 1998). Diabetes is difficult to assess as an aetiological factor, since it frequently develops after the diagnosis of the tumour, but it has been suggested that pre-existing diabetes doubles the risk of pancreatic cancer, at least in females. A recent meta-analysis showed a positive association between long-standing diabetes mellitus and pancreatic cancer (Everhart and Wright, 1995). Obesity has now been proposed as an aetiological factor (Ji et al., 1996; Ogren et al., 1996). Chronic pancreatitis does not appear to predispose to pancreatic cancer but it does pose a difficult differential diagnosis in many cases and acts as a confounding factor in epidemiological studies (Andren-Sandberg et al., 1997; Karlson et al., 1997; Bartsch et al., 1998). Recently, this association has also been shown for chronic calcific pancreatitis of the tropics (Mori et al., 1999). Even after correction for smoking, there appears to be a 2–5 times increased risk of pancreatic cancer 15–20 years after total gastrectomy (Warshaw and Fernandez-del Castillo, 1992). Recent studies have rekindled the controversial concept of cholecystectomy increasing the risk of cancer at the ampulla of Vater and pancreas (Schattner et al., 1997; Chow et al., 1999).

GENETICS

There is no apparent familial trend for this tumour. However, with the complete typing of human genome, more loci for pancreatic carcinogenesis regulator genes will be identified. Genetic syndromes associated with pancreatic cancer are hereditary pancreatitis, hereditary non-polyposis colon cancers (HNPCC or Lynch syndrome II), familial atypical mole-malignant syndrome (FAMMM) (all autosomal dominant) and ataxia telangiectesia (autosomal recessive) (Lynch et al., 1985; Lynch and Fusaro, 1991; Lowenfels et al., 1993; Ekbom et al., 1994; Lynch, 1994).

Already, there is growing evidence of pancreatic cancer in those with hereditary pancreatitis (cationic trypsinogen gene) (Gress et al., 1998). Human pancreatic cancers overexpress a number of important tyrosine growth factor receptors and their ligands (Korc, 1998). These include the epidermal growth factor receptor (EGFR) and related receptors, multiple ligands that bind to EGFR, certain fibroblast growth factor receptors (FGFR) and ligands, and insulin-like growth factor I (IGF-I) and its receptor. The excessive activation of mitogenic signalling cascades that are modulated by these overexpressed ligands and receptors is compounded by the presence of mutations in the K-ras oncogene. Pancreatic cancers also overexpress transforming growth factor-β (TGF-β) that usually inhibits the growth of epithelial cells. Pancreatic cancers, however, underexpress the type I TGF-β receptor and harbour mutations in the smad4 gene, alterations that prevent TGF-β from inhibiting cancer cell growth. Together, these perturbations confer onto pancreatic cancer cells a tremendous growth advantage (Korc, 1998).

The oncogenes involved in pancreatic cancer have thus far been identified as Ki-ras, p53 and MTS1 mutations (Grunewald et al., 1989; Kalthoff et al., 1993; Caldas et al., 1994). The frequent finding of Ki-ras mutations in various epithelial lesions of the ducts at similar sites as the pancreatic adenocarcinoma cells suggests a precursor lesion and a multi-hit hypothesis (Yanagisawa et al., 1993).

ANATOMY

In a survey of more than 500 patients at the Memorial Sloan-Kettering Cancer Centre, 66 per cent of tumours were found in the head and 20 per cent in the body and tail of the pancreas, with multiple deposits in 14 per cent (Cubilla and Fitzgerald, 1975). The size of tumours in the body and tail of the pancreas tends to be double that in the head, probably due to later presentation. Care must be exercised in the definition of 'periampullary' tumours. In a strictly anatomical sense, this definition would include cancers of the head of the pancreas, which arise in a juxta-ampullary position. However, tumours arising from the papilla of Vater itself, from adjacent duodenal mucosa or from distal bile duct epithelium, have a markedly different prognosis from pancreatic cancers in this region; it is, therefore, important to regard these as a distinct subgroup. Unfortunately, in most of the older surgical literature this distinction has not been made and has led to much difficulty in interpretation of results.

LYMPHATIC DRAINAGE

This is to the nodes around the inferior pancreatico-duodenal artery and superior mesenteric artery on the caudal border of the pancreas, those associated with the gastroduodenal and common hepatic artery leading to the coeliac axis nodes and those in the hepatoduodenal ligament associated with the proper hepatic artery, bile duct and portal vein. Tumours in the distal body and tail also drain towards the splenic hilus. While many of these nodes will be removed by conventional pancreato-duodenal resection (Whipple procedure), nodes along the superior pancreatic body are not removed in this operation. This has been one of the arguments in favour of total pancreatectomy for cancer of the head of the pancreas, although this procedure has not found wide favour. The better prognosis following resection of periampullary tumours may reflect their tendency to spread mainly to the posterior pancreato-duodenal group rather than to multiple areas

(Cubilla and Fitzgerald, 1975). Recent Japanese work has also highlighted the presence of metastasis in para-aortic lymph nodes; however, the benefit in terms of survival from radical resections involving such nodes remains to be proved (Nagai *et al.*, 1986; Ishikawa *et al.*, 1988; Nagakawa *et al.*, 1994; Kayahara *et al.*, 1999).

METASTASES AND NATURAL HISTORY

Less than 20 per cent of patients have disease confined to the pancreas at the time of presentation: 40 per cent of patients present with locally advanced disease and 40 per cent will have visceral metastases, usually involving the liver. Peritoneal implants are found at presentation in 35 per cent of patients: these are seldom more than a few millimetres in size, making detection extremely difficult with any of the conventional imaging techniques (Reznek and Stephens, 1993). The advent of diagnostic laparoscopy as an adjunctive staging procedure along with laparoscopic ultrasound would detect these visceral metastases and prevent these patients from undergoing open-and-close laparotomy (Espat *et al.*, 1999; Baron *et al.*, 1999; Catheline *et al.*, 1999; Gouma *et al.*, 1999; Reddy *et al.*, 1999). However, its exact importance has been questioned because of low yield as a diagnostic test in some series (Friess *et al.*, 1998). The question of multi-centricity remains controversial. It has been suggested that as many as 40 per cent of pancreatic cancers may be multi-centric. This may be due to field changes within the ductal epithelium, and indeed severe dysplasia is often noted in association with established ductal cancer. It may also be due to retrograde seeding of pancreatic cancer down an obstructed duct. Tryka and Brooks (1979) showed in a series of 25 patients who underwent total pancreatectomy that 38 per cent had tumour outwith the area normally resected by the Whipple procedure. While in seven cases this was due to direct extension up the common bile duct or along the neck of the pancreas, in five there was apparently true multi-focal disease.

PATHOLOGY

The majority (90 per cent) of tumours are adenocarcinomas of ductal origin, and possibly 10 per cent are acinar tumours. Endocrine tumours of the pancreas are described in Chapter 20, but it is important to note that some quite large tumours of neuroendocrine origin may be amenable to resection, either for long-term palliation or cure; this diagnosis should be considered in patients with apparently atypical or long-standing pancreatic tumours. The common type of ductal adenocarcinoma produces an intense scirrhous reaction and often leads to dilatation of the distal pancreatic duct. Those in the head almost invariably produce common bile duct obstruction, but this feature may be late or absent in cases of endocrine tumour. Cystadenocarcinoma of the pancreas is another variant, which may remain confined to the gland, grow to a considerable size and remain amenable to curative resection despite its bulk. It is frequently misdiagnosed as a benign pseudocyst: 15 per cent of cysts are neoplastic rather than inflammatory and these cysts must be excised (Warshaw and Rutledge, 1987).

There is a growing body of evidence to suggest that the atypical ductal lesions such as ductal hyperplasia, papillary adenomatosis and atypical papillary hyperplasia are precursor lesions to pancreatic ductal adenocarcinoma (Brat *et al.*, 1998).

SYMPTOMS AND PRESENTATION

Most patients (90 per cent) present with obstructive jaundice (Howard and Jordan, 1977), commonly associated with weight loss, anorexia and fatigue. Abdominal pain occurs in 50–90 per cent of cases. Back pain may represent a late stage of the disease, with deep retroperitoneal and neural invasion. 'Painless jaundice' has been classically ascribed to victims of pancreatic cancer, but is only true in the sense of lack of long-standing pain associated with gallstone disease, as a differential diagnosis in the jaundiced patient. 'Courvoisier's sign' may present in only 25 per cent of patients with malignant obstruction of the bile duct. Other late signs described for pancreatic cancer include Virchow's node or Troisier's sign (palpable left supraclavicular lymph node), Sister Mary Joseph's nodule (metastasis to umbilicus), Trousseau's sign (migratory thrombophlebitis) and Blumer's shelf (deposits in the peritoneal pouch in front of the rectum). A small number of cases present *de novo* with an attack of acute pancreatitis (Trapnell, 1972; Blumgart and Imrie, 1985). Thrombophlebitis migrans probably occurs in less than 10 per cent of cases and is relatively non-specific (Brooks and Culebras, 1976). Recent experimental work has shown that tissue factor expression (a procoagulant) may have a role in the thrombotic state of pancreatic cancer as well as helping the pancreatic cancer cells to invade other tissues (Kakkar *et al.*, 1999). In one series, 15 per cent of patients had new onset of diabetes mellitus during the year before the diagnosis of malignancy (Ona *et al.*, 1973). Sadly, most signs and symptoms of the disease are late and the tumour is advanced on presentation.

DIAGNOSIS

Examination

The principal sign is obstructive jaundice. Weight loss is usually evident and abdominal examination may reveal a palpable gall bladder (Courvoisier's sign). The sign of an intermittently palpable gall bladder may suggest a periampullary tumour.

Investigation

There are no specific laboratory tests. The liver function tests reveal the picture of obstructive jaundice. Pancreatic secretory tests are not helpful and although glucose tolerance may be abnormal, this does not aid diagnosis. Tumour markers have been studied extensively. Carcinoembryonic antigen (CEA) is elevated in 85–100 per cent of cases (Ona et al., 1973; Mackie et al., 1980). Pancreatic oncofetal antigen (POA) is more specific, with false-positive results only in severe pancreatitis. However, the sensitivity is only 60 per cent. POA tends to be associated with tumour differentiation rather than tumour mass and it is not associated with endocrine tumours or lymphomas of the pancreas. Mackie et al. (1980), in Chicago, evaluated prospectively a number of tumour markers in pancreatic cancer. The tests of greatest diagnostic value were POA, fasting plasma glucose and serum alkaline phosphatase. The two most widely used tumour markers are CA 19-9 and DU PAN 2. They can be detected in the serum of 70–90 per cent of patients with pancreatic carcinoma. Their levels correlate with the tumour burden and are often normal in patients with small tumours (Mahvi et al., 1985; Parker et al., 1992). However, CA 19-9 may be non-specifically elevated in biliary obstruction.

Ultrasound is the most valuable non-invasive method and contributes in three ways: first, in the diagnosis of obstructive jaundice; second, in demonstrating a mass in the pancreas; and third, as a guide for fine-needle aspiration cytology (FNAC). Ultrasound has a failure rate of around 10 per cent, mostly due to obesity or to bowel gas. CT scanning is complementary to ultrasound, rather than superior, and the failure rate is about the same, although not necessarily in the same patients (Reznek and Stephens, 1993). The availability of spiral CT scan and ultrafast MRI has shown that the pancreas can now be imaged with reasonable anatomic accuracy, especially with reference to encroachment on adjoining vessels (Ichikawa et al., 1997; Trede et al., 1997; Bluemke and Fishman, 1998; Yamaguchi et al., 1998; Nishiharu et al., 1999). The heavily T_2-weighted MRI pictures (named as magnetic resonance cholangiopancreatography; MRCP) give very good three-dimensional imaging of the biliary and pancreatic ducts (Yamaguchi et al., 1998). However, all scanning modalities are of limited value in detecting lymph node involvement, and when seen on scans, in the absence of prior biliary invasive intervention in the form of ERCP or percutaneous transhepatic cholangiography (PTC), this usually represents advanced disease.

Of the invasive tests, endoscopy may show extrinsic compression of the stomach or duodenum by a mass in the head of the pancreas, or indeed mucosal invasion by tumour. Endoscopy is of particular importance in identifying tumours of the ampulla of Vater. ERCP is probably the single most valuable test, with an overall success rate of 85–90 per cent. In obstructive jaundice, the 'double duct' sign – stenosis of the distal common bile duct and pancreatic duct at adjacent points – is almost diagnostic. Cytology is commonly obtained by brushings on ERCP but may also be obtained either by direct suction with the cannula in the pancreatic duct or by duodenal juice aspiration; both of these may be helped by intravenous injection of secretin to stimulate the flow of pancreatic juice. Biopsies of ampullary lesions may be obtained at ERCP. Overall, Moossa and Levin (1979) found the predictive value of positive ERCP to be 85 per cent and that of a negative test 91 per cent, in the presence of a prevalence rate for pancreatic cancer of 39 per cent. Cytology obtained at the time of cholangiography may clinch the diagnosis (Kurzawinski et al., 1993). In jaundiced patients, if a cholangiogram cannot be obtained by ERCP then PTC should be undertaken.

This will show the site of the obstruction but may not be diagnostic of pancreatic cancer. Chronic pancreatitis may produce a long rat-tail stricture in the head of the pancreas, with a characteristically (but not diagnostically) smooth tapered appearance. Arteriography is of less value as a diagnostic tool than ERCP but may provide additional information in patients who are being considered for resection. Freeney et al. (1993) compared contrast-enhanced CT and angiography and showed that in over 70 per cent of patients both techniques give similar information about vascular involvement, but routine preoperative angiography is practised by some (Appleton et al., 1989). In comparing both investigations Warshaw et al. (1990) showed that neither technique was as good as both together and recommended using both as complementary investigations. Angiography may be of value as a 'road map' for surgery, and in particular to identify anomalous arterial anatomy.

Endoscopic ultrasound (EUS) is a relatively new technique and, combined with the use of endoscopic Doppler evaluation and ultrasound guided FNAC, it is a useful adjunct in diagnosing vascular involvement and obtaining accurate biopsy tissue for small tumours (Soreide, 1987; Rosch et al., 1992; Brugge, 1995; Chang, 1995; Snady, 1995; Baarir et al., 1998).

Preoperative fine-needle aspiration cytology has become increasingly popular. The results in more than 800 patients in 12 collected series are reported by Soreide (1987). The average sensitivity was 71 per cent with a false-positive rate when adequately assessed of less than 1 per cent. Overall results for preoperative and intraoperative cytology in our own experience have been similar (Desa et al., 1991). The risks appear to be very low, and in particular only five cases of needle-track tumour seeding have been reported in more than 64 000 biopsies. Aspiration cytology is also applicable in the evaluation of a pancreatic mass found at surgery; the differentiation between cancer and chronic pancreatitis may not be easy.

Laparoscopy can detect small peritoneal nodules that elude ultrasound and CT detection, and may eliminate an unnecessary laparotomy in a number of patients (Friess *et al.*, 1998; Catheline *et al.*, 1999; Gouma *et al.*, 1999; Reddy *et al.*, 1999). More recently the combination of laparoscopy and laparoscopic ultrasound has been reported to be of value in the staging of pancreatic neoplasms and assessment of resectability (Fernandez-del Castillo and Warshaw, 1998; Friess *et al.*, 1998; Catheline *et al.*, 1999; Gouma *et al.*, 1999; Reddy *et al.*, 1999).

CLINICAL INVESTIGATION AND STAGING

Investigation is aimed, first, at elucidating the site of obstruction in the case of the jaundiced patient and, second, at determining the degree of advancement of the tumour. In patients presenting with non-specific symptoms, ultrasound, CT scan and ERCP together give the maximum diagnostic yield. The recent advent of MRI, helical CT scan, endoscopic ultrasound scan (USS) and laparoscopy has changed the algorithm in centres dealing with pancreatic cancer with a view to resection. An abdominal USS followed by MRI with MRCP, associated with endoscopic USS with laparoscopic assessment of peritoneum and liver, prevents any invasion of the biliary tree and allows operation to proceed with adequate imaging of all the concerned areas. However, it is true that most symptomatic tumours of the body and tail of the pancreas are large and irresectable at presentation.

A widely used staging system in the older literature is that of Hermreck *et al.* (1974). The staging system published by Sobin and Wittekind (Sobin and Wittekind, 1997) based on the TNM staging is similar, and is shown in Table 25.1. One of the problems with this scheme is that the stages are not necessarily sequential and patients may have lymphatic spread without involvement of neighbouring structures.

TREATMENT

Indications

Patients with pancreatic cancer will present in one or more of three ways: with obstructive jaundice and pruritus, pain in the abdomen or back, or with the systemic effects of advanced malignancy. In the last category, once the diagnosis has been established there may be little indication for any treatment other than symptomatic control. Non-surgical methods are available for treating the pain and these are referred to below. Pruritus and pain are distressing symptoms, which should be palliated, whether by operative or non-operative means. Beyond these broad principles there is no general agreement as to the optimum method for treating pancreatic cancer.

Techniques of treatment

SURGERY

Pancreato-duodenectomy, perhaps one of the most demanding elective general surgical procedures, was put on the surgical map by A.O. Whipple in 1935 (Chen and Chen, 1993). Opinions have swung periodically as to whether or not the operation should be preceded by biliary decompression. Although Whipple performed a two-stage procedure, from 1940 until the 1970s it was done as one-stage procedure. In the 1970s preoperative PTC or ERCP and stenting was in vogue, but now preoperative decompression has become less popular in many centres, primarily because of the risk of infection due to stenting.

Although there were initial criticisms of the mortality and morbidity of the Whipple procedure (Crile, 1970), these have largely been put to rest by reviews from both the USA and the UK showing that, if concentrated in expert hands, surgical treatment of pancreatic cancers would achieve acceptable results, both in terms of low perioperative mortality and morbidity and improved survival prospects (Aston and Longmire, 1973; Brooks and Culebras, 1976; Moossa and Levin, 1979; Pellegrini *et al.*, 1989; Trede *et al.*, 1990; Cameron *et al.*, 1993; Neoptolemos *et al.*, 1997). The increasing evidence that complications and morbidity are inversely related to caseload has put to rest the claim of the occasional pancreatectomist (Hannan *et al.*, 1989; Edge *et al.*, 1993; Brahmall *et al.*, 1995; Gordon *et al.*, 1995; Lieberman *et al.*, 1995; Neoptolemos *et al.*, 1997; Begg *et al.*, 1998).

The plethora of resectional and reconstructive possibilities advocated by various groups has made effective comparisons of studies for even standard pancreatic resection difficult. Nevertheless, single- and multi-institutional studies have shown that with lesser blood loss and fewer transfusions intra-operatively, and early detection of complications and their effective management by a dedicated multidisciplinary team of nutritionist, interventional radiologist and intensivist, along with better postoperative

Table 25.1 *Staging system for pancreatic carcinoma (Sobin and Wittekind, 1997: 88–90)*

Stage I	T1–2, N0, M0	No direct extension and no regional lymph node involvement
Stage II	T2, N0, M0	Direct extension into adjacent tissue; no lymph node involvement
Stage III	T1–3, N1, M0	Regional lymph node involvement with or without direct tumour extension
Stage IV	T1–3, N0–1, M1	Distant metastatic spread

adjuvant therapy, have all led to better postoperative survival, 5-year survival and median survival (Cameron *et al.*, 1993; Geer and Brennan, 1993; Neoptolemos *et al.*, 1997; Gordon *et al.*, 1995; Yeo *et al.*, 1995, 1997).

More extensive resections, such as total pancreatectomy, have been advocated, primarily based on the fact that the pancreatic cancer is a multi-focal disease and to achieve better locoregional clearance in the soft tissue surrounding the pancreas (Fortner, 1973, 1981; Tryka and Brooks, 1979; van Heerden *et al.*, 1981; Hiraoka and Kanemitsu, 1994; Moossa and Romeo, 1994). This has to be balanced against the fact that after total pancreatectomy the patient becomes a brittle diabetic, and moreover most reviews have not shown better survival than standard resection. The average survival was only 16 months.

The arguments for thorough lymphatic dissection are less easy to evaluate. The Japanese, in particular, are advocates of radical lymphadenectomy as part of pancreatic resection procedures (Nagai *et al.*, 1986; Ishikawa *et al.*, 1988; Nagakawa *et al.*, 1994; Kayahara *et al.*, 1999). They showed that, even for the small tumours (<2 cm), node positivity dropped the 1-year survival likelihood from 89 per cent to 59 per cent (Tsuchiya *et al.*, 1985). They have promoted the concept of resecting even the para-aortic lymph nodes right up to the origin of the inferior mesentric artery. Radical operations for pancreatic cancer have yielded 13 per cent 5-year survival after amalgamating various Japanese series, while in the United States the figure was 19 per cent (Livingstone *et al.*, 1991), although all the series are not strictly comparable because of the various definitions of postoperative adjuvant therapy.

The morbidity associated with pancreato-duodenectomy in various series is, on an average, around 19 per cent, but can reach up to 50 per cent (Miedema *et al.*, 1992; Cameron *et al.*, 1993). The common complications include early delayed gastric emptying, pancreatic fistula, intra-abdominal abscess formation, haemorrhage, wound infection and metabolic disorders.

Distal pancreatic tumours present late because of their relative lack of symptoms, and therefore, more often than not, they are not amenable to resectional procedures. However, a small series in a selected group of patients has shown good results (Johnson *et al.*, 1993).

Although preoperative imaging has improved the pick-up rate of irresectable tumours, occasionally after trial dissection a tumour previously deemed resectable, may not be so, especially if the concept of regional pancreatectomy or vascular reconstruction is not viewed as helpful. In such cases, surgical biliary bypass is indicated. The modern trend of pre-laparotomy laparoscopy may detect such cases. Two options exist at such a stage. Either laparoscopic biliary bypass if expertise exists (Franklin and Balli, 1998), or postoperative endoscopic biliary stenting (if there was no stent preoperatively).

Prophylactic gastric bypass as well, previously called a triple bypass (gastric, biliary and a jejuno-jejunal bypass), is not indicated because as few as 15 per cent of patients go on to develop duodenal obstruction before succumbing to irresectable pancreatic head adenocarcinoma (Brooks *et al.*, 1981). Also gastric bypass may be accompanied by delayed gastric emptying and increased time in hospital (Sarr and Cameron, 1982; Gompertz *et al.*, 1990).

Preoperative measures, such as good nutrition, upgrading of immunity (Rege *et al.*, 1993) and prevention of biliary sepsis or dehydration (renal failure), will help in a jaundiced patient. Preoperative biliary drainage may help in improving nutrition and restoring liver function to near normal. However, the introduction of infection limits the advantages, especially of the external drainage procedures (Hatfield *et al.*, 1982; McPherson *et al.*, 1982; Sarr and Cameron, 1982).

Preoperative preparation of the jaundiced patient by means of temporary endoscopic stenting or naso-biliary drainage, or by percutaneous transhepatic drainage, has remained a controversial area since enthusiastic reports in the late 1970s (Nakayama *et al.*, 1978). Controlled trials of percutaneous drainage have not shown any survival advantage and produced a high incidence of complications (Hatfield *et al.*, 1982; McPherson *et al.*, 1982; Norlander *et al.*, 1982). Endoscopic stenting probably has a lesser complication rate than percutaneous transhepatic external drainage, and many surgeons adopt this as a routine. A compromise has to be carefully judged between improvement in liver function by a period of drainage, and the risk of infection of the intrahepatic biliary tree. There is uniform agreement that the patient who is deeply jaundiced, with incipient renal failure and severe coagulopathy, is not a suitable candidate for major resectional surgery without some form of preoperative preparation.

NON-SURGICAL PALLIATION

Endoscopic biliary stenting of irresectable pancreatic tumours for the relief of jaundice (Fig. 25.1) is almost as good, if not better, than surgical bypass (Bornman *et al.*, 1986; Shepherd *et al.*, 1988; Anderson *et al.*, 1989; Dowsett *et al.*, 1989). It was first described in 1980 by Soehendra and Reynders-Frederix and has received a unanimous verdict of acceptability for palliation. Plastic stents have relieved jaundice in approximately 88 per cent of patients, but require stent exchange in 21–30 per cent of patients, due to either failure or complications of stenting (Siegel and Snady, 1986; Speer and Cotton, 1988). With the advent of new metallic self-expanding endoprosthesis, one can achieve larger-calibre drainage, and therefore obviate the need for stent exchange (Adam, 1990; Adam *et al.*, 1991). Recent multivariate analysis has shown that patients with tumours larger than 30 mm are more likely to survive more than 6 months and therefore would be suitable for metallic stenting over the plastic counterparts (Adam, 1990). The development of expandable Teflon stents may have advantages over the metallic stent, since they could be exchanged (Haringsma and Huibregtse, 1998). All these stents could be placed via a percutaneous transhepatic

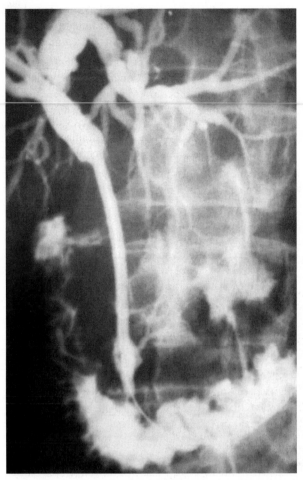

Figure 25.1 *A long 'double-mushroom' endoprosthesis in place through an extensive cancer in the head of the pancreas. The guide-wire used to place this stent can still be seen entering the duodenum.*

route, if there were any complication or contraindication for endoscopic stenting. Up to 7.5 per cent of the patients with palliative biliary stents will require palliation for gastric outlet obstruction (Siegel and Snady, 1986). This can be palliated endoscopically as well (Venu *et al.*, 1998).

PALLIATION OF PAIN

In addition to palliation of jaundice and duodenal obstruction, pain relief is important in the palliation of pancreatic cancer. Coeliac plexus blockade by injection of alcohol may be very effective for a number of months. This can be performed percutaneously under fluoroscopic or CT guidance, or intra-operatively. Leung *et al.* (1983) and Lillemoe *et al.* (1993) reported pain relief in 80–90 per cent of patients with unresectable pancreatic carcinoma so treated. Thoracoscopic splanchnicectomy has achieved similar results (Le Pimpec Barthes *et al.*, 1998; Worsey *et al.*, 1993). External-beam radiotherapy may also be effective in pain control for advanced cancers (Whittington *et al.*, 1981).

RADIOTHERAPY

The deep location of the pancreas and its close proximity to radiosensitive structures (spinal cord, kidneys, duodenum and liver) make delivery of full doses of conventional external-beam radiation (5000–6000 cGy) hazardous. Several early reports of 'cure' of pancreatic cancer were unsubstantiated by histological diagnosis (Dobelbower, 1979). Moertel *et al.* (1969) showed no survival improvement in 62 patients treated with 35 Gy and 5-fluorouracil (5-FU). Attempts to improve survival or secure a higher rate of remission by use of other supervoltage techniques have had no conspicuous success (Dobelbower, 1979). Intra-operative radiotherapy, pioneered by the Japanese (Abe *et al.*, 1969), has been adopted in some centres in the United States. Preoperative or intra-operative radiation therapy (IORT) is under investigation for its possible use in combination with resection (Jessup *et al.*, 1993). A controlled prospective trial of adjuvant IORT combined with curative resection (carried out by the National Cancer Institute) found that although overall survival time was unchanged, local control was better (Warshaw and Swanson, 1988). Although local control may be improved by IORT, this has no effect on disease at distant sites and many patients succumb from metastases (Jessup *et al.*, 1993). These methods may be combined, and the use of external-beam radiotherapy and electron-beam IORT allows delivery of a higher dose of radiation without damage to adjacent organs or tissues (Warshaw and Swanson, 1988). Complications have been reported in up to 35 per cent of cases, and include gastrointestinal bleeding, obstruction and perforation. Some centres have tried implantation of ^{125}I and have suggested that a degree of local control may be achieved (Jessup *et al.*, 1993), as well as pain relief (Fortner *et al.*, 1970). Recent reviews have pointed out that while external-beam radiotherapy (EBRT) may be a useful adjunct in palliation of pain in patients with pancreatic cancer, IORT may be useful for improving local control in patients with resectable disease (Gunderson *et al.*, 1999; Sindelar and Kinsella, 1999).

CHEMOTHERAPY

The response to single-agent chemotherapy has generally been poor. Combination chemotherapy has been reported to have slightly higher response rates and may increase median survival. However, only one good trial in the UK has compared therapy to supportive management in a randomized manner (Mallinson *et al.*, 1980), and this trial showed only a modest improvement in survival. FAM (5-FU, Adriamycin® and mitomycin C) produced a partial response in 73 per cent of patients in a small trial from Washington (Smith *et al.*, 1980). The median survival of responders was 12 months, compared with 3.5 months in non-responders. Epirubicin has been studied in 34 patients with pancreatic cancer, with a response rate of 24 per cent (Wils *et al.*, 1985). A further trial in New York showed a 19 per cent partial response rate in

16 patients (Hochster *et al.*, 1986). A more recent trial from Edinburgh has shown improved survival using 5-FU, Adriamycin® and mitomycin in patients with irresectable pancreatic cancer. Median survival in treated patients was 33 weeks, compared with 15 weeks in those who did not receive chemotherapy (Palmer *et al.*, 1994). Combination chemotherapy using FAM or epirubicin has shown some improvement in response rates, but little improvement in median survival (Smith *et al.*, 1980; Wils *et al.*, 1985; Hochster *et al.*, 1986; Palmer *et al.*, 1994). 5-FU seemed to be the only drug of some benefit till the arrival of gemcitabine.

Other therapeutic modalities that have been tried include the combined use of radiotherapy and chemotherapy with radiosensitizers. Cisplatin, 5-FU and mitomycin have some activity against pancreatic cancer and they have a synergistic effect when combined with radiotherapy. While conventional radiotherapy does not improve survival, with combined treatment an improvement in survival from 5 months (using radiotherapy alone) to 10 months has been reported (Warshaw and Swanson, 1988). These results are not dramatic, but they do show some promise. The Gastrointestinal Tumour Study Group demonstrated that chemoradiation after curative resection doubled the median survival of patients, from 11 months to 20 months (Jessup *et al.*, 1993). Bruckner *et al.* (1993) has used a regimen with split-course radiotherapy and simultaneous multidrug chemotherapy with continuous 5-FU, streptozotocin and cisplatin, and achieved a median survival of 1 year in a group of 20 patients with unresectable disease. The results of Radiation Therapy Oncology Group (RTOG) studies such as the RTOG 97-04 and RTOG 98-12, examining the question of chemoradiation with newer chemotherapeutic agents such as gemcitabine and paclitaxel, are eagerly awaited (Kroep *et al.*, 1999; Rich, 1999).

A recent trial by The European Study Group for Pancreatic Cancer (ESPAC) trialists has suggested that there is a role for adjuvant chemotherapy in resectable pancreatic cancer. However, there is no role for adjuvant radiotherapy or chemo-radiotherapy (Neoptolemos *et al.*, 2001). The same group of trialists (ESPAC) are investigating the role of new chemotherapeutic agents in resectable pancreatic cancer.

END RESULTS

Because most patients present with advanced disease, the overall results remain poor for this condition. Surgical treatment is the only chance for long-term survival. However, improvements in operative safety and better patient selection have allowed some degree of optimism in the approach to individual patients. It remains true that the overall resectability rate is no more than 25 per cent, despite improvements in diagnostic tools. Nevertheless, operative mortality is now low, typically below 5 per cent, and the 5-year survival figures have improved significantly

in recent times. Trede *et al.* (1990) reported a 5-year survival of 24 per cent and Cameron *et al.* (1993), 19 per cent. The figures are even better for those patients with stage I disease. While few centres will be equipped to make use of IORT, it may be that a combination of resection with postoperative chemoradiotherapy will improve these figures still further. While there remains no room for complacency in this highly lethal tumour, there are some grounds for increased optimism. Genetic breakthroughs, especially with imminent availability of human genome blueprint, may hold the key to therapy in this cancer, which is seldom diagnosed early enough to give cure.

SIGNIFICANT POINTS

- Cancer of the pancreas is increasing in incidence and surgical attitudes are changing.
- With careful evaluation, resectability rates are rising and 5-year survival following radical resection, along with lower operative risks, makes consideration of surgery worthwhile.
- Advances in chemotherapy and radiotherapy have been slow, and their role is still in doubt.

KEY REFERENCES

Manu, M., Buckels, J. and Bramhall, S. (2000) Molecular technology and pancreatic cancer. *Br. J. Surg.* **87**, 840–53.

Scrio, G., Huguet, C. and Williamson, R.C.N. (1994) *Hepatobiliary and pancreatic tumours* Edinburgh: Graffam Press.

Trede, M., Schwall, G. and Saeger, H.D. (1990) Survival after pancreatoduodenectomy: 118 consecutive resections without an operative mortality. *Ann. Surg.* **211**, 447–58.

Tytgat, G.N.J., Gouma, D.J., Offerhaus, G.J.A., Peters, G.J., Pinedo, H.M. and Bartelink, H. (1999) Biliopancreatic malignancy: from gene to cure. *Ann. Oncol.* **10**(suppl. 4).

REFERENCES

Abe, M., Yamano, K., Imura, T. *et al.* (1969) Intraoperative radiotherapy of abdominal tumours. Part I Intraoperative irradiation to a carcinoma of the pancreas head and biliary system. *Nippon Acta Radiol.* **29**, 75–85.

Adam, A. (1990) Percutaneous biliary drainage for malignancy (Editorial). *Clin. Radiol.* **41**, 225–7.

Adam, A., Chatty, N., Rode, N. *et al.* (1991) Self expanding stainless steel endoprosthesis for treatment of malignant bile duct obstruction. *Am. J. Roentology* **156**, 321–5.

Anderson, J.R., Sorenson, S.M., Kruse, A. *et al.* (1989) Randomised trial of endoscopic endoprosthesis versus operative bypass in malignant obstructive jaundice. *Gut* **30**, 1132–5.

Andren-Sandberg, A., Dervenis, C. and Lowenfels, B. (1997) Etiologic links between chronic pancreatitis and pancreatic cancer. *Scand. J. Gastroenterol.* **32**(2), 97–103.

Appleton, G.V.N., Bathurst, N.C.G., Virjee, J. *et al.* (1989) The value of angiography in the surgical management of pancreatic disease. *Ann. R. Coll. Surg. Engl.* **71**, 92–6.

Aston, S.J. and Longmire, W.P. Jr (1973) Pancreaticoduodenal resection: twenty years' experience. *Arch. Surg.* **106**, 813–17.

Baarir, N., Amouyal, G., Faintuch, J.M., Houry, S. and Huguier, M. (1998) Comparison of color Doppler ultrasonography and endoscopic ultrasonography for preoperative evaluation of the mesenteric-portal axis in pancreatic lesions. *Chirurgie* **123**(5), 445–9.

Baron, P.L., Kay, C. and Hoffman, B. (1999) Pancreatic imaging. *Surg. Oncol. Clin. N. Am.* **8**(1), 35–58.

Bartsch, H., Malaveille, C., Lowenfels, A.B., Maisonneuve, P., Hautefeuille, A. and Boyle, P. (1998) Genetic polymorphism of *N*-acetyltransferases, glutathione S-transferase M1 and NAD(P)H: quinone oxidoreductase in relation to malignant and benign pancreatic disease risk. The International Pancreatic Disease Study Group. *Eur. J. Cancer Prev.* **7**(3): 215–23.

Begg, C.B., Cramer, L.D., Hoskins, W.J. and Brennan, M.F. (1998) Impact of hospital volume on operative mortality for major cancer surgery. *JAMA* **280**(20), 1747–51.

Bluemke, D.A. and Fishman, E.K. (1998) CT and MR evaluation of pancreatic cancer. *Surg. Oncol. Clin. N. Am.* **7**(1), 103–24.

Blumgart, L.H. and Imrie, C.W. (1985) Tumours of the extrahepatic biliary tree and pancreas. In Wright, R., Millward-Sadler, G.H., Alberti, K.G.M.M. and Karran, S. (eds), *Liver and biliary disease*. London: Baillière Tindall, 1495–522.

Boring, C.C., Squires, T.S., Tong, T. *et al.* (1994) Cancer Statistics 1994. *CA Cancer J. Clin.* **44**, 7.

Bornman, P.C., Harries-Jones, E.P., Tobias, R. *et al.* (1986) Prospective controlled trial of transhepatic biliary endoprosthesis versus bypass surgery for incurable carcinoma of the head of the pancreas. *Lancet* **i**, 69–71.

Brahmall, S.R., Allum, W.H., Jones, A.G., Allwood, A., Cummins, C. and Neoptolemos, J. (1995) Treatment and survival in 13 560 patients with pancreatic cancer and the incidence of the disease in the West Midlands: an epidemiological study. *Br. J. Surg.* **82**, 111–15.

Brat, D.J., Lillemoe, K.D., Yeo, C.J., Warfield, P.B. and Hruban, R.H. (1998) Progression of pancreatic intraductal neoplasias to infiltrating adenocarcinoma of the pancreas. *Am. J. Surg. Pathol.* **22**(2), 163–9.

Brooks, D.C., Osteen, R.T., Gray, E.B. *et al.* (1981) Evaluation of palliative procedures for pancreatic cancer. *Am. J. Surg.* **141**, 430–3.

Brooks, J.R. and Culebras, J.M. (1976) Cancer of the pancreas: palliative operation, Whipple procedure, or total pancreatectomy? *Am. J. Surg.* **131**, 516–20.

Bruckner, H.W., Dalton, J., Schwartz, G.K. *et al.* (1993) Survival after combined modality therapy for pancreatic cancer. *J. Clin. Gastroenterol.* **16**, 199–203.

Brugge, W.R. (1995) Pancreatic cancer staging. Endoscopic ultrasonography criteria for vascular invasion. *Gastrointest. Endosc. Clin. N. Am.* **5**(4), 741–53.

Caldas, C., Hahn, S.A., Costa, L.T. *et al.* (1994) Frequent somatic mutations and homozygous deletions of the p16 (MTS1) gene in pancreatic adenocarcinoma. *Nat. Genet.* **8**, 27.

Calvert, G.M., Ward, E., Schnorr, T.M. and Fine, L.J. (1998) Cancer risks among workers exposed to metalworking fluids: a systematic review. *Am. J. Ind. Med.* **33**(3), 282–92.

Cameron, J.L., Pitt, H.A., Yeo, C.J. *et al.* (1993) One hundred and forty five consecutive pancreato-duodenectomies without mortality. *Ann. Surg.* **217**, 430–8.

Carter, D.C. (1990) Cancer of the pancreas. *Gut* **31**, 494–6.

Catheline, J.M., Turner, R., Rizk, N., Barrat, C. and Champault, G. (1999) The use of diagnostic laparoscopy supported by laparoscopic ultrasonography in the assessment of pancreatic cancer. *Surg. Endosc.* **13**(3), 239–45.

Chang, K.J. (1995) Endoscopic ultrasound-guided fine needle aspiration in the diagnosis and staging of pancreatic tumors. *Gastrointest. Endosc. Clin. N. Am.* **5**(4), 723–34.

Chen, T.S.N. and Chen, P.S.Y. (1993) The Whipples and their legacies in medicine. *Surg. Gynecol. Obstet.* **176**, 501–6.

Chow, W.H., Johansen, C., Gridley, G., Mellemkjaer, L., Olsen, J.H. and Fraumeni, J.F. Jr (1999) Gallstones, cholecystectomy and risk of cancers of the liver, biliary tract and pancreas. *Br. J. Cancer* **79**(3–4), 640–4.

Crile, G. Jr (1970) The advantages of bypass operations over radical pancreatoduodenectomy in the treatment of pancreatic carcinoma. *Surg. Gynecol. Obstet.* **130**, 1049–53.

Cubilla, A.L. and Fitzgerald, P.J. (1975) Morphological patterns of primary non-endocrine human pancreas carcinoma cancer. *Cancer Res.* **35**, 2234–48.

Desa, L.A., Akosa, A.B., Lazzara, S. *et al.* (1991) Cytodiagnosis in the management of extrahepatic biliary stricture. *Gut* **32**, 1188–91.

Dhir, V. and Mohandas, K.M. (1999) Epidemiology of digestive tract cancers in India IV. Gall bladder and pancreas. *Indian J. Gastroenterol.* **18**(1), 24–8.

Dobelbower, R.R. Jr (1979) The radiotherapy of pancreatic cancer. *Sem. Oncol.* **6**, 378–89.

Doll, R. and Peto, R. (1976) Mortality in relation to smoking: 20 years observations on male British doctors. *BMJ* **2**, 1525–36.

Dowsett, J.F., Russell, R.C.G. and Hatfield, A.R.W. (1989) Malignant obstructive jaundice. A prospective randomised trial of bypass surgery versus endoscopic stenting. *Gastroenterology* **96**, 128A.

Edge, S.B., Schmieg, R.E. Jr, Rosenlof, L.K. and Wilhelm, M.C. (1993) Pancreas cancer resection outcome in American University centers in 1989–1990. *Cancer* **71**(11), 3502–8.

Ekbom, A., McLaughlin, J.K., Karlsson, B. *et al.* (1994) Pancreatitis and pancreatic cancer: a population based study. *J. Natl Cancer Inst.* **86**, 625–7.

Espat, N.J., Brennan, M.F. and Conlon, K.C. (1999) Patients with laparoscopically staged unresectable pancreatic adenocarcinoma do not require subsequent surgical biliary or gastric bypass. *J. Am. Coll. Surg.* **188**(6), 649–55.

Everhart, J. and Wright, D. (1995) Diabetes mellitus as a risk factor for pancreatic cancer. A meta-analysis. *JAMA* **273**(20), 1605–9.

Fernandez, E., La Vechia, C., Porta, M., Negri, E., Lucchini, F. and Levi, F. (1994) Trends in pancreatic cancer mortality in Europe, 1955–89. *Int. J. Cancer* **57**(6), 786–92.

Fernandez-del Castillo, C.L. and Warshaw, A.L. (1998) Pancreatic cancer. Laparoscopic staging and peritoneal cytology. *Surg. Oncol. Clin. N. Am.* **7**(1), 135–42.

Fontham, E.T.H. and Correr, P. (1989) Epidemiology of pancreatic cancer. *Surg. Clin. North Am.* **69**, 551–67.

Fortner, J.G. (1973) Regional resection of cancer of the pancreas: a new surgical approach. *Surgery* **73**, 307–20.

Fortner, J.G. (1981) Surgical principles for pancreatic cancer: regional total and subtotal pancreatectomy. *Cancer* **47**, 1712–18.

Fortner, J.G., D'Angio, G.J., Hilaris, B.S. *et al.* (1970) Iodine 125 implantation for unresectable cancer of the pancreas. *Postgrad. Med.* **47**, 226–30.

Franklin, M.E. and Balli, J.E. (1998) Laparoscopic choledochoenterostomy. *Semin. Laparosc. Surg.* **5**(3), 180–4.

Freeney, P.C., Traverso, W. and Ryan, I.A. (1993) Diagnosis and staging of pancreatic adenocarcinoma with dynamic computed tomography. *Am. J. Surg.* **165**, 600–6.

Friess, H., Kleeff, J., Silva, J.C., Sadowski, C., Baer, H.U. and Buchler, M.W. (1998) The role of diagnostic laparoscopy in pancreatic and periampullary malignancies. *J. Am. Coll. Surg.* **186**(6), 675–82.

Geer, R.J. and Brennan, M.F. (1993) Prognostic indicators for survival after resection of pancreatic adenocarcinoma. *Am. J. Surg.* **165**, 68–73.

Gold, E.B. and Goldin, S.B. (1998) Epidemiology of and risk factors in pancreatic cancer. In Cameron, J.L. (ed.), Pancreatic neoplasms. *Surg. Oncol. Clin. North Am.* **7**(1), 67–91.

Gompertz, R.H., Benjamin, I.S., Yip, A. *et al.* (1990) Hilar cholangiocarcinoma: a 10-year experience. *Gut* **31**, A589.

Gordon, T.A., Burleyson, G.P., Tielsch, J.M. *et al.* (1995) The effects of regionalisation on cost and outcome for one high risk surgical procedure. *Ann. Surg.* **221**, 43–9.

Gouma, D.J., Nieveen van Dijkum, E.J. and Obertop, H. (1999) The standard diagnostic work-up and surgical treatment of pancreatic head tumours. *Eur. J. Surg. Oncol.* **25**(2): 113–23.

Gress, T.M., Micha, A.E., Lacher, U. and Adler, G. (1998) Diagnosis of a 'hereditary pancreatitis' by the detection of a mutation in the cationic trypsinogen gene. *Deutsche Medizinische Wochenschrift* **123**(15), 453–6.

Grunewald, K., Lynos, J., Frohlich, A. *et al.* (1989) High frequency of Ki-ras codon 12 mutations in pancreatic adenocarcinomas. *Int. J. Cancer* **43**, 1037.

Gunderson, L.L., Haddock, M.G., Burch, P., Nagorney, D., Foo, M.L. and Todoroki, T. (1999) Future role of radiotherapy as a component of treatment in biliopancreatic cancers. *Ann. Oncol.* **10**(suppl. 4), 291–5.

Hannan, E.L., O'Donnell, J.F., Kilburn, H. Jr, Bernard, H.R. and Yazici, A. (1989) Investigation of the relationship between volume and mortality for surgical procedures performed in New York State hospitals. *JAMA* **262**(4), 503–10.

Haringsma, J. and Huibregtse, K. (1998) Biliary stenting with a prototype expandable Teflon endoprosthesis. *Endoscopy* **30**(8), 718–20.

Hatfield, A.R.W., Terblanche, J., Fataar, S. *et al.* (1982) Preoperative external biliary drainage in obstructive jaundice. A prospective controlled clinical trial. *Lancet* **ii**, 896–9.

Hermreck, A.S., Thomas, C.Y. and Friesen, S.R. (1974) Importance of pathologic staging in the surgical management of adenocarcinoma of the exocrine pancreas. *Am. J. Surg.* **127**, 653.

Hiraoka, T. and Kanemitsu, K. (1994) Subtotal pancreatectomy and extended lymphadenectomy with intraoperative radiotherapy for pancreatic cancer. In Serio, G., Huguet, C. and Williamson, R.C.N. (eds), *Hepatobiliary and pancreatic tumours.* Edinburgh: Graffham Press, 20–5.

Hochster, H., Green, M.D., Speyer, J.L. *et al.* (1986) Activity of epirubicin in pancreatic carcinoma. *Cancer Treat. Rep.* **70**, 299–300.

Howard, L.M. and Jordan, G.L. (1977) Cancer of the pancreas. In Hickey, R.C. (ed.), *Current problems in cancer*, Vol. II, No. 3. Chicago: Yearbook Medical Publishers, 1.

Howe, G.R. and Burch, J.D. (1996) Nutrition and pancreatic cancer. *Cancer Causes Control* **7**(1), 69–82.

Ichikawa, T., Haradome, H., Hachiya, J. *et al.* (1997) Pancreatic ductal adenocarcinoma: preoperative assessment with helical CT versus dynamic MR imaging. *Radiology* **202**(3), 655–62.

Ishikawa, O., Ohhigashi, H., Sasaki, Y. *et al.* (1988) Practical usefulness of lymphatic and connective tissue clearance for the carcinoma of the pancreas head. *Ann. Surg.* **208**, 215–20.

Jessup, I.M., Steele, G., Mayer, R.I. *et al.* (1993) Neoadjuvant therapy for unresectable pancreatic adenocarcinoma. *Arch. Surg.* **128**, 559–64.

Ji, B.T., Hatch, M.C., Chow, W.H. *et al.* (1996) Anthropometric and reproductive factors and the risk of pancreatic cancer: a case-control study in Shanghai, China. *Int. J. Cancer* **66**(4), 432–7.

Ji, B.T., Silverman, D.T., Dosemeci, M., Dai, Q., Gao, Y.T. and Blair, A. (1999) Occupation and pancreatic cancer risk in Shanghai, China. *Am. J. Ind. Med.* **35**(1), 76–81.

Johnson, C.D., Schwall, G., Flechton-Macher, J. *et al.* (1993) Resection for adenocarcinoma of the body and tail of the pancreas. *Br. J. Surg.* **80**, 1177–9.

Kakkar, A.K., Chinswangwatanakul, V., Lemoine, N.R., Tebbutt, S. and Williamson, R.C. (1999) Role of tissue factor expression on tumour cell invasion and growth of experimental pancreatic adenocarcinoma. *Br. J. Surg.* **86**(7), 890–4.

Kalthoff, H., Schmeigel, W., Roeder, C. *et al.* (1993) p53 and K-ras alterations in pancreatic epithelial cells. *Oncogene* **8**, 289.

Karlson, B.M., Ekbom, A., Josefsson, S., McLaughlin, J.K., Fraumeni, J.F. Jr and Nyren, O. (1997) The risk of pancreatic cancer following pancreatitis: an association due to confounding? *Gastroenterology* **113**(2), 587–92.

Kayahara, M., Nagakawa, T., Ohta, T. *et al.* (1999) Analysis of paraaortic lymph node involvement in pancreatic carcinoma: a significant indication for surgery? *Cancer* **85**(3), 583–90.

Korc, M. (1998) Role of growth factors in pancreatic cancer. *Surg. Oncol. Clin. N. Am.* **7**, 25–41.

Kroep, J.R., Pinedo, H.M., van Groeningen, C.J. and Peters, G.J. (1999) Experimental drugs and drug combinations in pancreatic cancer. *Ann. Oncol.* **10**(suppl. 4), 234–8.

Kurzawinski, T., Deery, A. and Davidson, B.R. (1993) Diagnostic value of cytology for biliary stricture. *Br. J. Surg.* **80**, 414–21.

Le Pimpec Barthes, F., Chapuis, O., Riquet, M. *et al.* (1998) Thoracoscopic splanchnicectomy for control of intractable pain in pancreatic cancer. *Ann. Thorac. Surg.* **65**(3), 810–13.

Leung, J.W.C., Bower-Wright, M., Aveling, W. *et al.* (1983) Coeliac plexus block for pain in pancreatic cancer and chronic pancreatitis. *Br. J. Surg.* **70**, 730–2.

Lieberman, M.D., Kilburn, H., Lindsey, M. and Brennan, M.F. (1995) Relation of perioperative deaths to hospital volume among patients undergoing pancreatic resection for malignancy. *Ann. Surg.* **222**(5), 638–45.

Lillemoe, K.D., Cameron, J.L., Kaufman, H.S. *et al.* (1993) Chemical splanchnicectomy in patients with unresectable pancreatic cancer. A prospective randomized trial. *Ann. Surg.* **217**, 447–57.

Lin, Y., Tamakoshi, A., Wakai, K. *et al.* (1998) Descriptive epidemiology of pancreatic cancer in Japan. *J. Epidemiol.* **8**(1), 52–9.

Livingstone, E.H., Welton, M.L. and Reber, H.A. (1991) Surgical treatment of pancreas: the United States experience. *Int. J. Pancreatol.* **8**, 153–7.

Lowenfels, A.B., Maissonneuve, P., Cavallini, G. *et al.* (1993) Pancreatitis and risk of pancreatic cancer. *N. Engl. J. Med.* **328**, 1433–7.

Lynch, H.T. (1994) Genetics and pancreatic cancer. *Arch. Surg.* **129**, 266–8.

Lynch, H.T. and Fusaro, R.M. (1991) Pancreatic cancer and familial atypical multiple mole melanoma (FAMMM) syndrome. *Pancreas* **6**, 127–31.

Lynch, H.T., Voorhees, G.J., Lanspa, S.J. *et al.* (1985) Pancreatic carcinoma and hereditary non-polyposis colorectal cancer: a family study. *Br. J. Cancer* **52**, 271–3.

Mackie, C.R., Moossa, A.R., Go, V.L.W. *et al.* (1980) Prospective evaluation of some candidate tumour markers in the diagnosis of pancreatic cancer. *Dig. Dis. Sci.* **25**, 161–72.

Mahvi, D.M., Meyers, W.C., Bast, R.C. *et al.* (1985) Carcinoma of the pancreas. Therapeutic efficacy as defined by a serodiagnostic test utilizing a monoclonal antibody. *Ann. Surg.* **202**, 440–5.

Mallinson, C.N., Rake, M.O., Cocking, J.B. *et al.* (1980) Chemotherapy in pancreatic cancer: results of a controlled, prospective, randomised multi-centre trial. *BMJ* **281**, 1589–91.

Maruchi, W., Brian, D., Ludwig, J. *et al.* (1979) Cancer of the pancreas in Olmstead county, Minnesota, 1935–1974. *Mayo Clin. Proc.* **54**, 245.

McMahon, B. (1982) Risk factors for cancer of the pancreas. *Cancer* **50**, 2676–80.

McPherson, G.A.D., Benjamin, I.S., Habib, N.A. *et al.* (1982) Percutaneous transhepatic drainage in obstructive jaundice: advantages and problems. *Br. J. Surg.* **69**, 261–4.

Miedema, B.W., Sarr, M.G., van Heerden, J.A. *et al.* (1992) Complications following pancreaticoduodenectomy: current management. *Arch. Surg.* **127**, 945–50.

Moertel, C.G. and Gildorf, N. (1969) Combined 5-FU and radiation therapy of locally unresected gastrointestinal cancer. *Lancet* **ii**, 865–7.

Moossa, A.R. and Levin, B. (1979) Collaborative studies in the diagnosis of pancreatic cancer. *Sem. Oncol.* **6**, 298–308.

Moossa, A.R. and Romeo, O. (1994) Role of total pancreatecomy for carcinoma of the head of the pancreas. In Serio, G., Huguet, C. and Williamson, R.C.N. (eds), *Hepatobiliary and pancreatic tumours*. Edinburgh: Graffham Press, 15–19.

Mori, M., Hariharan, M., Anandakumar, M. *et al.* (1999) A case-control study on risk factors for pancreatic diseases in Kerala, India. *Hepato-Gastroenterology* **46**(25), 25–30.

Nagai, H., Kuroda, A. and Morioka, Y. (1986) Lymphatic and local spread of T1 and T2 pancreatic cancer. *Ann. Surg.* **204**, 65–71.

Nagakawa, T., Kobayashi, H., Ueno, K., Ohta, T., Kayahara, M. and Miyazaki, I. (1994) Clinical study of lymphatic flow to the para-aortic lymph nodes in the carcinoma of the head of the pancreas. *Cancer* **73**(4), 1155–62.

Nakayama, T., Ikeda, A. and Okuda, K. (1978) Percutaneous transhepatic drainage of the biliary tree. *Gastroenterology* **74**, 554–9.

Neoptolemos, J.P., Russell, R.C., Bramhall, S. and Theis, B. (1997) Low mortality following resection for pancreatic and periampullary tumours in 1026 patients: UK survey of specialist pancreatic units. UK Pancreatic Cancer Group. *Br. J. Surg.* **84**(10), 1370–6.

Neoptolemos, J.P., Dunn, J.A., Stocken, D.D. *et al.* (2001) Adjuvant chemoradiotherapy and chemotherapy in resectable pancreatic cancer: a randomised controlled trial. *Lancet* **358**(9293), 1576–85.

Nishiharu, T., Yamashita, Y., Abe, Y. *et al.* (1999) Local extension of pancreatic carcinoma: assessment with thin-section helical CT versus with breath-hold fast MR imaging–ROC analysis. *Radiology* **212**(2), 445–52.

Norlander, A., Kahin, B. and Sundblad, R. (1982) Effect of percutaneous transhepatic drainage upon liver function and postoperative mortality. *Surg. Gynecol. Obstet.* **155**, 161–6.

Ogren, M., Hedberg, M., Berglund, G., Borgstrom, A. and Janzon, L. (1996) Risk of pancreatic carcinoma in smokers enhanced by weight gain. Results from 10-year follow-up of the Malmo preventive Project Cohort Study. *Int. J. Pancreatol.* **20**(2), 95–101.

Ona, F.V., Zamcheck, N., Dhar, P. *et al.* (1973) CEA in the diagnosis of pancreatic cancer. *Cancer* **31**, 324.

Palmer, K.R., Kerr, M., Knowles, G. *et al.* (1994) Chemotherapy prolongs survival in inoperable pancreatic carcinoma. *Br. J. Surg.* **81**, 882–5.

Parker, N., Makin, C.A., Ching, C.K. *et al.* (1992) A new enzyme linked lectin/mucin antibody sandwich assay (CAM 17. 1/WGA) assessed in combination with CA 19-9 and peanut lectin binding assay for the diagnosis of pancreatic cancer. *Cancer* **70**, 1062–8.

Partanen, T., Hemminki, K., Vainio, H. and Kauppinen, T. (1995) Coffee consumption not associated with risk of pancreas cancer in Finland. *Prev. Med.* **24**(2), 213–16.

Pellegrini, C.A., Heck, C.F., Raper, S. *et al.* (1989) An analysis of the reduced morbidity and mortality rates after pancreaticoduodenectomy. *Arch. Surg.* **124**, 778–87.

Rattner, D.W. (1992) Pancreatic cancer in 1992: has any progress been noted? *Mayo Clin. Proc.* **67**, 907–9.

Reddy, K.R., Levi, J., Livingstone, A. *et al.* (1999) Experience with staging laparoscopy in pancreatic malignancy. *Gastrointest. Endosc.* **49**, 498–503.

Rege, N., Bapat, R.D., Koti, R., Desai, N.K. and Dahanukar, S. (1993) Immunotherapy with *Tinospora cordifolia*: a new lead in the management of obstructive jaundice. *Indian J. Gastroenterol.* **12**(1), 5–8.

Reznek, R.H. and Stephens, D.H. (1993) The staging of pancreatic adenocarcinoma. *Clin. Radiol.* **47**(6), 373–81.

Rich, T.A. (1999) Chemoradiation for pancreatic and biliary cancer: current status of RTOG studies. *Ann. Oncol.* **10**(suppl. 4), 231–3.

Rosch, T., Braig, C., Gain, T. *et al.* (1992) Staging of pancreatic and ampullary carcinoma by endoscopic ultrasonography. Comparison with conventional sonography, computed tomography, and angiography. *Gastroenterology* **102**(1), 188–99.

Sarr, M.G. and Cameron, J.L. (1982) Surgical management of unresectable carcinoma of the pancreas. *Surgery* **91**, 123–33.

Schattner, A., Fenakel, G. and Malnick, S.D. (1997) Cholelithiasis and pancreatic cancer. A case-control study. *J. Clin. Gastroenterol.* **25**(4), 602–4.

Schwartz, G.G., Skinner, H.G. and Duncan, R. (1998) Solid waste and pancreatic cancer: an ecologic study in Florida, USA. *Int. J. Epidemiol.* **27**(5), 781–7.

Selenskas, S., Teta, M.J. and Vitale, J.N. (1995) Pancreatic cancer among workers processing synthetic resins. *Am. J. Ind. Med.* **28**(3), 385–98.

Shepherd, H.A., Royhe, G., Ross, A.P.R. *et al.* (1988) Endoscopic biliary endoprosthesis in the palliation of malignant obstruction of the distal common bile duct: a randomised trial. *Br. J. Surg.* **75**, 1166–8.

Siegel, J.H. and Snady, H. (1986) The significance of endoscopically placed prostheses in the management of biliary obstruction due to carcinoma of pancreas: results of non-operative decompression of 227 patients. *Am. J. Gastroenterol.* **81**, 634.

Sindelar, W.F. and Kinsella, T.J. (1999) Studies of intraoperative radiotherapy in carcinoma of the pancreas. *Ann. Oncol.* **10**(suppl. 4), 226–30.

Smith, F.P., Hoth, D.F., Levin, B. *et al.* (1980) 5-Fluorouracil, adriamycin and mitomycin-C (FAM) chemotherapy for advanced adenocarcinoma of the pancreas. *Cancer* **46**, 2014–18.

Snady, H. (1995) Pancreatic cancer. Influence of endoscopic ultrasonography on management and outcomes. *Gastrointest. Endosc. Clin. N. Am.* **5**(4), 755–62.

Sobin, L.H. and Wittekind, C. (eds) (1997) *TNM classification of malignant tumours*, 5th edn. USA: Wiley-Liss.

Soehendra, N. and Reynders-Frederix, V. (1980) Palliative bile duct drainage – a new endoscopic method of introducing a transpapillary drain. *Endoscopy* **12**, 8.

Soreide, O. (1987) Percutaneous aspiration cytology for biliary obstruction and liver masses. In Bhumgart, L.H. (ed.), *Surgery of the liver and biliary tract*, Vol. 1. Edinburgh: Churchill Livingstone, 327.

Speer, A.G. and Cotton, P.B. (1988) Endoscopic treatment of pancreatic cancer. *Int. J. Pancreatol.* **3**, S147–58.

Stensvold, I. and Jacobsen, B.K. (1994) Coffee and cancer: a prospective study of 43 000 Norwegian men and women. *Cancer Causes Control* **5**(5), 401–8.

Tolbert, P.E. (1997) Oils and cancer. *Cancer Causes Control* **8**(3), 386–405.

Trapnell, J. (1972) The natural history and management of acute pancreatitis. *Clin. Gastroenterol.* **1**, 147–66.

Trede, M., Schwall, G. and Saeger, H.D. (1990) Survival after pancreatoduodenectomy. 118 consecutive resections without an operative mortality. *Ann. Surg.* **211**, 447–58.

Trede, M., Rumstadt, B., Wendl, K. (1997) Ultrafast magnetic resonance imaging improves the staging of pancreatic tumors. *Ann. Surg.* **226**(4), 393–405.

Tryka, A.F. and Brooks, J.R. (1979) Histopathology in the evaluation of total pancreatectomy for ductal carcinoma. *Ann. Surg.* **190**, 373–81.

Tsuchiya, R., Oribe, T. and Noda, T. (1985) Size of tumour and other factors influencing the prognosis of carcinoma of the head of the pancreas. *Am. J. Gastroenterol.* **80**, 459–62.

Van Heerden, J.A., ReMine, W.H., Weiland, L.H. *et al.* (1981) Total pancreatectomy for ductal adenocarcinoma of the pancreas. Mayo Clinic experience. *Am. J. Surg.* **142**(3), 308–11.

Venu, R.P., Pastika, B.J., Kini, M. *et al.* (1998) Self-expandable metal stents for malignant gastric outlet obstruction: a modified technique. *Endoscopy* **30**(6), 553–8.

Warshaw, A.L. and Fernandez-del Castillo, C. (1992) Pancreatic carcinoma. *N. Engl. J. Med.* **326**, 455–65.

Warshaw, A.L. and Rutledge, P.L. (1987) Cystic tumours mistaken for pancreatic pseudocysts. *Ann. Surg.* **205**, 393–8.

Warshaw, A.L. and Swanson, R.S. (1988) Pancreatic cancer in 1988. Possibilities and probabilities. *Ann. Surg.* **208**, 541–53.

Warshaw, A.L., Gu, Z.-Y., Wittenberg, J. *et al.* (1990) Preoperative staging and assessment of resectability of pancreatic cancer. *Arch. Surg.* **125**, 230–3.

Whittington, R., Dobelbower, R.R. and Mohiuddin, M. (1981) Radiotherapy of unresectable pancreatic carcinoma: a six-year experience with 104 patients. *Int. J. Radiat. Oncol. Phys.* **7**, 1639–44.

Wils, J., Bleiber, H., Blijham, G. *et al.* (1985) Phase II study of epirubicin in advanced adenocarcinoma of the pancreas. *Eur. J. Cancer Clin. Oncol.* **21**, 191–4.

Worsey, J., Ferson, P.F., Keenan, R.J., Julian, T.B. and Landreneau, R.J. (1993) Thoracoscopic pancreatic denervation for pain control in irresectable pancreatic cancer. *Br. J. Surg.* **80**(8), 1051–2.

Yamaguchi, K., Chijiwa, K., Shimizu, S., Yokohata, K., Morisaki, T. and Tanaka, M. (1998) Comparison of endoscopic retrograde and magnetic resonance cholangiopancreatography in the surgical diagnosis of pancreatic diseases. *Am. J. Surg.* **175**(3), 203–8.

Yanagisawa, A., Ohtake, K., Ohashi, K. *et al.* (1993) Frequent c-Ki-*ras* oncogene activation in mucous cell hyperplasia of pancreas suffering from chronic inflammation. *Cancer Res.* **53**, 953.

Yeo, C.J., Cameron, J.L., Lillemoe, K.D. *et al.* (1995) Pancreaticoduodenectomy for cancer of the head of the pancreas. 201 patients. *Ann. Surg.* **221**(6), 721–31.

Yeo, C.J., Cameron, J.L., Sohn, T.A. *et al.* (1997) Six hundred fifty consecutive pancreaticoduodenectomies in the 1990s: pathology, complications, and outcomes. *Ann. Surg.* **226**(3): 248–57.

Biliary tract

HEMANT M. KOCHER AND IRVING S. BENJAMIN

TUMOURS OF THE BILE DUCT (CHOLANGIOCARCINOMA)

Incidence

Tumours of the biliary tract can be divided into those of the intrahepatic bile ducts, extrahepatic bile ducts and those of the gall bladder (GB) (the first of these are similar in presentation and surgical management and are discussed in Chapter 25, but a brief review of relevant literature is done in this chapter). Biliary-tract tumours account for 10–15 per cent of all primary hepato-biliary cancers worldwide (Parkin *et al.*, 1993). An incidence of between 1500 and 3000 new cases per annum (1.2/100 000, equally distributed between the male and the female population) has been reported in the United States (Cameron, 1988; Landis *et al.*, 1998; Carriaga and Henson, 1995). The 1992 data from the Office of National Statistics, showed that for England and Wales, there were 1489 (919 men) new cases of cancers of the liver and intrahepatic bile ducts, while for that of the extrahepatic bile ducts and GB there were 1321 (578 men) new cases (Cancer Statistics Registration, 1998). Age-standardized rates in England and Wales vary from 1.5 to 3.4 per 100 000 population. It has been suggested that the incidence is increasing, but it seems more probable that the tumour is being diagnosed more frequently. These figures are in remarkable contrast to those reported from some other areas of the world, notably north-east Thailand, where minimum age-standardized annual incidence rates of 135.4 per 100 000 men and 43.0 per 100 000 women have been reported (Green *et al.*, 1991); comparable figures from French studies were 1.7 and 0.5 per 100 000, respectively (Renard *et al.*, 1987). Other high-risk areas

include Japan, Korea, Eastern Europe (European Russia, Czech republic, Poland) and American Indians, with age-adjusted incidence rates of 4–12 per 100 000 men or women (Parkin *et al.*, 1997). In most areas, biliary tumours have a higher incidence in women than men. These differences must carry important messages about aetiology, and may relate to parasitic infestations (*see* below).

Aetiology

This is essentially unknown, although a number of important correlations have been observed. While there is a close relationship between gallstones and GB cancer (70–98 per cent of cases) (Lowenfels *et al.*, 1985; Zatonski *et al.*, 1997), this association is much less clear-cut with cancer of the bile ducts (Ekbom *et al.*, 1993). Of cases treated at Hammersmith Hospital, 37 per cent had cholelithiasis (Blumgart *et al.*, 1984) and 50 per cent at the Lahey Clinic had had a previous cholecystectomy (Alexander *et al.*, 1984). An increased incidence of cholangiocarcinoma is noted with intrahepatic bile-duct stones, possibly those associated with recurrent pyogenic cholangitis (Kubo *et al.*, 1995; Lee and Sheen, 1995). A decrease in lectin affinity (decrease in the lectin-binding carbohydrate structures) has been attributed to tumour progression in such cases (Lee and Sheen, 1995). A stepwise progression from hyperplasia, dysplasia, carcinoma *in situ* and adenocarcinoma has been shown in patients with hepatolithiasis (Terada *et al.*, 1992). Caroli's disease, a rare congenital disorder, has been shown to predispose to bile-duct cancer (Dayton *et al.*, 1983; Fozard *et al.*, 1989). Choledochal cysts have a high incidence of malignant change, particularly when they present in adult life (Voyles *et al.*, 1983a). The common factor may be biliary stasis with associated changes in bile composition. It is now also clear that this condition is related to an anomalous junction between the pancreatic and biliary ductal systems. The type I anomaly (pancreatic duct joining bile duct) is associated with GB cancer, while the type II anomalous pancreatical biliary duct (APBD) junction (bile duct joining pancreatic duct) is the one commonly associated with cysts of the biliary tree, and their associated malignancy. The biliary amylase level is extremely high in both types of anomaly. Ohta *et al.* (1990) showed epithelial mucosal atypia with papillary or papillotubular proliferation and epithelial hyperplasia in patients with both anomalies. Kato *et al.* (1990) found mutagenic bile in 6/12 type I patients, and a high incidence of polyploid DNA in the GB epithelium of 2/4 patients, both of whom had mutagenic bile. Suda *et al.* (1987) found an APBD junction in 14.2 per cent of cases of biliary-tract carcinoma, and in all four cases of congenital biliary dilatation. However, Sharma (1994) did not find any correlation between a long common channel and risk of cholangiocarcinoma.

In South-East Asia biliary infestation with liver flukes (*Clonorchis sinensis* in China and Korea and *Opisthorchis viverrini* in Thailand, Laos and Cambodia) are associated with bile-duct cancer (Parkin *et al.*, 1993; Haswell-Elkins *et al.*, 1994). A higher incidence of cholangiocarcinomas is found in those males infected with *Opisthorchis viverrini* who smoke handmade cigarettes (Haswell-Elkins *et al.*, 1994; Mitacek *et al.*, 1999). For *Clonorchis sinensis* an association with heavy drinking has been shown to increase the risk for cholangiocarcinoma (Shin *et al.*, 1996). There is an association between cholangiocarcinoma and ulcerative colitis (Roberts-Thompson *et al.*, 1973). Primary sclerosing cholangitis (PSC) is a well-documented risk factor for cholangiocarcinoma, with a cumulative risk of 11.2 per cent for cholangiocarcinoma, 10 years after diagnosis of PSC (Kornfeld *et al.*, 1997). Monitoring with tumour markers has not been able to identify early cholangiocarcinomas (Hultcrantz *et al.*, 1999). Patients undergoing liver transplantation for PSC are known to have poorer survival in the presence of incidental cholangiocarcinomas (Knechtle *et al.*, 1995). A higher incidence of bile-duct cancer was also reported in patients who had received thorium dioxide in the past (Altmann, 1978). Methylene chloride and vinyl chloride monomer factory workers in the USA may also have a higher risk of biliary cancer (Bond *et al.*, 1990; Lanes *et al.*, 1990). Cirrhotics are at tenfold increased risk for cholangiocarcinomas, as compared to 60-fold for hepatocellular carcinoma (Sorensen *et al.*, 1998). Association of cholangiocarcinoma with haemoglobin E trait and beta-thalassaemia trait has also been postulated in Thailand (Insiripong *et al.*, 1997). Anecdotal reports of association with prior external-beam radiotherapy (EBRT), and with Wilson's disease have been described (Burmeister and Turner, 1995; Kosminkova *et al.*, 1995).

Molecular biology and genetics

A multi-hit hypothesis has been suggested for carcinogenesis in the bile ducts (Holzinger *et al.*, 1999). It has been suggested that this occurs in four stages:

1 predisposition and risk factors of biliary cancer;
2 genotoxic events and alterations leading to specific DNA damage and mutation patterns;
3 dysregulation of DNA repair mechanisms and apoptosis, permitting survival of mutated cells; and
4 morphological evolution from premalignant biliary lesions to cholangiocarcinoma.

Mutations in *p53* and K-*ras* oncogene have been the two most commonly studied genetic defects for cholangiocarcinomas (Petmitr, 1997; Sturm *et al.*, 1998; Holzinger *et al.*, 1999). K-*ras* mutation has not been found with uniformly high frequency (Petmitr, 1997; Sturm *et al.*, 1998).

The link between liver fluke infestation and carcinogenesis is provided by increased *in vivo* production of *N*-nitrosamines and DNA alkylation damage due to induction of cytochromal enzymes in macrophages (Satarug *et al.*, 1996).

Anatomy

Cancer of the extrahepatic biliary tree may be classified into three zones: the upper third, including the confluence of the hepatic ducts as far as the level of the cystic duct; the middle third, between the cystic duct and the upper border of the duodenum; and the lower third, from that level to the papilla of Vater. Weinbren and Mutum (1983) observed variations in the gross appearance of the tumour related to the anatomical site. Papillary lesions predominate in the distal segment, and sclerotic stenosing lesions in the upper third, while those in the central portion of the ducts tend to be nodular. However, some tumours are diffuse, and the papillary form of tumour may also be found in the proximal ducts. The difficult tumours at the confluence of the right and left ducts are sometimes eponymously referred to as Klatskin tumours, after Klatskin's report of 13 cases in 1965. The importance of the location of these tumours is their propensity to invade deeply into liver substance by direct extension proximally and also to involve the portal vein and hepatic artery in the region of the hilus, features that may preclude resection. The gross appearance of the tumour may be related to its prognosis (Yamamoto *et al.*, 1998). Formal pathological staging is by the TNM system (Table 26.1). Full staging can only be made following surgery and pathological examination of the resected specimen. Evaluation of the extent of disease at laparotomy is most important for staging, but in the first instance staging depends on imaging, which often defines the limits of the tumour, and this practical clinical staging based on imaging is discussed below.

Table 26.1 *TNM definitions for extrahepatic bile-duct cancer (from Sobin and Wittekind, 1997: 81–3)*

Primary tumour (T)	
Tx	Primary tumour cannot be assessed
T0	No evidence of primary tumour
Tis	Carcinoma *in situ*
T1	Tumour invades the mucosa or muscle layer
T1a	Tumour invades the mucosa
T1b	Tumour invades the muscle area
T2	Tumour invades perimuscular connective tissue
T3	Tumour invades adjacent structures: liver, pancreas, duodenum, GB, colon, stomach
Regional lymph nodes (N)	
Nx	Regional lymph nodes cannot be assessed
N0	No regional lymph node metastasis
N1	Metastasis in cystic duct, pericholedochal and/or hilar lymph nodes (i.e. in the hepatoduodenal ligament)
N2	Metastasis in peripancreatic (head only), periduodenal, periportal, coeliac and/or superior mesenteric lymph nodes
Distant metastasis (M)	
Mx	Presence of distant metastasis cannot be assessed
M0	No distant metastasis
M1	Distant metastasis
Stage grouping	
Stage 0	Tis, N0, M0
Stage I	T1, N0, M0
Stage II	T2, N0, M0
Stage III	T1, N1, M0
	T2, N1, M0
Stage IVa	T3, any N, M0
Stage IVb	Any T, any N, M1

Lymphatic drainage

This is to the lymph-node groups along the proper and common hepatic arteries, the coeliac nodes and, for distally placed lesions, the retropancreatic and superior mesenteric nodes. It is important to sample lymph nodes when considering curative resection and, when resecting tumours, to skeletonize the hepatic artery and remove all lymphatic tissues and associated neural tissue. These tumours have a propensity for longitudinal perineural invasion, both proximally and distally, and such invasion has a negative impact on survival (Bhuiya *et al.*, 1992). Bile-duct cancer may give rise to very well-differentiated nests of biliary epithelial cells within lymph nodes. The authors would regard such deposits as a contraindication to major liver resection for attempted cure, although they should not preclude local resection for palliation.

Metastases and natural history

Untreated, most patients with bile-duct cancer die within 6 months to a year of diagnosis, from a combination of local tumour spread and cholangitis. As well as lymph-node metastases, the tumours tend to spread along the subepithelial planes, and perineural invasion is common (Bhuiya *et al.*, 1992). This produces difficulty in operative diagnosis, since choledochoscopic biopsies may underestimate the extent of tumour. Direct spread to the liver is the rule, but distant involvement of intrahepatic bile radicles may also be found, and may represent a field change. In rare cases, distant metastases occur and the authors have seen one patient with metastatic deposits in bone.

Pathology

This has been well described by Weinbren and Mutum (1983). The tumours are generally well-differentiated adenocarcinomas (cholangiocarcinoma). They form acini in which mucin secretion is almost invariable and mucin lakes occur in 50 per cent of cases; this feature may help to distinguish cholangiocarcinomas from hepatocellular carcinoma at the hilus. A dense fibrous reaction surrounds the hilar tumours, which may be indistinguishable from tumour radiologically or even at operation. Even histological differentiation of this desmoplastic reaction from tumour requires careful and experienced examination of multiple sections. Invasion of nerve trunks occurs in 80 per cent.

The macroscopically papillary variety of tumour may arise in choledochal cysts, or from malignant change in cases of multiple biliary papillomatosis (Gouma et al., 1984). Immunocytochemical staining is positive for carcinoembryonic antigen (CEA) in 50 per cent and for epidermal keratin in 80 per cent, but negative for α-fetoprotein.

Proximal to the obstructed bile duct there are changes of cholestasis and acute inflammatory cell infiltrate, with marked perilobular fibrosis in long-standing cases. This fibrosis and the associated hepatocyte hyperplasia may contribute towards the portal hypertension, which may develop (Weinbren et al., 1985). Long-standing obstruction to one or more segmental hepatic ducts produces such intense ductal dilatation and fibrosis that segments or a lobe of the liver may become shrunken and functionally ineffective (Benjamin, 1983). This phenomenon may be compounded by hepatocyte atrophy if the portal vein to that segment of liver is also involved directly by tumour encasement. These features become important when determining the resectability of hilar cholangiocarcinomas and also in selecting ducts for non-operative decompression.

Symptoms and presentation

Most tumours occur between the ages of 50 and 70, but the authors have seen patients aged as young as 21 with extensive cholangiocarcinoma. Bile-duct cancer generally presents with obstructive jaundice. Differential diagnosis can be divided anatomically into diseases of the pancreatic head, bile duct and others. Pancreatic-head pathologies include malignancy, chronic pancreatitis and, rarely, pancreatic calculi. Biliary pathologies include common bile-duct stones, PSC, recurrent pyogenic cholangitis, iatrogenic injuries to bile duct and parasitic infestations. Other categories include metastasis to porta hepatis lymph nodes, periampullary and duodenal carcinoma. Rarely, hepatitis can masquerade as obstructive jaundice.

If a tumour arises eccentrically in the right or left hepatic duct, there may already be well-established sectoral or lobar obstruction by the time the tumour reaches the confluence and causes jaundice. Subtle symptoms of cholangitis during that time may draw early attention to the tumour, and papillary tumours of the ducts, particularly at the distal end, may cause intermittent obstruction. Pain consistent with a biliary-tract origin had been present for some time before diagnosis in 40 per cent of patients with biliary cancer seen at Hammersmith Hospital (Beazley et al., 1984). Pain may be the only symptom in those with pure intrahepatic cholangiocarcinomas (IHCC) (Chu et al., 1997). Other symptoms include anorexia and weight loss.

Apart from obstructive jaundice, examination may be unhelpful. Hepatomegaly may be found in up to 75 per cent of patients (Chu et al., 1997), and a hard, right-hypochondrial mass should raise the suspicion of a GB cancer, particularly in the older patient. Ascites may be present in advanced tumours.

Diagnosis

Of 13 cases reported by Klatskin (1965), none was diagnosed before operation, and the diagnosis was missed in nine of these cases at initial laparotomy. By 1981, a change in pattern was evident: of 37 patients referred to Hammersmith Hospital, 21 had a preoperative diagnosis (Voyles et al., 1983b), and the current trend is for almost all patients to have preoperative histological diagnosis – except those difficult cases with PSC, which may still spring a histological surprise of incidental cholangiocarcinoma, after resection or even liver transplant (Knechtle et al., 1995). This change reflects both an increased awareness and improvements in biliary imaging techniques.

Examination may not provide specific features. Investigation relies heavily on ultrasound and contrast cholangiography. Ultrasound is the initial examination of choice, and will establish the presence of biliary obstruction in more than 90 per cent of cases. Modern ultrasound technology, however, can provide even more detailed information. In one prospective study, ultrasound defined the level of obstruction in 95 per cent of the authors' patients (Gibson et al., 1986), a performance better than that of CT scanning in the same patients. It was also better in suggesting the cause of the obstruction and gave valuable information about invasion or encasement of the portal vein by tumour. Sensitivity has continued to improve, particularly in providing precise definition of the proximal level of tumour. It has frequently been stated that a hilar mass can rarely be identified by scanning. However, more recent experience has allowed identification of a hilar mass at ultrasound in 95 per cent of 57 consecutive patients referred with this diagnosis (Yeung et al., 1989). Ultrasound may also be used as a guide for fine-needle aspiration cytology. A major difficulty is the differentiation of carcinoma at the confluence from benign sclerosing lesions, and up to 13 per cent of such lesions may be misdiagnosed (Wetter et al., 1991). The addition of colour Duplex can diagnose vascular involvement in nearly 85–91 per cent of tumours (Triller et al., 1994).

Following ultrasound and possibly CT scanning, cholangiography is essential. Endoscopic retrograde cholangio pancreatography (ERCP) is frequently the first direct cholangiography obtained, although this may fail to give complete information about the extent of involvement of the hilar and segmental ducts (Fig. 26.1). A case may be made for earlier use of the percutaneous route (percutaneous transhepatic cholangiography, PTC) for hilar lesions, since this gives the most complete definition of

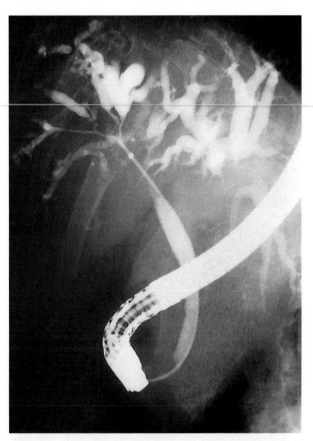

Figure 26.1 *An ERCP showing hilar cholangiocarcinoma infiltrating both right and left ductal systems. There is atrophy on the right side, but hypertrophy on the left side: a phenomenon seen with long-standing biliary obstruction.*

the hepatic ducts (Fig. 26.2). Often a combination of the two may be required for full staging. Magnetic resonance cholangiopancreatography (MRCP) may ultimately replace these invasive imaging methods, but often does not reach the degree of fine anatomical definition required for determination of resectability and operative planning. The importance of confirming the presence of malignancy preoperatively has already been referred to above. Many lesions may masquerade as biliary malignancy (Desa *et al.*, 1991), including localized strictures in PSC, benign iatrogenic biliary strictures and a group of apparently benign idiopathic inflammatory strictures. Cytology is valuable in this regard. We found, in 167 patients with suspected malignant biliary stricture, a sensitivity of 60 per cent, with only one false-positive result (cytology suspicious but not diagnostic of cancer) out of 216 specimens. The sensitivity of the technique is proportional to the precision with which targeting of the lesion can be obtained. Brushings or biopsy can be obtained at ERCP or at the time of PTC, aiming for the stricture or, if a stent has been placed, aiming at the stent as it passes through the tumour (Sakaguchi and Nakamura, 1986).

The use of angiography is of value for bile-duct lesions, both in identifying portal venous and hepatic arterial involvement with tumour and in providing a 'road map' for surgical intervention. This can be provided effectively by non-invasive techniques such as Duplex ultrasound scan (Triller *et al.*, 1994), helical CT (CT arterial portography) (Hommeyer *et al.*, 1995; Chong *et al.*, 1998) or MRI (MR arteriography and MR venography) (Shirkhoda *et al.*, 1997, 1998). Many surgeons would accept that involvement of the main stem of the portal vein indicates irresectability. However, this may not be so, both because the portal vein can be resected and reconstructed in some cases (Sakaguchi and Nakamura, 1986; Nishio *et al.*, 1999) and because apparent tumour involvement on a portogram may be artefactual or may represent compression rather than tumour invasion (Williamson *et al.*, 1980; Voyles *et al.*, 1983b).

Tumour markers are of limited value: CA 19-9 is frequently elevated in the serum of patients with jaundice, but this is not specific (Paganuzzi *et al.*, 1988). CEA is expressed in the cells of bile-duct cancer (Davis *et al.*, 1988) and may be elevated in the serum.

Staging

The TNM system described above is of limited value for clinical staging (Table 26.1). Bismuth *et al.* (1992) have published a gross descriptive staging for the primary tumours of the hepatic hilus: stage I tumours are entirely below the confluence, stage II tumours involve one main hepatic duct and stage III indicates invasion of both hepatic ducts. This is a practical surgical classification, which is cited by many surgical authors. It should not, however, be mistaken for an attempt to describe staging of the tumours, as it is unlikely that the majority of cases follow this sequence of progression. The available techniques for staging hilar tumours preoperatively, with the principal objective of defining cases that are potentially resectable, have been reviewed by Adam and Benjamin (1992). The use of cholangiography and angiography together has allowed definition of groups of patients who would be conventionally regarded as irresectable. These features include:

- involvement of second-order intrahepatic ducts on both sides of the liver, or multi-focal tumour;
- involvement of the main-stem portal vein (although see above);
- contralateral involvement of vessels or ducts on opposite sides of the liver.

With the advent of non-invasive modalities to study the vascular and biliary tree (*see* above), more information can be gained preoperatively, with reasonable accuracy, without resorting to angiography or cholangiography. This provides the surgeon with the road map as well as segmental anatomy to plan any resectional surgery, in addition to excluding irresectable cases.

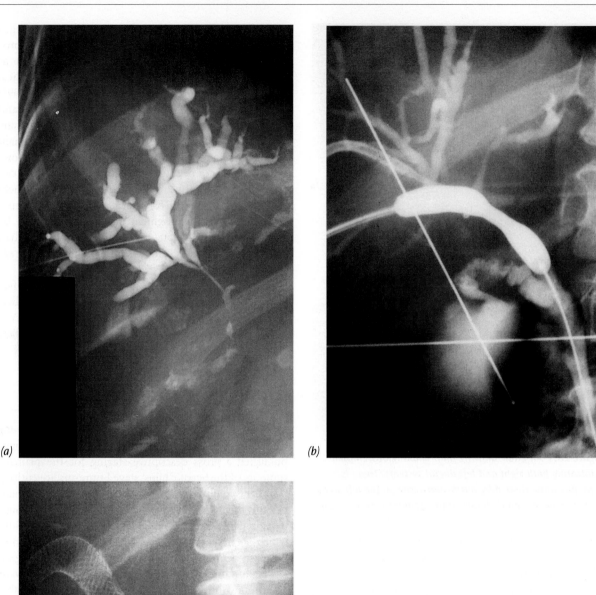

(a)

(b)

(c)

Figure 26.2 *(a) A PTC showing cannulation of the biliary tree in a patient where ERCP was not successful due to hilar cholangiocarcinoma. This film shows only the right-sided ductal system as the right and left side are disconnected. (b) The hilar stricture is now being dilated by means of a balloon, which shows the central compression due to the tumour. (c) Finally a metallic, self-expanding stent straddles the stricture and palliates jaundice.*

Some more recent reports have described refinement of these clinical staging methods. Laparoscopy and laparoscopic ultrasound have been discussed in relation to pancreatic cancer (Chapter 25). Percutaneous cholangioscopy has been reported, particularly by Japanese workers (Nimura *et al.*, 1988; Nimura, 1993), but has not gained wide acceptance, mainly because of its

invasive nature and the long time required to dilate the tract.

IHCCs, based on macroscopic appearances, have been further re-classified as: mass forming, periductal-infiltrating type, intraductal type (Nozaki *et al.*, 1998). A group in Thailand has proposed a different classification: type I, peripheral; type II, intermediate; type III, central; and type IV, diffuse (Uttaravichien *et al.*, 1999). The Japanese, on the other hand, have questioned the pattern of lymph-node metastasis for cholangiocarcinomas as proposed by the TNM staging (Nozaki *et al.*, 1998).

Treatment

The treatment options for cholangiocarcinoma are essentially:

1 no treatment;
2 palliative non-operative intubation;
3 operative intubation;
4 operative biliary-enteric bypass; and
5 resection of the tumour.

Because these tumours are generally regarded as slow growing and only locally invasive, the availability of non-operative methods of palliation has led some authors to suggest that these tumours are generally unsuitable for surgical management. However, resection is clearly the only management to offer a serious prospect of cure, so discussion will begin with consideration of this modality. Resection may be divided into conventional (including liver resections or pancreatico-duodenectomy) or extensive (radical: involving major vascular resection and reconstruction, including liver transplantation).

Purely IHCC may be regarded as a primary liver tumour and is treated as other liver tumours (*see* below). The distal bile-duct cholangiocarcinomas are treated as pancreatic tumours, usually with pancreatico-duodenectomy.

RESECTION

Worldwide experience of resection of hilar cholangiocarcinomas remains modest. With the emergence of liver resection as an acceptable surgical treatment with low morbidity and mortality, resection series have been increasingly reported, particularly from the East. Western series remain comparatively few. Recently cumulative experiences from various countries have been published, making comparisons feasible, even though not all use the same staging or classification.

Intrahepatic cholangiocarcinoma

The Thailand and the Taiwan groups have recently published two of the largest series of IHCC (Chen *et al.*, 1999; Uttaravichien *et al.*, 1999). The Thai group had a resectability rate of 65.2 per cent (90 of the 138 patients seen over a 5-year period) (Uttaravichien *et al.*, 1999). They found the mean survival time for right-lobe surgery to be significantly better than that for left-lobe surgery (582 days versus 458 days). On the other hand, the Taiwanese group resected 162 IHCC, with hepatolithiasis in a large number of cases (Chen *et al.*, 1999). The postoperative mortality was 3.7 per cent, and the

postoperative morbidity was worse for those with hepatolithiasis than without (37.7 per cent versus 16.7 per cent). The 1-, 3- and 5-year survival rates were 35.5 per cent, 20.5 per cent and 16.5 per cent in patients with hepatolithiasis, and 27.2 per cent, 8.8 per cent and 7.8 per cent in those without hepatolithiasis. Following curative resections (no microscopic disease left behind) an average median survival of 24 months was reported in most series (Lamesch *et al.*, 1997; Burke *et al.*, 1998; Harrison *et al.*, 1998; Lieser *et al.*, 1998; Madariaga *et al.*, 1998; Nozaki *et al.*, 1998; Roayaie *et al.*, 1998; Chen *et al.*, 1999; Chu and Fan, 1999; El Rassi *et al.*, 1999; Isaji *et al.*, 1999; Kim *et al.*, 1999; Sano *et al.*, 1999; Uttaravichien *et al.*, 1999; Valverde *et al.*, 1999; Yamamoto *et al.*, 1999). Two American series in a selected group of patients have reported median actuarial survivals of 42.9 and 59 months, respectively (Harrison *et al.*, 1998; Madariaga *et al.*, 1998). This is a remarkable advance since the nihilistic attitude towards this cancer in the 1960s. The prime reason for the increased survival may be the reduction in the operative mortality, ranging between 3 and 6 per cent in various series for curative resections for this tumour (Harrison *et al.*, 1998; Madariaga *et al.*, 1998; Chen *et al.*, 1999). Nevertheless, morbidity remains high, of the order of 37–47 per cent (Chen *et al.*, 1999; Chu and Fan, 1999; El Rassi *et al.*, 1999). Though surgery gives the only hope of cure, liver transplantation does not improve survival. Of the 50 patients undergoing resection with curative intent in one German centre (Lamesch *et al.*, 1997), 32 had curative liver resection alone, with a median survival of 13.9 months, as compared to a median survival of 5 months in 18 undergoing liver transplantation. Lymph nodal metastasis, especially to the N2 stations, can adversely affect prognosis (Burke *et al.*, 1998). This may indicate a need for adjuvant therapy.

The data on palliative procedures for IHCC is scarce. The Hong Kong group performed palliative procedures in 32 of 101 patients over 22 years (Chu and Fan, 1999). However, the median survival was only 3.3 months, as compared to 2.5 months in 21 patients treated without operation. The difference in those undergoing palliative and curative resection is also remarkable. A small Korean series of 28 patients over 7 years reported a median survival of 24 months in 15 patients undergoing resection with curative intent, as compared to 3 months in 10 patients who had palliative resection (Kim *et al.*, 1999). This probably makes the case for surgical resection for only those patients where curative resection can be achieved. However, there is a practical limitation due to the pre- and intra-operative imaging techniques for these cases, and clearance can sometimes only be distinguished on final histology.

Hilar cholangiocarcinoma

The reported experience with hilar cholangiocarcinoma is much greater in the Western world than for IHCC, and the resectability rate for these tumours is higher. The largest series, however, is from Japan (Miyazaki *et al.*, 1998; Nagino *et al.*, 1998). Nimura and his colleagues (Nagino *et al.*, 1998) reported 173 patients seen with hilar cholangiocarcinoma, 138 underwent resections, 124 including liver and 14 resecting bile duct only. These followed extensive staging and preoperative preparation, with percutaneous biliary drainage of multiple hepatic segments and cholangioscopy and biopsy in all cases. This approach was fairly aggressive, with 41 patients undergoing simultaneous resection and reconstruction of portal vein and/or hepatic artery and 16 patients undergoing simultaneous liver and pancreatic resections. All patients had wide lymphadenectomy. There was a hospital mortality of 9.7 per cent with a morbidity of 42.7 per cent. Of the 97 patients who left hospital after major liver resection, an unusually high 25.8 per cent survived 5 years. Other Japanese series and at least one German series (Klempnauer *et al.*, 1997; Miyazaki *et al.*, 1998) have reported comparable 5-year survival rates. Median survival remains at the best about 24 months (Klempnauer *et al.*, 1997). A Spanish series, albeit with small numbers, reported a median survival of 48 months in eight patients undergoing liver transplantation (Figueras *et al.*, 1998).

Palliative biliary bypass above the malignancy provides good relief of jaundice (Bismuth *et al.*, 1988; Guthrie *et al.*, 1994). But the advent of good endoscopic palliative stenting procedures has rendered surgery largely a complementary procedure (*see* below). Nevertheless, resection provides best palliation (Strasberg, 1998; Benjamin, 1999), with orthotopic liver transplantation giving some hope to these patients (Jonas *et al.*, 1998).

PALLIATION (NON-SURGICAL)

The advent of the biliary Wallstent endoprosthesis (Medinvent SA, Lausanne, Switzerland) has changed the nature and quality of palliation that can be offered to patients with hilar cholangiocarcinomas (Adam *et al.*, 1991; Rossi *et al.*, 1994). It offers better palliation than the plastic stents previously available, because it is self-expanding and is meshed and therefore not susceptible to frequent blockages (Fig. 26.2c). However, recent reports of intimal hyperplasia or tumour ingrowth through the mesh, causing blockage, in such stents have caused some concern (McKeown *et al.*, 1999). They can be introduced over a fine catheter by ERCP or PTC and thus can effectively palliate all types of extrahepatic cholangiocarcinomas. Greater details about stenting have been given in the section on non-surgical palliation of pancreatic cancer (Chapter 25).

RADIOTHERAPY

The beneficial effects of radiotherapy either as adjuvant or primary treatment for bile-duct cancer remain to be demonstrated in prospective randomized studies. A trial with chemoradiation has been proposed by the Radiation Therapy Oncology Group (RTOG), because of some initial success (Gonzalez Gonzalez *et al.*, 1999; Tyvin, 1999). EBRT, intra-operative radiotherapy (IORT) and intraluminal brachytherapy (ILBT) have all been tried in adjuvant and primary settings (Gonzalez Gonzalez *et al.*, 1999). The median survival in the adjuvant setting is unchanged from the 24 months discussed above, but those in the primary setting showed an improvement to 10.4 months (Gonzalez Gonzalez *et al.*, 1999). ILBT showed no improvement in either setting. Three-dimensional conformal radiotherapy promises to reduce adverse effects but may not show any improvement in survival. A recently published retrospective comparison of stenting with or without radiotherapy in non-resectable cholangiocarcinomas has shown little benefit of radiotherapy (Bowling *et al.*, 1996). Our local experience also shows that while EBRT and ILBT are well tolerated, they confer minimal survival benefit in patients with cholangiocarcinomas (Vallis *et al.*, 1996).

CHEMOTHERAPY

Even fewer studies have been conducted on chemotherapy for cholangiocarcinomas. Some benefit has been shown when 5-fluorouracil (FU) treatment has accompanied radiation (Whittington *et al.*, 1995). The Japanese experience with systemic or intra-arterial chemotherapy for recurrent cancer is disheartening (Ueska *et al.*, 1999), although it has not been evaluated systematically.

Authors' view on surgery

In summary, it is the authors' present policy to carry out surgical resection of cholangiocarcinomas whenever possible, and all patients undergo investigation for staging and assessment for resectability (scanning, cholangiography and angiography in selected cases) with this aim. Palliative local resection and hilar hepaticojejunostomy carries low morbidity and mortality, and is indicated whenever feasible. Extended resections including liver, portal vein and regional lymph nodes is only indicated for those with potentially curable lesions, since the morbidity of such procedures is higher, and the mortality not insignificant. For young and fit patients with irresectable lesions, or those that are found at operation to be irresectable, a biliary-enteric bypass is the treatment of choice. For most others, percutaneous transhepatic or endoscopic stent placement is preferred, whenever possible.

Recently the authors have referred most patients with irresectable or incompletely resected lesions for combination chemotherapy. The majority have been treated with continuous infusional 5-FU and intermittent epirubicin and cisplatin. Figures are not available for long-term follow-up, but there have been a number of apparent responses, including probable downstaging of local disease on subsequent radiological investigation: whether these results will translate into survival improvement remains to be seen.

GALL-BLADDER CANCER

Epidemiology

GB cancer is the most common biliary malignancy, with preponderance in Central and South America, Central and Eastern Europe, Japan and northern parts of India.

Aetiology

Gallstones are the single most important risk factor for GB cancer, though the aetiological link is not clear (Zatonski et al., 1997). Usually, patients with large stones of long duration are at increased risk for cancer. All the other risk factors associated with gallstone disease are also associated with GB cancer, such as elevated body mass index, high caloric and carbohydrate intake, female sex, high parity and young age at first childbirth. Patients with anomalous pancreatico-biliary ductal union are also known to be at increased risk for GB cancer (Chao et al., 1995). Single large (>1 cm) sessile polyps are more likely to be malignant (Aldridge and Bismuth, 1990).

Anatomy and lymphatic drainage

The lymphatic drainage follows the arterial supply, and is commonly to the cystic lymph node, pancreatico-duodenal lymph nodes (superior and posterior) and coeliac lymph nodes. Para-aortic and aorto-caval lymph nodes are also involved in advanced cases.

Metastasis and natural history

The most common mode of spread for GB cancer is contiguous spread to the liver, bile ducts, stomach, colon and duodenum, in that order. Distant metastasis occurs to liver, peritoneum and lungs. Usually patients succumb to the locally advanced disease rather than distant metastasis.

Pathology

Most cancers are adenocarcinomas, but adenosquamous and squamous cell carcinomas are also seen. Most tumours are of the flat, infiltrating variety, but polypoid and nodular tumours are also seen.

TNM staging is most commonly used. Lymphatic spread depends on the tumour stage, with T1 tumours having no lymphatic spread, and T3 and T4 tumours having up to 75 per cent lymphatic spread (Tsukada et al., 1996).

Symptoms and presentation

The most common presentation for GB cancers is pain, anorexia and weight loss, and obstructive jaundice (Kapoor and Benjamin, 1999). A GB mass may be palpable in half the patients on presentation (Kapoor and Benjamin, 1999).

Staging

TNM classification is the most used staging tool for the GB cancers (Table 26.2).

Investigations

Besides routine blood investigations, including liver function tests, the first investigation is ultrasound of the liver and biliary tract. Ultrasound is useful to detect the thickening of the wall of the GB (the differential diagnosis being inflammation of the GB), but polypoid lesions in the GB may also be detected.

Ultrasound also gives an estimate of the degree of the bile duct and liver involvement and, with Duplex, it may give an estimate of vascular involvement. The role of endoscopic ultrasound has yet to be fully evaluated for these cancers.

Spiral CT scan probably gives the best estimate of the locoregional disease (Fig. 26.3). However, MRI gives equally high-resolution images, with the additional benefit of providing MRCP, to give adequate ductal information. Nevertheless, most patients have ERCP just after ultrasound scan to relieve the obstructive jaundice, and therefore ERCP provides ductal information. In those cases where it is difficult to cannulate the bile duct from below,

Table 26.2 *Tumour node metastasis staging for GB carcinoma (Sobin and Wittekind, 1997: 78–80)*

TNM, tumour node metastasis	
T1	GB wall
T2	Perimuscular connective tissue
T3	Serosa and/or one organ, or liver ≤2 cm
T4	Two or more organs, or liver >2 cm
N1	Metastasis in the cystic duct, pericholedochal and/or hilar lymph nodes
N2	Metastasis in the peripancreatic, periduodenal, periportal, coeliac and/or superior mesenteric nodes
M	Distant metastasis
Stage grouping	
Stage I	T1, N0, M0
Stage II	T2, N0, M0
Stage III	T1, T2, N1, M0
	T3, N0, N1, M0
Stage IVa	T4, N0, N1, M0
Stage IVb	Any T, N2, M0
	Any T, any N, M1

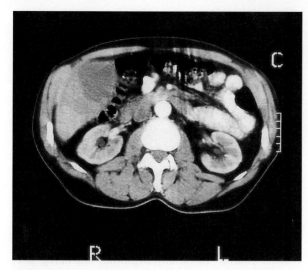

Figure 26.3 *A CT scan showing GB cancer invading the substance of the liver.*

PTC may be helpful. CT arterioportography and MR angiography usually give adequate information about the local vascular anatomy, but in selective cases hepatic angiography may be indicated.

Fine-needle aspiration cytometry (FNAC) is not recommended as routine because of the risk of peritoneal or needle-tract seeding, especially in curable cases, but is acceptable in irresectable cases being considered for palliative therapy.

The differential diagnosis of imaging on the GB is essentially stone disease and its sequelae, while those of obstructive jaundice are enumerated before. Mirrizzi syndrome may sometimes pose a particular problem in diagnosis.

Treatment

SURGERY

Radical surgery offers the only hope for cure, as adjuvant treatment gives little benefit. However, most patients have advanced disease on presentation and are unsuitable for surgery. Proposed therapeutic options for patients with GB cancer are shown in Table 26.3.

Surgery gives the best palliation of symptoms and hope for cure; however, views range from pessimism to aggressive resection. Advocates of aggressive surgical resection call for resection, even in locally advanced cancers, in the form of hepatico-pancreatico-duodenectomy, with some survival at 5 years (Miyazaki *et al.*, 1996). In patients with stage III and IV tumours the 5-year survival rate was 52 per cent after curative resection (*n* = 35). This was significantly better than the 5 per cent 5-year survival rate after a non-curative resection (*n* = 32) (Miyazaki *et al.*, 1996). This group recommended excision of the bile duct to ensure complete lymphatic clearance of the hepatico-duodenal ligament. Bile-duct and hepatic invasion (7/26)

Table 26.3 *Therapeutic options for patients with GB cancer*

Stage	Recommended surgical procedure
0 or I	Simple cholecystectomy (extended if T1b)
II	Extended cholecystectomy[a]
III	Extended cholecystectomy[a]
IV	Individualize: palliative bypass, extended hepatectomy, leave alone

[a] Extended cholecystectomy = cholecystectomy with radical lymph-node clearance and non-anatomical liver resection, may involve pancreatico-duodenectomy.

led to lesser curative resections, as compared to hepatic invasion alone (14/15) (Bartlett *et al.*, 1996).

Based on the tumour stage, the best results are reported for those tumours having no serosal invasion and undergoing adequate surgery (Yamaguchi *et al.*, 1997). Tumours with liver and biliary invasion have the poorest prognosis (Bartlett *et al.*, 1996; Shirai *et al.*, 1992).

Based on nodal involvement, patients with pancreatico-duodenal nodal involvement (N2) fare worst. Patients with no nodal involvement have better long-term prognosis after radical resection than those with just hepatico-duodenal ligament involvement (Nakamura *et al.*, 1995; Shimada *et al.*, 1997). The best policy would be to offer surgery only to those patients with tumour confined to the GB (T1 or T2) with spread to hepatico-duodenal ligament lymph nodes. Recent data from Japan have confirmed the dismal prognosis for patients with spread to the para-aortic lymph nodes, and this almost certainly contraindicates attempts at radical resection (Kondo *et al.*, 2000). However, since this tumour is relatively radioresistant and chemoresistant, surgery offers the best palliation, even in advanced cases, with a few reported long-term survivors (Todorki *et al.*, 1999).

RADIOTHERAPY

GB cancer is generally considered relatively radioresistant. Each study has too few patients enrolled to make any effective judgement of the value of various types of radiotherapy for this condition e.g. intra-operative or brachytherapy and conformal postoperative EBRT. Patients with advanced disease do have some survival benefit from radiotherapy, whether given as adjuvant or as primary treatment (Mehta *et al.*, 1996; Houry *et al.*, 1999; Todorki *et al.*, 1999).

CHEMOTHERAPY

Various agents in single-agent or combination chemotherapy have been tried, including paclitaxel, mitomycin C and 5-FU (Taal *et al.*, 1993; Gebbia *et al.*, 1996; Jones *et al.*, 1996). Thus far, 5-FU in combination with folinic acid seems to be the only regimen with any significant survival benefits (Gebbia *et al.*, 1996). Of the 30 patients studied, 30 per cent had a partial response while 27 per cent had stabilization of disease. Median overall survival was 8 months for these advanced GB cancers, with mild treatment-related toxicity. At present the authors' patients most frequently receive combination chemotherapy as for hilar cholangiocarcinomas (*see* above), although there is no clear evidence for the benefit of such a regimen.

FUTURE TRENDS

Cancer of the bile duct remains a difficult tumour to diagnose and to treat surgically, and has been a major site of attack for interventional radiologists and endoscopists, with a considerable widening of our therapeutic repertoire. The addition to this of internal and external radiotherapy may produce valuable information over the next decade and chemotherapy has yet to be fully investigated carefully for it to prove its value. Improvements in the results of major surgical resection has caused this approach to be re-evaluated and, although they still pose formidable surgical problems, much of the old nihilistic thinking about biliary cancer has been replaced by a more aggressive and somewhat more optimistic outlook.

SIGNIFICANT POINTS

- Tumours of the biliary tree and GB are now readily palliated by percutaneous or endoscopic stenting; but, again, the role of surgery is being increasingly emphasized.
- In particular, excellent recent results from Japan provide some optimism for cure of this tumour, although the surgery involved is technically very demanding.
- Modern chemotherapy regimens may have an increasing role, although the value of radiotherapy remains unproven.

KEY REFERENCES

Adam, A., Chetty, N., Roddie, M. *et al.* (1991) Self-expandable stainless steel endoprostheses for treatment of malignant bile duct obstruction. *Am. J. Roentgenol.* **156**, 321–5.

Scrio, G., Huguet, C. and Williamson, R.C.N. (1994) *Hepatobiliary and pancreatic tumours* Edinburgh: Graffam Press.

Tytgat, G.N.J., Gouma, D.J., Offerhaus, G.J.A., Peters, G.J., Pinedo, H.M. and Bartelink, H. (1999) Biliopancreatic malignancy: from gene to cure. *Ann. Oncol.* **10**(suppl. 4).

REFERENCES

Adam, A. and Benjamin, I.S. (1992) The staging of cholangiocarcinoma. *Clin. Radiol.* **146**(5), 299–303.

Adam, A., Chetty, N., Roddie, M., Yeung, E. and Benjamin, I.S. (1991) Self-expandable stainless steel endoprostheses for treatment of malignant bile duct obstruction. *Am. J. Roentgenol.* **156**, 321–5.

Aldridge, M.C. and Bismuth, H. (1990) Ball bladder cancer: the polyp-cancer sequence. *Br. J. Surg.* **77**, 363–4.

Alexander, F., Rossi, R.L., O'Bryan, M. *et al.* (1984) Biliary carcinoma: a review of 109 cases. *Am. J. Surg.* **147**, 503–9.

Altmann, H.W. (1978) Pathology of human liver tumours. In Remmer, H., Bolt, H.M., Bannasch, P. and Popper, H. (eds), *Primary liver tumours* MTP Press: Lancaster, 53–71.

Bartlett, D.L., Fong, Y., Fortner, J.G. *et al.* (1996) Long term results after resection for gall bladder cancer. *Ann. Surg.* **224**, 639–46.

Beazley, R.M., Hadjis, N., Benjamin, I.S. and Blumgart, L.H. (1984) Clinicopathological aspects of high bile duct cancer. Experience with resection and bypass surgical treatments. *Ann. Surg.* **199**(6), 623–36.

Benjamin, I.S. (1983) Biliary tract obstruction. *Surg. Gastroenterol.* **2**, 105–20.

Benjamin, I.S. (1999) Surgical possibilities for bile duct cancer: standard surgical treatment. *Ann. Oncol.* **10**(suppl. 4), 239–42.

Bhuiya, M.R., Nimura, Y., Kamiya, I. *et al.* (1992) Clinicopathologic studies on perineural invasion of bile duct carcinoma. *Ann. Surg.* **215**, 344–9.

Bismuth, H., Castaing, D. and Traynor, O. (1988) Resection or palliation: priority of surgery in the treatment of hilar cancer. *World J. Surg.* **12**, 39–47.

Bismuth, H., Nakache, R. and Diamond, T. (1992) Management strategies in resection for hilar cholangiocarcinoma. *Ann. Surg.* **215**, 31–8.

Blumgart, L.H., Benjamin, I.S., Hadjis, N.S. and Beazley, R.M. (1984) Surgical approaches to cholangiocarcinoma at confluence of hepatic ducts. *Lancet* **I**, 66–70.

Bond, G.G., McLaren, E.A., Sabel, F.L. *et al.* (1990) Liver and biliary tract cancer among chemical workers. *Am. J. Ind. Med.* **18**, 19–24.

Bowling, T.E., Galbraith, S.M., Hatfield, A.R., Solano, J. and Spittle, M.F. (1996) A retrospective comparison of endoscopic stenting alone with stenting and radiotherapy in non-resectable cholangiocarcinoma. *Gut* **39**(96), 852–5.

Burke, E.C., Jarnagin, W.R., Hochwald, S.N., Pisters, P.W., Fong, Y. and Blumgart, L.H. (1998) Hilar cholangiocarcinoma: patterns of spread, the importance of hepatic resection for curative operation, and a presurgical clinical staging system. *Ann. Surg.* **228**(3): 385–94.

Burmeister, B.H. and Turner, S.L. (1995) External beam radiation therapy as an agent in the aetiology of carcinoma of the bile duct: a report on two patients. *Clin. Oncol.* **7**(1): 48–9.

Cameron, J.L. (1988) Proximal cholangiocarcinomas. *Br. J. Surg.* **75**, 1155–6.

Cancer Statistics Registration (1998) Series: England and Wales. Series MB1 no. 25. London: Office of National Statistics.

Carriaga, M.T. and Henson, D.E. (1995) Liver, gallbladder, extrahepatic bile ducts, and pancreas. *Cancer* **75**, 171–90.

Chao, T.C., Jan, Y.Y. and Chen, M.F. (1995) Primary carcinoma of the gallbladder associated with anomalous pancreaticobiliary ductal junction. *J. Clin. Gastroenterol.* **21**(4), 306–8.

Chen, M.F., Jan, Y.Y., Jeng, L.B. *et al.* (1999) Intrahepatic cholangiocarcinoma in Taiwan. *J. Hepato-Biliary-Pancreatic Surg.* **6**(2), 136–41.

Chong, M., Freeny, P.C. and Schmiedl, U.P. (1998) Pancreatic arterial anatomy: depiction with dual-phase helical CT. *Radiology* **208**(2), 537–42.

Chu, K.M. and Fan, S.T. (1999) Intrahepatic cholangiocarcinoma in Hong Kong. *J. Hepato-Biliary-Pancreatic Surg.* **6**(2), 149–53.

Chu, K.M., Lai, E.C., Al-Hadeedi, S. *et al.* (1997) Intrahepatic cholangiocarcinoma. *World J. Surg.* **21**(3): 301–5.

Davis, R.I., Sloan, M.J.H., Hood, J.M. and Maxwell, P. (1988) Carcinoma of the extrahepatic biliary tract: a clinicopathological and immuno histochemical study. *Histopathology* **12**, 623–31.

Dayton, M.T., Longmire, W.P. Jr and Tompkins, R.K. (1983) Caroli's disease: a premalignant condition? *Am. J. Surg.* **145**(1), 41–8.

Desa, L.A., Akosa, A.B., Lazzara, S. *et al.* (1991) Cytodiagnosis in the management of extrahepatic biliary stricture. *Gut* **32**, 1188–91.

Ekbom, A., Hsieh, C.C., Yuen, J. *et al.* (1993) Risk of extra-hepatic bile-duct cancer after cholecystectomy. *Lancet* **342**(8882), 1262–5.

El Rassi, Z.E., Partensky, C., Scoazec, J.Y., Henry, L., Lombard-Bohas, C. and Maddern, G. (1999) Peripheral cholangiocarcinoma: presentation, diagnosis, pathology and management. *Eur. J. Surg. Oncol.* **25**(4), 375–80.

Figueras, J., Llado-Garriga, L., Lama, C. *et al.* (1998) Resection as elective treatment of hilar cholangiocarcinoma (Klatskin tumor). *Gastroenterol. Hepatol.* **21**(5), 218–23.

Fozard, J.B., Wyatt, J.I. and Hall, R.I. (1989) Epithelial dysplasia in Caroli's disease. *Gut* **30**(8), 1150–3.

Gebbia, V., Majello, E., Testa, A. *et al.* (1996) Treatment of advanced carcinomas of the exocrine pancreas and the gall bladder with 5-fluorouracil, high dose levofolinic acid and oral hydroxyurea on a weekly schedule. Results of multicentre study of the Southern Italy Oncology Group (GOIM). *Cancer* **78**(6), 1300–7.

Gibson, R.N., Yeung, E., Thompson, J.N. *et al.* (1986) Bile duct obstruction: radiologic evaluation of level, cause, and tumor resectability. *Radiology* **160**(1), 43–7.

Gonzalez Gonzalez, D., Gouma, D.J., Rauws, E.A.J., van Gulik, T.M., Bosma, A. and Koedooder, C. (1999) Role of radiotherapy, in particular intraluminal brachytherapy, in the treatment of proximal bile duct carcinoma. *Ann. Oncol.* **10**(suppl. 4), 215–20.

Gouma, D.J., Mutum, S.S., Benjamin, I.S. and Blumgart, L.H. (1984) Intrahepatic biliary papillomatosis. *Br. J. Surg.* **71**(1), 72–4.

Green, A., Uttaravichien, T., Bhudhisawasdi, V. *et al.* (1991) Cholangiocarcinoma in North East Thailand. A hospital-based study. *Trop. Geogr. Med.* **43**, 193–8.

Guthrie, C.M., Banting, S.W., Garden, O.J. and Carter, D.C. (1994) Segment III cholangiojejunostomy for palliation of malignant hilar obstruction. *Br. J. Surg.* **81**(11), 1639–41.

Harrison, L.E., Fong, Y., Klimstra, D.S., Zee, S.Y. and Blumgart, L.H. (1998) Surgical treatment of 32 patients with peripheral intrahepatic cholangiocarcinoma. *Br. J. Surg.* **85**(8), 1068–70.

Haswell-Elkins, M.R., Mairiang, E., Mairiang, P. *et al.* (1994) Cross-sectional study of *Opisthorchis viverrini* infection and cholangiocarcinoma in communities within a high-risk area in northeast Thailand. *Int. J. Cancer* **59**(4), 505–9.

Holzinger, F., Z'graggen, K. and Buchler, M.W. (1999) Mechanisms of biliary carcinogenesis: a pathogenetic multi-stage cascade towards cholangiocarcinoma. *Ann. Oncol.* **10**, 122–6.

Hommeyer, S.C., Freeny, P.C. and Crabo, L.G. (1995) Carcinoma of the head of the pancreas: evaluation of the pancreaticoduodenal veins with dynamic CT – potential for improved accuracy in staging. *Radiology* **196**(1), 233–8.

Houry, S., Haccart, V., Huguier, M. and Schlienger, M. (1999) Gall bladder cancer: role of radiation therapy. *Hepato-gastroenterology* **46**(27), 1578–84.

Hultcrantz, R., Olsson, R., Danielsson, A. *et al.* (1999) A 3-year prospective study on serum tumor markers used for detecting cholangiocarcinoma in patients with primary sclerosing cholangitis. *J. Hepatol.* **30**(4), 669–73.

Insiripong, S., Thaisamakr, S. and Amatachaya, C. (1997) Hemoglobin typing in cholangiocarcinoma. *Southeast Asian J. Trop. Med. Public Health* **28**(2), 424–7.

Isaji, S., Kawarada, Y., Taoka, H., Tabata, M., Suzuki, H. and Yokoi, H. (1999) Clinicopathological features and outcome of hepatic resection for intrahepatic cholangiocarcinoma in Japan. *J. Hepato-Biliary-Pancreatic Surg.* **6**(2), 108–16.

Jonas, S., Kling, N., Guckelberger, O., Keck, H., Bechstein, W.O. and Neuhaus, P. (1998) Orthotopic liver transplantation after extended bile duct resection as treatment of hilar cholangiocarcinoma. First long-terms results. *Transpl. Int.* **11**(suppl. 1), S206–8.

Jones, D.V., Lozano, R., Hoque, A., Markowitz, A. and Patt, Y.Z. (1996) Phase II study of paclitaxel therapy for unresectable biliary tree carcinomas. *J. Clin. Oncol.* **14**(8), 2306–10.

Kapoor, V.K. and Benjamin, I.S. (1999) Biliary malignancies. In Pitt, H.A. (ed.), *The biliary tract. Ballière's clinical gastroenterology*, vol. 11(4). London: Ballière Tindall.

Kato, I., Kuroishi, T. and Tominaga, S. (1990) Descriptive epidemiology of subsites of cancers of the liver, biliary tract and pancreas in Japan. *Jpn. J. Clin. Oncol.* **20**, 232–7.

Kim, H.J., Yun, S.S., Jung, K.H., Kwun, W.H. and Choi, J.H. (1999) Intrahepatic cholangiocarcinoma in Korea. *J. Hepato-Biliary-Pancreatic Surg.* **6**(2), 142–8.

Klatskin, G. (1965) Adenocarcinoma of the hepatic duct at its bifurcation within the porta hepatis: an unusual tumour with distinctive clinical and pathological features. *Am. J. Med.* **38**, 241–56.

Klempnauer, J., Ridder, G.J., von Wasielewski, R., Werner, M., Weimann, A. and Pichlmayr, R. (1997) Resectional surgery of hilar cholangiocarcinoma: a multivariate analysis of prognostic factors. *J. Clin. Oncol.* **15**(3), 947–54.

Knechtle, S.J., D'Alessandro, A.M., Harms, B.A., Pirsch, J.D., Belzer, F.O. and Kalayoglu, M. (1995) Relationships between sclerosing cholangitis, inflammatory bowel disease, and cancer in patients undergoing liver transplantation. *Surgery* **118**(4), 615–19.

Kondo, S., Nimura, Y., Hayakawa, J., Kamiya, J., Nagino, M. and Uesaka, K. (2000) Regional and para-aortic lymphadenectomy in radical surgery for advanced gall bladder carcinoma. *Br. J. Surg.* **87**, 418–22.

Kornfeld, D., Ekbom, A. and Ihre, T. (1997) Survival and risk of cholangiocarcinoma in patients with primary sclerosing cholangitis. A population-based study. *Scand. J. Gastroenterol.* **32**(10), 1042–5.

Kosminkova, E.N., Generalova, S.I.U. and Ponomarev, A.B. (1995) The development of diffuse cholangiocarcinoma in a female patient with long-term undiagnosed Wilson's disease. *Terapevticheskii Arkhiv* **67**(5), 85–7.

Kubo, S., Kinoshita, H., Hirohashi, K. and Hamba, H. (1995) Hepatolithiasis associated with cholangiocarcinoma. *World J. Surg.* **19**(4), 637–41.

Lamesch, P., Weimann, A., Hauss, J. and Pichlmayr, R. (1997) Surgical treatment of intrahepatic cholangiocarcinoma. *Chirurgie* **122**(2), 88–91.

Landis, S.H., Murray, T., Bolden, S. and Wingo, P.A. (1998) Cancer statistics, 1998. CA *Cancer J. Clin.* **48**, 6–29.

Lanes, S.F., Cohen, A., Rothman, K.J., Dreyer, N.A. and Soden, K.J. (1990) Mortality of cellulose fibre production workers. *Scand. J. Work Environ. Health* **16**, 247–51.

Lee, K.T. and Sheen, P.C. (1995) Lectin histochemical study of cholangiocarcinoma arising from stone-bearing intra-hepatic bile duct. *J. Surg. Oncol.* **59**(2), 131–5.

Lieser, M.J., Barry, M.K., Rowland, C., Ilstrup, D.M. and Nagorney, D.M. (1998) Surgical management of intrahepatic cholangiocarcinoma: a 31-year experience. *J. Hepato-Biliary-Pancreatic Surg.* **5**(1), 41–7.

Lowenfels, A.B., Lindstorm, C.G. and Conway, M.J. (1985) Gallstones and risk of gallbladder cancer. *J. Natl Cancer Inst.* **75**, 77–80.

Madariaga, J.R., Iwatsuki, S., Todo, S., Lee, R.G., Irish, W. and Starzl, T.E. (1998) Liver resection for hilar and peripheral cholangiocarcinomas: a study of 62 cases. *Ann. Surg.* **227**(1), 70–9.

McKeown, B.J., Wong, W.L., Jackson, B.T., Benjamin, I.S., Jeer, P. and Adam, A. (1999) Intimal hyperplasia within biliary Wallstents: failure of recanalisation by insertion of a second endoprosthesis. *Eur. Radiol.* **9**(4), 630–3.

Mehta, A., Bahadur, A.K., Aranya, R.C. and Jain, A.K. (1996) Role of radiation therapy in carcinoma of gall bladder – a preliminary Indian experience. *Trop. Gastroenterol.* **17**(1), 22–5.

Mitacek, E.J., Brunnemann, K.D., Hoffmann, D. *et al.* (1999) Volatile nitrosamines and tobacco-specific nitrosamines in the smoke of Thai cigarettes: a risk factor for lung cancer and a suspected risk factor for liver cancer in Thailand. *Carcinogenesis* **20**(1), 133–7.

Miyazaki, M., Itoh, H., Ambiru, S. *et al.* (1996) Radical surgery for advanced gall bladder carcinoma. *Br. J. Surg.* **83**, 478–81.

Miyazaki, M., Ito, H., Nakagawa, K. *et al.* (1998) Aggressive surgical approaches to hilar cholangiocarcinoma: hepatic or local resection? *Surgery* **123**(2), 131–6.

Nagino, M., Nimura, Y., Kamiya, J. *et al.* (1998) Segmental liver resections for hilar cholangiocarcinoma. *Hepatogastroenterology* **45**(19), 7–13.

Nakamura, S., Suzuki, S., Konno, H. *et al.* (1995) Ten-year survival after hepatectomy for advanced gall bladder carcinoma: a report of two cases. *Surgery* **117**, 232–4.

Nimura, Y. (1993) Staging of biliary carcinoma: cholangiography and cholangioscopy. *Endoscopy* **25**, 76–80.

Nimura, Y., Shionoya, S., Hayakawa, N. *et al.* (1988) Value of percutaneous transhepatic cholangioscopy (PTCS). *Surg. Endosc.* **2**, 213–19.

Nishio, H., Kamiya, J., Nagino, M. *et al.* (1999) Value of percutaneous transhepatic portography before hepatectomy for hilar cholangiocarcinoma. *Br. J. Surg.* **86**(11), 1415–21.

Nozaki, Y., Yamamoto, M., Ikai, I. *et al.* (1998) Reconsideration of the lymph node metastasis pattern (N factor) from intrahepatic cholangiocarcinoma using the International Union Against Cancer TNM staging system for primary liver carcinoma. *Cancer* **83**(9), 1923–9.

Ohta, T., Nagakawa, T., Ueno, K. *et al.* (1990) Clinical experience of biliary tract carcinoma associated with anomalous union of the pancreaticobiliary ductal system. *Jpn J. Surg.* **20**, 36–43.

Paganuzzi, M., Onetto, M., Marroni, P. *et al.* (1988) CA 19-9 and CA 50 in benign and malignant pancreatic and biliary diseases. *Cancer* **61**, 2100–8.

Parkin, D.M., Ohshima, H., Srivatanakul, P. and Vatanasapt, V. (1993) Cholangiocarcinoma: epidemiology, mechanisms of carcinogenesis and prevention. *Cancer Epidemiol. Biomarkers Prev.* **2**(6), 537–44.

Parkin, D.M., Whelan, S.I., Ferlay, J. *et al.* (eds) (1997) *Cancer incidence in five continents.* Lyon: IARC.

Petmitr, S. (1997) Cancer genes and cholangiocarcinoma. *Southeast Asian J. Trop. Med. Public Health* **28**(suppl. 1), 80–4.

Renard, P., Boutron, M.C., Faivre, J. *et al.* (1987) Biliary tract cancers in Cote d'Ore (France): incidence and natural history. *J. Epidemiol. Community Health* **41**, 344–8.

Roayaie, S., Guarrera, J.V., Ye, M.Q. *et al.* (1998) Aggressive surgical treatment of intrahepatic cholangiocarcinoma: predictors of outcomes. *J. Am. Coll. Surg.* **187**(4), 365–72.

Roberts-Thompson, I.C., Strickland, R.J. and MacKay, I.R. (1973) Bile duct carcinoma in chronic ulcerative colitis. *Aust. NZ J. Med.* **3**, 264–7.

Rossi, P., Bezzi, M., Rossi, M. *et al.* (1994) Metallic stents in malignant biliary obstruction: results of a multicenter European study of 240 patients. *J. Vasc. Interv. Radiol.* **5**(2), 279–85.

Sakaguchi, S. and Nakamura, S. (1986) Surgery of the portal vein in resection of cancer of the hepatic hihus. *Surgery* **99**, 344–9.

Sano, T., Kamiya, J., Nagino, M. *et al.* (1999) Macroscopic classification and preoperative diagnosis of intrahepatic cholangiocarcinoma in Japan. *J. Hepato-Biliary-Pancreatic Surg.* **6**(2), 101–7.

Satarug, S., Lang, M.A., Yongvanit, P. *et al.* (1996) Induction of cytochrome P450 2A6 expression in humans by the carcinogenic parasite infection, *Opisthorchiasis viverrini. Cancer Epidemiol. Biomarkers Prev.* **5**(10), 795–800.

Sharma, S.S. (1994) Pancreatobiliary ductal union in cholangiocarcinoma. *Gastrointest. Endosc.* **40**, 171–3.

Shimada, H., Endo, I., Togo, S. *et al.* (1997) The role of lymph node dissection in the treatment of gall bladder carcinoma. *Cancer* **79**, 892–9.

Shin, H.R., Lee, C.U., Park, H.J. *et al.* (1996) Hepatitis B and C virus, *Clonorchis sinensis* for the risk of liver cancer: a case-control study in Pusan, Korea. *Int. J. Epidemiol.* **25**(5), 933–40.

Shirai, Y., Yoshida, K., Tsukada, K. *et al.* (1992) Radical surgery for gall bladder cancer: long term results. *Ann. Surg.* **216**, 565–8.

Shirkhoda, A., Konez, O., Shetty, A.N., Bis, K.G., Ellwood, R.A. and Kirsch, M.J. (1997) Mesenteric circulation: three-dimensional MR angiography with a gadolinium-enhanced multiecho gradient-echo technique. *Radiology* **202**(1), 257–61.

Shirkhoda, A., Konez, O., Shetty, A.N., Bis, K.G., Ellwood, R.A. and Kirsch, M.J. (1998) Contrast-enhanced MR angiography of the mesenteric circulation: a pictorial essay. *Radiographics* **18**(4), 851–61.

Sobin, L.H. and Wittekind, C. (eds) (1997) *TNM classification of malignant tumours,* 5th edn. USA: Wiley-Liss.

Sorensen, H.T., Friis, S., Olsen, J.H. *et al.* (1998) Risk of liver and other types of cancer in patients with cirrhosis: a nationwide cohort study in Denmark. *Hepatology* **28**(4), 921–5.

Strasberg, S.M. (1998) Resection of hilar cholangiocarcinoma. *HPB Surg.* **10**(6), 415–18.

Sturm, P.D., Baas, I.O., Clement, M.J. *et al.* (1998) Alterations of the *p53* tumor-suppressor gene and K-*ras* oncogene in perihilar cholangiocarcinomas from a high-incidence area. *Int. J. Cancer* **78**(6), 695–8.

Suda, K., Miyano, T., Suzuki, F. *et al.* (1987) Clinicopathologic and experimental studies on cases of abnormal pancreato-choledocho-ductal junction. *Acta Pathol. Jpn* **37**, 1549–62.

Taal, B.G., Audisio, R.A., Bleiberg, H. *et al.* (1993) Phase II trial of Mitomycin C (MMC) in advanced gall bladder and biliary tree carcinoma. An EORTC Gastrointestinal Cancer Cooperative Group Study. *Ann. Oncol.* **4**(7), 607–9.

Terada, T., Nakanuma, Y., Ohta, T. and Nagakawa, T. (1992) Histological features and interphase nucleolar organizer regions in hyperplastic, dysplastic and neoplastic epithelium of intrahepatic bile ducts in hepatolithiasis. *Histopathology* **21**(3), 233–40.

Todorki, T., Kawamoto, T., Otsuka, M. *et al.* (1999) Benefits of combining radiotherapy with aggressive resection for stage IV gall bladder cancer. *Hepatogastroenterology* **46**(27), 1585–91.

Triller, J., Losser, C., Baer, H.U. *et al.* (1994) Hilar cholangiocarcinoma: radiological assessment of resectability. *Eur. J. Radiol.* **4**, 9–17.

Tsukada, K., Hatakeyama, K., Kurosaki, I. *et al.* (1996) Outcome of radical surgery for carcinoma of the gall bladder according to the TNM stage. *Surgery* **120**, 816–21.

Tyvin, R. (1999) Chemoradiation for biliary and pancreatic cancer: Current status of RTOG studies. *Ann. Oncol.* **10**, S231–3.

Ueska, K., Kamiya, J., Nagino, J. *et al.* (1999) Treatment of recurrent cancer after surgery for biliary malignancies. *J. Jpn. Surg. Soc.* **100**(2), 195–9.

Uttaravichien, T., Bhudhisawasdi, V., Pairojkul, C. and Pugkhem, A. (1999) Intrahepatic cholangiocarcinoma in Thailand. *J. Hepato-Biliary-Pancreatic Surg.* **6**(2), 128–35.

Vallis, K.A., Benjamin, I.S., Munro, A.J. *et al.* (1996) External beam and intraluminal radiotherapy for locally advanced bile duct cancer: role and tolerability. *Radiother. Oncol.* **41**(1), 61–6.

Valverde, A., Bonhomme, N., Farges, O., Sauvanet, A., Flejou, J.F. and Belghiti, J. (1999) Resection of intrahepatic cholangiocarcinoma: a Western experience. *J. Hepato-Biliary-Pancreatic Surg.* **6**(2), 122–7.

Voyles, C.R., Smadja, C., Shands, C. and Blumgart, L.H. (1983a) Carcinoma in choledochal cysts: age-related incidence. *Arch. Surg.* **118**, 986–8.

Voyles, C.R., Bowley, N.B., Allison, D.J. *et al.* (1983b) Carcinoma of the proximal extrahepatic biliary tree. Radiological assessment and therapeutic alternatives. *Ann. Surg.* **197**, 188–94.

Weinbren, K. and Mutum, S.S. (1983) Pathological aspects of cholangiocarcinoma. *J. Pathol.* **139**, 217–38.

Weinbren, K., Hadjis, N.S. and Blumgart, L.H. (1985) Structural aspects of the liver in patients with biliary disease and portal hypertension. *J. Clin. Pathol.* **38**, 1013–20.

Wetter, L.A., Ring, E.J., Pellegrini, C.A. and Way, L.W. (1991) Differential diagnosis of sclerosing cholangiocarcinomas of the common hepatic duct (Klatskin tumors). *Am. J. Surg.* **161**(1), 57–62.

Whittington, R., Neuberg, D., Tester, W.J., Benson, A.B. 3rd and Haller, D.G. (1995) Protracted intravenous fluorouracil infusion with radiation therapy in the management of localized pancreaticobiliary carcinoma: a phase I Eastern Cooperative Oncology Group Trial. *J. Clin. Oncol.* **13**(1), 227–32.

Williamson, B.W., Blumgart, L.H. and McKellar, N.J. (1980) Management of tumours of the liver. Combined use of arteriography and venography in the assessment of resectability especially in hilar tumours. *Am. J. Surg.* **139**, 210–15.

Yamaguchi, K., Chijiiwa, K., Saiki, S. *et al.* (1997) Retrospective analysis of 70 operations for gall bladder cancer. *Br. J. Surg.* **84**, 200–4.

Yamamoto, M., Takasaki, K. and Yoshikawa, T. (1999) Extended resection for intrahepatic cholangiocarcinoma in Japan. *J. Hepato-Biliary-Pancreatic Surg.* **6**(2), 117–21.

Yamamoto, M., Takasaki, K., Yoshikawa, T., Ueno, K. and Nakano, M. (1998) Does gross appearance indicate prognosis in intrahepatic cholangiocarcinoma? *J. Surg. Oncol.* **69**(3), 162–7.

Yeung, E., McCarthy, P., Gompertz, R.H. *et al.* (1989) Ultrasonic appearances of hilar cholangio-carcinoma (Klatskin tumours). *Br. J. Radiol.* **61**, 991–5.

Zatonski, W.A., Lowenfels, A.B., Boyle, P. *et al.* (1997) Epidemiologic aspects of gall bladder cancer: a case-control study of the SEARCH program of the International Agency for Research on Cancer. *J. Natl Cancer Inst.* **89**, 1132–8.

Stomach

MARIANNE C. NICOLSON

INCIDENCE

Gastric cancer accounted for approximately 6 per cent of all cancer deaths in the UK in 1990, a percentage which comprises almost 10 000 people. The mortality from gastric cancer worldwide is decreasing (Howson *et al.*, 1986) but the tumour is common enough in the high-risk populations of Latin America, North Europe and Japan to make it the world's second most common cancer (Parkin *et al.*, 1988). There is also a marked change in the most common site of primary gastric cancer, in that proximal tumours are much more common than previously. In Japan, gastric cancer accounts for 60 per cent of all cancers in men and 40 per cent of all cancers in women, thus explaining the early initiatives in that country, where significant energy and resources are being spent in an attempt to understand the causes, improve the treatment and prolong the life expectancy of people who develop the disease.

AETIOLOGY

Geographical factors do not, in themselves, provide an adequate explanation of the rates of gastric cancer. In a study of immigrant Japanese, the incidence of gastric cancer did not fall in the first generation, whereas in their offspring there was a decreased incidence in developing the disease (Haenzel, 1961). The theory of genetic predisposition does not therefore explain the high incidence of a disease in the Japanese. The risk factors are summarized in Table 27.1.

Reporting on a study of dietary details, Correa *et al.* (1983) concluded that several factors common to some populations were associated with a high risk. These were low intake of animal fat and protein, high intake of complex carbohydrates, nitrates or salt, and a low intake of salads, fresh greens and fruit. When the pH of the stomach is higher than usual, bacteria can survive and may reduce dietary nitrate to nitrite to form *N*-nitroso compounds through nitrosation of dietary amines. *N*-nitroso compounds are known to be carcinogenic in animals (Ogiu *et al.*, 1975). The source of dietary nitrites is preservatives and colouring agents, especially in home-cured meats, dried fish and sausages. Nitrates are found in crop fertilizers and recycled sewage and they can be converted to nitrites by bacterial action in the food or in the stomach. The protective effect of greens may be explained by the possibility that ascorbic acid may increase gastric

Table 27.1 *Risk factors for gastric cancer*

Diet	Low fresh fruit and vegetables
	Low animal fat
	Low protein
	High complex carbohydrate
	High nitrates
	High salt
Old age	Multifocal gastritis
	Previous partial gastrectomy
	Helicobacter pylori gastric infection
	Blood group A
	Genetic mutation in E-cadherin/*CDH1*
	Epstein–Barr virus infection

acidity and block the bacterial conversion of ingested nitrate to nitrite, thereby decreasing the concentration of nitrosamines.

Older age is one of the main risk factors for development of gastric cancer, with only 2 per cent of cases occurring in individuals of 30 years or younger (Tso *et al.*, 1987; Matley *et al.*, 1988; Okamoto *et al.*, 1988). The presence of a multifocal chronic gastritis has also been identified in patients who have a high risk of gastric cancer, and this appears to be more commonly associated with the disease than is auto-immune gastritis (pernicious anaemia). The main finding is of atrophic change in the gastric mucosa with replacement of glands by connective tissue and leucocytes. The secondary metaplasia or dysplasia results in the development of an intestinal-like mucosa with argentaffin cells, goblet and Paneth's cells. When the glandular structure is very bizarre there is an increased risk of transformation into gastric cancer (Correa, 1980).

There have been many reports of gastric cancer forming in the remnant following partial gastrectomy for both malignant and benign disease. A review of 51 such cases reported a difference in the types of tumour, depending on whether the initial partial gastrectomy had been performed for benign or malignant disease. In the study population, 35 patients had partial gastrectomy for gastric cancer and 16 were operated for benign disease. There was a well-defined pattern to the remnant cancer which developed following malignant disease treated with partial gastrectomy. Remnant cancer was more common following partial gastrectomy for neoplasia. The tumours were well defined, multifocal, located distant from the anastomosis and appeared within 5–14 years. The nature of the lesion was not typical of an aetiology related to reflux of bile or intestinal fluid, which are believed to be the initiating factors in tumours arising after partial gastrectomy for benign ulceration. In the latter case, the remnant tumour was typically diffuse, peri-anastomotic and of late onset (more than 20 years after partial gastrectomy) (Furukawa *et al.*, 1993).

Gastric infection with *Helicobacter pylori* is also believed to be a risk factor for gastric cancer through its association with atrophic gastritis (Correa *et al.*, 1990). The Eurogast Study Group (1993) reported on a study incorporating 17 populations from 13 countries where 100 per cent *H. pylori* infection was associated with a sixfold increase in gastric cancer, compared with those populations who had no such infection. Eradication of the infection is possible in 70 per cent of infected patients, using combination treatment with tripotassium dicitratobismuthate, amoxycillin and metronidazole for 1 week (Logan *et al.*, 1991). Abnormal variants in the interleukin-1B gene (genetic polymorphisms that enhance activity) are also associated with an increased risk of developing gastric cancer (El-Omar *et al.*, 2000). Infection with *H. pylori* in patients who have the polymorphism results in their producing more interleukin-1B, which can reduce

the expression of adhesion molecules such as E-cadherin (Bailey *et al.*, 1998). The E-cadherin gene is a cell adhesion molecule and a tumour suppressor gene which is underexpressed in advanced-stage and invasive gastric cancer.

Another infective agent which may increase the risk of gastric cancer is the Epstein–Barr virus (EBV). A study of EBV sequences detected by polymerase chain reaction revealed that 21 per cent of gastric adenocarcinomas in men in Los Angeles and 14 per cent in Hawaiian men were EBV associated (Shibata *et al.*, 1992). The figures were lower in the female population. EBV termini analysis indicated that the viral infection occurred early in transformation and was associated with an inflammatory component in the tumour.

There has been concern that prolonged ingestion of H_2-receptor antagonists could result in an increase in gastric cancer through the induction of hypergastrinaemia which causes fundal endocrine cell hyperplasia (Langman, 1985). Conversely, cimetidine was reported to enhance immune function and its use as an adjuvant therapy has been explored (*see* p. 592). Similarly, proton pump inhibitors (e.g. omeprazole) have been studied for any long-term effects in induction of gastric cancer: although there was an increase in subatrophic gastritis, there was no increase in gastric cancer.

There is evidence for genetic predisposition, and families with an autosomal dominant predisposition have been described in the literature. The Maori kindreds who developed early onset, diffuse gastric cancer were found to have mutation in the E-cadherin/*CDH1* gene, and there was subsequent realization that other ethnic groups may be affected. The likelihood of developing gastric cancer in these families is up to 70 per cent, similar to the situation with *MENII* and *BRCA1* genes and their association with phaeochromocytoma and breast cancer, respectively. Patients are often younger than the 'average' gastric cancer patient (38 versus 70 years) and linitis plastica is frequently the type of tumour seen. An overview of the situation and guidelines for management of such families has been produced to ensure early development of appropriate screening and treatment (Caldas *et al.*, 1999).

DIAGNOSIS

In Britain 1 in 50 patients presenting to the general practitioner for the first time with dyspepsia will have gastric cancer (OPCS, 1972). Up until 1980 only 1 per cent of cases in this country were diagnosed at an early stage – carcinoma confirmed within the submucosa (Fielding *et al.*, 1980). Conversely, the threefold higher incidence of the disease in Japan has encouraged screening of the population, which resulted in an increase in the proportion of early diagnoses, from 2 per cent in 1955

(Miwa, 1979) to 30 per cent in 1978 (Miwa, 1978). The Japanese mass screening was by indirect radiology (Hisamichi and Sugawara, 1984).

In Britain an improvement in the proportion of early tumours was seen when British dyspeptic patients over the age of 40 were referred for endoscopy following the first consultation with their general practitioner; 26 per cent of the gastric cancers found were early and 63 per cent of the cases were operable (Hallissey et al., 1990). The importance of detecting the disease at an early stage is emphasized in the 5-year survival figures for British patients presenting with advanced disease – 5 per cent (Allum et al., 1989b) – compared with 97 per cent for Japanese who are diagnosed and treated for early disease (Murakami, 1979). Several authors have suggested that gastric cancer in Japan is a different disease from that in the Western population, but the importance of diagnosing the condition in its early stage is not disputed.

In those patients who require investigation of upper gastrointestinal symptoms, initial assessment may either be with endoscopy or barium contrast studies. A review by Green et al. (1981) reported retrospectively on 27 cases of surgically proven gastric cancer. With conventional X-ray techniques, 44 per cent of cases were suspected or diagnosed, 19 were missed and 37 per cent were reported as benign. Endoscopy with biopsy and brushings is reported to have an overall sensitivity of 95 per cent in detecting gastric cancer (Llanos et al., 1982).

Computed tomography (CT) permits direct visualization of gastric lumen, wall and adjacent structures, to provide a more comprehensive picture of the disease, which is enhanced post-oral ingestion of contrast. It would be of significant benefit to patients if surgery could be avoided in cases where the tumour is not resectable, since in addition to preventing the trauma of an operation there would be no delay in initiating chemotherapy in order to attempt preoperative downstaging of the disease. A comparison of preoperative CT scanning and operative staging in 75 patients was disappointing in that it demonstrated understaging in 31 per cent and overstaging in 16 per cent of cases. The main failing seemed to be that the CT scan was unable to detect metastases in normal-sized lymph nodes and failed to detect peritoneal metastases in 30 per cent of patients (Sussman et al., 1988).

Endoscopic ultrasonography is available in few centres, but has been found to be accurate in measuring the depth of the tumour penetration in 92 per cent of cases, compared with 42 per cent accuracy with the use of CT scan (Botet et al., 1991). CT remains superior for detection of distant metastases. Gastric tumours staged at T3 and T4 have a significant risk for recurrence after 'curative' resection, and laparoscopy and laparoscopic ultrasound may add further information about T stage. Laparoscopy and laparoscopic ultrasound are best at evaluating the presence of peritoneal disease and allow direct visualization of the liver. In the latter, a sensitivity of 87 per cent has been reported for detection of liver metastases, with 83 per cent sensitivity for peritoneal deposits (Possik et al., 1986).

The usefulness of magnetic resonance imaging (MRI) in imaging gastric cancer is limited by motion artefacts from respiration and peristalsis, although there is a potential advantage of the ability to see normal layers within the gastric wall. The description of a low-signal band outside the gastric wall in the normal MRI pictures led to the idea that loss of the signal indicated tumour invasion to the fat layer (Matsushita et al., 1994). In that study, comprising 14 patients, the accuracy of MRI findings was 88 per cent when compared with histopathology.

Until better accuracy can be assured, laparotomy will remain the gold standard for staging gastric cancer, and the aim in all studies must be to have a standardized means of documenting the extent of disease, so enabling identification of clear prognostic indicators and selection of suitable patients for adjuvant studies.

PATHOLOGY

Ninety-seven per cent of stomach cancers are adenocarcinomas. The other 3 per cent – sarcomas and lymphomas – will not be discussed in this chapter. Several different histological subclassifications of adenocarcinoma are recognized. The intestinal and diffuse varieties were originally described by Lauren (1965) and are widely accepted, with good concordance in reports among pathologists – up to 80 per cent (Palli et al., 1991). In the infiltrative type of tumour, neoplastic cells adhere to each other to form gland-like structures. This is more common in elderly men in populations who demonstrate an increased incidence of gastric cancer. The pre-cancerous period is longer with this histological type, which occurs mainly in the body and fundus, along the greater curvature. Survival figures are slightly better for the intestinal than for the 'diffuse' tumour. The diffuse variety of gastric cancer shows less cohesion and causes thickening of the stomach wall by infiltration. It is found mainly in areas where gastric cancer is endemic and is associated with an over-representation of blood group A (Correa et al., 1973).

Lauren's differentiations had been fully described earlier by Borrman (1926), who described polypoid (I), ulcerating (II), combined (III) and infiltrating (IV) growth patterns, and these are easily recognized on endoscopy. The Japanese added early gastric cancer, which is also an endoscopic diagnosis, made on the discovery of discrete single or multiple lesions comfined to the mucosa (Johansen, 1976).

The site of most primary gastric cancers has changed in the recent past, with an increase in the incidence of proximal lesions and a smaller number of distal and antral tumours (Allum et al., 1989b). It is postulated that the increase in fruit and vegetable intake, with consequent reduction in exposure of the distal stomach to carcinogenic nitrates, may have led to the increase in the proportion of adenocarcinomas of the gastric cardia. The relevance of the change in anatomical site of stomach cancer is related to the associated poorer prognosis, possibly because disease at this site presents at a later stage or because surgery carries a higher morbidity due to the necessity for a thoracic approach.

Although it is important to establish the histological type of gastric cancer, there has been poor correlation between histology and prognosis in this tumour (Morson *et al.*, 1990) and newer, biological factors are now being investigated.

MOLECULAR BIOLOGY

Biological characteristics of gastric carcinoma have been studied with the aim of identifying new prognostic indicators and possible future targets for treatment.

The *c-erb-B2* oncogene is a member of the tyrosine kinase oncogene family. It codes for a 185 kDa transmembrane glycoprotein, and expression has been reported in gastric carcinomas (Park *et al.*, 1989). In one large study of 189 gastric carcinomas, 12.2 per cent of tumour specimens had evidence of the product of *c-erb-B2* localized to the cell membrane (Yonemura *et al.*, 1990). These tumours were more advanced and more commonly associated with serosal invasion, nodal involvement and peritoneal metastases, a finding confirmed by other authors (Yakota *et al.*, 1988; Falck and Gullick, 1989). There was a significant difference in 5-year survival between the two groups (11 per cent for *c-erb-B2*-positive versus 50 per cent for *c-erb-B2*-negative patients), indicating that expression of this protein correlates with poor prognosis, as has been shown in breast cancer (Slamon *et al.*, 1987).

Overexpression of the epidermal growth factor receptor (EGFR), which is encoded by the *erb-1* oncogene, was found in 18 per cent of tumour samples in one study. There was an increased frequency in intestinal tumours (27 per cent) compared with diffuse (12 per cent) (Lemoine *et al.*, 1991). Unlike *c-erb-2*, there was no association with overexpression and stage of disease in this study, but others have reported a range of overexpression, from 4 per cent (early disease) to 35 per cent (advanced disease) (Yasui *et al.*, 1988). There are some data suggesting that EGFR expression is associated with a worse prognosis in gastric cancer (Tahara *et al.*, 1986), which may be predicted from the data linking poor prognosis and presence of the antigen in patients with lung or head and neck cancers.

The H-*ras* oncogene has been found to be overexpressed both in primary stomach cancers and also in areas of gastric dysplasia (Ohuchi *et al.*, 1987). Enhanced expression of c-H-*ras* p21 in human stomach adenocarcinomas was defined by immunoassays using monoclonal antibodies

and *in-situ* hybridization. There was no correlation between expression and tumour depth or invasiveness.

The 5T4 antigen is a cell-membrane antigen found in few normal tissues but in a wide variety of transformed cell lines. In a study incorporating 99 gastrointestinal cancer specimens (27 gastric and 72 colorectal) a positive correlation was found between 5T4 and stage of disease but not cancer grade (Starzynska *et al.*, 1992). It is possible that if a monoclonal antibody were raised to 5T4, immunotherapy could be effective in gastrointestinal cancer.

Investigation and mutation of the *p53* gene in gastric cancer has found involvement mainly of exons 5 and 7 (codons 173 and 251), which occur most frequently in the advanced stages of disease. Exon 6 and 9 mutations of *p53* have also been recognized, but the relationship with pathological staging and prognosis has not been fully elucidated (Ficorella *et al.*, 1993). There may be an increased likelihood of lymph-node metastases in tumours which overexpress *p53* (85 per cent versus 64 per cent) (Kakeji *et al.*, 1993). It has been estimated that overexpression of *p53* may be present in up to 30 per cent of gastric cancers when immunohistochemical staining is used (Gamo *et al.*, 1993), but diffuse tumours with dispersed cells are less commonly associated with *p53* mutations (Matozaki *et al.*, 1992). Gastric cancers with *p53* abnormalities are more likely to be chemoresistant.

In addition to investigating molecular biology to allow prediction of overall prognosis in gastric cancer, there has been investigation of the role of the multi-drug resistant gene (*MDR-1*) in the tumour's resistance to chemotherapy. In a series of 22 patients, *MDR-1* was detected in 41 per cent, with high levels in 18 per cent (Wallner *et al.*, 1993). Although the study was small, the indication was clear that multi-drug resistance may be a feature in the relative lack of responsiveness to chemotherapy in gastric cancer.

STAGING

As in other tumours, the stage of disease at diagnosis is relevant both to the plan of management and to the prognosis. The gross appearance of early gastric tumours described by experienced endoscopists in Japan allows analysis of the extent of disease even where only mucosa and submucosa are involved. Subdivisions are as follows:

- I: Protruding type
- II: Superficial
  - elevated
  - flat
  - depressed
- III: Excavated

Types IIb and IIc predominate and are associated with a 95 per cent 5-year survival rate, possibly related to the

Table 27.2 *TNM classification in gastric cancer (1997)*

Stage		
I	IA	T1 N0 M0
	IB	T1 N1 M0
		T2 N0 M0
II		T1 N2 M0
		T2 N1 M0
		T3 N0 M0
III	IIIA	T2 N2 M0
		T3 N1 M0
		T4 N0 M0
	IIIB	T3 N2 M0
IV		T4 N1, N2, N3 M0
		T1, T2, T3 N3 M0
		Any T Any N M1

T, primary tumour; T1, lamina propria, submucosa;
T2, muscularis propria, subserosa; T3, penetrates serosa;
T4, adjacent structures; N1, 1–6 regional nodes; N2,
7–15 regional nodes; N3, >15 regional nodes;
M0, no distant metastases; M1, distant metastases.

fact the lymphatic channels are very rarely found in the gastric mucosa and submucosa.

In more advanced cases the preferred staging is the TNM system (Table 27.2). For operative purposes the stomach is divided anatomically into three sections: upper third (C), middle third (M) and lower third (A). The extent of stomach wall involvement is documented as S0 (no serosal involvement), S1 (suspected serosal involvement), S2 (definite serosal involvement) or S3 (invasion of contiguous structures). Lymph nodes are categorized as N1 (perigastric nodes along the lesser and greater curvature), N2 (paragastric nodes along the coeliac access and its trifurcation) or N3 (involvement of other intra-abdominal lymph nodes), which is now considered to signify distant metastasis. The curability of the tumour is directly related to its operability, and the exact nodal groups which must be removed to attempt cure depend on the location of the primary tumour.

Following resection, which may involve total or subtotal gastrectomy, accurate histological evaluation of tumour subtype and involvement of tumour margins complete the staging assessment. It is only when these procedures have been completed that a statement can be made on the curative or non-curative role of surgery in each particular case. Curative resection is possible when there are neither peritoneal nor hepatic deposits, and a tier of non-involved lymph nodes has been removed beyond those containing secondary tumour. Relating the staging to prognosis, serosal involvement predicts a 5-year survival of approximately 15 per cent, compared with 50 per cent when the serosa is free of tumour (Cunningham, 1990). Nodal involvement reduces the 5-year survival from 31 per cent to 17 per cent. The roles of surgery, radiotherapy and chemotherapy in stages I to IV will be discussed below.

TREATMENT

Surgery

A review of the surgical treatments of gastric cancer reported in eight papers dating from 1938 to 1982, incorporating more than 7000 patients, concluded that 80 per cent of patients underwent surgery (Cunningham, 1990). Approximately 50 per cent of procedures were considered to be curative, but operative mortality after total gastrectomy has until recently been high in the West, at 20–25 per cent, compared with <5 per cent in Japan, a finding partially explained by the greater experience of the Japanese in treating gastric cancer surgically. Akoh and Macintyre (1992) published a review of the outlook for patients with gastric cancer, including information from 100 English-language papers where the given data were adequate to allow a valid assessment of 5-year survival. The number of patients operated fell from 92 per cent before 1970 to 71 per cent by 1990, but the proportion of operated patients undergoing resection increased from 37 per cent to 48 per cent in the same period, suggesting an improvement in patient selection. The better staging and selection procedures, perhaps in combination with improved operative techniques, resulted in a larger number of patients being suitable for curative or radical resection (9 per cent before 1970 versus 31 per cent before 1990) with concurrent improvement in prognosis – 5-year survival rate 55.4 per cent, from 37.6 per cent in the period between 1940 and 1988.

Historically there have been several problems associated with the surgery for gastric cancer in the West. Accurate surgical staging was often not carried out, resections were not standardized between conservative (R1) and extended (R2,3), and there was frequently a lack of pathological data in the reporting of the surgical specimens (Cuschieri, 1986). The result of this was that, even in surgical procedures which were thought to be curative, the local regional relapse rate was around 85 per cent.

There is still controversy regarding the benefits of total over sub-total gastrectomy in treatment of gastric cancer. Some surgeons argue that the tumour is often multi-centric, and perform total gastrectomy as a matter of routine. While multi-centricity may be the norm for tumours which develop on a background of pernicious anaemia, severe dysplasia or multiple polyps, these aetiologies are in the minority. It could be argued that, for the most part, total gastrectomy is only necessary where the tumour is large, involving the middle third of the stomach, and adequate tumour clearance is not possible with a sub-total procedure. There is, to date, no evidence that survival is enhanced by performing total gastrectomy. One report on 402 patients (361 subtotal and 41 total gastrecomies) who had 'curative' resection for tumour in the lower two-thirds of the stomach, found a significant increase in 5-year survival for those patients aged over 60 years with nodal involvement who had sub-total gastrectomy (37 per cent versus 10 per cent) (Gennari *et al.*, 1986).

The overlap of lymphatic drainage in the stomach is one of the explanations for the difficulty in predicting the extent of disease. Japanese authors have recommended extended lymphadenectomy, but this practice is rare in America and Europe because of a lack of evidence of any benefit. The published Norwegian experience included 532 of a total 1165 patients with gastric cancer who were treated with potentially curative surgery which was defined as there being no macroscopic residual lesion and tumour-free margins (Haugstvedt *et al.*, 1993). The analysis failed to reveal any survival advantage for extensive resection, confirming the findings of Shiu *et al.* (1987). More recently the MRC randomized trial of D1 (standard perigastric nodal resection) versus D2 (extended to level 1 and 2 regional nodes) reported that, in their 400 patients, there was no difference in 5-year or relapse-free survival (Cuschieri *et al.*, 1999).

In the surgical management of locally advanced disease (where, by definition, there are involved regional lymph nodes, adjacent tissues or organs which preclude resection *en bloc*), the median survival is in the region of 5 months, with all patients dead by 2 years (Moertel *et al.*, 1969; Cunningham *et al.*, 1987). These poor figures belie the symptomatic benefit enjoyed by many patients, who obtain relief from the obstruction, bleeding or pain associated with their tumour preoperatively. It has been reported that resection should be attempted wherever possible because this confers both a greater palliative relief from gastrointestinal symptoms and an improved survival rate (Stern *et al.*, 1975). Total gastrectomy is not recommended as a palliative procedure because of the significant morbidity and high mortality from the procedure in this setting (Douglass and Nava, 1985). For tumours of the gastro-oesophageal junction, however, oesophagogastrectomy is the treatment of choice for fit patients. Although palliative gastrostomy and jejunostomy are practised in some centres, the poor response and high complication rates makes these unattractive options in the majority of cases (ReMine, 1979). The high morbidity and mortality associated with endoscopic insertion of a prosthetic stent make it a procedure suitable only for those with very poor prognosis who are unfit for surgery but who require palliation of salivary aspiration (Turnbull *et al.*, 1980).

Laser therapy is one of the most effective palliative treatments for gastric cancer. The acronym stands for 'light amplification by stimulated emission of radiation'. Endoscopically the laser light is converted into heat, which may coagulate bleeding points or vaporize neo-plastic tissue. It has been reported that bleeding lesions in the fundus and cardia are very difficult to treat, but effective palliation can be achieved in 80 per cent of patients (Mathus-Vliegen and Tytgat, 1990). Laser pallia-tion of cardiac stenosis was successful in 65 per cent of 11 patients, but less encouraging in distal (antral) lesions because of associated poor motility, resulting in pre-vention of gastric emptying despite formation of an adequate lumen (Suzuki *et al.*, 1989).

The conclusion on surgical management of gastric cancer is that only complete resection can currently offer a cure for the disease, and the trend towards more careful selection of patients suitable for curative resection must be welcomed. Meticulous documentation of the extent of disease by surgeons and pathologists will aid in deter-mining what constitutes a curative procedure, and spe-cialization of surgeons will also help to reduce operative mortality. In the palliative setting, development of new invasive techniques and improvement of those which are currently available will ensure maximum benefit with minimum morbidity for people with unresectable tumours. Those patients with incurable tumours who are not suffering from dysphagia, pain or bleeding should probably be spared surgery. In addition, the link between surgeons and oncologists should be encouraged, enabling all groups of patients with gastric cancer to have the oppor-tunity to participate in a clinical trial. As always, entering patients into trials for gastric cancer will expedite the accumulation of knowledge of the optimum treatment for different disease stages.

Radiotherapy

The pattern of local failure in gastric cancer following an attempt at curative resection (up to 85 per cent of patients) has led some specialists to suggest that intra- or postoperative radiotherapy should be of benefit in the adjuvant setting (Landry *et al.*, 1990).

In non-randomized studies of intra-operative radio-therapy, doses from 28 to 40 Gy were given, with the aim of delivering large doses of radiotherapy during the operation to sterilize the tumour bed. A slight benefit in survival was seen only in patients with stage IV disease (Abe *et al.*, 1981). In a randomized study of adjuvant treatment in gastric cancer, where no treatment was compared with adjuvant external-beam radiotherapy or adjuvant chemotherapy (5-fluorouracil, Adriamycin® and Mitomycin C®: FAM), no survival advantage was seen in the treated as opposed to the control group (Allum *et al.*, 1989a). No difference in survival was seen in a study of 115 patients who were randomized to receive postoperative radiotherapy alone or with 5-fluorouracil (5-FU) for varying periods of time (Bleiberg *et al.*, 1989). The study included patients who had undergone curative or palliative procedures, and no difference was seen in time to tumour progression.

External-beam irradiation used alone in the treatment of unresectable gastric cancer (at doses of 35–40 Gy) resulted in a median survival of approximately 5 months, with no patients alive at 15 months. In the alterna-tive arm of that randomized trial, the addition of the

Table 27.3 *Single-agent chemotherapy response in gastric cancer*

Drug	Response (%)
Epirubicin	36
5-Fluorouracil (infusional)	31
Mitomycin C®	30
Adriamycin®	25
CPT-11	23
Taxotere®	21
5-Fluorouracil (bolus)	21
Taxol®	
Cisplatin	19
BCNU	17

BCNU, 1,3-*bis*(2-chloroethyl)-1-nitrosurea (carmustine).

Table 27.4 *Combination chemotherapy response in gastric cancer*

Treatment	Response (%)	Reference
FAMTX	21–63	Wils *et al.* (1986, 1991) Waters *et al.* (1999)
ECF	40–70	Findlay *et al.* (1994) Ross *et al.* (1999)
FAM	9–40	Macdonald *et al.* (1980) Wils *et al.* (1991)
FAP	29–77	Wooley *et al.* (1981) Moertel *et al.* (1986) Tagliagambe *et al.* (1986) Wagener *et al.* (1985)
EAP	20–73	Preusser *et al.* (1988) Kelsen *et al.* (1981)
FEMTX	36	Pyrhonen *et al.* (1992)
5-FU + carboplatin	45	Shirai *et al.* (1993)
PELF	62	Cascinu *et al.* (1997)

FAMTX: 5-fluorouracil, Adriamycin® and sequential high-dose methotrexate; ECF: epirubicin, cisplatin and continuous-infusion 5-fluorouracil; FAM: 5-fluorouracil, Adriamycin® and Mitomycin C®; FAP: 5-fluorouracil, Adriamycin® and cisplatin; EAP: epirubicin, Adriamycin® and cisplatin; FEMTX: 5-fluorouracil, epirubicin and methotrexate; 5-FU: 5-fluorouracil; PELF: cisplatin, epirubicin, 5-FU and leucovorin.

radiosensitizing drug, 5-FU, to irradiation improved the median survival by 2 months (5 months versus 7 months), with an increase in 5-year survival from 0 per cent to 12 per cent (Holbrook, 1974).

The usefulness of radiotherapy in both advanced disease and the adjuvant setting is therefore debatable, but, in the former, the addition of radiosensitizing drugs may increase effectiveness. However, it is not a standard treatment.

Chemotherapy

Chemotherapy may have a role in early and advanced gastric cancer. Single-agent drug activity with conventional chemotherapy in gastric cancer may achieve objective responses in up to 36 per cent of patients (Table 27.3). Combination chemotherapy is generally more effective than single-agent treatment. Phase II studies of FAMTX (5-FU, Adriamycin® and sequential high-dose methotrexate) and ECF (epirubicin, cisplatin and continuous-infusion 5-FU) regimens reported responses in 58 per cent and 70 per cent, respectively, in advanced disease (Klein *et al.*, 1982; Findlay *et al.*, 1994). The small number of patients treated in phase II trials usually give an unrealisitically high overall response rate, and large randomized phase III studies are of more value. Logical, sequential randomized phase III studies have been performed in advanced gastric cancer to evaluate and compare the relative response rates and survival with different regimens. In addition to producing improvement in outcomes for patients with advanced disease, the aim is to bring the most effective and least toxic regimen forward to the adjuvant or neoadjuvant setting, as discussed below.

CHEMOTHERAPY IN ADVANCED DISEASE

There have been many phase II studies of combination chemotherapy in advanced gastric cancer since it was discovered that the effect may be synergistic rather than simply additive (Table 27.4). The FAM combination (5-FU, Adriamycin® and Mitomycin C®) achieved response rates of between 22 per cent and 40 per cent, but the duration of response and the median survival was only 6 months (Macdonald *et al.*, 1980). In a randomized study involving patients with both gastric and pancreatic cancer, a three-way randomization to 5-FU, 5-FU and doxorubicin or FAM revealed no difference in response rates or median survival in the groups, suggesting that single-agent 5-FU was an adequate treatment. There were 51 patients in each of the groups of gastric cancer treated with 5-FU or FAM (Cullinan *et al.*, 1985).

FAMTX was initially thought to be more active, but response rates fell to 33–50 per cent, with median survival 9 months, when the regimen was tested by the Gastrointestinal Tract Cancer Cooperative Group (GTCCG) of the European Organization for the Research and Treatment of Cancer (EORTC) (Wils *et al.*, 1986). FAM and FAMTX were then compared in a randomized trial; response rates were 41 per cent (FAMTX) versus 9 per cent (FAM) with median survival 42 versus 29 weeks (*P* < 0.004). At 1 year, 41 per cent of FAMTX versus 22 per cent of FAM patients were alive (Wils *et al.*, 1991). There is some concern regarding toxicity from FAMTX and this limits is general use, although studies of drug scheduling are being investigated in an attempt to resolve the problems.

FAP (5-FU, Adriamycin® and cisplatin) is one of the second-generation regimens in gastric cancer. The response rates quoted ranged from 29 per cent to 55 per cent, with median survivals of 4 to 12 months, but most study populations have included fewer than 35 patients (Wooley et al., 1981; Wagener et al., 1985; Moertel et al., 1986; Tagliagambe et al., 1986). Histologically complete responses have been reported with this combination in advanced gastric cancer.

A similarly active regimen is EAP (epirubicin, Adriamycin® and cisplatin), which produced an overall response rate of 73 per cent (complete response 16 per cent) in a phase II trial of metastatic gastric cancer (Preusser et al., 1988). All patients were of WHO performance status 2 or better. One important factor was that omission of 5-FU from the combination was not detrimental, although it is considered to be the standard drug in gastrointestinal cancer. A randomized trial of EAP versus FAMTX revealed that the latter combination was less toxic although equally effective (response rates 20 per cent versus 33 per cent). There were four treatment-related deaths in the EAP group and none in the patients treated with FAMTX.

EAP and FAM have also been compared in a population of 90 patients with advanced gastric cancer who were treated until disease progression. The response rates were 55.6 per cent (EAP) versus 16.7 per cent (FAM), with the former regimen producing less toxicity. The median disease-free survival of complete responders was longer with EAP treatment (12 months versus 8 months) but no difference was seen in overall survival (7 months versus 5 months) (Icli et al., 1993).

ECF was developed to exploit both the increase in activity of 5-FU seen in infusional rather than bolus delivery and the synergy of cisplatin and 5-FU. The 5-FU–cisplatin synergy is believed to be mediated through the depletion of intracellular methiamine by cisplatin. This in turn leads to an increase in the reduced metabolite concentration, enhancing the binding of fluorodeoxidine monophosphate to thymidylate synthetase. There may also be a reduction in cisplatin-damaged DNA repair due to interruption of cellular thymidine utilization by 5-FU. Initial results using ECF in 128 patients with measurable advanced gastric cancer demonstrated an overall response rate of 70 per cent with median survival 8 months. The complete response rate was 15 per cent (Findlay et al., 1994). The randomized trial of ECF versus FAMTX demonstrated an improved response rate for ECF (46 versus 21 per cent) with significantly less toxicity. The long-term survival in these patients was 14 per cent (ECF) versus 5 per cent (FAMTX) at 2 years, the ECF thus affording a very significant improvement in survival (Waters et al., 1999).

Mitomycin® is one of the most commonly prescribed drugs in gastric cancer therapy, and a multicentre trial in advanced disease compared ECF with MCF, where epirubicin was replaced by Mitomycin C® and the infused 5-FU was increased from 200 mg/m^2 per day to 300 mg/m^2 per day. Although there was no significant difference in overall response rates (40 versus 39 per cent) or median

survival (9.4 versus 8.8 months), the patients treated with ECF enjoyed improved quality of life, a finding revealing the relative lack of importance of alopecia when compared with mucositis, which was more common with the MCF regimen.

FEMTX, a regimen compromising 5-FU, epirubicin and methotrexate, was randomized against best supportive care in patients with unresectable gastric cancer (Pyrhonen et al., 1992). With 41 patients randomized, the overall response rate was 36 per cent. Median time to progression was 5.4 months. The treated group demonstrated significantly longer survival compared with the control population (12.3 versus 3.1 months), and treatment was well tolerated.

An intensive, weekly delivered four-drug combination of cisplatin, epirubicin, 5-FU and leucovorin (PELF) was studied in a phase II trial recruiting 105 patients (Cascinu et al., 1997). Despite the good response rate of 62 per cent, it was necessary to give colony stimulating factors to reduce myelosuppression, and the latter fact may limit use of the regimen in the palliative setting of advanced gastric cancer.

The activity of carboplatin and combination with infusional 5-FU was studied in 22 patients with advanced disease, with the aim of delivering an active non-nephrotoxic treatment. The objective response rate was 45 per cent in the 20 evaluable patients and toxicity was mild, with no measured deterioration in renal function. Median survival was 9 months (Shirai et al., 1993). A summary of the key papers discussed above is given in Tables 27.5 and 27.6.

Single-agent oral etoposide was investigated in chemonaive patients with advanced gastric cancer, and there were responses in 4 of 21 patients, with median duration 3.5 months (Ajani et al., 1993). The treatment was well tolerated. However, chronic oral etoposide in combination with high-dose megesterol acetate to reverse P-glycoprotein-mediated drug resistance was unacceptably myelotoxic when used to treat patients with advanced gastric cancer (Higuchi and Isell, 1993). Reduction of the etoposide dose from 50 mg/m^2 daily for 21 days to 50 mg daily over 4 days did not prevent myelosuppression. No responses were seen in the four patients treated, and both poor efficacy and toxicity will seriously limit continued use of the regimen.

Biological response modifiers have also been investigated in conjunction with chemotherapy in advanced gastric cancer, in an attempt to emulate the successful biochemical modulation of 5-FU seen in colorectal tumours. A combination of 5-FU, folinic acid and interferon-α 2b resulted in an objective response in 17 of 36 (47 per cent) patients, with a significant reduction in tumour-related pain in 22 of 26 (85 per cent). Toxicity was acceptable and the median duration of response was 5.5 months (Jager-Arand et al., 1993). There may be also a role for immunotherapy given in combination with chemotherapy in gastric cancer. In a randomized trial incorporating 204 patients, where combined 5-FU and Adriamycin® (FA)

Table 27.5 *Details of chemotherapy phase II regimens in gastric cancer*

Regimen	No. of patients evaluable for response	Median age (range)	Median performance status; no. of patients	No. with locally advanced disease	Response				Overall response (%)	Median survival (months)
					CR	PR	NC	PD		
EAP (Preusser et al., 1988)	44	50 (18–65)	ECOG <2; 44	2	7	25	–	–	73	9
FAM (Macdonald et al., 1980)	62	62 (28–83)	ECOG <2; 46	0	0	26	–	–	42	5.5
FAP (Wagener et al., 1985)	18	51 (34–68)	Karnofsky 80–90; 11	8	0	9	8	1	50	12
FAMTX (EORTC) (Wils et al., 1986)	67	58 (36–75)	ECOG 1	6	9	13	17	11	33	6
ECF (Findlay et al., 1994)	133	60 (28–82)	ECOG <2; 116	35	15	80	24	13	71	8.2
PELF weekly (Cascinu et al., 1997)	105	61 (24–73)	ECOG <2; 65	11	18	47	20	20	62	11

Table 27.6 *Details of randomized phase III trials in gastric cancer*

Regimen	No. of patients evaluable for response	Median age (range)	Median performance status; no. of patients	No. with locally advanced disease	Response				Overall response (%)	Median survival
					CR	PR	NC	PD		
FEMTX versus	17				4	2	7	4	36	12.3 months
Best Supp. Care (Pyrhonen et al., 1992)	19				0	0	4	15	0	3.1 months
FAM versus 5-FU (Cullinan et al., 1985)	13	50–69	ECOG 0-1		NS	NS		38		No difference (29 weeks)
	11	50–69	ECOG 0-1						18	
FAMTX versus EAP (Kelsen et al., 1992)	30	56 (37–72)	Karnofsky 80	11	3				33	7.3 months
	30	57 (37–72)	Karnofsky 80	9	0				20	6.1 months
FAMTX versus FAM (Wils et al., 1991)	105	57 (28–77)	ECOG 0-1; 81	19	5	28	25	16	41	42 weeks
	103	58 (23–69)	ECOG 0-1; 79	13	0	7	25	34	9	29 weeks
EAP compared with FAM (Icli et al., 1993) NB: non-randomized	52	*	*		12.8%	27.7%			40.5	7 months
	48				2.3%	11.6%			13.9	5 months
ECF versus FAMTX (Webb, 1997)	126	59 (35–79)	ECOG 0-1; 96	47	7	43	23	22	45	8.9 months
	130	60 (29–78)	ECOG 0-1; 97	51	2	21	23	37	21	5.7 months
ECF versus MCF (Ross, 1999)	Total	NSA	NSA						40	9.4 months
	randomised = 580								39	8.8 months

*Details not stated; comparable
NS, Not stated; NSA, Not stated in abstract.

was compared with FA plus polyadenylic, polyuridylic acid given after a curative resection in locally advanced disease, the estimated 5-year disease-free survival after 20 months follow-up was 40 per cent in the FA arm compared with 70 per cent for the chemo-immunotherapy arm (Kim *et al.*, 1991). The predicted 5-year survival was 45 per cent versus 75 per cent.

The poor outlook for patients with advanced gastric cancer makes it a suitable tumour type for novel anti-cancer agents to be investigated as first-line treatment. Activity of Taxol® (paclitaxel), a tubulin binder which has demonstrated significant activity in ovarian cancer, was investigated in 25 chemo-naive patients with advanced upper gastrointestinal-tract tumours (Einzig *et al.*, 1993). Only one response was seen in the 20 evaluable patients who received doses of $250 \, mg/m^2$ over 24 hours delivered 3-weekly. Similar poor results were obtained with the novel DNA intercalator, Amonifide®. A phase II trial involving 12 patients with recurrent metastatic or inoperable gastric cancer showed no responses and significant toxicity (Schilsky *et al.*, 1993).

The camptothecin analogue CPT-11 has also been evaluated in a phase II study including 81 patients with advanced gastric cancer. Forty-five of 66 patients had previously been treated with chemotherapy and the response rate in this group was 20 per cent, with an overall response rate of 23.3 per cent. The median duration of response was 68 days and toxicity was said to be clinically tolerable. The primary tumour responded in only 4 per cent of patients, with best results seen in lung and lymph-node metastases (33 per cent and 36 per cent, respectively) (Kambe *et al.*, 1993).

The lack of significant overlap in toxicity profiles of docetaxel (Taxotere®) and cisplatin led to these being evaluated in combination in advanced gastric cancer. In the phase II study, Taxotere® was delivered at $85 \, mg/m^2$, increasing to $100 \, mg/m^2$ with cisplatin $75 \, mg/m^2$ on day 1 of a 3-week cycle in 48 patients with advanced gastric cancer, and 27 patients responded (56 per cent) although the median survival was 9 months (Roth *et al.*, 2000). The most common toxicity was neutropenia in 81 per cent of patients, but there were only nine episodes of febrile neutropenia and no treatment-related deaths, leading the authors to conclude that this is a well-tolerated, effective regimen. As stated above, the small numbers of selected patients included in most phase II trials make conclusions difficult, and further evaluation of the regimen is necessary.

Provided that response rates (especially complete responses) can be increased without inducing excessive toxicity, there is room for optimism that it may become possible to increase the duration of response in this chemosensitive disease with a view to achieving long-term survival. It is likely that most cures will be seen only if there is minimal residual disease postoperatively and effective chemotherapy can be given in the adjuvant setting.

ADJUVANT CHEMOTHERAPY

The main problem with adjuvant chemotherapy in gastric cancer is that the patients need time to recover from the major surgery and are often in a poor nutritional state until 6 weeks postoperatively. The delay in ability to deliver the drugs is as significant a problem as is the historical lack of efficacy of the chemotherapy.

Initial studies of adjuvant chemotherapy in gastric cancer involved drugs thio-Tepa and 5-fluorodeoxouri-dine. Neither drug prolonged survival in a series of 903 patients treated between 1957 and 1969 (Serlin *et al.*, 1977). Following the studies described above, where it was established that the combination of radiation and FU produced an improvement in survival of unresectable patients, the same combination was investigated for activity in resected gastric cancer (Moertel *et al.*, 1984). Although the study was small, the initial impression was of an improvement in 5-year survival (23 per cent versus 4 per cent in the control group); 39 per cent of treated patients had a locoregional component of first clinical relapse, compared with 54 per cent in the non-treatment cohort. However, further analysis of the study population found no significant difference in survival between patients treated, patients refusing treatment and controls.

Adjuvant therapy using cimetidine for 2 years after gastric surgery was initially reported to confer a survival benefit (Tonneson *et al.*, 1988). However, the British Stomach Cancer Group published a placebo-controlled randomized study involving more than 400 patients, where there was no difference in survival for patients receiving one of two doses of cimetidine or placebo (Langman *et al.*, 1999).

Studies of adjuvant Mitomycin C® versus no treatment following curative resection of gastric adenocarcinoma in a group of 525 Japanese patients demonstrated a significant improvement in survival for treated versus control groups at 3 years (12.4 per cent), 4 years (14 per cent) and 5 years (13.5 per cent) after surgery. In another Japanese study, patients with serosal infiltration who were undergoing gastrectomy were randomized to receive either no additional treatment or 50 mg intraperitoneal carbon-absorbed Mitomycin® (M-CH) preoperatively (Hagiwara *et al.*, 1992). Those patients who received the M-CH demonstrated better survival at 18 months after randomization (34.6 per cent increase), which increased to 41.7 per cent at 3 years. One Western group published data on single-agent adjuvant Mitomycin C® (Grau *et al.*, 1993). In all cases the Mitomycin C® was started within 6 weeks after surgery. There was an improvement in survival in the treated group ($P < 0.025$) with a reduction in liver metastases and less likelihood of dying from recurrence (74 per cent control versus 59 per cent treatment).

Further evaluation of Mitomycin® looked at randomization between its administration as a single agent or in combination with Ftorafur® (Tegafur®), an orally delivered derivative of fluorouracil (Grau *et al.*, 1998).

Eighty-five patients were randomized with the schedule Mitomycin® 10–20 mg/m^2 i.v. on day 1 every 6 weeks alone, or with Ftorafur® 500 mg/m^2 per day for 36 consecutive days. All courses were repeated four times. With a median follow-up of 62 months, there was a survival advantage for the combination group – 67 per cent versus 44 per cent.

A similar study including 148 patients with resected stage III gastric cancer compared no adjuvant therapy with Mitomycin® 20 mg/m^2 on day 1 followed 30 days later by Tegafur® 400 mg twice daily for 3 months (Cirera et al., 1999). The overall 5-year survival favoured the treated group – 56 per cent versus 46 per cent – with 5-year disease-free survival of 55 per cent versus 31 per cent. However, there was no stratification for nodal disease stage and 20 per cent of treated patients were of N0 status compared with 7 per cent of controls, thus possibly confounding the results in this modest-sized study.

It might be presumed that the results would be even better with combination chemotherapy known to be active in advanced disease. This has not been the case.

The FAM regimen (activity in advanced disease discussed above) was randomized against no postoperative treatment in a population of 315 patients. No difference in survival was seen in comparison with 281 assessable patients, but there was a trend in favour of treatment (Coombs et al., 1990). The South-west Oncology Group studied the same regimen in stage IB, IC, II and III tumours and reported no significant difference in 5-year survival in their population of 176 patients (MacDonald et al., 1992). Modified FAM – FAM2 with 30 per cent increase in 5-FU, 77 per cent increase in doxorubicin and 33 per cent increase in Mitomycin® given at a reduced cycle interval – was investigated by the EORTC Gastro-intestinal group (Lise et al., 1995). There were 314 patients in total – 159 'controls' receiving surgery alone and 155 receiving FAM2 – but 19 allocated to chemotherapy did not receive it. Toxicity was significant, there was a delay in time to progression in the treated group, but no statistically significant difference in survival could be demonstrated between the two arms of the study.

Other studies have compared against surgery only the combinations 5-FU plus methyl-CCNU for 2 years (Higgins et al., 1983; Gastro-Intestinal Study Group, 1982; Engstrom et al., 1985), 5-FU plus methyl CCNU plus levamisole (Italian Gastrointestinal Study Group, 1988) and 5-FU plus Adriamycin® (Krook et al., 1991). Even a large, randomized Japanese study of 579 patients evaluating protracted adjuvant chemotherapy using Mitomycin®, i.v. 5-FU and oral UFT (uracil/Tegafur®) in patients with T1–2 disease demonstrated no benefit (Nakajima et al., 1999).

The conclusion of a meta-analysis of adjuvant chemotherapy trials involving 2096 patients was that there was no survival benefit using current drug combinations, although there was a trend towards improved survival when further studies were included in the sample (Bonenkamp et al., 1993). A further review of all randomized adjuvant chemotherapy trials published since 1984 reported a difference between the West and Asia in that a no treatment control group is the norm in the former, whereas a treatment control is used in Asia and chemo-immunotherapy is more commonly prescribed (Shimada and Ajani, 1999). The results of adjuvant chemotherapy in the West remain largely negative, but although there is not a clear indication in the Asian trials, most patients receive post- or perioperative therapy. A further meta-analysis of 20 articles published before January 2000 and including 3658 patients (2180 deaths) found that chemotherapy reduced the risk of death by 18 per cent, without any evidence of difference between the efficacy of anthracyclines over 5-FU (Mari et al., 2000). However, the limitations of such a literature-based analysis led the authors to conclude that adjuvant therapy remains experimental in gastric cancer.

Delivery of adjuvant chemotherapy is not standard treatment in gastric cancer. Future studies should be targeted towards those patients who are at highest risk of relapse (serosal penetration, extensive nodal involvement), should contain a no-treatment control arm and be stratified for disease stage.

PERIOPERATIVE/NEOADJUVANT CHEMOTHERAPY

The aim of giving chemotherapy before surgery is to reduce the tumour bulk and also to 'sterilize' the surrounding tissue to prevent spread of the tumour cells at the time of operation. The practical problems with neoadjuvant treatment in gastric cancer include the relatively poor efficacy of established regimens and the difficulty in running studies with adequate controls. Ideally, one would wish to randomize patients to neoadjuvant chemotherapy or to initial surgery and although this study is now running (sponsored by the Medical Research Council), recruitment is slow.

Several studies of primary chemotherapy have been published. The EAP (etoposide, Adriamycin(and cisplatin) regimen was used to treat 34 patients with gastric cancer who had failed laparotomy (Wilke et al., 1989). Twenty-three patients achieved a major response and 20 then proceeded to definitive surgery, with resection possible in 15. Five of these patients had a pathologically complete response, two were unresectable and overall the relapse rate at 20 months was 60 per cent. Median survival was 18 months overall and 24 months in the disease-free group. In the EORTC study of FAM versus FAMTX in unresectable patients, 19 received FAMTX and 7 proceeded to second laparotomy. Three of these patients had complete resection of the residual disease (Wils et al., 1991).

Experience with ECF initially was that 28 of 35 unresectable patients achieved a response and 19 of these went to surgery (Findlay et al., 1994). Ten complete resections were possible, and of these, four patients had a pathologically complete response but six patients had unresectable disease.

Intra-arterial chemotherapy with 5-FU and Adriamycin® versus intravenous therapy with the same agents versus surgery alone was investigated in a randomized study incorporating 207 patients preoperatively (Shchepotin et al., 1993). Sixty-two per cent of patients had no residual tumour in the resected stomach following intra-arterial treatment. A further 19 per cent of patients had small residual foci of tumour cells. There was no significant response to intravenous preoperative chemotherapy. There was no improvement in 2-year survival between intravenous chemotherapy versus surgery, contrasting with an improvement of 29 per cent in the intra-arterial versus intravenous group and 45 per cent in the intra-arterial group versus surgery only.

Although these results are encouraging, there is to date no clear evidence that neoadjuvant therapy is of value in gastric cancer. Definitive trials results are awaited. As newer effective drug combinations are developed and response rates in advanced disease increase, perhaps more patients will be treated in the neoadjuvant setting within the context of clinical trials. It will surely be through rendering more people suitable for curative resection that the long-term survival rates for gastric cancer will be improved.

INTRAPERITONEAL THERAPY

Cytological examination of perioperative peritoneal washings in patients with gastric cancer reveals malignant cells in 20–30 per cent of patients considered to have a poor prognosis (Nakajima et al., 1978). Because of data in ovarian cancer where intraperitoneal therapy can salvage some patients with small-volume residual disease (Ten Bokkel Huinink et al., 1985; Howell et al., 1983), single-agent cisplatin 60 mg/m^2 was given as an intraperitoneal treatment via a Tenckhoff catheter to 18 patients within 8 weeks of complete resection of the gastric cancer tumour where there was serosal involvement, positive regional nodes or cytologically positive peritoneal washings (Jones et al., 1993). Of the treated population, 22 per cent had cytologically positive peritoneal washings before or during chemotherapy. The median survival of the group was 17 months and the pattern of relapse was similar to that of untreated historical controls. Six patients relapsed with local/peritoneal disease and four with liver metastases, suggestive either of cisplatin resistance or of poor drug penetration into peritoneal seedlings.

Postoperative intraperitoneal 5-FU and cisplatin following three cycles of neoadjuvant FAMTX has been studied in high-risk gastric cancer (defined by findings at endoscopic ultrasonography) (Schwartz et al., 1993). Of 23 patients treated, FAMTX was found to downstage the tumours, resulting in 70 per cent resectability. The combination of chemo-hyperthermia and Mitomycin C® was investigated in 42 patients who were known to have peritoneal metastases. Twelve patients had malignant ascites. Two patients died due to the procedure. Survival in patients with stage 3 and 4 carcinomatosis (granulations greater than 5 mm diameter) was 50 per cent at 6 months and only 10 per cent at 12 months (Sayag-Beaujard et al., 1999).

The administration of carbon-adsorbed Mitomycin® prior to abdominal closure following gastrectomy was studied in a controlled, randomized trial incorporating 91 patients (Rosen et al., 1998). All patients had involvement of the serosal layer, and the two arms were well matched for age, histological subtype, tumour site and extent of surgery. There was an increased risk of complications and death in the treated as opposed to the control group, with 6 versus 2 intra-abdominal abscesses, 4 versus 1 fistula, 6 versus 1 prolonged abdominal pain and 5 versus 1 deaths. The therapy should not be delivered outwith a controlled, randomized clinical trial.

FUTURE DIRECTIONS

Facilitation of the early diagnosis of gastric cancer is an obvious ambition of those whose aim it is to cure more people of the disease, but the incidence in this country is not high enough to warrant random screening. Certainly one can recommend that people over the age of 45 who develop dyspepsia for the first time should be referred for endoscopy by an experienced physician or surgeon. The role of genetic screening is yet to be established.

Development of new drugs to be tested in phase II studies is an essential factor in the attempt to increase the responsiveness to gastric cancer, and trials with different combinations of new and established drugs should continue with the same aim. Scheduling of drugs is an important avenue of research, and alternative modes of drug delivery (e.g. infusional treatment, intraperitoneal administration) may increase the overall response rates.

When more effective chemotherapy combinations have developed and there is more information on biological predictors of relapse, studies of adjuvant and neoadjuvant therapy should continue in large randomized trials. The question of remission maintenance, possibly using biological response modifiers, could be investigated when complete responses are achieved with the combinations of chemotherapy, radiotherapy and surgery.

SIGNIFICANT POINTS

- Gastric cancer accounts for 6 per cent of all cancer deaths.
- Incidence of proximal tumours is increasing, but overall the incidence is decreasing.

- The majority of patients are elderly with advanced disease at diagnosis.
- Autosomal dominant inheritance is related to mutations of the E-cadherin/*CDH1* germline.
- A 97 per cent 5-year survival is possible in early, operable disease (Japanese data).
- Total gastrectomy – as opposed to subtotal – does not enhance survival.
- Radiotherapy is of no proven benefit in the adjuvant or the advanced disease setting.
- Adjuvant combination chemotherapy with currently available drugs has not produced a survival benefit.
- Advanced disease responds to chemotherapy in up to 70 per cent of cases.
- Median survival with chemotherapy in advanced disease is around 8 months.
- Earlier diagnosis to facilitate complete resection and improved chemoresponsiveness (new drugs) would improve survival in gastric cancer.

KEY REFERENCES

Ahlgren, J.D. and Macdonald, J.S. (1992) *Gastric cancer in gastrointestinal oncology*. Philadelphia: J.B. Lippincott, 151–93.

Findlay, M. and Cunningham, D. (1993) Chemotherapy of carcinoma of the stomach. *Cancer Treat. Rev.* **19**, 29–44.

Kelsen, D. (1996) Gastric cancer. *Semin. Oncol.* **23**, 279–406.

Thompson, G.B., van Heerden, J.A. and Starn, M.G. (1993) Adenocarcinoma of the stomach: are we making progress? *Lancet* **342**, 713–18.

Wils, J. (1998) Treatment of gastric cancer. *Curr. Opin. Oncol.* **10**, 357–61.

REFERENCES

Abe, M. and Takahashi, M. (1981) Intraoperative radiotherapy: the Japanese experience. *Int. J. Radiat. Oncol. Biol. Phys.* **7**, 863–8.

Ajani, J., Dumas, P., Pazdur, R. *et al.* (1993) Phase II trial of oral etoposide in untreated patients with advanced gastric carcinoma. *Proc. Am. Soc. Clin. Oncol.* **659**, 217 (abstract).

Akoh, J.A. and Macintyre, I.M.C. (1992) Survival rates in gastric cancer. *Br. J. Surg.* **79**, 293–9.

Allum, W.H., Hallissey, M.T., Ward L.C. *et al.* (1989a) A controlled, prospective, randomised trial of adjuvant chemotherapy or radiotherapy in resectable gastric cancer: interim report. *Br. J. Cancer* **60**, 739–44.

Allum, W.H., Powell, D.J., McConkey, C.C. and Fielding, J.W.L. (1989b) Gastric cancer: a 25 year review. *Br. J. Surg.* **76**, 535–40.

Bailey, T., Biddlestone, L., Shepherd, N. *et al.* (1998) Altered cadherin and catenin complexes in the Barrett's oesphagus–dysplasia–adenocarcinoma sequence: correlation with disease progression and dedifferentiation. *Am. J. Pathol.* **152**, 135–44.

Bleiberg, H., Goffin, J.C., Dalesio, O. *et al.* (1989) Adjuvant radiotherapy and chemotherapy in resectable gastric cancer. A randomised trial of the gastrointestinal tract cancer cooperative group of the EORTC. *Eur. J. Surg. Oncol.* **15**, 535–43.

Bonenkamp, J.J., Hermans, J., Sasako, M. *et al.* (1993) Meta-analysis of adjuvant chemotherapy for gastric cancer. *Proc. Am. Soc. Clin. Oncol.* **12**, 191 (abstract).

Borrman, R. (1926) Geschwulste des Magens und Duodenums. In Henke, F. and Lunbarsch O. (eds), *Handbuch der Speziellen Pathologischen Anatomie und Histologie*, vol. 4. Berlin: Julius Springer, 812.

Botet, J.F., Lightdale, C.J., Zauber, A.G. *et al.* (1991) Preoperative staging of gastric cancer: comparison of endoscopic US and dynamic CT. *Radiology* **181**, 426–32.

Caldas, C., Carneiro, F., Lynch, H.T. *et al.* (1999) Familial gastric cancer: overview and guidelines for management. *J. Med. Genet.* **36**, 873–80.

Cascinu, S., Labianca, R., Alessandroni, P. *et al.* (1997) Intensive weekly chemotherapy for advanced gastric cancer using fluorouracil, cisplatin, epi-doxorubicin, 6S-leucovorin, glutathione and filgastrim: a report from the Italian Group for the Study of Digestive Tract Cancer. *J. Clin. Oncol.* **15**, 3313–19.

Cirera, L., Balil, A., Batiste-Alentorn, E. *et al.* (1999) Randomised clinical trial of adjuvant mitomycin plus tegafur in patients with resected stage III gastric cancer. *J. Clin. Oncol.* **17**, 3810–15.

Coombs, R.C., Schein, P.S., Chilvers, C.E.D. *et al.* (1990) A randomised trial comparing adjuvant fluorouracil, doxorubicin and mitomycin with no treatment in operable gastric cancer. *J. Clin. Oncol.* **8**, 1362–9.

Correa, P. (1980) The epidermiology and pathogenesis of chronic gastritis: three etiologic entities. *Front. Gastroenterol. Res.* **6**, 98–108.

Correa, P., Sasano, N., Stemmermann, G.N. *et al.* (1973) Pathology in gastric carcinoma in Japanese populations: comparisons between Miyagi Perfecture, Japan and Hawaii. *J. Natl Cancer Inst.* **51**, 1449–59.

Correa, P., Cuello, C., Fajardo, L.F. *et al.* (1983) Diet and gastric cancer: nutrition survey in a high risk area. *J. Natl Cancer Inst.* **70**, 673–8.

Correa, P., Haenszel, W., Cuello, C. *et al.* (1990) Gastric precancerous process in a high risk population: cohort follow-up. *Cancer Res.* **50**, 4737–40.

Cullinan, S.A., Moertel, C.G., Fleming, T.R. *et al.* (1985) A comparison of three chemotherapeutic regimens in the treatment of advanced pancreatic and gastric carcinoma. *JAMA*, **253**, 2061–7.

Cunningham, D. (1990) The management of gastric cancer. In McArdle C.S. (ed.), *Surgical oncology*. London: Butterworths, 28–52.

Cunningham, D., Hole, D., Carter, D.C. *et al.* (1987) An evaluation of the prognostic factors in gastric cancer: the effects of chemotherapy on survival. *Br. J. Surg.* **74**, 715.

Cuschieri, A. (1986) Gastrectomy for gastric cancer: definitions and objectives. *Br. J. Surg.* **73**, 513–14.

Cushieri, A., Weeden, S., Fielding, J. *et al.* (1999) Patient survival after D1 and D2 resections for gastric cancer: long-term results of the MRC randomised surgical trial. *Br. J. Cancer* **79**, 1522–30.

Douglass, H.O. and Nava, H.R. (1985) Gastric adenocarcinoma: management of the primary disease. *Semin. Oncol.* **12**, 32–45.

Einzig, A.I., Wiernik, P.H., Lipsitz, S. *et al.* (1993) Phase II trial of Taxol in patients with adenocarcinoma of the upper gastrointestinal tract (UGIT); The Eastern Cooperative Oncology Group (ECOG) Results. *Proc. Am. Soc. Clin. Oncol.* **12**, 194 (abstract).

El-Omar, E.M., Carrington, M., Chow, W. *et al.* (2000) Interleukin-1 polymorphisms associated with increased risk of gastric cancer. *Nature* **404**, 398–402.

Engstrom, P.F., Lavin, P.T., Douglass, H.O. and Brunner, K.W. (1985) Postoperative adjuvant 5-fluorouracol plus methyl-CCNU therapy for gastric cancer patients: Eastern Cooperative Oncology Group Study (EST 3275). *Cancer* **55**, 1868–73.

Eurogast Study Group (1993) An international association between *Helicobacter pylori* infection and gastric cancer. *Lancet* **341**, 1360–2.

Falck, V.G. and Gullick, W.J. (1989) C-erbB-2 oncogene product staining in gastric adenocarcinoma. An immunohistochemical study. *J. Pathol.* **159**, 107.

Ficorella, C., Ricevuto, E., Marchetti, P. *et al.* (1993) p53 gene mutations in human primary gastric cancer by polymerase chain reaction – single strand confirmation polymorphism analysis. *Proc. Am. Assoc. Cancer Res.* **34**, 222 (abstract).

Fielding, J.W.L., Ellis, D.J., Jones, B.G. *et al.* (1980) Natural history of 'early' gastric cancer: results of a 10 year regional survey. *BMJ* **281**, 965–7.

Findlay, M., Cunningham, D.C., Norman, A. *et al.* (1994) A phase II study in advanced gastro-oesophageal cancer using epirubicin and cisplatin in combination with continuous infusion 5-fluorouracil (ECF). *Ann. Oncol.* **5**, 609–16.

Furukawa, H., Iwanaga, T., Hiratsuka, M. *et al.* (1993) Gastric cancer as a metachronous multiple lesion. *Br. J. Surg.* **80**, 54–6.

Gamo, M., Suzuki, T. *et al.* (1993) Mutation and overexpression of p53 in gastric cancer. *Proc. Am. Assoc. Cancer Res.* **34**, 533 (abstract).

Gastrointestinal Tumor Study Group (1982) Controlled trial of adjuvant chemotherapy following curative resection for gastric cancer. *Cancer* **49**, 1116–22.

Gennari, L., Bozzetti, F., Bonfanti, G. *et al.* (1986) Subtotal versus total gastrectomy for cancer of the lower two-thirds of the stomach: a new approach to an old problem. *Br. J. Surg.* **73**, 534–8.

Grau, J.J., Estape, J., Alcobendas, F. *et al.* (1993) Positive results of adjuvant mitomycin-C in resected gastric cancer: a randomised trial on 134 patients. *Eur. J. Cancer* **3**, 340–2.

Grau, J.J., Estape, J., Fuster, J. *et al.* (1998) Randomised trial of adjuvant chemotherapy with mitomycin plus ftorafur versus mitomycin alone in resected locally advanced gastric cancer. *J. Clin. Oncol.* **16**, 1036–9.

Green, P.H.R., O'Toole, K.M., Weingberg, L.M. *et al.* (1981) Early gastric cancer. *Gastroenterology* **81**, 247–56.

Haenzel, W.M. (1961) Cancer mortality and incidence among the foreign born in the United States. *J. Natl Cancer Inst.* **26**, 37–132.

Hagiwara, A., Takahashi, T., Kojima, O. *et al.* (1992) Prophylaxis with carbon-adsorbed mitomycin against peritoneal recurrence of gastric cancer. *Lancet* **339**, 629–31.

Hallissey, M.T., Allum, W.H., Jewkes, A.J. *et al.* (1990) Early detection of gastric cancer. *BMJ* **301**, 513–15.

Haugstvedt, T.K., Viste, A., Eide, G.E. *et al.* (1993) Norwegian multicentre study of survival and prognostic factors in patients undergoing curative resection for gastric carcinoma. *Br. J. Surg.* **80**, 475–8.

Higgins, G.A., Amadeo, J.H., Smith, D.E. *et al.* (1983) Efficacy of prolonged intermittent therapy with combined 5FU and methyl-CCNU following resection for gastric carcinoma. *Cancer* **52**, 1105–12.

Higuchi, C.M. and Issell, B. (1993) High dose megestrol acetate plus chronic oral etoposide treatment of advanced gastric cancer: preliminary toxicity results. *Proc. Am. Soc. Clin. Oncol.* **12**, 227 (abstract).

Hisamichi, S. and Sugawara, N. (1984) Mass screening for gastric cancer by X-ray examination. *Jpn J. Clin. Oncol.* **14**, 211–23.

Holbrook, M.A. (1974) Gastric cancer treatment principles. *JAMA* **228**, 1289–90.

Howell, S.B., Pfeiffle, L.E., Wing, R.A. and Olshen, R.A. (1983) Intraperitoneal cisdiamminedichloroplatinum with systemic thiosulfate protection. *Cancer Res.* **43**, 142–3.

Howson, C.P., Hiyama, T. and Wynder, E.L. (1986) The decline in gastric cancer: epidemiology of an unplanned triumph. *Epidemiol. Rev.* **8**, 1–27.

Icli, F., Karaoguz, H., Dincol, D. *et al.* (1993) Comparison of EAP and FAM combination chemotherapies in advanced gastric cancer. *Proc. Am. Soc. Clin. Oncol.* **12**, 207 (abstract).

Italian Gastrointestinal Tumour Study Group (1988) Adjuvant treatments following curative resection for gastric cancer. *Br. J. Surg.* **75**, 100–4.

Jager-Arand, E., Bernhard, H., Klein, O. *et al.* (1993) Combination 5-fluorouracil (5-FU) folinic acid (FA) and ±-Interferon 2B (IFN) in advanced gastric cancer. *Proc. Am. Assoc. Clin. Oncol.* **12**, 192 (abstract).

Johansen, A.A. (1976) Early gastric cancer. *Curr. Top. Pathol.* **63**, 1–47.

Jones, A.L., Trott, P., Cunningham, D. *et al.* (1993) A pilot study of intra-peritoneal cisplatin in the management of gastric cancer. *Ann. Oncol.* **5**, 123–6.

Kakeji, Y., Korenaga, D., Tsujitani, S. *et al.* (1993) Gastric cancer with p53 overexpression has high potential for metastasising to lymph nodes. *Br. J. Cancer* **67**, 589–93.

Kambe, M., Wakui, A., Nakao, I. *et al.* (1993) A late phase II study of Irinotecan (CPT-11) in patients with advanced gastric cancer. *Proc. Am. Assoc. Clin. Oncol.* **12**, 198 (abstract).

Kelsen, D., Atiq, O.T., Saltz, L. *et al.* (1992) FAMTX versus etoposide, doxorubicin and cisplatin: a random assignment trial in gastric cancer. *J. Clin. Oncol.* **10**, 541–8.

Kim, B.S., Chung, H.C., Roh, J.K. *et al.* (1991) A controlled trial of 5-FU, Doxorubicin (FA) chemotherapy vs. FA-polyadenylic acid (POLY_AU) chemo-immunotherapy for locally advanced gastric cancer after curative resection: an interim report. *Proc. Am. Soc. Clin. Oncol.* **10**, 134 (abstract).

Klein, H.O., Dias, W., Dieterle, F. *et al.* (1982) Chemotherapieprotokoll zur Behandlunk des metastasierenden magenkarzinoms: methotrexate, adriamycin und 5-fluorouacil. *Deutsch Med. Wochenschr.* **107**, 1708–12.

Krook, J.E., O'Connell, M.J., Wieand, H.S. *et al.* (1991) A prospective randomised evaluation of intensive-course 5-fluorouracil plus doxorubicin as surgical adjuvant chemotherapy for resected gastric cancer. *Cancer* **67**, 2454–8.

Landry, J., Tepper, J., Wood, W. *et al.* (1990) Pattern of failure following curative resection of gastric carcinoma. *Int. J. Radiat. Oncol. Biol. Phys.* **19**, 1357–62.

Langman, M.J.S. (1985) Antisecretory drugs and gastric carcinoma: diffuse and so-called intestinal-type carcinoma: an attempt at histoclinical classification. *Acta Pathol. Microbiol. Scand.* **64**, 31–49.

Langman, M.J.S., Dunn, J.A., Whiting, J.L. *et al.* (1999) Prospective, double-blind, placebo-controlled randomised trial of cimetidine in gastric cancer *Br. J. Cancer* **81**, 1356–62.

Lauren, P. (1965) Two histological main types of gastric carcinoma: diffuse and so-called intestinal-type carcinoma: an attempt at a histoclinical classification. *Acta Pathol. Microbiol. Scand.* **64**, 31–49.

Lemoine, N.R., Jain, S., Silvestre, F. *et al.* (1991) Amplification and overexpression of the EGF receptor and c-erbB-2 proto-ongene in human stomach cancer. *Br. J. Cancer* **64**, 79–83.

Lise, M., Nitti, D., Marchet, A. *et al.* (1995) Final results of a phase III clinical trial of adjuvant chemotherapy with the modified fluorouracil, doxorubicin and mitomycin regimen in resectable gastric cancer. *J. Clin. Oncol.* **13**, 2757–63.

Llanos, O., Guzman, S. and Duarte, I. (1982) Accuracy of the first endoscopic procedure in the differential diagnosis of gastric lesions. *Ann. Surg.* **195**, 224–6.

Logan, R.P.H., Gummett, P.A., Misiewicz, J.J. *et al.* (1991) One week eradication regimen for *Helicobacter pylori*. *Lancet* **338**, 1249–52.

Macdonald, J.S., Schein, P.S., Woolley, P.V. *et al.* (1980) 5-Fluorouracil, doxorubicin and mitomycin (FAM) combination chemotherapy for advanced gastric cancer. *Ann. Intern. Med.* **93**, 533–6.

Macdonald, J.S., Gagliano, R., Fleming, T. *et al.* (1992) A phase III trial of FAM (5-fluorouracil., adriamycin, mitomycin-C) chemotherapy versus control as adjuvant treatment for resected gastric cancer (A Southwest Oncology Group Trial – SWOG7804). *Proc. Am. Soc. Clin. Oncol.* **11**, 168 (abstract).

Mari, E., Floriani, I., Tinazzi, A. *et al.* (2000) Efficacy of adjuvant chemotherapy after curative resection for gastric cancer: a meta-analysis of published randomised trials. *Ann. Oncol.* **11**, 837–42.

Mathus-Vliegen, E.M.H. and Tytgat, G.N.J. (1990) Analysis of failures and complications of Neo-dymium: YAG laser photocoagulation in gastro-intestinal tract tumours. A retrospective survey of 8 years' experience. *Endoscopy* **22**, 17.

Matley, P.J., Dent, D.M., Hadden, M.V. and Price, S. (1988) Gastric carcinoma in young adults. *Ann. Surg.* **208**, 593.

Matozaki, J., Sakmoto, C., Matsuda, R. *et al.* (1992) Missense mutations and a deletion of the p53 gene in human gastric carcinoma. *Biochem. Biophys. Res. Commun.* **182**, 215–23.

Matsushita, M., Oi, H., Murakami, T. *et al.* (1994) Extraserosal invasion in advanced gastric cancer: evaluation with MR imaging. *Radiology* **192**, 87–91.

Miwa, K. (1978) *Report of treatment results of stomach carcinoma in Japan*. Tokyo: National Cancer Centre (Japanese Research Society for Gastric Cancer Monograph).

Miwa, K. (1979) Cancer of the stomach in Japan. *GANN Monograph on Cancer Res.* **22**, 61–75.

Moertel, C.G., Childs, D.S., Reitemeier, R.J. *et al.* (1969) Combined 5-fluorouracil and super-voltage radiation therapy of locally unresectable gastrointestinal cancer. *Lancet* **2**, 865–7.

Moertel, C.G., Childs, D.S., O'Fallon, J.R. *et al.* (1984) Combined 5-fluorouracil and radiation therapy as a surgical adjuvant for poor prognosis gastric carcinoma. *J. Clin. Oncol.* **2**, 1249–54.

Moertel, C.G., Rubin, J., O'Connell, M.J. *et al.* (1986) A phase II study of combined 5-fluorouracil, doxorubicin and cisplatin in the treatment of advanced upper gastrointestinal adenocarcinomas. *J. Clin. Oncol.* **4**, 1053–7.

Morson, B.C., Dawson, I.M.P., Day, D.W. *et al.* (1990) *Morson and Dawson's Gastrointestinal Pathology*, (3rd edn). Oxford: Blackwell.

Murakami, T. (1979) Early cancer of the stomach. *World J. Surg.* **3**, 685–92.

Nakajima, T., Harashima, S., Hirata, H. and Kajitant, T. (1978) Prognostic and therapeutic values of peritoneal cytology in gastric cancer. *Acta Cytol.* **22**, 55–9.

Nakajima, T., Nashimoto, A., Kitamura, M. *et al.* (1999) Adjuvant mitomycin and fluorouracil followed by oral uracil plus tegafur in serosa-negative gastric cancer: a randomised trial. *Lancet* **354**, 273–7.

Ogiu, T., Nakadate, M. and Odashima, S. (1975) Induction of leukaemias and digestive tract tumours in Donryu rats by l-propyl-1-nitrosourea. *J. Natl Cancer Inst.* **54**, 887–93.

Ohuchi, N., Hand, P.H., Merlo, G. *et al.* (1987) Enhanced expression of c-Ha-vas P21 in human stomach adenocarcinomas defined by immunoassays using monoclonal antibodies and *in situ* hybridisation. *Cancer Res.* **47**, 1413–20.

Okamoto, T., Makino, M., Kawasumi, H. *et al.* (1988) Comparative study of gastric cancer in young and aged patients. *Eur. Surg. Res.* **20**, 149.

OPCS (1972) *Mortality statistics for general practice. Second National Study 1970–71*. London: HMSO.

Palli, D., Bianchi, S., Cipriani, F. *et al.* (1991) Reproducibility of histologic classification of gastric cancer. *Br. J. Cancer* **63**, 765–8.

Park, J.-B., Rhim, J.S., Park, S.-C. *et al.* (1989) Amplification, overexpression and rearrangement of the erbB-2 protooncogene in primary human stomach carcinomas. *Cancer Res.* **49**, 6605–9.

Parkin, D.M., Laara, E. and Muir, C.S. (1988) Estimates of the worldwide frequency of sixteen major cancers in 1980. *Int. J. Cancer* **41**, 184–97.

Possik, R.A., Franco, E.L., Pires, D.R. *et al.* (1986) Sensitivity, specificity and predictive value of laparoscopy for staging gastric cancer and for the detection of liver metastases. *Cancer* **58**, 1–6.

Preusser, P., Wilke, H., Achterrath, W. *et al.* (1988) Phase II study with EAP (etoposide, adriamycin, cisplatinum) in patients with primary inoperable gastric cancer and advanced disease. *Recent Results Cancer Res.* **110**, 198–206.

Pyrhonen, S., Kuitunen, T. and Kouri, M. (1992) A randomised, phase III trial comparing fluorouracil, epidoxorubicin and methotrexate (FEMTX) with best supportive care in non-resectable gastric cancer. *Ann. Oncol.* **3**(suppl. 5), 12.

ReMine, W.H. (1979) Palliative operations for incurable gastric cancer. *World J. Surg.* **3**, 721–9.

Rosen, H.R., Jazko, G., Repse, S. *et al.* (1998) Adjuvant intraperitoneal chemotherapy with carbon-adsorbed mitomycin in patients with gastric cancer: results of a randomised multicentre trial of the Austrian working group for surgical oncology. *J. Clin. Oncol.* **16**, 2733–8.

Roth, A.D., Maibach, R., Martinelli, G. *et al.* (2000) Docetaxel (Taxotere)–cisplatin (TC): an effective drug combination in gastric carcinoma. *Ann. Oncol.* **11**, 301–6.

Sayag-Beaujard, A.C., François, Y., Glehen, O. *et al.* (1999) Intraperitoneal chemohyperthermia with mitomycin C for gastric cancer patients with peritoneal carcinomatosis. *Anticancer Res.* **19**, 1375–82.

Schilsky, R., Mullane, M., Carroll, R. *et al.* (1993) A phase II study of Amonafide in gastric adenocarcinoma. *Proc. Am. Soc. Clin. Oncol.* **12**, 208 (abstract).

Schwartz, G., Kelsen, D., Christman, K. *et al.* (1993) A phase II study of neoadjuvant FAMTX (5-fluorouracil [5FU]/adriamycin/methotrexate) and post operative intraperitoneal (ip) 5-FU and cisplatin (CDDP) in high risk patients with gastric cancer. *Proc. Am. Soc. Clin. Oncol.* **12**, 195 (abstract).

Serlin, O., Keehn, R.J., Higgins, G.A. *et al.* (1977) Factors related to survival following resection for gastric carcinoma. *Cancer* **40**, 1318–29.

Shchepotin, I., Cherny, V., Ugrinuv, O. *et al.* (1993) Preoperative superselective intra-arterial chemotherapy in the radical treatment of gastric cancer. *Proc. Am. Assoc. Cancer Res.* **34**, 201 (abstract).

Shibata, D., Stemmermann, G.N. and Weiss, L.M. (1992) EBV-associated gastric adenocarcinoma. *Proceedings of the Vth International Symposium on EBV and Associated Disease* P-VIII-19, 179.

Shirai, M., Matsuura, A., Toda, N. *et al.* (1993) Infusional 5-Fluorouracil (f-FU) plus weekly carboplatin (CBDCA) chemotherapy for advanced gastric cancer (AGC). *Proc. Am. Soc. Clin. Oncol.* **12**, 207 (abstract).

Shiu, M.H., Moore, E., Sanders, M. *et al.* (1987) Influence of the extent of resection on survival after curative treatment of gastric carcinoma. *Arch. Surg.* **122**, 1347–51.

Slamon, D.J., Clark, G.M., Mong, S. *et al.* (1987) Human breast cancer: correlation of relapse and survival with amplification of the HER-2/neu oncogene. *Science* **235**, 177–82.

Starzynska, T., Rahi, V. and Stern, P.L. (1992) The expression of 5T4 antigen in colorectal and gastric carcinoma. *Br. J. Cancer* **66**, 867–9.

Stern, J.L., Denman, S., Elias, E.G. *et al.* (1975) Evaluation of palliative resection in advanced carcinoma of the stomach. *Surgery* **77**, 291–8.

Sussman, S.K., Halvorsen, R.A., Illescas, F.F. *et al.* (1988) Gastric adenocarcinoma: CT versus surgical staging. *Radiology* **167**, 335–40.

Suzuki, H., Miho, O., Watanabe, Y. *et al.* (1989) Endoscopic laser therapy in the curative and palliative treatment of upper gastrointestinal cancer. *World J. Surg.* **13**, 158.

Tagliagambe, A., Lombardi, M., Troiani, R. *et al.* (1986) FAP regimen in advanced gastric cancer our experience. *Cancer Chemother. Pharmacol.* **18** (suppl. 1), A67.

Tahara, E., Symiyoshi, H., Hata, J. *et al.* (1986) Human epidermal growth factor in gastric carcinoma as a biologic marker of high malignancy. *Jpn J. Cancer Res.* **77**, 145–52.

Ten Bokkel Huinink, W.W., Dubbelman, R., Aartsen, A. *et al.* (1985) Experimental and clinical results with intraperitoneal cisplatin. *Semin. Oncol.* **12**, 43–6.

Tonnesen, H., Bulow, S., Fisherman, K. *et al.* (1988) Effect of cimetidine on survival after gastric cancer. *Lancet* **ii**, 990–1.

Tso, P.L., Bringaze, W.L., Dauterive, A.H. *et al.* (1987) Gastric carcinoma in the young. *Cancer* **59**, 1362.

Turnbull, A., Kussin, S., Kurtz, R.C. *et al.* (1980) Palliative prosthetic intubation in gastric cancer. *J. Surg. Oncol.* **15**, 37–42.

Wagener, D.J.Th., Yap, S.H., Wobbes, T. *et al.* (1985) Phase II trial of 5-fluorouracil, adriamycin and cisplatin (FAP) in advanced gastric cancer. *Cancer Chemother. Pharmacol.* **15**, 86–7.

Wallner, J., Depisch, D., Gsur, A. *et al.* (1993) MDR1 gene expression and its clinical relevance in primary gastric carcinomas. *Cancer* **71**, 667–71.

Waters, J.S., Norman. A., Cunningham, D. *et al.* (1999) Long-term survival after epirubicin, cisplatin and fluorouracil for gastric cancer: results of a randomized trial. *Br. J. Cancer* **80**, 269–72

Wilke, P., Preusser, P., Fink, V. *et al.* (1989) Preoperative chemotherapy in locally advanced and non-resectable gastric cancer: a phase II study with etoposide, doxorubicin and cisplatin. *J. Clin. Oncol.* **7**, 1318–26.

Wils, J.A., Bleiberg, H., Dalesio, O. *et al.* (1986) An EORTC gastrointestinal evaluation of the combination of sequential methotrexate (MTX) and 5-fluorouracil (5-FU) combined with adriamycin (A) in advanced measurable gastric cancer *J. Clin. Oncol.* **4**, 1799–803.

Wils, J.A., Klein, H.O., Wagener, D.J.Th. *et al.* (1991) Sequential high dose methotrexate and fluorouracil combined with doxorubicin – a step ahead in the treatment of advanced gastric cancer: a trial of the European Organisation for the Research and Treatment of Cancer Gastrointestinal Tract Cooperative Group. *J. Clin. Oncol.* **9**, 827–31.

Wooley, P.V., Smith, F., Estevez, R. *et al.* (1981) A phase II trial of 5-FU, adriamycin and cisplatin (FAP) in advanced gastric cancer. *Proc. Am. Soc. Clin. Oncol.* **22**, 455.

Yakota, J., Yamamoto, T., Miyjima, N. *et al.* (1988) Genetic alterations of the c-erbB-2 oncogene occur frequently in tubular adenocarcinoma of the stomach and are often accompanied by amplification of the v-erbA homologue. *Oncogene* **2**, 283.

Yasui, W., Hata, J., Yokozaki, H. *et al.* (1988) Interaction between epidermal growth factor and its receptor in progression of human gastric carcinoma. *Int. J. Cancer* **41**, 211.

Yonemura, Y., Ninomiya, I., Ohoyama, S. *et al.* (1990) Expression of c-erbB2 oncoprotein in gastric carcinoma. *Cancer* **67**, 2914–18.

28

Bladder

PAULA WELLS, ROBERT HUDDART AND ALAN HORWICH

INTRODUCTION

Bladder cancer is a disease with significant heterogeneity of outcome, ranging from tumours involving mucosa, in which metastatic disease is rare, to muscle-invasive disease with poor prognosis. Management is further complicated as bladder cancer often occurs in the elderly, who frequently suffer concurrent medical conditions (often related to smoking) and may be of poor performance status, thus limiting treatment options.

Invasive bladder cancer, in particular, remains an area of controversy, with significant variability in management worldwide. As in many arenas where uncertainty exists, this controversy is fuelled by the paucity of available data from prospective randomized clinical studies. Consequently, fundamental questions regarding treatment selection for individual patients have not been answered definitively. The literature contains studies addressing the various issues in the field, but often with conflicting or inconclusive results. From these, a number of recommendations can be made, but there is still a pressing need for large randomized studies to be conducted so clear answers to these questions can be obtained. It must be emphasized, however, that despite this there have been significant advances in both operative technique, technical radiotherapy and in the administration of chemotherapy, with attendant reduction in morbidity related to treatment and improvements in survival in patients suitable for radical treatment. In addition, advances in molecular biology have provided us with further insights into the mechanism of bladder cancer pathogenesis, invasion and metastasis, from which new targets for therapy may be derived.

EPIDEMIOLOGY

In the UK an estimated 12 900 cases of bladder cancer are diagnosed, with 5400 deaths from the disease, each year (Black et al., 1997). The disease accounts for 7.9 per cent of all new cases of cancer among men and 3.2 per cent among women, and is associated with 4.4 per cent of cancer deaths among men and 2.4 per cent among women. Internationally, the incidence rate of bladder cancer among men varies more than tenfold (Parkin et al., 1997) and has been rising in many areas of the world (McCredie, 1994). High rates occur in western Europe and North America while the disease is less common in eastern Europe and Asia. The disease predominates in Caucasians and incidence rises sharply with age (about two-thirds of cases occurring from 65 years onwards). From the mid-1970s to 1990, rates increased most notably in Europe (particularly in western Scotland, eastern Germany and Finland), a trend that has not been reproduced in North America. This may be explained partly by changes in diagnostic practice (Hankey et al., 1991; Lynch et al., 1991) with increased diagnosis of localized disease and a decrease in unstaged bladder cancer. The incidence rates of advanced bladder cancer remain unchanged. Overall, survival is greater for men and women in affluent groups, and in contrast to most other common malignancies, there is a survival advantage for men (Coleman *et al.*, 1999).

AETIOLOGY

Industrial exposure

Environmental factors (particularly tobacco smoking and industrial carcinogens) are clearly implicated in the development of bladder cancer. A number of clinical studies and mortality surveys have resulted in the identification of hazards in the dye stuffs and rubber industries (Case and Hosker, 1954; Case *et al.*, 1954) associated with a 10- to 50-fold increased risk of bladder cancer, primarily attributed to exposure to the aromatic amines, 2-naphthylamine and benzidine (Case *et al.*, 1954; Rubino *et al.*, 1982; Decarli *et al.*, 1985). The risk of death from bladder cancer is associated with young age at first exposure and increasing duration of employment, while mortality decreases with increasing time from last exposure. This association has been supported by data from the UK, where reduced bladder cancer risk was demonstrated following the introduction of protective measures and subsequent banning of the industrial use of 2-naphthylamine and benzidine in 1950 and 1962 respectively (Boyko *et al.*, 1985; Morrison *et al.*, 1985). 2-naphthylamine is also implicated in the development of bladder cancer in the rubber, electric cable and chemical manufacturing industries. Subsequently, studies have suggested approximately 40 potentially high-risk occupations (but strong evidence of increased risk is apparent for very few of these) and the association of several other aromatic amines, (including 4-aminophenyl and 4-chloro-O-toluene) in development of bladder carcinoma.

Tobacco smoking

Cigarette smoking is a well-established cause of bladder cancer and its importance lies in the prevalence of the habit within the population. Overall, smokers have a two- to three-fold risk, with mortality rates paralleling smoking patterns (Hoover and Cole, 1971; McLaughlin *et al.*, 1995). The risk increases with smoking intensity (packs per day), and decreases with cessation of smoking (30–60 per cent reduction in risk of cancer) (Cancer IAFRO, 1986), although in the long term this does not decline to the level of a non-smoker (Hartge *et al.*, 1987; Augustine *et al.*, 1988).

Drugs

A number of drugs have also been identified as aetiological agents in bladder cancer. For instance, phenacetin,

which was in general use as an analgesic, has been linked to carcinoma of both the upper and lower urinary tracts (McCredie *et al.*, 1983; Piper *et al.*, 1985). Also cytotoxic drugs used in the treatment of cancer, such as the alkylating agent cyclophosphamide, are themselves carcinogenic, as are many of their metabolites. For cyclophosphamide the carcinogenic effect is dose dependent, with bladder cancer risk increasing with dose delivered (Pederson-Bjergaard *et al.*, 1988; Levine and Richie, 1989; Travis *et al.*, 1995).

Radiation

The risk of bladder cancer is also increased in individuals exposed to ionizing radiation, either following therapeutic pelvic radiotherapy for both benign (e.g. dysfunctional uterine bleeding) and malignant disorders (e.g. cervical cancer) (Boice *et al.*, 1988; Inskip *et al.*, 1990). In these studies, increased risk was experienced by women who were under 55 years when treated, with increasing dose to the bladder and time since exposure; the relative risk reaching 8.7 for patients treated at least 20 years earlier. A similar association has been noted after radioactive iodine (iodine-131) treatment for thyroid cancer and in the survivors of the atomic bombs of Hiroshima and Nagasaki.

Urinary stasis

Another important group of aetiological factors are those arising secondary to chronic irritation of bladder urothelium, most particularly chronic or repeated urinary tract infections, often associated with urinary stasis. The most important infective agent in the aetiology of bladder carcinoma is *Schistosoma haematobium*, which is endemic in developing countries and associated with high incidence of squamous cell carcinoma (SCC) (Badawi *et al.*, 1995). Furthermore, developmental abnormalities of the bladder, bladder diverticulae, chronic bladder stones or indwelling catheters may also predispose to chronic infection, inflammation and increased risk of bladder carcinoma (Dolin and Cook-Mozaffari, 1992).

Genetic predisposition

A number of studies have investigated whether a genetic predisposition to bladder cancer exists. On the whole these studies have shown an increased relative risk for developing bladder cancer in the relatives of bladder cancer patients (Kiemeney and Schoenberg, 1996). In studies in Utah Mormons there was also an increased degree of relatedness in bladder cancer patients (Goldgar *et al.*, 1994). A case-controlled study showed that the risk was greatest in smokers versus non-smokers. There is also evidence that patients with deficient detoxification mechanisms, such as those with slow acetylator phenotype associated with homozygosity for a mutated gene (*NAT2*) (Hein, 1988; Brockmoller *et al.*, 1996) or homozygous absence of a functional human glutathione transferase M1 (GST M1) gene (which code for family of enzymes that detoxify a spectrum of reactive carcinogenic metabolites by catalysing their conjugation to glutathione) (Ketterer, 1988), are at increased risk of bladder cancer.

GENETICS OF BLADDER CANCER

A number of different oncogenes and tumour suppressor genes have been implicated in the aetiology of bladder cancer (Knowles, 1999). The most consistent abnormality seen in the development of bladder cancer is hemizygous deletion of chromosome 9. Loss of the entire chromosome 9 allele has been reported in up to 30–75 per cent of clinical tumours, including small, localized papillary carcinoma. In some tumours the loss is restricted either to the short arm (especially at 9p21) or the long arm of chromosome 9 (at one of three loci: 9q13–31, 9q32–33 or 9q34). 9p21 is the site of the tumour suppressor p16^{INK4a} (and associated genes *p14 ARF* and *p15^{INK4b}*) which are now known to be homozygously deleted in at least 20–45 per cent of bladder tumours. A large number of other bladder genetic changes have been identified in bladder tumours by comparative genomic hybridization and other techniques. The retinoblastoma gene (*Rb*) is likely to be the target of the 13q deletion and has been shown to be frequently mutated/dysregulated in bladder tumours, particularly in tumours without the 9p21 abnormality. The *p53* gene (the probable target of the 17p deletion) is mutated in 10–70 per cent of bladder tumours. Both these changes are associated with increase in grade and stage, with increased risk of progression and poorer survival (Esrig *et al.*, 1994). This risk of poor outcome is particularly marked in the presence of abnormalities of both p53 and Rb (Cordon-Cardo *et al.*, 1997; Grossman *et al.*, 1998) and is seen in both patients with T1 and invasive bladder cancer. These findings suggest that *p53/Rb* mutations are late rather than initiating events in the genesis of bladder cancer.

In addition to these, a number of oncogenes have been shown to be amplified and mutated in a number of series, with varying frequencies, at least partly due to the case mix (increased frequency in advanced disease). These include the c-*erb-B2* (amplified in 10–14 per cent of bladder tumours), cyclin d1 (amplified in 10–20 per cent of tumours), H-*ras* (mutated in 6–44 per cent of tumours) and epidermal growth factor receptor (EGFR; overexpressed in 11–48 per cent of bladder cancers) (Reznikoff *et al.*, 1996; Knowles, 1999). EGFR has promoted most interest as, in at least one study, overexpression was an independent prognostic factor for survival and progression (Mellon *et al.*, 1995).

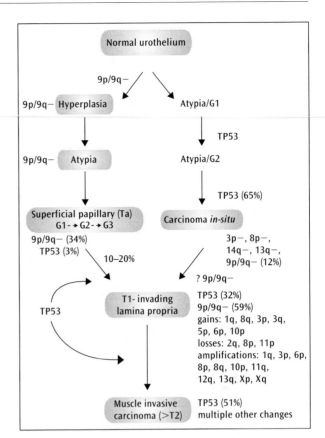

Figure 28.1 *Proposed model for the multiple genetic changes required to generate invasive bladder carcinoma. (From Knowles, 1999 with permission.)*

It is clear from this discussion that multiple genetic changes are required to generate an invasive bladder carcinoma. One possible model is illustrated in Figure 28.1. In addition to these genetic alterations, bladder cancers exhibit changes in microvasculature (Jaeger *et al.*, 1995), overexpression of vascular growth factors such as vascular endothelial growth factor (VEGF), changes in adhesion molecules such as E-cadherin, and re-expression of telomerase (Yoshida *et al.*, 1997).

PATHOLOGY

In Europe and the United States more than 90 per cent of tumours are of urothelial (transitional cell) origin and approximately 5 per cent are SCCs, except in areas where schistosomiasis is endemic (where they constitute up to 80 per cent of all urothelial malignancy). Primary adenocarcinoma of the bladder may arise from the urachal remnant or bladder exstrophy; while the remainder are rare tumours such as small cell carcinoma, sarcoma, lymphoma and melanoma.

Superficial bladder tumours

The term 'benign papillomas' (including the uncommon variants the inverted and everted papillomas) should be reserved for well-differentiated lesions that do not show evidence of invasion, abnormal mitotic activity or cellular atypia. The term 'papilloma' should not be used for superficial transitional cell carcinomas (TCC), even if they have a frond-like or papillary appearance. All superficial TCCs (Ta, T1 carcinoma *in-situ* (CIS)), are superficial to the deep muscle layer and exhibit evidence of invasion, abnormal mitotic activity or cellular atypia. Important prognostic differences exist between tumours confined by the basement membrane and those invading the lamina propria (which consists of loose connective tissue with its rich vascular and lymphatic channels). Within the lamina propria lies the muscularis mucosa, which some authors suggest has further prognostic significance, as invasion of this muscular layer is associated with a significantly higher incidence of tumour recurrence and progression (Hasui *et al.*, 1994). Unfortunately the muscularis mucosa is variably present, making it an unreliable landmark for diagnosis.

The prognosis of superficial bladder cancer is strongly correlated with tumour grade. Approximately 75–85 per cent patients with primary TCC present with low-grade tumours confined to superficial mucosa (Ta). Although up to 75 per cent of these recur, the majority remain amenable to transurethral resection and selective administration of intravesical therapy, with only 10 per cent of patients with recurrent lesions demonstrating invasion over a 10-year period (Bouffioux *et al.*, 1992). A proportion of papillary tumours will eventually invade superficial connective tissue (T1 disease) and are characterized by decreased survival. The 5-year survival is over 90 per cent for patients with Ta tumours (non-invasive) and 75 per cent for T1 tumours. High-grade superficial (T1) tumours are a considerably more aggressive entity, recurring in 80 per cent and progressing to invasive disease in more than 50 per cent of cases (Heney *et al.*, 1983; Herr, 2000).

Carcinoma *in-situ*

Carcinoma *in-situ* (CIS) is an important variant of superficial bladder cancer, characterized by a high propensity for progression to invasive disease (over 54 per cent of cases progressing within 5 years) (Lamm, 1992). It can be diffuse or focal, symptomatic or asymptomatic, and may or may not be associated with superficial papillary tumours. Diffuse CIS, particularly when associated with symptoms or identifiable papillary tumours, is an unfavourable prognostic finding. Riddle *et al.* (1975) reported a progression rate of 58 per cent in patients with diffuse CIS, while only 8 per cent of those with focal disease progressed. Furthermore, in a study of patients with CIS associated with low-grade papillary tumours, an incidence of subsequent muscle-invasive disease or metastases of 83 per cent was noted (Althausen *et al.*, 1976). Macroscopically the lesion is red and velvety, and

frequently extensive, involving prostatic urethra, prostate and ureters. The urothelium is markedly abnormal, showing marked lack of cellular cohesion, often resulting in very few malignant cells or only denuded mucosa. The tumour cells are often large with dysplastic nuclei and prominent nucleoli.

Invasive bladder carcinoma

The gross appearance of invasive TCC is variable, ranging from strikingly papillary, nodular or polypoid, to sessile and ulcerated lesions. Most frequently there are nests, small clusters or single cells irregularly dispersed in the lamina propria and muscularis propria, but occasionally a more diffuse pattern is present. The neoplastic cells are usually of moderate size, with modest amounts of pale to slightly eosinophilic cytoplasm, with at least moderate, if not marked, cellular atypia present. Approximately 10 per cent of TCCs, particularly high-grade tumours, contain foci of glandular or squamous differentiation, or even atypical spindle cells that mimic sarcomas. Other variants occur more rarely.

SCCs vary in morphological appearance, but are usually large and deeply invasive even when well differentiated. Their microscopic appearance is similar to that of lesions arising elsewhere in the body, most are moderately or well differentiated and often abundantly keratinized. Adenocarcinoma is generally of poor prognosis, with tumours arising from urachal remnants having the best outlook and signet-ring carcinomas (accounting for 3–5 per cent of tumours) the worst. The mucosa is usually oedematous and ulcerated in most cases of adenocarcinoma, but some develop the diffuse fibrosis and mural thickening similar to linitis plastica of the stomach. Small cell carcinoma is microscopically similar to its lung counterpart and carries a similarly gloomy outlook.

CLINICAL PRESENTATION AND INVESTIGATION

Approximately 80 per cent of cases of bladder cancer present with haematuria, which is usually painless and intermittent, and either visible (macroscopic) or detected on routine urinalysis (microscopic). The degree of haematuria does not correlate with disease extent, and therefore patients presenting in this way should be investigated as a matter of urgency. Fifteen per cent of patients presenting with macroscopic haematuria, and approximately 6 per cent with asymptomatic microscopic haematuria harbour bladder cancer. The presence of pain suggests an inflammatory component, most commonly associated with bacterial or interstitial cystitis, but it may also occur in up to 25 per cent of patients with bladder cancer. Irritative voiding symptoms, including urinary frequency, urgency and dysuria, are particularly associated with CIS and invasive bladder tumours (Farrow *et al.*, 1977). Bladder cancer may also present with bladder outlet obstruction or ipsilateral flank pain secondary to ureteral obstruction. Patients with advanced or metastatic disease often suffer constitutional symptoms, including anorexia, weight loss and pain arising from sites of metastasis such as bone. Physical examination is often unremarkable in these patients, but a careful pelvic examination should be undertaken to determine whether a mass is palpable, or to assess the fixity of tumour to adjacent organs. Urine microscopy and culture should be performed, and, if negative, repeated, in view of the intermittent nature of the haematuria.

Management of haematuria

Urological opinion should be sought in any case of macroscopic haematuria and persistent microscopic haematuria. Investigation of the upper urinary tract is obligatory and may be achieved with intravenous urography, or ultrasound of the kidneys and bilateral retrograde ureteropyelography performed at cystoscopy for patients allergic to intravenous contrast material or with a history of renal insufficiency. Ipsilateral hydronephrosis is often associated with muscle-invasive bladder carcinoma (approximately 90 per cent of cases), and its presence should prompt rigorous investigation (Hatch and Barry, 1986). The routine use of urinary cytology in all patients that are suspected of harbouring bladder carcinoma is debated. Cytology is most accurate for patients with high-grade tumours and CIS, but there remains a 20 per cent false-negative rate, while low-grade tumours are so frequently associated with a negative result that positive cytology should raise the suspicion of a concomitant high-grade lesion. Urine cytology should be obtained from a well-hydrated patient, as cellular degeneration occurs when urine remains in the bladder for prolonged periods. Other factors that may artefactually alter urinary cytology include the presence of urinary tract infection, indwelling catheters, bladder instrumentation, radiotherapy and intravesical immune or chemotherapy. Saline bladder washings may be employed to improve the accuracy and sensitivity of the technique.

Recently, several tests have been developed for the diagnosis or follow-up of recurrent bladder cancer on voided urine samples. Some including the BTA test (Bard Urological, Covington, GA, USA), the BTA Stat test (Bard Diagnostic Sciences, Inc., Redmond, WA, USA), the BTA TRAK assay (Bard Diagnostic Services, Inc.) and the urinary nuclear matrix protein NMP22 (Matritech Inc., Newton, MA, USA) are commercially available. The BTA test is a latex agglutination assay that detects the presence of basement membrane antigens isolated and characterized in the urine of patients with bladder cancer (Fradet and Cordon-Cardo, 1993). The BTA Stat and TRAK assays, on the other hand, are sensitive to human component factor H-related protein, produced *in vitro* specifically by human bladder cancer cell lines (Ellis *et al.*, 1997; Sarosdy, 1997). These tests were developed initially as a more sensitive alternative to urine cytology in detecting primary and recurrent superficial bladder cancer (Sarosdy *et al.*, 1995; D'Hallewin and Baert, 1996), but recent work has highlighted the risk of false-negative results and of false-positive reactions in patients with inflammatory bladder conditions or other genitourinary malignancy (Johnston *et al.*, 1997; Murphy *et al.*, 1997). Several other assays and techniques remain under development, including tests to identify nuclear matrix proteins (NMPs) (Soloway *et al.*, 1996), telomerase (Yoshida *et al.*, 1997) and other genetic alterations (Mao *et al.*, 1996). Most of these are limited in their detection of well-differentiated tumours and, because of this, none has sufficient accuracy to replace standard investigations, either for diagnosis or follow-up. It is possible that with more experience, one or a number of these markers may be shown to have a role in routine clinical practice.

Ultimately the diagnosis of bladder carcinoma is made on cystoscopy with pathological evaluation of a resected tumour specimen. The initial examination for patients with haematuria is often by flexible cystoscopy under local anaesthetic. Abnormal findings are confirmed under general anaesthetic with bimanual examination to confirm the presence, extent and fixation of a palpable bladder mass. The presence of induration or a palpable mass on bimanual examination following apparent complete resection of tumour implies extravesical extension, while resolution of these features implies organ-confined disease. Cystoscopic evaluation involves inspection of the entire urethra, prostate and bladder neck, with retrograde pyelography when the upper urinary tract has not already been satisfactorily visualized. The number, location, size and configuration of all tumours and any associated mucosal abnormalities should be noted, and documented on a bladder map. Biopsy or resection of a tumour should be accompanied by directed biopsies of adjacent and normal-appearing bladder mucosa, and should only be performed once satisfactory evaluation of the entire urinary tract has been undertaken. General assessment of the patient should include full blood count, biochemistry and a chest X-ray, and a bone scan when there is a history of bone pain.

Staging

The tumour node metastasis (TNM) system was adopted by the Union Internationale Contre Cancer (UICC) in 1963. By this, tumours are classified according to

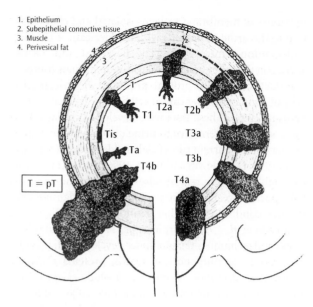

1. Epithelium
2. Subepithelial connective tissue
3. Muscle
4. Perivesical fat

T = pT

Figure 28.2 *Diagnostic representation of the 1997 TNM classification for bladder carcinoma.*

Table 28.1 *UICC TNM staging system for bladder carcinoma*

TX	Primary tumour cannot be assessed
T0	No evidence of primary tumour
TA	Non-invasive papillary carcinoma
Tis	Carcinoma *in-situ*: flat tumour
T1	Invades subepithelial connective tissue
T2A	Superficial (inner half) muscle invasion
T2B	Deep (outer half) muscle invasion
T3	Invades perivesical fat
T3A	Microscopic
T3B	Macroscopic
T4A	Invades prostate, uterus or vagina
T4B	Invades pelvic or abdominal wall
Lymph nodes	
N0	Is no regional node involvement
N1	Is a single node, less than 2 cm in largest diameter
N2	A single node 2–5 cm or multiple nodes less than 5 cm
N3	Nodal involvement greater than 5 cm

Primary tumour (G) suffix (m) should be added to the appropriate T to indicate multiple tumours. Suffix (IS) may be added to any T to indicate the presence of associated carcinoma *in-situ*. Provisional TX in regional lymph nodes cannot be assessed.

anatomical extent using data from examination under anaesthesia and radiological investigations. As accurate assessment of muscle invasion is not possible by clinical examination alone, a postoperative modification using the operative specimen is also required (pTNM). The latest modification, published in 1997, includes changes that reflect the prognostic implication of organ-confined muscle-invasive disease versus perivesical extension (Fig. 28.2) (Solbin, 1997). Tumours invading the superficial (inner half) of the muscle wall are now designated T2a and those of the deep (outer half) muscle layer, T2b, whereas any tumour penetrating muscle into perivesical fat is reclassified as stage T3 (Table 28.1). Support for the redefinition came from observations by Pearce *et al.* (1978) and Blandy *et al.* (1980), who noted little difference in survival between superficial and deep muscle invasion. Furthermore, the presence or absence of muscle invasion rather than its depth dictates management strategies for most centres.

Another area requiring clarification is the prognostic distinction between non-invasive tumour growing into the prostate from the urethra along the prostatic ducts, and direct invasion of a bladder tumour into prostatic stroma (a true T4a tumour). Pugh (1981) first drew attention to this problem with the UICC staging system, where non-invasive tumour was reclassified as P4aa and disease invading into prostatic stroma as P4ab. Similar observations have been made recently, confirming that prostatic stromal involvement adversely affects prognosis (Esrig *et al.*, 1996). The classification of nodal status has also been modified, from the 1978 system where they were staged according to site alone, to that of the 1987 edition where classification is according to number and size (Fig. 28.2).

Imaging of bladder cancer

Accurate staging of bladder cancer is important both to determine prognosis and for treatment decision making. Unfortunately, conventional imaging modalities are limited by inability to detect microscopic disease and inaccuracies in definition of macroscopic disease. Attempts to increase sensitivity compromise specificity, as interpretation of abnormalities as 'cancer' lead to increased detection of disease, but overestimate extent and presence of disease in many instances. However, radiological investigations form a vital part of tumour staging, and an understanding of the limitations of each modality is important to the interpretation of clinical data.

For many years the mainstay of pelvic staging has been computed tomography (CT). CT can identify tumours that extend into the bladder lumen and perivesical tissue, and the presence of bladder-wall thickening. However, these findings may reflect inflammatory processes rather than tumour infiltration, which limits the value of CT scans in defining depth of invasion and consequently stage of disease. A comprehensive review by MacVicar and Husband (1994) further addressed these issues, observing that CT was unable to demonstrate accurately deep muscle invasion, due to inability to distinguish between individual layers of the muscle wall, but it was useful in defining extension of disease through the bladder wall (T3). The ability of CT to detect involved lymph nodes is limited by size. Nodes of greater than 1–1.5 cm in diameter are considered abnormal, with a resulting sensitivity of between 50 and 85 per cent. However, nodal enlargement results from a number of other causes, resulting in false positives, such that specificity rates lie between 67 and 100 per cent (Walsh *et al.*, 1980; Koss *et al.*, 1981; Weinerman *et al.*, 1982).

Magnetic resonance imaging (MRI) is generally thought to offer advantages over CT in the staging of bladder cancer, but where perivesical tumour and advanced disease invading adjacent structures exist, CT may be adequate. CT is also equivalent in the definition of involved lymph nodes. MRI is superior to CT in the delineation of organ-confined tumour, due to an increased definition of superficial from deep muscle invasion. However, its ability to distinguish between T2a and T2b tumours is still limited, with accuracy increasing for the higher tumour stages (Kim *et al.*, 1994). The facility for multiplanar imaging is also particularly advantageous in the assessment of tumours of the bladder base. MRI is therefore recommended as the staging method of choice if facilities are available (Husband *et al.*, 1999). Gadolinium–DTPA enhancement improves assessment of bladder wall invasion but the technique is affected by late tissue changes resulting from radiotherapy (Hawnaur, 1993). Dynamic MRI with contrast enhancement has resulted in further improvement in image quality in the pelvis, which may translate into more accurate preoperative staging (Barentsz *et al.*, 1996). The recent development of iron oxide contrast agents for lymph node assessment may be a further step forward.

Transurethral ultrasound (TUUS) has been reported as the most sensitive method of staging bladder cancer locally, with a reported staging accuracy of 83 per cent (Schuller *et al.*, 1982). Koraitim *et al.* (1995) reported a 100 per cent correlation between preoperative TUUS and pathological staging from cystectomy specimens in non-invasive (Ta and T1) tumours, but the correlation fell with increasing depth of invasion, to 96 per cent for T2a and b, and 70 per cent for T3, disease. A major disadvantage of this technique is the need for general or spinal anaesthesia at the time of cystoscopy, limiting its use to specialist centres.

Screening

That patients with bladder carcinoma usually suffer haematuria at some point in their disease raises the possibility of testing for its presence as a screening test. Haematuria is, however, frequently intermittent and repeated testing is required to confirm its presence. Screening for haematuria can be achieved by microscopic analysis, or using a chemical reagent strip which detects the presence of haemoglobin. Two screening studies in the general population using home testing have reported similar findings (Britton *et al.*, 1992; Messing *et al.*, 1995). In these, 15–20 per cent of the screened population had haematuria, and of those who completed the evaluation, 6–8 per cent had urothelial cancers with 1.2–1.3 per cent arising in the bladder. It must be noted that neither study involved a randomized control population, and therefore results must be interpreted with caution. However, using age- and gender-matched unscreened controls derived from the tumour registry (Messing *et al.*, 1995), demonstrated that both populations had approximately the same proportions of superficial and high-grade carcinomas, but that the numbers of muscle-invasive tumours were much higher in the unscreened population. The time to death from bladder cancer was notably increased in the screened population, but this may reflect lead-time bias. Thus population screening may increase the probability of diagnosing disease at an earlier stage, but it remains unclear as to whether this affects survival. The positive predictive value (proportion of patients who test positively and are found to have disease) would be improved by limiting screening to those at high risk. For bladder cancer, this may mean restricting participation to people with occupational exposure to known bladder carcinogens and men aged 50 and over with smoking histories. Results of prospective randomized studies to determine the value of screening in this disease are awaited.

MANAGEMENT OF BLADDER CARCINOMA

Pathological examination of a cystectomy specimen provides the most reliable means of determining stage and patient prognosis for recurrence-free and overall survival. However, the clinical behaviour of bladder cancer is not adequately predicted by stage and grade alone, and the ability to define precisely the true biological potential of a tumour would facilitate better treatment selection, which may translate into improved survival figures. Our understanding of tumour biology has evolved rapidly over the past decade, prompted by advances in molecular biology, immunobiology and cytogenetics. From this, novel tumour markers have been identified and are being evaluated as potential prognostic indicators that may be applied in a clinical setting.

The main division in management is between tumours that invade muscle, where patients are at substantial risk of local and distant recurrence, and those which are restricted to the superficial lamina propria, with a good prognosis. We will therefore consider management in three groups: superficial, low-grade disease; superficial high-grade disease (including CIS); and, finally, muscle-invasive carcinoma.

Superficial low-grade tumours

SURGERY

The vast majority of superficial bladder cancers are amenable to transurethral resection (TUR). Full clinical

Table 28.2 *Prognostic factors for superficial bladder cancer*

EORTC trials			MRC trial
Time to first recurrence (univariate)	**Recurrence rate/year (multivariate)**	**Time to invasion (multivariate)**	**Recurrence rate at 2 years (univariate)**
Number of tumours[a]	Recurrence at 3 months	Recurrence at 3 months	Result of 3-month cystoscopy[b]
Grade[b]	Prior recurrence	Grade	Number of tumours[b]
Prior recurrence[b]	Number of tumours at entry	Prior recurrence	Grade[b]
Time from diagnosis[b]	Grade	Site of tumour	Maximum size[b]
Site of tumour[b]		Size of tumour	Site of tumour
		Sex	

[a] Included in multivariate analysis if site is excluded.
[b] Positive on multivariate analysis.

Table 28.3 *Risk of recurrence of patients with TaT1 bladder cancer according to prognostic groupings of Parmar* et al. *(1989)*

	Diagnosis	3-month cystoscopy	Proportion of patients (%)	2-year recurrence-free rate (%)
Group 1	Solitary	No recurrence	60	74
Group 2	Solitary	Recurrence	30–35	44
	or Multiple	No recurrence		
Group 3	Multiple	Recurrence	5–10	21

staging is undertaken prior to resection, including biopsies of apparently normal mucosa, particularly when urinary cytology is positive in the absence of an obvious bladder tumour and a normal upper tract. Finally tumour resection should be deep enough to obtain muscle as part of the evaluation of the T category.

Recurrent low-grade papillary tumours can also be treated by thermocoagulation using a neodymium-YAG (NdYAG) laser. This usually treats 3–5 mm, and although transmural coagulation of the bladder wall has occasionally been observed with higher energy systems, bladder integrity is usually preserved, and perforation with extravasation uncommon (Hofstetter *et al.*, 1981). Thus laser is considered a safe and effective treatment for papillary, low-grade tumours. Where high-grade disease or tumour invasion is suggested by a more sessile appearance, electrocautery resection is preferable, as an adequate specimen containing detrusor muscle for histological examination can be more readily assured.

PREDICTING RECURRENCE IN PATIENTS WITH SUPERFICIAL TUMOURS

Initial management of all patients with superficial bladder cancer involves complete resection of the tumour with subsequent treatment being dependent upon the predicted risk of recurrence and progression. Several studies have investigated factors that may predict recurrence and define patients requiring further treatment. Two of the largest series are those of the British Medical Research Council (MRC) (Parmar *et al.*, 1989) and of

the European Organization for Research and Treatment for Cancer (EORTC) (Kurth *et al.*, 1995), based on patients entered into their randomized trials of intravesical chemotherapy (*see* below). Although generalizations from these data must be interpreted with care, as only patients fulfilling the entry criteria for the studies are included, several important prognostic factors have been identified, as shown in Tables 28.2 and 28.3. Both studies highlighted the importance of grade and tumour number at presentation, but also 3-month cystoscopy as a predictor of subsequent recurrence. Indeed, in the MRC analysis when results from the 3-month cystoscopy were combined with the number of tumours at presentation, no other factor added significantly to the prediction of relapse. Not surprisingly, disease recurrence at cystoscopy continues to be highly predictive of future recurrence, with the probability of developing recurrence decreasing with each negative cystoscopy, reaching 8 per cent at 5 years and 0 per cent at 10 years (Fitzpatrick *et al.*, 1986). In these studies, T stages (Ta versus T1) were not strong predictors for recurrence, but it is likely, as shown by Kurth *et al.* (1995), that T stage does predict for risk of progression.

Over recent years a number of new biological factors have been identified as possible predictors of either recurrence of progression (Table 28.4). However, it is uncertain, with the possible exception of EGFR, whether they add predictive strength to the currently identified factors. Therefore further evaluation is required, including their use in large patient populations and inclusion into multivariate models, before any will be accepted into routine clinical practice.

Table 28.4 *Biological markers of recurrence and progression*

Marker	Advantages of monitoring	Disadvantages of monitoring	Reference
ABO blood antigen	Loss of expression with bladder cancer	20 per cent of normal cells do not express antigen	Montie *et al.* (1983)
M344 antigen	Decreased expression associated with increased grade. Rarely positive in G3 tumours	Adds little to grade	Sato *et al.* (1992)
Epidermal growth factor receptor	Overexpression linked to increased cancer-specific death rate, reduced recurrence-free survival, increased recurrence and progression (Cordon-Cardo *et al.*, 1992)	Overexpression associated with higher grade, stage and ploidy. Not conclusive predictive marker of superficial disease	Neal *et al.* (1989); Lipponen and Eskelinen (1994)
Acidic FGF	Expression correlates with tumour stage	Lacks specificity and is elevated in other disease processes, e.g. benign prostatic hypertrophy	Liukkonen *et al.* (1999)
Transforming growth factor-β	Highest levels found in low-grade and low-stage tumours (Chopin *et al.*, 1993; Izadifar *et al.*, 1999). Decreased expression associated with increased probability of progression and reduced survival (Eder *et al.*, 1997)	Not independent prognostic indicator of survival	
Rb and p53	Excellent outcome (Grossman *et al.*, 1998)	Not independent predictor of recurrence	Tokunaga *et al.* (1999)

FGF, fibroblast growth factor.

INTRAVESICAL THERAPY: CHEMOTHERAPY

Intravesical therapy can be given in the prophylactic, or adjuvant, setting, where it is intended to prevent recurrence after endoscopic resection of all visible tumours, or as definitive therapy, where it is designed to treat unresectable papillary tumours, or CIS. The advantages of the intravesical route are that high concentrations of agent are in contact with tumour-bearing mucosa or bladder epithelium at risk, with little or no systemic toxicity. Disadvantages include the local side-effects in the bladder due to high local drug concentrations and the need for transurethral manipulation. A variety of drugs of similar efficacy and toxicity have been used for prophylactic treatment of superficial bladder cancer, and are detailed in Table 28.5. In Europe, availability and practical considerations determine the choice of treatment, which lies between Adriamycin®, epirubicin and Mitomycin C®.

A number of randomized trials, including those of the EORTC and MRC, have addressed the optimal use of intravesical chemotherapy in the prophylactic treatment of stage Ta and T1 bladder cancer (Schulman *et al.*, 1982; Bouffioux *et al.*, 1992; Kurth *et al.*, 1997; van der Meijden, 1997). Most demonstrated that adjuvant treatment following TUR resulted in decreased recurrence rate or prolonged disease-free interval, but had insufficient statistical power to detect differences in time to progression and survival. A meta-analysis performed by the EORTC GU Group and the MRC Working Party on superficial

bladder cancer (Pawinski *et al.*, 1996) has confirmed the favourable impact on disease-free interval in these patients. However, no long-term benefit could be demonstrated in terms of increasing time to progression to invasive disease, duration of survival or progression-free survival.

The benefit of early versus more delayed chemotherapy, as well as short (sometimes single instillation) chemotherapy versus long-term adjuvant therapy has also been studied. Three trials investigating a single instillation of Mitomycin C® (40 mg in 40 ml saline) or epirubicin (80 mg in 40 ml of saline) given within 24 hours of TUR (Oosterlinck *et al.*, 1993; Tolley *et al.*, 1996) demonstrated a 40–50 per cent reduction of risk of recurrence, compared with TUR alone. This treatment has minimal toxicity and, as even the best prognostic groups have a 30 per cent risk of recurrence (*see* Fig. 28.3), these results suggest that a single instillation of Mitomycin C® (or epirubicin) may be advantageous at diagnosis.

Trials comparing single to more prolonged treatments suggest that additional benefit may be gained by repeated instillation of intravesical chemotherapy, although the majority of the benefit is gained from an early postoperative treatment. Such treatment is therefore advised for patients at high risk of recurrence at presentation or first cystoscopy (MRC groups 2/3; Table 28.6), patients with multiple tumours or frequently relapsing patients. A number of different regimes have been investigated,

Table 28.5 *Intravesical chemotherapy*

Agent	Mechanism of action	Absorption	Toxicity	Response rate
Thiotepa	Alkylating agent; interferes with protein synthesis	Molecular weight: 189 Da; systemic absorption high	Systemic: myelosuppression, rare and transient (Soloway and Ford, 1983). Local: chemical cystitis 12–69%, dependent on dose and instillation schedule (Thrasher and Crawford, 1992)	Definitive treatment: 38% (Bouffioux *et al.*, 1992). Adjuvant treatment: increased control rate of 17% over controls (Lamm, 1992); other studies, no statistical difference (Schulman *et al.*, 1982)
Doxorubicin	Anthracycline antibiotic; binds to DNA	Molecular weight: 580 Da; systemic absorption low	Systemic: very rare. Local: chemical cystitis 20–30% (Crawford *et al.*, 1986; Akaza *et al.*, 1987)	Definitive treatment: papillary tumours, 28–56% (Bouffioux *et al.*, 1992); CIS, CR 34% patients, median time to treatment failure 5 months (Lamm *et al.*, 1991). Adjuvant treatment: improved disease-free survival when given with MMC but no difference between short- and long-term schedules (Kurth *et al.*, 1997)
Mitomycin C®	Unknown mechanism of action, but produces a cytotoxic alkylating agent	Molecular weight: 329 Da; systemic absorption low	Systemic: rare. Local: chemical cystitis 6–41% (Thrasher and Crawford, 1992)	Definitive treatment: papillary tumours, 43% (Bouffioux *et al.*, 1992); CIS, CR 58% patients. Adjuvant treatment: reduced recurrence rates versus control (Huland *et al.*, 1984; Lamm, 1992); short-term adjuvant therapy (20 instillations of 20 mg MMC in 20 weeks) is as effective as maintenance therapy (Huland *et al.*, 1990)
Epirubicin	Anthracycline antibiotic; binds to DNA	Less toxicity than doxorubicin	Systemic: rare. Local: chemical cystitis 14% for 8 weekly instillations (Burk *et al.*, 1989); chemical cystitis 14% for single instillation (Oosterlinck *et al.*, 1993)	Definitive treatment: EORTC Study 30869, 56% CR in marker lesions (Lamm, 1992). Adjuvant treatment: EORTC Study 30863, single instillation of epirubicin significantly reduces recurrence (Oosterlinck *et al.*, 1993)

CR, complete remission; MMC, Mitomycin C.

varying from the MRC regime of five courses of treatment administered at 3-monthly intervals to the EORTC regime of weekly instillation for 4 weeks followed by monthly treatment for 11 months. The optimal duration of treatment has also been addressed by the EORTC. A 6-month course is usually sufficient, but 12 months provides better results for patients in whom early intravesical instillation is not possible (Bouffioux *et al.*, 1995). However, despite this there is little clear evidence that one regime is superior to another and a common pragmatic

regime is to treat with Mitomycin C® (40 mg in 40 ml saline) weekly for 6 weeks (side-effects allowing).

The use of bacille Calmette–Guérin (BCG) in low-grade superficial disease is controversial. Most commonly it is recommended in poor-risk patients, based on the suggestion of improved efficacy in randomized trials versus intravesical chemotherapy, and reduction in the incidence of progression, which is lacking for intravesical chemotherapy. As the majority of this patient group have a low risk for progression and recurrence, it would seem

Table 28.6 *Current guidelines for the treatment of patients with superficial bladder cancer*

Ta/T1	Grades 1–2 < 2 cm	Single, no indication
Ta/T1	Grades 1–2 > 2 cm	Single treatment of Mitomycin C® post TUR
Ta/T1	Grades 1–2	Single or multiple recurrences: Resect all tumours possible
		Intravesical chemotherapy for: (i) first relapse < 6/12 from original disease (ii) multiple relapses (iii) frequent relapses e.g. Single treatment Mitomycin C® for solitary recurrence < 6/12 from original disease.
		A course of Mitomycin C® (40 mg/40 ml) weekly × 6 or BCG weekly × 6
Tis		Intravesical BCG (consider maintenance) or cystectomy
T1	Grade 3	Intravesical BCG or cystectomy

TUR, transurethral resection; BCG, bacille Calmette–Guérin.

reasonable to use intravesical chemotherapy as first-line treatment, except perhaps in patients with a high risk of progression (including high grade and CIS), reserving the more toxic BCG for chemotherapy failures.

Superficial high-grade tumours (CIS and T1)

High-grade T1 tumours are considerably more aggressive than their lower-grade counterparts, with over one-third of patients progressing to invasive disease within a few years. The outcome is similar to CIS, which, in 90 per cent of cases, is found in association with visible bladder tumours. The lesion may be focal, but is usually diffuse, with only 10 per cent occurring as isolated pathological lesions. Even then, 20–34 per cent have concurrent microinvasive carcinoma at cystectomy (Lamm, 1992) and are at risk of developing muscle-invasive disease in 42–83 per cent of cases. CIS may not be visible endoscopically and even if lesions were seen, they are often too extensive to resect and have ill-defined margins. This, in association with the frequency of concomitant invasive carcinoma and high risk of progression to invasive disease, has resulted in a historical preference for cystectomy. However, the results of immediate cystectomy are not superior to cystectomy performed after failure of intravesical treatment (Lamm *et al.*, 1991), which has led to more widespread adoption of an organ-preserving approach.

CIS is the optimal target for intravesical therapy, as close contact between agent and tumour cell occurs and tumour burden is low. Initial response rates to chemotherapy are high but the long-term tumour-free response rates are disappointing. Recent data suggesting that intravesical chemotherapy has little impact on progression rates have led to increasing use of BCG as the first-line treatment of CIS and T1G3 tumours. BCG is currently the most active intravesical immunotherapy for bladder cancer, although its precise mechanism of

action is not well understood. However, it is known that direct contact between tumour cells and BCG is necessary and that T lymphocytes are required for BCG-mediated anti-tumour activity (Martinez-Pineiro and Martinez-Pineiro, 1997). A significant reduction in tumour recurrence and progression is noted in most prospective controlled studies comparing BCG with TUR alone. Nine trials have compared BCG and intravesical chemotherapy, of which four (3/6 versus Mitomycin C® (MMC) and 1/3 versus Adriamycin®/epirubicin) have demonstrated the superiority of BCG. However, these studies were too small to demonstrate a benefit for BCG over intravesical chemotherapy in reducing progression rates (Pagano *et al.*, 1992). Adjuvant therapy with BCG is frequently associated with significant toxicity that often results in early cessation of treatment. In an attempt to reduce toxicity and improve compliance, a prospective study of sequential chemotherapy and BCG versus BCG alone has been performed, which demonstrated comparable efficacy and superiority in terms of toxicity for the alternating regimen (Ali-El-Dein *et al.*, 1999). Primary CIS (no previous TCC), secondary CIS (occurring after previous TCC) and concurrent CIS (associated with superficial TCC) respond similarly to BCG treatment, and today BCG is recommended as first-line therapy for this disease.

Prescription of BCG is dependent upon the strain used, with different doses of each required for optimum effect. No consensus exists on the optimum schedule and strain to use; 50 mg of the Tice strain or 120 mg of the Connaught strain given weekly for 6 weeks would be common UK practice. The need for subsequent maintenance is controversial. A South-west Oncology Group (SWOG) trial of 'booster' treatment, with repeated 3-week courses at 3 months, 6 months and 6 monthly for 3 years, showed superior results to a single 6-week course (Lamm *et al.*, 1997). This is at the cost of significantly increased toxicity, and many urologists prefer to repeat the 6-week course at the time of treatment failure, as tested by Catalona *et al.* (1987). A reasonable compromise may be to follow the standard 6-week induction course, with monthly maintenance instillation for a further 3 months.

BCG causes a profound inflammatory reaction in bladder mucosa and results in more pronounced local toxicity than chemotherapy. Serious systemic symptoms are uncommon but do occur, and as many as 25 per cent of patients have an influenza-like syndrome, lasting between 12 and 24 hours after installation. Those patients suspected of contracting systemic tuberculosis are usually treated successfully with anti-tuberculous therapy. However, a number of deaths following intravesical treatment have been reported related to bladder trauma, either secondary to traumatic installation or where the installation has occurred immediately after TURBT. Some investigators have advised the use of prophylactic isoniazid prior to BCG treatment. The interim results of an EORTC Study (Protocol 30911) demonstrated a benefit in terms of local or systemic side-effects, but treatment was associated with transient liver dysfunction so prophylactic therapy with isoniazid is not recommended (Lamm *et al.*, 1992). BCG is contraindicated in immunocompromised patients, such as those with HIV, patients undergoing immunosuppressive therapy, in patients with coexistent malignancy such as leukaemia or Hodgkin's disease, and in pregnant or lactating women.

Intravesical BCG produces high and durable response rates in CIS, but 30 per cent of patients fail to respond to first-line treatment, while a further 30 per cent of patients achieving complete response with initial therapy relapse within 5 years. Overall only 31 per cent of patients treated with BCG for CIS remain tumour free at 10 years (Herr *et al.*, 1992). A considerable proportion of the failure is related to extravesical progression of disease, either to the lower ureters or prostatic urethra and duct. In the literature, reports of prostatic urethral involvement after BCG range from between 1.5 and 6.3 per cent, which is lower than that of chemotherapy (33 to 37 per cent) (Schelhammer, 1994).

The treatment of refractory CIS is still under debate. Opinions range from those who believe immediate cystectomy is the treatment of choice over conservative measures. However, many patients with relatively asymptomatic CIS may prefer to retain normal bladder function and therefore alternative conservative therapies are under investigation. Likewise, some urologists advocate total cystectomy after relapse following BCG, although the fact that progression usually occurs after 2 years means that in many cases a trial of second-line therapy is reasonable (Herr *et al.*, 1989). Although the number of patients treated in this way is small (Sarosdy and Lamm, 1989), they appear to respond to second-line treatment, and therefore management of such patients should be investigated in the context of a study. However,

consideration of early aggressive surgery should not be abandoned in all patients with CIS. In particular, the association of CIS and high-grade lamina propria invasive disease (T1G3) has substantial risk for progression and may be an indication for early cystectomy after failed intravesical therapy.

RADIOTHERAPY (RT) AND SYSTEMIC TREATMENTS FOR SUPERFICIAL DISEASE

RT is usually considered ineffective in superficial disease because, although it is effective in eradicating the primary, it has little impact in preventing recurrence. However, there has been some experience with T1G3 disease, and its role here is being tested in a randomized MRC trial where RT is being compared to TUR alone (solitary disease) or BCG (multiple tumours). As intravesical treatment is an attractive alternative for superficial disease, little exploration of systemic therapies in the prevention of recurrence has been undertaken. Two trials of oral systemic chemotherapy, methotrexate (Nogueira March *et al.*, 1985) and UFT (1:4 mixture of tegafur and uracil) (Kubota *et al.*, 1993), have shown reduced recurrence rates but not gained acceptance due to concerns regarding safety and systemic toxicity. Epidemiological evidence suggesting increased bladder cancer risk in populations with low vitamin A levels, and laboratory data demonstrating growth inhibition of retinoids (Nutting and Huddart, 2000), have led to the inception of two small randomized trials of retinoids as secondary prevention of bladder cancer, which both showed an advantage in terms of recurrence rates. A further small study of high-dose vitamins, including vitamin A, had similar results, with a 40 per cent reduction in recurrence when used in addition to BCG (Lamm *et al.*, 1994). Finally, the development of inhibitors of angiogenesis, and invasion inhibitors such as matrix metalloproteinase inhibitors, may be a fertile area for future research. The current guidelines for treatment of patients with superficial bladder cancer are outlined in Table 28.6

Management of invasive bladder cancer

PROGNOSTIC FACTORS

Stage and grade remain the most important prognostic factors for invasive disease, with the presence of extravesical extension (Wijkstrom *et al.*, 1998) and lymph node positivity (Skinner and Lieskovsky, 1984; Skinner *et al.*, 1991) having greatest impact on survival. The extent of lymph node involvement is also of prognostic significance, with survival decreasing with increasing numbers of positive nodes (Skinner *et al.*, 1991).

A number of potential biological prognostic markers have also been investigated in invasive bladder cancer, including the T138 antigen and the proliferative markers Ki-67 and proliferating cell nuclear antigen (PCNA).

However, although expression may correspond with tumour aggressiveness, their role in routine clinical practice awaits prospective evaluation in larger groups of patients (Fradet *et al.*, 1990; Okamura *et al.*, 1990; Bush *et al.*, 1991; Cohen *et al.*, 1993).

Useful prognostic information may also be gained by measuring changes in expression of molecules thought to be associated with invasion and metastasis. These include cellular adhesion molecules such as cadherins (Takeichi, 1991) and integrins (Edelman and Crossin, 1991), angiogenic stimulators such as the fibroblast growth factors (FGFs) (Jouanneau *et al.*, 1991) and epidermal growth factor (EGF) (Yura *et al.*, 1989) and angiogenic inhibitors such as thrombospondin-1 (TSP) and angiostatin (O'Reilly *et al.*, 1996). For instance, reduced expression of E-cadherin and loss of α_2-integrin expression have been associated with increasing stage, and preliminary data suggest a relationship between E-cadherin expression and prognosis (Lipponen and Eskelinen, 1995). As both tumour growth and invasion are dependent upon the process of new vessel formation (angiogenesis), the ability to quantitate angiogenesis within a tumour may also provide important prognostic information. To this end 'micro vessel density' (MVD) has been determined histochemically using antibodies to vascular endothelial cells, such as antibodies to Factor VIII and CD34. Furthermore, a positive correlation has been demonstrated between MVD, lymph node metastasis (Jaeger *et al.*, 1995) and tumour progression (Bochner *et al.*, 1995). Finally, reduced expression of the angiogenic inhibitor TSP has been significantly correlated with increased tumour recurrence and decreased survival (Grossfeld *et al.*, 1997). However, although these markers have provided insights into the biological behaviour of tumours, an inconsistent relationship exists between them and patient prognosis. Further studies are therefore required to clarify their role in the clinical setting.

SURGICAL TREATMENT

Radical cystectomy remains the treatment associated with highest local cure, with pelvic recurrence rates of less than 10 per cent in node-negative tumours, and 10–20 per cent in patients with resected pelvic nodal metastases (Montie *et al.*, 1984; Wishnow and Dmochowski, 1988; Roehrborn *et al.*, 1991; Lerner *et al.*, 1993). Initially cystectomy was associated with significant morbidity and high mortality, but improvements in operative technique have seen the perioperative complication rate fall from approximately 35 per cent prior to 1970 to less than 10 per cent reported currently, with a corresponding fall in operative mortality from nearly 20 per cent to less than 2 per cent (Skinner and Lieskovsky, 1988).

The operation involves *en bloc* removal of bladder, prostate and seminal vesicles in the male, or bladder, urethra, uterus, cervix, Fallopian tube, ovaries and anterior vaginal wall in the female, with surrounding perivesical fat, pelvic visceral peritoneum and lymph nodes. Following cystectomy the urine is either diverted into an incontinent stoma, a continent urinary reservoir or orthotopic bladder substitute (which allows the patient to void urethrally). The standard against which other techniques are compared is the ileal conduit, which involves formation of an ureteroileal anastomosis, and is associated with a lower incidence of long-term metabolic disturbance and renal deterioration than its predecessor the ureterosigmoidostomy. However, it is associated with significant physical and psychological morbidity and is therefore being superseded by continent diversions or orthotopic bladder substitutes. The continent urinary diversion is an intraabdominal urinary reservoir, which is catheterizable, or has an outlet controlled by the anal sphincter. The reservoir is usually fashioned from stomach, ileum or part of the large bowel with formation of some form of mechanism to prevent reflux of urine to the kidneys. Probably the best-studied ileal continent diversion is the Kock pouch (Kock *et al.*, 1989a), which uses intussuscepted ileum and has continent catheterizable stoma.

More recently, this technique been adapted for use as an orthotopic bladder substitute (Kock *et al.*, 1989b). Here a bladder is constructed using loops of ileum and re-anastomosed on to the urethra. The drawback of this approach is the longer operating time, with a high complication and re-operation rate and high incidence of urinary incontinence. This, in combination with the age and performance status of the average bladder cancer patient, means that this procedure is only suitable in a minority of cases.

Other more recent technical developments include the development of a nerve-sparing technique (Walsh and Mostwin, 1984) in the male, which has resulted in the preservation of sexual potency (Schoenberg *et al.*, 1996), and the urethra-sparing procedure in the female (Coloby *et al.*, 1994). By using a selective approach to urethrectomy, continence should be possible with an orthotopic bladder replacement, provided meticulous follow-up is employed to ensure early detection of recurrence. However, urethral preservation should be avoided in patients with multiple papillary tumours, tumours involving the bladder neck or posterior urethra (Hendry *et al.*, 1974) and in the presence of CIS.

Bladder-preserving surgery results in retention of physiological bladder function, continence, potency and the ability to sample regional pelvic lymph nodes. Partial cystectomy alone is only suitable for a minority of patients with invasive bladder cancer. Suitable patients have a solitary muscle-invasive primary, which is amenable to complete excision, and biopsy-proven absence of cellular atypia or CIS in the remaining bladder. High recurrence rates (38–78 per cent) have been reported in unselected cases (Sweeney *et al.*, 1992), but in carefully selected patients, 5-year survival figures comparable to contemporary series of radical cystectomy can be achieved (Sweeney *et al.*, 1992).

Bladder preservation rates of 53–77 per cent, with an overall survival of approximately 80 per cent, have been reported following radical TUR alone (Henry *et al.*, 1988; Herr, 1992; Solsona *et al.*, 1992). However, these were small studies in highly selected patients. Kondas and Szentgyorgyi (1992) have suggested, following analysis of their series of 761 patients, that the following criteria be applied in the selection of patients for curative TUR. The primary could be of any grade but should be solitary and organ confined, with a maximum diameter of 2–3 cm at the base and located at a fixed portion of the bladder. The completeness of resection is clearly an important factor in achieving control of the disease, which may be assessed by marginal and random biopsies following resection. Pathological confirmation of tumour clearance is also provided by negative urine cytology at 10 days and absence of disease at a secondary resection performed several weeks after the initial TUR (Herr, 1987; Koloszy, 1991; Alken and Kohrmann, 1994). Although by following these guidelines for bladder conservation high long-term control rates can be achieved, it is probably best to reserve such approaches for patients who are not fit enough for, or unable to have, local radical treatment. Local control of radical TUR may be improved by the use of chemotherapy (Martinez-Pineiro *et al.*, 1991; Thomas *et al.*, 1999) and/or RT in combination with radical TUR, and is discussed below.

RT IN THE MANAGEMENT OF MUSCLE-INVASIVE BLADDER CANCER

RT has been used in the successful treatment of bladder cancer, with overall 5-year survival figures ranging from 20 to 40 per cent reported (Duncan and Quilty, 1986; Blandy *et al.*, 1988; Gospodarowicz *et al.*, 1989; Davidson *et al.*, 1990; Smaaland *et al.*, 1991; Vale *et al.*, 1993; Pollack *et al.*, 1995). However, there is still resistance to bladder preservation using RT in some centres, related to the lack of well-executed trials comparing radical RT to cystectomy and apparent lack of survival benefit for surgery in the salvage setting (Bloom *et al.*, 1982; Barlebo *et al.*, 1990; Sell *et al.*, 1991). Comparisons between institutional studies and non-randomized data have consistently shown a higher local control rate for cystectomy and have led to fears of disease progression prior to salvage surgery, with a possible compromise in survival. However, when the effects of selection bias (e.g. fitter patients being selected for surgery), stage migration due to clinical versus pathological staging and differences in prognostic factors between patients selected for RT surgery are taken into consideration, there is little evidence with current data that overall survival is compromised. If relapse does occur after RT, the patient will require surgery in addition to their RT and this post-radiation cystectomy is a more difficult operation, associated with greater morbidity with little possibility of reconstructive surgery. All patients undergoing attempted bladder-preserving treatment should be counselled accordingly before commencing treatment. Despite these problems, the increasing interest in selective bladder preservation is likely to result in the more widespread use of RT as the primary treatment modality internationally.

CASE SELECTION FOR RADIOTHERAPY

In deciding to attempt bladder preservation using RT, careful case selection is required, as there are several situations in which primary cystectomy may be preferred. This is clearly the case for patients who have had previous pelvic RT. Another important group are those whose disease has resulted in irretrievable loss of bladder function, when there is little benefit from bladder preservation. RT does not improve incontinence or the capacity of a bladder damaged by previous interventions, and will exacerbate symptoms arising from a severely irritable bladder. Patients with active inflammatory bowel disease, extensive prior pelvic surgery or chronic pelvic infections are at high risk of severe bowel complications following RT. In these cases alternative treatment should be considered carefully. Surgery is preferred when tumours arise in bladder diverticulae, where there is increased risk of local failure both as a result of potential difficulties in patient set-up and inhomogeneity of dose distribution, but also due to the problem of adequate cystoscopic follow-up of the region. Finally, patients whose pattern of disease suggests a low possibility of control with RT alone should be considered for alternative therapies. These include those who have undergone multiple resections for recurrent superficial tumours or multiple courses of chemotherapy or BCG, patients with diffuse malignant involvement, multiple tumours, large tumours with extravesical masses >5 cm and tumours of squamous or adenocarcinoma histology. There are conflicting views as to the influence of coexistent CIS on local tumour control following RT (Wolf *et al.*, 1985; Quilty *et al.*, 1987; Gospodarowicz *et al.*, 1989; Fung *et al.*, 1991). Recent reports of the use of intravesical BCG for persistent or recurrent CIS post-RT suggest that high response rates can be achieved (Pisters *et al.*, 1991), but long-term follow-up is required to assess the true potential of this treatment.

RADIOTHERAPY TECHNIQUE

Our current RT technique utilizes CT scan-associated planning to visualize the bladder. The target volume comprises the empty bladder (to minimize the irradiated volume) and any extravesical disease with a 1.5–2 cm margin (to allow for microscopic disease and organ movement). In most instances an anterior and two lateral treatment fields encompass this. The pelvis is not routinely included in these treatments as this substantially adds to treatment toxicity without any clear evidence for improved pelvic control. The toxicity of treatment is cumulative and related to the dose and volume of normal tissue irradiated; the predominant acute symptoms being radiation cystitis associated with urinary frequency, urgency and dysuria, proctitis and lethargy. In the long term, bladder function may deteriorate as a result of organ shrinkage related to fibrosis. Superficial telangiectasia in the bladder may give rise to haematuria, while late bowel damage may result in bleeding, which may occasionally be profound and require operative intervention. Impotence may also occur although the precise incidence is not well documented.

There is a clear dose–effect relationship for RT, as demonstrated by the downstaging of the operative specimen after preoperative RT (Sagerman *et al.*, 1968; Prout, 1976; Miller, 1980) and improved local control and patient survival related to the total dose delivered to the primary (Morrison, 1975; Parsons and Million, 1988). On this basis doses in the region of 64 Gy in 2 Gy fractions are used at the Royal Marsden. Elsewhere in the UK shorter fractionation schemes, such as 55 Gy in 20 fractions, are used; which, although not tested against standard fractionation schedules, are thought to be of equivalent efficacy. The results of radical RT at the Royal Marsden Hospital are shown in Figures 28.3 and 28.4 in terms of survival according to stage and lymph node status. Significant proportions of patients are too frail or old to tolerate a standard course of RT. In such patients local control can be achieved by using weekly 6 Gy fractions to 30–36 Gy. This regime appears well tolerated with acceptable levels of late toxicity. This sort of schema can also be useful for control of local symptoms in patients with metastatic disease. A similar regime of 21 Gy in three fractions in one week has been tested in this setting, to 35 Gy in 10 fractions in a multicentre MRC trial of 500 patients. The results demonstrated no difference in efficacy, toxicity or survival between the two arms (Duchesne *et al.*, 2000).

PROGNOSTIC FACTORS FOR LOCAL CONTROL AFTER RADIOTHERAPY TREATMENT

A favourable response to RT may be expected in small-volume T2 (rather than T3/4) patients, in the absence of ureteral obstruction (Greiner *et al.*, 1977; van der Werf-Messing, 1979; Shipley *et al.*, 1985), in papillary rather than sessile tumours (van der Werf-Messing, 1979; Shipley *et al.*, 1985), with normal haemoglobin levels above 13 g/L (Quilty and Duncan, 1986; Cole *et al.*, 1995; Fossa *et al.*, 1996a; Overgaard and Horsman, 1996) and following a good response to the first 40 Gy of radical RT (Blandy *et al.*, 1980; Shipley *et al.*, 1985). Debulking of the tumour prior to RT also improves local control, both when RT is delivered as the sole modality (Fung *et al.*, 1991), or when administered concurrently with cisplatin (Sauer *et al.*, 1990). However, the excellent local control rates may be attributed partly to case selection (i.e. tumours are small enough to be debulked) rather than to the surgery itself.

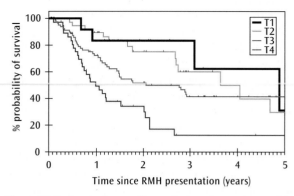

Figure 28.3 *Survival according to T stage for patients with bladder carcinoma treated at the Royal Marsden Hospital (RMH) between 1990 and 1999.*

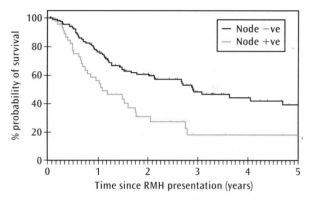

Figure 28.4 *Survival according to nodal status for patients with bladder carcinoma treated at the Royal Marsden Hospital (RMH) between 1990 and 1999.*

IMPROVING THE RESULTS OF RADICAL RADIOTHERAPY

In an attempt to improve the efficacy of RT, a number of strategies are being explored. Following the observation that treatment breaks are associated with impaired outcome and that bladder cancer has a short potential doubling time, accelerated fractionation has been explored. Despite promising pilot data, a recently completed randomized trial of 60.8 Gy in 32 fractions treating twice daily, versus a standard treatment of 64 Gy in 32 daily fractions, has failed to show any improvement in local control and enhanced acute toxicity (Horwich *et al.*, 1999).

The failure of RT to control disease may be related to the relative resistance of a hypoxic tumour fraction to therapy. Some data suggest that reversal of this tumour hypoxia using hyperbaric oxygen can improve local control (Overgaard and Horsman, 1996), but the difficulties of implementation of the technique in routine clinical practice have prevented its routine use. More recently, Carbogen (95 per cent O_2, 5 per cent CO_2) in combination with nicotinamide has been used to improve tumour oxygenation, with promising results in pilot studies

(Hoskin *et al.*, 1999). This is currently being tested in a phase III randomized trial.

Improved local control with acceptable local morbidity could also potentially be achieved by dose escalation. One way to achieve this is by using interstitial RT. This has been explored by several groups, most frequently in combination with TUR and low-dose external-beam RT (usually up to 30 Gy) (De Neve *et al.*, 1992; Rozan *et al.*, 1992; Moonen *et al.*, 1994; Pernot *et al.*, 1996; Wijnmaalen *et al.*, 1997). In most of these series impressive local control rates in excess of 80 per cent are reported, with acceptable toxicity levels, but despite this the need for the surgical placement of the implant restricts its use to a few specialist centres.

The dose of external-beam RT is limited by the tolerance of normal tissues and, in the bladder, retrospective data suggest that radiation tolerance is a function of the volume irradiated, with tolerance of part of the bladder being greater than that of the whole bladder. Interstitial RT data have shown that satisfactory local control can be achieved by treatment focused on the tumour (compared to treating the whole bladder). Reducing the volume of bladder irradiated could reduce toxicity, allowing the overall radiation dose to be increased, which should improve control rates. Potential problems of this approach arise from the fact that the bladder is not a fixed organ; so its location and size may vary. Studies comparing the CT-planned target volume before and during RT demonstrate that a shift of target volume may occur (Sur *et al.*, 1993). In one study, movement of the bladder wall was observed in 60 per cent of patients and, although movement tended to be towards the midline and hence into the target volume, a reduction in the margin around the tumour was seen in 33 per cent of patients (Turner *et al.*, 1997). Thus adequate margins around the tumour are required to ensure that geographical misses do not occur. Despite these problems, a small pilot study at the Royal Marsden Hospital with a modest decrease in the whole bladder dose has shown significant reduction in toxicity. This has formed the basis of more extensive prospective evaluation of this concept in the UK BC 2001 trial.

COMBINED-MODALITY TREATMENT

Selective bladder preservation

One approach to reconcile the advantages of bladder preservation with the efficacy of immediate cystectomy is in a programme of selective bladder preservation. This approach largely pioneered by Shipley and colleagues, involves the use of complete/radical TUR, followed by neoadjuvant chemotherapy and limited RT. Following this treatment, early cystoscopic reassessment is undertaken. Patients remaining in remission have consolidation RT to achieve bladder conservation, and patients with persistent or progressive disease undergo cystectomy. In the RTOG study of this approach (trial 8802) 75 per cent of patients achieved an initial complete remission (CR) and underwent conservative consolidation, a further 15 per cent required a salvage cystectomy, with the result that 60 per cent had bladder preservation with no obvious detriment to overall survival. A similar study is being conducted by the EORTC using complete TUR and three cycles of escalated MVAC, with reassessment prior to radiotherapy. If successful, these studies may form the basis of a future comparison of bladder conservation with cystectomy.

Preoperative and adjuvant RT

The rationale for use of preoperative RT is to prevent the intra-operative seeding of tumour cells, to sterilize microscopic tumour deposits in the perivesical tissues and, theoretically, to irradicate tumour that has not been rendered hypoxic secondary to surgically mediated changes in the surrounding vasculature. A number of retrospective reviews and non-randomized studies have suggested a benefit for preoperative RT over cystectomy alone (Whitmore and Batata, 1984; Parsons and Million, 1988; Cole *et al.*, 1994). However, the few randomized trials conducted showed no survival advantage to preoperative RT, although they suffered with poor accrual and had insufficient power to detect even a large treatment effect (Blackard and Byar, 1972; Slack *et al.*, 1977; Abrahamsen and Fossa, 1990). The most recently reported trial is that conducted by the South-west Oncology Group, which again did not demonstrate a benefit for preoperative irradiation and cystectomy. Despite being the largest study to date, with fewer than 150 patients randomized the power of the study is limited and the confidence intervals were wide (Crawford *et al.*, 1987; Smith *et al.*, 1988). Several other factors may contribute to this apparent lack of effect: the study used a short course of RT (20 Gy in 5 fractions over 1 week) and a large proportion of the patients had T2 tumours, which may not benefit from preoperative RT. Finally, the known difference in relapse between deeply muscle invasive (T2b) and extravesical (T3b) tumours was concealed by considering these patients as one group. It is probably best to conclude that the case for preoperative RT is not proven but may be an area for continued research. Limited examination of postoperative treatment has also been undertaken but is associated with too high an incidence of bowel toxicity to be considered routinely (Reisinger *et al.*, 1992).

Neoadjuvant chemotherapy

Neoadjuvant chemotherapy prior to surgery has been explored with the aim of improving the chances of bladder preservation, to provide potentially useful information as to the response to chemotherapy and to improve survival rates for patients with bladder cancer by the irradiation of micrometastases. A number of non-randomized studies have established the feasibility and safety of administering neoadjuvant chemotherapy, with response rates of 60–70 per cent and complete response rates of approximately 30 per cent reported

(Scher et al., 1989; Sternberg et al., 1995). To date definitive conclusions regarding their impact on survival are difficult. Randomized studies of neoadjuvant chemotherapy have tended to suffer from small sample size. Trials of single agent chemotherapy have shown no benefit (Table 28.7a). Most of the trials of multi-agent chemotherapy have tended to show a small benefit which has not been statistically significant (see Table 28.7). The Nordic I trial, conducted in Scandinavia, demonstrated an advantage to administering doxorubicin and cisplatin prior to preoperative RT and cystectomy in patients with advanced disease (T3 and T4) (Rintala et al., 1993; Malmstrom et al., 1996). However one must interpret these results with caution, as this trial was not designed to detect survival differences between patient subsets. The largest trial of neoadjuvant chemotherapy is the EORTC/MRC study of three cycles of CMV followed by either definitive RT or cystectomy. This study was designed to detect a 10 per cent difference in survival between treatment arms. The trial found a significant 8 per cent absolute advantage for metastasis-free survival (hazard ratio (HR) 0.79, 95 per cent confidence interval (CI) 0.66−0.93; p = 0.007) and a non significant improvement in locoregional control (HR 0.87, CI 0.73−1.02) for patients receiving chemotherapy. There was a 5.5 per cent absolute difference (HR 0.85, CI 0.71−1.02; p = 0.075) in overall survival benefit which did not attain statistical significance (Trialists, 1999). A further update on this data is expected in the future. The latest trial to report in abstract has been the South-west Oncology Group trial 8711. Patients receiving MVAC are reported as having a 15 per cent improvement in 5-year survival (one-sided t test p = 0.044). This analysis has been criticized as using a one-sided rather than (the more correct) two-sided statistical test. If a two-sided test is used, the difference is not significant (Natale et al., 2001). A meta-analysis including the Nordic I and MRC EORTC trial (but not the SWOG or an Egyptian trial) suggested a trend for improved survival (HR 0.73, CI 0.73−1.04) that failed to reach statistical significance (Parmar and Burdett, 1999). Taken together these trials may suggest a small benefit for neoadjuvant chemotherapy similar to that seen for other solid tumours but a definitive answer may depend on an update of the meta-analysis with the inclusion of more recent data.

Adjuvant postoperative chemotherapy has been less well studied. Some trials have suggested a possible benefit for this approach (Table 28.7c). These trials, however, are on the whole small and methologically flawed so this data should be treated cautiously. A large international study of this issue is currently being planned.

Concurrent chemotherapy and RT

In an attempt to improve the therapeutic ratio of RT, concurrent chemotherapy has been investigated as a radiosensitizer. The most frequently studied drug in this context is cisplatin as, in addition to its cytotoxicity,

it has been shown to enhance the radiation effect in vivo, in vitro and under hypoxic conditions. A large number of phase II studies have been performed, the majority utilizing cisplatin alone or in combination with 5-fluorouracil, which have demonstrated high complete responses with bladder preservation in over 60 per cent of patients (Jakse et al., 1985; Eapen et al., 1989; Rotman et al., 1990; Russell et al., 1990; Sauer et al., 1990; Shipley et al., 1990; Housset et al., 1993; Coppin et al., 1996). The National Cancer Institute of Canada has conducted a prospective trial (Coppin et al., 1996) examining the effect of the addition of concurrent cisplatin to preoperative or definitive RT on tumour control and overall survival. Despite the lack of power of this small study to detect any but large benefits, this trial demonstrated improved recurrence-free survival for the chemotherapy group and a non-significant trend to improved overall survival. Further confirmatory investigation of cisplatin is required to clarify this issue in the phase III setting. Work is also needed to address the issue of the optimum dose schedule for cisplatin, e.g. is daily administration better? Cisplatin is not necessarily the ideal agent for this form of treatment in this group of patients, who are often elderly and have renal impairment. It may be that using drugs that are less dependent on renal function, such as 5-fluorouracil (5-FU) alone or in combination, which have also shown promise in the phase II setting, or newer agents, such as gemcitabine, may be more practical. The combination of 5-FU and mitomycin C is being tested in a phase III trial in the UK (BC 2001).

THE MANAGEMENT OF ADVANCED DISEASE

Despite the recognized chemo- and radiosensitivity of TCC of the bladder, more than 5000 deaths are attributable to the disease in the UK each year. Approximately one-half of patients with muscle invasion ultimately succumb to metastatic disease. The most common sites of metastasis include the regional lymph nodes, bone, lung, skin and liver, and less frequently brain and meninges and the organs within the peritoneal cavity. The distribution of metastasis is important when considering treatment, as the site(s) of involvement correlate with prognosis, with improved survival in those with disease confined to the lymph nodes or skin and a substantially worse prognosis with liver and bone metastases (Geller et al., 1991). Consideration of these factors and other prognostic factors, especially performance status (Mead et al., 1998), is important when comparing the results of clinical trials in this setting.

Chemotherapy

Systemic chemotherapy is the main active treatment for patients with metastatic disease. Single-agent chemotherapy yields objective responses of the order of 10–20 per cent, with complete responses of <5 per cent (Turner et al., 1977; Blumenreich et al., 1982; Gagliano et al., 1983; Richards et al., 1983; Soloway et al., 1983;

Table 28.7 *Randomized trials of neoadjuvant and adjuvant chemotherapy in the treatment of invasive localized bladder cancer*

a) Trials of single agent adjuvant chemotherapy

Trial/author	Chemotherapy schedule	Local treatment	Number of patients	Survival (3 yrs unless stated) Chemotherapy	Control	Comments
Methotrexate						
CUCG (Shearer et al., 1988)	Methotrexate 100 mg/m^2 weekly $\times$ 3 100 mg q2 weeks $\times$ 6 100 mg q4 weeks $\times$ 9	Radiotherapy	376	37.3%	38.6%	n.s.
Cisplatin						
West Midlands (Wallace et al., 1991)	Cp 100 mg/m^2 $\times$ 3	Radiotherapy	159	39%	40%	
Australia (Wallace et al., 1991)	Cp 100 mg/m^2 $\times$ 2	Radiotherapy	137	38%	40%	
Spain (Martinez-Pineiro et al., 1995)	Cp 100 mg/m^2 $\times$ 3	Cystectomy	122	35.5%	37.3%	6.5 year survival

b) Trials of multi-agent neoadjuvant chemotherapy

Trial	Chemotherapy schedule	Number of patients	Survival (5 yrs) Chemotherapy	Control	Comments
MRC/EORTC (Trialists, 1999)	CMV	976	55.5%	50%	(3 yrs surv.)
Nordic I (Malmstrom et al., 1996)	AC	325	59%	51%	
Egypt (Abol-Enein et al., 1997)	CarbMV	196	62%*	42%	
RTOG (Shipley et al., 1998)	CMV	123	48%	49%	
SWOG (Natale et al., 2001)	MVAC	306	57%*	42%	

*Statistically significant ($p < 0.05$).

c) Trials of adjuvant (postoperative) chemotherapy

Trial	Chemotherapy schedule	Number of patients	Survival Chemotherapy	Control
Single agent (Studer et al., 1994)	C	80	54%	51%
Multiagent (Skinner, 1982)	CAP	91	51 months	29 months
(Stockle et al., 1993)	MVAC	49	62%	42%
(Freiha et al., 1996)	CMV	55	63 months	36 months
(Bono et al., 1997)	CM	125	No difference	

Al-Sarraf et al., 1985; van Oosterom et al., 1985; Troner et al., 1987; Hillcoat et al., 1989; Roth et al., 1994; Witte et al., 1997) but with a limited response duration of only 4–6 months (Soloway et al., 1983; Khandekar et al., 1985; Hillcoat et al., 1989; Loehrer et al., 1992). The most active agents in these studies include cisplatin, doxorubicin, Mitomycin C® and methotrexate, and then the vinca alkaloids and 5-fluorouracil.

Table 28.8 *Summary of the chemotherapy regimes used in the treatment of invasive bladder cancer*

CMV	Methotrexate 30 mg/m² days 1 and 8 Vinblastine 4 mg/m² days 1 and 8 Cisplatin 100 mg/m² day 2 Cycle repeated every 21 days
MVAC	Methotrexate 30 mg/m² days 1, 15 and 22 Vinblastine 3 mg/m² days 1, 15 and 22 Adriamycin® 30 mg/m² day 1 Cisplatin 70 mg/m² day 1 Cycle repeated every 28 days
HD-MVAC	Methotrexate 30 mg/m² day 1 Vinblastine 3 mg/m² day 1 Adriamycin 30 mg/m² day 1 Cisplatin 70 mg/m² day 1 G-CSF 7 days (day 4–11)
GC	Gemcitabine 1000 mg/m² days 1, 8 and 15 Cisplatin 70 mg/m² day 2 Cycle repeated every 28 days

Development of these single agents into two-, three- and four-drug combinations increased response rates and survival (Gagliano et al., 1983; Soloway et al., 1983; Al-Sarraf et al., 1985; Khandekar et al., 1985; Troner et al., 1987; Hillcoat et al., 1989). The best of which appear to be the MVAC and CMV regimes, incorporating methotrexate, vinblastine and cisplatin (with or without doxorubicin) (Harker et al., 1985; Sternberg et al., 1988, 1989) described in Table 28.8. For both these regimes high response rates, including a significant complete response rate, have been reported, for instance in the initial report on the MVAC regimen there was an overall response rate of 72 per cent, with a 36 per cent complete response (Sternberg et al., 1988, 1989), although subsequent reports, including multicentre studies, have shown that in an average patient population response rates of 40–50 per cent with 10 per cent complete response rate is more common (Loehrer et al., 1992; Cook et al., 2000). MVAC is now regarded as the gold standard chemotherapy against which other regimes have to be measured, but the high response rates do carry a price, with significant rates of toxicity. In Sternberg's initial work, there were significant rates of mucositis (40 per cent), renal toxicity (31 per cent) and neutropenic sepsis (20 per cent) with a toxic death rate of 4 per cent, which are similar to those seen in most subsequent studies.

The median survival of patients with metastatic uro-epithelial cancer not treated with chemotherapy is in the order of 3–6 months (Raghavan, 1990; Loehrer and De Mulder, 1997), which doubles to around 9–12 months with treatment (Young and Garnick, 1988; Raghavan, 1990; Loehrer and De Mulder, 1997). Although trials of multi-agent chemotherapy versus best supportive care

are not available, studies of more intensive versus less intensive chemotherapy, including MVAC versus cisplatin (Loehrer et al., 1992), MVAC versus cyclophosphamide, adriamycin and cisplatin (CAP) (Logothetis et al., 1990) and CMV versus methotrexate and vinblastine (MV) (Mead et al., 1998) have shown better response rates, progression-free survival and, in some cases, overall survival and symptomatic control for the more intensive regimen. The reports of a significant complete response rate raised the possibility of an increase in (up to 20 per cent) long-term survival, but more recent analysis suggests that survival at 5 years is unusual except in groups receiving chemotherapy for T4 or node-positive disease (who often receive additional RT) (Fossa et al., 1996b; Saxman et al., 1997).

In an attempt to improve these results, several trials have addressed the impact of moderate increases in dosing, using colony stimulating factors (Gabrilove et al., 1988; Logothetis et al., 1992; Moore et al., 1993; Seidman et al., 1993; Sternberg et al., 1993; Loehrer et al., 1994). In most cases this led to an increased intensity of the chemotherapy delivered and reduced haematological and mucosal toxicity (Gabrilove et al., 1988; Moore et al., 1993; Seidman et al., 1993; Sternberg et al., 1993). This approach has been tested in an EORTC phase III trial. This trial showed the high intensity MVAC produced better response rates, lower toxicity (less neuropenic sepsis and mucositis), a greater proportion of survivors at two years but similar median survival rates. The disparity of effect on median and two-year survival has led to a debate as to whether the differences are real or due to chance differences in prognostic factors. However, these results, allied to the shorter treatment time and lower toxicity of the high intensity MVAC, suggest that this may be a real advance on standard MVAC (Sternberg et al., 2001). The alternative approach of increasing dose intensity by acceleration of the chemotherapy schedule has not resulted in a major improvement in outcome and is associated with increased toxicity (Boshoff et al., 1995; Huddart et al., 2001).

The need for therapeutic improvements has led to the examination of several new agents. Of particular interest have been the taxanes paclitaxel (Taxol®) and docetaxel (Taxotere®) and the nucleoside analogue gemcitabine. Early studies of paclitaxel in chemotherapy naïve patients reported response rates of 42 per cent, with complete responses in 27 per cent of patients (Roth et al., 1994). However, although follow-up studies have confirmed activity, response rates were significantly lower, particularly in previously treated patients (Dreicer et al., 1996; Papamichael et al., 1997). Docetaxel has also shown activity in previously untreated patients with renal insufficiency (Dimopoulos et al., 1998) and as a second-line drug in patients who had failed post cisplatin (McCaffrey et al., 1997).

Gemcitabine, an analogue of cytosine arabinoside, first demonstrated activity in bladder cancer in early phase trials in Italy (Pollera *et al.*, 1994) in previously treated patients, and follow-up studies have demonstrated single-agent response rates of approximately 30 per cent (Stadler *et al.*, 1995; Moore *et al.*, 1997). In view of the activity of paclitaxel and gemcitabine, it is not surprising that a number of phase II studies of these agents in combination with cisplatinum/carboplatin and other active drugs have been performed (Redman *et al.*, 1998; Vaughn *et al.*, 1998; Zielinski *et al.*, 1998). A recently completed phase III trial has shown that gemcitabine and cisplatin (GC) achieves similar response rates and survival to MVAC, but with lower rates of treatment-related toxicity (von der Maase *et al.*, 2000). These results form the basis of further comparative studies of GC with the combination of both gemcitabine and paclitaxel with cisplatin.

Other agents that have shown moderate activity have included ifosfamide (with response rates of 20 per cent in previously treated patients) (Witte *et al.*, 1997) and gallium nitrate (Seligman and Crawford, 1991), although both of these drugs have considerable treatment-related toxicity, making them poor candidates for use in bladder cancer. The MRC is currently exploring whether infusional 5-fluorouracil has a better response rate than older studies of bolus doses.

Many patients are either too frail or have inadequate renal function to tolerate cisplatin-based treatment. Several groups have explored the use of the cisplatin analogue, carboplatin, in view of its more favourable toxicity profile and less renal dependence. Most studies have confirmed the activity of carboplatin but in the few comparative studies there is a tendency for lower efficacy (Bellmunt *et al.*, 1997). However, when cisplatin usage is not an option in combination with drugs such as methotrexate, use of carboplatin is a reasonable option.

Radiotherapy and surgery in the palliation of advanced disease

In patients with symptomatic advanced local disease, surgery and RT may be needed when conservative measures fail. When patients with urinary fistulas/leakage cannot be managed by simple conservative measures such as catheterization, supravesical bladder diversions (and occasionally cystectomy) can be an effective manoeuvre, particularly in patients of good performance status and reasonable life expectancy, to relieve the problems of bladder irritability and perineal excoriation caused by constant urinary leakage (Montie *et al.*, 1983). A further distressing symptom of bladder cancer is haematuria, which may be profound and associated with clot retention. Palliative RT may be very effective in controlling the bleeding using hypofractionated regimes, although the optimal treatment protocol has not been definitively ascertained. RT may also provide benefit for those patients with obstructive nephropathy, urinary incontinence and bone or brain metastases. In all cases, the expected benefit of any intervention in the palliative setting must be carefully weighed against its morbidity. Although treatment with surgery and multi-agent chemotherapy may result in excellent palliation for some patients, it must be remembered that this may be at the expense of significant toxicity. Most are too frail, and simple conservative measures or palliative RT in the setting of multidisciplinary care may be most appropriate.

SIGNIFICANT POINTS

- Bladder cancer is the fifth most common cancer in the UK, causing 5400 deaths per year.
- Risk of developing bladder cancer is increased by exposure to environment carcinogens (tobacco smoking, aromatic amines), drugs, radiation exposure and factors leading to chronic irritation of the bladder.
- The majority of bladder cancer presents with painless macroscopic haematuria and, in the UK, is largely due to transitional cell carcinomas subtypes.
- Superficial (non-invasive) tumours carry a good prognosis and can be controlled largely by local resection.
- Recurrence of superficial disease is, however, frequent following local treatment, especially if tumours are multiple or high grade. Risk of recurrence is reduced by intravesical chemotherapy or immunotherapy.
- Approximately 20 per cent of superficial disease may progress to invasive cancer. Progression is especially associated with high-grade disease. Progression risk may be reduced by BCG treatment.
- Invasive disease carries a worse prognosis. Radical cystectomy and radiotherapy (with salvage cystectomy for relapse or persistent disease) are alternative strategies with similar long-term survival outcomes.
- No clear advantages have been demonstrated for adjuvant radiotherapy or chemotherapy.
- Metastatic disease carries a poor prognosis. Multi-agent platinum-based chemotherapy is useful palliative treatment and carries survival and quality of life benefits.
- In patients with advanced disease, palliative radiotherapy and/or surgery may be of value.

KEY REFERENCES

Duchesne, G., Bolger, J., Griffiths, G.O. *et al.* on behalf of the Medical Research Council Bladder Cancer Working Party (2000). A randomized trial of hypofractionated schedules of palliative radiotherapy in the management of bladder carcinoma: results of Medical Research Council Trial BA09. *Int. J. Radiol. Oncol. Biol. Phys.* **47**(2), 379–88.

Hall, R.R. (ed.) (1999) *Clinical management of bladder cancer*. London: Arnold, Oxford University Press.

Lamm, D.L., Blumenstein, B.A., Crawford, E.D. *et al.* (1991) A randomized trial of intravesical doxorubicin and immunotherapy with bacille Calmette–Guérin for transitional-cell carcinoma of the bladder. *N. Engl. J. Med.* **325**(17), 1205–9.

Loehrer, P. and De Mulder, P. (1997) Management of metastatic bladder cancer. In Raghaven, D.S.H., Leibel, S. and Lange, P.H. (eds), *Principles and practice of genitourinary oncology*. Philadelphia: Lippincott–Raven.

Pawinski, A., Sylvester, R., Kurth, K.H., Bouffioux, C., van der Meijden, A., Parmar, M.K., Bijnens, L. (1996) A combined analysis of European Organization for Research and Treatment of Cancer, and Medical Research Council randomized clinical trials for the prophylactic treatment of stage TaT1 bladder cancer. European Organization for Research and Treatment of Cancer Genitourinary Tract Cancer Cooperative Group and the Medical Research Council Working Party on Superficial Bladder Cancer, *J. Urol.* **156**(6): 1934–1940, discussion 1940–1931 [82].

Skinner, D. and Lieskovsky, G. (1988) Management of invasive and high grade bladder cancer. In Skinner, D. and Lieskovsky, G. (eds), *Diagnosis and management of genitourinary cancer*. Philadelphia: WB Saunders.

Trialists ICo. (1999) Neoadjuvant cisplatin, methotrexate and vinblastine chemotherapy for muscle-invasive bladder cancer: a randomised controlled trial. *Lancet* **354**(9178); 533–40.

REFERENCES

Abol-Enein, H., El Makresh, M. and El-Baz, M.e.a. (1997) Neoadjuvant chemotherapy in the treatment of invasive transitional bladder cancer. A controlled, prospective randomised study. *Br. J. Urol.* **79**, 43.

Abrahamsen, J.F. and Fossa, S.D. (1990) Long-term morbidity after curative radiotherapy for carcinoma of the bladder. A retrospective study. *Strahlenther Onkol.* **166**(9), 580–3.

Akaza, H., Isaka, S., Koiso, K. *et al.* (1987) Comparative analysis of short-term and long-term prophylactic intravesical chemotherapy of superficial bladder cancer. Prospective, randomized, controlled studies of the Japanese Urological Cancer Research Group. *Cancer Chemother. Pharmacol.* **20**(suppl.), S91–96.

Ali-El-Dein, B., Nabeeh, A., Ismail, E.H. and Ghoneim, M.A. (1999) Sequential bacillus Calmette–Guérin and epirubicin versus bacillus Calmette–Guérin alone for superficial bladder tumors: a randomized prospective study. *J. Urol.* **162**(2), 339–42.

Alken, P. and Kohrmann, K.U. (1994) The essentials of transurethral resection of bladder tumours. *Arch. Ital. Urol. Androl.* **65**, 629–32.

Al-Sarraf, M., Frank, J., Smith, J.A. Jr *et al.* (1985) Phase II trial of cyclophosphamide, doxorubicin, and cisplatin (CAP) versus amsacrine in patients with transitional cell carcinoma of the urinary bladder: a Southwest Oncology Group study. *Cancer Treat. Rep.* **69**(2), 189–94.

Althausen, A.F., Prout, G.R. Jr and Daly, J.J. (1976) Non-invasive papillary carcinoma of the bladder associated with carcinoma *in situ*. *J. Urol.* **116**, 575–80.

Augustine, A., Hebert, J.R., Kabat, G.C. and Wynder, E.L. (1988) Bladder cancer in relation to cigarette smoking. *Cancer Res.* **48**(15), 4405–8.

Badawi, A.F., Mostafa, M.H., Probert, A. and O'Connor, P.J. (1995) Role of schistosomiasis in human bladder cancer: evidence of association, aetiological factors, and basic mechanisms of carcinogenesis. *Eur. J. Cancer Prev.* **4**(1), 45–59.

Barentsz, J.O., Jager, G.J., van Vierzen, P.B. *et al.* (1996) Staging urinary bladder cancer after transurethral biopsy: value of fast dynamic contrast-enhanced MR imaging. *Radiology* **201**(1), 185–93.

Barlebo, H., Steven, K. and Sprensen, B. (1990) Preoperative irradiation (40 Gy) and cystectomy versus radiotherapy (60 Gy) followed by salvage cystectomy in the treatment of advanced bladder cancer. *J. Urol.* **143**(suppl.), 291A.

Bellmunt, J., Ribas, A., Eres, N. *et al.* (1997) Carboplatin-based versus cisplatin-based chemotherapy in the treatment of surgically incurable advanced bladder carcinoma. *Cancer* **80**(10), 1966–72.

Black, R.J., Bray, F., Ferlay, J. and Parkin, D.M. (1997) Cancer incidence and mortality in the European Union: cancer registry data and estimates of national incidence for 1990 [*see* comments]. *Eur. J. Cancer* **33**(7), 1075–107 [published erratum appears in *Eur. J. Cancer* 1997, **33**(14), 2440].

Blackard, C.E. and Byar, D.P. (1972) Results of a clinical trial of surgery and radiation in stages II and 3 carcinoma of the bladder. *J. Urol.* **108**(6), 875–8.

Blandy, J.P., England, H.R., Evans, S.J. *et al.* (1980) T3 bladder cancer – the case for salvage cystectomy. *Br. J. Urol.* **52**(6), 506–10.

Blandy, J.P., Jenkins, B.J., Fowler, C.G. *et al.* (1988) Radical radiotherapy and salvage cystectomy for T2/3 cancer of the bladder. *Prog. Clin. Biol. Res.* **260**, 447–51.

Bloom, H.J., Hendry, W.F., Wallace, D.M. and Skeet, R.G. (1982) Treatment of T3 bladder cancer: controlled trial of pre-operative radiotherapy and radical cystectomy versus radical radiotherapy. *Br. J. Urol.* **54**(2), 136–51.

Blumenreich, M.S., Needles, B., Yagoda, A., Sogani, P., Grabstald, H. and Whitmore, W.F. Jr (1982) Intravesical cisplatin for superficial bladder tumors. *Cancer* **50**(5), 863–5.

Bochner, B.H., Cote, R.J., Weidner, N. *et al.* (1995) Angiogenesis in bladder cancer: relationship between microvessel density and tumor prognosis. *J. Natl Cancer Inst.* **87**(21), 1603–12.

Boice, J.D., Engholm, G., Kleinerman, R.A. *et al.* (1988) Radiation dose and second cancer risk in patients treated for cancer of the cervix. *Radiat. Res.* **116**, 3–55.

Bono, A., Benvenuti, C. and Gibba, A.e.a. (1997) Adjuvant chemotherapy in locally advanced bladder cancer. Final analysis of a controlled multicentre study. *Acta Urol. Ital.* **11**, 5–8.

Boshoff, C., Oliver, R.T., Gallagher, C.J. and Ong, J. (1995) Accelerated cisplatin-based chemotherapy for advanced bladder cancer. *Eur. J. Cancer* **31A**(10), 1633–6.

Bouffioux, C., Denis, L., Oosterlinck, W. *et al.* (1992) Adjuvant chemotherapy of recurrent superficial transitional cell carcinoma: results of a European organization for research on treatment of cancer randomized trial comparing intravesical instillation of thiotepa, doxorubicin and cisplatin. The European Organization for Research on Treatment of Cancer Genitourinary Group. *J. Urol.* **148**(2 Pt 1), 297–301.

Bouffioux, C., Kurth, K.H., Bono, A. *et al.* (1995) Intravesical adjuvant chemotherapy for superficial transitional cell bladder carcinoma: results of 2 European Organization for Research and Treatment of Cancer randomized trials with mitomycin C and doxorubicin comparing early versus delayed instillations and short-term versus long-term treatment. European Organization for Research and Treatment of Cancer Genitourinary Group. *J. Urol.* **153**(3 Pt 2), 934–41.

Boyko, R.W., Cartwright, R.A. and Glashan, R.W. (1985) Bladder cancer in dye manufacturing workers. *J. Occup. Med.* **27**, 799–803.

Britton, J.P., Dowell, A.C., Whelan, P. and Harris, C.M. (1992) A community study of bladder cancer screening by the detection of occult urinary bleeding. *J. Urol.* **148**(3), 788–90.

Brockmoller, J., Cascorbi, I., Kerb, R. and Roots, I. (1996) Combined analysis of inherited polymorphisms in arylamine *N*-acetyltransferase 2, glutathione *S*-transferases M1 and T1, microsomal epoxide hydrolase, and cytochrome P450 enzymes as modulators of bladder cancer risk. *Cancer Res.* **56**(17), 3915–25.

Burk, K., Kurth, K.H. and Newling, D. (1989) Epirubicin in treatment and recurrence prophylaxis of patients with superficial bladder cancer. *Prog. Clin. Biol. Res.* **303**, 423–34.

Bush, C., Price, P., Norton, J. *et al.* (1991) Proliferation in human bladder carcinoma measured by Ki-67 antibody labelling: its potential clinical importance. *Br. J. Cancer* **64**(2), 357–60.

Cancer IAfRo (1986) *Evaluation of carcinogenic risk of chemicals to humans: tobacco smoking.* Lyon: International Agency for Research on Cancer, 38.

Case, R.A.M. and Hosker, M.E. (1954) Tumour of the urinary bladder as an occupational disease in the rubber industry in England and Wales. *Br. J. Prev. Soc. Med.* **8**, 39–50.

Case, R.A.M., Hosker, M.E., McDonald, D.B. *et al.* (1954) Tumours of the urinary bladder in workmen engaged in the manufacture and use of certain dyestuff intermediates in the British chemical industry. *Br. J. Ind. Med.* **11**, 75–104.

Catalona, W.J., Hudson, M.A., Gillen, D.P., Andriole, G.L. and Ratliff, T.L. (1987) Risks and benefits of repeated courses of intravesical bacillus Calmette–Guérin therapy for superficial bladder cancer. *J. Urol.* **137**(2), 220–4.

Chopin, D.K., Caruelle, J.P., Colombel, M. *et al.* (1993) Increased immunodetection of acidic fibroblast growth factor in bladder cancer, detectable in urine. *J. Urol.* **150**(4), 1126–30.

Cohen, M.B., Waldman, F.M., Carroll, P.R., Kerschmann, R., Chew, K. and Mayall, B.H. (1993) Comparison of five histopathologic methods to assess cellular proliferation in transitional cell carcinoma of the urinary bladder [*see* comments]. *Hum. Pathol.* **24**(7), 772–8.

Cole, C.J., Pollack, A., Zagars, G.K., Dinney, C.P., Swanson, D.A. and von Eschenbach, A.C. (1994) Local control of muscle-invasive bladder cancer: preoperative radiotherapy and cystectomy versus cystectomy alone. *Int. J. Radiat. Oncol. Biol. Phys.* **30**(suppl. 1), 200.

Cole, C.J., Pollack, A., Zagars, G.K., Dinney, C.P., Swanson, D.A. and von Eschenbach, A.C. (1995) Local control of muscle-invasive bladder cancer: preoperative radiotherapy and cystectomy versus cystectomy alone. *Int. J. Radiat. Oncol. Biol. Phys.* **32**(2), 331–40.

Coleman, M.P., Babb, P., Damiecki, P. *et al.* (1999) *Cancer survival trends in England and Wales 1971–1995 deprivation and NHS Region.* London: The Stationary Office.

Coloby, P.J., Kakizoe, T., Tobisu, K. and Sakamoto, M. (1994) Urethral involvement in female bladder cancer patients: mapping of 47 consecutive cysto-urethrectomy specimens. *J. Urol.* **152**(5 Pt 1), 1438–42.

Cook, A., Huddart, R., Jay, G., Norman, A., Dearnaley, D. and Horwich, A. (2000) The utility of tumour markers in assessing the response to chemotherapy in advanced bladder cancer. *Br. J. Cancer* **82**(12), 1952–7.

Coppin, C.M., Gospodarowicz, M.K., James, K. *et al.* (1996) Improved local control of invasive bladder cancer by concurrent cisplatin and preoperative or definitive radiation. The National Cancer Institute of Canada Clinical Trials Group. *J. Clin. Oncol.* **14**(11), 2901–7.

Cordon-Cardo, C., Wartinger, D.D., Melamed, M.R., Fair, W. and Fradet, Y. (1992) Immunopathologic analysis of human urinary bladder cancer. Characterization of two new antigens associated with low-grade superficial bladder tumors. *Am. J. Pathol.* **140**(2), 375–85.

Cordon-Cardo, C., Zhang, Z.F., Dalbagni, G. *et al.* (1997) Cooperative effects of p53 and pRB alterations in primary superficial bladder tumors. *Cancer Res.* **57**(7), 1217–21.

Crawford, E.D., McKenzie, D., Mansson, W. *et al.* (1986) Adverse reactions to the intravesical administration of doxorubicin hydrochloride: report of 6 cases. *J. Urol.* **136**(3), 668–9.

Crawford, E.D., Das, S. and Smith, J.A. Jr (1987) Preoperative radiation therapy in the treatment of bladder cancer. *Urol. Clin. North Am.* **14**(4), 781–7.

Davidson, S.E., Symonds, R.P., Snee, M.P., Upadhyay, S., Habeshaw, T. and Robertson, A.G. (1990) Assessment of factors influencing the outcome of radiotherapy for bladder cancer. *Br. J. Urol.* **66**(3), 288–93.

Decarli, A., Peto, J., Piolatto, G. *et al.* (1985) Bladder cancer mortality of workers exposed to aromatic amines: analysis of models of carcinogenesis. *Br. J. Cancer* **51**, 707–12.

De Neve, W., Lybeert, M.L., Goor, C., Crommelin, M.A. and Ribot, J.G. (1992) T1 and T2 carcinoma of the urinary bladder: long term results with external, preoperative, or interstitial radiotherapy. *Int. J. Radiat. Oncol. Biol. Phys.* **23**(2), 299–304.

D'Hallewin, M.A. and Baert, L. (1996) Initial evaluation of the bladder tumor antigen test in superficial bladder cancer. *J. Urol.* **155**, 475–6.

Dimopoulos, M.A., Deliveliotis, C., Moulopoulos, L.A. *et al.* (1998) Treatment of patients with metastatic urothelial carcinoma and impaired renal function with single-agent docetaxel. *Urology* **52**(1), 56–60.

Dolin, P.J. and Cook-Mozaffari, P. (1992) Occupation and bladder cancer: a death-certificate study. *Br. J. Cancer* **66**(3), 568–78.

Dreicer, R., Gustin, D.M., See, W.A. and Williams, R.D. (1996) Paclitaxel in advanced urothelial carcinoma: its role in patients with renal insufficiency and as salvage therapy [*see* comments]. *J. Urol.* **156**(5), 1606–8.

Duchesne, G., Bolger, J., Griffiths, G. *et al.* (2000) A randomized trial of hypofractionated schedules of palliative radiotherapy in the management of bladder carcinoma: results of Medical Research Council Trial BA09. *Int. J. Radiol. Oncol. Biol. Phys.* **47**(2), 379–88.

Duncan, W. and Quilty, P.M. (1986) The results of a series of 963 patients with transitional cell carcinoma of the urinary bladder primarily treated by radical megavoltage X-ray therapy. *Radiother. Oncol.* **7**(4), 299–310.

Eapen, L., Stewart, D., Danjoux, C. *et al.* (1989) Intraarterial cisplatin and concurrent radiation for locally advanced bladder cancer. *J. Clin. Oncol.* **7**(2), 230–5.

Edelman, G.M. and Crossin, K.L. (1991) Cell adhesion molecules: implications for a molecular histology. *Annu. Rev. Biochem.* **60**, 155–90.

Eder, I.E., Stenzl, A., Hobisch, A., Cronauer, M.V., Bartsch, G. and Klocker, H. (1997) Expression of transforming growth factors beta-1, beta 2 and beta 3 in human bladder carcinomas. *Br. J. Cancer* **75**(12), 1753–60.

Ellis, W.J., Blumenstein, B.A., Ishak, L.M. and Enfield, D.L. (1997) Clinical evaluation of the BTA TRAK assay and comparison to voided urine cytology and the Bard BTA test in patients with recurrent bladder tumors. The Multi Center Study Group. *Urology* **50**(6), 882–7.

Esrig, D., Elmajian, D., Groshen, S. *et al.* (1994) Accumulation of nuclear p53 and tumor progression in bladder cancer [*see* comments]. *N. Engl. J. Med.* **331**(19), 1259–64.

Esrig, D., Freeman, J.A., Elmajian, D.A. *et al.* (1996) Transitional cell carcinoma involving the prostate with a proposed staging classification for stromal invasion [*see* comments]. *J. Urol.* **156**(3), 1071–6.

Farrow, G.M., Utz, D.C., Rife, C.C. and Greene, L.F. (1977) Clinical observations on sixty-nine cases of *in situ* carcinoma of the urinary bladder. *Cancer Res.* **37**(8 Pt 2), 2794–8.

Fitzpatrick, J.M., West, A.B., Butler, M.R., Lane, V. and O'Flynn, J.D. (1986) Superficial bladder tumors (stage pTa, grades 1 and 2): the importance of recurrence pattern following initial resection. *J. Urol.* **135**(5), 920–2.

Fossa, S.D., Aass, N., Ous, S., Waehre, H., Ilner, K. and Hannisdal, E. (1996a) Survival after curative treatment of muscle-invasive bladder cancer. *Acta Oncol.* **35**(suppl. 8), 59–65.

Fossa, S.D., Sternberg, C., Scher, H.I. *et al.* (1996b) Survival of patients with advanced urothelial cancer treated with cisplatin-based chemotherapy. *Br. J. Cancer* **74**(10), 1655–9.

Fradet, Y. and Cordon-Cardo, C. (1993) Critical appraisal of tumor markers in bladder cancer. *Semin. Urol.* **11**(3), 145–53.

Fradet, Y., Tardif, M., Bourget, L. and Robert, J. (1990) Clinical cancer progression in urinary bladder tumors evaluated by multiparameter flow cytometry with monoclonal antibodies. Laval University Urology Group. *Cancer Res.* **50**(2), 432–7.

Freiha, F., Reese, J. and Torti, F. (1996) A randomized trial of radical cystectomy versus radical cystectomy plus cisplatin, vinblastine and methotrexate chemotherapy for muscle invasive bladder cancer. *J. Urol.* **155**, 495–9.

Fung, C.Y., Shipley, W.U., Young, R.H. *et al.* (1991) Prognostic factors in invasive bladder carcinoma in a prospective trial of preoperative adjuvant chemotherapy and radiotherapy [*see* comments]. *J. Clin. Oncol.* **9**(9), 1533–42.

Gabrilove, J.L., Jakubowski, A., Scher, H. *et al.* (1988) Effect of granulocyte colony-stimulating factor on neutropenia and associated morbidity due to chemotherapy for transitional-cell carcinoma of the urothelium. *N. Engl. J. Med.* **318**(22), 1414–22.

Gagliano, R., Levin, H., El-Bolkainy, M.N. *et al.* (1983) Adriamycin versus adriamycin plus *cis*-diamminedichloroplatinum (DDP) in advanced transitional cell bladder carcinoma. A Southwest Oncology Group study. *Am. J. Clin. Oncol.* **6**(2), 215–18.

Geller, N.L., Sternberg, C.N., Penenberg, D., Scher, H. and Yagoda, A. (1991) Prognostic factors for survival of patients with advanced urothelial tumors treated with methotrexate, vinblastine, doxorubicin, and cisplatin chemotherapy. *Cancer* **67**(6), 1525–31.

Goldgar, D.E., Easton, D.F., Cannon-Albright, L.A. and Skolnick, M.H. (1994) Systematic population-based assessment of cancer risk in first-degree relatives of cancer probands. *J. Natl Cancer Inst.* **86**(21), 1600–7.

Gospodarowicz, M.K., Hawkins, N.V., Rawlings, G.A. *et al.* (1989) Radical radiotherapy for muscle invasive transitional cell carcinoma of the bladder: failure analysis. *J. Urol.* **142**(6), 1448–53.

Greiner, R., Skaleric, C. and Veraguth, P. (1977) The prognostic significance of ureteral obstruction in carcinoma of the bladder. *Int. J. Radiat. Oncol. Biol. Phys.* **2**(11–12), 1095–100.

Grossfeld, G.D., Ginsberg, D.A., Stein, J.P. *et al.* (1997) Thrombospondin-1 expression in bladder cancer: association with p53 alterations, tumor angiogenesis, and tumor progression. *J. Natl Cancer Inst.* **89**(3), 219–27.

Grossman, H.B., Liebert, M., Antelo, M. *et al.* (1998) p53 and RB expression predict progression in T1 bladder cancer. *Clin. Cancer Res.* **4**(4), 829–34.

Hall, R.R. (ed.) (1999) *Clinical management of bladder cancer.* London: Arnold, Oxford University Press.

Hankey, B.F., Edwards, B.K., Ries, L.A., Percy, C.L. and Shambaugh, E. (1991) Problems in cancer surveillance: delineating *in situ* and invasive bladder cancer [editorial]. *J. Natl Cancer Inst.* **83**(6), 384–5.

Harker, W.G., Meyers, F.J., Freiha, F.S. *et al.* (1985) Cisplatin, methotrexate, and vinblastine (CMV): an effective chemotherapy regimen for metastatic transitional cell carcinoma of the urinary tract. A Northern California Oncology Group study. *J. Clin. Oncol.* **3**(11), 1463–70.

Hartge, P., Silverman, D., Hoover, R. *et al.* (1987) Changing cigarette habits and bladder cancer risk: a case-control study. *J. Natl Cancer Inst.* **78**(6), 1119–25.

Hasui, Y., Osada, Y., Kitada, S. and Nishi, S. (1994) Significance of invasion to the muscularis mucosae on the progression of superficial bladder cancer. *Urology* **43**, 782–6.

Hatch, T.R. and Barry, J.M. (1986) The value of excretory urography in staging bladder cancer. *J. Urol.* **135**(1), 49.

Hawnaur, J.M. (1993) Staging of cervical and endometrial carcinoma. *Clin. Radiol.* **47**(1), 7–13.

Hein, D.W. (1988) Acetylator genotype and arylamine-induced carcinogenesis. *Biochim. Biophys. Acta* **948**, 37–66.

Hendry, W.F., Gowing, N.F. and Wallace, D.M. (1974) Surgical treatment of urethral tumours associated with bladder cancer. *Proc. R. Soc. Med.* **67**(4), 304–7.

Heney, N.M., Ahmed, S., Flanagan, M.J. *et al.* (1983) Superficial bladder cancer: progression and recurrence. *J. Urol.* **130**, 1083–6.

Henry, K., Miller, J., Mori, M., Loening, S. and Fallon, B. (1988) Comparison of transurethral resection to radical therapies for stage B bladder tumors. *J. Urol.* **140**(5), 964–7.

Herr, H.W. (1987) Conservative management of muscle-infiltrating bladder cancer: prospective experience. *J. Urol.* **138**(5), 1162–3.

Herr, H.W. (1992) Transurethral resection in regionally advanced bladder cancer. *Urol. Clin. North Am.* **19**(4), 695–700.

Herr, H.W. (2000) Tumour progression and survival of patients with high grade, noninvasive papillary (TaG3) bladder tumours: 15-year outcome. *J. Urol.* **163**(1), 60–1.

Herr, H.W., Badalament, R.A., Amato, D.A., Laudone, V.P., Fair, W.R. and Whitmore, W.F. Jr (1989) Superficial bladder cancer treated with bacillus Calmette–Guérin: a multivariate analysis of factors affecting tumor progression. *J. Urol.* **141**(1), 22–9.

Herr, H.W., Wartinger, D.D., Fair, W.R. and Oettgen, H.F. (1992) Bacillus Calmette–Guérin therapy for superficial bladder cancer: a 10-year followup. *J. Urol.* **147**(4), 1020–3.

Hillcoat, B.L., Raghavan, D., Matthews, J. *et al.* (1989) A randomized trial of cisplatin versus cisplatin plus methotrexate in advanced cancer of the urothelial tract. *J. Clin. Oncol.* **7**(6), 706–9.

Hofstetter, A., Frank, F., Keiditsch, E. and Bowering, R. (1981) Endoscopic Neodymium-YAG laser application for destroying bladder tumors. *Eur. Urol.* **7**(5), 278–82.

Hoover, R. and Cole, P. (1971) Population trends in cigarette smoking and bladder cancer. *Am. J. Epidemiol.* **94**, 409–18.

Horwich, A., Dearnaley, D.P., Huddart, R.A., Graham, J., Bessel, E., Mason, M. *et al.* (1999) A trial of accelerated fractionation (AF) in T2/3 bladder cancer. *The European Cancer Conference, Vienna.*

Hoskin, P.J., Saunders, M.I. and Dische, S. (1999) Hypoxic radiosensitizers in radical radiotherapy for patients with bladder carcinoma: hyperbaric oxygen, misonidazole, and accelerated radiotherapy, carbogen, and nicotinamide. *Cancer* **86**(7), 1322–8.

Housset, M., Maulard, C., Chretien, Y. *et al.* (1993) Combined radiation and chemotherapy for invasive transitional-cell carcinoma of the bladder: a prospective study. *J. Clin. Oncol.* **11**(11), 2150–7.

Huddart, R.A., Lau, F.N., Guerrero-Urbano, T. *et al.* (2001) Accelerated chemotherapy in the treatment of urothelial cancer. *Clin. Oncol.* **13**, 279–83.

Huland, H., Otto, U., Droese, M. and Kloppel, G. (1984) Long-term mitomycin C instillation after transurethral resection of superficial bladder carcinoma: influence on recurrence, progression and survival. *J. Urol.* **132**(1), 27–9.

Huland, H., Kloppel, G., Feddersen, I. *et al.* (1990) Comparison of different schedules of cytostatic intravesical instillations in patients with superficial bladder carcinoma: final evaluation of a prospective multicenter study with 419 patients. *J. Urol.* **144**(1), 68–71.

Husband, J.E.S., Johnson, R.J. and Reznek, R.H. (1999) *A guide to practical use of MRI in oncology.* London: Royal College of Radiologists.

Inskip, P.D., Monson, R.R., Wagoner, J.K. *et al.* (1990) Cancer mortality following radiotherapy for uterine bleeding. *Radiat. Res.* **123**, 331–44.

Izadifar, V., de Boer, W.I., Muscatelli-Groux, B., Maille, P., van der Kwast, T.H. and Chopin, D.K. (1999) Expression of transforming growth factor beta1 and its receptors in normal human urothelium and human transitional cell carcinomas. *Hum. Pathol.* **30**(4), 372–7.

Jaeger, T.M., Weidner, N., Chew, K. *et al.* (1995) Tumor angiogenesis correlates with lymph node metastases in invasive bladder cancer. *J. Urol.* **154**(1), 69–71.

Jakse, G., Frommhold, H. and zur Nedden, D. (1985) Combined radiation and chemotherapy for locally advanced transitional cell carcinoma of the urinary bladder. *Cancer* **55**(8), 1659–64.

Johnston, B., Morales, A., Emerson, L. and Lundie, M. (1997) Rapid detection of bladder cancer: a comparative study of point of care tests [*see* comments]. *J. Urol.* **158**(6), 2098–101.

Jouanneau, J., Gavrilovic, J., Caruelle, D. *et al.* (1991) Secreted or nonsecreted forms of acidic fibroblast growth factor produced by transfected epithelial cells influence cell morphology, motility, and invasive potential. *Proc. Natl Acad. Sci. USA* **88**(7), 2893–7.

Ketterer, B. (1988) Protective role of glutathione and glutathione transferases in mutagenesis and carcinogenesis. *Mutat. Res.* **202**(2), 343–61.

Khandekar, J., Elson, P., DeWys, W. *et al.* (1985) Comparative activity and toxicity of *cis*-diamminedichloroplatinum (DDP) and a combination of doxorubicin, cyclophosphamide and DDP in disseminated transitional cell carcinomas of the urinary tract. *J. Clin. Oncol.* **3**, 539–45.

Kiemeney, L.A. and Schoenberg, M. (1996) Familial transitional cell carcinoma. *J. Urol.* **156**(3), 867–72.

Kim, B., Semelka, R.C., Ascher, S.M., Chalpin, D.B., Carroll, P.R. and Hricak, H. (1994) Bladder tumor staging: comparison of contrast-enhanced CT, T1- and T2-weighted MR imaging, dynamic gadolinium-enhanced imaging, and late gadolinium-enhanced imaging. *Radiology* **193**(1), 239–45.

Knowles, M.A. (1999) The genetics of transitional cell carcinoma: progress and potential clinical application. *BJU Int.* **84**(4), 412–27.

Kock, N.G., Hulten, L. and Myrvold, H.E. (1989a) Ileoanal anastomosis with interposition of the ileal 'Kock pouch'. Preliminary results. *Dis. Colon Rectum* **32**(12), 1050–4.

Kock, N.G., Ghoneim, M.A., Lycke, K.G. and Mahran, M.R. (1989b) Replacement of the bladder by the urethral Kock pouch: functional results, urodynamics and radiological features. *J. Urol.* **141**(5), 1111–16.

Koloszy, Z. (1991) Histological 'self control' in transurethral resection of bladder tumours. *Br. J. Urol.* **67**, 162–4.

Kondas, J. and Szentgyorgyi, E. (1992) Transurethral resection of 1250 bladder tumours. *Int. Urol. Nephrol.* **24**(1), 35–42.

Koraitim, M., Kamal, B., Metwalli, N. and Zaky, Y. (1995) Transurethral ultrasonographic assessment of bladder carcinoma: its value and limitation [*see* comments]. *J. Urol.* **154**(2 Pt 1), 375–8.

Koss, J.C., Arger, P.H., Coleman, B.G., Mulhern, C.B. Jr, Pollack, H.M. and Wein, A.J. (1981) CT staging of bladder carcinoma. *Am. J. Roentgenol.* **137**(2), 359–62.

Kubota, Y., Hosaka, M., Fukushima, S. and Kondo, I. (1993) Prophylactic oral UFT therapy for superficial bladder cancer. *Cancer* **71**(5), 1842–5.

Kurth, K.H., Denis, L., Bouffioux, C. *et al.* (1995) Factors affecting recurrence and progression in superficial bladder tumours. *Eur. J. Cancer* **31**a(11), 1840–6.

Kurth, K., Tunn, U., Ay, R. *et al.* (1997) Adjuvant chemotherapy for superficial transitional cell bladder carcinoma: long-term results of a European Organization for Research and Treatment of Cancer randomized trial comparing doxorubicin, ethoglucid and transurethral resection alone. *J. Urol.* **158**(2), 378–84.

Lamm, D.L. (1992) Carcinoma *in situ. Urol. Clin. North Am.* **19**(3), 499–508.

Lamm, D.L., Blumenstein, B.A., Crawford, E.D. *et al.* (1991) A randomized trial of intravesical doxorubicin and immunotherapy with bacille Calmette–Guérin for transitional-cell carcinoma of the bladder. *N. Engl. J. Med.* **325**(17), 1205–9.

Lamm, D.L., van der Meijden, P.M., Morales, A. *et al.* (1992) Incidence and treatment of complications of bacillus Calmette–Guérin intravesical therapy in superficial bladder cancer. *J. Urol.* **147**(3), 596–600.

Lamm, D.L., Riggs, D.R., Shriver, J.S., vanGilder, P.F., Rach, J.F. and DeHaven, J.I. (1994) Megadose vitamins in bladder cancer: a double-blind clinical trial. *J. Urol.* **151**(1), 21–6.

Lamm, D.L., Blumenstein, B.A., Sarosdy, M. *et al.* (1997) Significant long term patient benefit with BCG maintenance therapy: a South-west Oncology Group study. *J. Urol.* 157.

Lerner, S.P., Skinner, D.G., Lieskovsky, G. *et al.* (1993) The rationale for *en bloc* pelvic lymph node dissection for bladder cancer patients with nodal metastases: long-term results. *J. Urol.* **149**(4), 758–64.

Levine, L.A. and Richie, J.P. (1989) Urological complications of cyclophosphamide [*see* comments]. *J. Urol.* **141**(5), 1063–9.

Lipponen, P.K. and Eskelinen, M.J. (1994) Expression of epidermal growth factor receptor in bladder cancer as related to established prognostic factors, oncoprotein (c-erbB-2, p53) expression and long-term prognosis. *Br. J. Cancer* **69**(6), 1120–5.

Lipponen, P.K. and Eskelinen, M.J. (1995) Reduced expression of E-cadherin is related to invasive disease and frequent recurrence in bladder cancer. *J. Cancer Res. Clin. Oncol.* **121**(5), 303–8.

Liukkonen, T., Rajala, P., Raitanen, M., Rintala, E., Kaasinen, E. and Lipponen, P. (1999) Prognostic value of MIB-1 score, p53, EGFr, mitotic index and papillary status in primary superficial (Stage pTa/T1) bladder cancer: a prospective comparative study. The Finnbladder Group. *Eur. Urol.* **36**(5), 393–400.

Loehrer, P. and De Mulder, P. (1997) Management of metastatic bladder cancer. In Raghaven, D.S.H., Leibel, S. and Lange, P.H. (eds), *Principles and practice of genitourinary oncology.* Philadelphia: Lippincott–Raven.

Loehrer, P.J. Sr, Einhorn, L.H., Elson, P.J. *et al.* (1992) A randomized comparison of cisplatin alone or in combination with methotrexate, vinblastine, and doxorubicin in patients with metastatic urothelial carcinoma: a cooperative group study. *J. Clin. Oncol.* **10**(7), 1066–73. [published erratum appears in *J. Clin. Oncol.* 1993 Feb; **11**(2), 384].

Loehrer, P.J. Sr, Elson, P., Dreicer, R. *et al.* (1994) Escalated dosages of methotrexate, vinblastine, doxorubicin, and cisplatin plus recombinant human granulocyte colony-stimulating factor in advanced urothelial carcinoma: an Eastern Cooperative Oncology Group trial. *J. Clin. Oncol.* **12**(3), 483–8.

Logothetis, C.J., Dexeus, F.H., Finn, L. *et al.* (1990) A prospective randomized trial comparing MVAC and CISCA chemotherapy for patients with metastatic urothelial tumors. *J. Clin. Oncol.* **8**(6), 1050–5.

Logothetis, C., Finn, L., Amato, R., Hassan, E. and Sella, A. (1992) Escalated MVAC ± rhGM-CSF in metastatic transitional cell carcinoma. *Proc. Am. Soc. Clin. Oncol.* **11**, 202.

Lynch, C.F., Platz, C.E., Jones, M.P. and Gazzaniga, J.M. (1991) Cancer registry problems in classifying invasive bladder cancer. *J. Natl Cancer Inst.* **83**(6), 429–33.

MacVicar, D. and Husband, J. (1994) Radiology in the staging of bladder cancer. *Br. J. Hosp. Med.* **51**, 454–8.

Malmstrom, P.U., Rintala, E., Wahlqvist, R., Hellstrom, P., Hellsten, S. and Hannisdal, E. (1996) Five-year followup of a prospective trial of radical cystectomy and neoadjuvant chemotherapy: Nordic Cystectomy Trial I. The Nordic Cooperative Bladder Cancer Study Group [*see* comments]. *J. Urol.* **155**(6), 1903–6.

Mao, L., Schoenberg, M.P., Scicchitano, M. *et al.* (1996) Molecular detection of primary bladder cancer by microsatellite analysis. *Science* **271**(5249), 659–62.

Martinez-Pineiro, J.A. and Martinez-Pineiro, L. (1997) BCG update: intravesical therapy. *Eur. Urol.* **31**(suppl. 1), 31–41.

Martinez-Pineiro, L., Gonzalez-Peramato, P., Hidalgo, L. *et al.* (1991) [Primary bladder adenocarcinoma: retrospective study of 11 cases and general review.] *Arch. Esp. Urol.* **44**(2), 131–8.

Martinez-Pineiro, J.A., Martin, M.G., Arocena, F. *et al.* (1995) Neoadjuvant cisplatin chemotherapy before radical cystectomy in invasive transitional cell carcinoma of the bladder: a prospective randomized phase II study. *J. Urol.* **153**, 964–73.

McCaffrey, J.A., Hilton, S., Mazumdar, M. *et al.* (1997) Phase II trial of docetaxel in patients with advanced or metastatic transitional-cell carcinoma. *J. Clin. Oncol.* **15**(5), 1853–7.

McCredie, M. (1994) Bladder and kidney cancers. *Cancer Surv.* **19–20**, 343–68.

McCredie, M., Stewart, J.H., Ford, J.M. and MacLennan, R.A. (1983) Phenacetin-containing analgesics and cancer of the bladder or renal pelvis in women. *Br. J. Urol.* **55**(2), 220–4.

McLaughlin, J.K., Zdenek, H., Blot, W.J. *et al.* (1995) Smoking and cancer mortality among U.S. veterans: a 26 year follow-up. *Int. J. Cancer* **60**, 190–3.

Mead, G.M., Russell, M., Clark, P. *et al.* (1998) A randomized trial comparing methotrexate and vinblastine (MV) with cisplatin, methotrexate and vinblastine (CMV) in advanced transitional cell carcinoma: results and a report on prognostic factors in a Medical Research Council study. MRC Advanced Bladder Cancer Working Party. *Br. J. Cancer* **78**(8), 1067–75.

Mellon, K., Wright, C., Kelly, P., Horne, C.H. and Neal, D.E. (1995) Long-term outcome related to epidermal growth factor receptor status in bladder cancer. *J. Urol.* **153**(3 Pt 2), 919–25.

Messing, E.M., Young, T.B., Hunt, V.B. *et al.* (1995) Hematuria home screening: repeat testing results. *J. Urol.* **154**(1), 57–61.

Miller, L.S. (1980) T3 bladder cancer: the case for higher radiation dosage. *Cancer* **45**(suppl. 7), 1875–8.

Montie, J.E., Whitmore, W.F. Jr, Grabstald, H.M. and Yagoda, A. (1983) Unresectable carcinoma of the bladder. *Cancer* **51**(12), 2351–5.

Montie, J.E., Straffon, R.A. and Stewart, B.H. (1984) Radical cystectomy without radiation therapy for carcinoma of the bladder. *J. Urol.* **131**(3), 477–82.

Moonen, L.M., Horenblas, S., van der Voet, J.C., Nuyten, M.J. and Bartelink, H. (1994) Bladder conservation in selected T1G3 and muscle-invasive T2–T3a bladder carcinoma using combination therapy of surgery and iridium-192 implantation. *Br. J. Urol.* **74**(3), 322–27.

Moore, M.J., Iscoe, N. and Tannock, I.F. (1993) A phase II study of methotrexate, vinblastine, doxorubicin and cisplatin plus recombinant human granulocyte-macrophage colony stimulating factors in patients with advanced transitional cell carcinoma. *J. Urol.* **150**, 1131–4.

Moore, M.J., Tannock, I.F., Ernst, D.S., Huan, S. and Murray, N. (1997) Gemcitabine: a promising new agent in the treatment of advanced urothelial cancer. *J. Clin. Oncol.* **15**(2), 3441–5.

Morrison, A.S., Ahlbom, A., Verhoek, W.G. *et al.* (1985) Occupation and bladder cancer in Boston, USA, Manchester, UK, and Nagoya, Japan. *J. Epidemiol. Community Health* **39**(4), 294–300.

Morrison, R. (1975) The results of treatment of cancer of the bladder – a clinical contribution to radiobiology. *Clin. Radiol.* **26**(1), 67–75.

Murphy, W.M., Rivera-Ramirez, I., Medina, C.A., Wright, N.J. and Wajsman, Z. (1997) The bladder tumor antigen (BTA) test compared to voided urine cytology in the detection of bladder neoplasms [*see* comments]. *J. Urol.* **158**(6), 2102–6.

Natale, R., Grossman, H., Blumenstein, B. *et al.* (2001) SWOG 8710 (INT-0080): randomized phase III trial of neoadjuvant MVAC + cystectomy versus cystectomy alone in patients with locally advanced bladder cancer. *Proc. Am. Soc. Clin. Oncol.* **20**, 2a abstract 3.

Neal, D.E., Smith, K., Fennelly, J.A., Bennett, M.K., Hall, R.R. and Harris, A.L. (1989) Epidermal growth factor receptor in human bladder cancer: a comparison of immunohistochemistry and ligand binding. *J. Urol.* **141**(3), 517–21.

Nogueira March, J.L., Ojea, A., Figueiredo, L., Jamardo, D., Diez, E. and Perez Villanueva, J. (1985) Evaluation of the efficacy of oral methotrexate in the prevention of recurrence of superficial bladder tumours. *Br. J. Urol.* **57**(3), 306–7.

Nutting, C. and Huddart, R.A. (2000) Rethinking the secondary prevention of superficial bladder cancer: is there a role for retinoids? *Br. J. Urol.* **85**, 1023–6.

Okamura, K., Miyake, K., Koshikawa, T. and Asai, J. (1990) Growth fractions of transitional cell carcinomas of the bladder defined by the monoclonal antibody Ki-67. *J. Urol.* **144**(4), 875–8.

Oosterlinck, W., Kurth, K.H., Schroder, F., Bultinck, J., Hammond, B. and Sylvester, R. (1993) A prospective European Organization for Research and Treatment of Cancer Genitourinary Group randomized trial comparing transurethral resection followed by a single intravesical instillation of epirubicin or water in single stage Ta, T1 papillary carcinoma of the bladder. *J. Urol.* **149**(4), 749–52.

O'Reilly, M.S., Holmgren, L., Chen, C. and Folkman, J. (1996) Angiostatin induces and sustains dormancy of human primary tumors in mice. *Nat. Med.* **2**(6), 689–92.

Overgaard, J. and Horsman, M.R. (1996) Modification of hypoxia-induced radioresistance in tumors by the use of oxygen and sensitizers. *Semin. Radiat. Oncol.* **6**(1), 10–21.

Pagano, F., Bassi, P., Milani, C., Piazza, N., Meneghini, A. and Garbeglio, A. (1992) BCG in superficial bladder cancer: a review of phase III European trials. *Eur. Urol.* **21**(suppl. 2), 7–11.

Papamichael, D., Gallagher, C.J., Oliver, R.T., Johnson, P.W. and Waxman, J. (1997) Phase II study of paclitaxel in pretreated patients with locally advanced/metastatic cancer of the bladder and ureter. *Br. J. Cancer* **75**(4), 606–7.

Parkin, D.M., Whelan, S.L., Ferlay, J. *et al.* (1997) *Cancer incidence in five continents*. Vol. VII. Lyon: International Agency for Research on Cancer, Scientific publications, No. 120.

Parmar, M.K.B. and Burdett, S. (1999) Neoadjuvant chemotherapy in the treatment of muscle invasive bladder cancer (commentary). In Hall, R.R. (ed.), *Clinical management of bladder cancer*. London: Arnold, 250–63.

Parmar, M.K., Freedman, L.S., Hargreave, T.B. and Tolley, D.A. (1989) Prognostic factors for recurrence and followup policies in the treatment of superficial bladder cancer: report from the British Medical Research Council Subgroup on Superficial Bladder Cancer (Urological Cancer Working Party). *J. Urol.* **142**(2 Pt 1), 284–8.

Parsons, J.T. and Million, R.R. (1988) Planned preoperative irradiation in the management of clinical stage B2-C (T3) bladder carcinoma. *Int. J. Radiat. Oncol. Biol. Phys.* **14**(4), 797–810.

Pawinski, A., Sylvester, R., Kurth, K.H. *et al.* (1996) A combined analysis of European Organization for Research and Treatment of Cancer, and Medical Research Council randomized clinical trials for the prophylactic treatment of stage TaT1 bladder cancer. European Organization for Research and Treatment of Cancer Genitourinary Tract Cancer Cooperative Group and the Medical Research Council Working Party on Superficial Bladder Cancer. *J. Urol.* **156**(6), 1934–40.

Pearce, H.D., Reed, R.R. and Hodges, C.V. (1978) Radical cystectomy for bladder cancer. *J. Urol.* **119**(2), 216–18.

Pederson-Bjergaard, J., Ersboll, J. and Hansen, V.L. (1988) Carcinoma of the urinary bladder after treatment with cyclophosphamide for non-Hodgkin's lymphoma. *N. Engl. J. Med.* **318**, 1028–32.

Pernot, M., Hubert, J., Guillemin, F. *et al.* (1996) Combined surgery and brachytherapy in the treatment of some cancers of the bladder (partial cystectomy and interstitial iridium-192). *Radiother. Oncol.* **38**(2), 115–20.

Piper, J.M., Tonascia, J. and Matanoski, G.M. (1985) Heavy phenacetin use and bladder cancer in women aged 20 to 49 years. *N. Engl. J. Med.* **313**(5), 292–5.

Pisters, L.L., Tykochinsky, G. and Wajsman, Z. (1991) Intravesical bacillus Calmette–Guérin or mitomycin C in the treatment of carcinoma *in situ* of the bladder following prior pelvic radiation therapy. *J. Urol.* **146**(6), 1514–17.

Pollack, A., Zagars, G.K., Cole, C.J., Dinney, C.P., Swanson, D.A. and Grossman, H.B. (1995) The relationship of local control to distant metastasis in muscle invasive bladder cancer. *J. Urol.* **154**(6), 2059–63.

Pollera, C.F., Ceribelli, A., Crecco, M. and Calabresi, F. (1994) Weekly gemcitabine in advanced bladder cancer: a preliminary report from a phase I study. *Ann. Oncol.* **5**(2), 182–4.

Prout, G.R. Jr (1976) The surgical management of bladder carcinoma. *Urol. Clin. North Am.* **3**(1), 149–75.

Pugh, R.C.B. (1981) Bladder Cancer. In Oliver, R.T.D., Hendry, W.F. and Bloom, H.J.G. (eds), *Principles in combination therapy*. London: Butterworths.

Quilty, P.M. and Duncan, W. (1986) The influence of hemoglobin level on the regression and long term local control of transitional cell carcinoma of the bladder following photon irradiation. *Int. J. Radiat. Oncol. Biol. Phys.* **12**(10), 1735–42.

Quilty, P.M., Hargreave, T.B., Smith, G. and Duncan, W. (1987) Do normal mucosal biopsies predict prognosis in patients with transitional cell carcinoma of bladder treated by radical radiotherapy? *Br. J. Urol.* **59**(3), 242–7.

Raghavan, D. (1990) Chemotherapy for advanced bladder cancer: 'Midsummer Night's Dream' or 'Much Ado About Nothing'? *Br. J. Cancer* **62**(3), 337–40.

Redman, B.G., Smith, D.C., Flaherty, L., Du, W. and Hussain, M. (1998) Phase II trial of paclitaxel and carboplatin in the treatment of advanced urothelial carcinoma. *J. Clin. Oncol.* **16**(5), 1844–8.

Reisinger, S.A., Mohiuddin, M. and Mulholland, S.G. (1992) Combined pre- and postoperative adjuvant radiation therapy for bladder cancer – a ten year experience [*see* comments]. *Int. J. Radiat. Oncol. Biol. Phys.* **24**(3), 463–8.

Reznikoff, C.A., Belair, C.D., Yeager, T.R. *et al.* (1996) A molecular genetic model of human bladder cancer pathogenesis. *Semin. Oncol.* **23**, 571–84.

Richards, B., Newling, D., Fossa, S. *et al.* (1983) Vincristine in advanced bladder cancer: a European organization for research on treatment of cancer (EORTC) phase II study. *Cancer Treat. Rep.* **67**(6), 575–7.

Riddle, P.R., Chisholm, G.D., Trott, P.A. and Pugh, R.C. (1975) Flat carcinoma *in situ* of bladder *Br. J. Urol.* **47**(7), 829–33.

Rintala, E., Hannisdahl, E., Fossa, S.D., Hellsten, S. and Sander, S. (1993) Neoadjuvant chemotherapy in bladder cancer: a randomized study. Nordic Cystectomy Trial I. *Scand. J. Urol. Nephrol.* **27**(3), 355–62.

Roehrborn, C.G., Sagalowsky, A.I. and Peters, P.C. (1991) Long-term patient survival after cystectomy for regional metastatic transitional cell carcinoma of the bladder. *J. Urol.* **146**(1), 36–9.

Roth, B.J., Dreicer, R., Einhorn, L.H. *et al.* (1994) Significant activity of paclitaxel in advanced transitional-cell carcinoma of the urothelium: a phase II trial of the Eastern Cooperative Oncology Group. *J. Clin. Oncol.* **12**(11), 2264–70.

Rotman, M., Aziz, H., Porrazzo, M. *et al.* (1990) Treatment of advanced transitional cell carcinoma of the bladder with irradiation and concomitant 5-fluorouracil infusion. *Int. J. Radiat. Oncol. Biol. Phys.* **18**(5), 1131–7.

Rozan, R., Albuisson, E., Donnarieix, D. *et al.* (1992) Interstitial iridium-192 for bladder cancer (a multicentric survey: 205 patients). *Int. J. Radiat. Oncol. Biol. Phys.* **24**(3), 469–77.

Rubino, G.F., Scansetti, G., Piolatto, G. *et al.* (1982) The carcinogenic effect of aromatic-amines: an epidemiological study on the role of *O*-toluidine and 4,4'-methylene-*bis*(2-methylaniline) in inducing bladder cancer in man. *Environ. Res.* **27**, 241–54.

Russell, K.J., Boileau, M.A., Higano, C. *et al.* (1990) Combined 5-fluorouracil and irradiation for transitional cell carcinoma of the urinary bladder [*see* comments]. *Int. J. Radiat. Oncol. Biol. Phys.* **19**(3), 693–9.

Sagerman, R.H., Veenema, R.J., Guttmann, R., Dean, A.L. Jr and Uson, A.C. (1968) Preoperative irradiation for carcinoma of the bladder. *Am. J. Roentgenol. Radium Ther. Nucl. Med.* **102**(3), 577–80.

Sarosdy, M.F. (1997) The use of the BTA Test in the detection of persistent or recurrent transitional-cell cancer of the bladder. *World J. Urol.* **15**(2), 103–6.

Sarosdy, M.F. and Lamm, D.L. (1989) Long-term results of intravesical bacillus Calmette–Guérin therapy for superficial bladder cancer. *J. Urol.* **142**(3), 719–22.

Sarosdy, M.F. and De Vere White, R.W. (1995) Results of a multicentre trial using the BTA test to monitor for and diagnose recurrent bladder cancer. *J. Urol.* **154**, 379–83.

Sato, N., Sumiya, H., Isaka, S., Shimazaki, J. and Matsuzaki, O. (1992) [Prognostic factors for progression of superficial bladder cancer]. *Nippon Hinyokika Gakkai Zasshi* **83**(8), 1263–9.

Sauer, R., Dunst, J., Altendorf-Hofmann, A., Fischer, H., Bornhof, C. and Schrott, K.M. (1990) Radiotherapy with and without cisplatin in bladder cancer [*see* comments]. *Int. J. Radiat. Oncol. Biol. Phys.* **19**(3), 687–91.

Saxman, S.B., Propert, K.J., Einhorn, L.H. *et al.* (1997) Long-term follow-up of a phase III intergroup study of cisplatin alone or in combination with methotrexate, vinblastine, and doxorubicin in patients with metastatic urothelial carcinoma: a cooperative group study. *J. Clin. Oncol.* **15**(7), 2564–9.

Schelhammer, P.F. (1994) Intravesical BCG treatment of superficial transitional cell carcinoma of the bladder and prostatic urethra. In Pagano, F.P. (ed.) *BCG immunotherapy in superficial bladder cancer.* Cleup: Badova.

Scher, H., Herr, H., Sternberg, C. *et al.* (1989) Neo-adjuvant chemotherapy for invasive bladder cancer. Experience with the M-VAC regimen. *Br. J. Urol.* **64**(3), 250–6.

Schoenberg, M.P., Walsh, P.C., Breazeale, D.R., Marshall, F.F., Mostwin, J.L. and Brendler, C.B. (1996) Local recurrence and survival following nerve sparing radical cystoprostatectomy for bladder cancer: 10-year followup [*see* comments]. *J. Urol.* **155**(2), 490–4.

Schuller, J., Walther, V., Schmiedt, E., Staehler, G., Bauer, H.W. and Schilling, A. (1982) Intravesical ultrasound tomography in staging bladder carcinoma. *J. Urol.* **128**(2), 264–6.

Schulman, C.C., Robinson, M., Denis, L. *et al.* (1982) Prophylactic chemotherapy of superficial transitional cell bladder carcinoma: an EORTC randomized trial comparing thiotepa, an epipodophyllotoxin (VM26) and TUR alone. *Eur. Urol.* **8**(4), 207–12.

Seidman, A., Scher, H., Gabrilove, J. *et al.* (1993) Dose-intensification of MVAC with recombinant granulocyte colony-stimulating factor as initial therapy in advanced urothelial cancer. *J. Clin. Oncol.* **11**, 408–14.

Seligman, P.A. and Crawford, E.D. (1991) Treatment of advanced transitional cell carcinoma of the bladder with continuous-infusion gallium nitrate. *J. Natl Cancer Inst.* **83**(21), 1582–4.

Sell, A., Jakobsen, A., Nerstrom, B., Sorensen, B.L., Steven, K. and Barlebo, H. (1991) Treatment of advanced bladder cancer category T2 T3 and T4a. A randomized multicenter study of preoperative irradiation and cystectomy versus radical irradiation and early salvage cystectomy for residual tumor. DAVECA protocol 8201. Danish Vesical Cancer Group, *Scand. J. Urol. Nephrol. Suppl.* **138**, 193–201.

Shearer, R.J., Chilvers, C.F., Bloom, H.J., Bliss, J.M., Horwich, A. and Babiker, A. (1988) Adjuvant chemotherapy in T3 carcinoma of the bladder. A prospective trial: preliminary report. *Br. J. Urol.* **62**(6), 558–64.

Shipley, W.U., Rose, M.A., Perrone, T.L., Mannix, C.M., Heney, N.M. and Prout, G.R. Jr (1985) Full-dose irradiation for patients with invasive bladder carcinoma: clinical and histological factors prognostic of improved survival. *J. Urol.* **134**(4), 679–83.

Shipley, W.U., Kaufman, D.S., Heney, N.M., Griffin, P.P., Althausen, A.F. and Prout, G.R. Jr (1990) The integration of chemotherapy, radiotherapy and transurethral surgery in bladder-sparing approaches for patients with invasive tumors. *Prog. Clin. Biol. Res.* **353**, 85–94.

Shipley, W.U., Winter, K.A., Kaufman, D.S. *et al.* (1998) Phase III trial of neoadjuvant chemotherapy in patients with invasive bladder cancer treated with selective bladder preservation by combined radiation therapy and chemotherapy: initial results of Radiation Therapy Oncology Group 89-03 [*see* comments]. *J. Clin. Oncol.* **16**(11), 3576–83.

Skinner, D.G. (1982) Management of invasive bladder cancer. A meticulous pelvic node dissection can make a difference. *J. Urol.* **145**, 459.

Skinner, D.G. and Lieskovsky, G. (1984) Contemporary cystectomy with pelvic node dissection compared to preoperative radiation therapy plus cystectomy in management of invasive bladder cancer. *J. Urol.* **131**(6), 1069–72.

Skinner, D. and Lieskovsky, G. (1988) Management of invasive and high grade bladder cancer. In Skinner, D. and Lieskovsky, G. (eds), *Diagnosis and management of genitourinary cancer.* Philadelphia: WB Saunders, 295–312.

Skinner, D.G., Daniels, J.R., Russell, C.A. *et al.* (1991) The role of adjuvant chemotherapy following cystectomy for invasive bladder cancer: a prospective comparative trial. *J. Urol.* **145**(3), 459–64.

Slack, N.H., Bross, I.D. and Prout, G.R. Jr (1977) Five-year follow-up results of a collaborative study of therapies for carcinoma of the bladder. *J. Surg. Oncol.* **9**(4), 393–405.

Smaaland, R., Akslen, L.A., Tonder, B., Mehus, A., Lote, K. and Albrektsen, G. (1991) Radical radiation treatment of invasive and locally advanced bladder carcinoma in elderly patients. *Br. J. Urol.* **67**(1), 61–9.

Smith, J.A.J., Crawford, E.D., Blumenstein, B. *et al.* (1988) A randomized prospective trial of preoperative irradiation plus radical cystectomy plus surgery alone for transitional cell carcinoma of the bladder. A Southwest Oncology Group Study. *J. Urol.* **139**, 266A.

Solbin, L.H. and Wittekind, C.H. (eds) (1997) Staging of urinary bladder cancer. *TNM classification of malignant tumours.* International Union Against Cancer 5th edn. New York: Wiley-Liss, 201–13.

Soloway, M.S. and Ford, K.S. (1983) Thiotepa-induced myelosuppression: review of 670 bladder instillations. *J. Urol.* **130**(5), 889–91.

Soloway, M.S., Einstein, A., Corder, M.P., Bonney, W., Prout, G.R. Jr and Coombs, J. (1983) A comparison of cisplatin and the combination of cisplatin and cyclophosphamide in advanced urothelial cancer. A National Bladder Cancer Collaborative Group A Study. *Cancer* **52**(5), 767–72.

Soloway, M.S., Briggman, J.V., Carpinito, G.A. *et al.* (1996) Use of a new tumor marker, urinary NMP22, in the detection of occult or rapidly recurring transitional cell carcinoma of the urinary tract following surgical treatment. *J. Urol.* **156**, 363–7.

Solsona, E., Iborra, I., Ricos, J.V., Monros, J.L. and Dumont, R. (1992) Feasibility of transurethral resection for muscle-infiltrating carcinoma of the bladder: prospective study. *J. Urol.* **147**(6), 1513–15.

Stadler, W., Kuzel, T., Raghavan, D., Levine, E., Vogelzang, N. and Dorr, F.A. (1995) A phase II study of gemcitabine in the treatment of patients with advanced transitional cell carcinoma. *Proc. Am. Soc. Clin. Oncol.* **14**, 241.

Sternberg, C. (1996) Neoadjuvant and adjuvant chemotherapy in locally advanced bladder cancer. *Semin. Oncol.* **23**, 621–32.

Sternberg, C.N., Yagoda, A. and Scher, H.I. (1988) Chemotherapy for advanced urothelial tract tumors: the M-VAC regimen. *Prog. Clin. Biol. Res.* **277**, 45–51.

Sternberg, C.N., Yagoda, A., Scher, H.I. *et al.* (1989) Methotrexate, vinblastine, doxorubicin, and cisplatin for advanced transitional cell carcinoma of the urothelium. Efficacy and patterns of response and relapse. *Cancer* **64**(12), 2448–58.

Sternberg, C.N., de Mulder, P.H.M., van Oosterom, A.T., Fossa, S.D., Giannarelli, D. and Soedirman, J.R. (1993) Escalated M-VAC chemotherapy and recombinant human granulocyte–macrophage colony-stimulating factor (rhGM-CSF) in patients with advanced urothelial tract tumours. *Ann. Oncol.* **4**, 403–7.

Sternberg, C.N., Raghaven, D., Ohi, Y. *et al.* (1995) Neoadjuvant and adjuvant chemotherapy in advanced disease – what are the effects on survival and prognosis? *Int. J. Urol.* **2**(suppl. 2), 76–88 [published erratum appears in *Int. J. Urol.* 1995 Jul; **2**(3), 214].

Sternberg, C.N., de Mulder, P.H., Schornagel, J.H. *et al.* (2001) Randomized phase III trial of high-dose-intensity methotrexate, vinblastine, doxorubicin, and cisplatin (MVAC) chemotherapy and recombinant human granulocyte colony-stimulating factor versus classic MVAC in advanced urothelial tract tumors. European Organization for Research and Treatment of Cancer Protocol No. 30924. *J. Clin. Oncol.* **19**, 2638–46.

Stockle, M., Myenburg, W., Wellek, S. *et al.* (1993) The role of M-VAC polychemotherapy in the treatment of advanced urothelial carcinoma of the bladder. *Ann. Urol.* **27**, 51–7.

Studer, U., Bacchi, M., Biedermann, C. *et al.* (1994) Adjuvant cisplatin chemotherapy following cystectomy for bladder cancer: results of a prospective randomized trial. *J. Urol.* **152**, 81–4.

Sur, R.K., Clinkard, J., Jones, W.G. *et al.* (1993) Changes in target volume during radiotherapy treatment of invasive bladder carcinoma. *Clin. Oncol.* **5**(1), 30–3.

Sweeney, P., Kursh, E.D. and Resnick, M.I. (1992) Partial cystectomy. *Urol. Clin. North Am.* **19**(4), 701–11.

Takeichi, M. (1991) Cadherin cell adhesion receptors as a morphogenetic regulator. *Science* **251**, 1451–5.

Thomas, D.J., Roberts, J.T., Hall, R.R. and Reading, J. (1999) Radical transurethral resection and chemotherapy in the treatment of muscle-invasive bladder cancer: a long-term follow-up. *BJU Int.* **83**(4), 432–7.

Thrasher, J.B. and Crawford, E.D. (1992) Complications of intravesical chemotherapy. *Urol. Clin. North Am.* **19**(3), 529–39.

Tokunaga, H., Lee, D.H., Kim, I.Y., Wheeler, T.M. and Lerner, S.P. (1999) Decreased expression of

transforming growth factor beta receptor type I is associated with poor prognosis in bladder transitional cell carcinoma patients. *Clin. Cancer Res.* **5**(9), 2520–5.

Tolley, D.A., Parmar, M.K., Grigor, K.M. *et al.* (1996) The effect of intravesical mitomycin C on recurrence of newly diagnosed superficial bladder cancer: a further report with 7 years of follow up. *J. Urol.* **155**(4), 1233–8.

Travis, L.B., Curtis, R.E., Glimelius, B. *et al.* (1995) Bladder and kidney cancer following cyclophosphamide therapy for non-Hodgkin's lymphoma. *J. Natl Cancer Inst.* **87**(7), 524–30.

Trialists ICo. (1999) Neoadjuvant cisplatin, methotrexate and vinblastine chemotherapy for muscle-invasive bladder cancer: a randomised controlled trial. *Lancet* **354**, 533–40.

Troner, M., Birch, R., Omura, G.A. and Williams, S. (1987) Phase III comparison of cisplatin alone versus cisplatin, doxorubicin and cyclophosphamide in the treatment of bladder (urothelial) cancer: a Southeastern Cancer Study Group trial. *J. Urol.* **137**(4), 660–2.

Turner, A.G., Hendry, W.F., Williams, G.B. and Bloom, H.J. (1977) The treatment of advanced bladder cancer with methotrexate. *Br. J. Urol.* **49**(7), 673–8.

Turner, S.L., Swindell, R., Bowl, N. *et al.* (1997) Bladder movement during radiation therapy for bladder cancer: implications for treatment planning. *Int. J. Radiat. Oncol. Biol. Phys.* **39**(2), 355–60.

Vale, J.A., A'Hern, R.P., Liu, K. *et al.* (1993) Predicting the outcome of radical radiotherapy for invasive bladder cancer. *Eur. Urol.* **24**(1), 48–51.

van der Meijden, A.P.M. (1997) Ta, T1 Bladder cancer: what can we learn from EORTC trials. *Urol. Int.* **4**, 15–19.

van der Werf-Messing, B. (1979) Preoperative irradiation followed by cystectomy to treat carcinoma of the urinary bladder category T3NX, 0–4M0. *Int. J. Radiat. Oncol. Biol. Phys.* **5**(3), 395–401.

van Oosterom, A.T., Fossa, S.D., Mulder, J.H., Calciati, A., de Pauw, M. and Sylvester, R. (1985) Mitoxantrone in advanced bladder carcinoma. A phase II study of the EORTC Genito-urinary Tract Cancer Cooperative Group. *Eur. J. Cancer Clin. Oncol.* **21**(9), 1013–14.

Vaughn, D.J., Malkowicz, S.B., Zoltick, B. *et al.* (1998) Paclitaxel plus carboplatin in advanced carcinoma of the urothelium: an active and tolerable outpatient regimen. *J. Clin. Oncol.* **16**(1), 255–60.

von der Maase, H., Hansen, S.W., Roberts, J.T. *et al.* (2000) Gemcitabine and cisplatin versus methotrexate, vinblastine, doxorubicin, and cisplatin in advanced or metastatic bladder cancer: results of a large randomized, multinational, multicenter, phase III study. *J. Clin. Oncol.* **17**, 3068–77.

Wallace, D.M., Raghavan, D., Kelly, K.A. *et al.* (1991) Neo-adjuvant (pre-emptive) cisplatin therapy in invasive transitional cell carcinoma of the bladder. *Br. J. Urol.* **67**(6), 608–15.

Walsh, J.W., Amendola, M.A., Konerding, K.F., Tisnado, J. and Hazra, T.A. (1980) Computed tomographic detection of pelvic and inguinal lymph-node metastases from primary and recurrent pelvic malignant disease. *Radiology* **137**(1 Pt 1); 157–66.

Walsh, P.C. and Mostwin, J.L. (1984) Radical prostatectomy and cystoprostatectomy with preservation of potency. Results using a new nerve-sparing technique. *Br. J. Urol.* **56**(6), 694–7.

Weinerman, P.M., Arger, P.H. and Pollack, H.M. (1982) CT evaluation of bladder and prostate neoplasms. *Urol. Radiol.* **4**(2–3), 105–14.

Whitmore, W.F. Jr and Batata, M. (1984) Status of integrated irradiation and cystectomy for bladder cancer. *Urol. Clin. North Am.* **11**(4), 681–91.

Wijkstrom, H., Norming, U., Lagerkvist, M., Nilsson, B., Naslund, I. and Wiklund, P. (1998) Evaluation of clinical staging before cystectomy in transitional cell bladder carcinoma: a long-term follow-up of 276 consecutive patients. *Br. J. Urol.* **81**(5), 686–91.

Wijnmaalen, A., Helle, P.A., Koper, P.C. *et al.* (1997) Muscle invasive bladder cancer treated by transurethral resection, followed by external beam radiation and interstitial iridium-192. *Int. J. Radiat. Oncol. Biol. Phys.* **39**(5), 1043–52.

Wishnow, K.I. and Dmochowski, R. (1988) Pelvic recurrence after radical cystectomy without preoperative radiation. *J. Urol.* **140**(1), 42–3.

Witte, R.S., Elson, P., Bono, B. *et al.* (1997) Eastern Cooperative Oncology Group phase II trial of ifosfamide in the treatment of previously treated advanced urothelial carcinoma. *J. Clin. Oncol.* **15**(2), 589–93.

Wolf, H., Olsen, P.R. and Hojgaard, K. (1985) Urothelial dysplasia concomitant with bladder tumours: a determinant for future new occurrences in patients treated by full-course radiotherapy. *Lancet* **1**(8436), 1005–8.

Yoshida, K., Sugino, T., Tahara, H. *et al.* (1997) Telomerase activity in bladder carcinoma and its implication for noninvasive diagnosis by detection of exfoliated cancer cells in urine. *Cancer* **79**(2), 362–9.

Young, D.C. and Garnick, M.B. (1988) Chemotherapy in bladder cancer: the North American experience. In Raghavan, D. (ed.), *The management of bladder cancer.* London: Edward Arnold.

Yura, Y., Hayashi, O., Kelly, M. and Oyasu, R. (1989) Identification of epidermal growth factor as a component of the rat urinary bladder tumor-enhancing urinary fractions. *Cancer Res.* **49**(6), 1548–53.

Zielinski, C.C., Schnack, B., Grbovic, M. *et al.* (1998) Paclitaxel and carboplatin in patients with metastatic urothelial cancer: results of a phase II trial. *Br. J. Cancer* **78**(3), 370–4.

29

Prostate

ROSHAN AGARWAL AND JONATHAN WAXMAN

INTRODUCTION

Prostate cancer is the second most common malignancy in men in most developed countries, and its incidence has increased significantly over recent years (Silverberg and Lubera, 1983). In the USA the lifetime probability of developing prostate cancer is 15.4 per cent, or one in six. In 1997, more than 209 900 American men were diagnosed with prostate cancer and more than 41 800 died from this disease (Parker *et al.*, 1997). In England and Wales death rates have trebled over the last 30 years. Carcinoma of the prostate is rare under the age of 40, and its incidence increases exponentially with age (Young *et al.*, 1981). There is a 10-fold geographical variation in the incidence of both incidental and clinically significant prostatic cancer (Yantani *et al.*, 1982). This chapter reviews the biology and management of prostate cancer.

AETIOLOGY

Genetic factors are though to be of little importance in the aetiology of prostate cancer. It is estimated that less than 5 per cent of all prostate cancer is hereditary. The risk of prostate cancer is increased by a factor of 1.3 if there is an affected father in the family, and by a factor of 2.5 if there is a brother who has prostate cancer (Hayes *et al.*, 1995).

Environmental factors are suggested by the higher incidence of prostate cancer in the successive generations of emigrants from low to high incidence areas, as shown by studies of Japanese migrants to North America (Buell and Dunn, 1965). Environmental factors such as chemical carcinogens or co-carcinogens may have a role in the aetiology of prostate cancer. A number of studies have evaluated the role of diet in the development of prostate cancer in which a high intake of saturated fat and low levels of dietary selenium, vitamin E and vitamin D have been associated with an increased risk of malignancy (Brawley and Parnes, 2000). Evidence supporting a role for infective agents, such as herpes simplex, cytomegalovirus and *Neisseria* gonococcus, in the aetiology of prostate cancer are inconclusive. Radiation exposure may be significant in the aetiology of prostate cancer. An analysis was performed of deaths reported amongst 39 546 people employed by the UK Anatomic Energy Authority between 1946 and 1979. The only malignancy clearly related to exposure to radiation was carcinoma of the prostate (Beral *et al.*, 1985).

Genetic abnormalities thought to predispose to the development of prostate cancer include those of the androgen receptor gene in exon A and the length of the CAG trinucleotide repeat sequence. This codes for glutamine residues in the N-terminal region of the androgen receptor, which affects its transcriptional activity. The number of CAG repeat dependent transcriptional activity and its variation among racial groups, such as African Americans, Caucasians, and Asian Americans, appears to reflect the incidence of prostate cancer in these groups (Coetzee and Ross, 1994). In addition, more recently, allelic variations of the vitamin D receptor have also been shown to be associated with alterations in the risk of prostate cancer (Brawley and Parnes, 2000).

Prostate cancer, in common with other malignancies, is thought to arise following a sequence of at least 8–10 genetic mutational events. A number of candidate chromosomal regions and genes involved in these events have been identified using classical cytogenetics, fluorescent in-situ hybridization, comparative genomic hybridization and studies of loss of heterozygosity. Early events in the development of prostate cancer appear to be the loss of tumour suppressive genes, such as p53, which is mutated in up to 64 per cent of tumours and p21 in up to 55 per cent (Burton et al., 2000). The p73 gene has recently been identified. This tumour suppressor gene has significant sequence homology to p53 and appears to be mutated in prostate cancer (Burton et al., 2000). MMAC1/p10, however, is the most widely mutated tumour suppressor gene in prostate cancer and may contribute to the acquisition of the metastatic phenotype (Teng et al., 1997). The development of the hormone refractory phenotype, however, appears to be related to the overexpression of the mutant p53 and Bcl-2 families of proteins as well as amplification of the androgen receptor (Apakama et al., 1996).

Premalignant change, carcinoma in-situ, precedes the development of many cancers. Intra-epithelial neoplasia is seen in the prostate, but unlike other cancers, the relationship of these changes to the development of invasive cancer is not clear. These changes may be present in the prostate of men from the age of 20 to 30. Prostatic intra-epithelial neoplasia (PIN) is divided into low and high grade, and includes the continuum from uncontrolled hyperplasia to the development of an anaplastic morphology with nuclear polymorphism and microinvasion of the basement membrane. PIN has been found in 4–16.5 per cent of needle biopsies of the peripheral zone of the prostate in various series (Bostwick et al., 1995).

PATHOLOGY

Over 70 per cent of tumours of the prostate arise from the acinar epithelium of the peripheral zone of the gland, and over 99 per cent are adenocarcinomas. Some carcinomas arise from the ductal epithelium and are transitional cell carcinomas. Only very rarely do malignant tumours arise from the fibromuscular stroma (less than 0.3 per cent). Equally rarely, tumours of other organs may metastasize or spread into the prostate. Apart from malignant lymphoma and carcinoma of the bladder, this is most unusual.

Histological recognition of prostatic cancer depends on the overall assessment of the architecture which, in cancer, loses the organized lobular arrangement seen in the benign gland and upon the cytology of individual cells. The prostatic cancer cell cytoplasm may contain large amounts of acid phosphatase and prostate-specific antigen (PSA) (Burton et al., 2000). Using immunohistochemistry for these antigens, it is possible to differentiate prostatic carcinoma cells from other tumour cells. In cases where the diagnosis of malignancy is unclear, a number of studies have demonstrated the utility of staining for high molecular weight cytokeratins, such as 34β E12 (Samaratunga and Singh, 1997).

In order to predict the clinical behaviour and aggressiveness of prostatic carcinoma, so that the most appropriate therapeutic regimen can be chosen and the prognosis determined, several grading systems have been developed by pathologists (Broders, 1926; Mostofi, 1975; Gleason et al., 1977; Brawn et al., 1982; Schroeder et al., 1985; Gaeta et al., 1986). The system in most common use is the Gleason method of grading. The Gleason combined grading allows the two most predominant forms of glandular differentiation to be scored separately for each section. The Gleason score correlates well with the prognosis in localized prostatic cancer where the treatment options are radiotherapy, surgery or observation (Ruijter et al., 1996). There is considerable inter- and intra-observer variation in the reporting of tumour grade.

SYMPTOMS AND PRESENTATION

Early prostatic cancer is usually asymptomatic and the only clinical manifestation may be induration within the substance of the prostate gland. As the tumour arises in the peripheral zone of the prostate, symptoms of prostatism are late events or may result from accompanying benign prostate hyperplasia. Haematuria is uncommon but may occur secondary to infection or erosion of the gland. Perineal pain may occur in late disease. Weight loss, cachexia, pain and neurological complications are late symptoms and related to metastases. The differential diagnosis of prostatic induration or hardness includes prostatitis, prostatic calculi, granulomatous prostatitis and tuberculosis.

DIAGNOSIS, EXAMINATION, INVESTIGATION AND BIOPSY

A diagnosis of prostate cancer will be suggested by the finding of a hard irregular gland on rectal examination, the presence of sclerotic lesions on a plain X-ray performed as part of the investigation of low back pain, or the detection of an elevated serum PSA. It is essential that the diagnosis is confirmed by histological or cytological examination of the prostatic tissue.

Fine-needle aspiration cytology of the prostate can be carried out as an outpatient procedure without anaesthetic, with minimal trauma to the prostate and a low incidence of complications. However, this technique has not gained widespread popularity, which is probably related to its limited sensitivity (approximately 80 per cent) when compared with needle biopsy (Engelstein et al., 1994).

Needle biopsy of the prostate with or without the assistance of transrectal ultrasound is the standard approach to the diagnosis of prostatic cancer. Needle biopsy may be performed under local anaesthetic as an outpatient procedure, using either a transperineal or a transrectal approach. The transperineal approach is associated with a slightly lower risk of complications such as sepsis (Thompson et al., 1982). In addition, in comparisons of 14 gauge and 18 gauge bioptic needles for biopsy, use of an 18 gauge needle with a bioptic gun is associated with less pain and lower risk of complications, and achieves an equivalent rate of tumour detection (Lessells et al., 1997). The current standard approach is to obtain sextant biopsies. In addition, any radiologically suspicious lesions on transrectal ultrasound are also biopsied. However, some authors have argued that the use of sextant biopsies may be inadequate for sampling the whole gland as it is associated with a false-negative rate of 10–13 per cent in various series (Lessells et al., 1997).

In addition to biopsy, newly diagnosed patients with prostate cancer should also undergo measurement of serum PSA, acid and alkaline phosphatase, chest X-ray, radionucleotide bone scan with appropriate skeletal X-rays, and an abdomino-pelvic computed tomography (CT) scan in patients with clinically localized prostate cancer.

PSA is the most sensitive and specific tumour marker for prostate cancer (Oesterling, 1991). It is a serine protease and causes liquefaction of seminal coagulum. However, PSA may have a role in the growth and progression of prostate cancer, acting as an autocrine factor, but this as yet remains unproven (Oesterling, 1991). In addition, the synthesis and secretion of PSA by prostatic carcinoma cells is androgen dependent and therefore changes in PSA should be interpreted in conjunction with the patient's clinical state in determining the response of prostate cancer to treatment (Ruckle et al., 1994).

CT scanning of the pelvis is currently the most commonly employed imaging modality for ascertaining the extent of local spread of prostate cancer. Despite initial enthusiasm, the use of transrectal ultrasound has not proved to be more useful at determining seminal vesicle involvement or extracapsular spread than digital rectal examinations (Smith et al., 1997). More recently, magnetic resonance imaging (MRI) has been used to evaluate these patients and appears to have equal sensitivity to CT for detection of pelvic lymph node involvement. However, with the use of endorectal coils, it may prove to have greater sensitivity in detecting non-organ-confined disease (Schiebler et al., 1993).

MRI is also the most sensitive technique for detecting bone metastases in prostate cancer. However, it is limited by its relative inability to image the whole skeleton. Radionucleotide bone scans are used routinely instead

and have a false-negative rate of 11 per cent in all patients. In some patients with advanced disease, the entire skeleton may appear abnormal due to metastatic disease and is often referred to as a 'super scan'. In this circumstance all tracer is taken up by bone and the kidneys are not outlined (McCarthy and Pollack, 1991).

A number of nomograms have been developed which combine information from the clinical tumour stage, serum PSA and Gleason score on biopsy to provide a risk estimate of organ-confined versus non-organ-confined disease (Partin et al., 1993). These are useful for selecting the optimal treatment strategy for individual patients.

CLINICAL CLASSIFICATION AND STAGING

The most frequently used classification systems are the revised 1997 TNM classification of the UICC and AJCC (Sobind and Wittekind, 1997) and the Whitmore–Jewett system which groups patients with prostate cancer into four categories, denoted by the letters A–D. A comparison of the two systems is shown in Table 29.1. The TNM classification has considerable advantages in separating the assessment of the primary tumour from that of nodal disease and metastatic state. In addition, the TNM system further substratifies patients in the broad T-stage categories as the Jewett system and therefore provides a more precise prognostic stratification. The revised 1997 TNM classification also includes the T1c category for patients identified by needle biopsy following detection of an elevated PSA.

The pathological classification of the TNM system corresponds to the clinical classification and is indicated by the prefix 'p'. There is, however, considerable discrepancy between clinical and pathological stage. Schroeder et al. (1978) found that 52.3 per cent of 262 tumours classified as T1 and T2 were upgraded to pT3 and 15.1 per cent of 152 T3 tumours were downstaged to pT2 following radical prostatectomy.

NATURAL HISTORY AND METASTASES

The natural history of prostate cancer is variable and often unpredictable. Historical control data from the era prior to the development of hormonal therapies provides information on the natural history of advanced disease. A collected series of 795 untreated patients reported by Nesbitt and Baum (1950) had a 5-year survival rate of 10 per cent without metastatic disease and 6 per cent if metastases were present. This is in contrast to current studies, which report a 10-year survival for patients with small bulk localized prostate cancer of up to 80–90 per cent (Chodak et al., 1994). Part of the explanation for these different results may be differences in methods of staging and the effect of stage migration.

Table 29.1 *Comparison of Whitmore–Jewett and AJCC/UICC (1997) TNM staging systems*

Whitmore–Jewett staging	AJCC/UICC (1997) TNM staging
A1 Microscopic focus of well-differentiated adenocarcinoma in up to three foci of transurethral specimens or enucleation; clinically not apparent on rectal examination	T1 Tumour not palpable nor visible by imaging: (a) incidental finding in ≤5% of resected tissue; (b) incidental finding in >5% of resected tissue; (c) tumour identified on needle biopsy due to raised PSA level
A2 Tumour not well differentiated or present in more than three areas	T2 Tumour confined to prostate: (a) involving 1 lobe only; (b) involving both lobes
B1 Asymptomatic palpable nodule <1.5 cm; normal surrounding prostate; no capsular extension; normal acid phosphatase	T3 Tumour extends through the prostatic capsule: (a) extracapsular extension (uni- or bi-lateral); (b) tumour invades seminal vesicles
B2 Diffuse involvement of gland; no capsular extension; normal acid phosphatase	T4 Tumour is fixed or invades adjacent structures other than seminal vesicles
C Extensive local tumour with penetration through the capsule, contiguous spread; may involve seminal vesicles, bladder neck, lateral side wall of pelvis; acid phosphatase may be elevated; normal bone scan	N1 Metastases in regional lymph node(s)
D1 Metastases to pelvic lymph nodes below aortic bifurcation; acid phosphatase may be elevated	M1 Distant metastases: (a) non-regional lymph nodes; (b) bone; (c) other sites
D2 Bone or lymph node metastases above aortic bifurcation or other soft tissue metastases	

With the introduction and routine use of PSA testing from the mid-1980s, increasing number of patients have been diagnosed with prostate cancer, many of whom would have remained undiagnosed in their lifetime (Kamoi and Babaian, 1999). In the USA, the incidence of prostate cancer rapidly rose with the introduction of PSA testing and peaked in 1992. Since then the incidence in some parts of the country have declined. It is difficult to ascribe this change solely to screening. This is because just 20 per cent of the target population for prostate cancer screening are tested in the USA (Kamoi and Babaian, 1999). This compares with <2 per cent in the UK.

A more important consequence of PSA testing, however, has been the increase in the numbers of patients with early prostate cancer. In the UK, it is estimated that 60 per cent of tumours diagnosed are metastatic. By contrast, in Canada and in the USA, this figure is reported to be between 20 and 40 per cent (Kamoi and Babaian, 1999).

In addition to tumour stage, a variety of other tumour factors affect the natural history of the disease. In 1999 the College of American Pathologists developed a consensus statement on prognostic factors in prostate cancer (Bostwick *et al.*, 2000), in which they ranked prognostic factors into three categories:

1 factors proven to be of prognostic importance;
2 factors extensively studied whose importance remains to be validated and statistically robust studies;
3 factors not sufficiently studied to demonstrate their prognostic value.

Factors of proven value were PSA level at diagnosis, histological grade as Gleason score and TNM stage grouping. In patients undergoing radical prostatectomy, surgical margin status is also of value. Factors included in category 2 were tumour volume, histological type and DNA ploidy. Although angiogenesis and microvessel density counts have received significant attention recently, their value is as yet unproven in the context of prostate cancer. None of the molecular markers of prostate cancer has been applied as clinical tools to routinely give prognostic information.

Race and age have also been suggested as influencing the natural history of advanced disease. However, stage for stage, grade for grade, and treatment for treatment, clinically manifest prostate cancer behaves identically among all races and in all age groups (Levine and Wilchinsky, 1979).

Prostate cancer can progress through local invasion to involve the seminal vesicles, ureters and the bladder base. Invasion of the external urethral sphincter by prostate carcinoma is often responsible for symptoms of prostatism. Lymphatic spread commonly occurs to the iliac chain initially and in more advanced disease may involve the para-aortic lymph nodes. Vascular spread of prostate carcinoma is responsible for metastases to bone, lung, liver and adrenals. Bone metastases generally involve the axial skeleton and are thought to occur via Batson's plexus of pre-sacral veins. Over 80 per cent of patients who die from prostate cancer have evidence of bone involvement. Pulmonary involvement is less common, and may occur in 15–20 per cent of patients. Involvement of the liver and adrenal glands occurs in between 5 and 15 per cent or patients and is thought to be related to the high lipid content of these tissues and consequent high local concentration of androgens (Long and Husband, 1999).

SCREENING

As metastatic prostate cancer is currently incurable, increasing efforts have been directed at the early detection of disease at an organ-confined stage when it is potentially curable. With the advent of PSA testing, a number of screening strategies for prostate cancer, which combine PSA with digital rectal examination (DRE) and transrectal ultrasound, have been devised (Kamoi and Babaian, 1999). Although preliminary data from the USA on the incidence and mortality from prostate cancer would suggest a beneficial effect of regular PSA testing, the results of randomized controlled trials being conducted in Holland, Canada and in the USA by the National Cancer Institute (NCI) are awaited (Kamoi and Babaian, 1999).

CHEMOPREVENTION

In 1993, the US NCI began the Prostate Cancer Prevention Trial (PCPT) in which a total of 18 882 healthy men aged 55 years and above were randomized to receive either finasteride 5 mg/day or placebo for 7 years (Lippman, 2000). The rationale for the study has been the accumulating evidence of the importance of long-term androgenic stimulation in prostate carcinogenesis. Finasteride is a 5α-reductase inhibitor which prevents the conversion of testosterone to dihydrotestosterone, which has a 10-fold higher potency in prostatic tissue and is physiologically the primary ligand for the androgen receptor. By inhibiting androgenic stimulation of the prostate gland, it is hypothesized that the incidence of biopsy-proven prostate cancer will be reduced by at least 25 per cent.

Another chemoprevention trial in prostate cancer called SELECT has been planned by the US NCI. It is likely to be a 2×2 factorial study in which patients will be randomized to selenium versus placebo and vitamin E versus placebo (Lippman, 2000). This trial is based on incidental findings from two previous studies (Brawley and Parnes, 2000), one of selenium supplementation and the other of α-tocopherol supplementation, which showed substantial reductions in prostate cancer incidence. However, these studies were not initially designed to assess their effects on prostate cancer.

Recent data suggest that chemoprevention trials aimed at modifying dietary intake of vitamin D and saturated fats may also be beneficial in reducing the incidence of prostate cancer (Ma et al., 1998).

TREATMENT OF PRIMARY TUMOUR

The median age of patients presenting with carcinoma of the prostate is 72 years and many will die from causes unrelated to their malignancy (Parker et al., 1997). Treatment of prostate cancer has significant side-effects and it should always be asked if it is necessary to treat those it is possible to treat and is it possible to treat those in whom it is necessary to treat. Indeed, in keeping with the long natural history of this disease, those patients with low-grade early-stage localized tumours with a life expectancy of <10 years may be treated by delaying intervention unless the patient is symptomatic. The indications for and against treatment and the rationale for various treatment policies are discussed below for each stage according to the TNM system.

Stage I and II prostatic carcinoma

With the advent of PSA testing over the past 20 years, the number of patients being detected with stage I and II disease has been increasing (Kamoi and Babaian, 1999). Although these groups of patients with organ-confined disease are potentially curable, there is considerable controversy as to their optimal management. This has arisen due to the long natural history of the disease, especially of small organ-confined, well- to moderately differentiated disease. A series of patient managed by watchful waiting, reported by Chodak et al. (1994), shows survival comparable to those of the most radical prostatectomy series and that of the age-matched population without prostate cancer. However, studies directly comparing the principal treatment modalities of radical prostatectomy, external-beam radiotherapy, interstitial radiotherapy and watchful waiting, have not yet been performed. Indeed, there has only been one study by Paulson et al. (1982) of only 96 patients comparing external-beam radiotherapy with radical prostatectomy, which suggested that surgery was associated with an increased time to disease progression.

The rates of radical prostatectomy have dramatically risen over the past two decades (Lu-Yao and Greenberg, 1994). Radical prostatectomy can be conducted either using a retropubic or perineal approach with equivalent rates of tumour control and complications (Sullivan et al., 2000). Patients undergoing radical prostatectomy routinely also undergo a pelvic lymphadenectomy to ascertain nodal involvement. Lymphadenectomy in these patients is not therapeutic and patients with evidence of nodal involvement in frozen section are spared further surgery. Recent surgical series have shown an equivalence between pelvic lymphadenectomy, done either at laparotomy or laparoscopically. The latter is usually performed in patients undergoing surgery using the perineal approach. Not all patients, however, may need a lymphadenectomy as patients with small, well-differentiated tumours with low preoperative PSAs are unlikely to have nodal metastases. Various nomograms have been developed which predict the likelihood of nodal involvement based on Gleason score, clinical T stage and PSA (Bluestein et al., 1994). Following radical prostatectomy, pathological evaluation stratifies patients into three categories: organ-confined, specimen-confined and margin-positive disease with recurrence-free survival rates of 85 per cent, 54 per cent and 42 per cent at 10 years, respectively. Patients with lymph node involvement recur in 85 per cent by 5 years and 100 per cent by 10 years (Pisters, 1999).

Radical prostatectomy can result in significant morbidity. The most favourable results of surgery are from single institution studies, which report potency preservation in about two-thirds of patients who were potent prior to surgery, and urinary incontinence with the requirement for pads in 6 per cent (Catalona and Basler, 1993). However, an analysis of Medicare records on over 101 000 patients who had undergone radical prostatectomies between 1991 and 1994 showed an operative mortality rate of 0.54 per cent and a major complication rate of 28.6 per cent. In addition, the morbidity and mortality were significantly higher in patients older than 75 years. In this series, 30 per cent of patients reported the need for pads or clamps for urinary incontinence and 60 per cent of patients reported loss of potency (Yao et al., 1999). Although a number of series have suggested a beneficial effect of nerve-sparing radical prostatectomy, this has not been proven in clinical trial. It should be noted that some patients may also develop faecal incontinence following radical prostatectomy. In a survey of 907 men, 14 per cent reported moderate to large amounts of faecal incontinence (Bishoff et al., 1998).

Prostate carcinoma is relatively radiation insensitive. The tumour has a low growth rate and this results in a slow response to radiotherapy. Clinical evidence of complete remission may take several months and PSA values at 6 months are taken as most significant in the prediction of future progression (Pollack et al., 1999).

Conventional radiotherapy for stage I and II disease has involved the delivery of 60 Gy over 6 weeks using a three-field technique with usual field sizes of 8 cm × 8 cm. The long-term results of radiotherapy in patients with T1 and T2 disease are similar to those reported with radical prostatectomy with 10-year relapse-free survival rates of 70–90 per cent with overall survival of 40–70 per cent (Pollack et al., 1999). It has been argued that surgery leads to better results than radiotherapy in patients with poorly differentiated tumours (Paulson et al., 1982).

Amongst the acute complications of radiotherapy for prostatic carcinoma are cystitis, proctitis and sometimes enteritis. This can usually be managed with a combination of loperamide and anticholinergics. Long-term side-effects, however, also occur and urinary incontinence requiring pads or clamps may be needed by 2–11 per cent of patients, which compares favourably with radical prostatectomy (Crook et al., 1996). Potency also appears to be better preserved following radiotherapy, with between 10 and 40 per cent of patients reporting loss of potency (Crook et al., 1996). However, this may be an effect of the duration of follow-up in these studies, because the effects of radiotherapy on potency are late, occurring

many years after treatment. Proctitis, however, is a more common complication with radiotherapy than surgery and in a Medicare survey, 10 per cent of patients reported specially frequent bowel movements following radiotherapy compared with 3 per cent after radical prostatectomy (Fowler et al., 1996). In other series, between 20 and 27 per cent of patients reported bowel dysfunction (Pollack et al., 1999).

The advent of three-dimensional (3-D) conformal radiotherapy has enabled dose escalation to the tumour bed with a concomitant sparing of normal tissue. Doses in excess of 70 Gy can be delivered to the prostate, which is likely to result in improved local tumour control based on current data on PSA response. In addition, for equivalent doses, randomized studies have demonstrated a reduction in the incidence of significant proctitis using 3-D conformal radiotherapy (Dearnaley et al., 1999). The introduction of intensity modulated radiotherapy (IMRT) has the potential to further enhance local tumour control without increasing normal tissue toxicity (Pollack et al., 1999).

Interstitial radiotherapy as an alternative to or in combination with external-beam radiotherapy has also been used for the treatment of stage I and II prostate carcinoma. Historically, radioactive gold or iodine-125 seeds were implanted at surgery using a freehand approach. However, significant variation in inter- and intra-prostatic dose delivered and the surgical morbidity associated with surgery necessary to implant these seeds retropubicly has led to a shift to the ultrasound-guided perineal approach.

Due to technical limitations of dose rate and delivery, it is not possible to treat patients with extracapsular disease and therefore the ideal candidate should have a PSA ≤10 mg/ml, Gleason score ≤6 and stage ≤T2b (Beahrs et al., 1992). Evidence of bulky tumours or bilateral involvement are also contraindications to brachytherapy. Short-term results based on rates of PSA relapse suggest rates of local control similar to that of radical prostatectomy and external-beam radiation therapy but preservation of sexual potency has been reported in 86–90 per cent of patients (Blasko et al., 1995). However, due to variations in delivered dose, higher rates of cystitis and proctitis of between 10 and 15 per cent have been reported (Ragde et al., 1997). The results of studies with longer-term follow-up will be required before the role of interstitial radiotherapy in the management of patients with stage I and II tumours can be fully ascertained.

The role of hormonal therapy in patients with stage I and II tumours is confined primarily to clinical trials of neoadjuvant or adjuvant androgen ablation in combination with either surgery or radiotherapy. The use of neoadjuvant hormonal therapy is associated with a 20–30 per cent reduction in tumour volume and approximately 2 per cent complete pathological response rate (Zelefsky et al., 1997). In addition, patients have a lower rate of margin-positive disease. However, the impact of this on survival is unclear and further follow-up is required. Neoadjuvant hormonal therapy prior to external-beam radiation has also been shown to reduce the volume of rectal tissue included in the treatment field with the consequent improvement in the incidence of proctitis (Zelefsky *et al.*, 1997). However, the follow-up in these studies is too short to assess its impact in stage I and II disease on overall survival.

Stage III prostatic carinoma

The results of radical prostatectomy and external radiotherapy are uniformly poor in patients with locally advanced disease. In patients with capsular penetration and low-grade tumours, following radical prostatectomy only 54 per cent will remain free of biochemical relapse at 10 years, whilst only 42 per cent of patients with extracapsular penetration and high-grade disease are relapse free (Duncan *et al.*, 1993). In patients treated with external-beam radiotherapy with clinical stage III disease, overall 10-year survival rates of between 35 and 45 per cent have been reported. The main reason for these results appears to be inadequate local control of tumour in over 80 per cent of patients in both radiotherapy and surgical series of patients with locally advanced disease. At present there is currently no standard treatment for such patients.

In patients with evidence of extracapsular disease following radical prostatectomy and raised PSAs, salvage external-beam radiotherapy has been advocated by some groups, and complete PSA responses reported in 10–55 per cent of patients (American Society for Therapeutic Radiology and Oncology Consensus Panel, 1999). Other groups have advocated early hormonal therapy of these asymptomatic patients. As yet no consensus exists on the optimum management of these patients. However, the long natural history of this disease cautions against adoption of unproven therapeutic approaches. Indeed, in a retrospective analysis of nearly 2000 men who underwent radical prostatectomy at Johns Hopkins, 15 per cent of patients had evidence of PSA relapse at 5 years (Pound *et al.*, 1999). However, only a third of patients with biochemical relapse developed evidence of clinical metastases at 8 years, with a median time to death from the development of metastatic disease of a further 5 years. This group of asymptomatic patients received hormonal therapy only if they had evidence of metastatic disease.

Neoadjuvant and adjuvant hormonal therapy in combination with external-beam radiotherapy for locally advanced prostatic carcinoma has been shown to be beneficial compared with external-beam radiotherapy alone. Trials by the Radiation Therapy Oncology Group (RTOG) and European Organization for the Research and Treatment of Cancer (EORTC) have consistently demonstrated an advantage in both local disease-control freedom from metastases and overall disease-free survival with combined therapy. A meta-analysis performed by the Agency for Healthcare Policy and Research (AHCPR) demonstrated a hazard ratio of 0.63 at 5 years in overall survival in favour of radiation therapy plus androgen ablation compared with radiotherapy alone (AHCPR, 1999).

However, in patients with a limited life expectancy and co-morbidity who are asymptomatic, it has been suggested that treatment may be delayed until symptoms develop. The results of a Medical Research Council (MRC) trial in patients randomized to immediate androgen ablation versus delayed treatment suggested an improvement in overall survival and a lower incidence of disease complications in those patients receiving immediate treatment (Medical Research Council Prostate Cancer Working Party Investigators Group, 1997).

Stage IV or metastatic prostate carcinoma

Hormone therapy has remained the gold standard for treatment of patients with metastatic disease since the demonstration in 1941 by Huggins and Hodges of the benefits of orchiectomy or diethylstilboestrol in the management of these patients. The results of hormonal therapy were not systematically analysed until the 1960s when the Veterans' Administration Co-operative Urological Research Group (VACURG) initiated a number of studies in this malignancy (Byar, 1972). The VACURG randomized 266 patients with stage III disease and 220 patients with stage IV disease to orchiectomy and compared their survival with 262 patients with stage III disease and 223 patients with stage IV disease randomized to receive placebo. There was no difference in long-term survival between the two groups, which was 50 per cent for stage III and 20 per cent for stage IV patients at 5 years (Blackard *et al.*, 1973). These findings have been criticized because of substantial proportion of patients with untreated prostatic cancer with disease progression eventually received hormonal treatment. Crude survival as quoted did not take this factor into account. However, despite this, the study was of great significance and its true finding is that delayed as compared to early treatment results in an equivalent survival.

The Veterans' Group also analysed the results of oestrogen therapy. They compared the survival of 265 patients with stage III disease and 211 patients with stage IV prostatic cancer who were treated with 5 mg diethylstilboestrol daily with 262 patients with stage III disease 223 patients with stage IV prostatic cancer who received placebo (Byar, 1972). This study produced the extraordinary finding of an increased risk of death in patients with stage III and stage IV disease from cardiovascular events. This reached significance in stage III disease alone (VACURG, 1967). In patients with previous cardiovascular problems, cardiac morbidity due oestrogen therapy may reach 66 per cent compared with 11 per cent in controls without cardiac histories (Coronary Drug Project Research Group, 1970). This is the result of the effects of oestrogen on antithrombin III levels and plasma volume.

Lower doses of oestrogen therapy have been investigated in patients with prostatic cancer. Both 0.2 mg daily and 1 mg daily of diethylstilboestrol are found to be as effective in terms of survival as 5 mg daily (Byar, 1972). It has not, however, been proved that these lower dosages of oestrogen are without an excess of cardiovascular side-effects as compared with control or orchiectomy-treated patients. Because of the side-effects of the oestrogen treatment and patients' dislike of orchiectomy, alternative medical treatments for prostate cancer have been developed.

Cyproterone acetate is a progestogenic anti-androgen. It acts by decreasing testosterone synthesis and by inhibiting secretion of the pituitary gonadotrophins. It also displaces and competes with testosterone for its cytoplasmic and nuclear receptors. This compound was introduced into clinical practice in 1966, and early studies showed response rates similar to that expected with orchiectomy or oestrogen therapy in patients with metastatic disease. In a randomized study conducted by the EORTC comparing the response of patients treated with cyproterone acetate or diethylstilboestrol, a slightly higher response rate was reported with diethylstilboestrol but survival was equivalent in both groups (Schroeder et al., 1984).

Flutamide is an anti-androgen thought to act by competing with testosterone for its peripheral receptor. However, its metabolic effects are complex. The original work on flutamide was performed at the Memorial Sloan Kettering and published in 1978. Follow-up of the work there showed responses in 63 of 72 patients treated (Sogani et al., 1984). Subsequently, two other longer-acting non-steroidal anti-androgens have been developed: nilutamide and bicalutamide. Both these compounds have the advantage of once-daily dosing and a greater affinity for the testosterone receptor. However, nilutamide is associated with a very high incidence of visual disturbance, especially night blindness, and therefore not commonly used (Janknegt et al., 1993).

The use of bicalutamide has increased over recent years. It is a purer anti-androgen than flutamide and does not have gastrointestinal toxicity. Bicalutamide monotherapy is reported to allow up to 60 per cent of patients to maintain potency. However, due to the peripheral conversion of testosterone to oestrogen, 30–40 per cent of patients develop breast tenderness or gynaecomastia (Boccardo et al., 1999). Despite these encouraging findings, trials of bicalutamide monotherapy versus medical or surgical castration in advanced prostatic cancer have shown inferior results with anti-androgen monotherapy (AHCPR, 1999).

Long-term administration of ketoconazole is associated with the development of gynaecomastia and this is due to an inhibition of testicular and adrenal steroidogenesis. This compound has been used to treat patients with prostate cancer. Castrate levels of testosterone, although achieved initially, are not maintained (Trachtenberg and Pont, 1984). This agent has been withdrawn from use in this condition also because of its side-effects which include septicaemia and abnormalities of renal and hepatic function in testosterone-suppressive dosages.

Gonadotrophin-releasing hormone agonists were introduced in the early 1980s for the treatment of sex-hormone-dependent malignancy. These compounds act by decreasing the release and synthesis of the pituitary gonadotrophins and this is due to downregulation of the pituitary gonadotrophin-releasing hormone receptor. Randomized studies have been initiated comparing response with these agents with conventional therapy. The Leuprolide Study Group compared the response of 101 patients treated with 3 mg daily oral diethylstilboestrol with 98 patients treated with 1 mg daily leuprolide subcutaneously. Response rates were identical: 1 per cent of those in the leuprolide group had a completed response and 37 per cent a partial response, 2 per cent of the diethylstilboestrol group had a complete response and 44 per cent a partial response (Leuprolide Study Group, 1984). The median duration of response was identical at 48 weeks and the median duration of survival not significantly different (Garnick, 1986).

Gonadotrophin-releasing hormone agonist treatment has been compared with orchiectomy and an identical response rate achieved (Parmar et al., 1987). These compounds are stimulatory in the initial phases of treatment and as a result an acute exacerbation of tumour symptoms and signs may occur (Waxman et al., 1985). Several studies have now demonstrated that this may be avoided by anti-androgens given to the patient prior to and continued for 2–3 weeks after the initiation of gonadotrophin-releasing hormone agonist therapy. One- and 3-monthly depot preparations are currently available and 6-monthly and yearly depot preparations under development. Several studies have now shown equivalence in terms of response and overall survival between gonadotrophin-releasing hormone agonists and orchiectomy or diethylstilboestrol (AHCPR, 1999). In addition, patients prefer medical castration to orchiectomy. In view of the cardiovascular morbidity associated with diethylstilboestrol, gonadotrophin-releasing hormone agonist treatment should presently be the therapy of first choice in patients with advanced prostatic cancer. However, the treatment of metastatic prostate cancer with medical or surgical castration is not curative and associated with a median duration of response of only one year (Schroeder, 1999). Several strategies have therefore been developed to try and improve survival, which are discussed below.

COMBINED ANDROGEN BOCKADE

It was suggested by Labrie that, in a disease which is androgen-sensitive, it is important to eliminate the effects of all sources of androgen, which includes adrenal as well as testicular sources, by the use of anti-androgens such as flutamide in combination with orchiectomy or an luteinizing hormone-releasing hormone (LH-RH) agonist. Several trials have been conducted using a variety of steroidal and non-steroidal anti-androgens combined with medical-surgical castration over the past decade. In 2000, the Prostate Cancer Triallists' Collaborative Study Group published their meta-analysis of all available trials, which showed a 2.3 per cent improvement in survival with the use of non-steroidal anti-androgens only. However, this was associated with an increased incidence of gastrointestinal toxicity. In addition, the cost of combined androgen blockade is substantially more than that of medical or surgical castration alone.

INTERMITTENT ANDROGEN BLOCKADE

The concept of intermittent androgen suppression was first described by Klotz et al. (1986). This involves medical castration until a PSA nadir is reached, followed by discontinuation of the LH-RH agonist with recommencement when the PSA rises to a specified level. *In-vitro* studies suggest that this approach has the potential to reduce the toxicity and cost of treatment, as well as possibly delay the development of hormone resistance. In the clinical setting, patients regain non-castrate testosterone level 3 months from cessation of LH-RH agonist therapy and therefore this strategy may also reduce the toxicity of castration. Recovery rates are variable. Early clinical trials using this approach have demonstrated its clinical feasibility; however, results of randomized comparisons with continuous androgen ablation are awaited.

SEQUENTIAL ANDROGEN BLOCKADE

Another approach that has been developed to minimize the toxicity associated with castration for metastatic disease has been the use of newer agents, such as finasteride. Finasteride is an 5α-reductase inhibitor which inhibits the conversion of testosterone to dihydrotestosterone, which has a 10-fold greater affinity for the androgen receptor, and is thought to be the principal physiological ligand. Early studies demonstrated a 30–40 per cent fall in PSA levels with finasteride therapy (Fleshner and Trachtenberg, 1995). Although significant, this is significantly inferior to castration, which results in a response in over 80 per cent of patients. Combinations of finasteride and anti-androgens, such as bicalutamide and flutamide, are currently in trial. As these therapies have the added advantage of maintaining potency, they may prove useful in the treatment of patients with evidence of biochemical relapse following radiotherapy or radical prostatectomy without evidence of symptomatic progression. Clinical trials evaluating these approaches are currently in progress.

ADJUVANT CHEMOTHERAPY

In a trial with limited numbers of patients, an advantage to adjuvant chemotherapy to those patients with localized prostate cancer treated with mitozantrone has been shown (Wang et al., 2000). These findings require confirmation in trials involving large numbers of patients.

TREATMENT OF RELAPSED PROSTATIC CANCER

The comparative lack of success of endocrine treatments for relapsed prostatic cancer is in stark contrast to the initial responsiveness sensitivity of this disease. Biochemical evidence of relapse occurs after a median duration of remission of approximately 1 year and symptom progression 2 years later (Goktas and Crawford, 1999). At symptomatic relapse, the median duration of survival is 6–8 months. During this period there are many effective treatments that produce useful symptomatic palliation of disease.

Endocrine therapy for relapsed prostatic cancer

A number of second-line hormonal therapies have been evaluated in patients with relapsed prostate cancer following initial medical or surgical castration. In patients who have been treated with combined androgen blockade, it is now recognized that withdrawal of the anti-androgen (flutamide, bicalutamide) may be associated with a withdrawal response in 10–40 per cent of patients with a median duration of response of 3 months (Oh and Kantoff, 1998). The addition of an anti-androgen at relapse in patients treated by the LH-RH agonist or castration alone also results in responses of 5–15 per cent, which is thought to be due to the blockade of adrenal androgens (Oh and Kantoff, 1998). Historically, aminoglutethimide in combination with hydrocortisone has been used to achieve a medical adrenalectomy with symptomatic responses in approximately 25 per cent of patients (Worgul et al., 1983). With the demonstration that similar suppression in testosterone levels could be achieved with hydrocortisone alone, aminoglutethimide is now rarely used. In a phase III study by Tannock et al. (1989), glucocorticoid therapy in patients with hormone-refractory prostate cancer showed response rates of 20 per cent, with significant improvement in quality of life over patients managed with best supportive care; however, a survival benefit was not seen. A more recent study has shown that the combination of steroids with mitozantrone chemotherapy can increase the response rate to 30 per cent and is associated with an improvement in quality of life (Tannock et al., 1996).

Radiotherapy for relapsed prostate cancer

Radiation treatment for relapsed prostate cancer is the most useful single agent treatment that can be offered to patients with this disease. Where there is a single area of bone pain, the choice is between a standard course of treatment of approximately 35 Gy over 2 weeks or a single large fraction of 8 Gy. Multiple areas of bone pain are also dealt with successfully with radiotherapy. There has recently been a trend towards the use of hemi-body irradiation. This involves treatment of the patient in two stages. With the use of lung shields, 8 Gy in a single fraction is delivered to the upper half of the patient's body. After a delay of 6 weeks, the lower half of the body is irradiated to the same dose. This seems to be very effective in palliation of bone pain and a degree of symptom relief is seen in virtually all patients. The duration of symptoms relief is variable, and most patients require further radiation therapy of bone metastases.

More recently, strontium has emerged as an alternative to hemi-body irradiation for patients with pain due to multiple bony metastases. Strontium localizes to the bone. Apart from a mild degree of myelosuppression seen in most patients, the treatment is extremely well tolerated. Its use currently is limited by cost.

Chemotherapy for recurrent prostatic cancer

Cytotoxic chemotherapy for prostatic cancer is said to be ineffective and this may relate to the limitations of dosage in frail patients with poor marrow reserve. However, with the demonstration by Tannock *et al.* (1996) of the significant palliation of symptoms that can be achieved using the combination of mitrozantrone and prednisolone over prednisolone alone, there has been renewed interest in the use of cytotoxic chemotherapy in this disease.

Single-agent treatment may produce response rates up to 30 per cent in some small series (Beedassy and Cardi, 1999). The most effective agents in these trials appear to be cyclophosphamide and the anthracyclines. Adriamycin given weekly in small dosages of 10–15 mg is said to lead to a response rate in the order of 20 per cent (Robinson *et al.*, 1983). Estramustine phosphate, which was originally developed as a targeted cytotoxic, does not show significant single-agent activity but does show significant toxicity. However, studies have shown that it has anti-microtubial effects and therefore has been evaluated in combination with other cytoskeletal toxins, such as paclitaxel and vinblastine (Beedassy and Cardi, 1999). Although these results appear promising, estramustine's oestrogen-related toxicity should be emphasized and this is very important in a situation where life quality is the major issue. Currently, the emphasis of these phase II studies is centred on quality of life because of the lack of success of chemotherapy in improving survival.

CONCLUSIONS

Prostatic cancer is an extraordinary disease, both in terms of its prevalence and its responsiveness to treatments. Over the past decade, significant advances have been made in the understanding of the biology of this condition. A number of new strategies such as inhibition of mitogenic signal transduction, gene therapy and tumour vaccination have emerged as potential treatments for the future of prostate carcinoma. The next few years will, we hope, see changes in our understanding of the biology of this condition such that the molecular control processes that lead to its development and to its regression will be unravelled.

SIGNIFICANT POINTS

- The majority of tumours are adenocarcinomas of the acinar epithelium of the peripheral zone of the gland.
- There is no clear-cut evidence that aggressive treatment either with surgery or radiotherapy affects survival in patients with localized, low-volume disease of well-differentiated histology.
- Endocrine therapy for metastatic disease produces remissions with a median duration of approximately 1 year.

KEY REFERENCES

Atzpodien, J., Korfer, A., Franks, C., Poliwoda, H. and Kirchner, H. (1990) Home therapy with recombinant interleukin-2 and interferon-α2β in advanced human malignancies. *Lancet* **335**, 1509–12.

Denis, L., Carneiro de Moura, J., Bono, A. *et al.* Goserelin acetate and flutamide versus bilateral orchiectomy: a phase III EORTC trial (30853). *Urology* **42**, 119–30.

Horwich, A., Mason, M. and Hendry, W. (1995) Testicular tumours. In Peckham, M., Pinedo, H.M. and Veronisi, U. (eds), *Oxford textbook of oncology*. Oxford: Oxford University Press.

Jeffery, G.M. and Mead, G.M. (1992) CMV chemotherapy for advanced transitional cell carcinoma. *Br. J. Cancer* **66**, 542–62.

Waxman, J. (2001) *Treatment options in urological oncology*. London: Edward Arnold.

REFERENCES

Agency for Healthcare Policy and Research (1999) *Relative effectiveness and cost-effectiveness of methods of androgen suppression in the treatment of advanced prostate cancer*. Summary Evidence Report/ Technology Assessment, Number 4. Rockville: AHPR.

American Society for Therapeutic Radiology and Oncology Consensus Panel (1999) Consensus statements on radiation therapy of prostate cancer: guidelines for prostate rebiopsy after radiation and for radiation therapy with rising PSA levels after radical prostatectomy. *J. Clin. Oncol.* **17**, 1155–63.

Apakama, I., Robinson, M.C., Walter, N.M. *et al.* (1996) *bcl-2* overexpression combined with p53 protein accumulation correlates with hormone-refractory prostate cancer. *Br. J. Cancer* **74**, 1258–62.

Beahrs, O.H., Henson, D.E., Hunter, R.V.P. *et al.* (eds) (1992) *Manual for staging of cancer*. American Joint Committee on Staging. Philadelphia, PA: Lippincott, 181–6.

Beedassy, A. and Cardi, G. (1999) Chemotherapy in advanced prostate cancer. *Semin. Oncol.* **26**, 428–38.

Beral, V., Inskip, H., Fraser, P. *et al.* (1985) Mortality of employees of the United Kingdom Atomic Energy Authority. *Br. Med. J.* **291**, 440–7.

Bishoff, J.T., Motley, J., Optenberg, S.A. *et al.* (1998) Incidenece of faecal and urinary incontinence following radical perineal and retropubic prostatectomy in a national population. *J. Urol.* **160**, 454–8.

Blackard, C.E., Byar, D.P. and Jordan, W.P. (1973) Orchiectomy for advanced prostatic cancer: a re-evaluation. *Urology* **1**, 553–60.

Blasko, J.C., Wallner, K., Grimm, P.D. *et al.* (1995) PSA based disease control following US guided 125-iodine implantation for T1/2 prostatic carcinoma. *J. Urol.* **154**, 1096–9.

Bluestein, D.L., Bostwick, D.G., Bergstrabl, E.J. and Oesterling, J.E. (1994) Eliminating the need for bilateral pelvic lymphadenectomy in select patients with prostate cancer. *J. Urol.* **151**, 1315–20.

Boccardo, F., Rubagotti, A., Barichello, M. *et al.* (1999) Bicalutamide monotherapy versus flutamide plus goserelin in prostate cancer patients: results of an Italian Prostate Cancer Project Study. *J. Clin. Oncol.* **17**, 2027–38.

Bostwick, D.G., Qian, J. and Frankel, K. (1995) The incidence of high grade prostatic intraepithelial neoplasia in needle biopsies. *J. Urol.* **154**, 1791–4.

Bostwick, D.G., Grignon, D.J., Hammond, E.H. *et al.* (2000) Prognostic factors in prostate cancer. *Arch. Pathol. Lab. Med.* **124**, 995–1000.

Brawley, O.W. and Parnes, H. (2000) Prostate cancer prevention trials in the USA. *Eur. J. Cancer* **36**, 1312–15.

Brawn, P.N., Ayala, A.G., Von Eschenbach, A.C., Hussey, D.H. and Johnson, D.E. (1982) Histologic grading study of prostate adenocarcinoma: the development of a new system and comparison with other methods – a preliminary study. *Cancer* **49**, 525.

Broders, A.C. (1926) Grading and practical application. *Arch. Pathol. Lab. Med.* **1**, 376–40.

Buell, P. and Dunn, J.E. (1965) Cancer mortality among Japanese Issei and Nisei of California. *Cancer* **18**, 656–64.

Burton, J.L., Oakley, N. and Anderson, J.B. (2000) Recent advances in the histopathology and molecular biology of prostate cancer. *BJU Int.* **85**, 87–94.

Byar, D.P. (1972) Treatment of prostatic cancer. Studies by the Veterans Administration Cooperative Urological Research Group. *Bull. N.Y. Acad. Med. Sci.* **48**, 751–66.

Catalona, W.J. and Basler, J.W. (1993) Return of erections and urinary incontinence following nerve sparing radical retropubic prostatectomy. *J. Urol.* **150**, 905–7.

Chodak, G.W., Thisted, R.A., Gerber, G.S. *et al.* (1994) Results of conservative management of clinically localized prostate cancer. *N. Engl. J. Med.* **330**, 242–8.

Coetzee, G.A. and Ross, R.K. (1994) Prostate cancer and the androgen receptor. *J. Natl Cancer Inst.* **86**, 872.

Coronary Drug Project Research Group (1970) The Coronary Drug Project. Initial findings leading to modifications of its research protocol. *J. Am. Med. Assoc.* **214**, 1303–13.

Crook, J., Esche, B. and Futter, N. (1996) Effet of pelvic radiotherapy for prostate cancer on bladder bowel and sexual function. *Urology* **47**, 387–94.

Dearnaley, D.P., Khoo, V.S., Norman, A.R. *et al.* (1999) Comparison of radiation side-effects of confomal and conventional radiotherapy in prostate cancer: a randomised trial. *Lancet* **353**, 267–72.

Duncan, W., Warde, P., Catton, C.N. *et al.* (1993) Carcinoma of the prostate: results of radical radiotherapy (1975–1985). *Int. J. Radiat. Oncol. Biol. Phys.* **26**, 203–10.

Engelstein, D., Mukamel, E., Cytron, S. *et al.* (1994) A comparison between digitally-guided fine needle aspiration and ultrasound-guided transperineal core needle biopsy of the prostate for the detection of prostate cancer. *Br. J. Urol.* **74**, 210–13.

Fleshner, N.E. and Trachtenberg, J. (1995) Combination finasteride and flutamide in advanced carcinoma of the prostate: effective therapy with minimal side effects. *J. Urol.* **154**, 1642–6.

Fowler, F.J., Barry, M.J., Lu-Yao, G. *et al.* (1996) Outcomes of external-beam radiotherapy for prostate cancer: a study of edicare beneficiaries in three surveillance, epidemiology and end result areas. *J. Clin. Oncol.* **14**, 2258–65.

Gaeta, J.F., Englander, L.C. and Murphy, G.P. (1986) Comparative evaluation of national prostatic cancer treatment group and Gleason systems for pathologic grading of prostatic cancer. *Urology* **27**, 306–8.

Garnick, M.B. (1986) Leuprolide versus diethylstilboestrol for previously untreated stage D2 prostate cancer. *Urology* **27**(suppl.), 21–6.

Gleason, D.F. and The Veterans' Co-Operative Urological Research Group (1977) Histologic grading and clinical staging of prostatic carcinoma. In Tannenbaum, M. (ed.), *Urologic pathology. The prostate*. Philadelphia: Lea and Febiger, 177–98.

Goktas, S. and Crawford, E.D. (1999) Optimal hormonal therapy for advanced prostatic carcinoma. *Semin. Oncol.* **26**, 162–73.

Hayes, R.B., Liff, J.M., Pottern, L.M., *et al.* (1995) Prostate cancer risk in U.S. blacks and whites with a family history of cancer. *Int. J. Cancer* **60**, 361.

Huggins, C. and Hodges, C.V. (1941) Studies on prostate cancer 1: the effect of castration, of oestrogen and of androgen injection on serum phosphatases in metastatic carcinoma of the prostate. *Cancer Res.* **1**, 293–7.

Janknegt, R.A., Abbou, C.C., Bartoletti, R. *et al.* (1993) Orchiectomy and nilutamide or placebo as treatment of metastatic prostate cancer in a multi-institutional double-blind randomised trial. *J. Urol.* **149**, 77.

Kamoi, K. and Babaian, R.J. (1999) Advances in the application of PSA in the detection of early stage prostate cancer. *Semin. Oncol.* **26**, 140–9.

Klotz, L.H., Kerr, H.W., Morse, M.J. *et al.* (1986) Intermittent endocrine therapy for advanced prostate cancer. *Cancer* **58**, 2546–50.

Lessells, A.M., Burnett, R.A., Howaston, S.R. *et al.* (1997) Observer variability in the histopathological reporting of needle biopsy specimens of the prostate. *Hum. Pathol.* **28**, 646–9.

Leuprolide Study Group (1984) Leuprolide versus diethylstilboestrol for metastatic prostate cancer. *N. Engl. J. Med.* **311**, 1281–6.

Levine, R.L. and Wilchinsky, M. (1979) Adenocarcinoma of the prostate. A comparison of the disease in blacks versus whites. *J. Urol.* **121**, 761–2.

Lippman, S.M. (2000) Phase III cancer chemoprevention: focus on the prostate. *J. Clin. Oncol.* **18**, 32–41.

Long, M.A. and Husband, J.E. (1999) Features of unusual metastases from prostate cancer. *Br. J. Radiol.* **72**, 933–41.

Lu-Yao, G.L. and Greenberg, E.R. (1994) Changes in prostate cancer incidence and treatment in the USA. *Lancet* **343**, 251.

Ma, J., Stampfer, M.J., Gann, P.H. *et al.* (1998) Vitamin D receptor polymorphisms, circulating vitamin D metabolites, and the risk of prostate cancer in US physicians. *Cancer Epidemiol. Biomark. Prev.* **7**, 385–90.

McCarthy, P. and Pollack, H.M. (1991) Imaging of patients with stage D prostate carcinoma. *Urol. Clin. North Am.* **18**, 35.

Medical Research Council Prostate Cancer Working Party Investigators Group (1997) Immediate versus deferred treatment for advanced prostatic cancer: initial results of the MRC trial. *Br. J. Urol.* **79**, 226–34.

Mostofi, F.K. (1975) Grading of prostatic carcinoma. *Cancer Chemother. Rep.* **59**, 111–17.

Nesbitt, R.M. and Baum, W.C. (1950) Endocrine control of prostatic carcinoma: clinical and statistical survey of 1818 cases. *J. Am. Med. Assoc.* **143**, 1317–20.

Oh, W.K. and Kantoff, P.W. (1998) Management of hormone refractory prostate cancer: current standards and future prospects. *J. Urol.* **160**, 1220–9.

Parker, S.L., Tong, T., Bolden, S. and Wingo, P.A. (1997) Cancer statistics 1997. *CA Cancer J. Clin.* **47**, 5–27.

Partin, A., Yoo, J., Carter, H.B. *et al.* (1993) The use of PSA, clinical stage and Gleason score to predict pathologic stage in men with localised prostate cancer. *J. Urol.* **150**, 110.

Parmar, H., Edwards, L., Phillips, R.H. *et al.* (1987) Orchiectomy versus long-acting D-Trp-6-LHRH in advanced prostatic cancer. *Br. J. Urol.* **59**, 248–54.

Paulson, D.F., Lin, G.H., Hinshaw, W., Stephani, S., and the Uro-Oncology Group (1982) Radical surgery versus radiotherapy for adenocarcinoma of the prostate. *J. Urol.* **128**, 502–4.

Pisters, L.L. (1999) The challege of locally advanced prostate cancer. *Semin. Oncol.* **26**, 202–16.

Pollack, A., Zagars, G.K. and Rosen, I.I. (1999) Prostate cancer treatment with radiotherapy: maturing methods that minimize morbidity. *Semin. Oncol.* **26**, 150.

Pound, C.R., Partin, A.W., Eisenberger, M.A. *et al.* (1999) Natural history of progression after PSA elevation following radical prostatectomy. *J. Am. Med. Assoc.* **281**, 1591–7.

Prostate Cancer Triallists' Collaborative Study Group (2000) Maximum androgen blockade in advanced prostate cancer: an overview of the randomised trials. *Lancet* **355**, 1491–8.

Ragde, H., Blasko, J.C., Grimm, P.D. *et al.* (1997) Interstitial iodine-125 radiation without adjuvant therapy in the treatment of localized prostate cancer. *Cancer* **80**, 442–53.

Robinson, M.R., Chandrgsekran, S., Newling, D.W. *et al.* (1983) Low dose doxorubicin in the management of advanced carcinoma of the prostate. *Br. J. Urol.* **55**, 747–53.

Ruijter, E.T., van de Kaa, C.A., Schalken, J.A. *et al.* (1996) Histological grade heterogeneity in multifocal prostate cancer. Biological and clinical implications. *J. Pathol.* **180**, 295–9.

Ruckle, H.C., Klee, G.G. and Oesterling, J.E. (1994) Prostate-specific antigen: concepts for staging prostate cancer and monitoring response to therapy. *Mayo Clin. Proc.* **69**, 69–79.

Samaratunga, H. and Singh, M. (1997) Distribution pattern of basal cells detected by cytokeratin 34 beta E12 in primary prostatic adenocarcinoma. *Am. J. Surg. Pathol.* **21**, 435–40.

Schiebler, M.L., Schnall, M.D., Pollack, H.M. *et al.* (1993) Current role of MR imaging in the staging of adenocarcinoma of the prostate. *Radiology* **189**, 339–52.

Schroeder, F.H. (1999) Endocrine treatment of prostate cancer – recent developments and the future. Part 1: maximal androgen blockade, early vs. delayed endocrine treatment and side-effects. *BJU Int.* **83**, 161–70.

Schroeder, F.H. and the EORTC Urological Group (1984) Treatment of prostatic cancer: the EORTC experience. *Prostate* **5**, 193–8.

Schroeder, F.H., Belt, E. and Mostofi, F.K. (1978) Prostatic carcinoma: late results on 484 patients treated by total perineal prostatectomy. Unpublished reference source.

Schroeder, F.H., Hop, W.C., Blom, J.H. and Mostofi, F.K. (1985) Grading of prostatic cancer: III. Multivariate analyses of prognostic parameters. *Prostate* **7**, 13–20.

Silverberg, E. and Lubera, J.A. (1983) A review of American Cancer Society estimates of cancer cases and deaths. *CA Cancer J. Clin.* **33**, 2–25.

Smith, J.A., Scardino, P.T., Resnick, M.I. *et al.* (1997) Transrectal ultrasound versus digital rectal examination for the staging of carcinoma of the prostate: results of a prospective multi-institutional trial. *J. Urol.* **157**, 902–6.

Sogani, P.C., Vagaiwala, M.R. and Whitmore, W.F. (1984) Experience with flutamide in patients with advanced prostate cancer without prior endocrine therapy. *Cancer* **54**, 744–50.

Sullivan, L.D., Weir, M.J., Kinahan, J.F. *et al.* (2000) A comparison of the relative merits of radical perineal and radical retropubic prostatectomy. *BJU Int.* **85**, 95–100.

Tannock, I., Gospodarowisez, M., Meakin, W. *et al.* (1989) Treatment of metastatic prostate cancer with low-dose prednisolone: evaluation of pain and quality of life as pragmatic indices of response. *J. Clin. Oncol.* **7**, 590.

Tannock, I., Osoba, D., Stockler, M.R. *et al.* (1996) Chemotherapy with mitoxantrone plus prednisolone or prednisolone alone for symptomatic hormone-resistant prostate cancer: a Canadian randomised trial with palliative end points. *J. Clin. Oncol.* **14**, 1756–64.

Teng, D.H.-F., Hu, R., Lin, H. *et al.* (1997) MMAC1/PTEN mutations in primary tumour specimens and tumour cell lines. *Cancer Res.* **57**, 5221–5.

Thompson, P.M., Pryor, J.P., Williams, J.P. *et al.* (1982) The problem of infection after prostatic biopsy. The case for the transperineal approach. *Br. J. Urol.* **54**, 736–40.

Trachtenberg, J. and Pont, A. (1984) Ketoconazole therapy for advanced prostate cancer. *Lancet* **2**, 433–5.

Sobin, L.H. and Wittekind, C. (1997) *TNM classification of malignant tumours*, 5th edn. New York/Chichester: Wiley.

Veterans Administration Co-operative Urological Research Group (1967) Treatment and survival of patients with cancer of the prostate. *Surg. Gynecol. Obstet.* **124**, 1011–17.

Wang, J., Halford, S., Rigg, A., Roylance, R., Lynch, M. and Waxman, J. (2000) Adjuvant mitozantrone chemotherapy in advanced prostate cancer. *BJU Int.* **86**, 675–80.

Waxman, J.H., Man, A., Hendry, W.F. *et al.* (1985) Importance of early tumour exacerbation in patients treated with long acting analogues of gonadotrophin releasing hormone for advanced prostatic cancer. *Br. Med. J.* **291**, 1387–8.

Worgul, T.J., Santen, R.J., Samajlik, E. *et al.* (1983) Clinical and biochemical effects of aminoglutethimide in the treatment of advanced prostatic carcinoma. *J. Urol.* **129**, 51–5.

Yantani, R. *et al.* (1982) Geographic pathology of latent prostatic carcinoma. *Int. J. Cancer* **29**, 611–16.

Yao, S.L. and Lu-yao, G. (1999) Population-based study of relationships between hospital volume of prostatectomies, patient outcomes, and length of hospital stay. *J. Natl Cancer Inst.* **91**, 1950–6.

Young, J.L., Jr, Percy, C.L. and Asire, A.J. (1981) Cancer incidence and mortality in the United States 1973–77. *Natl. Cancer Inst. Monogr.* **57**, 1–1081.

Zelefsky, M.J. and Harrison, A. (1997) Neoadjuvant androgen ablation prior to radiotherapy for prostate cancer: reducing the potential morbidity of therapy. *Urology* **49**(3A suppl.), 38–45.

30

Colon and rectum

RICHARD H.J. BEGENT, CHRISTOPHER H. COLLIS, TANYA LEVINE AND ADAM A.M. LEWIS

INTRODUCTION

Survival and quality of life of patients with colorectal carcinoma is improving as a result of enhanced understanding of the disease and introduction of new treatments. There is progress towards effective screening, earlier case finding, to adjuvant therapy and to intensive follow-up, with resection or chemotherapy for recurrence. There are improvements in palliative treatment and significant achievements in cytotoxic chemotherapy, targeted therapy and gene therapy, and diagnostic techniques. The field has become one of intense activity in which there is reason for optimism.

INCIDENCE AND CAUSE

In England and Wales in 1992, 29 664 people developed carcinoma of the colon or rectum. The male to female ratio was 1.27:1 for rectal and 0.82:1 for colon carcinoma. The incidence to mortality ratio for colon carcinoma was 1.47:1 for men and 1.49:1 for women and for carcinoma of the rectum it was 1.82 for men and 1.78 for women (OPCS, 1994). Colorectal cancer has an incidence of 54.7 per 100 000 of the population of men and 53.8 per 100 000 of women, and it is the second most common cause of death from cancer after lung carcinoma in men and after breast carcinoma in women

(OPCS, 1994). Survival has improved progressively in the UK, with a 6 per cent gain in age-standardized mortality from 1971–98 for men, and a 9 per cent gain for women. Five-year relative survival has increased steadily from 1971, at 23 per cent for 1971–75 compared with 39 per cent for 1986–90 for colon cancer, and from 28 per cent to 38 per cent for rectal cancer (ONS, 1998).

Comparisons with data from the USA appear to show 20 per cent higher 5-year survival rates in the USA (60 versus 39 per cent). The more active screening programmes in the USA are a possible contributor to this, although cancer registration is conducted differently.

Genetic damage causes colorectal cancer

Colorectal carcinoma appears to result from the accumulation of separate occurrences of genetic damage in a colonic epithelial cell. Genetic damage tends to accumulate with time, explaining the increasing incidence with age of sporadic cases and the rarity before 40 years of age. Figure 30.1 shows the relationship of incidence to age in England and Wales (derived from OPCS, 1994). The inheritance of specific gene defects accounts for 5–15 per cent of cases in recognized family cancer syndromes and results in development of a carcinoma at an earlier age, usually before 50 years. The molecular genetics by which colonic mucosa progresses through the normal–adenoma–carcinoma sequence was described by Fearon and Vogelstein (1990).

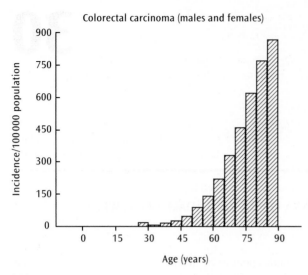

Figure 30.1 *Relationship between age and incidence of colorectal cancer. (Derived from OPCS, 1994).*

Diet

The association between a high-fibre diet and the low incidence of colorectal carcinoma has long been described. Possible explanations include a high-fibre diet leading to increased faecal bulk with possible dilution of any potential carcinogen and re-absorption and hydroxylation of bile acids (Jacobs, 1988). Some animal studies support this hypothesis, although it is doubtful whether results based on an animal being fed a single fibre component can be extrapolated to humans, given the range and complexity of our diet. Furthermore, the definition of a 'high-fibre diet' is not strict in the literature, and comprises a heterogeneous group of vegetable and plant polymers. However meta-analysis of over 60 human dietary studies did support the overall high-fibre hypothesis (Trock *et al.*, 1990).

Interest has also focused on diets rich in vegetables, fruit and plants. A prospective study of 764 343 subjects showed a reduced risk of colorectal cancer in 25 per cent of men and 38 per cent of women with the highest level of consumption of vegetables (Thun *et al.*, 1992). Interestingly, garlic has the strongest protective effect against distal colonic cancers in two large cohort series (Steinmetz and Potter, 1991; Giovannucci *et al.*, 1994). Potential anticarcinogens in such diets include folate, vitamins A, C and E, carotenoids, plant sterols and selenium.

A diet rich in red meat (Giovannucci *et al.*, 1994) and high in saturated fat (Willett *et al.*, 1990) is associated with increased risk of colorectal cancer, as is obesity (Giovannucci *et al.*, 1994) and reduced physical exercise (Gerhardsson *et al.*, 1988). Cigarette smoking is associated with colorectal adenoma formation (Peipins and Sandler, 1994). Regular aspirin consumption has been shown to confer a reduced cancer risk, although the exact dosage and duration is as yet unknown and must be balanced against possible side-effects of stroke and gastrointestinal haemorrhage (Greenberg and Baron, 1993).

DIAGNOSIS

Presentation by change in bowel habit, rectal bleeding, abdominal pain, weight loss or symptoms of anaemia is usually investigated by endoscopy. It is important that the whole colon is examined if a carcinoma is located in the lower bowel because of the possibility of a metachronous tumour elsewhere in the colon. In the elderly or frail, the use of air-contrast CT of the colon appears to be a reasonable alternative to colonoscopy (Domjan *et al.*, 1998). Spiral CT of the abdomen, pelvis and thorax, with intravenous contrast for the liver, provides the most accurate practical staging investigation. Failing this, liver ultrasound and chest X-ray are considered acceptable in some units. Serum carcinoembryonic antigen (CEA) should be measured as a prognostic indicator and as a basis for future monitoring.

PATHOLOGICAL FACTORS

Polyps

A polyp is a protrusion of a circumscribed lesion into a hollow viscus. Colorectal polyps may be classified according to their origin: epithelial (adenomatous and hyperplastic), hamartomatous (such as Peutz–Jeghers and juvenile polyps), inflammatory, lymphoid and mesenchymal, such as lipomas. The most common polyps reported by the pathologist are adenomatous and hyperplastic lesions.

Normal large-bowel epithelium has a turnover of approximately 6 days. The proliferative compartment is restricted to the lower third of the crypt. As cells divide and migrate from this zone, they differentiate and lose the ability to divide. In adenomatous lesions, the proliferative compartment enlarges so that the entire crypt and surface may be involved. The result of increased longevity of the cells and of reduced cell death, is crypt extension and branching, so producing a tubular architecture. In those lesions where there is mesenchymal proliferation as well, a villous architecture results. A combination of both processes results in a tubulovillous adenoma.

Adenomatous polyps are dysplastic by definition. While many polyps are stalked, some are sessile lesions. They are classified according to their architecture and degree of dysplasia. Tubular adenomas are composed of >75 per cent tubular glands, villous lesions >50 per cent villous architecture and tubulovillous adenomas

25–50 per cent villous pattern (Crawford, 1994). The degree of dysplasia is classified as mild, moderate or severe, and is based on the cytological features of the lining epithelial cells, along with the assessment of the neoplastic architecture. Severely dysplastic adenomas show loss of polarity, nuclear enlargement, prominent nucleoli, numerous mitoses and an often complex branching and cribriform pattern of the glands (Konishi and Morson, 1982).

Adenomas are benign neoplasms with a malignant potential. The risk of invasive malignancy is related to the size, architectural subtype, degree of dysplasia and number of adenomatous lesions in any one patient, although not all adenomas will develop into cancer and the exact risk and time course is not known (Morson and Bussey, 1985).

Those adenomas that are <1 cm in maximal dimension have <1 per cent risk of invasive malignancy, compared to 10 per cent of adenomas between 1 and 2 cm in diameter and 50 per cent of adenomas larger than 2 cm (Muto et al., 1975).

Increasing malignant potential is noted for those lesions with a villous architecture and severe dysplasia: the latter is associated with a greater incidence of aneuploidy (Goh and Jass, 1986). Any polyp removed endoscopically should always be submitted for histological examination. Those polyps classified as adenomatous should be categorized by the pathologist in terms of architecture and dysplasia. Completeness of excision cannot always be evaluated, due to poor orientation and fragmentation of the sample. The reporting pathologist should exclude coexistent invasive malignancy. Features favouring invasive transformation include a desmoplastic stroma surrounding infiltrating neoplastic glands with a destructive growth pattern, including invasion through the muscularis mucosae.

It is widely accepted that typical invasive colorectal carcinomas develop through the normal–adenoma–carcinoma sequence; a morphological corollary of the multistep theory of neoplasia. Evidence supporting this sequence includes:

1 Subjects with familial adenomatous polyposis (FAP) syndrome develop adenomas at an earlier age than development of carcinoma.
2 Adenomas are six times more common in colorectal cancer resections than in age-, sex- and segment-matched control subjects without carcinoma (Eide, 1986).
3 Adenomas are found in 75 per cent of resection specimens for synchronous cancers (Heald and Lockhart-Mummery, 1972), and patients with previous adenomas have a greater risk of metachronous cancer development (Bussey et al., 1967).
4 Residual adenomatous change may be found adjacent to invasive carcinoma. This is unusual when examining large tumours histologically, presumably reflecting destruction of the 'parent' adenoma by the infiltrating tumour edge.

Hyperplastic polyps are not neoplastic and result as a defect in epithelial cell maturation, producing their characteristic histological appearance. These are distinct from serrated adenomas (mixed hyperplastic adenomatous polyps) which combine the low-power architectural appearance of hyperplastic polyp with the cytological atypia of an adenoma. Longacre and Fenoglio-Preiser (1990) described malignant transformation in 10 per cent of serrated adenomas in a series of 110 cases. However, it must be stressed that these were described as 'intramucosal carcinomas', which is a term not recognized in the UK and is equivalent to severe dysplasia in our nomenclature. Consequently, the risk of invasive neoplastic transformation is still unknown.

Associated conditions

ULCERATIVE COLITIS

It is well recognized that patients with early onset, long-standing and extensive ulcerative colitis (UC) have an increased risk of colorectal carcinoma (Lennard-Jones et al., 1983). Tumours arising in this setting are multifocal, flat with a diffusely infiltrating edge and are poorly differentiated microscopically. Although these tumours typically arise from a pre-invasive dysplastic stage, over 95 per cent of dysplasias occur in endoscopically normal areas or foci with ill-defined velvety nodular mucosal thickening, and are quite distinct from adenomatous polyps (already described above) in the non-colitic population (Dhir and Gopinath, 1995). Microscopically these mucosal areas may be completely flat or have a mixed villiform and tubular architecture and are lined by variably dysplastic epithelium. Making a confident diagnosis of dysplasia can be difficult for the pathologist, as atypical areas often arise in bowel involved in active inflammation. In this situation, regenerative epithelial atypia may mimic dysplasia and the pathologist may be wise to issue a guarded report with advice to re-biopsy following treatment. A report of unequivocal high-grade dysplasia should prompt consideration of that patient for colectomy, so close liaison between pathologist and clinician is advisable.

Fewer than 5 per cent of patients with ulcerative colitis develop polypoid dysplasia, known as 'dysplasia-associated lesion or mass' (DALM). These are endoscopically complex villiform mucosal lesions and are distinct from the usual adenomatous polyps. Histologically they are characterized by a complex arborizing villiform and tubular structure, lined by variably dysplastic epithelium. Identification of DALM carries an ominous prognosis; Blackstone et al. (1981) described coexistent carcinoma in 67 per cent of patients with DALM, such that patients should be considered for urgent colectomy.

HEREDITARY NON-POLYPOSIS COLORECTAL CANCER (HNPCC)

This is an autosomal dominant hereditary disorder associated with cancers that may occur in multiple sites but which share the feature of DNA mismatch repair deficiency genes *hMSH2*, *hMLH1*, *hPMS1* and *hPMS2* on chromosomes 2p and 3p. Subjects are at an increased risk of developing colorectal cancer; the average age of diagnosis being 45 years and the overall lifetime risk 80 per cent in gene carriers (Vasen *et al.*, 1996). Although the disorder is not associated with the almost carpeting of adenomas seen in FAP, it is still thought that the tumours arise through the adenoma–carcinoma sequence; with the caveat that the adenomas appear more 'aggressive', with a higher incidence of large size, villous architecture and severe dysplasia (Jass *et al.*, 1994). In addition, the resultant invasive carcinoma tends to be right-sided with mucinous differentiation. In a young patient, tumour infiltrating lymphocytes on microscopic examination should prompt the reporting histopathologist to suggest a diagnosis of HNPCC, if not already considered clinically (Jass, 1998).

HNPCC is also associated with endometrial, ovarian, gastric, pancreatic and renal malignancies. The Muir–Torre syndrome is a particular variant in which colorectal cancer is associated with sebaceous tumours and keratoacanthomas (Burt, 1996).

FAMILIAL ADENOMATOUS POLYPOSIS SYNDROME

This is an autosomal dominant inherited disorder characterized by mutations in the *APC* gene located on chromosome 5. The function of the APC protein is unknown, although it does interact with the cell adhesion molecule, catenin (Burt, 1996). *APC* gene mutation is an early event in the development of colorectal cancer.

In FAP, the colorectum is literally carpeted with hundreds and thousands of adenomatous polyps. These typically occur at a mean age of 16 years and, unless prophylactic colectomy supervenes, 90 per cent of affected subjects will have one or more invasive cancers by 45 years of age (Burt *et al.*, 1995). FAP has three variants. In Gardner's syndrome colorectal adenomatous polyps are associated with osteomas and desmoid tumours. Turcot's syndrome is characterized by colonic polyposis associated with CNS tumours, which include medulloblastomas and ependymomas. Interestingly, one-third of these subjects have mutations in DNA mismatch repair genes and develop glioblastoma multiforme (Hamilton *et al.*, 1995). Attenuated FAP is a variant of FAP characterized by far fewer adenomas, which are typically right-sided (Spirio *et al.*, 1993). The risk of colonic cancer is high but not absolute, as compared to FAP.

In addition, colorectal cancer commonly occurs in families not otherwise affected by polyposis syndromes. There is a two- to fourfold increased risk for a family member if a first-degree relative has colorectal cancer (Fuchs *et al.*, 1994; Burt *et al.*, 1995), which is further increased if more than one first-degree relative is affected and they are below 50 years of age. As yet a specific genetic mutation(s) is not known.

MOLECULAR PATHOGENESIS OF COLORECTAL CARCINOMA

The histological progression of normal large bowel mucosa through adenoma to carcinoma is a morphological corollary of a multistep sequence of genetic mutations. The earliest mutation is that of the tumour suppressor gene *APC*, located on the long arm of chromosome 5. Wild-type *APC* encodes a cytoplasmic protein that is found in highest density in the upper portion of crypt epithelium. It interacts with β-catenin and is thought to be important in transmission of contact-inhibition stimuli into cells (Rubinfeld *et al.*, 1993). *APC* is a tumour suppressor gene and therefore acts in a recessive manner. FAP subjects inherit a germline mutation of one *APC* allele. The mutant *APC* gene protein product may form a heterodimer with the *APC* gene protein product from the unaffected allele, which prevents normal function. This mechanism may also occur in sporadic colorectal cancer cases following a somatic mutation of one allele. In addition, mutation of one *APC* gene allele may be followed by deletion of the other normal allele. This may be a consequence of genomic instability with flawed segregation of chromosomal material during mitosis. This 'loss of heterozygosity' (LOH) results in loss of normal tumour suppressor function with clonal expansion and proliferation. LOH is an important mechanism in the abolition of a normal tumour suppressor gene product function.

APC mutations have been found in adenomas <1 cm in size, and the rate of mutation is similar between adenomas and carcinomas, further endorsing the role of *APC* as the initial step in tumorigenesis (Powell *et al.*, 1992). This is then followed by mutation of the K-*ras* protooncogene. The wild-type gene encodes a protein with GDP/GTP binding domains and is important in intracellular signal transduction (Barbacid, 1987). As protooncogenes act in a dominant manner, mutation in only one allele is required to inhibit normal function (conversion to oncogene). Mutant K-*ras* protein permits stabilization of the active gene product with unregulated cell growth and therefore clonal expansion of the adenoma with an overall increase in size. Subclones then develop within this enlarging adenoma that contain further mutations, including deletion of the colorectal cancer gene (*DCC*) and *p53* genes. The *DCC* tumour suppressor gene is located on chromosome 18 and encodes a transmembrane protein with structural homologies to the cell adhesion molecule, neural cell adhesion molecule (NCAM) (Fearon *et al.*, 1990). Mutation in this gene confers a metastatic capacity to the tumour cells (Vogelstein *et al.*, 1988; Fearon *et al.*, 1990). Wild-type *p53* is a tumour suppressor gene and is the most widespread mutation found in human cancers (Greenblatt *et al.*, 1994). It is located on the short arm of chromosome 17 and is important in the control of the cell cycle, programmed cell death and DNA repair and synthesis (Lane, 1992). Thus mutation in *p53* allows unregulated cell growth. Genetic studies indicate that *p53* loss is a late event, occurring after mutation in *DCC* and corresponding histologically to the development of invasive carcinoma in an adenomatous polyp (Boland *et al.*, 1995).

PATHOLOGY OF INVASIVE COLORECTAL CANCERS

Macroscopic appearance

The gross morphology of colorectal cancers may be polypoid, fungating, ulcerative or diffusely infiltrating. Approximately 60 per cent of invasive carcinomas arise in the sigmoid colon and rectum, although an increase of right-sided colonic cancers from 18.7 to 27.5 per cent and a decrease in left-sided tumours from 72.1 to 62.5 per cent has been described in recent years (Slater *et al.*, 1984).

Microscopic appearance

Microscopically the tumours may be classified into well, moderately or poorly differentiated adenocarcinomas. Scattered neuroendocrine and Paneth cells may be evident, although typically they are few. Rare variants include the poor prognosis mucinous carcinoma, characterized by strips and sheets of neoplastic glandular epithelium bathed in lakes of mucin (the latter form more than 50 per cent of the tumour). Undifferentiated carcinoma, typically located in the caecum, is characterized by sheets of undifferentiated malignant cells with vesicular nuclei and prominent nucleoli. Despite its 'aggressive' microscopic appearance, the tumour has a good prognosis (Gibbs, 1977). Small cell carcinoma is an aggressive tumour, histologically indistinguishable from its pulmonary counterpart and with a similar biological profile (Mills *et al.*, 1983). Some 50 cases have been reported in the literature of primary colorectal signet cell carcinoma (Sasaki *et al.*, 1987). The more common gastric signet cell carcinoma or lobular carcinoma of the breast in women should be excluded before rendering a diagnosis.

Prognostic factors

STAGING

The mucosal origin allows the tumour to infiltrate circumferentially and longitudinally along the bowel.

Typically, however, macroscopic assessment correlates well with microscopic spread, such that a 2 cm distal margin of excision is adequate, as the risk of unrecognized tumour growth beyond this is negligible. Indeed, Royal College of Pathology recommendations state that distal resection margins >2 cm from the colorectal primary do not need to be sampled routinely by the pathologist (Quirke and Williams, 1998). The importance of complete circumferential excision for rectal tumours must be stressed and represents total mesorectal excision by the surgeon. The circumferential margin is the area below the peritoneal reflection anteriorly that continues on to the posterior wall, where it extends superiorly into the triangular 'bare area' that runs up to the sigmoid mesocolon. In pathological terms, the circumferential margin is said to be involved if the tumour is less than 1 mm from it, be it through direct continuity of spread from the main lesion, tumour emboli in lymphatics or lymph nodes or by tumour deposits discontinuous from the main growth (Quirke and Williams, 1998). Positive circumferential margin involvement is the main determinant of local recurrence in rectal carcinoma (Adam *et al.*, 1994). The 5-year survival rate of rectal carcinoma varies between 40 and 70 per cent and is due mainly to local recurrence, between 5 and 40 per cent, in potentially curative procedures (Quirke, 1998).

Colorectal cancer may spread by one of several routes, including locally with infiltration of contiguous tumour into adjacent organs, transcoelomically, and via lymphatics and veins. The vast majority of the colon, excepting part of the caecum, and a variable length of the anterior wall of the rectum is covered by serosa. Ulceration of this, either macroscopically or microscopically, by tumour constitutes a breach of the peritoneum and a route for dissemination of malignant cells into the abdominal cavity. Shepherd *et al.* (1997) showed that those colonic tumours with microscopic serosal surface ulceration by tumour resulted in peritoneal recurrence in 50 per cent of cases. Tumour spread via lymphatics to regional nodes forms an integral component of the various staging systems. Although, typically, metastases involve nodes in a sequential fashion corresponding to the anatomical sequence of drainage, in advanced carcinoma cases blockage 'upstream' by tumour of a node may result in retrograde lymph-node spread. The number of lymph nodes involved may affect the prognosis. The 5-year survival for Dukes C with one lymph node positive is 63.6 per cent, but falls to 2.1 per cent when more than 10 nodes are involved, and further endorses the care needed in initial sampling of the specimen by the pathologist (Dukes and Bussey, 1958). Although interest has recently focused on the use of ancillary techniques to detect nodal micrometastases, O'Brien *et al.* (1981) showed that routine analysis of haematoxylin and eosin sections of lymph nodes was equally sensitive in picking up tumour involvement as the use of CEA and EMA immunohistochemical techniques. Moreover those studies that have gone onto re-stage patients after immunohistochemical examination for micrometastases have failed to show any difference in 5-year survival (Cutait *et al.*, 1991). Furthermore, tumour may embolize via the portal system to the liver and, in low rectal carcinomas, via inferior haemorrhoidal veins, direct to the lungs. Prognosis is adversely affected when thick-walled extramural veins are involved, although this does not appear to be an independent prognostic variable (Jass *et al.*, 1986).

Dukes' staging is the most important prognostic indicator for subsequent patient management. This eponymous system, described in 1928, initally referred to rectal carcinomas (Dukes, 1932). It is now applied to all colorectal cancers. Dukes' A tumours refer to those invasive carcinomas that infiltrate into the submucosa or muscularis propria, but do not breach the bowel wall and are without lymph-node metastases (with a 93 per cent 5-year survival); Dukes' B refers to those tumours that extend into mesorectal or pericolic fat in continuity without lymph node involvement (associated 65 per cent 5-year survival) and Dukes' C to those tumours with regional lymph node involvement (23 per cent 5-year survival) (Dukes, 1940). Subsequent to this, the Dukes' classification has been modified. It is now accepted for all colorectal carcinomas. Dukes' C may be further subdivided into C1 (apical node negative) and C2 (apical node positive) tumours with concomitant 5-year survival of 40.9 per cent and 13.6 per cent, respectively (Dukes and Bussey, 1958). Turnbull *et al.* (1967) added the Dukes' D category, representing the presence or absence of distant metastases.

The American Joint Commission on Cancer (AJCC) has developed a staging system based on similar parameters and assessed by the extent of local invasion (T1, submucosa; T2, muscularis propria; T3, beyond muscularis propria; and T4, tumour cells breaching the peritoneal surface or invading adjacent organs), lymph node status (N0, no lymph nodes involved; N1, fewer than three lymph nodes involved; and N2, more than three lymph nodes positive) and presence or absence of distant metastases (M0/M1) (Beahrs *et al.*, 1992) (Tables 30.1 and 30.2).

The American Joint Committee on Cancer (AJCC, 2000) reported a multidisciplinary consensus conference

Table 30.1 *Staging systems for colorectal cancer*

Primary tumour (T)

TX	Primary tumour cannot be assessed
T0	No evidence of primary tumour
T1s	Carcinoma *in situ*
T1	Tumour invades submucosa
T2	Tumour invades muscularis propria
T3	Tumour invades through the muscularis propria into the subserosa, or into non-peritonealized pericolic or perirectal tissues
T4	Tumour perforates the visceral peritoneum or directly invades other organs or structures[a]

Regional lymph nodes (N)

NX	Regional lymph nodes cannot be assessed
N0	No regional lymph node metastasis
N1	Metastasis in 1 to 3 pericolic or perirectal nodes
N2	Metastasis in 4 or more pericolic or perirectal lymph nodes
N3	Metastasis in any lymph node along the course of a named vascular trunk

Distant metastasis (M)

MX	Presence of distant metastasis cannot be assessed
M0	No distant metastasis
M1	Distant metastasis

Stage grouping				Dukes'
Stage 0	Tis	N0	M0	
Stage I	T1	N0	M0	A
	T2	N0	M0	
Stage II	T3	N0	M0	B[b]
	T4	N0	M0	
Stage III	Any T	N1	M0	C[b]
	Any T	N2, N3	M0	
Stage IV	Any T	Any N	M1	D

T, primary tumours; N, regional lymph nodes; M, distant metastasis.
[a] Direct invasion of other organs or structures includes invasion of other segments of colorectum by way of serosa (e.g. invasion of the sigmoid colon by a carcinoma of the caecum).
[b] Dukes' B is a composite of better (T3, N0, M0) and worse (T4, N0, M0) prognostic groups, as is Dukes' C (any T, N1, M0) and (any T, N2, N3, M0).

which, using published literature, developed an arbitrary classification system of prognostic markers. They concluded that several T categories should be subdivided: pTis into intraepithelial carcinoma (pTie) and intramucosal carcinoma (pTim); pT1 into pT1a and pT1b, corresponding to the absence or presence of blood or lymphatic vessel invasion, respectively; and pT4 into pT4a and pT4b, according to the absence or presence of tumour involving the surface of the specimen, respectively.

OTHER PROGNOSTIC FACTORS

The AJCC working party (AJCC, 2000) also recommended that TNM groups be stratified based on the presence or absence of elevated serum levels of carcinoembryonic antigen (CEA) (≥ 5 ng/mL) on preoperative clinical examination (Table 30.3). In addition, the working party also concluded that carcinoma of the appendix should be excluded from the colorectal carcinoma staging system because of fundamental differences in natural history. Although many molecular and oncogenic markers showed promise to supplement or modify the current staging systems eventually, to the authors' knowledge none has yet been evaluated sufficiently to recommend their inclusion in the TNM system. Assessment of gene expression using oligonucleotide microarrays and of the differences in protein expression between cancer and normal cells by two-dimensional gel electrophoresis and

mass spectroscopy (proteomics) are yielding a systematic assessment of the biological basis of cancer, but are not sufficiently well developed at the time of writing to describe the patterns found in colorectal cancer. Tumour factors such as *p53* mutation, K-*ras* mutation, genomic instability, failure of mismatch repair, thymidilate synthase levels, proliferation rate, vessel counts and vascular endothelial growth factor (VEGF) expression levels influence prognosis, but the complexity of their interactions and the probability that important factors have yet to be identified makes it premature to define a prognostic system. However, it is likely that this will be elucidated in the next decade.

The pathologist plays a major role in the staging of colorectal cancers. It is only with meticulous examination of the gross specimen that all the prognostic parameters just described can be assessed. The most advanced molecular techniques employed on microscopic sections will not make up for poor sampling of the initial resection specimen.

TREATMENT

Preventative treatment

SIGMOIDOSCOPY

A case control study (Selby *et al.*, 1992) showed a 59 per cent reduction in mortality from bowel cancer in people screened by sigmoidoscopy, with the reduction only applying to tumours arising in the screened part of the bowel. The potential benefit comes largely from identifying and removing premalignant adenomas, although carcinomas may also be diagnosed. Evidence that sigmoidoscopy rather than colonoscopy is appropriate for initial screening comes from a study (Atken *et al.*, 1992) in which the standardized incidence ratio of colonic cancer was 3.6 if a single villous, tubulovillous or large (>1 cm) adenoma was found in the rectosigmoid by rigid sigmoidoscopy. If the adenomas were multiple, the standardized incidence ratio was 6.6. The presence of a large, tubulovillous or villous adenoma in the rectosigmoid appears to be predictive of carcinoma at remote proximal sites in the colon and identifies a group needing follow-up by colonoscopy. A pilot for a randomized British trial is re-examining this issue by performing a single flexible sigmoidoscopy between 55 and 64 years

Table 30.2 *Staging systems correlated with TNM*

Dukes' staging system correlated with TNM		
Dukes' A	T1N0M0	Stage I
	T2N0M0	Stage I
Dukes' B	T3N0M0	Stage II
	T4N0M0	Stage II
Dukes' C	T(any)N1M0, T(any)N2M0	Stage III
	T(any)N3M0	Stage III
Dukes' D	T(any)N(any)M1	Stage IV
Modified Astler–Coller (MAC) system correlated with TNM (AJCC stage)		
MAC A	T1N0M0	Stage I
MAC B1	T2N0M0	Stage I
MAC B2	T3N0M0, T4N0M0	Stage II
MAC B3	T4N0M0	Stage II
MAC C1	T2N1M0, T2N2M0, T2N3M0	Stage III
MAC C2	T3N1M0, T3N2M0, T3N3M0	Stage III
MAC C3	T4N1M0, T4N2M0, T4N3M0	Stage III

Table 30.3 *Incidence of positive tumour markers at different stages of disease*

Dukes' stage	5-year survival (%)	% raised CEA	% raised CA 19-9
A	80	4	11
B	50	26	31
C	30	44	26
Distant metastases	<5	65	49

of age. Preliminary data on 23 000 individuals screened reported good compliance rates, with the expected incidence of adenomas (9–10 per cent) and appropriate subsequent referral for colonoscopy. The incidence of cancers was higher than expected, at 7 per 1000. Fifty-five per cent of the cancers were Dukes' stage A, a higher proportion than in unscreened patients, and this suggests that the prospects of cure are higher. However, the generally accepted British (but not the North American) view is that it is still necessary to conduct a randomized clinical trial to investigate the effect of flexible sigmoidoscopy on survival before population screening is considered (Atken et al., 1998).

FAECAL OCCULT BLOOD

Three large randomized trials (Hardcastle et al., 1996; Kronborg et al., 1996; Mandel et al., 1999) show a survival advantage of up to 20 per cent for screening by faecal occult blood test every 2 years. The impact of a national screening programme in the UK would be to save about 1200 deaths a year with screening of people aged 50–69 and an expected compliance rate of 60 per cent (Atken, 1999). About 2 per cent of such individuals test positive, 10 per cent of these will be found to have a carcinoma, 30 per cent an adenoma >1 cm, 10 per cent a small adenoma and 50 per cent no abnormality. Those testing positive need either a colonoscopy or double-contrast barium enema and a flexible sigmoidoscopy. Colonoscopy in expert hands is probably the most sensitive, though it has a higher mortality (about 0.01 per cent) than the other investigations. Much of this risk is associated with polypectomy, which may, in any event, be required after a barium enema. The feasibility of a national screening programme is being investigated in a study of 100 000 people aged 50–69 in the UK.

Surgery

TREATMENT OF POLYPS

All polyps, with the exception of those that are sessile or very large, should be removed with a diathermy snare at the time of colonoscopy. Attempts to remove large sessile polyps may cause heavy bleeding or perforation. They are often malignant and should be treated by open surgery (Russell et al., 1990). Very small sessile polyps may be biopsied and destroyed with the 'hot biopsy' forceps. After colonoscopic removal of polyps, every effort should be made to retrieve them, as management thereafter will depend on histological examination. If a polyp is benign, no further surgical procedure is indicated. The patient should be followed up by colonoscopic screening, as the risk of further polyps may be as high as 40 per cent (Winawer et al., 1993a), although carcinoma after complete clearance of polyps is rare (Winawer et al., 1993b).

The principles for safe management of patients with malignant colonic polyps have been well established (Morson, 1984; Nivatvongs et al., 1991; Chantereau et al., 1992; Nozaki et al., 1997; Netzer et al., 1998). Endoscopic polypectomy must be complete. On histological examination, the excision margin or stalk must be free from invasion, the tumour moderately or well differentiated and with no evidence of malignant lymphatic or venous invasion. If the above criteria cannot be met, then formal surgical resection is indicated (Netzer et al., 1998), especially if the surgical risk is low. A better than 95 per cent 5-year survival rate has been achieved for malignant polyps removed by colonoscopic snaring, with no operative mortality, and a cumulative recurrence rate of 11.3 per cent after 5 years (Chantereau et al., 1992). After surgical excision, the corresponding recurrence rate was 8.9 per cent, with a 5-year survival rate of 86 per cent.

In the case of FAP, surgical resection is mandatory. Total colectomy and ileorectal anastomosis avoids the need for permanent ileostomy, but the lifetime risk of cancer in the rectal stump is at least 10 per cent and restorative proctocolectomy may be preferred. The choice of operation may be influenced by molecular genetic tests (Vasen, 1996).

OPERATIONS FOR CANCER

The purpose of surgical treatment is to remove the primary tumour, together with all lymph nodes following the course of the named arterial blood supply and any removable adjacent organs that have been directly invaded. Colorectal cancers can also be removed laparoscopically, but the place of this technique remains uncertain (Wexner and Cohen, 1995; Bokey et al., 1997; Kockerling et al., 1998).

For tumours involving the caecum and ascending colon, the ileocolic, right colic and right branch of the middle colic arteries are divided at their origins. The mesocolon is dissected from the right ureter, duodenum, pancreas and gonadal vessels and the entire right colon is then removed together with the greater omentum. An anastomosis is then made between the terminal ileum and mid-transverse colon. Similar principles govern the surgery for transverse and descending colon tumours, the anastomosis being made between ascending and descending colon or transverse and sigmoid colon, respectively. In the case of the sigmoid colon, the inferior mesenteric artery is ligated at its origin with the aorta and the anastomosis made, after mobilization of the splenic flexure, between the descending colon and the rectum.

The principles applied to curative surgery for rectal cancer are governed by the blood supply to the rectum. This is not only from the inferior mesenteric artery, but also from the middle rectal, branches of the internal iliac artery laterally and the pudendal vessels from below. There is a need to preserve anal sphincter function whenever possible and to avoid damage to the parasympathetic pelvic nerves which would result in impotence and bladder dysfunction.

Tumours lying above the levator ani muscle and anal sphincter are resected by anterior restorative resection through the abdomen. The operation involves ligation of the inferior mesenteric artery and removal of the rectum and the mesorectum, but without formal node dissection on the lateral pelvic wall. Local recurrence can be minimized by total mesorectal excision, although faecal continence may be impaired if the anastomosis is very low (Karanjia *et al.*, 1992). Construction of a colonic reservoir immediately proximal to the anastomosis may improve the functional results (Dehni *et al.*, 1998), although there may be some difficulty in spontaneous defaecation after this modification. The rectum is divided at least 1 cm below the tumour (Williams *et al.*, 1983) and an anastomosis made between the sigmoid colon and the rectum or anal canal. Most surgeons now use a circular stapler to achieve a secure low colo-rectal or colo-anal anastomosis, though excellent results may still be achieved by hand-sewn anastomosis (Matheson *et al.*, 1985). The place of protective colostomy or ileostomy after low anastomosis remain contentious. There appears to be little evidence that either the incidence of anastomotic leakage or the mortality following such a leakage is improved, but it is likely that pelvic floor contamination may impair later continence.

Low rectal carcinomas

Rectal cancers adjacent to or invading the levator ani and anal sphincter muscles can only be cured by removal of these structures. The operation of abdomino-perineal resection is identical to anterior restorative resection as far as the abdominal part of the operation is concerned. Synchronously, the anal canal, together with the contents of the ischio-rectal fossa and the entire levator ani muscle, is removed by a perineal approach and the perineal wound closed with suction drainage. A permanent colostomy is constructed, usually in the left iliac fossa, but preoperative fitting is essential so that the precise position of the stoma can be tailored to the needs of the patient.

Locally extensive tumour

About 10 per cent of large bowel tumours, particularly those within the pelvis, will be adherent to adjacent organs, either due to inflammatory fibrosis or malignancy. It has been shown that resection of adjacent organs may be achieved with reasonable safety in the absence of metastatic disease and the survival results can compare with those for tumours confined to the rectum or colon (Izbicki *et al.*, 1995; Poeze *et al.*, 1995). Complete pelvic exenteration has a high morbidity and mortality but careful selection may achieve worthwhile survival times (Shirouzu *et al.*, 1996). Preoperative radiotherapy may allow removal of advanced tumours with reduced morbidity (Saito *et al.*, 1998) and with a lower incidence of local recurrence (Marsh *et al.*, 1994).

Incompletely resectable tumour

The management of incurable or irremovable large bowel cancers is frequently difficult. In general, incurable disease should always be treated by palliative resection whenever possible, even if, in the case of rectal tumours, this requires a permanent colostomy. Reduction of tumour bulk and removal of tumour likely to cause obstruction or fungation provides the best palliation and allows radiotherapy and/or chemotherapy to be used with the best chance of benefit. In the presence of distant metastases, if the tumour is not removable or can only be removed by mutilating surgery then it is nearly always best to close the abdomen and rely on palliative non-surgical measures. Endoscopic laser ablation (Daneker *et al.*, 1991) may relieve obstruction, and promising early results have been achieved using expanding stents (Itabashi *et al.*, 1993; Saida *et al.*, 1996).

Operative mortality and morbidity

Operative mortality for non-emergency resections of potentially curable cancers lies between 1 and 10 per cent. Complications include those common to all surgery, but septic problems predominate. In particular, there is a wide variation in the rate of anastomotic leakage between surgeons, of between 1 and 10 per cent in most centres, according to whether is it measured radiologically or clinically. Temporary and rarely, permanent impotence in male patients may occur if there is damage to the pelvic parasympathetic nerves, and patients of both sexes may suffer bladder dysfunction for the same reason.

Obstructing and perforating cancers

Emergency operations for both obstructed and perforated carcinomas have a significantly higher perioperative mortality and worse long-term survival (Garcia Valdecasas *et al.*, 1991). The management of obstructing or perforated carcinoma of the left colon remains a controversial matter, with some preferring a staged resection and others a primary resection and anastomosis. The St Mary's Hospital Large Bowel Cancer Project (Phillips *et al.*, 1985) included 713 patients with malignant large bowel obstruction. Immediate anastomosis in the obstructed left colon had a high clinical leak rate but the mortality of primary resection was no greater than the cumulative mortality of the staged procedure. Primary resection has the advantage of a much reduced hospital stay in a group of patients with poor long-term survival prospects, and is now generally preferred (Anonymous, 1995; Lopez-Kostner *et al.*, 1997; Poon *et al.*, 1998). Better results are achieved by more experienced surgeons whichever policy is adopted (Anderson *et al.*, 1992; Sjodahl *et al.*, 1992; Deans *et al.*, 1994).

Local recurrence

Although the place of routine follow-up after surgery for colorectal cancer has been questioned (Bohm *et al.*, 1993), there is evidence that an aggressive approach and attempted surgical resection of any local recurrence can be worthwhile (Abulafi and Williams, 1994; Pietra *et al.*, 1998). In particular, a rise in CEA level above the baseline level established after a primary resection (Chu *et al.*, 1991; Rocklin *et al.*, 1991), seems to be a sensitive indicator of recurrence. 'Second-look' surgery, based on CEA monitoring, may lead to an improvement in the overall survival rate (Martin *et al.*, 1985; Hida *et al.*, 1996). The postoperative morbidity and mortality of re-operation is quite high, and the use of the gamma-detecting probe at surgery after intravenous administration of radiolabelled anti-tumour antibody to detect recurrence may improve selection of resectable tumours (Dawson *et al.*, 1991; Martin and Carey, 1991).

Local or anastomotic recurrence after operation for rectal cancer often presents with local symptoms such as recurrent bleeding, tenesmus, pain, incontinence and eventual obstruction. Many patients do not have disseminated cancer and CEA levels are often initially normal. If the initial procedure was an anterior restorative resection, these patients can sometimes be treated by abdomino-perineal resection (Rodriguez Bigas *et al.*, 1992), but often further radical surgery is impossible (Killingback, 1985). Small recurrences may be palliated with the neodymium yttrium–aluminium–garnet (NdYAG) laser, but poor results have been reported for large tumours, especially those associated with obstruction or involving the sphincters (Bright *et al.*, 1992). Other palliative measures include a stoma, radiotherapy and the use of stents (Itabashi *et al.*, 1993; Saida *et al.*, 1996).

Hepatic metastases

It is generally agreed that untreated multiple hepatic metastases lead to an inevitably fatal prognosis with an average survival of about 6 months from the time of diagnosis. However, there seems no doubt that surgical resection, in carefully selected patients, can offer long-term survival with acceptable morbidity and mortality (Taylor, 1996; Millikan *et al.*, 1997). Experienced hepatobiliary surgeons can achieve 5-year survival rates of 37 per cent after radical resection, with a 1 per cent mortality and 6 per cent serious complication rate. Results depend on the size of the tumour and resection margin (Rees *et al.*, 1997).

Lung metastases

Low rectal carcinomas may metastasize through the systemic circulation directly to the lung. This generally carries a poor prognosis but long-term survival is reported after resection when the number of metastases is small (August *et al.*, 1984).

Radiotherapy and chemotherapy

The potential clinical indications for radiotherapy and chemotherapy may be listed as follows:

1 To enhance the outcome of operable disease in terms of survival and local control.

2 To facilitate potentially difficult surgery.
3 To treat extensive inoperable disease:
   (a) to possibly render it operable;
   (b) to obtain long-term local control or possibly eradication;
   (c) purely for control of symptoms.
4 To conserve anal function:
   (a) as an adjunct to surgery;
   (b) as exclusive treatment.

These may be achieved by the following mechanisms:

1 Reduction of tumour mass (to facilitate surgery or palliate symptoms).
2 Local elimination of small-volume disease, to reduce local recurrence.
3 Local elimination of small-volume disease, a source of potential metastasis.
4 Elimination of micrometastases.

CARCINOMA OF THE RECTUM

Radiotherapy as the exclusive initial treatment

Radical radiotherapy is seldom used in the UK as the sole primary treatment, although it has a place if the patient is unfit for, or refuses, surgery. However, for low rectal tumours, 'contact' radiotherapy may be used, as popularized by Papillon (Papillon *et al.*, 1982) and as reported extensively from France and the USA. The tumour must lie within 10 cm of the anal verge and be less than 3×5 cm; there should be no extension beyond the bowel wall on digital nor on rectal ultrasound examination, and the anal canal should be uninvolved. Favourable features include exophytic and well- or moderately well-differentiated tumours.

Papillon used 50 kV X-rays at a dose rate of 1000 cGy/min, giving a 30 Gy application every 2 weeks for four applications. The overall 5-year survival was 76 per cent (11 per cent dying of carcinoma and 13 per cent with intercurrent disease), though locoregional failure was 11 per cent. Eleven per cent died of distant metastases (Papillon *et al.*, 1982). An update on the Lyon experience (Gerard *et al.*, 1998) reports a similar outcome. Of 62 cases reported from the Cleveland Clinic, only three died of cancer. Local failure occurred in 11 (18 per cent) and three had distant metastases, but the others with local disease only were successfully salvaged (Lavery *et al.*, 1987). Crile and Turnbull (1972) used teletherapy, 45 Gy, to the pelvis and after 6 weeks, brachytherapy with 1–3 applications of 30 Gy. All tumours were smaller than 3 cm and non-mobile, and the disease-free survival at 2 years was 42 per cent.

Radiotherapy in combination with surgery

Local recurrence in the pelvis and metastasis may be a major problem after anterior or abdomino-perineal resection. Reviewing his results for the likelihood of recurrence, Hager *et al.* (1983) found that patients with only mucosal involvement had a local recurrence rate of 8 per cent with a 90 per cent 5-year survival. Patients with muscular invasion had a recurrence rate of 15 per cent with a 58 per cent 5-year survival. A high-risk group, where there was incomplete resection, had a recurrence rate of 24 per cent with 61 per cent surviving at 4 years. Other studies show similar overall results. Approximately one-third of patients have Dukes' A (T1N0 and T2N0) tumours, where the local recurrence rate is less than 5 per cent. For non-adherent Dukes' B (again about a third of cases) the recurrence rate is approximately 10 per cent, and for adherent tumours or node-positive tumours (B3 and C), approximately the remaining third of cases, recurrence rates are reported to be 20–70 per cent. The desired effect of adjuvant treatment is to reduce local recurrence and increase survival. The former can be achieved, but the latter has proved more elusive.

Some argue that the very low recurrence rates achieved with excellent surgery mean that adjuvant radiotherapy is not justified, but as will be described below, there are many studies to indicate that, given adequate radiotherapy, local recurrence rates are reduced, and in one large study, a significant improvement in survival reported.

Adjuvant radiotherapy for operable disease

Radiotherapy is used in this group to facilitate surgery or shrink disease preoperatively, eliminating small-volume locoregional disease and sterilizing potential sources of metastases.

Postoperative radiotherapy

Many of the initial adjuvant studies involved postoperative radiotherapy, although there have been relatively few reports recently.

Postoperative radiotherapy to allow conservation of the anus For T1 and T2 tumours, when radical surgery is considered safe or practical, a conservative local resection followed by radiotherapy has been used. The radiotherapy follows the same principles used in the conservative treatment of breast carcinoma. Doses of 45–50 Gy have been given in a number of series, together with a boost of 5–20 Gy given where there was considered a particularly high risk of local recurrence, i.e. at the excision margins. If the results of 84 cases reported by Rich *et al.* (1985), Ellis *et al.* (1988), McCready *et al.* (1989) and Willett *et al.* (1989a) are summed, in those with positive margins the failure rate was 31 per cent, and in those with negative margins, 6 per cent. The local recurrence rate can be kept to about 15 per cent or less. In the great majority, sphincter function was very satisfactory. The highest failure rates (of the order of 56 per cent) were seen in those with positive margins and no boost. In conclusion, this conservative approach may well be reasonable, particularly for small (T1 and T2 tumours). The role of chemotherapy in this situation has not been fully evaluated.

Postoperative radiotherapy after radical surgery Compared with preoperative radiotherapy, the major benefit of postoperative radiotherapy is that patients with early tumours, and therefore with a known excellent prognosis (this may amount to some 30 per cent or more of cases) who are unlikely to benefit from radiotherapy, can be excluded. Also, those with intra-abdominal metastatic disease can avoid prolonged courses of radiotherapy. A further advantage of postoperative radiotherapy is that the radiotherapy programme can be accurately planned and tailored to the situation and principal risk sites, following a full surgical and pathological assessment of the disease.

Disadvantages are said to be the increased small bowel that fills the pelvis, although when postoperative radiotherapy is used we routinely construct an omental shelf to hold the small bowel out of the pelvis and out of the radiotherapy field, and with this procedure doses of 55–66 Gy are reported to have been tolerated satisfactorily (Lechner and Cesnik, 1992). An alternative procedure is to use a polyglycolic acid mesh, which also has been reported to minimize small bowel radiotherapy damage (Thom *et al.*, 1992). There is the further problem that bowel in the radiation field may be tethered, less mobile and more prone to radiotherapy damage. In patients treated postoperatively who have undergone an abdominoperineal resection, the perineum needs to be included, usually resulting in an unpleasant acute reaction. The perineum normally need not be included in preoperative fields. There is also the theoretical disadvantage that tissues are more likely to be hypoxic postoperatively and therefore any tumour contained in these tissues will be relatively more resistant to radiotherapy than if the radiotherapy is given preoperatively.

There have been several retrospective reports of non-randomized studies of postoperative radiotherapy. At the Massachusetts General, giving 45–55 Gy of pelvic irradiation to patients with extensive local disease or with positive lymph nodes, it was estimated that the local recurrence rate was reduced by 20 per cent (Hoskins *et al.*, 1985). This has also been shown in a number of other retrospective studies.

There remain three principal randomized studies from the US, comparing adjuvant postoperative radiotherapy with surgery alone (Table 30.4). In a randomized trial from the GITSG (Gastrointestinal Tumour Study Group, 1985) treating B2 to B3 and C1 to C3 tumours with 40–48 Gy, there was an improvement in survival and a reduction in the local failure rate, but this did not reach statistical significance. Chemotherapy (CT) with methyl CCNU and fluorouracil were also included in two arms of this four-arm trial and the best survival was in the combined treatment group. The local recurrence rates (differences did not reach statistical significance) were as shown in Table 30.5.

In a second randomized trial from the National Surgical Adjuvant Breast Programme (NSABP) (Fisher *et al.*, 1988), the three arms compared combination chemotherapy with fluorouracil, methyl CCNU and vincristine, with the radiotherapy and with surgery alone. Radiotherapy

Table 30.4 *Postoperative radiotherapy*

		Number of cases	Dose (Gy)	5-year local recurrence (%)		Survival (%)	
GITSG '84	Radiotherapy + surgery	50	40–48	20		43	At 8 years
	Surgery alone	58		24		27	
NSABP '87	Radiotherapy + surgery	184	46–47	16		41	At 5 years
	Surgery alone	184		25		43	
ODENSE '86	Radiotherapy + surgery	244	45–50	(B) 6	(C) 6	82	At 2 years
	Surgery alone	250		6	9	67	

Table 30.5 *Recurrence rates in the GITSG trial*

Treatment arm	Local recurrence (%)
CT + RT	11
RT alone	11
CT alone	27
Control	24

CT, chemotherapy; RT, radiotherapy.

significantly reduced the local failure rate to 16 per cent, compared with 21 per cent in the chemotherapy group and 25 per cent in the control group, but survival was only significantly improved by the chemotherapy arm and not by radiotherapy. In the third randomized study from Odense University (Balsev *et al.*, 1986), in which radiotherapy was given at a dose of 45–50 Gy, there was no significant difference in local failure, which was only 6 per cent compared with 9 per cent in the surgical arm, though the time to failure was significantly prolonged by radiotherapy.

Preoperative radiotherapy

Compared with postoperative radiotherapy this has the advantage of reducing tumour size, facilitating surgery and also increasing the proportion of patients in which the sphincter can be preserved. It also has the theoretical advantage of sterilizing the surgical resection margins and therefore reducing the risk of perioperative metastasis, as well as reducing the chance of marginal recurrence. It has also been argued that theoretically the tumour cells are less likely to be hypoxic preoperatively and therefore less likely to be radioresistant. It also has the advantage of being more sparing of normal tissues. Preoperatively the included bowel is likely to be mobile and therefore less susceptible to radiation damage than fixed postoperative loops of bowel. The perineum also seldom needs to be included, and this is a major source of unpleasant acute reaction when included in the field.

The major disadvantage is 'overtreatment' of very early tumours which would not otherwise have been selected for adjuvant radiotherapy, and possibly, at the other extreme, of treating patients with extensive intra-abdominal metastases who do not merit radical treatment

to the pelvis, who would have received adequate palliative treatment from surgery alone.

Preoperative radiotherapy to allow anus preservation
Preoperative radiotherapy for low and/or locally advanced (T3, T4) tumours has been reported by a number of groups to result in anal sphincter preservation in about 80 per cent of cases and a 5-year survival of about 80 per cent, as shown in Table 30.6. As will be discussed below and shown in Table 30.7, chemoradiation may well be even more effective.

Preoperative radiotherapy, 'adjuvant' to radical resection
A number of early trials used relatively low-dose radiotherapy, with 20 Gy or less, such as the Princess Margaret Hospital Study of 1977 (Rider *et al.*, 1977) and the 1988 MRC Study. Neither local control nor survival was affected.

Higher doses of radiotherapy were used in the EORTC Study (Gerard *et al.*, 1988) using 34.5 Gy in 15 fractions. There was reduced local recurrence, but survival was not significantly effected. The small study of 40 Gy in 20 fractions was particularly encouraging (Reis Neto *et al.*, 1989). This is a dose that is well tolerated, achieves a high response rate and a 5–10% complete response rate. As discussed above, a number of more recent studies have reported similar results (Table 30.6) (Bozzetti *et al.*, 1999; Ahmad and Nagle, 1997; Wagman *et al.*, 1998; Corsa *et al.*, 1997).

An outstanding report with positive outcome comes from the large study of the Swedish Rectal Cancer Trial (1997). This showed benefit both in terms of local control and survival. A short fractionation schedule was used and 1168 patients were randomized to receive either preoperative radiotherapy (25 Gy in five fractions) followed by surgery (within 7 days) or to surgery alone. At 5 years the local recurrence rate was reduced from 27 per cent in the surgery alone group to 11 per cent, and the 5-year survival was increased from 48 to 58 per cent. The group also reviewed 780 cases registered for the study, but not entered into the study. Of these, only 67 had radiotherapy and the 5-year survival was 48 per cent overall, i.e. identical to the no treatment group arm of the trial (40), confirming the truly representative nature of the control group. This is the first large trial to show clearly the benefit of preoperative radiotherapy in terms of survival as well as local control.

Table 30.6 *Preoperative radiotherapy alone*

Number of cases	Dose	CR (%)	5-year survival (%)	5-year anal function (%)	Reference
51	45 Gy	8.5	74 (2-year)	74	Bozzetti *et al.* (1999) (hyperfractionated)
48	40–45 Gy		82	86	Mohiuddin *et al.* (1998)
74	45 Gy	4	73	80	Ahmad and Nagle (1997)
35	46.8 + 3.6 Gy	14	64	79	Wagman *et al.* (1998)
56	36 Gy in 12 fractions	4	76	72	Corsa *et al.* (1997)

CR, complete remission.

Table 30.7 *Preoperative radiotherapy or chemoradiation (with 4- to 5-week fraction schedules)*

	Dose	CR (%)	Reference
I Radiotherapy alone	45 Gy (hyperfractionated)	8.5	Bozzetti *et al.* (1999)
	45 Gy	4	Ahmad and Nagle (1997)
	46.8 + 3.6 Gy	14	Wagman *et al.* (1998)
	36 Gy in 12 fractions	4	Corsa *et al.* (1997)
II Radiotherapy + 5-FU/FA (daily during weeks 1 and 5)	40 Gy	7	Kaminsky-Forrett *et al.* (1998)
	45 Gy (+hyperthermia)	14	Rau *et al.* (1998)
III Radiotherapy + MitoC day 1 + infusional 5-FU days 1–5	37.8 Gy	9	Valentini *et al.* (1997)
	40–60 Gy	20	Burke *et al.* (1998)
	50–54 Gy	19	Ch'ang *et al.* (1998)
IV Radiotherapy + continuous infusion 5-FU	45 Gy	30	Meterissian *et al.* (1994)
	45 Gy	29	Rich *et al.* (1995)
	45 Gy	27	Janjan *et al.* (1999)
	54 Gy	13	Videtic *et al.* (1998)
V Radiotherapy + 5-FU + cisplatin	45 Gy	27	Chari *et al.* (1995)

5-FU, fluorouracil; MitoC, Mitomycin C®.

There are considerable differences between the short and protracted fractionation approach. The short fractionation approach has been followed by early surgery, before there is much change in the normal tissues and before much reduction in tumour volume would be expected. Assessment of tumour response is therefore not a useful endpoint. The protracted fractionation schedules take advantage of radiobiological principles to maximize sparing of damage to normal tissue and would therefore be expected to cause less long-term normal-tissue damage. Furthermore, the protracted schedules allow assessment of tumour response since sufficient time has elapsed to allow for tumour regression.

Chemoradiation Chemoradiation has been shown to have a major impact on the management of anal, oesophageal or, more recently, cervical carcinoma, as well as improving the outcome of head and neck tumours. There has therefore been great interest in using chemoradiation with colorectal carcinoma. Used in the preoperative setting it is possible to assess the complete response rate and thus the efficacy of this compared to radiation alone. The principal and initial drug used was fluorouracil. Reported trials using fluorouracil are summarized in Table 30.7. Some used daily bolus injections. Fluorouracil has also been given as a 5-day infusion during the first and fifth week of a 5-week course of radiotherapy (Kaminsky-Forrett *et al.*, 1998). A similar protocol, but with Mitomycin C® on day 1, has been reported in three studies (Valentini *et al.*, 1997; Burke *et al.*, 1998; Ch'ang *et al.*, 1998), with complete remission rates of 7–28 per cent, almost twice that of radiotherapy alone. Alternatively, fluorouracil may be given as a continuous infusion, and the complete response rates of 13–30 per cent seem slightly better than with two 1-week infusions of fluorouracil (Meterissian *et al.*, 1994; Rich *et al.*, 1995; Videtic *et al.*, 1998; Janjan *et al.*, 1999). Cisplatin together with infusional fluorouracil has been reported by at least one group, with equally good results (Chari *et al.*, 1995).

In conclusion, it seems likely that chemoradiation may well give an additional benefit compared with radiotherapy alone, but there are few, if any, randomized trials assessing its efficacy, and the optimal schedule is not clear. Relevant results are summarized in Table 30.7.

Dose-response to radiotherapy The effect of dose has also been examined in a number of retrospective studies, and indeed, looking at the various studies presented here, those with low doses were generally ineffective compared with higher doses. In one report the relapse rate was only 10 per cent if the radiotherapy dose was equal to or greater than 45 Gy, but 50 per cent if the dose was less than 40 Gy (Brizel and Tepperman, 1984). Aleman *et al.* (1992), from the Netherlands Cancer Institute, reported 206 Stage B tumours that received 45 Gy in 25 fractions, 50 Gy in 25 fractions or 50 Gy in 25 fractions together with a 10 Gy boost because of positive margins. There was a significant correlation with dose, although this did not hold up for Dukes' C tumours. A recent report concluded that there seems little doubt that there is a dose–response effect (Ahmad and Nagle, 1997). On the other hand, this may not be apparent in individual studies. Guiney *et al.* (1999), when analysing results stage by stage, could find no correlation of dose with either local control or disease-free survival, although there was a reported improvement in both with concurrent 5-fluorouracil.

Timing of surgery following radiotherapy The optimal timing of surgery following radiotherapy is somewhat controversial. Where there is bulk tumour for which regression is required to facilitate surgery, it is important to leave at least 4–6 weeks for this to occur. However, if the tumour is operable, we have favoured surgery at 7–10 days after radiation, at which time the tissues are relatively easy to dissect, and the earlier timing ensures that any residual tumour is seen and resected. Likewise the Stockholm study recommends surgery at less than a week from completion of radiotherapy (Stockholm Rectal Cancer Study Group, 1990). On the other hand, many surgeons prefer to operate later, once the reaction has settled and the tumour has had a chance to shrink further.

Value of endo-anal ultrasound in assessing response and staging of disease prior to surgery, and to assess the need for preoperative treatment Endoanal and endorectal ultrasound should theoretically be a valuable tool to help to assess the stage of disease prior to preoperative treatment and prior to surgery. It might help, therefore, to assess which patients require preoperative treatment and also to assess their response to treatment and extent of disease prior to surgery. It has been studied particularly with preoperative radiotherapy and chemoradiation. Barbaro *et al.* (1999) concluded that it is an accurate staging technique with a 94 per cent positive predictive value and a 90 per cent negative predictive value. Likewise, Heriot *et al.* (1999) also describes it as the most effective method of local tumour staging, although they do point out it is poor at assessing tumour extension into adjacent organs, for which CT, and better still MRI, is more accurate. It has also been used to guide the choice between local resection and anterior resection (Lee *et al.*, 1999). On the other hand, Williamson *et al.* (1996) recommend caution, since it may not accurately predict the pathological stage. Furthermore, they concluded that the results were strongly related to the ultrasonographer and the ability to distinguish tumour from radiation-induced changes can be difficult.

Pre- or postoperative adjuvant radiotherapy The case for preoperative radiotherapy being preferable to postoperative radiotherapy is strong, although some still quote the option as debatable. A study of 471 patients from the Stockholm Group reported by Pahlman and Glimelius (1990), compared 25 Gy in five fractions given preoperatively with 50 Gy in 25 fractions plus a 10 Gy boost given postoperatively. The preoperatively treated group had a lower local recurrence rate (12 per cent) than the postoperative group (21 per cent) and the difference was statistically significant, although there was no overall significant 5-year survival difference. Pahlman is strongly of the opinion that preoperative radiotherapy should be used in preference to postoperative radiotherapy (Pahlman, 1998). A major current UK trial is again comparing preoperative radiotherapy with postoperative treatment (chemoradiation). The problem with these trials is that standard optimal preoperative and postoperative treatments are chosen and these can be quite different in nature and are likely to change as treatments improve. The outcomes are therefore likely to be limited to the optimal treatments chosen at the time of the study.

The potential for increased postoperative complications following preoperative radiotherapy has not been realized. The rate of anastomosis breakdown is not increased (Rau *et al.*, 1998). However, there may be further long-term effects that, as yet, have been poorly defined (Ooi *et al.*, 1999). It is important that quality of life and anal function are monitored carefully in all trials.

Pre- and postoperative treatment (or sandwich treatments) has been proposed to offer the advantages of both approaches. Early non-randomized study reports have reported its feasibility. However, for optimal downstaging, a moderately high preoperative dose is probably necessary, and for optimal tumour control, prolonged courses of treatment are likely to be adverse, due to the increased cell division rate of perturbed tumours. At present this approach is not recommended (Lusinchi *et al.*, 1997).

In conclusion, although the greatest experience has been with postoperative radiotherapy, preoperative radiotherapy is probably superior, as suggested by the one large study looking at this from Stockholm. In addition, preoperative radiotherapy has the potential of increasing the chance of sphincter preservation, allows a higher dose of combined chemotherapy and radiotherapy to be given preoperatively, and leaves a free hand for postoperative chemotherapy.

Adjuvant chemotherapy of rectal carcinoma

Survival is prolonged in rectal cancer when chemotherapy is given in addition to postoperative radiotherapy for patients at high risk of recurrence. In a randomized study (Krook *et al.*, 1991) patients with nodal involvement or infiltration through the muscle layers received radiation alone or radiation with chemotherapy: 5-Fluorouracil (fluorouracil) was given with radiotherapy, and fluorouracil with methyl CCNU before and after radiotherapy. There was a statistically significant reduction in local recurrence rate in the group receiving chemotherapy in addition to radiotherapy. It was speculated that this was the result of the radiosensitizing effect of fluorouracil given concurrently with radiotherapy. The overall death rate was reduced by 29 per cent with the addition of chemotherapy. This study is the most convincing to date, but before its publication a Consensus Statement from the National Cancer Institute in the United States (Office of Medical Applications of Research, 1990) considered the evidence in favour of this approach to Dukes' stage B and C carcinoma of the rectum to be strong.

Developments in therapy of rectal cancer

A number of trials of different aspects of adjuvant chemotherapy and radiotherapy for rectal cancer are in progress, and the most constructive approach is to enter patients into these. Some British surgeons have lower local recurrence rates than the American series reported here and have advocated that adjuvant therapy is not indicated for Dukes' stage B tumours. In the case of cancers high in the rectum, very low local recurrence rates can be obtained with surgery alone if adequate mesorectal excision is achieved.

The small bowel is more susceptible to damage from preoperative radiotherapy for tumours above the peritoneal reflection. Accordingly, there is a good argument for predominantly giving preoperative radiotherapy to lower rectal cancers, and limiting radiotherapy for high tumours to carefully selected, more advanced tumours. This should balance the limited potential for benefit with acceptable morbidity.

Localized inoperable tumours This is a rather heterogeneous group and includes both patients presenting with primary advanced disease previously untreated and also those with recurrent disease having received various treatment, either simply surgery alone or surgery and radiotherapy, or all three modalities, and the approach will clearly depend upon what treatment has already been given, as well as the disease extent and general status of the patient. Supra-radical surgery with extended dissections can be carried out to attempt to excise extensive tumour, and occasionally long-term control may be achieved.

Radical radiotherapy Radiotherapy alone may be as effective as surgery in controlling disease, and in one retrospective report of patients with recurrent disease both the time to recurrence and overall survival were similar in both groups, and therefore radiotherapy would seem to be a reasonable alternative to surgery if major surgery is contraindicated.

Preoperative radiotherapy and chemoradiation for localized inoperable tumours Doses of 45 Gy or more have been used, allowing resection in 50–75 per cent of cases, but long-term control is only achieved in 25–35 per cent. For example, Mendenhall *et al.* (1992b), using 33–60 Gy, reported that resection became possible in most cases (37 out of 42), half were complete and half incomplete, resulting in 5-year survivals of 14 per cent in those with incomplete resection and 29 per cent where a complete resection was achieved. Most would now use chemoradiation in the situation as described above.

Intra-operative radiotherapy Intra-operative radiotherapy has also been used for treatment of localized inoperable tumours, but facilities for this approach are limited. The Mayo Clinic (Gunderson *et al.*, 1988) used 45–55 Gy given by external radiotherapy and an intra-operative boost of 10–20 Gy. There was a local failure rate of 17 per cent and the overall 5-year survival rate of 25 per cent was not greatly enhanced compared with the previous studies of pre-operative external-beam therapy alone. Likewise the Massachusetts General Hospital report using 50.4 Gy in 5.5 weeks with an intra-operative boost of 10–20 Gy. Seventy per cent of patients went on to achieve complete surgical clearance and the early report of 3-year survival was 60 per cent (Tepper *et al.*, 1986). Both studies had worse results with recurrent disease than with primary locally advanced disease. More recent studies combined chemoradiation as primary treatment with intra-operative radiotherapy and report improved overall survival (Weinstein *et al.*, 1995; Lowy *et al.*, 1996).

Postoperative radiotherapy for residual macroscopic disease and/or recurrent inoperable disease Where residual disease remains apparent and pre-operative radiotherapy has not been given, radiotherapy can be offered. Many of the early studies of radiotherapy were related to treatment given in this way. There are no randomized studies. Reported local recurrence rates vary from 15 to 76 per cent, but the 5-year survival is more consistent, around 25 per cent (Whiting *et al.*, 1993).

Perhaps the most promising approach remains with preoperative radiotherapy and chemotherapy, but further randomized studies are needed to establish this.

COLONIC CARCINOMA

Adjuvant radiotherapy (postoperative)

No benefit from adjuvant radiotherapy has been shown for early colonic carcinoma. However, several studies have been performed, and the possibility of benefit has not been convincingly refuted. In general, local recurrence is less of a problem than with rectal carcinoma. Thus local radiotherapy has less theoretical opportunity for benefit. Whole abdominal irradiation, although tried, has been of minimal benefit, since the marked toxicity severely restricted the dose. However, with T3N0M0 tumours, where there may be a particularly high risk, radiotherapy may have a role. A study at the Massachussets General reported 133 cases of locally advanced tumours (T3 and T4) treated with radiotherapy to a dose of 45 Gy together with a boost of 5–10 Gy to the tumour bed (and 22 of these patients were given concurrent fluorouracil). Compared with 395 historical controls, the local failure rate was reduced from 26 to 18 per cent (Willett *et al.*, 1989b).

Adjuvant chemotherapy for colon carcinoma

Fluorouracil and folinic acid combinations are the most widely accepted treatment for advanced disease, prolonging survival compared with palliative measures. The addition of folinic acid approximately doubles the response rate compared with fluorouracil alone and this regimen is beneficial in adjuvant therapy after apparently curative resection of primary colon carcinoma.

Dukes' stage C Adjuvant chemotherapy with fluorouracil and folinic acid for 6 months significantly prolongs survival in patients with Dukes' stage C colon carcinoma (IMPACT group 1999). The use of this therapy is endorsed by the UK Department of Health Clinical Outcomes Group (Cancer Guidance Subgroup, 1997). The NCTG regimen (*see* Table 30.8) is commonly used, although a higher dose of folinic acid (leucovorin) ($200 \, mg/m^2$ instead of $20 \, mg/m^2$) was used in a number of the studies contributing to the IMPACT analysis. In this case the dose of fluorouracil is reduced from 425 to 370 or $400 \, mg/m^2$.

Dukes' stage B A survival advantage has not been shown unequivocally for fluorouracil and folinic acid for stage B. The relatively poor prognosis subgroup, B2 (T3–4, N0, M0) has been included in several randomized trials of adjuvant chemotherapy, along with stage C. Separate analysis of the B2 group in these studies does not give a clear answer as to the survival benefit. The IMPACT B2 investigators pooled data from five trials with 1016 patients (IMPACT B2, 1999). They found a hazards ratio for event-free survival and overall survival of 0.83 and 0.86, respectively, at 5 years. This benefit did not reach statistical significance. It leaves open the possibility that a larger trial would show a significant result.

The NSABP investigators (Mamounas *et al.*, 1999) analysed four trials, including 1565 patients with Dukes' B tumours. They compared the patient groups receiving the best regimen (usually fluorouracil and folinic acid) with the patients with the worst outcome (either no treatment or other chemotherapy regimens). The question addressed is complex and the general applicability of the result may be questioned, but the cumulative odds of death in the Dukes' B group was 0.7, which was statistically significant.

The rationale for effectiveness of chemotherapy is stronger in the Dukes' B group than in Dukes' C because

Table 30.8 *Chemotherapy regimens*

DeGramont (as used in MRC trials)
(well documented, 30% response rate in British trials)
Day 1: leucovorin 200 mg/m² (max. 350 mg) i.v. over 2 hours, then 5-fluorouracil 400 mg/m² i.v. bolus, then 400 mg/m² i.v. infusion over 22 hours.
Day 2: Repeat day 1.

Repeat whole cycle on day 15.

NCCTG regimen (considered standard treatment in USA; response rates lower than DeGramont but survival similar)
Day 1–5: leucovorin 20 mg/m² i.v. bolus immediately followed by 5-fluorouracil 425 mg/m² i.v. bolus.

Repeat whole cycle on day 25.

Weekly regimen (from QUASAR trial)
Fluorouracil 375 mg i.v. bolus followed by DL-folinic acid 50 mg i.v.

Lokich regimen
Hickman line inserted. 5-Fluorouracil administered at 300 mg/m² per 24 hours, using a continuous ambulatory pump. Warfarin, 1 mg daily, given prophylactically.

Irinotecan single agent
Irinotecan 350 mg/m² i.v. in 250 mL 0.9% sodium chloride over 30–90 minutes.
In the event of acute cholinergic symptoms after administration of irinotecan, atropine 0.25 mg is given subcutaneously. The relevant symptoms are early diarrhoea with abdominal cramps, sweating, myosis, salivation or lachrymation.

Repeat on day 21.

Irinotecan, fluorouracil, folinic acid (MRC CR08 trial)
Irinotecan 180 mg/m² i.v. in 250 mL 0.9% sodium chloride over 30–60 minutes.
In the event of acute cholinergic symptoms after administration of irinotecan, atropine 0.25 mg is given subcutaneously. The relevant symptoms are early diarrhoea with abdominal cramps, sweating, myosis, salivation or lachrymation.
Folinic acid 350 mg (flat dose) i.v. in 250 mL 0.9% sodium chloride over 2 hours.
Fluorouracil 400 mg/m² i.v. bolus.
Fluorouracil 2400 mg/m² i.v. via infusion pump over 46 hours.

Repeat on day 15.

Oxaliplatin, fluorouracil, folinic acid (MRC CR08 trial)
Oxaliplatin 85 mg/m² i.v. in 250 ml 5% dextrose over 2 hours, concurrent (but not mixed) with folinic acid.
Folinic acid 350 mg (flat dose) i.v. in 250 mL 0.9% sodium chloride over 2 hours.
Fluorouracil 400 mg/m² i.v. bolus.
Fluorouracil 2800 mg/m² i.v. via infusion pump over 46 hours.

Repeat on day 15.

Table 30.9 *Current recommendations for adjuvant therapy*

Site	Stage	Recommended adjuvant therapy
Rectum	A	None
Rectum	B	Radiotherapy and chemotherapy
Rectum	C	Radiotherapy and chemotherapy
Colon	A	None
Colon	B	Controversial
Colon	C	Chemotherapy

of the probability that tumour burden would be smaller. The power of this argument is frustrated by the rate of recurrence in Dukes' B being about half that in Dukes' C, so that many more patients would be required to demonstrate a benefit. It has been calculated that more than 15 000 patients would have to be enrolled in a trial to answer the question definitively in Dukes' B tumours (Harrington, 1999), and it is doubtful whether this could be done. Therapies with an anti-tumour effect greater than fluorouracil alone would require fewer patients, and selection of patients on the basis of more powerful prognostic markers than Dukes' staging would reduce the numbers of patients required for a trial to give a definitive answer. These are areas of active research. In the meantime, one could argue that, on the balance of probabilities, adjuvant chemotherapy in Dukes' B2 is justified, but this is not established beyond reasonable doubt.

Table 30.9 summarizes current recommendations for adjuvant therapy. New therapies being investigated in the adjuvant setting include antibody therapy, oxaliplatin or irinotecan with fluorouracil and folinic acid. The latter drugs are discussed under metastatic tumour therapy below.

17-1A antibody (Panorex) is a murine antibody directed against the EpCam antigen widely expressed on gastrointestinal and other carcinomas. It was largely ineffective against measurable metastatic colon carcinoma but was studied in adjuvant therapy of Dukes' stage C carcinoma by Riethmuller *et al.* (1998). It produced a 32 per cent reduction in mortality ($P < 0.01$ by log rank) compared to no treatment, at a level comparable to that with cytotoxic chemotherapy but with less toxicity. Distant metastases were significantly reduced in the treated group, whereas local recurrences were not. This was thought to be because distant metastases were likely to be present in more sensitive, smaller tumour deposits.

METASTATIC AND LOCALLY RECURRENT TUMOUR

Locally advanced disease: palliative radiotherapy
Patients with relapsed locally advanced disease may still achieve a good local response and good palliation. Even patients previously irradiated will tolerate up to 30 Gy, which may be usefully combined on occasion with other approaches, such as intra-arterial fluorouracil (Schnabel *et al.*, 1992).

Chemotherapy for metastatic and recurrent colonic or rectal carcinoma
Chemotherapy prolongs survival compared with palliative treatment (odds reduction 57 per cent) ($P = 0.00002$) in a meta-analysis of three trials of systemic and two of regional chemotherapy. Quality of life was at least as good in the treated patients (NHS Centre for Reviews and Dissemination, 1997). However, performance status does need to be at least moderate (ECOG 0, 1 or 2) for patients to have a reasonable prospect of response. In a Cochrane collaboration, meta-analysis of 13 randomized controlled trials, representing a total of 1365 randomized patients, met the inclusion criteria. Meta-analysis of a subset of trials that provided individual patient data demonstrated that palliative chemotherapy was associated with a 35 per cent (95 per cent CI, 24–44 per cent) reduction in the risk of death (Cochrane review, 2000). This translates into an absolute improvement in survival of 16 per cent at both 6 months and 12 months, and an improvement in median survival of 3.7 months. The overall quality of evidence relating to treatment toxicity, symptom control and quality of life was poor.

CHEMOTHERAPY REGIMENS

Chemotherapy regimens are summarized in Table 30.8.

Fluoropyrimidines
Fluorouracil has been the mainstay of chemotherapy for metastatic or locally recurrent colorectal cancer for three decades; it is now joined by promising new oral fluoropyrimidines. Response rates with fluorouracil alone are low (10–15 per cent). The effect is dose related and infusion over a few days increases response rates. The effect of fluorouracil is modulated by administration with leucovorin, which prolongs the inhibition of thymidylate synthase (TS) activity and hence DNA synthesis produced by fluorouracil through stabilization of the ternary complex of 5,10-methylene tetrahydrofolic acid with the fluorouracil metabolite, FdUMP and TS. Response rates are increased to 20–40 per cent and symptomatic relief is reported in up to 75 per cent. Prolongation of survival by comparison with fluorouracil alone has been reported. Meta-analysis has not confirmed this, although response rates were increased from 11 to 23 per cent, $P < 10^{-7}$ with fluorouracil and leucovorin compared with fluorouracil alone (Piedbois *et al.*, 1992). The relatively low overall response rate and crossover of patients from one regimen to the other may conceal a survival benefit. Typical chemotherapy regimens are shown in Table 30.8.

Meta-analysis of trials comparing fluorouracil alone with fluorouracil plus folinic acid show a significant improvement for patients receiving the combination (odds reduction 49 per cent) (ACCMP, 1992). The meta-analysis shows a higher response rate with high doses of folinic acid, but no survival benefit. The benefit from use of high doses is difficult to assess because of the different regimens used. There is evidence that the Lokich regimen has more severe toxicity than the high-dose DeGramont regimen (Maughan *et al.*, 1999).

Raltitrexed (Tomudex®) This synthetic fluoropyrimidine has been investigated in comparison with fluorouracil and appears to have similar effectiveness. Its 3-weekly intravenous administration is convenient and appeared to be cost-effective. The drug's development has been dogged by reports of higher death rates than with fluorouracil and folinic acid. This led to early cessation of the PETACC-1 trial, when the death rate appeared to be twice that of the conventional chemotherapy arm. The data are not statistically convincing but the level of concern is high enough for there to be reservations about the use of this drug when there are reasonable alternatives in the form of fluorouracil and folinic acid and new oral fluoropyrimidines.

Oral fluoropyrimidines Fluorouracil is absorbed erratically (0–80 per cent) and is not generally considered useful by this route. Capecitabine and UFT (uracil and Tegafur) with folinic acid have been developed to give sustained and predictable serum levels after oral administration. Preliminary results indicate that they give equivalent response rates and survival to intravenous fluorouracil with folinic acid, but with less mucositis and more hand–foot syndrome. On the basis of these data, it seems likely that oral fluoropyrimidines may replace fluorouracil because of greater patient convenience and reduction of hospital costs.

Capecitabine is an orally bioavailable prodrug of fluorouracil. Thymidine phosphorylase (TP) is required for activation, and this enzyme is overexpressed in some colorectal carcinomas, particularly in response to tumour hypoxia. This gives the prospect of selective generation in the tumour. Tumour levels of fluorouracil are reported to be 2–8 times higher than in normal tissues. Fluorouracil does not appear to be generated during absorption in the intestine and the incidence of diarrhoea is reported to be lower than with fluorouracil administration (Findlay *et al.*, 1997). Toxicity probably depends on the total amount of tumour and this needs to be borne in mind when treating patients with advanced disease. Capecitabine gave equivalent effectiveness to intravenous fluorouracil and folinic acid with reduced toxicity except for cutaneous hand foot syndrome (van Cutsem *et al.*, 2001).

Irinotecan

This topoisomerase I inhibitor blocks DNA replication mediated by the enzyme and induces single-strand DNA breaks which inhibit replication. It produces response rates of 11–23 per cent in phase II studies of patients with colorectal cancer whose tumours are resistant to fluorouracil. A further 40 per cent of patients showed stabilization of tumour for a median of 5 months. The most common adverse effects include diarrhoea, nausea and vomiting, myelosuppression, asthenia, alopecia and cholinergic syndrome, the latter occurring at, or soon after, the time of administration.

Two randomized trials of irinotecan have shown survival benefit (1-year survival increased by 13 and 22.4 per cent) compared with palliative therapy (Cunningham *et al.*, 1998) or with fluorouracil infusion (Rougier *et al.*, 1998). Patients whose tumours progressed within 6 months of fluorouracil showed a significant, though small, survival advantage for treatment with irinotecan.

Combination of irinotecan with fluorouracil and folinic acid shows synergy in preclinical studies, and clinical combination regimens have been developed. Randomized comparison of the combination with fluorouracil and folinic acid showed significantly higher response rates for the combination in two trials (Saltz *et al.*, 1999; Douillard *et al.*, 2000); the latter also showed a survival improvement of 17.4 versus 14.1 months. In previously untreated patients the weekly regimen reported by Saltz has produced severe toxicity and is probably best avoided.

Oxaliplatin

This drug belongs to a group of platinum compounds synthesized to include the 1,2-diaminocyclohexane (DACH) carrier ligand. Although they bind to DNA in a way broadly similar to cisplatin, they are effective in cisplatin-resistant cell lines, possibly through greater resistance to DNA repair. Development was delayed because of temperature-sensitive peripheral neuropathy. In phase I trials the reversible peripheral neuropathy was dose limiting, but oto-toxicity, renal and bone marrow toxicity were largely absent. Ten to 20 per cent single-agent response rates were reported. Synergy with thymidilate synthase inhibitors and with topoisomerase I poisons was reported in preclinical studies, and much of the subsequent clinical work has been with oxaliplatin in combination with fluorouracil and folinic acid. Response rates of 21–58 per cent have been reported in patients with advanced colorectal cancer relapsing after fluorouracil and folinic acid. In previously untreated patients, response rates were 34–67 per cent, and in randomized trials, by comparison with fluorouracil and folinic acid, statistically significantly higher response rates were seen than for fluorouracil and folinic acid. A small number of complete responses have been reported (for review see Raymond *et al.*, 1998). There is evidence that oxaliplatin given for metastases confined to the liver may increase survival when combined with subsequent resection of liver metastases (Giacchetti *et al.*, 1999).

The current Medical Research Council CR08 trial is designed to determine the best way of using the new agents. Patients will be randomized to one of five arms and response, quality of life and survival compared, as shown in Table 30.10.

Hepatic arterial infusion therapy

Floxuridine (FUDR), a fluorouracil analogue, has been investigated for hepatic arterial infusion, usually via an

Table 30.10 *MRC CR08 trial*

	Initial treatment	On tumour progression
1	FU and folinic acid	Irinotecan
2	FU and folinic acid	Irinotecan, FU and folinic acid
3	FU and folinic acid	Oxaliplatin, FU and folinic acid
4	Irinotecan, FU and folinic acid	–
5	Oxaliplatin, FU and folinic acid	–

FU, fluorouracil. Treatment regimens are shown in Table 30.8.

implanted pump. The drug is more readily concentrated in the small volume of the pump than fluorouracil and a greater proportion is extracted in the liver on the first pass. Randomized trials in patients with metastases confined to the liver showed improved survival for the hepatic artery infusion (15 months) compared with symptomatic treatment (7 months) (Allen-Mersh *et al.*, 1994). Quality of life was also significantly improved in the treatment group. Although this treatment can produce liver toxicity, this can generally be avoided as a significant problem by the protocols used by experienced groups. Patients treated this way usually die from extrahepatic tumour and, probably for this reason, a survival benefit over systemic fluorouracil and folinic acid has not been shown (Piedbois *et al.*, 1996).

PREDICTION OF RESPONSE TO CHEMOTHERAPY

High tumour thymidylate synthase (TS) levels predict poor prognosis independent of Dukes' stage. The effect of drugs acting on TS, particularly fluorouracil, may be expected to depend on the tumour concentration of the enzyme. In adjuvant chemotherapy, survival has been shown to correlate positively with TS expression measured by immuno-histochemistry (Johnston *et al.*, 1994). However, in patients with metastatic disease, low tumour TS levels predict for response to chemotherapy with fluorouracil (Leichman *et al.*, 1997). It follows that TS level is not a simple predictor of response, an understandable observation considering that its production is related to cell proliferation and high levels have been proposed as a marker of genetic instability in tumours.

Dihydropyrimidine dehydrogenase (DPD) activity may also be a potential factor controlling fluorouracil (FU) responsiveness at the tumour level (Sobrero *et al.*, 2000).

RADIOTHERAPY TECHNIQUES IN COLORECTAL CARCINOMA

Principles of radiotherapy

The treatment volume and dose given are dependent on the amount of tumour present and/or the risk of tumour recurrence, and the normal tissue tolerance. For 'standard' preoperative radiotherapy it has been usual to use a uniform dose to the whole pelvis. If there is a bulky or inoperable tumour, a proportionally higher dose may be needed for the tumour itself and this is achieved using a shrinking field technique. Likewise, if surgery cannot be contemplated, a shrinking volume technique is again appropriate.

For postoperative radiotherapy the treatment can be tailored to the operative findings. Where excellent local clearance is achieved, a uniform field to the pelvis to include the tumour bed and pelvic nodes at risk is appropriate, but again, if there is an area of high risk of local recurrence, this can be boosted by the shrinking field technique.

For palliative radiotherapy, lower doses such as 3000 cGy in 10 fractions or 2000 cGy in 5 fractions can be given by the simple technique of anterior and posterior fields.

For the treatment of colonic carcinoma, similar principles apply, although in general it is difficult to avoid small bowel and therefore either reduced doses or a reduced margin to the tumour has to be used so as to limit the exposure of the small bowel, but small bowel problems are likely to occur in some 5 per cent of patients (Duttenhaver *et al.*, 1986).

Regions at risk and tissue tolerance

Use of anterior and posterior fields for postoperative radiotherapy at the M.D. Anderson with the upper margin of the fields extending up to L2, resulted in a 17.5 per cent incidence of small bowel obstruction, compared with only 5 per cent in those who had surgery alone. When the fields were altered to an upper limit of just below L5, the incidence dropped to below 10 per cent (Withers *et al.*, 1981). At the Massachusetts General Hospital using multiple fields, the incidence of small bowel obstruction was only 6 per cent with radiotherapy, compared with 5 per cent with surgery alone (Hoskins *et al.*, 1985). In practice, therefore, the para-aortic and high pelvic nodes are seldom included unless there are special indications.

The internal iliac and pre-sacral nodes are at high risk of metastatic involvement and should be included in the radiotherapy field. External iliac nodes are not usually involved unless there has been invasion of pelvic organs such as the prostate, bladder, vagina or uterus.

Recommended treatment volume

To cover the regional nodes, the pelvic volume extends from the bottom of L5 to the upper side of the anal canal for high tumours, and to include the anal canal with lower tumours. The perineum need only be included if it is considered to be at special risk, or after an abdomino-perineal resection. If it is included, bolus may help to make the dose more uniform. Posteriorly, the field includes the sacrum, thus encompassing the pre-sacral nodes and sacral canal. Anteriorly, the margin may be more difficult to define with a plain film only. If the anterior margin is taken to just behind the symphysis pubis, this will ensure covering the primary lesion, the adjacent prostate, base of bladder and vagina and internal iliac nodes, although to include the external iliac nodes the field would generally need to come to the front of the symphysis pubis. The extent of the tumour and the localization of these areas at risk is more easily confirmed with CT planning.

If a high-risk area requires an additional dose over and above the small bowel tolerance of 40–50 Gy, or if palliative radiotherapy is the objective where minimal bowel toxicity is required, the reduced high-dose volume is best defined by CT planning.

Inclusion of the perineum adds considerably to the acute morbidity, but there has not been an increase in chronic complications reported. After abdomino-perineal resection without radiotherapy a perineal recurrence rate as high as 23 per cent has been reported, but following radiotherapy including the perineum, the incidence was only 2 per cent at the Mayo Clinic (Schild et al., 1989). In another series of 60 patients, only one recurrence occurred (Hoskins et al., 1985). It is wise, therefore, to include the perineum after abdomino-perineal resections, although for other low tumours, or for preoperative radiotherapy, the need is not established.

Radiotherapy planning, field arrangements and doses

Localization may be achieved by simulator or CT planning. The patient is best treated prone and the bladder should be full to minimize small bowel in the pelvis. A marker wire is placed over the lower anal margin to help identify the anal canal. On the lateral projection the rectum is generally clearly outlined by the normal rectal air, although a contrast tampon in the vagina may be a useful aid. Immobilization body moulds can also help with accuracy, and small-bowel contrast can help to identify small bowel where a large amount of small bowel is potentially being irradiated.

A direct posterior field and two lateral fields are commonly used, or two post-oblique fields may be used. Lateral fields allow perhaps slightly easier assessment of shielding of unnecessary normal tissues. Such areas prone to a brisk reaction and delayed healing include the natal cleft and perineum, and providing these areas are not at risk they can be easily shielded by appropriate leading of the lateral fields.

A wide range of doses has been used, as discussed above. Using fractionated radiotherapy, doses of 40 Gy in 20 fractions to 50 Gy in 30 fractions have been used, to which a boost to a reduced volume of a further 10–20 Gy may be added provided small bowel is excluded from the field.

COMPLICATIONS OF TREATMENT

Complications of radiotherapy

Perhaps the most frequent and serious complications of radiotherapy are to the small bowel, although particularly unpleasant and prolonged reactions can be seen in the perineum. Factors contributing to increased complications are shown in Table 30.11.

Acute reactions include the small bowel symptoms of diarrhoea and abdominal cramps, and the large bowel effects of acute proctitis with urgency and frequency, tenesmus and occasionally a bloody or mucus discharge. Urinary frequency and dysuria may occur. Skin erythema may be particularly troublesome in the skin folds of the natal cleft and perineum. These acute effects occur 2–3 weeks into a course of fractionated radiotherapy and generally resolve within a few weeks of stopping the treatment.

Most serious are the delayed reactions that may persist, carrying on from the acute reactions, or develop after a latent period of some 6–18 months (Table 30.12). In one retrospective study, ileus occurred in only 8 per cent of cases without radiotherapy, but in 23 per cent of those receiving radiotherapy, and surgery was required in only 4 per cent of those without radiotherapy versus 21 per cent of those receiving radiotherapy (Els et al., 1992). Infertility is inevitable if the gonads are included in the radiation field and may occur even if close to the edge of the field.

To minimize the risk of reactions, the factors listed in Table 30.11 should be taken into account. Total dose is the ultimate criterion, but for maximum therapeutic benefit and minimum toxicity fractions should probably

Table 30.11 *Factors increasing normal tissue damage from radiation*

RT related	Non-RT related
Total dose	Pelvic inflammatory disease
Large fraction size	Hypertension
Short overall treatment time	Diabetes mellitus
	Obesity
Low radiation energy	Prior pelvic irradiation
Large treatment volume	Concomitant radiotherapy
Poor planning techniques	

RT, radiotherapy.

Table 30.12 *Late radiation complications*

Chronic diarrhoea	Perineal and scrotal tenderness
Proctitis	Delayed perineal healing
Rectal blood loss	Bladder atrophy and bleeding
Rectal pain	Sacral necrosis
Small bowel obstruction	Infertility
Small bowel perforation	

be 200 cGy or less. A linear accelerator with 8–15 MV electrons is optimal and the treatment volume should be carefully assessed, being planned by computer to avoid hot spots and to limit the amount of bowel in the field. The other non-radiotherapy-related factors and medical conditions are difficult to quantify, but some allowance may need to be made.

Where radiation tissue damage has developed, a conservative approach is often successful. For radiation proctitis with troublesome intermittent bleeding, which may demand recurrent transfusions, local instillation of formalin has been reported to be effective and simple in controlling the bleeding (Seow Choen et al., 1993). If surgery has to be embarked upon, fresh tissues are needed to assist healing, such as unirradiated omentum or full-thickness pedicle skin flaps.

Complications of chemotherapy

Fluorouracil and folinic acid most commonly cause mucositis; this manifests principally as diarrhoea which may be severe and even life-threatening. It should be treated promptly and dehydration avoided. Modest dose reduction will normally prevent recurrence.

Myelosuppression is uncommon. Most patients become fatigued during chemotherapy lasting over 3–6 months. Fluorouracil infusion is associated with dermatitis involving the hands and feet, which may be alleviated by oral pyridoxine administration. Cardiac complications of fluorouracil indicate the need for caution when using it in patients with pre-existing heart disease. Adverse effects of irinotecan and oxaliplatin are dealt with under sections on the individual drugs, above.

FOLLOW-UP AFTER INITIAL TREATMENT

If there was no effective treatment for metastases or local recurrence, it could be argued that minimal follow-up is all that is necessary, and that if recurrence occurs, the symptoms should be treated palliatively. It was estimated in the 1980s (August et al., 1984) that as many as 20 per cent of patients relapsing after apparently curative resection can be cured by resection of hepatic or pulmonary metastases. Advances in imaging, surgical technique and supportive measures have probably improved on this. Results with liver metastases are best when there is a solitary liver deposit, but multiple deposits can be resected with long-term survival (Taylor, 1996; Millikan et al., 1997). The survival benefits of chemotherapy for metastatic disease are greatest when deposits are detected and treated at an early stage. There is therefore a strong case for early detection of either resectable or unresectable recurrence.

Intensive follow-up can usually detect recurrence before it produces symptoms. Monthly serum carcinoembryonic antigen (CEA) measurements predict clinically evident recurrence by an average of 6 months in about 60 per cent of patients, and trigger other investigations or exploratory laparotomy (Begent and Rustin, 1989). Routine chest radiographs, liver ultrasound and abdominal CT and colonoscopy are also used for early detection. A regimen of bi-annual spiral CT with intravenous contrast for 2 years is recommended. Immunoscintigraphy can be helpful in locating metastases when serum CEA levels rise (Begent et al., 1986, 1996). Fluorodeoxyglucose positron emission tomography (FDG-PET) appears particularly effective in locating recurrences which may be missed by CT or MRI (Ogunbiyi et al., 1997; Imdahl et al., 2000).

FUTURE DEVELOPMENTS

There has been an improvement in the outlook for people with colorectal cancer and a number of new approaches are in clinical trials which may have a further impact.

Surgery

It is possible that the frequency of local recurrence can be reduced by radioimmunoguided surgery. Antibody reacting with colorectal cancer antigens and radiolabelled with iodine-125 is given intravenously before surgery and a hand-held gamma-detecting probe is used to locate tumour at operation. Residual tumour, not detectable by conventional means, can be located in the tumour bed or at the margin of the resected specimen (Dawson et al., 1991; Mayer et al., 2000). Occult metastases have also been detected.

Potential advances in radiotherapy

Hyperfractionation has led to encouraging reports of responses in head and neck tumours and lung cancer. The theoretical advantage of this approach is to increase tumour cell kill by reducing the overall treatment time and therefore preventing proliferation during treatment, and yet sparing normal tissues by allowing repair of radiation reaction. Bozzetti et al. (1999) recently reported a moderately high complete response rate, using hyperfractionated treatment. Hyperthermia has also been assessed and appears to be tolerable and effective when used with radiotherapy (Rau et al., 1998). Trials have failed to show any significant benefit from neutron beam therapy (Duncan et al., 1987).

Antibody-targeted therapy

The field of antibody-targeted therapy is undergoing a period of renewed optimism as a result of tumour localization of radiolabelled anti-tumour antibodies being readily shown in the colorectal cancer (Begent *et al.*, 1996), and phase I and II trials have been conducted with various antibody specificities. Responses are reported in colorectal carcinoma with radioimmunotherapy in patients given anti-CEA antibodies labelled with iodine-131, which is effective via its β-emission (Lane *et al.*, 1994).

ANTIBODY-DIRECTED ENZYME PRODRUG THERAPY (ADEPT)

ADEPT uses the principle of pre-targeting, but adds augmentation of the therapeutic effect by targeting an enzyme, each molecule of which has the ability to activate many molecules of cytotoxic drug in the cancer. An antibody directed against a tumour-associated antigen is linked to an enzyme and given intravenously, resulting in selective accumulation of enzyme in tumour. When the discrimination between tumour and normal tissue enzyme levels is sufficient, a prodrug is given intravenously which is converted to an active cytotoxic drug by enzyme within the tumour. This gives higher tumour to normal tissue ratios at the time when therapy is given than can be achieved with direct tumour targeting. High levels of a cytotoxic drug are potentially generated in tumour through the capacity of each enzyme molecule to convert many molecules of prodrug into drug. Several enzyme and prodrug systems have been investigated.

There is clinical evidence that the mechanism functions as designed. Patients with colorectal carcinoma expressing carcinoembryonic antigen (CEA) received ADEPT with antibody to CEA conjugated to carboxypeptidase G2 (CPG2). A galactosylated antibody directed against the active site of CPG2 was then used to clear and inactivate circulating enzyme. A benzoic acid mustard–glutamate prodrug was given when plasma enzyme levels had fallen to a predetermined safe level and this was converted by CPG2 in the tumour into cytotoxic benzoic acid mustard. Tumour selectivity was shown, with high tumour to blood ratio of enzyme at the time of prodrug administration. Enzyme concentrations in the tumour were sufficient to generate cytotoxic levels of active drug. Prodrug was present at levels necessary for activation to generate tumour killing. There was evidence of tumour response in colorectal cancer (Napier *et al.*, 2000). Further advances are planned using an improved prodrug and a genetic fusion protein of a single-chain Fv and CPG2.

Gene therapy

Suicide gene therapy involves an enzyme such as CPG2, placed under control of the CEA promoter and expressed in CEA-positive tumour cells. A prodrug, such as that described above for ADEPT, is then activated at the tumour site after intravenous administration. This approach has been successful in experimental models and requires successful vector development for delivery of the enzyme gene to tumours in humans (Springer and Niculescu-Duvaz, 2000).

Vaccines

Vaccination against CEA using DNA or peptides is being investigated (Schlom *et al.*, 1999; Conry *et al.*, 2000). There is some evidence of clinical relevance in the generation of anti-CEA antibodies in a proportion of patients treated.

Future prospects

As post-genomic knowledge of the molecular basis of cancer develops, there is scope for novel therapies directed against many cell surface and intracellular targets, with a reasonable prospect of useful progress in the coming decade.

NHS GUIDELINES

There are key recommendations for colorectal cancer services (Cancer Guidance Subgroup of the Clinical Outcomes Group, 1997):

1 Patient focus. Patients should be offered full verbal and written information about their condition and about any treatment that may be offered. They should have continuing access to a member of the core team who can offer guidance and support.
2 Multidisciplinary teams. Management of cancer care by multidisciplinary teams, which work to agreed protocols, is likely to facilitate the implementation of the COG guidelines and improve the quality and co-ordination of care. These teams should include clinicians with up-to-date knowledge of diagnosis and treatment of colorectal cancer, and specialized nursing staff who can support and advise patients.
3 Endoscopy facilities. Adequate endoscopy facilities should be provided to help ensure accurate and timely diagnosis. The quality of endoscopy facilities, particularly colonoscopy completion and complication rates, should be monitored and staff given additional training when necessary to improve standards.
4 Surgery for rectal cancer. Surgery for rectal cancer should be concentrated in the hands of surgeons who can demonstrate good results, particularly in terms of low recurrence rates. Surgeons should monitor their response by working closely with histopathologists.
5 Improved pathology reporting. Pathology reporting should be sufficiently detailed to give comprehensive feedback on the adequacy of surgery, particularly for rectal cancer. Reports on surgical specimens should include data on the size, type, grade and Dukes' stage of tumour, and the involvement of lymph nodes and

surgical margins. This information is important to guide treatment decisions, for routine collection of data on case-mix by cancer registries, and for monitoring long-term outcomes.

6 Adjuvant therapies. Preoperative radiotherapy should be available for patients with rectal cancer. Adjuvant therapy can improve survival in some groups of patients and should be more widely available. Large-scale, nationally or internationally co-ordinated randomized trials should be supported in order to determine the best management of patients with colorectal cancer.

SIGNIFICANT POINTS

- Surgery followed only by simple palliation for symptoms caused by advanced disease is no longer sufficient in management of colorectal cancer.
- Early diagnosis through case finding and screening of high-risk groups can make it possible to treat at a stage when prognosis is relatively good.
- Adjuvant chemotherapy and radiotherapy have a place, but the best way of applying them is not clear and it is important that patients are entered into relevant clinical trials.
- There is clear evidence that early chemotherapy for recurrence can improve survival. This, and potential for cure of some metastases by surgical resection, justifies careful follow-up after initial surgery.
- Particular attention should be paid to measuring quality of life in clinical trials and in routine practice.
- Teams including the relevant specialists are likely to be most effective in implementing these measures in an efficient and cost-effective way.
- Improved understanding of cancer biology and of therapeutics promises continuing progress in diagnosis and management in the coming decade.

KEY REFERENCES

Atkin, W. (1999) Implementing screening for colorectal cancer. *BMJ* **319**, 1212–13.
Burt, R.W. (1996) Familial risk and colorectal cancer. *Gastroenterol. Clin. North Am.* **25**, 793–803.

Cancer Guidance Subgroup of the Clinical Outcomes Group (1997) *Improving outcomes in colorectal cancer.* Department of Health, Cat. Nos 97CV0119 and 97CC0120. London: HMSO.
Douillard, J.Y., Cunningham, D., Roth, A.D. *et al.* (2000) Irinotecan combined with fluorouracil compared with fluorouracil alone as first line treatment for metastatic colorectal cancer: a multicentre randomised trial. *Lancet* **355**, 1041–7.
Fearon, E.R. and Vogelstein, B. (1990) A genetic model of carcinogenesis. *Cell* **61**, 759–67.
IMPACT B2 investigators (1999) International multicentre pooled analysis of B2 colon cancer trials. Efficacy of adjuvant and folinic acid in B2 colon cancer. *J. Clin. Oncol.* **17**, 1356–63.
Swedish Rectal Cancer Trial (1997) Improved survival with preoperative radiotherapy in resectable rectal cancer. *N. Engl. J. Med.* **14**, 980–7. [Published erratum appears in *N. Engl. J. Med.* (1997) 22 May (336), **21**, 1539.]

REFERENCES

Abulafi, A.M. and Williams, N.S. (1994) Local recurrence of colorectal cancer: the problem, mechanisms, management and adjuvant therapy. [Review]. *Br. J. Surg.* **81**, 7–19.
ACCMP (Advanced Colorectal Cancer Meta-analysis Project) (1992) Modulation of fluorouracil with leucovorin in patients with advanced colorectal cancer. *J. Clin. Oncol.* **10**, 896–903.
Adam, I.J., Mohamdee, M.O., Martin, I.G. *et al.* (1994) Role of circumferential margin involvement in the local recurrence of rectal carcinoma. *Lancet* **344**, 707–10.
Ahmad, N.R. and Nagle, D. (1997) Long-term results of preoperative radiation therapy alone for stage T3 and T4 rectal cancer. *Br. J. Surg.* **84**(10), 1445–8.
AJCC (2000) American Joint Committee on Cancer Prognostic Factors Consensus Conference: Colorectal Working Group. *Cancer* **88**, 1739–57.
Aleman, B.M., Lebesque, J.V. and Hart, A.A. (1992) Postoperative radiotherapy for rectal and rectosigmoid cancer: the impact of total dose on local control. *Radiother. Oncol.* **25**(3), 203–6.
Allen-Mersh, T.G., Earlam, S., Fordy, C., Abrams, K. and Houghton, J. (1994) Quality of life and survival with continuous hepatic artery floxuridine infusion for colorectal liver metastases. *Lancet* **344**, 1255–60.
Anderson, J.H., Hole, D. and McArdle, C.S. (1992) Elective versus emergency surgery for patients with colorectal cancer. *Br. J. Surg.* **79**, 706–9.
Anonymous (1995) Single-stage treatment for malignant left-sided colonic obstruction: a prospective

randomized clinical trial comparing subtotal colectomy with segmental resection following intraoperative irrigation. The SCOTIA Study Group. Subtotal Colectomy versus On-table Irrigation and Anastomosis. *Br. J. Surg.* **82**(12), 1622–7.

Atkin, W. (1999) Implementing screening for colorectal cancer. *BMJ* **319**, 1212–13.

Atkin, W.S., Morson, B.C. and Cuzick, J. (1992) Long term risk of colorectal cancer after excision of rectosigmoid adenomas. *N. Engl. J. Med.* **326**, 658–62.

Atkin, W.S., Hart, A., Edwards, R. *et al.* (1998) Uptake, yield of neoplasia and adverse effects of flexible sigmoidoscopy screening. *Gut* **42**, 560–5.

August, D.A., Ottow, R.T. and Sugarbaker, A. (1984) Clinical perspective of human colorectal cancer metastasis. *Cancer Metastasis Rev.* **3**, 303–24.

Balsev, I., Pederson, M., Teglbjaerg, P.S. *et al.* (1986) Postoperative radiotherapy in Dukes' B and C carcinoma of the rectum and rectosigmoid: a randomized multicenter study. *Cancer* **58**, 22–8.

Barbacid, M. (1987) Ras genes. *Ann. Rev. Biochem.* **56**, 779–827.

Barbaro, B., Schulsinger, A., Valentini, V., Marano, P. and Rotman, M. (1999) The accuracy of transrectal ultrasound in predicting the pathological stage of low-lying rectal cancer after preoperative chemoradiation therapy. *Int. J. Radiat. Oncol. Biol. Phys.* **43**(5), 1043–7.

Beahrs, O.N., Henson, D.E., Hutter, R.V.P. *et al.* (1992) *Manual for staging for cancer*, (4th ed). Philadelphia: J.B. Lippincott, 69–73.

Begent, R.H.J., Keep, P.A., Searle, F. *et al.* (1986) Radioimmunolocalization and selection for surgery in recurrent colorectal cancer. *Br. J. Surg.* **73**, 64–7.

Begent, R.H.J. and Rustin, G.J.S. (1989) Tumour markers: from carcinoembryonic antigen to products of hybridoma technology. *Cancer Surv.* **8**, 108–21.

Begent, R.H.J., Verhaar, M.J., Chester, K.A. *et al.* (1996) Clinical evidence of efficient tumour targeting based on single-chain Fv antibody selected from a combinatorial library. *Nat. Med.* **2**, 979–84.

Blackstone, M., Riddell, R., Gerald Rogers, B.H. *et al.* (1981) Dysplasia-associated lesion or mass (DALM) detected by colonoscopy in long-standing ulcerative colitis: an indication for colectomy. *Gastroenterology* **80**, 366–74.

Bohm, B., Schwenk, W., Hucke, H.P. *et al.* (1993) Does methodic long-term follow-up affect survival after curative resection of colorectal carcinoma? *Dis. Colon Rectum* **36**, 280–6.

Bokey, E.L., Moore, J.W., Keating, J.P., Zelas, P., Chapuis, P.H. and Newland, R.C. (1997) Laparoscopic resection of the colon and rectum for cancer. *Br. J. Surg.* **84**(6), 822–5.

Boland, S.R., Sato, J., Appelman, H.D. *et al.* (1995) Microallelotyping defines the sequence and tempo of allelic losses at tumour suppressor gene loci during colorectal cancer progression. *Nat. Med.* **1**, 902–9.

Bozzetti, F., Baratti, D., Andreola, S. *et al.* (1999) Preoperative radiation therapy for patients with T2–T3 carcinoma of the middle-to-lower rectum. *Cancer* **86**(3), 398–404.

Bright, N., Hale, P. and Mason, R. (1992) Poor palliation of colorectal malignancy with the neodymium yttrium–aluminium–garnet laser. *Br. J. Surg.* **79**, 308–9.

Brizel, H.E. and Tepperman, B.S. (1984) Postoperative adjuvant irradiation for adenocarcinoma of the rectum and sigmoid. *Am. J. Clin. Oncol.* **28**, 3.

Burke, S.J., Percarpio, B.A., Knight, D.C. and Kwasnik, E.M. (1998) Combined preoperative radiation and mitomycin/5-fluorouracil treatment for locally advanced and rectal adenocarcinoma. *J. Am. Coll. Surg.* **187**(2), 164–70.

Burt, R.W. (1996) Familial risk and colorectal cancer. *Gastroenterol. Clin. North Am.* **25**, 793–803.

Burt, R.W., Di Sario, J.A. and Cannon-Albright, L. (1995) Genetics of colon cancer: Impact of inheritance on colon cancer risk. *Ann. Rev. Med.* **46**, 371–9.

Bussey, H.J.R., Wallace, M.H. and Morson, B.C. (1967) Metachronous carcinoma of the large intestine and intestinal polyps. *Proc. R. Soc. Med.* **60**, 208–10.

Cancer Guidance Subgroup of the Clinical Outcomes Group (1997) *Improving outcomes in colorectal cancer*. Department of Health, Cat. Nos 97CV0119 and 97CC0120. London: HMSO.

Ch'ang, H.J., Jian, J.J., Cheng, S.H. *et al.* (1998) Preoperative concurrent chemotherapy and radiotherapy in rectal cancer patients. *J. Formos. Med. Assoc.* **97**(1), 32–7.

Chantereau, M.J., Faivre, J., Boutron, M.C. *et al.* (1992) Epidemiology, management, and prognosis of malignant large bowel polyps within a defined population. *Gut* **33**, 259–63.

Chari, R.S., Tyler, D.S., Anscher, M.S. *et al.* (1995) Preoperative radiation and chemotherapy in the treatment of adenocarcinoma of the rectum. *Ann. Surg.* **221**, 778–86.

Chu, D.Z., Erickson, C.A., Russell, M.P. *et al.* (1991) Prognostic significance of carcinoembryonic antigen in colorectal carcinoma. Serum levels before and after resection and before recurrence. *Arch. Surg.* **126**, 314–16.

Cochrane review. Colorectal Meta-analysis Collaboration (2000) Palliative chemotherapy for advanced or metastatic colorectal cancer (Cochrane Review). *The Cochrane Library*, Issue 2. Oxford: Update Software.

Conry, R.M., Allen, K.O., Lee, S., Moore, S.E., Shaw, D.R. and LoBuglio, A.F. (2000) Human autoantibodies to carcinoembryonic antigen (CEA) induced by a vaccinia-CEA vaccine. *Clin. Cancer Res.* **6**(1), 34–41.

Corsa, P., Parisi, S. and Canistro, A. (1997) Preliminary results of preoperative radiotherapy schedule in the treatment of rectal tumors. *Radiol. Med. (Torino)* **94**(6), 658–63. Italian.

Crawford, J.M. (1994) The gastrointestinal tract. In Cotran, R.S., Kumar, V., Robbins, S. (eds), *Robbins pathologic basis of disease*, (5th edn). Philadelphia: W.B. Saunders, 811–13.

Crile, G. and Turnbull, R.B. (1972) Role of electrocoagulation in the treatment of carcinoma of the rectum. *Surg. Gynaecol. Obstet.* **135**, 391–6.

Cunningham, G., Pyrhonen, S., James, R. *et al.* (1998) Randomised trial of irinotecan versus supportive care alone after fluorouracil failure for patients with metastatic colorectal cancer. *Lancet* **352**, 1407–12.

Cutait, R., Alvee, V.A.F., Lopes, L.C. *et al.* (1991) Restaging of colorectal carcinoma based on the identification of lymph node micrometastases through immunoperoxidase staining of CEA and cytokeratins. *Dis. Colon Rectum* **34**, 917–20.

Daneker, G.W.J., Carlson, G.W., Hohn, D.C., Lynch, P., Roubein, L. and Levin, B. (1991) Endoscopic laser recanalization is effective for prevention and treatment of obstruction in sigmoid and rectal cancer. *Arch. Surg.* **126**, 1348–52.

Dawson, P.M., Blair, S.D., Begent, R.H.J. *et al.* (1991) The value of radioimmunoguided surgery in first and second look laparotomy for colorectal cancer. *Dis. Colon Rectum* **34**, 217–22.

Deans, G.T., Krukowski, Z.H. and Irwin, S.T. (1994) Malignant obstruction of the left colon. *Br. J. Surg.* **81**(9), 1270–6.

Dehni, N., Tiret, E., Singland, J.D. *et al.* (1998) Long-term functional outcome after low anterior resection: comparison of low colorectal anastomosis and colonic J-pouch-anal anastomosis. *Dis. Colon Rectum* **41**(7), 817–22 [discussion 822–3].

Dhir, V. and Gopinath, N. (1995) Endoscopic appearance of dysplasia and cancer in JBD Tytgat GNJ. *Eur. J. Cancer* **31**, 1174–7.

Domjan, J., Blaquiere, R. and Odurny, A. (1998) Is minimal preparation computed tomography comparable with barium enema in elderly patients with colonic symptoms? *Clin. Radiol.* **53**(12), 894–8.

Douillard, J.Y., Cunningham, D., Roth, A.D. *et al.* (2000) Irinotecan combined with fluorouracil compared with fluorouracil alone as first line treatment for metastatic colorectal cancer: a multicentre randomised trial. *Lancet* **355**, 1041–7.

Dukes, C.E. (1932) The classification of cancer of the rectum. *J. Pathol. Bacteriol.* **35**, 373.

Dukes, C.E. (1940) Cancer of the rectum: an analysis of 1000 cases. *J. Pathol. Bacteriol.* **50**, 527–39.

Dukes, C.E. and Bussey, H.J.R. (1958) The spread of rectal cancer and its effect on prognosis. *Br. J. Cancer* **12**, 309–20.

Duncan, W., Arnott, S.J., Jack, W.J.L. *et al.* (1987) Results of two randomized trials of neutron therapy in rectal adenocarcinoma. *Radiother. Oncol.* **8**, 191–8.

Duttenhaver, J.R., Hoskins, R.B., Gunderson, L.K. *et al.* (1986) Adjuvant postoperative radiation therapy in the management of adenocarcinoma of the colon. *Cancer* **57**, 955.

Eide, T.J. (1986) Prevalence and morphological features of adenomas of the large intestine with and without colorectal carcinoma. *Histopathology* **10**, 111–18.

Ellis, L.M., Menderhall, W.M., Bland, K.L. *et al.* (1988) Local excision and radiation therapy for early rectal cancer. *Am. Surg.* **54**, 217–20.

Els, M., Gross, T., Ackermann, C. and Tondelli, P. (1992) Incidence of ileus after rectal resection for rectal carcinoma, with and without adjunctive radiation therapy. *Schweiz. Med. Wochenschr.* **122**, 745–7.

Fearon, E.R. and Vogelstein, B. (1990) A genetic model for colorectal tumorigenesis. *Cell* **61**, 759–67.

Fearon, E.R., Cho, K.R., Nigro, J.M. *et al.* (1990) Identification of a chromosome 18q gene that is altered in colorectal cancers. *Science* **247**, 49–58.

Findlay, M.P., Van Cutsem, E., Kocha, W. *et al.* (1997) A randomised phase II study of Xeloda (capecitabine) in patients with advanced colorectal cancer. *Proc. Am. Soc. Clin. Oncol.* 16798.

Fisher, B., Wolmark, N., Rockette, H. *et al.* (1988) Postoperative adjuvant chemotherapy or radiation therapy for rectal cancer: Results from NSABP protocol R-01. *J. Natl Cancer Inst.* **80**, 21.

Fuchs, C.S., Giovannucci, E., Colditz, G.A. *et al.* (1994) A prospective study of family history and the risk of colorectal cancer. *N. Engl. J. Med.* **331**, 1669–94.

Garcia Valdecasas, J.C., Llovera, J.M., deLacy, A.M. *et al.* (1991) Obstructing colorectal carcinomas. Prospective study. *Dis. Colon Rectum* **34**, 759–62.

Gastrointestinal Tumour Study Group (1985) Prolongation of the disease-free interval in surgically treated rectal carcinoma. *N. Eng. J. Med.* **312**, 1465–72.

Gerard, A., Buyse, M., Nordlinger, B. *et al.* (1988) Preoperative radiotherapy as adjuvant treatment in rectal cancer. Final results of a randomized study of the European Organization for research and treatment of cancer (EORTC). *Ann. Surg.* **208**, 606–14.

Gerard, J.P., Baulieux, J., Francois, Y. *et al.* (1998) The role of radiotherapy in the conservative treatment of rectal carcinoma—the Lyon experience. *Acta Oncol.* **37**(3), 253–8.

Gerhardsson, M., Floderus, B. and Novell, S.E. (1988) Physical activity and colon cancer risk. *Int. J. Epidemiol.* **17**, 743–6.

Giacchetti, S., Itzhaku, M. and Gruia, G. (1999) Long-term survival of patients with unresectable colorectal cancer liver metastases following infusional chemotherapy with 5-fluorouracil, leucovorin, oxaliplatin and surgery. *Ann. Oncol.* **10**, 663–4.

Gibbs, N.M. (1977) Undifferentiated carcinoma of the large intestine. *Histopathology* **1**, 77–84.

Giovannucci, E., Rimm, E.B., Stampfer, M.J. et al. (1994) Intake of fat, meat and fiber in relation to risk of colon cancer in men. Cancer Res. 54, 2390–7.

Goh, H.S. and Jass, J.R. (1986) DNA content and the adenoma–carcinoma sequence in the colorectum. J. Clin. Pathol. 39, 387–92.

Greenberg, E.R. and Baron, J.A. (1993) Prospects for preventing colorectal cancer death. J. Natl Cancer Inst. 85, 1182–4.

Greenblatt, M.S., Bennett, W.P., Hollstein, M. et al. (1994) Mutations in the P53 tumour suppressor gene: clues to cancer etiology and molecular pathogenesis. Cancer Res. 54, 4855–78.

Guiney, M.J., Smith, J.G., Worotniuk, V. and Ngan, S. (1990) Results of external beam radiotherapy alone form incompletely resected carcinoma of rectosigmoid or rectum: Peter MacCallum Cancer Institute experience 1981–1990. Int. J. Radiat. Oncol. Biol. Phys. 43(3), 531–6.

Gunderson, L.K., Martin, J.K., Beart, R.W. et al. (1988) Intraoperative and external beam irradiation for locally advanced colorectal cancer. Ann. Surg. 207, 52.

Hager, T.H., Gall, F.P. and Hermanek, P. (1983) Local excision of cancer of the rectum. Dis. Colon Rectum 26, 149.

Hardcastle, J., Chamberlain, J., Robinson, M., Moss, S., Amar, S. and Balfour, T. (1996) Randomised controlled trial of faecal-occult-blood screening for colorectal cancer. Lancet 348, 1472–7.

Harrington, D.P. (1999) The tea leaves of small trials. J. Clin. Oncol. 17, 1336–8.

Heald, R.J. and Lockhart-Mummery, H.E. (1972) The lesion of the second cancer of the large bowel. Br. J. Surg. 59, 16–19.

Heriot, A.G., Grundy, A. and Kumar, D. (1999) Preoperative staging of rectal carcinoma. Br. J. Surg. 86(1), 17–28.

Hida, J., Yasutomi, M., Shindoh, K. et al. (1996) Second-look operation for recurrent colorectal cancer based on carcinoembryonic antigen and imaging techniques. Dis. Colon Rectum 39(1), 74–9.

Hoskins, R.B., Gunderson, L.L., Dosoretz, D.E. et al. (1985) Adjuvant postoperative radiotherapy in carcinoma of the rectum and recto-sigmoid. Cancer 55, 61.

Imdahl, A., Reinhardt, M.J., Nitzsche, E.U. et al. (2000) Impact of 18F-FDG-positron emission tomography for decision making in colorectal cancer recurrences. Langenbecks Arch. Surg. 385, 129–34.

IMPACT B2 investigators (1999) International multicentre pooled analysis of B2 colon cancer trials. Efficacy of adjuvant fluorouracil and folinic acid in B2 colon cancer. J. Clin. Oncol. 17, 1356–63.

Itabashi, M., Hamano, K., Kameoka, S. and Asahina, K. (1993) Self-expanding stainless steel stent application in rectosigmoid stricture. Dis. Colon Rectum 36(5), 508–11.

Izbicki, J.R., Hosch, S.B., Knoefel, W.T., Passlick, B., Bloechle, C. and Broelsch, C.E. (1995) Extended resections are beneficial for patients with locally advanced colorectal cancer. Dis. Colon Rectum 38(12), 1251–6.

Jacobs, L.R. (1988) Fiber and colon cancer. Gastroenterol. Clin. North Am. 17, 747–60.

Janjan, N.A., Abbruzzese, J., Pazdur, R. et al. (1999) Prognostic implications of response to preoperative infusional chemoradiation in locally advanced rectal cancer. Radiother. Oncol. 51(2), 153–60.

Jass, J.R. (1998) Diagnosis of hereditary non polyposis colorectal carcinoma. Histopathology 32, 491–7.

Jass, J.R., Atkin, W.S., Cuzick, J. et al. (1986) The grading of rectal carcinoma. Historical perspectives and a multi variate analysis of 447 cases. Histopathology 10, 437–59.

Jass, J.R., Smyrk, T.C., Stewart, S.M. et al. (1994) Pathology of hereditary non polyposis colorectal carcinoma. Anticancer Res. 14, 1631–4.

Johnston, P.G., Fisher, E.R. and Rockett, H.E. (1994) The role of thymidilate synthase expression prognosis and outcome of adjuvant chemotherapy in patients with rectal cancer. J. Clin. Oncol. 12, 2640–7.

Kaminsky-Forrett, M.C., Conroy, T., Luporsi, E. et al. (1998) Prognostic implications of downstaging following preoperative radiation therapy for operable T3–T4 rectal cancer. Int. J. Radiat. Biol. Phys. 42, 935–41.

Karanjia, N.D., Schache, D.J. and Heald, R.J. (1992) Function of the distal rectum after low anterior resection for carcinoma. Br. J. Surg. 79, 114–16.

Killingback, M.J. (1985) Indications for local excision of rectal cancer. Br. J. Surg. 72, S54–S56.

Kockerling, F., Reymond, M.A., Schneider, C. et al. (1998) Prospective multicenter study of the quality of oncologic resections in patients undergoing laparoscopic colorectal surgery for cancer. The Laparoscopic Colorectal Surgery Study Group. Dis. Colon Rectum 41(8), 963–70.

Konishi, F. and Morson, B.C. (1982) Pathology of colorectal adenomas. J. Clin. Pathol. 35, 830–41.

Kronborg, O., Fenger, C., Olsen, J., Jorgensen, O. and Sondergaard, O. (1996) Randomised study of screening for colorectal cancer with faecal-occult-blood test. Lancet 348, 1467–71.

Krook, J.E., Moertel, C.G., Gunderson, L.L. et al. (1991) Effective surgical adjuvant therapy of high risk rectal cancer. N. Engl. J. Med. 324, 709–45.

Lane, D.M., Eagle, K.F., Green, A.J., Keep, P.A. and Begent, R.H.J. (1994) Radioimmunotherapy of metastatic colorectal tumours with 131-Iodine antibody to CEA: Phase I/II study with comparative bio-distribution of intact and F(ab′)2 antibodies. Br. J. Cancer 70, 521–5.

Lane, D.P. (1992) Cancer, P53, guardian of the genome. Nature 358, 15–16.

Lavery, I.C., Jones, I.T., Weakley, F.L. et al. (1987) Definitive management of rectal cancer by contact (endocavitary) irradiation. Dis. Colon Rectum 30, 835.

Lechner, P. and Cesnik, H. (1992) Abdominopelvic omentopexy: preparatory procedure for radiotherapy in rectal cancer. Dis. Colon Rectum 35, 1157–60.

Lee, P., Oyama, K., Homer, L. and Sullivan, E. (1999) Effects of endorectal ultrasonography in the surgical management of rectal adenomas and carcinomas. *Am. J. Surg.* **177**(5), 388–91.

Leichman, C.G., Lenz, H. and Leichman, L. (1997) Quantitation of intratumoral thymidylate synthase expression predicts for response and resistance to protracted infusion fluorouracil and weekly leucovorin. *J. Clin. Oncol.* **15**, 3223–9.

Lennard-Jones, J.E., Morson, B.C., Ritchie, J.K. and Williams, C.B. (1983) Cancer surveillance in ulcerative colitis. Experience over 15 years. *Lancet* **2**, 149–52.

Longacre, T.A. and Fenoglio-Preiser, C.M. (1990) Mixed hyperplastic adenomatous polyps/serrated adenomas. *Am. J. Surg. Pathol.* **14**, 524–37.

Lopez-Kostner, F., Hool, G.R. and Lavery, I.C. (1997) Management and causes of acute large-bowel obstruction. *Surg. Clin. North Am.* **77**(6), 1265–90.

Lowy, A.M., Rich, T.A., Skibber, J.M., Dubrow, R.A. and Curley, S.A. (1996) Preoperative infusional chemoradiation, selective intraoperative radiation, and resection for locally advanced pelvic recurrence of colorectal adenocarcinoma. *Ann. Surg.* **2**, 177–85.

Lusinchi, A., Wibault, P., Lasser, P. *et al.* (1997) Abdominoperineal resection combined with pre- and postoperative radiation therapy in the treatment of low-lying rectal carcinoma. *Int. J. Radiat. Oncol. Biol. Phys.* **37**(1), 59–65.

Mamounas, E., Wieand, S., Wolmark, N. *et al.* (1999) Comparative efficacy of adjuvant chemotherapy in patients with Dukes' B versus Dukes' C colon cancer: results from four national adjuvant breast and bowel project adjuvant studies (C-01, C-02, C-03 and C-04). *J. Clin. Oncol.* **17**, 1349–55.

Mandel, J., Church, T., Ederer, F. and Bond, J. (1999) Colorectal cancer mortality: effectiveness of biennial screening for fecal occult blood. *N. Engl. J. Med.* **91**, 434–7.

Marsh, P.J., James, R.D. and Schofield, P.F. (1994) Adjuvant preoperative radiotherapy for locally advanced rectal carcinoma. Results of a prospective, randomized trial. *Dis. Colon Rectum* **37**(12), 1205–14.

Martin, E.W.J. and Carey, L.C. (1991) Second-look surgery for colorectal cancer. The second time around. *Ann. Surg.* **214**, 321–5.

Martin, E.W., Minton, J.P. and Carey, L.C. (1985) CEA-directed second-look surgery in the asymptomatic patient after primary resection of colorectal carcinoma. *Ann. Surg.* **202**, 310–14.

Matheson, N.A., McIntosh, C.A. and Krukowski, Z. (1985) Continuing experience with single layer appositional anastomosis in the large bowel. *Br. J. Surg.* **72**, S104–S106.

Maughan, T., James, R.D., and Kerr, D. (1999) Preliminary results of a multicentre randomised trial comparing 3 chemotherapy regimens (D Gramont, Lokich and raltitrexed) in metastatic colorectal cancer. *Proc. ASCO* **18**, abstract 1007.

Mayer, A., Tsiompanou, E., O'Malley, D. *et al.* (2000) Radioimmunoguided surgery in colorectal cancer using a genetically engineered, anti-CEA single chain Fv antibody. *Clin. Cancer Res.* **6**, 1711–19.

McCready, D.R., Ota, D.M., Rich, T.A. *et al.* (1989) Prospective phase 1 trial of conservative management of low rectal lesions. *Arch. Surg.* **124**, 67–70.

Mendenhall, W.M., Bland, K.I., Copeland, E.M. *et al.* (1992a) Does preoperative radiation therapy enhance the probability of local control and survival in high risk distal rectal cancer? *Ann. Surg.* **215**, 696–705.

Mendenhall, W.M., Souba, W.W., Bland, K.I., Million, R.R. and Copeland, E.M. (1992b) Preoperative irradiation and surgery for initially unresectable adenocarcinoma of the rectum. *Am. Surg.* **58**, 423–9.

Meterissian, S., Skibber, J., Rich, T. *et al.* (1994) Patterns of residual disease after preoperative chemoradiation in ultrasound T3 rectal carcinoma. *Ann. Surg. Oncol.* **1**(2), 111–16.

Millikan, K.W., Staren, E.D. and Doolas, A. (1997) Invasive therapy of metastatic colorectal cancer to the liver. *Surg. Clin. North Am.* **77**(1), 27–48.

Mills, S.E., Allen, M.S. Jr. and Cohen, A.R. (1983) Small cell undifferentiated carcinoma of the colon. *Am. J. Surg. Pathol.* **7**, 643–51.

Mohiuddin, M., Regine, W.F., Marks, G.J. and Marks, J.W. (1998) High-dose preoperative radiation and the challenge of sphincter-preservation surgery for cancer of the distal 2 cm of the rectum. *Int. J. Radiat. Oncol. Biol. Phys.* **40**(3), 569–74.

Morson, B.C. (1984) The polyp story. *Postgrad. Med. J.* **60**, 820–4.

Morson, B.C. and Bussey, H.J.R. (1985) Magnitude of risk for cancer patients and colorectal adenomas. *Br. J. Surg.* **72** (suppl.), 523–5.

Muto, T., Bussey, H.J.R. and Morson, B.C. (1975) The evaluation of cancer of the colon and rectum. *Cancer* **36**, 2251–70.

Napier, M.P., Sharma, S.K., Springer, C.J. *et al.* (2000) Antibody-directed enzyme prodrug therapy: efficacy and mechanism of action in colorectal carcinoma. *Clin. Cancer Res* **6**, 765–72.

Netzer, P., Forster, C., Biral, R. *et al.* (1998) Risk factor assessment of endoscopically removed malignant colorectal polyps. *Gut* **43**(5), 669–74.

NHS Centre for Reviews and Dissemination (1997) *Effective health care: The management of colorectal cancer.* York: University of York.

Nivatvongs, S., Rojanasakul, A., Reiman, H.M. *et al.* (1991) The risk of lymph node metastasis in colorectal polyps with invasive adenocarcinoma. *Dis. Colon Rectum* **34**, 323–8.

Nozaki, R., Takagi, K., Takano, M. and Miyata, M. (1997) Clinical investigation of colorectal cancer detected by follow-up colonoscopy after endoscopic polypectomy. *Dis. Colon Rectum* **40**(10), 516–22.

O'Brien, M.J., Zamcheck, N., Burke, B. *et al.* (1981) Immunocytochemical localisation of carcinoembryonic antigen in benign and malignant colorectal tissues. *Am. J. Clin. Pathol.* **75**, 283–90.

Office of Medical Applications of Research (1990) NIH consensus conference. Adjuvant therapy for patients with colon and rectal cancer. *J. Am. Med. Assoc.* **264**, 1444–50.

Ogunbiyi, O.A., Flanagan, F.L., Dehdashti, F. *et al.* (1997) Detection of recurrent and metastatic colorectal cancer: comparison of positron emission tomography and computed tomography. *Ann. Surg. Oncol.* **4**(8), 613–20.

ONS (1998) *Mortality Statistics: cause. England and Wales 1997* Series DH2 No. 24. London: HMSO.

Ooi, B.S., Tjandra, J.J. and Green, M.D. (1999) Morbidities of adjuvant chemotherapy and radiotherapy for resectable rectal cancer: an overview. *Dis. Colon Rectum* **42**(3), 403–18.

OPCS (1994) *1988 Cancer statistics: registrations, England and Wales*, Government Statistical Service Series MB1 No. 21. London: HMSO.

Pahlman, L. (1998) Radiochemotherapy as an adjuvant treatment for rectal cancer. *Recent Results Cancer Res.* **146**, 141–51.

Pahlman, L. and Glimelius, B. (1990) Pre or postoperative radiotherapy in rectal and rectosigmoid carcinoma: Report from a randomized multicenter trial. *Ann. Surg.* **211**, 187–95.

Papillon, J. (1982) *Rectal and oral cancers. Conservative treatment by irradiation – an alternative to radical surgery.* Berlin: Springer Verlag.

Peipins, L.A. and Sandler, R.S. (1994) Epidemiology of colorectal adenomas. *Epidemiol. Rev.* **16**, 273–97.

Phillips, R.K.S., Hittinger, R., Fry, J.S. *et al.* (1985) Malignant large bowel obstruction. *Br. J. Surg.* **72**, 296–302.

Piedbois, P., Buyse, M., Rustum, Y. *et al.* (1992) Modulation of fluorouracil by leucovorin in patients with advanced colorectal cancer: evidence in terms of response rate. Advanced Colorectal Cancer Meta-Analysis Project. *J. Clin. Oncol.* **10**(6), 896–903.

Piedbois, P., Buse, M., Kemeny, N. *et al.* (1996) Reappraisal of hepatic arterial infusion in the treatment of non-resectable liver metastases of colorectal cancer. *J. Natl Cancer Inst.* **88**, 252–8.

Pietra, N., Sarli, L., Costi, R., Ouchemi, C., Grattarola, M. and Peracchia, A. (1998) Role of follow-up in management of local recurrences of colorectal cancer: a prospective, randomized study. *Dis. Colon Rectum* **41**(9), 1127–33.

Poeze, M., Houbiers, J.G., van de Velde, C.J., Wobbes, T. and von Meyenfeldt, M.F. (1995) Radical resection of locally advanced colorectal cancer. *Br. J. Surg.* **82**(10), 1386–90.

Poon, R.T., Law, W.L., Chu, K.W. and Wong, J. (1998) Emergency resection and primary anastomosis for left-sided obstructing colorectal carcinoma in the elderly. *Br. J. Surg.* **85**(11), 1539–42.

Powell, S.M., Zilz, N., Beazer-Barclay, Y. *et al.* (1992) APC mutations occur early during colorectal tumourigenesis. *Nature* **359**, 235–7.

Quirke, P. (1998) Assessing the quality of rectal surgery. *Bull. R. Coll. Pathol.* **104**, abstract VII.

Quirke, P. and Williams, G.T. (co-ordinators) (1998) *Standards and minimum datasets for reporting common cancers. Minimum dataset for colorectal cancer histopathology reports.* London: Royal College of Pathologists.

Rau, B., Wurst, P., Hohenberger, P. *et al.* (1998) Preoperative hyperthermia combined with chemoradiotherapy in locally advanced rectal cancer: a phase II clinical trial. *Ann. Surg.* **227**, 380–9.

Raymond, E., Chaney, S., Taama, A. and Cvitcovic, E. (1998) Oxaliplatin: a review of clinical and preclinical studies. *Ann. Oncol.* **9**, 1053–71.

Rees, M., Plant, G. and Bygrave, S. (1997) Late results justify resection for multiple hepatic metastases from colorectal cancer. *Br. J. Surg.* **84**(8), 1136–40.

Reis Neto, J.A., Quilici, F.A. and Reis, J.A. Jr (1989) A comparison of non-operative vs preoperative radiotherapy in rectal carcinoma: A 10-year randomized trial. *Dis. Colon Rectum* **32**, 702–10.

Rich, T.A., Weiss, D.R., Mies, C. *et al.* (1985) Sphincter preservation in patients with low rectal cancer treated with radiation therapy with or without local excision or fulguration. *Radiology* **156**, 527–31.

Rich, T.A., Skibber, J.M., Ajani, J.A. *et al.* (1995) Preoperative infusional chemoradiation for therapy for stage T3 rectal cancer. *Int. J. Radiat. Oncol. Biol. Phys.* **32**, 1025–9.

Rider, W.D., Palmer, J.A., Mahoney, I.J. *et al.* (1977) Preoperative irradiation in operable cancer of the rectum. Report of the Toronto Trial. *Can. J. Surg.* **20**, 335–8.

Riethmuller, G., Holz, E., Schlimak, G. *et al.* (1998) Monoclonal antibody therapy for resected Dukes' C colorectal cancer: Seven year outcome of a randomised controlled trial. *J. Clin. Oncol.* **16**, 1788–94.

Rocklin, M.S., Senagore, A.J. and Talbott, T.M. (1991) Role of carcinoembryonic antigen and liver function tests in the detection of recurrent colorectal carcinoma. *Dis. Colon Rectum* **34**, 794–7.

Rodriguez Bigas, M.A., Stulc, J.P., Davidson, B. *et al.* (1992) Prognostic significance of anastomotic recurrence from colorectal adenocarcinoma. *Dis. Colon Rectum* **35**, 838–42.

Rougier, P., Van Cutsem, E., Bajetta, E. *et al.* (1998) Randomised trial of irinotecan versus fluorouracil by continuous infusion after fluorouracil failure in patients with metastatic colorectal cancer. *Lancet* **352**, 1407–12.

Rubinfeld, B., Souza, B., Albert, I. *et al.* (1993) Association of the APC gene product with β-catenin *Science* **262**, 1731–4.

Russell, J.B., Chu, D.Z., Russell, M.P. *et al.* (1990) When is polypectomy sufficient treatment for colorectal cancer in a polyp? *Am. J. Surg.* **160**, 665–8.

Saida, Y., Sumiyama, Y., Nagao, J. and Takase, M. (1996) Stent endoprosthesis for obstructing colorectal cancers. *Dis. Colon Rectum* **39**(5), 552–5.

Saito, N., Sarashina, H., Nunomura, M., Koda, K., Takiguchi, N. and Nakajima, N. (1998) Clinical evaluation of nerve-sparing surgery combined with preoperative radiotherapy in advanced rectal cancer patients. *Am. J. Surg.* **175**(4), 277–82.

Saltz, L., Locker, P. and Pirotta, N. (1999) Weekly irinotecan, leucovorin and fluorouracil is superior to daily × 5 LV-FU in patients with previously untreated metastatic colorectal cancer. *Proc. Am. Soc. Clin. Oncol.* **8**, 898.

Sasaki, O., Atkin, W.S. and Jass, J.R. (1987) Mucinous carcinoma of the rectum. *Histopathology* **11**, 259–72.

Schild, S.E., Martenson, J.A. Jr, Gunderson, L.L. and Dozois, R.R. (1989) Long-term survival and patterns of failure after postoperative radiation therapy for subtotally resected rectal adenocarcinoma. *Int. J. Radiat. Oncol. Biol. Phys.* **16**(2), 459–63.

Schlom, J., Tsang, K.Y., Kantor, J.A. *et al.* (1999) Strategies in the development of recombinant vaccines for colon cancer. *Semin. Oncol.* **26**(6), 672–82.

Schnabel, T., Zamboglou, N., Kuhn, F.P., Kolotas, C. and Schmitt, G. (1992) Intraarterial 5-FU-infusion and simultaneous radiotherapy as palliative treatment of recurrent rectal cancer. *Strahlenther. Onkol.* **168**(10), 584–7.

Selby, J.V., Friedman, G.D., Queensbury, C.P. *et al.* (1992) A case control study of screening sigmoidoscopy and mortality from colorectal cancer. *N. Engl. J. Med.* **326**, 653–5.

Seow Choen, F., Goh, H.S., Eu, K.W., Ho, Y.H. and Tay, S.K. (1993) A simple and effective treatment for hemorrhagic radiation proctitis using formalin. *Dis. Colon Rectum* **36**, 135–8.

Shepherd, N.A., Baxter, K. and Love, S. (1997) The prognostic importance of peritoneal involvement in colonic carcinoma: A prospective evaluation. *Gastroenterology* **112**, 1096–102.

Shirouzu, K., Isomoto, H. and Kakegawa, T. (1996) Total pelvic exenteration for locally advanced colorectal carcinoma. *Br. J. Surg.* **83**(1), 32–5.

Sjodahl, R., Franzen, T. and Nystrom, P.O. (1992) Primary versus staged resection for acute obstructing colorectal carcinoma. *Br. J. Surg.* **79**, 685–8.

Slater, G.I., Haber, R.H. and Aufses, A.H. (1984) Changing distribution of carcinoma of the colon and rectum. *Surg. Gynaecol. Obstet.* **158**, 716–18.

Sobrero, A., Kerr, D., Glimelius, B. *et al.* (2000) Cancer: a look to the future. New directions in the treatment of colorectal. *Eur. J. Cancer* **36**(5), 559–66.

Spirio, L., Olschwang, S., Groden, J. *et al.* (1993) Alleles of the APC gene: An attenuated form of familial polyposis. *Cell* **75**, 951–7.

Springer, C.J. and Niculescu-Duvaz, I. (2000) Prodrug-activating systems in suicide gene therapy. *J. Clin. Invest.* **105**(9), 1161–7.

Steinmetz, K.A. and Potter, J.D. (1991) Vegetables, fruit and cancer: II. Mechanisms. *Cancer Causes Control* **2**, 427–42.

Stockholm Rectal Cancer Study Group (1990) Preoperative short-term radiation therapy in operable rectal cancer: a randomized trial. *Cancer* **66**, 49–55.

Swedish Rectal Cancer Trial (1997) Improved survival with preoperative radiotherapy in resectable rectal cancer. *N. Engl. J. Med.* **14**, 980–7. [Published erratum appears in *N. Engl. J. Med.* (1997) May 22: 336, **21**, 1539.]

Taylor, I. (1996) Liver metastases from colorectal cancer: lessons from past and present clinical studies. *Br. J. Surg.* **83**(4), 456–60.

Tepper, J.E., Cohen, A.M., Wood, W.C. *et al.* (1986) Intraoperative electron beam radiotherapy in the treatment of unresectable rectal cancer. *Arch. Surg.* **121**, 421.

Thom, A., Baumann, J., Chandler, J.J. and Devereux, D.F. (1992) Experience with high dose radiation therapy and the intestinal sling procedure in patients with rectal carcinoma. *Cancer* **70**, 581–4.

Thun, M.J., Calle, E.E., Namboodiri, M.M. *et al.* (1992) Risk factors for fatal colon cancer in a large prospective study. *J. Natl Cancer Inst.* **84**, 1491–500.

Trock, B., Lanza, E. and Greenwald, P. (1990) Dietary fibre, vegetables and colon cancer: critical review and meta-analysis of the epidemiologic evidence. *J. Natl Cancer Inst.* **82**, 650.

Turnbull, R.B., Kyle, K., Watson, F.R. *et al.* (1967) Cancer of the rectum. The influence of the no touch isolation technique on survival rates. *Ann. Surg.* **166**, 420–7.

Valentini, V., Morganti, A.G., Luzi, S. *et al.* (1997) Is chemoradiation feasible in elderly patients? A study of 17 patients with anorectal carcinoma. *Cancer* **80**, 1387–92.

Van Cutsem, E., Findlay, M., Osterwalder, B. *et al.* (2000) Capecitabine, an oral fluoropyrimidine carbamate with substantial activity in advanced colorectal cancer: results of a randomized phase II study. *J. Clin. Oncol.* **18**(6), 1337–45.

Van Cutsem, E., Twelves, C., Cassidy, J. *et al.* (2001) Oral capecitabine compared with intravenous fluorouracil plus leucovorin in patients with colorectal cancer: results of a large phase III study. *J Clin Oncol.* **19**, 4097–5116.

Vasen, H.F.A., Wijnen, J.T., Menko, F.H. *et al.* (1996) Cancer risk in families with hereditary non polyposis colorectal cancer diagnosed by mutation analysis. *Gastroenterology* **110**, 1020–2.

Videtic, G.M., Fisher, B.J. and Perera, F.E. (1998) Preoperative radiation with concurrent 5-fluorouracil continuous infusion for locally advanced unresectable rectal cancer. *Int. J. Radiat. Oncol. Biol. Phys.* **42**(2), 319–24.

Vogelstein, B., Fearon, E.R., Hamilton, S.R. *et al.* (1988) Genetic alterations during colorectal tumour development. *N. Engl. J. Med.* **319**, 575–32.

Wagman, R., Minsky, B.D., Cohen, A.M., Guillem, J.G. and Paty, P.P. (1998) Sphincter preservation in rectal cancer with preoperative radiation therapy and coloanal anastomosis: long term follow-up. *Int. J. Radiat. Oncol. Biol. Phys.* **42**(1), 51–7.

Weinstein, G.D., Rich, T.A., Shumate, C.R. *et al.* (1995) Preoperative infusional chemoradiation and surgery with or without an electron beam intraoperative boost for advanced primary rectal cancer. *Int. J. Radiat. Oncol. Biol. Phys.* **32**, 197–204.

Wexner, S.D. and Cohen, S.M. (1995) Port site metastases after laparoscopic colorectal surgery for cure of malignancy. *Br. J. Surg.* **82**(3), 295–8.

Whiting, J.F., Howes, A. and Osteen, R.T. (1993) Preoperative irradiation for unresectable carcinoma of the rectum. *Surg. Gynaecol. Obstet.* **176**, 203–7.

Willett, C.G., Tepper, J.E., Donnely, S. *et al.* (1989a) Patterns of failure following local excision and local excision and postoperative radiation therapy for invasive rectal adenocarcinoma. *J. Clin. Oncol.* **7**, 1003–8.

Willett, C.G., Tepper, J.E., Shellito, P.C. *et al.* (1989b) Indications for adjuvant radiotherapy in extrapelvic colonic carcinoma. *Oncology* **3**, 25–33.

Willett, W.C., Stampfer, M.J., Colditz, G.A. *et al.* (1990) Relation of meat, fat and fiber intake to the risk of colon cancer in a prospective study amongst women. *N. Engl. J. Med.* **323**, 1664–72.

Williams, N.S., Dixon, M.F. and Johnston, D. (1983) Reappraisal of the 5 centimetre rule of distal excision for carcinoma of the rectum: A study of distal intramural spread and of patients survival. *Br. J. Surg.* **70**, 150–4.

Williamson, P.R., Hellinger, M.D., Larach, S.W. and Ferrara, A. (1996) Endorectal ultrasound of T3 and T4 rectal cancers after preoperative chemoradiation. *Dis. Colon Rectum* **39**(1), 45–9.

Winawer, S.J., Zauber, A.G., Ho, M.N. *et al.* (1993a) Prevention of colorectal cancer by colonoscopic polypectomy. The National Polyp Study Workgroup. *N. Engl. J. Med.* **329**(27), 1977–81.

Winawer, S.J., Zauber, A.G. and O'Brien, M.J. (1993b) Randomized comparison of surveillance intervals after colonoscopic removal of newly diagnosed adenomatous polyps. The National Polyp Study Workgroup. *N. Engl. J. Med.* **328**(13), 901–6.

Withers, H.R., Cuasay, L., Mason, K.A. *et al.* (1981) Elective radiation therapy in the curative treatment of cancer of the rectum and rectosigmoid colon. In Stroehlein, J.R. and Romsdahl, M.M. (eds), *Gastrointestinal cancer*. New York: Raven Press, 351.

Anus

BERNARD J. CUMMINGS

The objectives of cancer treatment include cure with as little interference with normal quality of life as possible. The effectiveness of a combination of radiation and cytotoxic drugs in producing complete regression of anal cancers, and the serious health and social disabilities associated with radical surgery and colostomy, have stimulated rapid changes in the treatment of anal cancers over the past two decades. Most patients who present with anal cancer now have good prospects for both cure and retention of anorectal function.

ANATOMY

The anal canal is defined in the major international cancer staging systems as that part of the intestine which extends from the rectum to the junction with the hair-bearing skin of the perianal region (Fleming et al., 1997; Sobin and Wittekind, 1997). The canal is 3–4 cm long, the superior limit being the palpable upper border of the anal sphincter and puborectalis muscle of the anorectal ring, and the distal limit the level at which the walls of the canal come into contact in their normal resting state (Fenger, 1988). The perianal area is the skin within a 5 cm radius of the anal verge or margin. The anal margin has had varying definitions, but may be considered the perianal skin immediately adjacent to the distal limit of the anal canal (Cummings, 1996b).

The perianal skin is similar histologically to hair-bearing skin elsewhere. At the anal verge, the skin blends with the modified squamous epithelium of the distal canal, which lacks hair or cutaneous glands. This modified squamous epithelium merges just below the pectinate or dentate line, the level of the anal valves, with a transitional-type epithelium that includes features of rectal, urothelial and squamous epithelia. The transitional zone extends proximally for about 2 cm, where it blends with the glandular mucosa of the rectum.

There are three major lymphatic pathways from the anal tissues. These pathways are not exclusive, and there are numerous lymphatic connections between the various levels of the canal and anal verge. Lymphatics from the uppermost part of the canal drain to the perirectal and superior haemorrhoidal nodes of the inferior mesenteric system. Those from the area around and above the dentate line flow to the internal pudendal, hypogastric and obturator nodes of the internal iliac system. Lymphatics from the distal canal, anal verge and perianal skin drain to the superficial inguinal nodes, and occasionally to the femoral nodes, of the external iliac system.

PATHOLOGY

Malignant tumours of the anal region arise in the canal about four times as frequently as in the perianal skin. When the origin is in doubt, it is usual to classify the tumour as an anal canal cancer.

About 90 per cent of primary cancers of the canal are squamous cell type. The major subtypes are large cell keratinizing, large cell non-keratinizing (transitional) and basaloid. The term 'cloacogenic' is often applied to the latter two subtypes, and may be used for all (Jass and Sobin, 1989). The prognostic value of histological subtyping of squamous cell cancers of the canal is moot, and they are often considered collectively as epidermoid cancers. The remaining 10 per cent of malignant anal canal tumours include adenocarcinomas of the anal glands, small cell and undifferentiated cancers and melanomas. Adenocarcinomas which arise in rectal-type mucosa in the proximal canal are usually classified as primary rectal cancers.

Primary cancers of the perianal skin are similar to cancers of the skin arising in other sites. Most are squamous cell cancers, with occasional basal cell cancers, skin adnexal adenocarcinomas and melanomas.

Anal dysplasia, or intra-epithelial neoplasia, has been recognized with increasing frequency. It has a spectrum similar to that seen in the uterine cervix. It is often multicentric and is considered precancerous (Jass and Sobin, 1989).

EPIDEMIOLOGY AND RISK FACTORS

Epidermoid cancers of the anus are about one-tenth as common as cancers of the rectum. The incidence has been rising in many countries over the past 30 years (Melbye et al., 1994b), but remains less than 1 per 100 000 according to most cancer registries. There is about a 1.5–3 to 1 female to male predominance for cancers of the canal, but perianal cancers are slightly more common in men than in women. The risk of anal cancer increases with age, the median age at diagnosis being about 60–65 years.

Epidemiological studies have identified a number of factors associated with epidermoid anal cancer, although no unequivocal aetiological pathway. Benign conditions such as fistulas, fissures and haemorrhoids do not predispose to anal cancer, and nor do inflammatory bowel diseases such as Crohn's disease and ulcerative colitis (Frisch et al., 1994a). Over the past decade, focus has fallen particularly on the potential of sexually transmitted factors as a cause of cancers of the anogenital area. The risk of anal cancer is increased in men, and to a lesser extent in women, who give a history of anoreceptive intercourse (Frisch et al., 1997). Other significant factors include multiple sexual partners, several sexually transmitted viral and bacterial infections (Frisch et al., 1997), and a history of cancer or intra-epithelial neoplasia of the vulva, vagina or cervix (Frisch et al., 1994b). Although anal cancer is not an AIDS-defining malignancy, an increased incidence of anal cancer has been reported for up to 5 years before the diagnosis of AIDS, and at and after AIDS diagnosis in homosexual men, and, to a lesser extent, non-homosexual men (Melbye et al., 1994a). Risk factors not associated directly with a potentially sexually transmitted agent include cigarette smoking (Daling et al., 1992) and iatrogenic immunosuppression for organ transplant (Penn, 1986).

The sexually transmissible agent implicated as the most likely basis for these various epidemiological observations is human papillomavirus (HPV), although it is at present thought that HPV infection is not, of itself, sufficient to cause malignant conversion (zur Hausen, 1999). Seventy per cent or more of anal canal and perianal cancers are HPV positive. Type 16 and, to a lesser extent, type 18 are the most commonly found genotypes, and the viral early genes E6 and E7 appear to play an important role in the initiation and maintenance of the malignant phenotype in HPV-positive cancers (zur Hausen, 1999). There is some geographic variation in the prevalence of the HPV types identified in anal cancer tissue (Scholefield et al., 1990). The presence of HPV genetic material in anal cancer cells does not appear to influence survival (Williams et al., 1996).

PRESENTATION

Most symptoms are non-specific. Bleeding, discharge and anal discomfort are reported by about half the patients with cancers of the canal, and about a quarter are aware of a mass. A palpable mass and discharge are the most common presenting features of perianal tumours. A few asymptomatic primary cancers are found during physical examinations for other conditions, or during investigation of an enlarged inguinal node. Unsuspected superficial cancer or high-grade dysplasia is sometimes found on histological examination of haemorroidectomy specimens or perianal condylomata. Gross fecal incontinence due to sphincter destruction or vaginal fistula formation occurs in fewer than 5 per cent, even in neglected cancers which may reach considerable size. Symptomatic extrapelvic metastases are a very rare first presenting indication of anal cancer.

DIAGNOSTIC WORK-UP AND STAGING

Anal canal cancers

The features of greatest prognostic significance for survival are the size of the primary cancer, and spread to regional lymph nodes or to extrapelvic sites. The factors that affect the probability of retaining anal function are sphincter competence at presentation, and the size of the primary cancer. Inguinal lymph-node metastases are clinically detectable in up to about 15 per cent of patients at presentation. In series managed by radical surgery, pelvic node metastases were found in about 30 per cent, with about equal risk of involvement in the internal iliac and perirectal–superior haemorrhoidal node pathways (Golden and Horsley, 1976; Boman et al., 1984). The reported incidence of palpable perirectal nodes varies considerably, ranging from as little as 0–1 per cent (Cummings et al., 1991) to as high as 34 per cent (Gerard et al., 1998). This variation is likely due to inconsistency

Table 31.1 *Anal canal TNM classification*

T – primary tumour

TX	Primary tumour cannot be assessed
T0	No evidence of primary tumour
Tis	Carcinoma *in situ*
T1	Tumour 2 cm or less in greatest dimension
T2	Tumour more than 2 cm but not more than 5 cm in greatest dimension
T3	Tumour more than 5 cm in greatest dimension
T4	Tumour of any size invades adjacent organ(s), e.g. vagina, urethra, bladder (involvement of sphincter muscle(s) *alone* is not classified as T4)

N – regional lymph nodes

NX	Regional lymph nodes cannot be assessed
N0	No regional lymph node metastasis
N1	Metastasis in perirectal lymph node(s)
N2	Metastasis in unilateral internal iliac and/or inguinal lymph node(s)
N3	Metastasis in perirectal and inguinal lymph nodes and/or bilateral internal iliac and/or inguinal lymph nodes

M – distant metastasis

MX	Distant metastasis cannot be assessed
M0	No distant metastasis
M1	Distant metastasis

Stage grouping

Stage 0	Tis	N0	M0
Stage I	T1	N0	M0
Stage II	T2	N0	M0
	T3	N0	M0
Stage IIIA	T1	N1	M0
	T2	N1	M0
	T3	N1	M0
	T4	N0	M0
Stage IIIB	T4	N1	M0
	Any T	N2, N3	M0
Stage IV	Any T	Any N	M1

Table 31.2 *Perianal skin TNM classification*

T – primary tumour

TX	Primary tumour cannot be assessed
T0	No evidence of primary tumour
Tis	Carcinoma *in situ*
T1	Tumour 2 cm or less in greatest dimension
T2	Tumour more than 2 cm but not more than 5 cm in greatest dimension
T3	Tumour more than 5 cm in greatest dimension
T4	Tumour invades deep extradermal structures, i.e. cartilage, skeletal muscle, or bone

N – regional lymph nodes (ipsilateral inguinal nodes)

NX	Regional lymph nodes cannot be assessed
N0	No regional lymph node metastasis
N1	Regional lymph node metastasis

M – distant metastasis

MX	Distant metastasis cannot be assessed
M0	No distant metastasis
M1	Distant metastasis

Stage grouping

Stage 0	Tis	N0	M0
Stage I	T1	N0	M0
Stage II	T2	N0	M0
	T3	N0	M0
Stage III	T4	N0	M0
	Any T	N1	M0
Stage IV	Any T	Any N	M1

A variety of other tumour marker, cellular, molecular and histopathological features have been studied, but at present none provides information to assess prognosis or guide the selection of treatment more effectively than the simple features of tumour size and the presence of lymph node or other metastases outlined above (Cummings, 1995).

The current International Union Against Cancer (UICC) staging system is shown in Table 31.1.

Perianal cancers

As with cancers of the canal, the strongest prognostic factors for survival are the size of the primary tumour, and the presence of inguinal node or more distant metastases. Sphincter competence at presentation and the size of the primary cancer affect the likelihood of preservation of anal function. Inguinal node metastases are found in no more than 5–10 per cent, and should be confirmed histologically. Computed tomography (CT) examination of the abdomen and pelvis is not indicated unless inguinal node metastases are present, or the cancer involves the anal canal. A chest X-ray is usually performed but rarely discloses metastases. The same panel of blood tests as for anal canal cancer should be obtained.

The staging system for cancers of the anal margin and perianal skin is the same as that for skin cancers elsewhere (Table 31.2).

in classifying nodules palpable in the anorectal wall as direct extensions of the primary cancer or as nodes. Extrapelvic metastases are uncommon at presentation, being found in no more than 5 per cent, usually in the liver or lungs and occasionally in bone.

The primary tumour, and suspected inguinal node metastases, should be biopsied, if necessary under general anaesthesia. Since non-specific or reactive enlargement of the inguinal nodes is common, metastasis should be confirmed by fine-needle aspiration or excision biopsy. Abdominal and pelvic computerized tomography scans will disclose liver and large nodal metastases, but small nodal metastases are not currently identified reliably by any available imaging modality. A standard chest X-ray is adequate to screen for pulmonary metastases. Localized skeletal symptoms should also be evaluated radiologically. Full blood count, renal and liver function tests, and, if risk factors are present, HIV antibody tests, should be performed.

MANAGEMENT

Anal canal cancers

COMBINED MODALITY TREATMENT

Primary tumour

Combined-modality radiation and chemotherapy, with radical surgery reserved for the management of recurrent cancer, is now firmly established as the initial treatment of choice for epidermoid cancers of the anal canal. Except where stated, the following comments address the management of epidermoid cancers. Prior to the adoption of combined-modality treatment, most patients were treated by radical surgery, such as abdomino-perineal resection, although some centres favoured radiation therapy. Radical resection has not been compared with radiation alone or with combined-modality treatment in formal randomized trials, but reviews of published results indicate that cure rates are comparable (Myerson *et al.*, 1997; Cummings, 1998a), and radiation-based treatment also permits preservation of anorectal function in the majority of patients (Cummings, 1998a).

A series of favourable reports, following the initial description in 1974 by Nigro, Vaitkevicius and Considine of the ability of concurrent radiation, 5-fluorouracil (5-FU) and Mitomycin C (MMC) to produce durable complete regression of anal cancers, led to the performance of three major randomized trials. These trials established that delivering 5-FU and MMC concurrently with radiation gave outcomes superior to those achieved by the same schedule of radiation alone or radiation and 5-FU (Flam *et al.*, 1996; UKCCCR Working Party, 1996; Bartelink *et al.*, 1997).

In the trial undertaken by the United Kingdom Co-ordinating Committee for Cancer Research (UKC-CCR), 577 patients with all stages of epidermoid cancer of the anal canal or anal margin were randomly assigned to receive radiation alone (45 Gy in 20–25 fractions in 4–5 weeks) or radiation plus 5-FU (1000 mg/m^2 per 24 hours for 96 hours, or 750 mg/m^2 per 24 hours for 120 hours) by continuous intravenous infusion in the first and final weeks of radiation treatment, and MMC (12 mg/m^2) by bolus injection on day 1 of the first course of 5-FU only (UKCCCR Working Party, 1996). Six weeks after the initial phase of treatment, patients received additional radiation without chemotherapy (15 Gy in six fractions by external-beam therapy or 25 Gy over 2–3 days by ^{192}Ir-implant). For those patients whose tumour showed less than a partial response at the 6 weeks evaluation point (about 10 per cent of those treated by either regimen), surgery was performed rather than additional radiation. Local failure was diagnosed by 3 years in 39 per cent of the patients treated by radiation and chemotherapy, compared to 61 per cent of those who received radiation only. The definition of local failure was broader in this trial than in most: in addition to the presence of

Table 31.3 *3-year results of randomized trials of radiation alone (RT) versus radiation, 5-fluorouracil and Mitomycin C (RTCT) (percentages)*

	UKCCCR (N = 557)			EORTC (N = 103)		
	RT	RTCT	P	RT	RTCT	P
Local control	39	61	<0.0001	55	65	0.02
Cause-specific survival	61	72	0.02	NA	NA	NA
Overall survival	58	65	0.25	65	70	0.17

NA, not applicable.

residual or recurrent cancer in the primary site or regional nodes, treatment-related morbidity requiring surgery or inability to close a pre-treatment colostomy were also considered as local failure. Surgery with colostomy was required for late treatment-related toxicity for 10 patients in each study arm. Six patients in the combined-modality group and two in the radiation-alone group died due to treatment-related morbidity. Primary tumour control, colostomy-free survival and cause-specific survival rates were all significantly improved by combined-modality treatment. The overall survival rate was also improved, although not to conventional levels of statistical significance (Table 31.3).

The European Organization for Research and Treatment of Cancer (EORTC) performed a similar study on 103 patients with advanced anal cancers (Bartelink *et al.*, 1997). Pelvic radiation treatment of 45 Gy in 25 fractions over 5 weeks was combined in half the patients with 5-FU (750 mg/m^2 per 24 hours for 120 hours by continuous intravenous infusion) in both the first and fifth weeks of radiation. In the first week only, a bolus injection of MMC (15 mg/m^2) was given on the first day of the 5-FU infusion. Six weeks later, additional radiation was delivered by external-beam or interstitial techniques (15 Gy if there had been complete clinical response to the initial course of treatment, 20 Gy if the response had been partial). Acute and late toxicity rates were similar in each treatment group. The local control and colostomy-free survival rates were significantly better following combined-modality treatment, but, as in the UK trial, the improvement in overall survival rates was not statistically significant (Table 31.3).

Two North American clinical trials groups, the Radiation Therapy Oncology Group (RTOG) and the Eastern Cooperative Oncology Group (ECOG), combined to determine whether MMC could be omitted from the treatment regimen (Flam *et al.*, 1996, 1999). In this trial, 291 patients with cancers of the anal canal of any T and N category, without evidence of extrapelvic metastases, were treated with external-beam pelvic radiation (45–50.4 Gy in 25–28 fractions over 5 weeks) plus two courses of 5-FU (1000 mg/m^2 per 24 hours by continuous intravenous infusion for 96 hours), with or without

Table 31.4 *5-year results of randomized trial of radiation and 5-fluorouracil with/without Mitomycin C (percentages)*

| | RTOG/ECOG (N = 291) | | |
	RT, 5-FU	RT, 5-FU, MMC	P
Biopsy negative at 6 weeks	85	92	0.13
Locoregional control	64	83	0.001
Disease-free survival	50	67	0.006
Overall survival	65	67	0.70

MMC ($10\,mg/m^2$ by bolus injection on the first day of each 5-FU infusion), in the first and fifth weeks of radiation treatment. Biopsy of the primary tumour site 6 weeks after radiation was a prescribed part of the protocol. Biopsies were positive in 15 per cent of those who received 5-FU only with radiation, and in 8 per cent of those treated with both 5-FU and MMC. Patients with residual cancer received additional radiation ($9\,Gy$ in 5 fractions in 1 week) concomitantly with a 96-hour infusion of 5-FU ($1000\,mg/m^2$ per 24 hours) and a short infusion of cisplatin ($100\,mg/m^2$ over 4–6 hours) on the second day of the infusion of 5-FU. Acute haematological toxicity was more common after MMC, but otherwise the rates of acute and late toxicity were comparable in each group. The rates of colostomy-free and disease-free survival were significantly better in those treated with radiation, 5-FU and MMC, but overall survival rates at 5 years were identical (Table 31.4).

The improvement in local control rates following treatment with combinations of radiation, 5-FU and MMC also resulted in a reduction in the need for colostomy and an increase in the numbers of patients who retained anorectal function. In general, these and other studies did not include detailed prospective evaluation of the quality of anorectal function. Investigators have recently indicated that function is impaired in some patients (Cummings, 1998b; Vordermark *et al.*, 1999). However, the general finding has been of 'adequate' function, and few patients have required surgery for incontinence. Low-grade symptomatic morbidity affecting the perianal skin, anorectum and other pelvic organs is usually managed medically, with varying levels of success (Cummings, 1998b).

The failure of the randomized trials to demonstrate statistically significant improvements in overall survival rates following combined-modality treatment has been taken, in part, as an indication of the effectiveness of surgical salvage of residual or recurrent cancer. Since local control rates were improved by radiation, 5-FU and MMC, this suggests that salvage was more successful in those patients who received the less intensive initial treatment. The effectiveness of surgical salvage in non-randomized series varies considerably, with very low rates of pelvic control after failure of combined-modality treatment being recorded by many. It is speculated that some anal cancers may acquire biological characteristics as a result of exposure to chemoradiation which render them difficult to eradicate, although overall pelvic failure rates following combined-modality treatment and salvage therapy are lower than those previously recorded with radical surgery alone. There is no evidence that efforts to identify radiation–chemotherapy-resistant cancers by elective biopsy or by evaluation of the extent of clinical response at about 6 weeks leads to a more successful outcome than delaying salvage surgery until cancer re-growth is clinically apparent.

Efforts have been made to improve local control rates by intensifying treatment, particularly radiation therapy. Radiation schedules can be intensified by increasing total dose and/or shortening the overall time in which treatment is delivered. Neither the randomized trials described earlier, nor the numerous non-randomized studies, have established the optimum schedules. When combined with 5-FU and MMC, radiation doses of as low as $30\,Gy$ in 15 fractions in 3 weeks have been reported capable of eradicating up to about 90 per cent of anal cancers 3 cm or less in size (Nigro, 1984; Cummings, 1998a). Higher doses, from $45\,Gy$ in 25 fractions in 5 weeks to $54\,Gy$ in 30 fractions in 6 weeks, often supplemented by further radiation after an interval of 6–8 weeks to a total of $60–65\,Gy$, have controlled from 65 to 75 per cent of primary tumours larger than 4 cm (Cummings, 1998a). Current studies of intensified treatment generally exclude small cancers (typically T1 category, up to 2 cm), but it is likely that the breakpoint could be set higher and that some patients are overtreated.

Interruptions in the radiation schedules, either elective or as clinically necessary, are common in the treatment of anal cancer. The shorter interruptions are related principally to the discomfort associated with acute dermatitis and anoproctitis. Longer intervals have been introduced where decisions regarding further treatment are predicated on the extent of clinical or histopathological response to the initial phase of combined radiation and chemotherapy. Interruptions run counter to radiobiological theory, in that extended overall time of treatment may increase the risk of cancer re-growth (Cummings, 1996a). Some investigators who have attempted to increase total radiation dose and shorten overall treatment time have encountered poor tolerance. For example, half the patients (9 of 18) in an RTOG Phase II trial of $59.4\,Gy$ in 33 fractions over 6.5 weeks required a break in treatment of 2 weeks or more (John *et al.*, 1996). Some current trials seek to shorten overall treatment time by allowing interruptions only for those patients who experience severe toxicity, or by incorporating briefer intervals than the 6–8 weeks before the second phase of treatment used in earlier studies.

Although many current protocols attempt to reduce overall treatment time, one of the more successful schedules reported included an extended interval. The schedule designed by Papillon combined a short, intensive 3-week radiation programme with an extended interval before interstitial brachytherapy (Papillon, 1982). The first stage of treatment delivered a minimum dose of 30 Gy (maximum dose 42 Gy) in 10 fractions in 19 days by cobalt-60 to a small volume of the posterior pelvis, which included the anal area and the presacral and posterior pelvic lymph nodes. Papillon favoured an 8-week interval, to allow shrinkage of the primary tumour, before implanting the residual cancer (20 Gy in 24 hours). Concurrent chemotherapy was later added to the initial phase of treatment (Papillon and Montbarbon, 1987). When combined with 5-FU (600 mg/m^2 per 24 hours for 120 hours) and MMC (12 mg/m^2 on day 1 of 5-FU and radiation), the local control rate of anal cancers more than 4 cm in size improved from 66 per cent (51 of 77) to 81 per cent (57 of 70) in a non-randomized series of patients (Papillon and Montbarbon, 1987).

The rationale for increasing the total radiation dose is based on analysis of non-randomized studies which suggest a dose–control relationship (Rich et al., 1993; Constantinou et al., 1997), and on subset analyses of the randomized trials which sometimes show relatively low control rates even for smaller tumours with the doses used. In the UKCCCR trial, there was a 3-year local failure rate of 25 per cent in the T1T2N0 cancers treated with chemotherapy and radiation doses of up to 60 Gy (external beam) or 70 Gy (external beam plus interstitial radiation) over 12 weeks (Northover et al., 1997). Some groups are now delivering up to 60 Gy in 7 weeks without interruption in the initial phase of treatment, particularly to patients with larger tumours (John et al., 1996; Martenson et al., 1996).

Most radiation protocols use techniques that encompass the whole lower pelvis, in order to include the inguinal and posterior pelvic lymph nodes and the primary cancer in a single radiation volume. The more limited posterior pelvic radiation volume favoured by Papillon (1982) is also effective, and the latter can be combined with separate radiation fields to the inguinal nodes if desired. There is some evidence that both acute and late morbidity are influenced by technique as well as by radiation dose–time–fractionation parameters, and the ideal technique has not yet been established (Cummings, 1998a).

It has been suggested that the dose intensity of chemotherapy may also affect outcome (Ceresoli et al., 1998). The three randomized trials described above used short continuous infusions of 5-FU. These 4- or 5-day infusions generally deliver more 5-FU in the same overall time period (and with much higher short-term serum and tissue levels) than infusions continued throughout the several weeks of radiation. Extended infusions are favoured by those who argue that it is desirable to seek a potentially synergistic radiosensitizing interaction with 5-FU for every radiation treatment (Rich et al., 1993). Most protocols continue to employ short-term infusions of 5-FU, although formal trials of protracted continuous infusions are in progress.

The cytotoxic drugs which have received the greatest attention are 5-FU and MMC, but other drugs have also been studied. Bleomycin (5 mg by intramuscular injection 1 h prior to radiation for the first 15 of 30 fractions) was given concurrently with radiation in Sweden, but the results of non-randomized studies did not suggest benefit (Glimelius and Pahlman, 1987). There is currently wide interest in the combination of radiation, 5-FU and cisplatin, based on its effectiveness against squamous cell cancers in other sites and on the potential of cisplatin as a radiation sensitizer. Non-randomized studies in anal cancer have reported levels of local tumour control comparable to those produced by 5-FU, MMC and radiation. For example, Gerard et al. (1998) treated 95 patients, of whom 42 had category T3 or T4 primary cancers. The most commonly used treatment schedule was a 30 Gy tumour dose at 6 cm depth (maximum dose 40 Gy) in 10 fractions in 17 days by cobalt-60 direct perineal and posterior pelvic fields (Papillon's technique; Papillon, 1982), with concurrent chemotherapy in the first week (5-FU 1000 mg/m^2 per 24 hours by continuous infusion for 96 hours, and bolus injections of cisplatin 25 mg/m^2 on each of the same 4 days), followed 8 weeks later by interstitial brachytherapy, 20 Gy in approximately 24 hours. The 5-year overall and colostomy-free survival rates were 84 per cent and 71 per cent, respectively. The RTOG is at present conducting a randomized trial in North America in which patients with primary cancers larger than 2 cm receive either 5-FU and MMC or 5-FU and cisplatin concurrently with radiation (59.4 Gy in 33 fractions in 6.5 weeks). In this protocol, cisplatin is given in a dose of 75 mg/m^2 on the first day of each 4-day infusion of 5-FU. The doses of 5-FU and MMC are those used in the previous RTOG trial (Flam et al., 1996). However, induction 5-FU–cisplatin is also given in the 5-FU–cisplatin arm, which will confound simple comparison of the relative merits of MMC and cisplatin administered concurrently with 5-FU and radiation.

Lymph-node metastases

Metastases in regional lymph nodes can be eradicated by the same chemotherapy and radiation schedules used to treat the primary anal cancer. When patients are first diagnosed with epidermoid anal canal cancers, pelvic node metastases are present in about 30 per cent and inguinal node metastases in about 15 per cent (Golden and Horsley, 1976; Boman et al., 1984). The probability of control of node metastases by radiation and chemotherapy is similar to that of the primary cancer, although some consider it preferable to locally excise inguinal node metastases prior to radiation and chemotherapy (Papillon, 1982; Cummings et al., 1991). Radical dissection of the inguino-femoral nodes either prior to or following high-dose radiation treatment should be avoided if possible, because of the risk of poor healing and persistent leg oedema. Although relapse of treated node masses is uncommon, patients with nodal metastases are at increased risk of extrapelvic metastases, and 5-year survival rates are usually

10–20 per cent less than in patients who do not have demonstrable inguinal or pelvic node metastases.

Late failure in inguinal nodes which were not enlarged at the time of first presentation has been reported in 15–25 per cent of patients whose primary cancer was treated surgically (Golden and Horsley, 1976; Stearns *et al.*, 1980). Elective irradiation of clinically normal inguino-femoral nodes causes little morbidity and reduces the risk of late recurrence in these nodes to less than 5 per cent (Cummings, 1998a).

Extrapelvic metastases

Extrapelvic metastases are found in 10–20 per cent of patients, and in the UKCCCR trial were the only recognized site of cancer in about one-quarter of those dying of anal cancer (UKCCCR Working Party, 1996). The median survival time after the diagnosis of metastases is from 8 to 12 months (Greenall *et al.*, 1985a; Tanum, 1993). Cisplatin and 5-FU produce responses more often than other drugs, although these responses are usually partial and short-lived (Flam, 1995). Combinations of radiation, 5-FU and MMC or cisplatin appear relatively ineffective when used to treat metastases, perhaps because the doses of radiation that can be given to organs such as the liver or lung are generally less than those directed to the pelvis. The role of adjuvant chemotherapy has not been determined, although studies of platinum-based induction and post-radiation chemotherapy are being undertaken, both to intensify treatment to the pelvic cancer and to evaluate the merits of systemic adjuvant therapy (Peiffert *et al.*, 1997a; Meropol *et al.*, 1999).

RADIATION THERAPY ALONE

The preference for combined-modality treatment has largely supplanted the use of radiation therapy alone. Combined-modality protocols have been shown to produce higher control rates than radiation alone for all sizes of anal canal tumours treated by the relatively protracted radiation schedules tested. However, uninterrupted courses of radical radiation, typically equivalent to 50 Gy in 4 weeks or 60–65 Gy in 6 weeks, control 80 per cent or more cancers up to about 4 cm in size and about 50 per cent of larger tumours (Cummings, 1998a). Radiation alone should be considered when chemotherapy is contraindicated, since survival rates are comparable to those of surgery, and anorectal function can be preserved (Cummings, 1998a).

SURGERY

The main role of surgery now is as salvage following unsuccessful radiation with/without chemotherapy, and as treatment for radiation-induced toxicity not amenable to conservative measures. Surgery is indicated for patients who cannot receive pelvic radiation, most commonly because of previous radiation for other cancers. Those few patients who present with incontinence due to destruction of the anal sphincters or to vaginal fistula are probably best managed surgically. Preoperative or postoperative adjuvant radiation with/without chemotherapy should be considered in order to reduce the risk of pelvic recurrence. In series managed exclusively by surgery, 5-year survival rates ranged from about 50–70 per cent, with locoregional recurrence rates of 25–35 per cent (Boman *et al.*, 1984; Greenall *et al.*, 1985a; Pintor *et al.*, 1989; Klas *et al.*, 1999). Most patients required excision of the anorectum and permanent colostomy. Local excision was generally considered only for superficial squamous cell cancers up to about 2–3 cm in size, since tumours of this size which have not penetrated the sphincter muscles are associated with a less than 10 per cent risk of nodal metastases (Boman *et al.*, 1984), and adequate resection margins can be established without sacrificing competence of the sphincters.

NON-EPIDERMOID CANCERS

Adenocarcinomas of the anal canal are usually managed surgically. The selection of abdomino-anal excision and colostomy or local excision is based on the size of the cancer and general principles of oncological surgery. Most series are small, but 5-year survival rates of less than 50 per cent, with local recurrence rates of about 25 per cent, are typical (Abel *et al.*, 1993; Tarazi and Nelson, 1994; Klas *et al.*, 1999). Because anal adenocarcinomas are encountered infrequently, they are often managed by the protocols in place for adenocarcinomas of the rectum, although the roles of adjuvant radiation and chemotherapy for anal cancers are uncertain. Some centres have treated anal adenocarcinomas by the protocols for epidermoid cancers, and have successfully preserved anorectal function in some patients (B.J. Cummings, unpublished data).

Melanomas of the anal canal have a poor prognosis. Surgery is the principal treatment. As with rectal melanomas, some authors recommend local excision rather than abdomino-anal excision and removal of regional lymph nodes, on the grounds that the very high risk of systemic metastases associated with nodal metastases renders radical excision of little value (Cooper *et al.*, 1982; Goldman *et al.*, 1990; Klas *et al.*, 1999).

Small cell and undifferentiated cancers metastasize early. No successful approach to treatment has been devised. Systemic chemotherapy similar to that used for small cell cancers which arise elsewhere is sometimes given, but is of unproven value. The primary cancer may be managed by local or radical surgery, according to the extent of involvement of the canal and adjacent tissues.

Perianal cancer

Local excision, sometimes coupled with skin graft, is the preferred treatment of all histological subtypes of perianal cancer when an adequate margin can be achieved without compromising anal function. The high local recurrence rates reported by some authors (Greenall *et al.*, 1985b) following resection of squamous cell cancers are likely due to failure to achieve clear resection margins and/or to multicentric intra-epithelial neoplasia. Further local excision of recurrence is often sufficient to effect local control (Greenall *et al.*, 1985b).

Radiation therapy is indicated when surgery would compromise anorectal function. While radiation therapy alone is effective for both limited and extensive squamous cell cancers (Papillon and Chassard, 1992; Touboul *et al.*, 1995; Peiffert *et al.*, 1997b), some centres prefer protocols of combined radiation and chemotherapy, identical to those used for anal canal cancer (Cummings *et al.*, 1986). The United Kingdom randomized trial included patients with cancers of the canal or anal margin (the latter when local excision was not possible). Results by site of origin were not reported, but local control and cause-specific survival rates in that trial favoured combined-modality treatment (UKCCCR Working Party, 1996).

Inguinal node metastases are uncommon, except from large squamous cell or poorly differentiated cancers, and may be managed by the same principles as node metastases from anal canal cancer. Elective treatment of the groin nodes is favoured by some when the primary tumour is larger than about 4 cm or poorly differentiated. Death from perianal cancer is uncommon, and is generally associated with large and deeply infiltrating primary cancers or with distant metastases, the latter often preceded by involvement of inguinal nodes.

Patients with HIV infection

Epidermoid cancers of the anal canal or perianal skin are more common in patients with HIV infection, both prior to and after the diagnosis of AIDS (Melbye *et al.*, 1994a). The treatment policies adopted for these patients are influenced not only by the presence and severity of any other illness affecting the patient, but also by the unusual sensitivity to radiation, and to a lesser extent to chemotherapy, demonstrated by many patients with AIDS. A policy of observation without specific intervention may be adopted for some patients, but local symptoms and the threat of loss of anorectal control may necessitate treatment of the anal cancer. An analysis of a small series of patients suggested that tumour control and acute treatment-related morbidity in patients with CD4 T-cell counts ≥200 were similar to those of the general population, but that patients with lower CD4 counts were more likely to require modifications of treatment (due to intense local reactions to radiation with/without chemotherapy) and later surgery to achieve local control (Hoffman *et al.*, 1999). The use of antiviral medications by patients with HIV infection may be associated with depressed haematological indices, and these patients often refuse cytotoxic chemotherapy because of concern that marrow reserves may be depleted. Management should be individualized, with judicious selection of observation, local excision and radiation therapy alone (or occasionally with chemotherapy), whenever possible reserving radical surgery for

persistent local cancer causing symptoms or affecting continence. Overall, local tumour control rates are variously reported as similar to, or a little less than, those for the general population with anal cancers of similar size. Prognosis for survival is generally determined by the course of AIDS.

SIGNIFICANT POINTS

- Separate cancers of the anal canal and perianal skin.
- Anal canal cancers:
  - most are squamous cell;
  - all variants of squamous cell cancer are managed similarly;
  - concurrent radiation, 5-fluorouracil and Mitomycin C is the standard treatment;
  - radical surgery is reserved for residual cancer, severe treatment-related toxicity, incontinence at presentation;
  - 5-year survival rates about 65 per cent;
  - local cancer control, with preservation of anal function, in about 75 per cent following radiation and chemotherapy;
  - current trials are investigating intensified radiation – higher doses, shorter overall time; cisplatin in place of Mitomycin C; induction and adjuvant chemotherapy.
- Perianal cancers:
  - most are squamous cell;
  - local excision is the standard treatment if anorectal function can be preserved;
  - radiation alone, or concurrent radiation, 5-fluorouracil and Mitomycin C is preferred for more extensive cancers;
  - radical surgery is reserved for residual cancer, severe treatment-related toxicity, incontinence at presentation;
  - 5-year survival rates about 80 per cent;
  - local cancer control, with preservation of anal function, in about 85 per cent.

KEY REFERENCES

Bartelink, H., Roelofsen, F., Eschwege, F. *et al.* (1997) Concomitant radiotherapy and chemotherapy is superior to radiotherapy alone in the treatment of locally advanced anal cancer: results of a phase III randomized trial of the European Organization for Research and Treatment of Cancer Radiotherapy and Gastrointestinal Cooperative Groups. *J. Clin. Oncol.* **15**, 2040–9.

Flam, M., John, M., Pajak, T.F. *et al.* (1996) Role of mitomycin in combination with fluorouracil and radiotherapy, and of salvage chemoradiation in the definitive nonsurgical treatment of epidermoid carcinoma of the anal canal: results of a phase III randomized intergroup study. *J. Clin. Oncol.* **14**, 2527–39.

UKCCCR Working Party (1996) Epidermoid anal cancer: results from the UKCCCR randomised trial of radiotherapy alone versus radiotherapy, 5-fluorouracil, and mitomycin. UKCCCR Anal Cancer Trial Working Party. UK Co-ordinating Committee on Cancer Research. *Lancet* **348**, 1049–54.

REFERENCES

Abel, M.E., Chiu, Y.S.Y., Russell, T.R. and Volpe, P.A. (1993) Adenocarcinoma of the anal glands. Results of a survey. *Dis. Colon Rectum* **36**, 383–7.

Bartelink, H., Roelofsen, F., Eschwege, F. *et al.* (1997) Concomitant radiotherapy and chemotherapy is superior to radiotherapy alone in the treatment of locally advanced anal cancer: results of a phase III randomized trial of the European Organization for Research and Treatment of Cancer Radiotherapy and Gastrointestinal Cooperative Groups. *J. Clin. Oncol.* **15**, 2040–9.

Boman, B.M., Moertel, C.G., O'Connell, M.J. *et al.* (1984) Carcinoma of the anal canal. A clinical and pathologic study of 188 cases. *Cancer* **54**, 114–25.

Ceresoli, G.L., Ferreri, A.J., Cordio, S. and Villa, E. (1998) Role of dose intensity in conservative treatment of anal canal carcinoma. Report of 35 cases. *Oncology* **55**, 525–32.

Constantinou, E.C., Daly, W., Fung, C.Y. *et al.* (1997) Time–dose considerations in the treatment of anal cancer. *Int. J. Radiat. Oncol. Biol. Phys.* **39**, 651–7.

Cooper, P.H., Mills, S.E. and Allen, M.S. (1982) Malignant melanoma of the anus. Report of 12 patients and analysis of 255 additional cases. *Dis. Colon Rectum* **25**, 693–703.

Cummings, B.J. (1995) Anal canal cancer. In: Hermanek, P., Gospodarowicz, M.K., Henson, D.E. *et al.* (eds), *Prognostic factors in cancer*. Berlin: Springer-Verlag, 80–7.

Cummings, B.J. (1996a) Anal canal cancer – to split or not to split? *Cancer J. Sci. Am.* **2**, 194.

Cummings, B.J. (1996b) Squamous cell carcinoma of the anal margin. *Oncology* **10**, 1853–4.

Cummings, B.J. (1998a) Anal cancer. In Perez, C.A. and Brady, L.W. (eds), *Principles and practice of radiation oncology* (3rd edn). Philadelphia: J.B. Lippincott, 1511–24.

Cummings, B.J. (1998b) Preservation of structure and function in epidermoid cancer of the anal canal. In Rosenthal, C.J. and Rotman, M. (eds), *Infusion chemotherapy–radiation therapy interactions:* its biology and significance for organ salvage and prevention of second primary neoplasms. Amsterdam: Elsevier Science, 167–78.

Cummings, B.J., Keane, T.J., Hawkins, N.V. and O'Sullivan, B. (1986) Treatment of perianal carcinoma by radiation plus chemotherapy (abstract). *Proc. Am. Soc. Therap. Radiol. Oncol., Int. J. Radiat. Oncol. Biol. Phys.* **12**(suppl. 1), 170.

Cummings, B.J., Keane, T.J., O'Sullivan, B. *et al.* (1991) Epidermoid anal cancer: treatment by radiation alone or by radiation and 5-fluorouracil with and without mitomycin C. *Int. J. Radiat. Oncol. Biol. Phys.* **21**, 1115–25.

Daling, J.R., Sherman, K.J., Hislop, T.G. *et al.* (1992) Cigarette smoking and the risk of anogenital cancer. *Am. J. Epidemiol.* **135**, 180–9.

Fenger, C. (1988) Histology of the anal canal. *Am. J. Surg. Pathol.* **12**, 41–55.

Flam, M.S. (1995) Chemotherapy of persistent, recurrent or metastatic cancer. In Cohen, A.M., Winawer, S.J., Friedman, M.A. and Gunderson, L.L. (eds), *Cancer of the colon rectum and anus*. New York: McGraw Hill, 1051–60.

Flam, M., John, M., Pajak, T.F. *et al.* (1996) Role of mitomycin in combination with fluorouracil and radiotherapy, and of salvage chemoradiation in the definitive nonsurgical treatment of epidermoid carcinoma of the anal canal: results of a phase III randomized intergroup study. *J. Clin. Oncol.* **14**, 2527–39.

Flam, M., John, M., Pajak, T.F. *et al.* (1999) Role of mitomycin in combination with fluorouracil and radiotherapy, and of salvage chemoradiation in the definitive nonsurgical treatment of epidermoid carcinoma of the anal canal: results of a phase III randomized intergroup study (author update). *Classic Papers and Current Comments. Highlights of Clinical Gastrointestinal Research* **3**, 539–52.

Fleming, I.D., Cooper, J.S., Henson, D.E. *et al.* (eds) (1997) *Manual for Staging of Cancer, American Joint Committee on Cancer Staging and End Results Reporting* 5th edn. Philadelphia: Lippincott–Raven.

Frisch, M., Olsen, J.H., Bautz, A. and Melbye, M. (1994a) Benign anal lesions and the risk of anal cancer. *N. Engl. J. Med.* **331**, 300–2.

Frisch, M., Olsen, J.H. and Melbye, M. (1994b) Malignancies that occur before and after anal cancer: clues to their etiology. *Am. J. Epidemiol.* **140**, 12–19.

Frisch, M., Glimelius, B., van den Brule, A.J. *et al.* (1997) Sexually transmitted infection as a cause of anal cancer. *N. Engl. J. Med.* **337**, 1350–8.

Gerard, J.P., Ayzac, L., Hun, D. *et al.* (1998) Treatment of anal canal carcinoma with high dose radiation therapy and concomitant fluorouracil-cisplatinum. Long-term results in 95 patients. *Radiother. Oncol.* **46**, 249–56.

Glimelius, B. and Pahlman, L. (1987) Radiation therapy of anal epidermoid carcinoma. *Int. J. Radiat. Oncol. Biol. Phys.* **13**, 305–12.

Golden, G.T. and Horsley, J.S., III. (1976) Surgical management of epidermoid carcinoma of the anus. *Am. J. Surg.* **131**, 275–80.

Goldman, S., Glimelius, B. and Pahlman, L. (1990) Anorectal malignant melanoma in Sweden: report of 49 cases. *Dis. Colon Rectum* **33**, 874–7.

Greenall, M.J., Quan, S.H. and Decosse, J.J. (1985a) Epidermoid cancer of the anus. *Br. J. Surg.* **72**(suppl.), S97–S103.

Greenall, M.J., Quan, S.H., Stearns, M.W. *et al.* (1985b) Epidermoid cancer of the anal margin. Pathologic features, treatment, and clinical results. *Am. J. Surg.* **149**, 95–101.

Hoffman, R., Welton, M.L., Klencke, B. *et al.* (1999) The significance of pretreatment CD4 count on the outcome and treatment tolerance of HIV-positive patients with anal cancer. *Int. J. Radiat. Oncol. Biol. Phys.* **44**, 127–31.

Jass, J.R. and Sobin, L.H. (1989) Anal canal. *Histological typing of intestinal tumours*. Berlin: Springer-Verlag.

John, M., Pajak, T., Flam, M. *et al.* (1996) Dose escalation in chemoradiation for anal cancer: preliminary results of RTOG 92-08. *Cancer J. Sc. Am.* **2**, 205–11.

Klas, J.V., Rothenberger, D.A., Wong, W.D. and Madoff, R.D. (1999) Malignant tumors of the anal canal. The spectrum of disease, treatment and outcomes. *Cancer* **85**, 1686–93.

Martenson, J.A., Lipsitz, S.R., Wagner, H. Jr *et al.* (1996) Initial results of a phase II trial of high dose radiation therapy, 5-fluorouracil, and cisplatin for patients with anal cancer (E4292): an Eastern Cooperative Oncology Group. *Int. J. Radiat. Oncol. Biol. Phys.* **35**, 745–9.

Melbye, M., Cote, T.R., Kessler, L. *et al.* (1994a) High incidence of anal cancer among AIDS patients. The AIDS/Cancer Working Group. *Lancet* **343**, 636–9.

Melbye, M., Rabkin, C., Frisch, M. and Biggar, R.J. (1994b) Changing patterns of anal cancer incidence in the United States, 1940–1989. *Am. J. Epidemiol.* **139**, 772–80.

Meropol, N.J., Niedzwiecki, D., Shank, B. *et al.* (1999) Combined modality therapy of poor risk anal canal carcinoma: A phase II study of the Cancer and Leukemia Group B (CALGB) (abstract). *Proc. Annual Meeting Am. Soc. Clin. Oncol.* **18**, A909.

Myerson, R.J., Karnell, L.H. and Menck, H.R. (1997) The National Cancer Data Base report on carcinoma of the anus. *Cancer* **80**, 805–15.

Nigro, N.D. (1984) An evaluation of combined therapy for squamous cell cancer of the anal canal. *Dis. Colon Rectum* **27**, 763–6.

Nigro, N.D., Vaitkevicius, V.K. and Considine, B. Jr (1974) Combined therapy for cancer of the anal canal: a preliminary report. *Dis. Colon Rectum* **15**, 354–6.

Northover, J., Meadows, H., Ryan, C. and Gray, R. (1997) Combined radiotherapy and chemotherapy for rectal cancer (letter). *Lancet* **349**, 205–6.

Papillon, J. (1982) *Rectal and anal cancers: conservative treatment by irradiation. An alternative to radical surgery*. Berlin: Springer-Verlag.

Papillon, J. and Chassard, J.L. (1992) Respective roles of radiotherapy and surgery in the management of epidermoid carcinoma of the anal margin. Series of 57 patients. *Dis. Colon Rectum* **35**, 422–9.

Papillon, J. and Montbarbon, J.F. (1987) Epidermoid carcinoma of the anal canal. A series of 276 cases. *Dis. Colon Rectum* **30**, 324–33.

Peiffert, D., Seitz, J.F., Rougier, P. *et al.* (1997a) Preliminary results of a phase II study of high-dose radiation therapy and neoadjuvant plus concomitant 5-fluorouracil with CDDP chemotherapy for patients with anal canal cancer: a French cooperative study. *Ann. Oncol.* **8**, 575–81.

Peiffert, D., Bey, P., Pernot, M. *et al.* (1997b) Conservative treatment by irradiation of epidermoid carcinomas of the anal margin. *Int. J. Radiat. Oncol. Biol. Phys.* **39**, 57–66.

Penn, I. (1986) Cancer is a complication of severe immunosuppression. *Surg. Gynecol. Obstet.* **162**, 603–10.

Pintor, M.P., Northover, J.M. and Nicholls, R.J. (1989) Squamous cell carcinoma of the anus at one hospital from 1948 to 1984. *Br. J. Surg.* **76**, 806–10.

Rich, T.A., Ajani, J.A., Morrison, W.H. *et al.* (1993) Chemoradiation therapy for anal cancer: radiation plus continuous infusion of 5-fluorouracil with or without cisplatin. *Radiother. Oncol.* **27**, 209–15.

Scholefield, J.H., Palmer, J.G., Shepherd, N.A. *et al.* (1990) Clinical and pathological correlates of HPV type 16 DNA in anal cancer. *Int. J. Colorectal Dis.* **5**, 219–22.

Sobin, L.H. and Wittekind, C.H. (eds) (1997) *TNM classification of malignant tumours*. International Union Against Cancer 5th edn. New York: Wiley-Liss.

Stearns, M.W. Jr, Urmacher, C., Sternberg, S.S. *et al.* (1980) Cancer of the anal canal. *Current Probl. Cancer* **4**, 1–44.

Tanum, G. (1993) Treatment of relapsing anal carcinoma. *Acta Oncol.* **32**, 33–5.

Tarazi, R. and Nelson, R.L. (1994) Anal adenocarcinoma: a comprehensive review. *Semin. Surg. Oncol.* **10**, 235–40.

Touboul, E., Schlienger, M., Buffat, L. *et al.* (1995) Epidermoid carcinoma of the anal margin: 17 cases treated with curative-intent radiation therapy. *Radiother. Oncol.* **34**, 195–202.

UKCCCR Working Party (1996) Epidermoid anal cancer: results from the UKCCCR randomised trial of radiotherapy alone versus radiotherapy, 5-fluorouracil, and mitomycin. UKCCCR Anal Cancer Trial Working Party. UK Co-ordinating Committee on Cancer Research. *Lancet* **348**, 1049–54.

Vordermark, D., Sailer, M., Flentje, M. *et al.* (1999) Curative-intent radiation therapy in anal carcinoma: quality of life and sphincter function. *Radiother. Oncol.* **52**, 239–43.

Williams, G.R., Lu, Q.L., Love, S.B. *et al.* (1996) Properties of HPV-positive and HPV-negative anal carcinomas. *J. Pathol.* **180**, 378–82.

zur Hausen, H. (1999) Papillomaviruses in human cancers. *Proc. Assoc. Am. Physicians* **111**, 581–7.

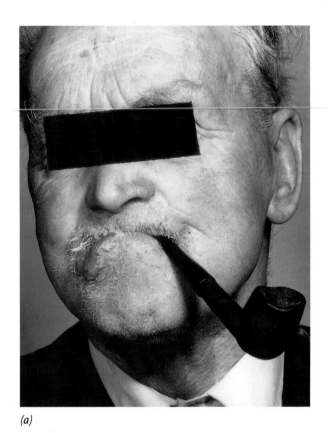

(a)

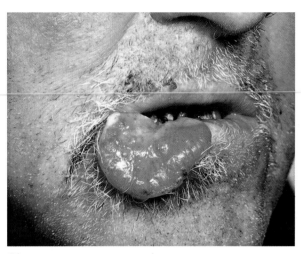

(b)

Plate 1 *(a) Squamous carcinoma of the lip in a pipe-smoker; note lateral transfer of pipe to permit continued smoking. (b) Close view of the tumour.*

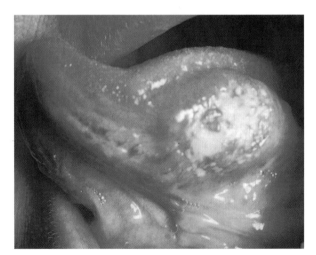

Plate 2 *Squamous carcinoma of the lateral border of the tongue.*

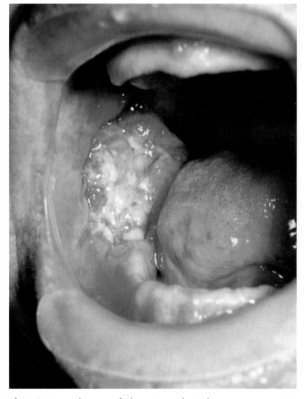

Plate 3 *A carcinoma of the retromolar trigone.*

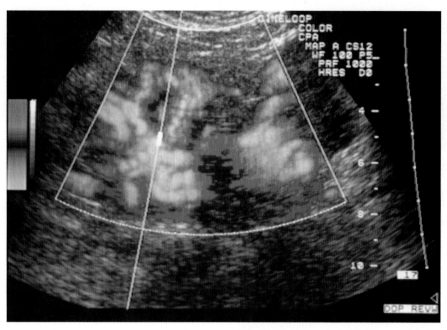

Plate 4 *Ultrasonography with colour Doppler showing persistent gestational trophoblastic disease following a CM within the body and wall of the uterus. A typical vesicular or 'snow storm' appearance of residual molar tissue can be seen within the uterus, together with a rich blood supply through the endometrium and myometrium. There is no evidence of a fetus.*

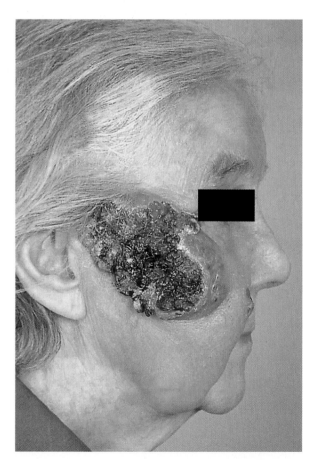

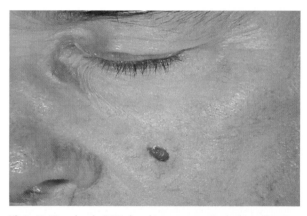

Plate 6 *Morphoeic BCC showing some central ulceration on the cheek of a 67-year-old man.*

Plate 5 *Large ulcerated BCC in an 82-year-old woman who was terrified that she had cancer and did not leave the house for 3 years.*

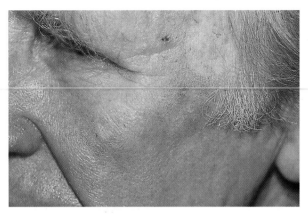

Plate 7 *Two atrophic pale patches on the forehead of a 70-year-old man who had received radiotherapy for BCCs 10 years earlier.*

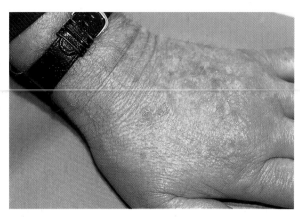

Plate 9 *Multiple actinic keratoses on the back of the hand of a 62-year-old woman.*

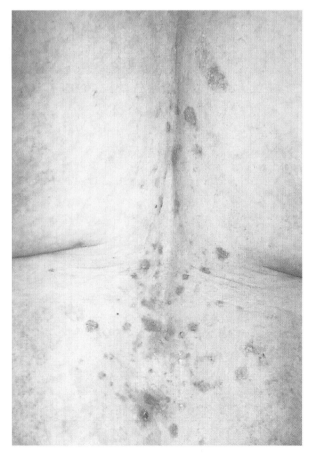

Plate 8 *Naevoid BCC syndrome multiple BCCs on the back of a 45-year-old woman.*

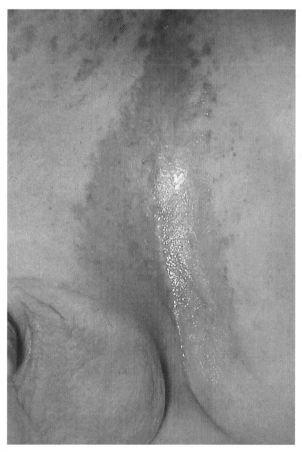

Plate 10 *LCH of the skin in a 13-month-old boy showing typical petechial, intertriginous involvement.*

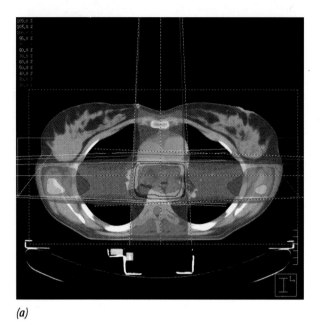

(a)

Plate 11 *(a) Transaxial CT slice used in planning radiotherapy for oesophageal cancer. (b) Three-dimensional reconstruction of CT data to show the relationship between the oesophageal target volume, lung, heart and spinal cord.*

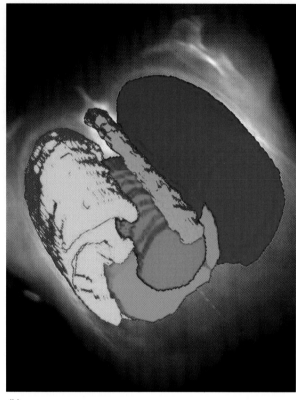

(b)

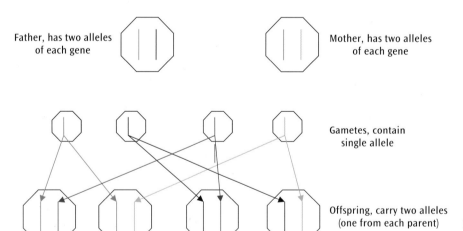

Father, has two alleles of each gene

Mother, has two alleles of each gene

Gametes, contain single allele

Offspring, carry two alleles (one from each parent)

Plate 12 *Principles of genetic inheritance.*

32

Germ-cell cancers of the testis and related neoplasms

GRAHAM M. MEAD

Germ-cell cancers are rare malignancies of young adult life which occur in males in 97–98 per cent of cases. Histologically identical neoplasms may arise in multiple sites, though by far the most common primary site is the testis. These neoplasms may also arise in the retroperitoneum, mediastinum, pineal/suprasellar area, the ovary and (in infants) the sacrococcygeal region. This chapter focuses predominantly on testicular germ-cell cancers but will also include sections on primary mediastinal and retroperitoneal disease. Over 95 per cent of patients presenting with a germ-cell tumour can expect to be cured.

TESTICULAR GERM-CELL TUMOURS

Incidence

Approximately one in 400–450 males in the UK will develop a testicular germ-cell cancer in their lifetime. This is the most common cancer of young men aged under 35 but still comprises of only 1 per cent of male cancers.

Germ-cell cancers of the testis are divided histologically into testicular seminoma and teratoma, these two subtypes occur with approximately equal incidence. The median age of onset of teratoma is 25–30 years, and of seminoma approximately a decade later. Germ-cell tumours of the testis are rare before the age of 15 and comparatively rare after the age of 60 when large-cell non-Hodgkin's lymphoma becomes the commonest type of testicular cancer.

Evidence from a variety of Western nations has shown a markedly increasing incidence of both types of germ-cell cancer in the last 40–50 years, with many countries reporting a two- to threefold increase in rates during this period (Senturia, 1987). Simultaneously there is strong evidence to suggest that sperm counts are falling and it seems likely that the same aetiological events underly both abnormalities.

Aetiological factors

Germ-cell tumours of the testis occur more commonly in white populations. The highest recorded incidence is seen in Nordic countries, in particular Denmark and Norway; however, paradoxically the incidence in Finland is low.

The main predisposing factor in the development of germ-cell cancer is testicular maldescent (Table 32.1).

Table 32.1 *Risk factors for testicular cancer[a]*

Factor	Approximate increase in risk
Unilateral testicular maldescent	×5
Bilateral testicular maldescent	×10
Family history (sib)	×10
Family history (father)	×2–3
Contralateral testicular cancer	×20
Mumps orchitis/testicular atrophy	?
Childhood inguinal hernia or hydrocoele	?
Down's syndrome	?

[a] Lifetime risk of testicular cancer in UK 1 in 450.

If either testis fails to descend normally, then the incidence of testicular cancer rises approximately fivefold (both testes are at increased risk) and if both are maldescended the incidence rises 10-fold. Patients undergoing orchidectomy for a germ-cell cancer have a markedly increased risk of developing contralateral disease – estimated at 4–5 per cent, and those with a family history of testicular germ-cell cancer (particularly siblings) have an increased risk of developing a tumour themselves of approximately five- to 10-fold (Forman *et al.*, 1992). Additional risk factors are Down's syndrome, the presence of testicular atrophy or dysgenesis, or a previous history of mumps orchitis. Other possible risk factors include higher social class and high maternal and low birth weight.

The incidence of testicular maldescent is rising in the UK. Whilst this abnormality is present in only 10 per cent of patients presenting with testicular cancer, it is thought that common prenatal influences underlie the rising incidence of both abnormalities. Interestingly, the incidence of testicular cancer among Danish males born during the period of invasion in World War II was markedly lower, suggesting a possible nutritional influence on the mother and developing male foetus.

Pathogenesis

Carcinoma *in-situ* (CIS), the presence of atypical intratubular germ cells (Fig. 32.1), is the uniform histological precursor of testicular germ-cell tumours (except for spermatocytic seminoma, a non-germ-cell cancer). CIS is present adjacent to recognizable cancer in almost all resected testes containing malignant germ-cell cancer. In addition, there is increased incidence of CIS (5 per cent of cases; Dieckmann and Loy, 1996) in the contralateral testis of men with testicular germ-cell tumours, particularly if the testis is atrophic. CIS generally occurs as a field change throughout the testis and can be detected by a biopsy of a single site. A longitudinal study on patients with this histological abnormality suggested an increasing incidence of invasive cancer with time, rising to 50 per cent by 5 years (von der Maase *et al.*, 1986). Testicular cancer is extremely rare in patients in whom a previous biopsy has demonstrated the absence of *in-situ* cancer. CIS has never been shown to resolve spontaneously, though the histological abnormalities will regress temporarily with chemotherapy and permanently with irradiation.

It is currently hypothesized that CIS develops in early (probably prenatal) life and that promotional events, probably associated with puberty, cause later development of testicular cancer.

CYTOGENETICS

Germ-cell cancers arising at any site are characterized, in a high proportion of cases (around 80 per cent), by the presence of an isochromosome of the short arm of chromosome 12 – denoted i(12p). The precise role of this

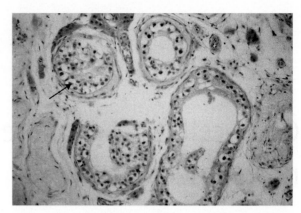

Figure 32.1 *H&E section of testicular biopsy. Areas of carcinoma* in-situ *are seen (ballooned germ cell arrowed).*

chromosomal abnormality in the pathogenesis of germ-cell tumours is at present unknown.

Pathology

Germ-cell tumours of the testis are histopathologically diverse and complex, and no entirely satisfactory classification exists which adequately describes the potential admixtures of malignant and benign elements which may be present (which are probably best described individually). Two histological classifications are in use at present and these are often used interchangeably. These are the British Testicular Tumour Panel and the World Health Organization classifications (used in the USA), (Table 32.2).

Both classifications describe four main malignant cell types which can be recognized cytologically: seminoma, malignant teratoma undifferentiated (also known as embryonal carcinoma), malignant teratoma trophoblastic (choriocarcinoma) and yolk-sac tumour. In addition, histologically 'benign' elements – teratoma differentiated (mature teratoma) – can commonly be recognized. Testicular germ-cell cancers can potentially contain any of these elements in any proportion. Whilst metastatic disease normally reflects the tissue types found in the primary, it is not rare for histologies to differ between the two sites.

Germ-cell cancers are commonly divided, for clinical purposes, into seminoma and non-seminomatous germ-cell tumours. In a proportion of cases (at least 15 per cent), elements of both tumour types are present in the primary. For practical purposes these patients are managed as non-seminoma. Available pathological and clinical data suggest that occasional patients with seminoma 'transform' histologically into teratoma, particularly of yolk-sac type.

Seminoma

Seminoma of the testis has a characteristic uniform, solid, greyish appearance (Fig. 32.2). Histologically, the appearances are quite characteristic and special stains are

Table 32.2 *Pathology of male germ-cell cancer*

UK	USA
Seminoma	Seminoma
Spermatocytic seminoma	Spermatocytic seminoma
Malignant teratoma	Non-seminomatous germ-cell cancer
differentiated (TD)	teratoma (mature, immature)
undifferentiated (MTU)	embryonal carcinoma
intermediate (MTI)	teratocarcinoma
trophoblastic (MTT)	choriocarcinoma
yolk-sac tumour (YST)	yolk-sac tumour (YST)
Combined tumour	Combined tumour
seminoma and teratoma	seminoma and teratoma

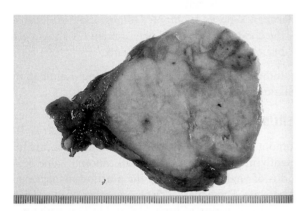

Figure 32.2 *Orchidectomy specimen. Typical cross-section of seminoma of the testis.*

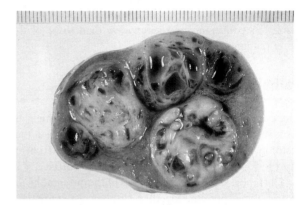

Figure 32.3 *Orchidectomy specimen. Typical teratoma of the testis. Complex cystic/solid tumour with areas of cartilage formation.*

not usually required. However, immunostains for placental alkaline phosphatase (staining seminoma) and cytokeratin and α-fetoprotein (AFP) (staining teratoma) will help distinguish difficult cases from teratoma. Anaplastic seminoma is a histologically less well-differentiated tumour; however, there are no clinical management implications in the recognition of such cases.

Spermatocytic seminoma has a different and also characteristic appearance. This is usually a tumour of elderly males, which rarely, if ever, metastasizes.

Non-seminomatous tumours

Malignant teratomas are commonly mixed tumours with different proportions of each malignant element (Fig. 32.3). In a proportion of cases with metastatic disease, spontaneous regression of the primary occurs, usually leaving a recognizable scar, though *in-situ* cancer may persist.

MALIGNANT TERATOMA UNDIFFERENTIATED (MTU)

MTU is known as embryonal carcinoma in the USA. This relatively featureless tumour is uncommonly found in pure form and has a higher propensity for vascular invasion and metastatic spread than the other tumour types.

TERATOMA DIFFERENTIATED (TD)

Teratoma differentiated – known as mature teratoma in the WHO classification – is commonly a cystic neoplasm containing mesodermal, endodermal and ectodermal elements which are histologically benign. Varying degrees of cellular atypia are usually present (immature teratoma). This tumour may be present in pure form in 2–3 per cent of cases (Simmonds *et al.*, 1996) but more commonly elements of TD are interspersed among malignant elements.

The component tissues of TD are clearly unstable and secondary (non-germ-cell) cancers are well described as arising within deposits of TD (Comiter *et al.*, 1998). TD may metastasize despite its benign appearance, most commonly to the retroperitoneum and should be regarded as malignant neoplasm (Simmonds *et al.*, 1996).

MALIGNANT TERATOMA INTERMEDIATE (MTI)

MTI is known as teratocarcinoma in the WHO classification and comprises a mixture of TD and MTU in varying degree.

MALIGNANT TERATOMA TROPHOBLASTIC (MTT)

In the UK classification of testicular teratoma, the presence of recognizable trophoblastic elements (cyto- and syncytiotrophoblast) is diagnostic of MTT. In the WHO classification the equivalent diagnosis is choriocarcinoma, but this implies the presence of a pure trophoblastic tumour (a rare, <1 per cent entity). Trophoblastic elements are responsible for human chorionic gonadotrophin (hCG) production (an essential marker of teratoma); they commonly spread widely via vascular channels (McKendrick et al., 1991).

YOLK-SAC TUMOUR (YST)

Yolk-sac elements may be present in any teratoma; in addition pure yolk-sac tumours are recognized, particularly in the testis of infants and as a primary tumour of the anterior mediastinum in adults. YST is responsible for the production of AFP. These tumours tend to metastasize less commonly and less widely than some of the other malignant components.

Pathological staging

The pathology report should include an assessment of gross tumour size. It is generally recommended that histological assessment should include examination of one block per cubic centimetre of resected cancer.

The report should include details of the different histological types present, together with an assessment of their proportion. Tumour extension through the tumour albuginea with involvement of the tumour vaginalis or rete testis should be reported, as should spermatic cord or scrotal invasion. An assessment should be made as to whether vascular/lymphatic invasion is present and a TNM stage should be allocated (Table 32.3).

Table 32.3 *TNM classification of primary tumour*

pT	Primary tumour
pTX	Primary tumour cannot be assessed (if no radical orchidectomy has been performed TX is used)
pT0	No evidence of primary tumour (e.g. histological scar in testis)
pTis	Intratubular germ-cell neoplasia (carcinoma *in-situ*)
pT1	Tumour limited to testis and epididymis without vascular/lymphatic invasion; tumour may invade tunica albuginea but not tunica vaginalis
pT2	Tumour limited to testis and epididymis with vascular/lymphatic invasion, or tumour extending through tunica albuginea with involvement of tunica vaginalis
pT3	Tumour invades spermatic cord with or without vascular/lymphatic invasion
pT4	Tumour invades scrotum with or without vascular/lymphatic invasion

Staging

Once a diagnosis of testicular cancer has been made the patient should be thoroughly staged. Staging should include:

- thorough clinical examination including a careful search for gynaecomastia (first apparent as a pre-areolar breast 'bud'), and for evidence of cervical, abdominal and inguinal masses. The remaining testis should also be examined.
- measurement of the serum markers AFP/hCG/lactate dehydrogenase (LDH). If these are found to be elevated, they should be repeated weekly to determine if they are rising or falling.
- a chest X-ray and computed tomography (CT) scan of the chest, abdomen and pelvis. Brain CT should also be performed in high-risk patients.

Individual components of the staging examinations will now be described in more detail.

SERUM MARKERS

Tumour marker (AFP, hCG, LDH) elevation occurs frequently in patients with germ-cell cancers (Table 32.4) and is of vital importance in the practical management of patients. These markers have a number of uses. Diagnostically, elevation of both AFP and hCG is pathognomonic of a diagnosis of malignant teratoma. The height of each tumour marker relates to prognosis in teratoma and helps to determine therapy; for example, very high and rising levels of any of the markers are an adverse feature in malignant teratoma which may indicate the need for a more intensive treatment approach. Markers are also used during therapy, to confirm response, and on follow-up should remain normal as useful (though not definitive) evidence of continued remission.

Tumour markers (at least AFP and hCG levels) should initially be measured before orchidectomy. The presence of an elevated AFP level indicates that elements of malignant teratoma are present in the tumour. Post-orchidectomy marker levels (if elevated pre-orchidectomy) should be measured at least weekly and should, of course, return rapidly to normal in the absence of metastatic disease. Marker levels should also be obtained immediately before and during chemotherapy as they provide an essential guide to response.

α-Fetoprotein (AFP)

AFP is an oncofetal antigen produced in the fetal liver, yolk sac and gastrointestinal tract. Elevated levels of AFP occur in malignant teratoma (produced by yolk-sac elements), in patients with malignant hepatoma and other gastrointestinal malignancies and in patients with liver cell damage and accompanying proliferation (e.g. cirrhosis with regeneration). Minor elevations of AFP can also occur after chemotherapy with the POMB/ACE chemotherapy regimen (cisplatin, vincristine, methotrexate and bleomycin alternating with dactinomycin, cyclophosphamide and etoposide), perhaps related to the use of methotrexate. AFP is never elevated in patients with pure seminoma.

AFP has a half-life of approximately 5–6 days. Elevation of AFP is found in approximately 70 per cent of teratoma patients pre-orchidectomy and a comparable number of cases pre-chemotherapy for metastatic disease.

β-Subunit of human chorionic gonadotrophin (hCG)

hCG is a glycopeptide secreted by the placenta in pregnancy. It consists of an α- and β-subunit, the former common to luteinizing hormone (LH), follicle stimulating hormone (FSH) and thyroid stimulating hormone (TSH), the latter specific to hCG only.

hCG elevation occurs in seminoma, usually at low levels (elevated in around 35 per cent of patients pre-orchidectomy) and malignant teratoma (elevated in approximately 70 per cent of patients pre-orchidectomy). hCG elevation also occurs in a variety of other cancers including lung cancer, stomach and bladder cancer; an elevated hCG is therefore not specific to germ-cell cancer. hCG is produced by the trophoblastic tumour elements; the half-life of hCG is 24–36 hours.

Placental alkaline phosphatase (PLAP)

PLAP is an isoenzyme of alkaline phosphatase which is normally expressed by placental syncytiotrophoblasts. PLAP has predominantly been used as a marker of seminoma; however, it has not found widespread use, particularly as its specificity is marred by an increase in levels in patients who are cigarette smokers.

Lactate dehydrogenase (LDH)

LDH (or its isoenzyme hydroxybutyrate dehydrogenase, HBD) is commonly elevated in both seminoma and teratoma. This glycolytic enzyme is present in all living cells, and the precise aetiology of its elevation in germ-cell tumours is unknown. The main use of LDH is in relationship to assessment of prognosis, particularly in malignant teratoma where increasing levels in patients with metastatic disease are related to a worsening outlook. LDH may be a useful marker in patients with stage I teratoma (particularly if AFP and hCG levels are normal pre-orchidectomy) and also in the follow-up of patients following chemotherapy for metastatic seminoma. Minor elevations of LDH are, however, rather non-specific and sensitivity and specificity tend to be low. LDH is not a useful marker during or shortly after chemotherapy as levels are increased at the time of bone marrow recovery.

LDH assays vary widely and are not standardized. It is conventional to quote the degree of elevation of LDH as a ratio when compared with the upper limit of normal of each laboratory (e.g. level 900, normal range 200–450, LDH ratio = 2).

RADIOLOGY

Chest X-ray

Patients with testicular cancer should all have a chest X-ray. Peripheral lung metastases may be evidence of metastatic teratoma (Fig. 32.4) and a mediastinal mass evidence of seminoma or teratoma. Lung metastases occur much less commonly in seminoma than in teratoma and this diagnosis should be reviewed if such lesions are present.

An association has been described between malignant germ-cell tumours and sarcoidosis. The presence of isolated and otherwise unexplained mediastinal or hilar nodal enlargement should raise suspicion of the possibility of this lesion and consideration should be given to a biopsy being performed if other confirmatory evidence of metastatic germ-cell cancer is unavailable (e.g. rising serum markers).

CT scanning

CT scanning remains the imaging method of choice in all patients with a germ-cell tumour. Abdominal lymphatic

Table 32.4 *Serum markers (AFP and hCG) in groups of 50 patients (Southampton data)*

	AFP		hCG	
	% elevated	Range (ku/L)	% elevated	Range (IU/L)
Seminoma				
Pre-orchidectomy				
All patients	–		36	4–77
Stage 1	–		31	4–77
Pre-chemotherapy				
Metastatic disease	–		63	4–1647
Teratoma				
Pre-orchidectomy				
All patients	68	11–33 000	70	4–57 000
Stage I	63	11–32 000	67	4–61 800
Pre-chemotherapy				
Metastatic disease	70	12–218 000	72	4–777 000

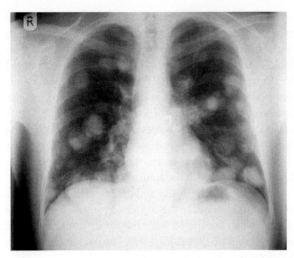

Figure 32.4 *Widespread lung metastases secondary to malignant teratoma of the testis.*

spread in both tumour types occurs to characteristic sites (the so-called 'landing zones') – these are the para-aortic area for left-sided primary tumours and the inter-aortocaval and para-caval area for right-sided tumours (Fig. 32.5). CT scanning is capable only of detecting nodal enlargement and interpretation of scans relies on assessment of nodal size and number. Using 10 mm as the upper limit of normal nodal size in the retroperitoneum results in acceptable sensitivity and specificity. Nodal enlargement in the 'landing zones' can be interpreted more definitely than that occurring elsewhere.

Equivocal or atypical retroperitoneal nodal enlargement may occur in patients with malignant teratoma and should not be over-interpreted. If supporting evidence for malignant spread is present (e.g. rising tumour markers), then the patient should proceed with treatment. If, however, doubt exists and tumour markers are normal or falling, it is reasonable to delay therapy and repeat the abdominal scan after 4–6 weeks with little adverse effect on the patient as treatment of these diseases is so effective.

Abdominal adenopathy may be massive and may then be associated with compression of one or both ureters or the inferior vena cava (characteristically occurring with right-sided tumours and sometimes associated with thrombosis and perhaps embolism). Contiguous spread may occur into the epidural space with spinal cord compression. Rarely, patients may develop high gastrointestinal obstruction or pancreatitis because of the size of tumour deposits.

CT scanning is also most effective at detecting lymphatic spread beyond the abdomen – characteristic initially to the retrocrural then posterior mediastinal nodes. This method of spread is most characteristic of seminoma, which tends to metastasize in a predictable and contiguous fashion.

Patients with retroperitoneal nodal spread may also develop retrograde spread to the contralateral landing

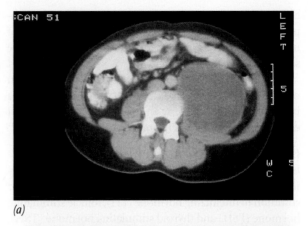

(a)

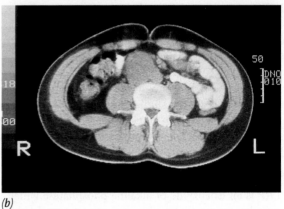

(b)

Figure 32.5 *Abdominal CT scans showing typical sites of spread of (a) left-sided and (b) right-sided metastatic disease.*

zone, iliac or even inguinal regions, which should be routinely scanned in all patients at presentation.

Whilst seminoma characteristically spreads by lymphatic routes, testicular teratoma commonly spreads by both lymphatic and vascular channels. Vascular spread occurs most commonly to the lungs but occasionally also to the liver, brain, gastrointestinal tract and bones. It is not unusual in patients with malignant teratoma for spread to occur exclusively to the lungs in the absence of retroperitoneal adenopathy. However small, single lung nodules should not be over-interpreted and repeat scanning may be necessary in the absence of diagnostic marker elevation to determine whether these are benign or malignant in nature.

A CT scan of the brain should be obtained in all patients with a high hCG level (e.g. >10 000 IU/L) and in those with florid lung metastases. Brain metastases are rare at presentation, but their early detection in high-risk cases is important.

Metastatic masses from both teratoma and seminoma may show low attenuation areas secondary to either necrosis or the presence of TD. Calcification may also be seen within either tumour type.

Magnetic resonance imaging (MRI)

MRI scanning is clearly the diagnostic imaging investigation of choice in patients with brain metastases or spinal cord compression. MRI is, however, not as effective as CT at examining the lungs – though there may be advantages in some cases with regard to the examination of mediastinal structures. No effective oral contrast medicine is available for MRI. This considerably reduces its usefulness for examining the retroperitoneum; the main sites of spread of germ-cell cancer are closely related to the gastrointestinal tract and oral contrast is used with CT scanning to aid differentiation from malignant masses.

Positron emission tomography (PET) scanning

PET scanning relies on the detection of enhanced uptake of radiolabelled fluorodeoxyglucose (FDG) by malignant tissue. A major advantage of this technique when compared with CT or MRI is the possibility of detecting malignant infiltration of normal size lymph nodes. Resolution is limited, however, as lesions <5 mm cannot be visualized. PET scanners are not presently widely available and scans are expensive. It is, however, clear that PET scans can be highly effective and superior to CT in detecting metastatic disease. Limited data from patients with stage I disease has shown that PET scanning can detect those patients destined to relapse as a result of low volume disease ahead of similar detection by CT (Lassen *et al.*, 1997). Similarly, metastatic sites can be detected in patients with elevated markers but normal CT scans.

PET has also been evaluated post-chemotherapy in an attempt to judge whether residual masses contain viable cancer or only TD/fibrosis. Results have been variable in this setting as necrotic tissue can occasionally be imaged by PET, as virtually always is cancer. TD, however, is not associated with increased FDG uptake. Early data suggests an important role for PET in the evaluation of residual masses following chemotherapy in patients with seminoma (vide infra). Positive FDG uptake appears to be associated with residual active seminoma.

Clinical presentation

The great majority of patients with a testicular germ-cell tumour present as a result of symptoms from their primary. Most commonly patients notice a lump or change of texture or weight of the testis, or generalized swelling which may be intermittently or progressively painful. Occasionally patients present with acute onset of local pain, swelling and infective symptoms, with failure of the testis to return to normal after antibiotics, or with a hydrocoele obscuring a tumour mass. An unusual though characteristic presentation is with a shrinking, usually painless, testis. Finally, the presence of a testicular cancer may first be manifest following trauma with associated swelling that may have failed to settle satisfactorily.

The duration of testicular symptoms varies from days to many years (the latter usually in patients with TD or seminoma). In approximately 10 per cent of patients there will be a previous history of testicular maldescent (of either the affected or the non-affected testis) and occasionally a

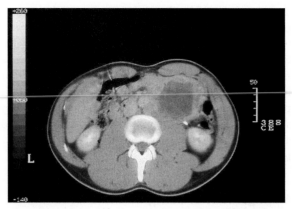

Figure 32.6 *Primary retroperitoneal choriocarcinoma. The patient presented with the abdominal mass shown and an hCG of 750 000 IU/L. Testicular ultrasound was normal. Chemotherapy resulted in cure.*

history of preceding childhood inguinal hernia repair or hydrocoele or a positive family history. Patients with an elevated hCG commonly notice nipple tenderness, sometimes together with gynaecomastia.

A number of patients with germ-cell tumours present with symptoms from extragonadal disease: the testicular primary may either not have been noticed, be clinically inapparent (and subsequently revealed by testicular ultrasound), or be absent (extragonadal primary, Fig. 32.6). The most common symptom in this situation is lumbar backache secondary to metastatic para-aortic lymphadenopathy. Where this disease is bulky, obstruction of the kidney(s), bowel or inferior vena cava may occur (with possible pulmonary emboli) with appropriate symptoms and signs.

Rarely, patients present with an inguinal lymph node mass – usually a result of previous inguinal/scrotal surgery with resulting anomalous lymphatic drainage – or with a cervical nodal mass. Patients with metastatic teratoma may present with lung metastases – manifest by chest pain, dyspnoea or haemoptysis. Metastatic disease in the lung can be rapidly progressive, particularly in the choriocarcinoma syndrome (McKendrick *et al.*, 1991) in which widespread vascular dissemination is common, and the outlook sometimes poor.

ASSESSMENT AND MANAGEMENT OF THE PRIMARY

Once the diagnostic suspicion of germ-cell tumour has been raised, all patients should have bilateral testicular ultrasound to assess testicular size, intra-testicular abnormalities (e.g. calcification) and to look for a neoplasm. The tumour markers AFP, hCG and LDH should be measured.

Where a suspicious lesion is present in the testis, then testicular exploration should be performed by an inguinal incision and orchidectomy performed if a tumour is found. Rarely, scrotal exploration will be performed in error as cancer has not been considered. In these cases the wound should be closed and inguinal orchidectomy performed. More radical surgery is not necessary.

Occasionally patients presenting with metastatic disease are diagnosed as a result of biopsy of one of these sites or are found to have diagnostic elevation of AFP or hCG. In such cases, particularly if performance status is poor or metastatic disease widespread, orchidectomy should be delayed and chemotherapy should be initiated at once. It is, however, recommended that orchidectomy is performed once treatment is completed.

Management of malignant teratoma (nonseminomatous germ cell tumour)

Forty-five to fifty per cent of patients with germ-cell cancer of the testis have either pure malignant teratoma or (in approximately 15 per cent of cases) a combined malignant teratoma and seminoma. These latter cases are managed exclusively as teratoma.

STAGE I TERATOMA

Approximately 40 per cent of patients with testicular teratoma will have stage I disease at first presentation, i.e. normal physical examination and CT scans of chest, abdomen and pelvis; serum markers, if initially elevated, should fall to within the normal range.

Management approaches for these patients vary and may include surveillance, adjuvant chemotherapy or retroperitoneal lymph node dissection (RPLND), though this latter approach is not used in the UK. There is no role for irradiation. Treatment is guided by the known risk factors for metastatic disease and patients are generally divided into high- or low-risk groups determined by the pathological features in the resected testis. The major factor predicting relapse is vascular (i.e. venous or lymphatic) invasion by cancer. This feature is present in approximately 25 per cent of cases and when present predicts a risk of subsequent relapse of approximately 40 per cent. Other risk features are the presence of MTU (embryonal carcinoma), with risk increasing with volume of this tumour type, and absence of yolk-sac tumour.

Surveillance

Following orchidectomy for stage I teratoma, the overall risk of relapse is 25–30 per cent (Read et al., 1992). Relapses usually occur within a few months and beyond 18–24 months relapse is rare. No standard surveillance protocol has been agreed; however, most oncologists recommend tumour marker measurements (AFP and hCG) and a chest X-ray monthly for one year then 2-monthly for one year. A CT scan of the abdomen should be performed at least at 3 months and one year following orchidectomy and the initial staging scan. Whilst CT scanning of the chest is conventionally performed at the same time as abdominal scanning, it is not clear whether this is necessary after initial staging or whether a chest X-ray will

suffice. Patients without evidence of relapse can be discharged after 5 years.

If patients without evidence of vascular invasion are selected for surveillance, the risk of relapse is only 15 per cent versus 40 per cent for those with this feature. Follow-up, however, should be the same. The overall cure rate should approach 100 per cent as salvage chemotherapy is highly effective (see 'Treatment of metastatic teratoma', below).

Adjuvant chemotherapy

Adjuvant chemotherapy has been tested in patients with stage I teratoma with a high risk of subsequent spread most commonly identified by the presence of vascular invasion. Two cycles of BEP (bleomycin, etoposide and cisplatin, see 'Treatment of metastatic teratoma', below) chemotherapy, given with a total dose of etoposide of $360 \, \text{mg/m}^2$ in each course, have been shown to reduce the relapse rate from 40 per cent to 1 per cent (Cullen et al., 1996). This treatment approach has been widely adopted in the UK, but should be regarded as a matter of choice for patients as cure rates should be exceptionally high whether or not this treatment approach is taken. Those rare patients relapsing after adjuvant chemotherapy are reported as having a poor prognosis but there are inadequate data in this area at present.

Retroperitoneal lymph node dissection (RPLND)

In the USA and many European countries RPLND remains a routine treatment approach to stage I teratoma (Donohue et al., 1993). The advent of more limited and therefore nerve-sparing surgery has dramatically reduced the previously common complication of retrograde ejaculation. Approximately 70–80 per cent of cases will have negative histology (pathological stage I), despite which finding 10 per cent of patients will relapse, almost always outside the abdomen. Patients in whom nodal disease is found and completely resected (stage II) have a 50 per cent relapse rate if no further treatment is given; the predominant risk factor for relapse is the presence of vascular invasion in the primary. Adjuvant chemotherapy (e.g. two cycles of BEP) or chemotherapy given at the time of relapse may be used for such cases with a high (>95 per cent) expectation of cure.

MANAGEMENT OF METASTATIC TERATOMA

In the USA and many European countries RPLND remains the treatment of choice for early stage II patients though increasingly patients with elevated serum markers, vascular invasion in the primary or tumour masses greater than 3 cm in diameter are treated with primary chemotherapy. In the UK combination chemotherapy is regarded as the treatment of choice; patients with residual masses at the completion of treatment have these surgically excised at that time.

Staging and prognostic factor classifications: teratoma

Metastatic testicular teratoma is a widely heterogeneous disease in which spread frequently occurs by lymphatic

Table 32.5 *Prognosis factors in metastatic teratoma IGCCC classification*

Good prognosis
56 per cent of cases
5-year progression-free survival 89%; survival 92%
- *testis/retroperitoneal primary* and
- *no non-pulmonary visceral metastases* and
- good markers: all of
  - *AFP <1000 ng/mL* and
  - *hCG <5000 IU/L* and
  - *LDH <1.5 × upper limit of normal*

Intermediate prognosis
28 per cent of cases
5-year progression-free survival 75%; survival 80%
- *testis/retroperitoneal primary* and
- *no non-pulmonary visceral metastases* and
- intermediate markers: any of
  - *AFP ≥1000 ng/mL and ≤10 000 ng/mL* or
  - *hCG ≥5000 IU/L and ≤50 000 IU/L* or
  - *LDH ≥1.5 × N and ≤10 × N*

Poor prognosis
16 per cent of cases
5-year progression-free survival 41%; survival 48%
- *mediastinal primary* or
- *non-pulmonary visceral metastases* or
- poor markers: any of
  - *AFP >10 000 ng/mL* or
  - *hCG >50 000 IU/L (10 000 ng/mL)* or
  - *LDH >10 × upper limit of normal*

and/or vascular routes. Unlike other malignancies, disease bulk may have no relevance to prognosis as many of the more bulky metastatic masses largely comprise TD. In addition, these neoplasms are characterized by elevation of serum markers (AFP, hCG and LDH); it has been known for many years that the degree of elevation of these markers relates to prognosis.

A wide variety of prognostic factor classifications were in use in the 1980s and 1990s. These bore little relationship to each other and it proved increasingly difficult to translate clinical trial data between groups because of the use of these different staging classifications. In 1997 this situation was finally resolved when the International Germ Cell Consensus Classification – a prognostic factor-based staging system – was introduced and widely adopted [International Germ Cell Cancer Collaborative Group (IGCCC), 1997]. This classification resulted from worldwide collaboration. Retrospective clinical data were collected on over 5000 patients with metastatic testicular teratoma, or primary mediastinal or retroperitoneal teratoma who had been treated with cisplatin-containing chemotherapy. The median follow-up time was 5 years. Extensive data were analysed with regard to tumour markers, site of primary and sites and extent of metastatic disease. It rapidly became apparent that the main determinant of prognosis was the degree of elevation of all three tumour markers. Two additional adverse features

were the presence of a mediastinal primary or spread to visceral sites (e.g. liver, bone and brain).

The IGCCC collaboration resulted in the staging classification shown in Table 32.5. Clinical trials initiated since the introduction of this classification have stratified patients using the criteria shown; however, studies completed prior to the introduction of this classification have used a wide variety of staging classifications, which have divided the metastatic testicular teratoma population into two or three groups. The older Royal Marsden Classification continues to be particularly helpful as a description of the extent of abdominal disease (stage IIA mass <2 cm, IIB 2–5 cm, IIC >5 cm) as larger tumour masses pre-chemotherapy more often require resection once chemotherapy is completed.

TREATMENT OF METASTATIC TERATOMA: BEP (BLEOMYCIN, ETOPOSIDE AND CISPLATIN) AS STANDARD THERAPY

Metastatic testicular teratoma is a highly chemosensitive disease. The introduction of PVB (cisplatin, vinblastine and bleomycin) by the Indiana group in the late 1970s ranks as one of the single most important advances in oncology. Twenty-five years ago 5–10 per cent of patients with metastatic teratoma were cured, whereas at present 85–90 per cent of such patients should be cured. This neoplasm is rare and its treatment complex. There is clear evidence that referral to specialist treatment centres, particularly for patients with intermediate and poor prognosis disease, improves survival (Mead, 1999). Chemotherapy protocols should be strictly adhered to and surgery considered in all cases post-chemotherapy where indicated. Patients with non-threatening metastatic disease will wish to consider banking sperm prior to chemotherapy, though sperm counts frequently recover despite such treatment.

The standard therapy for patients with all stages of metastatic testicular teratoma is BEP chemotherapy. This treatment was initially introduced by the Royal Marsden Hospital and in a landmark study by the South East Cancer Study Group (using a modified regimen) was shown not only to be much better tolerated than PVB, but also more effective (Williams *et al.*, 1987). BEP is given at 21-day intervals at a variety of doses and in a variety of schedules. This treatment is given for two courses (adjuvant therapy, Cullen *et al.*, 1996), three courses (good prognosis metastatic teratoma, Saxman *et al.*, 1998) or four courses (intermediate or poor prognosis teratoma) and requires inpatient admission, though the possibility of delivering this treatment on an outpatient basis is being explored.

BEP can almost always be delivered at full dose, on time (every 3 weeks), certainly full-dose therapy should be given on day 1 if the white cell count is $\geq 2.0 \times 10^9$/L with a platelet count $\geq 120 \times 10^9$/L.

Intravenous bleomycin can be given virtually regardless of blood counts but should be used with considerable

Table 32.6 *BEP or EP for good prognosis metastatic teratoma*

BEP × 3-weekly bleomycin (de Wit et al., 1999)
Three courses
- Bleomycin 30 000 units i.v./i.m. weekly × 9
- Etoposide 165 mg/m² i.v. daily × 3 every 3 weeks
- Cisplatin 50 mg/m² i.v. daily × 2 every 3 weeks

EP × 4 (Xiao et al., 1997)
Four courses
- Etoposide 100 mg/m² i.v. daily × 5 every 3 weeks
- Cisplatin 20 mg/m² i.v. daily × 5 every 3 weeks

---

care in older patients or if the serum creatinine is elevated (*see* below). There is no evidence that use of additional growth factors (e.g. filgrastim) are necessary or affect treatment results (Fossa *et al.*, 1998).

Good prognosis disease

Cure rates for good prognosis disease (Table 32.6) should exceed 95 per cent in the group defined by IGCCC criteria. Commencing from early studies in which four courses of BEP were regarded as standard, a number of important studies have attempted to reduce treatment toxicity while maintaining efficacy in these patients. These approaches have included the following.

Omission of bleomycin Bleomycin is a well-tolerated and long-established treatment for testicular teratoma. Whilst this drug is relatively non-myelosuppressive, a feared, though infrequent, complication of its use is pulmonary toxicity (*see* 'Chemotherapy-related toxicity', below). Because of this complication, attempts have been made to omit bleomycin from BEP chemotherapy. Indeed, a standard treatment approach advocated by the Memorial Sloan Kettering (Xiao *et al.*, 1997) is use of EP therapy (cisplatin 20 mg/m² daily × 5 together with etoposide 100 mg/m² daily × 5 on four occasions). Bleomycin toxicity occurs predominantly either when renal clearance is impaired (bleomycin should be given with caution in any patients with an elevated creatinine) or in older (>40 years) patients, where lower doses may be considered (*see* below).

Three large trials have examined the role of bleomycin in metastatic teratoma (e.g. de Wit *et al.*, 1997). In summary, these studies have shown that whilst bleomycin clearly increases myelotoxicity, and causes occasional mortality from bleomycin lung, overall survival is improved when this drug is used. It is now generally recommended that if three cycles of BEP are to be used, bleomycin be given weekly to a total dose of 270 000 units, a cumulative dose which should rarely be complicated by bleomycin lung.

Reduction in number of treatment courses from four to three The South Eastern Cancer Study Group (SECSG, Einhorn *et al.*, 1989) in a comparatively small study (184 patients) randomized between BEP × 4 and BEP × 3

courses. Three courses of treatment proved as effective as four, with reduced toxicity. Because of concerns about the statistical inadequacy of this result this trial was repeated by the MRC/EORTC group. The results of this study supported the SECSG result: 812 patients were randomized to BEP 3 or BEP 4. Failure-free and overall survival were, respectively, 90.4 per cent and 89.4 per cent and 90.2 per cent and 89.2 per cent (de Wit *et al.*, 2001). This study also examined whether cisplatin and etoposide should be administered over a 3- versus 5-day period and again found equivalent results.

Substitution of carboplatin for cisplatin Carboplatin is a much better tolerated drug than cisplatin and can be given on an outpatient basis. Preliminary phase II data suggested equivalence when carboplatin was substituted for cisplatin in BEP; however, two randomized trials (e.g. Horwich *et al.*, 1997) clearly demonstrated that carboplatin is inferior to cisplatin at the doses used in these studies. There is at present no role for carboplatin alone in the initial therapy of metastatic teratoma.

Good prognosis disease: summary The studies described above has clearly defined the BEP/EP regimens which can be used with good effect (Table 32.6). Each of these should produce a failure-free survival of around 90 per cent, with cure rates of over 95 per cent. The regimen including bleomycin is preferred in younger (age under 40 years) patients and the other regimen is preferred in older patients or those with chronic lung disease.

INTERMEDIATE AND POOR PROGNOSIS TERATOMA

Approximately 40–45 per cent of patients with teratoma fall into the intermediate and poor prognosis group. These patients often have rapidly progressive disease and treatment should proceed with relative urgency. Disease in the chest can be bulky and associated with intrapulmonary haemorrhage. Occasional patients have ensuing rapidly progressive dyspnoea and require urgent therapy, with careful attention to the avoidance of excess hydration. Abdominal disease can be associated with inferior vena cava (IVC) obstruction (particularly with right-sided tumours) or with ureteric obstruction which may require stenting. Clinicians should be aware of the possibility of central nervous system (CNS) disease in these patients.

Standard chemotherapy remains BEP (etoposide dose 500 mg/m² per course) given for four courses with a total bleomycin dose of 360 000 units. There is no evidence that filgrastim or other growth factors add to the efficacy of this regimen (Fossa *et al.*, 1998). A number of phase III trials have explored dose escalation of cisplatin, increased dose intensity and addition/substitution of other drugs (particularly ifosfamide), but have failed to improve on the results achieved with BEP, whilst at the same time increasing toxicity (Kaye *et al.*, 1998; Nichols *et al.*, 1998).

A number of more intensive treatment approaches to these patients have been explored. POMB/ACE chemotherapy has been extensively evaluated at Charing Cross Hospital with excellent results (Bower *et al.*, 1997) but has not been tested in a phase III trial. CBOP-BEP, a regimen employing initital intensive induction with both carboplatin and cisplatin with vincristine and infusional bleomycin has also given promising results, again only in phase II evaluation (Horwich *et al.*, 1994).

Further dose escalation has been explored in phase II studies. The Memorial Hospital have pioneered use of high-dose chemotherapy with stem cell support as part of the initial treatment approach. This group initially tried to identify a 'worst prognosis' group by evaluating the rate of fall of the tumour markers AFP and hCG following chemotherapy. When the rate of fall was deemed inadequate, this was used as a surrogate of an adverse outcome and patients were switched from BEP chemotherapy to high-dose chemotherapy with apparently favourable effect. A current Intergroup phase III study has built on this approach and seeks to compare four cycles of standard BEP with two cycles of BEP followed by two cycles of high-dose carboplatin, etoposide and cyclophosphamide with peripheral stem cell support. Eligible patients are those with a poor prognosis disease (IGCCC criteria) together with selected intermediate prognosis patients.

A German group have taken a different approach to this patient group by administering an initial cycle of VIP (etoposide, ifosfamide and cisplatin) with granulocyte colony stimulating factor (G-CSF) support followed by peripheral stem cell harvesting. Three more escalated cycles of chemotherapy with VIP are then given with stem cell and growth factor support. This approach enables considerable dose escalation to take place and in an ongoing phase III study four cycles of standard BEP chemotherapy is being compared with this regimen in patients with poor prognosis disease.

Management of CNS disease

Malignant teratoma can involve the CNS at presentation, or at relapse, then either in isolation (sanctuary site relapse) or in association with progressive systemic disease. Metastases may be single or multiple. Spinal cord compression may also occur, usually secondary to contiguous spread of tumour from an adjacent vertebral body or para-aortic mass. Meningeal disease occurs but is rare.

CNS disease is most commonly seen in patients with a high presenting hCG (e.g. >20 000 IU/L) or with multiple (>20) lung metastases, and a routine brain scan is indicated in such cases at initial evaluation.

Management of CNS disease at presentation is controversial (Fossa *et al.*, 1999a). If a single metastasis is present and potentially resectable, and the systemic disease is clinically non-threatening, then craniotomy and resection should be considered as an initial measure. This approach is used as these metastases are occasionally haemorrhagic and can bleed once chemotherapy has been commenced. Alternative approaches are the use of BEP chemotherapy or POMB/ACE (using methotrexate at

1 g/m^2); this latter regimen has been claimed to be more effective at penetrating the CNS. Chemotherapy is often supplemented by whole-brain radiation, but there is no evidence to support use of this treatment. Cure rates for patients presenting with CNS disease approach 50–60 per cent. Similar results should be achieved with isolated CNS relapse; patients with end-stage disease involving the CNS and peripheral sites should be treated palliatively.

MONITORING CHEMOTHERAPY RESPONSE

Patients receiving chemotherapy for metastatic teratoma should be monitored by sequential tumour marker measurements and simple radiological examinations (e.g. chest X-ray, abdominal ultrasound).

A common phenomenon following the first chemotherapy administration is for the tumour markers to rise for 7–10 days (tumour 'flare'), presumably as a result of tumour cell necrosis. Tumour markers should then fall consistently although not uncommonly marker levels do not fall at half-life rates. The tumour markers fall into the normal range in the great majority of patients.

However those patients with very high initial serum markers, particularly those with choriocarcinoma and a very high hCG, commonly develop a plateau in the range 10–50 IU/L. Whilst rising tumour markers clearly represent relapse of cancer, this is not necessarily the case with patients who have achieved a plateau. These patients can be observed – or where necessary operated upon – after which the tumour markers fall permanently to normal in around 50 per cent of cases despite the absence of histological evidence of cancer in resected masses.

Radiologically, tumour masses usually respond promptly to chemotherapy, though paradoxically those of choriocarcinoma are often slow to respond. This may be a particular problem where gross pulmonary disease is present.

It is important to be aware that growth of metastatic tumour (most commonly in the abdomen) may occur whilst tumour markers are falling. This is known as the 'growing teratoma syndrome' and is commonly due to expansion of masses of differentiated teratoma (Jeffery *et al.*, 1991; Fig. 32.7). This should not be regarded as failure of chemotherapy, and surgery is indicated. Timing this relative to chemotherapy administration must be subject to the site and extent of tumour masses, level of tumour markers and the response of disease at other sites.

POST-CHEMOTHERAPY SURGERY

Once chemotherapy is completed, then complete radiological and marker re-evaluation is indicated. Residual masses are common, particularly in patients with initially bulky disease and where elements of TD were present in the primary tumour (and thereby possibly in a proportion of metastases). It is not possible to absolutely predict the composition of residual masses; these may contain

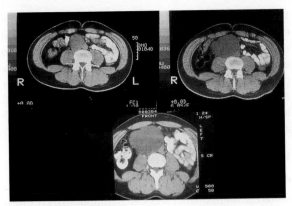

Figure 32.7 *Growing teratoma syndrome. The retroperitoneal mass shown in these X-rays continued to increase in size despite return of the serum markers to normal. The patient underwent thoracolaparotomy with removal of multiple lung metastases and the retroperitoneal mass illustrated. Pathologically all the resected tissue comprised TD.*

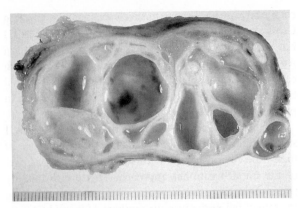

Figure 32.8 *Mass resected at post-chemotherapy laparotomy. Pathologically all the resected tissue comprised TD.*

necrotic tissue, TD or cancer (the latter is uncommon in the absence of rising serum markers). Except in special circumstances (marker plateau), surgery is not recommended in this latter group. In all other cases it is recommended that all abnormal masses visualized on abdominal CT scan be excised, certainly if these are >1.5 cm in diameter. However, clinical sense dictates that huge tumour masses at presentation which are resolving satisfactorily (e.g. 20 cm retroperitoneal mass reducing to 2 cm) may be observed for a short while to see if they regress further spontaneously.

In the UK, formal retroperitoneal lymph node dissection is not used. Though policies do vary worldwide, most surgeons in the UK remove abnormal residual masses visualized at laparotomy. When bulky disease is present, this surgery can be complex, patients occasionally requiring resection of a kidney, the inferior vena cava, or a length of aorta in order to achieve complete removal of tumour masses.

Residual lung masses seen on chest X-ray should also be resected if this is technically feasible, and combined thoracolaparotomy is a possibility if both abdominal and lung masses require resection. When this combined approach is not reasonable, then generally laparotomy is performed first with observation of the pulmonary masses during the time of recovery. If the primary tumour is still present, orchidectomy is recommended post-chemotherapy.

Careful histological evaluation of resected tissue by an experienced histopathologist is essential. Completely resected necrotic tissue or TD (which may appear quite dysplastic) requires no further therapy (Fig. 32.8). Patients in whom cancer is resected should probably receive further chemotherapy, generally with two more courses of BEP though this approach has not been well validated.

POST-TREATMENT FOLLOW-UP: TERATOMA

Following chemotherapy and surgery (where necessary), a baseline CT scan of all previously abnormal areas should be obtained. Further CT is not necessary if this study is normal. Patients should initially be monitored monthly with marker estimations and a chest X-ray.

Relapse from complete remission is relatively unusual (10 per cent of cases), occurring most commonly in patients with initial poor prognosis disease or with residual unresectable disease in the chest or abdomen. The great majority of relapses occur within 6 months; however, late relapses at up to 10–15 years post-chemotherapy have been recorded, particularly in patients with initial bulky disease or resected TD.

After an initial close surveillance policy, post-chemotherapy follow-up can be rapidly reduced to 6-monthly then yearly. Currently patients treated with chemotherapy alone should probably be followed for 5–10 years. Those in whom residual masses remain, or in whom TD has been resected, should probably be followed for life. It is not necessary to perform a chest X-ray at later evaluations, though all patients should have their serum markers checked.

MANAGEMENT OF RELAPSED TERATOMA

Teratoma relapse is often detected because of pathological marker elevation, or because of progression of residual masses or the appearance of new masses. In the latter cases, and if the tumour markers remain normal, biopsy or surgical removal (where technically feasible) should be considered as these may comprise TD, or, rarely, a new non-germ-cell malignant neoplasm, thought to be derived from residual elements of TD. Occasionally relapses occur in the CNS, which can act as a sanctuary site from chemotherapy; patients at risk are those with a very high presentation hCG or multiple (>20) lung metastases.

The prognosis at the time of relapse relates to initial response to chemotherapy (patients with primary refractory disease have a worse outlook than those with initial complete response), time to relapse (late relapses are more favourable), bulk of disease and height of serum tumour marker elevation at relapse (Fossa *et al.*, 1999c).

Patients with early progression and elevated serum markers should virtually always be managed initially with chemotherapy, though at all times the role of additional surgery should be considered. The most widely used regimen in patients developing progressive disease after treatment with BEP is VeIP (vinblastine, ifosfamide and cisplatin; Loehrer *et al.*, 1998). This regimen is particularly myelosuppressive but despite this should, where possible, be given at full dose and on time. An alternative regimen is POMB/ACE.

Patients responding to VeIP should receive four courses of treatment, after which complete re-evaluation should take place to see if salvage surgery is possible or necessary. Where tumour markers return to normal and residual masses remain, these should be resected. Patients with elevated markers and a single resectable site of disease (including an isolated brain metastasis, where present) should have this resected in this clinical setting as cure can occasionally result.

Occasional patients will relapse late (>2 years) following induction chemotherapy. These patients often have a pattern of relapse, particularly characterized by an elevated AFP. Current evidence suggests that these patients are relatively chemorefractory and that radical surgery, where possible, should be the initial treatment approach; this can result in cure. Where this is impossible, then initial chemotherapy should be given followed by surgery.

A number of treatment centres now manage patients with high-dose chemotherapy with stem cell support, rather than VeIP, as the initial treatment approach at the time of relapse. Certainly patients failing VeIP chemotherapy should be considered for high-dose chemotherapy.

HIGH-DOSE CHEMOTHERAPY AS SALVAGE TREATMENT

High-dose chemotherapy with stem cell rescue has been extensively evaluated as salvage treatment for relapsing teratoma. The results described are those of retrospective reviews (e.g. Rick *et al.*, 1998). A randomized trial comparing salvage therapy with VeIP (4 cycles) or VeIP (3 cycles) + high dose therapy has been completed in Europe, but not yet analysed.

A variety of chemotherapy regimens have been used. The most common is high-dose carboplatin and etoposide; other groups have, however, added either cyclophosphamide or ifosfamide to this regimen, though this clearly increases toxicity. The timing of high-dose therapy has been variable; more recent studies have used this treatment as initial salvage following failure of BEP. In older studies multiple chemotherapy regimens have been given

prior to high-dose chemotherapy. In addition, the number of cycles of high-dose therapy given has not been standardized. The great majority of centres use one or two courses of treatment but more have been evaluated.

There is no doubt that high-dose therapy can be curative in patients with relapsing germ-cell cancer. Beyer *et al.* (1996) determined the risk factors for failure following second-line chemotherapy as:

- progressive disease before high-dose therapy;
- mediastinal non-seminomatous primary tumour;
- refractory or absolutely refractory disease to conventional dose cisplatin (score 2 for the latter factor); and
- hCG level before high-dose therapy >1000 IU/L (score 2).

Patients with no risk factors were described as having a 2-year failure-free survival of 51 per cent, compared with 27 per cent and 5 per cent for those scoring 1 or 2 or >2, respectively.

High-dose chemotherapy is associated with considerable morbidity and an approximately 5 per cent mortality and should be confined to centres with extensive experience of this treatment modality. Residual masses should, where feasible, be resected following high-dose chemotherapy exactly as after initial chemotherapy.

NEW DRUGS

As over 85 per cent of patients with metastatic teratoma will be cured with combination chemotherapy, there are few circumstances in which new drugs can be tested. However, recent studies have provided clear evidence that paclitaxel is an effective agent (Motzer *et al.*, 1994). This drug is currently being tested in a randomized MRC/EORTC trial in which BEP is being compared with T-BEP (paclitaxel + BEP) in patients with an intermediate prognosis. Paclitaxel has also been used in combination (e.g. paclitaxel, ifosfamide and cisplatin) as a salvage regimen. More recently, gemcitabine has been shown to be active in patients with relapsed teratoma (Bokemeyer *et al.*, 1999); it is anticipated that this drug will also be used in combination in the future.

Management of malignant seminoma

Pure seminoma comprises approximately 50 per cent of testicular cancers; mixed tumours (seminoma + teratoma) should be managed as malignant teratoma.

STAGE I

Approximately 70 per cent of patients with seminoma have stage I disease at presentation. Patients with spermatocytic seminoma (a non-germ-cell tumour) have a very low risk of spread, and no further therapy is indicated. It is known from surveillance studies in classical seminoma that occult metastatic disease is present in

15–20 per cent of patients who in the absence of therapy developed subsequent relapse. A variety of management approaches have been used for stage I patients; cure rates for stage I disease should approach 100 per cent.

Adjuvant radiotherapy

Seminoma is a highly radiosensitive neoplasm, which tends to spread in an orderly and contiguous fashion, commencing in the para-aortic nodes. Adjuvant radiotherapy remains the standard treatment approach to the management of patients with stage I seminoma. The standard radiation dose in the UK is 30 Gy (25 Gy on mainland Europe) given in 15 fractions over a 3-week period. Until recently, the recommended treatment was a dog-leg field incorporating the para-aortic nodes and ipsilateral iliac nodes. This approach remains standard for patients with an increased risk of inguino/iliac disease (those with inguinal surgery or orchidopexy in childhood) but as a result of an MRC trial (Fossa *et al.*, 1999b) has been replaced by para-aortic radiotherapy for all other patients. In this randomized trial in 478 patients, treatment was given to either a para-aortic field or a dog-leg field. The 3-year relapse-free survival in both groups was 96–97 per cent. Only two relapses occurred within the radiation field and pelvic relapses were confined to the patients receiving para-aortic radiation (occurring in only 2 per cent of cases). The remaining relapses occurred in the posterior mediastinum, cervical area or lung. The overall cure rate was over 99 per cent. Toxicity was much less in the para-aortic radiation group and this field is now standard.

A new MRC randomized study, as yet not reported, has treated patients with stage I seminoma with radiation to the para-aortic strip to a dose of either 20 Gy or 30 Gy, and may further modify the treatment of this disease.

Short-term toxicities following radiotherapy include nausea, malaise, diarrhoea and infertility. In the longer term, there is an increased incidence of peptic ulceration and a small, but definite increase in second cancers.

Surveillance policy

Whilst adjuvant irradiation remains the recommended treatment for stage I seminoma, an alternative approach is surveillance, reserving treatment for patients who relapse. Approximately 15–20 per cent of patients will develop relapse of disease; however, seminoma is less commonly associated with marker elevation than teratoma, thereby placing an increased emphasis on radiological (CT scan) follow-up. In addition, relapse can occur late, and has been recorded >5 years following orchidectomy which means that follow-up needs to be prolonged. Finally, relapse can occur outside standard radiation fields and then involve treatment with chemotherapy. Surveillance is now rarely used, but is indicated when seminoma occurs in a patient who has been previously irradiated, or where this treatment is contraindicated.

Adjuvant chemotherapy

Seminoma is an exquisitely chemosensitive disease and in a number of studies in stage I disease one or two injections of intravenous carboplatin have resulted in a very low failure-free survival (0–5 per cent). Carboplatin treatment is well tolerated, though short-term nausea and vomiting and impairment of fertility can result.

In a completed MRC/EORTC randomized trial, carboplatin (at an area under the curve, AUC, dose of 7) was compared with para-aortic radiation in patients with stage I seminoma. Until results of this trial are available this treatment should be regarded as experimental.

STAGE IIA AND STAGE IIB SEMINOMA

In 10–15 per cent of patients with seminoma, evidence of low-volume para-aortic adenopathy (≤5 cm) will be found at presentation. For such patients radiotherapy remains the standard treatment; most radiotherapists treat a dog-leg field to a dose of 30 Gy (Warde *et al.*, 1998). Some radiotherapists also recommend treatment to the contralateral pelvic nodal field in such patients as there is a small risk of retrograde spread of tumour and subsequent relapse.

Residual masses present post-radiation are unusual, but are almost always sterile and can be watched. There is no indication for prophylactic treatment of the mediastinum, a common practice in the past.

Relapse rates after radiotherapy for stage IIA and B disease are certainly higher than those with stage I disease, but do not exceed 10–15 per cent. Relapses usually occur supradiaphragmatically and should be treated with combination chemotherapy.

An alternative approach to the management of stage IIB seminoma is combination chemotherapy with BEP (*see* below) and at least comparable results can be obtained with this treatment approach; this, however, exposes many more patients to the toxicity of chemotherapy.

PROGNOSTIC FACTORS: SEMINOMA

Patients with metastatic seminoma treated with platinum-containing chemotherapy were included in the IGCCC study (*see* 'Staging and prognostic factor classifications: teratoma', above), although because this clinical setting is comparatively rare only 660 cases were available for analysis (Table 32.7).

In marked contradistinction to malignant teratoma, seminoma arising in extragonadal sites (particularly the mediastinum) has no adverse prognostic implications and an identical prognosis to testicular seminoma. The main adverse features identified in this study were the presence of non-pulmonary visceral metastases. Patients were divided into a good or intermediate prognosis group using this factor alone. No poor prognosis group could be identified in this study.

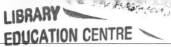

Table 32.7 *Prognosis factors in metastatic seminoma IGCCC classification*

Good prognosis
90 per cent of patients
5-year progression-free survival 82%; survival 86%
- *any primary site* and
- *no non-pulmonary visceral metastases* and
- *normal AFP, any hCG and LDH*

Poor prognosis
10 per cent of patients
5-year progression-free survival 67%; survival 72%
- seminoma
- any primary site and
- *non-pulmonary visceral metastases* and
  normal AFP, any hCG any LDH

STAGE IIC, D, RELAPSE POST-RADIOTHERAPY AND ALL OTHER METASTASTIC PATIENTS

It is generally accepted that all the above patients with seminoma should be treated with combination chemotherapy. Although radiotherapy was used in the past even for patients with extensive disease, this treatment has now been abandoned as patients with bulky disease suffered organ toxicity (e.g. nephrotoxicity) and relapses occurred commonly.

The great majority of patients with metastatic seminoma present with nodal disease in the retroperitoneum and/or posterior mediastinum and/or left cervical area. Occasionally, however, there has been spread to the lungs, pleura and bones, though these latter sites are most commonly seen at relapse after chemotherapy.

Metastatic seminoma is exquisitely sensitive to treatment with cisplatin and carboplatin used as single agents. In an MRC randomized trial, 130 patients with advanced seminoma were randomly assigned to treatment with either single agent carboplatin (400 mg/m^2 intravenously) or combination chemotherapy with etoposide and cisplatin. This trial was closed after 130 patients had been randomized. At a median follow-up time of 4.5 years, the failure-free survival and survival for patients allocated carboplatin or cisplatin and etoposide, respectively, were 71 per cent and 80 per cent and 84 per cent and 89 per cent (Horwich *et al.*, 2000). This trial was abandoned prematurely because of inferior treatment results seen in patients with metastatic teratoma. The treatment of choice for metastatic seminoma is regarded as treatment with cisplatin and etoposide ± bleomycin. Carboplatin is probably slightly less effective but has a role in special clinical circumstances, e.g. in patients with renal failure or profound learning difficulties (where cisplatin may be impractical), though it should be accepted that failure rates will be higher.

Virtually all patients with metastatic seminoma will respond rapidly and satisfactorily to chemotherapy, though a substantial proportion of patients (again particularly those with bulky disease) will have residual masses on completion of treatment, most commonly in the retroperitoneum. Attempts have been made to resect such disease; however, the desmoplastic response evoked by metastatic seminoma, and close relationship of such disease to vital retroperitoneal structures has rendered such surgery fraught with difficulties. In fact, approximately 90 per cent of resected masses have proved sterile histologically; this finding is confirmed by the very low relapse rate when such masses are observed rather than resected. Current consensus is that residual masses should be observed unless they increase in size, in which case a biopsy should be performed. PET scanning may, however, modify this approach in future. Adjuvant irradiation has also been used to treat masses but has been shown to be without benefit (Duchesne *et al.*, 1997). Overall, approximately 90 per cent of patients with metastatic seminoma should remain failure free after treatment with intravenous cisplatin and etoposide.

FOLLOW-UP OF SEMINOMA POST-TREATMENT

Patients with stage I seminoma have very low relapse rates and follow-up intervals of 3–4 months in the first 2 years should suffice, with less frequent follow-up thereafter. CT scanning is not routinely recommended as an intermittent chest X-ray, serum markers and clinical examination should suffice. Patients receiving radiotherapy for stage IIA and B seminoma should have a single post-treatment CT scan to ensure that disease has entirely resolved. Further abdominal scans should be considered if residual masses are present (though this is unusual).

Patients with bulky abdominal seminoma treated with chemotherapy require follow-up scans of residual abdominal masses, where present, until these have stabilized or resolved. These masses commonly calcify and remain present for years. Seminoma can be a very indolent disease and very late relapses have been reported; these, however, are extremely uncommon. Follow-up for 10 years is probably sufficient.

MANAGEMENT OF RELAPSED SEMINOMA

Patients relapsing after chemotherapy or radiotherapy for seminoma should have serum AFP and hCG levels measured and preferably a biopsy to confirm the relapsing masses comprise seminoma; histological 'progression' to teratoma or relapse of an occult mixed tumour can occur, often accompanied by a rising AFP level.

Patients relapsing after primary treatment with radiotherapy should be treated with cisplatin-containing combination chemotherapy as in the section above. Relapse of seminoma following chemotherapy is relatively uncommon, and therefore the available data are limited. Patients treated with carboplatin should receive a cisplatin-containing combination regimen and patients relapsing following cisplatin and etoposide should probably initially be treated with combination chemotherapy with VeIP. Radiotherapy to residual masses should be considered in all such patients with seminoma as this treatment remains highly effective. High-dose chemotherapy with stem cell rescue has also been used in a number of patients with seminoma with comparable results to patients with teratoma.

Chemotherapy-related toxicity

Treatment of germ-cell tumours with cisplatin-containing chemotherapy is associated with a wide range of toxicities, particularly for patients receiving salvage treatment for relapsed disease. Virtually all patients suffer problems with nausea and vomiting despite standard prophylactic treatment with a 5-HT$_3$ antagonist and dexamethasone; alopecia occurs universally. Myelosuppression is also virtually universal; this predominantly comprises neutropenia, sometimes complicated by a fever with the requirement for intravenous antibiotics (gentamicin should be avoided in these circumstances as nephrotoxicity may result).

Perhaps the most common life-threatening toxicity in relationship to BEP is bleomycin lung (Simpson *et al.*, 1998). Bleomycin causes pneumonitis and progressive pulmonary fibrosis with an overall incidence of 3–4 per cent in patients receiving BEP chemotherapy at full dose (360 000 units) with a mortality of 1–2 per cent. Bleomycin toxicity is dose related, but can occur after quite low doses have been given. Additional risk factors are increasing age (>40 years) and deteriorating renal function. Bleomycin should not be administered to patients with significant elevation of the serum creatinine. Bleomycin lung is difficult to anticipate; the finding of bilateral basal crepitations, bilateral basal changes on chest X-ray or persistent cough or dyspnoea may all indicate early toxicity and may be an indication for discontinuation of the drug.

Cisplatin commonly causes tinnitus and high-tone hearing loss which may become apparent during or after treatment. These symptoms tend to settle with time. In addition, impaired renal function, with an overall loss of 10–20 per cent of renal function, commonly occurs when BEP is given at full dose.

Once chemotherapy has been completed, recovery generally occurs rapidly and the great majority of patients resume their previous lifestyle. However, it is at this time that symptoms relating to peripheral neuropathy (caused by cisplatin) and sometimes transient L'hermitte's syndrome may occur.

Whilst infertility is probably universal during chemotherapy, sperm counts generally gradually recover to their previous levels, though this may take years if sperm counts are low at the initiation of chemotherapy or if more than four courses of cisplatin are given. There have been no reports of an increase in congenital abnormalities in the children of survivors of testicular cancer.

On long-term follow-up there may be a small increase in incidence of hypertension; hyperlipoproteinaemia has also been described.

Management of the contralateral testis

The lifetime risk of developing testicular cancer is one in 400–450. Patients diagnosed with a germ-cell cancer are, however, at much increased risk of contralateral disease. Rarely, patients present with synchronous bilateral tumours, much more commonly the second tumour is delayed by 5–10 years.

As discussed previously (*see* 'Pathogenesis', above) the underlying pathological event is the presence of carcinoma *in-situ* (CIS), recognizable only by testicular biopsy. In a large German series (Dieckmann and Loy, 1996), routine testicular biopsy was performed at the time of orchidectomy and CIS was detected in the contralateral testis in 4.9 per cent of cases, which equates approximately to the recognized risk of contralateral disease.

The main risk factor for contralateral CIS is the presence of an atrophic contralateral testis, probably best defined as a testicular volume of under 16 mL (measured by ultrasound). The second main risk factor is decreasing age, particularly <30 years. A history of testicular maldescent without accompanying atrophy is probably not a risk factor as was previously thought. In an MRC study (Harland *et al.*, 1998) a particularly high-risk group was identified: patients aged <30 years with a small remaining testis as defined above, were found to have a risk of contralateral CIS of over 30 per cent, for the remaining patients the risk was between 2 and 4 per cent.

There is strong clinical evidence that CIS carries a very high risk of subsequent malignancy (50 per cent risk by 5 years) and treatment is generally recommended once this abnormality is found. CIS is generally associated with poor sperm production and azoospermia is not unusual when CIS is gross.

CIS can be effectively treated with local radiation (current recommended dose 20 Gy in 10 daily fractions). Fertile patients may wish to bank sperm prior to such treatment, or may prefer to attempt to father children prior to treatment. In such cases a close watch on the remaining testis should be maintained with follow-up ultrasound. Radiotherapy uniformly causes sterility and probably causes Leydig cell damage as hypogonadism is not an uncommon late complication of treatment in these patients.

It was previously thought that treatment with chemotherapy reduced the risk of subsequent contralateral testicular cancer. There is, however, no evidence that this is true, though contralateral disease may be delayed.

Contralateral testicular cancer

When patients present with contralateral testicular tumour, urgent sperm banking should be offered where appropriate. Small clinical series have described attempts at testicular conservation; a partial orchidectomy is performed with irradiation of the remaining testis to abolish residual CIS. This approach is, in practice, rarely applicable and orchidectomy is necessary for the majority of patients.

Following bilateral orchidectomy, hormonal replacement treatment is essential. Hypogonadism is commonly manifest by flushes, sweats, swinging mood and impotence. A long-term complication of inadequate androgen levels is osteoporosis.

Hormone replacement can be achieved by a number of means. Perhaps the most effective is a subcutaneous testosterone implant; this is inserted via a cannula at 4-monthly intervals and provides effective and even testosterone replacement. Many patients are, however, treated with intramuscular testosterone (Sustanon 250) given every 3 weeks. Patches are now available but many patients find these unsatisfactory as they tend to be noisy, leak or cause irritation.

Patients on hormonal replacement treatment should have follow-up LH and testosterone levels measured to ensure that hormone replacement is adequate.

EXTRAGONADAL GERM-CELL TUMOURS

Mediastinal germ-cell tumour

Approximately 2–3 per cent of germ-cell tumours apparently arise in the mediastinum. Testicular biopsies in such patients are normal (and unnecessary if testicular ultrasound is normal). Patients with mediastinal germ-cell tumours commonly have gross advanced disease at presentation (Fig. 32.9); the common presenting features include dyspnoea, chest pain (often pleuritic), superior vena caval obstruction or pericardial tamponade.

Mediastinal seminoma and teratoma occur; the latter is most common. Mediastinal seminoma carries no increased risk of death when compared with comparable patients with testicular seminoma and should be routinely treated with four cycles of EP or BEP alone. There is no evidence to support the additional use of post-chemotherapy surgery or irradiation.

Mediastinal teratoma is an aggressive and relatively poor prognosis form of germ-cell cancer (Fizazi et al., 1998). A variety of histologies may be seen, including pure yolk-sac tumour or choriocarcinoma. Mediastinal teratoma is particularly associated with the development of a second malignancy (e.g. angiosarcoma) within the tumour mass.

These cases are rarely associated with Klinefelter's syndrome. In addition the coexistence of mediastinal teratoma and haematological malignancy (myelodysplasia, acute myeloid leukaemia or malignant histiocytosis) is well recorded (Nichols et al., 1985), both diseases arising from a common malignant clone characterized by i(12p). Haematological malignancy in these cases generally presents either simultaneously with the mediastinal tumour or within 18 months to 2 years. Prognosis is extremely poor.

As mediastinal teratoma usually presents with gross advanced disease, urgent therapy is necessary and the

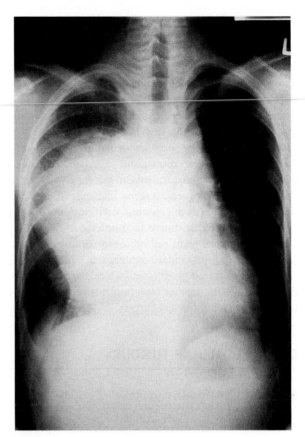

Figure 32.9 *Chest X-ray showing very large anterior mediastinal mass. The patient's serum AFP was grossly elevated and biopsy was considered unnecessary. BEP chemotherapy was given.*

diagnosis can often be based on serum marker elevations alone in a patient with a large anterior mediastinal mass. Mediastinal teratoma has the worst prognosis of any form of germ-cell cancer with a cure rate of approximately 50 per cent in most studies. BEP chemotherapy remains the standard treatment, although some authorities believe that more intensive chemotherapy regimens may produce better results. Following four courses of chemotherapy patients should be re-evaluated, virtually all have residual masses in the anterior mediastinum which should always, where technically feasible, be resected. These masses may comprise necrosis, differentiated teratoma or active cancer (areas of sarcoma may also be seen).

Post-chemotherapy follow-up should be close. Unfortunately, those patients that develop relapse of their disease manifest by increasing masses or elevated markers have an extremely poor prognosis as they are particularly refractory to salvage therapy. High-dose therapy with stem cell support is largely ineffective and experimental treatment protocols are appropriate.

Retroperitoneal primary germ-cell tumours

A small proportion of patients with germ-cell cancer present as a result of retroperitoneal lymph node enlargement. This is often massive and sometimes associated with obstruction of one or both ureters or the inferior vena cava.

Biopsy may reveal that the tumour is either a seminoma or malignant teratoma. Testicular ultrasound should be performed in all such cases. It is often possible from the presenting CT scan to determine whether the metastatic disease has derived from the left or right testis; ultrasound will commonly show abnormalities on this side. Even when testicular ultrasound is normal, bilateral testicular biopsies have shown an incidence of CIS of approximately 50 per cent. It seems likely that the testis is the primary site in such cases and orchidectomy should be performed once treatment is completed.

Retroperitoneal germ-cell cancers are managed in the same way as their testicular counterparts. The prognosis relates to recognized prognostic factors, particularly the degree of tumour marker elevation. Many patients will require post-chemotherapy surgery.

OTHER TESTICULAR TUMOURS

Sertoli cell tumour

Sertoli cell tumours comprise approximately 1 per cent of testicular malignancies. They occur at any age and in approximately 75 per cent of cases are benign. It is, however, not possible pathologically to absolutely differentiate benign from malignant cases, the latter ultimately being diagnosed when metastasis occurs.

Most cases of Sertoli cell tumour present with testicular swelling and orchidectomy is the treatment of choice. These tumours can occasionally be hormone secreting and associated with gynaecomastia.

Post-orchidectomy CT scanning should be performed. Most patients are stage I and will be cured by orchidectomy. Where retroperitoneal masses are apparent, surgery has usually been performed (commonly a RPLND). Long-term survival after this procedure has been reported. Prognosis is generally poor for those with widespread metastatic disease.

Leydig cell tumours

Leydig cell tumour also comprises approximately 1 per cent of testicular tumours and can also occur at any age, though childhood cases are rare (Bertram *et al.*, 1991). It is difficult to distinguish malignant from benign Leydig cell tumours on routine pathology. The main findings which should arouse suspicion of malignancy are larger tumour size ($\geqslant 5$ cm) and lymphatic or vascular invasion.

The treatment of choice is orchidectomy; this will cure the great majority of patients in whom the disease is either benign or stage I. Staging with a CT scan should be performed. Those rare patients with metastatic disease

should be considered for surgical resection by RPLND. Prognosis is poor if widespread metastases are present as this is not a chemosensitive disease.

CONCLUSIONS

The germ-cell tumours are a complex and fascinating group of malignancies whose incidence is rapidly rising. Their modern interdisciplinary management represents a triumph of clinical science, and it is anticipated that cure rates should continue to improve whilst treatment-related morbidity lessens.

The challenges for the future are mainly epidemiological. We need to know the cause of the present surge in incidence of these cases, in the hope that they can be prevented. Testicular maldescent is now commonly detected and corrected at a much earlier age and it is hoped that this may contribute to a reduction in incidence of subsequent malignancy. This main clinical challenge is early identification and effective therapy of high-risk teratoma which will require future international co-operation.

SIGNIFICANT POINTS

- Testicular germ-cell cancers comprise 1 per cent of male malignancies but are the most common cancers in young men. Cure is possible in 95 per cent of cases.
- Pathologically cases can be divided into seminomas (50 per cent) and non-seminomas (teratoma, 50 per cent). Mixed tumours are handled clinically as teratoma.
- Post-orchidectomy staging should include measurement of the serum markers AFP, hCG and LDH, and CT scanning. Patients should be allocated to a prognostic group using the International Germ Cell Cancer Consensus classification.
- Stage I seminoma is usually managed with adjuvant radiotherapy. Cure rate should exceed 99 per cent. Stage I teratoma may be managed with surveillance or (in high-risk cases) with adjuvant chemotherapy. Cure rate again should exceed 99 per cent.
- Bulky metastatic seminoma is managed with combination chemotherapy using at least cisplatin and etoposide. Cure rates of 90 per cent should be achieved. The standard chemotherapy for metastatic non-seminoma is BEP (bleomycin, etoposide, and cisplatin). A variety of

different schedules are used. For good prognosis disease, cure rates of 95–100 per cent should be achieved.

- There is a 5 per cent risk of developing contralateral testicular cancer. Selected patients should be screened for CIS (carcinoma *in-situ*) with testicular biopsy.

KEY REFERENCES

De Wit, R., Roberts, J.T., Wilkinson, P.M. *et al.* (2001) Equivalence of three or four cycles of bleomycin, etoposide and cisplatin chemotherapy and of a 3- or 5-day schedule in good-prognosis germ cell cancer: a randomized study of the European Organization for Research and Treatment of Cancer Genitourinary Tract Cancer Co-operative Group and the Medical Research Council. *J. Clin. Oncol.* **19**, 1629–40.

Horwich, A., Sleijfer, D.T., Fossa, S.D. *et al.* (1997) Randomized trial of bleomycin, etoposide, and cisplatin compared with bleomycin, etoposide and carboplatin in good-prognosis metastatic nonseminomatous germ cell cancer: a multiinstitutional Medical Research Council/European Organization for Research and Treatment of Cancer Trial. *J. Clin. Oncol.* **15**, 1844–52.

International Germ Cell Cancer Collaborative Group (1997) International germ cell consensus classification: a prognostic factor-based staging system for metastatic germ cell cancers. *J. Clin. Oncol.* **15**, 594–603.

Mead, G.M. (1999) Who should manage germ cell tumours of the testis? *Br. J. Urol.* **84**, 61–7.

Williams, S.D., Birch, R., Einhorn, L.H. *et al.* (1987) Treatment of disseminated germ-cell tumors with cisplatin, bleomycin, and either vinblastine or etoposide. *N. Engl. J. Med.* **316**, 1435–40.

REFERENCES

Bertram, K.A., Bratloff, B., Hodges, G.F. *et al.* (1991) Treatment of malignant Leydig cell tumor. *Cancer* **68**, 2324–9.

Beyer, J., Kramar, A., Mandanas, R. *et al.* (1996) High-dose chemotherapy as salvage treatment in germ cell tumours: a multivariate analysis of prognostic variables. *J. Clin. Oncol.* **14**, 2638–45.

Bokemeyer, C., Gerl, A., Schoffski, P. *et al.* (1999) Gemcitabine in patients with relapsed or cisplatin-refractory testicular cancer. *J. Clin. Oncol.* **17**, 512–16.

Bower, M., Newlands, E.S., Holden, L. *et al.* (1997) Treatment of men with metastatic non-seminomatous germ cell tumours with cyclical POMB/ACE chemotherapy. *Ann. Oncol.* **8**, 477–83.

Comiter, C.V., Kibel, A.S., Richie, J.P. *et al.* (1998) Prognostic features of teratomas with malignant transformation: a clinicopathological study of 21 cases. *J. Urol.* **159**, 859–63.

Cullen, M.H., Stenning, S.P., Parkinson, M.C. *et al.* (1996) Short-course adjuvant chemotherapy in high-risk stage I nonseminomatous germ cell tumours of the testis: a Medical Research Council Report. *J. Clin. Oncol.* **14**, 1106–13.

de Wit, R., Stoter, G., Kaye, S.B. *et al.* (1997) Importance of bleomycin in combination chemotherapy for good-prognosis testicular nonseminoma: a randomized study of the European Organization for Research and Treatment of Cancer Genitourinary Tract Cancer Co-operative Group. *J. Clin. Oncol.* **15**, 1837–43.

de Wit, R., Roberts, J.T., Wilkins, P. *et al.* (1999) Is 3BEP equivalent to 3BEP-EP in good prognosis germ cell cancer? An EORTC/MRC phase III study. *Proc. ASCO* **18**, 118.

De Wit, R., Roberts, J.T., Wilkinson, P.M. *et al.* (2001) Equivalence of three or four cycles of bleomycin, etoposide and cisplatin chemotherapy and of a 3- or 5-day schedule in good-prognosis germ cell cancer: a randomized study of the European Organization for Research and Treatment of Cancer Genitourinary Tract Cancer Co-operative Group and the Medical Research Council. *J. Clin. Oncol.* **19**, 1629–40.

Dieckmann, K.P. and Loy, V. (1996) Prevalence of contralateral testicular intraepithelial neoplasia in patients with testicular germ cell neoplasms. *J. Clin. Oncol.* **14**, 3126–32.

Donohue, J.P., Thornhill, J.A., Foster, R.S. *et al.* (1993) Primary retroperitoneal lymph node dissection in clinical stage A non-seminomatous germ cell testis cancer. *Br. J. Urol.* **71**, 326–35.

Duchesne, G.M., Stenning, S.P., Aass, N. *et al.* (1997) Radiotherapy after chemotherapy for metastatic seminoma – a diminishing role. *Eur. J. Cancer* **33**, 829–35.

Einhorn, L.H., Williams, S.D., Loehrer, P.J. *et al.* (1989) Evaluation of optimal duration of chemotherapy in favorable-prognosis disseminated germ cell tumours: a Southeastern Cancer Study Group Protocol. *J. Clin. Oncol.* **7**, 387–91.

Fizazi, K., Culine, S., Droz, J.P. *et al.* (1998) Primary mediastinal nonseminomatous germ cell tumours: results of modern therapy including cisplatin-based chemotherapy. *J. Clin. Oncol.* **16**, 725–32.

Forman, D., Oliver, R.T.D., Brett, A.R. *et al.* (1992) Familial testicular cancer: a report of the UK family register, estimation of risk and an HLA class 1 sib-pair analysis. *Br. J. Cancer* **65**, 255–62.

Fossa, S.D., Kaye, S.B., Mead, G.M. *et al.* (1998) Filgrastim during combination chemotherapy of patients with poor-prognosis metastatic germ cell malignancy. *J. Clin. Oncol.* **16**, 716–24.

Fossa, S.D., Bokemeyer, C., Gerl, A. *et al.* (1999a) Treatment outcome of patients with brain metastases from malignant germ cell tumours. *Cancer* **85**, 988–97.

Fossa, S.D., Horwich, A., Russell, J.M. *et al.* (1999b) Optimal planning target volume for stage I testicular seminoma: a Medical Research Council randomized trial. *J. Clin. Oncol.* **17**, 1146–54.

Fossa, S.D., Stenning, S.P., Gerl, A. *et al.* (1999c) Prognostic factors in patients progressing after cisplatin-based chemotherapy for malignant non-seminomatous germ cell tumours. *Br. J. Cancer* **80**, 1392–9.

Harland, S.J., Cook, P.A., Fossa, S.D. *et al.* (1998) Intratubular germ cell neoplasia of the contralateral testis in testicular cancer: defining a high risk group. *J. Urol.* **160**, 1353–7.

Horwich, A., Dearnaley, D.P., Norman, A. *et al.* (1994) Accelerated chemotherapy for poor prognosis germ cell tumours. *Eur. J. Cancer* **30A**, 1607–11.

Horwich, A., Sleijfer, D.T., Fossa, S.D. *et al.* (1997) Randomized trial of bleomycin, etoposide, and cisplatin compared with bleomycin, etoposide and carboplatin in good-prognosis metastatic nonseminomatous germ cell cancer: a multiinstitutional Medical Research Council/ European Organization for Research and Treatment of Cancer Trial. *J. Clin. Oncol.* **15**, 1844–52.

Horwich, A., Oliver, R.T.D., Wilkinson, P.M. *et al.* (2000) A Medical Research Council randomised trial of single agent carboplatin versus etoposide and cisplatin for advanced metastatic seminoma. MRC Testicular Tumour Working Party. *Br. J. Cancer* **83**, 1623–9.

International Germ Cell Cancer Collaborative Group (1997) International germ cell consensus classification: a prognostic factor-based staging system for metastatic germ cell cancers. *J. Clin. Oncol.* **15**, 594–603.

Jeffery, G.M., Theaker, J.M., Lee, A.H.S. *et al.* (1991) The growing teratoma syndrome. *Br. J. Urol.* **67**, 195–202.

Kaye, S.B., Mead, G.M., Fossa, S.D. *et al.* (1998) Intensive induction-sequential chemotherapy with BOP/VIP-B compared with treatment with BEP/EP for poor-prognosis metastatic nonseminomatous germ cell tumour: a randomized Medical Research Council/European Organization of Research and Treatment of Cancer Study. *J. Clin. Oncol.* **16**, 692–701.

Lassen, U., Daugaard, G., Rorth, M. *et al.* (1997) Detection of metastatic disease with positron emission tomography in computed tomography negative non-seminomatous germ cell tumors. *Proc. ASCO* **16**, A1142.

Loehrer, P.J., Gonin, R., Nichols, C.R. *et al.* (1998) Vinblastine plus ifosfamide plus cisplatin as initial salvage therapy in recurrent germ cell tumor. *J. Clin. Oncol.* **16**, 2500–4.

McKendrick, J.J., Theaker, J. and Mead, G.M. (1991) Nonseminomatous germ cell tumor with very high serum human chorionic gonadotrophin. *Cancer* **67**, 684–9.

Mead, G.M. (1999) Who should manage germ cell tumours of the testis? *Br. J. Urol.* **84**, 61–7.

Motzer, R.J., Bajorin, D.F., Schwartz, L.H. *et al.* (1994) Phase II trial of paclitaxel shows antitumor activity in patients with previously treated germ cell tumors. *J. Clin. Oncol.* **12**, 2277–83.

Nichols, C.R., Hoffman, R., Einhorn, L.H. *et al.* (1985) Hematologic malignancies associated with primary mediastinal germ-cell tumors. *Ann. Intern. Med.* **102**, 603–9.

Nichols, C.R., Catalano, P.J., Crawford, D.E. *et al.* (1998) Randomized comparison of cisplatin and etoposide and either bleomycin or ifosfamide in treatment of advanced disseminated germ cell tumors: an Eastern Cooperative Oncology Group, Southwest Oncology Group, and Cancer and Leukemia Group B study. *J. Clin. Oncol.* **16**, 1287–93.

Read, G., Stenning, S.P., Cullen, M.H. *et al.* (1992) Medical Research Council prospective study of surveillance for stage I testicular teratoma. *J. Clin. Oncol.* **10**, 1762–8.

Rick, O., Beyer, J., Kingreen, D. *et al.* (1998) High-dose chemotherapy in germ cell tumours: a large single centre experience. *Eur. J. Cancer* **34**, 1883–8.

Saxman, S.B., Finch, D., Gonin, R. *et al.* (1998) Long-term follow-up of a phase III study of three versus four cycles of bleomycin, etoposide, and cisplatin in favorable-prognosis germ-cell tumors: the Indiana University Experience. *J. Clin. Oncol.* **16**, 702–6.

Senturia, Y.D. (1987) The epidemology of testicular cancer. *Br. J. Urol.* **60**, 285–91.

Simmonds, P.D., Lee, A.H.S., Theaker, J.M. *et al.* (1996) Primary pure teratoma of the testis. *J. Urol.* **155**, 939–42.

Simpson, A.B., Pau, J., Graham, J. *et al.* (1998) Fatal bleomycin pulmonary toxicity in the west of Scotland 1991–95: a review of patients with germ cell tumours. *Br. J. Cancer* **78**, 1061–6.

von der Maase, H., Rorth, M., Walbom-Jorgenson, S. *et al.* (1986) Carcinoma *in situ* of contralateral testis in patients with testicular germ cell cancer: study of 27 cases in 500 patients. *Br. Med. J.* **293**, 1398–401.

Warde, P., Gospodarowicz, M., Panzarella, T. *et al.* (1998) Management of stage II seminoma. *J. Clin. Oncol.* **16**, 290–4.

Williams, S.D., Birch, R., Einhorn, L.H. *et al.* (1987) Treatment of disseminated germ-cell tumors with cisplatin, bleomycin, and either vinblastine or etoposide. *N. Engl. J. Med.* **316**, 1435–40.

Xiao, H., Mazumdar, M., Bajorin, D.F. *et al.* (1997) Long-term follow-up of patients with good-risk germ cell tumors treated with etoposide and cisplatin. *J. Clin. Oncol.* **15**, 2553–8.

33

Ovary and Fallopian tube

HANNAH E. LAMBERT, HILARY THOMAS AND W. PAT SOUTTER

INTRODUCTION

Carcinoma of the ovary is most prevalent in developed areas of the world such as Europe and the USA. In the UK over 6000 cases are reported per annum. The estimated incidence in England and Wales in 1992 was 20.3 per 100 000 women and the death rate 15.0 per 100 000 women. The lifetime risk of developing ovarian cancer (1.4 per cent) is higher than that for either cancer of the cervix (1.25 per cent) or the endometrium (1.1 per cent) but lower than for cancer of the breast (7.1 per cent). Ovarian cancer is the fourth most common cause of cancer death in women after breast, lung and bowel.

The majority of women develop tumours of epithelial origin. These are rare before the menarche, but the incidence increases with age to a peak in the 50–70-year-old age group. Most epithelial tumours are advanced at diagnosis so only 25–30 per cent are surviving at 5 years. Eventually 75 per cent of women with ovarian cancer will die from their disease. Other tumour types, such as germ-cell tumours, are more common in children and young women.

AETIOLOGY

The factors that lead to the development of ovarian carcinoma are not known. Epithelial tumours are most frequently present in women who have never been pregnant, have an early menarche, a late age at menopause and a long estimated number of years of ovulation. The infrequent occurrence of carcinoma of the ovary in women of high parity is thought to be due to the suppression of continuous ovulation, and there is good evidence that oral contraceptives play a protective role (Vessey et al., 1987).

Genetic factors

INHERITED GENES

Inheritance plays a significant role in about 5 per cent of epithelial ovarian cancers. The lifetime risk for a woman with one affected close relative is 2.5 per cent, nearly twice the risk in the general population (Ponder et al., 1992; Bell et al., 1998). If there is more than one affected close relative, the relative risk increases to 11 and the estimated risk by age 75 for women younger than 45 is 14 per cent (Stratton et al., 1998). A particular feature of familial cancers is the relatively early age at which they occur. Families with multiple cases of only ovarian cancer are rare. More commonly, there are cases of breast or colorectal cancer in the family. The Lynch syndrome consists of families with colorectal cancer, endometrial cancer and ovarian cancer (Watson and Lynch, 1992). The ovarian cancers are usually serous adenocarcinomas.

BRCA1 mutation is the major genetic determinant of familial inheritance. It is located on chromosome

17q and is probably associated with one-third of families with multiple breast cancer and 80 per cent of families with both breast and ovarian cancer (Ponder, 1994). A woman belonging to one of these families who has inherited the *BRCA1* gene has a 60 per cent risk of breast cancer by 50 years of age and a 90 per cent lifetime risk. The risks for ovarian cancer are less than half these. The coding sequence mutations and allelic loss seen in affected relatives suggest that *BRCA1* is a tumour-suppressor gene.

Mutations of *BRCA1* are also found in some cases of sporadic ovarian cancers, but there is no evidence at present of *BRCA1* abnormalities in the majority of sporadic ovarian cancers. *BRCA1* mutation is present in 5 per cent of women with ovarian cancer diagnosed before the age of 70 years (Stratton *et al.*, 1997).

A second gene, *BRCA2*, located at 13q12–13 has been reported in some breast/ovarian cancer families not associated with *BRCA1* mutations.

MANAGEMENT OF WOMEN WITH A FAMILY HISTORY OF OVARIAN CANCER

Women at high risk of ovarian cancer (15 per cent or more lifetime risk), on the basis of their family history, should be offered referral to a cancer genetics clinic. An ongoing United Kingdom Co-ordinating Committee for Cancer Research (UKCCCR) trial of ovarian screening for such women commenced in 1998. The eligibility criteria are as follows:

1 Two or more individuals with ovarian cancer who are first-degree relatives.
2 One individual with ovarian cancer and one with breast cancer diagnosed before the age of 50 who are first-degree relatives.
3 One individual with ovarian cancer and two with breast cancer diagnosed before the age of 60 who are connected by first-degree relationships.
4 An affected individual with a mutation of one of the genes known to predispose to ovarian cancer.
5 Three individuals with colorectal cancer, with at least one diagnosed below the age of 50 years, as well as one case of ovarian cancer, and all these individuals are connected by first-degree relationships.

This study is collecting screening data (CA 125 and ultrasound) to develop a model for familial risk of ovarian cancer, in order to optimize a treatment strategy.

If genetic analysis of the relevant DNA samples from several affected members of a family is available, it may be possible to establish which family members have inherited the disease-linked chromosome. Genetic screening has ethical and psychological considerations, which must be considered carefully and discussed with the relevant family members.

Prophylactic bilateral oophorectomy, usually combined with hysterectomy, is also recommended for clearly defined high-risk women after completion of their family. This does not remove the risk entirely as cases of carcinoma of the peritoneum have occurred after this procedure.

Molecular biology

Much effort has been invested in studying the biology of ovarian cancer in the hope that improved understanding would lead to better treatment or prevention.

CYTOGENETICS

Gross cytogenetic alterations are often seen in ovarian cancer. Up to two-thirds of invasive tumours are aneuploid, compared to one in eight of borderline tumours. Aneuploid tumours have a much worse prognosis than diploid tumours and DNA ploidy is an independent prognostic sign in both invasive and borderline tumours. The S-phase fraction, a measure of the number of cells engaged in active DNA synthesis, is higher in malignant than in benign ovarian tumours. There is no consistent pattern of chromosomal alteration and no aberration is truly specific or diagnostic. However, portions of certain chromosomes (8, 13, 14, 17, 22 and X) are frequently found to be lost from tumours.

ONCOGENES

In recent years, the search has focused on the overexpression of potential oncogenes and on the role of cytokines. *HER-2/neu* (*c-erb-B2*) is an oncogene that codes for an epidermal growth factor (EGF) receptor-like molecule. It is overexpressed in about 30 per cent of ovarian carcinomas and may indicate a poor prognosis. Mutations in the tumour suppressor gene *p53* are observed in up to half of women with advanced disease (Marks *et al.*, 1991). The lower incidence of mutations in early stage disease may suggest that *p53* mutations are a late event in the development of ovarian cancer. Alternatively, such mutations may result in rapid progression of disease.

Most ovarian and endometrial tumours overexpress colony-stimulating factor-1 (CSF-1, M-CSF) and its receptor encoded by the proto-oncogene, *c-fms*. CSF-1 can stimulate the growth of tumour cell lines, and transfection of the cells with a dominant negative mutant *c-fms* gene inhibits cell growth. This suggests that CSF-1 and *c-fms* can cause an autocrine stimulation of tumour growth. There is also evidence of persistent autocrine stimulation by transforming growth factor-α (TGF-α) and epidermal growth factor (EGF), both acting through the EGF receptor (EGFR). Paracrine stimulation by cytokines produced by macrophages may also influence both the growth and invasiveness of tumour cells. Tumour necrosis factor (TNF) appears to be particularly potent in this regard (Naylor *et al.*, 1995).

ANATOMY

The structure and function of the ovary varies with age. It enlarges after menarche and becomes atrophic after the menopause. The ovaries are two almond-shaped bodies, dull white in colour, measuring approximately $2 \times 1.5 \times 1.0$ cm. During the childbearing years, follicular cysts and corpora lutea up to 5 cm in diameter are commonly seen on ultrasound examination. These may persist for 8–12 weeks in some cases.

The ovaries are situated on either side of the pelvis attached to the posterior layer of the broad ligaments and lying inside the peritoneal cavity below the bifurcation of the common iliac arteries and anterior to the sacroiliac joints. The attachment of the ovary to the posterior layer of the broad ligament is known as the mesovarium. The ovary is suspended from the uterine cornua by the ovarian ligament, which runs inside the broad ligament to the mesovarium. The lateral pole of the ovary is supported by the infundibulo-pelvic ligament, which runs to the side wall of the pelvis.

The ovary is related medially to the body of the uterus and the ovarian ligament, and laterally to the infundibulo-pelvic ligament and the side wall of the pelvis. The broad ligament and the mesovarium lie anteriorly and the peritoneal cavity, the rectum and sigmoid colon, and the sacroiliac joints lie behind.

The ovary consists of a medulla and a cortex, surrounded by a layer of germinal epithelium. The medulla is attached to the broad ligament by the mesovarium through which it receives the ovarian vessels, lymphatics and nerves, by way of the broad ligament. The cortex is the functional part of the ovary and consists of a dense stroma, primordial follicles and corpora lutea. The outer part of the cortex, which is formed by a dense fibrous coat, is known as the tunica albuginea. The germinal epithelium is a layer of cuboidal cells, which cover the tunica albuginea and is continuous with the peritoneum of the mesovarium. Epithelial ovarian carcinomas develop from the germinal layer.

The lymphatic drainage is to both pelvic and para-aortic nodes, the latter via the ovarian vessels. Rarely, ovarian cancer can spread to the inguinal nodes. The sub-diaphragmatic lymphatics, which drain the peritoneal cavity, are also important in the spread of ovarian cancer.

NATURAL HISTORY

Approximately two-thirds of patients present with disease spread beyond the pelvis. This is probably due to the insidious nature of the signs and symptoms of carcinoma of the ovary but may sometimes be due to a rapidly growing tumour. Patients may complain of indigestion, vague abdominal discomfort, a feeling of pressure in the pelvis, urinary frequency, weight loss and, most frequently, swelling of the abdomen. Rarely, patients may complain of abnormal menses or post-menopausal bleeding. Due to the non-specific nature of most of these symptoms, ovarian cancer is seldom considered. However, clinicians should be alert to the fact that ovarian cancer may be the underlying cause in any woman with persistent unexplained abdominal pain and that in such women a careful pelvic examination should be carried out.

Ovarian cancer spreads directly to the pelvic peritoneum and other pelvic organs. Malignant cells are carried upwards in peritoneal fluid to lymphatic channels on the undersurface of the diaphragm. Thus transcoelomic spread occurs to the omentum, the small and large bowel, the surface of the liver, the peritoneal surface throughout the abdominal cavity and the surface of the diaphragm. Unsuspected metastases on the undersurface of the diaphragm were found in 44 per cent of 16 patients whose disease was thought to be confined to the ovaries (stage I) or to the pelvis (stage II) (Rosenoff et al., 1975). Intraperitoneal metastases are superficial and seldom involve the substance of the organ beneath. Even when the surface of the bowel is extensively involved by tumour, the muscularis layer is seldom infiltrated.

Lymphatic spread is generally thought to be mainly along the lymphatics that run with the ovarian vessels to the para-aortic region at the level of the renal vessels. These nodes may be involved in 15 per cent of stages I–II and in 50 per cent of stages III–IV. However, pelvic lymph-node involvement occurs more often than previously reported, being 14–31 per cent in stages I–II and 65–78 per cent in stages III–IV (Burghardt et al., 1987). Spread may occur to nodes in the neck or groin.

Haematogenous spread usually occurs late in the course of the disease. The main areas involved are the liver and the lung, although metastases to bone and brain can occur.

PATHOLOGY

Ovarian tumours can be solid or cystic. They may be benign or malignant and, in addition, there are those which, while having some of the features of malignancy, lack any evidence of stromal invasion. These are called borderline tumours. There have been many different classifications of ovarian tumours, but the one most commonly used was defined by the World Health Organization, a modified version of which is shown in Table 33.1.

Epithelial tumours

Approximately 85 per cent of malignant ovarian carcinomas are epithelial in origin. They develop from the surface epithelium of the ovary. The most common are serous, followed by mucinous and endometrioid tumours. Most

Table 33.1 *Histological classification of ovarian tumours*

I		Common epithelial tumours (benign, borderline or malignant)
	A	Serous tumour
	B	Mucinous tumour
	C	Endometrioid tumour
	D	Clear cell (mesonephroid) tumour
	E	Brenner tumour
	F	Mixed epithelial tumour
	G	Undifferentiated carcinomas
	H	Unclassified tumour
II		Sex cord stromal tumours
	A	Granulosa stroma cell tumour
	B	Androblastoma: Sertoli–Leydig cell tumour
	C	Gynandroblastoma
	D	Unclassified tumour
III		Lipid cell tumours
IV		Germ cell tumours
	A	Dysgerminoma
	B	Endodermal sinus tumour (yolk-sac tumour)
	C	Embryonal cell tumour
	D	Polyembryoma
	E	Choriocarcinoma
	F	Teratoma
	G	Mixed tumours
V		Gonadoblastoma
VI		Soft-tissue tumours not specific to ovary
VII		Unclassified tumours
VIII		Metastatic tumours

of the remainder are clear cell, undifferentiated or unclassified. Mesonephroid and Brenner tumours are rare.

Ten per cent of all epithelial tumours of the ovary are of borderline malignancy (Ovarian Tumour Panel of RCOG, 1983). These show varying degrees of nuclear atypia and an increase in mitotic activity, multilayering of neoplastic cells and formation of cellular buds, but no invasion of the stroma. Most borderline tumours remain confined to the ovaries, and this may well account for their much better prognosis. Peritoneal lesions are present in some cases and, although a few are true metastases, many are not, but remain stationary and even regress after removal of the primary (Fox, 1985). The histological diagnosis of borderline malignancy can be difficult, particularly in mucinous tumours. Most borderline tumours are serous or mucinous in type. Other borderline tumours are rare.

Well-differentiated epithelial carcinomas tend to be more often associated with early stage disease, but the degree of differentiation does correlate with survival, except in the most advanced stages. Diploid tumours tend to be associated with earlier-stage disease and a better prognosis. Histological cell type is not of itself prognostically significant. However, mucinous and endometrioid lesions are likely to be associated with earlier stage and lower grade than serous cystadenocarcinomas.

Other malignant ovarian tumours

Metastatic carcinomas, for example from the breast, the endometrium and the gastrointestinal tract, account for most of the remaining ovarian carcinomas. Differentiation from primary disease can be difficult in advanced cases, especially in the case of colonic tumours. Malignant sex-cord stromal tumours and germ-cell tumours are uncommon. They are discussed later in this chapter. Sarcomas are very rare indeed, as is the mixed Müllerian mesodermal tumour, which contains both malignant epithelial and sarcomatous elements.

CLINICAL STAGING

The staging of ovarian cancer as defined by FIGO is shown in Table 33.2. This staging is primarily surgical and is based mainly on the findings at laparotomy. Peritoneal deposits on the surface of the liver do not make the patient stage IV, the parenchyma must be involved. Similarly, the presence of a pleural effusion is insufficient to put the patient in stage IV unless malignant cells are found on cytological examination of the pleural fluid.

DIAGNOSIS

Any woman presenting with a pelvic mass needs preoperative assessment to determine whether there is a high suspicion of ovarian cancer. This is best carried out using a combination of CA 125, vaginal ultrasound and the patient's age to calculate the risk of malignancy index (RMI) (Tingulstad *et al.*, 1996). This combination has a reported sensitivity of approximately 80–90 per cent and a specificity of at least 87 per cent. Women with a high RMI should be referred for their surgery to a gynaecological oncologist specializing in the treatment of ovarian cancer.

It is crucial to the management of carcinoma of the ovary that the full extent of disease is defined before treatment is commenced. Full clinical examination, including abdominal, vaginal and rectal examination, is essential. An abdominal mass may be present. A pelvic mass is usually felt best by combined vaginal and rectal examination. The neck and groin should also be examined for involved nodes.

Haematological investigations include estimation of the tumour marker CA 125, a full blood count, urea, electrolytes and liver function tests. A chest X-ray is essential. It is sometimes advisable to carry out a barium enema or a colonoscopy to differentiate between an ovarian and a colonic tumour and to assess bowel involvement from the ovarian tumour itself.

Table 33.2 *FIGO staging for primary ovarian carcinoma*

Stage		International Federation of Gynaecology and Obstetrics (FIGO) definition
I		Growth limited to ovaries
	Ia	Growth limited to one ovary; no ascites; no tumour on external surface; capsule intact
	Ib	Growth limited to both ovaries; no ascites; no tumour on external surfaces; capsule intact
	Ic	Tumour either stage ia or ib but tumour on surface of one or both ovaries; or with capsule ruptured; or with ascites present containing malignant cells; or with positive peritoneal washings
II		Growth involving one or both ovaries with pelvic extension
	IIa	Extension and/or metastases to the uterus or tubes
	IIb	Extension to other pelvic tissues
	IIc	Tumour either stage IIa or IIb but tumour on surface of one or both ovaries; or with capsule ruptured; or with ascites present containing malignant cells; or with positive peritoneal washings
III		Growth involving one or both ovaries with peritoneal implants outside the pelvis or positive retroperitoneal or inguinal nodes. Superficial liver metastases equals stage III
	IIIa	Tumour grossly limited to the true pelvis with negative nodes but with histologically confirmed microscopic seeding of abdominal peritoneal surfaces
	IIIb	Tumour with histologically confirmed implants on abdominal peritoneal surfaces, none exceeding 2 cm in diameter. Nodes are negative
	IIIc	Abdominal implants greater than 2 cm in diameter or positive retroperitoneal or inguinal nodes
IV		Growth involving one or both ovaries with distant metastases. If pleural effusion is present, there must be positive cytology to allot a case to stage IV. Parenchymal liver metastasis equals stage IV

Imaging techniques

Vaginal ultrasound can distinguish between benign and malignant cysts and is part of the RMI to identify patients at high risk of having a malignancy of the ovary. Abdominal ultrasonography may help to confirm the presence of ascites before it is clinically apparent. In addition, it is a relatively reliable technique for examining the hepatic parenchyma and may detect enlarged pelvic or para-aortic lymph nodes. Computerized axial tomography of the abdomen and pelvis is a commonly used imaging technique for investigating ovarian cancer and is particularly useful for examining the upper abdomen and detecting nodal enlargement, while magnetic resonance imaging is more accurate for examining the pelvis.

None of these imaging techniques will detect small peritoneal metastases visible to the naked eye at surgery. The most accurate method for assessing lymph-node involvement remains biopsy at the time of surgery.

Cytology

In those patients who present with pleural effusion or ascites, specimens of fluid may be examined cytologically for the presence of malignant cells. It is not justifiable to perform a paracentesis for cytology as it can be deferred until laparotomy. However, if surgery is to be delayed until after initial treatment with chemotherapy, cytology of ascitic fluid is carried out to help to establish the diagnosis. Fine-needle aspiration of clinically suspicious lymph nodes in the groin or neck can be very valuable.

SCREENING

Tumour markers

Because carcinoma of the ovary tends to be asymptomatic in the early stages and most patients present with advanced disease, efforts have been made to define a tumour marker which could be used for screening purposes. So far, none has become available which is truly specific and which is suitable for the early detection of epithelial carcinoma.

The most useful marker at the present time is CA 125, derived from a human ovarian cancer line. However, it may also be raised in women who do not have an ovarian malignancy, for example in the presence of endometriosis, menstruation and pelvic inflammatory disease. Carcinoembryonic antigen (CEA) is elevated most often in mucinous cystadenocarcinoma. Concentrations in excess of 20 ng/ml are suggestive of ovarian tumour. Other tumour-associated antigens include OCCA and OCA, which are raised in both serous and mucinous cystadenocarcinoma, OVX1 and serum inhibin. Inhibin levels are elevated in most postmenopausal women with mucinous carcinomas of the ovary, and in some women with other types of epithelial ovarian tumours. It is raised in almost all granulosa cell tumours (Healy *et al.*, 1999).

Serum CA 125 is not considered sufficiently specific or sensitive to be suitable on its own to screen the general population. Specificity refers to the ability to identify correctly all those without cancer of the ovary and sensitivity refers to the ability to identify correctly all those in whom ovarian cancer is present. Reduced sensitivity is present in stage I cancer of the ovary, where levels of serum CA 125 can be normal. CA 125 has lower specificity in premenopausal women where it can be raised in benign conditions, as previously discussed.

The sensitivity of CA 125 can be improved either by using a lower cut-off point as the accepted upper limit of normal or by using additional tumour markers such as OVX1. The specificity of serum CA 125 is also improved by taking serial measurements, as levels rise in patients with preclinical ovarian cancer but remain static or fall in those with false-positive results (Jacobs, 1995). Very high levels of serum CA 125 indicate a high risk of ovarian cancer in the following year (Jacobs et al., 1996).

Ultrasound

After very disappointing results with conventional ultrasound methods for screening asymptomatic women, colour flow transvaginal ultrasound was assessed in 1601 women with a family history of ovarian cancer (Bourne et al., 1993). A laparotomy or laparoscopy was performed in 61 of these women as a result of an abnormal scan. Six of these had ovarian cancer, five were stage Ia and three of these were borderline tumours. Ultrasound is a more sensitive but less specific screening test than CA 125, but the proportion of women found to have screen-detected cancers on abdominal or transvaginal ultrasound, has never reached 0.1 per cent despite multiple studies.

Combined approach

Jacobs et al. (1996) carried out a large study on 22 000 postmenopausal volunteers using both CA 125 and abdominal ultrasound. Yearly CA 125 serum estimations were carried out and abdominal ultrasound was confined to those women in whom the level of CA 125 was raised. Forty-nine cancers developed in the study population over a period of 7 years. The cumulative risk of developing ovarian cancer was considerably raised for those women with a CA 125 level of 30 units or more. On the basis of this study a further randomized trial was carried out on these women. The study group had annual serum CA 125 markers yearly for 3 years and was compared to a group that was not screened any further. On the basis of the levels of the tumour markers and age-adjusted ovarian cancer incidence rates, a risk score of cancer (ROC) was calculated for each woman. If the ROC exceeded the study threshold, vaginal ultrasound was performed. If ultrasound was abnormal, explorative surgery was carried out in most women. After 7 years there were 16 cancers in the screened group, of whom six were detected on screening, and 20 women in the unscreened group. Although there was a difference in mortality between the two groups in favour of the women who were screened, this did not quite reach statistical significance (Jacobs et al., 1999).

At present, with the available technology, while a few early cancers may be screen-detected, screening the general population is not effective in reducing death from cancer (Bell et al., 1998). Patients at high risk should be encouraged to take part in trials to assess new screening techniques, but should not be led to believe that these have proven value.

SURGERY

Surgery is the mainstay of both the diagnosis and the treatment of ovarian cancer. In order to obtain satisfactory exposure for an adequate exploration of the upper abdomen, a vertical incision is required. A sample of ascitic fluid or peritoneal washings with normal saline must be taken for cytology. These should be obtained before any manipulation of the tumour to avoid contamination. The pelvis and upper abdomen are explored carefully, including the omentum, subdiaphragmatic areas, the paracolic gutters, large and small bowel and small bowel mesentery. Such an exploration is not possible with a low transverse incision. In the absence of gross upper abdominal disease, suspicious areas should be biopsied. A sample for cytology may be taken from the diaphragm with an Ayre's spatula.

The therapeutic objective of surgery for ovarian cancer is the removal of all visible tumour deposits (cytoreduction or debulking surgery). While this is achieved in the majority of stage I cases and in some stage II, it is probably impossible in more advanced disease. Because of the diffuse spread of tumour throughout the peritoneal cavity and the retroperitoneal nodes, microscopic deposits will persist in almost all cases even when all macroscopic deposits appear to have been excised. Thus, while surgery alone may be curative in many stage I cases, additional therapy is essential for most of the remainder.

Cytoreductive surgery

For the past 20 years, gynaecological oncologists have been advocating maximal cytoreductive surgery in advanced ovarian cancer, in the belief that this would improve the prospects for survival and make tumours more amenable to chemotherapy.

Many studies show that those women with minimal, that is, under 2 cm, or no residual disease after surgery have a better prognosis than those women in whom there was more residual disease after surgery. However, it is likely that the latter group includes the more aggressive tumours with an intrinsically worse prognosis. Griffiths et al. (1979) showed that women with residual masses of <1.5 cm diameter following surgery did as well as those whose metastases were small from the outset. These data suggested that surgical intervention could indeed influence the prognosis. Unfortunately, an analysis of more modern data has failed to confirm these findings (Hoskins *et al.*, 1992).

It has become clear that the prognosis for ovarian cancer is adversely affected by the volume of metastatic disease at the outset, even when maximum cytoreduction has been performed successfully (Hacker *et al.*, 1983). Similarly, women who have undergone bowel surgery as part of successful cytoreduction have a poorer prognosis than those women who did not undergo bowel surgery even if cytoreduction was unsuccessful (Potter *et al.*, 1991).

No prospective, controlled trials of primary cytoreductive surgery have been reported. However, a study of two different chemotherapy regimens showed no survival advantage for those women operated upon in units with higher rates of successful cytoreduction (Bertelsen, 1990). A subsequent meta-analysis of over 6000 cases was based on the principle that groups of women with higher rates of successful cytoreduction should have better survival rates if the surgery was contributing to the outcome (Hunter *et al.*, 1992). In this study, maximal cytoreductive surgery had no significant effect on median survival once the effects of chemotherapy had been taken into account.

While it seems likely that cytoreductive surgery can improve the quality of life for women with advanced ovarian cancer, any effect on survival will probably be small. Removal of the majority of the tumour volume should always be attempted, and is likely to be successful in some 75 per cent of cases. However, resection of bowel should not be performed except when obstruction is imminent. The meticulous removal of all tiny tumour nodules is unlikely to be helpful. Similarly, radical lymphadenectomy cannot be recommended as it increases morbidity without altering the prognosis. A number of studies have shown lymph-node involvement in early stage ovarian cancer and one retrospective study has suggested that pelvic and para-aortic lymphadenectomy may improve survival when all intraperitoneal disease has been removed (Scarabelli *et al.*, 1997).

Conservative surgery in stage I disease

The resection of all visible cancer usually requires a total hysterectomy and bilateral salpingo-oophorectomy, but unilateral salpingo-oophorectomy may be justifiable to preserve fertility in a young, nulliparous woman with a unilateral tumour and no ascites, after careful exploration to exclude metastatic disease. Curettage of the uterine cavity should be performed to exclude a synchronous endometrial tumour. Some recommend that the normal-looking ovary is biopsied, but the risk of occult spread to that ovary is small, and biopsy may impair fertility, negating the purpose of the conservative operation. If, subsequently, the tumour is found to be a poorly differentiated adenocarcinoma, or if the washings are positive, a second operation to clear the pelvis will be necessary. Recurrence rates have been found to be 5–9 per cent after conservative surgery (Zanetta *et al.*, 1997; Marchetti *et al.*, 1998).

Interval debulking surgery

An alternative approach when initial surgery has left bulky disease is a planned second laparotomy after three courses of cytoreductive chemotherapy in those women who respond. The chemotherapy is then resumed as soon as possible after the second operation. The effect of interval debulking surgery has been assessed by a randomized European Organization for the Research and Treatment of Cancer (EORTC) study, comparing chemotherapy alone with chemotherapy and interval debulking surgery in 319 women with advanced ovarian cancer (Van der Berg *et al.*, 1995). This study demonstrated that median survival may be extended by 6 months, and survival at 3 years increased from 10 per cent to 20 per cent, in the group undergoing the additional surgery. A similar randomized trial, examining the role of interval debulking surgery for ovarian cancer, where primary surgery has failed to achieve optimal debulking, is being carried out in the UK.

Second-look surgery

Second-look surgery is defined as a planned laparotomy at the end of chemotherapy. The objectives are: firstly, to determine the response to prior therapy in order to document accurately its efficacy and to plan subsequent management; and, secondly, to excise any residual disease. There is no doubt that second-look surgery gives the most accurate indication of the disease status, laparotomy being more accurate in this respect than laparoscopy. However, the balance of evidence suggests that neither the surgical resection of residual tumour nor the opportunity to change the treatment has any effect whatever on the patient's survival. It would seem that, until an effective consolidation therapy becomes available, second-look procedures have no place outside clinical trials.

SELECTING PATIENTS FOR POSTOPERATIVE TREATMENT

In stage I carcinoma of the ovary, where the tumour is confined to the ovaries, there is a need to define those cases where adjuvant therapy is indicated to prevent recurrent disease. While FIGO stage Ic includes cases with capsular penetration by tumour, rupture of the capsule and ascites or positive peritoneal washings, there is little evidence that each of these has the same prognostic value.

Dembo (1992) considered that dense adherence of a malignant ovarian cyst should be considered as stage II disease. Thereafter, only differentiation of the tumour, large volume of ascites and positive peritoneal washings were of prognostic significance in stage I disease. Vergote *et al.* (1993) found that grade of tumour was the most important prognostic indicator for disease-free survival in 290 patients with stage I disease. The prognostic indicators, DNA ploidy and substage were next in importance. Poor differentiation of the tumour and aneuploidy indicated a poor prognosis. Dense adhesions, ascites, extracapsular growth and rupture during surgery were no longer prognostic once these factors had been accounted for. Rupture of the tumour capsule during surgery has no effect on survival, but the prognosis is much worse when rupture has occurred before the operation (Sjovall *et al.*, 1994).

A randomized trial by the Gynecological Oncology Group (GOG) found that the survival at 5 years was over 90 per cent in patients with low- to intermediate-grade tumours confined to the ovaries, whether or not they received adjuvant therapy (Young *et al.*, 1990). These data suggest that women with stage Ia or Ib disease and well or moderately differentiated tumours do not require further treatment following surgery. Whether other women with cancer of the ovary, stage I or IIa, should be deferred until recurrent disease is detected has been investigated. The International Collaborative Ovarian Neoplasm Group (ICON 1) carried out a randomized study to look at this issue, using platinum-based chemotherapy. This study showed an advantage from adjuvant chemotherapy (personal communication).

RADIOTHERAPY

External radiotherapy

Radiotherapy has only a small role to play in the management of ovarian carcinoma. It is no longer given even in early stage disease, where Dembo *et al.* (1979) found that adjuvant whole-abdominal radiotherapy improved survival, but has been superseded by the platinum drugs. This work remains of historical importance as it emphasized that the whole abdominal cavity is at risk of occult metastases.

The radiotherapy technique, which needed to encompass the whole of the peritoneal cavity, used open anterior and posterior fields extending from the diaphragm to the pelvic floor. These large volumes included radiosensitive vital organs such as the liver, kidneys, small bowel and bone marrow, and therefore great care was required in both total dose and dose per fraction to prevent permanent damage. The dose to the kidneys needed to be limited to 20 Gy and that to the liver to 30 Gy. The total dose to the abdomen was usually not more than 30 Gy given in 25 fractions. This is an inadequate radiation dose for any but microscopic disease.

Leucopenia and thrombocytopenia were common, as was nausea and vomiting. Late complications were mainly gastrointestinal and were particularly likely to occur following multiple abdominal operations. Surgical intervention was required for at least 5 per cent of patients, who developed severe problems such as bowel stenosis or haemorrhage.

Whole-abdominal radiotherapy has also been used as consolidation therapy following adjuvant chemotherapy in those patients who were found to have little or no residual disease at second-look surgery. Lambert *et al.* (1993) carried out a randomized study of over 200 patients who received five courses of platinum chemotherapy. This was followed, in responding patients, by either a further five courses of the same chemotherapy or by whole-abdominal radiotherapy. There was no overall or disease-free survival difference between the two groups, even when there was no evidence of macroscopic residual disease at second look. Although there was no significant morbidity in this study, that has not always been the case in other non-randomized studies. There is therefore no role for consolidation therapy using whole-abdominal radiotherapy.

Radiotherapy can be useful as a palliative treatment for recurrent ovarian cancer resistant to the platinum drugs, with nearly 70–80 per cent experiencing some relief of symptoms, and 40–50 per cent, complete relief (Corn *et al.*, 1994; Gelblum *et al.*, 1998). It is particularly useful where disease is localized, for example a pelvic mass – thereby obviating the toxicity of treating large abdominal fields. The treated symptoms included vaginal and rectal bleeding, pain, pulmonary and neurological problems.

Radioactive isotopes

Radioactive isotopes of either gold or phosphorus linked to carrier colloids have been used intraperitoneally for many years in early carcinoma of the ovary. They have been used alone and in combination with external radiotherapy.

When given intraperitoneally, radioactive isotopes or conjugates are absorbed directly on to the peritoneal surface and are taken up by macrophages lining the peritoneal cavity or floating free. This gives a high dose of radiation but only to an effective depth of 4–6 mm, thereby limiting therapy to the peritoneal surface and to small microscopic deposits on its surface. Colloid-linked isotopes (gold and phosphorus) enter the lymphatic circulation by the diaphragmatic lymphatics to reach the mediastinal lymphatics and then the general circulation. Very little of the radiation reaches the retroperitoneal nodes. These isotopes are both β emitters (0.96 MeV for ^{198}Au and 1.76 MeV for ^{32}P) and have short half-lives of 2.69 and 14.2 days, respectively. Radioactive phosphorus has replaced radioactive gold because it is safer. Ten per cent of the activity of radioactive gold is from γ rays and this can be a hazard both to patients and staff. In comparison, radioactive phosphorus has no γ irradiation.

An additional advantage of ^{32}P is that it emits more penetrating and more destructive radiation than ^{198}Au.

Intraperitoneal isotopes are delivered through one or more catheters kept patent with heparinized saline. The isotope is administered 2–3 hours postoperatively. Prior to the therapeutic dose an abdominal scan is recommended, using a small dose of technetium-99m to confirm that the isotope is well distributed and that no loculations are present which could lead to very high local doses.

Cure rates of approximately 90 per cent for stage I disease have been reported after treatment with intraperitoneal radioactive isotopes in non-randomized studies. Vergote *et al.* (1992a) carried out a randomized study of nearly 350 patients, without residual tumour after primary laparotomy, who were randomized to either six courses of 50 mg/m^2 cisplatin given 3-weekly or to intraperitoneal ^{32}P instilled on the first postoperative day. Both overall survival and disease-free survival rates were similar in the two groups, but there was a high incidence of late bowel complications in the radioactive phosphorus group. There are no reported studies comparing intraperitoneal ^{32}P with no treatment in early stage ovarian cancer. The combination of intraperitoneal and external radiotherapy gives rise to unacceptable morbidity.

The overall conclusion is that at present there are no published studies to show that the use of ^{32}P prolongs survival compared to no treatment in early ovarian cancer, but there is evidence of an increased incidence of bowel complications. Furthermore, intraperitoneal phosphorus is of no value when there is more than minimal residual disease, when adhesions are present preventing the isotope reaching the whole peritoneal surface, or when retroperitoneal nodes are involved.

Antibody-guided irradiation

A different approach to intraperitoneal radiotherapy is intraperitoneal radio-immunotherapy with yttrium-90 attached to monoclonal antibodies such as human milk factor globulin 1 (HMFG 1). This experimental technique looks promising as consolidation therapy in women in apparent remission after surgery and first-line chemotherapy (Hird *et al.*, 1993; Nicholson *et al.*, 1998). A randomized trial of no further treatment versus intraperitoneal therapy is in progress.

Conclusions

Postoperative abdomino-pelvic radiotherapy for early ovarian carcinoma has, for all practical purposes, been replaced by chemotherapy. It is ineffective in the treatment of advanced disease. Intraperitoneal, colloid-bound, radioactive phophorus has not been proven to have any advantage over chemotherapy for early stage disease and

can cause serious late bowel problems. Intraperitoneal radioactive antibody therapy is still a research tool. Radiotherapy has been found to have a useful role in palliating symptoms in relapsed patients resistant to the platinum drugs.

CHEMOTHERAPY

Chemotherapy plays a major role in treating all but the very earliest cases of ovarian carcinoma of epithelial origin. Chemotherapy is usually given following surgery, but when surgery cannot result in optimal debulking, chemotherapy may be given as primary treatment before interval debulking surgery. Chemotherapy is given using either a single drug or two or more in combination or sequentially.

Single agents

Historically the most commonly used chemotherapeutic agents in carcinoma of the ovary have been the alkylating agents. They have been in use for several decades, initially for palliation, with reported initial response rates of 35–65 per cent and 5–15 per cent still responding after 2 years. The most commonly used alkylating agents were chlorambucil, melphalan and cyclophosphamide, and later ifosfamide and treosulfan. Chlorambucil and melphelan are now seldom used and the use of cyclophosphamide has dimished in the aftermath of recent trials where it was used in conjunction with cisplatin as a control arm.

Altretamine (hexamethylmelamine), which is derived from melamine, is an arizidine alkylating agent. It is given orally and has been found to have activity in 15 per cent of patients who have a treatment-free interval of at least 6 months from prior chemotherapy.

Other drugs showing some activity in ovarian cancer include the antimetabolites, 5-fluorouracil and methotrexate, but these are now seldom used. The anthracyclines, doxorubicin and epirubicin, are used singly in recurrent disease or as first-line treatment in combination chemotherapy, particularly as part of CAP (cyclophosphamide, doxorubicin, cisplatin). The addition of doxorubicin to other drugs has been found to be beneficial in terms of survival in two meta-analyses (Ovarian Cancer Meta-analysis project, 1991; A'Hern and Gore, 1995). Doxorubicin is a very toxic drug, which affects the bone marrow and causes total alopecia of head hair unless scalp cooling is used. It also produces mucositis, severe nausea and vomiting, the latter being ameliorated by the use of 5-hydroxytryptamine (5-HT) antagonists. It is cardiotoxic, which limits its total dose. Epirubicin is less cardiotoxic but a higher dose may be required to achieve comparable efficacy.

The platinum drugs, cisplatin (*cis*-dichlorodiamineplatinum) and its analogue carboplatin, are heavy-metal compounds, which cause cross-linkage of DNA strands in a similar fashion to alkylating agents. These are considered to be the most effective drugs in the management of ovarian carcinoma, and are the most widely used, either alone or in combination.

Cisplatin was first prescribed in the 1970s for patients who had failed on alkylating therapy. It gave almost a 30 per cent response in previously treated patients (Wiltshaw and Kroner, 1976). This led to its use in previously untreated patients. A prospective randomized study (Lambert and Berry, 1985) compared cisplatin with cyclophosphamide in advanced ovarian cancer and found better response and survival rates with cisplatin. The dose of cisplatin as a single agent is from $75\,mg/m^2$. The effectiveness of cisplatin is dose dependent at least up to $100\,mg/m^2$, after which it may reach a plateau.

Cisplatin is a very toxic drug. Until the advent of the 5-HT antagonists (ganesetron and ondansetron), severe nausea and vomiting, sometimes lasting several days, was a serious problem. Permanent renal damage occurs unless cisplatin is given with adequate hydration. Peripheral neuropathy and hearing loss are reported with increasing cumulative doses. Electrolyte disturbances such as hypomagnesaemia are occasionally seen, but, unlike most chemotherapeutic agents, marrow toxicity is not usually a problem, with the exception of anaemia.

Carboplatin is an analogue of cisplatin and is as effective as cisplatin in the treatment of ovarian cancer (Advanced Ovarian Cancer Trialists Group, 1991). The advantage of carboplatin, compared to cisplatin, is that it causes less nausea and vomiting and has no significant renal toxicity. Neurotoxicity is rare and hearing loss is subclinical. The lack of significant renal toxicity means that, unlike cisplatin, there is no need to give carboplatin with intravenous hydration. It is given in an infusion of dextrose over 1 hour on an outpatient basis. The dose is calculated in relation to the glomerular filtration rate, derived from ethylenediaminetetraacetic acid (EDTA) clearance, using the area under the curve (AUC) formula devised by Calvert (Calvert et al., 1989). This method allows a higher dose of carboplatin to be given in the presence of normal renal function, as the myelotoxicity of carboplatin, in particular leucopenia and thrombocytopenia, is related to renal function. The dose of carboplatin usually uses an AUC factor of 5–7.

The taxanes, paclitaxel in particular, and docetaxol, have been found to be active in ovarian carcinoma. Paclitaxel (Taxol®), the first drug containing the taxane ring structure to be used, was found to be the most active drug ever tested in those patients who were resistant to platinum chemotherapy (Trimble et al., 1993). As a single agent, it is used for the treatment of patients with ovarian cancer who have failed standard platinum regimens, but it has a much greater role in combination as primary treatment for this tumour.

Paclitaxel is derived from the bark of the Pacific yew tree (Taxus brevifolia) and has a mechanism of action which is unique among cytotoxic drugs. It acts by promoting polymerization of microtubules making them excessively stable. This leads to blocking of cell division and tumour growth.

In addition to myelosuppression and sensory neuropathy, paclitaxel can cause severe hypersensitivity reactions. The latter can be prevented in the majority of patients by the routine use of premedication with dexamethasone, diphenhydramine and ranitidine or cimetidine. Hair loss from all parts of the body is usually total, irrespective of dose, but nausea and vomiting are mild in contrast to that caused by the platinum drugs.

A prospective randomized study in a Canadian–European trial (Swenerton et al., 1993) concluded that it was safe and equally effective to administer paclitaxel in a dose of $175\,mg/m^2$ over 3 hours with premedication as described above, to prevent hypersensitivity reactions. This 3-hour regimen is now the standard in Europe and North America.

Docetaxel (Taxotere®) is a semi-synthetic taxoid derived from the needles of the European yew tree (Taxus baccata). Taxotere has an unusual skin toxicity and can produce marked oedema. It has a role as second-line treatment.

Two other drugs have also shown useful activity in the treatment of cancer of the ovary. These are topotecan and gemcitabine. Topotecan is a topoisomerase I inhibitor, an enzyme essential for DNA synthesis. It has been shown to have activity in refractory ovarian cancer and appears to be at least as effective as paclitaxel in the relapsed setting. It is given as an intravenous infusion and its main toxicity is to the bone marrow. It also causes alopecia. Gemcitabine, which also shows some activity in cisplatin-resistant ovarian cancer, is a pyrimidine antimetabolite with a close resemblance to cytosine arabinoside, but differing in both biological and clinical effects. It is given intravenously.

A different approach is the use of 'old' drugs used in a different way. Liposomal doxorubicin in a PEG (polyethylene glycol)-olated form has been named Caelyx®. Because liposomes covered in PEG are trapped in the abnormal vasculature of tumours, the local half-life of doxorubicin is prolonged. Caelyx® is under investigation.

Other drugs under investigation in the management of advanced and recurrent ovarian cancer include the metalloproteinase inhibitors, of which the orally administered Marimastat® is an example. The matrix metalloproteinases are a group of enzymes thought to promote the growth and dissemination of tumours. Marimastat® and carboplatin are being compared to carboplatin alone in relapsed disease, and Marimastat® is also being given to relapsed patients following response to second-line chemotherapy, to try and prolong the symptom-free period.

Combination chemotherapy

The impetus to the use of combination chemotherapy came from Young who, before the advent of cisplatin, compared melphalan with a four-drug regimen HexaCaf (Young *et al.*, 1978). The latter included hexamethyl-melamine, cyclophosphamide, methotrexate and 5-fluo-rouracil. They found that this non-platinum combination of drugs gave significantly increased median survival, particularly marked in those patients with minimal residual disease. However, this finding in favour of a combination non-cisplatin regimen over a single alkylating agent has not been confirmed in a later meta-analysis (Advanced Ovarian Trialists Group, 1991). A more recent meta-analysis by the same group (1998) analysed outcomes in 37 randomized, controlled trials and over 5600 patients with advanced ovarian cancer, among whom there were over 4600 deaths. The analysis compared single-agent non-platinum- versus platinum-based combination chemotherapy; the addition of platinum to a regimen; single-agent versus platinum combination and carboplatin versus cisplatin. No taxanes were included in these trials. The results suggested that platinum-based combination chemotherapy had the greatest survival benefit, with a 5 per cent improvement in survival at both 2 years (45–50 per cent) and 5 years (25–30 per cent). However, the only statistically significant difference was between platinum-based chemotherapy and a similar drug combination which did not include platinum. There was no evidence of any difference in survival between cisplatin and carboplatin regimens when given singly or in combination.

An ICON trial (ICON 2), commenced in 1992, compared single-agent carboplatin with a combination of cyclophosphamide, doxorubicin and cisplatin in over 1500 women. There was no difference in survival between the two groups, but carboplatin was the better tolerated regimen (ICON Collaborators, 1998).

Paclitaxel in combination with cisplatin has been compared with cisplatin and cyclophosphamide in combination in two randomized trials – GOG111 and OV10 – in patients presenting with advanced ovarian cancer. The GOG study gave a dose of cisplatin of $75\,\mathrm{mg/m^2}$ with $135\,\mathrm{mg/m^2}$ of paclitaxel, the latter over 24 hours, compared to the same dose of cisplatin and $750\,\mathrm{mg/m^2}$ of cyclophosphamide (McGuire *et al.*, 1996). The OV10 study was similar, except that paclitaxel was given at a dose of $175\,\mathrm{mg/m^2}$ over 3 hours (Stuart *et al.*, 1998). Most of the women had residual macroscopic disease after surgery. Both these trials showed a survival advantage in favour of the cisplatin–paclitaxel combination, with median survival being approximately 3 years compared to 2 years for those receiving cisplatin–cyclophosphamide. A third study, GOG132, compared paclitaxel alone, cisplatin in combination with paclitaxel, and with a higher dose of cisplatin given as a single agent. This trial showed both reduced survival for paclitaxel compared to either cisplatin or the combination and no benefit for the combination over cisplatin (Muggia *et al.*, 1997). However, some of the patients receiving cisplatin crossed over to paclitaxel before disease progression, which throws some doubt on the results.

With over 2000 patients, ICON 3 is the largest trial to date comparing a taxane combination with a platinum regimen. This randomized study compared paclitaxel at a dose of $175\,\mathrm{mg/m^2}$ given over 3 hours with either carboplatin as a single agent (AUC 5-6) or with CAP (that is, cyclophosphamide, doxorubicin and cisplatin). Preliminary data, reported in 1999, based on a median follow-up of 18 months, showed no benefit to the addition of paclitaxel, but these data are insufficiently mature to be used as a guide to clinical practice. More mature information is awaited with interest, both on grounds of toxicity and cost. The cost per life year saved by a carboplatin/paclitaxel combination is estimated to be in the range £7000–£11 000 and the cost per progression-free year £20 000–£22 000 (Beard *et al.*, 1997, 1998).

A platinum drug in combination with paclitaxel is accepted as standard therapy, both in North America and Europe. Carboplatin–paclitaxel is the chemotherapy regimen of choice in the management of advanced ovarian cancer. It is preferable to cisplatin–paclitaxel as it is better tolerated, particularly in regard to peripheral neuropathy. The mature results from the ICON 3 randomized study of carboplatin, alone or in combination with paclitaxel, are awaited.

Duration of chemotherapy

Most prospective randomized trials of platinum-based chemotherapy use six cycles, and the evidence appears to indicate that further prolongation of treatment is of no clinical benefit. The North Thames Ovary Group, in over 200 patients with stages Ic–IV ovarian cancer, found no statistical difference in disease-free or overall survival in a randomized study comparing five with eight cycles of carboplatin (Lambert *et al.*, 1997). Similarly in a study by Hakes *et al.* (1992), comparing five cycles with 10 cycles of CAP in stages III–IV, median survival was similar in the two groups. Further chemotherapy in those with residual disease at laparotomy after five cycles was ineffective. At present most clinicians give six cycles of chemotherapy as their standard regimen.

Experimental studies to improve survival in advanced ovarian cancer

Despite improved results in the treatment of advanced ovarian cancer with platinum-based chemotherapy, particularly in combination with paclitaxel, which have led to useful prolongation of survival, the long-term survival rate after 3 years is not changing dramatically. Only 25–30 per cent will survive 5 years and approximately 15–20 per cent will be cured with the therapeutic approaches used at present. This is an improvement compared to the 5–10 per cent cure rate obtained with single alkylating agents, but shows that the outlook for patients with advanced ovarian cancer remains very poor.

As well as looking at newer drugs such as paclitaxel, other approaches that have been examined include dose intensification with platinum compounds, intraperitoneal chemotherapy and reversal of drug resistance.

DOSE INTENSIFICATION

There are no data at present to show that dose intensification of platinum drugs beyond the upper limits of standard therapy improves survival, and there may well be a plateau in the dose–response curve. Ultimately, toxicity will limit the dose of chemotherapy that can be tolerated. While colony stimulating factors can alleviate marrow toxicity to some extent, repeated high doses of carboplatin can cause cumulative toxicity which is resistant to treatment, particularly thrombocytopenia. Other methods of dealing with marrow toxicity with high-dose carboplatin have been autologous bone marrow transplantation or harvesting peripheral blood progenitor cells (PBP).

With dose intensification, non-haematological toxicity is also a problem, particularly nephrotoxicity and neurotoxicity, with high-dose cisplatin. As few as three cycles of cisplatin at a dose of 200 mg/m^2 have caused over 50 per cent of patients to develop grade 3–4 peripheral neuropathy, and nearly half to develop moderate to severe ototoxicity. The use of neuroprotective drugs is still largely experimental and includes sulphur-containing compounds, such as WR-2721 (etiofos), which is believed to inhibit directly the interaction between cisplatin and peripheral nerves and which has been shown to reduce neuropathy when given with cisplatin. A neurotrophic drug, ORG 2766, an anologue of adrenocorticotrophic hormone (ACTH), is thought to enhance recovery from nerve damage. Trials have shown equivocal results. No drugs have been found to combat ototoxicity caused by high cumulative doses of cisplatin.

INTRAPERITONEAL CHEMOTHERAPY

The intraperitoneal use of cytotoxic drugs is of particular interest in ovarian cancer, which tends to recur or persist within the peritoneal cavity, even at a late stage of the disease. With intraperitoneal therapy, the difference between the intraperitoneal and intravenous concentrations that can be obtained with drugs that are slowly cleared from the peritoneal cavity allows much higher doses to be used with less toxicity. Cisplatin is considered to be the best drug currently available because it is both effective, with a peritoneal/plasma AUC ratio of between 30 : 1 and 50 : 1, and lacks intraperitoneal toxicity, even at high doses. However, in the future, cisplatin may be replaced by paclitaxel for intraperitoneal therapy (IP) as the latter has been found to have a high volume of distribution within the peritoneal cavity, extremely low plasma levels and a peritoneal/plasma AUC of approximately 1000 : 1. Systemic toxicity with high doses of IP cisplatin remains a problem, and intravenous thiosulphate has been used to try to reduce this by chelating with plasma cisplatin to form a non-toxic compound. Various trials of intraperitoneal cisplatin, used as a single agent or combined with other drugs such as etoposide, have been performed. They have demonstrated that complete remission rates of approximately 30 per cent are obtainable in those patients who had both an initial response to the platinum analogues and who have small-volume peritoneal disease – less than 1–2 cm – at relapse or persisting after conventional systemic chemotherapy. The impact on long-term survival is unknown.

The role for intraperitoneal chemotherapy is probably small. Not only is this an invasive technique but its usefulness is restricted by the depth of penetration of the drug to a few millimetres, therefore being of benefit only for those patients with minimal residual disease. Even distribution of the drug is essential and therefore the treatment cannot be given in the presence of extensive abdominal adhesions. Disease beyond the peritoneal cavity will also not be affected, for example within the liver parenchyma or lymph nodes. It is therefore an unsuitable technique for the majority of patients. However, Alberts et al. (1996) used the intraperitoneal approach with cisplatin in a randomized study in those patients with stage III cancer of the ovary and residual disease of 2 cm or less following surgery. Intraperitoneal cisplatin plus intravenous cyclophosphamide was compared to intravenous cisplatin plus intravenous cyclophosphamide. This study found both improved median survival and lower toxicity for the intraperitoneal group. Further information from randomized studies using intraperitoneal chemotherapy is needed before this approach can be accepted for routine management of patients.

REDUCING DRUG RESISTANCE

There appear to be two forms of drug resistance, intrinsic and acquired. Once acquired, salvage therapy is relatively ineffective due to broad cross-resistance that develops after initial chemotherapy. There are multiple mechanisms of drug resistance and this subject is covered in detail in Chapter 8. One mechanism is multi-drug resistance (MDR). Exposure of tumour cells to one drug can lead to cross-resistance to other drugs to which the tumour has not been exposed, even though they may be structurally and mechanistically dissimilar.

This occurs with many of the drugs used to treat ovarian cancer, including the taxanes and anthracyclines. MDR can be caused by changes in membrane permeability due to P-Gp, an energy-dependent transporter pumping certain chemicals and hydrophobic drugs out of the cell, thus stopping the action of the cytotoxic drug on the cell. P-Gp is encoded by a group of closely related genes, known as mdr1, which are on chromosome 7q21-1. Overexpression of these genes is found in the MDR phenotype. There are usually low levels of mdr1 and P-Gp expression in ovarian cancer, indicating initial chemosensitivity.

MDR can be caused by other genetic factors, such as a gene that encodes a protein MRP (multi-drug resistance related protein), which is found in the endoplasmic reticulum as well as the plasma membrane.

Membrane-active pharmacological agents, themselves possessing negligible anti-cancer activity, may be used in combination with anti-cancer agents such as doxorubicin to reverse experimental multi-drug resistance. This has formed the basis for clinical trials using MDR-reversing agents such as the cyclosporin analogue PSC-833 (Valspodar®).

Chemotherapy – conclusions

Adjuvant chemotherapy is used after debulking surgery for advanced stages of cancer of the ovary but is not necessary for stage Ia and b with well- or moderately well-differentiated tumours. The platinum analogues are the most active cytotoxic drugs available for epithelial cancer of the ovary, but the addition of a taxane appears to increase their efficacy. The combination of carboplatin and paclitaxel is the recommended regimen for adjuvant therapy for advanced ovarian cancer at the present time.

HORMONAL THERAPY

Cytoplasmic oestrogen and progesterone receptors have been detected in malignant ovarian tumours, but the use of progestogens in recurrent disease has been disappointing, except for giving a feeling of well being (Soutter and Leake, 1987). Other hormones have also been of little value, but there is the occasional partial remission and disease is stabilized in approximately 14 per cent of cases. Tamoxifen, at a dose of 20–80 mg/day, can cause some partial response or stabilization of disease in some cases. The GnRH antagonists, goserelin and buserelin, given subcutaneously every month, have also been reported as showing anti-tumour effect in those patients with progressive disease.

Hormone replacement therapy (HRT) in premenopausal women treated for ovarian cancer does not appear to affect the prognosis adversely. A retrospective study assessed 373 patients given HRT. No detrimental effect on the prognosis of patients was found (Eeles et al., 1991).

IMMUNOTHERAPY

The role of immunotherapy in ovarian carcinoma has been evaluated over many years but must be considered of unproven benefit at the present time. Early investigations were concerned with non-specific immunotherapy using BCG (bacille Calmette–Guérin) or Corynebacterium

parvum. These, together with chemotherapy, appeared to lead to prolongation of response. Subcutaneous interferon-α is currently being assessed in a prospective study by The Yorkshire Ovarian Group, to evaluate its role in prolonging disease-free and overall survival following chemotherapy in advanced ovarian carcinoma. Intraperitoneal immunotherapy with interferon-α for residual disease following initial chemotherapy has also been investigated and has resulted in some complete responses.

TREATMENT OF RECURRENT AND PERSISTENT DISEASE

Most patients with advanced epithelial ovarian carcinoma will either not respond to initial treatment or will recur. In either case, cure is not a realistic goal and treatment must be considered to be palliative, with quality of life being the first consideration and with some prolongation of life being expected where second responses are obtained. The longer the interval between the end of postoperative chemotherapy and the recurrence of the neoplasm, the greater the likelihood of the patient responding to second-line chemotherapy. The first sign of recurrence may be an increase in the level of the tumour marker, CA 125. If this level continues to rise even in the absence of signs or symptoms, it is most probable that recurrence has occurred. Treatment, which cannot be curative, is usually delayed until the patient is symptomatic. However, a current MRC trial (OV5) aims to determine whether immediate second-line chemotherapy in women with persistently raised CA 125 measurements, but who are asymptomatic, is beneficial.

Second-line chemotherapy can produce worthwhile responses, but the choice and effectiveness of treatment depends on the length of remission after first-line chemotherapy. Women whose disease progresses after 6 months, and particularly if more than 12 months has elapsed, following response to a course of platinum-based chemotherapy are likely to respond again to similar drugs (Markman et al., 1991). In the opinion of Thigpen et al. (1993), increasing the dose intensity of platinum therapy in patients who have recurrent ovarian cancer cannot overcome true clinical resistance. In sensitive tumours, the results are no better than with conventional platinum therapy. Therefore re-treatment should be with standard-dose therapy.

A randomized trial (ICON 4) is being carried out in those patients treated initially with platinum-based chemotherapy who have recurred after a therapy-free interval of greater than 6 months. Patients receive platinum-based chemotherapy with or without paclitaxel. This trial is to determine whether the combination of a platinum drug and paclitaxel, with their different modes of action on the tumour cell, is more effective as second-line therapy than the platinum regimen alone.

Progression of disease on treatment or within 6 months of platinum-based chemotherapy presents a difficult problem. Paclitaxel is useful for platinum-resistant patients, with approximately one-third of patients responding, but unfortunately remissions are usually short, with a median duration of 4 months (Kohn *et al.*, 1994). Topotecan and gemcitabine both show responses in platinum-resistant disease. They are usually used when paclitaxel has failed. Topotecan was found to be significantly more effective than Taxol® in a randomized study of women who had progressed during or after platinum chemotherapy (ten Bokkel *et al.*, 1997). Oral altretamine (hexamethyl-melamine) has also shown activity in platinum-resistant ovarian cancer, but with only a 14 per cent objective response rate, compared with approximately 30 per cent for paclitaxel (Vergote *et al.*, 1992b). Oral etoposide has also been shown to have some efficacy as salvage treatment, and hormones are sometimes useful in stabilizing disease.

In those patients with minimal residual disease found at second-look surgery, experimental techniques, in particular intraperitoneal therapy with either chemotherapy, usually cisplatin, with or without concomitant intravenous chemotherapy, or immunotherapy, have been used, as described earlier. There is no evidence that whole-abdominal radiotherapy or intraperitoneal isotopes are effective in this situation.

PROGNOSTIC FACTORS AND RESULTS

Borderline ovarian epithelial tumours

Borderline ovarian epithelial tumours have a good 5-year prognosis, but the death rate continues to rise slowly thereafter (Fox, 1987). DNA ploidy appears to be the most important prognostic factor. Patients with diploid stage I tumours have a very good prognosis, but aneuploid tumours have a 19-fold increased risk of dying (Kaern *et al.*, 1993). Patients with aneuploid tumours are more likely to be older, to have mucinous tumours or severe atypia. The 5-year survival for serous borderline epithelial tumours is 90–95 per cent, and at 15 years is 72–86 per cent. For mucinous tumours the survival rates are 81–91 per cent at 5 years and 60–85 per cent at 15 years.

Invasive epithelial ovarian cancer

The 5-year survival rate overall for England is only about 26 per cent (Berrino *et al.*, 1996), but recent data from Yorkshire show a survival rate that is higher, at 32 per cent, probably reflecting the ongoing improvement in both the surgical and chemotherapeutic management of advanced ovarian cancer. However, survival is still dependent on the intrinsic characteristics of each tumour.

Table 33.3 *Results of treatment for ovarian cancer by stage (modified from FIGO, 1995)*

Stage	% of total	% alive at 3 years	% alive at 5 years
I	28	84	78
II	11	69	59
III	47	36	23
IV	14	20	14
Total	100		39

The important prognostic factors include stage, size of residual tumour at the end of initial surgery, grade of tumour, DNA ploidy, overexpression of some oncogenes, age over 50 years, performance status and clear-cell carcinoma. The importance of stage can be seen from the 5-year survival figures, as shown in Table 33.3. However, while stage I tumours with grade 1 or 2 histology have a 5-year survival rate of over 90 per cent (Young *et al.*, 1990), some other stage I cases have a worse prognosis, which may be identified by study of some of the factors mentioned above. The most important is poor differentiation of the tumour. Ploidy is also important in both early and advanced disease, with those with diploid tumours surviving significantly longer than those with aneuploid tumours.

In more advanced tumours, stage is more important than grade for even well-differentiated tumours. Size of residual tumour at the end of initial surgery was shown to be one of two main determinants of prognosis, the other being platinum chemotherapy, in a meta-analysis of 38 chemotherapy studies carried out by Voest *et al.* (1989). The size of residual tumour that is usually taken as indicating a poor prognosis is 2 cm and this observation was confirmed in the study undertaken by the North Thames Ovarian Group (Lambert *et al.*, 1997). Age is of little significance in terms of prognosis, but women aged 70 years or more have a poorer prognosis, probably related to their reduced ability to receive intensive chemotherapy. Overexpression of some oncogenes is also an indicator of survival in ovarian carcinoma. Five oncogenes were studied by multiparameter flow cytometry in 80 patients. The oncogenes were: epidermal growth factor receptor (EGFR), insulin-like growth factor-I receptor, c-erb-B2, c-ras and c-myc. Overexpression was present in up to one-third of patients, and EGFR, c-ras and c-myc indicated a worse prognosis for patients. EGFR was the most sensitive predictor (van Dam *et al.*, 1993). p53 gene mutations are found in half of the women who have advanced ovarian cancer (Marks *et al.*, 1991). There is a lower incidence of mutations in early stage disease, suggesting that the occurrence of mutated p53 is a late event in the development of ovarian cancer. Alternatively, such mutations may result in rapid progression of disease.

The survival figures for cancer of the ovary have changed little over the past 20 years and remain poor for more advanced disease despite more radical surgery and improvements in chemotherapy (Table 33.3). Most studies do show some prolongation of median survival in those patients who are left with minimal residual disease following surgery and who respond to postsurgical treatment. However, this benefit has not been sufficiently long lasting to affect 5-year survival rates to any great degree. Despite side-effects, modern cytotoxic therapy has improved the quality of life for many patients with advanced ovarian cancer.

NON-EPITHELIAL TUMOURS

Non-epithelial tumours constitute approximately 10 per cent of all ovarian cancers.

Sex-cord stromal tumours

GRANULOSA AND THECA CELL TUMOURS

The most common sex-cord stromal tumours, which account for 2–3 per cent of ovarian malignancies, are the granulosa and theca cell tumours. They often produce steroid hormones, in particular oestrogens, which can cause postmenopausal bleeding in older women and sexual precocity in prepubertal girls. The hormones may cause cystic glandular hyperplasia, or occasionally carcinoma of the endometrium. Theca cell tumours are usually benign. The majority of those that are malignant contain granulosa as well as theca cells, the malignant element originating in the granulosa cell.

Granulosa cell tumours occur at all ages, but are found predominantly in postmenopausal women. The staging system for these tumours is the same as for epithelial tumours. Most are stage I at presentation. Bilateral tumours are present in 4–26 per cent of cases. Inhibin, secreted by granulosa cells, inhibits follicle stimulating hormone (FSH). It is elevated in granulosa cell tumours and can therefore be used as a tumour marker, but it is not very specific as it can be raised in pregnancy and in the presence of other ovarian tumours, benign ovarian disease and in non-ovarian cancers (Healy et al., 1999).

Surgical treatment is the same as for epithelial tumours. Unilateral oophorectomy is indicated only in young women with stage Ia disease. The effect of adjunctive therapy is difficult to assess as granulosa cell tumours can recur up to 20 years after the initial diagnosis. Radiotherapy used to be the treatment of choice as granulosa cell tumours are thought to be moderately radiosensitive.

Because of the rarity of this tumour, the efficacy of chemotherapy is unknown, but treatment for advanced or recurrent disease is either with the regimens used for germ-cell tumours, such as BEP (bleomycin, etoposide and cisplatin), or with the platinum-based regimens used for advanced epithelial ovarian cancer (Bridgewater and Rustin, 1999). Anti-oestrogen therapy, such as medroxyprogesterone acetate, has been used for palliation because of the production of oestrogen by granulosa cell tumours, but oestrogen is seldom produced in recurrent disease. In cases of late recurrence, further surgery should be considered before any other therapy is given.

The 5-year survival is around 80 per cent overall, being 100 per cent in true stage Ia tumours but less than 50 per cent in more advanced disease. Early recurrence is associated with a high mortality.

SERTOLI–LEYDIG CELL TUMOURS

Sertoli–Leydig cell tumours are rare. About 50 per cent produce male hormones, which can cause virilization. Rarely, oestrogens are secreted. The prognosis is good for the majority of women who have localized disease, which behaves in a benign fashion, and surgery as for granulosa cell tumours is the treatment of choice. Chemotherapy may be used for metastatic or recurrent disease.

GYNANDROBLASTOMAS AND LIPID CELL TUMOURS

Both gynandroblastomas and lipid cell tumours are very rare. Gynandroblastomas are tumours with elements of both Sertoli–Leydig and granulosa cell tumours. They are benign. Lipid cell tumours have an endocrine-type architecture and are derived from Leydig, luteal or adrenocortical cells. They present with hormonal symptoms, and 20 per cent behave in a malignant fashion.

Germ-cell tumours

DYSGERMINOMAS

Dysgerminomas are uncommon ovarian tumours accounting for 2–5 per cent of all primary malignant ovarian tumours. Originating in the germ cells, they usually occur in young women less than 30 years old. They behave in a similar way to seminoma in men, spreading mainly by lymphatics to para-aortic, mediastinal and supra-clavicular glands. All cases need to be investigated by chest X-ray and CT scanning. To exclude the presence of elements of choriocarcinoma, endodermal sinus tumour or teratoma, serum α-fetoprotein (AFP) and β-human chorionic gonadotrophin (βhCG) must be assayed. Occasionally some cases of pure dysgerminoma have raised levels of βhCG. Pure dysgerminomas have a good prognosis, with a 5-year survival rate of 83–100 per cent. The majority are stage I tumours (75 per cent), most being stage Ia, and 15 per cent are bilateral.

Treatment is by surgery. Fertility-sparing surgery should be the rule even in the presence of metastases, as chemotherapy is able to cure this disease (Bridgewater and Rustin, 1999). The usual surgery is staging with removal of the ovary. Surgical staging is as for epithelial ovarian cancer, with peritoneal washings and full inspection of the abdomen.

Most true stage Ia dysgerminomas are cured by surgery alone and therefore surveillance alone is all that is necessary, with treatment reserved for relapse. Surveillance includes routine imaging of the remaining ovary and clinical examination, which is monthly for the first year, every 2 months for 2 years, every 4 months in the fourth year and then 6 monthly for a total of 10 years. Serum tumour markers, which include hCG, AFP, lactate dehydrogenase (LDH) and CA 125, should be carried out as frequently as every 2 weeks for the first 6 months, monthly for the next 6 months, two-monthly for the second year, after which tumour markers should be repeated at each clinic visit.

In the past, radiotherapy has been used for advanced, metastatic or recurrent disease, and good results have been obtained in cases of pure dysgerminoma with whole-abdominal radiotherapy. Mixed tumours, that is, where other malignant elements are present, are not radiosensitive. Dysgerminoma is similar to seminoma in being a very radiosensitive tumour, and therefore only doses in the region of 20–25 Gy in 2–3 weeks to the pelvis and para-aortic nodes are required, unless the nodes are grossly involved, when 30–40 Gy are needed.

However, chemotherapy has replaced radiotherapy in the treatment of advanced, metastatic and recurrent dysgerminoma. Chemotherapy, in contrast to radiotherapy, is likely to preserve fertility and this is an important consideration, as the women who develop dysgerminoma are usually very young. The regimens used are the same as for other germ-cell tumours and are discussed below.

OTHER GERM-CELL TUMOURS

Germ-cell tumours other than dysgerminoma also occur in young women under 30 years old. In the past they were considered to have a very poor prognosis, but the majority are now cured by combination chemotherapy. Their derivation from germ cells is shown in Figure 33.1 (Telium, 1965). Mature teratomas are benign, the most common being the cystic teratoma or dermoid cyst found at all ages but particularly in the third and fourth decades.

Tumour markers are of value in diagnosis, monitoring therapy and in early detection of recurrence. The two main markers are AFP, produced by yolk-sac cells, and βhCG from the syncytiotrophoblast. CA 125 and lactic dehydrogenase can also be useful serum markers in tumours that do not produce βhCG or AFP.

Following conservative surgery to establish the diagnosis, remove the primary lesion and to stage the disease, the main treatment is combination chemotherapy, except for stage I malignant teratomas, which may be followed up closely. Surveillance is as described under dysgerminoma, and repeat CT of the chest, abdomen and pelvis is carried out as appropriate. Approximately two-thirds of patients under surveillance will not relapse. In those patients who do relapse, chemotherapy is curative in most cases.

Many combinations of chemotherapy have been used, the most common being VAC (vincristine, actinomycin D and cyclophosphamide). These regimens, which were given for periods of up to 2 years, have been replaced by much shorter courses of cisplatin chemotherapy, which is more effective in advanced disease. Cisplatin is given in combination with bleomycin and etoposide (BEP), usually to a total of four courses given every 3 weeks. An alternative regime is POMB/ACE. This regimen alternates cisplatin, vincristine, methotrexate and bleomycin with actinomycin D, cyclophosphamide and etoposide. Cycles are repeated every 2 weeks for five courses. These combination regimens preserve fertility in most cases and children born to mothers who have received this chemotherapy develop normally with no evidence of endocrine dysfunction (Newlands and Bagshaw, 1987).

MIXED MESODERMAL TUMOURS OF THE OVARY

Less than 1 per cent of all ovarian malignancies are the highly malignant mixed mesodermal tumours. Both homologous and heterologous mixed mesenchymal tumours occur, similar to those in the uterus. The former has malignant mesenchymal elements derived from ovarian structures, for example, leiomyosarcoma or fibrosarcoma, while in the latter the mesenchymal element is not ovarian, for example, rhabdomyosarcoma. The prognosis for either type of mixed mesodermal tumour is very poor, with a 2-year survival of less than 20 per cent. Chemotherapy as for epithelial ovarian cancer is commonly given.

CANCER OF THE FALLOPIAN TUBE

Cancers of the Fallopian tube can be either primary or secondary. Most tumours involving the Fallopian tube are metastatic from ovarian cancer, but secondary spread from the breast and gastrointestinal tract can also occur. Primary carcinoma is extremely rare, comprising only 0.3 per cent of gynaecological malignancies. The main incidence is after the menopause and the tumour is usually unilateral. Tumour spread is identical to that of ovarian

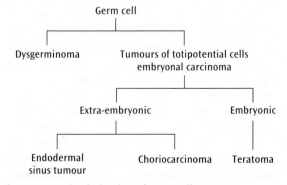

Figure 33.1 *The derivation of germ-cell tumours.*

cancer and metastases to pelvic and para-aortic nodes are common.

Pathology

The similarity in histology between serous adenocarcinoma of the ovary and primary tubal ovarian cancer, means that strict criteria must be applied before the diagnosis of tubal carcinoma can be made. The tumour usually distends the lumen of the tube and may protrude through the fimbrial end, and the tube may be retort-shaped, resembling a hydrosalpinx. The predominant histological pattern is papillary, with a gradation through alveolar to solid as the degree of differentiation decreases.

Staging

The clinical staging is the same as for ovarian cancer.

Diagnosis

Most cases of carcinoma of the Fallopian tube are diagnosed at laparotomy. The diagnosis is seldom considered preoperatively. The usual presenting symptom is postmenopausal bleeding, and there may also be a watery discharge and lower abdominal pain. Unexplained postmenopausal bleeding or abnormal cytology without an obvious cause should alert the clinician to the possible diagnosis of Fallopian tube carcinoma and a careful bimanual examination and pelvic ultrasound should be carried out.

Treatment

The management of cancer of the Fallopian tube is as for cancer of the ovary, with surgery to remove gross tumour. This should almost invariably involve total abdominal hysterectomy and bilateral salpingo-oophorectomy. Postoperative chemotherapy as for ovarian cancer will be required for all but the earliest cases.

Results

The overall survival rate at 5 years is around 35 per cent. The prognosis is improved if the tumour is detected early. The survival rate for stage I at 5 years is in the region of 70 per cent.

SIGNIFICANT POINTS

- Epithelial ovarian cancer usually presents when the disease is advanced. Screening of the general population to allow earlier diagnosis is not a feasible proposition at present.
- Except in borderline tumours and when the epithelial ovarian cancer is confined to the ovaries and is well or moderately well differentiated, it has a poor prognosis.
- Standard treatment for epithelial ovarian cancer is debulking surgery followed by a platinum drug, usually carboplatin, alone or with paclitaxel. The combination of a platinum drug with paclitaxel is considered to be the optimal therapy at present.
- The biological factors inherent in each malignant epithelial tumour are the main determinants for survival.
- Germ-cell tumours occur in young women. They have a good prognosis, with the majority being cured. Treatment is primarily by chemotherapy following minimal surgery to establish the diagnosis and remove the primary tumour. Fertility is usually preserved.

REFERENCES

Advanced Ovarian Cancer Trialists Group (1991) Chemotherapy in advanced ovarian cancer: an overview of randomised clinical trials. *BMJ* **303**, 884–93.

Advanced Ovarian Cancer Trialists Group (1998) Chemotherapy in advanced ovarian cancer: four systemic meta-analyses of individual patient data from 37 randomized trials. *Br. J. Cancer* **78**,1479–87.

A'Hern, R.P. and Gore, M.E. (1995) Impact of doxorubicin on survival in advanced ovarian cancer. *J. Clin. Oncol.* **13**, 726–32.

Alberts, D.S., Liu, P.Y., Hannigan, E.V. *et al.* (1996) Intraperitoneal cisplatin plus intravenous cyclophosphamide versus intravenous cisplatin plus intravenous cyclophosphamide for Stage III ovarian cancer. *N. Engl. J. Med.* **335**, 1950–5.

Beard, S.M., Coleman, R., Radford, J. *et al.* (1997) *Supplementary document: the use of cisplatin and paclitaxel as a first-line treatment in ovarian cancer.* Guidance note for puchasers: 98/10 (Supplement to 97/05), Trent Institute for Health Services Research.

Beard, S.M., Coleman, R., Radford, J. *et al.* (1998) *The use of cisplatin and paclitaxel as a first line treatment in ovarian cancer.* Guidance note for puchasers: 97/05, Trent Institute for Health Services Research.

Bell, R., Luengo, S. and Petticrew, M. (1998) *Screening for ovarian cancer: a systemic review*. CRD Report 13. York: NHS Centre for Reviews and Dissemination.

Berrino, F., Sant, M., Verdacchia, A. *et al.* (eds) (1996) *Survival of cancer patients in Europe: the EUROCARE study*. Lyon: International Agency for Research on Cancer.

Bertelsen, K. (1990) Tumour reduction surgery and long term survival in advanced ovarian cancer: a DACOVA study. *Gynecol. Oncol.* **38**, 203–9.

Bourne, T.H., Campbell, S., Reynolds, K.M. *et al.* (1993) Screening for early familial ovarian cancer with transvaginal ultrasonography and colour blood flow imaging. *BMJ* **306**, 1025–9.

Bridgewater, J. and Rustin, G.J.S. (1999) Management of non-epithelial ovarian tumours. *Oncology* **57**, 89–98.

Burghardt, E., Lahousen, M. and Stettner, H. (1987) The role of lymphadenectomy in the treatment of ovarian cancer. In Sharp, F. and Soutter, W.P. (eds), *Ovarian cancer – the way ahead*. The Seventeenth Study Group of the Royal College of Obstetricians and Gynaecologists. London: Royal College of Obstetricians and Gynaecologists, 257–74.

Calvert, A.H., Newell, D.R., Gumbrell, S. *et al.* (1989) Carboplatin dosage: prospective evaluation of a simple formula based on renal function. *J. Clin. Oncol.* **7**, 1748–56.

Corn, B.W., Lanciano, R.M., Boente, M. *et al.* (1994) Recurrent ovarian cancer. Effective radiotherapeutic palliation after chemotherapy failure. *Cancer* **74**, 2979–83.

Dembo, A.J. (1992) Epithelial ovarian cancer: the role of radiotherapy. *Int. J. Radiat. Oncol. Biol. Phys.* **22**, 835–45.

Dembo, A.J., Bush, R.S., Beale, F.A. *et al.* (1979) The Princess Margaret Hospital Study of ovarian cancer: staged I, II and asymptomatic III presentations. *Cancer Treat. Rep.* **63**, 249–54.

Eeles, R.A., Tan, S., Wiltshaw, E. *et al.* (1991) Hormone replacement therapy and survival after surgery for ovarian cancer. *BMJ* **302**, 259–62.

FIGO (1995) *22nd Annual Report*.

Fox, H. (1985) Pathology of surface epithelial tumours. In Hudson, C.N. (ed.), *Ovarian cancer*. Oxford: Oxford University Press, 72–93.

Fox, H. (1987) Prognostic indices in ovarian tumours of borderline malignancy with particular reference to morphometric analysis. In Sharp, F. and Soutter, W.P. (eds), *Ovarian cancer – the way ahead*. The Seventeenth Study Group of the Royal College of Obstetricians and Gynaecologists. London: Royal College of Obstetricians and Gynaecologists, 69–78.

Gelblum, D., Mychalczac, B., Almadrones, L. *et al.* (1998) Palliative benefit of external-beam radiation in the management of platinum refractory epithelial ovarian carcinoma. *Gynecol. Oncol.* **69**, 36–41.

Griffiths, C.T., Parker, L.M. and Fuller, A.F.J. (1979) Role of cytoreductive surgical treatment in the management of advanced ovarian cancer. *Cancer Treat. Rep.* **63**, 235–40.

Hacker, N.F., Berek, J.S., Lagasse, L.D. *et al.* (1983) Primary cytoreductive surgery for epithelial ovarian cancer. *Obstet. Gynecol.* **61**, 413–20.

Hakes, T.B., Chalas, E., Hoskins, W.J. *et al.* (1992) Randomised prospective trial of 5 versus 10 cycles of cyclophosphamide, doxorubicin and cisplatin in advanced ovarian carcinoma. *Gynecol. Oncol.* **45**, 284–9.

Healy, D.L., Burger, H.G. and Mamers, P. (1999) Elevated serum inhibin concentrations in postmenopausal women with ovarian tumours. *N. Engl. J. Med.* **329**, 1539–42.

Hird, V., Maraveyas, A., Snook, D., *et al.* (1993) Adjuvant therapy of ovarian cancer with radioactive monoclonal antibody. *Br. J. Cancer* **68**, 403–6.

Hoskins, W.J., Bundy, B.N., Thigpen, J.T. and Omura, G.A. (1992) The influence of cytoreductive surgery on recurrence-free interval and survival in small-volume stage III epithelial ovarian cancer: a Gynecologic Oncology Group study. *Gynecol. Oncol.* **47**, 159–66.

Hunter, R.W., Alexander, N.D.E. and Soutter, W.P. (1992) Meta-analysis of surgery in advanced ovarian carcinoma: is maximum cytoreductive surgery an independent determinant of prognosis? *Am. J. Obstet. Gynecol.* **166**, 504–11.

ICON Collaborators (1998) ICON 2: randomized trial of single-agent carboplatin aginst three-drug combination of CAP (cyclophosphamide, doxorubicin, and cisplatin) in women with ovarian cancer. *Lancet* **352**, 1571–6.

Jacobs, I. (1995) Screening for sporadic ovarian cancer. In Leak, R., Gore, M. and Ward, R.H. (eds), *The biology of gynaecological cancer*. London: RCOG Press, 231–344.

Jacobs, I., Skates, S., Prys Davies, A. *et al.* (1996) Risk of diagnosis of ovarian cancer after raised serum CA 125 concentration: a prospective study. *BMJ* **313**, 1355–8.

Jacobs, I.J., Skates, S.J., MacDonald, N. *et al.* (1999) Screening for ovarian cancer: a pilot randomised controlled trial. *Lancet* **353**, 1207–10.

Kaern, J., Tropé, C.G., Kristensen, V.M. *et al.* (1993) DNA ploidy; the most important prognostic factor in patients with borderline tumors of the ovary. *Int. J. Gynecol. Cancer* **3**, 349–58.

Kohn, E.C., Sarosy, G., Bicher, A. *et al.* (1994) Dose-intense Taxol: high response rate in patients with platinum-resistant recurrent ovarian cancer. *J. Natl Cancer Inst.* **86**, 18–24.

Lambert, H.E. and Berry, R.J. (1985) High dose cis-platinum compared with high dose cyclophosphamide in the management of advanced epithelial ovarian cancer stage III and IV: a report from the North Thames Co-operative Group. *BMJ* **290**, 889–93.

Lambert, H.E., Rustin, G., Gregory, W. and Nelstrop, A. (1993) A randomised trial comparing single agent carboplatin with carboplatin followed by radiotherapy for advanced ovarian cancer: a North Thames Ovary Study group. *J. Clin. Oncol.* **11**, 440–8.

Lambert, H.E., Rustin, G.J.S., Gregory, W.M. and Nestrop, A.E. (1997) A randomized trial of five versus eight courses of cisplatin or carboplatin in advanced ovarian carcinoma. A North Thames Ovary Group Study. *Ann. Oncol.* **8**, 327–33.

Marchetti, M., Padovan, P. and Fracas, M. (1998) Malignant ovarian tumours: conservative surgery and quality of life in young patients. *Eur. J. Gynaecol. Oncol.* **19**, 297–301.

Markman, M., Rothman, R., Hakes, T. *et al.* (1991) Second-line platinum therapy in patients with ovarian cancer previously treated with cisplatin. *J. Clin. Oncol.* **9**, 389–93.

Marks, J.R., Davidoff, A.M., Kerns, B.J.M. *et al.* (1991) Overexpression and mutation of p53 in epithelial ovarian cancer. *Cancer Res.* **51**, 2979–84.

McGuire, W.P., Hoskins, W.J., Brady, M.F. *et al.* (1996) Cyclophosphamide and cisplatin compared with paclitaxel and cisplatin in patients with Stage III and Stage IV ovarian cancer. *N. Engl. J. Med.* **334**, 1–6.

Muggia, F.M., Brady, P.S., Brady, M.F. *et al.* (1997) Phase III of cisplatin or paclitaxel versus the combination in suboptimal epithelial ovarian cancer: Gynaecological Oncology Group (GOG) study. *Proc. Ann. Meet. Am. Soc. Clin. Oncol.* **16**, abstract 1257.

Naylor, M.S., Burke, F. and Balkwill, F.R. (1995) Cytokines and ovarian cancer. In Sharp, F., Mason, P., Blackett, T. and Berek, J. (eds), *Ovarian cancer 3*. London: Chapman & Hall, 89–97.

Newlands, E.S. and Bagshaw, K.D. (1987) Advances in the treatment of germ cell tumours of the ovary. In Bonnar, J. (ed.), *Recent advances in obstetrics and gynaecology*. Edinburgh: Churchill Livingstone, 143–56.

Nicholson, S., Gooden, C.S.R., Hird, V. *et al.* (1998) Radioimmunotherapy after chemotherapy compared to chemotherapy alone in the treatment of advanced ovarian cancer: a matched analysis. *Oncol. Rep.* **5**, 223–6.

Ovarian Cancer Meta-analysis project (1991) Cyclophosphamide plus cisplatin versus cyclophosphamide, doxorubicin, and cisplatin chemotherapy of ovarian cancer: a meta-analysis. *J. Clin. Oncol.* **9**, 1668–74.

Ovarian Tumour Panel of the Royal College of Obstetricians and Gynaecologists (RCOG) (1983) Ovarian epithelial tumours of borderline malignancy: pathological features and current status. *Br. J. Obstet. Gynaecol.* **90**, 743–50.

Ponder, B. (1994) Breast cancer genes – searches begin and end. *Nature* **371**, 279.

Ponder, B.A.J., Peto, J. and Easton, D.F. (1992) Familial ovarian cancer. In Sharp, F., Mason, W.P. and Creasman, W. (eds), *Ovarian cancer 2, Biology, diagnosis and management*. London: Chapman & Hall, 3–7.

Potter, M.E., Partridge, E.E., Hatch, K.D., Soong, S.-J., Austin, J.M. and Shingleton, H.M. (1991) Primary surgical therapy of ovarian cancer: how much and when? *Gynaecol. Oncol.* **40**, 195–200.

Rosenoff, S.H., Devita, V.T., Hubbard, S. and Young, R.C. (1975) Peritoneoscopy in the staging and follow-up of ovarian cancer. *Semin. Oncol.* **2**, 223–8.

Scarabelli, C., Gallo, A., Visentin, M.C., Canzonieri, V., Carbone, A. and Zarrelli, A. (1997) Systematic pelvic and para-aortic lymphadenectomy in advanced ovarian cancer patients with no residual intraperitoneal disease. *Int. J. Gynecol. Cancer* **7**, 18–26.

Sjovall, K., Nilsson, B. and Einhorn, N. (1994) Different types of rupture of the tumour capsule and the impact on survival in early ovarian carcinoma. *Int. J. Gynecol. Cancer* **4**, 333–6.

Soutter, W.P. and Leake, R.E. (1987) Steroid hormone receptors in gynaecological cancers. In Bonnar, J. (ed.), *Recent advances in obstetrics and gynaecology*. Edinburgh: Churchill Livingstone, 175–94.

Stratton, J.F., Gayther, S.A., Russell, P. *et al.* (1997) Contribution of *BRCA1* mutations to ovarian cancer. *N. Engl. J. Med.* **336**, 1125–30.

Stratton, J.F., Pharoah, P., Smith, S.K. *et al.* (1998) A systemic review and meta-analysis of family history and risk of ovarian cancer. *Br. J. Obstet. Gynaecol.* **105**, 493–9.

Stuart, G., Bertelson, K., Mangioni, C. *et al.* (1998) Updated analysis shows a highly significant overall improved survival for cis-paclitaxel as first line treatment of advanced ovarian cancer: mature results of the EORTC–GCOG, NOCOVA, NCIC CTG and Scottish Intergroup trial. *Proc. Ann. Meet. Am. Soc. Clin. Oncol.* **17**, abstract 1394.

Swenerton, K., Eisenhauer, E., Huinink, W.T.B. *et al.* (1993) Taxol in relapsed ovarian cancer. High versus low dose and short versus long infusion: a European–Canadian study coordinated by the NCI Clinical Trials Group. *Proc. Am. Soc. Clin. Oncol.* **12**, 810.

Teilum, G. (1965) Classification of endodermal sinus tumours (mesoblastoma vitellinum) and so called 'embryonal carcinoma' of the ovary. *Acta Pathol. Microbiol.* **64**, 407.

ten Bokkel Huinink, W., Gore, M., Carmichael, J. *et al.* (1997) Topotecan versus paclitaxel for the treatment of recurrent epithelial ovarian cancer. *J. Clin. Oncol.* **15**, 2183–93.

Thigpen, J.T., Vance, R.B. and Khansur, T. (1993) Second-line chemotherapy for recurrent carcinoma of the ovary. *Cancer* **71**, 559–64.

Tingulstad, S., Hagen, B., Skjeldstad, F.E. *et al.* (1996) Evaluation of a risk of malignancy index based on serum CA 125, ultrasound findings and menopausal status in the pre-operative diagnosis of pelvic masses. *Br. J. Obstet. Gynaecol.* **103**, 826–31.

Trimble, E.L., Adams, J.D., Vena, D. *et al.* (1993) Paclitaxel for platinum-refractory ovarian cancer: results from the first 1,000 patients registered to National Cancer Institute Treatment Referral Centre 9103. *J. Clin. Oncol.* **11**, 2405–10.

Van Dam, P.A., Vergote, I.B., Lowe, D.G. *et al.* (1993) Epidermal growth factor receptor expression is an independent prognostic factor in ovarian cancer. *Int. J. Gynecol. Cancer* **3**(suppl. 1), 51.

Van der Berg, M.E.L., van Lent, M., Buyse, M. *et al.* (1995) The effect of debulking surgery after induction chemotherapy on the prognosis in advanced epithelial ovarian cancer. *N. Engl. J. Med.* **332**, 629–34.

Vergote, I.B., De Vos, L.N., Abeler, V.M. *et al.* (1992a) Randomized trial comparing cisplatin with radioactive phosphorus or whole abdominal irradiation as adjuvant treatment of ovarian cancer. *Cancer* **69**, 741–9.

Vergote, I., Himmelmann, A., Frankendal, B. *et al.* (1992b) Hexamethylmelamine as a second line therapy in platinum resistant ovarian cancer. *Gynecol. Oncol.* **47**, 282–6.

Vergote, I.B., Trope, C.G., Kaern, J. *et al.* (1993) Identification of high-risk Stage I ovarian carcinoma. Importance of DNA ploidy. *Int. J. Gynaecol. Cancer* **3**(suppl. 1), 51.

Vessey, M., Metcalfe, A., Wells, C. *et al.* (1987) Ovarian neoplasms, functional cysts and oral contraceptives. *BMJ* **294**, 1518–20.

Voest, E.E., Van Houwelingen, J.C., Neijt, J.P. (1989) A meta-analysis of prognostic factors in advanced ovarian cancer with median survival and overall survival (measured with the log (relative risk)) as main objectives. *Eur. J. Cancer Clin. Care* **25**, 711–20.

Watson, P. and Lynch, H.T. (1992) Hereditary ovarian cancer. In Sharp, F., Mason, W.P. and Creasman, W. (eds), *Ovarian cancer 2, Biology, diagnosis and management.* London: Chapman & Hall, 9–15.

Wiltshaw, E. and Kroner, T. (1976) Phase II study of *cis*-cishlorodiammine platinum (II) (RSC-119875) in advanced adenocarcinoma of the ovary. *Cancer Treat. Rep.* **60**, 55–60.

Young, R.C., Chabner, B.A., Hubbard, S.P. *et al.* (1978) Advanced ovarian adenocarcinoma: a prospective clinical trial of melphalan (L-PAM) versus combination chemotherapy. *N. Engl. J. Med.* **299**, 1261–6.

Young, R.C., Walton, L.A., Ellenberg, S.S. *et al.* (1990) Adjuvant therapy in stage I and stage II epithelial ovarian cancer: results of two prospective randomized trials. *N. Engl. J. Med.* **322**, 1021–7.

Zanetta, G., Chiari, S., Rota, S. *et al.* (1997) Conservative surgery for stage I ovarian carcinoma in women of childbearing age. *Br. J. Obstet. Gynaecol.* **104**, 1030–5.

Uterus

BLEDDYN JONES

EPIDEMIOLOGY

Cancers of the uterus show a marked increase in incidence and mortality with age, being commonest in the sixth and seventh decade with an approximate median age at presentation of 60. They account for approximately 3800 female deaths per year in England and Wales and are the fifth most common cause of cancer deaths in women (Cancer Survival Trends, 1999). The incidence figures are relatively stable over the past three decades, despite the increase in age distribution of the population. This fact is perhaps surprising, although the incidence figures may be further influenced by the protective effect of combined oral contraceptives, the increasing practice of prophylactic hysterectomies and exacerbated by oestrogen-only hormone replacement (HRT). The mortality rates are marginally greater in women from lower socio-economic groups. Uterine cancers are likely to become the most common curable cancers in women, due to the impact of screening on the incidence of invasive cervical cancer.

AETIOLOGY

The precise aetiology is unknown. There is little evidence of an inherited predisposition (Olson *et al.*, 1999). Environmental factors are therefore implicated, particularly the interaction between the promoter effect of oestrogens and environmental chemical carcinogens ingested in fat-rich foods. There are several predisposing factors, some of which are also recognized in the development of carcinoma of the breast, such as nulliparity. These include age, obesity, diabetes mellitus and hypertension. Polycystic ovarian disease can predispose younger women to develop endometrial cancer. Hormonal overstimulation of the endometrium by oestrogens, either endogenous or exogenous, for example by the use of oestrogen-only HRT prescriptions, predispose to the development of endometrial hyperplasias. Prolonged use of tamoxifen is associated with a sevenfold increase in the development of endometrial carcinoma and also of bowel cancer (Newcomb *et al.*, 1999) in those patients who have previously had a carcinoma of the breast. Other confounding variables (genetic, environmental carcinogens and similar risk factors, such as nulliparity) could partly explain this effect, although there is ample evidence that endometrial hypertrophy does develop after the long-term use of tamoxifen. Mutations of the genetic code can be produced by tamoxifen–DNA adducts (Terishima *et al.*, 1999). In recurrent endometrial cancer, tamoxifen can cause sustained tumour regression after failure of high-dose progestagen therapy, although these patients are normally tamoxifen naïve.

PATHOLOGY

Adenocarcinoma of endometrioid type (non-mucus-secreting) is typical. Squamous cell carcinoma can rarely occur. The histopathologist carefully determines:

1 Tumour grade (G1–3). This is the most important factor (Mundt and Condi, 2000). The higher grade

categories have an increased risk of local (vault) and pelvic nodal recurrence.

2 Extent of myometrial invasion: tumours invading the outer half are more likely to spread to pelvic nodes.
3 Vascular/lymphatic invasion.
4 Atypical histological types, such as clear cell and the serous papillary variant, confer a relatively poor prognosis. The latter frequently recur intra-abdominally and the natural history resembles that of ovarian cancer.

The position of the tumour, whether in the upper or lower segment may also influence outcome. The incidence of lymphatic spread is greater in the case of tumours in the lower segment of the uterus, which spread via the same lymphatic pathways as carcinoma of the cervix.

Sometimes there is diagnostic uncertainty if tumours of similar histology occur within the ovary and endometrium, due to either synchronous primaries or metastatic cancer. Where there is such doubt, clinicians tend to offer treatment based on the assumption that the primary tumour is ovarian, although the possibility of an endometrial primary should never be dismissed, particularly if the treatment response is not typical of ovarian cancer. The other important differential diagnosis is that of endocervical adenocarcinoma, which is normally mucus secreting, unlike endometrial carcinoma.

The role of peritoneal cytology as a strong independent prognostic factor remains to be determined in the case of stage I cancers but appears to be predictive with extrauterine cancer (Kadar *et al.*, 1992).

Some authorities classify the uterine cancers into the 'usual type' that are endocrine sensitive, while the other cancers are regarded as 'special variant' types and are oestrogen independent and poorly differentiated, arising in non-hyperplastic endometrium.

Genetic changes

Aneuploidy confers a poor prognosis (Larson *et al.*, 1999). Special variant tumours contain a far greater incidence of genetic changes, as assessed by loss of chromosomal heterozygosity (Tritz *et al.*, 1997). *p53* mutations are the most commonly reported genetic change, occurring in 20 per cent, but are probably not an early event in cancer evolution, since they are mainly found in more advanced tumours with a poor prognosis (Kihana *et al.*, 1995). Similarly, overexpression of *HER-2/neu* oncogene can be found in 10–15 per cent of advanced stages, whereas K-*ras* mutations are reported in 15 per cent of stage I–II cancers (Semczuk *et al.*, 1997).

Serum markers

CA 125 antigen is the marker of choice, being frequently raised at presentation. It is used to assess responses to therapy.

Tumour receptor status

There is evidence that higher nuclear progesterone receptor levels are associated with improved survival. In contrast, there is conflicting evidence as to the relevance of oestrogen receptors (Creasman, 1993).

Routes of spread

The tumour may extend to fill the endometrial cavity and prolapse beyond the os cervix as a pseudo-polyp. The depth of myometrial invasion correlates with an increase in pelvic lymph node spread. Approximately 9 per cent of patients in the stage I category have pelvic nodal involvement. Direct extension to the stroma of the cervix also results in increased pelvic lymphatic involvement. Very occasionally, submucosal vaginal extension may occur, resulting in an isolated metastatic deposit in the lower third of the vagina, usually in the suburethral region, which may cause urethral obstruction.

Para-aortic node spread occurs in only 6 per cent of stage I tumours but in 18 per cent of non-endometrioid adenocarcinoma variants and the incidence also increases with stage (Hicks *et al.*, 1993). Isolated relapse in the para-aortic region does infrequently occur after successful pelvic surgery and radiotherapy. Peritoneal spread may follow extension through the serosal surface of the uterus, as may direct infiltration of the surrounding pelvic tissues. Bloodstream spread is unusual but patients occasionally develop lung, liver and bone metastases. Rarely, a patient may develop a nodal metastasis in the inguinal region.

SYMPTOMS

The characteristic symptoms of post-menopausal bleeding and vaginal discharge should be investigated thoroughly in all women. Other symptoms due to a pelvic mass lesion (*see* Chapter 33) may occur in higher-stage tumours.

INVESTIGATION

Clinical assessment will include abdominal and pelvic examination. A direct biopsy (by Pipelle or other commercial aspirators) can be taken in the clinic. Should there be diagnostic difficulties, an examination under anaesthetic (EUA), hysteroscopy (and further biopsy) and curettage can be performed. Several imaging methods have also improved the diagnostic and staging accuracy of uterine tumours. Transvaginal ultrasound can be used to virtually exclude the presence of endometrial cancer and to assess the extent of myometrial invasion

(70–80 per cent accuracy). Greater accuracy (97–95 per cent) in staging, including the assessment of lymphadenopathy, may be obtained with magnetic resonance imaging (MRI) although very obese patients may not be accommodated within the scanner aperture. Pelvic computed tomography (CT) imaging is not as helpful as the above techniques in uterine tumour imaging, but abdominal CT imaging is more sensitive at the assessment of retroperitoneal lymphadenopathy.

STAGING

The current FIGO (Federation International Gynaecology Oncology) staging system differs in several ways from that of the uterine cervix. A simplified version is given in Table 34.1.

TREATMENT

Surgery

A total abdominal hysterectomy and bilateral salpingo-oophorectomy (TAH and BSO) is the cornerstone of management, being used in 90 per cent of patients and followed by average survival rates that exceed 70 per cent. Subtotal hysterectomy is sometimes performed, but this is not advisable as the uterine incision may contain cancer cells and subsequent radiotherapy may be compromised. These operations are normally done via a Pfannen–Stiel incision and there is virtually no risk of scar recurrence. The additional role of pelvic lymphadenectomy remains unproven (Kilgore *et al.*, 1995). In the UK, the MRC 'ASTEC' trial has been designed to determine whether this additional surgical procedure is of benefit.

Radiotherapy

Radiotherapy may be used in several circumstances (Thomas and Blake, 1996; Jones *et al.*, 1999).

Table 34.1 *FIGO staging system*

Stage	Anatomical description of involvement
IA	Limited to endometrium
IB	Invasion of inner half of myometrium
IC	Invasion of outer half of myometrium
IIA	Endocervical glandular extension
IIB	Cervical stromal invasion
IIIA	Invasion of serosa and/or adnexa and/or positive peritoneal cytology
IIIB	Pelvic or para-aortic lymph nodes
IV	Bladder/bowel/inguinal nodes/adominal or distant metastases

POSTOPERATIVE (ADJUVANT)

The rationale is to prevent local recurrence at:

- vaginal vault
- pelvic lymph nodes.

Vault brachytherapy alone

This technique will only prevent recurrence in the vaginal vault. This policy is advocated by some specialists for surgical stages IA, IB and G3 (Chadha *et al.*, 1999), for example by three 7 Gy fractions delivered at 0.5 cm from a vaginal applicator surface. The potential advantages are that patients who have a low risk of nodal metastases can be treated without external-beam radiotherapy and therefore avoid the potential side-effects. The disadvantages include the possibly poor intracavitary dose distribution at the vault, where there may be bilateral recesses, for which the use of two ovoid-shaped applicators may be preferable to the use of a conventional single vaginal cylinder technique. Another potential problem is that a later vault or isolated pelvic nodal relapse is difficult to treat, since the previously treated brachytherapy volume requires to be shielded.

External-beam and brachytherapy

A four-field treatment plan is usually used to deliver 40–45 Gy in 20–25 fractions over 4–5 weeks on a linear accelerator of at least 6 MV energy. The field dimensions are similar to those for carcinoma of the cervix, although the lateral field dimensions do not need to extend so far anteriorly since the uterine fundus is absent. Normally, the antero-posterior (AP) fields extend from the mid or lower border of the L5 vertebra to the lower aspect of the obturator foramen and laterally to 1 cm beyond the pelvic sidewall. The dimensions are normally 14 cm^2 or slightly larger. The lateral posterior field limit can be marked by a line positioned 2.5 cm anterior to the sacral hollow, or passing through the S2/3 junction where this is visible. The lateral anterior field limit normally passes through the mid symphysis pubis and should always pass just anterior to the acetabulum and provide a reasonable margin for lymph-node cover in front of the sacrum/L5 vertebra. The field width is usually 8–10 cm. Radiopaque vaginal and rectal markers are advocated by some specialists, but these are not essential as there is little risk of geographic miss in this situation. Shielding of the following regions is advisable:

- corners of anterior and posterior fields – this will reduce the integral dose to the intestine and hip joints; and
- posterior aspect of the sacrum in the lateral field – this will potentially reduce the risk of radiation-induced sacral insufficiency fractures.

Treatment difficulties can occur in very obese patients: additional applied dose, skin-fold reactions and difficulties in reproducing the daily set-up can be sufficient to restrict the prescribed dose to 30–40 Gy in some patients. After hysterectomy, there is a greater volume of small intestine within the pelvis and there may be postoperative adhesions. The bladder position is more posterior following hysterectomy and there may be incomplete emptying. These aspects, together with the associated medical conditions referred to, may all contribute to a reduction in pelvic radiation tolerance, such that doses higher than 40–45 Gy in 20–25 fractions should not be exceeded unless there are good reasons to do so. If there is definite inoperable malignant pelvic lymphadenopathy, an external-beam dose of 50.4 Gy in 28 fractions can be justified.

Intracavitary therapy following external-beam therapy

In this case, the effect of dose inhomogeneity in the vaginal vault is not likely to be as important as when brachytherapy only is used. It is reasonable to give either:

- a further 10–15 Gy using low/medium dose-rate caesium, provided the bladder or rectal dose estimates are not greater than 1 Gy/h; or
- a high dose rate (HDR), 6 Gy in one fraction or two fractions each of 4 Gy, at 0.5 cm from either the surface of a vaginal cylinder or an ovoid(s).

In these patients, the brachytherapy is intended to deliver a relatively small additional dose to the vault tissues that may potentially contain hypoxic scar tissue embedded with malignant cells following surgery. The technique most commonly used is that of a vaginal cylinder with radioactive loading of the upper 2–4 cm only. The volume of additional radiation is consequently kept small and the total dose (and biologically effective dose, BED) due to the summation of the external beam and brachytherapy at the prescription distance is assumed to represent the maximum possible normal tissue dose, which is kept within normal tissue tolerance. The total BED used in the UK in 1996 ranged between 90 and 124 Gy$_3$; doses at the lower end of this range appear to give satisfactory local control and no serious side effects in the author's present experience.

External-beam therapy alone following hysterectomy

Some authors prefer to avoid brachytherapy and report good results following external beam only (e.g. Weiss et al., 1999), although relatively high doses, such as 50.4 Gy in 28 fractions, are used. This may be satisfactory in fit patients, but there remains some concern as to the late side-effects of such doses to a large volume of pelvic tissues, particularly on the small intestine, in patient subgroups where pelvic tolerance may be compromised.

The alternative policy is frequent surveillance by means of pelvic examinations and biopsy where recurrent tumour is suspected. Prompt treatment, by external beam plus vaginal intracavitary brachytherapy, of recurrent pelvic carcinoma can be curative. A higher prescribed dose of radiotherapy is usually necessary: 45–50.4 Gy in 25–28 fractions plus two intracavitary HDR insertions of 5–6 Gy at 0.5 cm, or equivalent continuous radiation (e.g. 15–20 Gy at <1 Gy/h[1]). The intracavitary treatment length may need to be longer in these patients, depending on the extent of vaginal involvement. If two intracavitary fractions are used, a shrinking-volume brachytherapy

technique is possible. Such clinical management can only be followed confidently if adequate staff resources and reasonably rapid access to radiotherapy facilities are available.

Patients should be fully informed of the rationale for postoperative treatment and may have strong personal feelings as to whether they wish to proceed with adjuvant treatments. A full discussion, including risk of recurrence, assessment and explanation of the potential side-effects of radiotherapy, is useful in this context.

The reported outcomes vary, but there is a general consensus that overall pelvic recurrence rates are reduced from the 20–40 per cent range to around 1–5 per cent, although there is no proven influence on survival (Aalders et al., 1980; Lybert et al., 1998; Creutzberg et al., 2000). Side effects are significant in some series, although the BED values can be considered as excessive, particularly as far as the external radiotherapy is concerned. The results of further randomized trials, which use the dose fractionation recommended in this chapter, are awaited with interest.

RADICAL RADIOTHERAPY

Although infrequently performed, this can be effective in those patients deemed inappropriate for pelvic surgery due to medical or anatomical reasons. Treatment can be given by either intracavitary treatment alone or by combination of external-beam radiotherapy and intracavitary treatment.

The 5-year pelvic control rates are good (70–80 per cent at 5 years) for small tumours, but are less satisfactory (<50 per cent) in the higher stages. The tumour stage in this category can only be assessed by clinical and imaging techniques. Recent advances in pelvic imaging have allowed the oncologist to select a treatment dose that is appropriate to the dimensions of the uterus. For example, if there is a relatively small superficial cancer and the uterine wall thickness is only 1.5 cm, then the brachytherapy dose can be prescribed at this distance from the uterine canal, which represents the serosal surface, and this dose cannot then be exceeded in the surrounding normal tissues.

The intracavitary techniques are variable and include:

1 A single line source (Churn and Jones, 1999). This provides a high dose largely confined to the uterus and the length of treatment below the cervix can be adjusted according to the tumour extent. If there is cervical involvement, the activity is extended to include the upper 2 cm of vagina, and it may be necessary to include a longer portion of the vagina, or the whole vagina, according to degree of spread. Following 45 Gy in 25 fractions of external-beam radiotherapy, a dose of 6 Gy × 2 can be given at point A (see p. 748), provided that the rectal and bladder predicted doses are less than 80 per cent of the prescribed dose. A higher dose of 7–8 Gy per fraction may be prescribed at the distance of the uterine serosal surface from the uterine canal, if this is known with reasonable accuracy. The option of variable source positions or dwell times

allows for some degree of isodose curve variation, which can be useful if the tumour position is known with precision. For example, if the tumour is confined to the fundal region, then increased radiation loading at this level can be used (*see* Fig. 34.1).

2 A triple arrangement (uterine tube and ovoids) as in cervical cancer: the classical pear-shaped isodose distribution seems inappropriate, apart from in cases where there is direct tumour extension to the cervix.

3 A double line source in the uterus, one line per cornua.

4 The Heymans capsule, or equivalent technique, where multiple source carriers or catheters are used to fill the uterine cavity (Bond *et al.*, 1997).

5 The umbrella-type applicator, where several catheters splay outwards towards the uterine fundus. This technique requires wide dilatation of the endocervical and uterine canal (Bauer and Schulz-Wendtland, 1993).

The results of several reports of radical radiotherapy are summarized in Table 34.2.

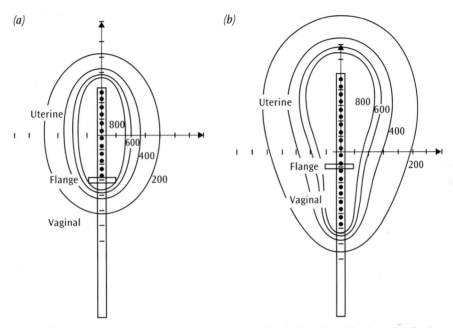

Figure 34.1 *Schematic diagram of source position (indicated by the black circles) and isodose distributions for a single intrauterine catheter. In (a) only the intrauterine portion of the catheter is loaded and each dwell position has an equal dwell time: this produces the cigar-shaped isodose distribution. In (b) the vagina is also included, but the intravaginal dwell times are 50 per cent of those in the intrauterine portion. Here, the isodose width is sufficient to cover the uterine fundus but narrower in order to cover a minimal amount of the paravaginal tissues. The dwell times at the fundal region may require to be increased relative to those in the centre of the catheter if there is a large fundal tumour.*

Table 34.2 *Inoperable uterine cancers treated only by radical radiotherapy*

Author(s)	5-year survival (%) (number of patients)	Grade 3 or severe toxicity (%)	Brachytherapy technique
Patanaphan *et al.* (1985)	46 (54)	N/A	Mainly intracavitary LDR
Wang *et al.* (1987)	46 (41)	N/A	Intracavitary radium
Fishman *et al.* (1996)	80–100 (54)	N/A	Intracavitary + external beam
Varia *et al.* (1987)	26–57 (73)	N/A	Intracavitary + external beam
Kupelian *et al.* (1993)	49–88 (152)	3	Intracavitary + external beam
Rouanet *et al.* (1993)	77 (250)	N/A	Intracavitary + external beam
Taghian *et al.* (1988)	52 (104)	17	LDR
Kukera *et al.* (1998)	53 (280)	<5	Single-line source, HDR
Grigsby *et al.* (1987)	77 (69)	16	Intracavitary ± external beam
Nguyen *et al.* (1995)	76 at 8 years (27)	11	HDR + external beam
Churn and Jones (1999)	Stage I + II = 64 Stage III + IV = 33 (37)	3	Single-line source; LDR or HDR + external beam

Ranges indicate spread of results with disease stage or grade; HDR and LDR, high and low dose rate brachytherapy, respectively; N/A, not applicable.
The references for the above are not in the Reference list, but can be searched individually for further information.

SIDE-EFFECTS

Doses equivalent to 75 Gy radium at point A appear to result in a 17 per cent severe complication rate (Taghian *et al.*, 1988). Techniques that attempt to give a high biological dose of external-beam and brachytherapy will also inevitably result in a high incidence of serious morbidity (Jereczek-Fossa *et al.*, 1998). HDR fraction sizes above 8 Gy are probably best avoided. Some series have used up to a 10 Gy boost after fractionated external radiotherapy, with reports of under 5 per cent severe complications at 5 years (Kucera *et al.*, 1998). Modest brachytherapy fractionation and care in choice of the prescription point may produce a further improvement in therapeutic ratio.

BED values of less than 110 Gy$_3$ appear to be safe in the context of cervical cancer (Leborgne *et al.*, 1997) and thus far BED doses within this range seem to be safe in intact uterine cancers. More recent use of lower prescribed doses and, in some instances, prescription at the serosal surface have produced a reduction in morbidity and adequate tumour control (e.g. Churn and Jones, 1999).

Where intracavitary techniques are not feasible after a standard dose of 45 Gy, it is reasonable to continue the prescription to 50.4 Gy (or higher, using smaller CT-planned fields). Following this, continuing tumour regression may permit successful brachytherapy, although to a lower dose than originally intended in order to respect pelvic tolerance. For extrauterine extension, the use of conformal or CT-planned therapy can, in principle, more safely deliver higher doses, provided the irradiated volume of normal tissue is sufficiently small.

In some patients, the para-aortic lymph nodes are the first site of relapse and these may be treated by radiotherapy with either radical or palliative intent; in the latter case neoadjuvant chemotherapy (e.g. using single-agent carboplatin) may be considered.

PALLIATION

Analgesics, steroids and other supportive medications and care will be necessary in some patients. Palliative radiotherapy can be applied to painful bone metastases and can sometimes, at relatively low dosage, reduce recurrent pelvic bleeding.

Hormones

Increasing concentrations of progestagens secreted by the corpus luteum of pregnancy allow atrophy and metaplasia of the endometrium to form the decidua. Similar effects, with complete remission of recurrent cancers in some patients, are seen in moderately well-differentiated endometrial cancers when supraphysiological doses of progestagens are prescribed (Megace® 160 mg daily; medroxyprogesterone acetate 200 twice or three times daily). Parenteral depot preparations are sometimes useful in relief of symptoms in patients who may not

be compliant or suitable for conventional treatment. The potent mineralocorticoid effect can cause sodium and water retention, and may precipitate hypertension and heart failure, and there is a risk of cerebrovascular accident (CVA). There is no evidence that adjuvant cytotoxic chemotherapy or high-dose progestagens improve survival. In the latter case, a meta-analysis and a large single randomized study have confirmed this (Martin-Hirsch *et al.*, 1996, COSA-NZ-UK Endometrial cancer study groups, 1998).

Studies of adjuvant progestagens following hysterectomy have, in some instances, led to increasing death rates due to side-effects in those treated versus control patients. Careful cardiovascular follow-up is essential in such patients. Obesity may be exacerbated due to appetite stimulation. Tamoxifen may sometimes cause remission, and aromatase inhibitors such as Arimidex® should, theoretically, also be effective. Newer non-steroidal pure anti-oestrogen compounds (Labrie *et al.*, 1999) and other derivatives of tamoxifen (O'Regan *et al.*, 1998) are under development and may have a future preventative and therapeutic role. Another approach has been the use of gonadotrophin-releasing hormones in recurrent cancers; the response rate of 28 per cent does not depend on tumour grade, but is paradoxically highest in previously irradiated sites (Jeyarajah *et al.*, 1996). Some authorities advocate the use of adjuvant progestagens where peritoneal cytology is positive, but there are no randomized trials that address this issue.

Cytotoxic chemotherapy

Younger and fitter patients with advanced tumour on presentation may benefit from initial chemotherapy and, if disease is confined to the pelvis and para-aortic nodes, this may be followed by radiotherapy. There are reports of possible improvements in survival when high-risk patients with papillary serous carcinoma of the uterus are given postoperative cisplatin/carboplatin plus cyclophosphamide (Bancher-Todesca *et al.*, 1998).

Palliation of metastatic disease is frequently disappointing (Muss, 1994). Adriamycin® is reported to be the best single agent (20–40 per cent response rates) and although response rates of up to 30–50 per cent have been reported following combination chemotherapy using Adriamycin® (up to 60 mg/m^2) and cisplatin (50 mg/m^2) given every 3 weeks, the duration of remissions is short. For older patients, the use of carboplatin (i.v. 350 mg/m^2 or AUC 5-6) should be considered, as this agent is fairly well tolerated and responses have been reported in stage IV patients (Cook *et al.*, 1999). There are also preliminary reports of responses using paclitaxel combinations.

Very young patients

Although rare, the condition can arise in premenopausal patients, where there are associations with polycystic ovaries, unopposed-oestrogen oral contraceptives and the use of oestrogens in gonadal dysgenesis. The cancers are usually well differentiated with minimal invasion and, in some instances, progestagens may be used to induce regression if fertility is to be preserved.

Follow-up

After standard adjuvant treatment: 3–6 monthly for 2 years then annually. Surveillance patients: 2–3 monthly for 2 years, then at longer intervals. Vault smears can be used in surveillance follow-up, but can cause diagnostic uncertainty after adjuvant radiotherapy. Where careful vaginal examination reveals an apparent recurrence, a formal incisional biopsy should be taken. Patients who have recurrent tumours should always see a clinical oncologist with an interest in this condition. CA 125 antigen levels are unhelpful, apart from in papillary serous variants.

Re-treatment

This can sometimes be attempted, particularly if previous treatment has not been given to a full radical dose or has been given to a limited volume. For example, if vaginal brachytherapy had previously been used to give vault irradiation only, a recurrence in the lower third of the vagina may be treated by further brachytherapy (or a combination of external beam and brachytherapy) with activity restricted to the tumour site and appropriate margin. Alternatively, interstitial brachytherapy combined with external-beam radiotherapy can be used to treat small-volume vault recurrences (Charra et al., 1998).

Limited doses of further external radiation may be given to palliate bleeding and pain, although the patient must understand that there is a relatively high risk of serious normal-tissue damage/reactions.

Future prospects

Greater use of imaging with conformal radiotherapy techniques may allow for safer and even more effective use of radiotherapy. The advent of CT/MRI-compatible applicators should enable much greater specificity of treatment volumes. Gene-specific therapies may allow effective tumour control with lower doses of radiation, as well as better control of metastatic spread.

SARCOMAS OF THE UTERUS

These rare tumours are managed by similar general principles as already discussed for epithelial malignant tumours of the uterus (Sevin and Angioli, 1996). There are several distinct pathological entities, which mainly comprise the carcinosarcomas or mixed mesodermal sarcomas, the leiomyosarcomas and the stromal carcinomas. Grading is as for sarcomas at other sites. Myxoid leiomyosarcomas appear to be of low grade but can behave in a malignant fashion. Positive peritoneal cytology appears to be prognostically important.

Patterns of spread may differ, but the adenocarcinomas within a mixed carcinosarcoma are associated with a greater tendency to spread via lymphatics rather than via the bloodstream.

There is no proven role for adjuvant cytotoxic chemotherapy, but chemotherapy may provide palliation of symptoms caused by systemic spread. Adriamycin® at a dose of up to 60 mg/m^2 is the best single agent, and there is insufficient evidence to support the use of combination chemotherapy. The uterine sarcomas should not be regarded as highly radioresistant, for although leiomyosarcomas are correctly included in this category, the other types may shrink in a slow but protracted manner after radical radiotherapy. Durable control of symptoms can occasionally be achieved after either conventionally fractionated or relatively low-dose hypofractionated palliative doses have been given.

In general, the local recurrence rates after surgery (approximately 50–80 per cent) are significantly greater than for carcinomas, even in the case of relatively well-differentiated sarcomas. Postoperative radiotherapy is usually given to prevent recurrence. Many retrospective series show a 15–30 per cent reduction in pelvic recurrence, but there is no definite evidence of enhanced survival. Care must be taken that there is no previous history of radiation exposure, which occurs in approximately 10 per cent of patients. Radical radiotherapy, rarely given in the case of inoperable or medically unfit patients, is reported to result in a 14 per cent 5-year survival for all stages, but 44 per cent in the stage I category, although the numbers of patients treated are small. It is important to remember that low-grade endometrial stromal sarcomas may regress with high-dose progestagen therapy.

SIGNIFICANT POINTS

- Because of age and co-morbidities, careful selection of patients is required for primary surgery or radical radiotherapy.
- After primary surgery, the indications for postoperative radiotherapy must be considered carefully.
- Recurrence at the vaginal vault following surgery alone is curable after radiotherapy in approximately 50 per cent of patients.

- Research for a safe form of adjuvant hormone therapy is required.
- Careful use of progestagens, or other alternatives, including tamoxifen, can provide valuable remissions.

KEY REFERENCES

Aalders, J., Abeler, V., Kolstad, P. et al. (1980) Postoperative external irradiation and prognostic parameters in stage I endometrial carcinoma; clinical and histopathological study of 540 patients. Obstet. Gynaecol. **56**, 419–27.

Creutzberg, C.I., Van Putten, W., Koper, P.C. et al. (2000) Surgery and post operative radiotherapy for patients with stage I endometrial carcinoma: multicentre randomised trial: PORTEC Study Group. Lancet **355**, 1404–11.

Thomas, R. and Blake, P. (1996) Endometrial carcinoma: adjuvant locoregional therapy. Clin. Oncol. **8**, 140–5.

Wylie, J., Irwin, C., Putulie, M. et al. (2000) Results of radical radiotherapy for recurrent endometrial cancer. Gynaecol. Oncol. **77**, 66–72.

REFERENCES

Aalders, J., Abeler, V., Kolstad, P. et al. (1980) Postoperative external irradiation and prognostic parameters in stage I endometrial carcinoma; clinical and histopathological study of 540 patients. Obstet. Gynaecol. **56**, 419–27.

Bancher-Todesca, D., Neunteufel, W., Williams, K.E. et al. (1998) Influence of postoperative treatment on survival in patients with uterine papillary serous carcinoma. Gynecol. Oncol. **71**, 344–7.

Bauer, M. and Schulz-Wendtland, R. (1993) Technical note: a new afterloading applicator for primary brachytherapy of endometrial cancer. Br. J. Radiol. **783**, 256–9.

Bond, M.G., Workman, G., Martland, J. et al. (1997) Dosimetric considerations of inoperable endometrial carcinoma by a high dose afterloading packing technique. Clin. Oncol. **9**, 41–7.

Cancer Survival Trends (1999) Cancer survival trends, 1971–1995. London: The Stationary Office.

Chadha, M., Nanavati, P.J., Liu, P., Fanning, J. and Jacobs, A. (1999) Patterns of failure in endometrial carcinoma stage IB grade 3 and IC patients treated with postoperative vaginal vault brachytherapy. Gynecol. Oncol. **75**, 103–7.

Charra, C., Roy, P., Coquard, R. et al. (1998) Outcome of treatment of the upper third vaginal recurrences of cervical and endometrial carcinomas with interstitial brachytherapy. Int. J. Radiat. Oncol. Biol. Phys. **40**(2), 421–6.

Churn, M. and Jones, B. (1999) Primary radiotherapy for carcinoma of the endometrium using external beam radiotherapy and single line source brachytherapy. Clin. Oncol. **11**, 255–62.

Cook, A.M., Lodge, N. and Blake, P.R. (1999) Stage IV endometrial cancer: a 10 year review of patients. Br. J. Radiol. **72**, 485–8.

COSA-NZ-UK Endometrial cancer study groups (1998) Adjuvant medroxyprogesterone acetate in high-risk endometrial cancer. Int. J. Gynaecol. Cancer **8**, 387–91.

Creasman, W.T. (1993) Prognostic significance of hormone receptors in endometrial cancer. Cancer **71**, 1467–70.

Creutzberg, C.I., Van Putten, W., Koper, P.C. et al. (2000) Surgery and post operative radiotherapy for patients with stage I endometrial carcinoma: multicentre randomised trial: PORTEC Study Group. Lancet **355**, 1404–11.

Hicks, M.L., Piver, M.S., Puretz, J.L. et al. (1993) Survival in patients with paraaortic lymph node metastasis from endometrial adenocarcinoma clinically limited to the uterus. Int. J. Radiat. Oncol. Biol. Phys. **26**, 607–11.

Jereczek-Fossa, B., Jassem, J., Nowak, R. and Badzio, A. (1998) Late complications after post operative radiotherapy in endometrial cancer: analysis of 317 consecutive cases with application of linear-quadratic model. Int. J. Radiat. Oncol. Biol. Phys. **41**, 329–38.

Jeyarajah, A.R., Gallagher, C.J., Blake, P.R. et al. (1996) Long term follow up of gonadotrophin-releasing hormone analog treatment for recurrent endometrial cancer. Gynecol. Oncol. **63**, 47–52.

Jones, B., Pryce, P.L., Blake, P.R. and Dale, R.G. (1999) High dose rate brachytherapy practice for the treatment of gynaecological cancers in the UK. Br. J. Radiol. **72**, 371–7.

Kadar, N., Holmesley, H.D. and Malfetano, J.H. (1992) Positive peritoneal cytology is an adverse fact in endometrial carcinoma only if there is other evidence of extrauterine disease. Gynecol. Oncol. **46**, 145–9.

Kihana, T., Hamada, K., Inoue, Y. et al. (1995) Mutation and allelic loss of the p53 gene in endometrial cancer. Cancer **76**, 72–8.

Kilgore, L.C., Partridge, E.E., Alvarez, R.D. et al. (1995) Adenocarcinoma of the endometrium: survival comparisons of patients with and without pelvic node sampling. Gynecol. Oncol. **56**, 29–33.

Kucera, H., Knokke, T.H., Kukera, E. and Potter, R. (1998) Treatment of endometrial carcinoma with high-dose-rate brachytherapy alone in medically inoperable patients. Acta Obstet. Gynaecol. Scand. **77**, 1008–12.

Labrie, F., Labrie, C., Belanger, A. *et al.* (1999) EM-652 (SCH 57069), a third generation SERM acting as pure antiestrogen in the mammary gland and endometrium. *J. Steroid Biochem. Mol. Biol.* **69**, 51–84.

Larson, D.M., Berg, R., Shaw, G. and Krawisz, B.R. (1999) Prognostic significance of DNA ploidy in endometrial cancer. *Gynecol. Oncol.* **74**, 356–60.

Leborgne, F., Fowler, J.F., Leborgne, J.H. *et al.* (1997) Biologically effective doses in medium dose rate brachytherapy of cancer of the cervix. *Radiat. Oncol. Invest.* **5**, 289–99.

Lybert, M.L., Van Putten, W.L., Brolmann, H.A. and Coeburgh, J.W. (1998) Postoperative radiotherapy for endometrial carcinoma, Stage I. Wide variation in referral patterns but no effect on long term survival in a retrospective study in the Southeast Netherlands. *Eur. J. Cancer* **34**, 586–90.

Martin-Hirsch, P.L., Lilford, R.J. and Jarvis, G.J. (1996) Adjuvant progestagen therapy for the treatment of endometrial cancer: review and meta-analyses of published randomised trials. *Eur. J. Obstet. Gynecol. Reprod. Biol.* **8**, 387–91.

Mundt, A.J. and Condi, P.P. (2000) Do conventional pathological factors lose their prognostic significance following postoperative radiation therapy in pathological stage I–II endometrial adenocarcinoma? *Int. J. Cancer* **90**, 224–30.

Muss, H.B. (1994) Chemotherapy of metastatic endometrial cancer. *Semin. Oncol.* **21**, 107–13.

Newcomb, P.A., Solomon, C. and White, E. (1999) Tamoxifen and risk of large bowel cancer in women with breast cancer. *Breast Cancer Res. Treat.* **53**, 271–7.

Olson, J.E., Sellars, T.A., Anderson, K.E. and Folsom, A.R. (1999) Does a family history of cancer increase the risk of postmenopausal endometrial cancer? *Cancer* **85**, 2444–9.

O'Regan, R.M., Cisneros, A., England, G.M. *et al.* (1998) Effects of the antioestrogens tamoxifen, toremifine and ICI 182, 780 on endometrial cancer growth. *J. Nat. Cancer Inst.* **90**, 1552–8.

Semczuk, A., Berbec, H., Kostuch, M. *et al.* (1997) Detection of K-*ras* mutations in cancerous lesions of human endometrium. *Eur. J. Gynaecol. Oncol.* **18**, 80–3.

Sevin, B.-U. and Angioli, R. (1996) In Sevin, B.-U., Knapstein, P.G. and Kochli, O.R. (eds), *Multimodality therapy in gynaecological oncology*. Stuttgart: N.Y. Thieme Press, 53–5.

Taghian, A., Pernot, M., Hoffstetter, S. *et al.* (1988) Radiotherapy alone for medically inoperable patients with inoperable carcinoma of the endometrium. *Int. J. Radiat. Oncol. Biol. Phys.* **15**, 1135–40.

Terishima, I., Suzuki, N. and Shibutani, S. (1999) Mutagenic potential of alpha-(N_2-deoxyguanosinyl) tamoxifen lesions, the major DNA adducts detected in endometrial tissues of patients treated with tamoxifen. *Cancer Res.* **59**, 2091–5.

Thomas, R. and Blake, P. (1996) Endometrial carcinoma: adjuvant locoregional therapy. *Clin. Oncol.* **8**, 140–5.

Tritz, D., Pieretti, M., Turner, S. and Powell, D. (1997) Loss of heterozygosity in usual and special variant carcinomas of the endometrium. *Hum. Pathol.* **28**, 607–12.

Weiss, M.F., Connell, P.P., Waggoner, S. *et al.* (1999) External pelvic radiotherapy in stage IC endometrial carcinoma. *Obstet. Gynecol.* **93**, 599–602.

35

Cervix

PETER BLAKE

INCIDENCE AND CAUSES

Incidence

INVASIVE CARCINOMA OF THE CERVIX

Invasive tumours of the female genital tract include those of the ovary, uterus, cervix, vagina and vulva and the rare gestational trophoblastic tumours. Worldwide, cervical cancer is the second most common female malignancy after breast cancer and far exceeds cancer of either the ovary or endometrium in incidence. In many developing countries it is the most common cancer in females, and in India cancer of the cervix is the most common cause of death in women aged between 35 and 45 years.

The incidence of cervical malignancy varies widely from one country to another, and between cultures and social classes within the same country. In Columbia, Central America, there is a 5.5 per cent lifetime risk of developing invasive carcinoma of the cervix. In England and Wales this risk is 1.25 per cent, and in Spain and Israel the risk is only 0.5 per cent. In the USA the incidence in African–American women is approximately twice that in Caucasian women. In the west of Scotland, there has been shown to be a clear association between socio-economic status and the incidence of invasive cervical carcinoma, with a threefold increased incidence in women from low socio-economic groups compared to more affluent women (Lammont et al., 1993).

In the UK gynaecological malignancies account for approximately 15 000 cases per annum of cancer in females and are second in incidence only to breast cancer, with an approximate incidence of 25 000 cases per annum. The incidence of invasive cervical cancer in the UK is about 4500 cases per annum, slightly less than that of ovarian cancer and slightly more than that of endometrial cancer (OPCS, 1989). The great majority are squamous tumours.

PRE-INVASIVE DISEASE OF THE CERVIX

Cervical intra-epithelial neoplasia precedes virtually every case of invasive squamous carcinoma of the cervix. This pre-invasive disease is commonly asymptomatic but may be detected by cytological examination of exfoliated cells taken from the transformation zone of the cervix at cervical smear. These cells are studied microscopically using the Papanicolau stain and an assessment made of the size, shape and mitotic activity of the nuclei and the nuclear–cytoplasmic ratio. On the basis of this assessment, the cells will be reported as being normal, as being inflammatory or showing mild atypia, as showing mild, moderate or severe dyskaryosis or as being characteristic of invasive disease. Those patients with moderate or severe changes require biopsy of the cervix for histological assessment (Anderson, 1985).

Abnormal glandular cells are much more difficult to sample and detect on exfoliative cytology due to their position higher in the endocervical canal and their situation deep within the glandular crypts of the endocervix. Criteria for the diagnosis of glandular intra-epithelial neoplasia and adenocarcinoma in-situ are similarly more complex than for the squamous counterparts.

The ease and reliability of exfoliative cytology has resulted in the establishment of many screening programmes for cervical squamous neoplasia. In some areas a well-organized programme with a high compliance rate has resulted in a large proportion of cases of cervical neoplasia being found in the pre-invasive stage or in the early, curable stages of invasive disease. This has reduced both the incidence of invasive cervical cancer and the mortality from the disease. This has been the result of cervical screening programmes in British Columbia, Iceland and Finland. In the UK, a decrease in mortality has only been seen due to improved coverage of the screening campaign. This was achieved in the early 1990s. Prior to that the poor compliance rate and a less well-organized service had produced little overall effect (Sigurdson, 1993). If screening is to have a major impact on disease incidence, an effective call and re-call system has to exist, in addition to a high-quality cytological service and adequate treatment facilities. Such a system can be difficult to operate in underdeveloped areas, where there are communication problems, and in developed areas where there is a large, shifting population of women at risk, as in metropolitan cities.

The use of screening programmes in some countries has altered the proportions of patients seen with pre-invasive and invasive neoplasia of the cervix, resulting in an overall drop in the incidence of invasive disease. However, in some subgroups of women, defined mainly by age and by sexual behaviour, there is a rising incidence of both pre-invasive and invasive cervical neoplasia. This is the case both within those countries with early detection programmes and in countries where screening is not yet established (Cook and Draper, 1984).

The peak incidence of cervical intra-epithelial neoplasia occurs between the ages of 25 and 40, whilst the peak incidence of invasive carcinoma occurs in a group of patients approximately 10 years older.

Causes of cervical neoplasia

There are several aetiological factors associated with carcinoma of the cervix, including sexual behaviour, parity, genital wart disease and smoking. The most marked of these is the sexual behaviour of both the woman and her partner.

SEXUAL BEHAVIOUR

Female behaviour

For many years an aetiological link between sexual intercourse and the development of cervical neoplasia has been recognized (Beral, 1974). Two aspects of sexual behaviour, the age at first intercourse and the number of sexual partners, have been studied extensively. There is a higher incidence of both pre-invasive cervical intra-epithelial neoplasia and of invasive disease in girls who commence regular intercourse in their teens compared with those who do not commence sexual activity until a later age. This suggests that the adolescent cervix is more vulnerable to potential oncogenic agents. In addition, the number of sexual partners appears to be important, with some studies having found a history of six or more sexual partners to be a significant risk factor.

Both low socio-economic status and multiparity are associated with a higher incidence of cervical neoplasia, but neither of these risk factors can probably be considered to be independent of age at first intercourse.

Male behaviour

The influence of the sexual histories of the women's partners has been less extensively studied than the sexual histories of the women themselves (Zunzunegui et al., 1986). In some studies, an association between cervical neoplasia and a history of the male partner having multiple other sexual partners has been noted. This gave rise, some years ago, to the concept of the 'high risk' male whose female partners are at a higher risk than average of developing cervical neoplasia due to the male being infected with a transmissible agent (Singer et al., 1976).

Contraception

A lower incidence of cervical neoplasia has been found in women using barrier methods of contraception than in those using the oral contraceptive pill. It is known that seminal fluid contains potent local immunosupressants, against which the cervix would be protected by barrier methods. Whilst this is further evidence of there being a transmissible agent in the aetiology of cervical neoplasia, it is not clear whether oral contraceptives themselves predispose to the development of cervical cancer.

All these observations would support the theory that there is at least one transmissible agent involved in cervical neoplasia.

SMOKING

The products of smoking are concentrated in cervical mucus and smoking produces changes in the DNA of cervical squamous cells. In addition, smoking decreases the population of Langerhan's cells responsible for cell-mediated immunity in the cervix. Both of these findings could indicate an important role for smoking in the development of cervical neoplasia, both by direct carcinogenesis and by rendering the cervix more vulnerable to infection by a transmissible agent (Barton et al., 1988).

IMMUNOSUPPRESSION

Smoking may cause some degree of local immunosuppression in the cervix, but systemic immunosuppression of patients who have undergone renal transplantation has been recognized for a considerable time as being a risk factor for cervical cancer. Cervical neoplasia is also more common in women with HIV, and the onset of invasive disease is an 'AIDS-defining illness' (Maiman et al., 1990).

TRANSMISSIBLE INFECTIVE AGENTS

Viruses

Most research in this area has concentrated in recent years on the roles of the herpes and papilloma viruses. Herpes simplex virus type 2 (HSV2) was shown to be weakly oncogenic in the laboratory, but analysis of many cervical tumours has failed to show that HSV2 is likely to be involved in carcinogenesis.

Human papillomaviruses (HPV), however, have attracted more attention in recent years, and there is a clear link between certain types of papilloma virus and cervical neoplasia. Over 70 types of HPV have now been isolated, and at least 20 of these infect the lower female genital tract. Several of these are associated with neoplasia, but type 16 and, to a lesser extent, type 18 are particularly associated with cervical intra-epithelial neoplasia and invasive disease. Both these viruses have the ability to transform cells in culture and these transformed cells can give rise to tumours in immunocompromised mice. It was initially tempting to think that HPV virus was the transmissible agent involved in cervical neoplasia and that infection with HPV ultimately gave rise to neoplasia. This theory was supported by finding HPV in a large proportion of cervical tumours and a much smaller incidence in normal cervical tissue (Baird, 1985).

Methods of detecting these viruses improved, most notably with the development of the polymerase chain reaction, which can detect a few copies of viral RNA. By this method the viruses could be found in small quantities in many more normal women than was previously the case. It appeared that HPV was almost ubiquitous in the female population and the relationship to neoplasia became obscure again. However, the presence of HPV may have been over-reported, due to poor laboratory practice, allowing the contamination of specimens with tiny quantities of virus.

Where stringent laboratory practices have been used, there is a clear difference in the prevalence of HPV in women with cervical neoplasia and in those without disease. In particular, it appears that normal women may well have episodes of infection with the virus which they then eradicate without neoplasia developing. Those women who fail to eradicate HPV infection, or who are repeatedly infected, may be at risk of developing cervical neoplasia (Munoz et al., 1988).

Further evidence for the role of HPV is the finding that those types associated with neoplasia may produce two proteins, E6 and E7, which bind to the protein p53, a product of the *p53* tumour supressor gene, and pRb, a product of the retinoblastoma gene, which is also involved in cell regulation (Tidy and Wrede, 1992). The normal function of these genes is to prevent cells with abnormal DNA from replicating, and DNA damage may be caused by several factors, most notably age and smoking.

It is likely that carcinogenesis in cervical squamous cells is a multi-factorial process. However, HPV now seems to

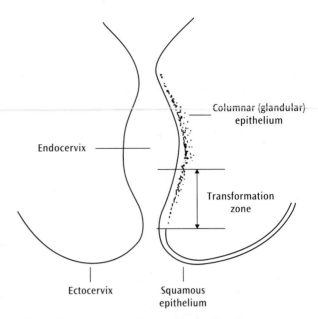

Figure 35.1 *Diagram of the cervix, showing the 'transformation zone', where the columnar epithelium of the endocervix meets the squamous epithelium of the ectocervix.*

be clearly implicated in this process, both by epidemiological and laboratory findings. Nevertheless, it is important for the patient and her partner that the medical profession resists the labelling of cervical neoplasia as simply another sexually transmitted disease, with the overtones that this label carries of sexual promiscuity and infidelity.

Site of action of the transmissible agent

The majority of neoplasias of the cervix arise at the squamo-columnar junction, an area known as the 'transformation zone', where columnar epithelium undergoes the metaplastic process of becoming squamous epithelium (Fig. 35.1). This transformation zone is larger in puberty, pregnancy and when taking the oral contraceptive pill. If this area of the cervix is seen as the 'target' on which a transmissible agent could work, then this could go some way to explain why sexual intercourse in puberty, when the transformation zone is large, is a risk factor. The importance of multiparity and the use of the oral contraceptive pill in cervical neoplasia could also be explained.

PATHOLOGY

Anatomy

ANATOMY OF THE CERVIX

The female reproductive organs comprise the vulva, vagina, uterus, Fallopian tubes and ovaries, and lie within the pelvis. They are represented in Figures 35.2 and 35.3. The uterus comprises of the uterine body, also known

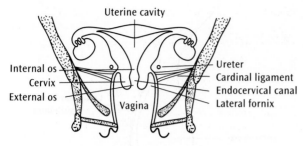

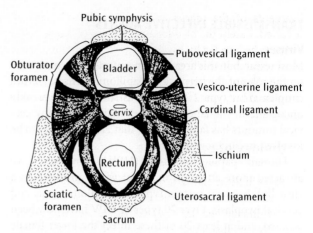

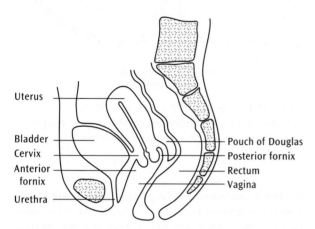

Figure 35.2 *Diagram of the cervix, showing the relationship to the ureters and the cardinal ligaments (parametria).*

Figure 35.4 *The ligaments supporting the uterus at the level of the cervix.*

Figure 35.3 *Lateral view of the pelvis, showing the relationship of the cervix to the bladder, rectum and pouch of Douglas.*

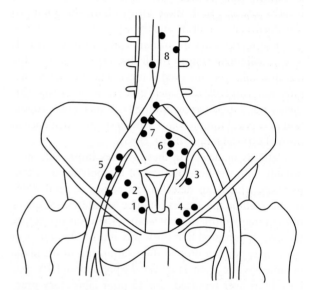

Figure 35.5 *The lymph node drainage of the cervix: (1) paracervical, (2) parametrial, (3) internal iliac, (4) obturator, (5) external iliac, (6) pre-sacral, (7) common iliac and (8) para-aortic nodes.*

as the corpus, and the cervix, which is the lower one-third and which enters the vagina. The relationship of the cervix to other structures in the pelvis is that it lies above and in continuity with the vagina, is posterior to the bladder, anterior to the rectum and pouch of Douglas and is related cranially to the body of the uterus, the peritoneum and the pelvic cavity. Laterally, the cervix abuts the paracervical tissues, the broad ligaments and the ureters, which run close to the lateral margins of the cervix (Fig. 35.2).

The cervix is supported by the cardinal ligaments laterally, the uterovesical ligaments anteriorly and the uterosacral ligaments posteriorly (Fig. 35.4). The endocervical canal connects the vagina with the uterine cavity and is lined by columnar epithelium. The part of the cervix protruding into the vagina, the exocervix, is covered by stratified squamous epithelium. The cervix and body of the uterus are small in childhood, enlarge during puberty and the reproductive years and then atrophy after the menopause. The junction between the columnar and squamous epithelium is called the 'transformation zone' and this zone enlarges in puberty, pregnancy and when taking the oral contraceptive pill (Fig. 35.1). The transformation zone also changes in position, being usually just inside the external cervical os in young women, but rising up the endocervical canal after the menopause.

LYMPHATIC DRAINAGE

There is a relatively well-defined pattern for the lymphatic drainage of the cervix, with direct drainage to the internal, external and common iliac nodes. Other node groups which may be involved by direct lymphatic spread are the parametrial, obturator and presacral nodes. Spread to the para-aortic nodes is uncommon without pelvic node involvement, and the supra-clavicular nodes may be involved subsequent to para-aortic node disease (Fig. 35.5).

Spread of disease

Cervical carcinoma spreads predominantly by direct invasion and lymphatic permeation. Direct spread is superiorly into the body of the uterus and inferiorly into the vaginal mucosa. Laterally, the parametrial tissues, ligaments of the uterus and pelvic side-wall may be involved. Rarely, the bladder anteriorly or rectum posteriorly can be invaded by advanced disease. Spread is usually continuous, but seedlings from cervical cancer can occasionally be noted in the lower vagina. Blood-borne spread is unusual but, when it does occur, is to the lungs, bone and liver.

Pathology of pre-invasive disease

Changes in the metaplastic process at the transformation zone may lead to dysplasia, which is known as cervical intra-epithelial neoplasia (CIN). The terms CIN1, CIN2 and CIN3 are histological terms used to describe increasing degrees of dysplasia from mild to moderate to severe. Cervical epithelium showing severe dysplasia (CIN3) was previously known as carcinoma *in-situ*.

It is known that a proportion of cases of CIN3 can develop into invasive carcinoma, whereas the great majority of CIN1 and most of CIN2 may revert to normal epithelium if left untreated. It is not known exactly what proportion of CIN3 may revert to normal and what proportion progresses to invasive disease, as ethical considerations dictate that all cases of CIN3 are treated. However, although the natural history of CIN is not entirely known, it is thought that, in most women, the transformation of benign epithelium to invasive cancer takes 10–15 years.

Micro-invasive carcinoma of the cervix

Once the basement membrane beneath the epithelium is breached by the neoplastic process the disease can no longer be termed pre-invasive and such disease is referred to as being microinvasive. In the FIGO (International Federation of Gynaecology and Obstetrics) classification (FIGO, 1992) this is stage Ia, which is subdivided into stage Ia1 and Ia2 (Table 35.1) according to whether the depth of invasion is up to 3 or 5 mm, respectively. When disease is more than 5 mm deep or wider than 7 mm, it is no longer referred to as microinvasive, but falls within the category of FIGO stage Ib invasive carcinoma of the cervix.

Invasive carcinoma of the cervix

Between 85 and 95 per cent of cervical carcinomas are squamous, the remainder being predominantly adenocarcinoma, adenosquamous carcinoma or, very rarely, sarcoma, lymphoma or melanoma.

SQUAMOUS CARCINOMA

Most squamous carcinomas involve the exocervix and are visible on a speculum examination. Some, however, develop within the endocervical canal and may remain occult until reaching quite a large size (a barrel carcinoma). Visible tumours may be either exophytic or ulcerating with underlying infiltration of surrounding structures.

Table 35.1 *Staging for carcinoma of the cervix (FIGO)*

Stage	Features
0	Pre-invasive carcinoma (CIN)
Ia1	Pre-clinical carcinoma, minimal microinvasion: diagnosed by microscopy only
Ia2	Pre-clinical carcinoma, microinvasion <5 mm deep and <7 mm wide: diagnosed by microscopy only
Ib1	Carcinoma more extensive than Ia2 but confined to the uterus (including the uterine body) <4 cm diameter
Ib2	Carcinoma more extensive than Ia2 but confined to the uterus (including the uterine body) >4 cm diameter
IIa	Carcinoma extending beyond the cervix into the upper two-thirds of the vagina
IIb	Carcinoma extending into the parametria but not reaching the pelvic side-wall
IIIa	Carcinoma involving the lower third of the vagina, but not reaching the pelvic side-wall
IIIb	Carcinoma extending to the pelvic side-wall or causing ureteric stenosis or obstruction
IVa	Carcinoma involving the mucosa of the bladder or rectum, or extending beyond the true pelvis
IVb	Distant metastasis

Commonly, tumours are graded as well differentiated (grade 1), moderately differentiated (grade 2) and poorly differentiated (grade 3). Alternatively, squamous tumours may be described as keratinizing, large-cell non-keratinizing and small cell non-keratinizing carcinomas. Occasionally, well-differentiated squamous carcinomas having the appearance of condylomata accuminata are seen, these are called verrucous carcinomas. Rarely, small cell neuroendocrine tumours similar to oat cell carcinoma of the bronchus are seen and these have a similar poor prognosis.

ADENOCARCINOMA

Adenocarcinomas arise from the glandular epithelium lining the endocervical canal and the endocervical glands. Because of the much more irregular nature of the boundary between the epithelium and the underlying stroma, it is much more difficult, in the case of adenocarcinoma, to define a pre-invasive, *in situ* stage equivalent to CIN3. However, pre-invasive forms of adenocarcinoma are being recognized with increasing frequency, and criteria are being developed to define glandular intra-epithelial neoplasia and adenocarcinoma *in-situ*. Adenocarcinoma has often been thought to carry a worse prognosis than squamous carcinoma, but this is probably due to the origin, deep in the endocervical canal, leading to a later presentation of disease on the exocervix and an increased bulk of tumour, stage for stage.

As the screening campaigns have reduced the incidence of squamous neoplasia, the incidence of adenocarcinoma has risen. However, this seems not simply to be due to the selective reduction in squamous neoplasia but also to a genuine increase in the incidence of glandular neoplasia, possibly associated with HPV type 18.

ADENOSQUAMOUS CARCINOMA

An increasing number of squamous carcinomas are being reported as showing glandular elements. While this may reflect a change in the incidence of adenosquamous carcinoma, it may also be a product of increasing use of histochemical stains for mucin production and recognition of an adenocarcinomatous component.

CLINICAL FEATURES OF INVASIVE CARCINOMA OF THE CERVIX

Symptoms

An increasing number of invasive cervical carcinomas are detected in the pre-symptomatic stages at cervical screening. However, the majority of patients still present with symptoms. The most common symptom of invasive cervical cancer is of bleeding, which may be post-coital, intermenstrual or postmenopausal. Vaginal discharge is the second most common symptom. These symptoms should always be investigated by clinical examination, inspection of the cervix and exfoliative cytology.

Although some women complain of a 'dragging' sensation in the pelvis, pain only occurs in advanced cases with nerve or muscle involvement. Similarly, rectal bleeding and haematuria are symptoms of locally advanced disease (stage IV).

Signs

Visual inspection of the cervix may reveal it to be enlarged, have obvious growth on the surface or to be ulcerated. In addition, node masses may be palpable in the groins or abdomen and in the left supra-clavicular fossa. Patients with advanced disease may have tumour in the vagina or vulva and may have symptoms and signs of anaemia, jaundice or uraemia.

INVESTIGATIONS

Investigations for pre-invasive neoplasia of the cervix

SCREENING

Effective screening of the cervix is carried out by obtaining a sample of cells from the endocervix, transformation zone and the exocervix by scraping the surface with a spatula. The most commonly used is Ayre's spatula which is made of wood (Fig. 35.6). The cells obtained on the spatula are spread on to a glass slide and fixed in 70 per cent alcohol immediately. They can then be stained later by the Papanicolau method. Cells are examined microscopically and are reported as being normal, inflammatory, showing mild atypia, mild dyskaryosis, moderate dyskaryosis, severe dyskaryosis, as being malignant or, finally, as being characteristic of invasive carcinoma. Cervical cytology can give rise to both false-negative and false-positive results, and confirmation of positive or unexpectedly negative cytological findings should be sought by colposcopy and biopsy.

The frequency of cervical screening is a matter for debate. In the UK the recommendation in most areas in the 1970s and early 1980s was that screening should be repeated every 5 years from the age of 35 to 60 years. However, it was recognized that sexually active women younger than 35 years were at risk and, moreover, it was these younger women who were more prepared to attend for screening, while the attendance rate in older women was poor (Cardiff Cervical Cytology Study, 1980). It was recognized that, to reduce the risk of developing invasive disease, screening should take place throughout a woman's sexually active life. Nowadays, many general practitioners take a smear every 3 years, at ante-natal assessments, or when clinically indicated. In some societies, especially where private medicine flourishes, cervical smears are taken annually.

More than 80 per cent of cases of pre-invasive disease will be detected at 5-yearly screening and, indeed, it is said that even one single cervical smear, taken at the age of 35–45 years, will reduce the lifetime risk of developing invasive cancer by 45 per cent. Increasing the frequency of screening increases the rate of detection only slightly. Therefore, the cost-effectiveness falls. In addition, with increased frequency of screening, lesser degrees of

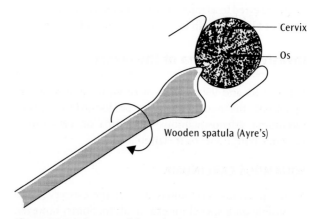

Figure 35.6 *Diagram of how the long tongue of an Ayre's spatula should be pushed well into the cervical os before rotating the spatula through 360 degrees to obtain cells from the transformation zone for exfoliative cytology.*

intra-epithelial neoplasia (CIN1 and CIN2) are found more often and are then treated. As it is known that many of these conditions return to normal if left untreated, this increased detection rate of low- or moderate-grade abnormalities may result in unnecessary treatment, morbidity and expense. A 3–5-yearly smear from the age of commencement of sexual activity to the age of 70 years is probably the most cost-effective programme (Benedet and Murphy, 1985).

COLPOSCOPY

This technique of examination involves looking at the cervix with a low-power microscope and can be carried out without the need for a general anaesthetic. By staining the cervix and upper vagina with acetic acid or iodine, areas of abnormal epithelium can be identified and biopsied precisely. In the case of extensive abnormalities or ones that extend up the endocervical canal and which cannot be entirely visualized, cone biopsy may be necessary.

Investigations for invasive disease

CLINICAL EXAMINATION

Clinical examination of the patient should involve palpation of the abdomen to detect enlarged kidneys, an enlarged or irregular liver, palpable para-aortic nodes or an enlarged bladder. The inguinal and supra-clavicular areas should be examined for metastatic lymph nodes. The vulva should be inspected and then the vagina and cervix examined using a speculum. If an abnormality is seen, a smear or punch biopsy should be taken for diagnosis. The cervix should be examined bimanually to assess the size, shape and mobility of the uterus and any extension of tumour into surrounding tissues. Rectal examination gives additional information on posterior spread along the uterosacral ligaments and lateral parametrial invasion and involvement of the pelvic side-wall.

EXAMINATION UNDER ANAESTHETIC

Investigations to assess the extent of disease must include an examination under anaesthetic, when both abdominal and pelvic examination will be carried out. In addition, a cystoscopy is necessary to rule out bladder involvement and, if there is any suspicion of posterior spread, proctoscopy and sigmoidoscopy should also be completed.

The endocervical canal should be dilated and curetted, following which there should be curettage of the endometrial cavity. The cervix itself is biopsied, if histological diagnosis has not already been made by punch biopsy, as is any other abnormality in the vagina or vulva.

HAEMATOLOGICAL AND RADIOLOGICAL TESTS

Serum electrolytes, a full blood count and renal and liver function tests will give an indication as to whether or not there is renal impairment by ureteric involvement, liver metastases or anaemia from tumour haemorrhage.

Further examination of the renal tract can be by intravenous urogram (IVU), ultrasound scan or computed tomography (CT) scan, and a chest X-ray can demonstrate metastatic disease. Nodal disease can be imaged by lymphography, CT scanning, ultrasound scanning or magnetic resonance imaging (MRI). Most commonly, a CT scan will be used to assess the state of the liver, renal tract, para-aortic and pelvic lymph nodes and direct spread within the pelvis. However, in the pelvis, MRI is a more effective method of imaging both primary disease and nodal involvement.

CLINICAL STAGING

Tumour staging

The most widely used staging system is that of FIGO, which is given in Table 35.1. Apart from microinvasive disease, which is defined histologically, the system depends largely on clinical examination under anaesthetic. The results of cystoscopy, proctoscopy, chest X-ray and IVU can all be used in determining FIGO stage, but other imaging techniques do not alter tumour staging.

Nodal status

Apart from FIGO stage IIIb, which may be used to describe the presence of a pelvic side-wall mass arising from involved nodes, the FIGO system does not take account of nodal involvement and this must be described separately. The TNM system describes regional (pelvic) nodes as N1 but no longer classifies para-aortic, supraclavicular or inguinal node involvement, which should be stated with the TNM stage.

PROGNOSTIC FACTORS

Approximately 50 per cent of patients with carcinoma of the cervix can be cured of their disease (Table 35.2). Most recurrences occur within the first 3 years, and 5-year survival rates are a good measure of the effectiveness of therapy. More than 90 per cent of patients with small

Table 35.2 *Results of treatment of cervical carcinoma (modified from FIGO, 1988)*

Stage	% of total	Five-year survival (%)
I	35	76
II	34	55
III	26	30
IV	4	7

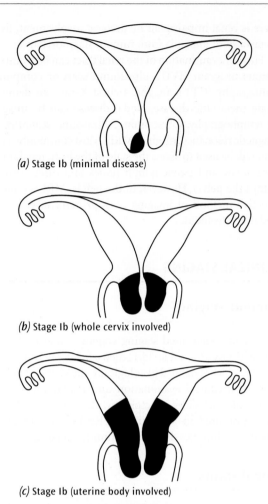

(a) Stage Ib (minimal disease)

(b) Stage Ib (whole cervix involved)

(c) Stage Ib (uterine body involved)

Figure 35.7 *Stage Ib carcinoma of the cervix, showing how this one stage includes a wide range of tumour volumes from minimal disease of just over 0.5 cm³ (a) to huge tumours involving the uterine body (c). Although the former would now be staged as Ib1 and the latter Ib2, there is still a wide range of tumour volumes within each substage.*

stage I tumours, with uninvolved lymph nodes, can be cured of their disease, but results remain disappointing for stage III and IV tumours, with 5-year survival rates of only approximately 30 per cent and 10 per cent, respectively. Results for stage II disease are, perhaps, the most variable between centres. Five-year survival rates of between 40 and 75 per cent are quoted.

Stage and tumour volume

Stage is the single most important factor related to prognosis (Table 35.2 and Figs 35.7 and 35.8). However, tumour bulk is also a major prognostic determinant and is obviously related to stage (Collins *et al.*, 1994).

The FIGO system divides cervical tumours into broad prognostic groups and now takes account of tumour volume in early stage disease. Tumour volume is one of the most important prognostic factors and a wide range of volumes can occur in any one FIGO stage. For example,

a stage Ib tumour can be anything from 0.25 cm³, for a tumour just exceeding the criteria for stage Ia (Fig. 35.7a), to as much as 100–200 cm³ for a 'barrel' tumour arising in the endocervical canal (Magee *et al.*, 1991). FIGO now divides stage Ib into Ib1 (tumours <4 cm diameter) and stage Ib2 (tumours >4 cm diameter). However, in addition to recording FIGO stage, it is also important to record tumour bulk as measured at the time of examination under anaesthetic.

Tumour volume can be measured accurately on reconstructed axial and sagital CT or MRI scans, using special computer programs, or can be estimated more crudely by calculating maximum height × width × depth.

In some centres local staging systems have been developed that reflect tumour volume more accurately by having substages for unilateral and bilateral disease and for uterine body involvement. Care must be taken when assessing the results of treatment from centres that do not explicitly state that they are using the FIGO system, as the quoted stage and substage may not reflect the same disease status in the local system as in the FIGO system.

Nodal status

Nodal status has a profound effect on survival. Those patients having stage Ib carcinoma of the cervix with positive pelvic nodes have a 5-year survival only half that of those with negative pelvic nodes. It is very unusual for patients with involved para-aortic nodes to survive 5 years, as this is commonly a marker of widespread dissemination (Shingleton and Orr, 1995).

In addition to the distribution of nodes, the total number of nodes involved is a powerful prognostic factor in surgically staged series (Inoue and Morita, 1990).

Lymphovascular permeation

Lymphovascular-space involvement has a prognostic significance in being an indicator of the likelihood of pelvic nodal involvement (Kamura *et al.*, 1993). However, it also appears to have a powerful prognostic effect even in the absence of pelvic nodal disease.

Histology

In some series the degree of differentiation of squamous cancers has been shown to be of prognostic significance, with patients with poorly differentiated tumours faring worse than those with moderately or well-differentiated tumours. However, this has not been a universal finding.

Adenocarcinomas and adenosquamous carcinomas have also been thought to have a worse prognosis, stage for stage, than squamous carcinomas. However, these histological types are often more bulky within any one stage, than squamous cancers, because of their site of origin

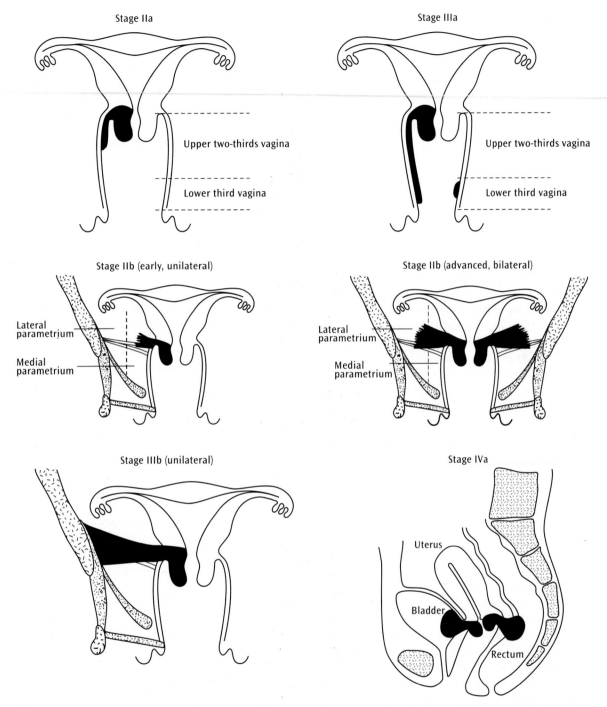

Figure 35.8 *Stages IIa–IVa carcinoma of the cervix. Stage IIa and IIIa tumours involve the vaginal mucosa only. Stage IIb and IIIb tumours involve the parametria and pelvic side-wall, respectively. A distinction is occasionally made between medial and lateral parametrial involvement and unilateral and bilateral fixation to the pelvic side-wall. Ureteric obstruction also stages a tumour as IIIb. Stage IVa tumours involve the rectum or bladder.*

being occult and high in the endocervical canal, with later presentation and a greater chance of involvement of the uterine body. It is the increased bulk of tumours of these histological types that causes them to have a worse prognosis.

Small cell neuroendocrine tumours of the cervix have a particularly bad prognosis because of their propensity to lymphatic and blood-borne spread, even in the early stages. As at other sites of the body, survival from this type of tumour is rare.

Human papillomavirus status

It has been found that patients with squamous carcinoma of the cervix that is positive for HPV, in which the

$p53$ tumour-supressor gene is blocked, have a better prognosis than patients who are HPV negative but who express an abnormal form of $p53$. This implies that a tumour arising from cells with an intrinsic abnormality removing all effective function of $p53$ behaves in a more malignant manner than a tumour in which normal $p53$ is still present but is blocked from action. It may be that such block-ing of the $p53$ gene by HPV proteins, E6 and E7, is not complete.

Age

Age as a prognostic factor in carcinoma of the cervix is a contentious issue. In some historical series young age has been shown to convey a survival advantage over old age. In other series no difference can be found between different age groups (Elliot *et al.*, 1989), while in other, modern series a poor prognostic effect of young age has been seen (Dattoli *et al.*, 1989). In addition, the incidence of nodal positivity in young patients appears to be higher, stage for stage, than in older patients, and to carry a worse prognosis. The impression is that cancer of the cervix in young women is occasionally a disease of rapid onset with a high propensity for metastasis and rapid progression (Lammont *et al.*, 1993).

TREATMENT

Cervical intra-epithelial neoplasia

Once diagnosed histologically, cervical intra-epithelial neoplasia may be removed under colposcopic control by laser vaporization, radical diathermy or surgical excision by scalpel, cutting laser or hot wire loop (LLETZ). Excision is increasingly favoured over destructive methods as it allows more accurate histological assessment of the entire abnormality than is possible on a biopsy alone. This relates particularly to occult foci of invasion which, if not recognized, may lead to undertreatment. Lesions that cannot be delineated on all sides, especially if they involve the endocervical canal, must be removed by cone biopsy (Fig. 35.9).

Stage Ia disease

Cone biopsy, completely excising a Ia1 lesion, should be adequate treatment for young women, providing that the depth of invasion is less than 3 mm with no lymphatic vessel involvement. If a cone biopsy cannot completely encompass a lesion, then simple hysterectomy should be undertaken with conservation of the ovaries in women not concerned about retaining fertility, or trachelectomy in those wishing to retain the chance of further pregnancy.

If the lesion invades further than 3 mm (stage Ia2), or if there is lymphatic space invasion, then the risk of

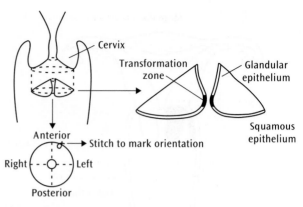

Figure 35.9 *A cone biopsy, cut either by laser or scalpel, must include all the transformation zone and be marked to allow orientation of the specimen in the pathology laboratory.*

involved lymph nodes rises and radical hysterectomy and lymphadenectomy is the treatment of choice for women not concerned about fertility. Where this is in issue, a large cone biopsy may suffice or a trachelectomy, but the pelvic lymph nodes should be assessed surgically either at an open retroperitoneal procedure or via a laparoscope. For older women or for those unfit for radical surgery, radiotherapy is an option.

Invasive cervical cancer

The treatment of invasive cervical cancer will depend on the stage of disease, the size of the tumour and the fitness of the patient. It can incorporate chemotherapy, radiotherapy and surgery. The treatment strategy for individual patients should be arrived at after discussion between specialists in all three disciplines.

SURGERY

Surgery is the treatment of choice for young patients with small-volume stage Ib disease in whom there is a low risk of nodal metastases. Good histological differentiation and the absence of lymphatic vessel invasion, small tumour volume and normal-sized nodes on imaging are indicators that lymph-node metastases are unlikely and surgery should be considered.

Surgery for invasive cervical carcinoma should include a radical hysterectomy and a pelvic lymphadenectomy (Fig. 35.10). This is often colloquially called a 'Wertheim's' hysterectomy, although this is a misnomer as Wertheim's original operation did not include a lymphadenectomy. A long vaginal cuff should be taken as a routine in this operation, but in a young woman with a squamous carcinoma it should be possible to conserve the ovaries and avoid the menopause. Advantages of surgery over radiotherapy, in young women, include the avoidance of further shrinkage of the vagina after treatment, and the maintenance of pliability and lubrication of the vaginal mucosa.

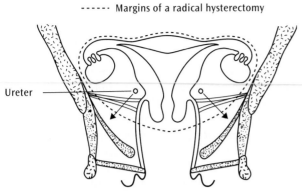

Figure 35.10 *A radical hysterectomy in which the ureters are mobilized to allow wide excision of the uterus and cervix. The cardinal ligaments and a wide cuff of vagina are also removed. A pelvic lymphadenectomy would usually accompany this procedure.*

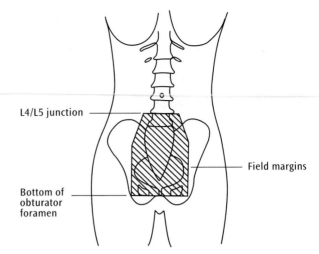

Figure 35.11 *The anterior external-beam radiotherapy field used to treat carcinoma of the cervix. To cover the 'first station' lymph nodes, the field extends from the junction of the fourth and fifth lumbar vertebrae to the bottom of the obturator foramina.*

In addition, the very small risk of late induction of a second malignancy is avoided.

A less extensive radical surgical technique is being developed for women of child-bearing age who want to preserve their fertility and whose tumours are small and limited to the cervix. This is radical trachelectomy, in which the cervix and paracervical tissues are removed together with a cuff of vagina. The body of the uterus is left in place and is anastomosed to the vagina. The new opening into the uterine cavity is narrowed with a circumferential stitch. This allows a pregnancy to be carried but requires delivery by caesarian section. The technique should be regarded as experimental as long-term resulted of tumour cure and successful pregnancies are still awaited. The procedure is usually accompanied by a pelvic lymphadenectomy carried out laparoscopically.

RADIOTHERAPY

For older women, or women with more bulky tumours, radiotherapy is the treatment of choice, as the results of treatment are equal to those of surgery and the treatment is better tolerated. However, there is morbidity in terms of fibrosis in the normal tissues, causing some reduction in the size of the vagina and its pliability and lubrication. Women with a high risk of nodal involvement because of large-volume disease, poor differentiation or lymphatic vessel involvement should also be treated by radiotherapy, often given with concomitant chemotherapy.

External-beam therapy

Carcinoma of the cervix is treated by a combination of both external and intra-cavitary radiotherapy. In some treatment centres patients with stage Ib tumours who are unfit for surgery are treated by intra-cavitary radiotherapy alone, provided that the tumours are not bulky. Commonly, a maximum diameter of 4 cm would be regarded as the upper limit of size for a tumour to be treated by intra-cavitary brachytherapy alone. More bulky tumours,

or those of higher stage, or with a high likelihood of pelvic lymph-node involvement, should be treated by external-beam radiotherapy to cover the lymph nodes draining the cervix. These include the external, internal and common iliac nodes (Fig. 35.5).

The volume encompassed by external radiotherapy should include these nodes with the primary tumour. This will commonly be from the junction of the fourth and fifth lumbar vertebrae to the bottom of the obturator foramina, and laterally to 1–2 cm outside the bony margin of the pelvis (Fig. 35.11). The volume may be more individually designed, with shielding of the upper corners of the antero-posterior fields to protect the small bowel. This volume can be encompassed by either a parallel opposed pair or, if it is appropriate to try to spare the posterior half of the rectum in the absence of uterosacral ligament involvement, then either a four-field 'box' technique or a technique using three fields, with an anterior and two wedged lateral fields, can be used. Ideally a 5–10 MeV linear accelerator should be used, in view of the depth of the tumour volume below the surface of the lateral fields (Fig. 35.12). Those patients with disease in the vaginal mucosa below the upper third should have the field extended to cover the full length of the vagina. This will involve marking the introitus with a lead marker inserted just inside the labia at the time of simulation.

If para-aortic nodes are involved then a long, 'spade-shaped' field may be used to cover the para-aortic nodes (usually with an upper border of T12/L1) and the pelvis. This volume is treated by a parallel opposed pair to a maximum dose of 45 Gy in 1.8–2 Gy fractions. Large volumes of small bowel will seldom tolerate doses in excess of this and treatment is, therefore, largely palliative. The borders of the para-aortic field should cover all enlarged nodes but should not encroach upon the kidneys, as outlined on an IVU, unless this cannot be avoided and there is thought to be some prospect of long-term disease control. There is no clear evidence that prophylactic para-aortic irradiation is of benefit (Haie *et al.*, 1988).

Intra-cavitary brachytherapy

Historically, cervical cancer was one of the first tumours to be treated by radiotherapy, when radium was inserted into the endocervical canal and upper vagina to irradiate local disease. Techniques were developed in several centres, notably Paris, Stockholm and Manchester, which allowed

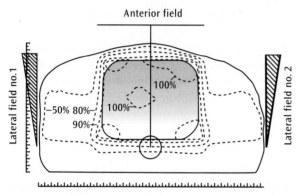

Figure 35.12 *The final plan, using an anterior and two wedged lateral fields, to deliver a homogeneous dose to the tumour volume to include the primary tumour and the draining lymph nodes.*

consistency in treatment and, therefore, enabled the effectiveness and morbidity of treatment to be measured. A technique commonly used these days is the 'Manchester' technique, involving an intra-uterine tube and two vaginal ovoids placed in the lateral vaginal fornices (Fig. 35.13). The proportions of radio-isotope, initially radium and more latterly caesium, within the intra-uterine tube and the vaginal ovoids, were calculated to give a constant dose rate to a geometrical point 'A' when using different lengths of intra-uterine tube and different sizes of vaginal ovoids. This constancy of dose rate when using applicators of different sizes is an important aspect of the Manchester system.

Point 'A' was originally defined as being 2 cm above the lateral fornix of the vagina, identified on check films as being the top of the 'ovoid', and 2 cm lateral to the axis of the intra-uterine sources. With modern afterloading applicators, the 'ovoids' may be radioluscent and may not be clearly seen on the check radiographs. It has become common practice, therefore, to position point 'A' 2 cm above the cervical flange on the intra-uterine tube at the cervical os and 2 cm lateral to the midline of the intra-uterine applicator. However, calculating the position of point 'A' in this way can lead to high dose rates at point 'A' if the cervix is long and the ovoids are high in relation to the flange. Judgement must be used in these situations in repositioning point 'A' more cranially while ensuring that the rectal dose remains within the tolerance range of two-thirds the point 'A' dose.

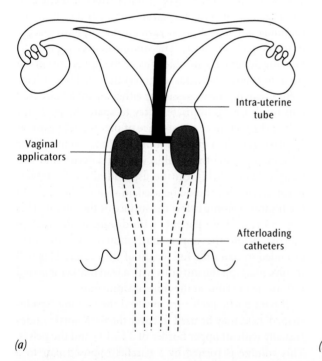

(a)

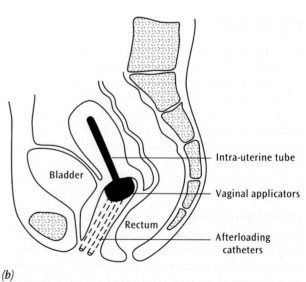

(b)

Figure 35.13 *(a) The arrangement of brachytherapy sources in the uterus and vagina for the treatment of cervical carcinoma. The sources may be active or, more usually these days, afterloaded into the applicators along catheters protruding from the vagina. (b) A lateral view of an intra-uterine tube and vaginal applicators for the treatment of carcinoma of the cervix.*

Active sources The radio-isotope used for intra-cavitary brachytherapy was initially radium which, because of its gaseous daughter product, radon, is hazardous. In most centres in developed countries radium has been replaced by caesium, which decays to solid, non-radioactive products. However, in developing countries and parts of Eastern Europe radium is still commonly used, as the cost of replacement with caesium sources is prohibitive. In addition, caesium sources require more frequent replacement because of the shorter half-life of the isotope.

The hazards of handling active sources have led to the development of after-loading techniques which aim to minimize source handling and staff exposure.

After-loading brachytherapy The basis of after-loading brachytherapy is that applicators are placed within the cervix and vaginal fornices. The radio-isotope is only introduced into these when the applicators are correctly positioned, check radiographs have been taken and the patient is comfortable and in a radiation-protected environment. The sources may then be inserted either manually or by remote control.

Manual methods were common and had the advantage of being relatively inexpensive. However, they did not entirely protect staff as the sources have to be inserted by staff and cannot be removed for short periods while attending to a patient's needs (Fig. 35.14). As a consequence, remote after-loading systems have been developed.

In these, the sources are driven into the applicators either pneumatically or on the end of cables. Cable-driven systems are generally motor-driven, although there are a few hand-driven systems for use in areas where the power supply is erratic. This process can only take place in a protected room when all staff are away from the area.

Although remote systems have the advantage of complete protection of staff, they do have the disadvantage of cost and the necessity for interlocking mechanisms. These ensure that the correct source has been inserted into the correct applicator for the programmed length of time and that the sources are withdrawn to a radiation-protected safe when the staff enter the treatment area.

Low dose rate after-loading Remote after-loading systems allow the dose rate of brachytherapy to be increased. Classically, the dose rate with the Manchester radium system was approximately 50 cGy/h to point 'A'. With modern engineering methods, caesium pellets can be produced which will allow a dose rate of between 150 and 200 cGy/h to point 'A'. As the dose needed to eradicate cervical carcinoma, when treated by intra-cavitary therapy alone, is in the region of 70–80 Gy to point 'A', therapy at standard (radium) dose rates would take approximately 6 days or, more commonly, two treatments of 3 days. By increasing the dose rate to point 'A' by a factor of three, the treatment time is reduced to two fractions, each of 1 day, allowing more patients to be treated in a week than was possible using standard sources. Equally, the intra-cavitary component of mixed external-beam and intra-cavitary treatment would seldom take more than 1 day at these higher dose rates and greatly improves the cost-effectiveness and patient acceptability of the treatment.

Many systems now use sources that deliver a higher than standard dose rate while remaining in the low dose-rate range as defined by the International Committee on Radiological Units (ICRU, 1984) (Table 35.3). While this has the advantage of reducing treatment time, it does have radiobiological consequences, necessitating a small reduction in dose of 10–15 per cent (Brenner and Hall, 1991).

High dose rate after-loading If the concept of increasing dose rate is taken further, then high dose rate (HDR) brachytherapy, delivering doses at rates in excess of 1 Gy/min to point 'A' gives the opportunity of very short treatment times. This allows complete geometrical stability of the applicator during the treatment and the possibility of a high patient throughput.

High patient throughput has obvious advantages in areas of high incidence of cervical cancer but requires that

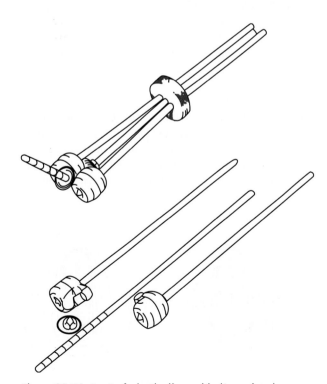

Figure 35.14 *A set of plastic disposable (Amersham) intra-cavitary applicators which are inserted individually and then locked together when correctly positioned. These applicators are manually after-loaded with caesium sources.*

Table 35.3 *ICRU definition of intra-cavitary dose rate to prescription point (ICRU, 1984)*

Dose rate	
Low	0.4–2 Gy/h
Medium	2–12 Gy/h
High	>0.2 Gy/min

there is a full and efficient infrastructure for the treatment process. In addition to the provision of a remote after-loading HDR facility, including machine, protected treatment room, control room and dosimetry facilities, consideration must be given to patient transport, waiting and recovery areas, the availability of staff and rapid treatment planning if a high throughput is to be realized.

Geometrical stability means that, if the applicator is well-positioned for the treatment, there is no change in the position during the few minutes that the treatment takes. This has consequent advantages, in terms of normal tissue sparing, over a low dose-rate insertion lasting several hours, during which time both the applicators and the tissues move. Equally, a bad insertion will remain bad throughout the short treatment time, whereas the more protracted low dose-rate insertion may allow some of the normal tissues in the high dose regions to move and thus be spared damage.

There is considerably less time for repair of radiation damage in the normal tissues in a high dose-rate treatment as opposed to during the continuous treatment given by a low dose-rate brachytherapy implant. Therefore, such treatments have to be fractionated over several days to allow repair in normal tissues between fractions. Apart from the operational consequences of this, in terms of the patient needing several treatment sessions instead of one or two, it also means that the applicators have to be positioned consistently for each fraction of intra-cavitary treatment, in order to take advantage of the geometrical stability. In addition, radiobiological models of repair predict that a dose reduction of 35–45 per cent from the dose that would be given at standard dose rates needs to be made in order to avoid excessive late normal tissue damage. This need for a dose reduction at high dose rates, together with the need to fractionate treatment over several days or weeks, introduces another area of uncertainty into intra-cavitary brachytherapy, a treatment modality that has been developed almost entirely empirically, by years of clinical experience, rather than by radiobiological considerations.

However, early clinical results show no difference between treatment at low dose rate and high dose rate in terms of local control of disease or late normal tissue complications (Fu and Philips, 1990; Patel *et al.*, 1993). This is in spite of mathematical modelling indicating that there is a theoretical increased risk of late normal tissue damage, for the same anti-tumour effect, from fractionated high dose rate brachytherapy compared to a continuous low dose rate insertion. This lack of difference may be due to the radiobiological disadvantages of HDR therapy being balanced by the geometrical and dosimetric advantages of a rigid applicator system.

The integration of external-beam therapy and intra-cavitary brachytherapy

Brachytherapy, used alone for the treatment of cervical cancer, is commonly given as two fractions when utilizing the Manchester system. At standard radium dose rates this involves two insertions, each lasting 3 days, spaced 1 week apart. More commonly a higher activity, low dose rate system would be used, reducing each fraction to 1 day. This allows a period of time between the first and second insertion for the tumour to shrink and for vaginal hygiene to be attended to. However, most patients suitable for brachytherapy alone would, nowadays, undergo surgery, and radiotherapy is used for more advanced tumours. Treatment is usually with external-beam therapy in addition to brachytherapy. The brachytherapy component can either precede or succeed the external-beam therapy.

Classically, intra-cavitary brachytherapy to central disease was carried out prior to external-beam therapy, which was given to treat the nodes on the pelvic side-wall. A dose was given from the brachytherapy that would be in excess of the tolerance dose to central pelvic tissues if the external-beam therapy, intended to top-up the dose to the pelvic side-walls, were given to the whole pelvis. Therefore, some central shielding was needed in the external-beam field to protect those tissues that had received a high brachytherapy dose. This was particularly the rectum and bladder. This shielding would take the form of a central lead block inserted in the anterior and posterior fields of a parallel opposed pair for all or part of the treatment. In some centres these blocks were custom-built for individual patients, to take account of the iso-dose pattern of the intra-cavitary therapy; more commonly the blocks were standard.

Standard shielding blocks have largely been rectangular, a shape which is suitable to shield tissues irradiated by a linear source arrangement, but which poorly matches the 'pear-shaped' isodose patterns created by the Manchester system (Fig. 35.15).

This programme of treatment has existed for many years and is still used in a number of centres for treating early carcinoma of the cervix. However, in addition to problems in shaping the shield, there can also be problems in locating this within the external-beam field. This is particularly so in cases where the intra-cavitary sources

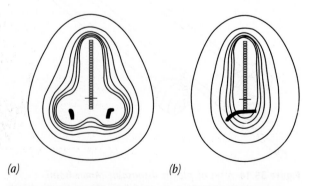

(a)   *(b)*

Figure 35.15 *(a) The classic 'pear-shaped' isodose curves produced in the lateral plane by 'Manchester' tube and ovoids. In the antero-posterior plane (b) there is little expansion of the isodose curves at the level of the cervix.*

have been pulled markedly away from the midline by tumour, or where two insertions have been carried out with different positioning of the applicators on each occasion. Mispositioning of an external-beam shield over the tissues irradiated by the intra-cavitary therapy could lead to relative underdosing on one side and overdosing on the other, which would have consequences both for recurrence and for complications of treatment.

Increasingly, external-beam therapy is used prior to intra-cavitary brachytherapy and the brachytherapy dose is reduced, so as to avoid the need for any central shielding in the external-beam fields. Typically, a dose of 45–50 Gy would be given over 4.5–5.5 weeks in 1.8 Gy or 2 Gy fractions to the pelvis, as described earlier. An intra-cavitary insertion would then be undertaken to give a further 25–30 Gy to point 'A' at standard dose rate. If higher than standard dose rates were used, then a lower dose would be delivered. Parametrial boosts may then be used to give a further 5 Gy to bulky disease within the parametria or involved nodes on the pelvic side-walls. These boost fields may have the medial edge, abutting the intra-cavitary treatment volume, shaped by rectangular blocks, custom-made blocks to match the intra-cavitary isodose curves or by a multi-leaf collimator to achieve approximately the same matching.

The dose to the rectum from the intra-cavitary insertion should not exceed two-thirds of the dose given to point 'A' and care must be taken, when using rigid applicators, that the uterus is not forcibly pushed posteriorly in the pelvis against the rectum, sigmoid colon or small bowel. Intra-uterine applicator tubes should either be made of flexible plastic, to conform to the curvature and anteversion of the uterus or, if made of metal, should have a forward curvature in the antero-posterior plane. Equally, an overly curved, rigid intra-uterine tube could overdose the dome of the bladder while sparing the bowel. A curvature of 20°–30° is probably suitable in most cases, depending on the patient's anatomy.

CHEMOTHERAPY FOR CARCINOMA OF THE CERVIX

Carcinoma of the cervix is not a highly chemosensitive tumour (Thigpen *et al.*, 1981). Response rates to single agents have seldom been reported in excess of 40 per cent and the most effective drugs appear to be cisplatin and ifosfamide. Currently, trials are under way into the role of these drugs, alone and in combination with others, for recurrent disease (Tutt *et al.*, 1999), in the neoadjuvant setting prior to surgery or radiotherapy (Hoskin and Blake, 1991; Sardi *et al.*, 1998) and during radiotherapy as concomitant therapy for advanced, bulky disease (Thomas, 1999).

Responses are seen to combination chemotherapy regimens including these drugs, and the best response rate is seen in primary untreated disease. However, the response rate in metastatic disease is lower and in recurrent disease,

within an irradiated area, is very low indeed. Therefore, the results of clinical trials are still awaited to prove the true benefit in survival brought about by these drugs, although they can be used judiciously for palliation of advanced and metastatic disease.

CONCOMITANT CHEMO-IRRADIATION

In 1999 the National Cancer Institute issued a statement that serious consideration should be given to the use of concomitant chemo-irradiation in the radical treatment of locally advanced carcinoma of the cervix (Thomas, 1999). This statement was based on three published papers and two abstracts reporting randomized controlled trials of therapies including chemo-irradiation in at least one arm (Keys *et al.*, 1999; Morris *et al.*, 1999; Rose *et al.*, 1999). All showed a statistically significant improvement in survival for patients in the chemo-irradiation arm in comparison to the standard therapy arm. Follow-up varied widely and toxicity data was reported in different ways. No study compared primary radiotherapy alone with the same regimen plus concomitant chemotherapy, and a wide range of drugs, doses and schedules was used in the five trials. Only three of the five trials related to radical non-surgical treatment alone and the other two were regimens delivered either pre- or postsurgery.

Despite this rather flimsy evidence, there has been a major change in practice in this area and concomitant chemo-irradiation has been adopted as standard therapy in many centres. Radiotherapy regimens have not been altered but chemotherapy, usually cisplatin, is given prior to several of the radiotherapy fractions. The frequency of administration has varied between once per week in the first 4 weeks to twice per week throughout the whole course of radiotherapy. Regimens are being studied of giving cisplatin at low dose prior to each fraction. In general, the total weekly dose of cisplatin is of the order of 40–60 mg/m^2.

Early data suggest that this addition of cisplatin has a marked effect on the haematological toxicity of treatment. In addition, some patients have experienced worse gastrointestinal toxicity than would be expected with radiotherapy alone. However, higher rates of complete response have been reported anecdotally, and it remains to be seen whether these are maintained in larger series of patients than were treated in the original trials. In addition, with careful toxicity recording, an increase in the incidence of late normal tissue reactions, in parallel with the increased acute reactions, should become apparent.

THE MAINTENANCE OF HAEMOGLOBIN LEVELS

Studies in the late 1970s had shown that women with a haemoglobin level below 10 g/dL had a lower cure rate of cervical cancer by radiotherapy than women with a higher haemoglobin level. However, it was not clear whether women had low haemoglobin levels because of more advanced tumours, which bled more, and therefore fared badly or whether the relative lack of oxygen in the tumour during radiotherapy conferred a radio-protective effect on the tumour. Further analysis of the chemo-radiotherapy trials had indicated a similar influence of anaemia. Women with a haemoglobin level above 12 g/dL fared better than those with a lower level and this appeared to be independent of tumour stage and size. This effect would therefore appear to be due to a radio-sensitizing effect of oxygen on the tumour and it is now recommended that the haemoglobin level is kept above 12 g/dL throughout radiotherapy.

Special situations

NON-SQUAMOUS CARCINOMA OF THE CERVIX

Adenocarcinoma and mixed carcinomas of the cervix have traditionally been thought to have a poor prognosis. However, tumour bulk is the most important prognostic factor and adenocarcinomas are frequently larger than squamous carcinomas, stage for stage, due to their origin being within the endocervical canal and their consequent late detection. Therefore, bulk for bulk, they probably fare no worse than squamous carcinomas.

Small cell neuroendocrine tumours of the cervix behave like small cell tumours at any other site. The most effective treatment is with chemotherapy (e.g. daunorubicin, cyclophosphamide and etoposide) followed by radiotherapy to the sites of bulk disease. There is usually a dramatic and rapid response, but the disease metastasizes and recurs equally rapidly. Therefore, the prognosis is very poor.

THE INCIDENTAL FINDING OF CERVICAL CANCER

Occasionally invasive cervical cancer is found in the specimen following a simple hysterectomy. If the depth of invasion indicates a risk of lymphatic spread (stage Ib or more, or if there are other poor prognostic features), then postoperative pelvic radiotherapy should be prescribed. If the cuff of vagina is inadequate, then vault brachytherapy also should be delivered. With this technique the results of treatment are no worse than those of radical surgery or radical radiotherapy alone.

Although the pelvis tolerates radiotherapy less well after surgery than when radiotherapy is given as primary treatment, it is usually possible to deliver 40–50 Gy over 5–6 weeks postoperatively without undue late morbidity. If there is residual disease at the vaginal vault or at the margins of excision, then a second phase of treatment is needed to take the total tumour dose to at least 60–65 Gy. In this circumstance it must be accepted that there is a greater likelihood of late morbidity. This may be minimized by restricting phase two to the smallest volume of tissue necessary to encompass the tumour, using a CT-planned small volume of external-beam therapy or intra-cavitary or interstitial brachytherapy, depending on the site and size of the residual disease.

CERVICAL CARCINOMA DURING PREGNANCY

This difficult situation arises uncommonly and treatment depends on the wishes of the parents as well as on the stage of disease. Treatment would be similar to that for non-pregnant patients in the first and second trimester of pregnancy, with treatment preceded by abortion or hysterotomy. Caesarean section should precede treatment in the third trimester when there is the chance of producing a viable child. The commonly perceived view that carcinoma of the cervix behaves more aggressively in pregnant patients than in non-pregnant patients is not proven in long-term studies taking account of the, usually young, age of the patients.

HAEMORRHAGE

Carcinoma of the cervix can present with severe haemorrhage, which should be treated in the first instance by firm vaginal packing, bed rest and a blood transfusion. Urgent external-beam radiotherapy may well produce haemostasis within 24–48 hours and, classically, large fractions of at least 4 Gy have been used, without any clear evidence that this is superior to standard sized fractions. Very occasionally, an intra-cavitary insertion is needed and, in intractable cases, embolization or ligation of the internal iliac arteries should be considered.

RECURRENT CARCINOMA OF THE CERVIX

Recurrence following either inadequate surgery or radical surgery can usually be treated by radiotherapy (possibly with concomitant chemotherapy) if a dose to the tumour in excess of 65 Gy can be achieved. This usually involves at least a two-phase approach to treatment with external radiotherapy followed by a CT-planned small volume boost, intra-cavitary brachytherapy or interstitial brachytherapy. Very occasionally the latter can be combined with debulking surgery as intra-operative interstitial brachytherapy, during which sensitive structures, such as the bowel, can be packed away from the high-dose regions and be spared damage.

Occasionally, recurrence after radical radiotherapy, if central, can be treated by either posterior, anterior or total pelvic exenteration involving diversion of the urinary and gastrointestinal tracts. Selection of patients for this procedure must include both the physical and psychological assessment of the patients' ability to cope with the resulting stomas.

Inoperable recurrent carcinoma of the cervix within a previously irradiated area has been referred to earlier as an indication for considering chemotherapy. In general, these tumours do not respond objectively, although there may be some subjective improvement. Therefore, with careful patient selection, chemotherapy may be used for palliation and, in a small number of patients, long-term control of disease can be achieved. As cure of recurrent disease by chemotherapy is virtually unheard of, it is most important to consider the toxicity of treatment in designing a palliative regimen for a patient.

COMPLICATIONS OF TREATMENT

Surgery

In addition to the morbidity and mortality associated with any major pelvic operation, radical hysterectomy can also cause specific problems in the pelvis. The most common of these is a degree of flaccidity of the bladder. This symptom is apparent soon after surgery and often improves with bladder drainage over a period of a few weeks. Very occasionally the bladder remains flaccid and the patient has to practice intermittent self-catheterization.

Other, more serious, problems that can arise are fistulas between the vagina, bladder and rectum. Very rarely such fistulas may also involve the ureters, small bowel or skin. These problems are much increased in incidence if surgery is as salvage for recurrence after radical radiotherapy.

Pelvic lymphocoeles may collect after a lymphadenectomy and may be asymptomatic or cause problems of pain or of obstruction to the ureters and bowel, if they are particularly large. If they become infected, after an attempt at drainage, then eradication of the infection may be difficult.

Radiotherapy

In general, treatment regimens are designed with the assumption that all patients have a similar sensitivity to therapeutic radiation. However, we know this not to be the case, as a wide range of both acute and late reactions are seen at standard doses. The prediction of individual normal tissue sensitivity is in its infancy but, when developed, should allow a degree of 'tailoring' of radiotherapy regimens to suit individual patients. In the meantime, only crude criteria can be used, with the exception of those very rare patients with conditions such as ataxia-telangiectasia or xeroderma pigmentosum, who are highly radiosensitive.

These crude criteria include identifying those who sunburn and blister without tanning, those who are of unusually fair complexion and those with rheumatoid arthritis or other connective tissue disorder. These latter groups may contain patients who have a defect of DNA damage repair who may show exaggerated radiation sensitivity (Harris et al., 1985). In addition, those patients with diabetic vascular changes and those with inflammatory bowel disease, such as Crohn's disease and ulcerative colitis, may also show excessive radiation reactions in the bowel.

EXTERNAL-BEAM THERAPY

Acute effects

At the dose levels necessary to treat carcinoma of the cervix with curative intent it is uncommon not to cause some degree of acute radiation reaction, usually in the bowel. In most patients this results in diarrhoea, which becomes apparent in the second or third weeks of a course of treatment. With fraction sizes of 1.8–2 Gy diarrhoea can usually be controlled by a low-roughage diet and an anti-motility drug such as codeine phosphate or loperamide, without any disruption to the course of treatment. Some patients find a bulking agent such as Isogel® helpful. In severe cases, when diarrhoea cannot be controlled, or if there is passage of copious mucus or blood, fraction size may have to be reduced or the treatment suspended. Very occasionally, in-patient care may be necessary, usually for older women or for those in whom large volumes of small bowel are being irradiated, as when the para-aortic nodes are treated.

Radiation cystitis occurs less commonly than bowel disturbance and must be distinguished from infection by culture of a specimen of urine. Treatment of any infection and the maintenance of a high urine output of an alkaline pH, which can be achieved with oral potassium citrate, may help to relieve symptoms.

With modern megavoltage radiotherapy it is unusual to cause skin reactions that are sufficient to warrant a delay in treatment. However, it is not uncommon for there to be an uncomfortable moist desquamation of the skin in the natal cleft. Topical steroids may be helpful before the skin is actually broken but, once this happens, soothing lotions, Geliperm® and antibacterial preparations may be necessary.

Late effects

If there are late radiation effects then these usually become apparent some months or years after treatment. They may arise gradually or acutely following some other pelvic event, such as a ruptured bowel diverticulum or appendicitis. These can affect any pelvic tissue but, most commonly, the bowel. Severe late effects should not occur in more than 2–5 per cent of patients treated with radical radiotherapy (Denton et al., 2000).

As with any external-beam treatment to the gastro-intestinal tract, bowel habit may be permanently altered. Such a change is usually towards looseness in the motions and increased frequency of evacuation. This may be due to decreased absorption of water in the large bowel and malabsorption of bile acids from the bowel contents, causing intestinal hurry. Both of these processes will lead to diarrhoea.

Some patients become intolerant of high-roughage, spicy or oily food and have a permanently restricted diet. These patients should be referred to a dietitian for specialist advice. Non-dietary methods, which may help, include medication with codeine phosphate or loperamide, to decrease bowel motility. Occasionally, Questran®, which binds to bile acids in the bowel, is also helpful.

Over a long period of time, malabsorption of vitamin B_{12} from the terminal ileum may become apparent by an increasing mean corpuscular volume (MCV), anaemia or, very rarely, neurological signs. If these symptoms occur, then serum B_{12} and folate levels should be estimated and any deficiency treated with parenteral B_{12} and oral folate.

Rectal bleeding may result from either ulceration of the bowel mucosa or from telangiectasia. Recurrent cervical cancer and primary carcinoma of the bowel, which may also cause bleeding, should be excluded by colonoscopy. Treatment of rectal bleeding may be attempted by the use of steroid enemas and, occasionally, tranexamic acid may help in intractable cases. However, in a very small number of patients the only effective cure is to completely rest the bowel by formation of a defunctioning colostomy.

Radiation damage may also cause stenosis or obstruction of the intestine, most commonly of the small bowel and, if present, this may occur at more than one level. Surgery to remove the affected bowel and anastomose the remaining lengths is skilled, as the vascularity of irradiated bowel is often poor, making the healing of anastomoses difficult.

Late damage to the bladder may result in only a small volume of urine being tolerated. This can be due not only to fibrosis in the bladder, restricting expansion, but also to a neurological disturbance resulting in lower pressures within the bladder triggering the desire to micturate.

Haematuria may be microscopic, occasional and mild or severe and intractable. Treatment with tranexamic acid may help lesser degrees of bleeding, once confirmed not to be due to recurrent tumour or to a new primary bladder cancer, but severe bleeding may only be treatable by urinary diversion.

Ureteric stenosis is a theoretical late effect of radiotherapy, which is always listed as a possible cause of post-radiotherapy ureteric stenosis. Unfortunately, this sign is far more often caused by recurrent tumour on the pelvic side-wall compressing or invading the ureter.

It is uncommon to have problems with avascular necrosis of the femoral heads with modern high-energy radiotherapy. High-energy X-rays are not absorbed to a significantly greater degree by bone than by soft tissue, unlike lower-energy orthovoltage X-rays. Nevertheless care should still be taken when planning patients, especially those that are overweight, to ensure that there is not a 'hot-spot' in the femoral head.

Lower limb oedema is seldom due to radiotherapy alone and is often a symptom of recurrent tumour in the pelvis or of a deep vein thrombosis. However, this symptom may occasionally be seen due to a combination of radiotherapy and radical surgery, especially if the latter was associated with any infection or with pelvic lymphoceles.

INTRA-CAVITARY THERAPY

Intra-cavitary brachytherapy produces a dose distribution which falls off rapidly with distance from the sources. Small changes in the relationship of normal tissues to the applicators may produce very large changes in the dose received by those tissues. Doses may be so large as to cause necrosis, which may not be functionally important

in some tissues, such as the cervix itself in women not concerned about fertility. However, it may provide a source of infection in devitalized pelvic tissues, which may produce an unpleasant discharge. Necrosis can be disastrous if it occurs in the vaginal mucosa, rectum, bladder or terminal ureter.

Attention to the accurate placement of the applicators and packing, together with a restriction on the total dose delivered to the sensitive tissues, such as the rectum and bladder, should help avoid these serious problems. Guidelines on these aspects of treatment are detailed earlier in this chapter. Dose reduction factors, to take account of non-standard dose rates, must also be used.

Chemotherapy

The toxic effects of cytotoxic drugs in the treatment of cancer of the cervix are no different from those caused in the treatment of other malignancies. The main toxicities experienced with the drugs commonly used in the treatment of carcinoma of the cervix are renal, haematological and neurological.

RENAL TOXICITY

The drugs most commonly used to treat cervical cancer – cisplatin, ifosfamide and methotrexate – deserve special mention as all are excreted, unchanged or as toxic metabolites, in the urine. Adequate renal function is, therefore, essential when using these drugs, in order to ensure that systemic effects are not exaggerated by delayed excretion. Renal function may be prejudiced by ureteric obstruction or bladder involvement by tumour. In addition, all three drugs can cause damage to the kidneys or urothelium and worsen renal function.

To avoid further damage to the renal system, cisplatin should only be given if a measure of the glomerular filtration rate shows there to be near-normal function. If not, then the dose of cisplatin should be reduced, and individual chemotherapy protocols have criteria for this. An example of criteria for dose reduction is shown in Table 35.4 for a regimen consisting of cisplatin, methotrexate and bleomycin.

Table 35.4 *Dose alteration of cisplatin, methotrexate and bleomycin (PMB) according to renal function (glomerular filtration rate)*

Creatinine or EDTA clearance (mL/min)	Cisplatin and methotrexate	Folinic acid
>80	100%	15 mg qds × 3 days
60–79	100%	15 mg qds × 4 days
40–59	50%	15 mg qds × 4 days
25–39	25%	15 mg qds × 4 days
<25	None	

qds, four times daily.

The damage that ifosfamide can cause to the urothelium, by its toxic metabolite acrolein, can be limited by the simultaneous administration of the drug mesna, which should be given for long enough to ensure complete excretion of acrolein. Methotrexate can damage renal tubules by crystallizing in acid urine and physically disrupting them. If the urine is maintained alkaline, by the oral administration of sodium bicarbonate, methotrexate is fully soluble and no crystals are formed.

MYELOSUPPRESSION

Both ifosfamide and methotrexate can cause myelosuppression. This toxic side-effect of methotrexate can be avoided by the administration of folinic acid, which must be given for sufficiently long to ensure that the serum level of methotrexate has dropped to a safe level, usually 48–72 hours. If there is a risk of the excretion of methotrexate being delayed by poor renal function, then serum methotrexate levels should be estimated and folinic acid continued until this has fallen into the safe range of $<0.05\,\mu$moles/L.

NEUROLOGICAL TOXICITY

Cisplatin toxicity also includes the induction of a peripheral neuropathy, tinnitus and damage to high-tone hearing. These symptoms must be enquired after before every course of cisplatin, and the drug stopped if they occur. Unfortunately, the peripheral neuropathy and hearing changes can sometimes not be evident until several weeks after finishing all cisplatin chemotherapy.

Ifosfamide can cause serious problems, ranging from mild irritability, through hallucinations to coma and death. Every patient receiving this drug should be questioned about their mental state regularly, as hallucinations are often the first signs of toxicity.

Hormonal changes

Surgical removal of the ovaries at radical hysterectomy for squamous carcinoma can usually be avoided in young women unless there is involvement of the body of the uterus by tumour. However, should removal be necessary, or should the ovaries lie within a radiation field, then an early menopause will occur in premenstrual women. There is no clear evidence that hormone replacement therapy (HRT) has an adverse effect on survival in patients who have been treated for squamous carcinoma, and it may be used to relieve menopausal symptoms. There is less certainty about the use of HRT in patients with adenocarcinoma, and some therapists believe that it should be withheld for at least 1 year following primary treatment.

While unopposed oestrogens may be used safely in patients who have undergone a hysterectomy, those who have not should be prescribed a cyclical oestrogen/progestogen preparation. Although radical radiotherapy ablates the endometrium in the great majority of patients, a few will still have withdrawal bleeds. In addition, a cyclical preparation is probably preferable to unopposed oestrogens for those patients with adenocarcinoma who do receive HRT.

Sexuality

Both the diagnosis and the treatment of carcinoma of the cervix can have a devastating effect on a patient's sexuality and sexual functioning. Many patients fear that the cancer has been caused by sexual intercourse and may return if they re-commence intercourse. In addition, they or their partners may fear that the disease is transmissible and that the male is at risk. Most of these fears are understandable and may be alleviated by discussion and explanation by medical and nursing staff. However, some patients may still choose not to resume sexual activity (Thranov and Klee, 1994).

Occasionally, a patient has a reaction to the diagnosis that is exaggerated and results in obsessional behaviour such as genital washing or isolation from her male partner. These patients may be helped by psychological counselling or, if the reaction is part of a depressive illness, by antidepressants.

Radical hysterectomy should not alter sexual function markedly, although patients do report altered sensation. However, radiotherapy can lead to shortening and drying of the vagina, with loss of lubrication and pliability. Shortening due to the formation of adhesions in the vagina can be avoided by regular douching during treatment and using a douche or dilator for a few months after treatment. However, radiation fibrosis in the walls of the vagina will still lead to some loss of length and pliability. Continued use of a vaginal dilator, with a lubricant gel, in those patients who have not resumed sexual activity, will maintain patency of the vagina, enabling resumption of sexual activity at a later date, and also examination in the follow-up clinic. Dryness of the vagina may be helped by a lubricant gel and also by HRT, which, in addition, can help increase libido which is often low in this group of patients.

POTENTIAL DEVELOPMENTS

Screening and diagnosis

Screening for cervical cancer is likely to become more widespread and more efficiently organized. Automated methods of assessing a Papanicolau smear already exist and will probably become the first stage in the interpretation of cervical smears. Automated methods of detecting human papillomavirus (HPV) in the smear are also being developed and may, again, be used as a first-stage test. Most importantly, public education is improving, both regarding the early symptoms of disease and the value of cervical screening. This education needs to be transferred to those areas of the developing world where cervical cancer is endemic.

Treatment

SURGERY

Laparoscopic surgery has been developed for several non-oncological procedures, with the intention of reducing operative morbidity and time in hospital. The technique is currently being developed for laparoscopic pelvic lymphadenectomy. This may allow early carcinoma of the cervix, stage Ia2 and very early stage Ib, to be staged and treated by radical trachelectomy and pelvic lymphadenectomy. Those patients who prove to have involved margins of excision in the cervix would proceed to radical hysterectomy and those with involved nodes would go on to radical radiotherapy. However, those patients with no involvement of either the margins of excision or pelvic lymph nodes would be spared the morbidity of a procedure that would necessarily render them infertile. Those who do require radical treatment would only need one modality and not two, as is presently the case when involved nodes are found at radical hysterectomy and postoperative radiotherapy is indicated. This approach should reduce the morbidity of treatment.

External-beam radiotherapy

Technical developments in radiotherapy are continually improving the accuracy of treatment. Those that are currently under development are collimation devices that aim to improve the ratio of tumour volume to normal tissue volume, and verification devices, to confirm that the treatment is being given to the intended volume.

In the first category is the development of multi-leaf collimators, which can obviate the need for lead blocks to shape fields. In addition to making treatment set-up much easier and more reproducible, these collimators also allow irregular fields to be treated. Current experience is largely in static fields. However, with appropriate computer software to drive the movement of the collimators, it may be possible to use them in a dynamic way, with changing field shape and size during rotational treatment. This technique of intensity-modulated radiotherapy (IMRT) could allow very complex tumour volumes to be treated with sparing of normal tissues. In the pelvis, the simplest use of multi-leaf collimators is to match the medial edge of the external-beam pelvic side-wall boosts to the shape of the intra-cavitary therapy isodoses. At the other end of the spectrum it may be possible, ultimately, to irradiate tumour volumes that follow the lymphatic drainage of the cervix up the pelvic side-walls, over the sacral promontory and into the lower para-aortic region, sparing rectum, bladder and bowel.

In the category of treatment verification devices fall 'beams-eye view' and 'transmission dose' devices. The former images each treatment field and compares the image taken with that of the confirmatory planning film. Any deviation from a pre-set norm would be signalled to the therapy radiographers to allow checking of the patient set-up. Transmission dose devices similarly measure the exit dose of each field and may be used to both calculate absorbed dose in tissues of different density and to confirm consistent patient set-up. Again, a significant deviation from a pre-set norm would alert radiographers to check the set-up and, if necessary because of patient weight loss or change in patient contour, replan the patient. This system may, with a multi-leaf collimator, allow tissue compensation to be made on a day-to-day basis.

INTRA-CAVITARY THERAPY

New applicator design, to improve stability and dose distribution, is an area of constant progress in intra-cavitary brachytherapy. However, the major advances are likely to occur in source distribution within the applicators, to allow 'optimization' of brachytherapy dose distributions. With computer-controlled microsources, as used in high dose rate therapy, it is possible to create novel dose distributions to spare sensitive tissues. Clinical experience is needed to find how far from the classical dose distributions brachytherapy can deviate in order to decrease morbidity without sacrificing effectiveness. Accurate recording of both treatment parameters and complications is essential for this process.

CHEMOTHERAPY

Studies into the role of existing drugs, alone or in combination, for the palliation of advanced disease, as neoadjuvant therapy prior to radiotherapy or surgery, and as concomitant chemo-irradiation, are likely to continue, especially the latter, which looks most promising.

The role of HPV in the development of cervical neoplasia and the recognition of the role that this virus may have in inactivating the tumour supressor gene *p53*, may provide a new avenue of research involving antiviral therapy and gene therapy (Khan, 1993). Vaccines against HPV and its products are already being tested clinically.

CONCLUSIONS

Cytological screening programmes and colposcopy should reduce the incidence of invasive carcinoma of the cervix, and appear to have done so in some populations of older women. However, overall there is an increasing incidence in pre-invasive neoplasia of the cervix and, in young women, there is also an increasing incidence of invasive disease. A transmissible agent, the human papillomavirus, is implicated in the aetiology of cervical cancer, but is unlikely to be the only causative agent.

Treatment of early disease with both radiotherapy and surgery is equally effective, but for more advanced tumours radiotherapy is preferable. Radiotherapy should consist of both an external-beam phase and an intra-cavitary brachytherapy phase if curative doses are to be delivered without major normal-tissue toxicity. Concomitant chemotherapy may benefit patients. Brachytherapy may be at high or low dose rate and, so far, little difference has been seen between the two when the high dose rate regimen is fractionated and the total dose reduced from that given at low dose rate.

Neoadjuvant chemotherapy still does not have a proven place in the treatment of cancer of the cervix. Currently, concomitant chemo-irradiation is the main area for study. Palliation of metastatic and recurrent disease may be achieved with carefully chosen chemotherapy regimens.

SIGNIFICANT POINTS

- Early sexual intercourse and multiple partners are predisposing factors to cervical neoplasia. Several human papillomaviruses, but particularly type 16, may inactivate tumour suppressor genes in infected cells. Other factors, such as smoking, may also be implicated in lowering local immunity to infection and in causing direct damage to DNA within the cervical epithelium.
- Cervical neoplasia usually starts in the 'transformation zone' and pre-invasive disease may be detected by exfoliative cytology of the cervix. For an asymptomatic woman with a normal smear history smears should be repeated every 3–5 years. Invasive disease is usually preceded by CIN for several years and spreads predominantly by direct invasion and lymphatic spread to pelvic nodes.
- The FIGO staging system is the most commonly used system, based on clinical examination, chest X-ray and imaging of the renal tract. However, other prognostic variables, such as nodal status and tumour bulk, should be determined and recorded in addition to FIGO stage.
- Stage is the most significant prognostic factor as it probably represents tumour bulk, which is often poorly measured and recorded. Pelvic node metastasis halves the prognosis of patients with early stage disease,

while para-aortic disease is often a marker of widespread dissemination. Lymphovascular permeation increases the likelihood of nodal metastases and may be a prognostic factor in itself.
- Excision of pre-invasive disease is preferable to ablation if occult invasive disease is not to be missed. Stage I disease may be treated by cone biopsy, total hysterectomy, radical trachelectomy with node sampling or radical hysterectomy and lymphadenectomy, depending on the size of tumour, depth of invasion, the presence of lymphovascular permeation and the patient's wishes to preserve fertility. Apart from a few patients with stage IIa disease with minimal involvement of the fornices of the vagina, all patients with more advanced tumours, and those unfit for surgery, should be treated with primary radiotherapy. Chemo-irradiation using concomitant cisplatin and radiotherapy, is currently undergoing investigation and would appear to offer a benefit in survival over radiotherapy alone.
- External radiotherapy should be individually planned for each patient, to take account of the size and distribution of disease and the nodal groups at risk of metastasis. Intra-cavitary therapy is vital if the primary tumour is to be controlled, as cure without this modality is unusual, even in early stage disease. Low, medium or high dose rate intra-cavitary systems may be used, but radiation dose and fraction size and number must be adjusted according to the most recent evidence if adverse effects are not to result.
- Apart from chemotherapy as concomitant treatment for cervical cancer, the only other proven use is as palliation for advanced and, occasionally, recurrent disease. Considerable care should be taken to ensure that the toxicity of treatment does not outweigh the benefit, as the prognosis of these patients is usually of the order of a few months only. However, response rates of up to 70 per cent can be seen in previously untreated disease in irradiated sites when using cisplatin-based combination therapy. Ifosfamide is probably too toxic for use in this palliative setting.

KEY REFERENCES

Anderson, M.C. (1985) The pathology of cervical cancer. *Clin. Obstet. Gynaecol.* **12**, 87–119.

Fu, K. and Philips, T. (1990) High dose-rate versus low dose-rate intracavitary brachytherapy for carcinoma of the cervix. *Int. J. Radiat. Biol. Oncol. Phys.* **19**, 791–6.

Khan, S.A. (1993) Cervical cancer, human papilloma virus and vaccines. *Clin. Oncol.* **5**, 386–90.

Sigurdson, K. (1993) Effect of organised screening on the risk of cervical cancer. Evaluation of screening activity in Iceland, 1964–1991. *Int. J. Cancer* **54**, 563–70.

Thomas, G. (1999) Improved treatment for cervical cancer – concurrent chemotherapy and radiotherapy. *N. Engl. J. Med.* **340**, 1198–200.

Tidy, J.A. and Wrede, D. (1992) Tumour supressor genes: new pathways in gynaecological cancer. *Int. J. Gynaecol. Cancer* **2**, 1–8.

REFERENCES

Anderson, M.C. (1985) The pathology of cervical cancer. *Clin. Obstet. Gynaecol.* **12**, 87–119.

Baird, P.J. (1985) The causation of cervical cancer. II: The role of human papilloma and other viruses. *Clin. Obstet. Gynaecol.* **12**, 10–32.

Barton, S.E., Maddox, P.H., Jenkins, D., Edwards, R., Cuzick, J. and Singer, A. (1988) Effect of cigarette smoking on cervical epithelial immunity: a mechanism for neoplastic change? *Lancet* **2**, 652–4.

Benedet, J.L. and Murphy, K.J. (1985) Cervical cancer screening. Who needs a Pap test? How often? *Postgrad. Med.* **78**, 69–71.

Beral, V. (1974) Cancer of the cervix: a sexually transmitted infection? *Lancet* **1**, 1037–42.

Brenner, D.J. and Hall, E.J. (1991) Fractionated high dose versus low dose rate regimens for intracavitary brachytherapy of the cervix. 1: General considerations based on radiobiology. *Br. J. Radiol.* **64**, 133–41.

Cardiff Cervical Cytology Study (1980) Enumeration and definition of population and initial acceptance rates. *J. Epidemiol. Community Health* **34**, 9–13.

Collins, C.D., Constant, O., Fryatt, I., Blake, P.R. and Parsons, C.A. (1994) Relationship of computed tomography tumour volume to patient survival in carcinoma of the cervix treated by radical radiotherapy. *Br. J. Radiol.* **67**, 252–6.

Cook, G.A. and Draper, G.J. (1984) Trends in cervical cancer and carcinoma *in situ* in Great Britain. *Br. J. Cancer* **50**, 367–75.

Dattoli, M.J., Gretz, H.F., Seller, U.*et al.* (1989) Analysis of multiple prognostic factors in patients with stage Ib cervical cancer: age as a major determinant. *Int. J. Radiat. Oncol. Biol. Phys.* **17**, 41–7.

Denton, A.S., Bond, S.J., Matthews, S., Bentzen, SM., Maher, E.J. and the UK Link Gynaecology–Oncology Group (2000) Short report: national audit of the management and outcome of carcinoma of the cervix treated with radiotherapy in 1993. *Clin. Oncol.* **12**, 347–53.

Elliot, P.M., Tattersall, M.H., Coppleson, M.*et al.* (1989) Changing character of cervical cancer in young women. *BMJ* **298**, 288–90.

FIGO (1988) *Report of the International Federation of Gynaecology and Obstetrics.* Radiumhemmet, S104.01, Stockholm, Sweden.

FIGO (1992) In UICC, *TNM atlas* (3rd edn). Heidelberg: Springer-Verlag, 196.

Fu, K. and Philips, T. (1990) High dose-rate versus low dose-rate intracavitary brachytherapy for carcinoma of the cervix. *Int. J. Radiat. Biol. Oncol. Phys.* **19**, 791–6.

Haie, C., Pejovic, M.H., Gerbaulet, A.*et al.* (1988) Is prophylactic para-aortic irradiation worthwhile in the treatment of advanced carcinoma of the cervix? Results of a controlled clinical trial of the EORTC radiotherapy group. *Radiother. Oncol.* **11**, 101–12.

Harris, G., Cramp, W.A., Edwards, J.C.*et al.* (1985) Radiosensitivity of peripheral blood lymphocytes in autoimmune disease. *Int. J. Radiat. Biol.* **47**, 689–99.

Hoskin, P.J. and Blake, P.R. (1991) Cisplatin, methotrexate and bleomycin (PMB) for carcinoma of the cervix; the influence of presentation and previous treatment upon response. *Int. J. Gynaecol. Cancer* **1**, 75–80.

ICRU (1984) *Dose and volume specification for reporting intracavitary radiotherapy in gynaecology.* International Commission on Radiation Units and Measurements, Report 38, Washington, DC.

Inoue, T. and Morita, K. (1990) The prognostic significance of number of positive nodes in cervical carcinoma stages IB, IIA and IIB. *Cancer* **65**, 1923.

Kamura, T., Tsukamoto, N., Tsuruchi, N. *et al.* (1993) Histopathological prognostic factors in stage IIb cervical carcinoma treated with radical hysterectomy and pelvic node dissection: an analysis with mathematical statistics. *Int. J. Gynaecol. Cancer* **3**, 219–25.

Keys, H.M., Bundy, B.N., Stehman, F.B.*et al.* (1999) Cisplatin, radiation and adjuvant hysterectomy compared with radiation and adjuvant hysterectomy for bulky stage Ib cervical carcinoma. *N. Engl. J. Med.* **340**, 1154–61.

Khan, S.A. (1993) Cervical cancer, human papilloma virus and vaccines. *Clin. Oncol.* **5**, 386–90.

Lammont, D.W., Symonds, R.P., Brodie, M.M., Nwabineli, N.J. and Gillis, C.R. (1993) Age, socio-economic status and survival from cancer of the cervix in the West of Scotland 1980–87. *Br. J. Cancer* **67**, 351–7.

Magee, B.J., Logue, J.P., Swindell, R. and McHugh, D. (1991) Tumour size as a prognostic factor in carcinoma of the cervix: assessment by transrectal ultrasound. *Br. J. Radiol.* **64**, 812–15.

Maiman, M., Fruchter, R.F. and Serur, E. (1990) Human immunodeficiency virus infection and cervical neoplasia. *Gynaecol. Oncol.* **38**, 377–82.

Morris, M., Eifel, P.J., Lu, J.*et al.* (1999) Pelvic radiation with concurrent chemotherapy compared with pelvic and para-aortic radiation for high-risk cervical cancer. *N. Engl. J. Med.* **340**, 1137–43.

Munoz, N., Bosch, X. and Kaldor, J.M. (1988) Does human papilloma virus cause cervical cancer? The state of the epidemiological evidence. *Br. J. Cancer* **57**, 1–5.

OPCS (Office of Population Censuses and Surveys) (1989) OPCS Monitor DH2 89/3.

Patel, F.D., Sharma, S.C., Negi, P.S., Ghoshal, S. and Gupta, B.D. (1993) Low dose rate vs. high dose rate brachytherapy in the treatment of carcinoma of the uterine cervix: a clinical trial. *Int. J. Radiat. Oncol. Biol. Phys.* **28**, 335–41.

Rose, P.G., Bundy, B.N., Watkins, E.B.*et al.* (1999) Concurrent cisplatin-based radiotherapy and chemotherapy for locally advanced cervical cancer. *N. Engl. J. Med.* **340**, 1144–53.

Sardi, J.E., Snaanes, C.E., Giaroli, A.A.*et al.* (1998) Neoadjuvant chemotherapy in cervical carcinoma stage IIB: a randomised controlled trial. *Int. J. Gynecol. Cancer* **8**, 441–50.

Shingleton, H.M. and Orr, J.W. (1995)*Cancer of the cervix*. Edinburgh: Churchill Livingstone, 191.

Sigurdson, K. (1993) Effect of organised screening on the risk of cervical cancer. Evaluation of screening activity in Iceland, 1964–1991. *Int. J. Cancer* **54**, 563–70.

Singer, A., Reid, B.L. and Coppleson, M. (1976) A hypothesis: the role of a high risk male in the aetiology of cervical carcinoma. A correlation of epidemiology and molecular biology. *Am. J. Obstet. Gynaecol.* **126**, 110–15.

Thigpen, T., Vance, R.E., Balducci, L. and Blessing, J. (1981) Chemotherapy in the management of advanced and recurrent cervical and endometrial cancer. *Cancer* **48**, 658–65.

Thomas, G. (1999) Improved treatment for cervical cancer – concurrent chemotherapy and radiotherapy. *N. Engl. J. Med.* **340**, 1198–200.

Thranov, I. and Klee, M. (1994) Sexuality among gynaecologic cancer patients – a cross-sectional study. *Gynaecol. Oncol.* **52**, 14–19.

Tidy, J.A. and Wrede, D. (1992) Tumour supressor genes: new pathways in gynaecological cancer. *Int. J. Gynaecol. Cancer* **2**, 1–8.

Tutt, A.N.J., Lodge, N. and Blake, P.R. (1999) Palliative chemotherapy in recurrent carcinoma of the cervix: an audit of the use of ifosfamide and review of the literature. *Int. J. Gynecol. Cancer* **9**, 12–17.

Zunzunegui, M.V., King, M.C., Coria, C.F. and Charlet, J. (1986) Male influences on cervical cancer risk. *Am. J. Epidemiol.* **123**, 302–7.

36

Vagina and vulva

W. PAT SOUTTER, HANNAH E. LAMBERT AND HILARY THOMAS

CARCINOMA OF THE VAGINA

Invasive vaginal cancer is rare, only 209 women developed this cancer in England and Wales in 1992. It comprises 1–2 per cent of all gynaecological malignancies, the incidence being 0.8 per 100 000 women in England and Wales in 1992. However, like the cervix, the vagina has a range of premalignant lesions, many of which may be previously unrecognized extensions of cervical abnormalities. Coincident with the rise in prevalence of cervical intra-epithelial neoplasia (CIN) is an increase in the frequency with which vaginal intra-epithelial neoplasia (VAIN) is seen.

Aetiology

There is little firm evidence of aetiological agents. The irritation caused by procidentia and vaginal pessaries has been suggested, but this is an infrequent association. A field effect, in the lower genital tract, has been suggested by the observation of multicentric neoplasia involving cervix, vagina and vulva (Hopkins and Morley, 1987), and both immunosuppression and infection with human papilloma virus have been impugned (Weed et al., 1983; Carson et al., 1986).

Previous radiotherapy for cervical cancer in young women has been suggested as a cause of cancer of the vagina. Three small studies suggested that young women treated with radiotherapy for cervical cancer might be at greater risk of developing vaginal cancer (Barrie and Brunschwig, 1970, Futoran and Nolan, 1976; Choo and Anderson, 1982). However, a huge international collaborative study of 25 995 women followed for more than 10 years after treatment with radiotherapy for cervical cancer recorded only 48 cancers of the vulva or vagina. This was

not significantly different from the seven such women out of 5125 treated with surgery. These data suggest that if vaginal cancer is induced by radiotherapy, it is a very rare event.

For some time the prevalence of clear-cell adenocarcinoma of the vagina was thought to be increased by intra-uterine exposure to diethylstilboestrol (DES), but with the accrual of more information the risks now seem to be very low and lie between 0.1 and 1.0 per 1000 (Coppleson, 1984; Herbst, 1984). While vaginal adenosis and minor anatomical abnormalities of no significance (e.g. cervical cockscomb) are common following intra-uterine DES exposure, the only lesion of any significance that is seen more commonly is CIN (Robboy et al., 1984).

Anatomy

The upper two-thirds of the vagina are derived from the Müllerian duct and the lower third from the ectoderm of the cloaca. The vagina is related anteriorly to the bladder above and the urethra below. Posteriorly, the vault of the vagina is covered with the peritoneum of the pouch of Douglas. It thus becomes closely related to loops of small or large bowel. Below this, it is closely related to the anterior wall of the rectum until the perineal body separates it from the anal canal. The ureters run close to the cervix over each side of the vaginal vault to the bladder. Laterally, the vagina is supported by the lower portion of the cardinal ligaments until it reaches the pelvic floor, where it is invested by the medial part of the levator ani muscles (pubococcygeus). Lateral to the vagina, most of the tissue is areolar except at the level of the perineal body.

The vagina is lined by stratified squamous epithelium. When the transformation zone of the cervix has extended on to the vagina, clefts or glands partly lined by columnar epithelium will be seen deep to the squamous epithelium.

Pathology

Vaginal intra-epithelial neoplasia (VAIN) is character-ized by loss of stratification and polarity of the cells and by nuclear atypia. The great majority (92 per cent) of primary vaginal cancers are squamous. Clear cell adeno-carcinomas, malignant melanomas, embryonal rhabdo-myosarcomas and endodermal sinus tumours are the most common of the small number of other tumours seen very rarely in the vagina. These are discussed separately.

Natural history

VAIN is seen most commonly in the upper vagina and is unusual in the mid and lower parts. The malignant poten-tial for VAIN is not as well documented as that of CIN, but it is clearly not a completely benign disease. It would seem sensible to treat it with the same respect accorded to CIN.

Although the upper vagina is the most common site for invasive disease, about 25–30 per cent of cases have disease confined to the lower vagina, usually the anterior wall. Squamous vaginal cancer spreads by local invasion initially. Lymphatic spread occurs by tumour emboli-zation to the pelvic nodes from the upper vagina and to both pelvic and inguinal nodes from the lower vagina. Haematogenous spread is unusual.

Clinical staging

The modified clinical staging suggested by Perez and colleagues (1973) has been widely adopted (Table 36.1).

Diagnosis and assessment

VAIN is usually a cytological or colposcopic diagnosis. Dyskaryosis in cervical or vaginal cytology is an indica-tion for colposcopy to determine the location and nature of the abnormality that is giving rise to the abnormal cells. As a substantial proportion of these women have undergone hysterectomy prior to the detection of VAIN, and as the majority of the lesions are in the vaginal vault,

Table 36.1 *Modified FIGO staging of vaginal cancer*

Stage 0	Intra-epithelial neoplasia
Stage I	Invasive carcinoma confined to the vaginal mucosa
Stage IIa	Subvaginal infiltration not extending to the parametrium
Stage IIb	Parametrial infiltration not extending to the pelvic side-wall
Stage III	Extends to pelvic side-wall
Stage IVa	Involves mucosa of bladder or rectum
Stage IVb	Spread beyond the pelvis

straddling the suture line or in the angles of the vault, assessment and biopsy can be difficult (Soutter, 1993). General anaesthesia is required for most cases. It should also be remembered that abnormal epithelium or inva-sive cancer can lie buried behind the sutures closing the vault.

Before making a diagnosis of primary vaginal cancer, the following criteria must be satisfied: the primary site of growth must be in the vagina; the uterine cervix must not be involved, and there must be no clinical evidence that the vaginal tumour is metastatic disease (International Federation of Obstetrics and Gynaecology, 2001).

The most common presenting symptom is vaginal bleeding (53–65 per cent) with vaginal discharge (11–16 per cent) and pelvic pain (4–11 per cent) being less common (Gallup *et al.*, 1987). The rate of detection of asymptomatic cancer with vaginal cytology varies greatly (10–42 per cent), depending on the patient population studied. Most of the disease thus detected is at an early stage.

The most important part of the pre-treatment assess-ment of invasive cancer of the vagina is a careful exam-ination under anaesthesia. A combined vaginal and rectal examination will help to detect extravaginal spread. Cysto-scopy, proctosigmoidoscopy and colposcopy may be indi-cated, the latter to identify coexisting VAIN. A generous, full-thickness biopsy is essential for adequate histological evaluation. Other investigations include a chest X-ray. Magnetic resonance imaging (MRI) with an endovaginal coil can be invaluable in showing disease spread outside the vagina. Transrectal ultrasound or computed tomog-raphy (CT) imaging may help to define the size and extent of the lesion.

Treatment and complications – vaginal intra-epithelial neoplasia

The treatment of VAIN includes local ablation with the carbon dioxide laser, local excision, partial and total vaginectomy and radiotherapy. Occasionally, in a post-menopausal woman, the abnormality resolves with oestrogen therapy.

Local ablation with the carbon dioxide laser is used for small lesions where there is no suspicion of invasion. Local excision is sufficient for small lesions, otherwise partial or total colpectomy (vaginectomy) is necessary. Surgery can give rise to severe coital problems, even when only partial vaginectomy is performed. In the young, sex-ually active woman these may be overcome by the con-struction of a neovagina but even this is not immune from later developing cancer (Hopkins and Morley, 1987).

Intra-cavitary radiotherapy is an option for lesions in the vaginal vault following a hysterectomy, but this will have the disadvantage that radiotherapy can cause vaginal stenosis or ovarian failure in a premenopausal woman.

Treatment of invasive cancer

RADIOTHERAPY

Invasive vaginal cancer is usually treated with radiotherapy, which is given either as a combination of external radiation and brachytherapy (interstitial or intra-cavitary) or by brachytherapy alone.

Early cases of vaginal cancer occurring in the lower vagina may be treated entirely with interstitial brachytherapy, usually with iridium-192. A template, for example, the Syed–Neblett applicator, which is after-loaded, allows an even distribution of radiation to the lesion. The objective is to achieve a tumour dose of 70–80 Gy in two fractions, 2 weeks apart. The radiation is given at a rate of 10 Gy/day.

Tumours of the upper two-thirds of the vagina are treated in an identical fashion to cancer of the cervix, either by radiotherapy or by chemoradiotherapy, usually with cisplatin given concurrently. External radiotherapy to the pelvis includes the parametria and the pelvic nodes, followed by brachytherapy. The lower end of the radiation field must cover the lesion in the vagina plus a 2 cm margin. If the lesion extends into the lower third of the vagina, the inguino-femoral nodes must also be included in the treatment volume. A total dose of 45–50 Gy in 25–28 fractions in 5–6 weeks is given to the pelvis. External radiotherapy is followed by intracavitary therapy. This is with an intra-uterine tube and ovoids, for lesions limited to the vaginal vault. For lesions below the vault the treatment boost is given with interstitial brachytherapy, which has been found to be more effective than intra-cavitary brachytherapy (Stock *et al.*, 1992). However, if the tumour has completely regressed following external irradiation, brachytherapy, using a vaginal obturator, will give a sufficient dose to the vaginal mucosa. The total dose from both external radiotherapy and low dose rate brachytherapy, is 70–75 Gy to the vaginal mucosa, or its equivalent using a high dose rate system.

Complications of radiotherapy

Vaginal stenosis may occur and is more likely when advanced tumours are treated. The overall prevalence of vaginal stenosis is around 30 per cent and is an undoubted problem for sexually active patients. This complication can be reduced by the use of vaginal douches during treatment and vaginal dilators afterwards. Mucosal ulceration, either immediate or delayed, can be a distressing complication but conservative therapy is usually effective. Vesicovaginal and rectovaginal fistulas and small bowel complications can occur but are rare. The risk of fistula formation is higher in advanced disease.

SURGERY

A stage I lesion in the upper vagina can be adequately treated by radical hysterectomy (if the uterus is still present), radical vaginectomy and pelvic lymphadenectomy. Exenteration is required for more advanced lesions and carries the problems of stomas. However, surgery may be the treatment of choice for women who have had prior pelvic radiotherapy.

RESULTS

Owing to the rarity of vaginal cancer there is a wide range of reported results. Probably the most reliable figures are from Kucera and Vavra (1991), who reported on 460 women with cancer of the vagina. They found that 77 per cent of the women with stage I disease were alive at 5 years, compared to 45 per cent of those with stage II, 31 per cent with stage III, and 18 per cent with stage IV.

Uncommon vaginal tumours

CLEAR CELL ADENOCARCINOMA

The relation of this rare tumour to intra-uterine exposure to DES is discussed above. The histology is characterized by vacuolated or clear areas in the cytoplasm and a hob-nail appearance of the nuclei of cells lining the lumen of glands. Radical surgery or radical radiotherapy is required for invasive lesions. As most are situated in the upper vagina, they may be treated as cervical lesions. Lymph-node metastases and 5-year survival figures are equivalent to those for cervical cancer.

MALIGNANT MELANOMA

Vaginal melanoma has a 5-year survival rate of less than 10 per cent. Vaginal bleeding and discharge are the most common presenting symptoms. The prognosis depends upon the depth of epithelial invasion. Radical surgery and radiotherapy are of little value if the lesion is deeply invasive because of its propensity to metastasize early via the bloodstream. There is, at present, no effective chemotherapy.

RHABDOMYOSARCOMA (SARCOMA BOTRYOIDES)

Ninety per cent of these rare tumours occur in children less than 5 years old. They present with vaginal bleeding and a grape-like mass in the vagina. The appearance of cross-striations in the rhabdomyoblasts is characteristic of this tumour. Treatment is with combination chemotherapy, which is carried out in specialist centres. When chemotherapy produces only a partial response, local surgery is carried out. Occasionally exenteration is required for resistant disease. Radiotherapy is restricted to patients with unresectable tumour, in view of the deleterious effects on bone growth. The overall survival rate is over 80 per cent.

ENDODERMAL SINUS TUMOURS

These very rare tumours may resemble rhabdomyosarcomas, but histology shows a primitive adenocarcinoma.

Most occur in infants under the age of 2 years. Treatment with chemotherapy is as for germ-cell tumours of the testis or ovary.

CARCINOMA OF THE VULVA

Invasive vulval cancer is not a common gynaecological cancer. There are about 800 new cases each year in England and Wales, and the annual incidence is approximately 3.1/100 000. The majority of these women are elderly, less than 10 per cent are under 55 years of age and 80 per cent are over 65, and with increased life expectancy this cancer is seen more often.

Cancer of the vulva is unpleasant, but potentially curable even in elderly, unfit ladies if referred early and managed correctly from the outset. It is essential that patients are referred to a multidisciplinary team in a cancer centre for treatment as soon as vulval cancer is suspected. Surgery for this condition needs special expertise and should only be undertaken by gynaecological oncologists. Initial, inappropriate surgery leads to a poor outcome.

Aetiology

Little is known of the aetiology of vulvar cancer. A viral factor has been suggested as DNA from human papillomavirus (HPV) types 16 and 18 has been detected in vulval intra-epithelial neoplasia (VIN). The type 2 herpes simplex virus (HSV) may be a co-factor.

Anatomy

The vulva includes the mons pubis, the labia majora and minora, the clitoris, the vestibule of the vagina, the bulb of the vestibule and the greater vestibular glands (Bartholin's). The mons pubis is a pad of fat anterior to the pubic symphysis and covered by hair-bearing skin. The labia majora extend posteriorly from the mons on either side of the pudendal cleft into which the urethra and vagina open. They merge with one another and the perineal skin anterior to the anus. They consist largely of areolar tissue and fat. On their lateral aspects the skin is pigmented and covered with crisp hairs. On the medial side the skin is smooth and has many sebaceous glands. The labia minora are small folds of skin that lie between the labia majora and divide anteriorly to envelope the clitoris. The medial surfaces contain many sebaceous glands. The clitoris is an erectile structure analogous to the male penis. Partly hidden by the anterior folds of the labia minora, the clitoris consists of a body of two corpora cavernosa lying side-by-side and connected to the pubic and ischial rami, and a glans of sensitive, spongy erectile tissue. The vestibule is that area between the labia minora into which the urethra and vagina open. The bulbs of the vestibule are elongated masses of erectile tissue lying on either side of the vaginal opening. The greater vestibular glands lie posterior to the bulbs of the vestibule and are connected to the surface by short ducts.

Lymphatic drainage

The lymph drains from the vulva to the inguinal and femoral glands in the groin and then to the external iliac glands. Drainage from the perineum and the clitoris is to both groins but some contralateral spread occurs from other sites on the vulva. Direct spread to the pelvic nodes along the internal pudendal vessels occurs only very rarely and no direct pathway from the clitoris to pelvic nodes has been consistently demonstrated.

Pathology

Both squamous vulval intra-epithelial neoplasia (VIN) and Paget's disease occur on the vulva. The histological features of VIN are analogous to those seen in CIN and VAIN. In the same way, the histological appearance of Paget's disease is similar to the lesion seen in the breast. In a third of cases of Paget's disease, there is an adenocarcinoma in underlying apocrine glands and these carry an especially poor prognosis. Most invasive cancers (85 per cent) are squamous. Some 5 per cent are melanomas and the remainder are made up of carcinomas of Bartholin's gland, other adenocarcinomas, basal cell carcinomas, and the very rare verrucous carcinomas, rhabdomyosarcomas and leiomyosarcomas.

Natural history

More women are developing VIN. Of these a large proportion – 40 per cent – are less than 40 years of age. VIN is histologically very similar to CIN and often occurs in association with it. It used to be said that its malignant potential is less than 5 per cent. However, this opinion is based largely on studies of women who have been treated by excision biopsy or vulvectomy. This may not be true of untreated or inadequately treated patients, as progression to invasive cancer in 2–8 years has been reported (Jones and McLean, 1986).

The definition of 'microinvasion' of the vulva has proved extremely problematical. The purpose is to identify a group of women with invasive carcinoma who could safely be treated with a less mutilating procedure than radical vulvectomy. Although it was initially suggested that up to 5 mm invasion into the stroma might be acceptable (Rutledge et al., 1970; Wharton et al., 1974), subsequent reports have suggested lower limits. Some have suggested 2 mm (Friedrich and Wilkinson, 1982), others preferred 1 mm (Iversen et al., 1981), while further reports emphasize the importance of lymphatic or vascular invasion and the degree of differentiation (Parker *et al.*, 1975) or confluence (Hoffman *et al.*, 1983). It seems that the safest course to follow is to perform groin node dissection in all cases with more than 1 mm stromal invasion without attempting to differentiate between superficial and deep inguinal nodes (Hacker *et al.*, 1984a; Monaghan, 1985).

Invasive disease involves the labia majora in about two-thirds of cases and the clitoris, labia minora, or posterior fourchette and perineum in the remainder. The tumour usually spreads slowly, infiltrating local tissue before metastasizing to the groin nodes. Spread to the contralateral groin occurs in about 25 per cent of those cases with positive groin nodes, so bilateral groin node dissection is required in almost all cases. Pelvic node involvement is not common and is usually secondary to groin node involvement but, rarely, there is direct spread to the pelvic nodes via the internal pudendal vessels. Blood spread to bone or lung is rare.

Death can be a long, unpleasant process and is often due to sepsis and inanation or haemorrhage. Uraemia from bilateral ureteric obstruction may supervene first. Such is the abject misery of this demise that all patients with resectable vulval lesions should be offered surgery regardless of their age and general condition.

Clinical staging

The FIGO classification is shown in Table 36.2. In spite of the apparent limitations of this classification, it does give

Table 36.2 *The FIGO staging of vulvar cancer (1995)*

Stage	Definition
Stage Ia	Confined to vulva and/or perineum, 2 cm or less maximum diameter. Groin nodes not palpable. Stromal invasion no greater than 1 mm[a]
Stage Ib	As for Ia but stromal invasion greater than 1 mm
Stage II	Confined to vulva and/or perineum, more than 2 cm maximum diameter. Groin nodes not palpable
Stage III	Extends beyond the vulva, vagina, lower urethra or anus; or unilateral regional lymph-node metastasis
Stage IVa	Involves the mucosa of rectum or bladder; upper urethra; or pelvic bone; and/or bilateral regional lymph node metastases
Stage IVb	Any distant metastasis including pelvic lymph node

[a] Depth of invasion is measured from the epithelial stromal junction of the adjacent most superficial dermal papilla to the deepest point of invasion.

a reasonable guide to the prognosis. Formerly, the main drawback was a reliance on clinical palpation of the groin nodes, which is notoriously inaccurate (Monaghan, 1985). Now that the surgical findings are incorporated in the staging evaluation, the prognostic value is greatly improved.

Diagnosis and assessment

Intra-epithelial disease of the vulva often presents as pruritus vulvae but 20–45 per cent are asymptomatic and frequently are found after treatment of other genital-tract malignancies, particularly cervical carcinoma. These lesions are often raised above the surrounding skin and have a rough surface, variable colour – white, due to hyperkeratinization; red, due to immaturity of the epithelium; or dark brown, due to increased melanin deposition in the epithelial cells. However, the full extent of the abnormality is often not apparent until 5 per cent acetic acid is applied. After 2 minutes, VIN turns white and mosaicism or punctation may be visible. All of these changes are best examined colposcopically. Toluidine blue is also used as a nuclear stain, but areas of ulceration give false-positive results and hyperkeratinization gives false negatives. Biopsies must be taken from abnormal areas. This can usually be done under local anaesthesia in the outpatient clinic using a disposable 4 mm Stiefel biopsy punch or a Keyes punch.

While vulval cancer can be asymptomatic, over 70 per cent of patients with invasive disease complain of irritation, pruritus, pain or soreness, and over half note a mass in the vulva or an ulcer. It is usually not until the mass appears that medical advice is sought. Bleeding and discharge are less common presentations. One of the major problems in invasive vulval cancer is the delay between the first appearance of symptoms and referral for a gynaecological opinion. This is only partly due to the patients' reluctance to attend. In many cases the doctor fails to recognize the gravity of the lesion and prescribes topical therapy, sometimes without examining the woman.

Because of the multicentric nature of female lower genital tract cancer, the investigation should include inspection of the cervix and cervical cytology. The groin nodes must be palpated carefully and any suspicious nodes may be sampled by fine-needle aspiration. A chest X-ray is always required and a CT scan may be helpful. Thorough examination under anaesthesia and a full-thickness biopsy are the most important investigations. The examination under anaesthesia should note particularly the size and distribution of the primary lesion, especially the involvement of the urethra or rectum, and secondary lesions in the vulval or perineal skin must be sought. The groin should be re-examined under general anaesthesia, as previously undetected nodes may be palpated at that time.

Treatment of VIN

The treatment of vulval intra-epithelial neoplasia is difficult. Uncertainty about the malignant potential, the multifocal nature of the disorder and the discomfort and mutilation resulting from therapy suggest that recommendations should be cautious and conservative, in order to avoid making the treatment worse than the disease. The youth of many of these patients is a further, important consideration. None the less, the documented progression of untreated cases to invasive cancer underlines the potential importance of these lesions. If the patient has presented with symptoms, therapy is required. Asymptomatic patients, particularly under the age of 50 years, are probably best observed closely, with biopsies repeated if there are any suspicious changes (Soutter, 1993).

If the lesion is small, an excision biopsy may be both diagnostic and therapeutic (Andreasson and Bock, 1985). If the disease is multifocal or covers a wide area, a skin graft may improve the cosmetic result of a skinning vulvectomy (Caglar et al., 1986). However, the donor site is often very painful and a satisfactory result can be obtained in many patients without grafting.

An alternative approach is to vaporize the abnormal epithelium with the carbon dioxide laser (Townsend et al., 1982). Given the very irregular surface of the vulva, it is very difficult to achieve a uniform depth of destruction. Moreover, the depth of treatment required for VIN is still unclear (Dorsey, 1986). In some cases hair follicles may be involved for several millimetres below the surface (Mene and Buckley, 1985). Even with carefully controlled depth of treatment, re-epithelialization of large areas treated with the laser will take several weeks. The other main disadvantage is not having histopathological assessment. The use of 5-fluorouracil (5-FU) cream is not widely recommended (Cavanagh et al., 1985).

Treatment of invasive disease

Surgery is the mainstay of treatment. The introduction of radical vulvectomy (complete removal of the vulva and bilateral inguino-femoral lymphadenectomy) reduced the mortality from 80 per cent to 40 per cent (Taussig, 1940; Way, 1960). However, to control lymphatic spread, these techniques removed large areas of normal skin from the groins and primary wound closure was rarely achieved. By using a modified incision, the same objectives can be accomplished without the removal of large areas of normal skin and with the enormous benefit that primary closure could be achieved in nearly all cases (Monaghan, 1986). A further refinement aimed at reducing still further the problems of wound healing was the use of separate groin incisions for stage I–II cases (Hacker et al., 1981). Studies comparing triple incision with en-bloc dissection have not shown any significant difference in either survival or recurrence (Helm et al., 1992; Siller et al.,

1995). Using the triple incision technique in 100 women with cancer of the vulva, Grimshaw et al. (1993) reported a 75 per cent 5-year survival corrected for death from intercurrent disease. The corrected survival for women with stage I disease was 95 per cent.

More recently there has been a move to an even more conservative approach. In early stage disease, in the absence of clinically suspicious or involved groin nodes, the surgery to the primary tumour should be 'radical to remove the tumour yet conservative to avoid unnecessary surgical and psychological morbidity' (Royal College of Obstetricians and Gynaecologists, 1999). The psychological morbidity of radical treatment has been reported by Andersen (1993). The management of the vulval lesion and treatment of the groins should be considered separately.

EXCISION OF THE VULVAL LESION

If the lesion is less than 2 cm in diameter, unifocal and if the rest of the vulva is healthy, radical local excision is the treatment of choice (Hacker, 1998). In all other cases, a radical removal of the whole vulva is required. The deep and the lateral surgical margins should be no less following radical local excision than after radical vulvectomy. The depth of resection should be to the fascia, and lateral margins should be 8 mm to minimize the risk of local recurrence. The distal 1 cm of the urethra can be excised safely to achieve an adequate margin without risking incontinence. If radical surgery is likely to cause sphincter damage, leading to urinary or faecal incontinence, preoperative radiotherapy or chemoradiotherapy should be considered to shrink the tumour.

GROIN NODE DISSECTION

Dissection of the groin nodes is carried out for all cases greater than stage Ia. The groin node dissection includes both the superficial inguinal and deep femoral nodes, as superficial groin node dissection alone is associated with a higher risk of groin node recurrence (Stehman et al., 1992b). If the nodes are not obviously clinically involved, separate incisions in the groin can be used (Hacker et al., 1981). In advanced disease, the triple incision technique may be inappropriate and a radical vulvectomy with an en-bloc groin node dissection may be required. Because of the extensive crossover of lymphatic channels from the vulva, bilateral groin node dissection is usually performed. However, in lateral tumours where the medial margin of the tumour is at least 2 cm from the mid-line, an ipsilateral groin node dissection is sufficient. However, if the nodes are found to be positive, the contralateral groin will need to be dissected at a second operation.

There is little value in performing a pelvic node dissection as postoperative radiation therapy to the groins and pelvis gives superior results when more than two groin nodes are involved (Homesley et al., 1986).

Complications

The most common complication is wound breakdown and infection. With the modified surgical techniques referred to above, this is seldom more than a minor problem. Conservative therapy with Eusol and liquid honey packs is all that is required. Lymphocyst formation can be very troublesome. Aspiration or secondary drainage is seldom helpful. Resolution usually occurs spontaneously. Osteitis pubis is a rare but very serious complication that requires intensive and prolonged antibiotic therapy. Thromboembolic disease is always a greatly feared complication of pelvic surgery for malignant disease but the combination of peroperative epidural analgesia to ensure good venous return with subcutaneous heparin begun postoperatively seems to reduce this risk. Secondary haemorrhage occurs from time to time. Leg oedema may be expected in about 30 per cent of women. Numbness and paraesthesia over the anterior thigh is common due to the division of small cutaneous branches of the femoral nerve. Loss of body image and impaired sexual function undoubtedly occur but the patients' responses to surgery are enormously variable and probably dependent on the woman's upbringing and attitudes to life.

Chemotherapy

Chemotherapy has not played a large role in the management of vulval carcinoma, because of the advanced age of most of the patients and the frequency of concurrent medical conditions. Chemotherapy has also been used for recurrent disease. Single agents that have been shown to be active include cisplatin, doxorubicin, bleomycin and methotrexate. Concomitant chemoradiotherapy regimens have been investigated but there are no randomized studies to show whether chemoradiotherapy is superior to radiotherapy alone (Thomas et al., 1989; Sebag-Montefiore et al., 1994).

Radiotherapy

While surgery is the mainstay of treatment for vulval carcinoma, adjuvant radiotherapy has a role in preventing recurrence. In the presence of advanced disease, with bowel or bladder involvement, surgery alone can result in poor function and cosmesis, and this has led to renewed interest in the use of non-surgical treatment modalities for this situation (Harrington and Lambert, 1994).

RADIOTHERAPY TECHNIQUE

External-beam radiotherapy has historically been considered too toxic a treatment to be tolerated by the epithelium of the vulva, leading to severe acute moist desquamation and severe late normal tissue damage (vulvar fibrosis, atrophy and necrosis, vaginal and urethral stenosis and fistula formation). However, these complications of radiotherapy are avoidable by using doses per fraction of no more than 1.8 Gy, and by limiting the overall total dose.

There is general agreement on a threshold dose for improved local control at about 50 Gy. Fraction size is important, with 1.7 Gy being close to tolerance. The doses which have been recommended by Royal College of Obstetricians and Gynaecologists (1999), based on the recommendations of Thomas et al. (1989, 1991), are 55 Gy as a maximum preoperatively (with or without concurrent 5-FU); 45–50 Gy as adjuvant postoperative treatment; 65 Gy as radical therapy. Higher doses can lead to severe morbidity. Hoffman et al. (1990) reported radionecrosis in 6 of 10 patients treated with more than 70 Gy.

The optimal fractionation regimen remains to be defined. Thomas et al. (1989), using daily fractions of 1.6–1.8 Gy to a total dose of 40–64 Gy to the vulva and 36–59 Gy to the nodes with concomitant 5-FU and Mitomycin C® chemotherapy in 27 patients found that 16 needed unplanned treatment breaks for periods of 10–34 days (median 19 days). This delay would only have been partly due to the additional use of the concomitant chemotherapy. The use of twice-daily fractionation, giving 1.5 Gy with a 6-hour gap has been reported from Hammersmith Hospital (Soutter et al., 1995). This regimen consists of 45 Gy in 30 fractions in 3 weeks and, in those patients not proceeding to surgery, is followed by a planned 2-week gap to allow skin healing before treatment is continued to a total of 64.5 Gy. Experience with this twice-daily treatment has shown that unplanned treatment breaks can be eliminated. Such a regimen offers obvious benefits in terms of ensuring overall treatment time is not prolonged.

Limitation of the size of the radiation field is also important. When radiotherapy is given with radical intent, it is given in two phases. The first phase treats the primary and nodal sites, using external irradiation, to a dose of 45–50 Gy. For the second phase the tumour is boosted using as small a field as possible. This is achieved by selecting the most appropriate technique, such as a direct field to the perineum using electron portals or interstitial radiotherapy or conformal radiotherapy. The total dose from both phases of treatment, as previously stated, is 65 Gy.

POSTOPERATIVE RADIOTHERAPY

Fifteen to 33 per cent of patients with advanced, operable vulval carcinoma recur after radical surgery – the majority (80–95 per cent) at locoregional sites in the first instance (Bryson et al., 1991).

A number of clinico-pathological variables have been defined which predict local recurrence and overall survival (Heaps et al., 1990; Hopkins et al., 1991). The clinically important features are FIGO stage, presence of clinically involved lymph nodes, tumour size independent of stage, tumour location (midline versus lateral, with midline tumours having a greater tendency to metastasize to bilateral inguinal nodes), age and performance status.

The significant pathological variables are the presence and number of pathologically involved lymph nodes, surgical excision margin less than 8 mm, depth of invasion, tumour grade, lymphatic vascular space invasion, perineural invasion and tumour border pattern (infiltrative versus pushing).

The most significant prognostic signs are size of tumour; inguinal node involvement and the width of the vulval tumour-free margin. Almost 1 in 5 patients found to have metastatic involvement of groin nodes removed at surgery will also have disease in the iliac nodes. In regard to tumour margin, there is no risk of recurrence if the tumour-free margin is 8 mm or more, but the risk of recurrence is 8 per cent if the margin is 4.8–8 mm, rising to 54 per cent if the margin is less than 4.8 mm (Heaps et al., 1990; Hacker and Van der Velden, 1993).

The criteria for postoperative radiotherapy to the inguinal and pelvic nodes have been specified as the presence of a single clinically involved node, more than two histologically involved inguinal nodes or extracapsular spread (Thomas et al., 1991). The dose for postoperative radiotherapy to the groins and pelvic nodes is 45–50 Gy at 1.8–2.0 Gy per fraction. The recommended depth is up to 8 cm, as the depth of the deep nodes will vary from patient to patient.

Adjuvant radiotherapy to the vulva is necessary where the disease-free margin is less than 8 mm, to prevent recurrence. This should be given to as small a field as possible to reduce morbidity. The recommended dose is 45–50 Gy.

RADIOTHERAPY AS AN ALTERNATIVE TO SURGERY FOR OCCULT NODAL DISEASE

Since 20–25 per cent of women with clinically stage I cancer of the vulva have occult nodal metastases, some form of local treatment is required to eradicate this potential source of recurrent (and metastatic) disease. The results of adjuvant nodal irradiation (Homesley et al., 1986) suggested the hypothesis that nodal irradiation could obviate the need for bilateral inguinal lymph-node dissection in low-risk groups. However, a randomized GOG study (Stehman et al., 1992a) did not confirm this. Fifty-two patients with clinically non-suspicious inguinal nodes undergoing radical vulvectomy were randomized to receive either node dissection or inguino-femoral nodal irradiation to a dose of 50 Gy at 2 Gy per fraction dosed at 3 cm depth. The study was closed prematurely when interim analysis revealed a significant advantage in favour of the surgical arm in terms of progression-free interval and survival. A criticism of this study is that treatment to the groins was only given to a depth of 3 cm. However, radiotherapy cannot be recommended at present as an alternative to surgery for occult nodal disease.

PREOPERATIVE RADIOTHERAPY

The use of preoperative neo-adjuvant therapies has been investigated in an attempt to downstage tumours and facilitate 'viscera-preserving' surgery. Small studies using preoperative radiotherapy have reported encouraging results in patients with advanced stage III and IV disease (Hacker et al., 1984b; Rotmensch et al., 1990). The largest study consisted of 48 cases, 11 of which had recurrent disease (Boronow et al., 1987). Some of these cases had radiotherapy after surgery but most were treated preoperatively. The projected 5-year survival for the 37 primary cases was 75.6 per cent and for the recurrent cases was 62.6 per cent. Only two patients subsequently underwent an exenterative procedure or stoma formation. The value of preoperative radiotherapy for involved inguinal nodes has also been demonstrated.

In recent years attention has focused on the use of neo-adjuvant chemoradiotherapy, with the chemotherapy being used as a radiosensitizer rather than as a cytotoxic agent. Most of these studies have been carried out on only small numbers of patients. Koh et al. (1993) treated 20 patients with bulky cancers of the vulva with radiation doses to a maximum of 70.4 Gy to bulk disease and 54 Gy to areas at risk of microscopic spread combined with 5-FU (six patients also received either cisplatin or Mitomycin C®). A response rate of 90 per cent was reported, with 10 pathological complete responses and 8 pathological partial responses at viscera-preserving surgery. It would therefore appear that preoperative radiotherapy may be useful for advanced tumours to try to downsize the tumour in order to preserve urinary and anal sphincter control.

PRIMARY RADICAL NON-SURGICAL THERAPY

The place of radiotherapy alone in the treatment of vulval carcinoma has not been studied systematically. Data accruing from reports of non-surgical management of squamous carcinoma of the anus have led to an evaluation of the possible role of primary radical non-surgical treatment of carcinoma of the vulva based on the treatment strategy for anal carcinoma (Nigro et al., 1974).

Thomas et al. (1989) treated nine patients with radiotherapy to a dose of 45–60 Gy with concomitant 5-FU and Mitomycin C®. Complete response was achieved in six of the women, although there were three local recurrences. After appropriate surgical salvage, seven of the nine patients remained disease free at a median of 20 months' follow-up. Two other studies have yielded equivalent results with similar treatment protocols, although cisplatin was substituted for Mitomycin C® by Berek et al. (1991) in 12 patients, and the majority of patients (14 of 20) received 5-FU alone in the study by Koh et al. (1993).

Based on the success of treating anal carcinoma, definitive radical radiotherapy to the vulva and inguinal nodes is usually given with concurrent 5-FU, the latter as a 4-day infusion in the first and fourth or fifth weeks of radiotherapy. The maximum radiation dose is 65 Gy.

CONCLUSIONS

Radiotherapy can be delivered safely to the vulva and regional lymph nodes with or without concomitant chemotherapy. The role of chemotherapy in the treatment of carcinoma of the vulva has not yet been clearly established.

The use of radiotherapy for early stage carcinoma of the vulva should be restricted to adjuvant therapy to the vulva and nodes in patients at high risk of local recurrence after surgery. There is no evidence to support the use of inguinal nodal irradiation as a replacement for bilateral inguinal lymph-node dissection.

In advanced FIGO stage III or IV disease the use of preoperative radiotherapy and chemoradiotherapy in an attempt to facilitate viscera-preserving surgery appears promising.

Results

Published 5-year survival rates for invasive cancer vary widely due to the low incidence of this tumour and the advanced age of the majority of these patients. Probably the most reliable information comes from a GOG study (Holmesley *et al.*, 1991) which defined risk groups for 377 women with cancer of the vulva, depending on size of tumour and groin node status, which on multifactorial analysis were the only variables associated with prognosis.

The risk was minimal in lesions measuring 2 cm or less and with no groin node involvement. Nearly all these patients were alive at 5 years. Women at low risk were those with lesions larger than 2 cm but less than 8.1 cm with no nodal involvement. They had a survival rate at 5 years of 87 per cent, as did those with lesions less than or equal to 2 cm in size but with a single node involved. Five-year survival dropped to 70 per cent for those at intermediate risk, which included those with lesions larger than 8 cm but with no groin node involvement and those with smaller lesions but with one or two nodes positive for metastatic disease. At high risk was any woman whose lesion was greater than 8 cm with two positive nodes, any size lesion with three or more ipsilateral nodes involved or with bilateral node involvement. The survival in this group at high risk was 29 per cent.

The effect on 5-year survival rate of lymph-node involvement, taken as a single prognostic variable, showed that a negative node status conferred a survival rate of 92 per cent, falling to 75 per cent with ipsilateral node involvement and 30 per cent with bilateral node involvement. If more than two nodes were involved, the survival rate was 25 per cent, falling to zero if more than six nodes were positive.

Uncommon tumours of the vulva

MELANOMA OF THE VULVA

Approximately 5 per cent of melanomas in women occur on the vulva and it is the second most common carcinoma of the vulva. Melanin production is variable and the lesions range from black to completely amelanotic. The most usual presenting complaint is of a lump or an enlarging mole. Pruritus and bleeding are less common.

The prognosis is strongly related to the depth of invasion (Clark *et al.*, 1969; Breslow, 1970; Podratz *et al.*, 1983). Because of the absence of a well-defined papillary dermis in much of the vulval skin, levels of invasion, as defined by Clark and co-workers (1969), are unsuitable and measurement of the thickness of the lesion, as suggested by Breslow (1970), is more commonly used. Breslow has five levels of invasion, from the surface epithelium to the point of deepest penetration. Level 1 is <0.76 mm in thickness, level 2 to 1.5 mm, level 3 to 3 mm, level 4 to 4 mm and level 5 deeper than 4 mm.

Local invasion occurs in an outward direction as well as downward, so excision margins must be very wide, 3–5 cm being suggested for all but the most superficial lesions. This usually requires a radical vulvectomy without lymphadenectomy, unless there is clinical evidence of groin disease. If the groin nodes are removed, the operation should be performed en bloc rather than through separate incisions, because of the melanoma's propensity to spread unseen by lateral intradermal infiltration.

Other forms of treatment, such as radiotherapy, chemotherapy and immunotherapy, have had very little impact on this disease.

The prognosis for level 1 melanoma of the vulva is very good as nodal involvement is unlikely. However, approximately one-third of patients have groin lymph-node metastases at presentation and 2.6 per cent have distant spread. While 5-year survival is approximately 56 per cent if the nodes are negative, the survival rate falls to 14 per cent when the nodes are positive (Morrow and DiSaia, 1976). Involvement of urethra or vagina, or the presence of satellite lesions, all worsen the prognosis.

PAGET'S DISEASE AND APOCRINE ADENOCARCINOMA OF THE VULVA

This is an uncommon condition, similar to that found in the breast. Pruritus is the presenting complaint. The lesion is indistinguishable clinically from squamous intraepithelial neoplasia and the diagnosis must be made by biopsy. In approximately one-third of patients there is an adenocarcinoma in the apocrine glands. This has a poor prognosis if the groin lymph nodes are involved, with no survivors at 5 years.

The treatment of Paget's disease is wide local excision, usually involving total vulvectomy because of the propensity of this condition to involve apparently normal skin. The specimen must be examined histologically, with great care to exclude an apocrine adenocarcinoma. Excluding underlying adnexal carcinomas, concomitant genital malignancies are found in 15–25 per cent of women with Paget's disease of the vulva (Degefu *et al.*, 1986). These are most commonly vulval or cervical, but transitional cell carcinoma of the bladder (or kidney), and ovarian, endometrial, vaginal and urethral carcinomas have all been reported.

VERRUCOUS CARCINOMA OF THE VULVA

This slowly growing neoplasm is rarely seen on the vulva. Both macroscopically and histologically it resembles condyloma accuminata, and the diagnosis can be difficult. Generous biopsies are required to provide sufficient material for the pathologist. The treatment is surgery, usually a radical vulvectomy but very occasionally wide local excision. The place of lymphadenectomy is debatable as lymph-node metastases are uncommon. Radiotherapy was considered to be contraindicated in verrucous carcinomas, as it was thought to result in dedifferentiation of the tumour, but this is no longer considered to be true.

BASAL CELL CARCINOMA

This tumour is rarely found on the vulva. Wide local excision gives excellent results in most cases.

BARTHOLIN'S GLAND CARCINOMA

Usually an adenocarcinoma, this tumour may be squamous, transitional cell type, or even mixed squamous and adenocarcinoma. It has often spread widely to pelvic and groin nodes before the diagnosis is made. It must be distinguished from adenoid cystic carcinoma, which is similar to the tumour found in salivary glands and which seldom gives rise to metastatic disease. The treatment is surgery but, because of its deep origin, part of the vagina, levatores ani and the ischio-rectal fat must be removed.

SARCOMAS

These rare tumours of the vulva include leiomyosarcomas, which tend to grow slowly and metastasize late, and rhabdomyosarcomas, which are rapidly growing, aggressive tumours. A radical vulvectomy and groin node dissection is the usual treatment but local recurrence and blood-borne metastases are common. The prognosis for sarcomas of the vulva is the same as for sarcomas in other parts of the body. There are very few long-term survivors.

SIGNIFICANT POINTS

Vaginal intra-epithelial neoplasia

- Vaginal intra-epithelial neoplasia is becoming more common.
- There is a risk in post-hysterectomy patients of disease hidden above the suture line in the vault.
- Surgical excision is the most effective treatment. Partial vaginectomy is often required for patients who have had a previous hysterectomy or radiotherapy.
- Brachytherapy has a place in women who have not had prior radiotherapy, but can cause ovarian failure and vaginal stenosis.

Invasive vaginal cancer

- Invasive vaginal cancer is a rare tumour, more often seen in association with an antecedent cervical malignancy.
- Radiotherapy is the main treatment method.
- Interstitial therapy alone offers good cure rates in early stages I–IIa occurring in the lower vagina. External radiotherapy is required for more advanced stages. Vaginal cancer occurring at the vault of the vagina is treated in a similar fashion to cancer of the cervix.

Carcinoma of the vulva

- Vulval intra-epithelial neoplasia is becoming more common, especially in young women.
- The treatment must be tailored carefully to the individual, to avoid mutilating therapy whenever possible.
- In view of the uncertainty about the malignant potential of these lesions, there may be a place for careful observation. However, it must not be forgotten that some of these patients will develop cancer of the vulva if untreated, so the importance of close follow-up must be emphasized to the patient and her general practitioner.
- The main problems with carcinoma of the vulva are delay in presentation and diagnosis, and inadequate initial therapy.

- Surgery remains the cornerstone of treatment but this can be made less extensive than in the past for early stage disease. Even when radical surgery is necessary, new techniques have reduced the morbidity enormously.
- Adjuvant radiotherapy is indicated for patients with metastatic groin node disease and to prevent local recurrence when the tumour-free margin is less than 8 mm.
- Radiotherapy will probably play a larger role in the future management of vulval carcinoma postoperatively, to prevent local recurrence, and preoperatively, to reduce tumour size in patients with advanced disease.

REFERENCES

Andersen, B.L. (1993) Predicting sexual and psychological morbidity and improving quality of life for women with gynaecological cancer. *Cancer* **71**,1678–90.

Andreasson, B. and Bock, J.E. (1985) Intraepithelial neoplasia in the vulval region. *Gynecol. Oncol.* **21**, 300–5.

Barrie, J.R. and Brunschwig, A. (1970) Late second cancers of the cervix after apparent successful initial radiation therapy. *Am. J. Roentgenol. Ther. Nucl. Med.* **108**, 109–12.

Berek, J.S., Heaps, J.M., Fu, Y.S. *et al.* (1991) Concurrent cisplatin and 5-fluorouracil chemotherapy and radiation therapy for advanced-stage squamous carcinoma of the vulva. *Gynecol. Oncol.* **42**, 197–201.

Boronow, R.C., Hickman, B.T., Reagan, M.T. *et al.* (1987) Combined therapy as an alternative to exenteration for locally advanced vulvovaginal cancer. *Am. J. Clin. Oncol.* **10**, 171–81.

Breslow, A. (1970) Thickness, cross-sectional areas and depth of invasion in the prognosis of cutaneous melanoma. *Ann. Surg.* **172**, 902–8.

Bryson, S.C., Dembo, A.J., Colgan, T.J. *et al.* (1991) Invasive squamous cell carcinoma of the vulva. Defining low and high risk groups for recurrence. *Int. J. Gynecol. Cancer* **1**, 25–31.

Caglar, H., Delgado, G. and Hreshchyshyn, M.M. (1986) Partial and total skinning vulvectomy in treatment of carcinoma *in situ* of the vulva. *Obstet. Gynecol.* **68**, 504–7.

Carson, L.F., Twiggs, L.B., Fukushima, M., Ostrow, R.S., Faras, A.J. and Okagaki, T. (1986) Human genital papilloma infections: an evaluation of immunologic competence in the genital neoplasia–papilloma syndrome. *Am. J. Obstet. Gynecol.* **155**, 784–9.

Cavanagh, D., Ruffolo, E.H. and Marsden, D.E. (1985) Cancer of the vulva. In Cavanagh, D., Ruffolo, E.H. and Marsden, D.E. (eds), *Gynecological cancer – a clinicopathological approach*. Connecticut: Appleton–Century–Crofts, 1–40.

Choo, Y.C. and Anderson, D.G. (1982) Neoplasms of the vagina following cervical carcinoma. *Gynecol. Oncol.* **14**, 125–32.

Clark, W.H., From, L., Bernadino, E.A. and Mihm, M.C. (1969) The histogenesis and biologic behaviour of primary human malignant melanomas of the skin. *Cancer Res.* **29**, 705–26.

Coppleson, M. (1984) The DES story. *Med. J. Aust.* **141**, 487–9.

Degefu, S., O'Quinn, A.G. and Dhurandhar, H.N. (1986) Paget's disease of the vulva and urogenital malignancies: a case report and review of the literature. *Gynecol. Oncol.* **25**, 347–54.

Dorsey, J.H. (1986) Skin appendage involvement and vulval intraepithelial neoplasia. In Sharp, F. and Jordan, J.A. (eds), *Laser surgery*. New York: Perinatology Press, 193–5.

Friedrich, E.G. and Wilkinson, E.J. (1982) The vulva. In Blaustein, A. (ed.), *Pathology of the female genital tract*. New York: Springer-Verlag, 13–58.

Futoran, R.J. and Nolan, J.F. (1976) Stage I carcinoma of the uterine cervix in patients under 40 years of age. *Am. J. Obstet. Gynecol.* **125**, 790–7.

Gallup, D.G., Talledo, O.E., Shah, K.J. and Hayes, C. (1987) Invasive squamous cell carcinoma of the vagina: a 14-year study. *Obstet. Gynecol.* **69**, 782–5.

Grimshaw, R.N., Murdoch, J.B. and Monaghan, J.M. (1993) Radical vulvectomy and bilateral inguinal–femoral lymphadenectomy through separate incisions – experience with a hundred cases. *Int. J. Gynecol. Cancer* **3**, 18–23.

Hacker, N.F. (1998) Current management of early vulvar cancer. *Am. Acad. Med. Singapore* **27**, 688–92.

Hacker, N.F. and Van der Velden, J. (1993) Conservative management of early vulvar cancer. *Cancer* **71**, 1673–7.

Hacker, N.F., Leuchter, R.S., Berek, J.S., Castaldo, T.W. and Lagasse, L.D. (1981) Radical vulvectomy and bilateral inguinal lymphadenectomy through separate groin incisions. *Obstet. Gynecol.* **58**, 574–9.

Hacker, N.F., Berek, J.S., Lagasse, L.D., Neiberg, R.K. and Leuchter, R.S. (1984a) Individualisation of treatment for stage I squamous cell vulvar carcinoma. *Obstet. Gynecol.* **63**, 155–62.

Hacker, N.F., Berek, J.S., Juillard, G.J.F. and Lagasse, L.D. (1984b) Preoperative radiation therapy for locally advanced vulvar cancer. *Cancer* **54**, 2056–61.

Harrington, K.J. and Lambert, H.E. (1994) Current issues in the non-surgical management of primary vulvar squamous cell carcinoma. *Clin. Oncol.* **6**, 331–6.

Heaps, J.M., Yao, S.F., Montz, F.J. *et al.* (1990) Surgical–pathologic variables predictive of local recurrence in squamous cell carcinoma of the vulva. *Gynecol. Oncol.* **38**, 309–14.

Helm, C.W., Hatch, K., Austin, J.M. *et al.* (1992) A matched comparison of single and triple incision techniques for the surgical treatment of carcinoma of the vulva. *Gynecol. Oncol.* **46**,150–6.

Herbst, A.L. (1984) Diethylstilboestrol exposure – 1984. *N. Engl. J. Med.* **22**, 1433–5.

Hoffman, J.S., Kuma, N.B. and Morely, G.W. (1983) Microinvasive squamous carcinoma of the vulva: search for a definition. *Obstet. Gynecol.* **61**, 615–18.

Hoffman, M., Greenberg, S., Greenberg, H. *et al.* (1990) Interstitial radiotherapy for the treatment of advanced or recurrent vulvar and distal vaginal malignancy. *Am. J. Obstet. Gynecol.* **162**, 1278–82.

Homesley, H.D., Bundy, B.N., Sedlis, A. and Adcock, L. (1986) Radiation therapy versus pelvic node resection for carcinoma of the vulva with positive groin nodes. *Obstet. Gynecol.* **68**, 733–40.

Homesley, H.D., Bundy, B.N., Sedlis, A. *et al.* (1991) Assessment of current International Federation of Gynecology and Obstetrics staging of vulvar carcinoma relative to prognostic factors for survival (a Gynecological Oncology Group Study). *Am. J. Obstet. Gynecol.* **164**, 997–1004.

Hopkins, M.P. and Morley, G.W. (1987) Squamous cell carcinoma of the neovagina. *Obstet. Gynecol.* **69**, 525–7.

Hopkins, M.P., Reid, G.C., Vettrano, I. *et al.* (1991) Squamous cell carcinoma of the vulva prognostic factors influencing survival. *Gynecol. Oncol.* **43**, 113–17.

International Federation of Obstetrics and Gynaecology (2001) Annual report on the results of treatment in gynaecological cancer, vol. 24. *J. Epidemiol. Biostat.* **6**, 141.

Iversen, T., Abeler, V. and Aalders, J. (1981) Individualised treatment of stage I carcinoma of the vulva. *Obstet. Gynecol.* **57**, 85–9.

Jones, R.W. and McLean, M.R. (1986) Carcinoma *in situ* of the vulva: a review of 31 treated and five untreated cases. *Obstet. Gynecol.* **68**, 499–503.

Koh, W.J., Wallace, H.J., Greer, B.E. *et al.* (1993) Combined radiotherapy and chemotherapy in the management of local-regionally advanced vulvar cancer. *Int. J. Radiat. Oncol. Biol. Phys.* **26**, 809–16.

Kucera, H. and Vavra, N. (1991) Primary carcinoma of the vagina: clinical and histopathological variables associated with survival. *Gynecol. Oncol.* **40**, 12–16.

Mene, A. and Buckley, C.H. (1985) Involvement of the vulval skin appendages by intraepithelial neoplasia. *Br. J. Obstet. Gynaecol.* **92**, 634–8.

Monaghan, J.M. (1985) Management of vulvar carcinoma. In Shepherd, J.H. and Monaghan, J.M. (eds), *Clinical gynaecological oncology*. London: Blackwells, 133–53.

Monaghan, J.M. (1986) Radical surgery for carcinoma of the vulva. In Monaghan J.M. (ed.), *Bonney's gynaecological surgery* (9th edn). Eastbourne: Baillière Tindall, 121–8.

Morrow, C.P. and DiSaia, P.J. (1976) Malignant melanoma of the female genitalia: a clinical analysis. *Obstet. Gynecol. Survey* **31**, 233–71.

Nigro, N.D., Vaitkevicius, V.K. and Considine, B. (1974) Combined therapy for cancer of the anal canal: a preliminary report. *Dis. Colon Rectum* **27**, 354–6.

Parker, R.T., Duncan, I., Rampone, J. and Creasman, W. (1975) Operative management of early invasive epidermoid carcinoma of the vulva. *Am. J. Obstet. Gynecol.* **123**, 349–55.

Perez, C.A., Arneson, A.N., Galakatos, A. and Samanth, H.K. (1973) Malignant tumours of the vagina. *Cancer* **31**, 36–44.

Podratz, K.C., Gaffey, T.A., Symmonds, R.E., Johansen, K.L. and O'Brien, P.C. (1983) Melanoma of the vulva: an update. *Gynecol. Oncol.* **16**, 153–68.

Robboy, S.J., Noller, K.L., O'Brien, P. *et al.* (1984) Increased incidence of cervical and vaginal dysplasia in 3,980 Diethylstilbestrol-exposed young women. *JAMA* **252**, 2979–83.

Rotmensch, J., Rubin, S.J., Sutton, H.G. *et al.* (1990) Preoperative radiotherapy followed by radical vulvectomy with inguinal lymphadenectomy for advanced vulvar carcinomas. *Gynecol. Oncol.* **36**, 181–4.

Royal College of Obstetricians and Gynaecologists (1999) *Clinical recommendations for the management of vulval cancer.* London: RCOG, 6.

Rutledge, F.N., Smith, J.P. and Franklin, E.W. (1970) Carcinomas of the vulva. *Am. J. Obstet. Gynecol.* **106**, 1117–30.

Sebag-Montefiore, D.J., McLean, C., Arnott, S.J. *et al.* (1994) Treatment of advanced carcinoma of the vulva with chemoradiotherapy – can exenterative surgery be avoided? *Int. J. Gynecol. Cancer* **4**, 150–5.

Siller, B.S., Alvarez, R.D., Connor, W.D. *et al.* (1995) T2/3 vulva cancer: a case-control study of triple incision versus en bloc radical vulvectomy and inguinal lymphadenectomy. *Gynecol. Oncol.* **57**, 335–9.

Soutter, W.P. (1993) Vaginal intraepithelial neoplasia and colposcopy of the vagina. In *A practical guide to colposcopy*. Oxford: Oxford Medical Publications, 144–60.

Soutter, W.P., Lambert, H.E. and McIndoe, G.A.J. (1995) Carcinoma of the vulva and its putative precursors. In Peckham, S.T., Pindeo, B. and Veronesi, U. (eds), *Oxford textbook of oncology*. Oxford: Oxford University Press, 1383–94.

Stehman, F.B., Bundy, B.N., Thomas, G. *et al.* (1992a) Groin dissection versus groin radiation in carcinoma of the vulva. A Gynecologic Oncology Group study. *Int. J. Radiat. Oncol. Biol. Phys.* **24**, 389–96.

Stehman, F.B., Bundy, B.N., Dvoretsky, P.M. and Creasman, W.T. (1992b) Early stage I carcinoma of the vulva treated with ipsilateral inguinal lymphadenectomy and modified radical hemivulvectomy. A prospective study of the Gynecologic Oncology Group. *Obstet. Gynecol.* **79**, 490–7.

Stock, R.G., Mychalczak, B., Armstrong, J.G. *et al.* (1992) The importance of brachytherapy technique in the management of primary carcinoma of the vagina. *Int. J. Radiat. Oncol. Biol. Phys.* **24**, 747–53.

Taussig, F.J. (1940) Cancer of the vulva – an analysis of 155 cases (1911–1940) *Am. J. Obstet. Gynecol.* **40**, 764–79.

Thomas, G., Dembo, A., DePetrillo, A. *et al.* (1989) Concurrent radiation and chemotherapy in vulvar carcinoma. *Gynecol. Oncol.* **34**, 263–7.

Thomas, G.M., Dembo, A.J., Bryson, S.C.P. *et al.* (1991) Changing concepts in the management of vulvar cancer. *Gynecol. Oncol.* **42**, 9–21.

Townsend, D.E., Levine, R.U., Richart, R.M., Crum, C.P. and Petrilli, E.S. (1982) Management of vulval intraepithelial neoplasia by carbon dioxide laser. *Obstet. Gynecol.* **60**, 49–52.

Way, S. (1960) Carcinoma of the vulva. *Am. J. Obstet. Gynecol.* **79**, 692–8.

Weed, J.C., Lozier, C. and Daniel, S.J. (1983) Human papilloma virus in multifocal, invasive female genital tract malignancy. *Obstet. Gynecol.* **62**, 83–87S.

Wharton, J.T., Gallagher, S. and Rutledge, F.N. (1974) Microinvasive carcinoma of the vulva. *Am. J. Obstet. Gynecol.* **118**, 159–62.

37

Gestational trophoblastic tumours

MICHAEL J. SECKL

INTRODUCTION

Gestational trophoblastic disease (GTD) was probably first described as 'dropsy of the uterus' around 400 BC by Hippocrates and his student, Diocles (Ober and Fass, 1961). In 1276 the attendants of Margaret Countess of Henneberg noticed that her abnormal delivery consisted of multiple hydropic vesicles. They probably believed that each vesicle was a separate conception, which led them to christen half John and half Mary. Marie Boivin (1773–1841), who worked as a Parisian midwife, was the first to document the chorionic origin of the hydatids (Ober and Fass, 1961). In 1895 Marchand described a malignant uterine disease of syncytial and cytotrophoblastic origin and made the link between hydatidiform mole and other forms of pregnancy (Ober and Fass, 1961).

Normal gestational trophoblast arises from the peripheral cells of the blastocyst in the first few days after conception. Trophoblastic tissue initially grows rapidly into two layers: (1) an inner cytotrophoblast of mononucleated cells which migrate out and fuse, forming (2) an outer syncytiotrophoblast of large multinucleated cells (Fig. 37.1). The latter subsequently aggressively invades the endometrium and uterine vasculature, generating an intimate connection between the fetus and the mother, known as the placenta. Invasion is, of course, one of the features of malignancy and, indeed, normal trophoblast can even be detected, by polymerase chain reaction, in the maternal circulation (Mueller *et al.*, 1990). Fortunately, complex biological and immunological mechanisms involved in controlling the relationship between the fetal trophoblast and the maternal host prevent such circulating trophoblast from producing metastases.

When GTD arises, the normal regulatory mechanisms controlling trophoblastic tissue are lost. Thus, the excessively proliferating trophoblast may invade through the myometrium, developing a rich maternal blood supply with tumour emboli and haematogenous spread occurring frequently. The World Health Organization has classified GTD into two premalignant diseases, termed complete and partial hydatidiform mole (CM and PM); and the three malignant disorders, or gestational trophoblastic tumours (GTT) – invasive mole, gestational choriocarcinoma and placental-site trophoblastic tumour (WHO, 1983). The origins, pathology and clinical behaviour of these various forms of GTD are different and will be discussed below. These tumours are important to recognize because they are nearly always curable and,

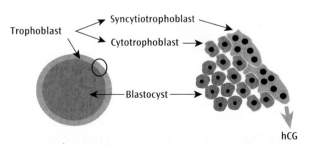

Figure 37.1 *Schematic diagram of an embryo at the blastocyst stage, demonstrating trophoblast development.*

in most cases, fertility can be preserved. This is mainly because:

1 GTTs are exquisitely chemosensitive;
2 they all produce human chorionic gonadotrophin (hCG), a serum tumour marker with a sensitivity and accuracy in screening, monitoring, management and follow-up of patients which is unparalleled in cancer medicine;
3 detailed prognostic scoring has permitted 'fine-tuning' of treatment intensity so that each patient only receives the minimum therapy required to eliminate their disease.

GENETICS AND PATHOLOGY

Complete hydatidiform mole

Genetic analysis of CMs has revealed that they nearly always only contain paternal DNA and are therefore androgenetic (Kajii and Ohama, 1977). This occurs in most cases because a single sperm bearing a 23X set of chromosomes fertilizes an ovum lacking maternal genes and then duplicates to form the homozygote, 46XX (Kajii and Ohama, 1977; Vassilakos et al., 1977; Lawler et al., 1979, 1982b; Jacobs et al., 1980; Fisher et al., 1982; Davis et al., 1984) (Fig. 37.2a). However, in up to 25 per cent of CMs fertilization can take place with two spermatozoa, resulting in the heterozygous 46XY or 46XX configuration

(Ohama et al., 1981; Fisher et al., 1989) (Fig. 37.2b). A 46YY conceptus has not yet been described and is presumably non-viable. Interestingly, some maternal elements are retained in CM, including the mitochondrial DNA (Edwards et al., 1984). Very rarely, a CM can arise from a fertilized ovum which has retained its maternal nuclear DNA and is therefore biparental in origin (Fisher and Newlands, 1998).

Macroscopically, the classical CM resembles a bunch of grapes, due to generalized (complete) swelling of chorionic villi. However, this appearance is only seen in the second trimester, and the diagnosis is usually made earlier these days, when not all the villi are so hydropic. Indeed, in the first trimester the villi microscopically contain little fluid, are branching and consist of hyperplastic syncitio- and cytotrophoblast with many vessels. This characteristic appearance is lost only with increasing gestational age, when the villi lose their vessels and the stromal cisterns fill with fluid. Although it was previously thought that CM produced no fetal tissue, histology from first-trimester abortions reveals evidence of embryonic elements, including fetal red cells (Paradinas, 1994; Paradinas et al., 1996, 1997). This has resulted in many CMs being incorrectly labelled as PMs. Consequently, the reported rates of persistent GTD after PMs has been artificially elevated and is probably less than 0.5 per cent (Paradinas, 1998). The presence of embryonic tissue from a twin pregnancy comprising a fetus and a CM is a further source of error which can lead to the incorrect diagnosis of PM.

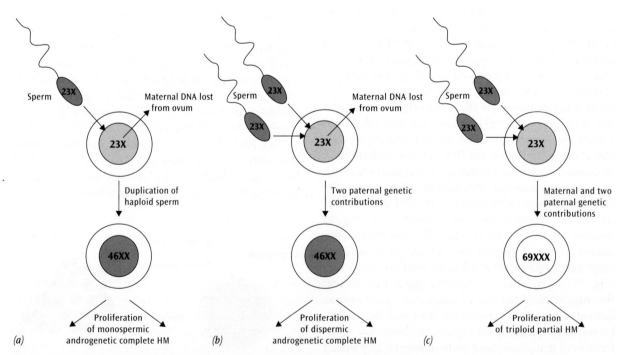

Figure 37.2 *Schematic diagram showing that the androgenetic diploid complete HM is formed either by duplication of the chromosomes from a single sperm (a) or by two sperm fertilizing the ovum (b) which, in both cases, has lost its own genetic component. The triploid genetic origin of a partial HM is demonstrated in (c).*

Partial hydatidiform mole

PMs are genetically nearly all triploid and, rarely, tetraploid, with at least two paternal chromosome sets but also some maternal contribution (Fig. 37.2c). Although triploidy occurs in 1–3 per cent of all recognized conceptions, and in about 20 per cent of spontaneous abortions with abnormal karyotype, triploids due to two sets of maternal chromosomes do not become PMs (Jacobs et al., 1982; Lawler et al., 1982a). Flow cytometry, which can now be done in formalin-fixed, paraffin-embedded tissues (Fisher et al., 1987), can therefore help in differentiating CM from PM, and PM from diploid non-molar hydropic abortions.

In PMs, swelling tends to be less intense and affects only some villi (partial). Both swollen and non-swollen villi can have trophoblastic hyperplasia, which is mild and focal (Szulman and Surti, 1978a, b). The villi have characteristic indented outlines and round inclusions (Paradinas, 1994; Paradinas et al., 1996). An embryo is usually present and can be recognized macroscopically or inferred from the presence of nucleated red cells in villous vasculature. It may survive into the second trimester, but in most cases it dies at about 8–9 weeks' gestation, and this is followed by loss of vessels and stromal fibrosis. In PMs evacuated early, villus swelling and trophoblastic excess can be so mild and focal that the diagnosis of PM may be missed (Paradinas, 1998). Indeed, at uterine evacuation for a 'miscarriage', it is likely that many PMs are misclassified as products of conception. Fortunately, we only see about one patient per year with persistent GTD related to a previously unrecognized PM. Of the increasing number of PMs that are correctly diagnosed, very few go on to develop persistent GTD. Indeed, in approximately 3000 PMs reviewed and followed at Charing Cross between 1973 and 1997, only 15 (0.5 per cent) have required chemotherapy. Consequently, it would be useful to have some way of identifying immediately post-evacuation which patients will subsequently require chemotherapy. This would avoid all patients with a PM undergoing hCG follow-up. Interestingly, our preliminary data suggest that the proliferation antigen Ki-67 may provide a solution, since this appears to be elevated only in those patients who develop persistent GTD.

Other pregnancies mistaken for PM

Over half of first-trimester non-molar abortions are due to trisomy, monosomy, maternally derived triploidy and translocations. These often develop hydrops, but this is small (<3 mm) and PM can be excluded if they are diploid on flow cytometry. Syndromes such as Turner's, Edward's and Beckwith–Wiedemann's can also cause histological confusion with PMs (Paradinas, 1998).

Invasive hydatidiform mole

This term is applied when a CM or, rarely, a PM invades into the myometrium. Invasive mole is common and is clinically identified by the combination of an abnormal uterine ultrasound (US) and a persistent or rising hCG level following uterine evacuation. The pathological confirmation of this condition is rarely required. Moreover, repeat dilatation and curettage (D&C) is often contraindicated because of the risks of uterine perforation, infection, life-threatening haemorrhage and subsequent hysterectomy. In occasional cases where histology is available, invasive mole can be distinguished from choriocarcinoma by the presence of chorionic villi.

Choriocarcinoma

Most choriocarcinomas have been shown to have grossly abnormal karyotypes with diverse ploidies and several chromosome rearrangements, none of which is specific for the disease (Arima et al., 1994). Studies of the origin of GTTs have confirmed that choriocarcinoma may arise from any type of pregnancy, including a normal term pregnancy (Wake et al., 1981; Chaganti et al., 1990; Osada et al., 1991; Fisher et al., 1992a), from a homozygous CM or from a heterozygous CM (Fisher et al., 1988, 1992a). Until recently, it has been thought that PMs cannot give rise to choriocarcinoma. However, recent work from our group has provided incontrovertible genetic evidence proving that PMs can indeed transform into choriocarcinomas. This is important as there are some centres that wrongly believe it is safe to discontinue hCG follow-up following the diagnosis of PMs.

Interestingly, choriocarcinoma may not always be due to the antecedent pregnancy. A patient with a history of a CM 4 years previously developed a choriocarcinoma following the delivery of a twin pregnancy. Using PCR to amplify short tandem repeat polymorphisms in DNA, this tumour was shown to be genetically identical with the previous CM (Fisher et al., 1995). Like invasive hydatidiform mole (HM), obtaining tissue to make a formal histological diagnosis of choriocarcinoma is often not appropriate and so doubt frequently exists whether patients have one or the other form of GTT.

Choriocarcinoma is highly malignant in behaviour, appearing as a soft, purple, largely haemorrhagic mass. Microscopically it mimics an early implanting blastocyst, with central cores of mononuclear cytotrophoblast surrounded by a rim of multinucleated syncytiotrophoblast and a distinct absence of chorionic villi. There are extensive areas of necrosis and haemorrhage and frequent evidence of tumour within venous sinuses. Interestingly, the disease fails to stimulate the connective tissue support normally associated with tumours and induces hypervascularity of the surrounding maternal tissues. This probably accounts for its highly metastatic and haemorrhagic behaviour.

Placental-site trophoblastic tumour

Placental-site trophoblastic tumour (PSTT) has been shown to follow term delivery, non-molar abortion, or CM. It is conceivable, although unproven, that PSTT might develop after a PM. Like choriocarcinoma, the causative pregnancy may not be the immediate antecedent pregnancy (Fisher *et al.*, 1995). Genetic analysis of some PSTTs has demonstrated that they are mostly diploid, originating from either a normal conceptus, and therefore biparental, or androgenetic from a CM (Lathrop *et al.*, 1988; Fisher *et al.*, 1992b; Kotylo *et al.*, 1992; Fukunaga and Ushigome, 1993; Arima *et al.*, 1994; Newlands *et al.*, 1998b). A tetraploid PSTT has been described (Kotylo *et al.*, 1992).

In the normal placenta, placental-site trophoblast is distinct from villous trophoblast and infiltrates the decidua, myometrium and spiral arteries of the uterine wall. PSTTs are rare, slow-growing malignant tumours composed mainly of intermediate trophoblast derived from cytotrophoblast, and so produce little hCG. However, they often stain strongly for human placental lactogen (hPL) and β1-glycoprotein. Elevated Ki-67 levels may help in distinguishing PSTT from a regressing placental nodule (Shih and Kurman, 1998). In contrast to other forms of GTT, spread tends to occur late by local infiltration and via the lymphatics, although distant metastases can occur. More than five mitoses per 10 high-power fields may predict tumours with metastasizing potential (Newlands *et al.*, 1998b).

EPIDEMIOLOGY AND AETIOLOGICAL FACTORS

Hydatidiform mole

INCIDENCE AND ETHNIC ORIGIN

From population-based studies, the incidence of CM in countries of the Western world is approximately 1/1000 pregnancies. Although the incidence was previously reported to be at least twofold higher in the Far East (Matsuura *et al.*, 1984), recent results indicate that this has fallen towards the stable levels found in Europe and North America (Hando *et al.*, 1998; Martin and Kim, 1998). The declining incidence in the Far East may be due to environmental factors, such as dietary change.

The incidence of PM has been underestimated in the past (Matsuura *et al.*, 1984; Lawler and Fisher, 1986). More recent studies indicate a much higher rate of PM relative to CM in patients presenting with spontaneous abortions (Jacobs *et al.*, 1982). Indeed, the incidence of triploidy amongst first-trimester spontaneous abortions suggests that as many as 90 per cent of PM could go undiagnosed (Newlands *et al.*, 1998a).

AGE

CMs are more frequent at the extremes of reproductive age, the lowest rate occurring between the ages of 25 and 29 years. In one study the relative increased risk, compared to the lowest rate between 25 and 29 years, was sixfold in girls under 15 years, threefold between 40 and 45 years, 26-fold between 45 and 49 years and more than 400-fold over 50 years of age (Bagshawe *et al.*, 1986). In contrast, the risk of developing a PM bears little or no relationship to age (Newlands *et al.*, 1998a).

PREVIOUS PREGNANCIES

There is no increased risk in CM associated with increasing gravidity. However, the risk of a subsequent pregnancy being a CM rises from 1 in 1000 to 1 in 76 with one previous CM and to 1 in 6.5 with two previous CMs (Bagshawe *et al.*, 1986). Therefore patients with a previous CM must be followed up after each subsequent pregnancy to confirm that their hCG levels return to normal. Although similar data for PMs is not yet available, we currently also follow up these patients in the same way.

Choriocarcinoma

The incidence of choriocarcinoma following term delivery without a history of CM is approximately 1 : 50 000. However, CM is probably the most common antecedent to choriocarcinoma, being 29–83 per cent in various studies across the world (WHO, 1983). onsequently, the overall incidence of choriocarcinoma is much higher. Proof of this is frequently difficult or inadvisable to obtain, but when histology has been available these tumours were identified as choriocarcinoma in 3 per cent and invasive mole in 16 per cent of previous CMs (rarely as PSTTs). Rarely, PMs can give rise to choriocarcinoma.

Unlike HM, choriocarcinoma does not exhibit any clear geographical trends in incidence but the effect of age remains important. Curiously, choriocarcinoma following a full-term pregnancy is more likely to be associated with a very aggressive disease course than after a CM. This may reflect the fact that some of the choriocarcinomas after a CM included cases of invasive mole.

Placental-site trophoblastic tumours

There are currently approximately 100 recorded cases of this tumour in the literature and so estimates of its true incidence may well be quite inaccurate (Newlands *et al.*, 1998b). Nevertheless, PSTT is thought to constitute about 1 per cent of all trophoblastic tumours (choriocarcinoma, invasive mole and PSTT).

Other factors with uncertain role

Several other factors have been examined for a possible aetiological role in the development of GTD. These include parity, smoking, contraceptive practice, dietary influences, herbicide and radiation exposure. None of these has been shown conclusively to play a role in this group of diseases (Palmer, 1994). However, a recent analysis has suggested that oral contraceptive use prior to conception slightly increases the risk of subsequently developing a gestational trophoblastic tumour (Palmer *et al.*, 1999).

Genetic factors

All autosomal genes consist of two alleles (paternal and maternal). Recent work has shown that some alleles are expressed only from one parent and not the other – a phenomenon called genomic imprinting. Interestingly, three closely related genes which are imprinted and located on chromosome 11p15 may be involved in GTT development and in other overgrowth syndromes (Li *et al.*, 1998). These are: H19, a putative tumour suppresser gene (Hao *et al.*, 1993) and p57^{kip2}, a cyclin-dependent kinase inhibitor (Matsuoka *et al.*, 1996), which are both normally expressed by the maternal allele; and the paternally expressed insulin-like growth factor-II (IGF-II), a growth factor commonly implicated in tumour proliferation (Ogawa *et al.*, 1993). While p57^{kip2} showed the expected pattern of expression in CM and choriocarcinoma (Chilosi *et al.*, 1998), CM and post-mole tumours were unexpectedly found to express H19 (Mutter *et al.*, 1993; Ariel *et al.*, 1994; Walsh *et al.*, 1995), and some post-term tumours showed biallelic expression of both H19 and IGF-II (Hashimoto *et al.*, 1995; Arima *et al.*, 1997). This suggests that loss of the normal imprinting patterns of these genes may be an important factor in the development of GTT.

The recent identification of rare families in which several sisters have repeat CMs which are biparental in origin (Fisher and Newlands, 1998) is likely to shed further light on the genes involved in CM formation. Indeed, linkage and homozygosity analysis suggested that in two families there is a defective gene located on chromosome 19q13.3–13.4 (Moglabey *et al.*, 1999). Interestingly, this is a region where at least one imprinted gene, PEG3 (Kim *et al.*, 1997), has already been mapped.

Other non-imprinted genes may be involved in the development of GTTs and carry prognostic significance. Patients whose blood group is B or AB, whose partners are either group O or A, may have a worse prognosis (Bagshawe, 1976). The reasons for this are not clear (Lawler *et al.*, 1976; Yamashita *et al.*, 1981). Loss of heterozygosity studies have shown that the putative tumour suppresser gene located on chromosome 7 is lost in GTTs (Matsuda *et al.*, 1997). This molecular approach can now be carried out on archival material (Fisher and Newlands, 1998), and so other genes important in the progression

of GTD may be discovered and found to play a critical role in the management of GTD.

Growth factors

There is considerable evidence implicating growth factors as important agents capable of driving tumour proliferation (Rozengurt, 1995). This has been particularly well defined for small cell lung cancer, where both neuropeptide and polypeptide growth factors may drive cell proliferation in an autocrine and paracrine fashion (Rozengurt, 1995; Seckl and Rozengurt, 1998). In contrast, the identity and role of growth factors in trophoblastic disease remains poorly understood. It is quite plausible that hCG may function as an autocrine/paracrine growth factor for GTTs. In addition, the ligands and/or the receptors for known growth factors, such as hepatocyte growth factor, platelet-derived growth factor, c-fms, cerbB2, IGF-II and granulocyte colony-stimulating factor (G-CSF), have been demonstrated in trophoblastic tissue or cell lines (Uzumaki *et al.*, 1989; Wolf *et al.*, 1991; Holmgren *et al.*, 1993; Fulop *et al.*, 1998a, b). Interestingly, we have frequently administered G-CSF to patients with GTD without any apparent compromise in therapeutic outcome, indicating that clinically important tumour growth is not induced by G-CSF. However, the role of these and other growth factors warrants further investigation in this group of diseases.

Risk of gestational trophoblastic tumours following complete or partial hydatidiform moles

The risk of malignant sequelae following evacuation of a PM is probably far less than 1 : 200, compared to 1 : 16 for a CM (Bagshawe *et al.*, 1990 and unpublished observations). Other workers have reported somewhat higher rates of persistent GTD developing after a PM, with values from 2 to 6 per cent (Rice *et al.*, 1990; Goto *et al.*, 1993). The differences in these studies may have arisen because the diagnosis was made using morphological criteria without the added benefit of cytogenetics to help discriminate between CM and PM. Since it is not yet possible to predict in advance which patients with a CM or PM will develop persistent GTD, all of them must be registered for hCG monitoring. Following this strict protocol enables the identification of individuals with persistent trophoblastic growth who could benefit from lifesaving chemotherapy.

HUMAN CHORIONIC GONADOTROPHIN

Molecular background and function

The family of pituitary/placental glycoprotein hormones includes hCG, follicle-stimulating hormone (FSH), lutenizing hormone (LH) and thyroid stimulating hormone (TSH). Each hormone comprises an α-subunit, which is common between the family members, and a distinct β-subunit, which is believed to confer receptor specificity. Consequently, assays to measure hCG are directed against the β-subunit. The crystal structures for both the α- and β-subunits of hCG have been solved (Lapthorn et al., 1994; Tegoni et al., 1999). The genes for βhCG and βLH have been mapped to a complex cluster of inverted and tandem genes on chromosome 19, of which six are for βhCG and the terminal seventh for βLH (Boorstein et al., 1982; Policastro et al., 1986). However, the precise role of each of the genes, which can all be transcribed, remains unclear (Bo and Boime, 1992). Interestingly the gene is highly conserved in nature, being found in prokaryotes (Grover et al., 1995). So far, only one receptor for βhCG has been identified in mammals, which also serves as the main receptor for LH (Tsai-Morris et al., 1991; Dufau, 1998). This, of course, raises the question of how hCG might exert specific effects distinct from LH. Furthermore, βhCG is now known to circulate in a variety of forms as a result of post-translational modifications of its structure (Cole, 1998). It is therefore possible that additional βhCG receptors exist. The function(s) of the intact and the modified forms of βhCG remain obscure. The fact that hCG production clinically indicates trophoblastic proliferation suggests that this molecule may be a growth factor for normal placenta, gestational trophoblastic disease and other hCG-producing tumours.

βhCG nassays

Many different βhCG assays are currently available. Some detect intact βhCG and others are either selective for individual fragments or detect various combinations of fragments. The mechanism of detection is also variable (e.g. complement fixation as opposed to radioimmunoassay) and this results in considerable differences in assay sensitivity. Thus pregnancy tests employing haemagglutination inhibition or complement fixation methods have a lower limit of sensitivity of only 2000 iu/L and may give false-negative results when values for hCG are very high. In contrast, the best radioimmunoassays use an antiserum recognizing all βhCG forms and are sensitive to 1 iu/L in serum and 20 iu/L in urine. Immunoenzymatic, immunochemiluminescent and fluoroimmunoassays have the potential to match or improve on this sensitivity. As we learn more about the various fragments of βhCG it may become apparent that certain fragments may be more sensitive for detection of small-volume disease or correlate with poor or good prognosis groups (Cole, 1998). Indeed, recent work has suggested that a hyperglycosylated form of βhCG may only be produced by GTT rather than by normal trophoblast (Birken et al., 1999). If this work is confirmed in larger studies, this could provide a major new tool to determine the presence of malignancy as opposed to normal pregnancy.

Use as a tumour marker

Human chorionic gonadotrophin, which has a half-life of 24–36 h, remains the most sensitive and specific marker for trophoblastic tissue. However, hCG production is not confined to pregnancy and GTD. Indeed, hCG is produced by any trophoblastic tissue found, for example, in germ cell tumours and in up to 15 per cent of epithelial malignancies (Vaitukaitis, 1979). The hCG levels in such cases can be just as high as those seen in GTD. Furthermore, the levels of hCG produced by GTD are frequently identical to those found in normal pregnancy, although very high levels outside the range for a twin pregnancy may lead to suspicion of a trophoblastic tumour. Consequently, hCG measurements per se do not reliably discriminate between pregnancy, GTD or non-gestational trophoblastic tumours. However, serial measurements of hCG have revolutionized the management of GTD, for several reasons. Thus, the amount of hCG produced correlates with tumour volume, so that a serum hCG of 5 iu/L corresponds to approximately 10^4–10^5 viable tumour cells. Consequently, these assays are several orders of magnitude more sensitive than the best imaging modalities available today. In addition, hCG levels can be used to determine prognosis (Bagshawe, 1976). Serial measurements allow progress of the disease or response to therapy to be monitored (Fig. 37.3). Development of drug resistance can be detected at an early stage, which facilitates appropriate management changes. Estimates may be made of the time for which chemotherapy should be continued after hCG levels are undetectable in serum, in order to reduce the tumour volume to zero. For these reasons hCG is the best tumour marker known, and is of wider interest as a model for the way in which tumour markers may be used in other diseases.

CLINICAL FEATURES

Complete and partial moles

These most commonly present towards the end of the first trimester as a threatened abortion with vaginal bleeding. Patients may notice the passing of grape-like structures (vesicles) and occasionally the entire mole may be spontaneously evacuated. The uterus may be of any size, but is commonly large for gestational age. Patients with marked trophoblastic growth and high hCG levels are particularly prone to hyperemesis, toxaemia and the development of theca lutein cysts, which may sometimes be palpable above the pelvis. Toxaemia was diagnosed in

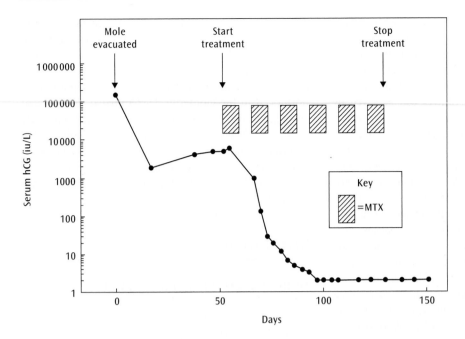

Figure 37.3 *The use of monitoring the serum hCG concentration following evacuation of a hydatidiform mole (HM). In this case, after an initial fall the hCG started to rise, indicating the development of invasive HM or choriocarcinoma, and so the patient was called up for staging. The prognostic score was low risk (see Table 37.5) and the patient was successfully treated with methotrexate (MTX) and folinic acid (see Table 37.6).*

27 per cent of patients with CM (Berkowitz and Goldstein, 1981), but is seen less frequently today because of early ultrasound diagnosis. Convulsions are rare. The high hCG levels may also produce hyperthyroidism because of cross-reactivity between hCG and TSH at the TSH receptor (Fradken *et al.*, 1989). Although pulmonary, vaginal and cervical metastases can occur, they may spontaneously disappear following removal of the mole. Thus the presence of metastases does not necessarily imply that invasive mole or choriocarcinoma has developed. Patients may present with acute respiratory distress not only because of pulmonary metastases and/or anaemia, but occasionally as a result of tumour embolization. The risk of embolization is reduced by avoiding agents that induce uterine contraction before the cervix has been dilated to enable evacuation of the CM.

Patients with PM usually do not exhibit the dramatic clinical features characteristic of CM (Goldstein and Berkowitz, 1994). The uterus is often not enlarged for gestational age and vaginal bleeding tends to occur later, so that patients most often present in the second trimester with a missed or incomplete abortion. In fact the diagnosis is rarely suspected until the histology of curettings is available. Clues to the diagnosis can occasionally be obtained by US (Fine *et al.*, 1989). The pre-evacuation hCG is <100 000 iu/L at diagnosis in over 90 per cent of cases.

Twin pregnancies

Twin pregnancies comprising a normal fetus and a hydatidiform mole are estimated to occur in between 1 : 20 000 and 100 000 pregnancies. Some probably abort in the first trimester and so go undiagnosed. However, some are discovered on US examination, either routinely or because

of complications such as bleeding, excessive uterine size or problems related to a high hCG.

Invasive moles

This is usually diagnosed because serial urine or serum hCG measurements reveal a plateaued or rising hCG level in the weeks after evacuation of the mole. Patients may complain of persistent vaginal bleeding or lower abdominal pains and/or swelling. This may occur as a result of haemorrhage from leaking tumour-induced vasculature as the trophoblast invades through the myometrium, or because of vulval, vaginal or intra-abdominal metastases. The tumour may also involve other pelvic structures, including the bladder or rectum, producing haematuria or rectal bleeding, respectively. Enlarging pulmonary metastases or tumour emboli growing in the pulmonary arteries can contribute to life-threatening respiratory complications (Seckl *et al.*, 1991). The risk of these complications is clearly higher in patients where the initial diagnosis of a molar pregnancy was missed and so are not on hCG follow-up.

Choriocarcinoma

Choriocarcinoma can present after any form of pregnancy, but most commonly occurs after CM. In the latter situation, it is often not practical to obtain histological proof of choriocarcinoma and so it is impossible to distinguish it from invasive mole. Choriocarcinoma following an apparently normal pregnancy or non-molar abortion usually presents within a year of delivery, but in the Charing Cross series the longest interval to date was 17 years (reviewed in Tidy *et al.*, 1995). The presenting features may be similar to those of HM, with vaginal bleeding, abdominal pain and a pelvic mass. However, one-third of all patients with choriocarcinoma present without gynaecological features, instead of suffering from symptoms of distant metastases (McGrath *et al.*, 1971; Tidy *et al.*, 1995). In these cases lives can be saved by remembering to include choriocarcinoma in the differential diagnosis of metastatic malignancy (particularly in lungs, brain or liver) presenting in a woman of childbearing age. Any site may be involved, including skin, producing a purple lesion, cauda equina and the heart. Pulmonary disease may be parenchymal, pleural or may result from tumour embolism and subsequent growth in the pulmonary arteries (Seckl *et al.*, 1991; Savage *et al.*, 1998). Thus respiratory symptoms and signs can include dyspnoea, haemoptysis and pulmonary artery hypertension. Cerebral metastases may produce focal neurological signs, convulsions, evidence of raised intracranial pressure and intracerebral or subarachnoid haemorrhage. Hepatic metastases may cause local pain or referred pain in the right shoulder. Although none of these presentations are specific to choriocarcinoma, performing a simple pregnancy test or quantitative hCG assay can provide a vital clue to the diagnosis. Other clues may come from features associated with a high circulating hCG level, including occasional thyrotoxicosis and ovarian theca lutein cysts.

Infantile choriocarcinoma

Choriocarcinoma in the fetus or new born is exceptionally rare, with approximately 17 reported cases (Belchis *et al.*, 1993; Kishkuno *et al.*, 1997). While a primary choriocarcinoma within the infant is possible, in 11 cases the mother also had the tumour. This suggests that the disease can cross the placenta, bypass an immature immune system in the fetus and flourish. Interestingly, the diagnosis was often made in the neonate before the mother. In all cases, the infant was anaemic and had a raised hCG, but the site of metastasis was variable, including brain, liver, lung and skin. Only one case has been treated successfully, the rest dying within weeks of initial diagnosis, which may have been delayed. Consequently, serum or urine hCG levels should be measured in all babies of mothers with choriocarcinoma. As the disease can present up to 6 months after delivery, an argument could be made for serial monitoring of hCG in these infants.

Placental-site trophoblastic tumour

The slow growth rate of PSTT means that it can present years after term delivery, non-molar abortion, or complete HM. Unlike choriocarcinoma, it tends to metastasize late in its natural history and so patients frequently present with gynaecological symptoms alone (Finkler *et al.*, 1988). In addition to vaginal bleeding, the production of

hPL by the cytotrophoblastic cells may cause hyperprolactinaemia, which can result in amenorrhoea and/or galactorrhoea. In some instances, presumably also as a result of tumour-secreted products, patients can develop nephrotic syndrome or haematuria with deposition of fibrinogen in the glomeruli. Disseminated intravascular coagulation has been reported in association with these features (Eckstein *et al.*, 1982; Young and Scully, 1984). Metastases may occur in the vagina, extrauterine pelvic tissues, retroperitoneum, lymph nodes, lungs and brain (Samlowski *et al.*, 1985; Hopkins *et al.*, 1992; Newlands *et al.*, 1998b).

INVESTIGATION

Human chorionic gonadotrophin

As already discussed above, this is an extremely useful marker of trophoblastic disease and its response to therapy.

Plain chest X-ray

All patients who are suspected of having gestational trophoblastic tumours should have a chest radiograph. The most common metastatic appearance is of multiple, discrete, rounded lesions (Fig. 37.4), but large solitary lesions or a miliary pattern can occur (Bagshawe and Noble, 1965). Furthermore, tumour emboli to the

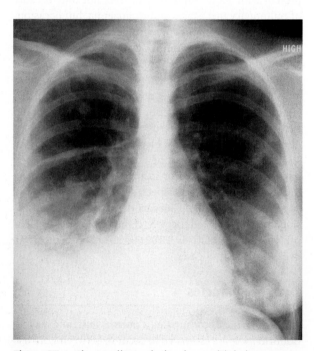

Figure 37.4 *Chest radiograph showing multiple lung metastases and a small right pleural effusion in a patient with choriocarcinoma.*

pulmonary arteries can produce an identical picture to venous thromboembolism, with wedge-shaped infarcts and areas of decreased vascular markings. Pulmonary artery hypertension can cause dilatation of the pulmonary arteries. Deposits affecting the pleural surfaces may result in haemorrhagic pleural effusions (Fig. 37.4). These diverse radiological appearances have been reviewed extensively (Bagshawe and Noble, 1965). Routine CT scanning of the chest does not add anything to the management of these cases.

Ultrasonography

Ultrasound and colour doppler imaging is not diagnostic but highly suggestive of persistent GTD when there is a combination of a raised hCG, no pregnancy and a vascular mass within the uterus (Plate 4). US permits accurate delineation of uterine volume, which correlates with the amount of disease and is a prognostic indicator (*see* GTT scoring system, pp. 786–7). In the Charing Cross Series, about 75 per cent of patients who require chemotherapy for molar disease have an enlarged uterus (>120 mL) (Boultebee and Newlands, 1995). The tumour is frequently confined to one area of uterine wall but diffuse uterine disease and extrauterine deposits may be visualized. Doppler frequently demonstrates a change in the waveform of the uterine arteries (Plate 4). This is attributed to large vascular channels forming in the myometrium, resulting in arteriovenous shunting (Long *et al.*, 1992). Furthermore, the increased sensitivity of modern colour Doppler US now reveals abnormal blood vessel encroachment through the myometrium into the endometrium (Plate 4). Although the uterine artery changes have no prognostic significance, the degree of vascular endometrial encroachment may aid in assessing the risk of major haemorrhage in patients with GTT (Boultebee and Newlands, 1995). Interestingly, these vascular abnormalities can persist long after the disease has been eradicated with chemotherapy. Patients with repeated vaginal haemorrhage from these vascular malformations may need arteriography and selective embolization (Fig. 37.5). This usually prevents subsequent bleeding but may need to be repeated. Importantly, embolization of these abnormal uterine vessels does not appear to affect fertility (Boultebee and Newlands, 1995).

Pelvic US can also demonstrate ovarian theca lutein cysts and other ovarian masses. Metastatic spread outside the pelvis, for example to the liver or kidneys, can also be identified and shown to have an abnormal Doppler signal. On completion of therapy, the US should be repeated to confirm that the masses have disappeared, or at least reduced in size. This ensures that the masses did not originate from some other pathology.

Investigation of patients with drug-resistant disease

When patients develop drug-resistant disease, further investigation is required to more accurately define where the residual tumour is located, as resection can be curative. Whole-body computed tomography (CT) is often helpful (Fig. 37.6) but, where available, MRI of the brain (Fig. 37.7) and pelvis is clearly superior to CT in these areas. Indeed, in our experience MRI of the head has revealed drug-resistant deposits of choriocarcinoma not seen on the CT, thus permitting curative surgery. If the

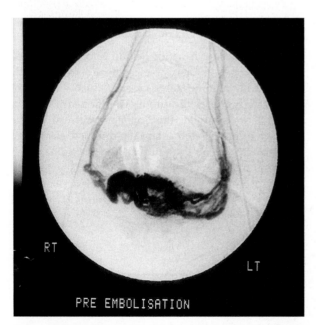
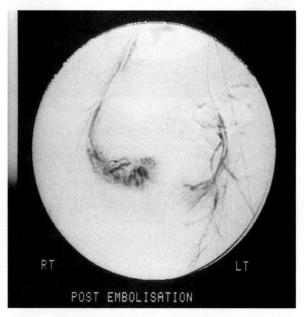

Figure 37.5 *Arteriographic appearance of a uterine arteriovenous malformation before (left) and after selective embolization (right) in a patient with repeated vaginal haemorrhages following previous curative treatment for invasive HM. The patient's bleeding subsequently stopped and she had a normal pregnancy.*

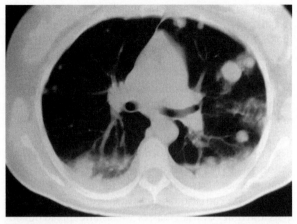

(a)

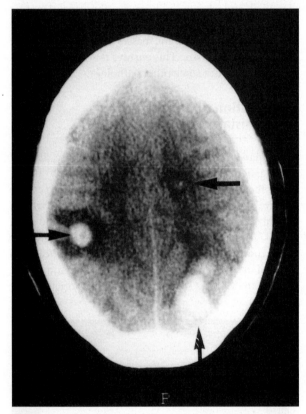

(b)

Figure 37.6 *CT scan demonstrating (a) lung and (b) brain metastases in a patient with choriocarcinoma.*

MRI/CT brain is normal, then a lumbar puncture to measure the hCG level in cerebrospinal fluid can be useful to detect disease in the central nervous system. An hCG ratio greater than 1 : 60 of that found in the serum is highly indicative of the presence of trophoblastic disease.

Experimental imaging techniques

Radiolabelled anti-hCG antibodies given intravenously can localize tumours producing hCG where other imaging techniques have failed, and has aided in the cure

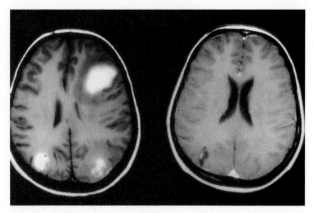

Figure 37.7 *The MRI appearances of the brain before (left) and after (right) EMA/CO chemotherapy (see Table 37.7) for metastatic choriocarcinoma.*

of patients (Begent *et al.*, 1987) (Table 37.1). This approach is most effective when there are $>10^6$–10^7 tumour cells, i.e. the serum hCG is >100 iu/L, but even then both false-positive and false-negative results occur. Thus, anti-hCG scanning should be regarded as complementary to other imaging investigations.

More recently, positron emission tomography (PET) has provided a novel approach to image many types of tumours using a variety of labels. Whole-body PET has already been reported to distinguish GTT emboli from blood clot in two patients with choriocarcinoma (Hebart *et al.*, 1996). Different PET compounds such as [^{18}F]fluorodeoxyglucose (^{18}FDG) PET, which can identify tumours missed by other techniques (Beets *et al.*, 1994), have yet to be shown to aid in the location of drug-resistant GTTs.

Genetic analysis

On some occasions it can be helpful to perform a comparative genetic analysis of the patient's trophoblastic tumour with their normal tissue and, if available, that of their partner. Thus, if the tumour is suspected of being of non-gestational origin, this can be confirmed by the presence of only maternal and the complete absence of paternal DNA. Genetic studies can also determine which of several antecedent pregnancies is the causal pregnancy of the current GTT. This can have an impact on determining appropriate therapy and prognosis (Fisher and Newlands, 1998).

MANAGEMENT

Molar evacuation

Evacuation of the uterine cavity using suction gives the lowest incidence of sequelae. When the molar trophoblast invades the myometrium, it is relatively easy to perforate

Table 37.1 *Surgery guided by immunoscintigraphy in gestational choriocarcinoma*

	Tumour site			
	Lung	Uterus	Brain	Total
Tumour located and resected	7	2	2	11
Relapse after resection or incomplete resection	2	1	1	4
Disease free when last seen	6	2	1	9

Reproduced with kind permission from Professor R.H.J. Begent (1995).

the uterus if a metal curette is used. Medical induction involving repeated contraction of the uterus induced by oxytocin or prostaglandin, or other surgical approaches including hysterectomy or hysterotomy, increases the risk of requiring chemotherapy by two- to threefold compared with suction evacuation. This is thought to be because tumour is more likely to be disseminated by uterine contraction and manipulation. For similar reasons, the use of prostanoids to ripen a nulliparous cervix is not recommended. If bleeding is severe immediately after suction evacuation, a single dose of ergometrine to produce one uterine contraction may stem the haemorrhage and does not appear to increase the chance of requiring chemotherapy.

In the past it has been common practice for gynaecologists to perform a second and sometimes a third evacuation of the uterine cavity in patients with a molar pregnancy. However, analysis of our data between 1973 and 1986 has shown that the chances of requiring chemotherapy after one evacuation is only 2.4 per cent but rises markedly to 18 per cent after two evacuations and 81 per cent after four evacuations (Table 37.2). Consequently, a second evacuation may be reasonable, if there is a clinical indication such as bleeding or if repeat US shows persisting molar trophoblast within the uterine cavity. The use of US control during this procedure may help to reduce the risk of uterine perforation. Further evacuations are not recommended because of the risk of complications and the high chance that the patient will require chemotherapy anyway.

Twin pregnancies

At Charing Cross Hospital in London, we have seen 73 confirmed cases of CM with a separate normal conceptus. Twenty-five per cent of these resulted in a live birth, while the remainder had non-viable pregnancies which ended mostly in spontaneous abortions or suction D&Cs. Interestingly, in both the viable and non-viable pregnancies, only 20 per cent of women subsequently needed chemotherapy to eliminate persistent GTD and none of these died of resistant disease. Thus, it appears reasonably safe to allow patients with twin pregnancies in which one of the conceptions is a CM to continue to term provided there are no other complications.

Table 37.2 *Correlation between the number of evacuations performed following a HM and the subsequent requirement for chemotherapy at Charing Cross Hospital (1973–86)*

Number of evacuations	Patients not treated	Patients treated	% Patients treated
1	4481	109	2.4
2	1495	267	18
3	106	106	50
4	5	22	81

Registration and follow-up after uterine evacuation

The majority of patients require no more treatment after evacuation but 16 per cent of patients with CM and <0.5 per cent with PM develop persistent GTD. In the case of CM this can be invasive mole, choriocarcinoma or, very rarely, PSTT, while with PMs this has only ever been shown to be invasive mole. It is vital that patients with persistent GTD are identified, as virtually all of them can be cured with appropriate therapy. In 1973, under the auspices of the Royal College of Obstetricians and Gynaecologists, a national follow-up service was instituted in the United Kingdom, whereby patients with GTD are registered with one of three laboratories, located in Dundee, Sheffield and London. Approximately 1400 women are registered per annum, and of these we treat 110–120 patients per annum. After registration, the patient's details and pathology, together with two weekly blood and urine samples, are sent through the post to one of the reference laboratories for confirmation of diagnosis and serial hCG estimations. Following the success of this scheme, other countries have now established, or are attempting to establish, a similar registration programme to reduce their GTT mortality rates.

Since a molar pregnancy is a premalignant condition, in the majority of cases the molar tissue dies out spontaneously. Consequently, the hCG concentration returns to normal. Once the hCG is within the normal range (≤4 iu/L), our recommendation is that the patient should not start a further pregnancy until the hCG has been normal for 6 months. We have found that the rate of fall of hCG can predict the likelihood of subsequently developing a trophoblastic tumour. If the hCG has fallen to normal within 8 weeks of evacuation, then marker follow-up can be safely reduced to 6 months, as none of these patients have required chemotherapy. However, in patients whose hCG levels are still elevated beyond 8 weeks from the date of evacuation, follow-up should continue for 2 years. Since patients who have had a previous mole or GTT are more at risk of having a second, all patients should have a further estimation of hCG at 6 and 10 weeks following the completion of each subsequent pregnancy.

Indications for chemotherapy

Factors associated with an increased risk of requiring chemotherapy are summarized in Table 37.3. The hormones in the oral contraceptive pill are probably growth factors for trophoblastic tumours and for this reason patients are advised not to use the pill until the hCG levels have returned to normal.

The indications for intervention with chemotherapy in patients who have had a CM or PM are shown in Table 37.4. Human chorionic gonadotrophin values $\geq 20\,000$ iu/L 4 weeks after evacuation of a mole, or rising values in this range at an earlier stage, indicate the patient is at increased risk of severe haemorrhage or uterine perforation with intraperitoneal bleeding. These complications can be life-threatening and their risk can be reduced by starting chemotherapy. Metastases in the lung, vulva and vagina can only be observed if the hCG levels are falling. However, if the hCG levels are not dropping, or the patient has metastases at another site, which can indicate the development of choriocarcinoma, chemotherapy is required.

Prognostic factors/scoring versus FIGO staging

The principal prognostic variables for GTTs, which were originally identified by Bagshawe (1976) and since modified by the WHO and our own experience, are summarized in Table 37.5. Each variable carries a score which, when added together for an individual patient, correlates with the risk of the tumour becoming resistant to single-agent therapy. Thus, the most important prognostic variables carry the highest score and include:

1 the duration of the disease, because drug resistance of GTTs varies inversely with time from the original antecedent pregnancy;
2 the serum hCG concentration, which correlates with viable tumour volume in the body;
3 the presence of liver and/or brain metastases.

Recent evidence demonstrates that liver metastases correlates with a worse prognosis than brain metastases (Bower *et al.*, 1997). Consequently, patients with liver

Table 37.3 *Factors increasing the risk of requiring chemotherapy following evacuation of a HM*

Factor	Reference
Uterine size > gestational age	Curry *et al.* (1975)
Pre-evacuation serum hCG level >100 000 iu/L	Berkowitz and Goldstein (1981)
Oral contraceptives given before hCG falls to normal	Stone *et al.* (1976)
Bilateral cystic ovarian enlargement	Berkowitz and Goldstein (1981)

Table 37.4 *Indications for chemotherapy*

1. Evidence of metastases in brain, liver or gastrointestinal tract, or radiological opacities >2 cm on chest X-ray
2. Histological evidence of choriocarcinoma
3. Heavy vaginal bleeding or evidence of gastrointestinal or intraperitoneal haemorrhage
4. Pulmonary, vulval or vaginal metastases unless hCG falling
5. Rising hCG after evacuation
6. Serum hCG $\geq 20\,000$ iu/L more than 4 weeks after evacuation, because of the risk of uterine perforation
7. Raised hCG 6 months after evacuation even if still falling

Any of the above are indications to treat following the diagnosis of GTD.

involvement now score six points rather than four. Future modifications of the scoring system may include removal of the ABO blood groups, since it contributes little to the overall scoring and it may be difficult to have complete data on both patients and relevant partners.

Anatomical staging systems such as that of the International Federation of Gynaecology and Obstetrics (FIGO) are used by several centres managing gestational trophoblastic tumours. Surgery is virtually never indicated in the initial management of this disease and the FIGO system does not appear to add anything in treatment planning to the existing scoring system. Furthermore, the original FIGO staging system did not always correctly predict prognosis, so that some patients were under- or overtreated (Smith *et al.*, 1992). This problem has recently been overcome by modifying the FIGO system to include some of the WHO variables (Goldstein *et al.*, 1998). However, the scoring system in Table 37.5 is easier to use, the most important variables being established from the history, examination, chest radiograph, US and a quantitative hCG estimation. Currently, an international committee has been established to develop a new combined FIGO/scoring system so that all centres managing this rare group of diseases can more easily compare their results. In the meantime, we continue to use the scoring system outlined in Table 37.5.

Table 37.5 *Scoring system for gestational trophoblastic tumours*

Prognostic factor	Score[a]			
	0	1	2	6
Age (years)	<39	>39		
Antecedent pregnancy (AP)	Mole	Abortion or unknown	Term	
Interval (end of AP to chemo at CXH in months)	<4	4–7	7–12	>12
hCG (iu/L)	10^3–10^4	<10^3	10^4–10^5	>10^5
ABO blood group (female × male)		A × O O × A O or A × unknown	B × A or O AB × A or O	
No. of metastases	Nil	1–4	4–8	>8
Site of metastases	Not detected, lungs, vagina	Spleen, kidney	GI tract	Brain, liver
Largest tumour mass		3–5 cm	>5 cm	
Prior chemotherapy			Single drug	2 or more drugs

[a] The total score for a patient is obtained by adding the individual scores for each prognostic factor. Low risk, 0–5; medium risk, 6–8; high risk, ≥9. Patients scoring 0–8 currently receive single-agent therapy with methotrexate and folinic acid, while patients scoring ≥9 receive combination drug therapy with EMA/CO (see Table 37.7). CXH, Charing Cross Hospital; hCG, human chorionic gonadotrophin; GI, gastrointestinal.

Chemotherapy

At Charing Cross Hospital, we have used the prognostic scoring system in Table 37.5 to subdivide the patients into three groups, termed low, medium and high risk, depending on their overall score. Formerly, each risk group corresponded with a separate treatment regimen and so there were three types of therapy, termed low, medium and high risk. Several years ago, we discontinued the medium-risk treatment for three reasons:

1 the short- and long-term toxicity of this treatment is probably not significantly different from that of high-risk therapy;
2 some patients treated with medium-risk therapy have developed drug resistance and subsequently required high-risk therapy anyway; and
3 about 30 per cent of medium-risk patients can still be cured on low-risk chemotherapy, which is less toxic than either medium- or high-risk chemotherapy (Rustin et al., 1996).

Moreover, there is no evidence that prior treatment failure with methotrexate is an adverse prognostic variable (Bower et al., 1997). Accordingly, patients who score between 5 and 8 are now offered the possibility of receiving low-risk chemotherapy, which was previously only given to those with a score ≤5. Patients scoring ≥9 are given high-risk treatment. The details of both low- and high-risk treatment are discussed below. Patients are admitted for the first 3 weeks of either therapy principally because the tumours are often highly vascular and may bleed vigorously in this early period of treatment.

Table 37.6 *Chemotherapy regimen for low-risk and intermediate risk patients*

Methotrexate (MTX)	50 mg by intramuscular injection repeated every 48 h × 4
Calcium folinate	7.5 mg orally 30 h after each injection of MTX (folinic acid)

Courses repeated every two weeks, i.e. days 1, 15, 29, etc.

LOW- AND MEDIUM-RISK PATIENTS

The regimen used since 1964 at Charing Cross Hospital and widely followed in other centres is shown in Table 37.6. A patient's response to this therapy is shown in Figure 37.3. This schedule is in general well tolerated, with no alopecia. Some patients develop mucosal ulceration affecting the mouth and, much more rarely, the vaginal and perianal areas. This can be prevented partly by a high fluid intake of 3 L/day while on treatment. However, if this approach fails, then either increasing the dose of the folinic acid or giving it earlier, at 24 hours after methotrexate, can be helpful. Methotrexate can induce serositis, resulting in pleuritic chest pain or abdominal pain. Myelosuppression is rare, but a full blood count should be obtained before each course of treatment. Liver and renal function should also be monitored regularly. All patients are advised to avoid sun exposure or use complete sun block for 1 year after chemotherapy because the drugs can induce photosensitivity.

About 25 per cent of low-risk patients need to change treatment: 5 per cent because of toxicity (usually severe pleuritic pain or drug-induced hepatitis), and 20 per cent as a result of drug resistance, which occurs despite the patients being correctly scored as low risk. In the middle-risk group >69 per cent of patients will develop drug resistance (Newlands *et al.*, 1986; Bagshawe *et al.*, 1989). Thus, careful monitoring for disease response and treatment-induced toxicity is required to ensure that these women achieve complete remission.

Survival in these patients is excellent, even though they may need to change treatment. The only deaths in patients treated with this schedule following the introduction of the prognostic scoring system were one from concurrent but not therapy-induced non-Hodgkin's lymphoma and one from hepatitis (Bagshawe *et al.*, 1989). Indeed, in a more recent analysis we found no evidence that single-agent therapy with methotrexate increases the risk of developing a second cancer (Rustin *et al.*, 1996).

HIGH-RISK PATIENTS

These patients are at risk of developing drug resistance and we have therefore treated them since 1979 with an intensive regimen consisting of etoposide, methotrexate and actinomycin D (EMA), alternating weekly with cyclophosphamide and vincristine, otherwise known as Oncovin® (CO). Table 37.7 gives details of this therapy, which can be given to most patients with only one overnight stay in hospital every 2 weeks. A patient's response to this therapy is shown in Figure 37.8. The regimen is myelosuppressive but prolonged gaps in therapy which

can permit tumour regrowth can usually be avoided by the following measures: continuing to treat unless the white cell count is less than 1.5×10^9/L and/or platelets fall below 60×10^9/L and/or mucosal ulceration develops. The introduction of G-CSF in patients who have a low neutrophil count also helps to maintain treatment intensity and has reduced the number of neutropaenic febrile episodes.

The cumulative 5-year survival of patients treated with this schedule is 86 per cent, with no deaths from GTT beyond 2 years after the initiation of chemotherapy (Bower *et al.*, 1997). While these results are good, significant adverse prognostic variables continue to be a problem in subgroups of patients: presence of liver metastases, the longer the interval from the antecedent pregnancy, brain metastases and term delivery in the antecedent pregnancy. Early deaths accounted for a significant proportion of the overall mortality, the causes being: respiratory failure, cerebral metastases, hepatic failure and pulmonary embolism. None of these women had a HM and so were not registered for follow-up and close monitoring to prevent them presenting with extensive disease. Clearly, it will be difficult to improve the survival of this particular subgroup. However, any woman of childbearing age presenting with widespread malignancy should have an hCG measurement, as very high levels of this hormone are highly suggestive of choriocarcinoma. Earlier recognition of choriocarcinoma will help to reduce disease extent and consequent mortality.

Surprisingly, previous chemotherapy was a good prognostic factor in our high-risk patients (Bower *et al.*, 1997). This can be explained partly by the fact that these patients were all on follow-up and so the disease extent was less than that of many who had not had previous treatment.

The long-term risk of chemotherapy-induced second tumours in patients treated for GTTs in our centre has recently been reviewed (Rustin *et al.*, 1996) and is discussed below (p. 792).

Management of drug-resistant disease

Frequent measurement of the serum hCG is a simple way to detect drug resistance at an early stage as the hormone levels will stop falling and may start to rise long before there are other clinical changes. However, it is important that decisions to alter treatment are not made on the basis of a single hCG result but on a progressive trend over two to three values. In patients receiving methotrexate for low-/middle-risk disease, if the hCG is ≤100 iu/L when drug resistance occurs, the disease can often be cured simply by substituting actinomycin D (0.5 mg i.v. total dose daily for 5 days in every 2 weeks). This drug is more toxic than methotrexate, inducing some hair thinning (occasional complete alopecia), myelosuppression and more oral ulceration.

Table 37.7 *Chemotherapy regimen for high-risk patients*

EMA		
Day 1	Etoposide	100 mg/m² by i.v. infusion over 30 min
	Actinomycin D	0.5 mg i.v. bolus
	Methotrexate	300 mg/m² by i.v. infusion over 12 h
Day 2	Etoposide	100 mg/m² by i.v. infusion over 30 min
	Actinomycin D	0.5 mg i.v. bolus
	Folinic acid rescue starting 24 h after commencing the methotrexate infusion	15 mg i.m. or orally every 12 h × 4 doses
CO		
Day 8	Vincristine	1 mg/m² i.v. bolus (max. 2 mg)
	Cyclophosphamide	600 mg/m² i.v. infusion over 30 min

EMA alternates with CO every week. To avoid extended intervals between courses caused by myelosuppression, it may occasionally be necessary to reduce the EMA by omitting the Day 2 doses of etoposide and actinomycin D.

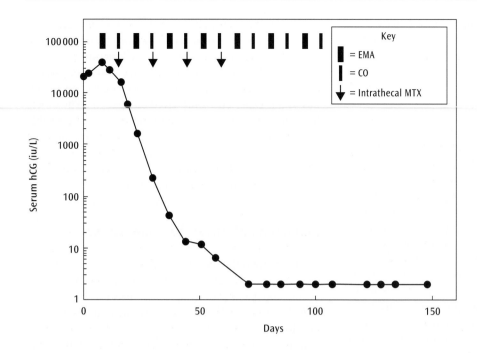

Figure 37.8 *The fall in hCG and, by inference, the tumour response to EMA/CO chemotherapy in a patient with choriocarcinoma who scored within the high-risk group. The patient has pulmonary metastases and received intrathecal methotrexate with each course of CO (cyclophosphamide and vincristine) until the hCG levels were within the normal range.*

Both low-risk and medium-risk patients failing methotrexate whose serum hCG is >100 iu/L are now all treated with the EMA/CO regimen outlined above. While this treatment has saved all low-risk patients, occasional middle-risk and some high-risk patients develop drug-resistant disease. Fortunately, 70 per cent of the 47 patients who have failed EMA/CO were still salvaged by further chemotherapy and/or surgery (Bower *et al.*, 1997). Indeed, the combination of surgical removal of the main site of drug resistance (usually in the uterus, lung or brain), together with chemotherapy, is particularly effective. Preoperative investigations include transvaginal or abdominal US Doppler of the pelvis, plain chest radiography, whole-body CT scan and MRI of the brain, lumbar puncture to measure hCG levels in the cerebrospinal fluid, and experimental imaging techniques such as anti-hCG or ^{18}FDG-PET scanning. If all these investigations are negative, hysterectomy should be considered. When multiple possible sites of resistant disease are found, anti-hCG or ^{18}FDG-PET imaging can potentially distinguish the biologically active from dead/necrotic lesions and so guide appropriate surgery. Following surgery, or when surgery is not appropriate, we use the *cis*-platinum-containing regimen, EP (etoposide 150 mg/m^2 and *cis*-platinum 75 mg/m^2 with hydration) alternating weekly with EMA (omitting Day 2 except the folinic acid). This is not an easy schedule to administer clinically, owing to both myelosuppression and complications associated with even minor renal impairment.

Other options that can be considered include use of some of the new anti-cancer agents such as the taxanes, topotecan, gemcitabine and temozolomide. Paclitaxel has been shown to have activity in patients with germ-cell tumours that have failed on prior treatment (Motzer

et al., 1994). Interestingly, two cases of drug-resistant GTT responded to paclitaxel, with one remaining in remission (Jones *et al.*, 1996) and, in another report, a third patient remains in remission following high-dose paclitaxel (250 mg/m^2 repeated three-weekly) (Termrungruanglert *et al.*, 1996).

Another approach in patients with refractory disease involves high-dose chemotherapy with autologous bone marrow or peripheral stem-cell transplantation. Patient selection here is probably important in determining outcome. We know from experience with refractory germ-cell tumours that patients with drug-sensitive disease are the ones that stay in remission (Beyer *et al.*, 1996; Lyttelton *et al.*, 1998). Recently, there have been two encouraging case reports of remissions following high-dose chemotherapy with cyclophosphamide, etoposide and melphalan (Giacalone *et al.*, 1995) and chemotherapy with ifosfamide, carboplatin and etoposide (van Besien *et al.*, 1997).

Management of acute disease-induced complications

HAEMORRHAGE

Heavy vaginal or intraperitoneal bleeding is the most frequent immediate threat to life in patients with trophoblastic tumours. The bleeding mostly settles with bed rest and after starting chemotherapy appropriate to the risk group. However, occasionally the bleeding can be torrential, requiring massive transfusion. In this situation if the bleeding is coming from the uterus, it may be necessary to consider a uterine pack or emergency embolization of the tumour vasculature. Fortunately, hysterectomy is rarely required. If the bleeding is intraperitoneal and does not settle with transfusion and chemotherapy, laparotomy may be required. Indeed, patients occasionally present this way.

RESPIRATORY FAILURE

Occasionally patients present with respiratory failure due to multiple pulmonary metastases or, more rarely, as a result of massive tumour embolism to the pulmonary circulation (Seckl *et al.*, 1991; Savage *et al.*, 1998). Fever with or without purulent sputum may be present and, in these cases, blood and sputum cultures should be obtained and antibiotics started to treat potential infection. If tumour embolus is suspected, a ventilation/perfusion scan, MRI or dynamic CT chest (Fig. 37.9) and electrocardiogram should be obtained and a heparin infusion started. Pulse oximetry and/or arterial blood gas should be regularly measured to allow appropriate adjustment of oxygen therapy and to monitor any deterioration in pulmonary function that may occur following the start of chemotherapy. The latter occurs probably because of oedema and inflammation around tumour deposits that

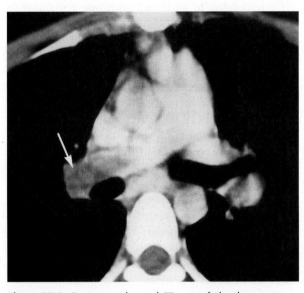

Figure 37.9 *Contrast-enhanced CT scan of the thorax at the level of the main pulmonary arteries, showing a filling defect in the right main pulmonary artery (arrow). The patient presented with a brief history of increasing shortness of breath which had suddenly worsened. During the previous 18 months she had suffered from irregular heavy bleeding per vagina, had four separate positive pregnancy tests and two normal pelvic ultrasound investigations. She was successfully treated with EMA/CO chemotherapy, with some resolution of the changes seen on CT and ventilation perfusion scanning. Post-mortem examinations of similar cases have revealed that the filling defect in the main pulmonary artery is tumour embolus and not clot. (Reproduced from Seckl* et al.*, 1991 with permission from Elsevier Science.)*

are becoming necrotic. To prevent this we usually commence therapy with only one or two drugs and introduce the other drugs once pulmonary function is stable. Occasionally patients require masked continuous positive airway pressure ventilation but mechanical ventilation has in our experience only saved one patient. The others have died from intrapulmonary haemorrhage probably as a result of trauma to the tumour vasculature induced by high positive airway pressures generated on mechanical ventilation. For this reason extracorporeal oxygenation has been proposed (Kelly *et al.*, 1990).

Management of cerebral metastases

Involvement of the central nervous system (CNS) by GTT may either be overt and require intensive therapy or occult and need prophylaxis. Any patient with a GTT who has lung metastases is at risk of either having or developing CNS disease. Furthermore, the second most common site of metastases in high-risk patients is the CNS and nearly all these individuals had lung deposits (Athanassiou *et al.*, 1983). The presence of neurological symptoms and signs may alert the clinician to the presence of brain metastases. However, some high-risk patients do not have either overt pulmonary or CNS disease at presentation but subsequently develop cerebral metastases which are then drug resistant. Consequently, careful investigation of patients at risk of developing brain metastases is warranted so that appropriate CNS-penetrating chemotherapy is given rather than the standard low- or high-risk treatments. Investigations include CT and/or MRI of the brain and, in patients who do not have raised intracranial pressure, measurement of the hCG levels in cerebrospinal fluid. A cerebrospinal fluid : serum ratio greater than 1/60 suggests the presence of CNS disease.

Prophylaxis against possible CNS disease (MRI brain normal) is given to patients from all risk categories with lung metastases and all high-risk patients regardless of the absence or presence of lung deposits. The prophylaxis consists of 12.5 mg methotrexate administered intrathecally, followed 24 hours later by 15 mg of folinic acid orally. This is given with every course of low-risk therapy, or with each CO in the high-risk therapy for three doses. Since the introduction of this policy, the development of brain metastases without evidence of drug resistance elsewhere has been much less frequent (Athanassiou *et al.*, 1983).

Overt CNS disease requires careful management as therapy can induce haemorrhage into the tumour, leading to a rise in intracranial pressure and subsequent loss of life (Athanassiou *et al.*, 1983). We and others have found that early resection of solitary brain deposits in patients with serious neurological signs can sometimes be life saving (Ishizuka, 1983; Song and Wu, 1988; Rustin *et al.*, 1989). In this respect, early consideration of the diagnosis may be helpful. Cerebral oedema can be reduced with high-dose corticosteroids and so patients are given 24 mg of dexamethasone in divided doses before starting chemotherapy. The EMA/CO regimen is modified by increasing the dose of methotrexate to $1 g/m^2$, given as a 24-h infusion on Day 1. The folinic acid rescue is increased to 30 mg given 8 hourly intravenously for 3 days, commencing 32 hours after the start of the methotrexate infusion. Provided there is no evidence of raised intracranial pressure, 12.5 mg of methotrexate is given intrathecally with each CO until the hCG in serum is normal. Modified EMA/CO is then continued for a further 6–8 weeks. Patients who survive the first 3 weeks of such treatment have a good prognosis, with an 89 per cent chance of cure (Athanassiou et al., 1983; Rustin et al., 1989).

Patients who develop cerebral tumour during chemotherapy have a poor prognosis because their disease is almost certainly drug resistant. Nevertheless, a combination of immediate surgery to remove the deposit(s) and modified chemotherapy designed to provide better CNS penetration can be curative in this situation (Athanassiou et al., 1983; Rustin et al., 1989). Radiotherapy has been advocated as an alternative therapeutic approach. However, it has not been shown to eradicate tumour in its own right, and in combination with chemotherapy has produced less effective results than chemotherapy alone (Athanassiou et al., 1983; Rustin et al., 1989). Nevertheless, stereotactic radiotherapy probably has a role in the treatment of isolated deep lesions that cannot be removed surgically.

Management of PSTTs

PSTTs are biologically quite different from the other forms of GTD, producing little hCG, growing slowly, metastasizing late and being relatively resistant to combination chemotherapy regimens. Therefore, hysterectomy remains the treatment of choice, provided the disease is still localized to the uterus. When metastatic disease is present, despite reports to the contrary (Lathrop et al., 1988), individual patients can respond and be apparently cured by chemotherapy (EP/EMA), either alone or in combination with surgery (Newlands et al., 1998b). The most important prognostic variable in these patients is the interval from the last pregnancy: where this is less than 2 years the prognosis is good, and where greater than 2 years the outlook is poor. Radiotherapy has produced mixed results and has not yet been proven to cure the disease. Because PSTT is so rare, it is unlikely that its treatment will ever be optimized.

Patient follow-up after chemotherapy

On completion of their chemotherapy, patients need to be followed up regularly for life, with hCG estimations to confirm that their disease is in remission. Initially the follow-up is with serum and urine samples (Table 37.8), but in due course the follow-up is only on urine samples. In the UK this is computerized and automatic reminders are sent to patients so that they do not get lost to follow-up. Patients are advised not to become pregnant until 12 months after completing their chemotherapy. This minimizes the potential teratogenicity of treatment and avoids confusion between a new pregnancy or relapsed disease as the cause of a rising hCG. Despite this advice, 230 women on follow-up at our centre between 1973 and 1997 have become pregnant during the first year. Fortunately, this did not appear to be associated with an increased risk of relapse or fetal morbidity and there were no maternal deaths. Indeed, 75 per cent of women continued their pregnancy to term. Consequently, although we continue to advise women to avoid pregnancy for 1 year after completing chemotherapy, those that do become pregnant can be reassured of a likely favourable outcome. Similar results have been reported by others (Fan et al., 1999). When a patient becomes pregnant, it is important to confirm by US and other appropriate means that the

Table 37.8 *Follow-up of patients with gestational trophoblastic tumours who have been treated with chemotherapy*

	Low/medium/high risk post-chemotherapy patients, hCG concentration sampling	
	Urine	**Blood**
Weekly for the first 6 weeks (outpatient follow-up consultation at 6 weeks post-chemotherapy)	✓	✓
Then every 2 weeks until 6 months	✓	✓
Then fortnightly until 1 year	✓	✗
Then monthly × 12	✓	✗
Then 2 monthly × 6	✓	✗
Then 3 monthly × 4	✓	✗
Then 4 monthly × 3	✓	✗
Then 6 monthly for life	✓	✗

pregnancy is normal. Follow-up is then discontinued until 3 weeks after the end of pregnancy when the hCG due to the pregnancy should have returned to normal. Patients who do not require chemotherapy following evacuation of their first mole, although not on life-long follow-up, should have their hCG levels measured 3 weeks and then 3 months after the end of any subsequent pregnancy. This is because they are at increased risk compared to the general population of a further molar pregnancy. In addition, with a subsequent pregnancy there is a small risk of reactivation of 'dormant' residual molar tissue, even if the pregnancy itself is normal.

The follow-up of PSTT differs from that of other GTD variants, since serum hCG is a less reliable tumour marker and late recurrences are probably more common (Newlands et al., 1998b). Indeed, these tumours may fail to secrete hCG at relapse despite an extensive tumour burden (Hopkins et al., 1992). Consequently, patients in remission from PSTT are followed up serologically and at regular intervals in the clinic for 5 years.

Contraceptive advice

Patients using oral contraceptives before the hCG is normal following evacuation of a HM have an increased incidence of sequelae requiring chemotherapy (Stone et al., 1976). In a more recent analysis of our patients registered between 1973 and 1989, we have found that the proportion of patients requiring chemotherapy after evacuation of their HM is 30.7 per cent, compared with 8 per cent in the overall population. For this reason, patients are advised to avoid the oral contraceptive pill until the hCG has returned to normal after removal of a HM. Patients who have had chemotherapy for their GTT are advised not to use the oral contraceptive pill until their hCG is normal and chemotherapy is completed. More data are needed about the importance of oral contraceptives but, until these are available, we feel that this is reasonable practice.

Long-term complications of therapy

Most patients, including those who have received intensive chemotherapy, return to normal activity within a few months, and the majority of the side-effects are reversible. Complete hair regrowth is seen in all patients with chemotherapy-induced alopecia, although sometimes it may be initially curly rather than straight. Late sequelae from chemotherapy have been remarkably rare. We have recently analysed 15 279 patient years of follow-up for the late sequelae from chemotherapy and this confirms that patients treated with methotrexate and folinic acid in the low-risk category have no significant increase in the incidence of second tumours (Rustin et al., 1996). In contrast, 26 patients receiving intensive combination chemotherapy for their gestational trophoblastic tumours developed another cancer, when the expected rate was only 16.45; a significant difference (Rustin et al., 1996). Acute myeloid leukaemia (AML) (relative risk 16.6) accounted for the early tumours up to 5 years after completing chemotherapy. Subsequently, at 5–9 years an increase was seen in colorectal cancer (relative risk 4.6), at 10–14 years in melanomas, and beyond 25 years in breast cancer (relative risk 5.8). The increased risk of AML probably reflects the rising use of etoposide, which is now well recognized to induce this form of leukaemia (Pui et al., 1991; Whitlock et al., 1991; Hawkins et al., 1992; Rustin et al., 1996).

Fertility is an important issue in the management of patients with GTTs. Although chemotherapy appears to induce a menopause 3 years earlier than would normally be expected (Bower et al., 1998), fertility does not otherwise appear to be affected (Woolas et al., 1998). In 392 patients receiving single-agent methotrexate, 327 (83.4 per cent) had successful live births. Interestingly, in the 336 patients receiving multi-agent chemotherapy, including EMA/CO, 280 (83.3 per cent) also succeeded in having normal pregnancies. Importantly, in this and a previous analysis there was no increase in the incidence of congenital malformations compared to the general population (Rustin et al., 1984; Woolas et al., 1998).

PROGNOSIS

All patients in the low- and middle-risk groups can be expected to be cured of their GTTs since the introduction of etoposide (Bagshawe et al., 1986; Newlands et al., 1986). For high-risk patients, survival has progressively improved and is currently 86 per cent (Bower et al., 1997). The diagnosis of choriocarcinoma is often not suspected until the disease is advanced. As a result, some deaths occur before chemotherapy has a chance to be effective. The number of such patients can be diminished by a greater awareness of the possibility that multiple metastases in a woman of childbearing age may be due to choriocarcinoma. The simple measurement of the hCG level in such individuals is a very strong indicator of choriocarcinoma and could help to hasten referrals for life-saving chemotherapy. However, patients in the high-risk group still die from drug-resistant disease and there remains a need to develop novel therapeutic approaches.

SUMMARY

In the past, many women have died from GTD. However, during the past 50 years we have learnt much about the biology, pathology and natural history of this group of disorders. Furthermore, accurate diagnostic and monitoring methods have been developed, together with effective treatment regimens. As a result, the management of GTD today represents one of the modern success stories in oncology, with few women dying from their trophoblastic tumours.

SIGNIFICANT POINTS

- While it is well known that CMs can transform into choriocarcinomas, it had previously been thought that PMs do not do this. Recent work, however, has conclusively shown that PMs can also transform into choriocarcinoma, so all patients with PMs require hCG follow-up.
- All patients with suspected GTT should be discussed with a gestational trophoblastic disease centre and have their histology centrally reviewed.
- The use of serum and urine hCG measurements to follow the disease course has been a key feature in the successful management of women with GTT. However, recent work has shown that care is required in the interpretation of hCG values obtained from commercial kit assays. This is because (a) only a single epitope of hCG is detected in most kit assays and this epitope may be lost in some GTTs; and (b) some patients have anti-mouse antibodies which bind to the mouse monoclonal antibody used in kit assays, generating a false-positive hCG.
- Currently the most reliable hCG assay involves the use of a polyclonal rabbit antisera used in a radioimmunoassay which detects many different epitopes of hCG.
- Middle-risk, like low-risk, patients with GTT are now initially treated with MTX/FA as this regimen has no long-term sequelae.
- Patients relapsing on MTX/FA are switched to actinomycin D if their hCG level is <100 iu/L or EMA/CO combination chemotherapy if the hCG is >100 iu/L.
- EMA/CO, like MTX/FA, does not appear to impair fertility, but there is a small increased risk of second tumours with EMA/CO.
- The long-term outcome for patients with GTT is excellent, with all low- and middle-risk patients and approximately 90 per cent of high-risk patients being cured.

KEY REFERENCES

Newlands, E.S., Paradinas, F.J. and Fisher, R.A. (1998) Recent advances in gestational trophoblastic disease. *Hematol. Oncol. Clin. North Am.* **13**, 225–44.

Paradinas, F.J. (1998) The diagnosis and prognosis of molar pregnancy. The experience of the National Referral Centre in London. *Int. J. Gynaecol. Obstet.* **60**, S57–64.

Rotmensch, S. and Cole, L.A. (2000) False diagnosis and needless therapy of presumed malignant disease in women with false positive hCG concentrations. *Lancet* **355**, 712–15.

Seckl, M.J., Fisher, R.A., Salerno, G.A. et al. (2000) Choriocarcinoma and partial hydatidiform moles. *Lancet* **356**, 36–9.

REFERENCES

Ariel, I., Lustig, O., Oyer, C.E. et al. (1994) Relaxation of genomic imprinting in trophoblastic disease. *Gynaecol. Oncol.* **53**, 212–19.

Arima, T., Imamura, T., Amada, S., Tsuneyoshi, M. and Wake, N. (1994) Genetic origin of malignant trophoblastic neoplasms. *Cancer Genet. Cytogenet.* **73**, 95–102.

Arima, T., Matsuda, T., Takagi, N. and Wake, N. (1997) Association of IGF2 and H19 imprinting with choriocarcinoma development. *Cancer Genet. Cytogenet.* **93**, 39–47.

Athanassiou, A., Begent, R.H.J., Newlands, E.S., Parker, D., Rustin, G.J.S. and Bagshawe, K.D. (1983) Central nervous system metastases of choriocarcinoma: 23 years' experience at Charing Cross Hospital. *Cancer* **52**, 1728–35.

Bagshawe, K.D. (1976) Risk and prognostic factors in trophoblastic neoplasia. *Cancer* **38**, 1373–85.

Bagshawe, K.D. and Noble, M.I.M. (1965) Cardiorespiratory effects of trophoblastic tumours. *QJM* **137**, 39–54.

Bagshawe, K.D., Dent, J. and Webb, J. (1986) Hydatidiform mole in the United Kingdom 1973–1983. *Lancet* **ii**, 673.

Bagshawe, K.D., Dent, J., Newlands, E.S., Begent, R.H.J. and Rustin, G.J.S. (1989) The role of low dose methotrexate and folinic acid in gestational trophoblastic tumours (GTT). *Br. J. Obstet. Gynaecol.* **96**, 795–802.

Bagshawe, K.D., Lawler, S.D., Paradinas, F.J., Dent, J., Brown, P. and Boxer, G.M. (1990) Gestational trophoblastic tumours following initial diagnosis of partial hydatidiform mole. *Lancet* **334**, 1074–6.

Beets, G., Penninckx, F., Schiepers, C. et al. (1994) Clinical value of whole body positron emission tomography with [^{18}F]fluorodeoxyglucose in recurrent colorectal cancer. *Br. J. Surg.* **81**, 1666–70.

Begent, R.H.J. (1995) Gestational trophoblastic tumours. In Peckham, M., Pinedo, H. and Veronesi, U. (eds), *Oxford textbook of oncology*. Oxford: Oxford University Press, p. 1369.

Begent, R.H.J., Bagshawe, K.D., Green, A.J. and Searle, A.J. (1987) The clinical value of imaging with antibody to human chorionic gonadotrophin in the detection of residual choriocarcinoma. *Br. J. Cancer* **55**, 657–60.

Belchis, D.A., Mowry, J. and Davis, J.H. (1993) Infantile choriocarcinoma. Re-examination of a potentially curable entity. *Cancer* **72**, 2028–32.

Berkowitz, R.S. and Goldstein, D.P. (1981) Pathogenesis of gestational trophoblastic neoplasms. *Pathol. Annu.* **11**, 391.

Beyer, J., Kramar, A., Mandanas, R. *et al.* (1996) High-dose chemotherapy as salvage treatment in germ cell tumors: a multivariate analysis of prognostic variables. *J. Clin. Oncol.* **14**, 2638–45.

Birken, S., Krichevsky, A., O'Connor, J. *et al.* (1999) Development and characterization of antibodies to a nicked and hyperglycosylated form of a hCG from a choriocarcinoma patient: generation of antibodies that differentiate between pregnancy hCG and choriocarcinoma hCG. *Endocrine* **10**, 137–44.

Bo, M. and Boime, I. (1992) Identification of the transcriptionally active genes of the chorionic gonadotropin beta gene cluster *in vivo*. *J. Biol. Chem.* **267**, 3179–84.

Boorstein, W.R., Vamkakopoulos, N.C. and Fiddes, J.C. (1982) Human chorionic gonadotropin beta subunit is encoded by at least eight genes arranged in tandem and inverted pairs. *Nature* **300**, 419–22.

Boultebee, J.E. and Newlands, E.S. (1995) New diagnostic and therapeutic approaches to gestational trophoblastic tumours. In Bourne, T.H., Jauniaux, E. and Jurkovic, D. (eds), *Transvaginal colour doppler. The scientific basis and practical application of colour doppler in gynaecology*. Berlin: Springer, 57–65.

Bower, M., Newlands, E.S., Holden, L. *et al.* (1997) EMA/CO for high-risk gestational trophoblastic tumours: results from a cohort of 272 patients. *J. Clin. Oncol.* **15**, 2636–43.

Bower, M., Rustin, G.J.S., Newlands, E.S. *et al.* (1998) Chemotherapy for gestational trophoblastic tumours hastens menopause by 3 years. *Eur. J. Cancer* **34**, 1204–7.

Chaganti, R.S.K., Kodura, P.R.K., Chakraborty, R. *et al.* (1990) Genetic origin of trophoblastic choriocarcinoma. *Cancer Res.* **50**, 6330–3.

Chilosi, M., Piazzola, E., Lestani, M. *et al.* (1998) Differential expression of p57^{kip2}, a maternally imprinted cdk inhibitor, in normal human placenta and gestational trophoblastic disease. *Lab. Invest.* **78**(3), 269–76.

Cole, L.A. (1998) hCG, its free subunits and its metabolites. Roles in pregnancy and trophoblastic disease. *J. Reprod. Med.* **43**, 3–10.

Curry, S.L., Hammond, C.B., Tyrey, L., Creasman, W.T. and Parker, R.T. (1975) Hydatidiform mole: diagnosis, management, and long-term follow up of 347 patients. *Obst. Gynaecol.* **45**(1), 1–8.

Davis, J.R., Surwit, E.A., Garay, J.P. and Fortier, K.J. (1984) Sex assignment in gestational trophoblastic neoplasia. *Am. J. Obstet. Gynecol.* **148**, 722–5.

Dufau, M.L. (1998) The luteinizing hormone receptor. *Annu. Rev. Physiol.* **60**, 461–96.

Eckstein, R., Paradinas, F. and Bagshawe, K.D. (1982) Placental site trophoblastic tumour (trophoblastic pseudotumour): a study of four cases requiring hysterectomy including one fatal case. *Histopathology* **6**, 211–26.

Edwards, Y.H., Jeremiah, S.J., McMillan, S.L., Povey, S., Fisher, R.A. and Lawler, S.D. (1984) Complete hydatidiform moles combine maternal mitochondria with paternal nuclear genome. *Ann. Hum. Genet.* **48**, 119–27.

Fan, X., Yan, L., Jia, S., Ma, A. and Qiao, C. (1999) A study of early pregnancy factor activity in the sera of women with trophoblastic tumor. *Am. J. Reprod. Immunol.* **41**, 204–8.

Fine, C., Bundy, A.L., Berkowitz, R.S., Boswell, S.B., Berezin, A.F. and Doubilet, P.M. (1989) Sonographic diagnosis of partial hydatidiform mole. *Obstet. Gynaecol.* **73**, 414–18.

Finkler, N.J., Berkowitz, R.S., Driscoll, S.G., Goldstein, D.P. and Bernstein, M.R. (1988) Clinical experience with placental site trophoblastic tumours at the New England Trophoblastic Disease Center. *Obstet. Gynaecol.* **71**, 854–7.

Fisher, R.A. and Newlands, E.S. (1998) Gestational trophoblastic disease: molecular and genetic studies. *J. Reprod. Med.* **43**, 81–97.

Fisher, R.A., Sheppard, D.M. and Lawler, D.W. (1982) Twin pregnancy with complete hydatidiform mole (46,XX) and fetus (46,XY): genetic origin proved by analysis of chromosome polymorphisms. *BMJ* **1**, 1218–20.

Fisher, R.A., Lawler, S.D., Ormerod, M.G., Imrie, P.R. and Povey, S. (1987) Flow cytometry used to distinguish between complete and partial hydatidiform moles. *Placenta* **8**, 249–56.

Fisher, R.A., Lawler, S.D., Povey, S. and Bagshawe, K.D. (1988) Genetically homozygous choriocarcinoma following pregnancy with hydatidiform mole. *Br. J. Cancer* **58**, 788–892.

Fisher, R.A., Povey, S., Jeffreys, A.J., Martin, C.A., Patel, I. and Lawler, S.D. (1989) Frequency of heterozygous complete hydatidiform moles, estimated by locus-specific minisatellite and Y chromosome-specific probes. *Human Genet.* **82**, 259–63.

Fisher, R.A., Newlands, E.S., Jeffreys, A.J. *et al.* (1992a) Gestational and non-gestational trophoblastic

tumours distinguished by DNA analysis. *Cancer*
69, 839–45.

Fisher, R.A., Paradinas, F.J., Newlands, E.S. and
Boxer, G.M. (1992b) Genetic evidence that placental
site trophoblastic tumours can originate from a
hydatidiform mole or a normal conceptus.
Br. J. Cancer **65**, 355–8.

Fisher, R.A., Soteriou, B.A., Meredith, L., Paradinas, F.J.
and Newlands, E.S. (1995) Previous hydatidiform
mole identified as the causative pregnancy of
choriocarcinoma following birth of normal twins.
Int. J. Cancer **5**, 64–70.

Fradken, J.E., Eastman, R.C., Lesniak, M.A. and
Roth, J. (1989) Specificity spillover at the hormone
receptor – exploring its role in human disease.
N. Engl. J. Med. **320**, 640–5.

Fukunaga, M. and Ushigome, S. (1993) Malignant
trophoblastic tumours: immunohistochemical
and flow cytometric comparison of choriocarcinoma
and placental site trophoblastic tumours.
Human Pathol. **24**, 1098–106.

Fulop, V., Mok, S.C., Genest, D.R., Szigetvari, I., Cseh, I.
and Berkowitz, R.S. (1998a) c-myc, c-erbB2, c-fms and
bcl-2 oncoproteins. Expression in normal placenta,
partial and complete mole, and choriocarcinoma.
J. Reprod. Med. **43**, 101–10.

Fulop, V., Mok, S.C., Genest, D.R., Gati, I., Doszpod, J.
and Berkowitz, R.S. (1998b) p53, p21, Rb and mdm2
oncoproteins. Expression in normal placenta,
partial and complete mole, and choriocarcinoma.
J. Reprod. Med. **43**, 119–27.

Giacalone, P.L., Benos, P., Donnadio, D. and Laffargue, F.
(1995) High-dose chemotherapy with autologous bone
marrow transplantation for refractory metastatic
gestational trophoblastic disease. *Gynaecol. Oncol.*
58, 383–5.

Goldstein, D.P. and Berkowitz, R.S. (1994) Current
management of complete and partial molar
pregnancy. *J. Reprod. Med.* **39**, 139–46.

Goldstein, D.P., Zanten-Przybysz, I.V., Bernstein, M.R. and
Berkowitz, R.S. (1998) Revised FIGO staging system for
gestational trophoblastic tumors. *J. Reprod. Med.*
43, 37–43.

Goto, S., Yamada, A., Ishizuka, T. and Tomoda, Y. (1993)
Development of postmolar trophoblastic disease
after partial molar pregnancy. *Gynaecol. Oncol.*
48, 165–70.

Grover, S., Woodward, S.R. and Odell, W.D. (1995)
Complete sequence of the gene encoding a chorionic
gonadotrophin-like protein from *Xanthomonas
maltophilia*. *Gene* **156**, 75–8.

Hando, T., Masaguki, O. and Kurose, T. (1998) Recent
aspects of gestational trophoblastic disease in Japan.
Int. J. Gynaecol. Oncol. **60**, S71–76.

Hao, Y., Crenshaw, T., Moulton, T., Newcomb, E. and
Tycko, B. (1993) Tumor suppressor activity of H19 RNA.
Nature **365**, 764–7.

Hashimoto, K., Azuma, C., Koyama, M. *et al.* (1995)
Loss of imprinting in choriocarcinoma. *Nat. Genet.*
9, 109–10.

Hawkins, M.M., Kinnier Wilson, L.M., Stovall, M.A. *et al.*
(1992) Epipodophyllotoxins, alkylating agents, and
radiation and risk of secondary leukaemia after
childhood cancer. *BMJ* **304**, 951–8.

Hebart, H., Erley, C., Kaskas, B. *et al.* (1996) Positron
emission tomography helps to diagnose tumor
emboli and residual disease in choriocarcinoma.
Ann. Oncol. **7**, 416–18.

Holmgren, L., Flam, F., Larsson, E. and Ohlsson, R. (1993)
Successive activation of the platelet-derived
growth factor beta receptor and platelet-derived
growth factor B genes correlates with the genesis
of human choriocarcinoma. *Cancer Res.* **53**,
2927–31.

Hopkins, M.P., Drescher, C.W., McQuillan, A., Keyser, J.
and Schmidt, R. (1992) Malignant placental site
trophoblastic tumour associated with placental
abruption, fetal distress, and elevated CA-125.
Gynecol. Oncol. **47**, 267–71.

Ishizuka, T. (1983) Intracranial metastases of
choriocarcinoma: a clinicopathologic study.
Cancer **52**, 1896–903.

Jacobs, P.A., Wilson, C.M., Sprenkle, J.A., Rosenshein, N.B.
and Migeon, B.R. (1980) Mechanism of origin of
complete hydatidiform mole. *Nature* **286**, 714–16.

Jacobs, P.A., Hunt, P.A., Matsuuro, J.S. and Wilson, C.C.
(1982) Complete and partial hydatidiform mole in
Hawaii: cytogenetics, morphology and epidemiology.
Br. J. Obstet. Gynaecol. **89**, 258–66.

Jones, W.B., Schneider, J., Shapiro, F. and Lewis, J.L.J.
(1996) Treatment of resistant gestational
choriocarcinoma with taxol: a report of two cases.
Gynaecol. Oncol. **61**, 126–30.

Kajii, T. and Ohama, K. (1977) Androgenetic origin of
hydatidiform mole. *Nature* **268**, 633–4.

Kelly, M.P., Rustin, G.J.S., Ivory, C., Phillips, P. and
Bagshawe, K.D. (1990) Respiratory failure due to
choriocarcinoma: a study of 103 dyspneic patients.
Gynaecol. Oncol. **38**, 149–54.

Kim, J., Ashworth, L., Branscomb, E. and Stubbs, L.
(1997) The human homolog of a mouse-imprinted
gene, Peg3, maps to a zinc finger gene-rich region
of human chromosome 19q13.4. *Genome Res.*
7, 532–40.

Kishkuno, S., Ishida, A., Takahashi, Y. *et al.* (1997) A case
of neonatal choriocarcinoma. *Am. J. Perineonatol.*
14, 79–82.

Kotylo, P.K., Michael, H., Davis, T.E., Sutton, G.P., Mark, P.R.
and Roth, L.M. (1992) Flow cytometric DNA analysis of
placental-site trophoblastic tumours. *Int. J. Gynaecol.
Pathol.* **11**, 245–52.

Lapthorn, A.J., Harris, D.C., Littlejohn, A. *et al.* (1994)
Crystal structure of human chorionic gonadotropin.
Nature **369**, 455–61.

Lathrop, J., Lauchlan, S., Nayak, R. and Ambler, M. (1988) Clinical characteristics of placental site trophoblastic tumour (PSTT). *Gynaecol. Oncol.* **31**, 32–42.

Lawler, S.D. and Fisher, R.A. (1986) Genetic aspects of gestational trophoblastic tumours. In Ichinoe, K. (ed.), *Trophoblastic diseases.* Tokyo: Igaku-Shoin, 23–33.

Lawler, S.D., Klouda, P.A. and Bagshawe, K.D. (1976) The relationship between HLA antibodies and the causal pregnancy in choriocarcinoma. *Br. J. Obstet. Gynaecol.* **83**, 651–5.

Lawler, S.D., Pickthall, V.G., Fisher, R.A., Povey, S., Wyn Evans, M. and Szulman, A.E. (1979) Genetic studies of complete and partial hydatidiform mole (letter). *Lancet* **ii**, 580.

Lawler, S.D., Fisher, R.A., Pickthall, V.G., Povey, S. and Wyn Evans, M. (1982a) Genetic studies on hydatidiform moles I: the origin of partial moles. *Cancer Genet. Cytogenet.* **4**, 309–20.

Lawler, S.D., Povey, S., Fisher, R.A. and Pickthall, V.G. (1982b) Genetic studies on hydatidiform moles II: the origin of complete moles. *Ann. Hum. Genet.* **46**, 209–22.

Li, M., Squire, J.A. and Weksberg, R. (1998) Overgrowth syndromes and genomic imprinting: from mouse to man. *Clin. Genet.* **53**, 165–70.

Long, M.G., Boultbee, J.E., Langley, R., Newlands, E.S., Begent, R.H.J. and Bagshawe, K.D. (1992) Doppler assessment of the uterine circulation and the clinical behaviour of gestational trophoblastic tumours requiring chemotherapy. *Br. J. Cancer* **66**, 882–7.

Lyttelton, M.P., Newlands, E.S., Giles, C. *et al.* (1998) High-dose therapy including carboplatin adjusted for renal function in patients with relapsed germ cell tumor: outcome and prognostic factors. *Br. J. Cancer* **77**, 1672–6.

Martin, B.H. and Kim, J.H. (1998) Changing face of gestational trophoblastic disease. *Int. J. Gynaecol. Oncol.* **60**, S111–20.

Matsuda, T., Sasaki, M., Kato, H. *et al.* (1997) Human chromosome 7 carries a putative tumor suppressor gene(s) involved in choriocarcinoma. *Oncogene* **15**, 2773–81.

Matsuoka, S., Thompson, J.S., Edwards, M.C. *et al.* (1996) Imprinting of the gene encoding a human cyclin-dependent kinase inhibitor, p57^{kip2}, on chromosome 11p15. *Proc. Natl Acad. Sci. USA* **93**, 3026–30.

Matsuura, J., Chiu, D., Jacobs, P.A. and Szulman, A.E. (1984) Complete hydatidiform mole in Hawaii: an epidemiological study. *Genet. Epidemiol.* **1**, 271–84.

McGrath, I.T., Golding, P.R. and Bagshawe, K.D. (1971) Medical presentations of choriocarcinoma. *BMJ* **2**, 633–7.

Moglabey, Y.B., Kircheisen, R., Seoud, M., El Mogharbel, N., Van den Veyver, I. and Slim, R. (1999) Genetic mapping of a maternal locus responsible for familial hydatidiform moles. *Hum. Mol. Genet.* **8**, 667–71.

Motzer, R.J., Bajorin, D.F., Schwartz, L.H. *et al.* (1994) Phase II trial of paclitaxel shows antitumour activity in patients with previously treated germ cell tumours. *J. Clin. Oncol.* **12**, 2277–83.

Mueller, U.W., Hawes, C.S., Wright, A.E. *et al.* (1990) Isolation of fetal trophoblast cells from peripheral blood of pregnant women. *Lancet* **336**, 197–200.

Mutter, G.L., Stewart, C.L., Chaponot, M.L. and Pomponio, R.J. (1993) Oppositely imprinted genes H-19 and insulin-like growth factor 2 are co-expressed in human androgenetic trophoblast. *Am. J. Hum. Genet.* **53**, 1096–102.

Newlands, E.S., Bagshawe, K.D., Begent, R.H.J., Rustin, G.J.S., Holden, L. and Dent, J. (1986) Development of chemotherapy for medium- and high-risk patients with gestational trophoblastic tumours (1979–1984). *Br. J. Obstet. Gynaecol.* **93**, 63–9.

Newlands, E.S., Paradinas, F.J. and Fisher, R.A. (1998a) Recent advances in gestational trophoblastic disease. *Hematol. Oncol. Clin. North Am.* **13**, 225–44.

Newlands, E.S., Bower, M., Fisher, R.A. and Paradinas, F.J. (1998b) Management of placental site trophoblastic tumours. *J. Reprod. Med.* **43**, 53–9.

Ober, W.B. and Fass, R.O. (1961) The early history of choriocarcinoma. *Ann. NY Acad. Sci.* **172**, 299–426.

Ogawa, O., Eccles, M.R., Szeto, J. *et al.* (1993) Relaxation in insulin-like growth factor II gene imprinting implicated in Wilm's tumour. *Nature* **362**, 749–51.

Ohama, K., Kajii, T., Okamoto, E. *et al.* (1981) Dispermic origin of XY hydatidiform mole. *Nature* **292**, 551–2.

Osada, H., Kawata, M., Yamada, M., Okumura, K. and Takamizawa, H. (1991) Genetic identification of pregnancies responsible for choriocarcinomas after multiple pregnancies by restriction fragment length polymorphism analysis. *Am. J. Obstet. Gynaecol.* **165**, 682–8.

Palmer, J.R. (1994) Advances in the epidemiology of gestational trophoblastic disease. *J. Reprod. Med.* **39**, 155–62.

Palmer, J.R., Driscoll, S.G., Rosenberg, L. *et al.* (1999) Oral contraceptive use and risk of gestational trophoblastic tumors. *J. Natl Cancer Inst.* **91**, 635–40.

Paradinas, F. (1994) The histological diagnosis of hydatidiform moles. *Curr. Diagn. Pathol.* **1**, 24–31.

Paradinas, F.J. (1998) The diagnosis and prognosis of molar pregnancy. The experience of the National Referral Centre in London. *Int. J. Gynaecol. Obstet.* **60**, S57–64.

Paradinas, F.J., Browne, P., Fisher, R.A., Foskett, M., Bagshawe, K.D. and Newlands, E. (1996) A clinical, histopathological and flow cytometric study of 149 complete moles, 146 partial moles and 107 non-molar hydropic abortions. *Histopathology* **28**, 101–10.

Paradinas, F.J., Fisher, R.A., Browne, P. and Newlands, E.S. (1997) Diploid hydatidiform moles with fetal red blood cells in molar villi: I. Pathology, incidence and prognosis. *J. Pathol.* **181**, 183–8.

Policastro, P.F., Daniels-McQueen, S., Carle, G. and Boime, I. (1986) A map of the hCG beta-LH beta gene cluster. *J. Biol. Chem.* **261**, 5907–16.

Pui, C.H., Ribeiro, R.C., Hancock, M.L. *et al.* (1991) Acute myeloid leukaemia in children treated with epipodophyllotoxins for acute lymphoblastic lymphoma. *N. Engl. J. Med.* **325**, 1682–7.

Rice, L.W., Berkowitz, R.S., Lage, J.M., Goldstein, D.P. and Bernstein, M.R. (1990) Persistent gestational trophoblastic tumour after partial hydatidiform mole. *Gynaecol. Oncol.* **36**, 358–62.

Rozengurt, E. (1995) Polypeptide and neuropeptide growth factors: signalling pathways and role in cancer. In Peckham, M., Pinedo, H.M. and Veronesi, U. (eds), *Oxford textbook of oncology.* Oxford: Oxford Medical Publications, 12–20.

Rustin, G.J.S., Booth, M., Dent, J., Salt, S., Rustin, F. and Bagshawe, K.D. (1984) Pregnancy after cytotoxic chemotherapy for gestational trophoblastic tumours. *BMJ* **288**, 103–6.

Rustin, G.J.S., Newlands, E.S., Begent, R.H.J., Dent, J. and Bagshawe, K.D. (1989) Weekly alternating chemotherapy (EMA/CO) for treatment of central nervous systems of choriocarcinoma. *J. Clin. Oncol.* **7**, 900–3.

Rustin, G.J.S., Newlands, E.S., Lutz, J.-M. *et al.* (1996) Combination but not single agent methotrexate chemotherapy for gestational trophoblastic tumours (GTT) increases the incidence of second tumours. *J. Clin. Oncol.* **14**, 2769–73.

Samlowski, W.E., Abbott, T.M., Kepas, D.E. and Eyre, H.J. (1985) Placental-site trophoblastic tumor (trophoblastic pseudotumor): case report demonstrating failure of chemotherapy, surgery, and radiotherapy to control metastatic disease. *Gynaecol. Oncol.* **21**, 111–17.

Savage, P., Roddie, M. and Seckl, M.J. (1998) A 28-year-old woman with a pulmonary embolus. *Lancet* **352**, 30.

Seckl, M.J. and Rozengurt, E. (1998) Neuropeptides, signal transduction and small cell lung cancer. In Martinet, Y., Hirsch, F.R., Martinet, N., Vignaud, J.-M. and Mulshine, J.L. (eds), *Clinical and biological basis of lung cancer prevention.* Basel: Birkhäuser Verlag, 129–42.

Seckl, M.J., Rustin, G.J.S., Newlands, E.S., Gwyther, S.J. and Bomanji, J. (1991) Pulmonary embolism, pulmonary hypertension, and choriocarcinoma. *Lancet* **338**, 1313–15.

Shih, I.M. and Kurman, R.J. (1998) Ki-67 labelling index in the differential diagnosis of exaggerated placental site, placental site trophoblastic tumour, and choriocarcinoma: a double staining technique using Ki-67 and Mel-CAM antibodies. *Hum. Pathol.* **29**, 27–33.

Smith, D.B., Holden, L., Newlands, E.S. and Bagshawe, K.D. (1992) Correlation between clinical staging (FIGO) and prognostic groups in gestational trophoblastic disease. *Br. J. Obstet. Gynaecol.* **100**, 157–60.

Song, H.Z. and Wu, P.C. (1988) Treatment of brain metastases in choriocarcinoma and invasive mole. In Song, H.Z. and Wu, P.C. (eds), *Studies in trophoblastic disease in China.* Oxford: Pergamon, 231–7.

Stone, M., Dent, J., Kardana, A. and Bagshawe, K.D. (1976) Relationship of oral contraceptive to development of trophoblastic tumour after evacuation of hydatidiform mole. *Br. J. Obstet. Gynaecol.* **86**, 913–16.

Szulman, A. and Surti, U. (1978a) The syndromes of hydatidiform mole. I. Cytogenetic and morphological correlations. *Am. J. Obstet. Gynaecol.* **13**, 665–71.

Szulman, A. and Surti, U. (1978b) The syndromes of hydatidiform mole. II. Morphological evidence of the complete and partial mole. *Am. J. Obstet. Gynaecol.* **132**, 20–7.

Tegoni, M., Spinelli, S., Verhoveyen, M., Davis, P. and Cambillau, C. (1999) Crystal structure of a ternary complex between human chorionic gonadotropin (hCG) and two Fv fragments specific for the alpha and beta-subunits. *J. Mol. Biol.* **289**, 1375–85.

Termrungruanglert, W., Kudelka, A.P., Piamsomboon, S. *et al.* (1996) Remission of refractory gestational trophoblastic disease with high-dose paclitaxel. *Anti-Cancer Drugs* **7**, 503–6.

Tidy, J.H., Rustin, G.J.S., Newlands, E.S. *et al.* (1995) Presentation and management of choriocarcinoma after nonmolar pregnancy. *Br. J. Obstet. Gynaecol.* **102**, 715–19.

Tsai-Morris, C.H., Buczko, E., Wang, W., Xie, X.Z. and Dufau, M.L. (1991) Structural organization of the rat lutenizing hormone (LH) receptor gene. *J. Biol. Chem.* **266**, 11355–9.

Uzumaki, H., Okabe, T., Sasaki, N. *et al.* (1989) Identification and characterization of receptors for granulocyte colony-stimulating factor on human placenta and trophoblastic cells. *Proc. Natl Acad. Sci. USA* **86**, 9323–6.

Vaitukaitis, J.L. (1979) Human chorionic gonadotrophin – a hormone secreted for many reasons. *N. Engl. J. Med.* **301**, 324–6.

van Besien, K., Verschraegen, C., Mehra, R. *et al.* (1997) Complete remission of refractory gestational trophoblastic disease with brain metastases treated with multicycle ifosfamide, carboplatin and etoposide (ICE) and stem cell rescue. *Gynecol. Oncol.* **65**, 366–9.

Vassilakos, P., Riotton, G. and Kajii, T. (1977) Hydatidiform mole: two entities. A morphologic and cytogenic study with some clinical considerations. *Am. J. Obstet. Gynaecol.* **127**, 167–70.

Wake, N., Tanaka, K.-I., Chapman, V., Matsui, S. and Sandberg, A.A. (1981) Chromosomes and cellular origin of choriocarcinoma. *Cancer Res.* **41**, 3137–43.

Walsh, C., Miller, S.J., Flam, F., Fisher, R.A. and Ohlsson, R. (1995) Paternally derived H19 is differentially expressed in malignant and non-malignant trophoblast. *Cancer Res.* **55**, 1111–16.

Whitlock, J.A., Greer, J.P. and Lukens, J.N. (1991) Epipodophyllotoxin-related leukaemia. Identification of a new subset of secondary leukaemia. *Cancer* **68**, 600–4.

WHO (1983) *Gestational trophoblastic diseases*. Technical Report series 692. Geneva: WHO, 7–81.

Wolf, H.K., Zarnegar, R., Oliver, L. and Michalopoulos, G.K. (1991) Hepatocyte growth factor in human placenta and trophoblastic disease. *Am. J. Pathol.* **138**, 1035–43.

Woolas, R.P., Bower, M., Newlands, E.S., Seckl, M.J., Short, D. and Holden, L. (1998) Influence of chemotherapy for gestational trophoblastic disease on subsequent pregnancy outcome. *Br. J. Obstet. Gynaecol.* **105**(9), 1032–5.

Yamashita, K., Ishikawa, M., Shimizu, T. and Kuroda, M. (1981) HLA antigens in husband–wife pairs with trophoblastic tumour. *Gynecol. Oncol.* **12**, 68–74.

Young, R. and Scully, R. (1984) Placental site trophoblastic tumour: current status. *Clin. Obstet. Gynaecol.* **27**, 248–58.

38

Non-melanoma skin cancer

SUNIL CHOPRA AND ANTHONY C. CHU

INTRODUCTION

Skin cancer is the commonest neoplastic condition presenting to the physician in the Caucasian population. Although each cell type in the skin is liable to give rise to a different type of neoplastic tumour, it is convenient to classify skin cancer into non-melanoma skin cancers and malignant melanoma, which will be discussed in a separate chapter.

In common with other neoplasms in the body, carcinogenesis of the skin is thought to be a multistep process. It is now generally agreed that a tumour results from the progeny of a single cell having acquired one or more somatic mutations (Knudson, 1985). The likelihood of acquiring these mutant clones depends on a complex interplay between genetic susceptibility of the individual and a wide range of environmental factors on the one hand and normal function of an intact immune system to rectify them on the other. In hereditary skin cancers such as Gorlin's syndrome and xeroderma pigmentosum, individuals are predestined to develop skin cancer because of their genetic constitutions, whereas the greatly increased incidence of skin cancer in the older population is seen as a culmination of oncogenic events and a diminished ability of the body to destroy the transformed cells with age.

The most potent environmental agent capable of inducing skin cancer is ultraviolet light (UV) exposure. The incidence of non-melanoma skin cancer increases with decline in latitude (Giles *et al.*, 1988; Scotto *et al.*, 1988), being highest in Australia with an annual incidence rate per million population of 1372 for men and 702 for women. Ozone depletion in the atmosphere allowing more harmful radiation to reach the human skin is probably partly responsible for the alarming increase in incidence. This is compounded by the popularity of sunny holidays abroad, outdoor recreational activities and the culture of the 'bronzed body beautiful'.

Melanin affords some protection against UV skin damage and explains the high incidence of skin tumours in Caucasian populations, particularly those of Celtic and Caledonian ancestry, and the low incidence in the more pigmented ethnic groups. Other environmental factors known to induce skin cancer include arsenic, ionizing radiation, human papillomavirus and polycyclic aromatic hydrocarbons.

BASAL CELL CARCINOMA (BCC)

Basal cell carcinoma (rodent ulcer or basal cell epithelioma) is a malignancy derived from the keratinocytes and stroma of the pilosebaceous follicle (Milne, 1972; Jih *et al.*, 1999; Kruger *et al.*, 1999).

Incidence

Basal cell carcinoma (BCC) is the most common human cancer affecting an estimated 750 000 Americans per year (Miller and Weinstock, 1994). The incidence of BCC has been shown to double every 10 years with the rapid rise attributed to the current fashion of 'bronze body beautiful'. Widespread use of sun beds and solariums and the popularity of sun-bathing holidays have resulted in more

BCCs and a younger population of affected patients (Wallberg and Skog, 1991). Estimates predict that 28 per cent of Caucasians born after 1994 will develop a BCC in their lifetime (Miller and Weinstock, 1994).

Aetiology

There is compelling epidemiological data implicating UV radiation exposure in BCC tumorigenesis. Sixty-six per cent of BCCs occur on the head and neck. The incidence is much greater in those with fair skin and skin type I, the tumour only very rarely occurring in African Americans (Aszterbaum et al., 1999). The incidence of BCCs in Caucasian patients increases with decline in latitude, being highest in Australia (Giles et al., 1988). However, the anatomical distribution of BCCs does not correspond well to the area of maximum exposure to UV. BCC is very common on the head and neck but unusual on other light-exposed areas such as the backs of the hands and forearms, unlike solar keratoses and squamous cell carcinomas, which occur on all light-exposed areas. The inner canthus and eyelids, which are more shielded from sunlight than other parts of the face, are frequently involved. Rare cases of vulval BCC also occur. This occurrence of BCCs in relatively sun-protected sites suggests that other cofactors may be important such as regional concentration of sebaceous glands. In one series, Noodleman and Pollack (1986) found that 7.3 per cent of 1774 cases of BCC had a previous history of trauma to the site of the BCC. BCCs may arise in congenital naevus sebaceus, skin damage by X-irradiation, burns or vaccination scars. Arsenic salts are also an important aetiological factor. Arsenic-induced tumours are usually multiple and occur mainly on the trunk (Yeh, 1973).

Advances in molecular genetics have provided a better understanding of the role of proto-oncogenes and tumour suppressor genes in skin carcinogenesis. Proto-oncogenes encode proteins involved in the series of events leading to cellular proliferation and also for growth factors, growth factor receptors and transcription factors. The mutation of a single copy of a proto-oncogene can lead to unrestricted cell growth. Tumour suppressor genes control critical points in cell growth and division. In most cases inactivation is required of both copies of a tumour suppressor gene for unrestricted cell growth to occur. Molecular studies of the basal cell naevus syndrome and BCCs have led to the identification of an important candidate tumour suppressor gene – the *Patched* gene, which is thought to be crucial in the pathogenesis of BCCs (Knudson, 1985). The *Patched* gene is the human homologue of the *Drosophila* segment polarity gene, which is also called *Patched*. *Patched* is now known to act as a tumour suppressor gene, requiring mutations in both inherited alleles in order to be inactivated (Johnson et al., 1996a). Studies on the *Patched* gene in patients with basal cell naevus syndrome and in sporadic BCC have demonstrated abnormalities in both copies of *Patched* in the vast majority of tumours. This consistent observation of *Patched* mutation in familial and sporadic BCCs has led to suggestions that inactivation of *Patched* is a necessary step in the evolution of BCC.

Study of the regulatory pathway controlled by *Patched* has led to the identification of a protein known to control growth and patterning, called Sonic Hedgehog, and demonstrated interaction with another transmembrane protein called Smoothened. Binding of Sonic Hedgehog to *Patched* disrupts the normal inhibition of Smoothened and this has been shown to result in the activation of transcription factors involved in stem cell proliferation (Riddle et al., 1993; Roelink et al., 1995). Smoothened mutations have been identified in some cases of sporadic BCC and BCC-like skin lesions have been demonstrated in transgenic mice overexpressing mutant Smoothened (Xie et al., 1998). Sporadic BCCs may result from either an acquired mutation in both copies of *Patched* or an acquired activation mutation of a single copy of the Smoothened allele (Fig. 38.1).

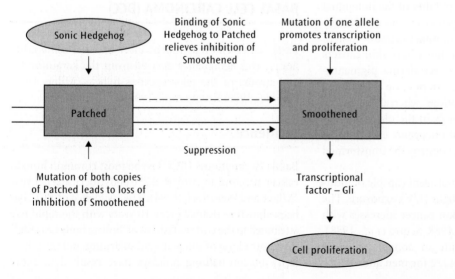

Figure 38.1 *Schematic mechanism of interaction between Sonic Hedgehog, Patched and Smoothened.*

p53 is a tumor suppressor gene. *p53* arrests cells, is G1, and thus regulates DNA repair in cells with damaged DNA. If the DNA change cannot be repaired *p53* will induce apoptosis of the cells. Up to half of all human tumours have mutations of the *p53* gene and in skin tumours, these have been shown to be UV related. Mutation of a single *p53* allele leads to the production of mutant p53 protein which will inactivate wild-type *p53*, allowing cells that have DNA damage to proliferate. One study demonstrated that phenotypically normal UV-exposed human epidermal cells show islands of keratinocytes which show mutant *p53* on immunostaining (Johason *et al.*, 1996). Such islands suggest that these cells are clonally expanded and therefore selectively outgrow those keratinocytes without mutation for *p53* (Johason *et al.*, 1996). Indeed, 30 per cent of sporadic BCCs show UV-type mutations of the *p53* gene (Johason *et al.*, 1996).

Polymorphisms in the gene for glutathione reductase, which is important in the detoxification of active oxygen species, have been linked to BCC as have polymorphisms in the cytochrome P450 genes, which are important in metabolizing environmental carcinogens (Lear *et al.*, 1997).

Organ transplant recipients on immunosuppressive therapy are prone to developing BCCs. In one Australian study, 10 per cent of patients developed BCC within 10 years of transplant. Caucasian origin, increasing age at transplantation, and time from transplant were significantly associated with occurrence of BCC. Such tumours are more aggressive than in the immune-intact patient (Ong *et al.*, 1999).

Anatomy

The majority of BCCs occur on the head and neck, especially the upper central portion of the face. It is a common tumour on the eyelid, the inner canthus of the eye and behind the ear. The palm of the hand, sole of the foot and vermilion of the lip are never involved. The morphoeic type occurs almost exclusively on the face, whilst the superficial type is more common on the trunk (MacKie, 1998). An aggressive form may occur on the occiput.

Metastasis and natural history

The course of BCCs is one of slow but steady progression, resulting in local destruction of structures if left untreated. In immunosuppressed patients, tumours may be more aggressive (Gormley and Hirsch, 1978). Metastasis is extremely rare, with an estimated risk of developing metastasis being as low as 0.1 per cent (Cotran, 1961). Metastasis develops only in long-standing lesions and spread is to regional lymph nodes or lung. Rare haematogenous spread has been reported. Death may occur by local invasion of tissues such as major blood vessels and the brain.

Clinico-pathological subtype of BCCs

The typical histology of BCC consists of clumps of darkly staining basaloid cells with characteristic palisading at the periphery. The tumours tend to infiltrate laterally rather than deeply and this, in conjunction with central ulceration, is responsible for the rolled border which is seen on examination of many BCCs. As well as keratinocyte proliferation, the stroma proliferates to a varying degree according to the clinico-pathological subtype of the BCC. The stroma appears as fine cellular connective tissue, which may show degenerative or metaplastic changes. There may also be inflammatory infiltration of the stroma by lymphocytes, histiocytes and occasionally plasma (Milne, 1972).

The six clinico-pathological subtypes of BCC are (du Vivier, 1993):

- nodular BCC
- pigmented BCC
- cystic BCC
- morphoeic (sclerosing) BCC
- superficial BCC
- linear BCC (Lewis, 1985).

NODULAR BCC

Clinical features

This tumour starts as a small papule which subsequently becomes nodular and undergoes central ulceration. The margins of the tumour are well defined, slightly raised with a rolled border and with a pearly shiny appearance. Blood vessels traversing over the margin give it a telangiectatic appearance (Fig. 38. 2). In larger lesions, ulceration may be the prominent feature but the raised, rolled border is always obvious (Plate 5).

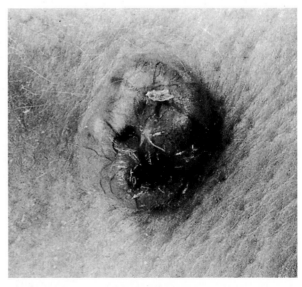

Figure 38.2 *Typical nodular basal cell carcinoma on a patient's face.*

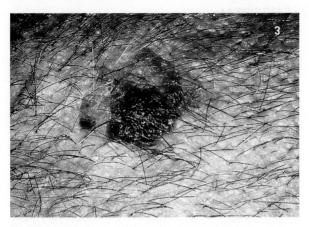

Figure 38.3 *Pigmented BCC on the chest of a 35-year-old man.*

Histopathology

This tumour is composed of discreet islands of darkly staining cells with uniform nuclei and scant cytoplasm. Typically, peripheral palisading is present. An actively proliferating connective tissue stroma is an integral part of the tumour.

PIGMENTED BCC

Clinical features

This type of BCC is clinically similar to the nodular BCC but the margins of the tumour are pigmented. Such pigmented BCCs may easily be mistaken clinically for malignant melanoma (Fig. 38.3).

Histopathology

The small cells with darkly staining uniform nuclei and scant ill-defined cytoplasm may contain granules of melanin and in such tumours large collections of melanophages may be found in the stroma.

CYSTIC BCC

Clinical features

This is a well-defined papule which attains a pearly coloured lobulated appearance with a telangiectatic surface. The central part of the tumour ulcerates later in its evolution.

Histopathology

The hallmark of this tumour is the presence of cystic foci creating a lace-like pattern of small, darkly staining cells. It is thought that the cystic spaces may be due to the cells outgrowing their nutritional supply and appearance of necrotic areas in the centre of the epithelial strands. However, some cystic spaces may be a manifestation of sweat duct differentiation. If mucinous degeneration of the stroma occurs, as well as degeneration of the basal cells themselves, this may give rise to the appearance of the adenocystic variety of BCC which appears as a large cystic space caused by necrosis of tumour cells with

a peripheral lace-like pattern caused by mucoid degeneration of the stroma.

MORPHOEIC (SCLEROSING) BCC

Clinical features

These tumours clinically appear as sclerotic, slightly depressed areas of skin with prominent telangiectasia (Plate 6). It is often difficult to determine the margins of the tumour.

Histopathology

The stromal element predominates and thin epithelial cords and strands of basal cells are seen embedded in dense, sometimes hyalinized connective tissue.

SUPERFICIAL BCC

Clinical features

This often occurs on the trunk or limbs. It is a well-defined, erythematous patch which may grow to several centimetres across. The surface is telangiectatic and may become eroded. A thread-like margin of the tumour is present, often with a pearly appearance. Most lesions are solitary and may be pigmented. Over many years, the lesion may thicken and ulcerate. Multiple surface BCCs have been associated with arsenic ingestion (Yeh, 1973).

Histopathology

There are small nests of cells along the dermal/epidermal junction with an overlying atrophic epidermis. It has been demonstrated that tumour nests form direct contact with each other in three-dimensional space.

LINEAR BCC

Clinical features

This is an uncommon variant of BCC and was first described in 1985 (Lewis, 1985). Clinically it is a linear, pearly and telangiectatic lesion and is located most often on the head and neck. On average this variant is thought to belong to a more aggressive subtype and is more likely to have subclinical spread (Lim *et al.*, 1999). Various mechanisms have been postulated to account for this morphological variant including a Koebner phenomenon or limited lateral spread of the cancer secondary to dermal fibrosis, or both (Chopra *et al.*, 1997).

Histopathlogy

Nodular masses of basal neoplastic cells are present in the dermis typical of basal cell epithelioma. In the tumour and in the stroma, deposits of melanin may be found, some of which are seen in melanophages (Chopra *et al.*, 1997).

Diagnosis

The diagnosis of BCCs is primarily a clinical diagnosis supported by a histopathological examination. If clinical doubt exists, a diagnostic biopsy is advised. There are four generally accepted methods for obtaining tissue for diagnosis. These are: shave biopsy, punch biopsy, cytology or by definitive surgery. A comparison of shave biopsy versus punch biopsy was performed retrospectively in 86 cases showing that the two techniques have equivalent diagnostic accuracy rates. Cytology provides a rapid alternative to either punch biopsy or shave biopsy and it can yield a diagnosis during the initial outpatient appointment. Barton and colleagues (1996) assessed the accuracy of cytology in eyelid lesions suspected clinically to be BCCs. The cytological and histopathological diagnoses were compared retrospectively in 20 lesions from 17 consecutive patients who underwent cytology followed by excision biopsy. The sensitivity of cytology for the diagnosis of BCC was 92 per cent. This was compared with a second group of 26 clinical BCCs from 22 consecutive patients who had an incisional biopsy and histological examination followed by excision with histological confirmation, in which the sensitivity was 100 per cent and the accuracy was 96 per cent. Cytology is sufficiently accurate to plan excision and reconstructive surgery when the diagnosis can be confirmed histologically but it is not sufficiently sensitive for conservative regimens such as radiotherapy because of the small risk of false-negative diagnosis (Barton *et al.*, 1996).

Management

A number of factors have a direct influence on the prognosis of BCC. Patients can be defined in terms of low- or high-risk categories by considering prognostic factors including tumour size, tumour site, tumour type and definition of margins, growth pattern/histological subtype, failure of previous treatment/recurrent tumours and those in immunocompromised patients (Telfer *et al.*, 1999).

Once a BCC has been diagnosed, histologically confirmed and the assessment of high-risk or low-risk tumour made, it is important to critically assess the most appropriate treatment for the patient. The obvious aim is to completely eradicate the BCC with the best possible cosmetic outcome and the least chance of tumour recurrence and the minimum of long-term side-effects. Some patients may be reluctant to consider surgery, in which case radiotherapy may be a suitable alternative.

MANAGEMENT OPTIONS

Many series have shown that treatment by curettage and cautery, surgical excision, radiotherapy, cryotherapy and Mohs' chemosurgery all have cure rates of well over 90 per cent. Tumours in certain sites have a greater risk of recurrence, namely the nasal alae, nasolabial fold, tragus and post-auricular area. This may be due to the fusion of embryonal planes at these sites allowing covert migration of tumour cells (Albright, 1982). Whilst most BCCs are treated by one of three methods – surgery, cryotherapy

or radiotherapy – a number of more novel treatment modalities are being developed.

Curettage and cautery

The tumour and 2–4 mm of adjacent normal tissue are removed by curettage under local anaesthesia and haemostasis is secured by cautery (Spiller and Spiller, 1984). The wound is left to heal by secondary intention. Topical antibiotics may reduce infection of the open wound. The main indication for this treatment is for selective low-risk lesions (small, well-defined primary lesions with non-aggressive histology in non-critical sites) where 5-year cure rates of up to 97 per cent are possible (Telfer *et al.*, 1999). However, a study using Mohs' technique (Edens *et al.*, 1983) found that residual tumour was left in at least 30 per cent of cases following curettage, which is far higher than the actual recurrence rate. It is possible that debulking of the tumour allows the immune response to clear the residual tumour (Nouri *et al.*, 1999).

Cryotherapy

Liquid nitrogen is used to produce tissue destruction by reducing the temperature to tumoricidal levels. A fine, intermittent spray is preferred as a continuous one produces a rapid lateral extension of the ice front rather than penetration to the bottom of the tumour. A safe margin of 3–5 mm is first drawn around the tumour, as its edges are difficult to see once frozen. Several methods are available to monitor that a temperature adequate for cryonecrosis, in the region of −50°C is achieved. In one method a thermocouple needle is inserted using a template until it is just below the tumour about 3–4 mm below the surface. Le Pivert (1997) designed an instrument to measure electrical impedance between electrodes inserted around the tumour and found that readings between 500 000 and 10 000 000 ohms indicated adequate freezing. There is a known interrelationship between the depth of freeze and the width of the freeze beyond the side margins of the tumour, the time of thawing from the freeze margin to the tumour margin and the time it takes for the whole tumour area to thaw. It is recommended a margin thaw time of at least 120 seconds be used (Albright, 1982).

Satisfactory results may be obtained by spraying the centre of the lesion until the ice front is maintained for 3–4 mm beyond the visible edge of the lesion for 30 seconds. After the tumour is frozen, it is allowed to thaw and then the freeze cycle is repeated at least once (McLean *et al.*, 1978).

Cryotherapy is suitable for BCCs with clinically well-defined borders, non-aggressive histology and exclusion of those tumours that are in critical facial sites (Telfer *et al.*, 1999). With well-selected cases, cure rates of up to 99 per cent can be achieved (Kuflik and Gage, 1991). Cryotherapy is particularly useful for the inner canthus of the eye where, unlike radiotherapy or surgical excision, the lacrimal apparatus is spared. Cryotherapy around the eye requires an appropriate shield of the eyeball, and the eardrum should be protected using dry cotton wool when the ear is being treated. Cryotherapy is not suitable for lesions bordering on the lip or eyelid as scarring leads to a contraction deformity at these sites. Use of cryotherapy is contraindicated in thick lesions as the borders of these are poorly defined and may be inadequately treated. It is also absolutely contraindicated in patients with abnormal cold tolerance, e.g. cryoglobulinaemia. After treatment there is often considerable oedema followed by a serous discharge, which may last 2–3 weeks. The site should be kept clean until the eschar separates.

Hyperpigmentation occurs at the site of freezing and is more obvious the darker the skin of the patient. Scarring tends to be minimal and this technique has rarely been associated with nerve damage.

Cryotherapy has many advantages as it is quick to perform, requires no hospitalization and most patients require less than two outpatient treatment sessions. Some studies have suggested that it is the most cost-effective method and, indeed, even gave the best cosmetic result (Fraunfelder *et al.*, 1984).

Curettage and cryotherapy

Excellent results have been obtained by careful curettage of the BCC followed by cryotherapy in a double freeze–thaw cycle. Nordin *et al.* (1997) followed up 50 patients with morphoeic type BCCs, which were 10 mm or larger in diameter, and were sited either on the nose or perinasally, treated by curettage and cryotherapy. The cosmetic result was found to be good and acceptable in all patients with only one recurrent BCC. Indeed, the authors suggested that this may be a cheap and cosmetically acceptable alternative to Mohs' micrographic surgery.

Radiotherapy

Ionizing radiations, since their discovery in 1895, have played an important role in the treatment of skin disorders, none more so than the BCC. Radiotherapy of skin cancer yields excellent results and the cure rates for primary BCC are above 90 per cent (Caccialanza *et al.*, 1999).

Critical organs near irradiation fields are protected by lead/rubber shields. To minimize the potential of additive effect of sun exposure in later years, patients under 45 years of age are not usually treated with radiotherapy when other alternatives are available (Goldschmidt and Sherwin, 1983a, b).

Radiotherapy allows greater preservation of normal tissue than surgical excision and so is useful for areas where tissue cannot be readily sacrificed because of cosmetic or functional importance. It is therefore particularly useful for tumours of the eyelids and canthi of the eyes, the nose, ears and lips. Large lesions on the cheek often respond with minimum scarring but radiation sequelae, particularly telangiectasia, pigment changes and ulceration, can cause problems on the limbs and trunk so radiotherapy is less popular for tumours on these sites. Radiotherapy is not suitable for tumours extending to underlying bone or cartilage.

Table 38.1 *Radiotherapy schemes for skin tumours*

Dose (cGy)	Time (weeks)	Fractions
2000	0	1
2700	2	3
4500	2	10
5000	3	15
5000	5	15
6000	6	30

In practice, the energy of the radiation beam is selected so that the dose to the base of the lesion is half that to the surface. This can be accurately determined from measurements of the half-value layer (thickness of the material, which reduces the intensity of the X-ray beam to 50 per cent). If skin is directly over bone or cartilage, the radiation is reduced as these structures have increased absorption in the orthovoltage range.

High-energy electron-beam therapy has certain advantages over conventional radiotherapy in treating large thick, or deeply infiltrating skin cancers. Electron-beam therapy delivers a high dose of radiation to superficial skin lesions with a rapid falloff in depth, so causing minimal damage to underlying normal structures such as bone or cartilage. Good results have been obtained for BCCs difficult to treat by other methods (Miller and Spittle, 1982).

A margin of at least 5 mm of clinically normal skin is included in the field of radiation. The target to skin distance should be at least twice as large as the diameter of the field to achieve uniform radiation over the area to be treated, and a cone is used to reduce scattered radiation. Fractionated dose schedules are preferred to a single large dose as these have been found to give rise to better cure rates and better cosmetic results since tumour tissue recovers more slowly than normal tissue (Reisner and Haase, 1990).

Table 38.1 provides a variety of dose schedules currently in use. The schedule chosen for a particular patient will depend on the site and size of the tumour, its relationship to other structures such as the eye, ear and nose, the age of the patient and the ease in getting the patient to the radiotherapy centre. Erythema usually develops in the first week of treatment followed by an exudative reaction (Fig. 38.4). Healing is completed about 3 weeks after the first dose. Comedones may appear several weeks after treatment, but usually resolve spontaneously. Long-term side-effects include atrophy, hyper- and hypopigmentation, telangiectasia and alopecia (Plate 7). Non-healing skin ulceration, persistent pain and secondary skin cancers are the more severe side-effects that may result from radiology. The cosmetic acceptability of radiology is high at 84 per cent, with cosmetic acceptability being higher for smaller fields irradiated. The incidence of acute complications is normally low at 2 per cent and that of chronic complications is even lower at 0.3 per cent (Caccialanza *et al.*, 1999).

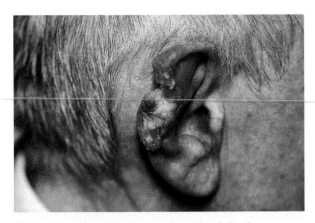

Figure 38.4 *Post-radiotherapy ulceration following treatment of a BCC of the pinna.*

Surgical excision of BCC

Surgical treatment of primary BCCs is highly effective. The major advantage of such an excision is that the excised tissue can be examined histologically and the surgical margins can also be assessed. In general, the cosmetic results are excellent but the major problem confronting the surgeon is defining the margins of the BCC prior to excision. The definition of such a margin is made more difficult as 15 per cent of BCCs show subclinical spread beyond 3 mm and 5 per cent show subclinical spread beyond 4 mm. Morphoeic BCCs are even more difficult to define with 18 per cent showing subclinical spread beyond 5 mm and 5 per cent showing subclinical spread beyond 13 mm (Breuninger *et al.*, 1991).

The excision of BCCs needs to take into account possible subclinical spread as well as the limitations of the tumour size and tumour site. Although histologically a BCC may not be completely excised, its actual clinical recurrence is much lower than would be expected. Therefore, it is a matter of controversy as to whether an incompletely excised BCC needs to be re-excised. A large study of re-excisions after incomplete excision of BCCs has revealed that in most cases re-excision will reveal residual tumour (Griffiths, 1999) and recurrence is most likely when both lateral and deep margins are involved. Therefore, if only a lateral margin is involved in a BCC that has a non-aggressive histology and is away from a critical site, it is reasonable to take a conservative approach (Telfer *et al.*, 1999). However, if the BCC involves a deep margin at a critical site then re-excision would be advised.

Mohs' micrographic surgery

In this technique, the tumour is debulked with a scalpel or curette with the scalpel angled at 45 degrees to the skin. A saucer of tissue is then removed. Anatomical orientation is carefully maintained by scoring the remaining skin edge and surface of the tissue removed. The tissue is divided along the scored lines, inverted and the edges marked with coloured stains. The tissue is embedded and horizontal frozen sections cut and stained so that the whole of the undersurface of the removed tissue is examined for residual tumour. The surgeon then returns to the patient and removes tissue only in areas where tumour is microscopically persistent. This process is repeated until the tumour is totally removed. This technique means that the normal surrounding tissue can be preserved while the whole of the tumour is removed. The defect can be left to heal by secondary intention or reconstruction can commence immediately (Mohs, 1991).

Mohs' micrographic surgery is regarded as a gold standard treatment for BCC and can give cure rates of 99 per cent in primary and 96–98 per cent in recurrent BCCs (Cottell and Proper, 1982). It is, however, very expensive in both time and support facilities compared with conventional methods of treatment. Therefore, the main indications for Mohs' micrographic surgery are for those BCCs in critical sites such as the eyes, ears, lips, nose and nasolabial folds, morphoeic or infiltrated histological subtype and patients with recurrent BCC especially after radiotherapy. It may also be used in tumours that are large and in high-risk sites (Smith and Grande, 1991; Telfer *et al.*, 1999).

Laser treatment

High-energy pulsed carbon dioxide (CO_2) lasers have been used extensively to resurface wrinkled and photo-damaged skin with a low risk of scarring. Results of histological studies demonstrate precise ablation depths in treated skin with minimal thermal damage to underlying tissue. The ultrapulse CO_2 laser with high energy and short pulses achieves char-free ablation of the tumours, bloodless surgical field, minimal non-specific thermal damage, rapid healing and diminished postoperative pain. Also, a number of lesions can be removed in a single session. Pulsed CO_2 laser treatment can be effective in ablating superficial BCC with one study showing complete histological clearance in nine of nine BCCs. CO_2 laser surgery has also been successfully combined with a micrographic approach similar to Mohs' micrographic surgery in order to increase its cure rate in a patient with a large BCC but as yet there have been no trials comparing this modality with the established ones (Humphreys *et al.*, 1998; Krunic *et al.*, 1998). Since scarring is minimized with this technique, it has been particularly advocated in eyelid BCCs. One study reported only one recurrence in a 72-month follow-up in 27 superficial primary eyelid BCCs (Bandieramonte *et al.*, 1997).

Photodynamic therapy

In a prospective clinical trial of photodynamic therapy in primary non-melanomatous skin tumours of the head and neck (BCC, squamous cell cancer), temoporfin (mTHPC), a second-generation systemic photosensitizer, was used intravenously 96 hours prior to argon-dye laser treatment. Within several days tumour necrosis appeared followed by wound healing within 4–8 weeks, leaving only minor scars. A complete response with an excellent cosmetic outcome was shown in 92.7 per cent and in only seven tumours was response partial due to low light dosage. The cosmetic outcome was very good and the therapy was supported by a high degree of patient satisfaction (Kubler *et al.*, 1999). The second generation of photosensitizers tend to reduce the risk of persistent generalized cutaneous photosensitivity. The advantages of photodynamic therapy for cutaneous malignancies include the ability to treat numerous lesions at the same time, in a non-invasive manner (Allison *et al.*, 1998).

Drug treatment

Topical 5-fluorouracil (5-FU) Topical 5-fluorouracil (5-FU) has been used for treatment of BCCs. Concentrations of up to 20 per cent can produce cure rates of up to 95 per cent in the superficial type of BCCs. The common type of nodular tumour is, however, too deep for 5-FU to penetrate adequately and results in these tumours are poor. It may, however, be used to palliate tumours where a patient may be too debilitated for other treatments.

In trials to improve and standardize topical fluorouracil therapy, thin BCCs have been treated with 25 per cent fluorouracil in petrolatum under occlusion for 3 weeks using weekly dressing changes. Of 44 thin BCCs treated, the 5-year cumulative recurrence rate was 21 per cent. In a second series of 244 BCCs, light curettage preceded the 25 per cent fluorouracil treatment to yield a 5-year cumulative recurrence rate of 6 per cent. Cosmetic results were good to excellent in more than 80 per cent in both series.

Isotretinoin Isotretinoin has been used in the treatment of BCCs but the results have been very disappointing (Craven and Griffiths, 1996). Although isotretinoin has been shown to be effective in chemoprevention in those patients at high risk of recurrent BCCs, most of such advantage is lost after the isotretinoin is stopped. A large number of patients withdraw from therapy due to the side-effects such as mucocutaneous irritation, arthralgia and myalgia. Therefore, isotretinoin is not used routinely either in the treatment or in the chemoprophylaxis of BCCs.

Interferon-2α and 2β Interferon-2α and 2β have been used in the treatment of BCCs but prospective studies show complete response rates as low as 66 per cent (Alpsoy *et al.*, 1996). The incidence of the side-effects of fever and malaise are also very common (Wickramasinghe *et al.*, 1989).

Imiquimod Since BCC responds, albeit partially, to interferon therapy, imiquimod, a cytokine and interferon inducer, has been used topically in a randomized, double-blind trial in the treatment of 35 patients with BCC. BCC cleared (on the basis of histological examination) in all patients dosed twice daily, once daily, and three times weekly. Adverse events are predominantly local reactions at the target tumour site, with the incidence and severity of local skin reactions being low in groups dosed less frequently (Beutner *et al.*, 1999).

Follow-up

The main aims of follow-up are detection of tumour recurrence and early detection and treatment of new lesions. Thirty-six per cent of the patients who have had a previous BCC will go on to develop a further BCC. Those especially at risk of BCCs are those with very fair skin and excess sun exposure. These patients go on to develop multiple BCCs and such multiple BCCs are found in as high as 20 per cent of such high-risk patients (Robinson, 1987).

Most BCCs that will recur will recur within 3 years. It is a matter of the resources available in an outpatient dermatology department or in general practice as to how frequent or for how long the follow-up surveillance should be. Obviously patients with multiple BCCs and at high risk of developing further BCCs should be followed-up at least 6-monthly for the patients' remaining lifetime. However, it may not be economically justifiable to follow-up every BCC, especially if it is a single isolated BCC in the older age group. One major advantage of regular follow-up is continued patient education as regards to sun avoidance.

NAEVOID BASAL CELL CARCINOMA SYNDROME (GORLIN'S SYNDROME)

Naevoid basal cell carcinoma syndrome (NBCCS) or Gorlin syndrome is an autosomal dominant disorder. Most cases show clear linkage to chromosome 9q22 (Wicking *et al.*, 1997). It is characterized by BCCs and multiple developmental defects (Levanat *et al.*, 2000).

Incidence

This is a rare genodermatosis. The sexes are equally affected. Most patients are Caucasian, but cases have been reported in Afro-Caribbeans and Asians (Cohen, 1999).

Aetiology

The syndrome is caused by mutations in *Patched*, a tumour suppressor gene. A single point mutation in one *Patched* allele may be responsible for the malformations found in the syndrome. Inactivation of both *Patched* alleles results in the formation of tumours and cysts (Cohen, 1999). However, there is, at the moment, poor correlation between identifiable genetic mutations and the resulting clinical phenotype, suggesting phenotypic variability in NBCCS is a complex genetic event (Wicking *et al.*, 1997).

Pathology

The skin lesions are indistinguishable from BCC but a broader spectrum of histological subtypes is found in tumours from patients with the syndrome. Multiple, keratinizing odontogenic and epidermal cysts are often seen in the NBCCS and such multiple keratinizing cysts within BCCs have been recorded (Lindeberg and Jepsen, 1983).

Clinical features (Kimonis *et al.*, 1997)

SKIN TUMOUR

Eighty per cent of Caucasians have at least one BCC, with the first tumour occurring at a mean age of 23 years. The number of BCCs can range from one to more than 1000 (Plate 8).

JAW CYSTS

These are odontogenic keratocysts (OKCs) and occur in 74 per cent of patients with the first cysts occurring in 80 per cent by the age of 20 years. The number of total jaw cysts can range from 1 to 28. Most sporadically occurring OKCs behave in a benign manner; however, those associated with NBCCS are clinically more aggressive in their behaviour (Lo Muzio *et al.*, 1999b). OKCs are often the first signs of NBCCS and can occasionally be detected in patients younger than 10 years of age. It is suggested that early onset of an OKC should prompt investigation for NBCCS (Lo Muzio *et al.*, 1999a). Cutaneous cysts may be found with an identical histology to those found in the jaw (Barr *et al.*, 1986).

PALMAR PITS AND PLANTAR PITS

These are seen in 87 per cent of patients and have vertical sides, are up to several millimetres in diameter and have an erythematous base. They are said to result from impaired maturation of the basal cells resulting in defective keratin, which is shed.

CENTRAL NERVOUS SYSTEM

Patients with NBCCS have a predisposition for the development of medulloblastoma and primitive neuroectodermal tumours of the central nervous system (Wolter *et al.*, 1997).

CARDIAC TUMOURS

There now appears to be an established association between cardiac tumours and NBCCS and evaluation of cardiac status is recommended in all patients with NBCCS (Barr *et al.*, 1986).

PHYSICAL FINDINGS

Patients with NBCCS may exhibit coarse facies, cleft lip or palate, relative macrocephaly, hypertelorism, frontal bossing, pectus deformity or Sprengel deformity.

RADIOLOGICAL SIGNS

Calcification may be observed in various sites including the falx cerebri and tentorium cerebelli. Other abnormalities include bridged sella, hemivertebrae, fusion of the vertebral bodies, and flame-shaped lucencies of the phalanges, metacarpal and carpal bones of the hands (Kimonis *et al.*, 1997).

LABORATORY ABNORMALITIES

There are no routine abnormalities apart from a possible raised alkaline phosphatase. It is postulated that elevated serum alkaline phosphatase in patients with NBCCS is correlated to the presence of growing odontogenic keratocysts (Lindeberg *et al.*, 1982).

Treatment

The first aim of treatment is to educate patients and parents as to the importance of avoiding known carcinogenic factors with sun avoidance being of paramount importance. The BCCs may be more aggressive than their sporadic counterparts and are best treated early. Radiotherapy is best avoided as this may lead to the development of further more aggressive BCCs (Golitz *et al.*, 1980) and may also accelerate the appearance of primitive neuroectodermal tumours of the central nervous system (O'Malley *et al.*, 1997). Retinoids have a therapeutic effect on existing BCCs and a prophylactic effect in inhibiting new tumour formation. However, to be of any major benefit, retinoids have to be maintained long term (Craven and Griffiths, 1996), and in view of the need to start such therapy at an early age, the patient would be subject to long-term rheumatological complications such as diffuse idiopathic skeletal hyperostosis (DISH) and pseudo-coxarthritis (Theiler *et al.*, 1993).

Success has been reported with a combination of topical 5-FU and topical tretinoin, which may prevent the development of new tumours, inhibit the growth of existing tumours and cause the regression of superficially invasive BCCs (Strange and Langm, 1992).

SQUAMOUS CELL CARCINOMA (SCC)

SCC is also known as epidermoid, spindle cell or prickle cell carcinoma. It is a malignant tumour that arises from epithelial keratinocytes whose cells usually show some degree of maturation toward keratin formation.

Incidence

There are approximately 200 000 new cutaneous SCCs each year in the USA and between 1300 and 2300 people die each year as a result of non-melanoma skin cancer, mostly metastatic SCC (Salasche, 2000).

The common pre-SCC lesion is the actinic keratoses. It is estimated that 11.5 per cent of all visits to a dermatologist in the USA are for actinic keratoses (Feldman *et al.*, 1998).

The incidence of actinic keratoses and SCCs are dependent on cumulative sun exposure and the individual's sun sensitivity. Both are more common in fair-skinned persons with light coloured eyes and fair hair.

Although actinic keratoses and SCCs are more prevalent in male subjects and tend to occur earlier in male subjects, with age, rates become more equal between the sexes (Holman *et al.*, 1984).

Aetiology

Ultraviolet (UV) light is the most important aetiological agent in SCC and the incidence rate directly correlates with the amount of UV light exposure that the individual has been subjected to. Most SCCs occur in sun-exposed areas of the skin. In conditions where the skin is more sensitive to UV damage, i.e. albinism, or where the skin is unable to repair UV-induced damage to DNA such as in xeroderma pigmentosum, there is an increased incidence of non-melanoma skin cancer.

The UV-induced premalignant lesion is the actinic keratosis (Mittelbronn *et al.*, 1998) and those induced by tar or pitch are called pitch warts. The malignant potential of actinic keratoses is probably quite low but given time, many will transform into SCC (Montgomery and Dorffel, 1932). Bowen's disease or SCC *in situ* of the skin may progress to invasive SCC if left untreated. Bowen's disease may occur anywhere on the skin or mucous membranes and is erythematous, slightly raised and scaly with a sharp margin (Fig. 38.5). When SCC *in situ* is found on the penis, the term erythroplasia of Queyrat is used. Known aetiological agents that induce Bowen's disease include UV light and chronic arsenic ingestion. In lesions due to arsenic exposure, associated pigmentation or punctate palmoplantar keratoses may be present. It is estimated that about 5 per cent of Bowen's disease become invasive SCCs; these tumours tend to be aggressive and about 30 per cent metastasize.

Most actinic keratoses and SCCs will contain mutations of the *p53* tumour suppressor gene and these mutations are usually UV induced. *p53* is a negative cancer regulator and normally acts to prevent cells from proliferating uncontrollably. *p53* also is responsible for apoptosis of keratinocytes that are genetically defective. Thus, *p53* is responsible for ensuring that cells with abnormal DNA do not replicate (Ziegler *et al.*, 1994).

Human papillomaviruses (particularly types 16 and 18) have been identified in SCC cells by *in situ* hybridization and polymerase chain reaction, commonly in lesions affecting the genitals, oral and periungual areas. Human papillomavirus has been advocated as a possible aetiological factor in some cases of SCC in patients who were immunosuppressed due to cardiac or renal transplantation (Pieceall *et al.*, 1991; Shamanin *et al.*, 1996). However, no such role for the human papillomavirus has been found in those patients infected with the HIV virus (Maurer *et al.*, 1997).

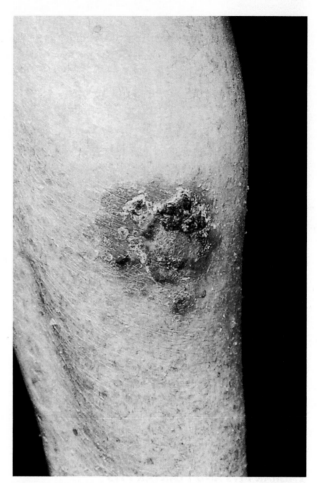

Figure 38.5 *Bowen's disease on the lower leg of a patient with a history of arsenic ingestion.*

A naturally occurring model for the association of human papillomavirus and SCC is seen in epidermodysplasia verruciformis. In this autosomal recessive condition, patients develop widespread and extensive warty lesions identical to those of the common wart and these patients ultimately develop intra-epithelial neoplasia and SCC following UV exposure. Human papillomavirus types 3, 5, 8–10, 12, 14, 15, 17, 19–25, 28, 29, 36–38, 47, 49 and 50 have been identified in lesions from patients with epidermodysplasia verruciformis. Types 5 and 8 are most commonly associated with malignancy but types 14, 17, 20 and 47 are occasionally involved (Ostrow *et al.*, 1987; Pfister, 1987; Yutsudo *et al.*, 1994).

Patients on long-term immunosuppressive therapy regimens for kidney and heart transplants have an increased risk of developing cutaneous SCCs, malignant melanoma and Kaposi's sarcoma. The risk of post-transplant cutaneous SCC is related to the degree of immunosuppression caused by long-term immuno-suppressive therapy (Jensen *et al.*, 1999).

Such tumours occurring in immunosuppressed patients are invariably more aggressive, invading locally as well as metastasizing earlier than in the non-immunosuppressed.

Metastases and natural history

Invasive SCC may grow slowly or rapidly and may metastasize, usually to the regional lymph nodes. In a review of 695 cases of cutaneous SCC of the trunk and limbs, metastases occurred in 34 cases, with a metastatic rate of 5 per cent, an overall mortality of 3 per cent, and a mortality in the metastatic group of 70 per cent (Joseph *et al.*, 1992). Local recurrence and regional metastasis is dependent on treatment used, prior treatment of the lesion, location, size, depth, histological differentiation, histological evidence of perineural involvement and host immunosuppression (Rowe *et al.*, 1992). Lesions found on the ears and lip are known to be at higher risk of local recurrence and metastasis. SCCs presenting on the lip have an especially high local and metastatic rate (Antoniades *et al.*, 1995) with 8 per cent of patients presenting with clinically positive lymph-node involvement and an overall 5-year mortality rate of 17 per cent (Breuninger *et al.*, 1991).

SCC arising from scar tissue is rare but has a higher rate of recurrence than SCC arising in UV-damaged skin. At least 25 per cent of such tumours may recur in 30 months. Female sex, large tumour size, and histological tumour grade are associated with recurrent disease. Therefore careful follow-up after treatment is recommended, especially for female patients, those with large tumours and those with high-grade tumours (Eroglu and Camlibe, 1997).

Pathology

The diagnosis of actinic keratosis is usually a clinical one. However, biopsy may be required to exclude an invasive component, especially if the lesion is symptomatic or becomes indurated. Pathological variants including hypertrophic, atrophic, acantholytic, Bowenoid and pigmented types have been described. The characteristics of all these pathological subtypes are atypical keratinocyte proliferation within the epidermis. Initially, dysplastic changes are confined to small foci in the epidermis in which there are aggregates of atypical pleomorphic keratinocytes at the basal layer. The epidermis shows an abnormal architecture and there may be irregular acanthosis and a digitate surface. The dermoepidermal junction is irregular and small round buds protrude into the upper papillary dermis from the basal layer. There may be hyperkeratosis and parakertosis with the areas of parakeratosis overlying the dysplastic keratinocytes in the epidermis. Since actinic keratoses and squamous cell carcinomas are almost always associated with solar elastosis in the dermis, if such a feature is not found one must seriously reconsider the diagnosis. The atypical keratinocytes themselves show loss of polarity, nuclear pleomorphism, disordered maturation and increased numbers of mitotic figures.

Invasive SCC consists of irregular masses, composed of a mixture of anaplastic and differentiated squamous cells, growing downwards into the dermis from the epidermis. In early tumours there may be an associated lymphocytic infiltrate. Special histological variants include the adenoid type (or acantholytic variant), which occurs mainly on the head in the elderly, the verrucous type, which occurs mainly in the oral mucosa, penis or sole of the foot and spindle cell type. Certain benign skin tumours such as keratoacanthomas may mimic the appearance of SCC; indeed, some authorities consider the keratoacanthoma as an immunologically controlled SCC.

The terms actinic keratoses and Bowen's disease reflect the same oncological process but to different degrees and it has been proposed that the term keratinocyte, intraepidermal neoplasia be adopted for such lesions (Yansos *et al.*, 1999; Cockerell, 2000). This would mean that Bowen's disease would be defined as keratinocyte, intraepithelial neoplasia grade III (Brodland and Zitelli, 1992) (Table 38.2).

Table 38.2 *Grading of keratinocyte intra-epithelial neoplasia*

Grade	Clinical appearance	Histology
1	Flat, pink macule or patch on solar damaged skin, no roughness	Focal atypia of basal keratinocytes of lower one-third of epidermis
2	Pink to red papule or plaque with rough surface and variable induration	Focal atypia of basal keratinocytes of lower two-thirds of the epidermis, focal hyperkeratosis, alternating hyperkeratosis and parakeratosis with sparing of adnexal structures apart from involvement of the upper epidermal adnexal structures, prominent acanthosis with buds of keratinocytes into the upper papillary dermis
3 (Bowen's disease)	Red, indurated plaques on sun-damaged skin. Scaling of the surface with variable pigmentation	Diffuse atypical keratinocyte proliferation involving the full thickness of the epidermis, parakeratosis, acanthosis, papillomatosis, involvement of adnexal structures

Diagnosis

The most common clinical presentation of an actinic kera-tosis is a red, scaling papule or plaque on a sun-exposed area. It may appear as discreet papule but may progress to become a nodule. The surrounding skin shows evidence of chronic solar irradiation with telangiectasia, yellowish discoloration and non-uniform pigmentation (Plate 9). The scaliness is best assessed by touch. The scale is adher-ent and attempts to remove it will lead to bleeding.

The first sign of change from intra-epithelial neopla-sia to SCC is induration followed by the development of a papular lesion with a keratotic surface which may break down to an ulcer with ill-defined margin (Fig. 38.6). The diagnosis is confirmed by biopsy or surgical excision of the lesion.

Treatment

KERATINOCYTE INTRA-EPIDERMAL NEOPLASM (ACTINIC KERATOSIS AND BOWEN'S DISEASE)

There are many treatments that are highly effective for actinic keratoses and Bowen's disease, with cryosurgery being the most common treatment in the UK. For a description of how to use cryotherapy see above. Curettage and cautery may be used, particularly in those lesions which are hypertrophic or where the diagnosis is in doubt. However, this method has no advantage over cryosurgery and requires the use of local anaesthetic. Topical 5-FU is a very convenient and cosmetically acceptable treatment of actinic keratoses and Bowen's disease. The most com-mon regimen is one of applying the cream daily to the affected region for 4 weeks. The patient should be warned that the skin will become inflamed as the dysplastic lesions are destroyed and they will experience pain, pruritus and burning at the site of application. With repeated use, some patients may develop an allergic dermatitis in response to the vehicle of the cream (Dinehart, 2000).

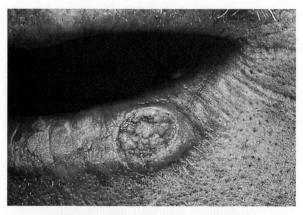

Figure 38.6 *Squamous cell carcinoma on the lower lip of a patient.*

SCC

The methods of treatment of SCC are similar to those described for BCC. However, SCC has a much greater metastatic potential and therefore it is important to ensure that all of the tumour is removed and if this is not the case that further therapy is instituted to eradicate the tumour. High-risk tumours, especially those on the lips and ears, are treated more aggressively as the risk of local recurrence and distant metastases are higher. Like BCCs, the treatments are highly effective and can achieve cure rates of 95 per cent.

Surgical excision

Margins of 4 mm are adequate for most SCCs. However, certain tumour characteristics are associated with a greater risk of subclinical tumour extension and include size of 2 cm or larger, aggressive histology – especially invasion of the subcutaneous tissue and perineural spread, and location in high-risk areas. In such cases, at least a 6-mm margin is recommended (Brodland and Zitelli, 1992; Lawrence and Cottel, 1994). SCCs with a diameter of more than 2 cm have a much higher risk of local recur-rence and an excision margin of 10 mm has been recom-mended for these tumours (Breuninger et al., 1991).

Mohs' micrographic surgery

Mohs' micrographic surgery offers the best chance of cure of high-risk tumours (Rowe et al., 1992). However, most surgeons are able to estimate the margin of most tumours clinically and 90 per cent of SCCs are excised during the first excision phase of the Mohs' procedure. Those lesions that are not removed completely with the initial excision tend to be those located on the periorbital region, forehead and cheeks (Ghauri et al., 1999).

Curettage and cautery

This technique is likely to result in inadequate clearance and it should not be regarded as an adequate form of treatment for SCC.

Cryotherapy

Kuflik and Gage (1991) claim a 5-year tumour-free rate of 96 per cent in a group of 52 SCCs using cryotherapy alone. Obviously such treatment would not be recom-mended for high-risk tumours but would have obvious advantages for low-risk tumours as it can be performed in outpatients without a local anaesthetic. Indeed, in elderly patients this modality may be ideal.

Radiotherapy

In the treatment of SCC, radiotherapy is generally reserved for patients over 45 years old because of theoretical risk of inducing further malignancies. It is not suitable for tumours invading underlying cartilage where radiother-apy may produce radiochondritis, and poorly differenti-ated tumours are treated by excision where possible. There is a relative contraindication to treating SCCs in cardiac or renal transplant patients as these patients may be particularly susceptible to further cutaneous malignancies.

The 5-year cure rate for treating non-melanoma skin cancer with radiotherapy is as high as 90 per cent and the cosmetic results have been evaluated as good or acceptable in 84 per cent of treated lesions. The acute complication rate is low and the chronic complication rate is even lower (Caccialanza et al., 1999).

Treatment schedules are similar to those of BCC with fractionated dose schedules. Electron-beam therapy is very good for lesions in sites difficult to treat by more conventional methods (Miller and Spittle, 1982).

Chemotherapy

For patients with extensive SCC which has relapsed after conventional surgery or radiotherapy or for metastatic disease, a variety of drugs including bleomycin, methotrexate, actinomycin, vincristine, vinblastine, 5-FU and hydroxyurea have been used with varying degrees of success (Stephens and Harker, 1979). Cisplatin has been used as monotherapy and in combination with other cytotoxic drugs in advanced lesions and metastatic cutaneous SCC. Eleven patients with advanced BCC or SCC of the skin were treated with cisplatin (75 mg/m^2, i.v.) + doxyrubicin (50 mg/m^2, i.v.) at 3-week intervals. Responses were seen after 10–12 courses and five of the 11 patients were in remission at the time of report (Stephens and Harker, 1979). A combination of cisplatin, 5-FU and bleomycin produced partial or complete remission in 11 of 14 patients with advanced cutaneous SCC (Sadek et al., 1990).

Follow-up

Patients with a previous history of SCC of skin are more likely to develop similar lesions. In a follow-up study of 101 patients with SCC, 52 per cent developed subsequently non-melanoma skin cancers within 5 years of therapy for the first lesion (Frankel et al., 1992). It is recommended that patients should be followed up every 3 months for the first year and every 6 months thereafter, for a minimum of 5 years after initial treatment. Patients should be examined for local recurrence, metastatic spread and new lesions. Recurrent lesions are treated where possible with cryotherapy or excision surgery and Mohs' surgery is particularly suitable to ensure complete clearance of recurrent tumour. Patients with recurrent lesions should be followed up indefinitely. All patients should be taught to self-examine regularly for local and regional recurrence.

XERODERMA PIGMENTOSUM

Incidence

Xeroderma pigmentosum is found worldwide, in all races with an equal sex incidence. The incidence is said to be higher in Japan and Libya. Interestingly, the spectrum of disease manifestations in different countries is quite varied (Jacyk, 1999; Khatri et al., 1999). The incidence in Europe and American are 1 : 250 000, 1 : 40 000 in Japan and 15–20 per million in Libya (Khatri et al., 1999).

Aetiology

Xeroderma pigmentosum is a group of autosomal recessive disorders the genetic loci of which all have recently been elucidated. The manifestations of xeroderma pigmentosum occur as a result of a defect in excision repair of UV-induced pyrimidine dimers from their DNA (Clever, 1968; Reed et al., 1969).

Nucleotide excision repair (NER) is one of the most studied DNA repair systems. The consequences of a defect in one of the NER proteins are manifested in three rare, recessive photosensitive syndromes: xeroderma pigmentosum, Cockayne's syndrome and a photosensitive form of brittle-hair disorder, trichodystrophy (TTD).

NUCLEOTIDE EXCISION REPAIR (NER)

NER is the most flexible of all DNA repair mechanisms because of its ability to eliminate a plethora of structurally unrelated DNA lesions. NER-deficient cells are sensitive to insults which cause a significant DNA helical distortion. The clinically most relevant NER substrates are *cis-syn*-cyclobutane dimers (CPDs) and pyrimidine(6–4)pyrimidone photoproducts. Both are formed between adjacent pyrimidines and they constitute the two major classes of DNA lesions induced by solar UV light. NER process involves the action of around 30 proteins, which enable damage recognition, local opening of DNA double helix around the injury and incision of the damaged strand on either side of the lesion. After excision of damage containing oligonucleotide the resulting gap is closed by DNA repair synthesis, followed by strand ligation (De Boer and Hoeijmakers, 2000).

Using the unscheduled DNA synthesis (UDS) assay, eight complementation groups of xeroderma pigmentosum have been identified: groups A, B, C, D, E, F, G and V (Lambert et al., 1999). The UDS measures DNA synthesis during G_1- and G_2-phase, which is negative unless nucleotide excision or base excision repair is taking place. The test is performed on normal and xeroderma pigmentosum cells following UV irradiation and DNA synthesis is assessed by [^{3}H]thymidine uptake and autoradiography.

Clinical features

The clinical expression of the disease depends on the complementation group, the race of the patient and geographic environment. At birth the skin is normal. However, freckling and xerosis of light-exposed sites begin between 6 months and 3 years of age. This process may extend to non-light-exposed areas. Variation in UV exposure will

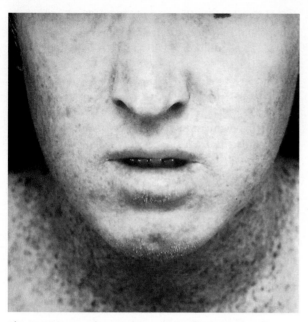

Figure 38.7 *Xeroderma pigmentosum in a young patient with severe freckling and pigmentary skin changes.*

cause such freckles to fluctuate in the intensity of colour. The skin becomes atrophic and telangiectasias appear and atrophy of the skin may cause superficial ulcers, which heal with great difficulty and leave significant scarring (Fig. 38.7). This process is particularly troublesome around the eyes where it may cause ectropion. The development of premalignant and malignant skin tumours will depend on the complementation group and the level of UV exposure that the patient is subjected to. Often there are numerous actinic keratoses as well as cutaneous horns and keratoacanthomas. SCC and BCCs may appear from an early age (Jacyk, 1999; Khatri *et al.*, 1999). Melanomas occur in up to 5 per cent of Caucasian xeroderma pigmentosum patients but studies of patients in Libya and South Africa have not shown a greater incidence of malignant melanoma in Libyans and black South Africans (Jacyk, 1999; Khatri *et al.*, 1999).

The commonest eye manifestation is photophobia with telangiectasia of the conjunctiva. There is gross hyperpigmentation of the eyelids and severe ectropion can result from superficial ulceration of the skin around the eye. Scarring of the cornea and pinguecula-like growths may occur. Patients are particularly prone to SCC of the lip and this has a particularly poor prognosis.

Eighteen per cent of xeroderma pigmentosum patients display progressive neurological abnormalities. The most severe are seen in group A patients, with mild disease seen in group D patients. This is caused by primary neuronal degeneration with loss of neurons.

Treatment

The most important single measure is UV avoidance with the patient forbidden to go out during the peak periods of sun exposure and advised to completely cover up in the sun and to always wear a high-factor sunblock. Occasionally patients have been treated with systemic retinoids with variable responses, but tumours tend to recur when the dose of the drug is reduced (Guillot *et al.*, 1984; Somos *et al.*, 1999).

Patients require regular follow-up and dysplastic and neoplastic lesions treated as described in sections on BCC and SCC. Radiotherapy is contraindicated in these patients due to the risk of inducing further malignancy.

MERKEL CELL CARCINOMA

Merkel cell carcinoma (MCC) is malignant neuro-endocrine cells. Recent studies have shown that MCC shares pathogenetic mechanisms with other neoplasms of neural crest derivation, such as malignant melanoma and neuroblastoma (Vortmeyer *et al.*, 1998).

Aetiology

Merkel cells are specialized sensory cells present in the basal or suprabasal layers of the epidermis. They are believed to be neurosensory cells which are derived from amine precursor uptake and decarboxylation system (APUD) cell series.

Cytogenetic and molecular studies have shown evidence of genetic changes on the distal portion of chromosome 1p in different tumours with well-established neuroendocrine origins, specifically neuroblastomas, malignant melanomas, and phaeochromocytomas. Involvement of chromosome 1 in MCC has been demonstrated by cytogenetic analysis and analysis of loss of heterozygosity in metastatic tumor tissue (Vortmeyer *et al.*, 1998).

The anti-apoptotic gene *bcl-2* is strongly expressed in metastatic MCC (Feinmesser *et al.*, 1999). *bcl-2* is capable of blocking programmed cell death and has been shown to play an important role in normal cell turnover, tumour biology, and chemoresistance. High *bcl-2* expression leading to prolonged survival of cells may therefore be of importance in the biological and clinical characteristics of MCC. Indeed, in a SCID mouse xenotransplantation model for human MCC, administration of *bcl-2* antisense oligonucleotide resulted in either a dramatic reduction of tumour growth or complete remission (Schlagbauer-Wadl *et al.*, 2000).

MCC shares many aetiological factors with BCCs and SCCs as it occurs mainly on sun-exposed sites and the role of chronic arsenic ingestion may be similar, as MCC has been documented in Taiwanese patients who resided in an endemic area of black foot disease, a condition found in patients with chronic arsenicism (Lien *et al.*, 1999). MCC seems to be common in transplant recipients and is more aggressive in these patients, indicating an aetiological role for immunosuppression (Penn and First, 1999).

Natural history

Most MCCs occur in patients over 65 years of age. They present as solitary dome-shaped lesions on the head and neck regions, but may be seen on the trunk and extremities. Multiple tumours, at presentation, have been reported.

MCC resembles malignant melanoma in several ways. Both are cutaneous lesions of the same embryonic origin. Both have an unpredictable biological behaviour, early regional lymph-node involvement, early distant metastases, and high recurrence rate (Wasserberg et al., 2000). However, if MCC is recognized and excised early, and if recurrences are sought and treated early, the prognosis for patients is favourable. Even after recurrence, the majority of patients experience long-term survival.

The overall 5-year disease-free survival rate is 70 per cent for all patients. The only independent predictor of survival is the tumour stage at presentation. For patients with stage I disease, the tumour size at presentation is also an independent predictor of survival.

Recurrence of disease occurs in 55 per cent, and the most common site of first recurrence is within the draining lymph nodes. Elective lymph node dissection is the only parameter independently predictive of improved relapse-free survival but it does not improve overall survival. The overall disease-free survival rate after recurrence is 60 per cent. Predictors of improved disease-free survival after recurrence include nodal as compared to local or distant recurrence, the ability to render the patient free of disease after recurrence, and a disease-free interval of >8 months (Allen et al., 1999).

Pathology

The majority of MCCs are dermal nodules with a clear Grenz zone separating the tumour from the epidermis. There are sheets of small, undifferentiated and tightly packed rounded cells that possess only scanty cytoplasm. The MCC may be histopathologically difficult to differentiate from other small cell neoplasms. Immunohistochemically, the MCC cells stain positive for neurofilament, cytokeratin, neuron-specific enolase, and epithelial membrane antigen. Leukocyte common antigen, S-100, 013 and chromogranin are negative. Karyotyping of neoplastic cells show loss of chromosome Y, the significance of which is unknown (Tope and Sangueza, 1994).

Treatment

The most important objective is to completely excise the tumour at its earliest stage. Treatment for localized disease without nodal involvement is surgical excision of the primary tumour with an adequate margin of clearance of 2.5–3.0 cm. Elective lymph-node dissection alone improves the length of the disease-free period but does not improve the overall survival (Allen et al., 1999). Post-excision radiotherapy is known to improve survival (Ott et al., 1999) and should be given to the site of the original tumour and the primary draining lymph nodes. Fractionated doses of 5000–6000 cGy given over 4–6 weeks is recommended (Ratner et al., 1993). MCC is chemosensitive but rarely curable in patients with metastasis or locally advanced tumours. A high incidence of mortality directly related to chemotherapy has been reported (Voog et al., 1999). However, orally administered etoposide has been used with great success in advanced MCC, even in patients previously treated intravenously with the same drug (Fenig et al., 2000).

LANGERHANS CELL HISTIOCYTOSIS

Langerhans cell histiocytosis (LCH) previously known as histiocytosis X, eosinophilic granuloma, Hand–Schüller–Christian disease or Letterer–Siwe disease, is now the preferred term as it unifies this group of histiocytic diseases involving cells of the Langerhans cell lineage under one heading. LCH is defined as a condition characterized by an abnormal accumulation and/or proliferation of cells expressing the phenotypic markers of normal epidermal Langerhans cells in various organs. The cellular infiltrate results in damage to the respective organ; subsequently, dysfunction or even complete failure of that organ may occur. Although most patients with single-system disease do well without the need for treatment, patients with multi-system disease may develop fulminant disease, which may be fatal.

Incidence

LCH is an uncommon disease, with an estimated 50 new cases a year in England and Wales (Broadbent and Pritchard, 1985). There is a geographically random distribution and little month-to-month variation. In childhood disease there is a male-to-female ratio of 2:1, but in adults the sex incidence is equal.

Aetiology

The cause of LCH is unknown. Several theories including viral, immune defects, dysregulation of cytokine gene and oncogene expression have been suggested. The findings of Birbeck granules in the cytoplasm of cells involved in LCH under transmission electron microscopy (Basset and Turiaf, 1965) and the presence of a membrane-bound glycoprotein, CD1a complex (Beckstead et al., 1984; Groh et al., 1988), have firmly placed the cell type involved as the epidermal Langerhans cells. Functionally, LCH cells are defective as antigen-presenting cells when compared to epidermal Langerhans cells on a per cell basis (Yu *et al.*, 1992). Loss of this primary function suggests that a biological insult(s) occurring in Langerhans cell progenitor cells results in a diversion from the normal maturation pathway into a less specialized form of differentiation. Although LCH is generally regarded as a reactive condition, recent studies have demonstrated that the LCH cells represent a clonal expansion of cells with a Langerhans cell phenotype (Willman *et al.*, 1994; Yu *et al.*, 1994). Clonal populations of cells have been identified in contact allergic dermatitis and benign tumours such as lymphomatoid papulosis, but clonality is one of the cardinal features of malignancy. In LCH, the cells are clonal regardless of the extent or severity of the disease, i.e. from single organ disease to multiple organ disease. It appears that clonal expansion of Langerhans cells is the first biological event in LCH, with further biological events determining the course of the disease.

Natural history

The natural history of LCH is extremely variable. In single-system disease, particularly of bone, LCH may be an incidental radiological finding that resolves without causing any disability to the patient. At the other extreme, multi-system disease presenting in early infancy may rapidly progress to death, whilst intermediate cases may continue to progress over decades with substantial morbidity or may rapidly burn themselves out without residual defect. The number of systems involved by LCH is the most reliable prognostic factor. When either one or two systems is involved, mortality is rare; when three or more systems are involved mortality rates rise to 30 per cent or higher. Other poor prognostic factors include early age of disease onset before 2 years of age, internal organ involvement and male gender. The most aggressive form of LCH presents in the first few months of life with multi-system involvement and behaves like an aggressive malignancy and prognosis is extremely poor.

Pathology

The characteristic cell seen in LCH lesions is the LCH cell. This is a large cell with an indented nucleus. The cells are non-specific esterase, surface ATP-ase and α-D-mannosidase positive, and alkaline phosphatase and non-specific esterase negative. The cells characteristically contain the S100 protein and produce dense cell surface and paranuclear staining with peanut agglutinin. Immunohistochemistry shows that the LCH cells are CD1a and CD4 positive (Harrist *et al.*, 1983) and exhibit the phenotype of a Langerhans cell that has been arrested at an early stage of maturation (Chu and Jaffe, 1994). On electron microscopy Birbeck granules identical to those described in Langerhans cells are seen. There is no histological difference between lesions in multi-system compared with localized disease. Organs commonly affected by LCH, in descending order of frequency, are: the skin (including external ear and gum), cortical bone, lymph nodes, central nervous system, liver/spleen, bone marrow, intestines and thymus. Single cases of LCH involvement of the eye and pancreas have been reported. Organs in which LCH involvement have not been reported are the heart and kidneys.

Clinical presentation and diagnosis

LCH has protean manifestations and patients may present to many different medical and surgical specialities. Lesions in bone may be asymptomatic or cause pathological feature, and are seen as lucent areas on radiography. Skin rashes may be initially mistaken for seborrhoeic dermatitis, particularly in the scalp and napkin areas (Plate 10). Pituitary involvement initially causes diabetes insipidus but may progress to anterior pituitary failure. Lung involvement produces diffuse upper zone shadowing on X-ray. The liver and spleen may be involved, causing organ enlargement, and bone marrow infiltration may produce anaemia, leucopenia or thrombocytopenia. Intermittent pyrexia may occur in patients and may be due to increased levels of interleukin-1 (IL-1) and tumour necrosis factor-α (TNF-α) production rather than secondary infection.

A diagnosis of LCH can only be made on tissue biopsy of clinically suspicious lesions. The typical appearance of LCH cells in affected lesions is a large cell with coffee-bean-shaped nuclei and abundant vacuolated cytoplasm. The diagnostic confidence is enhanced by positive staining of the putative LCH cells using antibodies against S100 or peanut agglutinin. A definitive diagnosis is made when Birbeck granules are seen under transmission electron microscopy or positive immunostaining to CD1a determinant in lesional cells (Chu *et al.*, 1987). Radioactively labelled monoclonal antibodies against the CD1a molecule is currently being tested for diagnosis of lesions in inaccessible sites.

Clinical grading

The total number of systems involved, age of disease onset and the presence of 'vital organ' involvement are the important prognostic factors in LCH. The Lahey scoring system (Lahey, 1962) where one point is allocated for each organ system involved by clinical assessment or simple laboratory investigation, is still the most widely used (Table 38.3). More recently the Histiocyte Society has simplified the staging of a patient with LCH to three groups:

- single-system disease;
- multi-system disease;

Table 38.3 *Lahey scoring system for LCH*

One point is awarded for evidence of involvement of the following:
- Skeleton
- Skin
- Liver
- Spleen
- Lung
- Pituitary
- Hb <10.5 g/dL, WBC <3000/mm^3 or >14 000/mm^3
- Platelets <2 000 000/mm^3

- multi-system disease with evidence of organ dysfunction.

Organ dysfunction is taken as abnormal liver function tests, abnormal blood film, failure to thrive or abnormal lung function tests. Prognosis decreases with more advanced disease.

Treatment

In each patient the likely natural history of the disease should be assessed so the benefits of treatment can be weighed against the risks. For treatment purposes, LCH can be divided into single- and multi-system disease. In single-system disease, there is an excellent prognosis so local measures only are indicated. Intralesional steroids (Broadbent and Pritchard, 1985) are effective in bone disease. In isolated skin disease, topical nitrogen mustard, 2 mg/100 mL tap water and PUVA (psoralen with ultraviolet A) are the treatments of choice (Munn and Chu, 1998).

In multi-system disease, local treatment may reduce the need for systemic treatment. Steroid injection into bony lesions may be useful and it has been claimed that low-dose radiotherapy to the pituitary can reverse early diabetes insipidus (Greenberger *et al.*, 1979). This study was, however, based on clinical rather than laboratory findings and children with LCH have been observed to have episodes of polyuria and polydipsia without biochemical evidence of diabetes insipidus (McLelland *et al.*, 1987).

There is much controversy over how aggressive chemotherapy should be. There have been no trials that show combination chemotherapy to be more effective than single-agent treatment but toxicity is certainly greater. A recent study, however, suggests that the incidence of diabetes insipidus may be reduced by combination treatment.

Conservative groups (Broadbent and Pritchard, 1985) avoid systemic chemotherapy if possible, but use prednisolone for courses of 2–3 months, starting at 2 mg/kg for the first month then reducing to 1 mg/kg for the second and tailing off over the third. Although this is effective in children, adults with LCH do not respond well to systemic steroids and frequently develop side-effects from the treatment. Cytotoxic drugs carry the risks of myelosuppression,

immunosuppression and organ-specific toxicity. The vinca alkaloids, methotrexate and 6-mercaptopurine are effective agents but the epidophyllotoxin, etoposide (VPI6) may be more effective than any of them. Some patients resistant to other forms of chemotherapy have responded to etoposide whilst others, with steroid-resistant disease, have become steroid sensitive after etoposide (two to six courses of 150 mg/m^2 intravenously for 3 days or 300 mg/m^2 orally for 3 days) (McLelland *et al.*, 1987).

In some patients, response to etoposide is good but the patient then relapses once the treatment is stopped. In our experience, maintenance treatment with azathioprine or 6-mercaptopurine with or without weekly methotrexate has proved very effective in maintaining disease remission and after 6–12 months can be stopped without recurrence of disease.

Osband *et al.* (1981) treated 17 patients with injections of calf thymic extract and reported the response to be at least as good as that of historical controls treated with more conventional chemotherapy. Subsequent clinical trials have failed to substantiate earlier claims. Immunotherapy has now fallen out of favour.

Treatment requires careful balance of the risk versus benefit to the individual patient. As the disease is uncommon and the manifestations very variable, careful multi-centre trials need to be performed to assess alternative approaches to treatment.

CUTANEOUS T-CELL LYMPHOMA (CTCL)

Epidemiology

CTCL is usually a disease of older patients with a peak incidence in the fourth to sixth decades. Any age group can be affected with documented cases as young as 10 years.

The epidemiology of CTCL is poorly described and population-based registries often fail to completely register patients with CTCL. It is estimated that there are approximately 1000 new cases of CTCL a year in the USA with the highest incidence being among the black population. The incidence is lower among Hispanics and Asians than among non-Hispanic whites. The USA has a higher reported incidence than Europe and Australia, and China has a very low reported incidence. It is known that there is a greater frequency of CTCL among men than among women and risk increases with advancing age, although childhood cases are well documented (Howard *et al.*, 1995).

Aetiology

The cause of CTCL is unknown. A large number of theories about its pathogenesis have been put forward, with the most enduring and most attractive being that CTCL is a disease of antigen persistence within the skin, causing chronic lymphocyte stimulation and the transformation of benign lymphocytes into a low-grade T-cell malignancy (Tan et al., 1974). This theory was based on the histological observation that in the early phases of CTCL, the cellular infiltrate is mixed and looks benign with marked epidermotropism. As the lymphoma becomes more advanced and more aggressive, the infiltrate becomes more monomorphous with obvious cellular atypia and loss of epidermotropism.

Studies have now demonstrated that the neoplastic cell in CTCL is a Th2 cell. In the early stages of the disease, reactive T cells with a Th1 phenotype predominate as part of an anti-tumour response. As the disease progresses, the malignant Th2 cells become dominant with loss of epidermotropism (Vowels et al., 1992, 1994; Saed et al., 1994). This helps to explain the histological features of CTCL as it develops.

Migration of T cells to the epidermis is mediated by the Th1 cytokine interferon-γ (IFNγ) as well as TNF-α. The initial binding of T cells to keratinocytes is mediated by intracellular adhesion molecule-1 (ICAM-1; as well as other selectins such as E selectin), which is induced on keratinocytes by IFNγ (Sugerman and Bigby, 2000). As the malignant cells proliferate in CTCL, the immune response switches from a Th1 anti-tumour response to a Th2 response related to the functional activity of the malignant cells, with loss of migration and retention of T cells into the epidermis and downregulation of the Th1 response by cytokines such as IL-10.

Since the theory of antigen persistence was proposed in 1974 (Tan et al., 1974) there has been no clear consensus on the nature of the antigen. Detailed investigation of pre-existing allergies, atropy or biological, physical or chemical exposure has failed to demonstrate a correlation between these factors and CTCL (Howard et al., 1995).

The association of CTCL with the human T-cell lymphoma/leukaemia virus I and II (HTLV-I and II) remains controversial. Clinically, cutaneous lesions of CTCL and adult T-cell leukaemia/lymphoma are similar, which fuelled speculation that classic CTCL could be caused by a retrovirus. No consistent results from exhaustive searches for a retrovirus have been forthcoming (Lisby et al., 1992; Pancake et al., 1995).

Recent studies have suggested that superantigens could be implicated in the pathogenesis of CTCL. Superantigens are proteins produced by some bacteria and viruses that bind directly to the T-cell receptor, resulting in T-cell stimulation and proliferation. Staphylococcus aureus, a common constituent of the skin flora, is well known to produce superantigens. Twenty-six per cent of new CTCL patients are culture positive for Staphylococcus aureus and patients with Sézary syndrome also harbour the toxic shock staphylococcal toxin 1 (TSST-1) strains of Staphylococcus aureus (Madeleine and Cather, 2000). Interestingly, the human leucocyte antigen DR5 is significantly associated with CTCL and HLA-DR5 is particularly susceptible

to staphylococcal superantigen stimulation (Madeleine and Cather, 2000).

Classification of CTCL

New advances in immunohistochemistry and molecular biology have led to a move away from the many different designations given to each of the many clinical expressions of CTCL, including mycosis fungoides, parapsoriasis on plaque, parapsoriasis variegata, parapsoriasis lichenoides, xanthoerythroderma perstans, poikiloderma vasculare atrophicans, Woringer–Kolopp disease (pagetoid reticulosis), granulomatous slack skin syndrome and Sézary syndrome. Today many authorities acknowledge that this variety of designations confuses the fact that they are all manifestations of a single pathological process (Ackerman, 1996).

The term latent lymphoma has been suggested for those disorders where the risk of systemic spread is limited, the disease is slowly progressive or locally self-regressing. This category would include large plaque parapsoriasis, self-regressing CTCL and lymphomatoid papulosis (Willemze and Meijer, 1999).

A number of classifications of cutaneous lymphoma have been proposed including the European Organization for Research and Treatment of Cancer (EORTC), Revised European–American Classification for Lymphoid Neoplasms (REAL) and Kiel classifications, all of which are still being used. For the cutaneous lymphomas, the EORTC is the most appropriate as this takes into account the clinical behaviour of the tumour as well as the cell type involved.

In 1997 the Cutaneous Lymphoma Study Group of EORTC published a proposal for a classification of the primary cutaneous lymphomas (Willemze et al., 1997). The EORTC classification is the first and only classification that is designated exclusively for the group of primary cutaneous lymphomas (Table 38.4).

Clinical features of CTCL

LYMPHOMATOID PAPULOSIS

This disease is characterized by recurrent crops of self-healing, red-brown, centrally necrotic, asymptomatic papules and nodules. The lesions may vary in number from a few to more than 100 at a time and may resolve spontaneously within 3–4 weeks, leaving hyperpigmentation and/or small atrophic scars. The disease is more frequent in the third and fourth decades. Around 15 per cent of patients ultimately progress to frank CTCL. However, some studies have found a cumulative risk over time of developing CTCL approaching 80 per cent after 15 years with the median time of development of lymphoma being 12 years. Although CTCL is the most common lymphoma to which lymphomatoid papulosis progresses, transition

Table 38.4 *EORTC classification for cutaneous lymphomas*

Primary cutaneous T-cell lymphoma	Primary cutaneous B-cell lymphoma
Indolent	*Indolent*
Mycosis fungoides	Follicle centre cell lymphoma
Pagetoid reticulosis	Immunocytoma/marginal zone B-cell lymphoma
Large cell CTCL, CD30+	Large B-cell lymphoma of the leg
Aggressive	
Sézary syndrome	
Large cell CTCL, CD30−	
Provisional	*Provisional*
Granulomatous slack skin	Intravascular CBCL
CTCL, pleomorphic small/medium sized	Plasmocytoma
Subcutaneous panniculitis-like T-cell lymphoma	

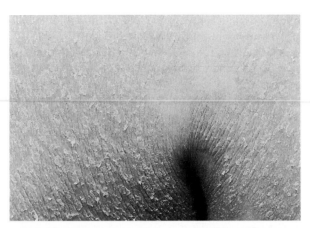

Figure 38.8 *Patch stage of CTCL, of the poikiloderma atrophicans vasculare type.*

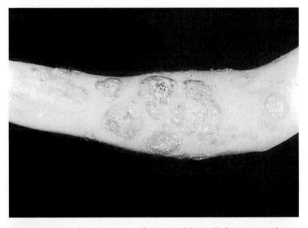

Figure 38.9 *Plaque stage of CTCL with well demarcated papillosquamous lesions on forearms.*

to Hodgkin's disease and undifferentiated lymphoma have also been reported. Typically, the eruption follows a chronic course of remissions and relapses over months and years. Lymphomatoid papulosis is believed to represent the indolent end of the spectrum of CD30+ lymphoproliferative disorders (Howard *et al.*, 1995).

MYCOSIS FUNGOIDES

This is the most common clinical variant of CTCL. This is conventionally divided into early patch, plaque and nodular disease, depending on the stage of disease.

Patch stage (poikiloderma atrophicans vasculare, large-plaque parapsoriasis)

This commonly affects the body creases and buttocks but any site of the body can be affected although more rarely the head, hands and feet. The lesions are round or oval usually along the axis of extremities or parallel to the ribs with the borders of the lesions being ill defined. They are rose to yellowish pink and the surface is slightly scaly. A characteristic clinical feature is variability of the colour of the patches from one patch to the next and even within a patch (Fig. 38.8). Reticulate hyperpigmentation and hypopigmentation, telangiectasia and skin atrophy characterize the poikiloderma atrophicans vasculare variant. Hypopigmented macular lesions can be observed in dark-skinned patients as a manifestation of patch stage CTCL (Akaraphanth *et al.*, 2000).

Plaque stage

After a period ranging from months to years, patch stage disease may progress into plaque stage disease. Plaques are well demarcated, elevated and feel infiltrated (Fig. 38.9). They are erythematous, thick plaques. Some have an irregular shape often appearing annular, serpiginous.

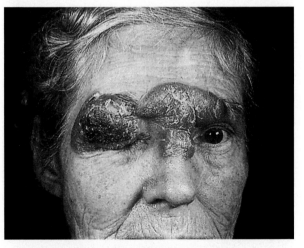

Figure 38.10 *Tumid CTCL arising from long-standing plaque stage disease on forehead and supraocular region.*

The palms and soles may develop a verrucous crusted surface.

Nodular stage

The appearance of dome-shaped, red-brown nodules in pre-existing plaques heralds the tumour stage (Fig. 38.10).

In the *tumeur d'emblée* form of CTCL, such nodules may also occur in previously uninvolved skin.

Nodules and tumours have a predilection for the face and flexures and may become ulcerated and secondarily infected.

As CTCL advances, autopsy studies have shown that every organ can be secondarily affected. The most common extracutaneous site of involvement are the lymph nodes followed by the lungs, spleen, liver and the gastrointestinal tract. Bone marrow involvement is more likely to occur in the advanced stage of the disease. Malignant T cells in the peripheral circulation may be found in 15–20 per cent of patients with plaque and tumour-stage CTCL.

SÉZARY SYNDROME

Sézary syndrome is the erythrodermic, leukaemic variant of CTCL representing only 5 per cent of new cases of CTCL. At its most advanced form patients may present with leonine facies, hyperkeratosis and fissuring of the palms and soles and severe pruritus (Fig. 38.11). The disease must be distinguished from other causes of erythroderma such as drug eruptions, atopic dermatitis, contact dermatitis and erythrodermic psoriasis. Recently it has been proposed that minimal criteria for diagnosis of Sézary syndrome should be erythroderma, compatible skin pathology, more than 5 per cent circulating atypical mononuclear cells and evidence of a peripheral blood T-cell clone detected by polymerase chain reaction (PCR) for the T-cell receptor (TCR) gene (Russell Jones and Whittaker, 1999).

Sézary syndrome is an aggressive disease and patients with this syndrome have a median survival of less than 3 years (Russell Jones and Whittaker, 1999).

ALOPECIA MUCINOSA

This clinically manifests as grouped erythematous follicular papules or indurated nodular plaques associated with alopecia. The head and neck are the major sites of involvement but more widespread disease can affect the trunk and extremities. Surprisingly the resultant alopecia is often clinically not apparent unless the lesions affect the scalp or eyebrow. Up to 30 per cent of such patients may have an associated CTCL. The lymphoma may precede the development of alopecia mucinosa or it may be identified on biopsy of alopecia mucinosa. There is no reliable criterion for predicting which patients will progress to develop CTCL (Howard *et al.*, 1995).

WORINGER–KOLOPP DISEASE

Typically lesions present as solitary or a few plaques on acral sites (Fig. 38.12). It shows an indolent clinical course. There have been isolated reports of histologically similar lesions of Woringer–Kolopp disease following insults such as spider bites, burns or trauma. Clonal T-cell receptor rearrangements have been identified in increasing numbers of cases designated with this disease. Patients with a small number of lesions have the smallest tumour burden and therefore have the best outcome. Immunophenotyping in Woringer–Kolopp disease have demonstrated that in some cases, the epidermal T cells are γδT cells, suggesting that this type of CTCL is biologically different from normal CTCL (Alaibac and Chu, 1992).

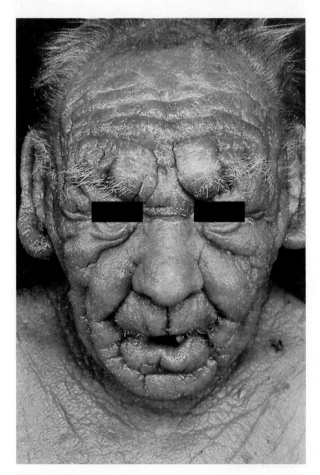

Figure 38.11 *Erythrodermic CTCL in an elderly man with diffuse infiltration of the skin giving rise to a leonine facies.*

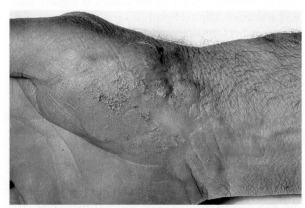

Figure 38.12 *Woringer–Kolopp disease presenting as an isolated plaque on the hand of a 30-year-old man.*

GRANULOMATOUS SLACK SKIN DISEASE

This is a rare variant of CTCL characterized by the development of bulky and pendulous skin. It affects mainly young individuals of both sexes with a male predominance. It has a slowly progressive but relentlessly chronic course leading to the development of extracutaneous lymphoma and also to other types of malignancy such as Hodgkin's disease. A clonal rearrangement of the T cells has been reported in this disease and its pathogenesis in clinical terms corresponds to a granulomatous process with secondary elastolysis provoked by the underlying lymphoma (Le Boit et al., 1987).

PRIMARY CUTANEOUS ANAPLASTIC LARGE CELL LYMPHOMA (CD30+, KI-1)

The primary cutaneous anaplastic large cell lymphoma usually presents as a solitary nodule in the seventh or eighth decade of life. Dissemination to extracutaneous sites occurs in less than 25 per cent of patients and even if extracutaneous spread does occur, the 4-year survival rate exceeds 90 per cent. Therefore, this is a tumour of a very favourable prognosis (Willemze et al., 1997).

Prognosis and staging

In 1979, the Mycosis Fungoides Co-operative Group adopted a TNM classification including both clinical evaluation of skin and nodes and extent of histopathological lymph node involvement (Table 38.5). The staging

Table 38.5 *TNM classification of CTCL*

T	*Skin*
T0	Clinically and/or histopathologically suspicious lesions
T1	Limited plaques, papules or patches covering <10% skin surface
T2	Plaques, papules or patches covering >10% skin surface
T3	Tumours
T4	Erythroderma
N	*Lymph nodes*
N0	No palpable lymph nodes and negative histology
N1	Palpable lymph nodes but negative histology
N2	No palpable lymph nodes but positive histology for CTCL
N3	Palpable lymph nodes and positive histology for CTCL
B	*Peripheral blood*
B0	Atypical circulating cells absent or <5%
B1	Atypical circulating cells at 5% or more of total lymphocytes
M	*Visceral organs*
M0	No organ involvement
M1	Visceral involvement

classification also takes into account whether there are less than 5 per cent atypical circulating cells or more than 5 per cent atypical circulating cells. Visceral organ involvement is divided into those who have evidence of such involvement and those who do not.

Although erythrodermic CTCL is classified as T4 disease, recent large studies have shown that tumour stage CTCL (T3) has a worse prognosis than erythrodermic CTCL (Diamandidou et al., 1999). This suggests that the currently used TNM staging system is less than ideal and a revised TNM staging system is under proposal.

The clinical stage at presentation has been found to be the most important independent prognostic factor for CTCL. The other poor prognostic factors include age above 60, a high serum lactate dehydrogenase, a β_2-microglobulin level above 2 mg/L and transformation to large cell lymphoma. Several staging systems have evaluated the importance of the type and degree of the lymph-node involvement but there is no general consensus about the best way to characterize lymph-node involvement. Most investigators would agree, however, that lymph-node involvement confers a poor prognosis in patients with CTCL (Diamandidou et al., 1999).

Patients with T1 disease have similar survivals to that of an age-, sex- and race-matched population. Survival of T2, T3 and T4 patients is significantly shorter than that of a similar control population, with T2 showing a moderate, and T3 and T4 showing a marked decrease in relative survival. In addition, the relative survival of T2 patients with plaque stage disease as defined by histology is significantly less than that of similar stage patients with patch stage disease. This is probably a reflection of the influence of the depth of the infiltrate and cytological atypia and is in keeping with findings that survival of patients with T1 and T2 CTCL who have an infiltrate thicker than 1 mm have an inferior survival compared to those patients with a thinner infiltrate.

A recent large study showed that the percentage of patients still alive after 5 years with stage T2 disease was 70 per cent, with stage T4 disease 60 per cent and with stage T3 disease 30 per cent. In those patients with lymph-node involvement at presentation, only 40 per cent were alive at 5 years compared with those without lymph-node involvement where 75 per cent were alive after 5 years (Diamandidou et al., 1999).

Recent studies have focused on the immunocompetence of the patient with regard to prognosis. Compromise of the immune system in CTCL may lead to increased infection rate and the occurrence of secondary malignancies (Heald et al., 1994). Enumeration of the peripheral CD8+ cell count can be used as a measure of anti-tumour response in CTCL patients.

Pathology

The histopathological diagnosis of CTCL is perhaps one of the most difficult to make (Earl et al., 1999).

This is true not only of early disease but also in advanced cases (Hermann *et al.*, 1994).

The earliest histological changes are a sparse superficial perivascular infiltrate of lymphocytes and slight epidermotropism associated with a lack of spongiosis. The cornified layer is slightly thickened or laminated with subtle foci of parakeratosis. Lymphocytic atypia is present and consists of slight nuclear enlargement, nuclear convolution and mild hypochromasia. The most significant feature indicative of CTCL is the presence of haloed lymphocytes which are retraction-induced vacuoles surrounding lymphocytic nuclei within the epidermis. Five or more such cells per $\times20$ field are strongly indicative of CTCL. Prominent haloed lymphocytes are seen in approximately 60 per cent of cases of CTCL but only in 13 per cent of non-CTCL cases (Sanchez and Ackerman, 1979).

A specific feature of CTCL is the presence of epidermal lymphocytes that are larger than dermal lymphocytes (Smoller *et al.*, 1995, 1998). Within the epidermis, T cells may be observed singly or forming Pautrier's microabscesses, which are collections of at least four atypical lymphocytes within an intra-epidermal vacuole.

Diagnosis

The diagnosis of CTCL is based on the clinical finding with supporting histology. The diagnostic confidence is greatly enhanced using T-cell gene rearrangement studies and immunohistochemistry (Fucich *et al.*, 1999). Although initially Southern blot analysis of the β-TCR gene was thought to be the most specific method of detection of clonal T-cell populations, it is not very sensitive, demanding that at least 5 per cent of the infiltrating cells are clonal. PCR-based detection methods are just as specific and may be sensitive to 0.1 per cent of the infiltrating cells (Russell Jones and Whittaker, 1999).

An aberrant T-cell immunophenotype, in particular, the loss of one or more pan-T-cell antigens (CD2, CD3, CD5 or CD7) supports a diagnosis of CTCL. The most common pan-T-cell antigen to be lost is CD7. Loss of more than one marker adds further support to the diagnosis of a neoplastic process. However, CD7-negative T cells have occasionally been identified in reactive processes (Willemze *et al.*, 1997).

Treatment

Patients with CTCL should be managed by a multidisciplinary team with the involvement of dermatologists, medical oncologists, radiation oncologists, dermatopathologists and haematologists (Parry *et al.*, 1999). The modern therapy for CTCL includes not only therapy directed towards the skin itself, but also therapies which aim to modify the host's immune system in order to reverse the immunosuppressive responses of the tumour cells in the later stages of the disease. Therapy may be divided into skin-directed therapy and biological response modifiers, which are treatments that aim to boost the normally functioning immune system and correct immunological and cellular abnormalities or defects (Sinha and Heald, 1998).

SKIN-DIRECTED TREATMENT

Topical therapy

High-potency topical corticosteroids have been used for many years in CTCL. Response rate in early CTCL or small plaque parapsoriasis may be as high as 94 per cent with up to 63 per cent achieving complete remission in patients with T1 disease. Side-effects include reversible serum cortisol depression, minor skin irritation, skin atrophy and striae (Zackheim *et al.*, 1998).

Mechlorethamine is an alkylating agent, which alkylates DNA guanine residues leading to mispairing of guanine with thymine, imidazole re-opening and inter-strand cross-linking as well as cross-linkage to nearby proteins. Mechlorethamine seems to exert its effects most predominantly on cells in the late G_1-phase or S-phase of the cell cycle. Mechlorethamine hydrochloride is available in powder form and patients are instructed to dissolve the drug in tap water. Dilutions may vary between 10 and 20 mg drug dissolved in 40–60 mL water. In our practice, we generally use 10 mg of the drug in 60 mL water and only increase the concentration if no clinical response has occurred after 2 months. Therapy is carried out daily for 3–6 months. Response rates vary from 50 to 75 per cent in T1 patients and from 25 to 50 per cent in T2 patients (Ramsay *et al.*, 1995). There are no systemic side-effects from this therapy but more than 50 per cent of patients experience an allergic or irritant dermatitis that normally develops between 1 and 3 months of therapy (Esteve *et al.*, 1999). In addition, studies performed in mice show that the skin of hairless mice exposed to both UVB light and topical mechlorethamine resulted in a significant increase in the rate of appearance of skin tumours.

Carmustine is a nitrosurea alkylating agent which is used topically in early-stage CTCL. It is available in both solution and ointment form. The aqueous solution is normally used as 10 mg carmustine in 60 mL of an ethanol and water solution and it is used daily for at least 3 months. If the response is inadequate, the concentration is increased to 20 mg carmustine in 60 mL water and ethanol solution. With the solution, 86 per cent of T1 and 48 per cent of T2 patients achieve clinical remission. Side-effects include erythema of the skin accompanied by skin tenderness, persistent telangiectasia and mild leucopenia in 3–5 per cent of patients. There is no evidence that topical carmustine causes skin carcinogenesis. Generally, carmustine is used when the patient cannot tolerate mechlorethamine.

UVB radiation therapy is an agent used for the treatment of patch stage but not for plaque stage CTCL due to its limited penetration through the skin. Clinical remissions of up to 74 per cent may be achieved with a follow-up period of 12.8 years. The duration of response may last up to 51 months. It is the treatment of choice in small plaque parapsoriasis. In the past, broad-band UVB therapy was the main form of UVB therapy. However, narrow-band UVB therapy (311 nm) has been shown to be a more effective, short-term treatment modality for clearing small plaque parapsoriasis and early-stage CTCL (Hofer and Cerroni, 1999).

Although UVB phototherapy is very useful for patch stage CTCL, treatment of plaque stage CTCL requires modalities of therapy capable of penetrating into the dermis – a quality that UVB does not have. Therefore, PUVA treatment is the treatment of choice for plaque stage CTCL (Hermann *et al.*, 1994). Treatment in Europe is normally given three to four times a week until the cutaneous lesions clear. Maintenance therapy is advised once complete clearance has occurred and it is recommended that maintenance therapy be given once weekly for 2–6 weeks, then once every 2 weeks for 8 weeks, once every 3 weeks for 9–12 weeks, and finally once every 4 weeks indefinitely. If CTCL recurs, the frequency of treatment is increased to between one and three times per week until complete clearing is again achieved and then treatment is gradually tapered to once monthly maintenance (Johnson *et al.*, 1996b). Patients with early-stage disease 1A or 1B respond well to PUVA with 90 per cent of stage 1A patients and 76 per cent of stage 1B patients achieving a complete response. The response to PUVA of more extensive disease is much reduced. Although 59 per cent of tumour stage (2B) patients achieve a complete response, many patients require additional localized radiation therapy.

A new form of UVA treatment called UVA 1 with a wavelength of 340–400 nm has been used to treat CTCL. UVA 1 has been proposed as an alternative to PUVA for stage IA and IB CTCL for the following reasons:

- UVA 1 reaches deeper layers of the dermis at higher intensities compared to PUVA;
- UVA 1 is capable of inducing both protein-synthesis-independent and dependent T-cell apoptosis, whereas PUVA therapy can only induce the latter;
- UVA 1 phototherapy avoids the unwanted side-effects resulting from the photosensitizing methoxypsoralen;
- UVA 1 phototherapy works in a similar way to PUVA, inducing apoptosis of malignant T-cell clones.

Resolution of CTCL with UVA 1 radiation occurs after 16–20 exposures. The dose of irradiation is increased sequentially up to a dose of 130 J/cm². However, large-scale studies are still required to measure the true efficacy of UVA 1 therapy in CTCL (Plettenberg *et al.*, 1999).

Photodynamic therapy has recently been adapted for CTCL. Photodynamic therapy involves the uptake of a non-toxic photosensitizer in a selective manner by malignant tissue. With subsequent exposure to visible light, a photochemical reaction is initiated which destroys the malignant cells. The sensitizer used is topical 20 per cent δ-aminolaevulinic acid which is applied for 10–20 minutes, 4–6 hours before irradiation with visible light. More than one treatment may be required to clear skin lesions and local anaesthetic cream is recommended to reduce any discomfort during treatment. As little as three treatment sessions can lead to significant resolution of CTCL lesions (Warrell *et al.*, 1991).

Radiotherapy

CTCL cells are very radiosensitive. Individual skin lesions can be treated by orthovoltage X-irradiation (60–140 kV) using fractionated doses of 75–500 cGy and a total dose of 800–1500 cGy. This is useful in controlling locally aggressive tumours and recurrent disease in covered areas in patients treated with PUVA.

Total skin electron-beam (TSEB) therapy has been developed to treat wide areas of skin and to maintain radiotherapy to the epidermis and dermis only, thereby decreasing the chances of bone marrow suppression and long-term malignancy. It has been found that the entire target volume for most patients with patch and plaque stage CTCL is within 5 mm of the skin surface (Bittoun *et al.*, 1990). However, inflammatory and malignant tumours or ulcers may extend further. Modern TSEB therapy exploits the convex circumference of the patients to bring the peak dose of radiation to the surface of the skin. Most centres now use dual fixed-angle, fixed-field or rotation methods of delivering the electron beams of up to 4–9 MeV electrons. Total doses given are typically 2400–3600 cGy. The composite 80 per cent depth dose produced by these methods is within the maximum 5-mm edge of the suggested target volume for patch and plaque stage disease. However, several factors contribute to the fact that different parts of the body actually receive variable doses of electrons, which can limit the efficacy of this form of treatment. The scalp is commonly under-dosed, as are those areas that are shielded, which include the ventral penis, the perineum, the upper medial thighs, perianal skin and inframammary folds (Jones *et al.*, 1995). The face, upper chest and pelvis may receive uncertain doses and any areas where the skin is especially concave, such as the midline groove of the spine, may receive lower doses and disease recurrence at these sites is common. During the process of TSEB treatment, the hands, feet, genitalia and scalp may be shielded as well as sites of prior radiation and the area of a cardiac pacemaker. Thick plaques, infiltrating tumours and malignant ulcers may contain malignant cells at depths greater than those treated with standard TSEB treatment and in these patients some centres have developed electron beams capable of penetrating up to 8 mm deep (Jones *et al.*, 1995).

At Stanford University, clinical remission has been achieved using a regimen of TSEB treatment of 6 MeV electrons given 4 days/week to a total of 3600 cGy in

10 weeks. Such remission was 98 per cent in stage T1, 71 per cent in T2, 36 per cent in T3 and 64 per cent in T4 CTCL. Five-year relapse-free rates were 55 per cent for T1, 25 per cent for T2 and none for T3. There were insufficient data published for T4. The side-effects of TSEB include erythema, desquamation, peripheral oedema, bullae, alopecia, xerosis, nail dystrophy and telangiectasia (Hoppe, 1991). TSEB treatment is generally only given to a patient once in a lifetime, but recent evidence suggests that repeat courses can be given but at a reduced dose (Wilson et al., 1996).

SYSTEMIC TREATMENT

Chemotherapy

Traditionally, systemic chemotherapy has been reserved for those patients with CTCL who have relapsed or have refractory disease to skin-directed therapies, or those with nodal or visceral disease at the time of diagnosis. Both single-agent chemotherapy and combination chemotherapy have been tried but most studies include few patients at differing stages of disease and with differing previous treatments. The majority of patients respond, with complete response rates ranging from 20 to 60 per cent. The duration of response is often short, often only averaging several months. However, when CTCL exhibits marked atypia and higher proliferation indices, it may be more responsive to chemotherapy.

Oral methotrexate with doses as high as 50 mg/week has been shown to be safe and can achieve improvement in different stages of CTCL. Zakheim et al. (1996) treated 29 patients with erythrodermic CTCL with low-dose methotrexate and achieved a total response rate of 58 per cent. The median disease-free period was 31 months and median survival was 8.4 years.

Doxorubicin is an anthracycline that has been shown to be active in the treatment of advanced CTCL with a high response rate. However, myelotoxicity and cardiotoxicity limit its use. The development of liposomal encapsulated doxyrubicin reduced such toxicity and also improved its efficacy. A pilot study on six patients with relapsing or recalcitrant CTCL showed an overall response rate of 83 per cent. The most frequent side-effects are mild anaemia and lymphopenia (Wollina, 2000).

CTCL is not particularly responsive to chemotherapy and patients rapidly become refractory to chemotherapy. In an attempt to avoid such resistance, combination chemotherapy regimens have been used. The most effective seems to be a combination of etoposide, vincristine, doxorubicin, bolus cyclophosphamide and oral prednisolone (EPOCH). Fifteen patients with CTCL, refractory to mono-chemotherapy, were treated with this combination, resulting in an overall response rate of 80 per cent. The median progression-free survival was 8 months, and the median patient survival was 13.5 months. Toxicity occurred in 60 per cent of patients and this comprised neutropenia, staphylococcal bacteraemia, disseminated herpes infection, Pneumocystis carinii pneumonia, neurotoxicity and cardiac dysfunction (Akpek et al., 1999).

A number of combination chemotherapy regimens have been tried in CTCL with the best results observed to a combination of cyclophosphamide, doxorubicin, vincristine, prednisolone/doxorubicin, vincristine, prednisolone (CHOP/HOP). This combination was shown to give a partial response in 100 per cent of patients with 42 per cent of these achieving a complete response but with a median duration of response of only 5 months. Another combination that gives 100 per cent partial response and a 57 per cent complete response is a combination of cyclophosphamide, vincristine, methotrexate and prednisolone (COMP) (Rosen et al., 1995).

Denileukin diftitox (DAB interleukin-2) T-cell-targeted therapy

Denileukin diftitox (DAB interleukin-2; Ontak) is a recently FDA-approved fusion of diphtheria toxin and IL-2, which has undergone phase II trials for use in CTCL. The fusion molecule binds to the IL-2 receptor on the T cell, is endocytosed and the diphtheria toxin is released into the T cell (Olson et al., 2001). In a clinical trial of patients with refractory CTCL, the fusion product was administered intravenously, daily for 5 days at 9 and 18 μ/kg per day and repeated every 3 weeks. Partial or complete responses for a median duration of 6.8 months were achieved in these patients. Side-effects include chills, fever and nausea and occurred in 60 per cent of patients. At day 10 of treatment, vascular capillary leak syndrome was seen in 10 per cent of patients.

Biological response modifiers

Biological response modifiers aim to boost the normal functioning immune system and correct immunological and cellular abnormalities or defects present in the disease.

Extracorporeal photophoresis Extracorporeal photophoresis is an immunomodulatory therapy that was approved by the United States Food and Drug Administration in 1988 for the treatment of CTCL. In many institutions, this therapy combined with other biological response modifiers has become the primary therapy for erythrodermic forms of CTCL, in particular for Sézary syndrome.

Extracorporeal photophoresis consists of the administration of oral methoxypsoralen and removal of one unit of blood, which is centrifuged to separate it into its components. The leucocytes and plasma are recombined and a thin film of the leucocyte suspension is passed through a clear plastic canal between two banks of high-intensity UVA lamps. After irradiation, the erythrocytes are replaced and the blood is transfused back into the patient. Patients generally receive treatments on two successive days each month.

Long-term follow-up of patients who have undergone such therapy have shown that even advanced forms of erythrodermic CTCL have a clinical remission rate of

25 per cent with as many as 10 per cent having no detectable residual disease for up to 11 years (Rook *et al.*, 1999). However, some studies have shown an insignificant effect on the survival of patients with Sézary syndrome (Andrews *et al.*, 1998). The main reason for such different results in the use of extracorporeal photophoresis is the patient selection in the different studies. In the study by Andrews *et al.* (1998), the patients all had classical Sézary syndrome whereas the studies showing successful use of the treatment have treated patients with erythrodermic CTCL, not all of which had classical Sézary syndrome.

Extracorporeal photophoresis appears to be most effective (Rook *et al.*, 1999) in patients where:

- only modest or small numbers of peripheral blood Sézary cells (10–20 per cent of mononuclear cells) are present;
- disease is of short duration (<2 years);
- there are normal or near normal numbers of cytotoxic T cells;
- there is normal natural killer activity;
- there is no prior history of intensive chemotherapy;
- there is absence of bulky lymphadenopathy or overt visceral disease.

The mechanism of action of extracorporeal photophoresis is unknown but it is postulated that the treatment immunizes patients to tumour-specific peptides on the CTCL cells (Heald *et al.*, 1992). It has been demonstrated that extracorporeal photophoresis induces release of certain monocytic cytokines such as TNF-α, IL-12, and IL-6 (Gottlieb *et al.*, 1996).

Interferon-α This is given systemically at doses from 3 to 20 million units daily, three times weekly. A response rate of 70 per cent may be achieved and the best results are observed in those patients with early CTCL. Unfortunately, the median duration of response can be as short as 6 months. Side-effects include malaise, low-grade fever, gastrointestinal complaints, bone marrow depression and elevated transaminase levels (Madeleine and Cather, 2000).

Interleukin-12 IL-12 may augment Th1 responses by the induction of IFNα and IL-2 expression. In a multicentre, phase II trial, doses of 300 ng/kg IL-12 were administered subcutaneously twice weekly. Partial responses were observed in several patients who improved initially but later relapsed (Bright *et al.*, 1999).

Retinoid therapy Isotretinoin and etretinate at doses of 1 mg/kg per day have response rates of about 60 per cent in CTCL but their use is limited because of the side-effect of mucocutaneous dryness that most patients suffer. Interestingly, although clinical remission may be evident on retinoid therapy, biopsy of areas of previous skin involvement show the persistence of atypical cells.

Targretin (Bexarotene) is the first retinoid X-receptor (RXR) nuclear receptor selective retinoid to enter clinical trials in humans. In patients with early-stage plaque or patch disease an 80 per cent response rate may be achieved. Several patients with extensive disease may achieve almost complete remissions. Indeed, complete response may be seen in patients with large cell transformation and in Sézary syndrome. Targretin causes a rapid response with improvement in CTCL lesions as early as 4–8 weeks (Madeleine and Cather, 2000). Toxicity includes increased lipids resulting in pancreatitis but this may be avoided by the use of lipid-lowering drugs. Fatigue and cold intolerance caused by central hypothyroidism were experienced in the majority of CTCL patients. Prolonged use of oral targretin is well tolerated but is associated with lymphopenia.

Tagretin has been formulated as a 1 per cent cream and has undergone phase I and II trials. It was found to be effective in CTCL and its use was accompanied by decreased T-cell infiltrates.

Combination therapies

Several treatment modalities may have additive clinical efficacy when combined. The combination of retinoids with PUVA showed little difference in response rates but patients receiving the retinoid with PUVA required fewer PUVA treatments and a significantly lower dose of UVA than those on PUVA alone (Thomsen *et al.*, 1989).

A prospective randomized multi-centre clinical trial comparing the use of IFNα-2a with acitretin versus IFNα-2a with PUVA in patients with CTCL stages I and II showed that the latter combination was far superior, resulting in a 70 per cent complete remission rate compared with 38 per cent in the IFN/acetretin group (Stadler *et al.*, 1998).

Follow-up

A prospective study by Epstein *et al.* (1972) of 144 patients with CTCL over a 15-year period showed a mean survival of 8.8 years, 50 per cent of the patients dying in the first 5 years.

The experience we have of CTCL in the UK is different and we see a number of patients with relatively nonaggressive disease who have a long clinical course and may die of unrelated causes. The discrepancy between the UK and the USA may be that we see a less aggressive variant of the disease in the UK or that we diagnose patients earlier or with milder disease.

Early stages of CTCL are amenable to a large number of therapies which give good results with little morbidity. Later-stage disease, however, is resistant to treatment and we have little to offer patients with visceral involvement.

Patients with CTCL need to be reviewed regularly and many patients will be on maintenance treatment. Careful examination should assess the extent and nature of the cutaneous involvement and the presence of lymphadenopathy or organomegaly. There is now compelling evidence to suggest that a CD8 T-cell count should be included as the routine test in all patients with CTCL.

SIGNIFICANT POINTS

- Skin cancer is the commonest neoplastic condition presenting to the physician in the white population.
- The most important environmental agent capable of inducing skin cancer is exposure to ultraviolet light.
- Selection of treatment modality for skin cancers depends on a number of different factors, such as age of patient, site, size, tumour type and whether one is dealing with a primary or recurrent lesion.
- Mohs' micrographic surgery is best reserved for recurrent tumours and subgroups of primary tumours that have a high incident of local recurrence or metastasis.
- Prognosis in cutaneous T-cell lymphoma is related to the degree of immunosuppression of the patient. A key test is a CD8— positive cell count.

KEY REFERENCES

Azterbaum, M., Beech, J., Ervin, H. et al. (1999) Ultraviolet radiation mutagenesis of hedgehog pathway genes in basal cell carcinomas. J. Invest. Dermatol. Symp. Proc. **4**, 41–5.

Chu, A.C. and Jaffe, N. (1994) The normal Langerhans cell and the LCH cell. Br. J. Cancer **70**, S4–10.

De Boer, J. and Hoeijmakers, J.H.J. (2000) Nucleotide excision repair and human syndromes. Carcinogenesis **21**, 453–60.

Jensen, P., Hansen, S., Moller, B. et al. (1999) Skin cancer in kidney and heart transplant recipients and different long term immunosuppressive therapy regimens. J. Am. Acad. Dermatol. **40**, 177–86.

Saed, G., Fivenson, D.P., Naidu, T. et al. (1994) Mycosis fungoides exhibits a Th1-type cell mediated cytokine profile, whereas Sézary syndrome expressed a Th1 type profile. J. Invest. Dermatol. **103**, 29–33.

Telfer, N.R., Colver, G. and Bowers, P.W. (1999) Guidelines for the management of basal cell carcinoma. Br. J. Dermatol. **141**, 415–23.

Willemze, R., Keri, H., Sterry, W. et al. (1997) EORTC classification of primary cutaneous lymphomas: a proposal from the Cutaneous Lymphoma Study Group of the European Organisation for Research and Treatment of Cancer. Blood **90**, 354–71.

REFERENCES

Ackerman, A.B. (1996) If small plaque (digitate) parapsoriasis is a cutaneous T-cell lymphoma, even an 'abortive' one, it must be mycosis fungoides. Arch. Dermatol. **132**, 562–6.

Akaraphanth, R., Lim, H.W. and Douglass, M.C. (2000) Hypopigmented mycosis fungoides. J. Am. Acad. Dermatol. **42**, 33–9.

Akpek, G.M., Koh., H.K., Bogin, S. et al. (1999) Chemotherapy with etoposide, vincristine, doxorubicin, bolus cyclophosphamide, and oral prednisone in patients with refractory cutaneous T-cell lymphoma. Cancer **86**, 1368, 1376.

Alaibac, M. and Chu, A.C. (1992) Pagetoid reticulosis: γδT-cell lymphoma? Eur. J. Dermatol. **2**, 109–11.

Albright, S. (1982) Treatment of skin cancer using multiple modalities. J. Am. Acad. Dermatol. **7**, 143–71.

Allen, P.J., Zhang, Z.F. and Coit, D.G. (1999) Surgical management of Merkel cell carcinoma. Ann. Surg. **229**, 97–105.

Allison, R.R., Mang, T.S. and Wilson, B.D. (1998) Photodynamic therapy for the treatment of non-melanomatous cutaneous malignancies. Semin. Cutan. Med. Surg. **17**, 153–63.

Alpsoy, E., Yilmaz, E., Basaran, E. et al. (1996) Comparison of the effects of intralesional interferon alfa-2a, 2b and the combination of 2a and 2b in the treatment of basal cell carcinoma. J. Dermatol. **23**, 394–6.

Andrews, E.F., Seed, P., Whittiker, S. et al. (1998) Extracorporeal photopheresis on Sézary syndrome: no significant effect in the survival of 44 patients with a peripheral blood T-cell clone. Arch. Dermatol. **134**, 1001–5.

Antoniades, D.Z., Styanidis, K., Papanayotou, P. et al. (1995) Squamous cell carcinoma of the lips in a northern Greek population. Evaluation of prognostic factors on 5-year survival rate. Eur. J. Cancer **31B**, 333–9.

Aszterbaum, M., Beech, J., Ervin, H. et al. (1999) Ultraviolet radiation mutagenesis of hedgehog pathway genes in basal cell carcinomas. J. Invest. Dermatol. Symp. Proc. **4**, 41–5.

Bandieramonte, G., Lepera, P., Moglia, D. et al. (1997) Laser microsurgery for superficial T1-T2 basal cell carcinoma of the eyelid margins. Ophthalmology **104**, 1179–84.

Barr, R.J., Headley, J.L., Jensen, J.L. and Howell, J.B. (1986) Cutaneous keratocysts of nevoid basal cell carcinoma syndrome. J. Am. Acad. Dermatol. **14**, 572–6.

Barton, K., Curling, O.M., Paridaens, A.D. et al. (1996) The role of cytology in the diagnosis of periocular basal cell carcinomas. Ophthal. Plast. Reconstr. Surg. **12**, 190–4. Discussion 195.

Basset, F. and Turiaf, J. (1965) Identification par la microscopic électronique de particules de nature probablement virale dans les lesions granulomateuses d'une hystiocytose X pulmonaire. *C.R. Acad. Sci. (Paris)* **261**, 3701–3.

Beckstead, J., Wood, G.S. and Turner, R.R. (1984) Histiocytosis X cells and Langerhans cells: enzyme histochemical and immunological similarities. *Hum. Pathol.* **15**, 826–33.

Beutner, K.R., Geisse, J.K., Helman, D. *et al.* (1999) Therapeutic response of basal cell carcinoma to the immune response modifier imiquimod 5 per cent cream. *J. Am. Acad. Dermatol.* **41**, 1002–7.

Bittoun, J., Saint-Jalmes, H., Querieux, B.G. *et al.* (1990) *In vivo* high resolution MR imaging at the skin in a whole-body system at 1.5 Tl. *Radiology* **176**, 457–60.

Breuninger, H., Gutknecht, M., Dietz, K. *et al.* (1991) Locally infiltrative growth of squamous cell carcinoma of the skin and treatment guidelines resulting from it. *Hautarzt* **42**, 559–63.

Bright, J.J., Xin, Z. and Sriram, S. (1999) Superantigens augment antigen-specific Th1 responses by including IL-12 production in macrophages. *J. Leukoc. Biol.* **65**, 665–70.

Broadbent, V. and Pritchard, J. (1985) Hystiocytosis X – current controversies. *Arch. Dis. Child.* **60**, 605–7.

Brodland, D.G. and Zitelli, J.A. (1992) Surgical margins for excision of primary cutaneous squamous cell carcinoma. *J. Am. Acad. Dermatol.* **27**, 241–8.

Caccialanza, C., Piccinno, R. and Beretta, M. (1999) Results and side effects of dermatologic radiotherapy: a retrospective study of irradiated cutaneous epithelial neoplasms. *Am. Acad. Dermatol.* **41**, 589–94.

Chopra, K.F. and Cohen, P.R. (1997) Linear basal cell carcinomas: report of multiple sequential tumors localized to a radiotherapy port and review of the literature. *Tex. Med.* **93**, 57–9.

Chu, A., D'Angio, G.J., Favara, B. *et al.* (1987) Histiocytosis syndromes in children. Lancet **1**, 208–9.

Chu, A.C. and Jaffe, N. (1994) The normal Langerhans cell and the LCH cell. *Br. J. Cancer* **70**, S4–10.

Clever, J. (1968) Defective repair replication of DNA in xeroderma pigmentosum. *Nature* **218**, 652–6.

Cockerell, C.J. (2000) Histopathology of incipient intraepidermal squamous cell carcinoma ('actinic keratosis'). *J. Am. Acad. Dermatol.* **42**, 117.

Cohen, M.M. Jr (1999) Nevoid basal cell carcinoma syndrome: molecular biology and new hypotheses. *Int. J. Oral Maxillofac. Surg.* **28**, 216–23.

Cotran, R. (1961) Metastasizing basal cell carcinomas. *Cancer* **14**, 1036–40.

Cottell, W.I. and Proper, S. (1982) Mohs' surgery, fresh tissue technique: our technique with a review. *J. Dermatol. Surg. Oncol.* **8**, 576–87.

Craven, N.M. and Griffiths, C.E.M. (1996) Retinoids in the management of non-melanoma skin cancer and melanoma. *Skin Cancer* **26**, 275–6.

De Boer, J. and Hoeijmakers, J.H.J. (2000) Nucleotide excision repair and human syndromes. *Carcinogenesis* **21**, 453–60.

Diamandidou, E., Colome, M., Fayad, L. *et al.* (1999) Prognostic factor analysis in mycosis fungoides/Sézary syndrome. *J. Am. Acad. Dermatol.* **40**, 914–24.

Dinehart, S.M. (2000) The treatment of actinic keratoses. *J. Am. Acad. Dermatol.* **42**, 25–8.

du Vivier, A. (1993) *Atlas of Clinical Dermatology*, 2nd edn. New York: Mosby Wolfe, 9.17–9.22.

Earl, J., Glusac, M.K., Shapiro, P.E. *et al.* (1999) Cutaneous T-cell lymphoma, refinement in the application of controversial histologic criteria. *Dermatol. Clin.* **17**, 601–13.

Edens, R.L., Bartlow, G.A., Haghighi, P. *et al.* (1983) Effectiveness of curettage and electrodessication in the removal of basal cell carcinoma. *J. Am. Acad. Dermatol.* **9**, 383.

Epstein, E., Levin, D.L., Croft, J.D. *et al.* (1972) Mycosis fungoides. Survival, prognostic factors, response to therapy and autopsy findings. *Medicine* **51**, 61–72.

Eroglu, A. and Camlibe, S. (1997) Risk factors for locoregional recurrence of scar carcinoma. *Br. J. Surg.* **12**, 1744–6.

Esteve, E., Bagot, M., Joly, P. *et al.* (1999) A prospective study of cutaneous intolerance to topical mechlorethamine therapy in patients with cutaneous T-cell lymphomas. French Study Group of Cutaneous Lymphomas. *Arch. Dermatol.* **135**, 1349–53.

Feinmesser, M., Halpem, M., Fenig, E. *et al.* (1999) Expression of the apoptosis-related oncogenes *bcl-2*, *bax*, and *p53* in Merkel cell carcinoma: can they predict treatment response and clinical outcome? *Hum. Pathol.* **30**, 1367–72.

Feldman, S.R., Fleischer, A.B. Jr, McConnell, C. *et al.* (1998) Most common dermatologic problems identified by internists 1990–1994. *Arch. Intern. Med.* **158**, 726–30.

Fenig, E., Brenner, B., Njuguna, E., Katz, A., Schachter, J. and Sulkes, A. (2000) Oral etoposide for Merkel cell carcinoma in patients previously treated with intravenous etoposide. *Am. J. Clin. Oncol.* **23**, 65–7.

Frankel, D., Hanusa, B.H. and Zitalli, J.A. (1992) New primary non-melanoma skin cancer patients with a history of squamous cell carcinoma of the skin. Implications and recommendations for follow-up. *J. Am. Acad. Dermatol.* **26**, 720–6.

Fraunfelder, F.T., Zacarian, S.A., Limmer, B.L. *et al.* (1984) Results of cryotherapy for eyelid malignancies. *Am. J. Ophthalmol.* **97**, 184–8.

Fucich, L.F., Freeman, S.F., Boh, E.E. *et al.* (1999) Atypical cutaneous lymphocytic infiltrate and a role for quantitative immunohistochemistry and gene rearrangement studies. *Int. J. Dermatol.* **38**, 749–56.

Ghauri, R.R., Gunter, A.A. and Weber, R.A. (1999) Frozen section analysis in the management of skin cancers. *Ann. Plast. Surg.* **43**, 156–60.

Giles, G.G., Mark, R. and Foley, P. (1988) Incidence of non-melanocytic skin cancer treated in Australia. *Br. Med. J.* **296**, 13–17.

Goldschmidt, H. and Sherwin, W.K. (1983a) Office radiotherapy of cutaneous carcinomas. I. Radiation techniques, dose schedules, and radiation protection. *J. Dermatol. Surg. Oncol.* **9**, 31–46.

Goldschmidt, H. and Sherwin, W.K. (1983b) Office radiotherapy of cutaneous carcinomas. II. Indications in specific anatomic regions. *J. Dermatol. Surg. Oncol.* **9**, 47–76.

Golitz, L.E., Norris, D.A., Luekens, C.A. Jr, *et al.* (1980) Nevoid basal cell carcinoma syndrome. Multiple basal cell carcinomas of the palms after radiation therapy. *Arch. Dermatol.* **116**, 1159–63.

Gormley, D.P. and Hirsch, P. (1978) Aggressive basal cell carcinoma of the scalp. *Arch. Dermatol.* **114**, 782–3.

Gottlieb, S.L., Wolfe, J.T., Fox, F.E. *et al.* (1996) Treatment of cutaneous T-cell lymphoma with extra-corporal photophoresis monotherapy and in combination with recombinant interferon alfa: a ten year experience at a single institution. *J. Am. Acad. Dermatol.* **35**, 946–57.

Greenberger, J., Cassady, J.R., Jaffe, N. *et al.* (1979) Radiation therapy in patients with histiocytosis: management of diabetes insipidus and bone lesions. *Int. J. Radiat. Oncol. Biol. Phys.* **5**, 1749–55.

Griffiths, R.W. (1999) Audit of histologically incompletely excised basal cell carcinomas: recommendations for management by re-excision. *Br. J. Plast. Surg.* **52**, 24–8.

Groh, V., Gadner, H., Radaszkiewicz, T. *et al.* (1988) The phenotypic spectrum of histiocytosis X cells. *J. Invest. Dermatol.* **90**, 441–7.

Guillot, B., Favoer, C., Guilhou, J.J. *et al.* (1984) Xeroderma pigmentosum. Un case traité par l'association betacarotene – canthaxanthine et retinoide aromatique. *Arch. Dermatol. Venereol.* **111**, 65–6.

Harrist, T., Bahn, A.K., Murphy, G.F. *et al.* (1983) Histiocytosis X. *In situ* characterization of cutaneous infiltrates with monoclonal antibodies. *Am. J. Clin. Pathol.* **79**, 294–300.

Heald, P., Rook, A., Perez, M. *et al.* (1992) Treatment of erythrodermic cutaneous T-cell lymphoma with extracorporeal photochemotherapy. *J. Am. Acad. Dermatol.* **27**, 427–33.

Heald, P.W., Yan, S.L. and Edelson, R. (1994) Profound deficiency in normal circulating T-cells in erythrodermic cutaneous T cell lymphoma. *Arch. Dermatol.* **130**, 198–203.

Hermann, J.J., Kuzel, T.M., Rosen, S.T. *et al.* (1994) Proceedings of the second international symposium on cutaneous T-cell lymphoma. *J. Am. Acad. Dermatol.* **31**, 819.

Hofer, A. and Cerroni, L. (1999) Narrowband (311-nm) UV-B therapy for small plaque parapsoriasis and early-stage mycosis fungoides. *Arch. Dermatol.* **135**, 1377–80.

Holman, C.D., Armstrong, D.K., Evans, P.R. *et al.* (1984) Relationship of solar keratosis and history of skin cancer to objective measures of actinic skin damage. *Br. J. Dermatol.* **110**, 129–38.

Hoppe, R.T. (1991) Total skin electron beam therapy in the management of mycosis fungoides. *Front. Radiat. Ther. Oncol.* **25**, 80–9.

Howard, K., Charif, M., Martin, A. *et al.* (1995) Epidemiology and clinical manifestations of cutaneous T-cell lymphoma. *Hematol. Oncol. Clin. North Am.* **9**, 5–11.

Humphreys, T.R., Malhotra, R., Scharf, M.J. *et al.* (1998) Treatment of superficial basal cell carcinoma and squamous cell carcinoma *in situ* with a high-energy pulsed carbon dioxide laser. *Arch. Dermatol.* **134**, 1247–52.

Jacyk, W.K. (1999) Xeroderma pigmentosum in black South Africans. *Int. J. Dermatol.* **39**, 511–14.

Jensen, P., Hansen, S., Moller, B. *et al.* (1999) Skin cancer in kidney and heart transplant recipients and different long term immunosuppressive therapy regimens. *J. Am. Acad. Dermatol.* **40**, 177–86.

Jih, D.M., Lyle, S., Elenitsan, R. *et al.* (1999) Cytokine 15 expression in trichoepitheliomas and a subset of basal cell carcinomas suggests they originate from hair follicle stem cells. *J. Cutan. Pathol.* **26**, 113–18.

Johason, A.S., Kunala, S., Price, G.J. *et al.* (1996) Frequent clones of P53-mutated keratinocytes in normal human skin. *Proc. Natl Acad. Sci. USA* **93**, 14025–9.

Johnson, R.L., Rothman, A.L., Xie, J. *et al.* (1996a) Human homolog of *patched*, a candidate gene for the basal cell nevus syndrome. *Science* **14**, 1668–71.

Johnson, R., Staiano-Coico, L., Austin, L. *et al.* (1996b) PUVA treatment selectively induces a cell cycle block and subsequent apoptosis in human T-lymphocytes. *Photochem. Photobiol.* **65**, 566–71.

Jones, G.W., Hoppe, R.T. and Glatstein, E. (1995) Electron beam treatment for cutaneous T-cell lymphoma. *Hematol. Oncol. Clin. North Am.* **9**, 1057–76.

Joseph, M.G., Zulueta, W.P. and Kennedy, P.J. (1992) Squamous cell carcinoma of the skin of the trunk and limbs: the incidence of metastases and their outcome. *Aust. N. Z. J. Surg.* **62**, 697–701.

Khatri, M.L., Bemghazil, M., Shafi, M. *et al.* (1999) Xeroderma pigmentosum in Libya. *Int. J. Dermatol.* **38**, 520–4.

Kimonis, V.E., Goldstein, A.M., Pastakia, B. *et al.* (1997) Clinical manifestations in 105 persons with nevoid basal cell carcinoma syndrome. *Am. J. Med. Genet.* **31**, 299–308.

Knudson, A. (1985) Hereditary cancer, oncogenes and anti oncogenes. *Cancer Res.* **45**, 1437–43.

Kruger, K., Blume-Peytavi, U. and Orfanos, C.E. (1999) Basal cell carcinoma possibly originates from the outer root sheath and/or the bulge region of the vellus hair follicle. *Arch. Dermatol. Res.* **29**, 253–9.

Krunic, A.L., Viehman, G.E., Madani, S. *et al.* (1998) Microscopically controlled surgical excision combined with ultrapulse CO_2 vaporization in the management of a patient with the nevoid basal cell carcinoma syndrome. *J. Dermatol.* **25**, 10–12.

Kubler, A.C., Haase, T., Staff, C. *et al.* (1999) Photodynamic therapy of primary non-melanomatous cutaneous skin tumours of the head and neck. *Lasers Surg. Med.* **25**, 60–8.

Kuflik, E.G. and Gage, A.A. (1991) The five-year cure rate achieved by cryosurgery for skin cancer. *J. Am. Acad. Dermatol.* **24**, 1002–4.

Lahey, M. (1962) Prognosis in reticuloendotheliosis in children. *J. Pediatr.* **60**, 664–71.

Lambert, W.C., Kuo, H.R. and Lambert, M.W. (1999) Xeroderma pigmentosum. In Chu, A.C. and Edelson, R.L. (eds), *Malignant tumours of the skin*. London: Arnold, 119–37.

Lawrence, N. and Cottel, W.I. (1994) Squamous cell carcinoma of skin with perineural invasion. *J. Am. Acad. Dermatol.* **31**, 30–3.

Lear, J.T., Smith, A.G., Heagerty, A.H.M. *et al.* (1997) Truncal site and detoxifying enzyme polymorphisms significantly reduce time to presentation of further primary cutaneous basal cell carcinoma. *Carcinogenesis* **18**, 1499–503.

Le Boit, P.E., Becktead, K., Atkin, E. *et al.* (1987) Granulomatous slack skin: clonal rearrangement of the T-cell receptor beta gene is evidence for the lymphoproliferative nature of the cutaneous elastolytic disorder. *J. Invest. Dermatol.* **120**, 807–9.

Le Pivert, P. (1977) The measurement of low frequency electrical impedance as a guide to effective cryosurgery. *J. Dermatol. Surg. Oncol.* **3**, 395–7.

Levanat, S., Mubrin, M.K., Crnic, I. *et al.* (2000) Variable expression of Gorlin syndrome may reflect complexity of the signalling pathway. *Pflugers Arch.* **439**, 31–3.

Lewis, J.E. (1985) Linear basal cell epithelioma. *Int. J. Dermatol.* **24**, 124–5.

Lien, H.C., Tsai, T.F., Lee, Y.Y. *et al.* (1999) Merkel cell carcinoma and chronic arsenicism. *J. Am. Acad. Dermatol.* **41**, 641–3.

Lim, K.K., Randle, H.W., Roenig, R.K. *et al.* (1999) Linear basal cell carcinoma: report of seventeen cases and review of the presentation and treatment. *Dermatol. Surg.* **25**, 63–7.

Lindeberg, H. and Jepsen, F.L. (1983) The nevoid basal cell carcinoma syndrome. Histopathology of the basal cell tumors. *J. Cutan. Pathol.* **10**, 68–72.

Lindeberg, H., Halaburt, H. and Larsen, P.O. (1982) The naevoid basal cell carcinoma syndrome. Clinical, biochemical and radiological aspects. *J. Maxillofac. Surg.* **10**, 246–9.

Lisby, G., Reitz, M.S., Vejlsgaard, G.L. and Reitz, M.S. Jr (1992) No detection of HTLV-1 DNA in punch biopsies from patients with cutaneous T-cell lymphoma by the polymerase chain reaction. *J. Invest. Dermatol.* **98**, 417–20.

Lo Muzio, L., Nocini, P. and Bucci, P. (1999a) Early diagnosis of nevoid basal cell carcinoma syndrome. *J. Am. Dent. Assoc.* **130**, 669–74.

Lo Muzio, L., Staibano, S., Pannone, G. *et al.* (1999b) Expression of cell cycle and apoptosis-related proteins in sporadic odontogenic keratocysts and odontogenic keratocysts associated with the nevoid basal cell carcinoma syndrome. *J. Dent. Res.* **78**, 1345–53.

MacKie, R. (1998) Epidermal skin tumours. In Champion, R.H., Burton, R.H., Burns, D.A. and Breathnach, S.M. (eds), *Textbook of dermatology*, 6th edn. Oxford: Blackwell Scientific, 1651–93.

Madeleine, D. and Cather, J.C. (2000) Emerging new therapies for cutaneous T-cell lymphoma. *Dermatol. Clin.* **18**, 147–56.

Maurer, T.A., Christian, K.V., Kerschmann, R.L. *et al.* (1997) Cutaneous squamous cell carcinoma in human immunodeficiency virus-infected patients. A study of epidemiologic risk factors, human papillomavirus, and p53 expression. *Arch. Dermatol.* **133**, 577–83.

McLean, D., Haynes, H.A., McCarthy, P.I. *et al.* (1978) Cryotherapy of basal cell carcinoma by a simple method of standardized freeze-thaw cycles. *J. Dermatol. Surg. Oncol.* **4**, 175–7.

McLelland, J., Pritchard, J. and Chu, A.C. (1987) Current controversies in histiocytosis X. *Hematol. Oncol. Clin. North Am.* **1**, 147–62.

Miller, D.L. and Weinstock, M.A. (1994) Non-melanoma skin cancer in the United States: incidence. *J. Am. Acad. Dermatol.* **30**, 774–8.

Miller, R.A. and Spittle, M.F. (1982) Electron beam therapy for difficult cutaneous basal and squamous cell carcinomas. *Br. J. Dermatol.* **106**, 429–36.

Milne, J.A. (1972) *An introduction to the diagnostic histopathology of the skin*. London: Edward Arnold, 261–2.

Mittelbronn, M.A., Mullins, D.L., Ramos-Caro, F.A. *et al.* (1998) Frequency of pre-existing actinic keratosis in cutaneous squamous cell carcinoma. *Int. J. Dermatol.* **37**, 677–81.

Mohs, F. (1991) Chemosurgery: a microscopically controlled method of cancer excision. *Arch. Surg.* **42**, 279–95.

Montgomery, H. and Dorffel, J. (1932) Verruca senilis und keratoma senile. *Arch. Dermatol. Syph.* **166**, 286–9.

Munn, S. and Chu, A.C. (1998) Langerhans cell histiocytosis of the skin. *Hematol. Oncol. Clin. North Am.* **12**, 269–86.

Noodleman, F.R. and Pollack, S.V. (1986) Trauma as a possible etiologic factor in basal cell carcinoma. *J. Dermatol. Surg. Oncol.* **12**, 841–6.

Nordin, P., Larko, O. and Stenquist, B. (1997) Five-year results of curettage-cryosurgery of selected large primary basal cell carcinomas on the nose: an alternative treatment in a geographical area underserved by Mohs' surgery. *Br. J. Dermatol.* **136**, 180–3.

Nouri, K., Spencer, J.M., Taylor, J.R. *et al.* (1999) Does wound healing contribute to the eradication of basal cell carcinoma following curettage and electrodessication? *Dermatol. Surg.* **25**, 183–7; discussion 187–8.

Olson, E.A., Duvic, M., Frankel, A. *et al.* (2001) Pivotal phase III trial of two dose levels of denileukin diftitox for the treatment of cutaneous T-cell lymphoma. *J. Clin. Oncol.* **19**, 376–88.

O'Malley, S., Weitman, D., Olding, M. *et al.* (1997) Multiple neoplasms following craniospinal irradiation for medulloblastoma in a patient with nevoid basal cell carcinoma syndrome. *J. Neurosurg.* **86**, 286–8.

Ong , C.S., Keogh, A.M., Kossaro, S. *et al.* (1999) Skin cancer in Australian heart transplant recipients. *J. Am. Acad. Dermatol.* **40**, 27–34.

Osband, M., Lipton, J.M., Lavin, P. *et al.* (1981) Histiocytosis X. Demonstration of abnormal immunity, T-cell histamine H2-receptor deficiency and successful treatment with thymic extract. *N. Engl. J. Med.* **304**, 146–53.

Ostrow, R.R., Manias, D., Mitchell, A.J. *et al.* (1987) Epidermodysplasia verruciformis. *Arch. Dermatol.* **123**, 1511–16.

Ott, M.J., Tanabe, K.K. and Gadd, M.A. (1999) Multimodality management of Merkel cell carcinoma. *Arch. Surg.* **134**, 388–92.

Pancake, B.A., Zucker-Franklin, D., Coutavas, E.E. (1995) The cutaneous T-cell lymphoma, mycosis fungoides, is a human T-cell lymphotrophic virus-associated disease. *J. Clin. Invest.* **95**, 547.

Parry, E.J., Stevens, S.R., Gilliam, A.C. *et al.* (1999) Management of cutaneous lymphomas using a multidisciplinary approach. *Arch. Dermatol.* **135**, 907–11.

Penn, I. and First, M.R. (1999) Merkel's cell carcinoma in organ recipients: report of 41 cases. *Transplantation* **68**, 1717–21.

Pfister, H. (1987) Human papilloma virus and impaired immunity vs epidermodysplasia verruciformis. *Arch. Dermatol.* **123**, 1469–70.

Pieceall, W.E., Goldberg, L.H. and Ananthaswarry, H.N. (1991) Presence of human papilloma virus type 16 DNA sequences in human non-melanoma skin cancers. *J. Invest. Dermatol.* **97**, 880–4.

Plettenberg, H., Stege, H. and Megahed, M. (1999) Ultraviolet cutaneous T-cell lymphoma. *J. Am. Acad. Dermatol.* **41**, 47–50.

Ramsay, D., Meller, J.A. and Zackheim, H.S. (1995) Topical treatment of early cutaneous T-cell lymphoma. *Hematol. Oncol. Clin. North Am.* **9**, 1031–55.

Ratner, D., Nelson, B.R., Brown, M.D. and Johnson, T.M. (1993) Merkel cell carcinoma. *J. Am. Acad. Dermatol.* **29**(2, Pt 1), 143–56.

Reed, W., Landing, B., Sugarman, G. *et al.* (1969) Xeroderma pigmentosum: clinical and laboratory investigations of its basic defect. *J. Am. Med. Assoc.* **207**, 2073–9.

Reisner, K. and Haase, W. (1990) Electron beam therapy of primary tumors of the skin. *Radiol. Med. (Torino)* **80**(4, suppl. 1), 114–15.

Riddle, R.O., Johnson, R.L., Laufer, E. *et al.* (1993) Sonic hedgehog mediates the polarising activity of the ZPA. *Cell* **75**, 1401–16.

Robinson, J.K. (1987) Risk of developing another basal cell carcinoma. *Cancer* **60**, 118–20.

Roelink, H., Porter, J.A., Chiang, C. *et al.* (1995) Floor plate and motor neuron induction by different concentrations of the amino-terminal cleavage product of sonic hedgehog autoproteolysis. *Cell* **81**, 445–55.

Rook, A.H., Suchin, K.R., Kao, D.M.F. *et al.* (1999) Photopheresis: clinical applications and mechanism of action. *J. Invest. Dermatol. Symp. Proc.* **4**, 85–90.

Rosen, S.T. and Foss, F.M. (1995) Chemotherapy for mycosis fungoides and the Sézary syndrome. *Hematol. Oncol. Clin. North Am.* **9**, 1109–16.

Rowe, D.E., Carroll, R.J. and Day, C.L. Jr (1992) Prognostic factors for local recurrence, metastasis, and survival rates in squamous cell carcinoma of the skin, ear, and lip. Implications for treatment modality selection. *J. Am. Acad. Dermatol.* **26**, 976–90.

Russell Jones, R.R. and Whittaker, S. (1999) T-cell receptor gene analysis in the diagnosis of Sézary syndrome. *J. Am. Acad. Dermatol.* **41**, 254–9.

Sadek, H., Azli, N., Wendling, J.L. *et al.* (1990) Treatment of advanced squamous cell carcinoma of the skin with cisplatin 5-fluorouracil and bleomycin. *Cancer* **66**, 1692–6.

Saed, G., Fivenson, D.P., Naidu, T. *et al.* (1994) Mycosis fungoides exhibits a Th1-type cell mediated cytokine profile, whereas, Sézary syndrome expresses a Th1-type profile. *J. Invest. Dermatol.* **103**, 29–33.

Salasche, S.J. (2000) Epidemiology of actinic keratoses and squamous cell carcinoma. *J. Am. Acad. Dermatol.* **42**, 4–7.

Sanchez, J.L. and Ackerman, A.B. (1979) The patch stage of mycosis fungoides. *Am. J. Dermatopathol.* **1**, 5–11.

Schlagbauer-Wadl, H., Klosner, G. and Heere-Ress, E. (2000) Bcl-2 antisense oligonucleotides (G3139) inhibit Merkel cell carcinoma growth in SCID mice. *J. Invest. Dermatol.* **114**, 725–730.

Scotto, J., Fears, T.R. and Fraumeni, J.F. Jr (1983) Incidence of non-melanoma skin cancer in the United States. Publication No. 83-2433. Bethesda, Md: National Institutes of Health.

Scotto, J., Cotton, G., Urbach, F., Berger, D. and Fears, T. (1988) Biologically effective ultraviolet radiation: surface measurements in the United States, 1974 to 1985. *Science* **239**, 762–4.

Shamanin, V., Zur Hausen, H., Lavergne, D. *et al.* (1996) Human papillomavirus infections in non-melanoma skin cancers from renal transplant recipients and non-immunosuppressed patients. *J. Natl Cancer Inst.* **88**, 802–11.

Sinha, A.A. and Heald, P. (1998) Advances in the management of cutaneous T-cell lymphoma. *Dermatol. Clin.* **16**, 301–11.

Smith, S.P. and Grande, D.J. (1991) Basal cell carcinoma recurring after radiotherapy: a unique, difficult treatment subclass of recurrent basal cell carcinoma. *J. Dermatol. Surg. Oncol.* **17**, 26–30.

Smoller, B.R., Bishop, K., Glusac, E., Kim, Y.H. and Hendrickson, M. (1995) Reassessment of histological parameters in the diagnosis of mycosis fungoides. *Am. J. Surg. Pathol.* **19**, 1423–30.

Smoller, B.R., Detwiler, S.P., Kohler, S. *et al.* (1998) Role of histology in providing prognostic information in mycosis fungoides. *J. Cutan. Pathol.* **25**, 311.

Somos, S., Farkas, B. and Schneider, I. (1999) Cancer protection in xeroderma pigmentosum variant (XP-V). *Anticancer Res.* **3**, 2195–9.

Spiller, W.F. and Spiller, R.F. (1984) Treatment of basal cell epithelioma by curettage and electro dessication. *J. Am. Acad. Dermatol.* **11**, 808–14.

Stadler, R., Otte, H.-G., Luger, T. *et al.* (1998) Prospective randomized multicenter clinical trial on the use of Interferon alpha-2a plus PUVA Acitretin versus Interferon alpha-2a plus PUVA in patients with cutaneous T-cell lymphoma stages I and II. *Blood* **92**, 3578–81.

Stephens, F.O. and Harker, G.J.S. (1979) The use of intra-arterial chemotherapy for treatment of malignant skin neoplasms. *Australas. J. Dermatol.* **20**, 99–107.

Strange, P.R. and Langm, P.G. Jr. (1992) Long-term management of basal cell nevus syndrome with topical tretinoin and 5-fluorouracil. *J. Am. Acad. Dermatol.* **27**, 842–5.

Sugerman, G. and Bigby, M. (2000) Preliminary function analysis of human epidermal T-cells. *Arch. Dermatol. Res.* **292**, 9–15.

Tan, R., Butterworth, C.M., McLaughin, H. *et al.* (1974) Mycosis fungoides – a disease of antigen persistence. *Br. J. Dermatol.* **91**, 607–16.

Telfer, N.R., Colver, G. and Bowers, P.W. (1999) Guidelines for the management of basal cell carcinoma. *Br. J. Dermatol.* **141**, 415–23.

Theiler, R., Hubscher, E., Wagenhauser, F.J., Panizzon, R. and Michel, B. (1993) Diffuse idiopathic skeletal hyperostosis (DISH) and pseudo-coxarthritis following long-term etretinate therapy. *Schweiz. Med. Wochenschr.* **123**, 649–53.

Thomsen, K., Hammar, H., Molin, L. *et al.* (1989) Retinoids plus PUVA (REPUVA) in mycosis fungoides, plaque stage. *Acta Derm. Venereol.* **69**, 536–8.

Tope, W.D. and Sanguexa, O.P. (1994) Merkel cell carcinoma. Histopathology, immunohistochemistry, and cytogenetic analysis. *J. Dermatol. Surg. Oncol.* **20**, 648–52; quiz 653–4.

Voog, E., Biron, P., Martin, J.P. *et al.* (1999) Chemotherapy for patients with locally advanced or metastatic Merkel cell carcinoma. *Cancer* **85**, 2589–95.

Vortmeyer, A.O., Merino, M.J., Boni, R. *et al.* (1998) Genetic changes associated with primary Merkel cell carcinoma. *Am. J. Clin. Pathol.* **109**, 565–70.

Vowels, B.R., Cassin, M., Vonderheid, E.C. *et al.* (1992) Aberrant cytokine production by Sézary syndrome patients: cytokine secretion pattern resembles murine Th2 cells. *J. Invest. Dermatol.* **99**, 90–8.

Vowels, B.R., Lessin, S.R., Cassin, M. *et al.* (1994) Th2 cytokine mRNA expression in skin in cutaneous T cell lymphoma. *J. Invest. Dermatol.* **103**, 29–32.

Wallberg, P. and Skog, E. (1991) The incidence of basal cell carcinoma in an area of Stockholm county during the period 1971–1980. *Acta Derm. Venereol. (Stockh.)* **71**, 134–7.

Warrell, R.P., Franke, S.R.I., Miller, W.H. *et al.* (1991) Differentiation therapy of acute promyelocytic leukaemia with tretinoin (all trans-retinoic acid). *N. Engl. J. Med.* **324**, 1385.

Wasserberg, N., Schachter, J., Fenig, E. *et al.* (2000) Applicability of the sentinel node technique to Merkel cell carcinoma. *Dermatol. Surg.* **26**, 138–41.

Wicking, C., Shanley, S. and Smyth, I. (1997) Most germ-line mutations in the nevoid basal cell carcinoma syndrome lead to a premature termination of the PATCHED protein, and no genotype-phenotype correlations are evident. *Am. J. Hum. Genet.* **60**, 21–6.

Wickramasinghe, L., Hindson, T.C. and Wacks, M. (1989) Treatment of neoplastic skin lesions with interferon. *J. Am. Acad. Dermatol.* **204**, 71–4.

Willemze, R. and Meijer, C.L. (1999) EORTC Classification for primary cutaneous lymphomas: the best guide to good clinical management. *Am. J. Dermatopathol.* **21**, 265–73.

Willemze, R., Kerl, H., Sterry, W. *et al.* (1997) EORTC classification of primary cutaneous lymphomas: a proposal from the Cutaneous Lymphoma Study Group of the European Organization for Research and Treatment of Cancer. *Blood* **90**, 354–71.

Willman, C.L., Busque, L., Griffith, B.B. *et al.* (1994) Langerhans cell histiocytosis (histiocytosis X): a clonal proliferative disorder. *N. Engl. J. Med.* **331**, 154–60.

Wilson, L.D., Quiros, P.A., Kolenik, S.A. *et al.* (1996) Additional courses of total skin electron beam therapy in the treatment of patients with recurrent cutaneous T-cell lymphoma. *J. Am. Acad. Dermatol.* **35**, 69–73.

Wollina, U. (2000) Treatment of relapsing of recalcitrant cutaneous T-cell lymphoma with pegylated liposomal doxorubicin. *J. Am. Acad. Dermatol.* **42**, 40–60.

Wolter, M., Reifenberger, J., Sommer, C. *et al.* (1997) Mutations in the human homologue of the *Drosophila* segment polarity gene patched (PTCH) in sporadic basal cell carcinomas of the skin and primitive neuroectodermal tumors of the central nervous system. *Cancer Res.* **57**, 2581–5.

Xie, J., Murone, M., Luoh, S.M. *et al.* (1998) Activating Smoothened mutations in sporadic basal-cell carcinoma. *Nature* **391**, 90–2.

Yansos, V.A., Conrad, N., Zabawski, E. *et al.* (1999) Incipient intraepidermal cutaneous squamous cell carcinoma: a proposal for reclassifying and grading solar (actinic) keratoses. *Semin. Cutan. Med. Surg.* **18**, 3–14.

Yeh, S. (1973) Skin cancer in chronic aresenicism. *Hum. Pathol.* **4**, 469–85.

Yeh, S., How, S.W. and Lin, C.S. (1986) Arsenic cancer of the skin. Histological study with special reference to Bowen's disease. *Cancer* **21**, 312–39.

Yu, R., Morris, J.F., Pritchard, J. *et al.* (1992) Defective alloantigen presenting capacity of Langerhans cell histiocytosis cells. *Arch. Dis. Child.* **67**, 1370–2.

Yu, R., Chu, C., Buluwela, L. *et al.* (1994) Clonal proliferation of Langerhans cells in Langerhans cell histiocytosis. *Lancet* **343**, 767–8.

Yutsudo, M., Tangigaki, T., Kanda, R. *et al.* (1994) Involvement of human papilloma virus type 20 in epidermodysplasia verruciformis skin carcinogenesis. *J. Clin. Microbiol.* **32**, 1076–8.

Zackheim, H.S., Kashani-Sabet, M. and Hwang, S.T. (1996) Low dose methotrexate to treat erythrodermic cutaneous T-cell lymphoma: results in twenty-nine patients. *J. Am. Acad. Dermatol.* **34**, 626–31.

Zackheim, H.S., Kashani-Sabet, M. and Amin, S. (1998) Topical corticosteroids for mycosis fungoides. *Arch. Dermatol.* **134**, 949–54.

Ziegler, A., Jonason, A.S., Leffell, D.J. *et al.* (1994) Sunburn and p53 in the onset of skin cancer. *Nature* **372**, 773–6.

39

Malignant melanoma

JAMES F. SPICER AND MARTIN E. GORE

INTRODUCTION

Malignant melanoma arises from melanocytes and makes up 2 per cent of all cancers. Five thousand cases are diagnosed in the UK each year (CRC, 1999a). In recent decades the incidence of melanoma has risen faster than that of any other malignancy, except lung cancer in women, increasing at 3–7 per cent per year in white populations (Rees, 1996). Incidence in the UK rose by 84 per cent from 1980 to 1989, and in 1995 was 6.7 and 8.5 per 100 000 in males and females, respectively. This amounts to a lifetime risk in excess of 1 in 200. Reasons for the increasing frequency of melanoma may include changes in recreational sun exposure, a rise in ambient solar radiation resulting from stratospheric ozone depletion and increasing detection of early disease. Another possible factor to explain the dramatic rise in incidence may be the increasing recognition and removal of an indolent non-metastasizing but invasive form of melanoma (Rees, 1996).

There were 1378 deaths from cutaneous melanoma in England and Wales during 1997. Mortality has not risen as fast as incidence, and has peaked among Scottish women (MacKie *et al.*, 1997). A similar trend is seen worldwide, mortality in the USA rising much less dramatically than incidence (Fig. 39.1), and decreasing among Australian women (Giles *et al.*, 1996). A review of histopathology over a 20-year period did not find a significant decrease in the average thickness of invasive malignant melanoma (MacKie *et al.*, 1997). This suggests that the discrepancy between trends in incidence and mortality cannot be explained entirely by early detection of melanoma of lesser thickness.

Five-year all-stage survival for patients diagnosed in the UK in the period 1986–90 was 79 per cent. This represents an improvement of 20 per cent over those diagnosed between 1971 and 1975 (CRC, 1999b). However, the largest contribution to these encouraging average figures is from the great majority of newly diagnosed melanomas which are less than 0.75 mm thick, and the outlook for advanced disease is much poorer.

AETIOLOGY

It seems likely that both sun exposure and genetic predisposition have important aetiological roles in melanoma (Table 39.1).

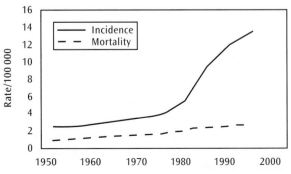

Figure 39.1 *Melanoma incidence and mortality in the USA (redrawn from Rigel* et al.*, 1996).*

Table 39.1 *Risk factors for malignant melanoma*

Sun exposure	History of severe sunburn, propensity to burn
	Duration and intensity of exposure aged <20 years
Phenotype	Pale skin, freckling
	Number common naevi >2 mm; >4 clinically atypical naevi
	Giant pigmented hairy naevus
Medical history	Changing mole
	Non-melanoma skin cancer
	Previous melanoma
Family history	At least 2 first-degree relatives with melanoma

Sun exposure

Evidence for the role of sunlight is largely epidemiological (Boyle *et al.*, 1995). Melanoma is 12 times more common in white individuals, and six times more common in those of hispanic origin, than in black-skinned races living the same lifestyle. Those of European descent living in Australia have a significantly greater risk of melanoma than those remaining in northern Europe, and residence in more equatorial latitudes in early life is associated with increased risk of melanoma (Weinstock *et al.*, 1989). Sun exposure during childhood is the most important non-genetic risk factor. As already indicated, the influence of climate may have been exacerbated recently by a rise in recreational sun exposure and by ozone depletion. The disease occurs more commonly on sun-exposed parts of the body, and the ear is the site of highest incidence per unit area. However, the link between site of lesion and sun exposure is less straightforward than for other cutaneous malignancies. The proposed role for incident light receives support from animal models (Noonan *et al.*, 2001) and from the observation that psoralen and ultraviolet A (PUVA) photochemotherapy used in the treatment of psoriasis is associated with a five times relative risk of melanoma approximately 15 years after treatment (Stern *et al.*, 1997).

Several observations emphasize the complexity of the relationship between sun exposure and melanoma. The disease is relatively common in younger patients without a long cumulative exposure, and is more common among indoor than outdoor workers in the same socio-economic class. Most melanomas occur on anatomical sites which are only intermittently exposed. Case-control studies also provide conflicting evidence of sunscreen efficacy, some even suggesting sunscreen use is associated with increased risk (English *et al.*, 1997). However, these sunscreen studies are very susceptible to confounding effects because the sun-seeking and sun-sensitive are more likely to use sunscreens (Finkel, 1998).

An overview of 29 epidemiological studies suggests an association between melanoma and intermittent sun exposure, a model which accommodates the apparently conflicting observations outlined above (Elwood and Jopson, 1997). An association with sunburn *per se* has been questioned (Autier *et al.*, 1998), and sunburn may be just a marker of both intermittent intense sun exposure and genetic susceptibility (Finkel, 1998). Despite growing acceptance of this intermittent exposure model, there remain uncertainties. The damaging wavelength in this context may or may not be ultraviolet, and the mechanisms of tumorigenesis are not understood and may include both direct DNA damage and cutaneous immuno-suppression. There is some concern that the marketing of sunscreens promotes increased sun exposure, and randomized evidence suggests that rather than reducing exposure, sunscreen use increases time spent in the sun (Autier *et al.*, 1999). Definitive evidence of the effectiveness of sunscreens is awaited, but protective sun-avoidance measures should be encouraged in the meantime.

Genetics

There is a strong family history in 5–7 per cent of melanoma patients (Lindor and Greene, 1998). Many of these patients have atypical mole syndrome (AMS), with a large number of naevi, some of atypical appearance and with dysplastic histological features. The presence of four or more atypical moles, compared with none, is associated with a relative risk for melanoma of 29 (Bataille *et al.*, 1996). Familial cases also occur in the absence of atypical moles. Studies of melanoma-prone kindreds suggest linkage to at least three independent loci, namely 9p21–22, 1q36 and 6p21–23 (Castellano and Parmiani, 1999). Linkage to the 9p region is seen in about 50 per cent of families, and genetic abnormalities in a large proportion of sporadic melanomas also map to this locus. The tumour suppressor gene *INK4a* maps to 9p21–22, and inactivating germline mutations have been detected in this gene which affect one or both of alternative transcripts encoding p16 and p14ARF. p16 is a cyclin-dependent kinase inhibitor, and p14ARF inhibits cell cycle progression by mechanisms which include stabilization of p53. The distinct locus *INK4b* at 9p encodes p15, another cyclin-dependent kinase inhibitor. Specific genes mutated at the 1p and 6p loci have not yet been identified, but the site on chromosome 1p is associated with AMS rather than with melanoma alone.

PREVENTION

Primary prevention

Recommendations have been made to ensure that potentially harmful sun exposure is minimized. Use of protective clothing, shade and sunscreen with a sun protection factor (SPF) of at least 15 are important, especially in early childhood (Donawho and Wolf, 1996). There is some case-control data linking the use of sunbeds and sunlamps with an increased risk of melanoma (Walter *et al.*, 1990; Westerdahl *et al.*, 2000).

Although 20 per cent of malignant melanomas arise in association with apparently benign moles (Marks *et al.*, 1990) there is no role for the prophylactic removal of benign naevi, as the risk of malignant progression in an individual mole is extremely small.

Secondary prevention

It is likely that the development of metastatic melanoma is preceded by a radial growth phase, of variable duration, which has no metastatic potential. Screening for this lesion allows early diagnosis, which should be of survival benefit as tumours in this phase tend to be thin. Individuals at very significantly increased risk who may benefit from screening include those with giant pigmented hairy naevus (greater than 20 cm in diameter, or 5 per cent of body surface area) or a strong family history of melanoma. Referral of these patients to a specialist dermatology or cancer genetics clinic is warranted for counselling, investigation and follow-up. Patients with AMS or a previous history of melanoma are at moderately increased risk, and counselling about risk and the teaching of self-examination is appropriate. There is case-control evidence for a reduction in mortality in those who practice self-examination (Berwick *et al.*, 1996). A large English and Scottish pilot screening programme was instituted over a period of 2 years in regions of England and Scotland covering a population of 3.6 million people. This public health education programme resulted in a fall in the proportion of thick tumours amongst Scottish women, but not men (Melia *et al.*, 1995). Additional pigmented lesion clinics were set up to cope with the increased number of patients referred by general practitioners during the period of the study.

DIAGNOSIS AND PATHOLOGY

Signs and symptoms

For the purposes of primary care and public education four major clinical characteristic features of malignant melanoma have been described, known as the 'ABCD' of melanoma; Asymmetry, Border irregularity, Colour variation and Diameter greater than 6 mm (NIH, 1992). Other features suggesting the diagnosis are inflammation and spontaneous bleeding. It may be argued that any significant change in a pigmented lesion is an indication for excision biopsy.

Table 39.2 *Anatomical distribution of melanoma according to sex (CRC, 1995)*

	Male (%)	Female (%)
Head and neck	25	14
Upper limb	17	18
Trunk	37	14
Lower limb	21	53

The typical location of melanoma shows marked differences between the sexes (Table 39.2), occurring in many males on the trunk and on the legs in the majority of females.

Patterns of growth

Classification according to macroscopic appearance is useful because of differences in the natural history of these lesions. Superficial spreading melanoma makes up 70 per cent of the total. These often arise as a dark area in a pre-existing junctional naevus. Progression is slow at first, the surface subsequently becoming raised and irregular with indentation of the perimeter. Nodular melanomas (20 per cent) are usually darker than superficial spreading tumours (blue/black, occasionally amelanotic), uniform in colour, and often dome-shaped. They usually arise from apparently normal skin. Lentigo maligna melanoma (5 per cent) generally occurs on the face or neck of older patients. This lesion is always associated with pathological features of sun damage to adjacent skin. Progression may be more indolent in the elderly and overall survival is much higher than other growth patterns. Acral lentiginous melanoma is also relatively uncommon (5 per cent), but occurs as a higher proportion amongst dark-skinned older patients. Palms, soles of the feet and nailbeds are affected. These are generally large, flat and fast-growing. Malignant melanoma also occurs on mucosal surfaces. Intra-ocular melanoma will be discussed separately.

Histopathology

A description of the detailed histopathological features of melanoma is beyond the scope of this discussion. Pathology reporting of an excised primary lesion should include margins of excision, Breslow thickness, Clark's level, growth pattern and presence or absence of ulceration, lymphocytic infiltrate, mitotic count and vascular or lymphatic invasion. Special stains in general use include S100, which is present on almost all melanomas but not specific, and HMB45, which is more specific but less sensitive for melanoma. Both radial and vertical growth phases are recognized, although the distinction is not always clear in individual cases. The radial phase has a better prognosis but is believed to progress with variable delay to a vertical growth phase.

STAGING AND PROGNOSIS

Tumour stage at presentation is the most significant determinant of prognosis (Fig. 39.2). The American Joint Committee on Cancer (AJCC) staging classification has recently been revised (Balch *et al.*, 2001). Stage grouping is compared with thickness and TNM staging in Table 39.3.

Multivariate analysis suggests several major contributors to prognosis in early stage disease. Microstage is best categorized by Breslow thickness, which is defined as the total vertical height of the invasive lesion. It defines subgroups with significantly different survivals. Correlation between Breslow thickness and survival is better than Clark's level, which classifies primary tumours according to histological depth of dermal invasion. Ulceration is a very significant prognostic indicator, as recognized by the recent staging classification review (Balch *et al.*, 2001). Stage I and II disease with and without ulceration is associated with 50 per cent and 79 per cent 10-year survival, respectively (Balch, 1992). Vascular invasion and lymphocytic infiltration are also significant predictors of prognosis.

Molecular markers differentially expressed in advanced disease include integrins and CD44 splice variants, which are associated with a highly metastatic phenotype in melanoma cell lines (De Wit *et al.*, 1996). The melanosomal proteins MART1, gp100 and tyrosinase have been identified as antigens important in the recognition of melanoma cells by tumour-infiltrating lymphocytes. Reverse transcriptase polymerase chain reaction (RT-PCR) detection of tyrosinase, MAGE3 and MART1 mRNA has been used in excised sentinel lymph nodes to increase the sensitivity of diagnosis of regional lymph-node disease. In addition, circulating melanocytes are detectable using this method (Hoon *et al.*, 1995), although the prognostic significance of this finding remains uncertain.

Other adverse prognostic influences in localized melanoma include increased age, male sex, growth pattern and primary anatomical site (head, neck and trunk worse than limb). There is no good evidence that pregnancy, hormone replacement therapy and oral contraceptives affect outcome.

The most common first site of relapsed disease is the regional lymph-node basin. The number of involved nodes correlates with survival (Morton *et al.*, 1991). Ninety-nine per cent of clinically detectable distant metastases occur at the following sites, in descending order of frequency: skin, subcutaneous tissue and lymph nodes; lung; liver; brain; bone; bowel (Balch and Milton, 1985). In patients with distant metastases, soft-tissue disease,

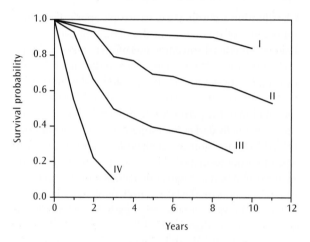

Figure 39.2 *Survival curves by AJCC stage (redrawn from Ketcham and Balch, 1985).*

Table 39.3 *American Joint Committee on Cancer (AJCC) staging (Balch* et al.*, 2001)*

Thickness or metastasis	Ulceration	Stage grouping	TNM		
In-situ melanoma		0	T_{IS}	N0	M0
1.0 mm or less	No	IA	T1a	N0	M0
	Yes	IB	T1b	N0	M0
1.01–2.0 mm	No	IB	T2a	N0	M0
	Yes	IIA	T2b	N0	M0
2.01–4.0 mm	No	IIA	T3a	N0	M0
	Yes	IIB	T3b	N0	M0
>4.0 mm	No	IIB	T4a	N0	M0
	Yes	IIC	T4b	N0	M0
1 node		III	Any T	N1	M0
2–3 nodes		III	Any T	N2	M0
4 or more nodes		III	Any T	N3	M0
Distant metastasis		IV	Any T	Any N	M1

Nodal metastases are further classified as 'a' (micrometastatic) or 'b' (clinically detectable, or extracapsular extension). Distant metastases are designated 'a' (distant skin, subcutaneous or nodal), 'b' (lung) or 'c' (all other visceral sites, or elevated LDH).

single visceral metastasis, normal serum lactate dehydrogenase (LDH) and normal albumin level are all favourable factors (Eton *et al.*, 1998).

Staging investigations for patients with moderate or high risk of systemic disease (AJCC stages IIB, III) should include full blood count, biochemistry including liver enzymes, chest X-ray and ultrasound of the liver. A bone scan is only indicated if symptoms suggestive of bony metastases are present. The role of sentinel lymph-node biopsy in stage II disease is rapidly gaining acceptance and is discussed later.

SURGICAL MANAGEMENT OF PRIMARY TUMOUR

Full-thickness biopsy is essential for microstaging, and shave biopsy is contraindicated in suspected melanoma (Ball and Thomas, 1995). Excision is preferred but incision or punch biopsies may be considered if the surgical field is limited by anatomy, as may occur on the face. There is no evidence that incision promotes seeding of melanoma cells. The initial excision should be elliptical with minimal margins of about 2 mm. A subsequent re-excision with wider margins is required if a diagnosis of melanoma is confirmed.

The margin of re-excision depends upon thickness of the lesion. A 1 cm margin is adequate for primary tumours of 0.75 mm or less; 2 cm margins are considered necessary for lesions between 0.75 and 1.9 mm. There is no indication for the traditional wider margins of excision for melanomas less than 2 mm thick, which are not associated with any improvement in local or distant recurrence rates or survival (Veronesi *et al.*, 1988). However, wider excisions increase the incidence of skin grafting, which is both a costly and morbid procedure. There is an ongoing UK Melanoma Study Group/British Association of Plastic Surgeons trial comparing 1 and 3 cm excision margins for tumours thicker than 2 mm.

Primary closure is often achievable, and where it is not, the increasing use of cutaneous flaps has resulted in a decreased need for skin grafts. Primary melanomas at some sites require special consideration. For example, subungual melanomas are treated by amputation, usually at the distal interphalangeal joint, and in many head and neck primaries a conservative approach is dictated by the anatomy.

SURGICAL MANAGEMENT OF REGIONAL NODES

Therapeutic lymph-node dissection

This procedure is always indicated in cases of confirmed regional lymph-node involvement in the absence of distant metastases. The number of involved nodes correlates with outcome in melanoma (Morton *et al.*, 1991). Fine-needle aspiration cytology with immunocytochemistry using antibodies such as S100 is diagnostically accurate when nodal metastases are suspected, but clinical findings are equivocal. Open biopsy is contraindicated because it compromises the efficacy of subsequent lymph-node dissection. Thus, in a patient with suspected lymph-node involvement, the initial investigation is always fine-needle aspiration cytology and not lymph-node excision biopsy.

There is controversy over whether patients with clinically involved superficial groin nodes should undergo a superficial dissection alone or an *en bloc* dissection, including external iliac and obturator nodes (Fraker, 1997). In a conservative approach, patients first undergo superficial inguinal dissection and then those with a histologically positive Cloquet's node at the junction of deep and superficial groups can proceed to a deep dissection. However, some argue for the more aggressive deep as well as superficial inguinal dissection for all patients with clinically involved groin nodes. Overall, patients with either superficial inguinal or deep groin lymph-node involvement have a 39 per cent and 20 per cent disease-free survival rate at 5 years, respectively (Karakousis *et al.*, 1991). Complete dissection to include level III nodes medial to pectoralis minor is indicated for axilliary involvement. Lymphatic drainage of the head and neck is unpredictable and lymphoscintigraphy may be used to identify involved nodal groups. There are no trial data comparing radical with modified neck dissection in melanoma, but the radical approach is thought preferable, with reference to data available for squamous cell carcinoma. The only significant complication of lymphadenectomy is limb oedema, which is much more common in the lower limb, especially in patients who have had an ilioinguinal block dissection (26 per cent in one series), but may even occur following sentinel biopsy.

Elective lymph-node dissection

The majority of melanomas develop secondary spread via the lymphatics and the most common site of first relapse is the locoregional lymph-node basin. The practice of elective lymph node dissection (ELND) was developed because of this, and involves lymphadenectomy in the absence of evidence for regional lymph node involvement. Two large randomized trials comparing ELND with observation showed no survival advantage (Veronesi *et al.*, 1977; Balch *et al.*, 1996). Retrospective analysis of the later of these two studies suggested that patients younger than 60 benefited, while those older than 60 had a reduced survival. A WHO study comparing immediate ELND with dissection delayed until detection of clinically apparent lymph-node metastases also showed no survival benefit for ELND (Cascinelli *et al.*, 1998). There is currently no role for ELND outside a clinical trial. Only one-third of patients undergoing ELND were found to have occult disease in the operative specimen, and so the majority underwent surgery without any likelihood of benefit. Lymphoscintigraphy and sentinel lymph-node biopsy may prove to be useful in identifying those with occult nodal metastases.

Sentinel lymph-node biopsy

Recognition of nodal spread is important because, as described above, some patients presenting with clinically negative lymph nodes in fact have occult regional lymph-node metastases. Accurate staging by determining true nodal metastatic status in patients without clinically obvious lymphatic spread identifies patients with thin primary lesions who have a relatively poor prognosis and may benefit from therapeutic lymph-node dissection and adjuvant treatment (McMasters et al., 2001). It also allows identification of a patient group that is unlikely to relapse and should not be exposed to the toxicity of systemic therapy. Intra-operative intra-dermal injection of blue dye and radiolabelled colloid allows the tracing of lymphatic channels to a sentinel lymph node (SLN), which is the first node in the regional lymphatic basin into which the primary site drains. The SLN can be identified in close to 100 per cent of cases, and the 3-year disease-free survival for patients with negative and positive SLNs is 88.5 per cent and 55.8 per cent ($P < 0.0001$), respectively (Gershenwald et al., 1999). A detailed histopathological analysis consisting of haematoxylin and eosin staining, with the use of S100 and HMB45 immunostains in equivocal cases, can be concentrated on this small specimen. RT-PCR may also have a role as it can detect expression of the melanoma-specific MAGE3, MART1 and tyrosinase in 36 per cent of patients with histopathologically negative SLNs (Bostick et al., 1999), and this group has been found to have a significantly increased risk of relapse. SLN biopsy is a minor surgical procedure, often performed in an outpatient setting. The false-negative rate compared with subsequent elective lymph node dissection as gold standard was only 0.7 per cent in one study (Morton et al., 1992).

Occult primary

Occasionally patients present with melanoma metastatic to lymph nodes without a detectable primary lesion. One-third of these patients have a history of previous non-diagnostic treatment for a pigmented lesion. In the case of cervical lymphadenopathy, a careful examination of the scalp and eyes is necessary and a mucosal melanoma of the head and neck region needs to be excluded. Whichever nodal group is involved, surgical treatment of the nodes is as outlined above, regardless of an inability to detect the primary tumour. Long-term survival is similar to stage-matched patients with known primary (Milton et al., 1977).

ADJUVANT TREATMENT

Patients with thick primary lesions, in-transit metastases or involved nodes are at high risk of relapse. The survival of patients with metastatic disease is poor and is not improved by any currently available treatments, therefore there is currently considerable interest in the development of successful adjuvant therapies.

Local adjuvant treatment

Regional modalities have not proved successful because they do not prevent patients from developing systemic disease. Isolated limb perfusion, a technique used in recurrent local disease and described below, is not useful in the adjuvant setting as it does not improve overall survival, although there is a small benefit in terms of disease-free survival (Koops et al., 1998). Radiotherapy, discussed more fully later, has been used in the adjuvant setting in both cutaneous and mucosal melanomas of the head and neck region, although no randomized evidence of its efficacy is available.

Cytotoxic chemotherapy and non-specific immune stimulants

Randomized trials with untreated control arms of single-agent chemotherapy using dacarbazine (DTIC), nitrosureas, vinca alkaloids, cisplatin and paclitaxel have failed to show any consistent survival benefit (Lee et al., 1995). Combination chemotherapy, non-specific immune stimulants (such as BCG, Corynebacterium parvum, transfer factor and levamisole), and chemo-immunotherapy regimes (such as DTIC plus BCG) have proved equally ineffective. A randomized trial involving high-dose chemotherapy with autologous bone-marrow transplantation has also been performed in node-positive melanoma, but no benefit was demonstrated (Meisenberg et al., 1993).

Neoadjuvant chemo-immunotherapy does have potential utility for shrinking the primary tumour prior to surgery, and for assessing in vivo sensitivity, but is applicable to bulky node-positive disease only. Good response rates have been seen in a phase II study of preoperative combination chemotherapy with cisplatin, vinblastine, DTIC with interleukin-2 (IL-2) and interferon-α (IFNα) (Buzaid et al., 1998). This strategy and regimen has the potential of being the experimental arm of a randomized controlled trial.

Interferons and other cytokines

Trials of IFNα in the adjuvant setting were initially stimulated by promising response rates seen in metastatic disease. A number of adjuvant therapy trials can be criticized for being underpowered and including

Table 39.4 *Completed randomized comparisons of adjuvant interferon with observation*

	n	Treatment	Result	*P*
Creagan 1995 (II, III) (NCCTG)	262	HD sc 3 months	DFS 10.8–17 months	Trend
Kirkwood 1996 (<4 mm, III) (ECOG 1684)	270	HD i.v. then MD sc 1 yr	DFS	0.002
			5 yr OS 26–37%	0.024
			MS 2.8–3.8 yr	0.02
Grob 1998 (>1.5 mm) (French)	499	LD sc 1 yr	4 yr DFS 53–60%	0.04
Pehamberger 1998 (>3.5 mm) (Austrian)	311	LD sc	DFS	<0.02
Kirkwood 2000 (>4 mm, III) (ECOG 1690)	642	HD i.v. then MD sc 1 yr vs LD sc 2 yr	DFS for HD only[a]	0.02
Cameron 2001 (>4 mm, III) (SMG)	95	LD sc	DFS, OS	Trend
Cascinelli 2001 (III) (WHO)	444	LD sc 1 yr	ND	ns
Hancock 2001 (>4 mm, III) (AIM-HIGH)	654	LD sc 2 yr	ND[a]	ns

Comparison in each case was with observation following surgery alone.
HD, MD, LD = high, medium and low dose; sc = subcutaneous; DFS = disease-free survival; MS, OS = median, overall survival; ND = no difference; ns = not significant; II, III = AJCC stage; [a] Further follow-up awaited.

heterogeneous risk groups (Sondak and Wolfe, 1997). Comparisons between trials of IFNα are difficult because of varying doses, durations and routes of administration, but there is the suggestion of greater activity for high-dose regimens, and greater benefit for node-positive over node-negative patients (Table 39.4).

The Eastern Co-operative Oncology Group (ECOG) trial 1684 (Kirkwood *et al.*, 1996) is the only study to have shown a survival advantage for any adjuvant therapy. A total of 287 patients with node-positive disease or primaries thicker than 4 mm were randomized to treatment or observation after surgery. A very high (maximum tolerable) dose of IFNα-2b was administered intravenously as an induction course (20 MU/m^2 daily) for 1 month, then patients received maintenance subcutaneously for one year (10 MU/m^2 three times per week). Significant toxicity was experienced, requiring dose reduction in the majority, with two treatment-related deaths. However, a strikingly positive result was seen, with significant improvement in both median relapse-free survival (from 1.0 to 1.7 years, $P = 0.002$) and overall survival (from 2.8 to 3.8 years, $P = 0.02$). There was no rise in relapse rate on discontinuing interferon, and the improved survival was sustained.

Several other trials failed to show a survival advantage for adjuvant IFNα, and differed in their effects on relapse-free survival. The North Central Cancer Treatment Group (NCCTG) treated stage II and III disease with high-dose intramuscular IFNα-2a for 3 months (Creagan *et al.*, 1995). There was no overall survival benefit but relapse-free survival was significantly improved (30–40 per cent at 5 years) for node-positive patients. WHO trial 16 studied low doses of IFNα-2a in node-positive melanoma, with no impact on relapse-free or overall survival (Cascinelli, 2001). The Scottish study compared low-dose IFNα-2b with observation in a small group of patients with high risk, including node positive, melanoma. No significant

differences in disease-free or overall survival were seen (Cameron *et al.*, 2001). The recent UKCCR AIM-HIGH study compared low-dose IFNα-2a with observation in a larger group of similar high risk patients (Hancock *et al.*, 2001). At four years' follow-up there were no significant survival differences between the two groups.

Neither NCCTG nor ECOG 1684 showed a benefit for node-negative patients, possibly because of the small number of patients in this group and their low event rate. However, two recent European studies compared low-dose IFNα-2a with observation in patients with thick primaries without nodal involvement, and both studies (Grob *et al.*, 1998; Pehamberger *et al.*, 1998) showed improved relapse-free survival for patients with interferon. No significant difference in overall survival was seen, although in one of the studies there was a strong trend towards significance in the treated group ($P = 0.059$).

Since the publication of ECOG 1684 IFNα has become standard therapy in some centres, particularly in the United States, for those at high risk of recurrence. However, most groups in Europe felt that confirmatory data were required before high-dose interferon became standard adjuvant therapy for this group of patients, not least because of the toxicity associated with this interferon regimen. A confirmatory study (ECOG 1690) has been undertaken and preliminary results published. This is a three-arm trial comparing high- and low-dose IFNα with observation. Analysis to date (Kirkwood *et al.*, 2000) shows improved relapse-free survival for high- but not for low-dose interferon, but does not confirm an impact on overall survival by either interferon regimen at median follow-up of 52 months. Interestingly, survival of patients in the observation arm of the confirmatory trial 1690 was significantly better than those in the observation arm of 1684. This may be the result of 'rescue' treatment with high-dose interferon in those patients in the control arm of 1690 who relapse. Further detailed analysis of this trial is awaited. A meta-analysis of published data from randomized trials of adjuvant IFNα in 3700 patients confirmed a clear disease-free survival benefit for IFN over observation ($P = 0.0001$), but although the odds ratio for overall survival was 0.9, the confidence intervals were consistent with no survival benefit (Wheatley et al., 2001). No statistically significant benefit of high- over lower-dose IFN was found. The result of the EORTC 19852 study comparing intermediate-dose IFN with observation in high-risk patients is awaited.

ECOG 1694, a comparison of high-dose IFNα-2b with G_{M2}-KLH vaccine in high-risk, including node positive, patients has generated recent controversy (Kirkwood et al., 2001). Both disease-free and overall survival were significantly superior in the IFN-treated group. Although no comparison with untreated patients was made the survival of the vaccinated group was similar to that of the observation arm of E1690. A detrimental effect of vaccination might be postulated but there was no evidence for this in earlier trials of G_{M2}-KLH vaccine (see below).

The activity of interferons may be related to an increase in expression of tumour antigens (Kirkwood, 1998), so they could prove useful in combination with anti-tumour vaccines. IL-2 is the only cytokine other than IFNα to have activity in advanced melanoma. One randomized trial of adjuvant treatment with a combination of IFNα and IL-2 has been carried out (Dummer et al., 1998). This included 225 patients with AJCC stage II melanoma who were randomized to receive the combination therapy or observation alone. There were no significant differences in relapse-free or overall survival, although there was a trend ($P = 0.07$) towards improved overall survival in the treated group.

Vaccines

Autologous tumour cell vaccines are useful in adjuvant treatment only following resection of bulky regional lymph nodes, because of a minimum requirement for tumour tissue to allow vaccine preparation. Allogeneic vaccines, in theory, have more application and are discussed below in the context of metastatic disease. There are four randomized trials of vaccination in the adjuvant setting (Table 39.7), none of which shows a survival benefit for vaccination (Morton et al., 1978; Livingston et al., 1994; Brystryn et al., 1998; Wallack et al., 1998). However, three of these trials have demonstrated a significant benefit in those patients who demonstrate an immune response to their vaccinations.

RECURRENT LOCAL DISEASE

Recurrent local disease is defined as any tumour occurring within 5 cm of a previous primary closure or skin graft. More distant locoregional lesions are satellite lesions and in-transit metastases, representing lymphatic permeation towards the regional lymph nodes. The risk of recurrence is very dependent on the thickness of the primary lesion, being low (0.2 per cent) for tumours less than 0.75 mm thick and significantly higher (13 per cent) for primary tumours greater than 4 mm (Urist et al., 1985). Other risk factors include ulceration, primary site (highest for hands, feet, and head and neck) and the presence of distant metastases. The majority of local recurrences occur within 5 years. Some investigators have suggested that local recurrence does not alter prognosis; however, in-transit metastases are often a harbinger of regional lymph node or distant metastasis, although these may occur many years later. Several palliative management options are available, but there has been no randomized comparison of these alternatives.

Surgery is the treatment of choice for single recurrences. Margins of 2 cm are recommended to achieve clear margins (Brown and Zitelli, 1995).

Isolated limb perfusion (ILP) is performed using an extracorporeal bypass circuit via the main artery and vein to the target limb. This delivers higher doses than are tolerated systemically, with a considerable rise in the area under the curve for the drug because it is not metabolized or excreted. Treatment periods of about 90 minutes are combined with limb hyperthermia (38–40°C), recent data suggesting that the best results are achieved at temperatures greater than 41°C. This technique is preferred to surgery when recurrences are multiple, frequent or large.

Good response rates are achievable with ILP, but no randomized studies have been undertaken to compare it with other modalities, and the technique requires major surgery. There is long experience with single-agent melphalan, but cisplatin and dactinomycin have also been used. DTIC is not useful in this context as it requires hepatic conversion to its active metabolite. The combination of melphalan with tumour necrosis factor-α (TNFα), with or without interferon-γ (IFNγ) (which increases tumour expression of TNF receptor), gives very high response rates, in excess of 70 per cent complete responses (Lienard et al., 1999). Results of this phase II study compared with historical controls suggest that ILP using TNFα and melphalan is superior to melphalan alone, but the addition of IFNγ did not significantly improve the response rate. Treatment complications of ILP can be severe, including acute respiratory distress syndrome and acute renal failure, because about 5 per cent of the perfusate escapes into the systemic circulation. An ongoing randomized National Cancer Institute trial is comparing hyperthermic ILP using melphalan or the combination of melphalan and TNF in patients with locally advanced melanoma of an extremity.

Laser ablation is useful for treating multiple small (<1.5 cm) lesions (Hill and Thomas, 1993). Recovery following treatment is much quicker than with ILP and treated areas are painless. The recurrence rate at treated sites is only 2 per cent, and although further crops of lesions are likely, these too are readily retreated with the CO_2 laser. Radiotherapy may have a role following multiple recurrences, but it is not generally used in the first instance. Intralesional therapy with BCG (widely used 30 years ago), purified protein derivative, IFNα and monoclonal antibodies produce responses of the order of 20 per cent, most often in small lesions, and systemic benefit has rarely been reported.

ROLE OF RADIOTHERAPY

Melanoma is generally regarded as relatively insensitive to radiotherapy, with a wide shoulder on the cell-survival curve. However, there are some situations in which radiotherapy can be a useful treatment modality, and there is some evidence that higher doses per fraction are more effective (Overgaard et al., 1985). Radiotherapy is rarely used for the treatment of a primary tumour, although it is a viable alternative for a few groups of patients in whom surgery would result in cosmetic or functional deformity, such as those with large facial lentigo maligna melanoma (Geara and Ang, 1996). Radiotherapy is also used in head and neck mucosal melanoma, where the prognosis is poor and surgery can be disfiguring.

A pilot study of the use of radiotherapy to local lymph nodes as adjuvant treatment of high-risk disease in the head and neck suggests benefit for those with primary tumours of 1.5 mm or thicker with clinically uninvolved nodes, or as an adjunct to the surgical treatment of involved nodes (Ang et al., 1990). A randomized study by the Radiation Therapy Oncology Group of adjuvant therapy in node-positive disease is under way in patients undergoing neck dissections, but accrual has been slow. There may be a potential role for combining radiotherapy with interferon in this setting.

Effective but short-lived palliation can be achieved in skin, soft-tissue and bony metastatic disease. It is especially useful for bone pain, with relief of symptoms lasting up to 6 months. Central nervous system metastases are common in melanoma and can sometimes be usefully treated with radiotherapy. Significant neurological improvement occurs in the majority following whole-brain irradiation but is short-lived, and is less likely if the patient has a poor performance status or a neurological deficit that is not responsive to steroids. Stereotactic radiotherapy may be more suitable for single intracranial metastases, although surgical removal must be considered in this situation, particularly when there are no other sites of disease. Spinal cord compression is best treated surgically, but radiotherapy should still be considered in patients who are not considered suitable for surgery. Radiolabelled antibodies have been used as a means of targeting radiation to metastatic melanoma, but this approach remains experimental.

The role of radiotherapy in ocular melanoma is being evaluated as part of the ongoing Collaborative Ocular Melanoma Study and is discussed below.

INTRA-OCULAR MELANOMA

This is the most common intra-ocular tumour, arising from uveal melanocytes. It is much less common than cutaneous melanoma, but occurs relatively more frequently in white- than in dark-skinned individuals. The incidence of intra-ocular melanoma has been stable over recent decades, in contrast to the dramatic rise in the frequency of cutaneous melanoma (Sahel et al., 1997).

The diagnosis is usually made without biopsy, the rate of correct clinical diagnosis using examination, ultrasound and fluorescein angiography being very high. Fine-needle aspiration can be useful in rare cases of doubt. Ultrasound is also useful for the detection of extrascleral extension and in post-enucleation follow-up. All patients with intraocular melanoma require investigation to exclude distant metastases, as for patients with high-risk cutaneous melanoma. Adverse prognostic features include age, tumour diameter greater than 10 mm, scleral involvement and high mitotic count.

Management is very dependent on tumour size. Small lesions (<8 mm) may be observed with careful follow-up, as these tumours can remain dormant for many years. They can be treated locally with laser photocoagulation, resection, external-beam radiation or brachytherapy. The more conservative options are preferred for smaller tumours with the aim of preserving sight in the affected eye. There is a consensus of opinion that large tumours (>16 mm) should be managed by enucleation. Patients treated in this way have a long-term survival rate of about 50 per cent. The Collaborative Ocular Melanoma Study (COMS) is addressing the question of whether external-beam radiotherapy should be added prior to surgery. The optimal treatment of medium-sized tumours (8–16 mm) is controversial, and alternatives to enucleation may be appropriate. The COMS investigators are randomizing patients with medium-sized tumours to either enucleation or brachytherapy (using isotope plaques sutured to the scleral surface of the eye over the tumour base). The prognosis for iris melanomas is generally better than for other ocular sites, and a conservative surgical approach avoiding enucleation is often taken.

No adjuvant systemic therapy has been shown to be of value in ocular melanoma and most patients with extrascleral involvement treated with enucleation subsequently die of metastatic disease. The prognosis of metastatic ocular melanoma is very poor, with median survival in the range of 2–5 months, and palliative treatment is appropriate (Albert et al., 1992). Response rates of approximately 20 per cent are seen using combination chemotherapy together with interferon (Pyrhonen, 1998).

METASTATIC DISEASE

Patients with metastatic melanoma have a poor prognosis, with a median survival of 6 months. The aim of therapy is palliation rather than cure. There is no consistent randomized evidence for a significant improvement in overall survival with any systemic therapy, but response to treatment can result in good palliation. Where possible, patients should be offered participation in clinical trials. Withholding treatment may be a valid option in the presence of slow-growing asymptomatic metastases, and deferment of treatment allows quality of life to be maintained. In patients with poor prognosis and widespread disease, treatment is unlikely to be of benefit.

Surgery and radiotherapy

Surgery can give long-lasting palliation for isolated metastases (Wornom et al., 1986) and is usually most appropriate for skin, soft-tissue and single brain lesions. Radiotherapy can also be useful in this context and has been discussed above.

Chemotherapy

Few cytotoxic drugs have significant activity in melanoma, but dacarbazine (DTIC), nitrosureas, platinum compounds and vinca alkaloids have established a role in single-agent treatment. The single most active drug is DTIC (Comis, 1976), with best responses in the range of 15–20 per cent. Principal side-effects are nausea and vomiting, fever, flu-like symptoms, occasional hepatotoxicity and moderate myelosuppression, but it is very well tolerated when given with a 5-hydroxytryptamine (5-HT_3) antagonist as an anti-emetic, and DTIC can usually be given as an outpatient treatment. Dosing regimens vary, but DTIC is typically given as a single dose of 850 mg/m^2 three weekly, or 250 mg/m^2 per day for 5 days three weekly. There is no good evidence for superiority of any particular dosing schedule. The nitrosureas, especially the newer agent fotemustine, readily penetrate the central nervous system and responses have been seen in patients with brain metastases. Principal toxicities are myelosuppression and pulmonary side-effects. Response rates of 10–15 per cent are observed with nitrosureas, platinum compounds, vinca alkaloids and the taxanes.

The median duration of response with single-agent chemotherapy is 6–10 months, and complete responses are uncommon (5 per cent with DTIC). Responses are usually limited to those without visceral metastases (liver, bone or brain), and are more common in women. Long-term survival is rare (<4 per cent) and there is no significant improvement in overall survival with chemotherapy.

There is a long history of promising activity suggested by single-institution studies of combination chemotherapy, but subsequently not confirmed in multicentre trials.

Combinations which have been used include CVD (cisplatin, vinblastine and DTIC) and BCDT (BCNU, cisplatin, DTIC and tamoxifen). These regimens have given response rates of 20–40 per cent in phase II trials. As with single agents, duration of response is usually short and complete responses are rare. BCDT, the 'Dartmouth' regimen, has been used commonly, and promising response rates (55 per cent) were seen in an early study, with 4/20 complete responses, including some in patients with visceral disease (Del Prete et al., 1984). However, response rates of only 20–25 per cent were observed in more recent phase II and phase III trials (Atkins, 1997). The CVD regimen has been compared prospectively with single-agent DTIC, without significant difference in outcome, and the results of a similar randomized comparison of BCDT with single-agent DTIC in 240 patients with metastatic disease also shows no advantage to combination therapy (Chapman et al., 1999). The response rate to the Dartmouth regimen was 18.5 per cent versus 10 per cent with DTIC alone ($P = 0.52$), and there was also no significant difference in overall survival. Toxicity was more common and more severe in the combination arm, and this should probably no longer be used routinely.

The place of tamoxifen in combination therapies for metastatic disease has been investigated over a number of years. It is responsible for some increase in morbidity as a result of thromboembolism in the context of the Dartmouth regimen. Initially a randomized study of 117 patients treated with either DTIC plus tamoxifen or with DTIC alone showed significantly improved response and median survival (69 versus 30 weeks, $P = 0.008$) in the combination arm (Cocconi et al., 1992). However, subsequent data failed to confirm this finding, as there was no survival advantage gained by adding tamoxifen to DTIC alone or to DTIC plus IFNα (Falkson et al., 1998) and two randomized comparisons in a total of 393 patients showed that the addition of tamoxifen to BCD (BCNU, cisplatin and DTIC) did not provide meaningful clinical advantage (Creagan et al., 1999; Rusthoven et al., 1996).

In summary, combination treatment has no convincing advantage over DTIC, the most active single-agent chemotherapy, and there is no place for the routine addition of tamoxifen to chemotherapy. Single-agent DTIC remains the standard treatment in metastatic disease.

Newer cytotoxic agents finding application in the treatment of melanoma include temozolomide, a pro-drug of MTIC, the active metabolite of DTIC. Temozolomide has excellent oral bioavailability and readily penetrates the central nervous system. Nausea and vomiting, and mild myelosuppression, are the main side-effects but, as with DTIC, the use of 5-HT_3 antagonists as anti-emesis means that treatment is very well tolerated. In a randomized prospective comparison with DTIC, temozolomide showed an equivalent response rate and overall survival, and superior disease-free survival (Middleton et al., 2000). Fotemustine, a chlorethyl nitrosurea, also has good central nervous system penetration with response rates in the range of 12–25 per cent. Docetaxel has also shown good responses in initial studies, including patients with bony metastases.

High-dose chemotherapy has been investigated using several single agents (BCNU, melphalan, thiotepa) and combinations such as DTIC with melphalan. Overall response rates of 40–60 per cent have been reported, but trials included small numbers of patients and there were few sustained remissions or long-term survivors. Toxicity was, predictably, significant, and treatment-related deaths occurred in up to one-third of patients in the very high-dose protocols. High-dose chemotherapy should still be considered experimental in the absence of randomized evidence of superiority over conventional doses.

Immunotherapy

Host immunity is believed to play an important role in melanoma. As a result there has been intense interest in the use of the biological response modifiers IFNα and IL-2 and, in biochemotherapy, their combination with chemotherapeutic agents.

INTERFERON-α

IFNα has a role in promoting tumour cell differentiation and the expression of major histocompatibility complex (MHC) and other antigens. It also has immunomodulatory effects via activation of natural killer (NK) cells, cytotoxic T lymphocytes and macrophages. An overview of trials using IFNα as a single agent in metastatic melanoma (Legha, 1997) showed a response rate of 15 per cent. Responses were seen in both previously treated and untreated patients, a third of responses were complete, but median survival was only 8 months. IFNα does not show cross-resistance with chemotherapy. There has been no randomized comparison of single-agent IFNα with chemotherapy or supportive care. Toxicity of IFNα is manageable and usually limited to nausea, flu-like symptoms and lethargy.

INTERLEUKIN-2

IL-2 also has immunomodulatory effects on NK cells and cytotoxic T lymphocytes, but no direct anti-tumour activity. A number of trials in the past decade of single-agent IL-2, using a wide range of dosing schedules, have been subjected to an overview (Philip and Flaherty, 1997). This shows an overall response rate of 15 per cent, with only 2 per cent of patients achieving complete remission. Responses are seen as frequently in patients with visceral metastases as in those without, in contrast to the effect of chemotherapy. It has been suggested that higher dose regimens are the most effective, and the largest study of single-agent IL-2 using high-dose bolus therapy (Rosenberg et al., 1994) reported a 7 per cent complete response rate, most of which were of considerably longer duration than seen with chemotherapy. The toxicity of IL-2 is significant at higher doses and includes hypotension, renal impairment and myelosuppression. Hospitalization for treatment is required, but with supportive care anticipating these toxicities even high doses can be administered safely.

The combination of IL-2 with further immunomodulatory measures, such as tumour-infiltrating lymphocytes (derived from the patient's own excised tumour) and lymphokine-activated killer cells, has been investigated, particularly by Rosenberg and co-workers at the National Cancer Institute (NCI). Despite promising enhancement of IL-2 activity in animal studies and phase II human trials, response rates have not been improved sufficiently to justify the complexity, toxicity and expense of this strategy.

COMBINATION OF IFNα AND IL-2

The combination of IFNα with IL-2 is suggested by laboratory evidence of synergistic activity. Despite initially promising phase II results, a meta-analysis of 911 patients gave an overall response rate of only 17 per cent, with a median survival of 11 months, which is not a significant improvement over chemotherapy regimens (Allen et al., 1997). The only randomized trial of high-dose IL-2 with or without IFNα (Sparano et al., 1993) showed no survival advantage in adding IFNα (10.2 months for IL-2 alone versus 9.7 months), and gave disappointing response rates of 5 per cent for IL-2 alone and 10 per cent for the combination.

Biochemotherapy

Five randomized trials published between 1990 and 1996 investigated the combination of IFNα with chemotherapy, using single-agent DTIC. Only one trial out of five suggested a significant improvement in response or survival with the addition of IFNα. This was a small, single-institution study of 61 patients (Falkson et al., 1991); those in the combination arm had a 53 per cent response rate and 18-month median survival, compared with 20 per cent ($P = 0.007$) and 10 months ($P < 0.01$) for the group receiving DTIC alone. This result has not been confirmed by four other studies in which a total of 589 patients were randomized. IFNα has also been added to combination chemotherapies such as CVD and the Dartmouth regimen, without significant improvement in response or survival compared to combination chemotherapy alone. Similarly, a variety of doses and administration methods for IL-2 combined with chemotherapy have not shown an advantage over immunotherapy or chemotherapy used alone.

Recently, the term 'biochemotherapy' has come to describe a combination of both IFNα and IL-2 with chemotherapy. The most effective biochemotherapy regimens appear to be those containing cisplatin. One of the earliest phase II trials of biochemotherapy, using single-agent cisplatin, IL-2 and IFNα showed a response rate of 54 per cent and a complete remission rate of 13 per cent (Khayat *et al.*, 1993). Similar response rates were seen with CVD chemotherapy in combination with IL-2 and IFNα, and a retrospective comparison of biochemotherapy with CVD combination chemotherapy suggested a statistically significant improvement in median survival and complete remission over CVD alone (Legha *et al.*, 1996). In this study, immunotherapy and CVD chemotherapy were combined by administering them alternately or sequentially; the highest median survival of 13 months was demonstrated in patients receiving sequential treatment, compared retrospectively with 9 months for a group treated with CVD alone (*P* = 0.04). As seen with other treatment modalities in metastatic melanoma, the duration of partial responses was short. However, complete remissions were seen in 23 per cent of patients treated with the sequential regimen, and the median duration of complete remissions was greater than 3 years, with some patients surviving disease-free for 6 years (Table 39.5). These durable complete remissions are one of the most characteristic and encouraging features of biochemotherapy.

Differential responses, in which not all lesions in a responding patient show signs of regression, are known to occur with chemotherapy and have been observed with biochemotherapy for metastatic melanoma. Responses were seen in 18 per cent of 27 patients treated with cisplatin, IFNα and IL-2, but 41 per cent of these were differential responses (Mainwaring *et al.*, 1997), with eight patients exhibiting a differential response in lesions at the same site. It is possible that this phenomenon explains in part the variable response rates reported for biochemotherapy regimens.

Five prospective randomized trials of biochemotherapy have been published (Table 39.6). A trial (Johnston *et al.*, 1998) from the Royal Marsden compared BCDT alone and in combination with IL-2 and IFNα. The response rates in 65 patients were not significantly different, 23 per cent for BCDT with IFNα/IL-2, and 27 per cent for BCDT alone. The relatively low response rates in the two arms can probably be explained by the low doses of immunotherapy used in this study. There were also no significant differences in progression-free survival or overall survival between the two groups, but biochemotherapy was associated with significantly more toxicity than combination chemotherapy alone. A subsequent NCI study of CDT (cisplatin, DTIC and tamoxifen) alone or in combination with IL-2 and IFNα similarly failed to show any significant response or survival benefit for biochemotherapy, which was again associated with more treatment-related toxicity (Rosenberg *et al.*, 1999). Responses were, however, numerically superior overall in patients treated with biochemotherapy (44 per cent, versus 27 per cent for CDT alone, *P* = 0.071). An EORTC trial demonstrated improved response (33 per cent compared to 18 per cent, respectively, *P* = 0.04) and disease-free survival for IFNα and IL-2 combined with cisplatin compared with immunotherapy alone, although overall survival was 9 months in both treatment arms (Keilholz *et al.*, 1997). A comparison of CVD (cisplatin, vinblastine and DTIC) alone or in combination with IL-2 and IFNα

Table 39.5 *Complete response rates (CR) to alternating or sequential biochemotherapy*

	n	CR	CR duration (months)
CVD	50	2 (4%)	Not stated
Alternating	39	2 (5%)	72+, 75+
Sequential	62	14 (23%)	8/14: 40+ to 52+

Patients receiving sequential biochemotherapy (cisplatin, vinblastine and DTIC with IFNα and IL-2) achieved more frequent and durable complete responses than those receiving alternating biochemotherapy or chemotherapy alone. Comparison with combination chemotherapy alone was retrospective (Legha *et al.*, 1996).

Table 39.6 *Randomized trials of biochemotherapy in metastatic melanoma*

	n	Regimen	Response (%)	Survival
Keilholz (1997)	138	IL-2/IFN ± C	33 vs 18 (*P* = 0.04)	ns
Johnston (1998)	65	BCDT ± IL-2/IFN	23 vs 27 (ns)	ns
Rosenberg (1999)	102	CDT ± IL-2/IFN	44 vs 27 (ns, *P* = 0.07)	ns
Eton (2000)	190	CVD ± IL-2/IFN	48 vs 25 (*P* = 0.001)	DFS (*P* = 0.0007)
Ridolfi (2001)	176	CD ± IL-2/IFN	25 vs 20 (ns)	ns

Response comparisons show biochemotherapy first.
C, cisplatin; B, BCNU; D, DTIC; T, tamoxifen; V, vinblastine; IL-2, interleukin-2; IFN, interferon; ns, not significant; DFS, disease-free survival.

(Eton *et al.*, 2000) demonstrated a significantly superior response rate for biochemotherapy (48 per cent, versus 25 per cent for CVD alone, $P = 0.001$). Disease-free survival ($P = 0.0007$), but not overall survival, was superior in the biochemotherapy group. However, an Italian trial comparing CD (cisplatin with DTIC) alone or in combination with a lower immunotherapy dose did not show a superior response rate or survival advantage for immunotherapy (Ridolfi *et al.*, 2001).

Regimens which include intravenous IL-2 require hospitalization, to monitor and treat hypotension and other side-effects, which include myelosuppression, cardiac toxicity and autoimmune phenomena. In general these side-effects are manageable in fit patients but biochemotherapy should not be considered in the elderly or otherwise frail.

Two further randomized studies are ongoing; an EORTC trial is treating patients with cisplatin, DTIC and IFNα with or without IL-2. An interim analysis (Keilholz *et al.*, 1999) does not show a significant difference in response rate (28 per cent without and 22 per cent with IL-2), but disease-free survival appears to be improved in the treatment arm including IL-2. The results of a similar American intergroup study are also awaited.

Vaccines

Vaccines have become a major area of interest in the development of new treatments for melanoma. The aim of these vaccines is to augment a specific host response to tumour antigens which may otherwise be only weakly immunogenic, present in small quantities, or not accessible on the cell surface. In general, a response to a therapeutic vaccine takes longer to develop than to chemotherapy (4–8 weeks), but as with other immunotherapies, there is evidence that vaccine responses may be more durable. Toxicity is generally low and usually confined to local irritation at the site of injection. Although little randomized data are available, the overall impression is of some degree of effectiveness for vaccines against melanoma. Vaccines are probably most effective in the presence of minimum tumour bulk or in the adjuvant setting. This is possibly because of the immunosuppressive effects of bulky tumour and the barrier presented by large disease volume to tumour clearance by the immune system. The use of vaccines in both adjuvant and metastatic settings will be discussed here. Vaccine material may be either cell-derived or recombinant.

Cell-derived vaccines may be autologous or allogeneic. Autologous tumour vaccines are made up of material from the patient's own tumour, which is treated to improve immunogenicity, for example by ultraviolet (UV) irradiation or digestion with neuraminidase, before being returned to the patient. This tailoring of vaccine to patient ensures that antigens present in the vaccine are expressed by the target tumour and are biologically relevant. This technique requires significant tumour volume to allow vaccine preparation and so is limited to the treatment of patients with bulky nodal or distant metastatic disease that is amenable to resection. However, patients in these groups have a poor prognosis and may not be those most likely to benefit from immunotherapy. A vaccine using autologous tumour cells modified with dinitrophenyl (DNP) as a hapten produced only four responses in 64 patients with metastatic melanoma (Berd *et al.*, 1998). This vaccine does seem more promising as adjuvant therapy; post-surgical administration of DNP vaccine to patients with nodal metastases at one site gave a projected 5-year survival of 45 per cent (Berd *et al.*, 1997). These results are better than historical figures for surgery alone, but randomized data are required to confirm these findings.

Allogeneic tumour vaccines are prepared from cultured cell lines and so are more available, cost effective and readily standardized than autologous tumour vaccines. Furthermore, allogeneic cells should be more immunogenic than autologous tissue. Allogeneic vaccines are available for patients with low disease burden, because tumour harvesting is not required for vaccine preparation. Phase II trials in both AJCC stage III and IV disease indicate a survival advantage over historical controls for CancerVax®, an irradiated mix of three melanoma cell lines. Two multicentre randomized trials of this vaccine are ongoing. Both are comparing groups treated with either CancerVax® plus BCG or with placebo plus BCG, the first trial in the adjuvant setting in patients with resected AJCC stage III disease, the second in patients with low-volume distant metastases following surgery.

The results of five randomized trials of vaccines in melanoma have been published (Table 39.7). Three of these trials used antigen derived from allogeneic tumour

Table 39.7 *Randomized trials of vaccines in malignant melanoma*

	Vaccine/AJCC stage	*n*	Survival
Morton* (1978)	Melanoma cell/III	134	ns
Livingston* (1994)	GM2/III	122	ns
Bystryn* (1998)	Shed antigen/III	38	77% vs 60% (ns)[a]
Wallack* (1998)	Vaccinia lysate/III	217	ns
Mitchell (1998)	Melacine/IV	140	ns

*Adjuvant trials. [a] Two year survival rate, compared with placebo. ns = not significant.

cells. A polyvalent shed antigen vaccine prepared from four melanoma cell lines was shown in a small (38 patients) randomized placebo controlled trial in stage III melanoma to improve 2-year survival to 77 per cent in the vaccinated group, from 60 per cent in the placebo-treated group (Bystryn et al., 1998). Viral lysates are reputed to provoke an intense anti-viral immune response which should also stimulate rejection of the tumour. A randomized trial of a vaccinia melanoma lysate in metastatic disease, however, failed to show a benefit despite promising results from phase II trials compared with historical controls (Wallack et al., 1998). A total of 217 patients were randomized to receive either lysate vaccine or vaccinia virus control with no significant differences in disease-free ($P = 0.61$) or overall survival (48 per cent 5-year survival in both groups, $P = 0.79$). Melacine®, a lyophilized preparation derived from two melanoma cell lines, has been administered with cyclophosphamide in a randomized comparison with combination chemotherapy (Mitchell, 1998). The response rates and survival were not significantly different but Melacine® was associated with fewer and milder side-effects.

Genetic modification of both autologous and allogeneic melanoma cells has been used to generate vaccines that overexpress a number of immunomodulatory agents, including IL-2, IFNγ and granulocyte/macrophage colony stimulating factor (GM-CSF). Overall response rates were low (Roth and Cristiano, 1997) but several investigators have demonstrated host responses to vaccination. These responses include expansion of cytotoxic T lymphocytes recognizing melanoma antigens, induction of melanoma-specific immunoglobulin, and enhancement of delayed-type hypersensitivity (DTH). In addition, some studies have shown a significant treatment benefit in those patients showing a host response. For example, autologous cells from 12 patients with metastatic disease were genetically engineered using recombinant retroviruses to secrete IL-2 (Palmer et al., 1999). No clinical responses were seen but DTH or CTL responses were seen in five patients and the median disease-free survival in this group was significantly improved (7 months versus 1 month, $P = 0.005$).

Several antigens associated with melanocytic lineage have been identified, and have allowed defined antigen vaccines to be developed (Restifo and Rosenberg, 1999). The ganglioside G_{M2}, expressed on most melanoma cells, has been used as a melanoma vaccine in a randomized trial in the adjuvant setting. Stage III patients were treated post-surgically with either G_{M2} and BCG or with BCG only. There were no significant differences in disease-free or overall survival when analysed on an intention-to-treat basis. However, some patients had detectable levels of anti-G_{M2} antibodies prior to vaccination, and when this group was excluded from the analysis, those patients who developed antibodies following treatment did show a significant improvement in survival (Livingston et al., 1994). This is a further example of the

importance of host response. The G_{M2} antigen has been shown to induce antibody production more effectively when linked to the carrier protein keyhole limpet haemocyanin (KLH). Multicentre randomized phase III trials comparing G_{M2}-KLH/BCG with placebo (in Europe and Australia) or with IFNα (in the United States) have been undertaken in patients with AJCC stage IIB (>4 mm thick) or III disease, and a trial in patients with thin stage II disease (stage IIA) is planned. Both disease-free and overall survival in patients with thick melanoma vaccinated with G_{M2}-KLH were inferior to those of a group treated with IFNα (Kirkwood et al., 2001).

Peptide melanoma antigens recognized by T cells have been identified. These include tyrosinase, gp100 and MART1 (for melanoma antigen recognized by T-cells), which can all produce clinical responses when processed by dendritic cells. These antigen-presenting cells have been extracted from peripheral blood and exposed in vitro to peptides prior to direct injection into lymph nodes, to maximize contact with circulating T cells. Responses, including some durable complete remissions, were seen in 5 of 16 patients with advanced melanoma (Nestle et al., 1998). Rosenberg and colleagues have taken the approach of altering the sequence of synthetic gp100 peptides to enhance their affinity for HLA molecules, so as to improve presentation to T cells. A modified peptide co-administered with IL-2 produced responses in 42 per cent of patients with metastatic disease (Table 39.8), a significant improvement over results from trials of high-dose IL-2 alone (Rosenberg et al., 1998). Randomized trials are awaited to confirm the efficacy of these new defined-antigen vaccines.

The importance of host response to melanoma vaccines has already been mentioned in the context of both genetically modified and defined antigen vaccines. The survival benefit to the subset of patients exhibiting a host response can be significant. As an example, the 5-year survival rate among patients ($n = 29$) demonstrating a strong IgM and DTH response to the CancerVax® allogeneic vaccine was 75 per cent, compared with 8 per cent ($P < 0.0001$) for those patients ($n = 13$) with neither strong IgM nor DTH responses (Hsueh et al., 1998). However, the generation of a host response is not sufficient for clinical benefit, as demonstrated by the NCI experience with synthetic gp100 peptide vaccines (Table 39.8). Modification of gp100 greatly enhances

Table 39.8 *Clinical and host responses to gp100 peptide vaccines in metastatic melanoma (Rosenberg et al., 1998)*

Vaccine	*n*	Clinical response (%)	Host CTL response (%)
gp100	9	11	25
Modified gp100	11	0	91
Modified gp100 + IL-2	19	42	16

CTL, cytotoxic T lymphocytes.

CTL host response but reduces clinical response, and addition of IL-2 improves clinical response despite a poorer host response.

Differential response, seen with chemotherapy and biochemotherapy, also occurs following vaccine therapy for melanoma. Tumour escape, a term describing the evasion of immune recognition by tumour cells, is a further phenomenon associated with currently available vaccines. It may be that selective loss of β_2-microglobulin, class I MHC or antigen-processing machinery by subclones of melanoma cells within the tumour provide a mechanism for this process (Restifo and Rosenberg, 1999), analagous to the expression of the multidrug resistance gene in the development of resistance to chemotherapy.

improvement in overall survival with any systemic therapy. DTIC has an established palliative role; several novel therapies, including molecularly defined vaccines, are in development.

SIGNIFICANT POINTS

- Sunlight is an important aetiological factor in malignant melanoma; protective measures to reduce exposure are recommended, particularly during childhood.
- Incidence and mortality have risen sharply over the past two decades, but in some countries the death rate is starting to fall in females.
- Excision with a 1 cm margin is adequate treatment for primary tumours 0.75 mm thick or less, and 2 cm is considered necessary for lesions between 0.75 and 1.9 mm; ongoing trials aim to determine appropriate margins for thicker melanomas. Cutaneous flaps and skin grafting are used when primary closure is not possible.
- There is no survival advantage to elective lymph-node dissection. Sentinel lymph-node biopsy (SLNB) is an accurate predictor of nodal metastasis, and may have a role in the management of patients with lesions thicker than 1 mm without clinically obvious nodal involvement, as a more accurate staging method. SLNB guides therapeutic lymph-node dissection and helps to select candidates for entry to trials of adjuvant therapy.
- The roles of IFNα and vaccines in the adjuvant setting require further randomized trials.
- There is no consistent randomized evidence in metastatic disease for a significant

KEY REFERENCES

Berd, D. (1998) Cancer vaccines: reborn or just recycled? *Semin. Oncol.* **25**(6), 605–10.
Berwick, M. and Halpern, A. (1997) Melanoma epidemiology. *Curr. Opin. Oncol.* **9**(2), 178–82.
Fraker, D.L. (1997) Surgical issues in the management of melanoma. *Curr. Opin. Oncol.* **9**(2), 183–8.
Punt, C.J. (1998) The use of interferon-alpha in the treatment of cutaneous melanoma: a review. *Melanoma Res.* **8**(2), 95–104.
Restifo, N.P. and Rosenberg, S.A. (1999) Developing recombinant and synthetic vaccines for the treatment of melanoma. *Curr. Opin. Oncol.* **11**(1), 50–7.

REFERENCES

Albert, D.M., Niffenegger, A.S. and Willson, J.K. (1992) Treatment of metastatic uveal melanoma: review and recommendations. *Surv. Ophthalmol.* **36**, 429–38.
Allen, I.E., Kupelnick, B., Kumashiro, M. *et al.* (1997) The combination of chemotherapy with IL-2 with or without IFN-alfa is more active than chemotherapy or immunotherapy alone in patients with metastatic melanoma: a meta-analysis of 7711 patients with metastatic melanoma. *Proc. Am. Soc. Clin. Oncol.* **16**, 494.
Ang, K.K., Byers, R.M., Peters, L.J. *et al.* (1990) Regional radiotherapy as adjuvant treatment for head and neck malignant melanoma. Preliminary results. *Arch. Otolaryngol. Head Neck Surg.* **116**, 169–72.
Atkins, M.B. (1997) The treatment of metastatic melanoma with chemotherapy and biologics. *Curr. Opin. Oncol.* **9**, 205–13.
Autier, P., Boyle, P. and Dore, J.F. (1998) Sorting the hype from the facts in melanoma. *Lancet* **352**, 738–9.
Autier, P., Dor, J.F., Lienard, D. *et al.* (1999) Sunscreen use and duration of sun exposure: a double-blind, randomized trial. *J. Natl Cancer Inst.* **91**, 1304–9.
Balch, C. (1992) An analysis of prognostic factors in 8500 patients with cutaneous melanoma. In Balch, C. (ed.), *Cutaneous melanoma*. Philadelphia: JB Lippincott, 200.
Balch, C.M. and Milton, G.W. (1985) Diagnosis of metastatic melanoma at distant sites. In Balch, C.M.

and Milton, G.W. (eds), *Cutaneous melanoma: clinical management and treatment results worldwide.* Philadelphia: JB Lippincott, 221–50.

Balch, C.M., Soong, S.J., Bartolucci, A.A. *et al.* (1996) Efficacy of an elective regional lymph node dissection of 1 to 4 mm thick melanomas for patients 60 years of age and younger. *Ann. Surg.* **224**, 255–63.

Balch, C.M., Buzaid, A.C., Soong, S.J. *et al.* (2001) Final version of the American Joint Committee on Cancer staging system for cutaneous melanoma. *J. Clin. Oncol.* **19**, 3635–48.

Ball, A.S. and Thomas, J. (1995) Surgical management of malignant melanoma. *Br. Med. Bull.* **51**, 584–608.

Bataille, V., Bishop, J.A., Sasieni, P. *et al.* (1996) Risk of cutaneous melanoma in relation to the numbers, types and sites of naevi: a case-control study. *Br. J. Cancer* **73**, 1605–11.

Berd, D., Maguire, H.C. Jr, Schuchter, L.M. *et al.* (1997) Autologous hapten-modified melanoma vaccine as postsurgical adjuvant treatment after resection of nodal metastases. *J. Clin. Oncol.* **15**, 2359–70.

Berd, D., Maguire, H.C., Bloome, E., Clark, C., Medley, W. and Mastrangelo, M.J. (1998) Regression of lung metastases after immunotherapy with autologous DNP modified melanoma vaccine. *Proc. Am. Soc. Clin. Oncol.* **17**, 434.

Berwick, M., Begg, C.B., Fine, J.A., Roush, G.C. and Barnhill, R.L. (1996) Screening for cutaneous melanoma by skin self-examination. *J. Natl Cancer Inst.* **88**, 17–23.

Bostick, P.J., Morton, D.L., Turner, R.R. *et al.* (1999) Prognostic significance of occult metastases detected by sentinel lymphadenectomy and reverse transcriptase–polymerase chain reaction in early-stage melanoma patients. *J. Clin. Oncol.* **17**, 3238–44.

Boyle, P., Maisonneuve, P. and Dore, J.F. (1995) Epidemiology of malignant melanoma. *Br. Med. Bull.* **51**, 523–47.

Brown, C.D. and Zitelli, J.A. (1995) The prognosis and treatment of true local cutaneous recurrent malignant melanoma. *Dermatol. Surg.* **21**, 285–90.

Buzaid, A.C., Colome, M., Bedikian, A. *et al.* (1998) Phase II study of neoadjuvant concurrent biochemotherapy in melanoma patients with local-regional metastases. *Melanoma Res.* **8**, 549–56.

Bystryn, J.C., Oratz, R., Shapiro, R.L. *et al.* (1998) Phase III double-blind trial of a shed polyvalent melanoma vaccine in stage III melanoma. *Proc. Am. Soc. Clin. Oncol.* **17**, 434.

Cameron, D.A., Cornbleet, M.C., Mackie, R.M. *et al.* (2001) Adjuvant interferon alpha 2b in high risk melanoma – the Scottish study. *Br. J. Cancer* **84**(9), 1146–9.

Cascinelli, N., Belli, F., MacKie, R.M. *et al.* (2001) Effect of long-term adjuvant therapy with interferon alpha-2a in patients with regional node metastases from cutaneous melanoma: a randomised trial. *Lancet* **358**, 866–9.

Cascinelli, N., Morabito, A., Santinami, M., MacKie, R.M. and Belli, F. (1998) Immediate or delayed dissection of regional nodes in patients with melanoma of the trunk: a randomised trial. WHO Melanoma Programme. *Lancet,* **351**, 793–6.

Castellano, M. and Parmiani, G (1999) Genes involved in melanoma: an overview of INK4a and other loci. *Melanoma Res.* **9**, 421–32.

Chapman, P.B., Lawrence, H.E., Meyers, M.L. *et al.* (1999) Phase III multicenter randomized trial of the Dartmouth regimen versus dacarbazine in patients with metastatic melanoma. *J. Clin. Oncol.* **17**, 2745–51.

Cocconi, G., Bella, M., Calabresi, F. *et al.* (1992) Treatment of metastatic malignant melanoma with dacarbazine plus tamoxifen. *N. Engl. J. Med.* **327**, 516–23.

Comis, R.L. (1976) DTIC (NSC-45388) in malignant melanoma: a perspective. *Cancer Treat. Rep.* **60**, 165–76.

CRC (1995) *Cancer Research Campaign Factsheet 4.1: Malignant melanoma.* London: CRC.

CRC (1999a) *Cancer Research Campaign Factsheet 1.1: Incidence – UK.* London: CRC.

CRC (1999b) *Cancer Research Campaign CancerStats: Survival England & Wales 1971–95.* London: CRC.

Creagan, E.T., Dalton, R.J., Ahmann, D.L. *et al.* (1995) Randomized, surgical adjuvant clinical trial of recombinant interferon alfa-2a in selected patients with malignant melanoma. *J. Clin. Oncol.* **13**, 2776–83.

Creagan, E.T., Suman, V.J., Dalton, R.J. *et al.* (1999) Phase III clinical trial of the combination of cisplatin, dacarbazine, and carmustine with or without tamoxifen in patients with advanced malignant melanoma. *J. Clin. Oncol.* **17**, 1884–90.

De Wit, P.E., Van Muijen, G.N., De Waal, R.M. and Ruiter, D.J. (1996) Pathology of malignant melanoma, including new markers and techniques in diagnosis and prognosis. *Curr. Opin. Oncol.* **8**, 143–51.

Del Prete, S.A., Maurer, L.H., O'Donnell, J., Forcier, R.J. and LeMarbre, P. (1984) Combination chemotherapy with cisplatin, carmustine, dacarbazine, and tamoxifen in metastatic melanoma. *Cancer Treat. Rep.* **68**, 1403–5.

Donawho, C. and Wolf, P. (1996) Sunburn, sunscreen, and melanoma. *Curr. Opin. Oncol.* **8**, 159–66.

Dummer, R., Hauschild, A., Henseler, T. and Burg, G. (1998) Combined interferon-alpha and interleukin-2 as adjuvant treatment for melanoma. *Lancet* **352**, 908–9.

Elwood, J.M. and Jopson, J. (1997) Melanoma and sun exposure: an overview of published studies. *Int. J. Cancer* **73**, 198–203.

English, D.R., Armstrong, B.K., Kricker, A. and Fleming, C. (1997) Sunlight and cancer. *Cancer Causes Control* **8**, 271–83.

Eton, O., Legha, S.S., Moon, T.E. *et al.* (1998) Prognostic factors for survival of patients treated systemically for disseminated melanoma. *J. Clin. Oncol.* **16**, 1103–11.

Eton, O., Legha, S., Bedikian, A. *et al.* (2000) Phase III randomized trial of cisplatin, vinblastine and dacarbazine (CVD) plus interleukin-2 and interferon-alpha-2b versus CVD in patients with metastatic melanoma. *Proc. Am. Soc. Clin. Oncol.* **18**, 2174a.

Falkson, C.I., Falkson, G. and Falkson, H.C. (1991) Improved results with the addition of interferon alfa-2b to dacarbazine in the treatment of patients with metastatic malignant melanoma. *J. Clin. Oncol.* **9**, 1403–8.

Falkson, C.I., Ibrahim, J., Kirkwood, J.M., Coates, A.S., Atkins, M.B. and Blum, R.H. (1998) Phase III trial of dacarbazine versus dacarbazine with interferon alpha-2b versus dacarbazine with tamoxifen versus dacarbazine with interferon alpha-2b and tamoxifen in patients with metastatic malignant melanoma: an Eastern Cooperative Oncology Group study. *J. Clin. Oncol.* **16**, 1743–51.

Finkel, E. (1998) Sorting the hype from the facts in melanoma. *Lancet* **351**, 1866.

Fraker, D.L. (1997) Surgical issues in the management of melanoma. *Curr. Opin. Oncol.* **9**, 183–8.

Geara, F.B. and Ang, K.K. (1996) Radiation therapy for malignant melanoma. *Surg. Clin. North Am.* **76**, 1383–98.

Gershenwald, J.E., Thompson, W., Mansfield, P.F. *et al.* (1999) Multi-institutional melanoma lymphatic mapping experience: the prognostic value of sentinel lymph node status in 612 stage I or II melanoma patients. *J. Clin. Oncol.* **17**, 976–83.

Giles, G.G., Armstrong, B.K., Burton, R.C., Staples, M.P. and Thursfield, V.J. (1996) Has mortality from melanoma stopped rising in Australia? Analysis of trends between 1931 and 1994. *BMJ* **312**, 1121–5.

Grob, J.J., Dreno, B., de la Salmoniere, P. *et al.* (1998) Randomised trial of interferon alpha-2a as adjuvant therapy in resected primary melanoma thicker than 1.5 mm without clinically detectable node metastases. French Cooperative Group on Melanoma. *Lancet* **351**, 1905–10.

Hancock, B.W., Wheatley, K., Harrison, G. and Gore, M. (2001) Aim High-Adjuvant Interferon in Melanoma (High Risk), a United Kingdom Co-ordinating Committee on Cancer Research (UKCCCR) randomised study of observation versus adjuvant low dose extended duration interferon alpha-2a in high risk resected malignant melanoma. *Proc. Am. Soc. Clin. Oncol.* **19**, 1393a.

Hill, S. and Thomas, J.M. (1993) Treatment of cutaneous metastases from malignant melanoma using the carbon-dioxide laser. *Eur. J. Surg. Oncol.* **19**, 173–7.

Hoon, D.S., Wang, Y., Dale, P.S. *et al.* (1995) Detection of occult melanoma cells in blood with a multiple-marker polymerase chain reaction assay. *J. Clin. Oncol.* **13**, 2109–16.

Hsueh, E.C., Gupta, R.K., Qi, K. and Morton, D.L. (1998) Correlation of specific immune responses with survival in melanoma patients with distant metastases receiving polyvalent melanoma cell vaccine. *J. Clin. Oncol.* **16**, 2913–20.

Johnston, S.R., Constenla, D.O., Moore, J. *et al.* (1998) Randomized phase II trial of BCDT [carmustine (BCNU), cisplatin, dacarbazine (DTIC) and tamoxifen] with or without interferon alpha (IFN-alpha) and interleukin (IL-2) in patients with metastatic melanoma. *Br. J. Cancer* **77**, 1280–6.

Karakousis, C.P., Emrich, L.J., Driscoll, D.L. and Rao, U. (1991) Survival after groin dissection for malignant melanoma. *Surgery* **109**, 119–26.

Keilholz, U., Goey, S.H., Punt, C.J. *et al.* (1997) Interferon alfa-2a and interleukin-2 with or without cisplatin in metastatic melanoma: a randomized trial of the European Organization for Research and Treatment of Cancer Melanoma Cooperative Group. *J. Clin. Oncol.* **15**, 2579–88.

Keilholz, U., Punt, C.J.A., Gore, M. *et al.* (1999) Dacarbazine, cisplatin and interferon alpha with or without interleukin-2 in advanced melanoma: interim analysis of EORTC trial 18951. *Proc. Am. Soc. Clin. Oncol.* **18**, 530.

Ketcham, A.B. and Balch, C.M. (1985) Classification and staging systems. In Balch, C.M. and Milton, G.M. (eds), *Cutaneous melanoma: clinical management and treatment results worldwide.* Philadelphia: JB Lippincott, 55–62.

Khayat, D., Borel, C., Tourani, J.M. *et al.* (1993) Sequential chemoimmunotherapy with cisplatin, interleukin-2, and interferon alfa-2a for metastatic melanoma. *J. Clin. Oncol.* **11**, 2173–80.

Kirkwood, J.M. (1998) Adjuvant IFN alpha2 therapy of melanoma. *Lancet* **351**, 1901–3. [*See* comments.]

Kirkwood, J.M., Strawderman, M.H., Ernstoff, M.S., Smith, T.J., Borden, E.C. and Blum, R.H. (1996) Interferon alfa-2b adjuvant therapy of high-risk resected cutaneous melanoma: the Eastern Cooperative Oncology Group Trial EST 1684. *J. Clin. Oncol.* **14**, 7–17.

Kirkwood, J.M., Ibrahim, J.G., Sondak, V.K. *et al.* (2000) High- and low-dose interferon alfa-2b in high-risk melanoma: first analysis of intergroup trial E1690/S9111/C9190. *J. Clin. Oncol.* **18**, 2444–58.

Kirkwood, J.M., Ibrahim, J.G., Sosman, J.A. *et al.* (2001) High-dose interferon alfa-2b significantly prolongs relapse-free and overall survival compared with the GM2-KLH/QS-21 vaccine in patients with resected stage IIB-III melanoma: results of intergroup trial E1694/S9512/C509801. *J. Clin. Oncol.* **19**, 2370–80.

Koops, H.S., Vaglini, M., Suciu, S. *et al.* (1998) Prophylactic isolated limb perfusion for localized, high-risk limb melanoma: results of a multicenter randomized phase III trial. European Organization for Research and Treatment of Cancer Malignant Melanoma Cooperative Group Protocol 18832, the World Health Organization Melanoma Program Trial 15, and the

North American Perfusion Group Southwest Oncology Group-8593. *J. Clin. Oncol.* **16**, 2906–12.

Lee, S.M., Betticher, D.C. and Thatcher, N. (1995) Melanoma: chemotherapy. *Br. Med. Bull.* **51**, 609–30.

Legha, S.S. (1997) The role of interferon alfa in the treatment of metastatic melanoma. *Semin. Oncol.* **24**, S24–31.

Legha, S.S., Ring, S., Bedikian, A. *et al.* (1996) Treatment of metastatic melanoma with combined chemotherapy containing cisplatin, vinblastine and dacarbazine (CVD) and biotherapy using interleukin-2 and interferon-alpha. *Ann. Oncol.* **7**, 827–35.

Lienard, D., Eggermont, A.M.M., Schraffordt Koops, H. *et al.* (1999) Isolated limb perfusion with tumour necrosis factor-alpha and melphalan with or without interferon-gamma for the treatment of in-transit melanoma metastases: a multicentre randomised phase II study. *Melanoma Res.* **9**, 491–502.

Lindor, N.M. and Greene, M.H. (1998) The concise handbook of family cancer syndromes. Mayo Familial Cancer Program. *J. Natl Cancer Inst.* **90**, 1039–71.

Livingston, P.O., Wong, G.Y., Adluri, S. *et al.* (1994) Improved survival in stage III melanoma patients with G_{M2} antibodies: a randomized trial of adjuvant vaccination with G_{M2} ganglioside. *J. Clin. Oncol.* **12**, 1036–44.

MacKie, R.M., Hole, D., Hunter, J.A. *et al.* (1997) Cutaneous malignant melanoma in Scotland: incidence, survival, and mortality, 1979–94. The Scottish Melanoma Group. *BMJ* **315**, 1117–21.

Mainwaring, P.N., Atkinson, H., Chang, J. *et al.* (1997) Differential responses to chemoimmunotherapy in patients with metastatic malignant melanoma. *Eur. J. Cancer* **33**, 1388–92.

Marks, R., Dorevitch, A.P. and Mason, G. (1990) Do all melanomas come from 'moles'? A study of the histological association between melanocytic naevi and melanoma. *Australas. J. Dermatol.* **31**, 77–80.

McMasters, K.M., Reintgen, D.S., Ross, M.I. *et al.* (2001) Sentinel lymph node biopsy for melanoma: controversy despite widespread agreement. *J. Clin. Oncol.* **19**, 2851–5.

Meisenberg, B.R., Ross, M., Vredenburgh, J.J. *et al.* (1993) Randomized trial of high-dose chemotherapy with autologous bone marrow support as adjuvant therapy for high-risk, multi-node-positive malignant melanoma. *J. Natl Cancer Inst.* **85**, 1080–5.

Melia, J., Cooper, E.J., Frost, T. *et al.* (1995) Cancer Research Campaign health education programme to promote the early detection of cutaneous malignant melanoma. II. Characteristics and incidence of melanoma. *Br. J. Dermatol.* **132**, 414–21.

Middleton, M.R., Grob, J.J., Aaronson, N. *et al.* (2000) Randomized phase III study of temozolomide versus dacarbazine in the treatment of patients with advanced metastatic malignant melanoma. *J. Clin. Oncol.* **18**, 158–66.

Milton, G.W., Shaw, H.M. and McCarthy, W.H. (1977) Occult primary malignant melanoma: factors influencing survival. *Br. J. Surg.* **64**, 805–8.

Mitchell, M.S. (1998) Perspective on allogeneic melanoma lysates in active specific immunotherapy. *Semin. Oncol.* **25**, 623–35.

Morton, D.L., Eilber, F.R., Holmes, E.C. and Ramming, K.P. (1978) Preliminary results of a randomized trial of adjuvant immunotherapy in patients with malignant melanoma who have lymph node metastases. *Aust. N. Z. J. Surg.* **48**, 49–52.

Morton, D.L., Wanek, L., Nizze, J.A., Elashoff, R.M. and Wong, J.H. (1991) Improved long-term survival after lymphadenectomy of melanoma metastatic to regional nodes. Analysis of prognostic factors in 1134 patients from the John Wayne Cancer Clinic. *Ann. Surg.* **214**, 491–9.

Morton, D.L., Wen, D.R., Wong, J.H. *et al.* (1992) Technical details of intraoperative lymphatic mapping for early stage melanoma. *Arch. Surg.* **127**, 392–9.

Nestle, F.O., Alijagic, S., Gilliet, M. *et al.* (1998) Vaccination of melanoma patients with peptide- or tumor lysate-pulsed dendritic cells. *Nat. Med.* **4**, 328–32.

NIH (1992) Diagnosis and treatment of early melanoma. National Institutes of Health Consensus Development Conference Statement, Bethesda, MD.

Noonan, F.P., Recio, J.A., Takayama. H. *et al.* (2001) Neonatal sunburn and melanoma in mice. *Nature* **413**, 271–2.

Overgaard, J., von der Maase, H. and Overgaard, M. (1985) A randomized study comparing two high-dose per fraction radiation schedules in recurrent or metastatic malignant melanoma. *Int. J. Radiat. Oncol. Biol. Phys.* **11**, 1837–9.

Palmer, K., Moore, J., Everard, M. *et al.* (1999) Gene therapy with autologous, interleukin 2-secreting tumor cells in patients with malignant melanoma. *Hum. Gene Ther.* **10**, 1261–8.

Pehamberger, H., Soyer, H.P., Steiner, A. *et al.* (1998) Adjuvant interferon alfa-2a treatment in resected primary stage II cutaneous melanoma. Austrian Malignant Melanoma Cooperative Group. *J. Clin. Oncol.* **16**, 1425–9.

Philip, P.A. and Flaherty, L. (1997) Treatment of malignant melanoma with interleukin-2. *Semin. Oncol.* **24**, S32–38.

Pyrhonen, S. (1998) The treatment of metastatic uveal melanoma. *Eur. J. Cancer,* **34**(suppl. 3), S27–30.

Rees, J.L. (1996) The melanoma epidemic: reality and artefact. *BMJ* **312**, 137–8.

Restifo, N.P. and Rosenberg, S.A. (1999) Developing recombinant and synthetic vaccines for the treatment of melanoma. *Curr. Opin. Oncol.* **11**, 50–7.

Ridolfi, R., Romanini, A., Labianca, R. *et al.* (2001) Chemotherapy vs. biochemotherapy: phase III trial in outpatients with advanced melanoma. *Proc. Am. Soc. Clin. Oncol.* **19**, 1392.

Rigel, D.S., Friedman, R.J. and Kopf, A.W. (1996) *J. Am. Acad. Dermatol.* **34**, 839–47.

Rosenberg, S.A., Yang, J.C., Topalian, S.L. *et al.* (1994) Treatment of 283 consecutive patients with metastatic melanoma or renal cell cancer using high-dose bolus interleukin 2. *JAMA* **271**, 907–13.

Rosenberg, S.A., Yang, J.C., Schwartzentruber, D.J. *et al.* (1998) Immunologic and therapeutic evaluation of a synthetic peptide vaccine for the treatment of patients with metastatic melanoma. *Nat. Med.* **4**, 321–7.

Rosenberg, S.A., Yang, J.C., Schwartzentruber, D.J. *et al.* (1999) Prospective randomized trial of the treatment of patients with metastatic melanoma using chemotherapy with cisplatin, dacarbazine, and tamoxifen alone or in combination with interleukin-2 and interferon alfa-2b. *J. Clin. Oncol.* **17**, 968–75.

Roth, J.A. and Cristiano, R.J. (1997) Gene therapy for cancer: what have we done and where are we going? *J. Natl Cancer Inst.* **89**, 21–39.

Rusthoven, J.J., Quirt, I.C., Iscoe, N.A. *et al.* (1996) Randomized, double-blind, placebo-controlled trial comparing the response rates of carmustine, dacarbazine, and cisplatin with and without tamoxifen in patients with metastatic melanoma. National Cancer Institute of Canada Clinical Trials Group. *J. Clin. Oncol.* **14**, 2083–90.

Sahel, J.A., Steeves, R.A. and Albert, D.M. (1997) Intraocular melanoma. In Devita, V.T., Hellman, S. and Rosenberg, S.A. (eds), *Cancer: principals and practice of oncology*. Philadelphia: JB Lippincott, 1995–2011.

Sondak, V.K. and Wolfe, J.A. (1997) Adjuvant therapy for melanoma. *Curr. Opin. Oncol.* **9**, 189–204.

Sparano, J.A., Fisher, R.I., Sunderland, M. *et al.* (1993) Randomized phase III trial of treatment with high-dose interleukin-2 either alone or in combination with interferon alfa-2a in patients with advanced melanoma. *J. Clin. Oncol.* **11**, 1969–77.

Stern, R.S., Nichols, K.T. and Vakeva, L.H. (1997) Malignant melanoma in patients treated for psoriasis with methoxsalen (psoralen) and ultraviolet A radiation (PUVA). The PUVA Follow-Up Study. *N. Engl. J. Med.* **336**, 1041–5.

Urist, M.M., Balch, C.M., Soong, S. *et al.* (1985) The influence of surgical margins and prognostic factors predicting the risk of local recurrence in 3445 patients with primary cutaneous melanoma. *Cancer* **55**, 1398–402.

Veronesi, U., Adamus, J., Bandiera, D.C. *et al.* (1977) Inefficacy of immediate node dissection in stage 1 melanoma of the limbs. *N. Engl. J. Med.* **297**, 627–30.

Veronesi, U., Cascinelli, N., Adamus, J. *et al.* (1988) Thin stage I primary cutaneous malignant melanoma. Comparison of excision with margins of 1 or 3 cm. *N. Engl. J. Med.* **318**, 1159–62. [Published erratum appears in *N. Engl. J. Med.* **325**(4), 292.]

Wallack, M.K., Sivanandham, M., Balch *et al.* (1998) Surgical adjuvant active specific immunotherapy for patients with stage III melanoma: the final analysis of data from a phase III, randomized, double-blind, multicenter vaccinia melanoma oncolysate trial. *J. Am. Coll. Surg.* **187**, 69–77.

Walter, S.D., Marrett, L.D., From, L., Hertzman, C., Shannon, H.S. and Roy, P. (1990) The association of cutaneous malignant melanoma with the use of sunbeds and sunlamps. *Am. J. Epidemiol.* **131**, 232–43.

Weinstock, M.A., Colditz, G.A., Willett, W.C. *et al.* (1989) Nonfamilial cutaneous melanoma incidence in women associated with sun exposure before 20 years of age. *Pediatrics* **84**, 199–204.

Westerdahl, J., Ingvar, C., Masback, A., Jonsson, N. and Olsson, H. (2000) Risk of cutaneous malignant melanoma in relation to use of sunbeds: further evidence for UV-A carcinogenicity. *Br. J. Cancer* **82**, 1593–9.

Wheatley, K., Hancock, B., Gore, M., Suciu, S. and Eggermont, A. (2001) Interferon-α as adjuvant therapy for melanoma: a meta-analysis of the randomised trials. *Proc. Am. Soc. Clin. Oncol.* **19**, 1394a.

Wornom, I.L., Smith, J.W., Soong, S.J., McElvein, R., Urist, M.M. and Balch, C.M. (1986) Surgery as palliative treatment for distant metastases of melanoma. *Ann. Surg.* **204**, 181–5.

40

Bone

JEREMY S. WHELAN, JUSTIN P. COBB AND ANNA M. CASSONI

INTRODUCTION

Cancers which arise in bone are exceptionally uncommon. Several discrete diseases can be identified through their differing clinico-pathological features, but for all bone tumours pain is the most common presenting symptom. As this is a feature of a vast array of musculoskeletal disorders, delay in diagnosis is a well-recognized problem.

Principles of management, particularly surgical, are broadly applicable across the different histological types. Osteosarcoma and Ewing's tumours together constitute the greatest numbers of cases. Occurring most often in adolescence and young adults, both diseases are now curable in a significant proportion of cases with modern multimodality treatment. For chondrosarcoma, a locally aggressive tumour of adults, there have been fewer advances in either our knowledge of the underlying biology or treatment of recurrent disease.

Advances in surgical techniques have been substantial. Thus amputation is now uncommonly performed for extremity tumours. As improvements in systemic therapy have increased the number of survivors, so attention has turned to improving long-term functional improvements.

Of critical importance in the care of these diseases is close co-operation between experienced surgeons, radiologists and oncologists. Appropriate supportive care facilities and experienced nursing staff are necessary for those receiving intensive chemotherapy and, as many are children and teenagers, a multidisciplinary approach is required to meet the additional needs which arise, including educational provision and psychosocial support for both patient and family. All those with suspected primary bone tumours should therefore be referred quickly to a recognized specialist centre.

INCIDENCE AND AETIOLOGY

A classification of primary bone tumours is shown in Table 40.1. These diseases do not appear to share a common aetiology, although several aetiological factors are apparent, particularly for osteosarcoma.

Table 40.1 *Classification of malignant primary bone tumours*

A	Osteosarcoma	
	1	High-grade central
	2	Mixed, fibroblastic, osteoblastic, chondroblastic, osteoclast-rich, small cell
	3	Low-grade central
	4	Surface
	5	High-grade surface, periosteal, parosteal
B	Ewing's family of tumours	
C	Chondrosarcoma	
	1	Chondrosarcoma (grades 1–3)
	2	Dedifferentiated chondrosarcoma
	3	Mesenchymal chondrosarcoma
D	Malignant fibrous histiocytoma of bone	
E	Other spindle cell tumours of bone	
		Fibrosarcoma, leiomyosarcoma, liposarcoma, haemangiopericytoma, haemangioendothelioma
F	Primary bone lymphoma	
G	Post-radiation sarcoma	
H	Paget's sarcoma	

Accurate date for the incidence of these diseases is not readily available. Cancer registry data may not always contain accurate histological information, particularly for tumours occurring in adults. On the other hand, specialist bone tumour registers may not give a true reflection of population incidence, but rather of referral patterns, especially when a registry is located in a specialist centre.

The patterns of incidence differ between the diseases shown in Table 40.1. Both osteosarcoma and Ewing's tumour have a peak incidence early in adolescence. This occurs slightly earlier in girls, and the association with a pubertal growth spurt, plus the common location of tumours around the knee and in the proximal humerus, indicate an aetiological association with rapid bone growth.

While Ewing's tumours occur very uncommonly after the age of 40 years, there is a low incidence of osteosarcoma throughout adulthood and, indeed, a second peak of incidence in the elderly, which is explained in part by an association with Paget's disease. Both osteosarcoma and Ewing's tumours tend to have a male preponderance when occurring early in life, and Ewing's tumours have an unexplained racial pattern, being exceptionally uncommon in Africans and African-Americans.

In the majority, the occurrence of any of the tumours shown in Table 40.1 is a sporadic event. However, there are some well-recognized aetiological factors, of which the most important is radiation. More recently, a number of genetic abnormalities associated with the development of bone tumours have been identified. These factors are summarized in Table 40.2.

Radiation was identified as an important causative factor for bone tumours from observations of luminous dial painters after the First World War. Large-scale production of instrument dials and watches took place in Canada and the United States. The dials were hand painted, most often by young female workers using paint containing radium and mesothorium mixed with zinc sulphide. The practice of pointing the paintbrushes in the workers' mouths led to widespread ingestion of radium. Radionecrosis, primarily of the jaw but also occurring in other bones, resulted and over the next 40 years, osteosarcomas frequently developed, those ingesting more than 700 μCi having a cumulative incidence as high as 70 per cent during this period (Polednak, 1978).

Sarcomas are a recognized late complication of therapeutic radiation. The most common histological subtype is osteosarcoma, and tumours arise after a latent period averaging between 8 and 20 years. Of greatest concern is the development of a radiation-induced sarcoma as a consequence of successful treatment of childhood malignancy. Although the overall incidence is low, it has become an important factor to consider in the development of new treatments which now attempt to limit use of radiation. Exposure to alkylating agents may add to this risk of sarcoma development. Radiation used in the treatment of breast and gynaecological cancers in adults is also associated with the development of sarcomas, although the risk appears to be less than that in children. Such tumours often pose considerable management problems.

Survivors of retinoblastoma have a striking vulnerability to subsequent development of osteosarcoma. The excess risk (variously estimated as between 150- and 400-fold) is principally in those with familial retinoblastoma and is especially associated with prior treatment with radiotherapy, with most, but not all, these secondary osteosarcomas arising within a field of previous irradiation (Draper et al., 1986). The identification of the retinoblastoma gene as a tumour suppressor gene altered in a wide range of cancers had led to insights into osteosarcoma pathogenesis. Loss of heterozygosity for Rb is a frequent finding, possibly associated with an adverse prognosis.

A further key genetic discovery was made by Li and Fraumeni, who discovered families with an inherited predisposition to specific cancers, of which sarcomas in childhood and adolescence are particularly notable. This predisposition arises as a consequence of a germline mutation in another tumour suppressor gene, p53 (Li, 1993). Tumours arising in Li–Fraumeni families account for only a tiny proportion of osteosarcoma and, indeed, sporadic mutations in p53 are thought to account for less than 3 per cent of osteosarcomas. Thus, for most osteosarcomas the underlying pathogenesis remains obscure.

The discovery of a chromosomal translocation specific to Ewing's sarcoma, (t11;22), has provided important insights, particularly in identifying primitive neuroectodermal tumours which share this translocation as having a common lineage. These related diseases are now usefully referred to as Ewing's family of tumours (EFT). Although presumed to be neural, the identification of an originating cell for these tumours remains elusive.

Other factors associated with the development of bone tumours include Paget's disease and some rare familial syndromes (Price and Goldie, 1969). Malignant fibrous histiocytoma of bone often arises in an area of pre-existing abnormal bone, such as an infarct.

Table 40.2 *Aetiology of malignant primary bone tumours*

A	Genetic
	Familial retinoblastoma
	Li–Fraumeni syndrome
	Multiple enchondromata (diaphyseal achalasia)
B	Radiation
C	Paget's disease
D	Miscellaneous e.g. polyostotic fibrous dysplasia

GENERAL PRINCIPLES OF MANAGEMENT

A broad framework of management, from initial evaluation to treatment, is appropriate for all patients with primary bone tumours. At all stages, specialist experience and liaison between disciplines is essential.

Initial evaluation

The most common presenting symptom is pain, often characterized by a gradual increase in intensity. An important distinguishing feature is that of night pain of sufficient severity to disturb sleep. This symptom should always be taken seriously and investigated appropriately. Swelling often accompanies pain, and again is a feature that demands rapid and careful investigation.

Most patients, even those with high-grade tumours, have no systemic symptoms. When these occur, the manifestations are most often fever, weight loss and even sweats, usually as a consequence of metastatic EFT. Like soft-tissue sarcomas, the principle site of metastatic spread is to the lung, but this is only present in some 10–15 per cent of patients at diagnosis, and symptoms from lung metastases are much less frequent.

Plain radiographs in two planes are the essential first investigation. As described in the section on individual tumour types, radiological features are often characteristic. Further evaluation of a primary tumour can then be undertaken with magnetic resonance imaging and, particularly for lesions on the surface of the bone, computed tomography. Radiological evaluation is mandatory before diagnostic biopsy is undertaken.

Biopsy

Two key components of a successful biopsy are appropriate siting of the biopsy and evaluation by a pathologist experienced in the pathology of malignant bone tumours. The first is important because inappropriate placement of the biopsy may compromise future surgery as the biopsy tract is presumed to be contaminated and must be excised. Also, bone tumours are often heterogeneous, so the placement of the biopsy should take into account radiological changes that may indicate areas of higher- or lower-grade of malignancy within the same tumour.

Expert interpretation of the biopsy is also essential as most pathologists will be unfamiliar with primary bone tumours and the appearances are often misleading, for instance when distinguishing reactive from tumour bone in bone-forming tumours such as osteosarcoma.

If a lesion is small, conveniently located, appears relatively benign radiologically and excision biopsy is considered to be technically straightforward, this should be the first surgical procedure. In all other cases the lesion should be biopsied before any treatment is undertaken. For diagnostic purposes, a core biopsy, using a disposable bone-marrow biopsy trephine, provides adequate tissue for the diagnosis of all musculoskeletal lesions (Stoker et al., 1991).

Very hard lesions, such as periosteal osteosarcomas, may require a fine-toothed trephine, and intra-osseous lesions may require the proximal cortex of bone to be drilled. There is, however, no place for incisional biopsy in musculoskeletal oncology. Movement of tissue planes hampers subsequent effective excision of the biopsy scar and its contaminated field. The use of conventional histopathological techniques, together with immunocytochemistry, are now sufficiently advanced to provide a reliable diagnosis. Touch preparations are particularly important for staining for alkaline phosphatase. The presence of this enzyme in malignant cells is a hallmark of osteosarcoma. Tissue for chromosomal and molecular genetic studies is extremely helpful, but is only rarely needed for diagnostic purposes in primary malignant bone tumours.

Staging

The staging system recognized throughout the world is that published by Enneking and his associates in 1980 (Enneking et al., 1980). Two grades of tumour are recognized and two extents, within and without the cortex. As defined by these workers, this implied that almost all osteosarcoma are stage IIb as they almost invariably spread on both sides of the bone. Despite this 'extra compartmental extent', at operation these lesions are very well defined by pseudoperiosteum. We would therefore re-interpret Enneking's definition of the compartment to be that bounded by the pseudo-periosteum as demonstrated on initial MRI scan, and often more obvious after two courses of chemotherapy. Interpreted in this way, the great majority of osteosarcomas would be stage II and have much less risk of local recurrence than the very occasional tumour which does burst out and frankly invade muscle, unaided by biopsy. A practical staging notation used within the London Bone and Soft Tissue Tumour Service is found in Table 40.3.

The patterns of spread of primary bone tumours are well characterized. Appropriate staging investigations are shown in Table 40.4. For those tumours with metastatic potential, the lungs and other sites in the skeleton are most often affected. Thus, computed tomography (CT) of the chest and an isotope bone scan are necessary. Bone-marrow biopsy is required for the assessment of Ewing's tumours, when approximately 10 per cent will have evidence of bone-marrow involvement.

Treatment

The integration of local and systemic therapies is an important feature of the management of high-grade tumours, where most will begin treatment with chemotherapy, local therapy being carried out anywhere between 6 and 20 weeks later. Other tumours may be managed by definitive surgery alone, after biopsy and staging as described above.

Table 40.3 *Staging notation*

Stage	Grade	Site	Treatment	Example
Ia	Low	Within pseudoperiosteum	Wide local excision	Low-grade central osteosarcoma
Ib	Low	Invading muscle	Wide local excision	Parosteal osteosarcoma, chondrosarcoma
IIa	High	Within pseudoperiosteum	Chemotherapy, local excision	Most high-grade osteosarcoma
IIb	High	Invading muscle	Chemotherapy, local excision or radiotherapy if inaccessible	Ewing's tumour
IIIa	High	Oligometastatic	Chemotherapy, local excision, metastatectomy	Any sarcoma with few metastases
IIIb	High	Polymetastatic	Palliative chemotherapy and radiotherapy	Inoperable metastatic sarcoma

Table 40.4 *Staging investigations*

	Plain radiographs	MRI of primary	Isotope bone scan	Thorax CT	Bone-marrow biopsy	Others
Osteosarcoma	Y	Y	Y	Y	N	
Ewing's tumours	Y	Y	Y	Y	Y	
Chondrosarcoma	Y	Y	Y	Y	N	
MFH	Y	Y	Y	Y	N	
Bone lymphoma	Y	Y	Y	Y	Y	Abdomen CT, LDH

CT, computed tomography; LDH, lactate dehydrogenase; MFH, malignant fibrous histiocytoma; MRI, magnetic resonance imaging.

Local therapy

SURGERY

The guiding principles in sarcoma surgery are:

1 High-grade sarcoma is usually systemic at presentation. Surgery is therefore aimed at local disease control.
2 The safe margin of resection includes a biologically competent barrier.
3 A tissue plane that has normal mobility is not crossed by the tumour.
4 Neo-adjuvant chemotherapy may improve the local grade.

Margins

The safe margin of resection should be decided upon clinical grounds. This may be a layer of fascia, or epineurium. Within a compartment such as a bone or muscle, this margin is less obvious. There remains a spread of opinion across the world in this regard, with the Japanese Musculoskeletal Oncology Society recommending 5 cm of normal tissue, at one extreme, and the British Orthopaedic Oncology Society using 2 cm as the margin of error. Imaging modalities help decide this margin within the bone or muscle, while the mobility of tissues is a better guide to involvement by tumour across adventitial layers. The surgeon is therefore the one who makes this decision, by observing that the structure is uninvolved and by the normal mobility of the adventitia, thus frequently saving a vessel or nerve which is close to the tumour, and may be deflected by it, but is not involved. This is at present a superior strategy than simple acceptance of MRI scanning information. The partial volume effects at the junction of different tissue types are indistinguishable from tumour involvement at our current level of understanding.

Limb salvage versus amputation

At present, there is no agreement regarding the place of limb salvage in paediatric and adolescent sarcoma surgery. Massive replacement, which is the mainstay of reconstructive surgery, has a significant re-operation rate, with a significant human and financial cost, although the costs of amputation are also considerable (Grimer *et al.*, 1997).

It remains difficult to justify this on quality-of-life terms alone (Postma *et al.*, 1992), but more and more surgeons do attempt to save limbs rather than amputate, even in the young. Amputation is only reserved for those cases in whom there is segmental involvement of the neurovascular bundle as well as bone and muscle.

Local recurrence

Local recurrence is often cited as a very major cause of relapse, with the implication that inadequate surgery is a cause of death. There is no controlled data to confirm this, only the observation that the mortality rate in those centres with very aggressive surgeons is not significantly better than those with more conservative ones. In multivariate analysis, it is the size of the tumour and associated chemosensitivity that dictate this, not the type of surgery. Skip lesions may commonly be the cause of local recurrence, having developed early in the disease process as a result of a failure of cell-mediated control mechanisms. Thus local recurrence is usually a marker of disease activity, and a failure of host tumour control mechanisms at a cellular level, rather than a cause of it.

Resection strategy

The surgical strategy combines both the resection and the reconstruction. The surgeon will plan his resection according to the examination and imaging, and the reconstruction according to the tools he has available. Resection of a sarcoma in the limbs depends upon the extent of the tumour, in both the longitudinal and axial directions,

Table 40.5 *Criteria for deciding operative margin*

Intra-osseous/ intramuscular extent	MRI: T_1 weighting
Soft-tissue extent	Examination and operative findings
Margin of excision	Grade

Table 40.6 *Surgical grade of tumour*

Histological grade	Surgical margins
Low	Narrow
Intermediate with no adjuvants	Wide
Intermediate with adjuvants available	Narrow: may save vessels and nerves
High with no preoperative treatment	Wide
High with response to chemotherapy	Intermediate or narrow in axial plane
	Still wide within bone or muscle

and the response to neo-adjuvant treatment. Neo-adjuvant chemotherapy may allow the surgeon to save structures that would have been sacrificed to avoid doubt. The local extent is decided by imaging studies and clinical findings, as shown in Table 40.5.

Surgical grade

The surgical grade of a lesion will determine how much margin the surgeon should use. In Table 40.6, the margin is seen to be as wide in an intermediate-grade lesion such as parosteal osteosarcoma as in a high-grade lesion. With effective neoadjuvant chemotherapy, however, a high-grade Ewing's sarcoma, for instance, may be treated with significantly smaller margins than a chondrosarcoma of much lower grade for which no adjuvant therapies are effective.

Reconstructive strategy

At present, reconstructive options wordwide vary according to availability of technology, surgical tradition, and the expectations of the patient group. Table 40.7 shows how such options are used in Europe today.

Axial tumours

The surgery of axial tumours follows the same strategy as that for limb tumours. The surgeon and the patient have to make even harder choices regarding the sacrifice of function. Once again, the aggressive surgical choices of resection and reconstruction are often reserved for the intermediate-grade lesion with longer life expectancy but no effective adjuvant: a chordoma or chondrosarcoma should be considered for wide local surgery even if mutilatory, while a high-grade Ewing's tumour or osteosarcoma would be restaged after chemotherapy, and limb salvage might be applicable. In these circumstances, it may be appropriate to give all the chemotherapy preoperatively to minimize the impact of surgery, by improving the margins.

RADIOTHERAPY

Indications

There are indications for radiotherapy that are common to several tumour types. Inappropriateness of surgery is

Table 40.7 *The indications for different reconstructive methods*

Reconstruction method	Indications
Massive replacement	When a joint is involved
	When immediate strength is desirable
Expanding massive	If growth in that limb segment is anticipated
Biological replacement	
Pedicled graft, e.g. fibula	Diaphyseal resection close to donor site
Free vacularized graft, e.g. fibula, iliac crest, rib	Diaphyseal resection with no local donor site
Exo-grafts	
Irradiated/pasteurized resection specimen	<10 cm metadiaphyseal resection, with well-preserved bone at site of lesion
Allograft bone	<10 cm metadiaphyseal resection, with bone destruction
Combination graft (e.g. irradiated autograft and vascularized fibula)	>10 cm metadiaphyseal resection, allowing joint-sparing solution

the most common. Clearly, inaccessibility to surgery is also common. However, the decision on what is and what is not operable will depend on the likely success of any available alternative, as well as the risk of metastatic spread. Considerable loss of function from surgery may be acceptable in tumours such as chondrosarcoma, less so in Ewing's tumours where the results of radiotherapy are good. Factors such as skeletal maturity and the consequences on growth and function of surgery and radiotherapy, success of prosthetic replacement at each site and extent of soft-tissue involvement must be considered in every case.

Where the aim of treatment is curative, residual microscopic disease remaining at the site of radical surgery is generally an indication for radiotherapy, as it will be associated with an increased risk of recurrence. Exceptions to this are when there is highly effective chemotherapy yet to be used, as in lymphoma, where the tumour is extremely indolent at a site where recurrences would be amenable to further surgery, or where the risk of radiation-induced damage is considered inappropriate to the eventual risk of recurrence. Although no residual microscopic disease may have been detected at operation, in some circumstances there is a recognized increased risk of local recurrence and these are also indications for adjuvant radiotherapy. Open biopsy carries the risk of implantation along the biopsy track. Where this cannot be excised during definitive surgery, postoperative radiotherapy is indicated. Displaced pathological fracture before surgery carries an increased risk of recurrence and may also be considered an indication for postoperative radiotherapy.

Principles of planning

The general principles of planning radiotherapy for bone tumours are similar to those for soft-tissue sarcomas (Table 40.8). Meticulous immobilization, wedge compensation of beams and individual compensation, if necessary in the long axis of the limb, should be provided. All radical treatments should be CT planned and preferably with conformal techniques. The influence on local control rates of radiotherapy technique and the value of modern diagnostic imaging have been reported (Dunst *et al.*, 1991; Donaldson *et al.*, 1998).

In the treatment of limbs, a strip of unirradiated skin and subcutaneous tissue sufficient to allow lymphatic drainage must be left. Where possible, the spared strip should be medial and joint spaces excluded or shielded. The traditional recommendation is that the whole scar and the full length of the prosthetic material should be included in the target volume. However, the length of scars often reflect the requirements of inserting the prosthesis and may be difficult to cover without compromising function.

As a general principle, the volume selected should be on the basis of the pre-chemotherapy extent, with margins along relevant tissue planes depending on the histology of the tumour and the precise anatomy of the part. This maybe modified; for example, when a bulky tumour protruded into a body cavity but has subsequently regressed. As much bowel as possible should be excluded from the treatment volume by positioning, treating with a full bladder if appropriate or, on occasion, displacement with a gel-filled prosthesis or an omental sling.

Radical treatments are given in two phases: the first volume includes a margin of some 5 cm, and in the second

Table 40.8 *Principles of radiotherapy for bone tumours*

Action	Comment
Plan with MRI and CT and after discussion with musculoskeletal radiologist and, if after surgery, the surgeon	Definition of extent difficult, especially where there is oedema
GTV based on largest tumour extent (except where originally protruded into body cavity and has regressed)	Risk of microscopic contamination after surgery or chemotherapy-induced regression
Margin along *relevant* tissues planes	Risk of spread along marrow cavity and especially in soft tissues along muscles planes. Intact fascia form an effective barrier to spread
Include scar and all prosthetic material, but as this may considerably extend volume, consider risk of contamination in individual cases	There is a risk of microscopic disease here. However, the size of this risk with chemotherapy and good surgical technique is not known
Spare a 'corridor' for lymphatic drainage	High doses are used for these tumours. Failure to provide for lymphatic drainage will produce very severe effects
Without compromising on target volume: Spare as much of joint as possible	The more spared, the less the risk of stiffness; however, disability can be minimized by exercise
Spare epiphyses if possible	10 Gy will probably stop growth
Avoid gonads	Careful technique may sometimes allow this

GTV, gross tumour volume.

phase this is reduced to 2 cm. In the pelvis or spine, smaller margins are sometimes necessary to minimize toxicity. Where radiotherapy is adjuvant to surgery, the initial wide volume only may be used. Certain areas produce particular problems. In the pelvis, while shielding the gonads should be considered, this may not be possible because of the site and extent of the tumour. In the lumbar spine, effective shielding of the kidneys may prove difficult where there has been extensive paravertebral spread into the psoas. Consideration must always be given to spinal cord tolerance. Doses for cure should be at a level to carry only a small risk of cord damage. In more resistant tumours, such as chondrosarcoma or osteosarcoma, the dose per fraction should be reduced in order to achieve the highest possible dose. The presence of a metal-based limb prosthesis will perturb the dose distribution, producing areas of dose reduction along the axis of the incident beam (Hudson *et al.*, 1984). This effect may be minimized by using multiple beams, but this is often not possible in a limb while maintaining effective sparing for lymphatic drainage.

Adverse consequences of radiotherapy

On the whole, acute complications are mild to moderate with conventional fractionation. However, when it is necessary to include perineum or significant amounts of bowel within the field, these may produce severe acute toxicity. Of greater concern are the long-term effects. These relate primarily to abnormalities of growth and limb function and to induction of second malignancies. The risk of impaired function of organs such as kidney or heart from the radiotherapy must be added to the organ-specific toxic effects of chemotherapy used in multimodality treatment.

High-dose radiotherapy to long bones is associated with a higher frequency of fracture, especially where the full circumference must be irradiated, or where there has been extensive cortical bone destruction or biopsy. Effective chemotherapy used before radiotherapy may allow considerable resolution of tumour and healing of bone before radiotherapy is introduced, and it is anticipated that this will result in a reduced risk of fracture.

Reports of effects on late function vary considerably in their frequency and severity. They are related to technique, volume, dose, patient age, pre-treatment function and the use of physiotherapy. While older series report complications in up to 30 per cent of cases, more recent studies suggest that 80 per cent of patients have normal or minimally affected limb function (Jentzsch *et al.*, 1981). Active physiotherapy, particularly aimed towards developing and maintaining joint extension and flexion, should be instituted early and continued for 1–2 years, during which time the maximum radiation-induced fibrosis develops.

Of greater concern is the risk of second malignancy, primarily solid tumours. Several studies show an increased risk, quantifying this at 2.7 times greater after radiotherapy

Table 40.9 *Advantages of neo-adjuvant chemotherapy for bone tumours*

1	Rapid improvement in symptoms
2	Early treatment of micrometastatic disease
3	Facilitation of resection in responding tumours
4	Time to manufacture customized endo-prosthesis
5	Prognostic information from assessment of histological response

and a 33 per cent cumulative risk at 10 years (Tucker *et al.*, 1987; Hawkins *et al.*, 1996). Risks are higher at doses of 60 Gy and when alkylating agents are also used. The risk persists even in the megavoltage era, but appears to be less in patients treated more recently.

Chemotherapy

Osteosarcoma and Ewing's tumours are fatal as a consequence of metastatic spread, principally to the lungs. Advances in chemotherapy over the past 30 years are largely responsible for the dramatic improvements in survival from these tumours. Significant proportions of patients remain incurable, often those who have advanced disease at presentation. Furthermore, current chemotherapy regimens are associated with considerable morbidity, both in the short and long term. As many survivors of bone tumours are young, late toxic effects, particularly cardiotoxicity and infertility, are of great concern to investigators planning effective treatments.

Chemotherapy is often given after biopsy has established an appropriate diagnosis and before definitive local therapy, so-called neo-adjuvant therapy. This practice began in the 1970s as orthopaedic techniques to avoid amputation improved. While rates of conversion of tumours from only suitable for amputation to suitable for limb-salvage surgery may be low (<10 per cent), operability is certainly facilitated in many tumours. Additionally, the prognostic information gained from histological scoring of chemotherapy response in the resected tumour remains a very valuable clinical tool. Other advantages of neo-adjuvant chemotherapy are shown in Table 40.9.

The role of chemotherapy in the management of less common high-grade primary bone tumours is not clearly defined and is discussed as appropriate in specific sections below.

OSTEOSARCOMA

This is the most common high-grade primary tumour of bone. Survival has improved dramatically since the introduction of chemotherapy. Many of the principles underpinning the treatment of osteosarcoma are applicable to other bone tumours.

Subtypes of osteosarcoma

HIGH-GRADE CENTRAL OSTEOSARCOMA

This variant accounts for most cases. Histologically there are areas of spindle-cell formation and variable amounts of tumour bone formation. In other areas of the tumour there may be malignant cartilage or fibroblastic differentiation. Occasionally there is dense osteoblast activity giving rise to a great deal of new bone formation and radiological appearances of dense tumour bone. The malignant osteoblasts make alkaline phosphatase and this is a useful cytological stain for confirmation that the tumour is, in fact, an osteosarcoma. An uncommon variant is an aggressive form of osteosarcoma known as telangiectatic osteosarcoma. There is a lytic process radiologically, with little evidence of new bone formation. Histologically there are vascular spaces and the tumour can be mistaken for an aneurysmal bone cyst.

Typically high-grade tumours start at the epiphysis. They expand within the bone and break through the cortex to lift the periosteum. The elevated periosteum is associated with new bone formation, giving rise to the typical Codman's triangle. The tumour finally erupts through the periosteal boundary and impinges on the adjacent soft tissues. When very large, the tumour extends to the skin and incorporates the neurovascular bundle behind the knee or in the axilla. At this stage endoprosthetic replacement may be extremely difficult.

LOW-GRADE CENTRAL OSTEOSARCOMA

This tumour has a slower rate of progression and is better demarcated radiologically. Histologically, it can be difficult to distinguish from fibrous dysplasia, but the cellular pleomorphism will usually give the diagnosis. It is rare and has a good prognosis when treated by surgery alone.

SURFACE OSTEOSARCOMAS

Some osteosarcomas arise on the surface of the bone rather than centrally. Occasionally, these are high-grade tumours but two other variants are more commonly recognized. Periosteal osteosarcoma appears to carry an intermediate course between high-grade tumours and the low-grade surface tumour, parosteal osteosarcoma. Although the prognosis is better than with classic central osteosarcoma, both parosteal and periosteal osteosarcomas may contain areas of high-grade tumour within them. They tend to arise in a more diaphyseal site than the central osteosarcomas, and the medulla of the bone is not involved until late. In parosteal tumours there is intense formation of trabecular bone and the tumour becomes heavily calcified with a lobulated appearance. The periosteal osteosarcoma contains more cartilage and the calcification is more punctate. Histologically, tumour cells which are making tumour bone and which have alkaline phosphatase in the cytoplasm help to differentiate the tumour from chondrosarcoma.

Clinical presentation

The two major clinical features are pain and swelling. Typically pain precedes the swelling by weeks or months. It starts as an intermittent pain, partially relieved by the usual analgesics but not relieved by rest. After a few weeks the pain intensifies and becomes constant. A characteristic feature, and one which would lead to earlier diagnosis if it were better appreciated, is that patients complain of intensification of pain at night time. After several weeks the second symptom appears, which is swelling. At first this may not be obvious since the soft tissues of the muscle and subcutaneous fat conceal the swelling. At this point the patients or parents become alarmed and usually insist on X-rays if these have not already been arranged.

Sadly, several months often elapse before the diagnosis of a malignant bone tumour is made. This is due to the rarity of the tumours and because in the young, musculoskeletal pains, trivial injuries and strains are common. Very often the patients will have had physiotherapy for some weeks without avail and, indeed, physiotherapy may make symptoms worse. A long period of delay in diagnosis

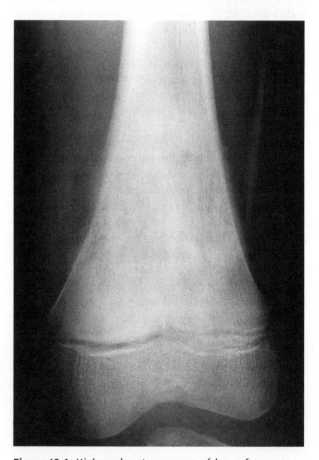

Figure 40.1 *High-grade osteosarcoma of lower femur. A diffuse permeating lesion is seen with elevation of the periosteum (Codman's triangle).*

may create great tension in the family and sometimes considerable difficulties for the relationship between the patient and the family practitioner.

Occasionally patients with osteosarcoma may have a very aggressive tumour that is accompanied by fever and constitutional malaise, anaemia and weight loss. This always implies an extremely bad prognosis and is usually associated with multiple bone or lung metastases. Osteosarcoma nearly always metastasizes to the lung in the first instance. However, bone metastases also occur and, with increasing experience of combination chemotherapy, recurrence at other sites such as skin, brain, and intra-abdominally, is increasingly recognized.

In the lung, metastases are usually asymptomatic. They are typically situated subpleurally where they may give rise to pneumothorax. If the metastasis involves the pleural space a pleural effusion develops. Centrally located metastases may compress one or other main bronchus and give rise to breathlessness, chest pain or haemoptysis.

Investigations

Plain X-rays are essential. The characteristic features of a malignant bone tumour are a permeating, lytic lesion without any clear dividing boundary. When the tumour has broken through the cortex of the bone the periosteum is lifted and there may be formation of a Codman's triangle (Fig. 40.1). In osteosarcoma there may be varying degrees of tumour bone formation leading to dense sclerosis (Fig. 40.2a) or small areas of spiculation of bone, sometimes arranged at right angles to the long axis of the bone (Fig. 40.2b – 'sunray spiculation'). Surface osteosarcomas are associated with the typical radiological appearances shown in Figure 40.3a and b. An isotopic bone scan will typically show an area of increased uptake of isotope at the site of the lesion, and may show bone metastases if present. A CT scan of the chest is essential and may show pulmonary metastases (Fig. 40.4). Magnetic resonance imaging (MRI) is now used to determine both the extent

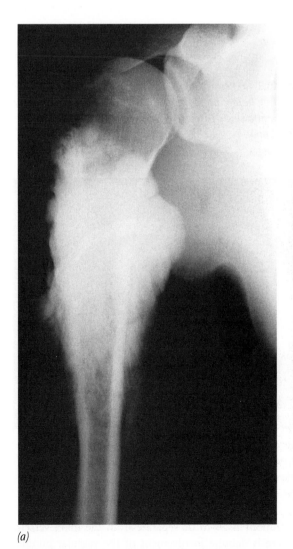

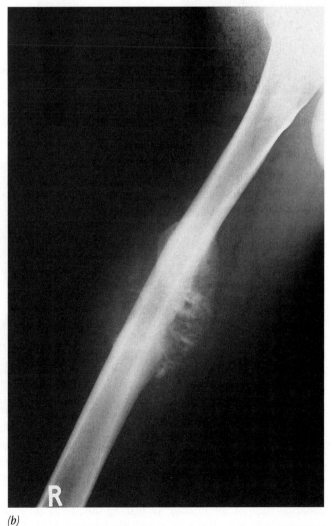

(a)   *(b)*

Figure 40.2 *(a) Plain X-ray of osteoblastic osteosarcoma, showing dense tumour bone surrounding the metaphysis of the upper humerus. (b) Plain X-ray of osteosarcoma of the lower third of the femur, showing 'sunray spiculation'.*

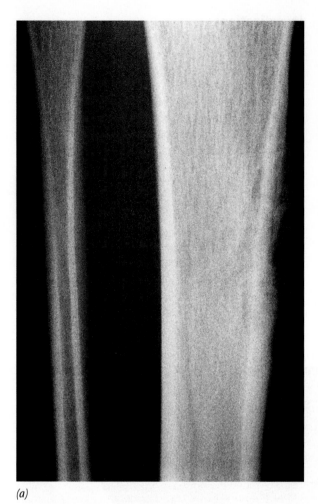

(a)

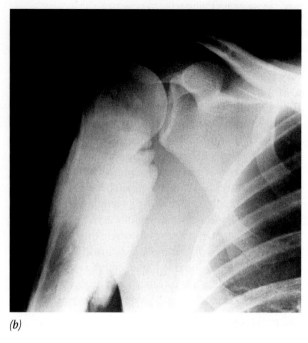

(b)

Figure 40.3 *(a) Periosteal osteosarcoma, showing a permeating lesion in the upper tibia cortex. (b) X-ray of upper humerus, showing dense calcification in a parosteal osteosarcoma.*

of the intramedullary component of the tumour and the soft-tissue extension of the mass (Fig. 40.5).

Accurate assessment of audiological, cardiac, renal glomerular and tubule function should be carried out in all newly diagnosed patients with osteosarcoma. Periodic re-assessment during therapy is indicated, as nephrotoxicity due to agents such as cisplatin and ifosfamide or anthracycline-induced cardiotoxicity may require adjustments in treatment to minimize the risks of permanent damage.

Surgery

Osteosarcoma is usually a tumour involving the limbs, so the lesion is always close to blood vessels. Using MRI scanning to define the intra-osseous extent, it is only necessary to excise sufficient normal bone to account for the surgical error in measuring the levels of bony resection. The vascular bundles close to the tumour may need to be excised with the tumour and replaced, or they can be dissected clear of the tumour. In making this decision preoperatively, it is often wise to wait for a second MRI scan after the preoperative chemotherapy cycles, since the situation may change. This second scan will often show

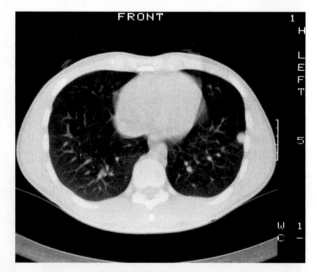

Figure 40.4 *CT scan of the chest in a patient with osteosarcoma and a normal chest X-ray. A single subpleural metastasis is seen on the left. This is a typical position for bone sarcoma metastases.*

the tumour itself to be separate from the main vessels. If there is definite involvement of the vascular bundle, this will need to be sacrificed. Sarcomas rarely invade peripheral nerves and excision is not usually needed.

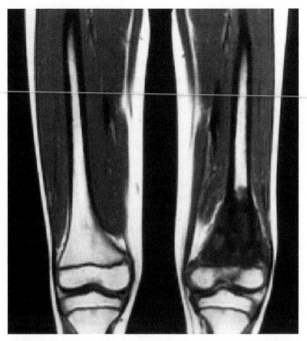

Figure 40.5 *MRI scan showing osteosarcoma of the left lower femur. The tumour has extended into the soft tissues.*
Typically, it has stopped at the level of the unfused epiphysis.

Epineural dissection of the nerves may be undertaken instead, although this means a marginal excision of the tumour.

Reconstruction is planned after using MRI scans to determine the safe level of bone section and soft-tissue dissection. Occasionally amputation may be the only possible procedure because of extensive soft-tissue and skin involvement. However, the limb can usually be saved by use of a massive endoprosthesis. Because the tumour usually arises close to joints, the joint must often be excised and an artificial joint on the end of the titanium shaft will be substituted for the bone segment. The use of allograft bone as an alternative has not provided the long-term stability obtained with endoprostheses, and so is less favoured at the present time, although it is still an option. When circumstances allow, the joint closest to the tumour may be saved and a so-called 'intercalary' prosthesis used to take the place of the bone segment that has been excised.

Limb segments may be reconstituted using vascularized fibular grafts or by means of bone transport, but both of these techniques require very extensive operative intervention. In these patients with high-grade tumours we would recommend the use of massive prostheses because of the rapid rehabilitation. This allows chemotherapy to begin again within 2–3 weeks of the surgery.

Chemotherapy

Before the 1970s osteosarcoma was a devastating disease, treatable only by amputation, with more than 80 per cent of patients succumbing rapidly due to lung metastases. Subsequent developments have transformed this appalling outlook. Firstly, cytotoxic agents were identified which induced responses in advanced osteosarcoma. The most important of these were methotrexate given at very high doses, doxorubicin and cisplatin. Secondly, was the observation that resection of pulmonary metastases was both technically possible and profitable in terms of survival. Finally, improving surgical techniques allowed limb preservation in some cases. This last development led to the concept of preoperative chemotherapy, response to which seemed to facilitate 'limb salvage' surgery and which allowed time to manufacture custom-measured metallic endoprostheses.

After 1975, evidence of a survival advantage for adjuvant chemotherapy grew, in particular through a series of uncontrolled studies conducted at the Memorial Sloan Kettering hospital of combination chemotherapy given after surgery. These drug regimens used doxorubicin, high-dose methotrexate, and bleomycin, cyclophosphamide and actinomycin D – a combination known as BCD. These programmes evolved to produce a regimen called T10, for which impressive 2-year survival rates were claimed (Rosen *et al.*, 1982). At the time, these studies were difficult to interpret because of the lack of any concomitant control and the very short follow-up period. Alterations in selection criteria which had occurred during the 1970s – particularly the introduction of CT scanning – made firm assessment of the results difficult.

The doubts were allayed to a considerable extent by two randomized studies. Link and co-workers compared T10-based chemotherapy with no chemotherapy. There was a clear difference in relapse-free survival in favour of chemotherapy at diagnosis (Link *et al.*, 1986). A further study from Eilber and colleagues randomized patients to receive no further chemotherapy following initial intra-arterial doxorubicin and tumour irradiation. The other arm of the randomization was to receive postoperative treatment with BCD and high-dose methotrexate. There was a significant improvement in relapse-free survival and overall survival in the small number of patients who were randomized (Eilber *et al.*, 1987).

Since then, adjuvant chemotherapy has been accepted as part of standard management for high-grade osteosarcoma. Chemotherapy given prior to surgery for the primary has also become accepted, offering the advantages outlined in Table 40.9. Assessment of the histological response to chemotherapy has been identified as the most powerful prognostic factor in this disease; those patients who experience very extensive necrosis (in excess of 90 per cent) have an overall survival in excess of 70 per cent at 5 years, while those in whom the degree of necrosis falls short of this have a significantly inferior survival. There are theoretical disadvantages associated with preoperative chemotherapy, namely that poorly or non-responsive tumours may grow during treatment, increasing the risk of amputation and of distant spread. The single randomized trial to address this issue showed that those receiving preoperative chemotherapy enjoyed a significantly higher rate of limb salvage surgery without any survival disadvantage (Goorin *et al.*, 1996).

The most active cytotoxic agents include methotrexate, doxorubicin, cisplatin, ifosfamide and etoposide. There have been no important recent additions to this list and clinical studies have been aimed at definition of optimal treatment schedules. Intra-arterial chemotherapy has been shown to produce high rates of histological necrosis but does not improve survival and is not routinely indicated. There are relatively few randomized trials of chemotherapy for osteosarcoma which have sufficient statistical power to provide firm evidence for best practice. Important studies have been carried out by the European Osteosarcoma Intergroup (EOI), the first of which aimed to define the importance of high-dose methotrexate, and the second of which compared a prolonged multi-drug regimen, similar to T10, to a two-drug combination given for just six cycles (Bramwell *et al.*, 1992; Souhami *et al.*, 1997). The EOI studies are summarized in Table 40.10.

The first of these studies has been used to support arguments against the inclusion of high-dose methotrexate in regimens. However, the study design was flawed as patients in the methotrexate arm received significantly less doxorubicin and cisplatin than those in the control arm. The second study, however, clearly demonstrated equivalent survival for the two-drug combination compared with a more complex and toxic regimen based on the T10 programme, widely accepted as a standard protocol.

The results of multi-centre randomized studies have consistently fallen short of those reported from single centres for this disease. The overall survival for the combined data from the above two studies is 56 per cent, while single centres, such as the Memorial Sloan Kettering Hospital, consistently report survival in the order of 70 per cent (Meyers *et al.*, 1992). The explanation for this is complex and multifactorial, but a major component will relate to case mix. Greater collaboration between co-operative groups is needed.

Adaptation of therapy according to risk factors remains insufficiently developed for patients with extremity osteosarcoma. This is because the most powerful indicator of outcome, histological response, is only available well into any programme of systemic therapy. Furthermore, no study has clearly identified that alteration of therapy on the basis of histological response can improve survival for those with poor rates of necrosis. It is hoped that newer biological markers, such as *c-erb-B2* expression, may provide earlier indications of outcome that can be used to plan individualized treatment. This is anticipated to be an important focus for clinical research in the future.

Radiotherapy

The role of radiotherapy in this tumour is confined to adjuvant treatment for risk of microscopic disease and operability. This relatively radioresistant tumour does have a degree of response to radiotherapy if high doses are given. Long-term control doses of 70 Gy or more have been used (Cade, 1955). This produced, in unresected tumours, a reported local control rate of 20–25 per cent, and reports of tumour sterilization in amputation specimens of 33 per cent. Radical radiotherapy alone is used for inoperable tumours, usually of the axial skeleton, which are associated with poor prognosis. High-dose radiotherapy is required to control local symptoms for the remainder of the patient's life. Symptomatic improvement is produced in approximately 50 per cent of patients.

Treatment of metastases

Presentation with pulmonary metastasis is a grave prognostic sign and almost no patients are cured if they present with bone metastases. Patients who present with one or two pulmonary metastases should be treated with chemotherapy. If they respond completely, a very close surveillance policy must be followed and resectable metastases should be removed if they re-appear on CT scanning. Patients presenting with multiple pulmonary metastases will almost certainly not be cured even if there is complete response to chemotherapy. Nevertheless treatment is worthwhile and very durable responses may be obtained.

The more common situation is for metastases to appear after chemotherapy has been completed. Some patients are certainly cured by thoracotomy. Good prognostic factors for the success of thoracotomy are few metastases, unilateral rather than bilateral disease, a long period of freedom from relapse following the cessation

Table 40.10 *European Osteosarcoma Intergroup randomized studies of chemotherapy for extremity osteosarcoma*

Study	Number of patients	Arms	Outcome
1 (accrual 1983–86)	179	Doxorubicin + cisplatin versus doxorubicin + cisplatin + methotrexate	Equivalent overall survival
2 (accrual 1988–92)	391	Doxorubicin + cisplatin versus 'T10'	Equivalent overall survival
3 (1993–)	400+	Doxorubicin + cisplatin, 3-weekly versus doxorubicin + cisplatin, 2-weekly with GCSF	Awaited

GCSF, granulocyte colony stimulating factor.

of chemotherapy, and the peripheral location of the metastases (Ward *et al.*, 1994). Patients who develop pulmonary metastases while on chemotherapy have a very bad prognosis indeed. Although the introduction of new agents may produce responses, and is worthwhile, the chances of cure are very small. Similarly, relapse immediately, or a few months after, the cessation of chemotherapy is also very adverse. Pleural effusion is an extremely adverse sign and nearly always indicates intra-pleural spread of the tumour, which is incurable.

There are many questions still to be asked about optimum management of pulmonary metastases. It is not clear how often repeated thoracotomies are successful. Some patients have multiple thoracotomies, each of which appears justified but which fails to produce lasting benefit. Occasionally freedom from disease may be achieved, especially when the intervals between surgery are relatively long. Prophylactic pulmonary irradiation after metastatectomy has never been investigated appropriately to determine whether it might confer a lasting benefit.

Variants of osteosarcoma

Small cell osteosarcoma and telangiectatic osteosarcoma are high-grade tumours which should be treated as for conventional osteosarcoma. Parosteal osteosarcoma is of low-grade malignancy and is not usually treated with chemotherapy unless there is clear evidence of high-grade dedifferentiation within the tumour (Sheth *et al.*, 1996). Periosteal osteosarcoma is of higher grade than parosteal osteosarcoma but still with a lower risk of metastasis than conventional osteosarcoma (Ritts *et al.*, 1987). There is little definite evidence that chemotherapy benefits these patients, but it is usually given, especially if there are extensive areas of high-grade tumour.

Post-irradiation and Paget's osteosarcoma are always of high grade histologically and may have an appearance more like malignant fibrous histiocytoma. The main treatment is surgical resection, but this is often very difficult in view of their location. There are no survivors of Paget's sarcoma but other secondary osteosarcomas are frequently cured if complete excision is possible.

EWING'S FAMILY OF TUMOURS

James Ewing's original descriptions of this disease remain pertinent today. It is a member of the group of small, round, blue cell tumours of childhood, with neuroblastoma, rhabdomyosarcoma and some lymphomas, distinguishable only by immunocytochemistry or biological markers. Its aetiology and cell of origin remain obscure despite the demonstration of characteristic chromosomal translocations, t(11;22) and, less commonly, t(21;22). These translocations have illuminated the close relationship between classical Ewing tumour and other related tumours, primitive neuroectodermal tumours of bone and soft tissue which share the same cytogenetic abnormality but may express more neural markers.

Clinical features and diagnosis

The presentation is as for osteosarcoma. The main symptoms are pain and swelling, and the location of the tumour is usually diaphyseal rather epiphyseal. Unlike osteosarcoma, EFTs are much more commonly found in the pelvis, the ribs and the axial skeleton. The most common sites are femur, humerus, ilium, other regions of the pelvis, ribs, skull and jaw, and small bones of the hands and feet. The tumour is typically permeating, spreading widely within the medulla and the vascular spaces of the bone cortex. It causes necrosis of bone, and the tumour itself may be necrotic.

New bone is often laid down around the site of the tumour, giving rise, radiologically, to the typical 'onion skin' appearance. There is often thickening and sclerosis of the cortex of the bone, although occasionally Ewing's tumours are purely destructive with widespread bone lysis (Fig. 40.6).

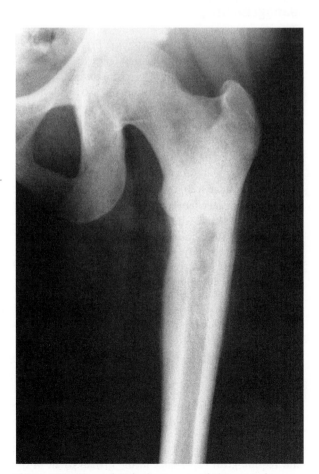

Figure 40.6 *X-ray of Ewing's sarcoma of the upper femur. Dense cortical thickening is present with 'onion-skin' periosteal reaction.*

Diagnosis is by biopsy, and it is important that the specimen is examined by a skilled pathologist in conjunction with the X-rays. The differential diagnosis will include non-malignant conditions such as osteomyelitis. An appropriate panel of immunocytochemical markers must be used to exclude lymphomas and carcinomas. Various degrees of neural differentiation will be indicated by markers such as S100 and chromogranin, and expression of CD99, although not specific for EFT, is usually strongly positive.

Investigations

Investigations should include plain radiographs of the affected bone. An isotope bone scan will confirm the increased uptake in the presence of the primary tumour and may show other bone metastases. A CT scan of the lungs is essential to confirm or exclude visible pulmonary metastases and an MRI of the affected bone is useful both in assessing tumour size (and thus prognosis, *see* below) and in planning primary treatment. Staging is completed by examination of a bone marrow aspirate and trephine biopsy. Investigations of organ function should be carried out as for osteosarcoma.

Management

When a patient with Ewing's sarcoma first presents it is essential that a thorough discussion takes place about the way in which management is to be conducted. This discussion must involve medical oncologists, radiotherapists and surgeons. The first decision to be made will be concerning the local treatment. Essentially there will be two choices, either that the lesion can be removed surgically or that the patient will have to receive radiation. Occasionally it will not be possible to decide definitively at the outset between these two alternatives, but the response to initial chemotherapy will have to be awaited in order to determine whether surgical resection is feasible. The decision will be based on several factors:

- Is the lesion likely to be resectable in its entirety with uninvolved resection margins?
- Will radiotherapy be thereby avoided?
- Will the functional results of surgery be acceptable?
- Will the functional results of radiotherapy be acceptable?
- What is likely to be the long-term local control rate with either surgery or radiation?
- Will a synchronous combined programme of chemotherapy and radiation be feasible over the size of the planned radiation field?

The answers to these questions are extremely difficult and require great experience in the management of the tumours. On the one hand, small expendable bones can be easily resected and the rate of local recurrence will be low. On the other hand, massive tumours in the pelvis which cannot be resected have to be treated with radiation, with a high risk of local recurrence because of the tumour size. In between, there will be highly complex decisions where the balance of advantages must be carefully assessed. The problem with radiation is that local control may not always be achieved, and that the risk of second cancer in the radiated bone is significant. In the case of surgery, functional results may be really quite poor and, if the resection margins are involved, the need for radiation will not have been avoided. On the other hand, the local recurrence rates with surgical resection with or without radiation are probably lower than with radiation alone. Finally, it should be noted that isolated local relapse is relatively uncommon in EFS, with most patients having distant metastases at relapse.

Chemotherapy

Alkylating agents were among the first drugs used in Ewing's sarcoma, and cyclophosphamide was the standard agent for many years. Early combination therapy comprised vincristine, actinomycin D and cyclophosphamide (VAC). A randomized study carried out by the American co-operative group (IESS) demonstrated that the addition of doxorubicin to this combination led to a significant survival advantage, superior to that provided by pulmonary irradiation. More recently, ifosfamide has been shown to be a highly active drug, and many current regimens use ifosfamide as the alkylating agent of choice.

Combination chemotherapy regimens are based on combinations of vincristine, actinomycin and cyclophosphamide, or vincristine, doxorubicin and cyclophosphamide. More recently, the combinations have substituted ifosfamide for cyclophosphamide and there has been increased interest in the use of etoposide as part of more intensive programmes.

A recently completed study between the UK and the Cooperative Ewing's Sarcoma Studies from West Germany has compared predominantly ifosfamide-based chemotherapy with chemotherapy based on ifosfamide and cyclophosphamide in low-risk Ewing's sarcomas. In another group of patients, the ifosfamide-based chemotherapy was compared with the same chemotherapy with the addition of etoposide. Follow-up in this study is still short but there appears to be no clear advantage in favour of etoposide in this schedule. Overall survival is similar to earlier studies and there remains considerable room for improvement, particularly in patients presenting with adverse features.

Prognosis in this disease can be related to several features. The most important of these is the presence of metastatic disease. It is evident that a proportion of patients with metastatic disease confined to the lungs will be cured by conventional chemotherapy, but there are virtually no survivors if the bone marrow or other bones are involved. Tumour volume can all be used to stratify patients, with those with tumours larger than 1–200 ml faring less well. Finally, in patients who undergo surgery, the response to preoperative chemotherapy appears to be an important factor, as in osteosarcoma.

There has been considerable interest in dose-escalated therapy using peripheral stem-cell rescue for those with an adverse prognosis. Although studies so far are small and uncontrolled, the evidence is such that the value of this approach is now being addressed in a large randomized study.

Radiotherapy

The aim of local treatment is to achieve control while preserving function. Before effective multi-agent chemotherapy, radiation alone cured approximately 15 per cent of patients, the remainder dying of metastatic disease. Reported local control produced by radiotherapy ranged from 50 to 75 per cent (Horowitz et al., 1993). Multiagent chemotherapy, in addition to improving the survival rate, contributed to an improvement in local control rate which was achieved in approximately 85 to 90 per cent (Nesbit et al., 1990), with single-institution studies generally reporting better results than multicentre groups. Tumours greater than 100 ml^3 in volume and those in the pelvis are associated with higher local failure rates and also lower survival rates. The observation of lower survivals in patients treated with radiotherapy rather than surgery, the finding of unexpectedly high local recurrence rates in autopsy series, and the risk of second malignancy has led to the increasing use of surgery. The majority of studies show that improved local control is associated with the use of surgery and this is generally the local modality of choice, except where it would produce significant morbidity (Dunst et al., 1995; Donaldson et al., 1998; Carrie et al., 1999). Comparison of the efficacy of the two modalities is not appropriate because of different selection criteria. The most difficult decisions relate to bulky pelvic primaries, where the 5-year survival is less than 50 per cent and it is not clear whether combined surgery and radiotherapy improves outcome. The approach in the UK has generally been for surgery if clearly operable with radiotherapy added for positive or close margins, especially with poor chemotherapy response, and radiotherapy for the remainder. In Europe preoperative radiotherapy is preferred. The latter approach is associated with increased but manageable postoperative toxicites and increases the resection rate, but a clear benefit on survival has not been demonstrated (Dunst et al., 1995). Doses for Ewing's are 40–45 Gy for microscopic disease and 55–60 Gy for bulk disease.

Local control is dependent upon technique and dose. The CESS 86 study had a much lower failure rate when central planning was introduced (Sauer et al., 1987). In the past, recommendations have been to treat the whole cavity because of the risk of skip lesions within the marrow of tumour-bearing bones. With modern modality therapy the use of more limited fields does not compromise in-field control. There is no evidence of a dose response above 55 Gy, although numbers in each dose group are small. Radiotherapy for Ewing's is administered during chemotherapy. This can increase both acute and late effects and some modification is usually introduced. Doxorubicin and actinomycin may be omitted during radiotherapy, or a protocol using hyperfractionation and planned gaps is used. This reduces late effects and allows manageable acute toxicity while not significantly extending the period of radiotherapy (Bolek et al., 1996).

Surgery

The surgery of Ewing's sarcoma is much more demanding than that of osteosarcoma because the tumour is almost always stage IIb rather than IIa (using the modified staging notation described for osteosarcoma). The margins of resection are thus much more difficult to define. Surgery is reserved for those cases in whom cure is a probability. In the limbs this will often involve the resection of the greater part of the long bone. In the pelvis and axial skeleton, these lesions can only rarely be excised with confidence about the resection margins, and are sometimes too extensive for reasonable functional reconstruction. However, it is in just these sites that radiation has proved less efficient in providing local control of a very large lesion. Increasingly, combined surgical and radiation approaches are being used for large pelvic Ewing's tumours.

While it is sometimes possible to avoid postoperative radiotherapy by careful planning, the tumour is highly permeative and presents considerable technical problems. The aim, where possible, is to avoid the combined affects of surgery and radiation.

Results and prognosis

Approximately 60 per cent of all patients with Ewing's sarcoma will be cured of their disease. However, this overall figure is a simplification, since patients with small tumours have a better prognosis than those with very large lesions (Cotterill et al., 2000). The outlook for Ewing's sarcoma of the small bones of the hands, feet and jaw is already excellent. On the other hand, the prognosis of Ewing's sarcoma in the pelvis, treated with combination chemotherapy and radiation, has remained unsatisfactory. At this site, with these very large tumours, local control with surgery or radiation is difficult to achieve.

MALIGNANT FIBROUS HISTIOCYTOMA OF BONE

Malignant fibrous histiocytoma (MFH) is a distinct clinico-pathological entity which was first described by

Feldman and Norman (1972). It accounts for approximately 5 per cent of primary malignant bone tumours. The cell of origin is unclear. The peak incidence is in middle age, although it tends to occur slightly later in women. In approximately 20 per cent of patients MFH arises in an area where the bone has been previously abnormal, such as fibrous dysplasia, bone infarction, or Paget's disease or radiation. The primary site is usually the femur or tibia, although the humerus and pelvis are sometimes affected.

Until the past decade, treatment for MFH of bone has been with surgery, sometimes combined with local radiation. However, it is now clear that only 30 per cent of patients will survive 5 years if local treatment is given alone. More recently, adjuvant chemotherapy has been used, either preoperatively, as in osteosarcoma, or after the primary surgical excision. No randomized trials of chemotherapy have been conducted, but it is clear that the tumour is chemosensitive, as judged by both clinical response and by histopathological evidence of tumour necrosis in the resection specimen (Earl et al., 1993; Bacci et al., 1997).

The chemotherapeutic agents which should be used have not been defined systematically but, in general, treatment programmes have followed those for osteosarcoma (Bramwell et al., 1999). Cisplatin, doxorubicin and ifosfamide have been the agents used in these studies. However, large-scale studies, where patients are followed over a long period of time, are necessary to define the current cure rate in this condition.

PRIMARY NON-HODGKIN'S LYMPHOMA OF BONE

This tumour accounts for about 4 per cent of primary bone tumours. Although nodal non-Hodgkin's lymphomas may spread to the bone marrow, and occasionally present with bone metastasis, the primary tumour is defined as a presentation with a malignant bone tumour where staging investigations fail to reveal generalized spread of the disease in the marrow or distant lymph-node sites.

The mainstay of local treatment for primary non-Hodgkin's lymphoma of bone (PBL) is radiation treatment. Using doses of at least 20 Gy, few patients will relapse at the local site. Although local radiation may produce cure in patients who have a localized and low-grade PBL, many patients do develop more systemic spread, and the present management consists of both radiation treatment and chemotherapy. The results have been encouraging, with approximately 50 per cent of patients with the more advanced (stage III and IV) tumours being alive at 5 years. Patients with stage I and stage II disease, who have been treated with chemotherapy and radiation, have a better 5-year survival rate, with more than 82 per cent of patients disease-free at 5 years (Fairbanks et al., 1994; Heyning et al., 1999). Prognostic factors include not only stage of disease, but also the histological type of lymphoma. The higher grade, pleomorphic tumours have a worse prognosis and tend to be more permeating and lytic radiologically. Occasionally patients present with multifocal primary bone lymphoma and these patients are treated with intensive combination chemotherapy.

CHONDROSARCOMA

Pathology

Chondrosarcomas are malignant tumours of cartilage. Histological grading based on cellularity and grading is reflected by clinical behaviour. Frank dedifferentiation to a high-grade tumour is also recognized and such tumours have a high metastatic potential and a poor overall survival.

The tumour is rare before the third decade and more common in the fourth and fifth decades. It has predilection for the girdles and proximal long bones, but may arise at any site. The tumours are usually slow growing and, particularly in the pelvis, may reach a great size before detection. The principal presentation is with a painful lump.

Investigation

The radiographic features are usually diagnostic. However, thorough preoperative assessment is essential. A CT and MR scan of the lesion should be performed and subsequent needle biopsy of the most malignant-looking area should be undertaken. This will prevent a high-grade tumour which has developed in an osteochondroma from being treated inadequately.

Surgical management

Chondrosarcoma does not respond to chemotherapy or radiotherapy except when dedifferentiated. These tumours should be resected after meticulous imaging to determine the levels and planes of resection. Wide local excision should be performed. Like other musculoskeletal sarcomas, these tumours invade neither peripheral nerves nor dura and so they may be resected without causing serious mutilation, even when awkwardly sited. However, vascular grafts might be necessary. Reconstruction of the limb segments that have been removed is as for osteosarcoma. Chemotherapy (using cisplatin/doxorubicin/ifosfamide combinations) may produce responses in dedifferentiated lesions.

Prognosis

The prognosis of chondrosarcoma depends on its grade and site (Lee et al., 1999). The resection margin depends entirely on the size and site of the lesion and the adequacy of preoperative planning. With meticulous planning of approach and planes of dissection, even very large tumours in the pelvis may be removed with minimal risk of local contamination. Curettage of these lesions is never curative and prevents secondary surgery from ever being successful. In the elderly and debilitated, intra-lesional surgery may be contemplated for palliation where the physical cost of curative surgery is too great. In the young, however, where cure is essential, ablative surgery with reasonable margins must be undertaken to prevent a distressing prolonged illness consisting of progressive locally recurrent disease.

SIGNIFICANT POINTS

- Primary tumours of bone are uncommon but share similar clinical features of pain and swelling. These are often ignored for a considerable time.
- Initial evaluation should be conducted in specialist centres. Appropriate imaging should be carried out before planned biopsy.
- Diagnosis can usually be made by core needle biopsy. Placement of the biopsy track should be determined after consideration of future surgery.
- Histological interpretation requires special expertise and should take account of clinical and radiological features.
- Many primary bone tumours, particularly osteosarcoma and Ewing's sarcoma, may be cured by appropriate multimodality therapy. Such treatment is intensive and complex. It requires close communication between surgical and non-surgical oncology teams.
- Further advances in treatment are likely to come through a growing understanding of the unusual biological features of these disease.

KEY REFERENCES

Campanacci, M. (1986) *Bone and soft tissue tumours.* Vienna: Springer Verlag.

Mirra, J.M., Picci, P. and Gold, R.H. (1989) *Bone tumours. Clinical, radiologic and pathologic correlations.* Philadelphia: Lea and Febiger.

Whelan, J.S. (1997) Osteosarcoma. *Eur. J. Cancer* **33**, 1611–19.

REFERENCES

Bacci, G., Ferrari, S., Bertoni, F. *et al.* (1997) Neoadjuvant chemotherapy for osseous malignant fibrous histiocytoma of the extremity: results in 18 cases and comparison with 112 contemporary osteosarcoma patients treated with the same chemotherapy regimen *J. Chemother.* **9**, 293–9.

Bolek, T.W., Marcus, R.B. Jr, Mendenhall, N.P. *et al.* (1996) Local control and functional results after twice-daily radiotherapy for Ewing's sarcoma of the extremities *Int. J. Radiat. Oncol. Biol. Phys.* **35**, 687–92.

Bramwell, V.H.C., Burgess, M., Sneath, R. *et al.* (1992) A comparison of two short intensive adjuvant chemotherapy regimens in operable osteosarcoma of limbs in children and young adults: the first study of the European Osteosarcoma Intergroup. *J. Clin. Oncol.* **10**, 1579–91.

Bramwell, V.H., Steward, W.P., Nooij, M. *et al.* (1999) Neoadjuvant chemotherapy with doxorubicin and cisplatin in malignant fibrous histiocytoma of bone: a European Osteosarcoma Intergroup study. *J. Clin. Oncol.* **17**, 3260–9.

Cade, S. (1955) Osteogenic sarcoma: a study based on 133 patients. *J. R. Coll. Surg. Edin.* **1**, 79–111.

Carrie, C., Mascard, E., Gomez, F. *et al.* (1999) Nonmetastatic pelvic Ewing sarcoma: report of the French society of pediatric oncology. *Med. Pediatr. Oncol.* **33**, 444–9.

Cotterill, S.J., Ahrens, S., Paulussen, M. *et al.* (2000) Prognostic factors in Ewing's tumor of bone: analysis of 975 patients from the European Intergroup Cooperative Ewing's Sarcoma Study Group. *J. Clin. Oncol.* **18**, 3108–14.

Donaldson, S.S., Torrey, M., Link, M.P. *et al.* (1998) A multidisciplinary study investigating radiotherapy in Ewing's sarcoma: end results of POG #8346. Pediatric Oncology Group. *Int. J. Radiat. Oncol. Biol. Phys.* **42**, 125–35.

Draper, G.J., Sanders, B.M. and Kingston, J.E. (1986) Second primary neoplasms in patients with retinoblastoma. *Br. J. Cancer* **53**, 661–71.

Dunst, J., Sauer, R., Burgers, J.M. *et al.* (1991) Radiation therapy as local treatment in Ewing's sarcoma. Results of the Cooperative Ewing's Sarcoma Studies CESS 81 and CESS 86. *Cancer* **67**, 2818–25.

Dunst, J., Jurgens, H., Sauer, R. *et al.* (1995) Radiation therapy in Ewing's sarcoma: an update of the CESS 86 trial [*see* comments]. *Int. J. Radiat. Oncol. Biol. Phys.* **32**, 919–30.

Earl, H.M., Pringle, J., Kemp, H.B. *et al.* (1993) Chemotherapy for malignant fibrous histiocytoma of bone. *Ann. Oncol.* **4**, 409–15.

Eilber, F., Giuliano, A., Eckardt, J. *et al.* (1987) Adjuvant chemotherapy for osteosarcoma: a randomised prospective trial. *J. Clin. Oncol.* **5**, 21–6.

Enneking, W.F., Spanier, S.S. and Goodman, M.A. (1980) A system for the surgical staging of musculoskeletal sarcomata. *Clin. Orthop.* **153**, 106–20.

Fairbanks, R.K., Bonner, J.A., Inwards, C.Y. *et al.* (1994) Treatment of stage IE primary lymphoma of bone. *Int. J. Radiat. Oncol. Biol. Phys.* **28**, 363–72.

Feldman, F. and Norman, D. (1972) Intra- and extraosseous malignant histiocytoma (malignant fibrous xanthoma). *Radiology* **104**, 497–508.

Goorin, A., Gieser, P., Schwartzentruber, D. *et al.* (1996) No evidence for improved event-free survival with presurgical chemotherapy for non-metastatic extremity osteosarcoma: preliminary results of a randomised non-metastatic pediatric oncology group trial 8651. *Med. Ped. Oncol.* **27**, 263.

Grimer, R.J., Carter, S.R. and Pynsent, P.B. (1997) The cost-effectiveness of limb salvage for bone tumours. *J. Bone Joint Surg. Br.* **79**, 558–61.

Hawkins, M.M., Wilson, L.M., Burton, H.S. *et al.* (1996) Radiotherapy, alkylating agents, and risk of bone cancer after childhood cancer. *J. Natl Cancer Inst.* **88**, 270–8.

Heyning, F.H., Hogendoorn, P.C., Kramer, M.H. *et al.* (1999) Primary non-Hodgkin's lymphoma of bone: a clinicopathological investigation of 60 cases. *Leukemia* **13**, 2094–8.

Horowitz, M.E., Delaney, T.F., Malawar, M.M. and Tsolos, M.G. (1993) In Pizzo, P.A. and Poplack, D.G. (eds), *Principles and practice of pediatric oncology.* Philadelphia: Lippincott.

Hudson, F.R., Crawley, M.T. and Samarasekera, M. (1984) Radiotherapy treatment planning for patients fitted with prostheses. *Br. J. Radiol.* **57**, 603–8.

Jentzsch, K., Binder, H., Cramer, H. *et al.* (1981) Leg function after radiotherapy for Ewing's sarcoma. *Cancer* **47**, 1267–78.

Lee, F.Y., Mankin, H.J., Fondren, G. *et al.* (1999) Chondrosarcoma of bone: an assessment of outcome. *J. Bone Joint Surg. Am.* **81**, 326–38.

Li, F.P. (1993) Molecular epidemiology studies of cancer in families. *Br. J. Cancer* **68**, 217–19.

Link, M.P., Goorin, A.M., Miser, M.D. *et al.* (1986) The effect of adjuvant chemotherapy on relapse-free survival in patients with osteosarcoma of the extremity. *N. Engl. J. Med.* **314**, 1600–606.

Meyers, P.A., Heller, G., Healey, J. *et al.* (1992) Chemotherapy for nonmetastatic osteogenic sarcoma: the Memorial Sloan-Kettering experience. *J. Clin. Oncol.* **10**, 5–15.

Nesbit, M.E. Jr, Gehan, E.A., Burgert, E.O. Jr *et al.* (1990) Multimodal therapy for the management of primary, nonmetastatic Ewing's sarcoma of bone: a long-term follow-up of the First Intergroup study. *J. Clin. Oncol.* **8**, 1664–74.

Polednak, A.P. (1978) Bone cancer among female radium dial workers. Latency periods and incidence rates after exposure: brief communication. *J. Natl Cancer Inst.* **60**, 77–82.

Postma, A., Kingma, A., De Ruiter, J.H. *et al.* (1992) Quality of life in bone tumor patients comparing limb salvage and amputation of the lower extremity. *J. Surg. Oncol.* **51**, 47–51.

Price, C.H. and Goldie, W. (1969) Paget's sarcoma of bone. A study of eighty cases from the Bristol and the Leeds bone tumour registries. *J. Bone Joint Surg. Br.* **51**, 205–24.

Ritts, G.D., Pritchard, D.J., Unni, K.K. *et al.* (1987) Periosteal osteosarcoma. *Clin. Orthop.* June (219), 299–307.

Rosen, G., Caparros, B., Huvos, A.G. *et al.* (1982) Preoperative chemotherapy for osteogenic sarcoma: selection of postoperative adjuvant chemotherapy based on the response of the primary tumor to preoperative chemotherapy. *Cancer* **49**, 1221–30.

Sauer, R., Jurgens, H., Burgers, J.M. *et al.* (1987) Prognostic factors in the treatment of Ewing's sarcoma. The Ewing's Sarcoma Study Group of the German Society of Paediatric Oncology CESS 81. *Radiother. Oncol.* **10**, 101–10.

Sheth, D.S., Yasko, A.W., Raymond, A.K. *et al.* (1996) Conventional and dedifferentiated parosteal osteosarcoma. Diagnosis, treatment, and outcome. *Cancer* **78**, 2136–45.

Souhami, R.L., Craft, A., van der Eiken, J. *et al.* (1997) A randomised trial of two regimens of chemotherapy in operable osteosarcoma: a study of the European Osteosarcoma Intergroup. *Lancet* **350**, 911–17.

Stoker, D.J., Cobb, J.P. and Pringle, J.A.S. (1991) The needle biopsy of musculoskeletal lesions: a review of 208 cases. *J. Bone Joint Surg. Br.* **23**, 498–500.

Tucker, M.A., D'Angio, G.J., Boice, J.D. *et al.* (1987) Bone sarcomas linked to radiotherapy and chemotherapy in children. *N. Engl. J. Med.* **317**, 588–93.

Ward, W.G., Mikaelian, K., Dorey, F. *et al.* (1994) Pulmonary metastases of stage IIB extremity osteosarcoma and subsequent pulmonary metastases. *J. Clin. Oncol.* **12**, 1849–58.

41

Soft tissue sarcomas

THOMAS F. DELANEY, ANDREW E. ROSENBERG, DAVID C. HARMON, HENRY J. MANKIN,
IRA J. SPIRO, DANIEL ROSENTHAL AND HERMAN D. SUIT

Sarcomas of the soft tissues constitute a highly hetero-geneous group of tumours with respect to histological type and anatomical distribution. The term sarcomas of soft tissues embraces all the malignant tumours that arise from the mesenchymal tissues excluding bone, i.e. malignant fibrous histiocytoma, liposarcoma, leiomyosarcoma, syn-ovial sarcoma, rhabdomyosarcoma, epithelioid sarcoma, angiosarcoma, fibrosarcoma, etc. In addition, malignant tumours of peripheral nerve sheaths are included despite being ectodermal in origin, as their clinical behaviour is not measurably different from the other sarcomas. On the other hand, tumours of the lymphoid tissues (mesenchymal) are discussed in other sections.

Sarcomas of the soft tissues are quite uncommon, with an estimated 8100 newly diagnosed patients per year in the USA (Greenlee *et al.*, 2000); this represents 0.66 per cent of the invasive malignant neoplasms diagnosed per year. More than half that number will die of this disease. Review of the statistics of recent years suggests an increase in the incidence of soft tissue sarcomas, although it is not clear whether this represents a true increase or merely reflects more accurate diagnosis and increasing interest in these tumours (Enzinger and Weiss, 2001). Although the malignant tumours of soft tissue are rare, benign tumours are common. Enzinger and Weiss estimate that the frequency is 100 times that for the malignant lesions (Enzinger and Weiss, 2001).

To appreciate the rarity of the sarcomas, note that during the same period and among the same US popula-tion, there were 184 200 patients diagnosed with carcinoma of the breast. Thus, women are approximately 48 times more likely to develop a carcinoma of the breast than a sarcoma.

A large proportion of the sarcoma patients are referred to major centres with subspecialist teams because of the following factors:

- the relative rarity;
- appearance at all body sites;
- occurrence at all ages; and
- broad spectrum of histological types.

This has resulted in a rather greater clinical and laboratory research activity than might be expected for tumours of this low frequency. This is reflected in the large number of papers (more than 2600 in 1999) being published each year in the general area of sarcoma.

Although these lesions are uncommon, there has been a considerable increase in general medical interest over recent years in the management presented by these patients. This is due to rapidly changing management strategies and improvements in clinical results. In particu-lar, solid evidence has accumulated that, in addition to surgery, there are important roles for radiation therapy and chemotherapy in the management of some groups of these patients. Until the early 1960s, the medical con-sensus was that surgery offered the only serious prospect for cure of patients with soft tissue sarcomas. Radical sur-gery, particularly amputation, produced an impressive gain over simple local excision, but at the cost of major functional loss or cosmetic disfigurement. Clinical stud-ies over the last three decades have demonstrated that more conservative surgical approaches combined with radiation therapy, infusional chemotherapy or tumour necrosis factor (TNF-α) may be as effective as the more classical radical surgical procedures with respect to disease-free survival and provide superior functional and cosmetic results. Furthermore, there is some evidence that aggressive chemotherapy given to patients who are free of clinically evident metastatic tumour produces a disease-free survival and possibly higher cure rate. This, clearly, has been achieved for rhabdomyosarcoma of childhood (*see* Chapter 47).

The excellent results currently being obtained by more conservative treatment strategies are through a multi-disciplinary approach to the overall management of these patients (diagnostic evaluation, biopsy, treatment, rehabilitation and follow-up). The multidisciplinary team includes not only the surgeon but also the radiotherapists, medial and paediatric oncologists, pathologists and diagnostic radiologists. The pathologist is an extremely valuable member of the team because the staging system now employed (for other than childhood rhabdomyosarcoma) utilizes histopathological grade as the principal determinant of stage. Assessment of the local extent of the sarcoma and the search for evidence of distant metastatic tumour is conducted with the diagnostic radiologist.

This chapter discusses current practice in the management of patients with soft tissue sarcoma other than rhabdomyosarcoma of the paediatric age group.

During the last three decades, there have been large changes in the clinical management of patients with soft tissue sarcoma. The pathological diagnosis is now based on much more objective criteria with the introduction of immunohistochemistry and, to a lesser extent, cytogenetics. Modern imaging techniques, computed tomography (CT) and magnetic resonance imaging (MRI), have made enormous improvements in the ability to define the size, precise anatomical site, local invasion and the pattern of spread of the sarcoma. Positron emission tomography (PET) scanning and Magnetic Resonance Spectroscopic Imaging (MRSI) are now being evaluated in several centres with serious expectation for gains in the assessment of the magnitude of response to treatment. The strategies for the control of the primary/regional lesion are, in most patients, combined modality and this is achieving greatly enhanced functional and cosmetic outcomes. These gains have stemmed largely from the integration of radiation with surgery. Despite serious and sustained efforts in the form of phase III trials, the efficacy of chemotherapy to prolong survival has not been shown with the drug protocols tested to date. A meta-analysis of the phase III trials suggests an improvement in disease-free survival and a small but not statistically significant survival gain with the use of adjuvant chemotherapy in resectable, high-grade soft tissue sarcoma in adults (Sarcoma Meta-analysis Collaboration, 1997). There are several important developments being evaluated in the laboratory and the clinic, which offer the potential of further large gains.

AETIOLOGY

Genetic

Involvement of genetic factors in the genesis of soft tissue sarcoma is manifest by the strong hereditary tendency for certain sarcomas (Strong, 1977; Littlefield, 1984; Li *et al.*, 1988; Rowley, 1998). Gardner's syndrome is an hereditary disease, one feature of which is desmoid tumours (McAdam and Goligher, 1970); neurofibromatosis I also features tumour of the soft tissues: neurofibromas and neurofibrosarcoma. A significant proportion of these patients ultimately exhibit transformation of the neurofibroma into neurofibrosarcoma (Fraumeni, 1973; Strong, 1977; Zoller *et al.*, 1997). This disorder is associated with a mutation in the NF1 gene. It has been proposed that malignant degeneration reflects the two-hit hypothesis in which one allele is constitutionally inactivated in the germline while the other allele undergoes somatic inactivation (the second hit) (Colman *et al.*, 1995). Sarcomas of soft tissue and bone, particularly osteosarcoma, have been observed later in life in surviving patients with familial or bilateral retinoblastoma (Derkinderen *et al.*, 1988; Wong *et al.*, 1997). In one study of 1604 patients with retinoblastoma, the cumulative incidence of a second cancer at 50 years after diagnosis was 51 per cent for hereditary retinoblastoma (which is associated with mutations in the retinoblastoma tumour suppressor gene; *see* below), and 5 per cent for non-hereditary (sporadic) retinoblastoma (Wong *et al.*, 1997). More than 60 per cent of the cancers were a form of sarcoma. Malignant schwannoma may complicate the multiple endocrine neoplasia syndrome (Pizzo *et al.*, 1985). Patients with Li–Fraumeni syndrome often develop sarcomas (Li and Fraumeni, 1969; Li *et al.*, 1988). The Li–Fraumeni syndrome is inherited as an autosomal recessive trait, and is primarily characterized by soft tissue and bone sarcomas and breast cancer; other features include brain tumour, leukaemia and adrenocortical cancer occurring before the age of 45 (Li and Fraumeni, 1969; Li *et al.*, 1988). Some patients develop multiple malignancies (Hisada *et al.*, 1998). A germline mutation in the *p53* tumour suppressor gene is found in most affected families (*see p53* gene below) (Malkin, 1993; Evans and Lozano, 1997; Varley *et al.*, 1997). In one series of 151 children with soft tissue sarcoma, five of the families (3.3 per cent) manifested the classic Li–Fraumeni familial cancer syndrome, another ten (6.6 per cent) had features consistent with the syndrome, and 16 (10.5 per cent) had one parent with a possible hereditary cancer syndrome or with cancer before the age of 60 (Hartley *et al.*, 1993). In an analysis of 754 first-degree relatives of 177 children with sarcomas of soft tissue, Birch *et al.* (1990) found an increased incidence of malignant tumours in relatives of patients who were male, <2 years of age, and with an embryonal rhabdomyosarcoma.

Molecular biology

Changes in the genome are basic to the cellular transformation and the subsequent progression into the malignant phenotype. The malignant cell displays heritable alterations in its pattern of growth, ability to produce a continuously expanding progeny, relative independence of host growth regulating factors and the capacity to establish metastatic foci. These alterations in the genes include amplification, overexpression, positional rearrangement, deletion, etc. The first demonstration of a specific gene abnormality associated with malignant transformation in man was the loss of the *RB* gene, a tumour suppressor gene (Cavanee *et al.*, 1985; Friend *et al.*, 1987) and retinoblastoma. Knudsen had earlier proposed the genetic basis for hereditary and sporadic retinoblastoma, positing the loss or inactivation of both tumour suppressor genes as a requirement for tumour development (Knudsen, 1971). Even before the *Rb* gene had been identified, it was recognized that some sporadic sarcomas had deletions on chromosome 13 similar to those observed in some patients with retinoblastoma. Deletions or mutations of the tumour suppressor retinoblastoma (*Rb*) gene are critical in the pathogenesis of retinoblastoma and a variety of solid tumours. Alterations in the *Rb* gene are common in soft tissue sarcoma (Cance *et al.*, 1990; Wunder *et al.*, 1991; Karpeh *et al.*, 1995), occurring in up to 70 per cent of tumours (Cance *et al.*, 1990; Karpeh *et al.*, 1995). It has been proposed that *Rb* alterations are primary events in human sarcomas and may be involved in tumorigenesis or the early phases of tumour progression (Karpeh *et al.*, 1995). The *Rb* gene is critical for proper entry and transition through the cell cycle. Mutations are believed to perturb normal cell cycle function. This change has been shown to be associated with infrequent osteogenic or other sarcomas as second malignant neoplasms in patients with hereditary retinoblastoma (Friend *et al.*, 1987). Furthermore, the absence of detectable RB protein is associated with a small proportion of apparently sporadic sarcomas (Shew *et al.*, 1989). In an examination of 43 sarcomas of bone and soft tissues, Wunder *et al.* (1991) found alteration in the *RB* gene in approximately 40 per cent of the tumours.

The gene *p53* is also a 'tumour suppressor gene' and mutation on this gene and/or absence of its protein is associated with the development of sarcomas and other malignancies. The p53 protein is a transcriptional activator that plays a key role in the integration of signals inducing cell division, arrest of DNA synthesis following DNA damage, and programmed cell death (apoptosis). DNA damage results in increased levels of p53 protein which induces cell cycle arrest at the G_1/S interface, thereby permitting the cell to repair genomic damage or to initiate apoptosis (Lane, 1992; El-Deiry *et al.*, 1993; Levine *et al.*, 1994). The wild-type *p53* in normal tissue has a short half-life and is not detectable by immunohistochemical methods; by comparison, mutations of the gene result in a stabilized p53 protein that accumulates in the cell and often becomes detectable by immunohistochemistry. Gross rearrangements and nonsense mutations, however, may show no immunostaining for p53, indicating that this technique fails to identify a significant proportion of tumours with p53 alterations (Toguchida *et al.*, 1992b). Animal models are compatible with p53 defects having a pathogenetic role in sarcoma development. Mice deficient for p53 also develop a variety of neoplasms including bone and soft tissue sarcomas (Donehower *et al.*, 1992). Similarly, irradiated transgenic mice harbouring mutant *p53* show higher frequencies of sarcomas (Lee *et al.*, 1994). On the other hand, transduction of wild-type *p53* genes into soft tissue sarcomas bearing mutated *p53* genes restores enhanced cell cycle control and suppresses sarcoma growth (Pollock *et al.*, 1998).

Somatic mutations in the *p53* gene are the most frequently detected molecular alteration in sporadic soft tissue sarcoma. These mutations have been detected in a variety of soft tissue sarcomas including malignant fibrous histiocytoma (MFH), leiomyosarcoma, liposarcoma, and rhabdomyosarcoma (Mulligan *et al.*, 1990; Stratton *et al.*, 1990; Porter *et al.*, 1992; Soini *et al.*, 1992; Toguchida *et al.*, 1992b; Andreassen *et al.*, 1993; Wadayama *et al.*, 1993; McIntyre *et al.*, 1994; Patterson *et al.*, 1994; Simms *et al.*, 1995; Pollock *et al.*, 1996; Blom *et al.*, 1998). Germline mutations of *p53* are also found in most families with the Li–Fraumeni syndrome (Malkin, 1993). Germline mutations in this gene also may occur in other patients with soft tissue sarcoma, particularly those with other cancers which are not considered indicative of the Li–Fraumeni syndrome (Malkin *et al.*, 1992; Toguchida *et al.*, 1992a; McIntyre *et al.*, 1994).

The *MDM2* gene, located at 12q13–14, is overexpressed in a variety of human tumours including soft tissue sarcomas (Oliner *et al.*, 1992; Khatib *et al.*, 1993; Florenes *et al.*, 1994; Nilbert *et al.*, 1994). Its gene product localizes predominantly to the nucleus, where it acts as an inhibitor of the *p53* tumour suppressor gene product. The gene *SAS* has been observed to be amplified in a high proportion of malignant fibrohistocytomas and liposarcomas (Smith *et al.*, 1992). Furthermore, Duda *et al.* (1993) reported that approximately 40 per cent of sarcomas were found to have an increased expression of c-erb-B2 oncogene and epidermal growth factor receptor (EGFR). Additional gene mutations or other alterations in sarcomas include: *CDK4* (Kanoe *et al.*, 1998), *ras*, *myc*, and c-*fos* (Brown *et al.*, 1984; Chardin *et al.*, 1985). There are reports regularly appearing with accounts of other genetic abnormalities in sarcomas; for recent reviews see Milas *et al.* (1998) and Gebhardt (1996).

Cytogenetics

Genetic abnormalities evidenced by non-random chromosomal aberrations in sarcomas are well established and are being increasingly utilized in the definitive diagnosis. Furthermore, these chromosomal abnormalities have been characterized at the molecular level and many of the chimeric genes have been identified, providing clues to the molecular alterations that are fundamental for the development of soft tissue sarcomas. The best recognized and frequently employed are mentioned here briefly. Most synovial cell sarcomas are characterized by the translocation t(x;18)(p11.2;q11.2) (Turc-Carel *et al.*, 1986). In fact, this aberration is considered sufficiently specific that, in the instance of a differential diagnostic problem, the presence of the t(X;18) would be accepted as decisive. For example, based on this translocation, a synovial sarcoma has been diagnosed in the base of the tongue and other sites not known to have synovial tissue. The presence of this translocation is, however, not accepted as definitive in the presence of typical histopathological appearance of other pathological types, i.e. there are tumours that have the typical appearance of malignant fibrous histiocytoma and this chromosomal abnormality. These are not currently accepted as synovial sarcoma. This indicates that a single chromosomal abnormality does not explain fully the neoplastic phenotype. The breakpoint of this translocation fuses the *SVT* gene from chromosome 18 to one of two homologous genes, *SSX1* or *SSX2* on the X chromosome (Clark *et al.*, 1994; Kawai *et al.*, 1998). The *SVT-SSX* gene is thought to function as an aberrant transcriptional regulator. The nature of the chimeric gene appears to have prognostic and pathogenetic importance, as metastasis-free survival is much higher (relative risk 3.0) with *SVT-SSX2* compared to *SVT-SSX1* (Kawai *et al.*, 1994). *SVT-SSX1* is associated with biphasic tumours (glandular epithelial differentiation on a background of spindle tumour cells), while *SVT-SSX2* is associated with monophasic tumours that lack glandular epithelial differentiation.

Other chromosomal changes characteristic of specific sarcoma type include the reciprocal exchange t(11;22)(q24;q12) seen in approximately 85–90 per cent of Ewing's sarcoma and primitive neuroectodermal tumours (PNET) (Turc-Carel *et al.*, 1988; Ladanyl *et al.*, 1990; Delattre *et al.*, 1994). In this translocation, the *EWS* gene from chromosome 22q12 is covalently linked to the ETS family member, FLI-1 (Zucman *et al.*, 1993). The chimeric proteins that result from this translocation may alter transcription of an unidentified gene on chromosome 22 (Delattre *et al.*, 1992; Zucman *et al.*, 1993). A less common translocation t(21;22)(q22;q12) has also been identified and links *EWS* to a different ETS family member, ERG (Sorensen *et al.*, 1994).

Myxoid and round cell subtypes of liposarcomas display a reciprocal translocation t(12;16)(q13;p11) (Crozat *et al.*, 1993; Rabbitts *et al.*, 1993). In this translocation, the CHOP (cyclophosphamide, doxorubicin, vincristine and prednisolone; induced by DNA damage) gene is inserted adjacent to a novel gene called *FUS*. The fusion gene, called *TLS-CHOP*, shows sequence homology to the Ewing's fusion gene (Aman *et al.*, 1992; Crozat *et al.*,

1993; Rabbitts *et al.*, 1993; Hisaoka *et al.*, 1998). It fails to induce G_1/S arrest, which is one of the functions of the non-oncogenic form of CHOP (*GADD153*) (Barone *et al.*, 1994). Identification of the fusion gene has been used as a diagnostic aid for these subtype of liposarcoma (Hisaoka *et al.*, 1998).

Alveolar rhabdomyosarcomas show a translocation at t(2;13)(q35;q14) or less often t(1;13)(p36;q14); the chimeric genes have been cloned and have been termed *PAX3-FKHR* and *PAX7-FKHR*, respectively (Davis and Barr, 1997; Barr *et al.*, 1998). These translocations are associated with overexpression of the fusion product (Davis and Barr, 1997). *PAX7-FKHR* tumours more often present with extremity lesions, are more likely to be localized, and are less likely to metastasize widely than *PAX3-FKHR* tumours (Kelly *et al.*, 1996b). A downstream target of *PAX3-FKHR* may be *MET*, which encodes a receptor involved in growth and motility signalling (Ginsberg *et al.*, 1998). Molecular determination of minimal residual disease in alveolar rhabdomyosarcoma is possible but the clinical significance of this finding is uncertain (Kelly *et al.*, 1996a).

Clear cell sarcoma is usually classified as a malignant melanoma, although cytogenetically the tumours are distinct. Clear cell sarcomas often exhibit a translocation at t(12;22)(q13–14;q12), which is not seen in malignant melanoma (Fletcher, 1992). Trisomy of chromosome 8 is also observed in clear cell sarcoma (Travis and Bridge, 1992). Alterations in the 12q13–15 region has been described in a subgroup of haemangiopericytomas (Sreekantaiah *et al.*, 1991; Mandahl *et al.*, 1993). Multiple chromosomal abnormalities have also been seen in some of these tumours (Sreekantaiah *et al.*, 1991).

The trend of recent advances is that diagnoses will increasingly be made on the basis of specific immunohistochemistry and cytogenetics. Furthermore, molecular assays for fusion genes provide a genetic approach to the differential diagnosis of soft tissue sarcomas (Barr *et al.*, 1995).

Environmental factors

Radiation is recognized as capable of inducing sarcoma of bone and soft tissue. The frequency increases with radiation dose and with the post-radiation observation period (Kim, 1978; Sadove *et al.*, 1981; Robinson *et al.*, 1988). The most frequent histopathological type of radiation-induced sarcoma arising in soft tissues is malignant fibrous histiocytoma (approximately 70 per cent) (Laskin, 1988). Taghian *et al.* (1991) studied 7620 patients treated for carcinoma of the breast; the rate of induced tumours at 10 years was 0.2 per cent. Karlsson *et al.* (1996) have presented the findings of an analysis of 13 patients who developed soft tissue sarcoma out of a total of 13 490 women treated by surgery ± radiation in the West of Sweden Health Care Region. Although seen rarely after low doses (<40 Gy), this is predominantly a complication of high-dose treatment. The actuarial frequency at 15–20 years is approximately 0.5 per cent for radiation of normal bone and soft tissue in the adult treated with radiation alone to full dose.

The frequency is higher following treatment of children, especially with radiation and chemotherapy; the frequency may be as high as 20–30 per cent at remote times (Strong, 1977). This is further supported by the analysis of 1458 patients followed after treatment for retinoblastoma for 17 years. The cumulative mortality from second primary neoplasms at 40 years was 26 per cent and 1.5 per cent among patients with bilateral and unilateral disease, respectively (Eng et al., 1993). Within the bilateral population, the figures were 30 per cent and 6.4 per cent for irradiated and non-irradiated patients. For sarcomas (including those which arose within and without the irradiated field), the observed/expected ratios were 61 and 22 for patients with bilateral disease. The comparable figures for patients with unilateral disease were 5 and 2. There was a difference in the use of chemotherapy in patients treated for bilateral and unilateral retinoblastoma, viz. 48 per cent and 13 per cent, respectively. The UK Registry of Childhood Tumours have investigated a cohort of 13 175 paediatric patients who had survived for ≥3 years for secondary bone neoplasms (Hawkins et al., 1996). These patients had been seen over the time period 1940–1983. A total of 55 patients had developed secondary bone tumours. Among these ≥3 years survivors, there were 0.9 per cent who developed bone tumours within 20 years. There was an increasing frequency with radiation dose. In addition, there was also an increasing frequency with dose of alkylating agent. In an analysis at Memorial Hospital of 130 long-term survivors after treatment for rhabdomyosarcoma (>2 years off chemotherapy) and a median follow-up period of 9 years, three patients developed leukaemia and four developed a solid tumour (Scaradavou et al., 1995). Of the latter, three were in the radiation field; the fourth appeared in a non-irradiated subject. This experience is rather more favourable than that with retinoblastoma.

Chemotherapeutic agents are likewise associated with risks of sarcoma induction. For example, there are two reports that describe the appearance of osteosarcoma in children treated for leukaemia by drugs alone (Shaw et al., 1988). Tucker et al. (1987) analysed the late sequelae in 9170 long-time survivors of childhood cancer. Chemotherapy alone was concluded to be an independent risk factor.

Exposure to a few selected industrial chemicals including vinyl chloride, phenoxyacetic acid, arsenic and phenoxy herbicides may be followed by the appearance of sarcomas. There are, however, a number of inherent problems in occupational epidemiology with small numbers of patients in any given series and the difficulty in isolating a single agent (Sathiakumar and Delzell, 1997). For these reasons, few associations can be considered established and causal (Dich et al., 1997). For example, there is a clear association between vinyl chloride and hepatic angiosarcoma (Lee et al., 1996). Phenoxyacetic acid (Hardell and Eriksson, 1988) and arsenic (Lander et al., 1975) are also implicated as inducing agents for hepatic sarcomas in humans. Wingren et al. (1990) reported an increased incidence of soft tissue sarcomas in gardeners (phenoxy herbicides), railroad workers, construction workers exposed to impregnating agents or asbestosis and unspecified chemical workers. The association between exposure to phenoxy herbicides and soft tissue sarcoma has been corroborated (Vineis et al., 1991). The last risk may be greater with exposure to phenoxy herbicides contaminated with 2,3,7,8-tetrachlorodibenzo-p-dioxin (TCDD) or higher chlorinated dioxins (Fingerhut et al., 1991; Kogevinas et al., 1997). A role for dioxin per se is controversial. A population-based case control study, however, found no increased risk for soft tissue sarcoma among Vietnam veterans, including those exposed to Agent Orange, which contains dioxin (The Selected Cancers Cooperative Study Group, 1990). High intensity chlorophenol exposure in jobs involving wood preservation, machinists and the use of cutting fluids may increase the risk of soft tissue sarcoma, independent of phenoxy herbicides (Wingren et al., 1990; Hoppin et al., 1998). However, some studies have not confirmed this association (Hardell and Eriksson, 1988).

Chronic oedema and trauma may also be contributing factors to the malignant transformation. Sarcomas of soft tissue (primarily lymphangiosarcomas) may be observed following massive and quite protracted oedema. Classically, this has been seen in the post-mastectomy, lymphoedematous arm (Stewart–Treves syndrome) (Stewart and Treves, 1948; Tomita et al., 1988). It has also been described following chronic lymphoedema due to filarial infection (Muller et al., 1987). Chronic irritation secondary to foreign bodies may be a factor in the induction of sarcomas. We have observed one patient in whom a fibrosarcoma appeared at 15 years at the site of a plastic tube insertion through the scalp for control of hydrocephalus. Trauma is rarely a factor in the development of these tumours with the exception of desmoid tumours. There are occasionally patients with a history of major trauma to the affected site many months prior to the appearance of local symptoms of tumour. The usual history is of a traumatic incident occurring shortly prior to the awareness of the mass, suggesting that the trauma merely brought the patient's attention to the presence of the mass.

CLINICAL EVALUATION

Clinical history

The most frequent initial complaint is that of a painless lump of a few weeks to several months' duration. Occasionally, pain or tenderness precedes the detection of a lump. With progressive growth of tumour, symptoms appear which are secondary to infiltration of or pressure on adjacent structures (e.g. tendons, muscles, nerves) or organs. Occasionally symptoms secondary to the metabolic effects of the tumour products are seen, e.g. fever, anaemia, lethargy, weight loss, histamine-like reactions. These are not rare in patients with malignant fibrous histiocytoma (Enzinger and Weiss, 2001). To accrue clinical genetic data in sarcoma patients, the history should include details of the cause of death and history of malignant disease in siblings, parents, grandparents and progeny.

Anatomical site, sex and age

Sites of appearance of soft tissue sarcoma in order of frequency are: lower extremity, upper extremity, torso, head/neck, retroperitoneum (Table 41.1). There is only a very slight preponderance of soft tissue sarcoma in males. They are more common in older people, with 40 per cent in persons >55 years of age and 15 per cent in patients <15 years of age (Enzinger and Weiss, 2001). Rhabdomyosarcomas almost always arise in children, synovial sarcomas develop in late adolescence and young adulthood and liposarcoma and malignant fibrous histiocytoma usually occur during mid- and late adulthood.

Physical examination

There must be a complete physical examination with particular attention paid to the region of the primary lesion: definition of size, site of origin (superficial or deep, attached to or fixed to deep structures), solitary or multinodular, involvement or discoloration of overlying skin, functional status of vessels and nerves, presence of distal oedema, muscular strength, range of motion of affected part, etc. If the patient has had prior excision, the operated site should be examined for presence of ecchymosis, status of wound healing, palpable evidence of residual tumour and location of drain site. The regional and distant lymph-node groups need to be examined with care

Table 41.1 *Distribution (%) of sarcoma of soft tissue according to anatomical site in three US surveys*

	MGH[a] (n = 788)	Russell (n = 1215)	Lawrence (n = 4550)
Lower extremity	44	40	46
Upper extremity	21	13	13
Head and neck	12	15	8
Torso	10	18	18
Retroperitoneum	6	13	12
Other	7	1	1

[a]All patients seen 1971–1993 and treated by radiation surgery for stage M0 disease.

in all patients, especially those with large grade 2 and 3 (on a three-step grading scale) sarcomas. In an analysis of the experience at Massachusetts General Hospital (MGH), no patient with grade 1 sarcoma developed regional node involvement. The incidence in patients with grades 2 and 3 sarcomas were 2 per cent and 12 per cent, respectively. Of the patients with grade 3 sarcoma, the incidences were 3 per cent and 15 per cent for lesions <5 cm and >5 cm, respectively (Mazeron and Suit, 1987). Fong et al. (1993) found a slightly lower frequency of metastasis to regional nodes in the Memorial Hospital series. Involvement of regional nodes is relatively frequent in patients with rhabdomyosarcoma and epithelial sarcoma, but uncommon in patients with fibrosarcoma and malignant fibrous histiocytoma. Myxoid liposarcoma not uncommonly metastasizes first to soft tissue or bone.

Laboratory investigations

Laboratory studies need not go beyond a complete blood count and urinalysis for all but the exceptional patient. For patients with lesions in the abdomino-pelvic cavity, liver function and/or liver scan should be obtained as involvement of liver is not rare in such patients.

Radiographic evaluation

For the primary site, the radiographic evaluation should include plain films and CT or MRI scanning. The most useful radiological study to evaluate the primary site is the MRI (Bland et al., 1987); CT is of particular value in assessing retroperitoneal tumours, bony involvement and the presence of lung metastases. Plain radiographs are helpful in the evaluation of soft tissue tumours by demonstrating bone involvement and soft tissue masses arising from bone tumours. However, unlike bone tumours, imaging studies cannot be used to assess the biological behaviour of soft tissue tumours (Kransdorf et al., 1993). Indeed, specific diagnosis remains impossible for many soft tissue lesions regardless of the choice of imaging (O'Keefe et al., 1990). Imaging studies alone cannot definitively distinguish malignant from benign soft tissue lesions. MRI may prove of clinical value in planning the biopsy site, either using needle or incisional techniques. Furthermore, the demonstration of necrotic regions appears to be of diagnostic importance in discrimination between benign and malignant tumours (Gustafson et al., 1992). PET scanning (Fig. 41.1a, b) has been shown to be useful in discriminating between benign and high-grade lesions although it is unsuitable for distinguishing between benign and low-to-intermediate grade lesions (Nieweg et al., 1996). In the future, PET may be of substantial value in defining response to preoperative therapy (Jones et al., 1996). MRI studies should always include T_2-weighted sequences as these provide the optimum contrast between lesion and muscle. Contrast enhanced T_1-weighted images (especially with fat suppression techniques) are also helpful. MRI often provides a clearer demonstration of the anatomical location of the lesion and the pattern of local extensions (Fig. 41.2a, b). The findings from these scans should be correlated with those of the physical examination to assess the details of the anatomical site of the tumour. It should be determined whether the lesion is in the subcutaneous tissue, transgressing the fascia, intermuscular or intramuscular, displacing or enveloping major vessels or nerves, abutting or invading bone, etc. Depending upon the pattern of presentation and the nature of any planned surgery, an arteriogram may be of value. For rhabdomyosarcoma, epithelioid sarcoma, high-grade synovial and unclassified sarcomas, CT or lymphangiographic evaluation of the regional nodes should be obtained. Bone scans need not be performed unless specifically indicated. We do not consider a positive bone scan of bone near or

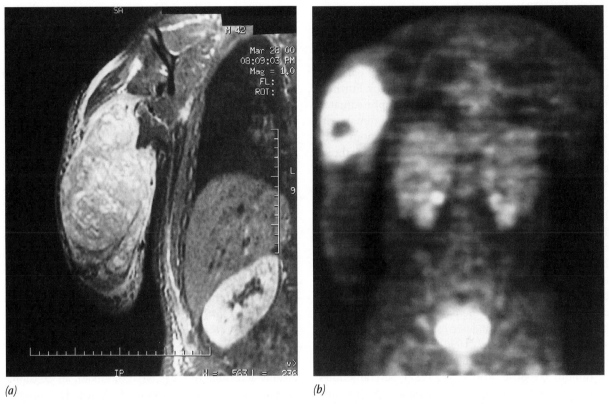

(a)

(b)

Figure 41.1 (a) Stir pulse, inversion recovery sequence MRI with fat suppression shows a large malignant fibrous histiocytoma arising in the triceps. The tumour is readily distinguishable from fat and muscle by its extremely bright signal. (b) Corresponding whole-body fluorodeoxyglucose positron emission tomography (FDG-PET) images of the patient showing intense uptake in the proximal right upper extremity.

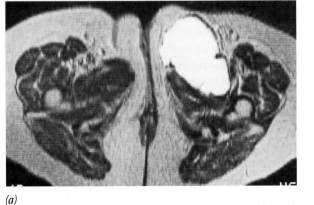

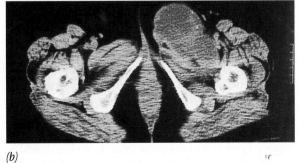

(a)

(b)

Figure 41.2 (a) T_2-weighted MR scan (TR = 2500, TE = 96) shows a large synovial sarcoma arising on the anterior aspect of the adductor muscle group. The tumour is readily distinguishable from fat and muscle by its extremely bright signal. (b) CT scan at this level also shows the tumour clearly, but the contrast with muscle is far less.

adjacent to a soft tissue sarcoma to be proof of invasion of periosteum or bone. For a diagnosis of invasion of bone there must be clear radiographic evidence of destruction of cortical bone. The single most important examination for distant metastasis is whole-lung CT; this should be obtained in all patients. We have had several patients where metastatic disease in lung was diagnosed on CT and not seen on good quality chest X-rays. This has been extensively confirmed by the study of Peuchot and Libshitz (1987) who reported that, of the nodules detected by CT but not by chest X-ray and those biopsied, 94 per cent were metastatic tumour.

Imaging of the response to treatment has been disappointing up to the present. Decrease in tumour size may occur (Sanchez et al., 1990), but does not correlate well with successful radiation or chemotherapy. Furthermore, although tumour volume can be approximated from two-dimensional images (CT or plain films), reliable algorithms to distinguish objectively tumour from surrounding tissues are not available, and thus three-dimensional imaging techniques have, as yet, not found a role. Changes in MRI signal characteristics have been unreliable. Absence of high-signal intensity on T_2 images has been shown to indicate freedom from tumour. However, residual high signal may be due to tumour, oedema or fibrosis (Vanel et al., 1987). MRI spectroscopy has been used to detect high-energy phosphate metabolism in the lesions. This has helped in the distinction between malignant and benign tumours (Negendank et al., 1989). In one study there was a negative correlation between changes in pH and necrosis as seen in the surgical specimen (Dewhirst et al., 1990). Other early studies of bone sarcomas have not been promising in the prediction of tumour response (Ross et al., 1987). Several studies with phosphorus-31 magnetic resonance spectroscopy have shown changes in high-energy phosphate metabolism after effective chemotherapy (Dewhirst et al., 1990; Koutcher et al., 1990; Redmond et al., 1992), but the range of variation in sarcoma is large, and because of limitations in spatial resolution the procedure cannot be reliably done unless a large soft tissue mass is present.

Biopsy

An adequate biopsy must be obtained in order that the best feasible histopathological diagnosis as to tumour type and grade be made. The optimal treatment strategy is based on the correct diagnosis. Under optimal conditions, the biopsy procedure should be performed by an experienced surgeon who is part of the multidisciplinary caretaking team and will be responsible for the definitive surgery. Prior to the biopsy, the imaging studies should be carefully studied to ascertain the most logical approach to the lesion, with explicit consideration of the regions to be traversed in subsequent surgical procedures (including marginal or wide resection or amputation) so that the biopsy track will not interfere with either surgery or radiation field.

The incision for the biopsy of lesions on an extremity should be longitudinal (there is almost never a reason for a transverse incision on an extremity). The incision should be as short as possible, yet long enough to avoid excessive retraction of tissue or to make dissection and haemostasis difficult. The biopsy track should go through a muscle belly rather than along fascial planes (the former tends to keep the tumour 'spill' within an anatomical compartment whilst the latter allows transgression of two or more compartments) and careful attention should be paid to achieve haemostasis in order to avoid ecchymosis or a haematoma. The wound should be closed in layers with a narrow skin closure; as a rule, drains should not be utilized (the tract of the drain is considered to be contaminated with tumour and may greatly extend the planes of subsequent surgery or the radiation treatment volume).

There are some circumstances where a needle biopsy, either using a trucut or even an aspiration 'skinny' needle, is advantageous. For lesions that are readily palpable such a procedure can be done without imaging, but for tumours located at depth a CT-directed approach is advocated. The amount of tissue obtained by such a procedure is limited and this should be considered before deciding which procedure to perform. At our hospital, needle biopsy is also frequently employed to confirm metastatic or recurrent tumour. Biopsy by the needle technique may also be used in those anatomical situations where incisional biopsy would require a major procedure.

Incisional biopsies are almost always advocated for soft tissue tumours. Occasionally, for a small lesion in a readily accessible site (e.g. wrist or ankle), an excisional biopsy may be the approach of choice. The surgeon should adhere to the same principles as for the definitive surgery (see below) if complications are to be avoided.

The biopsy specimen needs to be of sufficient volume to be certain that it is representative. A pathological assessment of a frozen section is useful in assuring that the tissue obtained is from the lesion and is adequate for the diagnostic evaluation. Cultures should always be obtained. In our institution specimens are processed for haematoxylin and eosin staining and various immunohistochemical stains considered necessary to aid in the diagnosis. A small portion of the tissue is set aside for electron microscopy. Furthermore, we subject the biopsy specimen from sarcomas to flow cytometric analysis for DNA content.

HISTOPATHOLOGICAL DIAGNOSIS

Practical concepts

The pathologist needs to be aware of the clinical and radiographic findings and the diagnostic considerations of each case. In this way the pathologist will be best prepared to choose the appropriate methodology needed to make a complete and accurate assessment of tissue specimens.

THE BIOPSY

Ideally, the tissue should be in the fresh state when received by the pathologist so that a portion can be used to perform a frozen section. Frozen section analysis can determine if there is adequate material for diagnosis and if the lesion is non-neoplastic or a benign or malignant neoplasm. It may even permit the rendering of a specific diagnosis. Depending on the results of the frozen section, the pathologist can then triage the tissue as necessary and submit samples for electron microscopy, DNA flow cytometry, cytogenetics, or keep tissue frozen for immunoperoxidase or molecular studies. If a needle biopsy is performed, then three cores of tumour-bearing tissue are usually required; if an open biopsy is performed, 0.5 cm^3 of tumour is sufficient to perform the needed studies. The accuracy of obtaining diagnostic tissue by needle biopsy is reported to be 96 per cent (Shives, 1993), with a 94 per cent accuracy in diagnosing the tumour as malignant, an 85 per cent accuracy of subtyping the sarcoma, and an 88 per cent accuracy of grading the sarcoma (Ball *et al.*, 1990). All tissue not used for special studies should be examined by light microscopy. We recommend that the entire tumour, if less than 5 cm, be studied histologically if removed as an excisional biopsy.

THE RESECTION SPECIMEN

At the Massachusetts General Hospital the pathologist goes into the operating room to receive the resection specimen and assess the margins of excision. At this time the pathologist orientates the specimen with the surgeon and discusses potentially close or positive margins. If necessary, a frozen section to confirm the status of a margin is performed. Once the specimen is in the pathology laboratory, it is carefully dissected to determine the size of the sarcoma, its gross characteristics, its relationship to normal structures, pattern of invasion and the adequacy of excision. All portions of the sarcoma are thoroughly sampled for study by light microscopy. The final analysis includes classification and grading, determination of vascular invasion, status of the margins, proximity to normal structures, and cytotoxic therapy effect as seen by percentage necrosis.

Classification

The rationale for developing a well-defined, comprehensive and flexible classification system of soft tissue tumours is to provide morphological guidelines which expand our understanding of neoplasia, predict biological behaviour and facilitate the development of more effective treatment. Originally, classification schemes were descriptive in nature and based on tumour cell configuration. Subsequently they have evolved through the concept of histogenesis or 'cell of origin' to the current belief that a primitive or stem-like mesenchymal cell undergoes neoplastic transformation and, depending on the genetic code translated, differentiates along one or multiple cell lines. Currently, the most widely used classification system is the Enzinger and Weiss (2001) modification of the World Health Organization formulation. In this system, soft tissue tumours, including non-neoplastic tumour-like lesions, are categorized into three broad groups:

1 tumours which differentiate along cell or tissue lines that have normal counterparts, i.e. fibrous tissue, fat, vessels, smooth muscle, skeletal muscle, nerve, ganglia, synovium, bone and cartilage;
2 tumours whose lines of differentiation have no normal counterpart but which are consistent and recognized by a distinctive morphology, i.e. myxoma, epithelioid sarcoma, and alveolar soft part sarcoma; and
3 tumours which are so poorly differentiated and morphologically unique that they defy classification.

In our experience, the vast majority of tumours fall into the first two groups. Overall, there are approximately 200 different entities, of which 80 are malignant.

As intensive study of these tumours is rapidly expanding and new diagnostic procedures are increasingly employed, there is inevitably some flux in the diagnostic criteria for the diverse groups of soft tissue tumours. Examples include:

- the reclassification of most adult pleomorphic rhabdomyosarcomas and many pleomorphic liposarcomas to malignant fibrous histiocytoma;
- the recognition that a granular cell tumour is a schwann cell neoplasm;
- the recognition that clear cell sarcoma is a malignant melanoma primary to the soft tissues; and
- the recognition that extraskeletal Ewing's sarcoma is a primitive neuroectodermal tumour.

The distribution of histological types of sarcoma of soft tissue from several large series is presented in Table 41.2.

GRADING

The histological typing of soft tissue tumours does not *per se* provide sufficient information on which to base therapeutic decisions. Tumour grading is based on the concept that morphology reflects biological behaviour. The specific microscopic characteristics of soft tissue tumours that best predict their aggressiveness, i.e. the

Table 41.2 *Distribution (%) of histological types of sarcoma of soft tissues at four US hospitals*

	MGH, 1994 ($n = 738$)	Russell, 1987 ($n = 1215$)	Coindre, 1993 ($n = 761$)	Lawrence, 1987 ($n = 5885$)
Fibrosarcoma/spindle cell sarcoma	11.2	19.0	4.9	8.3
Liposarcoma	16.0	18.2	13.7	19.7
Malignant fibrohistiocytoma	21.9	10.5	30.4	21.2
Unclassified	8.5	10.0	12.4	5.3
Leiomyosarcoma	10.3	6.5	10.4	14.2
Neurosarcoma	9.6	4.9	7.2	3.6
Synovial sarcoma	7.8	6.9	8.4	3.6
Rhabdomyosarcoma	3.1	19.2	2.4	4.9
Other	11.6	4.6	10.2	19.1

potential for regional and distant metastasis, can be identified, integrated and represented by grade.

The 1997 American Joint Committee on Cancer (AJCC) and International Union Against Cancer (IUCC) staging system for sarcoma of soft tissue (Fleming *et al.*, 1997) is based upon a four-step grading, i.e. low-, intermediate-, high-grade and undifferentiated neoplasms (*see* Table 41.4). In this grading system, grade 1 and 2 tumours are considered low grade lesions with minimal metastatic potential; grade 3–4 neoplasms are high grade tumours that carry a significant risk of metastasis. Many institutions continue to employ a three-step grading scale consisting of low (G1), intermediate (G2) and high (G3) grades. In this grading scale G1 lesions are considered to have minimal metastatic potential and are analogous to the G1 and G2 designations on the four-step scale for staging purposes. The G2 and G3 tumours on the three-step scale are analogous to the G3 and G4 on the four-step scale. The designation of grade is based upon a consideration and integration of each of these morphological features: degree of cellular differentiation, extent of necrosis, number of mitoses, cellularity, pleomorphism or anaplasia, quantity of matrix, vascularity, haemorrhage, vascular invasion and encapsulation (Suit *et al.*, 1975; Myhre-Jensen *et al.*, 1983; Costa *et al.*, 1984; Rydholm *et al.*, 1984; Trojani, 1984; Kulander *et al.*, 1989; Lack *et al.*, 1989). Among these variables, necrosis, mitoses and degree of differentiation appear to be the best predictors of outcome. Despite some lack of agreement on the number of grades employed and the significance of individual morphological parameters (there is inevitably a subjective component in assigning grade and only a part of the tumour is examined), grading, more than any clinical and pathological parameter available, is the most important prognosticator (Russell *et al.*, 1977). High-power views of myxoid liposarcoma grades 1, 2 and 3 (on a three-step scale) are shown in Figure 41.3a–c. The problems with current grading systems are that their criteria are not precisely defined, application and interpretation is subjective and implementation is complex. Consistent grading requires adequate tissue and experienced pathologists.

The pathologist's armamentarium in diagnosing and grading sarcomas

Light microscopy in most instances is the modality of choice for determining whether a soft tissue tumour is benign or malignant, subtype, grade, margins and presence or absence of vascular invasion. However, electron microscopy (EM), immunohistochemistry, DNA flow cytometry, cytogenetics and molecular analysis can provide valuable information that substantiates the histological interpretation.

EM is particularly helpful for differentiating amongst poorly differentiated tumours, the various spindle cell sarcomas and malignant round-cell tumours. In some cases the presence of single ultrastructural features such as Z-bands in rhabdomyosarcomas may be diagnostic. EM, however, is frequently not reliable in distinguishing benign from malignant soft tissue tumours (Angervall and Kindblom, 1993). Immunohistochemistry has become increasingly important in diagnosing sarcomas (Ushigome *et al.*, 1992). This technique is based on the utilization of visually tagged monoclonal or polyclonal antibodies directed against proteins found in specific cell types. If a tumour expresses certain proteins as detected by this method, then its phenotype or line of differentiation can be identified (Table 41.3). The more important antibodies include those that recognize some of the different intermediate filaments (vimentin, keratin, desmin, neurofilament), leucocyte common antigen, S-100 protein, myoglobin, and Factor VIII-related antigen. For some antigens (e.g. neurofilament and surface antigens to lymphocytes), frozen tissue is clearly superior to formalin-fixed tissue (Miettinen, 1988). For other antigens, such as S-100 protein, peptide hormones, neuron-specific enolase, and α1-antitrypsin, formalin fixation is optimal (Miettinen, 1988). It is important to remember that there is no antibody that distinguishes a benign from a malignant soft tissue tumour and that there are a multitude of exceptions to the expected distribution of antigens. Consequently there can be significant overlap in the immunohistochemical profile of various sarcomas (Wick *et al.*, 1988).

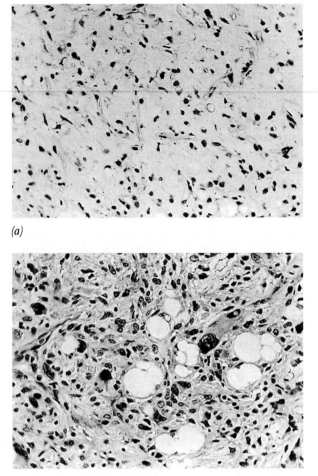

(a)

(b)

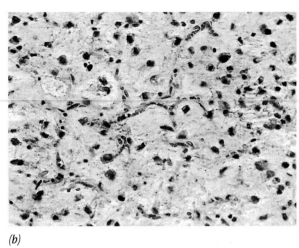

(c)

Figure 41.3 *(a) Myxoid liposarcoma, grade 1/3 (well differentiated with characteristic plexiform capillary pattern and scattered mono- and multivacuolated lipoblasts (H&E, ×313). (b) Myxoid liposarcoma, grade 2/3 (moderately differentiated). In comparison with the grade 1/3 myxoid liposarcoma, there is increased cellularity, hyperchromasia and pleomorphism (H&E, ×313). (c) Myxoid liposarcoma, grade 3/3 (poorly differentiated). There is dense cellularity, marked hyperchromasia and pleomorphism and atypical mitoses (upper left). Scattered multivacuolated lipoblasts are present. The myxoid stroma and plexiform and vascular patterns are less apparent (H&E, ×313).*

Table 41.3 *Immunohistochemistry in soft tissue sarcomas*

Antibody	Distribution
Vimentin	Almost all sarcomas and some carcinomas
Keratin	Almost all carcinomas and some sarcomas (epithelioid sarcoma, synovial sarcoma)
Desmin	Leiomyosarcoma, rhabdomyosarcoma and occasionally MFH
Neurofilament	Primitive neuroectodermal tumour, neuroblastoma
Leucocyte common antigen	Lymphoma
S-100 protein	Malignant schwannoma, melanoma, clear cell (melanoma of soft parts), chondrosarcoma, leiomyosarcoma, rhabdomyosarcoma, liposarcoma
Myoglobin	Rhabdomyosarcoma
Factor VIII-related antigen	Angiosarcoma, Kaposi's sarcoma
Actin	Leiomyosarcoma, rhabdomyosarcoma (MFH)
EMA	Carcinomas, synovial sarcoma, meningioma
Leu 7	Malignant schwannoma, leiomyosarcoma, synovial sarcoma, rhabdomyosarcoma

MFH, malignant fibrohistiocytoma.

In addition to identifying antigens associated with a specific phenotype, immunohistochemistry has been used to evaluate the drug resistance and proliferative rate of sarcomas and their expression of growth factors. P-glycoprotein is a plasma membrane glycoprotein which appears to play a role in multidrug chemotherapy resistance (Weinstein *et al.*, 1990) and can be detected by immunohistochemistry. Investigations have tried to determine whether the level of P-glycoprotein expression predicts the type of response to chemotherapy. High levels of P-glycoprotein expression may adversely affect the chemosensitivity of sarcomas, which correlates with a worse prognosis (Elias, 1993). Similarly, the absence of P-glycoprotein in some sarcomas portends a favourable outcome (Elias, 1993; Chan et al., 1990). Ki-67, a nuclear antigen expressed in all phases of cell proliferation except the resting phase (Sahin et al., 1991), is a recognized marker of cell proliferation. Demonstration of Ki-67 appears to measure the number of proliferating cells in a tumour more accurately than does DNA flow cytometry (Sahin et al., 1991). In malignant fibrous histiocytoma, the expression of Ki-67, as determined by immunohistochemistry, has shown that proliferative activity is independent of grade (Swanson and Brooks, 1990). Some studies have demonstrated a correlation between Ki-67 and prognosis in general (Ueda et al., 1989), but further investigation is warranted before firm conclusions can be established (Zehr et al., 1990).

Mutations of p53, a tumour suppressor gene, have been shown to play an important role in the development of a variety of neoplasms including soft tissue tumours. The abnormal accumulation of p53 indicates that a mutation has occurred. p53 can be visualized by immunohistochemistry and it has been detected in both benign and malignant soft tissue neoplasms (Dei Tos et al., 1993). In sarcomas, p53 has been associated with specific subtypes, a high histological grade and poor prognosis (Kawai et al., 1994).

Finally, several growth factors including platelet-derived growth factor (Palman et al., 1992), insulin growth factor (Roholl et al., 1990) and epidermal growth factor (Duda et al., 1993) have been identified in a variety of benign and malignant soft tissue tumours. The significance of their presence is unclear but may relate to both cell differentiation and tumour growth.

DNA flow cytometry can play a role in determining the prognosis of sarcomas; however, it still cannot replace diagnosis by light microscopy. DNA flow cytometry measures the amount of DNA in cells. Generally, the cells in reactive processes, benign tumours and low-grade sarcomas have normal amounts of DNA and are termed diploid. By contrast, the neoplastic cells in high-grade sarcomas have a tendency to contain abnormal amounts of DNA and are termed aneuploid. Some studies have shown a statistically significant relationship between aneuploidy of sarcomas and poor clinical outcome (Agarwal et al., 1991). There also appears to be a relationship in some cases between tumour grade and ploidy level; higher proportions of aneuploid tumours are found amongst the higher-grade sarcomas (Kroese et al., 1990). Besides 'ploidy' of a tumour, flow cytometry can perform cell cycle analysis and determine the number of cells that are synthesizing DNA in preparation for cell division. In general, malignant tumours have a higher proportion of cells that are undergoing mitosis than benign tumours (Bodensteiner et al., 1991). Similarly, high-grade sarcomas usually have a greater number of cycling cells than

low-grade sarcomas (Bodensteiner et al., 1991). The problem with flow cytometry is that there are many exceptions to the rules: benign tumours may be aneuploid and actively growing; high-grade sarcomas may be diploid with a relatively low proportion of cycling cells.

Cytogenetic analysis is now being performed more frequently on sarcomas. It is a diagnostically useful technique because some sarcomas have specific cytogenetic alterations that appear to be pathognomonic. For instance, 83 per cent of Ewing's sarcoma/primitive neuroectodermal tumours have a characteristic t(11;22) translocation and 50 per cent of alveolar rhabdomyosarcomas show a t(2;13) translocation (DeChiara et al., 1993; Delattre et al., 1994; Parham et al., 1994). Myxoid liposarcomas have been found to have a t(12;16) translocation, clear cell sarcoma a t(12;22) translocation; extraskeletal myxoid chondrosarcoma a t(9;22) translocation; and synovial sarcomas a t(x;18) translocation (Angervall and Kindblom, 1993). Structural abnormalities of chromosome 1p have been found in 70–80 per cent of neuroblastomas. They are often associated with double minute chromosomes and/or homogeneously staining regions (sites of amplification of complex rearranged genes), including a core of multiple copies of N-myc oncogene. Aside from being helpful in diagnosis, the findings of these 1p rearrangements and double minute chromosomes further denote a poor clinical outcome (Sainati et al., 1992).

Molecular biology will play a more important role in evaluating soft tissue sarcomas in the near future as the technology becomes more available. The identification of specific DNA and RNA gene sequences and oncogenes will help to diagnose and predict the biological behaviour of sarcomas. For example, the expression of the gene product MYO D1 has already proved to be helpful in recognizing tumours showing skeletal muscle differentiation (Angervall and Kindblom, 1993; Dias et al., 1994).

STAGING

The Task Force on Soft Tissue Sarcomas of the American Joint Committee on Cancer (AJCC) Staging and End Result Reporting and the Union Internationale Contre le Cancer (UICC) have established a staging system for soft tissue sarcomas which is an extension of the TNM system to include G for histological grade (Table 41.4, Fleming et al., 1997). Grade, size, depth and presence of nodal or distant metastases are the determinants of stage. This staging system is applied to all sarcomas of soft tissue except rhabdomyosarcoma (for which there is a special staging system), Kaposi's sarcoma, dermatofibrosarcoma, desmoid, and sarcoma arising from the dura mater, brain, parenchymatous organs or hollow viscera. The staging system was revised in 1997 with the addition of subgroupings of the T stage to designate superficial and deep lesions and the assignment of patients with nodal

Table 41.4 *AJCC staging system for sarcoma of soft tissues (AJCC Staging Manual, 1997)*

Histological grade of malignancy

GX	Grade cannot be assessed
G1	Well differentiated
G2	Moderately differentiated
G3	Poorly differentiated
G4	Undifferentiated

T Primary tumour

TX	Primary tumour cannot be assessed
T0	No evidence of primary tumour
T1	Tumour 5 cm or less in greatest dimension T1a: superficial tumour T1b: deep tumour
T2	Tumour greater than 5 cm in greatest dimension T2a: superficial tumour T2b: deep tumour

N Regional lymph nodes

NX	Regional lymph nodes cannot be assessed
N0	No histologically verified metastases to regional lymph nodes
N1	Histologically verified regional lymph node metastasis

M Distant metastasis

MX	Distant metastasis cannot be assessed
M0	No distant metastasis
M1	Distant metastasis

Stage I

A	Low-grade, small, superficial and deep: G1–2 T1a–1b N0 M0
B	Low-grade, large, superficial: G1–2 T2a N0 M0

Stage II

A	Low-grade, large, deep: G1–2 T2b N0 M0
B	High-grade, small, superficial and deep: G3–4 T1a–1b N0 M0
C	High-grade, large, superficial: G3–4 T2a N0 M0

Stage III	High-grade, large, deep: G3–4 T2b N0 M0
Stage IV	Any metastasis: any G any T N1 M0; any G any T N0 M1

Table 41.5 *Five-year actuarial distant metastasis (DM) probability in 501 consecutive local control patients as a function of tumour size for grades 2 and 3 (on a three-step scale) in series from Massachusetts General Hospital (treatment by radiation and surgery)*

Size (mm)	No. of patients	DM (%)
>25	58	3
26–50	128	22
51–100	177	34
101–150	68	43
151–200	49	58
200	21	57
Total	501	35

Analysis: August 1994.

T stage is determined on the basis of size and depth. As evidence for the importance of size as a determinant of frequency of distant metastasis, we present in Table 41.5 an analysis of distant metastasis versus tumour size among patients who have achieved local control. For patients with grade 1 sarcomas, distant metastases are quite uncommon. The pooled data for G2 and G3 lesions (on a three-step scale) show regular increases in distant metastases with tumour size. From these data there clearly is importance in stratification of patients according to grade and size in attempts to compare efficacy of different modes of treatment, defining the natural history of various histological types, or assessing the role of site, patient age, sex, etc. In our judgement, the staging system, which is useful in predicting distant failures has to include tumour size. The staging system which places primary emphasis on extension beyond compartment is useful for planning surgical approach (Enneking *et al.*, 1980). Compartmental status in combined modality treatment does not affect outcome to an important degree.

MANAGEMENT OF THE PRIMARY LESION

Our goal in devising a management strategy for the patient with soft tissue sarcoma is to achieve a tumour-free and morbidity-free patient.

Surgery alone

Until the 1950s, treatment protocols for soft tissue tumours often consisted of marginal local surgical extirpation of the lesion ('shelling out') or, for larger or more extensive tumours, amputation. The former procedures were done without a clear understanding of the nature of the composition of the compressed 'pseudocapsule' or recognition of the presence of daughter nodules within or just outside this region, so that the local recurrence rates for such limited procedures were extraordinarily high. In the 1960s, many

involvement to stage IV. Superficial lesions do not involve the superficial investing fascia in extremity lesions. For practical purposes, all retroperitoneal and visceral lesions would be deep lesions. The current system is outlined in Table 41.4. Grade of sarcoma is determined on the basis of the histological features of the individual tumour. No tumour is assigned to a grade because of the histological type. Various grading systems exist. Some institutions will assign grades 1–3, where grade 1 lesions are considered low grade with minimal metastatic potential and the intermediate-grade 2 and high-grade 3 lesions are considered high grade and capable of metastatic disease. Other institutions have used a four-tiered system, with grades 1 and 2 considered low grade and grades 3 and 4 considered high grade. The grading system cited in the AJCC UICC staging manual is outlined in Table 41.4.

authors were able to demonstrate improved results by a more radical resection in which the surgical resection was through normal tissue in three dimensions; the local recurrence rate was drastically reduced from 75–90 per cent to 10–30 per cent (Martin *et al.*, 1965; Cantin *et al.*, 1968). By the early 1980s better imaging led to improved staging methodology and a clearer understanding of the pattern of local extension of sarcoma by invasion through the pseudocapsule (Enneking *et al.*, 1981) and most surgeons advocated wide or even radical margins for the management of soft tissue tumours with vast improvement in local control (Markhede *et al.*, 1981).

The technique utilized to achieve a wide or radical extirpation of the tumour will vary considerably with anatomical site and anatomical details of prior surgical procedures (especially the biopsy). The surgery is heavily dependent on the knowledge of anatomy of the part and careful study of the imaging studies is an essential part of the preparation for the procedure. The surgery, in theory at least, if it is to be successful in avoiding a local recurrence, must include not only the complete tumour and the track of the prior biopsy, but as wide a cuff of normal tissue as is possible without compromising function so severely as to make the procedure of limited value as limb-sparing surgery. Thus, if one is treating a tumour of the vastus lateralis by surgery alone, not only should that muscle be at least partially resected but prudence dictates that the underlying vastus intermedius, the lateral intermuscular septum and the adjacent portions of the biceps femoris and rectus femoris should be included in the specimen. Provided the surgical margins are proved to be clear, the procedure is usually successful (a local recurrence rate of 5 per cent). Despite the mass of muscle removed from that site, the patient demonstrates only modest disability in normal activities.

The surgical procedure as described above is an effective solution to the problem in sites such as the fleshy parts of the thigh or the calf, or even some parts of the arm in selected patients, but is usually unsatisfactory and more complex when the tumour lies close to vital structures or in an anatomical site where a wide margin is difficult to obtain. Tumours which lie in the popliteal or antecubital fossae are particularly problematic as are those lesions arising in the soft tissues of the volar aspects of the forearm, hands and feet.

In general, the results of surgery alone, even with the best techniques, have a local failure rate of 10–20 per cent when all patients on whom the surgery is performed, including those with unsatisfactory margins, are considered (Enneking *et al.*, 1981; Markhede *et al.*, 1981). The local control rate after surgery alone was 67 per cent in a recent phase III trial of surgery versus surgery and brachytherapy (Harrison *et al.*, 1993). A local failure not only enormously compounds the management problems at the site of the original lesion, but also increases the risk of distant metastases. This has been a problem, especially for sarcomas of the head and neck region.

Surgery combined with radiotherapy

Although wide resection or amputation is often effective in achieving local control, there is usually a significant functional and cosmetic loss. Despite careful preoperative evaluation, a portion of the resected specimen will be found to have unsatisfactory margins and mean that additional treatment is essential. The consequence is that those patients experience both radical surgery and radiation.

Until the early 1960s, the prevailing medical opinion was that the sarcomas were radiation-resistant and that radiation had little to offer these patients (Suit *et al.*, 1985). This opinion was based upon the observation that patients treated by radiation during the 1930s and 1940s fared poorly. This was due to the fact that treatment was by radiation alone, tumours were large, radiation doses were low due to the availability of X-rays of energy of ≤300 kVp, and the clinicians expected a prompt regression. More recent clinical experience and laboratory research has shown without ambiguity that radiotherapy combined with surgery is a highly effective modality (*see* below). Further, radiation sensitivity of cell lines from human sarcomas is comparable to that of epithelial tumours as determined by *in vitro* assays using colony-forming ability as the end point for cell viability. This is illustrated by Figure 41.4 which shows the cumulative distribution of the SF2 (proportion of cells which survive a dose of 2 Gy) for sarcoma cell lines to be no less favourable than that for squamous cell carcinoma cell lines. The available evidence indicates that the tumour control probability for a soft tissue sarcoma and an epithelial tumour of the same size and treated to the same radiation dose are similar. For example, the 5-year local control results of treatment of a patient with carcinoma of the breast or soft tissue sarcoma by resection with negative margins and radiation are essentially the same (approximately 0.9), despite the latter tumour being much the larger.

The rationale for utilizing radiotherapy with a conservative surgical procedure is that radiotherapy in less than radical doses eradicates the small number of tumour cells remaining after a less extensive excision, i.e. those which would be removed in the grossly normal tissue included in the radical surgical specimen but not in that from the simple excision. Thus, moderate radiation doses can be expected to provide the gain over simple surgery that has been shown for radical surgery. An attractive feature of radiotherapy is the relative ease with which the treatment volume can be designed to include tissues suspected of involvement without concern for the position of nerves, vessels and tendons. Results from several clinical studies demonstrate that this approach is clinically practical, and has achieved local control and survival results equal to those obtained by radical surgery with the important gain in cosmetic and functional results (*see* below).

Patients whose sarcomas are so extensive that even a conservative resection would result in a minimally useful limb would be best served, in most instances, by a prompt

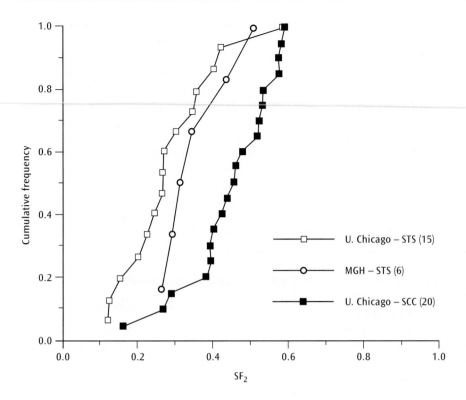

Figure 41.4 *Cumulative distribution of measured SF2 values for cell lines derived from human soft tissue sarcoma and squamous cell carcinoma of head and neck region. SF2, proportion of cells which survive a dose of 2 Gy.*

amputation. For example, the elderly patient with a large sarcoma on the ankle and who has poor vascular supply is a poor candidate for an attempted limb salvage procedure. At the opposite extreme are patients with small sarcomas of the subcutaneous tissue or other anatomical sites that can be resected with wide margins and negligible functional consequences. They need only surgery.

For the more frequent deeply sited lesions, there is usually a close margin at some point on the resected specimen; hence, a combined radiation and surgical approach is required to realize a very low likelihood of local failure.

Radiotherapy alone

Prior to the discussion of combined radiotherapy and surgery, it is useful to document that radiotherapy alone can be effective in achieving cures of patients with soft tissue sarcomas. Our clear preference is to combine limited surgery with radiotherapy. Radiotherapy alone is used for those patients who, for reasons of anatomical location, medical inoperability, or refusal of any surgery, are not candidates even for a conservative surgical procedure. In 1951, Cade described 22 patients who, for a variety of reasons, were treated by radiation alone. Six survived for 5–26 years. Windeyer *et al.* (1966) described results of radiotherapy alone in fibrosarcoma; of eight patients available for 5-year follow-up, four were free of local disease, although one had required surgery for a recurrence. McNeer *et al.* (1968) reported their analysis of the results of treatment of 653 patients with sarcomas of soft tissue treated at the Memorial Hospital. Twenty-five

of the 653 patients were treated by radiotherapy alone; 15 of the 25 were surviving at 5 years, and eight of 20 were surviving at 10 years. Local control was achieved in 14 of the 25 patients.

To achieve a high probability of local control, high doses are essential; this is not different from the treatment of epithelial tumours treated by radiation alone. For example, for consistently good results with radiotherapy of a 5-cm, squamous cell carcinoma, ≈60 ml, the dose needs to be 70–75 Gy. As the pattern of spread requires rather generous margins, clinically appreciable late tissue atrophy may follow such high-dose treatments. This would be an increasingly significant concern in the treatment of even larger lesions. The combined modality strategy provides for the patient a high probability of satisfactory local outcome while avoiding the problems inherent in either radical surgery or ultra-high-dose radiation.

Sequence of radiotherapy and surgery

For patients who are likely to require radiation, our preference is for the radiation to be administered before rather than after the surgical resection. In particular, we suggest that, for the large sarcomas, radiotherapy is more effective if it precedes surgery. Randomized, controlled data comparing the long-term efficacy of preoperative versus postoperative radiotherapy are unfortunately not available. The one phase III clinical trial to evaluate this question was only designed to evaluate the incidence of acute wound healing complications in patients with curable extremity soft-tissue sarcoma (O'Sullivan *et al.*,

1999). One hundred and ninety patients were randomized to either preoperative or postoperative radiotherapy. Complications were defined as secondary wound surgery, hospital admission for wound care, or deep packing or prolonged wound dressings within 120 days of tumour resection. The study was terminated when a highly significant result was obtained at the time of a planned interim analysis. Of 88 evaluable patients, 31 (35 per cent) had wound complications with preoperative radiotherapy compared to 16 of 94 cases (17 per cent) treated postoperatively ($P = 0.01$). Other factors associated with wound complications were the volume of tissue resected and lower limb location of tumour. No difference in local control, disease-free survival or overall survival was noted. It is no surprise that preoperative radiotherapy is associated with more acute wound complications. Because preoperative radiation therapy fields are smaller, and doses are lower (50 Gy versus 60 Gy), it was anticipated that late effects might be fewer and functional results better in the preoperative group. Indeed, patients treated with postoperative radiotherapy were found to have more grade 2 or greater subcutaneous fibrosis and limb oedema. No differences in skin, bone or joint toxicity were seen (O'Sullivan and Davis, 2001).

PREOPERATIVE RADIOTHERAPY

Treatment volumes for radiation administered prior to surgery are planned solely on the basis of known and likely extent of disease. By contrast, postoperative irradiation fields must include not only the site of the tumour, but also all tissues handled during the surgical procedure including the stab wound for the drain tube(s). Therefore, the treatment volume for postoperative radiotherapy will usually be larger than for preoperative irradiation. Nielsen *et al.* (1991) reported a prospective study of radiation field size in a series of 26 patients who were planned for radiation to be given preoperatively and then following surgery were re-planned: the field sizes were 241 cm^2 and 391 cm^2, respectively. The consequence of the smaller treatment volumes means that late radiation reactions are expected to be less severe in patients who receive radiation preoperatively. However, there is a modest increase in the acute reaction as manifest by a delay in the healing of the surgical wound.

Preoperative radiotherapy facilitates the development of an overall treatment plan by the surgeon, radiation therapist, and medical/paediatric oncologist before any therapeutic manoeuvre is implemented.

Initiation of radiotherapy is not delayed when given preoperatively. Where radiotherapy is given postoperatively, delays of 10–14 days or even longer may occur before the treatment is started. This means that residual tumour cells are in a tumour bed flooded with growth factors and, hence, have an opportunity to increase in number. Where wound healing delays treatment further,

recurrent tumour may be grossly evident at the time of initiation of irradiation (especially where surgery was not complete and the lesion was high grade).

At the time of surgery, the tumour is usually smaller and surrounded by a relatively dense pseudocapsule if radiotherapy has been given preoperatively. This means that the margins can be reduced and, hence, a more conservative approach is feasible. This should be associated with lesser disability. In addition, a lesion previously considered inoperable may regress to such an extent that it becomes operable.

Radiation given preoperatively reduces the number of viable tumour cells to such small absolute levels that the likelihood of autotransplantation in the surgical bed is virtually eliminated.

POSTOPERATIVE RADIOTHERAPY

Postoperative radiotherapy has the following advantages:

- Histopathological diagnosis/grade is made from tissue samples taken throughout the entire tumour rather than an incisional biopsy specimen.
- Surgery is immediate. This is important to some patients.
- There is delay in wound healing caused by prior radiation therapy.
- Initial surgery is the only feasible sequence for quite small lesions removed by excisional biopsy, often judged to be benign. This has rarely led to problems other than the occasionally poorly placed incision by a non-oncological surgeon.

On the negative side, however, the treatment volume is larger.

Radiotherapy treatment planning

The principal tasks in treatment planning are:

- definition of the target volume in three dimensions;
- determination of the portal arrangements, portal weighting, and beam characteristics which yield the treatment volume most closely approaching the target volume;
- procedure for immobilization of the anatomical part and confirmation that the target is on the beam line; and
- decision as to dose and fractionation.

The target volume is that volume of tissue which is demonstrated to contain tumour by clinical or radiological examination and which is judged to have a significant probability of involvement by tumour on a subclinical basis. As the distribution of radiation dose throughout the affected region is to be planned on the basis of the estimated distribution of the tumour clonogen number/unit volume of tissue, there will be successive reductions in the treatment volume so that the final dose is given to the grossly evident tumour mass. Specification of these volumes will be based upon analysis of the details of the clinical history and physical examination, histopathological type and grade, the nature of prior surgery and interpretation of the various radiographic procedures (especially CT and/or MRI). The radiation oncologist is better informed if the radiographic studies are reviewed with the radiologist and histopathological material with the pathologist. Similarly, if there has been prior surgery, treatment planning will be facilitated by discussing the operative findings with the surgeon.

After study of the defined target volume, the radiation oncologist, working in conjunction with the radiation physicist, assesses which of the various treatment modalities, used alone or in combination, will produce the smallest treatment volumes for each of the two or three target volumes. Use of more than one treatment modality should be considered, e.g. external photons or electron beam, interstitial therapy, intraoperative electron beam, etc. Three-dimensional treatment planning software using data obtained from a CT scan of the patient immobilized in the treatment position on a flat couch is now available to make the planning process much more accurate and achieve smaller treatment volumes. MRI and CT images can be fused with treatment planning software to optimize target definition. The clinician defines the target and non-target structures on each section of the CT and/or MRI scans and defines the dose constraints for each of the normal structures. The expectation from the use of smaller treatment volumes is an important gain: there is only a disadvantage to the patient in having non-involved tissue irradiated. Although there is no certain means for defining the exact limit of extension along the path of invasion, e.g. a muscle bundle, the clinician can define structures which are non-target with high confidence, e.g. bowel, in planning treatment of a pelvic side wall lesion.

Every possible technical effort should be made to reduce the treatment volume toward target volume (Suit et al., 1988). Where appropriate, the treatment plan should include the use of wedge filters, compensating filters, patient immobilization devices, side lights, tattoo marks, secondary collimation (cerrobend cut-outs, multi-leaf collimators), on-line portal imaging, etc. The tattoo marks are placed, wherever possible, on skin that is relatively fixed, e.g. over the anterior iliac crest, over the greater trochanter, etc. An example of a patient immobilization device is shown in Figure 41.5. Here the leg is rigidly locked into position so that there is virtually no motion during the course of an individual treatment and there is great reproducibility in repositioning of the patient at each treatment session. To increase the reproducibility of the set-up, the position of the patient's head, arms and legs should be comfortable and their position at simulation defined in the record either by diagrams or photographs. In general terms, for patients in a supine position, the

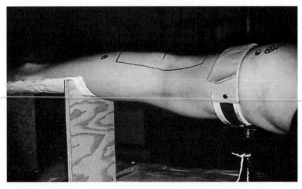

Figure 41.5 *Example of an immobilization system employed in radiation therapy of a lesion in the lateral knee region. Here, an extremely tight immobilization was achieved. Treatment was administered by a pair of anterior and posterior oblique wedge fields.*

head should be straight, arms by the side, heels together; patient position is checked to make sure that the midline of the patient is parallel to the long axis of the couch.

A valuable point to keep in mind in planning treatment is that there may be a failure (recurrence or necrosis) and the plan should, if feasible, allow for potential sites for flaps, surgical incision, etc., if salvage surgery is necessary.

Comments made here regarding radiation dose levels are meant to serve only as guidelines. The dose for the individual patient must be based on assessment of the planned field size, treatment volume, general condition of patient, prior surgery, status of wound, concurrent medical diseases (diabetes, lupus erythematosis, etc.), which reduce tolerance of normal tissues included in the treatment volume. Our general approach has been to employ two or three treatment volumes. The first treatment volume includes all tissues suspected to be involved by subclinical disease. Treatments are administered in five fractions per week giving 1.8–2.0 Gy per fraction to a dose of 50 Gy. All fields are irradiated on each treatment session. During this component of treatment, a bolus is applied over the biopsy or surgical scar (the bolus is usually 1–2 cm wide and thick enough to achieve approximately a 90 per cent dose level on the skin). At the 50-Gy point, the treatment volume is reduced to cover the grossly involved tissues with a narrow margin. Where radiotherapy alone is used, the dose is then carried to approximately 75 Gy, usually with an intermediate field size reduction at the 65-Gy level. For patients treated postoperatively, treatment, of course, is not started until the wound is healed. The dose is ≈60 Gy if the margins were negative, 66 Gy for positive margins and 75 Gy for gross residual sarcoma. For patients treated preoperatively, our radiation dose is 50 Gy. A boost dose is administered for patients with positive margins or gross residual disease (Sadoski et al., 1993). We consider a margin to be positive provided tumour cells are identified at the inked margin. Some centres class margins as positive when cells

Table 41.6 *Local control results in patients treated by surgery and radiation*

Centre	No. patients	Local failure (%)	Reference
Postop radiation			
MGH	176	14	Spiro *et al.* (1997)
MDAH	300	22	Lindberg *et al.* (1981)
IGR	89	14	Abbatucci *et al.* (1986)
RPMI	53	14	Karakousis *et al.* (1986)
NCI	128	10	Potter *et al.* (1985)
Toronto	23	9	Wilson *et al.* (1994)
St. Louis	35	14	Pao and Pilepich (1990)
Amsterdam	64	8	Keus *et al.* (1994)
U. Penn/Fox Chase	67	13	Fein *et al.* (1995)
U. Chicago	50	24	Mundt *et al.* (1995)
Preop radiation			
MGH	181	10	Spiro *et al.* (1997)
MDAH	110	10	Barkley *et al.* (1988)
Toronto	39	3	Wilson *et al.* (1999)
U. Fla	58	9	Brant *et al.* (1990)
Intra-op BRT			
Memorial	55	18	Harrison *et al.* (1993)
Mayo	63	8[a]	Schray *et al.* (1990)
i.a./i.v. Adriamycin + radiation			
UCLA	371	≈10	Eilber *et al.* (1993)
U. Virginia	55	2	Wanebo *et al.* (1995)

[a]Mean follow-up was 20 months. MGH, Massachusetts General Hospital; MDAH, M.D. Anderson Hospital; IGR, Institut Gustav Roussy; RPMI, Roswell Park Memorial Institute; NCI, US National Cancer Institute; U. Fla, University of Florida.

are within 1–2 mm from the inked margin. For most patients, the boost dose is given by external-beam radiotherapy techniques using small fields directed at the clip-defined tumour bed. In some instances the boost dose is given by intraoperative electron beam or by catheters placed into the tumour bed for brachytherapy when there is concern regarding the adequacy of the resection. For either approach the total dose is also ≈64–66 Gy for positive margin and 75 Gy for gross residue.

Several centres combine wide resection and intra-operative brachytherapy as the complete treatment, i.e. no external-beam radiation. The catheters are placed into the tumour bed and not loaded for 4 days; the dose is 45–50 Gy (Harrison *et al.*, 1993).

Results of radiotherapy combined with surgery

The 5-year results of treatment of patients with soft tissue sarcoma of the extremities by radiotherapy and surgery are presented in Table 41.6. These results from 15 institutions document that long-term local control is achieved in 82–92 per cent of patients. This is the equivalent of the local control rates following modern surgical procedures. For example, in the phase III trial of brachytherapy at the Memorial Hospital, the local control result in the surgery alone group of 70 patients was 67 per cent (Harrison *et al.*, 1993). That interstitial therapy is an effective modality in the treatment of these patients is shown by that trial. Five-year actuarial local control rates were 82 per cent and 67 per cent for the surgery + brachytherapy and the surgery alone arms, respectively. Likewise, high local control rates for brachytherapy have been obtained at the Mayo Clinic (Schray *et al.*, 1990).

For consideration of the results according to stage and treatment method, we describe results achieved at Massachusetts General Hospital in the treatment of 367 consecutive patients by radiotherapy and resectional surgery for sarcoma of soft tissue of the extremities, torso and head and neck region during the period from September 1971 to June 1988. Current status and 5-year actuarial local control and overall survival results are given in Tables 41.7 and 41.8. Results were good among patients with stage IA, IB, IIA and IIIA disease. However, for patients with stage IIB and IIIB, treatment was clearly less successful. This experience emphasizes the great importance of grade and size of sarcoma on prognosis.

Results obtained for the postoperative and preoperative groups who had high-grade sarcoma according to size of sarcoma are presented in Table 41.9. There appears to be an important gain in local control of the large sarcomas (>10 cm) by preoperative radiotherapy. The good results obtained in the preoperative radiation group are derived from large patient numbers (123 patients in stage IIB and IIIB compared with 67 for the postoperative treatment group).

Table 41.7 *Current status and 5-year actuarial results in 176 consecutive patients treated at Massachusetts General Hospital by surgery and postoperative radiotherapy according to 1988 AJCC stage (1971–1988)*

Stages	No. patients	NED	LF + DM	DM	ID	Local control (%)	OS (%)
IA	18	16	1	0	1	100	100
IB	21	18	1	0	2	95	94
IIA	39	25	6	5	3	84	91
IIB	34	16	7	9	2	77	72
IIIA	30	22	1	4	3	95	88
IIIB	33	11	7	15	0	73	49
IVA	1	1	0	0	0	100	100
Total	176	109	23	33	11	86	80

NED, no evident disease; LF, local failure; DM, distant metastasis; ID, dead of intercurrent disease; OS, overall survival.

Table 41.8 *Current status and 5-year actuarial results in 181 consecutive patients treated at Massachusetts General Hospital by preoperative radiotherapy and conservative surgery according to stage (1971–1988)*

Stages	No. patients	NED	LF + DM	DM	ID	Local control (%)	OS (%)
IA	6	6	0	0	0	100	100
IB	15	10	3	1	1	86	93
IIA	23	18	1	4	0	91	81
IIB	64	35	2	26	1	96	66
IIIA	12	9	2	1	0	79	91
IIIB	59	21	5	28	5	88	52
IVA	2	2	0	0	0	100	100
Total	181	101	13	60	7	90	70

NED, no evident disease; LF, local failure; DM, distant metastasis; ID, dead of intercurrent disease; OS, overall survival.

Table 41.9 *Five-year actuarial local control results according to size of primary soft tissue sarcoma (Massachusetts General Hospital)*

Size (mm)	Postoperative		Preoperative	
	No. patients	LC (%)	No. patients	LC (%)
25	20	100	11	80
26–49	45	95	16	100
50–100	64	83	63	93
101–150	12	91	34	100
151–200	6	50	25	79
200	3	67	11	100
Total	150	87	160	93

Postoperative radiotherapy has been highly effective in the treatment of small sarcomas (<5 cm). For these lesions treated by local excision, the wounds heal rapidly and radiotherapy can be started promptly. From our perspective, where radiotherapy is to be employed it should be given preoperatively except for the small lesions.

Preoperative radiotherapy in the treatment of patients with sarcoma of soft tissue is not new. Atkinson *et al.* reported in 1963 on 15 patients with operable sarcoma of soft tissue who were treated by preoperative radiotherapy (45 Gy in 4–5 weeks) followed 4–6 weeks later by 'block resection'. The tumours were 4–20 cm in size; 10 were recurrent lesions. There had been one local failure and no distant metastases in these patients. Median follow-up was 3 years and 5 months. In the same clinic there had been 40 local recurrences following block resections alone performed on 54 patients with 'comparable' lesions. Barkley *et al.* (1988) have reported on 110 patients with locally advanced lesions treated by preoperative irradiation and resection; their local control rate was 90 per cent.

Intra-arterial infusion chemotherapy, radiotherapy and resection

Eilber and Morton have been strong proponents of a programme that has consisted of intra-arterial doxorubicin followed by rapid fraction radiation therapy (3.5 Gy per fraction) and subsequent local excision (Eilber *et al.*,

1993, 1984). Their data has shown local recurrence rates of <10 per cent with survival rates of 74 per cent in stage III tumours. Among these patients there was a 5 per cent amputation rate. They have since shown that it is not necessary to provide the doxorubicin by an intra-arterial route. This approach is fully competitive with the straight surgery and radiation protocols.

Isolated limb perfusion with TNF-α

Hyperthermic isolated limb perfusion with chemotherapeutic agents has been tried as another way to control very large tumours that would otherwise require amputation because of proximity to nerve or blood vessels. Most such regimens do not appear superior to surgery plus radiotherapy. However, hyperthermic TNF-α plus melphalan has achieved complete response rates of approximately 30 per cent, partial remission rates of 50 per cent with overall limb-salvage rates over 80 per cent (Schraffordt Koops et al., 1998).

This work was initiated by Lejeune et al. (1989) and has been extended to several other centres. TNF-α has long been known to be a potent non-specific tumour cell cytotoxic agent with demonstrated high efficacy in treatment of tumour-bearing rodents. Application in man has been severely restricted due to systemic toxicity. However, by the use of the isolated limb perfusion technique, the systemic toxicity has been effectively bypassed. Eggermont et al. (1996) reported the results from a multi-centre study of isolated limb perfusion with TNF-α, interferon-γ (IFNγ) and melphalan for extremity sarcomas. The complete response (CR) and partial response (PR) rates were 18 per cent and 64 per cent; limb salvage was achieved in 84 per cent of patients. Of 39 patients who also had conservative resection, there have been five local failures. Vaglini et al. (1994) reported from Milan a high response rate using the same protocol. Olieman et al. (1998) reported the results of a series of 34 patients treated by this isolated limb perfusion with TNF-α, IFNγ and melphalan followed by resection and radiation in 15 patients. Limb salvage was realized in 85 per cent. Local recurrence developed in 26 per cent of patients treated by perfusion alone and in none of the perfusion + radiation patients. The two groups sustained approximately equivalent treatment-related morbidity. There is one report indicating an increase in severe morbidity when radiation is combined with the perfusion (Vrouenraets et al., 1997). The mechanism of action of the TNF-α is not fully understood. Its efficacy is reported to be reduced in hypoxic cells (Lynch et al., 1995). Gutman et al. (1997) report a 37 per cent CR rate using TNF-α and melphalan.

Surgical margins and local control

Sadoski et al. (1993) have analysed 132 consecutive patients with soft tissue sarcoma of the extremities treated with

Table 41.10 *Five-year actuarial local control (LC) results and margin status after preoperative radiotherapy for extremity soft tissue sarcoma (Massachusetts General Hospital)*

Margin	No. patients	LC (%)
+	27	81
−	106	97
<1mm	27	96
>1 mm	36	97
Undefined	21	94
No tumour[a]	22	100

[a] Specimen negative for tumour.

preoperative radiotherapy and resectional surgery and found that (Table 41.10):

- the 5-year actuarial local control rates were 97 per cent and 81 per cent for patients with negative margins and positive margins, respectively (this difference is highly significant);
- there was no difference between the various subcategories of negative margins [negative at <1 mm (96 per cent), negative at >1 mm (97 per cent), not measured (94 per cent) and no tumour in the specimen (100 per cent)];
- there was no difference in local control for treatment of primary and locally recurrent lesions (after previous surgery alone) when the tumours were stratified for margin status; and
- for the patients with negative margin local control was not a function of sarcoma size.

Tanabe et al. (1994) reported the margin status of 95 patients treated by preoperative radiotherapy (50–60 Gy) and limb sparing surgery for their high-grade soft tissue sarcoma at the M. D. Anderson Hospital. They observed local control in 91 per cent and 62 per cent of patients with margins negative and positive, respectively.

Fagundes et al. (1992) reported that patients treated by resection and postoperative radiation for malignant fibrous histiocytoma failed locally in nine of 23 (39 per cent) and one of 11 instances for positive and negative margins, respectively. Among 26 patients treated with resection, doxorubicin and postoperative radiation [51 Gy (3 Gy ×17)] for positive margins (Wiklund et al., 1993), local failure was observed in six (23 per cent). Herbert et al. (1993) observed local control in 50 per cent of patients with positive margins compared with 100 per cent in those with negative margins. These reports indicate that positive margins are associated with a reduced local control rate. The experience at the Princess Margaret Hospital (LeVay et al., 1993) strongly supports efforts to achieve negative margins. Local relapse rates at 5 years were 13 per cent, 24 per cent and 77 per cent for negative margins, micropositive margins and gross residual disease in the wound, respectively. Our policy is to make serious efforts to achieve negative margins.

Wound healing after surgery and radiation

Bujko et al. (1992) have analysed the wound healing in 202 patients treated by preoperative radiotherapy. The overall wound complication rate was 37 per cent. One patient died because of necrotizing fasciitis. In 33 (16.5 per cent) cases, secondary surgery was necessary, including six patients (3 per cent) who required amputation. The wounds in the remaining 40 patients (20 per cent) were treated without surgery. Multivariate analyses of the data showed that the following factors were significantly associated with wound morbidity: tumour in the lower extremity ($P < 0.001$), increasing age ($P = 0.004$) and postoperative boost with interstitial implant ($P = 0.016$). Accelerated fractionation (twice daily) reached border-line statistical significance ($P = 0.074$). Two other factors showed association with wound morbidity by univariate analysis but not in multivariate model: high pathological grade ($P = 0.02$) and estimated volume of resected specimen $>200 \, cm^3$ ($P = 0.065$). We have observed this to be a problem, especially for the elderly obese patients with large sarcomas in the proximal thigh.

Quantitation of the impact of preoperative radiation dose on wound healing in patients with soft tissue sarcomas is difficult because wound complications are also seen in patients treated by surgery alone. Furthermore, there is tremendous heterogeneity among sarcoma patients with respect to anatomical site, histological type, lesion size, prior surgery, medical status and age. In the series of patients managed by surgery alone and reported by Arbeit et al. (1987), the incidences of all categories of wound complication were 27.5 per cent (8/29) and 33 per cent (21/64), respectively. This is comparable to 37 per cent observed in our study. However, in neither surgical series were amputations performed for wound-related morbidity and the percentage of patients requiring a secondary procedure was lower than in our irradiated patients (3.5 per cent and 3 per cent versus 16.5 per cent).

Higher wound complication rates are reported for patients treated with radiotherapy preoperatively compared with postoperatively. Schray et al. (1990) observed wound morbidity in 25 per cent of patients treated with preoperative external-beam radiotherapy and brachytherapy, whereas only a 5 per cent complication rate was seen in those treated postoperatively. Bell et al. (1991) described a series of 19 patients with 'difficult' sarcomas from 52 registered patients. Criteria for selection were one or more of the following: tumour size $>20 \, cm$, extension to true pelvis, involvement of great vessel and bone. Among 13 patients who had preoperative radiation, six (46 per cent) developed wound complications that required a secondary surgical procedure. In a report by Bryant et al. (1985), 32 patients were managed with preoperative radiation. Those treated by an accelerated fractionation protocol (two fractions of 1.8 Gy/day) suffered more complications than patients irradiated on a one fraction per day schedule (56 per cent versus

46 per cent). All four major complications (one leading to amputation and three to death) were in the twice-daily group. Mansson et al. (1983) studied 22 patients irradiated preoperatively: two patients had a complicated wound healing. The total preoperative dose was 40 Gy in all but two patients and no postoperative boost was given. Goodnight et al. (1985) reported a 24 per cent wound complication rate requiring secondary surgery following preoperative radiation (35–40 Gy total dose, 3.5 Gy and 2 Gy dose per fraction) and intra-arterial doxorubicin. A similar schedule of treatment was utilized by Denton et al. (1984) and 13 per cent of patients sustained severe wound morbidity; two required amputation and two needed reconstructive surgery. In the report of a series of 100 patients treated with a similar approach by Eilber et al. (1988), wound complication was reported in 13 per cent of cases. None of their patients needed secondary surgery for closure. The randomized trial described above also documented a higher rate of acute wound complications in patients treated preoperatively (O'Sullivan et al., 1999).

Based on our current results and the experience of others as described in the literature, we suggest the following strategies which may lead to reduced wound morbidity:

- more gentle handling of tissue during surgery;
- meticulous attention to achieve haemostasis before wound closure;
- avoid closure under tension;
- eliminate all dead space in the wound. If rotation of a flap is needed to fill the space, it should be used;
- drain the wound and leave the tubes in place until the drainage is $\approx 10 \, mL/day$;
- in many situations use of a compression dressing is advantageous;
- immobilize the affected part for 7–10 days;
- special attention needs to be directed towards defining the subgroup(s) of patients in whom the postoperative boost dose could be omitted. For example, in those patients at MGH whose specimen have negative histological margins, the addition of the postoperative boost did not demonstrate any additional gain over the excellent local control achieved with $\approx 50 \, Gy$ of preoperative radiotherapy. Hence, the postoperative boost is no longer used in such patients (Sadoski et al., 1993).

Functional outcome

Data regarding the functional outcome of patients undergoing limb-salvage procedures are limited. In a series of 88 patients treated with either preoperative or postoperative radiation therapy, 68 patients had acceptable functional results and 61 of these patients returned to work (Bell et al., 1991). In this series large tumours, neural sacrifice, proximal thigh tumours and postoperative complications were associated with a poor outcome. The authors suggested that limiting wound healing complications would impact favourably on functional outcome. Robinson *et al.* (1991) evaluated a group of patients with lower limb sarcomas and concluded that radiotherapy was associated with reduced muscle power and range of motion, compared with patients treated with surgery alone. However, most patients retained excellent limb function and quality of life. These authors also noted that large doses per fraction were associated with increased fibrosis and poorer outcome.

Long-term treatment complications were analysed in sarcoma patients undergoing limb-sparing therapy at the National Cancer Institute (Stinson *et al.*, 1991). All patients received radiotherapy and surgery. Bone fracture was observed in 6 per cent, contracture in 20 per cent, oedema greater than 2+ in 19 per cent, moderate-to-severe decrease in strength in 20 per cent and induration in 57 per cent. The percentage of patients ambulating without assistive devices with mild or no pain was 84 per cent. Higher nominal standard doses (>1760 rets) were associated with a greater incidence of late complications.

Two studies have assessed psychosocial outcome in amputees compared with patients undergoing limb salvage (Sugarbaker *et al.*, 1982; Weddington, 1985). Neither study showed a difference in the two groups, although in the study by Sugarbaker *et al.*, patients in the limb-salvage group received chemotherapy and radiotherapy. Patients who had radical surgery/amputation adapted quite well to the imposed disability.

Salvage surgery after local recurrence

Twenty seven patients with locally recurrent extremity soft tissue sarcoma following initial conservative surgery and radiotherapy were analyzed and reported by the Musculoskeletal Oncology Unit at Princess Margaret Hospital (Catton *et al.*, 1996). Two patients with concurrent systemic relapse were treated palliatively. Seven patients were not candidates for conservative re-excision and underwent amputation. Eleven underwent conservative resection without radiation; seven of these relapsed again and five went on to receive combined conservative surgery and re-irradiation. A further five underwent conservative resection with radiation, for a total of ten patients treated with excision and re-irradiation. Six of these ten underwent brachytherapy, one was treated with combined brachytherapy and external beam therapy, and three received external beam radiotherapy. Median re-treatment radiotherapy dose was 2/9.5 Gy. Overall local control was 19/23 (91 per cent). The local control after re-excision alone was 4/11 (36.7 per cent), while that for re-excision with re-irradiation was 10/10 (100 per cent). Six of these ten patients experienced significant post irradiation wound healing problems, but three recovered fully, of the twenty five patients, fourteen are alive and disease-free, two are alive with local disease and four with systemic disease, and five are dead of disease.

Potter *et al.* (1985) have reviewed the results of salvage surgery in patients with local and distant failures among a total of 307 patients with sarcomas located in the extremities, trunk, breast, or head/neck region who were completely resected in the initial treatment at NCI (there was no preoperative radiation). Disease recurred in 107/307 patients (35 per cent). Twenty one of the 107 (20 per cent) had an isolated local recurrence. Twenty of twenty one (96 per cent) were rendered disease-free with salvage surgery.

Summary of indications for radiotherapy in soft tissue sarcoma

Grade 1 lesions, so situated anatomically that they can be approached with virtual certainty that the lesion and a generous margin of grossly normal tissue can be resected and yet provide the patient with a good functional and cosmetic result, should be treated by radical surgery alone (Baldini *et al.*, 1999). Selected patients with superficial sarcomas may also be treated with surgery alone (Rydholm *et al.*, 1991; Baldini *et al.*, 1999). There would be no indication for radiation therapy provided histological study of the specimen shows that good margins were obtained. For many grade 1 lesions these requirements will not be satisfied. For such patients and also all patients with grade 2 or 3 lesions, our policy would be to recommend preoperative radiotherapy for lesions diagnosed by incisional biopsy and postoperative radiotherapy for small lesions removed by excisional biopsy.

ROLE OF ADJUVANT CHEMOTHERAPY

Although surgery and radiotherapy achieve control of the primary tumour and cure most adult patients with soft tissue sarcomas, many patients, especially those with large grade 2 or 3 primaries, die of metastatic disease not evident at diagnosis. Several studies have shown chemotherapy to be effective against clinically evident metastases (Gottlieb *et al.*, 1972; Townsend *et al.*, 1976; Rosenberg *et al.*, 1978; Sordillo *et al.*, 1978; das Gupta *et al.*, 1982; Antman, 1983). This has suggested to many that chemotherapy used as an adjuvant therapy (in high-risk stage M0 patients) would inactivate micrometastases and increase long-term survival.

The first prospective randomized trial of adjuvant chemotherapy for this group of tumours was reported from the M. D. Anderson Hospital (Lindberg *et al.*, 1977); they failed to demonstrate any advantage of vincristine, cyclophosphamide, Adriamycin and dactinomycin chemotherapy over untreated controls. Similarly, a randomized Mayo Clinic series (Edmonson *et al.*, 1984) found a slight extension of disease-free survival with no increase in overall survival for patients receiving vincristine, cyclophosphamide and dactinomycin alternating with vincristine, doxorubicin and dacarbazine (DTIC).

However, using Adriamycin (530 mg/m^2) and cyclophosphamide (500–700 mg/m^2) followed by high-dose methotrexate, Rosenberg *et al.* (1983) demonstrated a significantly improved disease-free survival for patients with extremity lesions randomized to adjuvant chemotherapy (92 per cent versus 60 per cent at 3 years with a survival advantage of 95 per cent versus 74 per cent). Some serious cardiotoxicity was encountered. With longer follow-up in this small randomized trial, the survival advantage was no longer significant (Chang *et al.*, 1988). Single-agent doxorubicin has failed to show an improvement in disease-free or overall survival in patients receiving postoperative chemotherapy compared with surgery alone (Picci *et al.*, 1988). Studies from Dana Farber Cancer Institute, Massachusetts General Hospital and the Eastern Co-operative Oncology Group (ECOG) (Wilson *et al.*, 1986) and from UCLA (Eilber *et al.*, 1988) and the Scandinavian Sarcoma Group (Alvegaard *et al.*, 1989) showed similar results.

The very large EORTC study of adjuvant chemotherapy has employed CYVADIC, consisting of cyclophosphamide, vincristine, Adriamycin and DTIC. Results reported by Bramwell *et al.* in 1994 demonstrated a significant delay in the appearance of relapse: in 317 patients the relapse-free survival rates at 7 years were 56 per cent for the treated group and 43 per cent for controls ($P = 0.007$). However, survival rates were not significantly different at 63 per cent and 56 per cent. There were fewer local failures among the CYVADIC-treated head, neck and trunk patients ($P = 0.002$) but not among those with extremity tumours. There was no difference in distant metastasis (32 per cent versus 36 per cent, $P = 0.42$). A summary of randomized trials is presented in Table 41.11.

A meta-analysis of 13 randomized trials of adjuvant chemotherapy versus control in soft tissue sarcomas demonstrated that Adriamycin-based chemotherapy yielded an absolute gain in overall recurrence-free survival of 10 per cent from 45 per cent to 55 per cent ($P = 0.0001$) and a trend for improvement of overall survival of 4 per cent from 50 to 54 per cent ($P = 0.12$). For local control

the gain was 6 per cent at 10 years, viz. 75 per cent → 81 per cent, $P = 0.016$. The most clear evidence of a gain in survival obtained for patients 31–60 years old, recurrent lesions, extremity and high grade (Sarcoma Meta-analysis Collaboration, 1997). Encouraging results with more intense adjuvant therapy was reported by investigators at Massachusetts General Hospital who evaluated doxorubicin, ifosfamide and DTIC chemotherapy and radiation in adult patients with >8 cm AJCC (1992) stage IIB or IIIB soft tissue sarcomas of the extremity (Spiro *et al.*, 1996; DeLaney *et al.*, 2001). Moreover, a newer randomized trial of more intense adjuvant chemotherapy with epirubicin, ifosfamide, mesna and granulocyte colony stimulating factor (G-CSF) also seems to show a possible further advantage in disease-free and overall survival (Frustaci *et al.*, 2001).

METASTATIC DISEASE (STAGE IVB)

Chemotherapy

Doxorubicin and ifosfamide have been demonstrated to be the most active chemotherapy agents in widely disseminated soft tissue sarcoma. For doxorubicin, objective response rates between 20 per cent and 40 per cent for the single agent have been reported. A steep dose–response curve for objective responses was described by O'Bryan *et al.* (1977): 0 per cent at 25 mg/m^2, 18 per cent at 45 mg/m^2, 20 per cent at 60 mg/m^2 and 37 per cent at 75 mg/m^2. Complete responses were few, durations averaged 8 months with little survival advantage conferred by single-agent treatment. DTIC by itself has a modest response rate around 16 per cent (Gottlieb *et al.*, 1976). Methotrexate was described as active in 36 per cent of 41 patients with six complete responders (Subramanian and Wiltshaw, 1978) but as inactive by Pinedo and Verweij (1986). High-dose methotrexate may be active as initial therapy but of limited value in pre-treated patients

Table 41.11 *Randomized adjuvant trials in soft tissue sarcomas (modified from Antman, 1997)*

| Investigator | No. patients | Drugs | DFS (%) | | Survival (%) | |
			Treated	Control	Treated	Control
Lindberg *et al.* (1977)	47	V, C, Ad/Ac	77	83		
Edmonson *et al.* (1984)	61	V, Ac, C/V, Ad, D	67	63	71	71
Rosenberg *et al.* (1983)	67	C, Ad/M	54[a]	28	65	46
Omura (1985)	156	Ad	59	47	68	65
Eilber (1986)	119	Ad	56	54	78	74
Gherlinzoni (1986)	77	Ad	73[a]	45	91[a]	70
Antman (1990)	168	Ad	66	53	68	65
Bramwell *et al.* (1994)	468	Ad, C, V, D	56[a]	43	63	56
Frustaci *et al.* (2001)	104	Ad, I	50[a]	37	69	50

DFS, disease-free survival at various time periods; V, vincristine; C, cyclophosphamide; Ad, Adriamycin; Ac, actinomycin; D, DTIC; M, methotrexate; I, ifosfamide. [a] Significant difference.

(Karakousis *et al.*, 1980). Cyclophosphamide appears less active in adults than in children and less active than the related compound ifosfamide (Bramwell *et al.*, 1993). High doses of ifosfamide may be particularly active (Christman *et al.*, 1993). Cisplatin may have a role (Karakousis *et al.*, 1979; Grabois *et al.*, 1994). Pinedo and Verweij (1986) and Greenall *et al.* (1986) have reviewed numerous other agents evaluated in small trials.

Many combination chemotherapy regimens for metastatic disease have been studied in phase II trials. Most of these trials include doxorubicin (or epirubicin) and an alkylating agent. Adding DTIC to doxorubicin improved the response rate to 41 per cent as described by Gottlieb *et al.* (1972), but the response rate has decreased over time (Gottlieb *et al.*, 1976). Randomized trials (Omura *et al.*, 1983; Borden *et al.*, 1987) found some gain for the combination. A South-west Oncology Group (SWOG) phase III trial compared bolus versus infusional administration of doxorubicin plus DTIC and reported no diffeences in overall response (17 per cent in both arms) or complete responses (5 per cent in both arms). Additionally, there was no difference in the median survival, 10.5 months in both groups (Zalupski *et al.*, 1991). Adding cyclophosphamide to the basic duo was reported to raise the response rate to 56 per cent (Blum *et al.*, 1980) and this was confirmed by a randomized trial (Baker, 1987). Comparisons have shown that the addition of less active drugs necessitate lower doses of doxorubicin and, accordingly, reduces overall effectiveness (Cruz *et al.*, 1979; Schoenfeld *et al.*, 1982). Adding ifosfamide seems to be clearly beneficial as reported by Blum *et al.* (1993) and Schutte *et al.* (1993).

The ECOG conducted a three-arm trial comparing doxorubicin alone, doxorubicin plus ifosfamide, and mitomycin plus doxorubicin plus cisplatin. Objective tumour regression occurred more frequently in the combination arms than in the single-agent arm (20 per cent with doxorubicin alone, 34 per cent in doxorubicin plus ifosfamide, and 32 per cent in the mitomycin plus doxorubicin plus cisplatin arm). However, the combination regimens resulted in significantly greater myelosuppression, e.g. 80 per cent of the doxorubicin/ifosfamide group had grade 3 or greater myelosuppression. Most notably, no significant survival differences were observed between the three treatment regimens (Edmonson *et al.*, 1993).

The extensively utilized CYVADIC regimen has evolved from the sequential trials sponsored by SWOG (Gottlieb *et al.*, 1975). Greenall *et al.* (1986) reviewed studies reporting response rates of 15–60 per cent, the average being 41 per cent. Noteworthy is that up to 15 per cent of the responses have been scored as complete. The median response was longer (13 months) and 21 per cent of complete responders described by Yap *et al.* (1983) achieved 5-year disease-free status. Pinedo and Verweij (1986) have also reviewed alternative regimens. A popular regimen adds ifosfamide to Adriamycin and DTIC (Elias and

Antman, 1986). A combination of ifosfamide with mesna, doxorubicin and DTIC has resulted in response rates in measurable metastatic sarcomas as high as 47 per cent with complete response rates as high as 10 per cent (Chang *et al.*, 1989; Elias *et al.*, 1989). Another protocol describes activity with DTIC and cisplatin in pretreated patients (Piver *et al.*, 1986).

Dose intensity may be extremely important as described by Zaninelli *et al.* (1993). Very high-dose ifosfamide had been used by Rosen *et al.* (1994) with high response rates despite some toxicity. Higher-dose therapy with standard agents (Bodey, 1981) may require special supportive care such as bone marrow transplantation (Kessinger *et al.*, 1994), but may offer a chance for higher complete response rates and longer response duration. There has been a considerable interest focused on maintaining dose intensity of chemotherapy using colony stimulating factors to alleviate myelosuppression. Granulocyte/macrophage colony stimulating factor (GM-CSF) has been used with a variety of regimens to help maintain dose intensification. In a few studies this has resulted in improved response rates (Mertens and Bramwell, 1993). Even higher dose chemotherapy, as used at M. D. Anderson, seems to result in higher response rates (59–69 per cent) (Pisters *et al.*, 1997; Patel *et al.*, 1998).

Pulmonary surgery for metastatic disease

Distant metastases usually present 2 years after the initial diagnosis. Patients with high-grade sarcomas have a higher risk of developing distant disease compared with low-grade extremity sarcomas (Donohue *et al.*, 1988). For patients with extremity tumours, metastatic disease most frequently appears in the lungs (Gadd *et al.*, 1993). Evidence is now available that resection of pulmonary metastases may be worthwhile in selected patients. In one study, resection of all visible tumour was possible in 86 of 102 patients with pulmonary metastases from sarcomas, and overall 5-year survival was 26 per cent (Martini *et al.*, 1974). In another series of 40 patients, pulmonary lesions were completely resectable in 34 and 5-year survival was 33.8 per cent (Feldman and Kyriakos, 1972). Factors such as disease-free interval (time elapsing between resection of the primary tumour and appearance of pulmonary metastases) and tumour doubling time (calculated from measurements of the diameter of pulmonary nodules seen on serial chest X-rays) influence prognosis. The following criteria for selection of patients for surgery have been suggested (Joseph, 1974):

- control of the primary tumour has been achieved;
- there is no evidence of extrapulmonary metastases;
- pulmonary lesions should be resectable; multiple lesions are not a contraindication but if extensive multiple resections are necessary the failure rate rises;

- the patient should be fit for surgery as regards general condition and respiratory status;
- tumour doubling time should be at least 40 days.

Complete resection of pulmonary lesions is possible in some patients who have limited disease and adequate pulmonary function. While individual clinical trials indicate improved survival rates, overall, a large review found that fewer than 10 per cent of patients undergoing pulmonary resection for metastatic disease were long-term survivors (Brennan *et al.*, 1997).

DESMOID TUMOURS

Desmoid tumours are benign, slowly growing fibroblastic neoplasms arising from fibroblastic stromal elements. Although neoplastic and locally aggressive, desmoids do not have the capacity to establish metastatic lesions. Histologically, the lesions are characterized by small numbers of slender, bland fibroblasts in an abundant fibrous stroma that is locally infiltrating adjacent tissues. There are usually few mitotic figures and necrosis is absent.

Desmoid tumours are uncommon, with an estimated incidence in the USA of two to four per million inhabitants per year or 900 new tumours per year (Reitamo *et al.*, 1982). Desmoids are slightly more common in females than males (Enzinger and Weiss, 2001). These tumours are uncommon in the young and in the elderly and occur predominantly in individuals of 15–60 years of age. There is no significant racial or ethnic distribution. The aetiology of desmoid tumours is not known.

There are clonal chromosomal changes and the incidence of desmoids is much higher in patients with familial adenomatous polyposis (FAP, Gardner's syndrome) (Jarvinen, 1987). There also appears to be an association with antecedent trauma in some patients. Clonal chromosomal changes, particularly trisomy 8 and 20, occur in many desmoid tumours and appear to be non-random aberrations (Fletcher *et al.*, 1995; Kouho *et al.*, 1997). The presence of these trisomies appears to be associated with a higher risk of recurrence (Fletcher *et al.*, 1995; Kouho *et al.*, 1997). One study used the double FISH (fluorescence *in situ* hybridization) technique to assay the frequency of trisomy in single cell suspensions of desmoid tumours (Qi *et al.*, 1996). Three positive signals for chromosome 8 or 20 were seen in at least 1 per cent of 200 counted cells in 16 cases. More than 20 per cent of cells were positive for trisomy 8 in six cases and for trisomy 20 in four cases. In two cases, more than 20 per cent of the cells were positive for both. In another report, trisomy 8 and/or trisomy 20 were observed in cells cultured from 6 of 13 desmoid tumours (Qi *et al.*, 1996). FISH analysis performed on the nuclei from 25 desmoid tumours from paraffin blocks or frozen tissue suggested a possible relationship with recurrence. In patients followed for more than one year, local recurrence was observed in four of six trisomy 8 positive tumours compared with two of 17 trisomy 8 negative tumours.

This finding of individual trisomies and even more their association in the same cell is rare in solid tumours, particularly mesenchymal tumours (Qi *et al.*, 1996; Bridge *et al.*, 1999). However, these aberrations are known to occur in related benign, fibrous lesions arising in both soft tissue and bone (Bridge *et al.*, 1999) and in infantile fibrosarcoma (Mertens *et al.*, 1995; Qi *et al.*, 1996).

One feature of many proliferative tissues is re-expression of telomerase. Telomerase activity may be required for unlimited growth of cells and is repressed in most somatic tissues; in comparison, it is detectable in immortal cell lines, germ cells, many malignancies, and some benign lesions. However, one study could not detect telomerase activity in any of 21 desmoids, suggesting that alternative mechanisms may operate in these proliferative neoplasms (Scates *et al.*, 1998).

Gardner's syndrome has traditionally been distinguished from FAP by the presence of prominent extraintestinal lesions, such as desmoid tumours, osteomas and cysts. The desmoid tumours in these patients often occur in the mesentery or abdominal wall following surgery that is usually performed for treatment of carcinoma of the colon, such as ileal pouch-anal anastomosis (Penna *et al.*, 1993; Church, 1998; Sagar *et al.*, 1998). The estimated risk of developing desmoid tumours in patients with FAP is 10 per cent (Jarvinen, 1987; Tsukada *et al.*, 1992; Hizawa *et al.*, 1997; Griffioen *et al.*, 1998). Until the extensive employment of elective colectomy, the dominant cause of death in patients with FAP was carcinoma of the colon. With the increasing use of prophylactic colectomy in these patients, desmoid tumours have become an important cause of morbidity (Penna *et al.*, 1993; Church, 1998; Sagar *et al.*, 1998) and among the major causes of mortality (Kadmon *et al.*, 1995).

Mutations of the adenomatous polyposis coli (APC) gene are responsible for FAP. This gene is complex and several different mutations have been observed. These mutations are likely to participate in the development of desmoids in patients with Gardner's syndrome but not those that develop sporadically in patients without Gardner's syndrome (Halling *et al.*, 1999; Giarola *et al.*, 1998). In one series, for example, *APC* germline mutations were identified in four of four FAP-associated desmoids but in none of 16 sporadic cases (Giarola *et al.*, 1998).

There appears to be a relationship between the development of desmoid tumours and antecedent trauma, particularly surgical trauma in patients with FAP. In one report, 16 of 56 (29 per cent) desmoid tumours developed at the site of earlier surgery (Goy *et al.*, 1997). In another series, prior abdominal surgery had been performed in 68 per cent of patients with FAP and abdominal desmoid tumours; the lesions developed within 5 years after surgery in approximately one-half of patients (Lynch and Fitzgibbons, 1996). A similar relationship has been observed in some sporadically occurring desmoid tumours. In one series, an antecedent history of trauma at the tumour site was elicited in 28 per cent of 32 primary desmoid tumours (Enzinger and Weiss, 2001).

Desmoid tumours usually present as a painless or minimally painful mass with a history of slow growth. Abdominal desmoids can be associated with intestinal obstruction, mucosal ischaemia and functional deterioration in ileoanal anastomoses (Penna et al., 1993; Church, 1998; Sagar et al., 1998). Desmoid tumours occur at virtually all body sites, most commonly in the torso (shoulder girdle and hip-buttock region) and the extremities. The location is usually deep in the muscles or along fascial planes. Multiple lesions at distant sites are infrequent; however, additional lesions are not rare on the same extremity following the initial treatment.

The diagnosis of a desmoid tumour is established by histological examination of a biopsy specimen. Incisional biopsy is preferred because of the need to distinguish between a benign and malignant process. Intra-abdominal desmoids can be detected by CT. However, we prefer MRI for definition of the pattern and extent of involvement. There are no radiographic characteristics that can reliably distinguish between sporadic intra-abdominal desmoids and tumours associated with Gardner's syndrome (Kawashima et al., 1994).

Desmoid tumours are locally progressive with infiltration of adjacent normal tissues and structures. They can also be locally malignant and highly destructive of normal tissue, leading to the death of the patient. In a report of 138 patients managed at one institution between 1965 and 1984, 11 died of their disease (Posner et al., 1989). Factors associated with a poor outcome in this study were: age 18–30 years, presentation with local recurrence, incomplete excision and no postoperative radiation therapy. However, this series may not be representative since many patients had advanced disease. In a review of the experience of other centres, we found few deaths and estimate the overall mortality rate of patients with desmoid tumours at other than intra-abdominal sites to be approximately 1 per cent. Thus, even though desmoids are benign in the sense that they cannot produce distant metastases, the disease process may occasionally be devastating. Fortunately, the pace of progression is commonly relatively slow, with periods of comparative stability or even temporary regression. Spontaneous regressions have been observed and re-growth is not observed in all patients following grossly incomplete surgical resection (Jenkins et al., 1986; Spear et al., 1998). In one series, for example, only three of six such patients had subsequent growth (Spear et al., 1998).

Desmoid tumours should be treated by surgical resection with a wide margin when medically and technically feasible. Since these tumours are benign, treatments with potentially serious late sequelae should be avoided if at all possible. Radiation therapy is an effective option for patients who are not good surgical candidates or decline surgery and, as an adjunctive therapy, for patients with grossly or microscopically positive margins. There is increasing evidence for a role for systemic therapy, especially chemotherapy.

Results from a number of centres demonstrate that radiation alone (50–60 Gy) or combined with surgery in patients with positive margins achieves permanent control of desmoid tumours in approximately 70–80 per cent of patients (Acker et al., 1993; Kamath et al., 1996; Goy et al., 1997; Ballo et al., 1998; Spear et al., 1998). The results of a review of the Massachusetts General Hospital experience are consistent with those reported by others in the literature (Spear et al., 1998). One hundred and seven patients were treated with surgery alone (51 patients), radiation alone (15 patients), or surgery with radiation (41 patients). The 5-year actuarial local control rates were 69, 93 and 72 per cent in the three groups. Patients treated with surgery alone had control rates of 50 per cent (three of six) for gross residual disease, 56 per cent for microscopically positive margins, and 77 per cent for negative margins. Local control with radiation alone was achieved in five of five patients with a primary tumour and nine of 10 with recurrent lesions. Others have reported similar experiences. The pooled rate of local control for radiation alone was 85 per cent in 114 patients from nine centres. A recent review of the literature reported improved local control with the use of radiotherapy in patients with desmoid tumours (Nuyttens et al., 2000). The local control achieved with surgery alone in patients with (−), (+) and unknown margins was 72 per cent, 41 per cent and 61 per cent, respectively. The rates for surgery and radiotherapy were significantly superior at 94 per cent, 75 per cent and 75 per cent. For the radiotherapy alone group, the local control was 78 per cent, which was statistically superior to that of 61 per cent achieved by surgery alone. Although most patients respond, the time to regression after radiation alone is often quite long and several years may elapse before regression is complete.

Recurrences occur after radiation therapy in some patients. In one study, for example, 23 patients were treated with radiation for unresectable disease; the actuarial relapse rate at 5 years was 31 per cent (Ballo et al., 1998). Radiation doses above 56 Gy did not improve the outcome but were associated with increased complications (30 versus 5 per cent with lower doses at 15 years). Positive resection margins were not an adverse prognostic factor.

Increasing experience is accumulating with systemic agents in patients with advanced or recurrent disease, especially at intra-abdominal and abdominal wall sites. There are, for example, a number of anecdotal reports of excellent response to tamoxifen, the anti-oestrogen toremifine, and progestational agents (Thomas et al., 1990; Wilcken and Tattersall, 1991; Tsukada et al., 1992; Izes et al., 1996; Gelmann, 1997). There are also documented responses to non-steroidal anti-inflammatory drugs (NSAIDs; most often sulindac), alone or often in combination with tamoxifen (Waddell *et al.*, 1983; Tsukada *et al.*, 1992; Izes *et al.*, 1996; Lackner *et al.*, 1997). Regression is usually partial and may take many months after an initial period of tumour enlargement. Long-term complete response data are not yet available, but this appears to be a potentially attractive treatment option. NSAID therapy also appears to protect against colon cancer.

Low-dose chemotherapy based upon methotrexate and vinblastine has obtained worthwhile response rates in patients with desmoid tumours, particularly children (Weiss and Lackman, 1989; Skapek *et al.*, 1998). In a study of 10 children with primary or recurrent desmoid tumour, five patients had clinical evidence of response to therapy with complete resolution or partial resolution of the physical findings and radiographic abnormalities (Skapek *et al.*, 1998). Three patients had stable disease during 10–35 months of treatment. There is also experience with other chemotherapeutic regimens. The combination of methotrexate and vinorelbine may produce a similar response to methotrexate and vinblastine with less neurotoxicity (Weiss *et al.*, 1999). In addition, there are anecdotal reports of much more aggressive doxorubicin-based drug protocols with good responses (Patel *et al.*, 1993; Seiter and Kemeny, 1993; Lynch *et al.*, 1994).

It is important that treatment recommendations for desmoid tumours be based upon analysis of the risk-to-benefit ratio because of the inconsistent nature and response to treatment of this tumour. Surgical excision alone is the procedure of choice for patients with a resectable lesion who are medically able to tolerate surgery. Radiation is an effective alternative when surgery would result in major functional or cosmetic defects. We do not recommend adjunctive radiation therapy in patients with microscopically positive margins. Since the incidence of re-growth is low (i.e. less than 50 per cent), patients without recurrence will be spared the long-term sequelae from radiation doses of 50–60 Gy. Furthermore, effective treatment is available if re-growth does occur. For gross residual disease of a primary desmoid, we recommend resection or radiation. For a recurrent desmoid tumour, our preference is surgical resection. However, radiation alone may be considered as the initial procedure in selected patients due to the higher morbidity of surgery and the increased probability of positive margins. For patients with intra-abdominal desmoid tumour complicating FAP (Gardner's syndrome), we recommend a more conservative strategy due to the relatively poor results of surgery and the higher rate of recurrence (Kawashima *et al.*, 1994). Such patients can be treated with tamoxifen or low-dose chemotherapy such as methotrexate and vinblastine. Surgery is the second option if there is no response. The follow-up protocol for patients with desmoid tumours includes examination every 6 months for the first 2 years, every 12 months to year 6, and then biannually.

SIGNIFICANT POINTS

- The introduction into clinical pathology of immunohistochemistry and cytogenetics has made the designation of the histological type much more objective. This means a greatly increased uniformity of diagnostic criteria being applied in all centres. This should be of value in analysis of clinical trials and patient series from diverse institutions.
- MRI is now accepted as the best imaging system for the delineation of the anatomical site and the pattern of extension of the soft tissue sarcoma.
- Determination of the inherent radiation sensitivity of human sarcoma cell lines *in vitro* has demonstrated that the cell lines derived from mesenchymal and epithelial tumours are of comparable radiation sensitivity, i.e. there is no evidence from *in vitro* experiments to support the older concept that the cells of sarcomas were exceptionally radiation-resistant.
- Data from many cancer centres document that the combination of relatively conservative surgery with moderate dose radiotherapy yields local control rates at least as high as that achieved by modern radical surgery alone. This is associated with an important gain in cosmetic and functional result. For sarcomas of the extremities, primary amputation has been reduced from 50–70 per cent to ≈5 per cent.
- The rationale for this combination is that the surgical procedure removes the gross disease (nearly all of the tumour clonogens) and the radiation is needed only to inactivate those cells which have extended beyond the evident lesion. Thus, the addition of radiotherapy to the treatment strategy achieves the same or better result as extension of the resection from a simple to a radical one, i.e. inclusion of a large amount of grossly normal tissue in the surgical specimen so as to remove the microscopic extensions of disease into the apparently normal adjacent tissue.
- There are several conservative treatment strategies currently being employed against the soft tissue sarcomas. These

include administration of the radiation either preoperatively, postoperatively, intraoperatively (electron beam or brachytherapy) and the combination of intra-arterial chemotherapy and radiation preoperatively. These various approaches in most centres realize local control rates of ≈90 per cent. There are few data upon which an assessment of the functional and cosmetic results can be compared for the different approaches.

- Preoperative radiotherapy has two large advantages over postoperative radiotherapy for soft tissue sarcoma: the treatment volume is smaller (the radiation need be given only to those tissues suspected of involvement by tumour whereas radiation administered postoperatively must cover all tissues handled during the resection) and there is no delay in the start of the radiation (there is a delay of 2–4 weeks for the start of the postoperative irradiation during which time the remaining cells are exposed to high levels of cytokines/growth factors such that there would be expected in an increase clonogen number).
- There is some delay in the healing of the surgical wound due to the radiation given before the resection. This can be kept to a minimum by elimination of the dead space, closure with no tension, drains in place until collection ≥15 mL/day and minimal undermining of skin.
- Adjuvant chemotherapy has not been unequivocally shown to be effective in increasing the distant metastasis-free survival rate for patients with soft tissue sarcoma. This is a major puzzle as adjuvant chemotherapy has a well-established and large efficacy against occult metastatic disease in patients with osteogenic sarcoma and Ewing's sarcoma.
- Desmoid tumours are not true malignant neoplasms. Local control after margin-positive resection of primary desmoid tumours is appreciable. Further, there are well-documented accounts of substantial tumour masses exhibiting complete regression following metabolic and or hormonal medication. However, some are very aggressive and locally widely invasive; there is a recognizable probability of fatal outcome of desmoid tumours, especially for those arising in the root of the neck, intra-abdominal/pelvic regions. The treatment of desmoid tumours is surgical where this is technically and medically feasible. For those patients for whom resection would be associated with major morbidity, radiotherapy has been shown to be a highly effective alternative. The local control rate is 80 per cent, which is approximately the same as for treatment by radiotherapy alone or after incomplete resection.

KEY REFERENCES

Cancer Treatment Symposia (1985) vol. 3.

Enneking, W.F. (1987) *Limb salvage in musculoskeletal oncology*. New York: Churchill Livingstone.

Enzinger, F.M. and Weiss, S.W. (2001) *Soft tissue tumors*, 4th edn. St. Louis: C.V. Mosby.

Hajdu, S.I. (1986) *Differential diagnosis of soft tissue and bone tumors*. Philadelphia: Lea and Febiger.

Heppner, G.H. (1984) Tumor heterogeneity. *Cancer Res.* **44**, 2259–65.

Knudson, A.G. (1985) Hereditary cancer, oncogenes, and antioncogenes. *Cancer Res.* **45**, 1437–43.

Lawrence, W. (ed.) (1993) *Surgical oncology clinics of North America. Soft tissue sarcomas of the limbs*. Philadelphia: W.B. Saunders.

Proceedings of International Symposium on Sarcomas Tarpon Springs, Florida (1987) Amsterdam: Martinus Nijhoff.

Verweij, J., Pinedo, H.M. and Suit, H.D. (eds) (1997) Soft tissue sarcomas: present achievements and future prospects. Dordrecht: Kluwer Academic Publishers.

REFERENCES

Abbatucci, J.S., Boulier, N., de Ranieri, J. *et al.* (1986) Local control and survival in soft tissue sarcomas of the limbs, trunk walls and head and neck: a study of 113 cases. *Int. J. Radiat. Oncol. Biol. Phys.* **12**, 579–86.

Acker, J.C., Bossen, E.H. and Halperin, E.C. (1993) The management of desmoid tumors. *Int. J. Radiat. Oncol. Biol. Phys.* **26**, 851.

Agarwal, V., Greenebaum, E. and Wersto, R. (1991) DNA ploidy of spindle cell soft-tissue tumors and its relationship to histology and clinical outcome. *Arch. Pathol. Lab. Med.* **115**, 558–62.

Alvegaard, T.A., Sigurdsson, H., Mouridsen, H. *et al.* (1989) Adjuvant chemotherapy with doxorubicin for high-grade soft tissue sarcoma: a randomized trial of the Scandinavian Sarcoma Group. *J. Clin. Oncol.* **7**, 1504–13.

Aman, P., Ron, D., Mandahl, N. *et al.* (1992) Rearrangement of the transcription factor gene CHOP in myxoid liposarcomas with t(12;16)(q13;p11). *Genes Chromosomes Cancer* **5**, 278.

Andreassen, A., Oyjord, T., Hovig, E. *et al.* (1993) p53 abnormalities in different subtypes of human sarcomas. *Cancer Res.* **53**, 468.

Angervall, L. and Kindblom, L.G. (1993) Principles for pathologic-anatomic diagnosis and classification of soft-tissue sarcomas. *Clin. Orthop.* **289**, 9–18.

Antman, K.H. (1983) Survival of patients with localized high-grade soft tissue sarcoma with multimodality therapy. A matched control study. *Cancer* **51**, 396–401.

Antman, K.H., Ryan, L., Borden, E. *et al.* (1990) Pooled results from three randomized adjuvant studies of doxorubicin versus observation in soft tissue sarcoma: 10 year results and review of the literature. In Salmon, S. (ed), *Adjuvant Therapy of Cancer VI.* Philadelphia: P.A. Saunders, 529–44.

Antman, K.H. (1997) Adjuvant therapy of sarcomas of the soft tissue. *Semin. Oncol.* **24**, 556–60.

Arbeit, J.M., Hilaris, B. and Brennan, M.F. (1987) Wound complications in the multimodality treatment of extremity and superficial truncal sarcomas. *J. Clin. Oncol.* **5**, 480–8.

Atkinson, L., Garvan, J.M. and Newton, N.C. (1963) Behavior and management of soft connective tissue sarcomas. *Cancer* **16**, 1552–62.

Baker, A.R. (1987) NIH experience in the management of extremity soft tissue sarcomas. *Proceedings of the International Symposium on Sarcomas, Tarpon Springs, Florida.* Amsterdam: Martinus Nijhoff.

Baldini, E.H., Goldberg, J., Jenner, C. *et al.* (1999) Long-term outcomes after function-sparing surgery without radiotherapy for soft tissue sarcoma of the extremities and trunk. *J. Clin. Oncol.* **17**, 3252–9.

Ball, A.B.S., Fisher, C. and Pittam, M. (1990) Diagnosis of soft tissue tumours by Tru-Cut biopsy. *Br. J. Surg.* **77**, 756–8.

Ballo, M.T., Zagars, G.K. and Pollack, A. (1998) Radiation therapy in the management of desmoid tumors. *Int. J. Radiat. Oncol. Biol. Phys.* **42**, 1007.

Barkley, H.T., Martin, R.G., Romsdahl, M.M., Lindberg, R. and Zagars, G.K. (1988) Treatment of soft tissue sarcomas by preoperative irradiation and conservative surgical resection. *Int. J. Radiat. Oncol. Biol. Phys.* **14**, 693–9.

Barone, M.V., Crozat, A., Tabaee, A. *et al.* (1994) CHOP(GADD153) and its oncogenic variant, TLS-CHOP, have opposing effects on the induction of G1/S arrest. *Genes Dev.* **8**, 453.

Barr, F.G., Chatten, J., DCrus, C.M. *et al.* (1995) Molecular assays for chromosomal translocations in the diagnosis of pediatric soft tissue sarcomas. *J. Am. Med. Assoc.* **273**, 553.

Barr, F.G., Nauta, L.E. and Hollows, J.C. (1998) Structural analysis of PAX3 genomic rearrangements in alveolar rhabdomyosarcoma. *Cancer Genet. Cytogenet.* **102**, 32.

Bell, R.S., O'Sullivan, B., Davis, A. *et al.* (1991) Functional outcome in patients treated with surgery and irradiation for soft tissue tumors. *J. Surg. Oncol.* **48**, 224–31.

Birch, J.M., Hartley, A.L., Blair, V. *et al.* (1990) Cancer in the families of children with soft tissue sarcoma. *Cancer* **66**, 2239–48.

Bland, K.I., McCoy, D.M., Kinard, R.E. and Copeland, E.M.R. (1987) Application of magnetic resonance imaging and computerized tomography as an adjunct to the surgical management of soft tissue sarcomas. *Ann. Surg.* **205**, 473–81.

Blom, R., Guerrieri, C., Stål *et al.* (1998) Leiomyosarcoma of the uterus: a clinicopathologic, DNA flow cytometric, p53 and mdm-2 analysis of 49 cases. *Gynecol. Oncol.* **68**, 54.

Blum, R.H., Corson, J.M., Wilson, R.E., Greenberger, J.S., Canellos, G.P. and Frei, E., 3d (1980) Successful treatment of metastatic sarcomas with cyclophosphamide, adriamycin and DTIC (CAD). *Cancer* **46**, 1722–6.

Blum, R.H., Edmonson, J., Ryan, L. and Pelletier, L. (1993) Efficacy of ifosfamide in combination with doxorubicin for the treatment of metastatic soft-tissue sarcoma. The Eastern Cooperative Oncology Group. *Cancer Chemother. Pharmacol.* **31**(suppl. 2), S238–40.

Bodensteiner, D., Reidinger, D., Rosenfeld, C. *et al.* (1991) Flow cytometry of needle aspirates from bone and soft tissue tumors. *South. Med. J.* **84**, 1451–4.

Bodey, G.P. (1981) Protected environment prophylactic antibiotic program for malignant sarcoma: randomized trial during remission induction chemotherapy. *Cancer* **47**, 2422–9.

Borden, E.C., Amato, D.A., Rosenbaum, C. *et al.* (1987) Randomized comparison of three adriamycin regimens for metastatic soft tissue sarcomas. *J. Clin. Oncol.* **5**, 840–50.

Bramwell, V., Rouesse, J., Steward, W. *et al.* (1994) Adjuvant CYVADIC chemotherapy for adult soft tissue sarcoma-reduced local recurrence but no improvement in survival: a study of the European Organization for Research and Treatment of Cancer Soft Tissue and Bone Sarcoma Group. *J. Clin. Oncol.* **12**, 1137–49.

Bramwell, V.H., Mouridsen, H.T., Santoro, A. *et al.* (1993) Cyclophosphamide versus ifosfamide: a randomized phase 11 trial in adult soft-tissue sarcomas. The European Organization for Research and Treatment of Cancer [EORTC], Soft Tissue and Bone Sarcoma

Group. *Cancer Chemother. Pharmacol.* **31**(suppl. 2), S180–4.

Brant, T.A., Parsons, J.T., Marcus, R.B. *et al.* (1990) Preoperative irradiation for soft tissue sarcomas of the trunk and extremities in adults. *Int. J. Radiat. Oncol. Biol. Phys.* **19**, 899–906.

Brennan, M.F., Casper, E.S. and Harrison, L.B. (1997) Soft tissue sarcoma. In DeVita, V.T., Hellman, S. and Rosenberg, S.A. (eds). *Cancer: principles and practice of oncology.* New York: Lippincott-Raven Publishers, 1738–88.

Bridge, J.A., Swarts, S.J., Buresh, C. *et al.* (1999) Trisomies 8 and 20 characterize a subgroup of benign fibrous lesions arising in both soft tissue and bone. *Am. J. Pathol.* **154**, 729.

Brown, R., Marshall, C.J., Pennie, S.G. and Hall, A. (1984) Mechanism of activation of an N-*ras* gene in the human fibrosarcoma cell line HT1080. *EMBO J.* **3**, 1321–6.

Bryant, M., Martinez, A., Pritchard, D. *et al.* (1985) Soft tissue sarcomas of the extremities: morbidity of combined radiation and limb salvage with special emphasis on twice a day fractionation (Abstract). *Int. J. Radiat. Oncol. Biol. Phys.* **11**(suppl. 1), 87.

Bujko, K., Suit, H.D., Springfield, D.S. and Convery, K. (1992) Wound healing after surgery and preoperative radiation for sarcoma of soft tissues. *Surg. Gynecol. Obstet.* **176**, 124–34.

Cade, S. (1951) Soft tissue tumours: their natural history and treatment. *Proc. R. Soc. Med.* **44**, 1936.

Cance, W.G., Brennan, M.F., Dudas, M. *et al.* (1990) Altered expression of the retinoblastoma gene product in human sarcomas. *N. Engl. J. Med.* **323**, 1457.

Cantin, J., McNeer, G.P., Chu, F.C. and Booker, R.J. (1968) The problem of local recurrence after treatment of soft tissue sarcoma. *Ann. Surg.* **168**, 47–53.

Catton, C., Davis, A. and Bell, R.I. (1996) Soft tissue sarcoma of the extremity. Limb salvage after failure of combined conservative therapy. *Radiother. Oncol.* **41**, 209–14.

Cavanee, W.K., Hansen, M.F., Nordenskjold, M. *et al.* (1985) Genetic origin of mutations predisposing to retinoblastoma. *Science* **228**, 501–3.

Chan, H.S.L., Thorner, P.S., Haddad, G. *et al.* (1990) Immunohistochemical detection of P-glycoprotein: prognostic correlation in soft tissue sarcoma of childhood. *J. Clin. Oncol.* **8**, 689–704.

Chang, A.E., Kinsella, T., Glatstein, E. *et al.* (1988) Adjuvant chemotherapy for patients with high-grade soft-tissue sarcomas of the extremity. *J. Clin. Oncol.* **6**, 1491–500.

Chang, A.E., Rosenberg, S.A., Glatstein, E.J. and Antman, K.H. (1989) Sarcomas of soft tissues. In DeVita, V.T., Hellman, S. and Rosenberg, S.A. (eds), *Cancer: principles and practice of oncology.* Philadelphia: J.B. Lippincott, 1345.

Chardin, P., Yermian, P., Madaule, P. and Tavitian, A. (1985) N-*ras* gene activation in the RD human rhabdomyosarcoma cell line. *Int. J. Cancer* **35**, 647–52.

Christman, K.L., Casper, E.S. and Schwartz, G.K. (1993) High-intensity scheduling of ifosfamide in adult patients with soft-tissue sarcoma. *Proc. ASCO* **12**, A1642.

Church, J.M. (1998) Mucosal ischemia caused by desmoid tumors in patients with familial adenomatous polyposis: report of four cases. *Dis. Colon Rectum* **41**, 661.

Clark, J., Rocques, P.J., Crew, A.J. *et al.* (1994) Identification of novel genes, SYT and SSX, involved in the t(X;18)(p11.2;q11.2) translocation found in human synovial sarcoma. *Nat. Genet.* **7**, 502.

Colman, S.D., Williams, C.A. and Wallace, M.R. (1995) Benign neurofibromas in type 1 neurofibromatosis (NF1) show somatic deletions of the NF1 gene. *Nat. Genet.* **11**, 90.

Costa, J., Wesley, R.A., Glatstein, E. and Rosenberg, S.A. (1984) The grading of soft tissue sarcomas. Results of a clinicohistopathologic correlation in a series of 163 cases. *Cancer* **53**, 530–41.

Crozat, A., Aman, P., Mandahl, N. and Ron, D. (1993) Fusion of CHOP to a novel RNA binding protein in human myxoid liposarcoma. *Nature* **363**, 640.

Cruz, A.B., Thames, E.A., Aust, J.B. *et al.* (1979) Combination chemotherapy for soft-tissue sarcomas: a phase III study. *J. Surg. Oncol.* **11**, 313–23.

das Gupta, T.K., Patel, M.K., Chaudhuri, P.K. and Briele, H.A. (1982) The role of chemotherapy as an adjuvant to surgery in the initial treatment of primary soft tissue sarcomas in adults. *J. Surg. Oncol.* **19**, 139–44.

Davis, R.J. and Barr, F.G. (1997) Fusion genes resulting from alternative chromosomal translocations are overexpressed by gene-specific mechanisms in alveolar rhabdomyosarcoma. *Proc. Natl Acad. Sci. USA* **94**, 8047.

DeChiara, A., T'Ang, A. and Triche, T. J. (1993) Expression of the retinoblastoma susceptibility gene in childhood rhabdomyosarcomas. *J. Natl Cancer Inst.* **85**, 152–7.

Dei Tos, A.P., Doglioni, C., Laurino, L. *et al.* (1993) p53 protein expression in non-neoplastic lesions and benign and malignant neoplasms of soft tissue. *Histopathology* **22**, 45–50.

DeLaney, T.F., Spiro, I.J., Suit, H.D. *et al.* (2001) Neoadjuvant chemotherapy and radiotherapy for large extremity soft tissue sarcomas (abs). *Proc. Am. Soc. Ther. Radiol. Onc.* **51**, 148.

Delattre, O., Zucman, J., Plougastel, B. *et al.* (1992) Gene fusion with an ETS DNA binding domain caused by chromosome translocation in human tumours. *Nature* **359**, 16.

Delattre, O., Zucman, J., Melot, T. *et al.* (1994) The Ewings family of tumors – a subgroup of small round cell tumors defined by specific chimeric transcripts. *N. Engl. J. Med.* **331**, 294–9.

Denton, J.W., Dunham, W.K., Salter, M., Urist, M.M. and Balch, C.M. (1984) Preoperative regional chemotherapy and rapid fraction irradiation for sarcomas of the soft tissue and bone. *Surg. Gynecol. Obstet.* **158**, 545–51.

Derkinderen, D.J., Koten, J.W., Nagelkerke, N.J.D. *et al.* (1988) Non-ocular cancer in patients with hereditary retinoblastoma. *Int. J. Cancer* **41**, 499–504.

Dewhirst, M.W., Boatman, H.D., Leopold, K.A. *et al.* (1990) Soft-tissue sarcomas: MR imaging and MR spectroscopy for prognosis and therapy monitoring. *Radiology* **174**, 847–53.

Dias, P., Dealing, M. and Houghton, P. (1994) The molecular basis of skeletal muscle differentiation. *Semin. Diagn. Pathol.* **11**, 3–14.

Dich, J., Zah, S.H., Hanberg, A. and Adami, H.O. (1997) Pesticides and cancer. *Cancer Causes Control* **8**, 420.

Donehower, L.A., Harvey, M., Slagle, B.L. *et al.* (1992) Mice deficient for p53 are developmentally normal but susceptible to spontaneous tumours. *Nature* **356**, 215.

Donohue, J.H., Collin, C., Friedrich, C., Godbold, J., Hajdu, S.I. and Brennan, M.F. (1988) Low-grade soft tissue sarcomas of the extremities: analysis of risk factors for metastasis. *Cancer* **62**, 184–93.

Duda, R.B., Cundiff, D., August, C.Z., Wagman, E.D. and Bauer, K.D. (1993) Growth factor receptor and related oncogene determinations in mesenchymal tumors. *Cancer* **71**, 3526–30.

Edmonson, J.H., Fleming, T.R., Ivins, J.C. *et al.* (1984) Randomized study of systemic chemotherapy following complete excision of nonosseous sarcomas. *J. Clin. Oncol.* **2**, 1390–6.

Edmonson, J.H., Ryan, L.M., Blum, R.H. *et al.* (1993) Randomized comparison of doxorubicin alone versus ifosfamide plus doxorubicin or mitomycin, doxorubicin and cisplatin against advanced soft tissue sarcomas. *J. Clin. Oncol.* **11**, 1269–75.

Eggermont, A.M.M., Schraffordt Koops, H., Lienard, D. *et al.* (1996) Isolated limb perfusion with high-dose tumor necrosis factor-α in combination with interferon-γ and melphalan for nonresectable extremity soft tissue sarcomas: a multicenter trial. *J. Clin. Oncol.* **14**, 2653–65.

Eilber, F.R., Morton, D.L., Eckardt, J., Grant, T. and Weisenburger, T. (1984) Limb salvage for skeletal and soft tissue sarcomas. Multidisciplinary preoperative therapy. *Cancer* **53**, 2579–84.

Eilber, F.R., Giuliano, A.E., Huth, J.F. and Morton, D.L. (1988) A randomized prospective trial using postoperative adjuvant chemotherapy (adriamycin) in high-grade extremity soft-tissue sarcoma. *Am. J. Clin. Oncol.* **11**, 39–45.

Eilber, F.G., Giuliano, A., Huth, J. *et al.* (1988) Neoadjuvant chemotherapy, radiation and limited surgery for high grade soft tissue sarcoma of the extremity. Recent concepts in sarcoma treatment. In Ryan, J.R. and Baker, L.H. (eds), *Proceedings of International Symposium on Sarcomas, Tarpon Springs, Florida, 1987.* Dordrecht: Kluwer Academic Publishers, 115–22.

Eilber, F.R., Eckardt, J.J., Rosen, G., Fu, Y.S., Seeger, L.L. and Selch, M.D. (1993) Neoadjuvant chemotherapy and radiotherapy in the multidisciplinary management of soft tissue sarcomas of the extremity. *Surg. Oncol. Clin. North Am.* **2**, 611–20.

El-Deiry, W.S., Tokino, T. and Velculesco, V.E. (1993) WAF1, a potential mediator of p53 suppression. *Cell* **75**, 817.

Elias, A., Ryan, L., Sulkes, A., Collins, J., Aisner, J. and Antman, K.H. (1989) Response to mesna, doxorubicin, ifosfamide and dacarbazine in 108 patients with metastatic or unresectable sarcoma and no prior chemotherapy. *J. Clin. Oncol.* **7**, 1208–16.

Elias, A.D. (1993) Chemotherapy for soft-tissue sarcomas. *Clin. Orthop. Relat. Res.* **289**, 94–105.

Elias, A.D. and Antman, K.H. (1986) Doxorubicin, ifosfamide and dacarbazine (AID) with mesna uroprotection for advanced untreated sarcoma: a phase I study. *Cancer Treat. Rep.* **70**, 827–33.

Eng, C., Li, F.P., Abramson, D.H., Ellsworth, R.M. *et al.* (1993) Mortality from second tumors among long-term survivors of retinoblastoma. *J. Natl Cancer Inst.* **85**, 1121–8.

Enneking, W.F., Spanier, S.S. and Goodman, M.A. (1980) A system for the surgical staging of musculoskeletal sarcoma. *Clin. Orthop.* **153**, 106–20.

Enneking, W.F., Spanier, S.S. and Malawar, M.D. (1981) The effect of anatomic setting on the results of surgical procedures for soft parts sarcoma of the thigh. *Cancer* **47**, 1005.

Enzinger, F.M. and Weiss, S.W. (2001) *Soft tissue tumors,* 4th edn. St. Louis: C.V. Mosby.

Evans, S.C. and Lozano, G. (1997) The Li-Fraumeni syndrome: an inherited susceptibility to cancer. *Mol. Med. Today* **13**, 390.

Fagundes, H.M., Lai, P.P., Dahmer, L.P. *et al.* (1992) Postoperative radiotherapy for malignant fibrous histiocytoma. *Int. J. Radiat. Oncol. Biol. Phys.* **23**, 615–19.

Fein, D.A., Lee, W.R., Lanciano, R.M. *et al.* (1995) Management of extremity soft tissue sarcomas with limb-sparing surgery and postoperative irradiation: do total dose, overall treatment time and the surgery-radiotherapy interval impact on local control? *Int. J. Radiat. Oncol. Biol. Phys.* **32**, 969–76.

Feldman, P.H.S. and Kyriakos, M. (1972) Pulmonary resection for metastatic sarcoma. *J. Thorac. Cardiovasc. Surg.* **64**, 784–99.

Fingerhut, M.A., Halperin, W.E., Marlow, D.A. *et al.* (1991) Cancer mortality in workers exposed to 2,3,7,8-tetrachlorodibenzo-*p*-dioxin. *N. Engl. J. Med.* **324**, 212.

Fleming, I.D., Cooper, J.S., Henson, D.E. *et al.* (eds) (1997) *American Joint Committee on Cancer staging manual,* 5th edn. Philadelphia: Lippincott-Raven, 149.

Fletcher, J. (1992) Translocation (12;22)(q13–14;q12) is a nonrandom aberration in soft-tissue clear-cell sarcoma. *Genes Chromosomes Cancer* **5**, 184.

Fletcher, J.A., Naeem, R., Xiao, S. and Corson, J.M. (1995) Chromosome aberrations in desmoid tumors. Trisomy 8 may be a predictor of recurrence [*see* comments]. *Cancer Genet. Cytogenet.* **79**, 139.

Florenes, V.A., Maelandsmo, G.M., Forus, A. *et al.* (1994) MDM2 gene amplification and transcript levels in human sarcomas: relationship to TP53 gene status. *J. Natl Cancer Inst.* **86**, 1297.

Fong, Y., Coal, D.G., Woodruff, J.M. and Brennan, M.F. (1993) Lymph node metastasis from soft tissue sarcoma in adults. Analysis of data from a prospective data base of 1772 sarcoma patients. *Ann. Surg.* **217**, 72–7.

Fraumeni, J.F. (1973) Genetic factors in the etiology of cancer. In Holland, J.F. and Frei, E.M. (eds), *Cancer medicine*. Philadelphia: Lea and Febiger, 7–15.

Friend, S.H., Horowitz, J.M., Gerber, M.R. *et al.* (1987) Deletions of a DNA sequence in retinoblastomas and mesenchymal tumors: organization of the sequence and its encoded protein. *Proc. Natl Acad. Sci. USA* **84**, 9059–63.

Frustaci, S., Gherlinzoni, F., De Paoli, A. *et al.* (2001) Adjuvant chemotherapy for adult soft tissue sarcomas of the extremities and girdles: results of the Italian randomized cooperative trial. *J. Clin. Oncol.* **19**, 1238–47.

Gadd, M.A., Casper, E.S., Woodruff, J., McCormack, P.M. and Brennan, M.F. (1993) Development and treatment of pulmonary metastases in adult patients with extremity soft tissue sarcoma. *Ann. Surg.* **218**, 705.

Gebhardt, M.C. (1996) Molecular biology of sarcomas. *Orthop. Clin. North Am.* **27**(3), 421–9.

Gelmann, E.P. (1997) Tamoxifen for the treatment of malignancies other than breast and endometrial carcinoma. *Semin. Oncol.* **24**, S1.

Gherlinzoni, F., Bacci, G., Picci, P. *et al.* (1986) A randomized trial for the treatment of high grade soft tissue sarcomas of the extremities: preliminary observations. *J. Clin. Oncol.* **4**, 552–8.

Giarola, M., Wells, D., Mondini, P. *et al.* (1998) Mutations of adenomatous polyposis coli (APC) gene are uncommon in sporadic desmoid tumours. *Br. J. Cancer* **78**, 582.

Ginsberg, J.P., Davis, R.J., Bennicelli, J.L. *et al.* (1998) Up-regulation of MET but not neural adhesion molecule expression by the PAX3-FKHR fusion protein in alveolar rhabdomyosarcoma. *Cancer Res.* **58**, 3542.

Goodnight, J.E., Bargar, W.L., Voegeli, T. and Blaisdell, F.W. (1985) Limb-sparing surgery for extremity sarcomas after preoperative intraarterial doxorubicin and radiation therapy. *Am. J. Surg.* **150**, 109–13.

Gottlieb, J.A., Baker, L.H., Quagliana, J.M. *et al.* (1972) Chemotherapy of sarcomas with a combination of adriamycin and dimethyl triazeno imidazole carboxamide. *Cancer* **30**, 1632–8.

Gottlieb, J.A. *et al.* (1975) Adriamycin (NCS-123127) used alone and in combination for soft tissue and bone sarcomas. *Cancer Chemother. Rep.* **6**, 271–82.

Gottlieb, J.A., Benjamin, R.S., Baker, L.H. *et al.* (1976) Role of DTIC (NSC45388) in the chemotherapy of sarcomas. *Cancer Treat. Rep.* **60**, 199–203.

Goy, B.W., Lee, S.P., Eilber, F. *et al.* (1997) The role of adjuvant radiotherapy in the treatment of resectable desmoid tumors. *Int. J. Radiat. Oncol. Biol. Phys.* **39**, 659.

Grabois, M., Frappaz, D. and Bouffet, E. (1994) High-dose VP-16 cisplatinum in soft tissue sarcoma of children. *Cancer Chemother. Pharmacol.* **33**, 355–7.

Greenall, M.J., Magill, G.B., DeCosse, J.J. and Brennan, M.F. (1986) Chemotherapy for soft tissue sarcoma. *Surg. Gynecol. Obstet.* **162**, 193–8.

Greenlee, R.T., Murray, T., Bolden, S. and Wingo, P.A. (2000) Cancer statistics, 2000. *CA Cancer J. Clin.* **50**, 7–33.

Griffioen, G., Bus, P.J., Vasen, H.F. *et al.* (1998) Extracolonic manifestations of familial adenomatous polyposis: desmoid tumors and upper gastrointestinal adenomas and carcinomas. *Scand. J. Gastroenterol. Suppl.* **225**, 85.

Gustafson, P., Herrlin, K., Biling, L., Willen, H. and Rydholm, A. (1992) Necrosis observed on CT enhancement is of prognostic value in soft tissue sarcoma. *Acta Radiol.* **33**, 474–6.

Gutman, M., Inbar, M., Lev-Shiush, D. *et al.* (1997) High dose tumor necrosis factor-α and melphalan administered via isolated limb perfusion for advanced limb soft tissue sarcoma results in a >90% response rate and limb preservation. *Cancer* **79**, 1129–37.

Halling, K.C., Lazzaro, C.R., Honchel, R. *et al.* (1999) Hereditary desmoid disease in a family with a germline Alu I repeat mutation of the APC gene. *Hum. Hered.* **49**, 97.

Hardell, L. and Eriksson, M. (1988) The association between soft tissue sarcoma and exposure to phenoxyacetic acids. *Cancer* **62**, 652–6.

Harrison, L.B., Franzese, F., Gaynor, J.J. and Brennan, M.F. (1993) Long-term results of a prospective randomized trial of adjuvant brachytherapy in the management of completely resected soft tissue sarcomas of the extremity and superficial trunk. *Int. J. Radiat. Oncol. Biol. Phys.* **27**, 259–65.

Hartley, A.L., Birch, J.M., Blair, V. *et al.* (1993) Patterns of cancer in the families of children with soft tissue sarcoma. *Cancer* **72**, 923.

Hawkins, M.M., Wilson, L.M., Burton, H.S. *et al.* (1996) Radiotherapy, alkylating agents and risk of bone cancer after childhood cancer. *J. Natl Cancer Inst.* **88**, 270–8.

Herbert, S.H., Corn, B.W., Solin, L.J. *et al.* (1993) Limb-preserving treatment for soft tissue sarcomas of the extremities. *Cancer* **72**, 1230–8.

Hisada, M., Garber, J.E., Fung, C.Y. *et al.* (1998) Multiple primary cancers in families with Li–Fraumeni syndrome. *J. Natl Cancer Inst.* **90**, 606.

Hisaoka, M., Tsuji, S., Morimitsu, Y. et al. (1998) Detection of TLS/FUS-CHOP fusion transcripts in myxoid and round cell liposarcomas by nested reverse transcription-polymerase chain reaction using archival paraffin-embedded tissues. *Diagn. Mol. Pathol.* **7**, 96.

Hizawa, K., Iida, M., Mibu, R. et al. (1997) Desmoid tumors in familial adenomatous polyposis/Gardner's syndrome. *J. Clin. Gastroenterol.* **25**, 334.

Hoppin, J.A., Tolbert, P.E., Herrick, R.F. et al. (1998) Occupational chlorophenol exposure and soft tissue sarcoma risk among men aged 30–60 years. *Am. J. Epidemiol.* **148**, 693.

Izes, J.K., Zinman, L.N. and Larsen, C.R. (1996) Regression of large pelvic desmoid tumor by tamoxifen and sulindac. *Urology* **47**, 756.

Jarvinen, H. (1987) Desmoid disease as a part of the familial adenomatous polyposis coli. *Acta Chir. Scand.* **153**, 379.

Jenkins, N.H., Freedman, L.S. and McKibbin, B. (1986) Spontaneous regression of a desmoid tumour. *J. Bone Joint Surg. [Br.]* **68**, 780.

Jones, D.N., McCowage, G.B., Sostman, H.D. et al. (1996) Monitoring of neoadjuvant therapy response of soft-tissue and musculoskeletal sarcoma using fluorine-18-FDG PET. *J. Nucl. Med.* **37**, 1438–44.

Joseph, W.L. (1974) Criteria for resection of sarcoma metastatic to the lung. *Cancer Chemother. Rep.* **58**, 285–90.

Kadmon, M., Moslein, G., Buhr, H.J. and Herfarth, C. (1995) Desmoid tumors in patients with familial adenomatous polyposis (FAP). Clinical and therapeutic observations from the Heidelberg polyposis register. *Chirurg* **66**, 997.

Kamath, S.S., Parsons, J.T., Marcus, R.B. et al. (1996) Radiotherapy for local control of aggressive fibromatosis. *Int. J. Radiat. Oncol. Biol. Phys.* **36**, 325.

Kanoe, H., Nakayama, T., Murakami, H. et al. (1998) Amplification of the CDK4 gene in sarcomas: tumor specificity and relationship with the RB gene mutation. *Anticancer Res.* **18**(4A), 2317–21.

Karakousis, C.P., Holtermann, O.A. and Holyoke, E.D. (1979) Cis-dichlorodiammineplatinum(II) in metastatic soft tissue sarcomas. *Cancer Treat. Rep.* **63**, 2071–5.

Karakousis, C.P., Rao, U. and Carlson, M. (1980) High dose methotrexate as secondary chemotherapy in metastatic soft-tissue sarcomas. *Cancer* **46**, 1345–8.

Karakousis, C.P., Emrich, L.J., Rao, U. and Krishnamsetty, R.M. (1986) Feasibility of limb salvage and survival in soft tissue sarcomas. *Cancer* **57**, 484–91.

Karlsson, P., Holmberg, E., Johansson, K.A. et al. (1996) Soft tissue sarcoma after treatment for breast cancer. *Radiother. Oncol.* **38**, 25.

Karpeh, M.S., Brennan, M.F., Cance, W.G. et al. (1995) Altered patterns of retinoblastoma gene product expression in adult soft-tissue sarcomas. *Br. J. Cancer* **72**, 986.

Kawai, A., Noguchi, M. and Beppu, Y. (1994) Nuclear immunoreaction of p53 protein in soft tissue sarcomas. A possible prognostic factor. *Cancer* **73**, 2499–505.

Kawai, A., Woodruff, J., Healey, J.H. et al. (1998) SVT-SSX gene fusion as a determinant of morphology and prognosis in synovial sarcoma. *N. Engl. J. Med.* **338**, 153.

Kawashima, A., Goldman, S.M., Fishman, E.K. et al. (1994) CT of intraabdominal desmoid tumors: is the tumor different in patients with Gardner's disease? *AJR Am. J. Roentgenol.* **162**, 339.

Kelly, K.M., Womer, R.B. and Barr, F.G. (1996a) Minimal disease detection in patients with alveolar rhabdomyosarcoma using a reverse transcriptase polymerase chain reaction method. *Cancer* **78**, 1320.

Kelly, K.M., Womer, R.B., Sorensen, P.H. et al. (1996b) Common and variant gene fusions predict distinct clinical phenotypes in rhabdomyosarcoma. *J. Clin. Oncol.* **15**, 1831.

Kessinger, A., Petersen, K., Bishop, M. and SchmitPokorny, K. (1994) High dose therapy (HDT) with autologous hematopoietic stem cell rescue (HSCR) for patients with metastatic soft tissue sarcoma. *Proc. ASCO* **13**, 1674.

Keus, R.B., Rutgers, E.J., Ho, G.H., Gortzak, E., Albus-Lutter, C.E. and Hart, A.A.M. (1994) Limb-sparing therapy of extremity soft tissue sarcomas: treatment outcome and long-term functional results. *Eur. J. Cancer* **30**, 1459–63.

Khatib, Z.A., Matsushime, H., Valentine, M. et al. (1993) Coamplification of the CDK4 gene with MDM2 and GLI in human sarcomas. *Cancer Res.* **53**, 5535.

Knudsen, A.G. (1971) Mutation and cancer: statistical study of retinoblastoma. *Proc. Natl Acad. Science USA* **68**, 820–3.

Kim, J.H. (1978) Radiation induced soft tissue sarcoma and bone sarcoma. *Radiology* **129**, 501–8.

Kogevinas, M., Becher, H., Benn, T. et al. (1997) Cancer mortality in workers exposed to phenoxy herbicides, chlorophenols and dioxins. An expanded and updated international cohort study. *Am. J. Epidemiol.* **145**, 1061.

Kouho, H., Aoki, T., Hisaoka, M. and Hashimoto, H. (1997) Clinicopathological and interphase cytogenetic analysis of desmoid tumours. *Histopathology* **31**, 336.

Koutcher, J.A., Ballon, D., Graham, M. et al. (1990) ^{31}P NMR spectra of extremity sarcomas: diversity of metabolic profiles and changes in reponse to chemotherapy. *Magn. Reson. Med.* **16**, 19–34.

Kransdorf, M.J., Jelinek, J.S. and Moser, R.P. (1993) Imaging of soft tissue tumors. *Radiol. Clin. North Am.* **31**, 359–71.

Kroese, M.C.S., Rutgers, D.H., Wils, I.S. et al. (1990) The relevance of the DNA index and proliferation rate in the grading of benign and malignant soft tissue tumors. *Cancer* **65**, 1782–8.

Kulander, B.G., Polissar, L., Yang, C.Y. *et al.* (1989) Grading of soft tissue sarcomas: necrosis as a determinate of survival. *Mod. Pathol.* **2**, 205–8.

Lack, E.E., Steinberg, S.M., White, D.E. *et al.* (1989) Extremity soft tissue sarcomas: analysis of prognostic variables in 300 cases and evaluation of tumor necrosis as a factor in stratifying higher grade sarcomas. *J. Surg. Oncol.* **263**, 73.

Lackner, H., Urban, C., Kerbl, R. *et al.* (1997) Noncytotoxic drug therapy in children with unresectable desmoid tumors. *Cancer* **80**, 334.

Ladanyl, M., Heinemann, F.S., Huvos, A.G. *et al.* (1990) Neural differentiation in small round cell tumors of bone and soft tissue with the translocation t(11;22)(q24;q12): an immunohistochemical study of 11 cases. *Hum. Pathol.* **21**, 1245.

Lander, J.J., Stanley, R.J., Sumner, H.W., Boswell, D.C. and Aach, R.D. (1975) Angiosarcoma of the liver associated with Fowlers solution (potassium arsenite). *Gastroenterology* **68**, 1582–6.

Lane, D.P. (1992) p53, guardian of the genome. *Nature* **358**, 15.

Laskin, T. (1988) Postradiation soft tissue sarcomas, an analysis of 53 cases. *Cancer* **62**, 2330–40.

Lee, F.I., Smith, P.M., Bennett, B. and Williams, D.M. (1996) Occupationally related angiosarcoma of the liver in the United Kingdom 1972–1994. *Gut* **39**, 312.

Lee, I.M., Abrahamson, J.L., Kandel, R. *et al.* (1994) Susceptibility to radiation carcinogenesis and accumulation of chromosomal breakage in p53 deficient mice. *Oncogene* **9**, 3731.

Lejeune, F.J., Lienard, D., el Douaihy, M., Seyedi, J.V. and Ewalenko, P. (1989) Results of 206 isolated limb perfusions for malignant melanoma. *Eur. J. Surg. Oncol.* **15**, 510–19.

LeVay, J., O'Sullivan, B., Catton, C. *et al.* (1993) Outcome and prognostic factors in soft tissue sarcoma in the adult. *Int. J. Radiat. Oncol. Biol. Phys.* **27**, 1091–100.

Levine, A.J., Pery, M.E. and Chang, A. (1994) The 1993 Walter Hubert Lecture: The role of the p53 tumour-suppressor gene in tumorigenesis. *Br. J. Cancer* **69**, 409.

Li, F.P. and Fraumeni, J.F. Jr (1969) Soft tissue sarcomas, breast cancer and other neoplasms. *Ann. Intern. Med.* **71**, 747.

Li, F.P., Fraumeni, J.F. Jr, Mulvihill, J.J. *et al.* (1988) A cancer family syndrome in twenty-four kindreds. *Cancer Res.* **48**, 5358–62.

Lindberg, R.D., Murphy, W.K., Benjamin, R.S. *et al.* (1977) Adjuvant chemotherapy in the treatment of primary soft tissue sarcomas: a preliminary report. In *Management of primary bone and soft tissue tumors*, Chicago:Year Book Medical Publishers, 343–52.

Lindberg, R.D., Martin, R.G., Romsdahl, M.M. and Barkley, H.T. Jr (1981) Conservative surgery and postoperative radiotherapy in 300 adults with soft-tissue sarcomas. *Cancer* **47**, 2391–7.

Littlefield, J.W. (1984) Genes, chromosomes and cancer. *J. Pediatr.* **104**, 489–94.

Lynch, E.M., Sampson, L.E., Khalil, A.A., Horsman, M.R. and Chaplin, D.J. (1995) Cytotoxic effect of tumour necrosis factor-α on sarcoma F cells at tumour relevant oxygen tensions. *Acta Oncol.* **34**, 423–7.

Lynch, H.T. and Fitzgibbons, R.J. (1996) Surgery, desmoid tumors and familial adenomatous polyposis: case report and literature review. *Am. J. Gastroenterol.* **91**, 2598.

Lynch, H.T., Fitzgibbons, R., Chong, S. *et al.* (1994) Use of doxorubicin and dacarbazine for the management of unresectable intra-abdominal desmoid tumors in Gardner's syndrome. *Dis. Colon Rectum* **37**, 260.

Malkin, D. (1993) p53 and the Li-Fraumeni syndrome. *Cancer Genet. Cytogenet.* **66**, 8392.

Malkin, D., Folly, K.W., Barbier, N. *et al.* (1992) Germline mutations of the p53 tumor suppressor gene in children and young adults with second malignant neoplasms. *N. Engl. J. Med.* **326**, 1309.

Mandahl, N., Orndal, C., Heim, S. *et al.* (1993) Aberrations of chromosome segment 12q13–15 characterize a subgroup of hemangiopericytomas. *Cancer* **71**, 3009–13.

Mansson, E., Willems, J., Aparisi, T. *et al.* (1983) Preoperative radiation therapy of high malignancy grade soft tissue sarcoma. *Acta Radiol. Oncol.* **22**, 461–4.

Markhede, G., Angervall, L. and Stener, B. (1981) A multivariate analysis of the prognosis after surgical treatment of malignant soft tissue tumors. *Cancer* **40**, 1721–33.

Martin, R.G., Butler, J.J. and Albores-Saavedra, J. (1965) Soft tissue tumors – surgical treatment and results. In *Tumors of bone and soft tissue*. Chicago: Year Book Medical Publishers, Chicago, 333–48.

Martini, N., Bains, M.S., Huvos, A.G. and Beattie, E.J. (1974) Surgical treatment of metastatic sarcoma to the lung. *Surg. Clin. North Am.* **54**, 841–8.

Mazeron, J.J. and Suit, H.D. (1987) Lymph nodes as sites of metastasis from sarcomas of soft tissue. *Cancer* **60**, 1800–8.

McAdam, W.A.F. and Goligher, J.C. (1970) The occurrence of desmoids in patients with familial polyposis coli. *Br. J. Surg.* **57**, 618–31.

McIntyre, J.F., Smith-Sorensen, B., Friend, S.H. *et al.* (1994) Germline mutations of the p53 tumor suppressor gene in children with osteosarcoma. *J. Clin. Oncol.* **12**, 925.

McNeer, G.P., Cantin, J., Chu, F. and Nickson, J.J. (1968) Effectiveness of radiation therapy in management of sarcoma of soft somatic tissues. *Cancer* **22**, 391–7.

Mertens, F., Willen, H., Rydholm, A. *et al.* (1995) Trisomy 20 is a primary chromosome aberration in desmoid tumors. *Int. J. Cancer* **63**, 527.

Mertens, W.C. and Bramwell, V.H. (1993) Soft tissue sarcoma in adults. *Curr. Opin. Oncol.* **5**, 678–85.

Miettinen, M. (1988) Immunohistochemistry of soft-tissue tumors. Possibilities and limitations in surgical pathology. *Pathol. Annu.* **25**, 1–36.

Milas, M., Yu, D. and Pollock, R.E. (1998) Advances in the understanding of human soft tissue sarcomas: molecular biology and therapeutic strategies (Review). *Oncol. Rep.* **5**(5), 1275–9.

Muller, R., Hajdu, S.I. and Brennan, M.F. (1987) Lymphangiosarcoma associated with chronic filarial lymphedema. *Cancer* **59**, 179.

Mulligan, L.M., Matlashewski, G.I., Scrable, H.I. and Cavenee, W.K. (1990) Mechanisms of p53 loss in human sarcomas. *Proc. Natl Acad. Sci. USA* **87**, 5863.

Mundt, A.J., Awan, A., Sibley, G.S. *et al.* (1995) Conservative surgery and adjuvant radiation therapy in the management of adult soft tissue sarcoma of the extremities: clinical and radiobiological results. *Int. J. Radiat. Oncol. Biol. Phys.* **32**, 977–85.

Myhre-Jensen, O., Kaae, S., Madsen, E.H. and Sneppen, O. (1983) Histopathological grading in soft tissue tumors. Relation to survival in 261 surgically treated patients. *Acta Pathol. Microbiol. Immunol. Scand. [A]* **91**, 145–50.

Negendank, W.G., Crowley, M.G., Ryan, J.R., Keller, N.A. and Evelhoch, J.L. (1989) Bone and soft tissue lesions: diagnosis with combined H-1 MR imaging and P-31 spectroscopy. *Radiology* **173**, 181–7.

Nielsen, O.S., Cummings, B., O'Sullivan, B. *et al.* (1991) Preoperative and postoperative irradiation of soft tissue sarcomas: effect on radiation field size. *Int. J. Radiat. Oncol. Biol. Phys.* **21**, 1595–9.

Nieweg, O.E., Pruim, J., van Ginkel, R.J. *et al.* (1996) Fluorine-18-flurodeoxyglucose PET imaging of soft-tissue sarcoma. *J. Nucl. Med.* **37**, 257–61.

Nilbert, M., Rydholm, A., Willen, M., Mitelman, F. and Mandahl, N. (1994) MDM2 gene amplification correlates with ring chromosomes in soft tissue tumors. *Genes Chromosomes Cancer* **9**, 261–5.

Nuyttens, J.J., Rust, P.F., Thomas, C.R. Jr and Turrisi, A.T., 3rd (2000) Surgery versus radiation therapy for patients with aggressive fibromatosis or desmoid tumors. A comparative review of 22 articles. *Cancer* **88**, 1517–23.

O'Bryan, R.M., Baker, L.H., Gottlieb, J.E. *et al.* (1977) Dose response evaluation of adriamycin in human neoplasia. *Cancer* **39**, 1940–8.

O'Keefe, F., Lorigan, J.G. and Wallace, S. (1990) Radiological features of extraskeletal Ewing sarcoma. *Br. J. Radiol.* **63**, 456–60.

Olieman, A.F., Pras, E., van Ginkel, R.J. *et al.* (1998) Feasibility and efficacy of external beam radiotherapy after hyperthermic isolated limb perfusion with TNF-α and melphalan for limb-saving treatment in locally advanced extremity soft-tissue sarcoma. *Int. J. Radiat. Oncol. Biol. Phys.* **40**, 807–14.

Oliner, J.D., Kinzler, K.W., Meltzer, P.S. *et al.* (1992) Amplification of a gene encoding a p53-associated protein in human sarcomas. *Nature* **358**, 80.

Omura, G.A., Major, F.J., Blessing, J.A. *et al.* (1983) A randomized study of adriamycin with and without dimethyl triazeno-imidazole carboxamide in advanced uterine sarcomas. *Cancer* **52**, 626–32.

Omura, G.A., Major, F.J., Blessing, J.A. *et al.* (1985) A randomized trial of adjuvant adriamycin in uterine sarcomas: a Gynecologic Oncology Group study. *J. Clin. Oncol.* **3**, 1240–5.

O'Sullivan, B. and Davis, A. (2001) A randomized phase III trial of pre-operative compared to post-operative radiotherapy in extremity soft tissue sarcoma. *Proc. Am. Soc. Ther. Radiol. Oncol.* **51**, 151.

O'Sullivan, B., Davis, A., Bell, R. *et al.* (1999) Phase III randomized trial of pre-operative versus post-operative radiotherapy in the curative management of extremity soft tissue sarcoma. A Canadian Sarcoma Group and NCI Canada Clinical Trials Group study. *Proc. ASCO* **18**, 2066A.

Palman, C., Bowen-Pope, D.F. and Brooks, J.J. (1992) Platelet-derived growth factor receptor (P-subunit) immunoreactivity in soft tissue tumors. *Lab. Invest.* **66**, 108–15.

Pao, W.J. and Pilepich, M.V. (1990) Postoperative radiotherapy in the treatment of extremity soft tissue sarcomas. *Int. J. Radiat. Oncol. Biol. Phys.* **19**, 907–11.

Parham, D.M., Shapiro, D.N., Downing, J.R. *et al.* (1994) Solid alveolar rhabdomyosarcomas with the t(2;13). Report of two cases with diagnostic implications. *Am. J. Surg. Pathol.* **18**, 474–8.

Patel, S., Vadhan-Raj, S., Burgess, M.A. *et al.* (1998) Results of two consecutive trials of dose-intensive chemotherapy with doxorubicin and ifosfamide in patients with sarcomas. *Am. J. Clin. Oncol.* **21**, 317–21.

Patel, S., Evans, H. and Benjamin, R. (1993) Combination chemotherapy in adult desmoid tumors. *Cancer* **72**, 3244.

Patterson, H., Gill, S., Fisher, C. *et al.* (1994) Abnormalities of the p53, MDM2 and DCC genes in human leiomyosarcomas. *Br. J. Cancer* **69**, 1052.

Penna, C., Tiret, E., Parc, R. *et al.* (1993) Operation and abdominal desmoid tumors in familial adenomatous polyposis. *Surg. Gynecol. Obstet.* **177**, 263.

Peuchot, M. and Libshitz, H.I. (1987) Pulmonary metastatic disease: radiologic-surgical correlation. *Radiology* **164**, 719–22.

Picci, P., Bacci, G., Gherlinzoni, F. *et al.* (1988) Results of a randomized trial for the treatment of localized soft tissue sarcoma (STS) of the extremities in adult patients. In Ryan, J.R. and Baker, L.O. (eds), *Recent concepts in sarcoma treatment*. Boston: Kluwer Academic Publishers, 144–8.

Pinedo, H.M. and Verweij, J. (1986) The treatment of soft tissue sarcomas with a focus on chemotherapy: a review. *Radiother. Oncol.* **6**, 193–205.

Pisters, P.W., Patel, S.R., Varma, D.G. *et al.* (1997) Preoperative chemotherapy for stage IIIB extremity soft tissue sarcoma: long-term results from a single institution. *J. Clin. Oncol.* **15**, 3481–7.

Piver, M.S., Lele, S.B. and Patsner, B. (1986) cis-Diamminedichloroplatinum plus dimethyl-triazenoimidazole carboxamide as second- and third-line chemotherapy for sarcomas of the female pelvis. *Gynecol. Oncol.* **23**, 371–5.

Pizzo, P.A., Miser, J.S., Cassady, J.R. and Filler, R.M. (1985) Solid tumors in childhood. In DeVita, V.T., Hellman, S. and Rosenberg, S.A. (eds), *Cancer: principles and practice of oncology*. Philadelphia: Lippincott, 1511–89.

Pollock, R., Lang, A., Ge, T. *et al.* (1998) Wild-type p53 and a p53 temperature-sensitive mutant suppress human soft tissue sarcoma by enhancing cell cycle control. *Clin. Cancer Res.* **4**, 1985.

Pollock, R.E., Lang, A., Luo, J. *et al.* (1996) Soft tissue sarcoma metastasis from clonal expansion of p53 mutated tumor cells. *Oncogene* **12**, 2063.

Porter, P.L., Gown, A.M., Kramp, S.G. and Coltrera, M.D. (1992) Widespread p53 overexpression in human malignant tumors. *Am. J. Pathol.* **140**, 145.

Posner, M.C., Shiu, M.H., Newsome, J.L. *et al.* (1989) The desmoid tumor. Not a benign disease. *Arch. Surg.* **124**, 191.

Potter, D.A., Glenn, J., Kinsella, T. *et al.* (1985) Patterns of recurrence in patients with high-grade soft tissue sarcomas. *J. Clin. Oncol.* **3**, 353–66.

Qi, H., Dal Cin, P., Hernandez, J.M. *et al.* (1996) Trisomies 8 and 20 in desmoid tumors [see comments]. *Cancer Genet. Cytogenet.* **92**, 147.

Rabbitts, T.H., Forster, A., Larson, R. and Nathan, P. (1993) Fusion of the dominant negative transcription regulator CHOP with a novel gene FUS by translocation t(12;16) in malignant liposarcoma. *Nat. Genet.* **4**, 175.

Redmond, O.M., Bell, E., Stack, J.P. *et al.* (1992) Tissue characterization and assessment of preoperative chemotherapeutic response in musculoskeletal tumors by in vivo 31p magnetic resonance spectroscopy. *Magn. Res. Med.* **27**, 226–37.

Reitamo, J.J., Hayry, P., Nykyri, E. and Saxen, E. (1982) The desmoid tumor. I. Incidence, sex-, age- and anatomical distribution in the Finnish population. *Am. J. Clin. Pathol.* **77**, 665.

Robinson, E., Neugut, A. and Wylie, P. (1988) Clinical aspects of post-irradiation sarcomas. *J. Natl Cancer Inst.* **80**, 233–40.

Robinson, M.H., Spruce, L., Eeles, R. *et al.* (1991) Limb function following conservation treatment of adult soft tissue sarcoma. *Eur. J. Cancer* **27**, 1567–74.

Roholl, P.J.M., Skottner, A., Prinsen, I. *et al.* (1990) Expression of insulin-like growth factor I in sarcomas. *Histopathology* **16**, 455–60.

Rosen, G., Forscher, C., Lowenbraun, S. *et al.* (1994) Synovial sarcoma. Uniform response of metastases to high dose ifosfamide. *Cancer* **73**, 3506–11.

Rosenberg, S.A., Kent, H., Costa, J. *et al.* (1978) Prospective randomized evaluation of the role of limb-sparing surgery, radiation therapy and adjuvant chemoimmunotherapy in the treatment of adult soft-tissue sarcomas. *Surgery* **84**, 62–9.

Rosenberg, S.A., Tepper, J., Glatstein, E. *et al.* (1983) Prospective randomized evaluation of adjuvant chemotherapy in adults with soft tissue sarcomas of the extremities. *Cancer* **52**, 424–34.

Ross, B., Helsper, J.T., Cox, J. *et al.* (1987) Osteosarcoma and other neoplasms of bone: magnetic resonance spectroscopy to monitor therapy. *Arch. Surg.* **122**, 1464–9.

Rowley, J.D. (1998) The critical role of chromosome translocations in human leukemias. *Annu. Rev. Genet.* **32**, 495–519.

Russell, W.O., Cohen, J., Enzinger, F. *et al.* (1977) A clinical and pathological staging system for soft tissue sarcomas. *Cancer* **40**, 1562–70.

Rydholm, A., Berg, N.O., Gullberg, B., Thorngren, K.G. and Persson, B.M. (1984) Epidemiology of soft tissue sarcoma in the locomotor system. A retrospective population-based study of the inter-relationships between clinical and morphologic variables. *Acta Pathol. Microbiol. Immunol. Scand. [A]* **92**, 363–74.

Rydholm, A., Gustafson, P., Rooser, B., Willen, H., Akerman, M., Herrlin, K. and Alvegard, T. (1991) Limb-sparing surgery without radiotherapy based on anatomic location of soft tissue sarcoma. *J. Clin. Oncol.* **9**, 1757–65.

Sadoski, C., Suit, H., Rosenberg, A., Mankin, H. and Convery, K. (1993) Preoperative radiation, surgical margins and local control of extremity sarcomas of soft tissues. *J. Surg. Oncol.* **52**, 223–30.

Sadove, A.M., Block, M. and Rossof, A.H. (1981) Radiation carcinogenesis in man: new primary neoplasms in fields of prior therapeutic radiation. *Cancer* **48**, 1139–43.

Sagar, P.M., Moslein, G. and Dozois, R.R. (1998) Management of desmoid tumors in patients after ileal pouch-anal anastomosis for familial adenomatous polyposis. *Dis. Colon Rectum* **41**, 1350.

Sahin, A.A., Ro, J.Y., El-Naggar, A.K. *et al.* (1991) Tumor proliferative fraction in solid malignant neoplasms. A comparative study of Ki-67 immunostaining and flow cytometric determinations. *Am. J. Clin. Pathol.* **96**, 512–19.

Sainati, L., Stella, M., Montaldi, A. *et al.* (1992) Value of cytogenetics in the differential diagnosis of the small round cell tumors of childhood. *Med. Pediatr. Oncol.* **20**, 130–5.

Sanchez, R.B., Quinn, S.F., Walling, A., Estrada, J. and Greenberg, H. (1990) Musculoskeletal neoplasms after intraarterial chemotherapy: correlation of MR images with pathologic specimens. *Radiology* **174**, 237–40.

Sarcoma Meta-analysis Collaboration (1997) Adjuvant chemotherapy for localised resectable soft-tissue sarcoma of adults: meta-analysis of individual data. *Lancet* **350**, 1647–54.

Sathiakumar, N. and Delzell, E. (1997) A review of epidemiologic studies of triazine herbicides and cancer. *Crit. Rev. Toxicol.* **27**, 599.

Scaradavou, A., Heller, G., Sklar, C.A. *et al.* (1995) Second malignant neoplasms in long-term survivors of childhood rhabdomyosarcoma. *Cancer* **76**, 1860–7.

Scates, D., Clark, S.K., Phillips, R.K. and Venitt, S. (1998) Lack of telomerase in desmoids occurring sporadically and in association with familial adenomatous polyposis. *Br. J. Surg.* **85**, 965.

Schoenfeld, D.A., Rosenbaum, C., Horton, J. *et al.* (1982) A comparison of adriamycin versus vincristine and adriamycin and cyclophosphamide versus vincristine, actinomycin-D and cyclophosphamide for advanced sarcoma. *Cancer* **50**, 2757–62.

Schraffordt Koops H., Eggermont, A.M., Lienard, D. *et al.* (1998) Hyperthermic isolated limb perfusion for the treatment of soft tissue sarcomas. *Semin. Surg. Oncol.* **14**, 210–14.

Schray, M.F., Gunderson, L.L., Sim, F.H., Pritchard, D.J., Shives, T.C. and Yeakel, P.D. (1990) Soft tissue sarcomas. Integration of brachytherapy, resection and external irradiation. *Cancer* **66**, 451–6.

Schutte, J., Mouridsen, H.T., Steward, W. *et al.* (1993) Ifosfamide plus doxorubicin in previously untreated patients with advanced soft-tissue sarcoma. *Cancer Chemother. Pharmacol.* **31**(suppl. 2), S204–9.

Seiter, K. and Kemeny, N. (1993) Successful treatment of a desmoid tumor with doxorubicin. *Cancer* **71**, 2242.

Shaw, P.J., Bergin, M. and Stevens, M. (1988) Osteogenic sarcoma following acute lympholastic leukemia. *Am. J. Pediatr. Hematol. Oncol.* **10**, 81–7.

Shew, J.Y., Ling, N., Yang, X., Fodstad, O. and Lee, W.H. (1989) Antibodies detecting abnormalities of the retinoblastoma susceptibility gene product (pplIORB) in osteosarcomas and synovial sarcomas. *Oncogene Res.* **1**, 205–14.

Shives, T.C. (1993) Biopsy of soft-tissue tumors. *Clin. Orthop. Relat. Res.* **289**, 32–5.

Simms, W.W., Ordonez, N.G., Johnston, D., Ayala, A.G. and Czerniak, B. (1995) p53 expression in dedifferentiated chondrosarcoma. *Cancer* **76**, 223–7.

Skapek, S.X., Hawk, B.J., Hoffer, F.A. *et al.* (1998) Combination chemotherapy using vinblastine and methotrexate for the treatment of progressive desmoid tumor in children. *J. Clin. Oncol.* **16**, 3021.

Smith, S.H., Weiss, S.W., Jankowski, S.A. *et al.* (1992) SAS amplification in soft tissue sarcomas. *Cancer Res.* **52**, 3746.

Soini, Y., Vahakangas, K., Nuorva, K. *et al.* (1992) p53 immunohistochemistry in malignant fibrous histiocytomas and other mesenchymal tumours. *J. Pathol.* **168**, 2933.

Sordillo, P.P, Magill, G.B., Shiu, M.H., Lesser, M., Hajdu, S.I., and Golbey, R.B. (1981) Adjuvant chemotherapy of soft-part sarcomas with ALOMAD (S4). *J. Surg. Oncol.* **18**, 345–53.

Sorensen, P.H., Lessnick, S.L., Lopez-Terrada, D. *et al.* (1994) A second Ewing's sarcoma translocation, t(21;22), fuses the EWS gene to another ETS-family transcription factor, ERG. *Nat. Genet.* **6**, 146.

Spear, M.A., Jennings, L.C., Mankin, H.J. *et al.* (1998) Individualizing management of aggressive fibromatoses. *Int. J. Radiat. Oncol. Biol. Phys.* **40**, 637.

Spiro, I.J., Suit, H., Gebhardt, M. *et al.* (1996) Neoadjuvant chemotherapy and radiotherapy for large soft tissue sarcomas. *Proc. ASCO* **15**, 524 (Abstr. 168).

Spiro, I.J., Gebhardt, M.C., Jennings, L.C., Mankin, H.J., Harmon, D.C. and Suit, H.D. (1997) Prognostic factors for local control of sarcomas of the soft tissues managed by radiation and surgery. *Semin. Oncol.* **24**(5), 540–6.

Sreekantaiah, C., Bridge, J.A., Rao, U.N. *et al.* (1991) Clonal chromosomal abnormalities in hemangiopericytoma. *Cancer Genet. Cytogenet.* **54**, 173.

Stewart, F.W. and Treves, N. (1948) Lymphangiosarcoma in postmastectomy lymphedema: a report of six cases in elephantiasis chirurgica. *Cancer* **1**, 64–81.

Stinson, S.F., DeLaney, T.F., Greenberg, J. *et al.* (1991) Acute and long term effects on limb function of combined modality limb sparing therapy for extremity soft tissue sarcomas. *Int. J. Radiat. Oncol. Biol. Phys.* **21**, 1493–9.

Stratton, M.R., Moss, S., Warren, W. *et al.* (1990) Mutation of the p53 gene in human soft tissue sarcomas: association with abnormalities of the RB1 gene. *Oncogene* **5**, 1297.

Strong, L.C. (1977) Genetic considerations in pediatric oncology. In Sutow, W.W., Fernbach, D.J. and Vietti, T.J. (eds), *Clinical pediatric oncology*. St. Louis: C.V. Mosby, 16–32.

Subramanian, S. and Wiltshaw, E. (1978) Chemotherapy of sarcoma. *Lancet* **1**, 683–6.

Sugarbaker, P.H., Barofsky, I., Rosenberg, S.A. and Gianola, F.J. (1982) Quality of life assessment of patients in extremity sarcoma clinical trials. *Surgery* **91**, 17–23.

Suit, H.D., Russell, W.O. and Martin, R.G. (1975) Sarcoma of soft tissue: clinical and histopathologic parameters and response to treatment. *Cancer* **35**, 1478–83.

Suit, H.D., Mankin, H.J., Wood, W.C. and Proppe, K.H. (1985) Radiation and surgery in the treatment of primary sarcoma of soft tissue: pre-operative, intra-operative and post-operative. *Cancer* **55**, 2659–67.

Suit, H.D., Mankin, H.J., Wood, W.C. *et al.* (1988) Treatment of the patient with stage M0 sarcoma of soft tissue. *J. Clin. Oncol.* **6**, 854–62.

Swanson, S.A. and Brooks, I.J. (1990) Proliferation markers Ki-67 and p105 in soft-tissue lesions. Correlation with DNA flow cytometric characteristics. *Am. J. Pathol.* **137**, 1491–500.

Taghian, A., de Vathaire, F., Terrier, M. *et al.* (1991) Long-term risk of sarcoma following radiation treatment for breast cancer. *Int. J. Radiat. Oncol. Biol. Phys.* **21**, 361–7.

Tanabe, K.K., Pollock, R.E., Ellis, L.M. *et al.* (1994) Influence of surgical margins on outcome in patients with preoperatively irradiated extremity soft tissue sarcomas. *Cancer* **73**, 1652–9.

The Selected Cancers Cooperative Study Group (1990) The association of selected cancers with service in the US military in Vietnam. II. Soft tissue and other sarcomas. *Arch. Intern. Med.* **150**, 2485.

Thomas, S., Datta-Gupta, S. and Kapur, B.M. (1990) Treatment of recurrent desmoid tumor with tamoxifen. *Aust. N. Z. J. Surg.* **60**, 919.

Toguchida, J., Yamaguchi, T., Dayton, S.H. *et al.* (1992a) Prevalence and spectrum of germline mutations of the p53 gene among patients with sarcoma. *N. Engl. J. Med.* **326**, 1301.

Toguchida, J., Yamaguchi, T., Ritchie, B. *et al.* (1992b) Mutation spectrum of the p53 gene in bone and soft tissue sarcomas. *Cancer Res.* **52**(22), 6194–9.

Tomita, K., Yokogawa, A., Oda, Y. and Terahata, S. (1988) Lymphangiosarcoma in postmastectomy lymphedema (Stewart-Treves syndrome): ultrastructural and immunohistologic characteristics. *J. Surg. Oncol.* **38**, 275.

Townsend, C.M., Eilber, F.R. and Morton, D.L. (1976) Skeletal and soft tissue sarcomas. Results of surgical adjuvant chemotherapy. *Proc. Am. Assoc. Cancer Res.* **17**, 265.

Travis, J.A. and Bridge, J.A. (1992) Significance of both numerical and structural chromosomal abnormalities in clear cell sarcoma. *Cancer Genet. Cytogenet.* **64**, 104.

Trojani, M. (1984) Staging system for soft tissue and bone. *Int. J. Cancer* **33**, 37–42.

Tsukada, K., Church, J.M., Jagelman, D.G. *et al.* (1992) Noncytotoxic drug therapy for intra-abdominal desmoid tumor in patients with familial adenomatous polyposis. *Dis. Colon Rectum* **35**, 29.

Tucker, M.A., D'Angio, G.J., Boice, J.D., Strong, L.C. *et al.* (1987) Bone sarcomas linked to radiotherapy and chemotherapy in children. *N. Engl. J. Med.* **317**, 588–93.

Turc-Carel, C., Dalcin, P. and Limon, J. (1986) Translocation of x;18 in synovial sarcoma. *Cancer Genet. Cytogenet.* **22**, 93–4.

Turc-Carel, C., Aurias, A., Mugneret, F. *et al.* (1988) Chromosomes in Ewing's sarcoma. I. An evaluation of 85 cases and remarkable consistency of t(11;22) (q24;q12). *Cancer Genet. Cytogenet.* **32**, 229–38.

Ueda, T., Aozasa, K., Tsujimoto, M. *et al.* (1989) Prognostic significance of Ki-67 reactivity in soft tissue sarcomas. *Cancer* **63**, 1607–11.

Ushigome, S., Shimoda, T., Nikaido, T. *et al.* (1992) Histopathologic diagnostic and histogenetic problems in malignant soft tissue tumors. Reassessment of malignant fibrous histiocytoma, epithelioid sarcoma, malignant rhabdoid tumor, neuroectodermal tumor. *Jpn. Soc. Pathol.* **42**, 691–706.

Vaglini, M., Belli, F., Ammatuna, M. *et al.* (1994) Treatment of primary or relapsing limb cancer by isolation perfusion with high-dose alpha-tumor necrosis factor, gamma interferon and melphalan. *Cancer* **73**, 483–92.

Vanel, D., Lacombe, M.J., Couanet, D. *et al.* (1987) Musculoskeletal tumors follow-up with MR imaging after treatment with surgery and radiation therapy. *Radiology* **164**, 243–5.

Varley, J.M., McGown, G., Thorncroft, M. *et al.* (1997) Germ-line mutations of TP53 in Li-Fraumeni families: an extended study of 39 families. *Cancer Res.* **57**, 3245.

Vineis, P., Faggiano, F., Tedeschi, M. and Ciccone, G. (1991) Incidence rates of lymphomas and soft tissue sarcomas and environmental measurements of phenoxy herbicides. *J. Natl Cancer Inst.* **83**, 362–3.

Vrouenraets, B.C., Keus, R.B., Nieweg, O.E. and Kroon, B.B. (1997) Complications of combined radiotherapy and isolated limb perfusion with tumor necrosis factor alpha + interferon gamma and melphalan in patients with irresectable soft tissue tumors. *J. Surg. Oncol.* **65**, 88–94.

Wadayama, B., Toguchida, J., Yamaguchi, T., Sasaki, M.S. and Yamamuro, T. (1993) p53 expression and its relationship to DNA alterations in bone and soft tissue sarcomas. *Br. J. Cancer* **68**(6), 1134–9.

Waddell, W.R., Gerner, R.E. and Reich, M.P. (1983) Nonsteroid anti-inflammatory drugs and tamoxifen for desmoid tumors and carcinoma of the stomach. *J. Surg. Oncol.* **22**, 197.

Wanebo, H.J., Temple, W.J., Popp, M.B. *et al.* (1995) Preoperative regional therapy for extremity sarcoma. A tricenter update. *Cancer* **75**, 2299–306.

Weddington, W.W. (1985) Psychological outcomes in survivors of extremity sarcomas following amputation or limb salvage. *J. Clin. Oncol.* **3**, 1393–9.

Weinstein, R.S., Kuszak, J.R., Klaskens, L.F. *et al.* (1990) P-glycoproteins in pathology: the multidrug resistance gene family in humans. *Hum. Pathol.* **21**, 34–48.

Weiss, A.J. and Lackman, R.D. (1989) Low-dose chemotherapy of desmoid tumors. *Cancer* **64**, 1192.

Weiss, A.J., Horowitz, S. and Lackman, R.D. (1999) Therapy of desmoid tumors and fibromatosis using vinorelbine. *Am. J. Clin. Oncol.* **22**, 193.

Wick, M.R., Swanson, P.E. and Manivel, J.C. (1988) Immunohistochemical analysis of soft tissue sarcomas. *Appl. Pathol.* **6**, 169–96.

Wiklund, T.A., Alvegard, T.A., Mouridsen, H.T. *et al.* (1993) Marginal surgery and postoperative radiotherapy in soft tissue sarcomas. *Eur. J. Cancer* **29**, 306–9.

Wilcken, N. and Tattersall, M.H. (1991) Endocrine therapy for desmoid tumors. *Cancer* **68**, 1384.

Wilson, A.N., Davis, A., Bell, R.S. *et al.* (1994) Local control of soft tissue sarcoma of the extremity:

the experience of a multidisciplinary sarcoma group with definitive surgery and radiotherapy. *Eur. J. Cancer* **30A**, 746–51.

Wilson, R.B., Crowe, P.J., Fisher, R., Hook, C. and Donnellan, M.J. (1999) Extremity soft tissue sarcoma: factors predictive of local recurrence and survival. *Aust. N. Z. J. Surg.* **69**(5), 344–9.

Wilson, R.E., Wood, W.C., Lerner, H.L. *et al.* (1986) Doxorubicin chemotherapy in the treatment of soft-tissue sarcoma. Combined results of two randomized trials. *Arch. Surg.* **121**, 1354–9.

Windeyer, B., Dische, S. and Mansfield, C.M. (1966) The place of radiotherapy in the management of fibrosarcoma of the soft tissues. *Clin. Radiol.* **17**, 32–40.

Wingren, G., Fredrikson, M., Brage, N., Nordenskjold, B. and Axelson, O. (1990) Soft tissue sarcoma and occupational exposures. *Cancer* **66**, 806–11.

Wong, F.L., Boice, J.D. Jr, Abramson, D.H. *et al.* (1997) Cancer incidence after retinoblastoma. Radiation dose and sarcoma risk. *J. Am. Med. Assoc.* **278**, 1262.

Wunder, J.S., Czitrom, A.A., Kandel, R. and Andrulis, I.L. (1991) Analysis of alterations in the retinoblastoma gene and tumor grade in bone and soft-tissue sarcomas. *J. Natl Cancer Inst.* **83**, 194.

Yap, B.S. *et al.* (1983) The curability of advanced soft tissue sarcomas in adults with chemotherapy. *Proc. ASCO* **2**, 239.

Zalupski, M., Metch, B., Balcerzak, S. *et al.* (1991) Phase III comparison of doxorubicin and dacarbazine given by bolus versus infusion in patients with soft-tissue sarcomas: a Southwest Oncology Group study. *J. Natl Cancer Inst.* **83**(13), 926–32.

Zaninelli, M., Pasini, F., Pancheri, F. *et al.* (1993) Dose intensity influences the response rate in metastatic or locally advanced unresectable soft-tissue sarcoma (STS). *Cancer* **73**, 1644–51.

Zehr, R.J., Bauer, T.W., Marks, K.E. *et al.* (1990) Ki-67 and grading of malignant fibrous histiocytomas. *Cancer* **66**, 1984–90.

Zoller, M.E., Rembeck, B., Oden, A. *et al.* (1997) Malignant and benign tumors in patients with neurofibromatosis type 1 in a defined Swedish population. *Cancer* **79**, 2125.

Zucman, J., Melot, T., Pesmaz, C. *et al.* (1993) Combinatorial generation of variable fusion proteins in the Ewing family of tumours. *EMBO J.* **12**, 4481.

42

Leukaemias

TARIQ I. MUGHAL AND JOHN M. GOLDMAN

INTRODUCTION

Human leukaemias comprise a heterogeneous group of clonal disorders which are characterized by an excessive accumulation of abnormal haemopoietic cells in the bone marrow and peripheral blood. The past two decades have witnessed an enormous increase in our understanding of the pathogenesis, in particular of the molecular genetics, prognosis and treatment of leukaemia (Lowenberg et al., 1999). Genes implicated in many of these leukaemias are now well characterized (Rowley, 1980; Fourth International Workshop on Chromosomes in Leukemia, 1984). For convenience, leukaemias are often broadly considered as 'acute' and 'chronic'. Acute leukaemias are often of short duration or rapid onset, whereas chronic leukaemias are of long duration or gradually evolve. Neither term refers to the severity of the disease.

The clinical manifestations of leukaemias are usually due to the proliferation of the abnormal cells and the infiltration of the bone marrow, with resultant features of marrow failure. It is not uncommon to encounter various degrees of anaemia, neutropenia and thrombocytopenia amongst patients with leukaemias. Often leukaemic infiltration of other normal tissues also occurs, resulting in a variety of well-characterized signs, including hepatomegaly, splenomegaly, lymphadenopathy and leukaemia cutis.

The leukaemias are classified in accordance with salient pathological features of the abnormal excessive haemopoietic cells. The principal purpose of this is an attempt to collate conditions which might share similar molecular pathogenesis, and thereby reduce the effects of the groups' heterogeneity. The acute leukaemias are divided into acute myeloid leukaemia (AML) and acute lymphoblastic leukaemia (ALL); the chronic leukaemias are divided into chronic myeloid leukaemia (CML) and chronic lymphoid leukaemia (CLL). Undoubtedly as our understanding of the molecular mechanism of malignant transformation in leukaemias improves, the recognition of more homogeneous subgroups should be possible. Recent work suggests that gene arrays can be used to determine a set of genes that distinguish AML from ALL (Golub et al., 1999). This should facilitate a better classification and management strategy for individual patients. The French–American–British (FAB) classification for acute leukaemias remains the most widely used format, despite having been developed entirely on morphology (Bennett et al., 1976). Various revisions and modifications have maintained the usefulness of this system (Bennett et al., 1985; Bloomfield and Brunning, 1985). The FAB group has also defined criteria for the myelodysplastic syndromes (MDS), a morphologically heterogeneous group of clonal disorders with a potential to evolve into AML (Bennett et al., 1982). The group has also formulated a classification for CLL and CML, based on morphology, membrane markers and, in some categories, cytogenetic abnormality (Bennett et al., 1989, 1994).

In this chapter we review the current scenario with emphasis on recent therapeutic advances.

ACUTE LEUKAEMIAS

Acute myeloid leukaemia

Acute myeloid leukaemia is characterized by the malignant transformation of myeloid stem cells in the bone marrow, which are incapable of normal differentiation and maturation. Since normal haematopoieisis is organized hierarchically, the malignant transformation can occur at several levels, and AML may arise in a stem cell capable of differentiating into cells of erythroid, granulocytic, monocytic and megakaryocytic lineages, or in a lineage-restricted stem cell. Rarely, the transformation may occur in a stem cell capable of differentiating into both lymphoid and myeloid lineages and a hybrid, or biphenotypic leukaemia, where the leukaemic cell may demonstrate both lymphoid and myeloid markers, could result.

AML accounts for nearly 80 per cent of all adult acute leukaemias with an annual incidence of approximately 2.3 per 100 000 adults, and it increases progressively with age to approximately 10 per 100 00 adults 60 years of age or older. In contrast, AML accounts for 10–15% of childhood leukaemias with an annual incidence of less than 1 per 100 000 children (Kosary *et al.*, 1995). In most cases the aetiology is not obvious, but some constitutional and acquired disorders do predispose to AML. Children with Down's syndrome, Bloom's syndrome or Fanconi's anaemia have an extraordinarily high risk of acute leukaemias. Many studies of causality suggest the small risk of radiation and aromatic hydrocarbons, in particular benzene is a well-recognized factor contributing to the risk of leukaemia (Ichimaru *et al.*, 1978; Austin *et al.*, 1988). More recently, the serious risk of a therapy-related acute leukaemia has been described, especially when exposed to leukaemogenic agents such as an alkylating agent. The risk of this serious complication appears to be 3–10 per cent and peaks 5–10 years after the start of therapy. Some of these patients initially develop MDS with deletions of chromosomes 5 and 7 (Kaldor *et al.*, 1990; van Leeuwen, 1996). A second distinct therapy-related AML has been recognized as a complication of certain drugs that inhibit topoisomerase II. In contrast to the previously described therapy-related AML, this type develops after a relatively short latency period of 2–3 years, is not preceded by MDS, and is often associated with abnormalities of chromosome 11q23 (Pui *et al.*, 1991; Greaves, 1997).

Most patients with AML present with signs and symptoms arising from bone marrow failure and organ infiltration by leukaemic cells. Pallor, lethargy, dyspnoea, infections and bleeding manifestations are not uncommon. Occasionally patients may present as a consequence of hyperleucostasis. The diagnosis of AML is made when more than 30 per cent leukaemic cells (blasts; also known as myeloblasts) are found in the bone marrow or peripheral blood (Fig. 42.1). Conventional morphological investigations should determine reactivity of the myeloblasts with myeloperoxidase, Sudan black, and the non-specific esterases α-naphthylacetate and naphthylbutyrate. These may allow distinction of AML from ALL and MDS and preliminary classification in accordance to the FAB group, but further characterization and distinction from MDS-related AML (secondary AML) often require additional

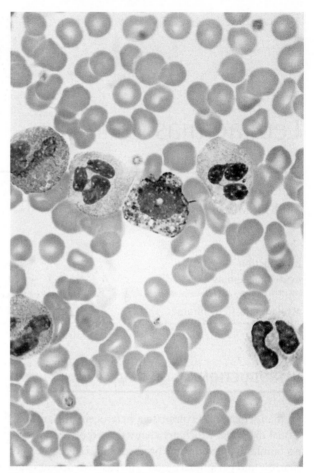

Figure 42.1 *A peripheral blood film of a patient with acute myeloid leukaemia, FAB subtype M1, showing Type I and Type II blasts (×960). Kindly provided by Professor Barbara Bain, Imperial College School of Medicine, London.*

investigations. These include immunological and cytogenetic or direct molecular genetic analysis of the leukaemic blasts. The most recent revision of the FAB classification incorporates immunological and molecular genetic abnormalities into the diagnostic criteria for some FAB subtypes (Bennett *et al.*, 1991).

FAB CLASSIFICATION OF AML

The FAB classification of acute leukaemias was first described in 1976, based solely on morphological studies identifying the lineage of the leukaemic cells and the degree of differentiation present. The current version, shown in Table 42.1, divides AML into nine distinct subtypes that differ morphologically and histochemically; immunological and genetic differences are also incorporated in some subtypes. The most common subtypes are M2 and M4, followed by M1, and then by M5 and M4Eo; M3, M6 and M7 are relatively rare. In the subtype M1 the blasts, which account for over 90 per cent of non-erythroid cells, show minimal evidence of differentiation. Two types of M1 blasts have been categorized: Type I lack granules

Table 42.1 *The French–American–British (FAB) classification of AML and associated genetic abnormalities*

FAB subtype	Common name (% of cases)	Results of staining			Associated translocations and rearrangements (% of cases)	Genes involved
		Myeloperoxidase	Sudan black	Non-specific esterase		
M0	Acute myeloblastic leukaemia with minimal differentiation (3%)	−	−	−[a]	inv(3q26) and t(3;3) (1%)	EV11
M1	Acute myeloblastic leukaemia without maturation (15–20%)	+	+	−		
M2	Acute myeloblastic leukaemia with maturation (25–30%)	+	+	−	t(8;21) (40%), t(6;9) (1%)	AMLI-ETO, DEK-CAN
M3	Acute promyelocytic leukaemia (5–10%)	+	+	−	t(15;17) (98%), t(11;17) (1%), t(5;17) (1%)	PML-RARα, PLZF-RARα, NPM-RARα
M4	Acute myelomonocytic leukaemia (20%)	+	+	+	11q23 (20%), inv(3q26) and t(3;3) (3%), t(6;9) (1%)	MLL, DEK-CAN, EV11
M4EO	Acute myelomonocytic leukaemia with abnormal eosinophils (5–10%)	+	+	+	inv(16) and t(16;16) (80%)	CBFα-MYH11
M5	Acute monocytic leukaemia (2–9%)	−	−	+	11q23 (20%), t(8;16) (2%)	MLL, MOZ-CBP
M6	Erythroleukaemia (3–5%)	+	+	−		
M7	Acute megakaryocytic leukaemia (3–12%)	−	−	+[b]	t(1;22) (5%)	Unknown

[a] Cells are positive for myeloid antigen (e.g. CD13 and CD33).
[b] Cells are positive for α-naphthylacetate and platelet glycoprotein IIb/IIIa pr factor VIII-related antigen and negative for naphthylbutyrate.

and Type II contain granules and have a somewhat lower nucleocytoplasmic ratio. In the sub-type M2 the blasts account for 30–90 per cent of non-erythyroid cells and there is evidence of maturation to the promyelocytic stage or beyond; Auer rods are common. Subtype M3 cells are heavily granulated promyelocytes, often with bundles of Auer rods (Fig. 42.2); M3v cells are the hypogranular variant. Disseminated intravascular coagulation (DIC) is common at presentation in both varieties of M3. Subtype M4 is characterized by myelomonocytic morphology and a monocytosis is common; a variant of M4, M4Eo is recognized when more than 5 per cent dysplastic eosinophils are seen. Two variants of subtype M5 are recognized: M5a, in which more than 80 per cent of the non-erythroid cells are monoblasts, and M5b, in which less than 80 per cent of the non-erythroid cells are monoblasts and the rest are promonocytes and monocytes. Infiltration of tissues, in particular gums, perianal area and skin with blasts are frequent in subtypes M4 and M5.

In the subtypes M6 and M7, the malignant transformation occurs at the level of the stem cells committed to

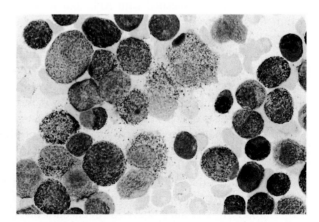

Figure 42.2 *A peripheral blood film from a patient with acute myeloid leukaemia, FAB subtype M3, showing Auer rods (×960). Kindly provided by Professor Barbara Bain, Imperial College School of Medicine, London.*

the erythroid and megakaryocytic lineages, respectively. In the subtype M6, over 30 per cent of non-erythroid cells are Type I or II blasts and over 50 per cent of all marrow cells are erythroblasts. Subtype M7 is characterized by marrow fibrosis and large polymorphic blasts with cytoplasmic blebs are often seen (these are CD41 positive).

MOLECULAR PATHOGENESIS

The past two decades have witnessed the emerging role of cytogenetic analysis of leukaemic cells in stratifying patients into risk-based categories and facilitating treatment in accordance to the risk category (Rowley, 1990). Patients with inv(16), t(8;21) or t(15;17) have the best prognosis after treatment with an anthracycline and standard-dose cytarabine, with 70–90 per cent entering complete remission (CR) and 40–50 per cent remaining so at 5 years (Keating *et al.*, 1988). Patients with +8, 20q− and the −5/−7 abnormalities have a poor prognosis, with 30–50 per cent being able to enter CR and less than 5 per cent remaining so at 5 years. These observations have firmly established correlations between the cytogenetic and clinical phenotypes of AML. The implication of being able to apply this information to improve the prognosis of patients has been exemplified by the use of all-*trans* retinoic acid (ATRA) to treat patients with AML, FAB subtype M3 (also known as acute promyelocytic leukaemia; APL). In APL a balanced reciprocal translocation results in the fusion of portions of the promyelocytic leukaemia (PML) gene on chromosome 15 with the gene for retinoic acid receptor alpha (RARα) on chromosome 17 (Grimwade and Solomon, 1997). This chimeric gene encodes the PML–RARα fusion protein, which retains the RA ligand-binding domain and may account for the unique sensitivity of APL to differentiation by retinoids such as ATRA (Lin *et al.*, 1998). It has now been established that at least three further reciprocal translocations involving the RARα gene (17q21) but not the PML gene, are associated with APL, and it is the nature of the fusion protein that determines the degree of responsiveness to ATRA (Grigani *et al.*, 1998). Recently it has also been observed that arsenic-based compounds can also exert a differentiation effect on APL cells and therefore reverse the leukaemic phenotype (Steven *et al.*, 1998). Arsenic trioxide has also been shown to induce apoptosis with caspase activation in leukaemic cells.

Other well-characterized genetic abnormalities pertain to the acute myeloid leukaemia 1 (AML1) and the mixed-lineage leukaemia (MLL) genes. The AML1 gene is involved in three different chromosomes translocations which share a breakpoint at its locus on chromosome 21q22: t(8;21), t(3;21) and t(12;21). AML1 encodes the α subunit of core-binding factor (CBF), a multicomponent transcription-factor complex that regulates a number of haematopoiesis-specific genes and is essential for normal haematopoiesis. The t(8;21) translocation is found in 40 per cent of patients with AML, FAB subtype M2; the t(3;21) is found in some patients with MDS and also myeloid blast transformation of CML, and t(12;21) is found in childhood ALL (Sawyers, 1997). The fusion proteins show a common theme of transcription-factor-domain swaps and the normal function of the AML1 gene is disrupted. Further insights into AML1 function have been gained by examining its binding partners in the CBF; in particular CBFβ, which is targeted in AML, associated chromosomal rearrangement inv(16) or its variant t(16;16) (Liu *et al.*, 1993). Collectively these data suggest the AML1 pathway as a common target for leukaemia-specific translocations. MLL gene rearrangements occur in structural abnormalities of chromosome 11q23 which are found in about 10 per cent of patients with AML, FAB subtypes M4 or M5, and about 85 per cent of patients with secondary AML that develops after exposure to topoisomerase II inhibitors (Waring and Cleary, 1997). Many efforts are currently being directed in the search for other consistent molecular abnormalities that might act as therapeutic targets (Rubnitz *et al.*, 1996).

PROGNOSTIC FACTORS

A number of clinical and morphological features of AML, combined with the additional information available from the routine use of immunological and genetic analysis, have enabled the stratification of patients in risk categories based on prognosis which is largely dependent on being able to achieve a CR. The speed of the initial response to induction therapy and the leukaemia burden (white-cell count of greater than $20\,000/mm^3$) are also useful in assessing risk of relapse.

The good-risk category includes patients under the age of 60 years, have genetic evidence of t(15;17), t(8;21) or inv(16) and FAB subtypes M1 or M2. These patients have a greater than 85 per cent rate of CR, 30–40 per cent risk of relapse and 40–50 per cent event-free survival at 5 years. The poor-risk category includes patients who are older than 60 years, have abnormalities involving chromosome 5(−5 or 5q−), chromosome 7(−7 or 7q−) or chromosome 3, and have a poor performance status. Patients who require more than one induction treatment to achieve CR, have an elevated serum lactate dehydrogenase and secondary AML (MDS-related or therapy-related) also belong to this category, with a 30–50 per cent rate of CR and less than 20 per cent event-free survival at 5 years. The standard (intermediate) risk category includes patients with a normal karyotype and has a 50–85 per cent rate of CR and about 30 per cent event-free survival at 5 years.

TREATMENT

For patients with AML there are two sequential objectives of current standard treatment. The first is to induce CR and the second is to prevent relapse. Conventionally haematological CR has been defined by a full recovery of peripheral blood counts. The use of immunological and molecular genetic markers should improve on these definitions of CR in the future. Thus the conventional treatment plan for all patients with AML consists of remission induction followed by consolidation therapy. It is now appropriate not to consider all patients with AML as a single entity for the post-remission therapy, but rather tailor this according to the individual risk category defined by cytogenetic criteria. It is also appropriate to consider separately the treatment of patients with APL, which is now the most curable subtype.

Remission induction

Substantial improvements have been made during the past two decades with regards to the proportion of patients under the age of 60 years who are able to achieve CR (Mayer et al., 1994; Rees et al., 1996). These improvements appear to be largely due to better supportive care, which has enabled the safer delivery of more intensive remission induction, particularly with high doses of cytarabine (Bishop et al., 1999). A variety of induction regimens followed by consolidation treatment with or without prolonged maintenance have been investigated extensively and the results suggest that about 70 per cent achieve a CR and with postremission therapy, 25–30 per cent will remain in CR at 5 years. For patients who receive less intensive postremission therapy, only 10–15 per cent will remain in CR at 5 years (Buchner et al., 1985). The major unresolved issue for patients under the age of 60 years is that of remaining in continuous CR.

The most common remission induction consist of two courses of an anthracyline, usually daunorubicin or doxorubicin at 40–60 mg/m^2 per day for 3 days and a continuous infusion of cytarabine at 100–200 mg/m^2 per day for 7 days. Several recent randomized trials of alternatives to daunorubicin or doxorubicin have suggested that both idarubicin and mitozantrone are more effective, although both result in longer periods of pancytopenia (Arlin et al., 1990; Berman et al., 1991). There is, however, some debate with regards to the equivalent doses and further studies are in progress. In the recently completed MRC AML 10 trial, 1820 patients under the age of 56 years were randomized to either daunorubicin, cytarabine and 6-thioguanine or daunorubicin, cytarabine and etoposide chemotherapy as induction treatment for two courses (Burnett et al., 1998). After the two induction courses, patients in CR received a third induction course consisting of amsacrine, cytarabine and etoposide, following which bone-marrow stem cells were harvested and patients who lacked an HLA-matched sibling donor, or who did not wish to receive an allograft, were randomized to receive a further course of induction treatment consisting of mitozantrone and cytarabine (at 1 g/m^2, every 12 h for 3 days), followed by either autologous stem-cell transplant (SCT) or no further treatment. In this trial, 80 per cent of patients achieved CR and the overall survival at 7 years was 40 per cent. In an attempt to improve the overall survival, several recently completed studies have incorporated high-dose cytarabine (3 g/m^2) in the induction phase (Weick et al., 1996). The overall survival in such studies, as in the MRC AML 12 trial which recruited 2400 patients, has improved to 49 per cent, but the toxicity from the high-dose cytarabine is considerable

(Burnett et al., 1999a). In an attempt to add further anti-leukaemic treatment while limiting further toxicity, current trials such as the MRC AML 15 trial use antibody-directed chemotherapy. Gemtuzumab ozogamicin (mylotarg) is a novel agent, which comprises a humanized anti-CD33 monoclonal antibody that is linked to a potent antitumour antibiotic calicheamicin. The monoclonal antibody is directed against the CD33 epitope expressed on the surface of leukaemic blasts in over 90 per cent of patients with AML (Sievers et al., 1999).

For patients with APL, ATRA should be used incorporated in induction therapy. There is some uncertainty as to how best to combine ATRA with chemotherapy. Current evidence appears compelling that an anthracycline (daunorubicin or idarubicin) should be included in induction in contrast to cytarabine which probably can be omitted (Tallman et al., 2002). A recent study has shown that patients with APL fare just as well without cytarabine as part of their induction or consolidation treatment (Sanz et al., 1999). The European APL group is addressing this issue further with patients being randomized to ATRA plus daunorubicin or to ATRA plus daunorubicin and cytarabine. There have been no randomized trials addressing the choice of anthracyclines so far, although there is agreement about the dose. It is reasonable to commence induction with ATRA alone for 2–4 days, provided the white blood count is not high, as it is remarkably effective in controlling the characteristic coagulopathy which can often be life threatening, and then commence anthracycline treatment. Earlier studies did suggest CR rates of 80–90 per cent with ATRA alone, but the remissions were shorter than those produced by ATRA followed by chemotherapy or chemotherapy alone (Fenaux et al., 1992; Tallman et al., 1997). Despite the qualified success of ATRA, the mortality associated with the induction therapy remains at around 10 per cent and an acquired retinoid resistance contributes to relapse in about 20–30 per cent of patients (Burnett et al., 1999b). ATRA does have a serious side-effect of capillary leak syndrome often associated with leucocytosis (referred to as the 'ATRA syndrome'). Current studies should show how best to integrate this novel molecular targeting into conventional chemotherapy.

Postremission therapy

All patients under the age of 60 years who achieve a CR following induction therapy require further treatment in order to improve their chances of remaining in continuous CR. Currently there are three well-defined and intensively investigated options: either receiving an allograft from an HLA-matched donor (sibling or unrelated) or an autograft, or further intensive chemotherapy.

Allogeneic SCT from an HLA-matched sibling donor has been standard treatment for AML in first CR for two decades (Thomas et al., 1979; Appelbaum et al., 1984). It offers a 50–60 per cent chance of long-term remission. The risk of relapse following an allograft is 20 per cent.

This reduced relapse rate is largely due to the anti-leukaemic effect of the allograft against residual leukaemia cells, the graft-versus-leukaemia (GvL) effect. The toxicity of the procedure and mortality related to transplant-related complications, such as immunosuppression and graft-versus-host disease (GvHD), accounts for 20–25 per cent. There have been no prospective randomized trials of allografting, but comparative analysis of patients with suitable donors versus those without such donors have confirmed the survival benefits conferred by allografting in first CR (Zittoun *et al.*, 1995; Keating *et al.*, 1998). In recent years, results from intensive chemotherapy have improved (as discussed above) and there has been a better stratification of patients' risk of relapse.

Autologous SCT has also been used widely for the past two decades, and data from the European Blood and Marrow Transplantation Registry (EBMT) suggests a long-term survival rate of 45–55 per cent (Gorin, 1998). Relapse is the most common reason for failure, possibly because of residual disease and the loss of a putative GvL effect in the autograft procedure. This is offset by the appreciably lower risk of transplant-related mortality, but it is noteworthy that 5–8 per cent of patients die in CR, often because of poor engraftment. There is no evidence that *in vitro* purging of the harvested stem cells confers additional benefit (Gorin *et al.*, 1991). The MRC AML 10 trial assessed the value of adding autologous SCT to a cohort of patients who had already received intensive postremission therapy (Burnett *et al.*, 1998). This trial showed a substantial reduction in risk of relapse with autologous SCT (37 per cent versus 58 per cent; $P = 0.0007$), resulting in a superior 7-year event-free survival (53 per cent versus 40 per cent; $P = 0.04$), despite a higher mortality rate in the transplantation group. Parenthetically, the event-free survival advantage was only in patients who lived beyond 2 years of the transplant. Several other European comparative studies reveal similar findings (Harousseau *et al.*, 1997). A US Intergroup trial comparing high-dose cytarabine ($3 \, g/m^2$ every 12 h for 12 doses) with autologous or allogeneic SCT during first remission of AML showed an equivalent event-free survival and a better overall survival with chemotherapy than autologous or allogeneic SCT (Cassileth *et al.*, 1998). A further recent study has demonstrated evidence of a dose–response effect of cytarabine in patients with AML, including those in the poor-risk group (Kern *et al.*, 1998).

These studies have introduced an element of uncertainty as to how best to treat patients under the age of 60 years who are in first CR. It would appear reasonable not to offer allografting as first-line postremission treatment to all patients, but rather in accordance to their risk category and, preferably, in the context of clinical trials. Current comparative trials are assessing the potential improvements in autologous SCT by better engraftment with the use of peripheral blood stem cells and it should be possible to better identify patients who can benefit from salvage transplantation.

For patients who relapse with AML, the treatment options are few. For patients in the good-risk group who relapse following a remission of at least 12 months, the survival rate following subsequent chemotherapy treatment is about 20 per cent (Grimwade *et al.*, 1998). For these reasons every effort is directed to prevent relapse. For children and adults younger than 40 years of age, it is reasonable to proceed with a SCT, either an autograft or an allograft using an HLA-matched sibling donor. It is uncertain as to whether these patients should first receive induction therapy or proceed directly with transplantation. An earlier study from the Seattle group assessed these aspects and showed an equivalent survival with either option (Petersen *et al.*, 1993). Current EBMT registry data suggest a survival rate of about 30 per cent for patients with AML in first relapse or second CR treated by an autologous or allogeneic SCT, using an HLA-identical sibling donor (EBMT, 1998).

For patients with APL who enter CR, anthracycline-consolidation therapy is required, although there is some uncertainty with regard to the number of cycles needed. Studies have also suggested that all patients should receive maintenance therapy with ATRA, with or without low-dose chemotherapy (Fenaux *et al.*, 1999). There is some concern with regard to the possible increased neurotoxicity associated with ATRA maintenance therapy, particularly in children (Mahmoud *et al.*, 1993). Therapy-related MDS and secondary AML are also being recognized increasingly in APL patients and better risk-stratification and monitoring of residual disease by polymerase chain reaction should facilitate better individualization of therapies (Latagliata *et al.*, 2002). Arsenic trioxide is now considered effective treatment for those patients who relapse or are refractory to ATRA-based therapy (Soignet *et al.*, 1998). The role of arsenic trioxide during the induction phase is currently being investigated, based on possible synergism with ATRA (Jing *et al.*, 2001). Allogeneic SCT has no role in the management of APL in first remission since the results from current induction treatments are excellent. There are, however, no studies that have compared the results of SCT in relation to the induction therapy containing ATRA. The EBMT retrospective registry data on 362 patients with APL treated in the pre-ATRA era, who received SCT in first CR, suggested that 45 per cent of such patients had long-term remissions and possible cure (Mandelli *et al.*, 1994). Allogeneic SCT may be useful for patients who relapse following an arsenic trioxide induced second CR. Impressive results have also been observed in patients with relapsed disease who receive an autograft using stem cells which are molecularly negative for the PML-RARα gene product (Meloni *et al.*, 1997).

TREATMENT OF PATIENTS OLDER THAN 60 YEARS OF AGE WITH AML

This age group accounts for about 75 per cent of all newly diagnosed AML, the majority of whom are in the poor-risk group (Lowenberg, 1996). Furthermore, older patients are less able to tolerate the rigours associated with the intensive induction regimens, leave alone transplantation. The incidence of significant co-morbid medical conditions is also high in this cohort. Unfortunately, a nihilistic approach results in a poor quality of life and very poor survival. Patients who are younger than 80 years of age, have no significant medical history and have a good performance status have an approximately 50 per cent chance of achieving CR with conventional induction treatment and an event-free survival of about 20 per cent at 2 years (Lowenberg et al., 1989). A minority may benefit from low-dose maintenance therapy, in particular from a quality-of-life perspective. Many efforts are being devoted to improve the supportive care of these patients and to use haematopoietic growth factors, in particular granulocyte colony stimulating factor (G-CSF), as an adjunct to induction therapy (Dombret et al., 1995). The current MRC AML 14 trial evaluates two treatment strategies in patients aged 60 years or over with AML or high-risk myelodysplastic syndrome. The trial has an 'intensive' and a 'non-intensive' approach; where there is uncertainty, patients are randomized between the 'intensive' and 'non-intensive' treatments. The 'intensive' treatment arm compares two doses of daunorubicin, the addition of the multi-drug resistance modulator PSC833, two doses of cytarabine, and three versus four courses of treatment in total. The 'non-intensive' chemotherapy treatment arm compares hydroxyurea control with low-dose cytarabine, with or without ATRA. In older patients with APL, it may be worthwhile considering less toxic consolidation treatment such as liposomal ATRA or anti-CD33 monoclonal antibody-based strategies (Latagliata et al., 1997; Jurcic et al., 2000).

CONCLUSIONS

Considerable advances have been made in the molecular understanding of AML and some of this progress has resulted in being able to target the leukaemic cells with molecular and immunological strategies. The first successful example of this has been the use of ATRA in the treatment of APL. It is likely that novel agents targeting the P-glycoprotein and the multidrug resistance (MDR1) gene will enter clinics in the near future. The impressive results obtained with the tyrosine kinase inhibitor, STI571, for the treatment of patients with CML suggest that with further characterization of the different signalling pathways, other novel therapies should emerge (Druker and Lydon, 2000). Another tyrosine kinase inhibitor, SU5416, which blocks the activity of the vascular endothelial growth factor receptor-2 (VEGFR-2) and the stem-cell factor (SCF) receptor c-kit, was recently shown to result in a durable remission in a patient with AML in second relapse which was refractory to conventional therapy (Mesters et al., 2001). A farnesyltranferase inhibitor, R115777, which targets RAS inhibition, has recently

entered clinical studies, with encouraging preliminary results (Karp et al., 2001). Other current investigational approaches include the use of radioimmunoconjugates, thalidomide and vaccine strategies (Ruffner and Matthews, 2000; Steins et al., 2002). Further improvements in peripheral-blood stem-cell transplant technology and the revised focus of stem-cell transplant as potential immunotherapeutic approach using methods designed to augment the GvL effect may improve the cure rates for patients under 60 years of age, while new approaches are needed for treating patients over 60 years of age (Appelbaum, 2002).

Acute lymphoblastic leukaemia

Acute lymphoblastic leukaemia (ALL) most commonly affects children, particularly those between 2 and 10 years of age. It accounts for 80 per cent of all childhood leukaemias and is the most common type of cancer in children (Parker et al., 1997). It also affects adults, mainly those between 30 and 50 years of age, accounting for 20 per cent of all adult acute leukaemias. It is characterized by abnormalities of the lymphoid cell precursors, leading to excessive accumulation of leukaemic lymphoblasts in the marrow and other organs, in particular the spleen and liver.

The annual worldwide incidence of ALL among children is probably about 2 per 100 000 children and in adults about 0.7 per 100 000 adults. The peak incidence in the UK and the US appears to be between the ages of 3 and 5 years. It is of interest to note that in some less affluent countries, such as Turkey, ALL might be less prevalent than AML in children. The disease appears to afflict more males than females and there appears to be a higher prevalence in Caucasians. ALL has been linked more often than AML to a possible infectious aetiology, in particular Epstein–Barr virus (EBV) and malaria, but no firm proof has transpired (Greaves, 1997). There is, however, a firm association between one of the several known strains of the human T-cell lymphotropic virus (HTLV), HTLV-1, and adult T-cell leukaemia/lymphoma (ATL). Epidemiological studies have suggested that a subtype of childhood ALL, common ALL, may arise as a consequence of rare and immunologically abnormal response to a common infection in genetically susceptible children (Kinlen, 1995).

Most patients with ALL present with features resulting from organ infiltration by leukaemic lymphoblasts, in particular bone pain. Lymphadenopathy, hepatosplenomegaly, testicular enlargement or a meningeal syndrome is not uncommon. Rarely, patients may present with respiratory difficulties as a consequence of a mediastinal mass. The diagnosis of ALL is made from a combination of morphological features, cytochemical reactions and immunological markers. The disease is biologically and clinically heterogeneous. The prognosis in childhood ALL is good, but in contrast, adults with ALL have a poor prognosis. This appears to be due to a much higher frequency

Table 42.2 *FAB classification in acute lymphocytic leukaemia*

Subtype	Description	Incidence (%)	CR (%)	3-year remission (%)
L1	Small homogeneous, high nuclear : cytoplasmic ratio, small nucleoli	20	85	40
L2	Larger, pleomorphic, low nuclear : cytoplasmic ratio, prominent nucleoli	70	75	36
L3	Larger, vacuolated basophilic cytoplasm, large vesicular nucleus, large nucleoli	10	65	10

CR, complete response; FAB, French–American–British.

of poor risk factors and the likelihood of an intrinsically different biological disease, since age appears to be an independent prognostic factor (Cortes and Kantarjian, 1995).

FAB CLASSIFICATION OF ALL

The FAB classification recognizes three distinct subtypes solely on morphological studies: L1, L2 and L3 (Table 42.2). In the subtype L1, the lymphoblast is relatively small with scanty cytoplasm and inconspicuous nucleoli. In the subtype L2, the lymphoblast is larger with more abundant cytoplasm and, in the subtype L3, the lymphoblast is mature and resembles the Burkitt's lymphoma cell (Fig. 42.3). Since there is no clear relationship between the FAB subtypes and the immunological markers, a parallel immunological classification attempted to categorize the lymphoblast by analogy with its normal counterpart in the B- or T-lymphoid lineages. Moreover, in contrast to AML, ALL lymphoblasts lack significant cytochemical features, emphasizing the diagnostic role of immunophenotyping. Cytogenetic analysis of the lymphoblasts has revealed an abnormal karyotype in more than 90 per cent of cases studied and led to the adoption of an integrated classification based on FAB subtype, immunophenotype and cytogenetic category (First MIC Co-operative Study Group, 1986). This modified classification appears to be much more clinically useful and also facilitates the addition of new categories as they are recognized. Approximately 20 per cent of all ALL lymphoblasts are T cell in origin, 75 per cent are precursor B cell, and 5 per cent are more mature B cells (usually FAB subtype L3). Acute undifferentiated leukaemia (AUL) is uncommon. In 25 per cent of children and about 35 per cent of adults with ALL, the lymphoblasts express both lymphoid and myeloid antigens. This feature was previously associated with a poorer prognosis; it is now considered to have no prognostic or therapeutic implication (Uckun *et al.*, 1997).

MOLECULAR PATHOGENESIS

The recognition of genetic abnormalities in the majority of lymphoblasts has contributed enormously to understanding the molecular pathogenesis and prognosis of

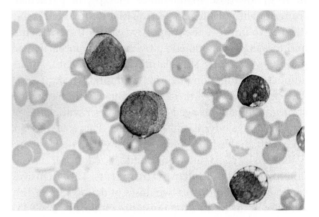

Figure 42.3 *A peripheral blood film from a patient with acute lymphoblastic leukaemia, FAB subtype L3, showing vacuolated lymphoblasts (×960). Kindly provided by Professor Barbara Bain, Imperial College School of Medicine, London.*

ALL. Hyperdiploidy (more than 50 chromosomes) found in up to 25 per cent of children and 6 per cent of adults with ALL is characterized by lymphoblasts of an early pre-B immunophenotype and an excellent prognosis, with the lymphoblasts demonstrating unique susceptibility to antimetabolites. The observation that about half of these patients develop additional genetic abnormalities, in particular duplications of chromosome 1q and isochromosome of 17q, has led to the hypothesis of a probable 'two-hit' genetic event, resulting in a transformed phenotype which may not respond to therapy as well (Kaspers *et al.*, 1995). Approximately 25 per cent of adults and 4 per cent of children have the Philadelphia (Ph) chromosome [t(9;22)(q34;q11)], one-third of patients have BCR–ABL transcripts indistinguishable from those found in CML. The remaining two-thirds have a breakpoint in the first intron of the BCR gene (between e1 and e2) in an area designated the minor breakpoint cluster region (m-bcr); this is transcribed as an e1a2 mRNA which encodes for a 190 kD protein (p190$^{BCR-ABL}$), in contrast to the p210$^{BCR-ABL}$ found in CML (Melo, 1996). About a fifth of all children with ALL have been shown to have t(12;21)(p12;q22) which results in the formation of a chimeric gene consisting of the 5′ portion of the TEL (also known as ETV6) gene linked to an almost complete AML1 gene. The resultant chimeric oncoprotein acts as a putative transcriptional repressor of the interleukin-3 (IL-3) promoter, thought to be central to leukaemogenesis (Uchida *et al.*, 1999). A recent report of the finding of the t(12;21) *in utero* by an elegant analysis of neonatal Guthrie blood-spot cards for children aged between 2 years and 5 years, who had newly diagnosed common B-cell precursor ALL, suggests that this subtype of childhood ALL may have a prenatal origin (Wiemels *et al.*, 1999). However, studies in identical twins show that an additional postnatal genetic event is also required for clinical evidence of the leukaemia (Ford *et al.*, 1998).

Structural abnormalities involving chromosome 11q23, which targets the MLL gene, account for approximately 6 per cent of children and adults with ALL, but are the most frequent genetic abnormalities observed in infants. The most frequent 11q23 abnormality, the t(4;11), is associated with mixed-lineage disease and usually carries a dire prognosis. Translocations involving t(1;19), found in 5 per cent of children and 3 per cent of adults with ALL, result in the fusion of the gene encoding the E2A transcription factor on chromosome 19 and the PBX1 transcription factor on chromosome 1. The resulting chimeric protein has been shown in mice to lead to leukaemias that are characterized by a block in differentiation and growth factor dependence (Dedre *et al.*, 1993). An uncommon translocation, t(11;17) results in the fusion gene E2A–HLF, which is known to inhibit apoptosis (Inaba *et al.*, 1996).

In ALL with mature B- or T-lineage immunophenotypes, chromosomal translocations often result from errors in antigen receptor gene rearrangements and so become inappropriately expressed. This is exemplified in patients with B-lineage ALL and Burkitt's lymphoma who usually have the t(8;14) translocation or its variant t(2;8) or t(8;22). As a consequence of these rearrangements, the c-*MYC* gene is dysregulated and in the presence of other co-operating mutations, such as k-*RAS* and n-*RAS*, results in the malignant process (Harris *et al.*, 1988). Genes which are affected in a similar manner in T-lineage ALL include SCL (TAL-1), LMO1 (TTG-1) and LMO2 (TTG-2), which are essential for the development of all haematopoietic lineages. In the translocation t(1;14) which is present in about 5 per cent of T-ALL, the SCL is rearranged into the TCRδ gene and carries a poor prognosis. The translocation t(11;14)(p15;q11) results in rearrangement of LMO1 into the TCRα/δ locus, whereas the t(11;14)(p13;q11) results in the rearrangement of LMO2 into this locus (Porcher *et al.*, 1996).

PROGNOSTIC FACTORS

Prior to the advent of molecular genetic analysis, a constellation of clinical, biological and morphological features were used for risk assessment, many of which were subsequently refuted. It is now possible to characterize subtypes of ALL into more homogeneous groups by means of the genetic features and then stratify patients into a low-, standard (intermediate)- or high-risk group in accordance to their molecular genetic, immunological and clinical features, as shown in Table 42.2. It is also useful to consider the degree of early responsiveness to therapy.

In general, balanced translocations in adult ALL have a worse prognosis than quantitative chromosomal abnormalities. Adults also have disproportionately high frequency of unfavourable genetic changes, and it is of interest that their prognosis is considerably worse compared to that of children with equivalent genetic changes and immunophenotype (Group Français de Cytogenetique Hematologique, 1996; Chessells *et al.*, 1998). The presence of the BCR–ABL gene in lymphoblasts usually confers a poor prognosis, but occasionally children who present with low initial leucocyte counts may fare reasonably well. Hyperploids (fewer than 45 chromosomes) almost always carry a grave prognosis, as do infants with t(4;11). In a recent study investigating the relationship between minimal residual disease status and clinical outcome and comparing this with age, gender, immunophenotype, and presenting white cell count, the minimal residual disease tests were found to be independent predictors of disease-free survival (Mortuza *et al.*, 2002).

TREATMENT

The conventional approach for all patients with ALL, except the mature B-cell subtype (FAB L3) and infants with ALL, is a treatment plan in three phases: remission induction, consolidation and maintenance. All patients with ALL who achieve CR should receive some form of central nervous system (CNS) prophylaxis. The mature B-cell ALL and infant ALL appear to be best treated with short term regimens of intensive therapy, and will be addressed separately.

Remission induction

The principal aim is to achieve CR with restoration of normal haematopoiesis. Better supportive care has made it safer for patients with standard and poor-risk ALL to receive more intensive induction regimens with four or more drugs. Current results suggest that over 95 per cent of children and 75–90 per cent of adults are able to achieve a CR, and with consolidation and maintenance therapy, about 70–80 per cent of children and 30–40 per cent of adults will remain in CR at 5 years (Larson *et al.*, 1995).

Universally, induction therapy includes a glucocorticoid, prednisolone or dexamethasone, vincristine and asparaginase. Very recently, the Italian GIMEMA group was able to demonstrate the usefulness of a 7-day prednisolone pre-treatment on predicting the outcome in adult ALL patients (Anino *et al.*, 2002). The realization of the rapid reduction of lymphoblasts following the initial therapy suggested that the intensity of this phase of the treatment plan is important and led to efforts to intensify it.

For this reason, an anthracycline, usually daunorubicin or doxorubicin, and sometimes cyclophosphamide have been added, in particular for the adult patients. Likewise the subsequent phases of the treatment plan were also made more intensive.

It is possible that dexamethasone may provide better protection than prednisolone against a CNS relapse, since it has a better penetration across the blood–brain barrier. Regardless, all patients with ALL who achieve CR should receive some form of proven CNS prophylaxis. The standard approach is to administer cranial irradiation totalling 1800 cGy in conjunction with intrathecal methotrexate. Recent experiences suggest that the dose of cranial irradiation can safely be reduced to 1200 cGy, even in patients at high risk (Conter et al., 1997). This lower dose of irradiation could be valuable in reducing the risk of late cerebral toxicity. Intrathecal methotrexate without irradiation has resulted in comparatively high rates of CNS relapse and it is possible that methotrexate in combination with cytarabine and dexamethasone (triple intrathecal therapy) might be better. Moreover, since most induction regimens nowadays include drugs which are able to cross the blood–brain barrier it is likely that the need for additional irradiation may have diminished (Cortes et al., 1995). Recently, however, the results of the Dana-Farber ALL consortium protocol at a median follow-up of 9.2 years suggested that eliminating cranial irradiation without a concomitant increased intensity of systemic or intrathecal therapy results in a marked increase in CNS relapse in standard-risk male children, but interestingly not female children (LeClerc et al., 2002).

Several forms of asparaginase, each with a different pharmokinetic profile, are currently available. In a single randomized study, patients treated with asparaginase derived from Escherichia coli fared better than that derived from Erwinia carotovora. Studies have also compared the efficacy of mitozantrone and daunorubicin and found them to be equivalent. Parenthetically it should be emphasized that as attempts have been made to increase the intensity of the remission induction, complex regimens using multiple drugs have entered the clinics at frequent intervals without being tested stringently in randomized trials. This has made it difficult to assess with any precision the results of the more intensive treatments, nor is it possible to draw firm opinions on the contributions of each individual drug. These points notwithstanding, most current treatment protocols are well received by the specialists in view of the improving outcomes of the patients.

For patients with mature B-cell ALL the prognosis is poor for both children and adults, and as recently as a decade ago, the probability of achieving a CR was about 35 per cent. Newer treatment strategies based on experiences from the treatment of children and young adults with Burkitt's lymphoma resulted in the inclusion of fractionated high-dose cyclophosphamide, high-dose methotrexate, and cytarabine (standard dose). These

modifications led to the CR rates improving to 75 per cent and the event-free survival to around 50 per cent. These improvements have been credited to the high-dose components of the protocols, although it is difficult to assess which of the high-dose combinations are more important and the optimal doses remain debatable. Further refinements have occurred since, and the currently reported CR rate is 85 per cent (Soussain et al., 1995; Hoelzer et al., 1996). For the moment the favoured dose of cyclophosphamide is 8 g/m^2 and that of methotrexate is 5 g/m^2. Once a CR is achieved it appears desirable to proceed with an intensive consolidation for about 8 months. Neither autologous nor allogeneic SCT have been tested adequately, but should be considered, in the context of a clinical trial, for patients who fail to achieve a CR with one or two induction treatments. Maintenance therapy appears to have no value in this disease. Since the high-dose drugs used are active in CNS disease, patients receive additional intrathecal methotrexate without cranial irradiation.

Patients with BCR–ABL positive ALL tend to have a very poor prognosis. Recently, the results of a small trial in which 20 patients with Ph-positive ALL or CML in lymphoid blast transformation were treated with the novel Abl tyrosine kinase inhibitor STI571 alone, revealed that 14 (70 per cent) had a haematological response, including 4 patients with a complete response (Druker and Lydon, 2000; Druker et al., 2001a). Most of the responses were short-lived, but the results are encouraging and further studies are in progress.

Postremission therapy

Once remission is achieved and normal haematopoiesis restored, therapy is continued in accordance with one or other established schedule. Most schedules incorporate the use of daily 6-mercaptopurine and weekly oral methotrexate concomitantly, with a once-monthly dose of alternating daunorubicin, vincristine and cyclophosphamide, or a similar alternative schedule. Some specialists prefer to use a more intensive regimen, in particular for the poor-risk category, and there is no definite agreement on the optimal schedule or the optimal duration, although the usefulness of this phase of the treatment is established, even in patients with low-risk disease. Its value, however, is less certain in adults with poor-risk disease and there is a trend to offer this cohort of patients a more intensive multidrug therapy (Chessells et al., 1995).

Following the completion of consolidation therapy, the optimal duration of which (as discussed above) remains uncertain, most patients in continuous CR, with the exception of those with mature B-cell phenotype, require prolonged continuation of treatment for a further few years. The validity of such an approach remains unclear but most specialists are of the opinion that long-term multidrug exposure may aid in destroying the residual lymphoblasts or assist in apoptosis. A recent meta-analysis of trials assessing the value of maintenance therapy concluded that it is of probable value but not beyond a period of 3 years (Childhood ALL Collaborative Group, 1996).

Treatment of relapsed ALL

Despite the significant improvement in the therapy of ALL, particularly in children, about 25 per cent of children and 50–60 per cent of adults experience a relapse. Remission can be regained in most of these patients, but in many cases it is not sustained. Factors that are associated with a poor outcome after a relapse include a shorter length of first remission, bone marrow as the initial site of relapse, older age, T-ALL, and male sex (Wheeler *et al.*, 1998). The MRC UKALLR1 study showed that patients who had a bone marrow relapse during the first 24 months following their initial diagnosis fared the worst (Lawson *et al.*, 2000). This study showed that patients with an isolated extramedullary relapse do have a better prognosis, even though many will have molecular evidence of bone marrow relapse (Neale *et al.*, 1994). The MRC UKALLX trial showed that only 3 per cent of patients with a bone marrow relapse are alive in second remission at 5 years, irrespective of the type of their second treatment. There is considerable uncertainty with regard to the appropriate further treatment once a second remission is established. There have been no prospective randomized trials of second post-remission chemotherapy versus stem-cell transplant and whatever evidence is available, is largely based on historical controls.

Stem-cell transplantation

Allogeneic SCT using an HLA-matched donor, preferably genotypically matched, is often offered to patients with ALL who have failed remission induction or have achieved a second CR (Appelbaum, 1997). Transplantation in first CR, as consolidation therapy, is considered unproved at present but may well be the desired treatment for those patients who fall in the poor-risk category (Sebban *et al.*, 1994). The role of autologous SCT remains unclear, despite encouraging preliminary results, with most comparative studies showing no major survival difference compared to chemotherapy (Billett *et al.*, 1993; Borgmann *et al.*, 1995). A small Italian study has suggested a possible role of autologous SCT in patients who sustain an early CNS relapse, but in general at present it is probably best to offer this treatment as part of a clinical trial (Messina *et al.*, 1998).

CONCLUSIONS

Notwithstanding the good results of intensive chemotherapy in children with good- and standard-risk ALL, the treatment of the remaining children and most adults remains relatively difficult. Substantial efforts are being directed to improve this scenario, both in terms of understanding the molecular pathogenesis better and new therapeutic agents, in addition to the potential role of SCT. One particular drug, arabinosylguanine (Compound

506U), has shown encouraging activity in T-cell ALL (Kurtzberg *et al.*, 1996). Targeted immunotherapy strategies are also being explored in an attempt to induce immune response against the lymphoblast (Braun *et al.*, 1997). Other new approaches include the use of immunotoxins and measures to enhance immune modulation, particularly following allogeneic SCT, in an attempt to reduce the risk of relapse (Ek *et al.*, 1998; Locatelli, 1998).

CHRONIC LEUKAEMIAS

Chronic myeloid leukaemia

CML is a clonal disease that results from an acquired genetic change in a pluripotential haemopoietic stem cell. The leukaemia cells have a consistent cytogenetic abnormality, the Ph chromosome, and contain a BCR–ABL fusion gene and its corresponding protein, which is considered to be the 'major' cause of chronic phase CML (Nowell and Hungerford, 1960; Rowley, 1973). This BCR–ABL oncoprotein has enhanced tyrosine kinase activity, which is considered responsible for its oncogenic activity (Groffen *et al.*, 1984). The discovery that this kinase activity could be inhibited in a highly specific manner has proved to be a major landmark in the treatment of patients with CML. CML was regarded as incurable for most of the last century, it gradually became clear in the 1980s that selected patients could indeed be accorded long-term remission and probably cure by allogeneic SCT (Goldman *et al.*, 1986; Mughal *et al.*, 2001). However, even today this treatment is available to only a minority of patients. In the last three years preliminary results of clinical studies using the Abl tyrosine kinase inhibitor, STI571 or imatinib mesylate, as a single-agent treatment for patients with CML have shown great promise but the follow-up is still too short for firm conclusions to be made (Druker *et al.*, 1996). Other important therapeutic advances include the introduction of interferon (IFN-α) and of adoptive immunotherapy with alloreactive lymphocytes, which can rescue patients who relapse following allogeneic SCT (Mughal and Goldman, 1995).

The incidence of CML is about 1–1.5 per 100 000 of population per annum. It represents approximately 15 per cent of all adult leukaemias and less than 5 per cent of all childhood leukaemias. The median age of onset is 50 years and there is slight male excess. Although in most cases there appears to be no predisposing factors, there is a marginally increased risk of developing CML following exposure to high doses of irradiation, as occurred in survivors of Hiroshima and Nagasaki atomic bombs in 1945 (Ichimaru *et al.*, 1978). A small number of families with a high incidence of the disease have been reported, and relapse of CML originating in donor cells following related allogeneic SCT has been recorded (Marmont *et al.*, 1984). Nevertheless it is extremely difficult

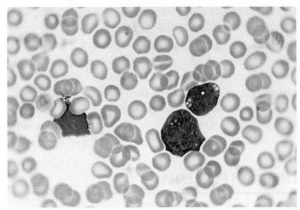

Figure 42.4 *A peripheral blood film from a patient with chronic myeloid leukaemia in the chronic phase (×960). Kindly provided by Professor Barbara Bain, Imperial College School of Medicine, London.*

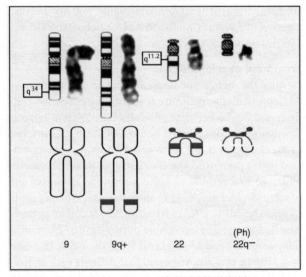

Figure 42.5 *Partial karyotype of the Philadelphia chromosome translocation t(9;22)(q34;q11) showing the breakpoints on chromosomes 9 and 22.*

to incriminate any aetiological factor in individual patients with CML.

Characteristically, CML is a biphasic or triphasic disease that is usually diagnosed in a stable or chronic phase (CP) which lasts typically 3–6 years. Figure 42.4 shows a peripheral blood film from a typical patient with CML in CP. About a third of such patients are diagnosed following a routine blood test and the remainder present with signs and symptoms related to anaemia and splenomegaly. The disease then spontaneously progresses to blast transformation with about 70–80 per cent of patients entering a myeloid blast transformation, and their survival is usually between 2 and 6 months; those entering a lymphoid blast transformation may have a slightly better survival. About half of the patients in the CP transform directly into blast transformation and the remainder do so following a period of accelerated phase.

MOLECULAR PATHOGENESIS

The Ph chromosome is an acquired cytogenetic abnormality present in all leukaemic cells of the myeloid lineage, and in some B cells and in a very small proportion of T cells in CML patients (Kurzrock *et al.*, 1988). It is formed as a result of a reciprocal translocation of the chromosomes 9 and 22, t(9;22)(q34;q11) (Fig. 42.5). The classical Ph chromosome is easily identified in 80 per cent of CML patients; in a further 10 per cent of patients, variant translocations which may be 'simple' involving chromosome 22 and a chromosome other than chromosome 9, or 'complex', where chromosome 9, 22 and other additional chromosomes are involved. About 8 per cent of patients with classical clinical and haematological features of CML lack the Ph chromosome and are referred to as cases of Ph-negative CML. About half of such patients have a BCR–ABL chimeric gene and are referred to as Ph-negative, BCR–ABL positive cases; the remainder are BCR–ABL negative and some of these have mutations in the *RAS* gene. It is probable that these latter

patients have a more aggressive clinical course. Some patients acquire additional clonal cytogenetic abnormalities, in particular +8, +Ph, iso17q− and +19, as their disease progresses. The emergence of such clones often heralds development of blastic transformation.

The various genomic events have now been elucidated and the chimeric BCR–ABL gene is believed to play a central role in the pathogenesis of CML, although the precise details are still not fully understood (Groffen and Heisterkamp, 1997; Sawyers, 1999). Three separate breakpoint locations on the BCR gene on chromosome 22 have been identified (Fig. 42.6). The break in the major breakpoint cluster region (M-BCR) occurs nearly always in the intron between exon e13 and e14 or in the intron between exon e14 and e15 (toward the telomere). By contrast, the position of the breakpoint in the ABL gene on chromosome 9 is highly variable and may occur at almost any position upstream of exon a2. The Ph translocation results in the juxtaposition of 5′ sequences from the BCR gene with 3′ sequences from the ABL gene. This event results in the generation of the chimeric BCR–ABL fusion gene transcribed as an 8.5 kb mRNA which encodes a protein of 210 kD (p210$^{BCR-ABL}$) that has a greater tyrosine kinase activity compared to the normal ABL protein. The different breakpoints in the M-BCR result in two slightly different chimeric BCR–ABL genes, resulting in either an e13a2 or e14a2 transcript. The type of BCR–ABL transcript has no important prognostic significance.

The second breakpoint location on the BCR gene occurs between exons e1 and e2 in an area designated the minor breakpoint cluster region (m-bcr) and forms a BCR–ABL transcript that is transcribed as an e1a2 mRNA which encodes for p190$^{BCR-ABL}$ (Ahuja *et al.*, 1991). This is found in about two-thirds of patients with Ph-positive ALL. A third breakpoint location is found in patients with

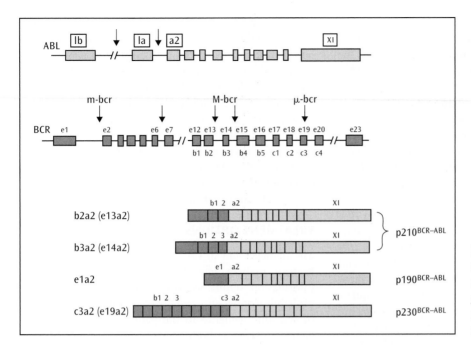

Figure 42.6 *A schematic representation of the various breakpoints in the ABL and BCR genes and the proteins encoded in BCR–ABL positive leukaemias.*

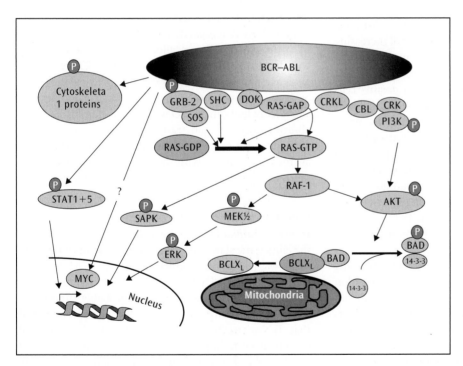

Figure 42.7 *Signal transduction pathways activated in BCR–ABL positive cells.*

the very rare Ph-positive chronic neutrophilic leukaemia (Pane *et al.*, 1996). This has been designated the micro breakpoint cluster region (μ-bcr) and results in e19a2 mRNA, which encodes a larger protein of 230 kD (p230^BCR–ABL).

The identification of several features in the BCR–ABL oncoprotein that are essential for cellular transformation led to the identification of signal transduction pathways activated in *BCR–ABL* positive cells (Fig. 42.7). Much attention has since focused on determining the precise role played by the various BCR–ABL proteins in the pathogenesis of CML (Deininger *et al.*, 2000). A number

of possible mechanisms of BCR–ABL mediated malignant transformation have been implicated, not necessarily mutually exclusive. These include constitutive activation of mitogenic signalling, reduced apoptosis, impaired adhesion of cells to the stroma and extracellular matrix, and proteasome-mediated degradation of ABL inhibitory proteins. The deregulation of the ABL tyrosine kinase facilitates autophosphorylation, resulting in a marked increase of phosphotyrosine on BCR–ABL itself, which creates binding sites for the SH2 domains of other proteins. A variety of such substrates, which can be tyrosine phosphorylated, have now been identified. Although much is known of the abnormal interactions between the BCR–ABL oncoprotein and other cytoplasmic molecules, the finer details of the pathways through which the 'rogue' proliferative signal is mediated, such as the RAS-MAP kinase, JAK-STAT, and the PI3 kinase pathways, are incomplete and the relative contributions to the leukaemic 'phenotype' are still unknown. Moreover, the multiple signals initiated by the BCR–ABL have both proliferative and anti-apoptotic qualities, which are often difficult to separate. Much remains to be learned about the significance of tyrosine phosphatases in the transformation process.

Normal haemopoietic stem cells survive in CML patients but they must presumably be maintained in a resting state (or 'deep' G_0 phase) as a result of the proliferation of CML cells. Under certain circumstances, however, these normal cells can be induced to proliferate and this provides the rationale for autografting as treatment for CML. There is also evidence for a profoundly quiescent subpopulation of primitive progenitor cells that are Ph-positive. This might be one reason why cycle-active cytotoxic drugs alone, even in high doses, may fail to eradicate the CML clone (Graham et al., 2002).

The Ph-positive cell is prone to acquire additional chromosomal changes, putatively as a result of increasing 'genetic instability', and this presumably underlies progression to advanced phases of the disease. The average length of chromosomal telomeres in the Ph-positive cells is generally less than that in corresponding normal cells and the enzyme telomerase, which is required to maintain the length of telomere, is upregulated as the patient's disease enters the advanced phases. About 25 per cent of patients with CML in myeloid transformation have point mutations or deletions in the p53 gene and about half of all patients in lymphoid transformation show homozygous deletion in the p16 gene (Epstein, 1999). There is some evidence supporting the role of the retinoblastoma (Rb) and the c-MYC genes.

At the cytokinetic level, the mechanism by which the BCR–ABL gene results in the preferential proliferation and differentiation of myeloid progenitors is also unclear. There is evidence for the presence of normal progenitors cells which are probably maintained in G_0 as a result of proliferation of leukaemic cells but can, under certain circumstances, be induced to proliferate (Graham et al., 2002; Holyoake et al., 1999).

PROGNOSTIC FACTORS

Various efforts have been made to establish criteria definable at diagnosis that may help to predict survival for individual patients (Sokal et al., 1984). The most frequently used method is that proposed by Sokal, whereby patients can be divided into various risk categories based on a mathematical formula that takes into account the patient's age, blast cell count, spleen size and platelet count at diagnosis. Stratifying patients into good-, intermediate- and poor-risk categories may assist in the decision-making

process regarding appropriate treatment options. Clinically, however, the best prognostic indicators seem to be the response to initial treatment with IFN-α, with those achieving haematological control of their disease having the best survival. The recently introduced Euro or Hasford system is an updated Sokal index, which includes consideration of response to IFN-α and basophils and eosinophils numbers (Hasford et al., 1998). Other possible prognostic factors are the presence or absence of deletions in the derivative 9q+ chromosome and the rate of shortening of telomeres in the leukaemia clone (Brümmendorf et al., 2000; Huntly et al., 2001).

TREATMENT OPTIONS

The management of CML epitomizes the art of shared decision-making, whereby the specialist gives factual information about available treatment options, the probability of benefits and the morbidity, and the degree of scientific evidence to the patient. This strategy has gained support as both transplant and non-transplant therapy for CML in CP has improved over the past decade and the real objective in the management needs to be addressed. It is prudent to discuss the relative merits of hydroxyurea, IFN-α, allografting and autografting with the patient at the time of diagnosis. There is good evidence that some patients can be cured by allogeneic SCT, and various methods have been designed to develop a risk score that can predict within broad limits the probability of survival and transplant-related mortality for individual patients (Gratwohl et al., 1998). The management of patients with the advanced phases of CML tends to be similar to that of those with poor-risk acute leukaemias.

Non-transplant treatment options

Interferon alpha Prior to the introduction of IFN-α into the clinics, the standard treatment for patients with CML in CP was hydroxyurea, which largely replaced busulphan in the early 1980s (Bolin et al., 1982). By the mid-1990s it was established that IFN-α was probably superior to either of these drugs and, more importantly, it appeared that IFN-α treatment resulted in a prolongation of overall survival, in particular for patients who achieved substantial cytogenetic responses (Allan et al., 1995). A meta-analysis of seven prospective randomized trials showed the superiority of IFN-α over both busulphan and hydroxyurea (Chronic Myeloid Leukemia Trialists' Collaborative Group, 1997). The analysis involved 1554 patients with CML in CP, and found a 5-year survival rate of 57 per cent for IFN-α-treated patients compared to 42 per cent for the chemotherapy-treated cohort. The absolute difference in 5-year survival for IFN-α against hydroxyurea and busulphan was 12 per cent and 20 per cent, respectively. It was observed that the disease duration may influence response rates and newly diagnosed patients fare best. The maximal cytogenetic response usually occurs by 12–18 months following IFN-α therapy

(European Study Group on Interferon in Chronic Myeloid Leukemia, 2002).

There are several important issues still unresolved with regard to IFN-α. The optimal dose remains a matter of some controversy, with the average weekly doses ranging from 9 to 35 MU or more (Silver *et al.*, 1999). A further area of increasing importance is the pharmaco-economic analysis of IFN-α usage in CML, since benefit appears to be marginal (Goldman, 1998). Moreover the duration of IFN-α treatment remains undefined. Toxicity is mild in general but is quite common. Most patients suffer from flu-like symptoms, lethargy and weight loss; less common side-effects include immune-mediated complications, such as thrombocytopenia and hypothyroidism. The notion of adding cytarabine to IFN-α appears attractive on the basis of several recent studies, and it may well be that initial treatment should be with IFN-α and cytarabine (Guilhot *et al.*, 1997; Tura, 1998).

STI571 (Imatinib mesylate) STI571 or imatinib mesylate is a 2-phenylaminopyrimidine, previously known as CGP 57148, which by occupying the kinase pocket of the BCR–ABL oncoprotein is able to block access to ATP, thereby preventing phosphorylation of any substrate (Fig. 42.8) (Goldman, 2000). Preclinical studies confirmed its efficacy in blocking the tyrosine kinase activity of ABL (Druker and Lydon, 2000). STI571 entered clinical trials in 1998 and current results are indeed quite impressive, with more than 90 per cent of patients in the CP refractory or resistant to IFN-α obtaining complete haematological responses (Druker *et al.*, 2001b; Goldman and Melo, 2001; Kantarjian *et al.*, 2002). About 40–45 per cent of these patients achieved cytogenetic responses, which were major in about 30 per cent. Both the haematological and cytogenetic responses occur much earlier than with IFN-α. Patients with CML in blast crisis, both myeloid and lymphoid, also responded, though less durably (Druker *et al.*, 2001a). STI571 was administered orally and so far side effects have been relatively minor. Despite the follow-up being still relatively short, this novel drug has already become the preferred non-transplant treatment option (Mughal and Goldman, 2001). Recent follow-up data suggest that responses (haematological and cytogenetic) are sustained but there are relatively few molecular remissions (Hochhaus, 2002). STI571 is currently being compared with IFN-α and low-dose cytarabine in a randomized trial of newly diagnosed patients. It is also likely to be tested in combination with various chemotherapeutic agents or IFN-α or pegylated IFN-α.

Acquired resistance to STI571 appears to result from some *BCR–ABL* positive cells evading its inhibitory effects by diverse mechanisms, including *BCR–ABL* overexpression as a possible consequence of *BCR–ABL* gene amplification, P-glycoprotein overexpression resulting in the reduction in the uptake of STI571, and possibly excessive degradation of the *BCR–ABL* protein. The acquisition of compensatory mutations in genes other than *BCR–ABL* may also contribute to STI571 resistance (Gorre *et al.*, 2001). Point mutations in the Abl kinase domain have been identified in some patients whose disease progressed after initial response to STI571.

Stem-cell transplantation

Allogeneic SCT using blood- or marrow-derived stem cells performed in the CP can cure selected patients with CML and cure depends on the contribution of graft versus leukaemia (GvL) effect (Thomas *et al.*, 1986; Barrett and Malkovska, 1996). A recent analysis of data collated by the International Bone Marrow Transplant Registry (IBMTR) revealed that the probability of event-free survival (EFS) at 5 years is 55–60 per cent (Horowitz *et al.*, 1996a). The probability of relapse at 5 years was 15 per cent. In contrast, the results of allogeneic SCT performed in more advance phases of the disease are generally poor. The major determinants for survival, other than the phase of the disease, include the patient's age at transplant and the cytomegalovirus (CMV) status of the patient, and the age and sex of the donor. Survival appears to be best for patients who are transplanted within 1 year of diagnosis, are less than 40 years of age, have a young male donor, and both patient and donor are CMV seronegative. For such a cohort, the 5-year EFS is probably around 70–80 per cent, and the relapse rate 10–20 per cent. It is possible that the precise details of the transplant procedure and the choice of stem cells (marrow versus peripheral blood) also influence the outcome. Following a peripheral-blood SCT, the patients appear to achieve rapid engraftment but there may be a slight excess of chronic GvHD, perhaps due to the increased T-cell numbers in the peripheral blood compared to bone marrow. There has also been some concern with regard to the effect of prior IFN-α therapy following an initial observation suggesting a possible detrimental effect, and further careful monitoring is warranted (Horowitz *et al.*, 1996b).

The best results from allogeneic SCT are from a HLA-identical sibling donor; such donors are available for less than 30 per cent of patients eligible for SCT. Many efforts

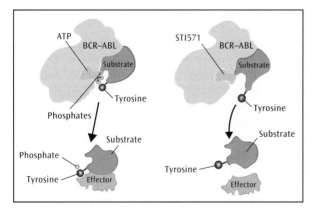

Figure 42.8 *Schematic representation of the mode of action of STI571 (imatinib mesylate). Adapted from Goldman* et al. *2001.*

have been directed toward the search for suitable volunteer unrelated donors (VUD). Newer molecular techniques for subtyping the class I antigens are now in the clinics and should improve the chances of finding such phenotypically matched or acceptably mismatched donors (Spencer *et al.*, 1995). The results of VUD SCT are inferior to those of sibling SCT due to the increased rate of graft failure, GvHD and transplant-related mortality (TRM). The presence of GvHD greatly increases the risk of TRM and morbidity post-SCT from infections. GvHD prophylaxis with the combination of cyclosporin and methotrexate has been shown to be superior to use of cyclosporin alone. Additional T-cell depletion of the graft is often used to prevent GvHD, in particular in VUD SCT. This is effective, but there is significant increase in the relapse rate of CML as the GvHD effect is accompanied by GvL, which both depend on T cells. Current results from the Seattle group suggest an EFS of 57 per cent at 5 years in patients who were under the age of 55 years, and an EFS of 74 per cent for patients under the age of 50 years who were transplanted within 1 year of diagnosis (Hansen *et al.*, 1998). Clearly these results are remarkable and approach the cure rates accorded by genotypically matched donors. Syngeneic SCT in CML has a comparable overall survival to sibling SCT, but due to the lack of a GvL effect, there is a higher relapse rate, resulting in lower EFS. Allo-SCT from other family members who are partially matched requires intensive conditioning regimens and has a higher toxicity from GvHD and graft failure.

Efforts to minimize the toxicity of conditioning regimens to make SCT more available to higher risk and perhaps older patients have been benefited by the advent of the purine analogues which are potent immunosuppressive agents. These regimens can therefore be non-myeloablative and yet, due to the addition of such immunosuppressive drugs as fludarabine, ensure adequate engraftment. These procedures have been termed mini-SCT or non-myeloablative SCT and signal the exciting advance in our understanding of how SCT actually works (Slavin *et al.*, 1998b).

Treatment for relapse of CML post-transplant

In the 10–20 per cent of patients who relapse post allo-SCT for CML, this occurs in the first 3 years. This relapse tends to follow an orderly progression, with the patient initially demonstrating evidence of a molecular relapse with increasing positivity of BCR–ABL transcripts by PCR, followed by a cytogenetic relapse when the Ph chromosome is found and then haematological and clinical relapse. Molecular monitoring of all SCT recipients is therefore valuable (Mughal *et al.*, 2001). For patients with molecular relapse, remission can be re-induced simply by withdrawal of immunosuppression or by the transfusion of donor lymphocytes (DLI), providing additional evidence of the potent role of GvL in CML (Collins *et al.*, 1997; Goldman, 1999). DLI can induce remissions in 60–80 per cent of patients with molecular

or cytogenetic relapse. The potential benefit of adding IFN-α to DLI is currently being assessed. Patients who fail to enter remission with DLI may be treated with imatinib mesylate. They may also be candidates for a second allo-SCT but the risk of TRM is relatively high.

Autologous stem-cell transplantation

Despite the qualified success associated with allo-SCT, the majority of CML patients are not eligible for this therapy and the vast majority have little cytogenetic response to IFN-α. Autologous SCT following high-dose chemotherapy has a lower TRM and is available to more patients. Retrospective analyses suggest that autografting with blood- or marrow-derived stem cells can prolong survival (Mughal *et al.*, 1993; McGlave *et al.*, 1994). It is now also widely recognized that some Ph-negative stem cells survive at the time of diagnosis in most patients, lending support to efforts being made to develop autografting techniques that favour reconstitution with Ph-negative haematopoiesis. The Genoa group has reported the results of harvesting predominantly Ph-negative stem cells following high-dose chemotherapy using a combination of idarubicin, cytarabine and etoposide (Carella *et al.*, 1997). Patients autografted with Ph-negative stem cells may achieve Ph-negative haematopoiesis, which is durable in some cases.

Other groups have attempted to isolate Ph-negative cells by *in vitro* marrow-purging methods, such as incubation with 4-hydroxyperoxycyclophosphamide and, more recently, antisense oligonucleotides and ABL-specific tyrosine kinase inhibitors, which uniquely inhibit the proliferation of CML but not of other myeloid cell lines from CML patients. Other *in vivo* purging methods being pursued include combinations of IFN-α and chemotherapy. In general, the clinical results appear to be better than when unmanipulated grafts are used, but most patients will ultimately develop 100 per cent Ph-positive haematopoiesis. The somewhat overdue randomized trials to establish the precise role of autografting are currently in progress.

CONCLUSIONS

The enormous understanding of the molecular anatomy and pathophysiology of CML has provided important insights into targeting the treatment to specific molecular defects. The successful introduction of STI571 as targeted therapy for CML has made the approach to management of the newly diagnosed patient fairly complex. It is useful to assess the various treatment options carefully in terms of the relative risk–benefit ratios and develop a management strategy accordingly. For the present such an approach should define a patient cohort in which the risk of transplant-related mortality is relatively low and for whom one can reasonably recommend an early allogeneic SCT as primary therapy, and defining another cohort for which allogeneic SCT should not be considered.

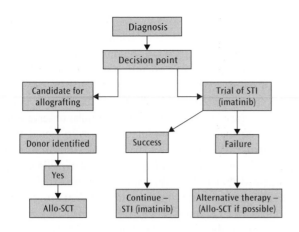

Figure 42.9 *A suggested therapeutic algorithm for the treatment of patients with chronic myeloid leukaemia in the chronic phase.*

This would leave an intermediate cohort for whom the advisability of early transplant is uncertain (Fig. 42.9). Such patients could reasonably receive an initial trial of STI571 or IFN-α and proceed to allogeneic SCT only if they are deemed to have failed the therapeutic trial. For patients over the age of 60 years, a similar approach can be adopted using a low-intensity SCT, possibly followed by DLI. It can be anticipated that should the current results obtained with STI571 prove to be durable, then perhaps all patients should be offered a trial of STI571 in the first instance, followed perhaps by some form of immunotherapy to eradicate residual disease. The current revised indications for allogeneic SCT, in particular for the molecularly matched unrelated recipients, will then need further revision. It is noteworthy that the total number of CML patients transplanted is already declining, ahead of firmly established evidence of the long-term efficacy of STI571 (Gratwohl *et al.*, 2001).

Chronic lymphocytic leukaemia

Chronic lymphocytic leukaemia (CLL) typically consists of a clonal expansion of mature, long-lived, functionally deficient B-lymphocytes that express high levels of the anti-apoptotic protein BCL-2 (Hanada *et al.*, 1993). The CLL malignant cells also characteristically express high levels of a further anti-apoptotic protein, BCL-XD, and low levels of the pro-apoptotic protein, BAX, and are therefore resistant to apoptosis (Pepper *et al.*, 1996). It is the most common type of leukaemia in the western world, accounting for more than 30 per cent of all leukaemias, and affects people over the age of 40 years. It is very rare in the orient, although the reason for this is unknown. It is more prevalent in males, with a male : female ratio of 2 : 1. The median age of occurrence is 60 years, and the incidence increases steadily with age, reaching 40 per 100 000 of adults in the eighth decade. In the US over 10 000 new cases are diagnosed each year.

Unlike the other leukaemias, CLL is not induced by exposure to any known chemicals or irradiation, although one study observed an increase in CLL among persons chronically exposed to electromagnetic fields (Feychting *et al.*, 1997). Should this latter observation be confirmed, it would have broad public health implications, in particular with the increasing technologies, such as cellular telephones, employing electromagnetic radiation. Recently there was some speculation that CLL might be causally linked to infection by HTLV-1, based upon a small Jamaican study, but this remains unconfirmed (Mann *et al.*, 1987). A second related retrovirus, HTLV-2, has been identified in some cases of T-cell prolymphocytic leukaemia (PLL) and T-cell hairy cell leukaemia (Kalyanaraman *et al.*, 1982).

DIAGNOSIS OF CLL

The characterization of CLL is based on cell morphology and immunological markers, as proposed by the FAB group (Bennett *et al.*, 1982). Immunophenotyping is useful in distinguishing B- from T-cell disorders and from a variety of the related lymphoproliferative disorders such as hairy cell leukaemia, PLL, lymphoplasmacytoid lymphomas and the leukaemic phase of follicular non-Hodgkin's lymphoma (Catovsky *et al.*, 1981). The first formal guidelines for the diagnosis of CLL were proposed in 1989 by a joint National Cancer Institute (US) and the International Workshop on Chronic Lymphoid Leukemia group (International workshop on Chronic Lymphocytic Leukemia, 1989). These guidelines were revised in 1996 and a minimum diagnostic criterion was suggested – a blood lymphocytosis (absolute lymphocyte count of at least 5000/mm³) with mature-appearing lymphocytes and a characteristic immunophenotype of monoclonal B cells, described as: surface immunoglobulin (most often IgM or IgM and IgD) of low intensity with either κ or λ light chain, expression of pan-B-cell antigens (CD19, CD20 and CD23) and the co-expression of CD5 on the leukaemic B cells (Cheson *et al.*, 1996). CLL cells are typically negative for surface CD22 and FMC7. Most cells are in the G_0 phase of the cell cycle and are unresponsive to standard mitogenic stimuli.

Over the past decade the overlap in the immunophenotypic features among the various B-cell disorders have been increasingly documented; in particular the expression of potential disease-specific markers such as CD5, considered to be CLL specific, is also positive in mantle-cell lymphoma (Pombo de Oliveira *et al.*, 1989). There also appears to be a degree of heterogeneity in the expression of certain markers within the specific disease category, which may well be useful prognostically (Legac *et al.*, 1991). The Royal Marsden group have examined these aspects and proposed a scoring system for the diagnosis of CLL based on reactivity with CD5, CD23 and FMC7 and the intensity of expression of membrane immunoglobulins and CD22 (Matutes *et al.*, 1994a). Each marker is assigned a value of 0 or 1 according to whether it is typical or not for CLL. Scores range from 5 (typical CLL) to 0 (atypical CLL). This method has been validated and is useful in facilitating the diagnosis and classification of CLL and related disorders.

About 40 per cent of all patients with CLL are diagnosed by a routine blood test for unrelated reasons. The remainder present with fever, weight loss, lymphadenopathy, hepatosplenomegaly and infections.

MOLECULAR PATHOGENESIS

Unlike other leukaemias, in which a variety of molecular events have been elucidated, CLL remains undefined at the molecular level for the moment. Small studies have demonstrated several molecular abnormalities, but these have not been confirmed (Gaidano et al., 1994). It is possible that the monotonous morphology of the CLL cells may represent the result of varying molecular events (Fig. 42.10). Cytogenetic abnormalities occur in about 50 per cent of all patients with CLL, with trisomy 12 and 13q14 deletions being the most frequent. The finding of these abnormalities is considered to be a poor prognostic feature (Matutes, 1996). Molecular evidence of a minimal region of deletion (MRD) spanning <300 kb and common to all CLL cell lines with 13q14 deletions has been identified, suggesting that the abnormalities at 13q14 may represent a common event in the pathogenesis of CLL (Kalachikov et al., 1997).

The potential role of the immunoglobulin (Ig) genes is expressed in CLL in the pathogenesis of the disease. CLL cells have been speculated in view of the somatically mutated Ig variable-region genes, despite having several features characteristic of naïve B cells, indicating that the cell of origin has passed through the germinal centre (Caligaris-Cappio, 1996). Rai's group in New York have recently established the presence of Ig V gene mutation and the expression of CD38 on CLL cells (Damle et al., 1999). These investigators found that those patients with unmutated V genes (both V_H and V_L) displayed higher percentages of CD38+ cells compared to those with mutated V genes. Patients in the unmutated and higher CD38+ groups were frequently noted to have trisomy 12 advanced stage and have a significantly poorer survival. These patients generally fared poorly with polychemotherapy, including fludarabine. Similar observations have been made by Hamblin's group, who noted that unmutated V_H genes also had atypical morphology (Hamblin et al., 1999). In a recent update, this group confirmed that CD38 expression and immunoglobulin variable region mutations are independent prognostic variables in CLL, but CD38 expression may vary during the course of the disease (Hamblin et al., 2002).

STAGING SYSTEMS AND PROGNOSTIC FACTORS

Rai's staging system, first introduced in 1975, is based on Dameshek's proposed model of orderly disease progression in CLL, and consists of five stages (Rai et al., 1975). The Rai stages were found to correlate with prognosis. Binet (also known as the International staging system for CLL) thereafter developed a similar system consisting of three stages and it largely superseded Rai's system (Binet et al., 1981). Both systems are shown in Table 42.3. Rai's system has been revised more recently to include three stages: low risk (Rai 0–1), intermediate risk (Rai 2) and high risk (Rai 3–4) (Rai, 1987). The poor prognosis associated with the unmutated V genes and an overexpression of CD38 are relatively new entrants to the list of other previously well-established prognostic factors, such as doubling of the lymphocyte counts in less than 12 months, a diffuse pattern of involvement on the trephine biopsy and an abnormal karyotype.

TREATMENT

It is prudent to recognize that some patients with CLL have an indolent disease and may not require any specific

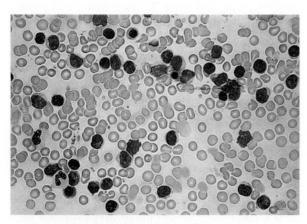

Figure 42.10 *A peripheral blood film from a patient with chronic lymphoid leukaemia (×960). Kindly provided by Professor Daniel Catovsky, Royal Marsden Hospital, London.*

Table 42.3 *Rai and Binet staging systems for chronic lymphocytic leukaemia*

Rai stage	
0	Lymphocytosis
1	Lymphocytosis and lymphadenopathy
2	Lymphocytosis and splenomegaly or hepatomegaly
3	Lymphocytosis and anaemia (haemoglobin < 11 g/dl)
4	Lymphocytosis and thrombocytopenia (platelets < 100 000/μl)
Binet stage	
A	Two or fewer lymphoid-bearing areas
B	Three or more lymphoid-bearing areas
C	Presence of anaemia (haemoglobin < 10 g/dl) and/or thrombocytopenia (platelets < 100 000/μl)

therapy, since this would not prolong survival, although over 50 per cent of all early-stage patients with CLL eventually progress and require treatment (Dighiero *et al.*, 1998). Most specialists offer treatment when patients present with more advanced disease (Rai high risk; Binet stage C). It may also be desirable to begin treatment when patients develop 'B' symptoms (weight loss, fevers, night sweats), there is progressive evidence of increasing tumour burden and the development of autoimmune anaemia or thrombocytopenia.

Chlorambucil, either alone or with a glucocorticoid steroid, usually prednisolone, has been the most frequently used first-line drug in the treatment of CLL for almost four decades. Cyclophosphamide orally is an equivalent drug. For patients presenting with more advanced disease, combination chemotherapy is often resorted to. The most common regimens are cyclophosphamide, vincristine and prednisolone; sometimes an anthracycline is also added. Although these latter regimens have resulted in higher responses, there are no major durable responses or survival advantages compared to chlorambucil. A recent meta-analysis on data collated by the CLL Trialists' Collaborative Group validates these observations and confirmed no survival advantages for immediate versus deferred chemotherapy in patients with early-stage CLL (Chronic Lymphocytic Leukemia Trialists' Collaborative Group, 1999). It is, however, important to note that this analysis is applicable to treatment with alkylating agents and may not be useful for newer drugs such as fludarabine.

Fludarabine (9-β-D-arabinofuranosyl-2-fluroadenine monophosphate) is a purine analogue, which has been found to be a remarkably effective treatment for CLL patients resistant to chorambucil (Keating, 1990). The drug is generally myelosuppressive and may be associated with an increased risk of viral infections. A recent randomized US trial comparing fludarabine with chorambucil in newly diagnosed patients with CLL has confirmed a higher incidence of CR (27 per cent versus 3 per cent), overall responses (70 per cent versus 43 per cent) and duration of these responses (2.75 years versus 1.4 years) in the fludarabine-treated cohorts, but no evidence of prolongation of survival (Rai *et al.*, 1996). A smaller French randomized study of fludarabine versus CAP (cyclophosphamide, Adriamycin and prednisolone) revealed similar findings (French Cooperative Group on CLL, 1996). Currently most specialists use fludarabine for second-line therapy of CLL patients. Other new drugs that have now entered the clinics include cladribine (2′-chlordeoxyadenosine) and pentostatin (5′-deoxycoformycin).

Preliminary results with allogeneic and autologous SCT for the treatment of advanced-stage CLL in young adults demonstrate high response rates with durable CR (Rabinowe *et al.*, 1993). Long-term follow-up, using PCR amplification and sequencing of the rearranged IgH from the original malignant clone, show that most of the patients remain disease free and free of PCR-detected MRD, suggesting that this treatment may offer the chance of cure to selected patients with poor-risk CLL (Provan *et al.*, 1996; Forsyth *et al.*, 2000). Recent results collated by the EBMT and IBMTR registries confirm the applicability of SCT, both allogeneic and autologous, for the treament of patients with Rai poor-risk CLL who are under the age of 50 years (Michallet, 1998). The 5-year EFS for the patients who were allografted was 34 per cent, and for autografted patients it was 28 per cent. The risk of relapse for the allografted group was 40 per cent and for the autografted group, 70 per cent. These preliminary experiences are encouraging and further studies are in progress. The concept of fludarabine-based non-myeloablative conditioning regimens being able to enhance the GvL effect and decrease toxicity attributed to conditioning has also been demonstrated (Khouri *et al.*, 1997; Esteve *et al.*, 2001). This latter experience suggests that standard-dose fludarabine-based chemotherapy is sufficiently immunosuppressive to allow engraftment, and subsequent DLI should enhance the GvL effect further.

Other investigational therapies include the use of monoclonal antibodies, in particular Campath 1-H (a mouse antibody against CD52) and the heavy- and light-chain constant regions of human IgG1 and kappa, respectively. Preliminary results from several small phase I/II studies have demonstrated its effectiveness as salvage therapy in about a third of patients who relapsed following an initial response with fludarabine (Bowen *et al.*, 1997). Some of the current studies are also assessing the role of Campath-1 H as first-line therapy compared to chorambucil. Combination therapy of fludarabine, Campath-1 H and rituximab (mabthera) is also being considered as potential investigational second-line treatment based on small pilot studies. Campath-1 H is also being investigated as an *in vivo* purging agent in patients being considered for autologous SCT. Gene transfer of CD40-ligand has been shown to induce autologous immune recognition of CLL cells and is being developed further for the treatment of CLL (Kato *et al.*, 1998).

LYMPHOPROLIFERATIVE DISORDERS RELATED TO CLL

T-cell chronic lymphocytic leukaemia

Epidemiology studies from the Far East suggest that T-cell CLL, which represents less than 3 per cent of all European and US CLL patients, is the dominant form of this disease in Asia. Morphological and immunophenotyping studies suggest this disease to be a PLL subtype. Patients often present with pancytopenia and prominent splenomegaly and the lack of lymphadenopathy is noteworthy. The general prognosis is similar to that of poor-risk CLL and most patients tend to be refractory to fludarabine treatment.

Prolymphocytic leukaemia

PLL can be *de novo* or arise as a consequence of CLL transformation. PLL cells are larger and less homogeneous than CLL cells, and have a clear and more abundant cytoplasm, clumped nuclear chromatin, and a single prominent nucleolus (Melo *et al.*, 1987). The immunophenotype of a PLL cell is FMC7+, CD22+ and surface IgM+. Cytogenetic analysis often reveals 14q+ and t(11;14) (q13;q32). Most patients have a clinical course similar to that of poor-risk CLL and do respond to fludarabine. A minority of patients have an indolent course.

Large granular lymphocytic leukaemia

Large granular lymphocytes (LGL) are a heterogeneous group of large lymphocytes, which express CD8 and CD56 (previously known as natural killer or NK) surface antigens and are associated with antibody-dependent cell-mediated cytotoxicity. LGL leukaemia, also described as Tγ lymphoproliferative disorder, has a varied natural history, ranging from an indolent condition to that of ALL (Catovsky and Foa, 1990). Most patients present with recurrent infections, anaemia and splenomegaly, and usually no significant lymphadenopathy.

The majority of patients with LGL leukaemia do not require any specific treatment at presentation and various strategies have been offered on an *ad hoc* basis, including prednisolone, cyclophosphamide (low dose), IFN-α, splenectomy and intensive chemotherapy for the more aggressive forms. The prognostic factors associated with poor prognosis are fever, low CD56 expression and low granular lymphocyte counts.

Hairy cell leukaemia

Hairy cell leukaemia (HCL) is a mature B-lymphoproliferative disorder characterized by distinct clinical, morphological and histological features (Matutes *et al.*, 1994b). It is characterized by splenomegaly and marrow failure in conjunction with infiltration of myeloid tissues by a lymphoid cell with villous processes that project from the cytoplasm of the cell. Immunophenotyping is useful to distinguish HCL from B-cell disorders with hairy or villous lymphocytes, such as the variant form of HCL or splenic lymphoma with villous lymphocytes (SLVL). Typically, HCL cells express the following markers: CD11c, CD25, HC2 and B-ly-7. The Royal Marsden group devised a scoring system based on these four markers, for a more accurate diagnosis of HCL (Mulligan *et al.*, 1991).

The identification and precise diagnosis of these disorders is important because of the prognostic and therapeutic implications. Whereas patients with typical HCL (Catovsky Score 4) respond to IFN-α and 5′-deoxycoformycin (pentostatin), these drugs are less useful in the variant form of HCL and splenectomy is the treatment of choice for SLVL (Wong-Staal and Gallo, 1985).

Adult T-cell leukaemia/lymphoma

Adult T-cell leukaemia/lymphoma (ATL) is a distinct form of leukaemia/lymphoma first described on the island of Kyushu in southern Japan and subsequently found to occur in the Caribbean, US and other countries (Morimoto *et al.*, 1985). Epidemiological studies have described the causal association between ATL and HTLV-I (van Leeuwen, 1996). It has a median age of occurrence of 40 years. ATL cells typically have the phenotype of mature helper T cells and express CD2, CD3 and CD4 antigen. They also express CD25 and clonal rearrangement of the T-cell receptor β chain is often present. Cytogenetic abnormalities are common and include trisomy 3q or 6q−, 14q and inv(14).

ATL is characterized by lymphadenopathy and hepatosplenomegaly. There is a high incidence of cutaneous involvement, which may take a variety of forms. Lytic bone lesions and hypercalcaemia occur commonly. Standard therapy is similar to that employed in the management of poor-prognosis high-grade lymphoma, but the outcome is generally unsatisfactory. Allogeneic SCT could be contemplated if a suitable donor is available.

MYELODYSPLASTIC SYNDROMES

The myelodysplastic syndromes (MDS) are clonal disorders characterized clinically and morphologically by ineffective haematopoiesis leading to bone-marrow failure and a high probability of malignant transformation at the level of a myeloid stem cell, resulting in AML (Koeffler and Golde, 1980). It has been proposed that MDS should be considered as a pre-leukaemic condition in which the malignant clone has the potential to evolve into AML or not; transformation into ALL is extremely rare. MDS generally affects patients over the age of 60 years; although an increasing number of younger adults are being reported, mostly with therapy-associated MDS (t-MDS). With the exception of the 5q− syndrome, men appear to be affected more often than women. Childhood MDS is rare and found in constitutional conditions such as Down syndrome.

MOLECULAR PATHOGENESIS AND DIAGNOSIS

The cytogenetic events that lead to MDS are heterogeneous but certain abnormalities, such as loss or gain of all or parts of chromosomes 5, 7, 8 and 20 tend to prevail (Pedersen-Bjergaard and Rowley, 1994). The precise molecular changes involved, in particular those that result in transformation into AML, has not been fully elucidated but a number of potential candidate genes have been identified (Davis and Greenberg, 1998). These include the N-*ras*, the *p53*, the *IRF-1*, the *bcl-2*, the *p15INK* and the *MLL* genes. It is likely that sequential mutations leading to genetic abnormalities are required. The natural history and biology of MDS, like that of AML, depends upon the nature of the underlying events. Those patients who have a balanced chromosomal translocation are more likely to present with frank transformation into AML in contrast to those with unbalanced translocation, who are likely to present in the 'earlier' stages of MDS with transformation occurring following further genetic events (Heaney and Golde, 1999). For example patients with the 5q− cytogenetic abnormality tend to have a rather benign clinical course and only about 25 per cent will transform into AML following additional genetic events.

Most patients are diagnosed as a consequence of pancytopenia on a routine examination, which are the result of ineffective haematopoiesis rather than a lack of haematopoietic activity. The diagnosis of MDS is often suspected on morphological grounds in a patient with cytopenias. The bone-marrow cellularity is either normal or increased. Characteristic morphological changes include mature hypogranular and hypolobulated (pseudo-Pelger–Huët) granulocytes, micromegakaryocytes and a variety of red-cell precursor abnormalities, ranging from ringed sideroblasts to megaloblastic changes. Dysplastic abnormalities in all cell lineages are prominent (Hofmann et al., 1996). Cytogenetic analysis using the fluorescence in situ hybridization technology and PCR studies on bone marrow samples is a useful tool in confirming the diagnosis and facilitating classification. Cytokinetic studies of bone marrow cells suggest a substantially higher rate of cell division and apoptosis is prominently increased. Other potentially useful studies currently being assessed include magnetic resonance imaging (Takagi et al., 1999).

CLASSIFICATIONS

The FAB classification, proposed in 1982, almost 30 years following the landmark description of MDS (when the term 'preleukaemia' was designated) by Matthew Block and colleagues, is intended for diagnostic and prognostic purposes (Table 42.4) (Block et al., 1953). The classification has several important limitations. Firstly, the term 'refractory anaemia' is imprecise and cannot be identified morphologically. Secondly, chronic myelomonocytic leukaemia is perhaps more closely related to the myeloproliferative disorders than to the other subtypes of MDS. Thirdly, the use of an arbitrary criteria, for example the

percentage of marrow blasts, to distinguish between an advanced MDS and a frank AML is often misleading. In general, the attempt by this FAB classification scheme to separate MDS as a distinct disorder from AML has been considered a significant negative. In an attempt to establish a scientifically more accepted classification, two alternative schema have been proposed. The WHO classification is based largely on the use of 20 per cent blasts in the bone marrow as a means to separate transforming MDS and AML (Harris et al., 1999). This classification also has severe limitations since there is little concordance for the clinical, molecular and biological features of the proposed sub-categories (Greenberg et al., 1997). An alternative classification proposed by the International Myelodysplastic Syndrome Risk Analysis Workshop has attempted to assign a score in accordance to the clinical and biological features (Estey et al., 1997). Patients are assigned a score based upon the cytogenetic abnormalities, the percentage of blasts in the marrow and the number of lineages affected in the cytopenia and stratified into four prognostic groups: low score (median survival 5.7 years), intermediate score subgroup 1 (median survival 3.5 years), intermediate score subgroup 2 (median survival 1.2 years) and high score (median survival 0.4 year). This system appears to have had an international approval and may well become the classification system of choice for the immediate future.

CLINICAL SYNDROMES

Among patients with MDS, those with certain associated or underlying genetic events appear to have a unique natural history and it is sometimes convenient to consider them as separate clinical entities. These include the 5q− syndrome, which is characterized by a relatively indolent clinical course (Van dern Berghe et al., 1974). Anaemia is often the major manifestation but mild neutropenia can also occur; thrombocytosis is also often present. Red cell support is often the sole treatment accorded. Hypoplastic

Table 42.4 *The FAB classification of the myelodysplastic syndromes*

Category	Peripheral blood	Bone marrow
Refractory anaemia (RA) or refractory cytopenia[a]	Anaemia[a], blasts <1%, monocytes <1 × 10⁹/1	AND Blasts <5%, ring sideroblasts <15% of erythroblasts
Refractory anaemia with ring sideroblasts (RARS)	Anaemia, blasts <1%, monocytes <1 × 10⁹/1	AND Blasts <5%, ring sideroblasts >15% of erythroblasts
Refractory anaemia with excess of blasts (RAEB)	Anaemia, blasts >1%, Monocytes <1 × 10⁹/1 blasts <5%	OR Blasts >5% AND Blasts >20%
Chronic myelomonocytic leukaemia (CMML)	Monocytes >1 × 10⁹/1, granulocytes often increased, blasts <5%	Blasts up to 20%, promonocytes often increased
Refractory anaemia with excess of blasts in transformation (RAEB-t)	Blasts >5% or Auer rods in blasts in bone or marrow	OR Blasts >20% BUT Blasts <30%

[a] Or, in the case of refractory cytopenia, either neutropenia or thrombocytopenia.

myelodysplasia tends to be unique, not so much from its clinical manifestations or its natural history, but rather from a diagnostic perspective since these patients can often be diagnosed as aplastic anaemia (Tuzuner et al., 1995). The demonstration of the characteristic MDS cytogenetic abnormalities allows the correct diagnosis to be made. Therapy-related myelodysplasia is caused by chemotherapy or radiotherapy that results in cytogenetic events which dictate its clinical course (Pedersen-Bjergaard et al., 1995). In general, the prognosis with t-MDS tends to be worse compared to the other subtypes of MDS since many of these patients have the cytogenetic abnormalities associated with a poor prognosis, in particular those in whom it is associated with high-dose chemotherapy followed by autologous SCT (Pedersen-Bjergaard et al., 2000). Deletions or loss of chromosome 5 and 7 are often associated with exposure to alkylating agents (Christiansen et al., 2001). Balanced translocations involving chromosomes 3, 11 and 21 are associated with topoisomerase II inhibitors, such as epipodophyllotoxins and anthracyclines.

TREATMENT

Chemotherapy

Standard AML-type chemotherapy, in general, has resulted in unsatisfactory results and it would be appropriate to treat patients with MDS in accordance to their prognostic score. It is of interest to note that when patients are stratified in this way, there are no major differences between the outcome of patients with MDS and AML with an equivalent genetic abnormality (Estey et al., 1998). Patients with deletions in chromosome 7 and trisomy 8 appear to fare particularly badly. In contrast, patients with 5q− syndrome can often be maintained on supportive red-cell transfusions alone for long periods. Induction regimens containing some of the newer drugs, such as topotecan, have shown encouraging responses (Morosetti and Koeffler, 1996).

Differentiating agents, such as low-dose cytarabine, 5-aza-2′-deoxycytidine, retinoids and cholecalciferols have been assessed extensively, based on in vitro observations that the myeloblasts in MDS might be induced to differentiate and that remission might be achieved without a marrow aplasia. The results, for the most part, have been disappointing (Matthews, 1998).

Haematopoietic growth factors

Haematopoietic growth factors, in particular G-CSF and granulocyte–macrophage colony stimulating factor (GM-CSF), have been investigated and found to be moderately useful in the correction of neutropenias, but most cytopenias returned to their pre-therapy levels once the growth factors were discontinued (Vadhan-Raj et al., 1987). Currently, combinations of G-CSF or GM-CSF, erythropoietin, stem-cell factor and, in some cases, differentiating agents are being evaluated. Parenthetically, some concern was expressed recently following the observation of

increasing blasts in a cohort of patients receiving G-CSF compared to a placebo. Erythropoietin leads to a reduced red cell transfusion requirement in about 25 per cent of patients, in particular those with low serum erythropoietin levels, but patients with high serum erythropoietin levels may also respond (Hellstrom-Lindberg, 1995).

Immunotherapy

Steroids have been used frequently either alone or in combination therapies and in general have been found to have a low response rate and increase risk to infection. The antithymocyte globulins (ATG) have been used to treat the hypoplastic MDS and small series suggest short-term responses in about two-thirds of the patients (Biesma et al., 1997). ATG therapy has also been investigated in patients with other subtypes of MDS and found to be of a modest benefit (Molldrem et al., 1997). Substantial haematological responses have been reported following treatment with cyclosporin A in patients with the refractory anaemia and refractory anaemia with excess blast subtypes of MDS (Jonasova et al., 1998). Currently a number of trials evaluating the combination of ATG, cyclosporin A and other forms of immunotherapy including interleukin-6, interleukin-3, interleukin-11 (thrombopoeitin) and IFN-α are in progress and should help define the potential benefits of such therapy. Recently there has also been interest in cytokine inhibition strategies. Amifostine, an agent which suppresses inflammatory cytokine release, including TNF-α and reduces apoptosis in MDS, has been evaluated in a small study and the preliminary results are encouraging, particularly in patients with single lineage cytopenias (List et al., 1999). It is also being combined with growth factors and chemotherapy. Pentoxifylline, another agent which can interfere with the signal pathways of the cytokines TNF-α, TGF-β and IL-1β is also being investigated in a variety of novel approaches (Raza et al., 2000). Studies with thalidomide are also in progress and early indications of an improvement of marrow function noted (Raza et al., 2001).

Stem-cell transplantation

Allogeneic SCT, using an HLA-matched sibling donor, offers the only chance of achieving a cure to a small proportion of patients with MDS. Historically, the results of allografting these patients have been considerably poorer than those with AML and no MDS due to a higher relapse rate (Demuynck et al., 1996). It has been speculated that the higher disease burden and poor prognosis cytogenetic features present in many of the MDS patients may be the major factors. There is, however, some uncertainty with regard to the use of chemotherapy prior to SCT and the importance of the disease burden. Current results of allografting such patients with more effective conditioning regimens have led to better results. The Seattle group has demonstrated a long-term EFS of about 75 per cent for patients under the age of 40 years (Appelbaum and Anderson, 1998). Results of allografting using a matched unrelated volunteer donor have also improved with transplantation earlier in the course of the disease and better conditioning (Anderson *et al.*, 1996). Recent results on 50 patients aged 55–66 years who received an allograft either from an HLA-identical sibling or a matched unrelated donor following conditioning with cyclophosphamide and busulphan show an EFS of 47 per cent at 3 years for the HLA-identical sibling cohort and 39 per cent for all the patients (Deeg *et al.*, 2000). It is possible that further progress may result from the use of non-myeloablative allogeneic SCT followed by donor lymphocyte infusions (Slavin *et al.*, 1998a). Such an approach should be particularly suitable for older patients.

Autologous SCT may be useful for patients who achieve a remission following chemotherapy and are not suitable for an allogeneic SCT. This concept gains support from the observation that some patients with MDS exhibit morphologically and cytogenetically normal haematopoiesis following chemotherapy. Several co-operative groups have assessed the value of autologous SCT following chemotherapy in patients with high-risk MDS and current results suggest EFS of about 30 per cent at 2 years, although the relapse rates were high (De Witte *et al.*, 1997). In two parallel studies, 184 patients from the EORTC–EBMT trials were compared with 216 patients from the MD Anderson Cancer Center in Houston, Texas receiving chemotherapy only and preliminary results support the use of autologous SCT (Oosterveld *et al.*, 1999).

CONCLUSIONS

Despite the significant increase in the understanding of the molecular pathogenesis of MDS, little is known about the various interactions between the immune system and the MDS stem cell and the bone marrow microenvironment. Further insights should facilitate a better application of the current and evolving treatments such as the use of CD33 monoclonal antibodies and non-myeloablative SCT (Caron *et al.*, 1998). Better biological understanding, classification and tools should help estimate the risk of transformation for individual patients and a risk-adapted therapeutic strategy can be offered.

SIGNIFICANT POINTS

Biology

- Cytogenetics are valuable for classifying acute leukaemia and for assessing prognosis.
- The AML-1, MLL and PML-RARα genes play a crucial role in pathogenesis of AML.

- The BCR–ABL fusion protein plays a central role in the pathogenesis of CML and other Philadelphia-positive leukaemias.
- Abnormalities in chromosome 13q14 are common in CLL.
- Some types of therapy-related acute leukaemia involve specifically chromosome 11q23.
- Several candidate genes are implicated in the transformation of MDS to AML.

Treatment

- Molecular and immunological strategies to target leukaemic cells are now in clinical trials.
- STI571, a new ABL-kinase inhibitor, is active in patients with CML in both chronic and advanced phases.
- ATRA is part of standard treatment for APL.
- Allo-SCT results in long-term remissions, perhaps 'cure', for the majority of eligible patients with CML.
- Allo-SCT established as 'post-remission' or 'consolidation' therapy for acute leukaemia.
- Non-myeloablative allogeneic SCT is now being tested for various forms of leukaemia.
- DLI is valuable for CML patients who relapse after allo-SCT and proves the existence of an allogeneic GvL effect.
- Remissions in MDS are difficult to achieve and in many cases supportive therapy is appropriate.
- Conventional treatment of CLL does not greatly prolong life.

KEY REFERENCES

Appelbaum, F.R. (1997) Allogeneic hematopoietic stem cell transplantation for acute leukemia. *Semin. Oncol.* **24**, 114–23.

Bennett, J.M., Catovsky, D., Daniel, M.T. *et al.* (1976) Proposals for the classification of the acute leukaemias. *Br. J. Haematol.* **33**, 451–8.

Chronic Lymphocytic Leukemia Trialists' Collaborative Group (1999) Chemotherapeutic options in chronic lymphocytic leukemia: a meta-analysis of the randomized trials. *J. Natl Cancer Inst.* **91**, 861–8.

Goldman, J.M. (2000) Tyrosine-kinase inhibition in treatment of chronic myeloid leukaemia. *Lancet* **355**, 1031–2.

Greenberg, P., Cox, C., LeBeau, M.M. *et al.* (1997) International scoring system for evaluating prognosis in myelodysplastic syndromes. *Blood* **89**, 2079–88 [Erratum: (1998) *Blood* **91**, 1100].

Lowenberg, B., Downing, R. and Burnett, A. (1999) Acute myeloid leukemia. *N. Engl. J. Med.* **341**, 1051–62.

Sawyers, C.L. (1999) Chronic myeloid leukemia. *N. Engl. J. Med.* **340**, 1330–40.

REFERENCES

Ahuja, H., Bar-Eli, M., Arlin, Z. *et al.* (1991) The spectrum of molecular alterations in the evolution of chronic myeloid leukemia. *J. Clin. Invest.* **87**, 2042–6.

Allan, N.C., Richards, S.M. and Shepherd, P.C.A. (1995) UK Medical Research Council randomised multicentre trial of interferon-αn1 for chronic myeloid leukaemia: improved survival irrespective of cytogenetic response. *Lancet* **345**, 1392–7.

Anderson, J.E., Anasetti, C., Appelbaum, F.R. *et al.* (1996) Unrelated donor marrow transplantation for myelodysplasia (MDS) and MDS-related acute myeloid leukaemia. *Br. J. Haematol.* **93**, 59–67.

Anino, L., Vegna, M.L., Camera, A. *et al.* (2002) Treatment of adult acute lymphoblastic leukemia (ALL): long-term follow-up of the GIMEMA ALL 028 randomized study. *Blood* **99**, 863–71.

Appelbaum, F.R. (1997) Allogeneic hematopoietic stem cell transplantation for acute leukemia. *Semin. Oncol.* **24**, 114–23.

Appelbaum, F.R. (2002) Hematopoietic cell transplantation as immunotherapy. *Nature*, in press.

Appelbaum, F.R. and Anderson, J. (1998) Allogeneic bone marrow transplantation for myelodysplastic syndromes: outcome analysis according to IPSS score. *Leukemia* **12**(suppl. 1), S25–S29.

Appelbaum, F.R., Dahlberg, S., Thomas, E.D. *et al.* (1984) Bone marrow transplantation or chemotherapy after remission induction for adults with acute nonlymphoblastic leukemia: a prospective comparison. *Ann. Intern. Med.* **101**, 581–8.

Arlin, Z., Case, D.C. Jr, Moore, J. *et al.* (1990) Randomized multicenter trial of cytosine arabinoside with mitoxantrone or daunorubicin in previously untreated adult patients with acute nonlymphocytic leukaemia (ANLL). *Leukemia* **4**, 177–83.

Austin, A., Delzell, E. and Cole, P. (1988) Benzene and leukemia: a review of the literature and risk assessment. *Am. J. Epidemiol.* **137**, 419.

Barrett, A.J. and Malkovska, V. (1996) Graft-versus-leukaemia: understanding and using the allo-immune response to treat hematological malignancies. *Br. J. Haematol.* **93**, 754–61.

Bennett, J.M., Catovsky, D., Daniel, M.T. *et al.* (1976) Proposals for the classification of the acute leukaemias. *Br. J. Haematol.* **33**, 451–8.

Bennett, J.M., Catovsky, D., Daniel, M.T. *et al.* (1982) Proposals for the classification of the myelodysplastic syndromes. *Br. J. Haematol.* **51**, 189–99.

Bennett, J.M., Catovsky, D., Daniel, M.T. *et al.* (1985) Proposed revised criteria for the classification of acute myeloid leukemia: a report of the French–American–British Co-operative Group. *Ann. Intern. Med.* **103**, 620–5.

Bennett, J.M., Catovsky, D., Daniel, M.T. *et al.* (1989) Proposals for the classification of chronic (mature) B and T lymphoid leukaemias. *J. Clin. Path.* **42**, 567–84.

Bennett, J.M., Catovsky, D., Daniel, M.T. *et al.* (1991) Proposal for the recognition of minimally differentiated acute myeloid leukaemia (AML-MO). *Br. J. Haematol.* **78**, 325–9.

Bennett, J.M., Catovsky, D., Daniel, M.T. *et al.* (1994) The chronic myeloid leukaemias: guidelines for distinguishing chronic granulocytic, atypical chronic myeloid and chronic myelomonocytic leukaemia. Proposals by the French–American–British Co-operative Leukaemia Group. *Br. J. Haematol.* **87**, 746–55.

Berman, E., Heller, G., Santorsa, J. *et al.* (1991) Results of a randomized trial comparing idarubicin and cytosine arabinoside with daunorubicin and cytosine arabinoside in adult patients with newly diagnosed acute myelogenous leukemia. *Blood* **77**, 1666–74.

Biesma, D.H., van den Tweel, J.G. and Verdonck, L.F. (1997) Immunosuppressive therapy for hypoplastic myelodysplastic syndrome. *Cancer* **79**, 1548–51.

Billett, A.L., Kornmehl, E., Tarbell, N.J. *et al.* (1993) Autologous bone marrow transplantation after a long first remission for children with recurrent acute lymphoblastic leukemia. *Blood* **81**, 1651.

Binet, J.L., Augier, A., Dighiero, G. *et al.* (1981) A new prognostic classification of chronic lymphocytic leukemia derived from a multivariate survival analysis. *Cancer* **48**, 198.

Bishop, J.F., Matthews, J.P., Young, G.A. *et al.* (1999) A randomized study of high-dose cytarabine in induction in acute myeloid leukaemia. *Blood* **87**, 1710–17.

Block, M., Jacobson, L.O. and Bethard, W.F. (1953) Preleukemic acute human leukemia. *JAMA* **152**, 361–5.

Bloomfield, C.D. and Brunning, R.D. (1985) The revised French–American–British classification of acute myeloid leukemia: is new better? *Ann. Intern. Med.* **103**, 614–16.

Bolin, R.W., Robinson, W.A., Sutherland, J. *et al.* (1982) Busulfan versus hydroxyurea in the long-term therapy of chronic myelogenous leukemia. *Cancer* **50**, 1683–7.

Borgmann, A., Schmid, H., Hartmann, R. *et al.* (1995) Autologous marrow transplants compared with chemotherapy for children with acute lymphoblastic leukaemia in a second remission: a matched pair analysis. *Lancet* **346**, 873.

Bowen, A.L., Zomas, A., Emmett, E. *et al.* (1997) Subcutaneous CAMPATH-1H in fludarabine-resistant/relapsed chronic lymphocytic and B-prolymphocytic leukaemia. *Br. J. Haematol.* **96**, 617–19.

Braun, S.E., Chen, K., Battiwalla, M. *et al.* (1997) Gene therapy strategies for leukemia. *Mol. Med. Today* **3**, 39–46.

Brümmendorf, T.H., Holyoake, T.L., Rufer, N. *et al.* (2000) Prognostic implications of differences in telomere length between normal and malignant cells from patients with chronic myeloid leukemia measured by flow cytometry. *Blood* **95**, 1883–90.

Buchner, T., Urbanitz, D., Hiddemann, W. *et al.* (1985) Intensive induction and consolidation with or without maintenance chemotherapy for acute myeloid leukaemia (AML): two multicenter studies of German AML Co-operative Group. *J. Clin. Oncol.* **3**, 1583–9.

Burnett, A.K., Goldstone, A.H., Stevens, R.M.F. *et al.* (1998) Randomised comparison of addition of autologous bone-marrow transplantation to intensive chemotherapy for acute myeloid leukaemia in first remission: results of MRC AML 10 trial. *Lancet* **351**, 700–8.

Burnett, A.K., Goldstone, A.H. and Milligan, D.W. (1999a) Daunorubicin versus mitoxantrone as induction for AML in younger adults given intensive chemotherapy: preliminary results of MRC AML 12 trial. *Br. J. Haematol.* **105**(suppl. 1), 67a.

Burnett, A.K., Grimwade, D., Solomon, E. *et al.* (1999b) Presenting white blood cell count and kinetics of molecular remission predict prognosis in acute promyelocytic leukemia treated with all-*trans*-retinoic acid: results of randomized MRC trial. *Blood* **94**, 3015–21.

Caligaris-Cappio, F. (1996) B-chronic lymphocytic leukemia: a malignancy of anti-self B cells. *Blood* **87**, 2615.

Carella, A.M., Cunningham, I., Lerma, E. *et al.* (1997) Mobilization and transplantation of Philadelphia-negative peripheral blood progenitor cells early in chronic myelogenous leukemia. *J. Clin. Oncol.* **15**, 1575.

Caron, P.C., Dumont, L. and Scheinberg, D.A. (1998) Supersaturating infusional humanized anti-CD-33 monoclonal antibody HuM195 in myelogenous leukemia. *Clin. Cancer Res.* **4**, 1421–8.

Cassileth, P.A., Harrington, D.P., Appelbaum, F.R. *et al.* (1998) Chemotherapy compared with autologous or allogeneic bone marrow transplantation in the management of acute myeloid leukemia in first remission. *N. Engl. J. Med.* **339**, 1649–56.

Catovsky, D. and Foa, R. (1990) *The lymphoid leukemias*, 1st edn. London: Butterworth.

Catovsky, D., Cherchi, M., Brooks, D. *et al.* (1981) Heterogeneity of B-cell leukemias demonstrated by the monoclonal antibody FMC7. *Blood* **58**, 406–8.

Cheson, B.D., Bennett, J.M., Grever, M. *et al.* (1996) National Cancer Institute-Sponsored Working Group guidelines for chronic lymphocytic leukemia: revised guidelines for diagnosis and treatment. *Blood* **87**, 4990.

Chessells, J.M., Bailey, C. and Richards, S.M. (1995) Intensification of treatment and survival in all children with lymphoblastic leukaemia: results of UK Medical Research Council trial UKALL X. *Lancet* **345**, 143–8.

Chessells, J.M., Hall, E., Prentice, H.G. *et al.* (1998) The impact of age on outcome in lymphoblastic leukaemia: MRC UKALL X and XA compared: a report from the MRC Paediatric and Adult Working Parties. *Leukemia* **12**, 463–73.

Childhood ALL Collaborative Group (1996) Duration and intensity of maintenance chemotherapy in acute lymphoblastic leukaemia: overview of 42 trials involving 12,000 randomised children. *Lancet* **347**, 1783–8.

Christiansen, D.H., Andersen, M.K. and Pedersen-Bjergaard, J. (2001) Mutations with loss of heterozygosity of p53 are common in therapy-related myelodysplasia and acute myeloid leukemia after exposure to alkylating agents and significantly associated with deletion or loss of 5q, a complex karyotype, and poor prognosis. *J. Clin. Oncol.* **19**, 1405–13.

Chronic Lymphocytic Leukemia Trialists' Collaborative Group (1999) Chemotherapeutic options in chronic lymphocytic leukemia: a meta-analysis of the randomized trials. *J. Natl Cancer Inst.* **91**, 861–8.

Chronic Myeloid Leukemia Trialists' Collaborative Group (1997) Interferon alpha versus chemotherapy for chronic myeloid leukemia: a meta-analysis of seven randomized trials. *J. Natl Cancer Inst.* **89**, 1616–20.

Collins, R.H., Shpilberg, O., Drobyski, W.R. *et al.* (1997) Donor leukocyte infusions in 140 patients with relapse malignancy after allogeneic bone marrow transplantation. *J. Clin. Oncol.* **15**, 433.

Conter, V., Schrappe, M., Arico, M. *et al.* (1997) Role of cranial radiotherapy for childhood T-cell acute lymphoblastic leukemia with high WBC count and good response to prednisolone. *J. Clin. Oncol.* **15**, 2786–91.

Cortes, J.E. and Kantarjian, H.M. (1995) Acute lymphoblastic leukemia: a comprehensive review with emphasis on biology and therapy. *Cancer* **76**, 2393–417.

Cortes, J., O'Brien, S., Pierce, S. *et al.* (1995) The value of high-dose systemic chemotherapy and intrathecal therapy for central nervous system prophylaxis in different risk groups of adult acute lymphoblastic leukemia. *Blood* **86**, 2091.

Damle, R.N., Wasil, T., Fais, F. *et al.* (1999) Ig V gene mutation status and CD38 expression as novel prognostic indicators in chronic lymphocytic leukemia. *Blood* **94**, 1840.

Davis, R.E. and Greenberg, P.L. (1998) Bcl-2 expression by myeloid precursors in myelodysplastic syndromes: relation to disease progression. *Leuk. Res.* **22**, 767–77.

Dedre, D.A., Waller, E.K., LeBrun, D.P. *et al.* (1993) Chimeric homeobox gene E2A-PBX1 induces proliferation, apoptosis, and malignant lymphomas in transgenic mice. *Cell* **74**, 833–43.

Deeg, H.J., Shulman, H.M., Andersen, J.E. *et al.* (2000) Allogeneic and syngeneic marrow transplantation for myelodysplastic syndromes in patients 55 to 66 years of age. *Blood* **95**, 1188–94.

Deininger, M.W., Goldman, J.M. and Melo, J.V. (2000) The molecular biology of chronic myeloid leukemia. *Blood* **96**, 3343–56.

Demuynck, H., Verhoef, G.E., Zachee, P. *et al.* (1996) Treatment of patients with myelodysplastic syndromes with allogeneic bone marrow transplantation from genotypically HLA-identical sibling and alternative donors. *Bone Marrow Transplant* **17**, 745–51.

De Witte, T., Van Biezen, A., Hermans, J. *et al.* (1997) Autologous bone marrow transplantation for patients with myelodysplastic syndrome (MDS) or acute myeloid leukemia following MDS. *Blood* **90**, 3853–7.

Dighiero, G., Maloum, K., Desablens, B. *et al.* (1998) Chlorambucil in indolent chronic lymphocytic leukemia. *N. Engl. J. Med.* **338**, 1506.

Dombret, H., Chastang, C., Fenaux, P. *et al.* (1995) A controlled study of recombinant human granulocyte colony-stimulating factor in elderly patients after treatment for acute myelogenous leukemia. *N. Engl. J. Med.* **332**, 1678–83.

Druker, B.J. and Lydon, N.B. (2000) Lessons learned from the development of an Abl tyrosine kinase inhibitor for chronic myelogenous leukemia. *J. Clin. Invest.* **105**, 3–7.

Druker, B.J., Tamura, S., Buchdunger, E. *et al.* (1996) Effects of a selective inhibitor of the Abl tyrosine kinase on the growth of BCR-ABL positive cells. *Nat. Med.* **2**, 561.

Druker, B.J., Sawyers, C.L., Kantarjian, H. *et al.* (2001a) Activity of a specific inhibitor of the BCR–ABL tyrosine kinase in blast crisis of chronic myeloid leukemia and acute lymphoblastic leukemia with the Philadelphia chromosome. *N. Engl. J. Med.* **344**, 1038–42.

Druker, B.J., Talpaz, M., Resta, D. *et al.* (2001b) Efficacy and safety of a specific inhibitor of the BCR–ABL tyrosine kinase in chronic myeloid leukemia. *N. Engl. J. Med.* **344**, 1031–7.

EBMT (1998) Allogeneic bone marrow transplantation for leukemia in Europe: report from the Working Party on Leukemia, European Group for Bone Marrow Transplantation. *Lancet* **1**, 1379–82.

Ek, O., Gaynon, P., Zeren, T. *et al.* (1998) Treatment of human B-cell precursor leukemia in SCID mice by using a combination of the anti-CD immunotoxin B43-PAP with the standard chemotherapeutic drugs vincristine, methylprednisolone, and L-asparaginase. *Leuk. Lymphoma* **31**, 143.

Epstein, F.H. (1999) The biology of chronic myeloid leukemia. *N. Engl. J. Med.* **341**, 164–72.

Esteve, J., Villamor, N., Colomer, D. *et al.* (2001) Stem cell transplantation for chronic lymphocytic leukemia: different outcome after autologous and allogeneic transplantation and correlation with minimal residual disease status. *Leukemia* **15**, 445–51.

Estey, E., Thall, P., Beran, M. *et al.* (1997) Effect of diagnosis (refractory anemia with excess blasts, refractory anemia with excess blasts in transformation, or acute myeloid leukemia [AML]) on outcome of AML-type chemotherapy. *Blood* **90**, 2969–77.

Estey, E., Kantarjian, H., Giles, F. *et al.* (1998) Treatment of newly diagnosed AML and MDS with cyclophosphamide, Ara-C, topotecan. *Blood* **92**(suppl. 1), 232a.

European Study Group on Interferon in Chronic Myeloid Leukemia (2002) Chronic myeloid leukemia and α-interferon. A study of complete cytogenetic responders. *Blood*, in press.

Fenaux, P., Castaigne, S., Dombret, H. *et al.* (1992) All-transretinoic acid followed by intensive chemotherapy gives a high complete remission rate and may prolong remissions in newly diagnosed acute promyelocytic leukemia: a pilot study on 26 cases. *Blood* **80**, 2176–81.

Fenaux, P., Chastang, C., Chevret, S. *et al.* (1999) A randomized comparison of all-*trans*-retinoic acid (ATRA) followed by chemotherapy and ATRA plus chemotherapy and the role of maintenance therapy in newly diagnosed acute promyelocytic leukemia. The European APL group. *Blood* **94**, 1192–200.

Feychting, B., Forssen, U. and Floderus, B. (1997) Occupational and residential magnetic field exposure and leukemia and central nervous system tumors. *Epidemiology* **8**, 384.

First MIC Co-operative Study Group (1986) Morphologic, immunologic and cytogenetics (MIC) working classification of acute lymphoblastic leukaemias. *Cancer Genet. Cytogenet.* **23**, 189–97.

Ford, A.M., Bennett, C.A., Price, C.M. *et al.* (1998) Fetal origins of the TEL-AML1 fusion gene in identical twins with leukemia. *Proc. Natl Acad. Sci. USA* **95**, 4584–8.

Forsyth, P.D., Milligan, D.W., Davies, F.E. *et al.* (2000) High-dose chemoradiotherapy with autologous stem cell rescue for patients with CLL is an effective and safe means of inducing molecular responses: an MRC pilot study. *Blood* **96**, 843a (abstract).

Fourth International Workshop on Chromosomes in Leukemia, 1982 (1984) Clinical significance of chromosome abnormalities in acute nonlymphoblastic leukemia. *Cancer Genet. Cytogenet.* **11**, 332–50.

French Cooperative Group on CLL (1996) Multicentre prospective randomized trial of fludarabine versus cyclophosphamide, doxorubicin, and prednislone (CAP) for treatment of advanced stage chronic lymphocytic leukaemia. *Lancet* **347**, 1432.

Gaidano, G., Newcomb, E.W., Gong, J.Z. *et al.* (1994) Analysis of alterations of oncogenes and tumor suppressor genes in chronic lymphocytic leukemia. *Am. J. Pathol.* **144**, 1312.

Goldman, J.M. (1998) Cost effectiveness of interferon-α for chronic myeloid leukaemia. *Ann. Oncol.* **9**, 351–2.

Goldman, J.M. (1999) Donor lymphocyte infusion for chronic myelogeneous leukemia. *Blood* **94**(10: suppl. 1), 60.

Goldman, J.M. (2000) Tyrosine-kinase inhibition in treatment of chronic myeloid leukaemia. *Lancet* **355**, 1031–2.

Goldman, J.M. and Melo, J.V. (2001) Targeting the BCR–ABL tyrosine kinase in chronic myeloid leukemia. *N. Engl. J. Med.* **344**, 1084–6.

Goldman, J.M., Apperley, J.F., Jones, L.M. *et al.* (1986) Bone marrow transplantation for patients with chronic myeloid leukemia. *N. Engl. J. Med.* **314**, 202.

Golub, T.R., Slonim, D.K., Tamayo, P. *et al.* (1999) Molecular classification of cancer: class discovery and class prediction by gene expression monitoring. *Science* **286**, 531–7.

Gorin, N.C. (1998) Autologous stem cell transplantation in acute myelocytic leukemia. *Blood* **92**, 1073–90.

Gorin, N.C., Labopin, M., Meloni, G. *et al.* (1991) Autologous bone marrow transplantation for acute myeloblastic leukemia in Europe: further evidence of the role of marrow purging by mafosfamide. *Leukemia* **5**, 896–904.

Gorre, M.E., Mohammed, M., Ellwood, K. *et al.* (2001) Clinical resistance to STI571 cancer therapy caused by BCR–ABL gene mutation or amplification. *Science* **293**, 876–80.

Graham, S.M., Jørgensen, H.G., Allan, E. *et al.* (2002) Primitive, quiescent, Philadelphia-positive stem cells from patients with chronic myeloid leukemia are insensitive to STI571 *in vitro*. *Blood* **99**, 319–25.

Gratwohl, A., Hermans, J., Goldman, J. *et al.* (1998) Risk assessment for patients with chronic myeloid leukaemia before allogeneic blood or marrow transplantation. *Lancet* **352**, 1078–92.

Gratwohl, A., Passweg, J., Baldomero, H. *et al.* (2001) Hematopoetic stem cell transplantation activity in Europe. *Bone Marrow Transplant* **27**, 899–916.

Greaves, M.F. (1997) Aetiology of acute leukaemia. *Lancet* **349**, 344–9.

Greenberg, P., Cox, C., LeBeau, M.M. *et al.* (1997) International scoring system for evaluating prognosis in myelodysplastic syndromes. *Blood* **89**, 2079–88 [Erratum: (1998) *Blood* **91**, 1100].

Grigani, F., De Matteis, S., Nervi, C. *et al.* (1998) Fusion proteins of the retinoic acid receptor-alpha recruit histone deacetylase in promyelocytic leukaemia. *Nature* **391**, 815–18.

Grimwade, D. and Solomon, E. (1997) Characterisation of the PML/RAR alpha rearrangement associated with t(15:17) acute promyelocytic leukaemia. *Curr. Top. Microbiol. Immunol.* **220**, 81–112.

Grimwade, D., Walker, H., Oliver, F. *et al.* (1998) The importance of diagnostic cytogenetics on outcome in AML: analysis of 1,612 patients entered into the MRC AML 10 Trial. *Blood* **92**, 2322–33.

Groffen, J. and Heisterkamp, N. (1997) The chimeric BCR–ABL gene. *Bailliere's Clin. Haematol.* **10**, 187.

Groffen, J., Stephenson, J.R., Heisterkamp, N. *et al.* (1984) Philadelphia chromosomal breakpoints are clustered within a limited region, bcr, on chromosome 22. *Cell* **36**, 93.

Group Français de Cytogenetique Hematologique (1996) Cytogenetic abnormalities in adult acute lymphoblastic leukemia: correlations with hematologic findings and outcome: a collaborative study of the Groupe Français de Cytogenetique Hematologique. *Blood* **87**, 3135–42 [Erratum: (1996) *Blood* **88**, 2818].

Guilhot, F., Chastang, C., Michallet, M. *et al.* (1997) Interferon alpha-2b combined with cytarabine versus interferon alone in chronic myelogenous leukemia. *N. Engl. J. Med.* **337**, 223.

Hamblin, T.J., Davis, Z., Gardiner, A. *et al.* (1999) Unmutated Ig V$_H$ genes are associated with a more aggressive form of chronic lymphocytic leukemia. *Blood* **94**, 1848–54.

Hamblin, T.J., Orchard, J.A., Ibbotson, R.E. *et al.* (2002) CD38 expression and immunoglobulin variable region mutations are independent prognostic variables in chronic lymphocytic leukemia, but CD38 expression may vary during the course of the disease. *Blood* **99**, 1023–9.

Hanada, M., Delia, D., Aiello, A. *et al.* (1993) bcl-2-gene hypomethylation and high-level expression in B-cell chronic lymphocytic leukemia. *Blood* **82**, 1820.

Hansen, J.A., Gooley, T.A., Martin, P.J. *et al.* (1998) Bone marrow transplantation from unrelated donors for patients with chronic myeloid leukemia. *N. Engl. J. Med.* **338**, 962.

Harousseau, J.L., Cahn, J.Y., Pignon, B. *et al.* (1997) Comparison of autologous bone marrow transplantation and intensive chemotherapy as postremission therapy in adult acute myeloid leukemia. *Blood* **90**, 2978–86.

Harris, A.W., Pinkert, C.A., Crawford, M. *et al.* (1988) The Emu-myc transgenic mouse: a model for high-incidence spontaneous lymphoma and leukemia of early B cells. *J. Exp. Med.* **167**, 353–71.

Harris, N.L., Jaffe, E.S., Diebold, J. *et al.* (1999) The World Health Organization classification of the hematologic malignancies report of the clinical advisory committee meeting, Airlie House, Virginia, November 1997. *J. Clin. Oncol.* **17**, 3835–49.

Hasford, J., Pfirrmann, M., Hehlmann, R. *et al.* (1998) A new prognostic score for survival of patients with chronic myeloid leukaemia treated with interferon alfa. *J. Natl Cancer Inst.* **90**, 850–8.

Heaney, M.L. and Golde, D.W. (1999) Myelodysplasia. *N. Engl. J. Med.* **340**, 1649–60.

Hellstrom-Lindberg, E. (1995) Efficacy of erythropoietin in the myelodysplastic syndromes: a meta-analysis of 205 patients from 17 studies. *Br. J. Haematol.* **89**, 831–7.

Hochhaus, A. (2002) Lack of a molecular remission in patients with chronic myeloid leukemia following a complete cytogenetic remission with STI571. Personal communication.

Hoelzer, D., Ludwig, W.D., Thiel, E. *et al.* (1996) Improved outcome in adult B-cell acute lymphoblastic leukemia. *Blood* **87**, 495–508.

Hofmann, W.K., Ottomann, O.G., Ganser, A. *et al.* (1996) Myelodysplastic syndromes: clinical features. *Semin. Hematol.* **33**, 177–85.

Holyoake, T., Jiang, X., Eaves, C. and Eaves, A. (1999) Isolation of a highly quiescent subpopulation of primitive leukemic cells in chronic myeloid leukemia. *Blood* **94**, 2056–64.

Horowitz, M.M., Rowlings, P.A. and Passweg, J.R. (1996a) Allogeneic bone marrow transplantation for chronic myeloid leukemia: a report from the International Bone Marrow Transplant Registry. *Bone Marrow Transplant* **17**(suppl. 3), S5–S6.

Horowitz, M.M., Giralt, S., Szydlo, R. *et al.* (1996b) Effect of prior interferon therapy on outcome of HLA-identical sibling bone marrow transplants for chronic myelogenous leukemia (CML) in first chronic phase. *Exp. Hematol.* **24**, 1143.

Huntly, B.L., Reid, A.G., Bench, A.J. *et al.* (2001) Deletions of the derivative chromosome 9 occur at the time of the Philadelphia translocation and provide a powerful and independent prognostic indicator in chronic myeloid leukemia. *Blood* **98**, 1732–8.

Ichimaru, M., Ishimaru, T. and Belsky, J.L. (1978) Incidence of leukemia in atomic bomb survivors belonging to a fixed cohort in Hiroshima and Nagasaki, 1950–1971: radiation dose, years after exposure, age at exposure, and type of leukemia. *J. Radiat. Res.* **19**, 262.

Inaba, T., Inukai, T., Yoshihara, T. *et al.* (1996) Reversal of apoptosis by the leukaemia-associated E2A-HLF chimaeric transcription factor. *Nature* **382**, 541–4.

International Workshop on Chronic Lymphocytic Leukemia (1989) Chronic lymphocytic leukemia: recommendations for diagnosis, staging and response criteria. *Ann. Intern. Med.* **110**, 236.

Jing, Y., Wang, R., Xai, L. *et al.* (2001) Combined effects of all-*trans*-retinoic acid and arsenic trioxide in acute promyelocytic leukemia cells *in vitro* and *in vivo*. *Blood* **97**, 264–9.

Jonasova, A., Neuwirtova, R., Cermak, J. *et al.* (1998) Cyclosporin A therapy in hypoplastic MDS patients and certain refractory anaemias without hypoplastic bone marrow. *Br. J. Haematol.* **100**, 304–9.

Jurcic, J.G., DeBlasio, T., Dumont, L. *et al.* (2000) Molecular remission induction with retinoic acid and anti-CD33 monoclonal antibody HuM195 in acute promyelocytic leukemia. *Clin Cancer Res.* **6**, 372–80.

Kalachikov, S., Migliazza, A., Cayanis, E. *et al.* (1997) Cloning and gene mapping of the chromosomes 13q14 region detected in chronic lymphocytic leukemia. *Genomics* **42**, 369.

Kaldor, J.M., Day, N.E., Clarke, E.A. *et al.* (1990) Leukemia following Hodgkin's disease. *N. Engl. J. Med.* **322**, 7.

Kalyanaraman, V.S., Sarnagadharan, M.G., Robert-Guroff, M. *et al.* (1982) A new subtype of human T-cell leukemia virus (HTLV-2) associated with a T-cell variant of hairy cell leukemia. *Science* **218**, 561.

Kantarjian, H., Sawyers, C., Hochhaus, A. *et al.* (2002) Hematologic and cytogenetic responses to imatinib mesylate in chronic myelogenous leukemia. *N. Engl. J. Med.* **346**, 645–52.

Karp, J.E., Lancet, J.E., Kaufmann, S.H. *et al.* (2001) Clinical and biologic activity of farnesyltransferase inhibitor R115777 in adults with refractory and relapsed acute leukemias: a phase I clinical-laboratory correlative trial. *Blood* **97**, 3361–9.

Kaspers, G.J., Smets, L.A., Pieters, R. *et al.* (1995) Favourable prognosis of hyperdiploid common acute lymphoblastic leukemia may be explained by sensitivity to antimetabolites and other drugs: results of an *in vitro* study. *Blood* **85**, 751–6.

Kato, K., Cantwell, M.J., Sharma, S. *et al.* (1998) Gene transfer of CD40-ligand induces autologous immune recognition of chronic lymphocytic leukemia B cell. *J. Clin. Invest.* **101**, 1133.

Keating, M.J. (1990) Fludarabine phosphate in the treatment of chronic lymphocytic leukemia. *Semin. Oncol.* **17**, 49.

Keating, M.J., Smith, T.L., Kanatarjian, H. *et al.* (1988) Cytogenetic pattern in acute myelogenous leukemia: a major reproducible determinant of outcome. *Leukemia* **2**, 403–12.

Keating, S., de Witte, T., Suciu, S. *et al.* (1998) The influence of HLA-matched sibling donor availability on treatment outcome for patients with AML: an analysis of the AML 8A study of the EORTC Leukemia Co-operative Group and GIMEMA. *Br. J. Haematol.* **102**, 1344–53.

Kern, W., Aul, C., Maschmeyer, G. *et al.* (1998) Superiority of high-dose over intermediate-dose cytosine arabinoside in the treatment of patients with high-risk acute myeloid leukemia: results of an age-adjusted prospective randomised comparison. *Leukemia* **12**, 1049–55.

Khouri, I., Przepiorka, D., Besien, K. *et al.* (1997) Allogeneic blood or marrow transplantation for chronic lymphocytic leukaemia: timing of transplantation and potential effect of fludarabine on acute graft-versus-host disease. *Br. J. Haematol.* **97**, 466–73.

Kinlen, L.J. (1995) Epidemiological evidence for an infective basis in childhood leukaemia. *Br. J. Cancer* **71**, 1–5.

Koeffler, H.P. and Golde, D.W. (1980) Human preleukemia. *Ann. Intern. Med.* **93**, 347–53.

Kosary, C.L., Ries, L.A.G., Miller, B.A., Hankey, B.F. and Edwards, B.K. (eds) (1995) *SEER cancer statistics review, 1973–1992L: tables and graphs*. Bethesda, MD.: National Cancer Institute (NIH publication no. 96-2789).

Kurtzberg, J., Keating, M., Moore, J.O. *et al.* (1996) 2-Amino-9-β-D-arabinosyl-6-methoxy-9H-guanine (GW 506U; compound 506U) is highly active in patients with T-cell malignancies: results of a phase 1 trial in pediatric and adult patients with refractory hematological malignancies. *Blood* **88**(suppl. 1), 669a.

Kurzrock, R., Gutterman, J.U. and Talpaz, M. (1988) The molecular genetics of Philadelphia chromosome positive leukemias. *N. Engl. J. Med.* **31**, 990.

Larson, R.A., Dodge, R.K., Burns, C.P. *et al.* (1995) A five-drug remission induction regimen with intensive consolidation for adults with acute lymphoblastic leukemia: Cancer and Leukemia Group B Study 8811. *Blood* **85**, 2025.

Latagliata, R., Avvisati, G. and Lo Coco, F. (1997) The role of all-*trans*-retinoic acid (ATRA) treatment in newly-diagnosed acute promyelocytic leukemia patients aged >60 years. *Ann. Oncol.* **8**, 1273–5.

Latagliata, R., Petti, M.C., Fenu, S. *et al.* (2002) Therapy-related myelodysplastic syndrome – acute myelogenous leukemia in patients treated for acute promyelocytic leukemia: an emerging problem. *Blood* **99**, 822–4.

Lawson, S.E., Harrison, G., Richards, S. *et al.* (2000) The UK experience in treating relapsed childhood acute lymphoblastic leukaemia: a report on the Medical Research Council UKALLR1 study. *Br. J. Haematol.* **108**, 531.

LeClerc, J.M., Billett, A.L., Gelber, R.D. *et al.* (2002) Treatment of childhood acute lymphoblastic leukemia: results of Dana-Farber ALL consortium protocol 87-01. *J. Clin. Oncol.* **20**, 237–46.

Legac, E., Chastang, C., Binet, J.L. *et al.* (1991) Proposals for a phenotype classification of B-chronic lymphocytic leukemia; relationship with prognostic factors. *Leuk. Lymphoma* **5**(suppl.), 53–8.

Lin, R.J., Nagy, L., Inoue, S. *et al.* (1998) Role of the histone deacetylase complex in acute promyeloctic leukaemia. *Nature* **391**, 811–14.

List, A.F., Holmes, H., Greenberg, P.L. *et al.* (1999) Phase II study of amifostine in patients with myelodysplastic syndromes. *Blood* **94**, 34a (abstract).

Liu, P., Tarle, S.A., Hajra, A. *et al.* (1993) Fusion between transcription factor CBFβ/PEBP2β and a myosin heavy chain in acute myeloid leukemia. *Science* **261**, 1041–4.

Locatelli, F. (1998) The role of repeat transplantation of haemopoietic stem cells and adoptive immunotherapy in treatment of leukaemia relapsing following allogeneic transplantation. *Br. J. Haematol.* **102**, 633.

Lowenberg, B. (1996) Treatment of the elderly patient with acute leukaemia. *Baillieres Clin. Haematol.* **9**, 147–59.

Lowenberg, B., Zittoun, R., Kerkhofs, H. *et al.* (1989) On the value of intensive remission-induction chemotherapy in elderly patients of 65+ years with acute myeloid leukemia: a randomised phase III study of the European Organisation for Research and Treatment of Cancer Leukemia Group. *J. Clin. Oncol.* **7**, 1268–74.

Lowenberg, B., Downing, R. and Burnett, A. (1999) Acute myeloid leukemia. *N. Engl. J. Med.* **341**, 1051–62.

Mahmoud, H.H., Hurwitz, C.A., Roberts, W.M. *et al.* (1993) Tretinoin toxicity in children with acute promyelocytic leukaemia. *Lancet* **342**, 1394–5.

Mandelli, F., Labopin, M., Granena, A. *et al.* (1994) European survey of bone marrow transplantation in acute promyelocytic leukemia (M3). Working Party on Acute Leukemia of the European Cooperative Group for Bone Marrow Transplantation (EMBT). *Bone Marrow Transplant* **14**, 293–8.

Mann, D.L., DeSantis, P. and Mark, G. (1987) HTLV-1 associated B-cell CLL: indirect role for retrovirus in leukemogenesis. *Science* **263**, 1103.

Marmont, A., Frassoni, F., Bacigalupo, A. *et al.* (1984) Recurrence of Ph′-leukemia in donor cells after marrow transplantation for chromosome g leukemia. *N. Engl. J. Med.* **310**, 903.

Matthews, D.C. (1998) Immunotherapy in acute myelogenous leukemia and myelodysplastic syndrome. *Leukemia* **100**, 304–9.

Matutes, E. (1996) Trisomy 12 in chronic lymphocytic leukaemia. *Leuk. Res.* **20**, 375.

Matutes, E., Owusu-Ankomah, K., Morilla, R. *et al.* (1994a) The immunological profile of B-cell disorders and proposal of a scoring system for the diagnosis of CLL. *Leukemia* **8**, 1640–5.

Matutes, E., Morilla, R., Owusu-Ankomah, K. *et al.* (1994b) The immunophenotype of hairy cell leukemia (HCL). Proposal for a scoring system to distinguish HCL from B-cell disorders with hairy or villous lymphocytes. *Leuk. Lymphoma* **14**(suppl. 1), 57–61.

Mayer, R.J., Davis, R.B., Schiffer, C.A. *et al.* (1994) Intensive postremission chemotherapy in adults with acute myeloid leukemia. *N. Engl. J. Med.* **331**, 896–942.

McGlave, P., De Fabritiis, P., Deisseroth, A. *et al.* (1994) Autologous transplant therapy for chronic myelogenous leukaemia prolongs survival: results from eight transplant groups. *Lancet* **343**, 1486.

Melo, J.V. (1996) The diversity of the BCR–ABL fusion proteins and their relationship to leukemia phenotype. *Blood* **88**, 2375.

Melo, J.V., Brito-Babapulle, V., Pombo de Oliveria, M.S. *et al.* (1987) The relationship between chronic lymphocytic leukemia and prolymphocytic leukemia. In Gale, R.P. and Rai, K.R. (eds), *Chronic lymphocytic leukemia. Recent progress and future direction.* New York: Alan R, Liss, 205–14.

Meloni, G., Diverio, D., Vignetti, M. *et al.* (1997) Autologous bone marrow transplantation for acute promyelocytic leukemia in second remission: prognostic relevance of pre-transplant minimal residual disease assessment by reverse-transcription polymerase chain reaction of the PML/RARα fusion in gene. *Blood* **90**, 1321–5.

Messina, C., Valsecchi, M.G., Arico, M. *et al.* (1998) Autologous bone marrow transplantation for treatment of isolated central nervous system relapse of childhood acute lymphoblastic leukemia. *Bone Marrow Transplant* **19**, 963.

Mesters, R.M., Padro, T., Bieker, R. *et al.* (2001) Stable remission after administration of the receptor tyrosine kinase inhibitor SU5416 in a patient with refractory acute myeloid leukemia. *Blood* **98**, 241–3.

Michallet, M. on behalf of IBMTR and EBMT registry (1998) The outcome of allogeneic and autologous transplants. In Barrett, A.J. and Treleavan, J. (eds), *The clinical practice of stem-cell transplantation,* vol. 1, 298–303.

Molldrem, J.J., Caples, M., Mavroudis, D. *et al.* (1997) Antithymocyte globulin for patients with myelodysplastic syndrome. *Br. J. Haematol.* **99**, 699–705.

Morimoto, C., Matsuyama, T., Oshige, C. *et al.* (1985) Functional and phenotypic studies of Japanese adult T-cell leukemia cells. *J. Clin. Invest.* **73**, 1771.

Morosetti, R. and Koeffler, H.P. (1996) Differentiation therapy in myelodysplastic syndromes. *Semin. Hematol.* **33**, 236–45.

Mortuza, F.Y., Papaioannou, M., Moreira, I.M. *et al.* (2002) Minimal residual disease tests provide an independent predictor of clinical outcome in adult acute lymphoblastic leukemia. *J. Clin. Oncol.* **20**, 1094–104.

Mughal, T.I. and Goldman, J.M. (1995) Chronic myeloid leukaemia: a therapeutic challenge. *Ann. Oncol.* **6**, 637–44.

Mughal, T.I. and Goldman, J.M. (2001) Chronic myeloid leukaemia: STI571 magnifies the therapeutic dilemma. *Eur. J. Cancer* **37**, 561–8.

Mughal, T.I., Hoyle, C. and Goldman, J.M. (1993) Autografting for patients with chronic myeloid leukemia – the Hammersmith experience. *Stem Cells* **11**, 20–2.

Mughal, T.I., Yong, A., Szydlo, R. *et al.* (2001) The probability of long-term leukaemia free survival for patients in molecular remission 5 years after allogeneic stem cell transplantation for chronic myeloid leukaemia in chronic phase. *Br. J. Hematol.* **115**, 569–74.

Mulligan, S., Matutes, E., Dearden, C. *et al.* (1991) Splenic lymphoma with villous lymphocytes: natural history response to therapy in 50 cases. *Br. J. Haematol.* **78**, 206–9.

Neale, G.A.M., Pui, C.-H., Mahmoud, H.H. *et al.* (1994) Molecular evidence for minimal residual bone marrow disease in children with 'isolated' extra-medullary relapse of T-cell acute lymphoblastic leukemia. *Leukemia* **8**, 768.

Nowell, P.C. and Hungerford, D.A. (1960) A minute chromosome in human chronic granulocytic leukemia. *Science* **132**, 1497.

Oosterveld, M., Estey, E., Muus, P. *et al.* (1999) Chemotherapy only versus chemotherapy followed by transplantation in high-risk MDS and s-AML: two parallel studies adjusted for various prognostic factors. *Blood* **94**, 2933 (abstract).

Pane, F., Frigeri, F., Sindona, M. *et al.* (1996) Neutrophilic-chronic myeloid leukemia: a distinct disease with a specific molecular marker. *Blood* **88**, 2410–4 [Erratum: (1997) *Blood* **89**, 4244].

Parker, S.L., Tong, T., Bolden, S. *et al.* (1997) Cancer statistics, 1997. *CA Cancer J. Clin.* **47**, 5–27 [Erratum: (1997) *CA Cancer J. Clin.* **47**, 68].

Pedersen-Bjergaard, J. and Rowley, J.D. (1994) The balanced and the unbalanced chromosome aberrations of acute myeloid leukemia may develop in different ways and may contribute differently to malignant transformation. *Blood* **83**, 2780–6.

Pedersen-Bjergaard, J., Andersen, M.K. and Christiansen, D.H. (2000) Therapy-related acute myeloid leukemia and myelodysplasia after high-dose chemotherapy and autologous stem cell transplantation. *Blood* **95**, 3273–9.

Pedersen-Bjergaard, J., Pederson, M., Roulston, D. *et al.* (1995) Different genetic pathways in leukemogenesis for patients presenting with therapy-related myelodysplasia and therapy-related acute myeloid leukemia. *Blood* **86**, 3542–52.

Pepper, C., Bentley, P. and Hoy, T. (1996) Regulation of clinical chemoresistance by bcl-2 and bax oncoproteins in B-cell chronic lymphocytic leukemia. *Br. J. Haematol.* **95**, 513.

Petersen, F.B., Lynch, M.H.E., Clift, R.A. *et al.* (1993) Autologous marrow transplantation for patients with acute myeloid leukemia in untreated first relapse

or in second complete remission. *J. Clin. Oncol.*
11, 353–60.

Pombo de Oliveira, M.S., Jaffe, E.S. and Catovsky, D.
(1989) Leukaemic phase of mantle-zone (intermediate)
lymphoma. Its characterisation in 11 cases. *J. Clin.
Pathol.* **42**, 962–72.

Porcher, C., Wojciech, S., Rockwell, K. *et al.* (1996)
The T cell leukemia oncoprotein SCI/tal-1 is essential
for development of all hematopoietic lineages.
Cell **86**, 47–57.

Provan, D., Bartlett-Pandite, L., Zwicky, C. *et al.* (1996)
Eradication of polymerase chain reaction-detectable
chronic lymphocytic leukemia cells is associated
with improved outcome after bone marrow
transplantation. *Blood* **88**, 2228–35.

Pui, C.H., Ribeiro, R.C., Hancock, M.L. *et al.* (1991)
Acute myeloid leukemia in children treated with
epipodophyllotoxins for acute lymphoblastic
leukemia. *N. Engl. J. Med.* **325**, 1682–7.

Rabinowe, S.N., Soiffer, R.J., Gribben, J.G. *et al.*
(1993) Autologous and allogeneic bone marrow
transplantation for poor prognosis patients with
B-cell chronic lymphocytic leukemia. *Blood*
82, 1366.

Rai, K.R. (1987) A critical analysis of staging in CLL. *1987
UCLA symposia on molecular and cellular biology*,
New Series 59, 253.

Rai, K.R., Sawitsky, A., Cronkite, E.P. *et al.* (1975) Clinical
staging of chronic lymphocytic leukemia. *Blood*
46, 219.

Rai, K.R., Peterson, B., Elias, I. *et al.* (1996) A
randomised comparison of fludarabine and
chlorambucil for patients with previously untreated
chronic lymphocytic leukemia. A CALBG, SWOG,
CTG/NCI-C and ECOG Intergroup study. *Blood*
88(suppl. 1), 141a.

Raza, A., Qawi, H., Lisak, L. *et al.* (2000) Patients with
myelodysplastic syndromes benefit from palliative
therapy with amifostine, pentoxifylline, and
ciprofloxacin with or without dexamethasone.
Blood **95**, 1580–7.

Raza, A., Meyer, P., Lisak, L. *et al.* (2001) Thalidomide
produces transfusion independence in long-standing
refractory anaemias of patients with myelodysplastic
syndromes. *Blood* **15**, 958–65.

Rees, J.K.H., Gray, R.G. and Wheatley, K. (1996) Dose
intensity in acute myeloid leukemia: greater
effectiveness at lower cost. Principal report of the
MRC's AML 9 Study. *Br. J. Haematol.* **94**, 89–98.

Rowley, J.D. (1973) A new consistent chromosomal
abnormality in chronic myelogenous leukaemia
identified by quinacrine fluorescence and Giemsa
staining. *Nature* **243**, 290.

Rowley, J.D. (1980) Chromosome changes in acute
leukaemia. *Br. J. Haematol.* **44**, 339–46.

Rowley, J.D. (1990) Recurring chromosome abnormalities
in leukemia and lymphoma. *Semin. Hematol.* **27**, 122.

Rubnitz, J.E., Behm, F.G. and Downing, J.R. (1996)
Rearrangements in acute leukemia. *Leukemia*
10, 74–82.

Ruffner, K.L. and Matthews, D.C. (2000) Current uses of
monoclonal antibodies in the treatment of acute
leukemia (Review). *Semin. Oncol.* **27**, 531–9.

Sanz, M.A., Martin, G., Rayon, C. *et al.* (1999) A modified
AIDA protocol with anthracycline-based consolidation
results in high antileukemic efficacy and reduced
toxicity in newly diagnosed PML/RAR-alpha-positive
acute promyelocytic leukemia. PETHEMA group.
Blood **94**, 3015–21.

Sawyers, C.L. (1997) Molecular genetics of acute
leukaemia. *Lancet* **349**, 196–200.

Sawyers, C.L. (1999) Chronic myeloid leukemia.
N. Engl. J. Med. **340**,1330–40.

Sebban, C., Lepage, E., Vernant, J.P. *et al.* (1994)
Allogeneic bone marrow transplantation in adult acute
lymphoblastic leukemia in first complete remission:
a comparative study. *J. Clin. Oncol.* **12**, 2580–7.

Sievers, E.L., Appelbaum, F.R., Speilberger, R.T. *et al.*
(1999) Selective ablation of acute myeloid leukemia
using antibody-targeted chemotherapy: a phase I study
of an anti-CD33 caliceamicin immunoconjugate.
Blood **93**, 3678–84.

Silver, R.T., Woolf, S.H., Hehlmann, R. *et al.* (1999)
An evidence-based analysis of the effect of busulfan,
hydroxyurea, interferon, and allogeneic bone marrow
transplantation in treating the chronic phase of chronic
myeloid leukemia: development for the American
Society of Hematology. *Blood* **94**, 1517–36.

Slavin, S., Nagler, A. and Naparstek, E. (1998a)
Nonmyeloablative stem cell transplantation and cell
therapy as an alternative to conventional bone
marrow transplantation with lethal cytoreduction
for the treatment of malignant and nonmalignant
hematological disease. *Blood* **91**, 756–63.

Slavin, S., Nagler, A., Naparstek, E. *et al.* (1998b)
Non-myeloablative stem cell transplantation with cell
therapy as an alternative to conventional bone marrow
transplantation with lethal cytoreduction for the
treatment of malignant and non-malignant
hematologic diseases. *Blood* **91**, 756.

Soignet, S.L., Maslak, P., Wang, Z.G. *et al.* (1998) Complete
remission after treatment of acute promyelocytic
leukemia with arsenic trioxide. *N. Engl. J. Med.*
339, 1341–8.

Sokal, J.E., Cox, E.B., Baccarani, M. *et al.* (1984)
Prognostic discrimination in 'good-risk' chronic
granulocytic leukemia. *Blood* **63**, 789.

Soussain, C., Patte, C., Ostronoff, M. *et al.* (1995) Small
noncleaved cell lymphoma and leukemia in adults:
a retrospective study of 65 adults treated with the
LMB pediatric protocols. *Blood* **85**, 664–74.

Spencer, A., Brookes, P.A., Kaminski, E. *et al.* (1995)
Cytotoxic T-lymphocyte precursor frequency analysis
in bone marrow transplantation with volunteer

unrelated donors: value in donor selection. *Transplantation* **59**, 1303.

Steins, M.B., Padro, T., Bieker, R. *et al.* (2002) Efficacy and safety of thalidomide in patients with acute myeloid leukaemia. *Blood* **99**, 834–9.

Steven, L., Signet, M.D., Peter, M. *et al.* (1998) Complete remission after treatment of acute promyelocytic leukemia with arsenic trioxide. *N. Engl. J. Med.* **339**, 1341.

Takagi, S., Tanaka, O., Origasa, H. *et al.* (1999) Prognostic significance of magnetic resonance imaging of femoral marrow in patients with myelodysplastic syndromes. *J. Clin. Oncol.* **17**, 277–83.

Tallman, M.S., Anderson, J.W., Schiffer, C.A. *et al.* (1997) All-*trans*-retinoic acid in acute promyelocytic leukemia. *N. Engl. J. Med.* **337**, 1021.

Tallman, M.S., Nabhan, C., Feusner, J.H. *et al.* (2002) Acute promyelocytic leukemia: evolving therapeutic strategies. *Blood* **99**, 759–67.

Thomas, E.D., Buckner, C.D., Clift, R.A. *et al.* (1979) Marrow transplantation for acute nonlymphoblastic leukemia in first remission. *N. Engl. J. Med.* **301**, 597–9.

Thomas, E.D., Clift, R.A., Fefer, A. *et al.* (1986) Marrow transplantation for the treatment of chronic myelogenous leukemia. *Ann. Intern. Med.* **104**, 155–63.

Tura, S. (1998) Cytarabine increases karyotypic response in alpha-IFN treated chronic myeloid leukemia patients: results of a national prospective randomized trial. *Blood* **92**, 317a.

Tuzuner, N., Cox, C., Rower, J.M. *et al.* (1995) Hypocellular myelodysplastic syndromes (MDS): new proposals. *Br. J. Haematol.* **91**, 612–17.

Uchida, H., Downing, J.R., Miyazaki, Y. *et al.* (1999) Three distinct domains in TEL-AMLI are required for transcriptional repression of the IL-3 promoter. *Oncogene* **18**, 1015–22.

Uckun, F.M., Sather, H.N., Gaynon, P.S. *et al.* (1997) Clinical features and treatment outcome of children with myeloid antigen positive acute lymphoblastic leukemia: a report from the Children's Cancer Group. *Blood* **90**, 28–35.

Vadhan-Raj, S., Keating, M., LeMaistre, A. *et al.* (1987) Effects of recombinant human granulocyte–macrophage colony stimulating factor in patients with myelodysplastic syndrome. *Blood* **73**, 31–7.

Van dern Berghe, H., Cassiman, I.J., David, G. *et al.* (1974) Distinct haematological disorder with deletion of long arm of no. 5 chromosome. *Nature* **251**, 437–8.

van Leeuwen, F.E. (1996) Risk of acute myelogenous leukaemia and myelodysplasia following cancer treatment. *Baillieres Clin. Haematol.* **9**, 57–8.

Waring, P.M. and Cleary, M.L. (1997) Disruption of a homolog of trithorax by 11q23 translocations: leukemogenic and transcriptional implications. *Curr. Top. Microbiol. Immunol.* **220**, 1–23.

Weick, J.K., Kopecky, K.J., Appelbaum, F.R. *et al.* (1996) A randomized investigation of high-dose versus standard cytosine arabinoside with daunorubicin in patients with previously untreated acute myeloid leukemia: a Southwest Oncology Group study. *Blood* **88**, 2841–51.

Wheeler, K., Richards, S., Bailey, C. *et al.* (1998) Comparison of bone marrow transplant and chemotherapy for relapsed childhood acute lymphoblastic leukaemia – the MRC UK ALL X experience. *Br. J. Haematol.* **101**, 94.

Wiemels, J.L., Cazzaniga, G., Daniotti, M. *et al.* (1999) Prenatal origin of acute lymphoblastic leukaemia in children. *Lancet* **354**, 1499–503.

Wong-Staal, F. and Gallo, R.C. (1985) The family of human T-lymphotropic leukemia/lymphoma virus: HTLV-I as the cause of adult T cell leukemia and HTLV-III as the cause of acquired immunodeficiency syndrome. *Blood* **65**, 253.

Zittoun, R.A., Mandelli, F., Willemze, R. *et al.* (1995) Autologous or allogeneic bone marrow transplantation compared with intensive chemotherapy in acute myelogenous leukemia. *N. Engl. J. Med.* **332**, 217–23.

43

Total body irradiation

DIANA M. TAIT

INTRODUCTION

Total body irradiation (TBI) has been used as a treatment approach for malignant disease since as early as 1900, although the concept of bone marrow transplantation (BMT) was introduced later. In 1905 Heineke reported favourable, although brief, responses in patients with leukaemia and round cell sarcoma. By today's standards the treatment methods were primitive; Hueblein (1932) described his technique at the Memorial Sloane–Kettering Hospital in New York in which up to four patients could be treated at a time, positioned between 5 and 7 m away from a single 'deep therapy' X-ray tube in a lead-lined room. Although the early results were poor, the practice became more common. By 1942 Medinger and Craver were able to publish a series of 270 patients with leukaemia and lymphoma who had received TBI at the Memorial. They found that 300 R (about 2.85 Gy), delivered over 10 days, was the maximum tolerable dose, and that this achieved, at best, only short remissions. In the light of these results, and with the introduction of cytotoxic drugs such as nitrogen mustard, interest in TBI waned.

However, experiments performed in the 1950s showed that it was possible for mice to survive significantly higher doses of TBI than was previously thought possible, provided irradiation was followed by the administration of fresh bone marrow cells (Lorenz et al., 1951). It could be demonstrated that improved survival was related to the engraftment of donor stem cells (Nowell et al., 1956). The subsequent development of TBI, in the setting of bone-marrow transplantation, owes a great deal to the work of Thomas, initially at Cooperstown and later in Seattle. He postulated that, using bone-marrow rescue, TBI doses could be escalated sufficiently to effectively treat human leukaemia (Thomas et al., 1957). In 1962 he was able to show that dogs could survive an otherwise lethal dose of 1200 R (11.5 Gy) by being given their own, previously harvested, bone marrow immediately afterwards (Thomas and Ferrebee, 1962). He then began to treat patients with end-stage leukaemia and, after the discovery of the human leukocyte antigens (1971), performed successful bone-marrow transplantation following TBI, using marrow from HLA-matched siblings (Thomas et al., 1971). Survival in these patients was still poor, but better results were obtained with the addition of cyclophosphamide to TBI in the conditioning regimen prior to BMT, and by treating better-risk patients who were in remission.

The role of TBI and BMT was established following the publication in 1979 by the Seattle group of 60 per cent actuarial survival at 3 years in patients with acute myeloid leukaemia treated in first remission (Thomas et al., 1979). This was at least comparable, and at best superior, to results achieved by conventional chemotherapy alone. Since then TBI has been used widely as part of the conditioning regimen for BMT in the treatment of haematological malignancies. Less commonly, it has been used in the treatment of solid tumours (Horovitz et al., 1993), and of a variety of non-malignant conditions, such as aplastic anaemia and certain inborn errors of metabolism. It has also been used, without marked success, as an immunosuppressive agent in the treatment of myasthenia gravis (Chassard et al., 1992; Durelli et al., 1993) and polymyositis (Cherin et al., 1992).

AIMS

The two major aims of TBI are to provide adequate immunosuppression to allow marrow engraftment, and to contribute to leukaemic cell kill. The relative importance of these two aims is a matter of controversy, but also one of relevance, as there are major implications for the choice of TBI regimen. What follows is an outline of this complex and controversial area which has been comprehensively reviewed (Gale *et al.*, 1991; Appelbaum, 1993; Weldon, 1997).

Immunosuppression

The immunosuppression provided by TBI contributes to the prevention of allograft rejection, but is obviously not a contributing factor in autografts where rejection is not a problem. Animal data show a steep TBI dose–response for successful engraftment (Vriesendorp, 1985), but engraftment depends not just on TBI. Other factors, such as drug treatment with cyclophosphamide and cyclosporin, the degree of HLA matching between host and donor, and whether or not the graft is T-cell depleted, impact on this process (Barrett *et al.*, 1989). In fact, it has not been possible in clinical practice to demonstrate any clear relationship between TBI parameters and the incidence of graft rejection, and, at least in the case of non-T-cell depleted transplants from matched sibling donors, sustained engraftment is achieved in more than 98 per cent of recipients. It would therefore seem possible to moderate commonly used TBI schedules to reduce toxicity without necessarily compromising marrow engraftment.

Cell kill

In practice, disease relapse is a much greater problem than failure to engraft. Most leukaemic cell lines are radiosensitive, so that TBI should add significantly to the cell kill achieved by cytotoxic drugs and by the graft versus leukaemia (GVL) effect. In addition, radiation might be particularly important for the eradication of disease from 'sanctuary' sites, such as the testes and the central nervous system. One approach has therefore been to intensify the TBI regimen, accepting major toxicity, in the hope of preventing relapse. However, this approach is not universally accepted. Some transplanters believe the anti-leukaemic effect of TBI is relatively unimportant compared with that of cytotoxic drugs and, in the case of allografts, GVL. The arguments on which this belief is based are complex and beyond the scope of this chapter, but are lucidly presented by Gale *et al.* (1991).

There are clinical data to support both of these schools of thought. The best evidence in favour of the theory that TBI cell kill really matters, comes from two randomized trials from Seattle which have looked at the effect of TBI dose escalation (Clift *et al.*, 1990, 1991). In both trials, fractionated TBI given as 12 Gy in six fractions was compared with 15.75 Gy in seven fractions, prior to allogeneic BMT. The first trial was composed of patients with acute myeloid leukaemia (AML), and the second those with chronic myeloid leukaemia (CML). In both there were significantly fewer relapses with the higher dose (Table 43.1). However, there was no survival benefit for dose escalation because of increased treatment-related mortality. Critics of the conclusion that there is a clinically important dose response for leukaemic cell kill point out that the relapse rates in the lower-dose arms were higher than would usually be expected (Gale *et al.*, 1991).

The argument that TBI cell kill is of relatively little importance comes from the higher relapse rate seen following syngeneic BMT (i.e. from an identical twin), in which there is no GVL. This observation suggests that GVL eradicates residual disease in the latter (Butturini *et al.*, 1987). Furthermore, the relapse rate after autografting is similar to that after syngeneic BMT. It can be inferred that most relapses after autografts arise from persistent leukaemic cells in the recipient rather than the infused marrow, thus reflecting the failure of the TBI to eradicate disease.

It is hard, therefore, to draw any definite conclusions about the role of TBI in preventing disease relapse, and, consequently, whether there is much to be gained by more intensive TBI schedules. The probability of relapse is related to many other factors, including patient characteristics, features of the leukaemia and other aspects of the BMT process. It is likely that the importance of TBI in preventing relapse, and therefore the potential benefit of more aggressive TBI, varies according to this probability.

Table 43.1 *Results from the only two randomized trials of TBI dose escalation (Clift et al., 1990, 1991)*

Study	AML (Clift *et al.*, 1990)		CML (Clift *et al.*, 1991)	
TBI protocol	12 Gy	15.7 Gy	12 Gy	15.7 Gy
Number	34	37	57	59
Treatment-related deaths	4	12	12	20
Disease-free survival	20	22	35	39

TECHNIQUE

Equipment

The technique used to deliver TBI varies considerably between centres. The ideal method would be comfortable for the patient, convenient for the department to administer alongside its routine workload, and would deliver an accurate dose to the entire body in a specified distribution at the desired dose rate. Most radiotherapy centres do not have dedicated TBI units and the techniques used tend, in practice, to reflect the facilities available, sometimes at the expense of some, or all, of these ideals. For example, difficulties in achieving a sufficiently large field size to irradiate the whole body has required, in some cases, the patient to assume the fetal position, often for long periods of time. Furthermore, these long treatment times on general purpose radiotherapy machines can seriously disrupt the overall workload of a department. In addition, even with the most sophisticated of equipment, the actual dose distribution delivered may depend as much on the shape of the particular patient as on any technical factors.

The Royal Marsden Hospital has a purpose-built TBI unit consisting of two parallel opposed cobalt-60 sources positioned 7 metres apart, with the treatment couch in between (Fig. 43.1). The maximum field size at the level of the couch is 200 cm × 65 cm, so that even the tallest of patients may lie full-length. The large source-to-patient distance helps to produce a relatively homogeneous dose distribution, and the dose rate may be varied by the use of attenuators placed in the beams. Because of the low energy of the cobalt sources compared with that of a linear accelerator, a light blanket placed over the patient provides sufficient build-up to avoid unwanted skin sparing. A dedicated unit such as this provides the luxury of treating patients independently of the general work of the department.

Patient selection and counselling

Before giving TBI it must be established that the patient is fit for the procedure. Possible contraindications to TBI include previous irradiation, impaired lung function and advanced age. Abnormalities of lung function have been shown to be significant risk factors for death following BMT conditioned with TBI (Crawford and Fisher, 1992). Patients are sometimes extremely wary of TBI, possibly associating it with unfavourable aspects of radiation, such as nuclear accidents. Proper counselling therefore takes considerable time and should include a description of the procedure and the associated risks (see later) before obtaining patient consent.

Conditioning and preparation

The most common conditioning regimen for BMT involves the use of TBI together with cyclophosphamide, the TBI being given the day after the chemotherapy. A few hours prior to TBI the patient is premedicated with an anti-emetic, usually a 5-HT$_3$ antagonist such as ondansetron. Where a single-fraction schedule is used, a sedative given just before, and if necessary at intervals during TBI, helps the patient to remain relatively still without compromising co-operation.

Fractionation

The question of whether or not to fractionate TBI has been debated and remains unresolved. Radiobiological theory predicts that, for a given leukaemic cell kill, fractionation of TBI should spare late normal tissue effects such as lung damage and growth impairment. Results from animal work (Appelbaum, 1993) and some retrospective clinical series are consistent with this theory (Deeg, 1983; Socie et al., 1991). However, it is hard to draw any conclusions from such series as results are drawn from many centres, with different patient selection criteria and TBI techniques which are likely to vary in ways other than fractionation. Unfortunately there are only very limited data on the question of fractionation. This includes a randomized trial of only 53 patients which was too small to provide any definitive answers

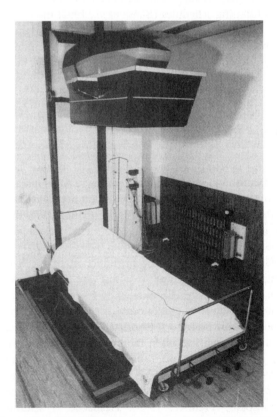

Figure 43.1 *The dedicated dual-headed cobalt TBI facility at the Royal Marsden Hospital.*

(Deeg *et al.*, 1986), and a non-randomized study from the Institut Gustave-Roussy (Cosset *et al.*, 1989). In practice, most centres are now using fractionated TBI, a choice which is probably based as much on convenience as it is on theoretical considerations or clinical data. Fractionated TBI is commonly given at a dose rate in the order of 0.15 Gy/min, so that each fraction takes about 20 minutes, allowing for time to change treatment position and to replace thermoluminescent dose meters or diodes. On the other hand, single fraction treatments are given at a rate of about 0.04 Gy/min, so the overall treatment time is 4–5 hours. With time added on for stoppages, single-fraction treatments usually take between 5 and 6 hours. Consequently, fractionation tends to cause less disruption to the routine workload of a department.

Dose distribution

It is generally considered desirable to deliver TBI with a homogeneous dose distribution. However, thinner parts of the body, such as the head and feet, will tend to receive a higher dose than wider parts, such as the trunk. These differences may be minimized by altering the proportion of time spent in each of the two treatment positions; supine and lateral. In this way it is usually possible to achieve less than 10 per cent dose variation across the body. Some centres restrict the dose to certain organs, such as lung, liver or kidneys, by the use of appropriate shielding, and thus aim to reduce toxicity. There are insufficient data to firmly establish the benefit of such shielding, but there are studies that point to an advantage. For example, use of blocking to alternate liver dose appears to reduce the incidence of veno-occlusive disease mortality from 15 to 5 per cent (Lawton *et al.*, 1989).

Dosimetry

For the treatment itself, the patient lies on the couch, either in the supine or lateral position, with hands across the chest, in order to spare the lungs to some extent (Fig. 43.2). The dosimetry may be based either on pre-treatment calculations using patient dimensions, or on *in vivo* measurements taken during part of the treatment itself. In the latter case thermoluminescent dose meters and/or semiconductor diodes are attached to the skin in specified positions to measure the dose received and its distribution.

At the Royal Marsden the prescription is specified at the maximum lung dose, on the premise that it is lung toxicity that is dose-limiting. Other centres use a different prescription point such as the pelvis where, if the separation is smaller than in the lungs, the dose absorbed may be higher. Typical dose prescriptions are 12 Gy in six fractions over 3 days, or 10 Gy in the case of single-fraction treatment.

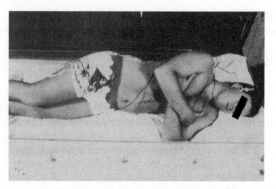

Figure 43.2 *Lateral treatment position with the arms folded across the chest. Semiconductor diodes and thermoluminescent dose meter drips can be seen applied to specific dose measurement points.*

TOXICITY

BMT is a toxic treatment which may cause numerous adverse effects. Undoubtedly, TBI contributes to this toxicity, but transplantation is a complex process, involving many potentially toxic components, to which it is difficult to attribute specific toxicity. However, careful analysis of toxicity is important; not least because it is now possible to condition patients for BMT with drugs alone, thus avoiding TBI. However, such comparative data as there is suggest an advantage to TBI-containing conditioning schedules (Blaise *et al.*, 1992; Inoue *et al.*, 1993). This evidence is strengthened by a meta-analysis of busulfan–cyclophosphamide versus a TBI-containing regime, which demonstrated less veno-occlusive disease and a better, but not statistically significant, overall survival with TBI (Hartman *et al.*, 1998).

Acute toxicity

Acute side-effects occurring during TBI include nausea and vomiting, headache and hyperpyrexia. Nausea and vomiting have been associated with anxiety (Westbrook *et al.*, 1987), movement during irradiation (Westbrook *et al.*, 1987), single-fraction treatment (Cosset *et al.*, 1989) and dose rates greater than 0.06 Gy/min (Barrett, 1982). However, since the introduction of the 5-HT$_3$ antagonists, nausea and vomiting are seldom severe. For example, Schwella *et al.* (1994) report 'sufficient emesis control' in 22 out of 25 patients given ondansetron prior to fractionated TBI. 5-HT$_3$ antagonists have been shown, in randomized controlled trials, to prevent TBI-induced nausea and vomiting more effectively than both placebo (Tiley *et al.*, 1992) and a combination of dexamethasone, metoclopramide and lorazepam (Prentice, 1993). Headache is seldom a problem and is associated with the use of 5-HT$_3$ antagonists (Prentice, 1993). Hyperpyrexia commonly occurs

(Chaillet *et al.*, 1993) but is rarely symptomatic and does not persist longer than 24 hours.

Other side-effects that occur within the first few days following TBI include xerostomia, jaw pain due to parotitis, diarrhoea, skin erythema and eye problems, including photophobia, dry eye syndrome and conjunctival oedema (Chaillet *et al.*, 1993). Parotid swelling and pain usually settle within 2–3 days, but xerostomia may persist for months. Diarrhoea is seen in about one-third of patients (Ozsahin *et al.*, 1992a), being more common in those who receive methotrexate as graft-versus-host prophylaxis. Skin erythema is inevitable except when very high energy photons (18–20 MV) are used (Chaillet *et al.*, 1993). The ocular problems have been reviewed by Spires (1993).

Intermediate toxicity

Adverse effects occurring within weeks or a few months of TBI include interstitial pneumonitis, hepatic veno-occlusive disease, somnolence syndrome and alopecia. The hair loss is usually of little significance because almost all patients already have complete alopecia from their chemotherapy, and re-growth normally occurs within months. However, permanent alopecia after BMT has been reported and is associated with chronic graft-versus-host disease and prior cranial irradiation (Vowels *et al.*, 1993). The somnolence syndrome is characterized by drowsiness, headache and anorexia coming on about 6 weeks after irradiation and lasting for 1–2 weeks. Pneumonitis and hepatic veno-occlusive disease are two of the most important causes of toxicity following BMT and will be discussed at more length.

Pneumonitis is common after BMT and is frequently fatal. Data from the International Bone Marrow Transplant Registry (Weiner *et al.*, 1986), based on 932 patients, show that pneumonitis occurred in 29 per cent and was fatal in 84 per cent of these cases. The precise role of radiation in the pathogenesis of pneumonitis remains unclear. Theory predicts that radiation pneumonitis would occur more commonly with higher radiation dose and dose rate, and would be spared by fractionation. Some retrospective series have, indeed, shown these associations (Weiner *et al.*, 1986; Socie *et al.*, 1991), but others have found no relationship between the incidence of pneumonitis and radiation parameters (Frassoni *et al.*, 1989; Kim *et al.*, 1990). Furthermore, the randomized trials of TBI dose escalation (Clift *et al.*, 1990, 1991), of different dose rates (Ozsahin *et al.*, 1992a), of fractionation (Deeg *et al.*, 1986) and of lung shielding (Labar *et al.*, 1992) failed to show any significant relationship between these variables and pneumonitis. However, these trials were small and therefore lacked the power to detect relatively small, but clinically important, differences in the frequency of pneumonitis.

Factors other than radiation certainly contribute to the pneumonitis seen after BMT. Evidence suggests that cytomegalovirus (CMV) infection (Winston *et al.*, 1990), graft-versus-host disease (GVH) (Weiner *et al.*, 1986), gangclovir prophylaxis (Schmidt *et al.*, 1991), type of transplant (allogeneic or autologous) (Deeg, 1988), cyclophosphamide dose (Ozsahin *et al.*, 1992b) and use of methotrexate (Weiner *et al.*, 1986) are all related to the incidence of pneumonitis. Pulmonary function in long-term survivors shows an initial decline in function with subsequent recovery, unless there is a further event such as infection or GVH (Gore *et al.*, 1996).

Hepatic veno-occlusive disease is another important cause of morbidity and mortality after TBI, incurring a mortality rate of 50 per cent. In severe cases it presents with jaundice, hepatomegaly and ascites, and is thought to account for up to 10 per cent of treatment-related deaths following BMT (Ganem *et al.*, 1988). Reports of its incidence vary from 6 to 52 per cent (Westbrook *et al.*, 1987; Ozsahin *et al.*, 1992a), the difference reflecting, at least in part, differences in diagnostic criteria. Elevated transaminases, female gender and the use of cytosine arabinoside all predispose to veno-occlusive disease, but it is generally accepted that TBI is an important contributor (McDonald *et al.*, 1984; Ganem *et al.*, 1988). Once again, as for pneumonitis, there are conflicting data regarding the relationship of TBI parameters to the incidence of veno-occlusive disease, although fractionated TBI appears to be better tolerated than single-fraction TBI in this respect. These data have recently been summarized by Ozsahin *et al.* (1994b). Liver blocks may reduce the incidence of veno-occlusive disease (Lawton *et al.*, 1989).

Late toxicity

Late effects of BMT which may be caused by TBI include endocrine failure, growth impairment, cataracts and second malignancies. A fuller list is given in Table 43.2. These effects have attracted a great deal of interest in recent years, partly because there has been increased data with the passage of time, and partly because of the hope of avoiding the effects by the use of conditioning regimens excluding TBI.

Endocrine late effects may be diverse but commonly present with hypothyroidism and gonadal failure. Hypothyroidism is frequent after BMT and is probably caused by TBI (Borgstrom and Bolme, 1994). It is, of course, easily treatable. BMT is almost always followed by primary ovarian failure in women (Sanders *et al.*, 1988), and azoospermia in men (Sanders *et al.*, 1983). In women menopausal symptoms and sexual dysfunction are very common and hormone replacement therapy for long-term survivors of BMT is strongly recommended, both to alleviate these symptoms and to prevent problems such as osteoporosis (Cust *et al.*, 1989). However, it is possible, especially for younger women, to retain ovarian function and there are at least six reported cases of women who have borne children after TBI

Table 43.2 *Toxicity of bone-marrow transplantation*

Early and intermediate
  Nausea and vomiting
  Xerostomia
  Skin erythema
  Parotitis
  Hypothermia
  Alopecia
  Interstitial pneumonitis
  Veno-occlusive disease
Late
  Endocrine
    infertility
    premature menopause
    hypothyroidism
    growth impairment
  Ocular
    cataracts
    dry eyes
  Neurological
    necrotizing leukoencephalopathy
    polyneuropathy
    intellectual impairment
  Renal
    impaired renal function
    haemolytic uraemic syndrome
  Skeletal
    exostoses
    osteoporosis
    aseptic necrosis
  Pulmonary
    bronchiolitis obliterans
  Second malignancies

(Buskard *et al.*, 1988; Russell and Hanley, 1989; Giri *et al.*, 1992; Samuelsson *et al.*, 1993). Ovarian recovery after TBI, in the setting of allogeneic transplantation, has been assessed by long-term follow-up of 79 patients (Spinelli *et al.*, 1994). There is also one case of a male, proved by genetic testing to have fathered a child, having previously received TBI (Pakkala *et al.*, 1994).

Using conditioning regimens not including TBI may not, in fact, help gonadal function significantly. In one series, pituitary and gonadal function were measured in women before, and 3–4 months after, BMT. As expected, the post-treatment results were abnormal, but no significant differences were found between those who had received radiation and those who had been conditioned with high-dose chemotherapy alone (Chattergee *et al.*, 1994).

BMT in children leads to significant growth impairment, which is associated with growth hormone deficiency, and is more marked with single-dose, than with fractionated TBI (Thomas *et al.*, 1993). It occurs sooner in those who have previously received prophylactic cranial irradiation (Bozzola *et al.*, 1993), and is less severe in those whose transplant schedule does not include TBI (Brauner *et al.*, 1993; Giri *et al.*, 1993). This growth impairment responds to therapeutic growth hormone (Bozzola *et al.*, 1993).

Cataract formation occurs in 15–50 per cent of those who survive 5 years after BMT, and may be inevitable with sufficiently long follow-up. The use of steroids for the treatment of GVH disease (Dunn *et al.*, 1993; Hamon *et al.*, 1993), high TBI dose rates (Fife *et al.*, 1994; Ozsahin *et al.*, 1994a) and single-fraction treatments (Fife *et al.*, 1994; Ozsahin *et al.*, 1994a) are associated with early cataractogenesis.

There is increasing concern, and emerging data, on the risk of second malignancy following BMT. Two broad categories of malignancy occur; lymphoproliferative disorders and solid tumours, and TBI seems to be one of several causative factors (Deeg and Witherspoon, 1993; Kulkarni *et al.*, 2000).

THE FUTURE

The role of TBI has been called into question by the advent of conditioning regimes for BMT that comprise drugs alone, usually a combination of busulfan and cyclophosphamide (BuCy). Clearly, TBI is no longer essential for BMT. Regimens based on BuCy, with some modifications, are currently being tested against TBI-containing protocols. However, of the three randomized trials that have been published so far, comparing TBI with BuCy, two have shown a survival benefit for TBI (Blaise *et al.*, 1992; Ringden *et al.*, 1994), and in the third there were no significant differences in outcome between the two treatments (Blume *et al.*, 1993). At present, therefore, TBI remains an established part of conditioning for BMT. There remains considerable uncertainty as to what constitutes the ideal TBI regimen. As has been discussed, this stems partly from the fact that the outcome of BMT depends on many factors other than TBI parameters and, consequently, comparison between centres and with historical controls is difficult to interpret. This difficulty is compounded by the paucity of good randomized trials comparing different TBI protocols. Significant improvements over conventional TBI regimens are unlikely to be made in the absence of large randomized trials, which would require the co-operation of many centres.

Progress may come from attempts to modify the dose distribution of radiation in order to target sites of disease, with sparing of normal tissues. Two methods are being investigated. The first relies on conjugating iodine-131 to antibodies directed against antigens expressed by haematopoietic cells (Amin *et al.*, 1993). The second uses bone-seeking radionuclides emitting radiation of the appropriate energy, such as samarium-153 or holmium-166, which are taken up by bone and act on disease in the marrow by virtue of its proximity. Dosimetric studies using radiolabelled anti-CD45 antibodies have demonstrated that at least twice as much radiation can be delivered to bone as to lungs or liver (Matthews *et al.*, 1992). This technique is now being tried in combination with conventional TBI and cyclophosphamide. If this approach proves successful, dose escalation of the radio-labelled antibodies may allow a dose reduction of conventional TBI, and therefore, the hope of a less toxic treatment with an increased anti-leukaemic effect.

SIGNIFICANT POINTS

- TBI is an important part of conditioning for BMT in the treatment of haematological malignancies.
- The major aims of TBI are leukaemic cell kill and, in the case of allografts, immunosuppression to prevent graft rejection.
- Care is needed in the selection and counselling of patients before TBI.
- TBI techniques vary between centres.
- Fractionated TBI is usually more convenient than treatment with a single fraction, and less toxic.
- It is usual to aim for a homogeneous dose distribution and to accept variation of less than 10 per cent.
- BMT is a toxic process, with important causes of treatment-related death being interstitial pneumonitis and hepatic veno-occlusive disease.
- Conditioning regimens with drugs alone may be less toxic than TBI, but have not yet been shown to be as effective.
- Combinations of TBI and radiolabelled antibody treatment may improve the outcome of BMT.

KEY REFERENCES

Appelbaum, F.R. (1993) The influence of total dose, fractionation, dose rate, and distribution of TBI on bone marrow transplantation. *Semin. Oncol.* **20**(suppl. 4), 3–10.

Gale, R.P., Butturini, A. and Bortin, M.M. (1991) What does TBI do in bone marrow transplants for leukemia? *Int. J. Radiat. Oncol. Biol. Phys.* **20**, 631–4.

Ozsahin, M., Pene, F., Cosset, J.M. and Laugier, A. (1994) Morbidity after TBI. *Semin. Radiat. Oncol.* **4**, 95–102.

REFERENCES

Amin, A.E., Wheldon, T.E., O'Donoghue, J.A. and Barrett, A. (1993) Radiobiological modeling of combined targeted ^{131}I therapy and total body irradiation for treatment of disseminated tumours of differing radiosensitivity. *Int. J. Radiat. Oncol. Biol. Phys.* **27**, 323–30.

Appelbaum, F.R. (1993) The influence of total dose, fractionation, dose rate, and distribution of TBI on bone marrow transplantation. *Semin. Oncol.* **20**(suppl. 4), 3–10.

Barrett, A. (1982) Total body irradiation before bone marrow transplantation in leukaemia: a cooperative study from the European Group for Bone Marrow Transplantation. *Br. J. Radiol.* **55**, 562–7.

Barrett, A.J., Horovitz, M.M., Gale, R.P. *et al.* (1989) Marrow transplantation for ALL: factors affecting relapse and survival. *Blood* **74**, 862–71.

Blaise, D., Maraninchi, D., Archimbaud, E. *et al.* (1992) Allogeneic BMT for AML in first remission: a randomized trial of busulfancytoxan versus cytoxan-TBI as preparative regimen: a report from the Group d'Etudes de la Greffe de Moelle Osseuse. *Blood* **79**, 2578–82.

Blume, K.G., Kopecky, I., Henslee-Downey, I.P. *et al.* (1993) A prospective randomized comparison of TBI-etoposide versus busulfan-cyclophosphamide as preparatory regimens for BMT in patients with recurrent leukemia: a Southwest Oncology Group Study. *Blood* **81**, 2187–93.

Borgstrom, B. and Bolme, P. (1994) Thyroid function in children after allogeneic BMT. *Bone Marrow Transplant.* **13**, 59–64.

Bozzola, M., Gorgiani, G., Locatelli, F. *et al.* (1993) Growth in children after BMT. *Horm. Res.* **39**, 1226.

Brauner, R., Fontoura, M., Zucker, I.M. *et al.* (1993) Growth and growth hormone secretion after BMT. *Arch. Vis. Child.* **68**, 458–63.

Buskard, N., Ballem, P., Hill, R. *et al.* (1988) Normal fertility after total body irradiation and chemotherapy in conjunction with a bone marrow transplant for acute leukaemia. *Clin. Invest.* **2**(suppl.), C57.

Butturini, A., Bortin, M.M. and Gale, R.P. (1987) Graft-versus-leukaemia following bone marrow transplantation. *Bone Marrow Transplant.* **2**, 233–42.

Chaillet, M.P., Cosset, I., Socie, G. *et al.* (1993) Prospective study of the clinical symptoms of therapeutic whole body irradiation. *Health Phys.* **64**, 370–4.

Chassard, I.L., Martinent, L., Bady, B. *et al.* (1992) Role of irradiation as a treatment for myasthenia gravis. A review of about 30 cases. *Bull. Cancer Radiother.* **79**, 137–48.

Chattergee, R., Mills, W., Katz, M. *et al.* (1994) Prospective study of pituitary–gonadal function to evaluate short-term effects of ablative chemotherapy or TBI with autologous or allogeneic marrow transplantation in post-menarcheal female patients. *Bone Marrow Transplant.* **13**, 511–17.

Cherin, P., Herson, S., Coutellier, A. *et al.* (1992) Failure of TBI in polymyositis: report of three cases (letter) *Br. J. Rheumatol.* **31**, 282–3.

Clift, R.A., Buckner, C.D., Appelbaum, F.R. *et al.* (1990) Allogeneic marrow transplantation in patients with AML in first remission: a randomized trial of two irradiation regimens. *Blood* **76**, 1867–71.

Clift, R.A., Buckner, C.D., Appelbaum, F.R. *et al.* (1991) Allogeneic marrow transplantation in patients with chronic myeloid leukaemia in the chronic phase: a randomized trial of two irradiation regimens. *Blood* **77**, 1660–5.

Cosset, J.M., Baume, D., Pico, J.L. *et al.* (1989) Single dose versus hyperfractionated total body irradiation before allogeneic bone marrow transplantation: a non-randomized comparative study of 54 patients at the Institut Gustave-Roussy. *Radiother. Oncol.* **15**, 151–60.

Crawford, S.W. and Fisher, L. (1992) Predictive value of pulmonary function tests before marrow transplantation. *Chest* **101**, 1257–64.

Cust, M.P., Whitehead, M.I., Powles, R. *et al.* (1989) Consequences and treatment of ovarian failure after TBI. *BMI* **299**,1494–7.

Deeg, H.J. (1988) Interstitial pneumonitis. In Deeg, H.J., Klingeimann, H.E. and Phillips, G.L. (eds), *A guide to bone marrow transplantation.* Berlin: Springer-Verlag, 114–22.

Deeg, H.J. and Witherspoon, R.P. (1993) Risk factors for the development of secondary malignancies after marrow transplantation. *Haematol. Oncol. Clin. North Am.* **7**, 417–29.

Deeg, H.J. for the Seattle Marrow Transplant Team (1983) Acute and delayed toxicities of TBI. *Int. J. Radial. Oncol. Biol. Phys.* **9**, 1933–9.

Deeg, H.J., Sullivan, K.M., Buckner, C.D. *et al.* (1986) Marrow transplantation for ANLL in first remission: toxicity and long term follow up of patients conditioned with single dose or fractionated TBI. *Bone Marrow Transplant.* **1**, 151–7.

Dunn, J.P., Jabs, D.A., Wingard, J. *et al.* (1993) Bone marrow transplantation and cataract development. *Arch. Ophthalmol.* **III**, 1367–73.

Durelli, L., Ferrio, M.F., Urgesi, A. *et al.* (1993) TBI for myasthenia gravis: a long term follow up. *Neurology* **43**, 2215–21.

Fife, F., Milan, S., Westbrook, K., Powles, R. and Tait, D.M. (1994) Risk factors for requiring cataract surgery following total body irradiation. *Radiother. Oncol.* **33**, 93–8.

Frassoni, F., Scarpati, D., Bacigalupo, A. *et al.* (1989) The effect of total body irradiation dose and chronic GVHD on leukaemic relapse after allogeneic BMT. *Br. J. Haematol.* **73**, 211–16.

Gale, R.P., Butturini, A. and Bortin, M.M. (1991) What does TBI do in bone marrow transplants for leukemia? *Int. J. Radiat. Oncol. Biol. Phys.* **20**, 631–4.

Ganem, G., Girardin, M.F.S.M., Kuentz, M. *et al.* (1988) Venoocclusive disease of the liver after allogeneic BMT in man. *Int. J. Radiat. Oncol. Biol. Phys.* **14**, 879–84.

Giri, N., Vowels, M.R. and Barr, A.L. (1992) Successful pregnancy after TBI and BMT for acute leukemia. *Bone Marrow Transplant.* **10**, 93–5.

Giri, N., Davis, E.A. and Vowels, M.R. (1993) Long term complications following BMT in children. *J. Paediatr. Child Health* **29**, 201–5.

Gore, E.M., Lawton, C.A., Ash, R.C. and Lipchick, R.J. (1996) Pulmonary function changes in long-term survivors of bone marrow transplantation. *Int. J. Radiat. Oncol. Biol. Phys.* **36**, 67–75.

Hamon, M.D., Gale, R.F., MacDonald, R.M. *et al.* (1993) Incidence of cataracts after single fraction total body irradiation: the role of steroids and GVHD. *Bone Marrow Transplant.* **12**, 233–6.

Hartman, A.-R., Williams, S.F. and Dillon, J.J. (1998) Survival, disease-free survival and adverse effects of conditioning for allogenic bone marrow transplantation with busulfan/cyclophosphamide vs total body irradiation: at meta-analysis. *Bone Marrow Transplant.* **22**, 439–43.

Heineke, H. (1905) Experimentelle Untersuchungen uber die Einwirkund der Rontgenstrahlen auf das Knochenmark, nebst einige Bemerkungen uber die Rontgentherapie der Leukamie und Pseudoleukamie und des Sarcoms. *Deutsche Zeitschr. Chirurgie* **78**, 196–231.

Horovitz, M.E., Kinsella, T.J., Wexler, L.H. *et al.* (1993) TBI and autologous bone marrow transplant in the treatment of high-risk Ewing's sarcoma and rhabdomyosarcoma. *J. Clin. Oncol.* **II**, 1911–18.

Hueblein, A.C. (1932) A preliminary report on continuous irradiation of the entire body. *Radiology* **18**, 1051–62.

Inoue, T., Ikeda, H., Yamazaki, H. *et al.* (1993) Role of total body irradiation as based on the comparison of preparation regimes for allogeneic bone marrow transplantation for acute leukemia in first complete remission. *Strahlenther Onkol.* **169**, 25.

Kim, T.H., McGlave, P.B., Ramsay, N. *et al.* (1990) Comparison of two TBI regimens in allogeneic bone marrow transplantation for ANLL in first remission. *Int. J. Radiat. Oncol. Biol. Phys.* **19**, 889–97.

Kulkarni, S., Powles, R., Treleaven, S. *et al.* (2000) Melphalan/TBI is not more carcinogenic than cyclophosphamide/TBI for transplant conditioning: follow-up of 725 patients from a single centre over a period of 26 years. *Bone Marrow Transplant.* **25**, 365–70.

Labar, B., Bogdanic, V., Nemet, D. *et al.* (1992) TBI with or without lung shielding for allogeneic BMT. *Bone Marrow Transplant.* **9**, 343–7.

Lawton, C.A., Barber-Derus, S., Murray, K.J. *et al.* (1989) Technical modifications in hyperfractionated total body irradiation for T-lymphocyte deplete bone marrow transplant. *Int. J. Radiol. Oncol. Biol. Phys.* **17**, 319–22.

Lorenz, E., Uphoff, D., Reid, T.R. *et al.* (1951) Modification of irradiation injury in mice and guinea pigs by bone marrow injections. *J. Natl Cancer Inst.* **12**, 197–201.

Matthews, D.C., Appelbaum, F.R., Eary, J.F. *et al.* (1992) Use of radioiodinated anti-CD45 monoclonal antibody to augment marrow irradiation prior to marrow transplantation or acute leukaemia (abstract). *Blood* **80**(suppl. 1), 335a.

McDonald, G.B., Sharma, P., Matthews, D.E. *et al.* (1984) VOD after BMT: diagnosis, incidence and predisposing factors. *Hepatology* **4**, 116–22.

Medinger, F.C. and Craver, L.F. (1942) Total body irradiation. *Am. J. Roentgenol.* **48**, 651–71.

Nowell, P.C., Cole, L.J., Habermeyer, J.G. *et al.* (1956) Growth and continued function of rat marrow cells in X-irradiated mice. *Cancer Res.* **16**, 258–61.

Ozsahin, M., Pene, F., Touboul, E. *et al.* (1992a) Total body irradiation before bone marrow transplantation: results of two randomized instantaneous dose rates in 157 patients. *Cancer* **69**, 2853–65.

Ozsahin, M., Schwartz, L.H., Pene, F. *et al.* (1992b) Is body weight a risk factor of interstitial pneumonitis after BMT? *Bone Marrow Transplant.* **10**, 97.

Ozsahin, M., Belkacemi, Y., Pene, F. *et al.* (1994a) TBI and cataract incidence: a randomized comparison of two instantaneous dose rates. *Int. J. Radiat. Oncol. Biol. Phys.* **28**, 343–7.

Ozsahin, M., Pene, F., Cosset, J.M. and Laugier, A. (1994b) Morbidity after TBI. *Semin. Radiat. Oncol.* **4**, 95–102.

Pakkala, S., Lukka, M. and Helminen, P. (1994) Paternity after BMT following conditioning with TBI. *Bone Marrow Transplant.* **13**, 489–90.

Prentice, H.G. (1993) Efficacy and safety of granisetron in the treatment of emesis caused by TBI; a comparison with standard anti-emetic therapy. *Proc. Ann. Meet. Am. Soc. Clin. Oncol.* **12**, A1574.

Ringden, O., Ruutu, T., Remberger, R. *et al.* (1994) A randomized trial comparing busulphan with TBI as conditioning in allogeneic marrow transplant recipients with leukaemia; a report from the Nordic Bone Marrow Transplantation Group. *Blood* **83**, 2723–30.

Russell, J.A. and Hanley, D.A. (1989) Full term pregnancy after allogeneic transplantation for leukemia in a patient with oligomenorrhoea. *Bone Marrow Transplant.* **4**, 579–80.

Samuelsson, A., Fuchs, T., Simonsson, B. and Bjorkholm, M. (1993) Successful pregnancy in a 28-year-old patient autografted for ALL following myeloablative treatment including TBI. *Bone Marrow Transplant.* **12**, 659–60.

Sanders, J.E., Buckner, C.D., Leonard, J.M. *et al.* (1983) Late effects on gonadal function of cyclophosphamide, TBI and marrow transplantation. *Transplantation* **36**, 252–5.

Sanders, J.E., Buckner, C.D., Amos, D. *et al.* (1988) Ovarian function following marrow transplantation for acute leukaemia. *J. Clin. Oncol.* **6**, 813–18.

Schmidt, G.M., Horak, D.A., Niland, J.C. *et al.* (1991) A randomized controlled trial of prophylactic ganciclovir for CMV pulmonary infection in recipients of allogeneic bone marrow transplants. *N. Engl. J. Med.* **324**, 1005–11.

Schwella, N., Konig, V., Schwerdtfeger, R. *et al.* (1994) Ondansetron for efficient emesis control during TBI. *Bone Marrow Transplant.* **13**, 169–71.

Socie, G., Devergie, A., Girinsky, T. *et al.* (1991) Influence of the fractionation of TBI on complications and relapse rate for CML. *Int. J. Radiat. Oncol. Biol Phys.* **20**, 397–404.

Spinelli, S., Chiodi, S., Bacigalupo, A. *et al.* (1994) Ovarian recovery after total body irradiation and allogenic bone marrow transplantation: long-term follow up of 79 females. *Bone Marrow Transplant.* **14**, 373–80.

Spires, R. (1993) Ocular manifestations in bone marrow transplantation. *J. Ophthalmic Nurs. Technol.* **12**, 208–10.

Thomas, B.C., Stanhope, R., Plowmari, P.N. and Leiper, A.D. (1993) Growth following single fraction and fractionated TBI for BMT. *Eur. J. Paediatr.* **52**, 888–92.

Thomas, E.D. and Ferrebee, J.W. (1962) Transplantation of marrow and whole organs; experiences and comments. *Can. Med. Assoc. J.* **86**, 435–44.

Thomas, E.D., Lochte, H.L. Jr, Lu, W.C. *et al.* (1957) Intravenous infusion of bone marrow in patients receiving radiation and chemotherapy. *N. Engl. J. Med.* **257**, 491–6.

Thomas, E.D., Buckner, C.D., Rudolph, R.H. *et al.* (1971) Allogeneic marrow grafting for haematological malignancy using HLA-matched donor recipient sibling pairs. *Blood* **38**, 267–87.

Thomas, E.D., Buckner, C.D., Clift, R.A. *et al.* (1979) Marrow transplantation for acute non-lymphoblastic leukaemia in first remission. *N. Engl. J. Med.* **301**, 597–9.

Tiley, C., Powles, R., Catalano, J. *et al.* (1992) Result of a double blind placebo controlled study of odansetron as an antiemetic during total body irradiation in patients undergoing bone marrow transplantation. *Leukaemia and Lymphoma* **7**, 317–21.

Vowels, M., Chan, L.L., Giri, N. *et al.* (1993) Factors affecting hair re-growth after BMT. *Bone Marrow Transplant.* **12**, 347–50.

Vriesendorp, H.M. (1985) Engraftment of haemopoietic cells. In Van Bekkum, D.W. and Lowenberg, B. (eds), *Bone marrow transplantation, biological mechanisms and clinical practice.* New York: Dekker, 73–145.

Weiner, R.S., Bortin, M.M., Gale, R.P. *et al.* (1986) Interstitial pneumonia after bone marrow transplantation. Assessment of risk factors. *Ann. Intern. Med.* **104**, 168–75.

Westbrook, C., Glaholm, J. and Barrett, A. (1987) Vomiting associated with whole body irradiation. *Clin. Radiol.* **38**, 263–6.

Wheldon, T.E. (1997) The radiobiological basis of total body irradiation. *Br. J. Radiol.* **70**, 1204–7.

Winston, D.J., Ho, W.G. and Champlin, R.E. (1990) CMV infections after allogeneic BMT. *Rev. Infect. Dis.* **12**(suppl.), 776–92.

44

Hodgkin's disease

HELEN ANDERSON, RAJINISH K. GUPTA AND T. ANDREW LISTER

Hodgkin's disease (HD) is generally perceived to be a malignant disease of the lymphoid system. The morbid anatomy was first presented by Thomas Hodgkin in 1832 and named Hodgkin's disease by Wilks in 1865. The natural history is that of an inexorable progression towards death, survival rarely exceeding a few years and correlating with the extent of disease at the initial presentation. Beginning in the late 1950s and early 1960s, studies from Stanford and later elsewhere have led to a greater understanding of the disease process, the reasonably predictable pattern of spread and the principles of staging. As a consequence, the past three decades have witnessed the development of curative treatments, initially with radiotherapy, then with chemotherapy and more recently combination chemotherapy. This progress has transformed a nearly uniformly fatal disease to one that is often cured, even though the pathogenesis remains elusive. With an improving understanding of the disease, staging and prognostic evaluation in the last few years, survival rates are improving. However, long-term toxicities and complications continue to prevent further reductions in mortality and morbidity. The future goal is to reduce these effects whilst ensuring that the disease remains adequately treated.

EPIDEMIOLOGY

Hodgkin's disease is uncommon, accounting for about 1 per cent of malignant diseases diagnosed in countries in the Western world each year. The annual incidence in Europe and the USA is three new cases per 100 000 population and is slightly lower (2.4) in the UK. However, it has an unusual age distribution, distinct from other lymphomas, that makes it one of the most common malignant diseases in young people.

Three epidemiological patterns of Hodgkin's disease have been described. In so-called 'developed' countries, Hodgkin's disease has the classical bimodal age incidence, characterized by low rates in childhood with a rise to a peak in young adults and then a second peak in older adults, particularly in men. This pattern is in contrast to that seen in developing countries, which shows the first peak occurring in childhood, a lower incidence in the third decade and a second peak in the older age group. An intermediate pattern is found in rural areas of developed countries, in central Europe and in the southern USA. This may represent a transitional state. Many studies have shown that the risk of developing Hodgkin's disease is related to high socioeconomic status, at least in young adults, whilst older patients tend to be of lower socioeconomic class. Overall, there is a male to female preponderance of 1.5 : 1, although this changes with different age groups and histological subtypes. For example, females predominate in the nodular sclerosing form of the disease. Other studies have suggested correlation with race, sibship size, housing, parental education and family history all as independent factors in the risk of developing the disease. There is also some evidence that there is a seasonal variation in certain subtypes. The proposal that Hodgkin's disease is the result of an infectious agent was first indicated by Thomas Hodgkin himself in 1832, followed by Sternberg (1898) and Reed (1902). Seroepidemiological studies have suggested a potential role of viruses, particularly the Epstein–Barr virus (EBV), including the finding that EBV DNA is present in up to 50 per cent of tumour biopsies. In summary, epidemiological features of Hodgkin's disease and recent pathological findings suggest that it may be a heterogeneous condition with different aetiological factors in the different age groups.

PATHOLOGY

Histopathology and diagnosis

Hodgkin's disease is histologically characterized by the presence of a minority of characteristic 'malignant' cells in an appropriate background of essentially normal or reactive admixture of lymphocytes (mainly T cells), plasma cells, eosinophils, granulocytes and histiocytes with fibrous tissue. These cells are cytologically normal. The diagnostic malignant cells, often less than 1 per cent of the total cellular content of the tumour mass, may be the classical binucleated Sternberg–Reed cells or mononuclear variants (Hodgkin's cells), multinucleated, pleomorphic or 'L and H' variants. They are characterized by their large size with vesicular nuclei, pronounced nuclear membrane and prominent eosinophilic inclusion-like nucleoli (owl's eyes). It is generally accepted that the diagnosis of Hodgkin's disease requires the presence of Sternberg–Reed cells.

However, Sternberg–Reed cells are not pathognomonic of Hodgkin's disease and may be found in other lymphomas and in reactive lymphoproliferative disorders. At the Rye meeting in 1965, Hodgkin's disease was described as being characterized by lesions containing diagnostic Sternberg–Reed cells, in association with a cytological and architectural background, i.e. the characteristic milieu of one of the described histological subtypes (Lukes et al., 1966). Ultimately, an experienced histopathologist is essential to make the diagnosis.

Hodgkin's disease most frequently involves axial lymph nodes, particularly in the neck and mediastinum. Other nodal groups such as the mesenteric nodes are generally spared. Although not absolute, there is a tendency for each particular subtype to localize to particular nodal groups, e.g. mediastinal nodes are commonly affected by nodular sclerosing Hodgkin's disease and high neck and abdominal nodes by mixed cellularity and lymphocyte-depleted types. Extranodal dissemination is often of the nodular sclerosing type.

Classification

The classification of Hodgkin's disease was until recently based on the Rye modification of the Lukes and Butler classification (Butler, 1992). This classification has been most commonly used and most of the trial data currently available are based on this classification system. The Rye classification is based on the different morphological pictures observed on conventionally stained histological slides. The ratio of Sternberg–Reed cells to reactive cells and the composition of the non-neoplastic infiltrate is of critical importance [from the most cellular (lymphocytic predominance) to the least cellular (lymphocytic depleted)]. However, in 1994 the revised European-American classification of lymphoid neoplasms (REAL classification) was published (Harris et al., 1994). This attempted to refine the classification of all the lymphomas (and myeloma) according to the morphological, immunological and genetic techniques available at the time. Most of the subgroups defined in the Rye system are retained, but in addition, a provisional entity, lymphocyte-rich classical Hodgkin's disease, was included. The classification recognizes two main types of Hodgkin's disease: classical types [nodular sclerosis, mixed cellularity, lymphocyte-rich classical (HD), and lymphocyte depletion] and nodular lymphocyte predominance type (NLPHD). These types are thought to represent distinct biological entities.

LYMPHOCYTE PREDOMINANCE

This is a rare subtype (<5 per cent) and in recent years there has been much discussion as to whether this should be recognized as a distinct clinico-pathological entity. It resembles other types of HD in having a minority of malignant cells in an inflammatory cell background but it has a number of differing morphological and immunophenotypical features. Previously it was further subclassified into a nodular and diffuse type, but this subdivision has been dispensed with. It has a nodular growth pattern with or without diffuse areas. Diagnostic Sternberg–Reed cells are rarely seen and diagnosis relies on the presence of Sternberg–Reed-related polyploid cells known as 'L and H' (lymphocytic and/or histiocytic) or 'popcorn' cells (Fig. 44.1). The background is predominantly lymphocytes with or without histiocyte clusters. Immunophenotypically it reacts with B-cell antibodies but is usually Ig negative. Also of note, the popcorn malignant cells are usually EBV negative in contrast to classical HD where up to 70 per cent of Sternberg–Reed cells are positive for EBV DNA. Clinically, this subtype occurs in all ages, males more than females. It usually involves the peripheral lymph nodes and is localized at diagnosis. Survival is long, with or without treatment for localized cases.

NODULAR SCLEROSIS

This subtype is currently diagnosed in about 70 per cent of all cases in developed countries and is usually more common in females, particularly in the young age group. Often this subtype is found in mediastinal and neck disease. The histological appearance of nodular sclerosing

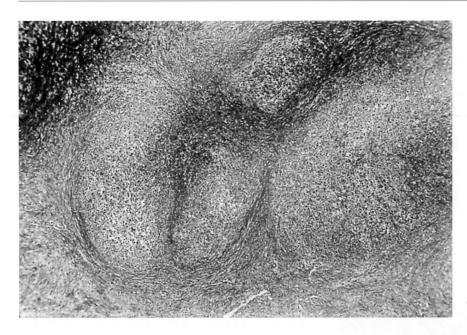

Figure 44.1 *Lymphocytic predominance Hodgkin's disease with typical 'L and H' cells.*

Hodgkin's disease is based on the presence of nodules of neoplastic and reactive cells, bands of birefringent collagen and lacunar cells (Figs 44.2 and 44.3). Lacunar cells are a variant of Sternberg–Reed cells which show contraction of their cytoplasm during fixation in formalin. The degree of fibrosis may vary greatly and, in those cases where sclerosis is sparse, absent or confined to a limited area, the term 'nodular sclerosis cellular phase' has been coined. Areas of necrosis of any amount are common in nodular sclerosis but rare in other types. Nodular sclerosis accounts for a large proportion of cases and attempts have been made to subclassify correlating with the prognostic behaviour of the disease. Two grades (I and II) of nodular sclerosis have been defined and correlated with the behaviour of the disease (grade II being more aggressive) (Ferry *et al.*, 1993). In addition, a 'syncytial' variant, characterized by sheets and cohesive clusters of Sternberg–Reed cells, is also described, equivalent to the grade II histology (Strickler *et al.*, 1986).

MIXED CELLULARITY

This subtype, found in 25 per cent of cases in developed countries, is often the most common in developing countries, e.g. Kenya. It is more common in males and is often associated with the EBV. In HIV-related Hodgkin's disease, mixed cellularity and nodular sclerosis (usually grade II) are the most frequent histological subtypes and are 'always' EBV positive. The mixed cellularity subtype is the commonest type to be found in the infradiaphragmatic area including the spleen. It can exhibit a variable appearance (as a consequence of being a diagnosis of exclusion) with mainly typical, sometimes lacunar, Sternberg–Reed cells and an abundant, variable, mixed cellular infiltrate in the absence of a sclerosing stromal reaction (Fig. 44.4), although a fine interstitial fibrosis may be present. It is important to realize that those cases that do not fit into

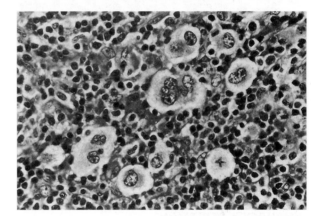

Figure 44.2 *Nodular sclerosing Hodgkin's disease. Low power.*

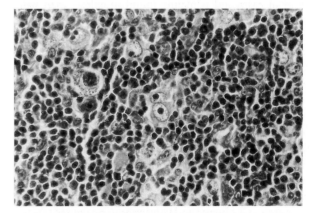

Figure 44.3 *Nodular sclerosing Hodgkin's disease with several lacunar cells. High power.*

the other types are included within this subtype. The possibility of peripheral T-cell lymphoma and T-cell-rich B-cell large cell lymphoma should also be considered when considering the differential diagnosis.

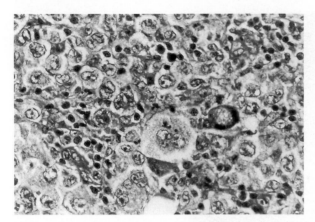

Figure 44.4 *Mixed cellularity Hodgkin's disease with a classical Sternberg–Reed cell in the centre of the field.*

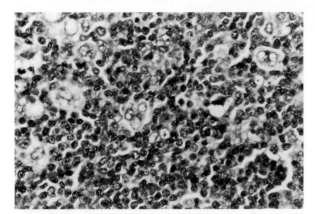

Figure 44.5 *Lymphocytic depletion Hodgkin's disease.*

LYMPHOCYTE DEPLETION

This is the rarest subtype, diagnosed in less than 5 per cent of cases and is mainly found in elderly men with advanced disease, in HIV-positive individuals and in developing countries. It frequently presents in extranodal sites (bone marrow, spleen, liver) or intra-abdominal lymphadenopathy without peripheral nodes. The infiltrate in this subtype is often diffuse and hypocellular with occasional fibroblasts and neutrophils (Fig. 44.5). There are often large numbers of Sternberg–Reed and variant cells, which may form confluent sheets. This has been subtyped as 'reticular' variant or 'Hodgkin's sarcoma', which is a particularly aggressive form of the disease with patients rarely surviving long enough to receive treatment. The borderline between this variant and anaplastic large cell lymphoma is blurred and continues to be refined.

PROVISIONAL ENTITY: LYMPHOCYTE-RICH CLASSICAL HD

This is a form of Hodgkin's disease that has been newly defined in the REAL classification system. It is a diffuse tumour with a rich background of lymphocytes with infrequent classic Sternberg–Reed cells. There is an overlap with diffuse forms of the lymphocyte predominant subtype, the cellular phase of nodular sclerosing and mixed cellularity. It is thought, however, that the Sternberg–Reed cells have classic forms, unlike those in lymphocyte predominant Hodgkin's disease, and so do not fall into this subgroup. The immunophenotype, genetic features and clinical course are similar to nodular sclerosing and mixed cellular Hodgkin's (Harris *et al.*, 1994).

Pathogenesis

There is no longer any apparent disagreement that Hodgkin's disease is anything other than a malignant condition. However, the heterogeneity of the disease, both histologically and clinically, has introduced the notion of several causative agents. Mueller in 1991 suggested that the malignant transformation occurs secondary to a sustained host response to chronic tissue-based antigenic stimulation. This is supported by more recent molecular biological studies. The current hypothesis is that cells in the majority of classical HD represent a monoclonal outgrowth of late germinal or post-germinal centre B cells that have lost their capacity to express immunoglobulin (Kanzler *et al.*, 1996; Stein and Hummel, 1999). In a minority of classic HD, the Sternberg–Reed cells are derived from cytotoxic T cells (Oudejans *et al.*, 1996). Normally B cells that are unable to express immunoglobulin apoptose. However, the fact that they do not supports a defect in the apoptotic pathway as an important feature in the pathogenesis of Hodgkin's disease. The presence of a predominant non-malignant infiltrate in the lesions of Hodgkin's disease is in part explained by the multiple cytokines that have been found to originate from the malignant Sternberg–Reed cell. These cytokines stimulate an inflammatory reaction, fibrosis, and may be responsible for the depressed immunity associated with Hodgkin's disease.

Immunohistochemistry (Harris *et al.*, 1994)

In the background of classical HD, T cells predominate the majority of which have a CD4 phenotype. There is no marker specific for the Sternberg–Reed cell but they express antigens usually found on activated lymphocytes. The Sternberg–Reed cells in classical HD, CD30$^+$, CD15$^\pm$, CD45$^-$, are usually B-cell and T-cell-associated antigen negative and EMA$^-$. CD15 and CD30 may be difficult to detect in paraffin sections. In nodular sclerosis, mixed cellularity and lymphocyte-rich Hodgkin's disease expression of B-cell and T-cell antigens may be present, usually in a minority of cells. In lymphocyte-depleted HD the absence of B-cell or T-cell antigens are usually required for the diagnosis because the histological differential diagnosis often includes B- or T-large cell lymphoma or anaplastic large cell lymphoma. Lymphocyte-predominant Hodgkin's disease has a unique phenotype expressing CD45, B-cell-associated antigens (CD19, 20, 22 79a) and CDw75. It is usually CD15 and Ig negative. In the background the small lymphocytes are predominantly B cells though T cells are present surrounding the L and H cells.

Molecular biology

GENE REARRANGEMENTS

Studies on the clonal rearrangement of the immunoglobulin gene during B-cell differentiation and the T-cell receptor genes during T-cell development are difficult to perform in Hodgkin's disease due to the scarcity of malignant cells. However, in all subtypes of Hodgkin's disease, Ig and TCR genes are usually germline (Harris *et al.*, 1994).

VIRAL ASSOCIATION (JARRETT, 1992)

An association between EBV and Hodgkin's disease has been suggested by serological findings, the increased risk of developing the disease after infectious mononucleosis and epidemiological evidence. With the development of the polymerase chain reaction (PCR), evidence of EBV DNA sequences have been reported in the majority of biopsies: 60–70 per cent in mixed cellularity, 40 per cent in nodular sclerosing Hodgkin's disease. Of note, malignant cells in lymphocyte-predominant HD are usually EBV negative.

In those cases of Hodgkin's disease that have EBV-positive Sternberg–Reed cells it has been confirmed that virtually all (if not all) of the malignant cells harbour the viral genome. This, along with the evidence of clonality of the EBV genome within the biopsy material and the persistence of viral DNA throughout the course of the Hodgkin's disease, suggests an aetiological role for EBV at the time of malignant transformation rather than it being a 'silent passenger'. However, the debate continues.

ONCOGENES

Immunohistochemistry on sections from primary biopsy material has demonstrated the presence of protein products of c-*myc*, bcl-2 , *LMP 1* and *p53* in a variable number of Sternberg–Reed cells in a proportion of cases. One postulated role of such oncogenes is in the blockage of the apoptotic pathway leading to the immortalization of the Sternberg–Reed cells. The full implications of such findings are unknown at present.

CYTOKINES

As haematopoiesis relies on a complex interaction of cytokines which have roles in activation, proliferation and differentiation of cells of various lineages, it has been suggested that cytokines are also involved in Hodgkin's disease. The expression of a variety of cytokines has been

demonstrated on Sternberg–Reed cells. It is also possible that systemic humoral factors such as interleukin-1 (IL-1), interleukin-6 (IL-6) and tumour necrosis factor-α could result in the systemic 'B' symptoms seen in some patients with Hodgkin's disease. Transforming growth factor (TGF)-Pi activity has been demonstrated in the Sternberg–Reed cells of cases of nodular sclerosing disease. This cytokine may be the stimulus for the sclerosis found in this particular subtype. Detectable levels of soluble CD30 antigen, soluble IL-2 receptor and IL-6 have been found in the serum of patients with Hodgkin's disease with some suggestion of prognostic value.

CYTOGENETICS

In contrast to non-Hodgkin's lymphomas, cytogenetic analysis in Hodgkin's disease is extremely difficult due to the small number of malignant cells and their fragility. Multiple non-random structural and numerical abnormalities have been reported. Essentially it appears that Sternberg–Reed cells are polyploid.

CLINICAL FEATURES

Clinical findings

LYMPH NODES

Painless enlargement of superficial lymph nodes is the most common presentation of Hodgkin's disease and is evident at the time of diagnosis in at least 70 per cent of patients. On examination there is usually a 'rubbery' consistency to the nodes which are non-tender; 60–80 per cent of patients have enlarged cervical nodes, 6–20 per cent have axillary and 6–15 per cent inguinal adenopathy. Exclusive infradiaphragmatic lymphadenopathy is seen only in up to 10 per cent of patients. At presentation mediastinal nodes will be involved in up to 60 per cent cases and retroperitoneal nodes in 25 per cent of cases. Occasionally, alcohol-induced lymph-node discomfort ranging to sharp pain may be noted (<10 per cent). Splenomegaly is found in 30 per cent of patients at presentation.

SYSTEMIC SYMPTOMS

Systemic symptoms, in particular low-grade fever and drenching night sweats, are present in about 40 per cent of patients at presentation, usually in those with more advanced disease. These symptoms, together with weight loss or generalized pruritus, may be the presenting complaint. The criteria for the classical 'B' symptoms, i.e. unexplained weight loss, fever and drenching night sweats, are defined under 'Staging'.

Other non-specific symptoms such as cough, chest pain, bronchial obstruction, superior vena caval obstruction, abdominal pain, ascites, jaundice, bone pain, spinal cord compression and peripheral oedema are all uncommon presenting features.

MODE OF SPREAD

Hodgkin's disease appears to begin in an area within the lymphatic system and to spread in an orderly manner to contiguous lymph nodes via lymphatic channels. Non-contiguous spread and haematological distribution are more common with recurrent disease. Non-contiguous spread is also said to be more common with certain histological types.

The criteria have been defined in the Cotswold report for organ involvement (Lister *et al.*, 1989). In advanced Hodgkin's disease (stages IIIB, IVA and 1VB), the liver is involved in 20 per cent of cases, bone marrow in 10 per cent of cases, and rarely other organs such as bone (7 per cent) and lung (5 per cent).

Differential diagnosis

The clinical differential diagnosis is between other causes of lymphadenopathy, both malignant and benign, causes of a raised ESR and rarely causes of isolated splenomegaly.

INVESTIGATIONS

The management of Hodgkin's disease begins with establishing the diagnosis, which can only be made on the basis of biopsy of involved tissue. Where possible, a whole lymph node should be taken fresh for pathological examination. When the diagnosis of Hodgkin's disease is made on the basis of a biopsy from an extranodal site, confirmation with a lymph-node biopsy is desirable unless the diagnosis is considered unequivocal.

Following confirmation of the diagnosis, further evaluation seeks to define the extent of the disease and to allocate a stage and hence plan treatment and advise on prognosis (Lister and Crowther, 1990).

A detailed history should be obtained and should include:

- presence or absence of unexplained fever and its duration;
- unexplained sweating, especially at night and its severity;
- unexplained weight loss as a percentage of usual body weight and the duration involved;
- unexplained pruritus, its extent and severity.

Performance status, alcohol-induced pain, family history of malignant disease, previous immunosuppressive illness, history of previous malignancy and prior treatment with chemotherapy or radiotherapy should be noted.

A complete physical examination must be performed with special attention to areas where lymphadenopathy

Table 44.1 *Cotswolds recommendations for investigation of patients with Hodgkin's disease*

Recommended
History and examination
    B symptoms: weight loss <10% during previous
    6 months, documented fever, night sweats
Radiology
    Plain chest radiography
    Computed tomography of the thorax
    Computed tomography of the abdomen and pelvis[a]
    Bipedal lymphograma[b]
Haematology
    Full blood count[d]
    Lymphocyte count[d]
    Erythrocyte sedimentation rate[d]
    Bone marrow biopsy[c]
Biochemistry
    Tests of liver function[d]
    Albumin, lactate dehydrogenase, calcium levels[d]

Under special circumstances
    Ultrasonographic scanning
    Magnetic resonance imaging

Other imaging techniques
    Isotope scanning
    Gallium
    Technetium

[a,b] Both not usually required.
[c] Not for stage IA of IIA with favourable features.
[d] Do not determine stage: may not influence management.
From Lister and Crowther (1990), with permission.

may occur. The largest mass in each region should be measured and recorded, together with the size of the liver and spleen, also measured in centimetres. Waldeyer's ring should be examined,

The recommended procedures and investigations for complete staging are listed in Table 44.1. Although these continue to be the accepted recommendations, the emphasis on certain procedures and the introduction of new procedures is slowly evolving. Other than histological examination of involved tissue with Hodgkin's disease, there are no diagnostic laboratory tests or markers.

Recommended procedures

HAEMATOLOGY

In most cases, haernatological tests are within the normal range, although an associated normochromic, normocytic anaemia is not uncommon. The erythrocyte sedimentation rate (ESR; Westergren method) at one hour is elevated in 30–50 per cent of cases and is associated with the presence of B symptoms. An absolute lymphocyte count is necessary as lymphopenia is associated with advanced disease and a poor prognosis. Eosinophilia is occasionally seen and, rarely, immune thrombocytopenia and neutropenia occur.

Bone marrow aspiration and trephine is also advised in high-risk cases and not in those patients with stage I or IIA, providing there are no 'adverse features'.

BIOCHEMISTRY

These should include biochemical tests of liver, bone and renal function. Abnormalities in liver function tests may be seen in Hodgkin's disease in the absence of liver infiltration. Proteinuria is occasionally seen and hypercalcaemia is rare. Although these investigations may not directly influence staging, they may influence modification of treatment and dosage and provide a guide to further investigations.

RADIOLOGY

Radiological investigation should include:

- chest radiograph (postero-anterior, penetrated anteroposterior and lateral). Mediastinal involvement, usually of the upper mediastinum is the most common finding. Hilar, subcarinal and posterior mediastinal lymphadenopathy is unusual without paratracheal node involvement. Involvement of the lung parenchyma may take several forms. There may be infiltration from adjacent lymph nodes or, less frequently, rounded opacities corresponding to nodules that may be single or multiple.
- computed tomography (CT) (thorax, abdomen and pelvis). CT scanning of the thorax is extremely sensitive in detecting mediastinal disease and delineates the nodal areas in the thorax as defined in the Cotswolds classification. In the abdomen, CT with intravenous contrast and images at 1 cm intervals will detect hepatosplenomegaly, abdominal masses and enlargement of lymph nodes.

Procedures to be considered under certain conditions

LYMPHOGRAGHY

Bipedal lymphography is the classical and the most sensitive method for demonstrating the involvement of retroperitoneal lymph nodes by distortion of the pattern of the architecture or increase in size. However, it is time consuming and relies on the experience and expertise of the radiologist. This investigation is becoming less commonly employed even though it is considered to be complementary to CT scanning and allows easy follow-up in positive cases.

ULTRASOUND SCANNING

This also is not routinely performed. It does, however, have a role in certain circumstances: it can assist confirmation of splenic or liver involvement in cases where this is not clear on CT scanning.

RADIOISOTOPE IMAGING

Gallium-67 citrate scanning has been used for some time particularly in the situation of determining whether active disease is present in a residual mass following treatment for Hodgkin's disease. It has been demonstrated that patients with a residual mass in the mediastinum have a higher chance of recurrence if the mass is positive on high-dose gallium scanning. The technique is less useful for abdominal disease. Its role in initial staging is also doubtful.

In recent years PET scanning using 2-fluorodeoxyglucose has become more popular in both the initial staging of Hodgkin's disease and in diagnosing residual disease or relapse in previously treated patients. Evidence is accumulating that it may be more sensitive that it may have greater sensitivity and specificity than standard imaging procedures.

Technetium bone scanning may be useful in certain clinical situations.

MAGNETIC RESONANCE IMAGING (MRI)

MRI may be used in particular situations for clarification when CT and/or isotope scanning is inconclusive, e.g. CNS involvement, bone involvement and residual abnormalities in the mediastinum.

STAGING LAPAROTOMY

Laparotomy was introduced in the late 1960s to increase the precision of staging the disease (Glatstein *et al.*, 1969). It became clear that in patients with clinical stage I and II disease occult abdominal disease was found in 25–30 per cent of cases, mostly in the spleen and seldom in the para-aortic region. After a period in which staging laparotomy was used routinely, a number of clinical factors were found to predict for a low or high risk of a 'positive' laparotomy. The same factors were also found to be predictive for a low or high long-term relapse-free survival if supradiaphragmatic radiotherapy only was given.

The late side-effects of splenectomy such as pneumococcal sepsis and a possibly higher risk of secondary leukaemia, as well as the surgical morbidity of the procedure, have since argued against the use of staging laparotomy. Over the years it has become apparent that there is little impact on overall survival of patients who underwent laparotomy compared with those who did not. With the increasing use of chemotherapy, adjuvant or otherwise, laparotomy and splenectomy are rarely employed and then only in very selected cases.

STAGING

Clinical staging is the outcome of investigation which defines the extent and distribution of Hodgkin's disease within an individual patient. This assessment allows consideration of the optimal treatment and possible prognosis (Lister and Crowther, 1990).

Pre-treatment staging

The staging system is an anatomical one that describes the sites of tumour in relation to the diaphragm. The Ann Arbor classification reported in 1971 modified the previous Rye system based on the developments in the preceding 5 years, namely, the introduction of the concept of extranodal extension and the use of staging laparotomy (Glatstein *et al.*, 1969). Stage of disease correlates with the natural history, choice of treatment and allows evaluation once therapy has been completed (Ultmann, 1992).

As a result of the development of successful chemotherapy regimens, the use of combined modality treatment, the declining use of laparotomy and the introduction of CT scanning as an alternative to lymphography, a further revision of the staging classification was undertaken in 1989.

The Cotswolds staging classification (Table 44.2) incorporated minor revisions but maintained the anatomically orientated nature of the Ann Arbor classification. There were five main changes:

1 CT scanning was accepted as an imaging investigation.
2 Involvement of liver and spleen was redefined.
3 The concept of 'tumour bulk' was clarified.
4 The concept of 'unconfirmed/uncertain' complete remission was introduced.
5 Hilar disease was separated from mediastinal nodal involvement.

Table 44.2 *The Cotswolds staging classification*

Stage I	Involvement of a single lymph node region or lymphoid structure (e.g. spleen, thymus, Waldeyer's ring)
Stage II	Involvement of two or more lymph node regions on the same side of the diaphragm (the mediastinum is a single site, hilar lymph nodes are lateralized). The number of anatomical sites should be indicated by a suffix (e.g. IIB)
Stage III	Involvement of lymph node regions or structures on both sides of the diaphragm
	III₁: with or without splenic hilar, coeliac, or portal nodes
	III₂: with para-aortic, iliac, mesenteric nodes
Stage IV	Involvement of extranodal site(s) beyond that designated 'E'
	A: no symptoms
	B: fever, drenching sweats, weight loss
	X: bulky disease:
	>1/3 widening of mediastinum
	>10 cm maximum dimension of nodal mass
	E: involvement of a single extranodal site, contiguous or proximal or known nodal site
	CS: clinical stage
	PS: pathological stage

STAGING CRITERIA

Thus, the anatomical staging criteria can be stated as follows.

Clinical stage (CS)

1 Lymph node involvement:
   (a) clinical enlargement of a node when alternative pathology may be excluded; and
   (b) enlargement on plain radiograph, CT or lymphography.
2 Splenic involvement: unequivocal, palpable splenomegaly alone, or equivocal, palpable splenomegaly, with radiological confirmation of either enlargement or multiple focal defects, which are neither cystic nor vascular. Radiological enlargement alone is inadequate.
3 Liver involvement: clinical liver enlargement alone with or without abnormalities of liver function tests, is no longer considered adequate in classifying the liver as involved. Thus, the liver is considered to be involved if there are multiple focal defects which are neither cystic nor vascular noted with at least two imaging techniques.
4 Bone involvement: history of pain or elevation of serum alkaline phosphatase, supported by changes on plain radiology or evidence from another imaging technique.
5 CNS involvement:
   (a) a spinal extradural deposit may be diagnosed on the basis of the clinical history and confirmation by myelography, CT or MRI; and
   (b) intracranial involvement will rarely be diagnosed clinically at presentation. Confirmation requires a space-occupying lesion with additional extranodal sites.
6 Other sites of involvement: clinical involvement of other extranodal sites may only be diagnosed if the site is contiguous or proximal to a known nodal site.

Pathological stage (PS)

The pathological stage depends on histological confirmation of specific sites of involvement including laparotomy.

CRITERIA FOR B SYMPTOMS

- Unexplained weight loss of more than 10 per cent of the body weight during the 6 months before initial staging investigation.
- Unexplained, persistent, or recurrent fever with temperatures above 38°C during the previous month; and
- Recurrent, drenching nights sweats during the previous month.

CRITERIA FOR BULK

Clinically palpable, largest single lymph node or conglomerate node mass, greater than 10 cm in the largest diameter. Mediastinal bulk disease is present when its maximum width is equal to or greater than one-third of the internal transverse diameter of the thorax at the level of T5/6 on a chest radiograph.

Nodal bulk in the abdomen is defined as the largest dimension of 10 cm or greater, independent of the radiological technique used.

CRITERIA FOR EXTRANODAL SPREAD

The E suffix used to indicate that limited extranodal involvement was retained, although there appears to be some diversity in its interpretation.

STAGING NOTATION

This is shown in Table 44.2.

Post-treatment evaluation

One month after the completion of planned therapy, response is documented on the basis of clinical examination, results of repeat radiology which was abnormal at presentation and re-biopsy of bone marrow and abnormal tissue if apparent and accessible. Following 'mantle' irradiation, a reassessment CT scan of the chest should be postponed until 3 months after treatment. The criteria for response are used and classified into complete remission (CR), unconfirmed/uncertain remission [CR(u)], partial remission or progressive disease. Subsequently, it is recommended that patients are seen at 3-monthly intervals during the first 2 years after therapy, 4-monthly intervals in the third year, 6-monthly in the fourth and fifth years and annually thereafter. Appropriate investigations should be performed in the light of any symptoms or signs and of the initial sites of disease. Assessment of the possible long-term complications should also be undertaken.

PROGNOSTIC FACTORS

Prognostic factors for the outcome of treatment in Hodgkin's disease have been studied more intensively in recent times with the tendency to tailor treatment more specifically to particular groups of patients. Also, since a small percentage of patients will die within 5 years of presentation with progressive disease, it may be possible to recognize those at risk on the basis of certain clinical and investigational factors. In the past, various publications included analysis of prognostic factors; besides the classical factors of Ann Arbor stage, systemic symptoms, histopathology, age and gender, a further collection of factors have been claimed to influence prognosis. Large databases have been co-ordinated to meta-analyse risk factors in order to enable better predictions of outcome. One such approach collated data in patients with advanced stage disease from 25 study groups or treatment centres (Hasenclever and Diehl, 1998). Twenty factors were considered and from these, seven factors were identified as having similar important prognostic effects: serum albumin <4 g/dL, haemoglobin <10.5 g/dL, male sex, 45 years old or older, stage IV disease, leucocytosis ($>15\,000$/mm^3) and lymphopenia (a lymphocyte count less than 600/mm^3). A score predicted the rate of freedom from progression of disease with each factor reducing tumour control by 7–8 per cent at 5 years. Other markers such as elevated ESR, lactate dehydrogenase (LDH), alkaline phosphatase (ALP) and creatinine, said to be of use, usually reflect disease activity and are rarely independent of other clinical markers.

Prognostic factors for achieving complete remission

If both clinical and serum parameters are considered together, then apparently Ann Arbor stage and B symptoms or the serum parameters (ESR and albumin) are the most reliable predictors.

Prognostic factors for freedom from recurrence

There are several more factors that appear to contribute to the prediction of the quality of a complete remission. Male gender and older age are well known to be unfavourable. Histology (mixed cellularity and lymphocytic depletion) also appears to play a role in all stages, but particularly in stages I and II. B symptoms and infradiaphragmatic disease appear to be associated with an unfavourable prognosis in stage I, whilst the number of involved sites plays a role in stages II and III. These findings may reflect the considerable heterogeneity of stages.

Prognostic factors for survival

There are few prognostic factors that appear to influence survival. However, it seems that increasing age, male gender, and histology (particularly the lymphocyte-depleted form) are all unfavourable factors. The number of involved sites may also be important, but there is no direct contribution from serum parameters or the presence of bulk disease.

There are several factors that have yet to be convincingly demonstrated to be reproducible and useful, such as tumour burden, bone marrow involvement, nodular sclerosing histology, soluble IL-2 receptor level and soluble CD30 concentration. These conclusions may allow consideration of factors other than stage alone for the selection of appropriate treatment strategy.

TREATMENT

The general principle governing the treatment of Hodgkin's disease is the same as for any other illness, namely, to achieve the desired effect with the minimum intervention. The success of modern therapy makes it very simple to recommend that cure should almost always be pursued aggressively at the time of initial diagnosis. However, failure of the treatment of first choice or recurrence, certainly the second or third time, makes the choice between increasingly intensive approaches with diminishing chances of success progressively more pertinent.

The specific options are between radiotherapy, chemotherapy and a combination of the two, the details depending on the prevailing circumstances. The perception that radiotherapy is less dangerous and less unpleasant than chemotherapy in the past led to a preference for its use if the anticipation of cure is high enough. This view may be reinforced by the observation that those with recurrence after irradiation may subsequently be cured with chemotherapy.

Despite this, the current general trend is for more patients to receive at least some chemotherapy as part of their initial management. This is a consequence of the persistent belief that the best opportunity for eliminating Hodgkin's disease completely is at the time of diagnosis, a reluctance to undertake surgical staging, the development of non-sterilizing and non-leukaemic chemotherapy and the emergence of results demonstrating the long-term complications associated with the extent and dose of radiotherapy. The impact of meticulous attention to detail upon outcome and side-effects, whether on radiation field or chemotherapy dose and schedule, cannot be overemphasized.

The use of high-dose (myeloablative) chemotherapy with haematopoietic stem cell rescue is becoming an increasingly used option in the management of patients with resistant Hodgkin's disease. There is accumulating evidence as to its benefit but definitive randomized control trials comparing its use with standard therapy are still lacking.

The choice of treatment will be influenced by several factors, such as the point in the course of the illness, the patient's wishes and the overall situation. The diagnosis and the likely outcome of whichever treatment is being considered need to be explained carefully to the patient and to the family, often more than once, at presentation and, in particular, as the situation changes. It is important to be clear as to whether treatment is being advised with curative intent, or whether the aim is to keep the person well for as long as possible. This is particularly important as some patients who have never had a remission from the disease may nonetheless remain relatively well for several years, although eventual death from Hodgkin's disease is inevitable.

Radiotherapy

Radiotherapy was introduced into the treatment of Hodgkin's disease at the turn of the century with some benefit but considerable toxicity. The concept of treating a wider field than the apparently involved nodes was first proposed by Finzi in 1913 and pursued with vitality. Gilbert (1939) employed segmental fields with obvious advantage and the subsequent use of even wider fields to incorporate all contiguous sites had a dramatic effect on the survival pattern of the disease, the most notable advances being recorded at the Princess Margaret Hospital, Toronto (Peters and Middlemiss, 1958) and Stanford (Kaplan, 1966). The philosophy of designing therapy on the presumption that this disease spreads contiguously was made practically much easier to apply without a great increase in toxicity by the invention of the linear accelerator. Radiotherapy remains the most effective single agent for the treatment of nodal Hodgkin's disease.

RADIATION FIELD AND DOSE

As described by Kaplan, careful attention must be paid to the use of a linear accelerator, large fields contoured to the patient's anatomy and tumour configuration, a tumoricidal dose, opposed field fractioned treatment and pre-treatment simulation with careful planning. Capable of producing 6–10 MV photons and permitting treatment to large fields with reasonable skin sparing, the linear accelerator, properly used, will allow the irradiation of involved and contiguous, supposedly uninvolved, lymphoid regions with a dose adequate to ensure tumour eradication. Techniques such as the use of non-divergent lead blocks and divergent blocks made from a low melting point alloy permit the shaping of large fields. An extended distance is usually required to achieve these large fields and, in most situations, opposed field treatment techniques are employed to ensure dose homogeneity.

Routine field simulation and port film (beam film) verification on the treatment machine aid optimal field design and recording that the prescribed treatment is properly given. The recommended dose is 35–40 Gy, fractionated over approximately 4 weeks. Evenly weighted, opposed field treatments are generally employed, both fields treated daily, with fractions of 1.5–2 Gy depending on field size, patient's tolerance and so on. The use of such fractions is vital to avoid pulmonary and gastrointestinal radiation damage. The dose for the prophylactic treatment of adjacent clinically uninvolved areas is uncertain but a minimum of 30–36 Gy is usually recommended.

INVOLVED FIELD

This is radiation to involved node groups only with a small margin of adjacent normal tissue.

EXTENDED FIELD

Extended field irradiation generally implies a field that encompasses all nodal sites either above or below the diaphragm.

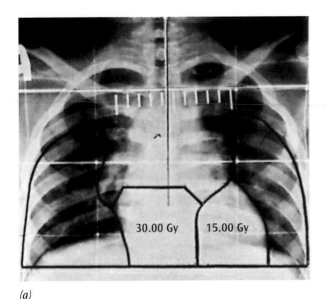
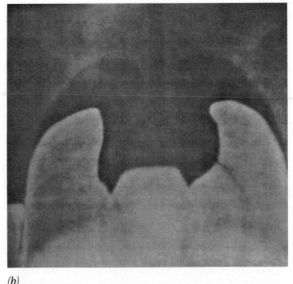

(a)   (b)

Figure 44.6 *(a) A typical anterior mantle set-up film for a patient with PSIIA Hodgkin's disease with a small mediastinal mass. Note that blocks are placed over the apex of the heart and the subcarinal portion of the heart at 15 and 30 Gy, respectively. (b) An anterior mantle port film, taken on the treatment machine, confirming the proper placement of blocks as defined on the set-up film. Note that blocks have been placed over the larynx, humeral heads and axillary skin folds. (Reproduced with permission from Hoppe, 1990).*

SUPRADIAPHRAGMATIC FIELDS

The 'mantle' field includes all the lymph-node areas below the base of the mandible and above the level of the insertion of the diaphragm. This incorporates the cervical, supraclavicular, axillary, infraclavicular, mediastinal and pulmonary hilar lymph nodes. Individually contoured lung blocks designed to protect the lungs allows treatment of the mediastinal and hilar lymphoid sites and conform to both the patient's anatomy and tumour distribution. Additional special blocks may be placed over particular areas depending upon the location of the disease in individual patients and the total dose of irradiation to be used, e.g. occiput, spinal cord posteriorly, larynx and humoral heads.

At Stanford if there is mediastinal disease, the entire cardiac silhouette is treated to 15 Gy. Thereafter, a block is placed over the apex to shield a portion of the pericardium and after a total dose of 30 Gy has been given a subcarinal block is placed 5 cm below the carina, protecting even more of the heart and pericardium (Hoppe, 1990). A different technique is used at St Bartholomew's Hospital, London where the lung block protects the apex of the heart and a subcarinal block is not routinely used.

Low-dose irradiation may be given to the lungs by the use of partial transmission blocks, e.g. when there is pulmonary hilar lymph node involvement, 15–16 Gy may be delivered by using a 37 per cent transmission lung block. Modifications to the mantle field are often undertaken during the course of therapy, e.g. the 'shrinking field technique', when wider blocks are made to protect more of the lungs as large mediastinal masses regress.

Essentially it is important to remember that each mantle field is tailored to an individual's requirements. If, for example, there is disease extending to the chest wall, then areas of involvement under the lung blocks will require a boost with electrons or tangential photon fields. Another example would be the use of opposed lateral Waldeyer fields to treat high cervical nodes that extend close to the upper border of the usual mantle field. The lower border of this field would oppose the upper border of the mantle.

A typical anterior mantle set-up film for a patient with stage IIA disease with a small mediastinal mass is shown in Figure 44.6.

SUBDIAPHRAGMATIC FIELDS

The classical subdiaphragmatic irradiation field is the inverted Y. This encompasses the para-aortic, splenic hilar, common iliac, external iliac and the inguinal femoral lymph nodes. It is, however, more common to limit the lower border of the subdiaphragmatic field to the level of the L4–5 interspace (para-aortic/splenic pedicle field) or to below the aortic bifurcation to include the common iliac nodes (spade field) (Fig. 44.7).

In a similar situation to the lungs, partial transmission block over the liver will allow a low dose of irradiation to the liver if required. Thus, a 50 per cent transmission block delivers 20–22 Gy to the liver during the same duration in which the para-aortic nodes are treated to 40–44 Gy.

Treating the pelvis requires two particular considerations, namely haematological and gonadal. Since there is a substantial volume of active bone marrow in the pelvis,

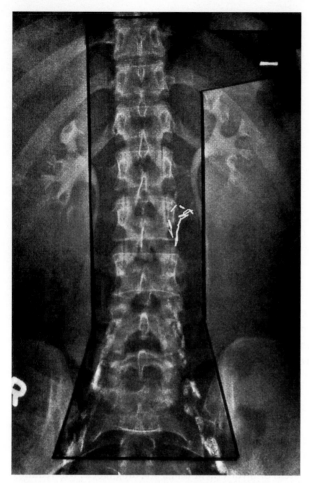

Figure 44.7 *A typical spade field as visualized using a simulator. Note the splenic pedicle clip and the extension of the field to encompass the splenic hilar lymph nodes. In this patient, IVP contrast has been administered and the position of the kidneys is readily apparent. (Reproduced with permission from Hoppe, 1990).*

fields must be carefully designed to minimize the amount of marrow subjected to irradiation. Lymphography may allow more precise delineation of a pelvic field and hence spare more of the bone marrow.

Gonadal toxicity is also extremely important. In women an oophoropexy may be performed to avoid irradiation damage. This may be carried out at the same time as staging laparotomy, radiopaque clips being placed to locate the ovaries. A double thickness block is then used to shield the organs. In men the risk of azoospermia is not negligible, particularly if no special blocking is employed as up to 10 per cent of the therapeutic dose may reach the testes. Again the use of a double thickness midline block and specially made testicular shield can reduce this to 0.75–3 per cent. Total nodal irradiation (TNI) refers to sequential treatment with mantle and inverted Y fields. The term sub-total nodal irradiation (STNI) is used to describe a standard mantle field with a subdiaphragmatic field that does not include the pelvis.

Chemotherapy

The indications for chemotherapy can be subdivided into the following categories (Oza *et al.*, 1991b):

- primary treatment for advanced disease;
- combined modality therapy;
- adjuvant to radiotherapy in early-stage disease;
- salvage therapy;
- high-dose therapy;
- palliative therapy.

Nitrogen mustard was the first compound to be assessed for a cytotoxic effect in patients with Hodgkin's disease following the observation that sulphur mustard gas induced neutropenia. Regression of lymphadenopathy was observed but no one was cured. For the next 20 years, many other agents were tried, but usually only with palliative intent after irradiation had failed. The considerable sensitivity of the disease to the sequential use of single-agent chemotherapy was demonstrated in 1966 by Hamilton Fairly *et al.* Cyclophosphamide induced remission in 69 per cent of patients. When failure occurred, 65 per cent responded to vinblastine, whilst at a fourth failure, 59 per cent responded to procarbazine. Cure was neither anticipated nor achieved.

By this time the first evidence that combining drugs improved the response rate was becoming available, with the demonstration that the combination of chlorambucil and vinblastine yielded a response rate of 73 per cent, much greater than the low rate obtained with either drug given alone (Lacher and Durrant, 1965). This paved the way for the design of quadruple combination chemotherapy, conceived at the National Cancer Institute in 1964. The MOPP programme, comprising nitrogen mustard, vincristine, prednisolone and procarbazine (derived from the more toxic initial combination that included methotrexate instead of procarbazine) was administered in 2-weekly cycles every month. It was an instant success, inducing complete remission of advanced disease in the majority of cases (DeVita *et al.*, 1980; Longo *et al.*, 1986).

MOPP has since been the yardstick against which all other chemotherapy regimens have been compared. Many variants have been introduced, including the substitution of vinblastine for vincristine (MVPP) to reduce the neurotoxicity of vincristine but accepting increased myelotoxicity and therefore a longer intercycle time. This programme of MVPP has been used at St Bartholomew's Hospital since 1968. The cycles were repeated every 6 weeks instead of 4 weeks because of the greater haematological toxicity associated with vinblastine. Results of the use of this regimen over a period of 20 years have been published. Chlorambucil was substituted for nitrogen mustard (ChIVPP) to reduce the severe vomiting and nausea associated with the latter. It appears that provided approximately six cycles of therapy are given as intended and without too much reduction in drug dose, all the variants yield the same proportion of patients alive after 10–20 years.

The immediate toxicity of this form of chemotherapy treatment is considerably greater than that of radiotherapy. All can induce nausea and vomiting, sometimes severe, and most induce alopecia. Bone marrow suppression is common, carrying the risk of potentially fatal infection. The psychological problems encountered by many patients should not be forgotten in addition to the probability of infertility, particularly for men, and the risk of second malignancy. However, these complications are far outweighed by the benefits of successful treatment for those with Hodgkin's disease.

The complete remission rate of 60–80 per cent, coupled with recurrence occurring in about one-third of patients within the first 3 years and the late side-effects still left considerable room for improvement. The next advance was the introduction of a 'non-cross-resistant' combination of doxorubicin (Adriamycin), bleomycin, vicristine and dacarbazine (ABVD) pioneered by Bonadonna et al., in Milan (1975, 1991). It was noted that ABVD was not associated with either permanent male infertility or secondary leukaemia and initial results suggested that this treatment could 'salvage' a proportion of patients in whom MOPP was failing, although this was not a universal finding. Subsequent randomized trials in newly diagnosed patients with Hodgkin's disease have shown ABVD to be superior with fewer toxic side-effects (Canellos et al., 1992).

Recently there has been a trend towards the use of non-alkylating agent-containing combinations because they appear to be both less sterilizing and associated with a much lower incidence of second malignancy. However, other potential side-effects are obviously a cause for concern, such as the potential cardiomyopathy associated with doxorubicin and pulmonary toxicity with the use of bleomycin. The demonstration that etoposide has activity against Hodgkin's disease has encouraged some to substitute it for bleomycin and dacarbazine (EVA) (Table 44.3).

Following the acknowledgement that ABVD was a less toxic and an effective alternative to MOPP, studies were performed incorporating so-called hybrid approaches which addressed the issue of whether alternating non-cross-resistant combinations, e.g. MOPP-ABVD, would increase complete remission rates and improve the fraction of patients cured of the disease. Most of these studies showed no significant advantage of hybrids over ABVD and many showed increased toxicity in the hybrid arm. Different chemotherapy regimens continue to be tested and, although ABVD remains the current standard, newer regimens such as the Stanford V and BEACOPP (bleomycin, etoposide, adriamycin, cyclophosphamide, vincristine, procarbazine and prednisone) show early promising results (Horning et al., 1996; Diehl et al., 1998).

Treatment guidelines

NEWLY DIAGNOSED PATIENTS

Clinical stage I and II

There was for a number of years reasonable agreement that for early stages, small volume, stage I and II disease, extended field radiotherapy was effective treatment (Hoppe et al., 1991). For example, at St Bartholomew's Hospital a full mantle field was prescribed after laparotomy (Ganesan et al., 1992) whilst at Stanford a full mantle plus spade field was irradiated in supradiaphragmatic disease, inverted Y ± splenic irradiation in subdiaphragmatic disease. However, many studies showing the favourable outcome for these approaches were based on pathologically staged patients. With the decrease in enthusiasm for staging laparotomy because of its attendant risks, and despite the usefulness of prognostic factors in defining risk of relapse, it is apparent that even patients with a very favourable prognosis who have high rates of complete remission (95 per cent) there is a significant risk of subsequent relapse (23 per cent; Carde et al., 1988). There is a move towards treating patients with early-stage disease with some chemotherapy. Some argue that not all patients who relapse enter a further remission. In addition, there is the psychological trauma of further treatment, the additive long-term complications and toxicities of full dose treatments and the reliance on meticulous staging and prognostic factor analysis, which can be simplified if all patients receive some chemotherapy. There are some rare exceptions where radiotherapy alone is advocated: non-bulky, stage IA epitrochlear or high-neck lymphocyte-predominant disease can be treated with involved-field irradiation only and also non-bulky stage IA nodular sclerosing disease of the mediastinum, which is virtually always confined to the site of presentation and can be treated with regional irradiation alone. There is, however, no significant difference in survival between those treated successfully with chemotherapy for recurrence after primary radiotherapy and those who received chemotherapy initially and the ultimate choice of therapy should always be tailored to the individual patient.

Most combined chemotherapy approaches to date use ABVD, as it is the most effective and least toxic in advanced disease studies combined with smaller, involved field irradiation only. This appears to produce excellent cure rates with the potential for reducing the long-term side-effects. Currently, four cycles of ABVD have been formally tested but even briefer chemotherapy and/or reduced doses of radiotherapy are being evaluated and may be found to work as effectively.

Stage IIIA

For patients with stage IIIA disease there are studies that advocate the use of combined modality regimens, chemotherapy alone or TNI alone. The only firm recommendation is that, in the absence of bulk disease, combined modality is probably unnecessary (Oza et al., 1991a) and

Table 44.3 *Programmes of combination chemotherapy effective in the treatment of advanced stage Hodgkin's disease*

Drug combination	Dose (mg/m²)	Route	Days given[a]	Complete remission	Disease-free survival
MOPP				84	60% at 20 years
Mechlorethamine (nitrogen mustard)	6	i.v.	1, 8		
Vincristine	1.4	i.v.	1, 8		
Procarbazine	100	p.o.	1–14		
Prednisone	40	p.o.	1–14		
ChIVPP				85	65% at 10 years
Chlorambucil	6	p.o.	1–14		
Vinblastine	6	i.v.	1, 8		
Procarbazine	100	p.o.	1–14		
Prednisone	40	p.o.	1–14		
MVPP				82	60% at 5 years
Mechlorethamine	6	i.v.	1, 8		
Vinblastine	6	i.v.	1, 8		
Procarbazine	100	p.o.	1–14		
Prednisone	40	p.o.	1–14		
ABVD				81	64% at 3 years
Doxorubicin	25	i.v.	1, 15		
Bleomycin	10	i.m.	1, 15		
Vinblastine	6	i.m.	1, 15		
Dacarbazine	375	i.v.	1, 15		
MOPP/ABVD				89	76% at 7 years
Alternating months of MOPP and ABVD					
MOPP/ABV hybrid				97[b]	77% at 7 years
Mechlorethamine	6	i.v.	1		
Vincristine	1.4 (max 2)	i.v.	1		
Procarbazine	100	p.o.	1–7		
Prednisone	40	p.o.	1–14		
Doxorubicin	35	i.m.	8		
Bleomycin	10	i.v.	8		
Vinblastine	6	i.v.	8		

[a] Drug combinations were given over a 28-day cycle. Numbers shown refer to days of the cycle.
[b] After chemotherapy in 84% and after chemotherapy plus radiotherapy in an additional 13%.
From Urba and Longo (1992), with permission.

may simply increase the probability of further complications. If a minimum of six cycles of chemotherapy is used, then laparotomy is not required.

Stage IIIB and IV

This is the group for whom prognosis has been improved dramatically during the past 20 years with the advent of combination chemotherapy. Thus, it is generally agreed that chemotherapy is the treatment of choice for advanced stage Hodgkin's disease; however, the current controversies debate the identification of the most effective and safe drug regimen. Results of a number of trials suggest that ABVD is as effective as the alternating combination of MOPP/ABVD and superior to MOPP alone, with fewer acute and long-term side-effects. Newer combinations such as the Stanford V and BEACOPP regimens are currently being tested. Early results are promising, particularly in high-risk patients, but await longer follow-up data. The role of radiotherapy combined with chemotherapy in advanced disease is limited to certain specific indications.

Massive mediastinal disease

Patients with bulky mediastinal disease, irrespective of stage, do not require surgical staging as they should be recommended to have combined modality therapy, i.e. initial combination chemotherapy followed by 'mantle' irradiation. A clear decrease in recurrence rate has been demonstrated for combined modality therapy in comparison with radiotherapy alone or chemotherapy alone. The choice of chemotherapy must take into consideration the potential additive toxicities such as pulmonary (bleomycin) and cardiac (doxorubicin) when radiotherapy is part of the planned treatment. The reduction in total radiation dose of a 'mantle' field or the use of involved field radiation, may be equally effective with a modest risk of long-term complications (Fig. 44.8).

RECURRENCE/PROGRESSION

Salvage chemotherapy

The term 'salvage' therapy is generally used to describe the use of intensive combination chemotherapy given at the time of recurrence still with curative intent. It is therefore assumed that the long-term complications and toxicities incurred are acceptable in the light of the potential benefit in relation to the risk of the illness. The type of treatment will obviously depend on the clinical situation, particularly in relation to the type(s) and timing of previous treatments.

Recurrent Hodgkin's disease

First recurrence Up to one-third of patients treated with Hodgkin's disease will require further therapy at some time for recurrent disease. The efficacy of combination chemotherapy following recurrence is said to be dependent upon the initial therapy, the duration of first remission, the extent of disease at the time of recurrence, choice of therapy and the patients' age (Longo *et al.*, 1992). However, others have stated that the only adverse factors are advanced age, male gender and the presence of B symptoms at the time of recurrence. An agreed list of prognostic factors in this circumstance, as in all other aspects of Hodgkin's disease, is lacking.

The use of combination chemotherapy following recurrence after initial radiotherapy alone is often successful in achieving a prolonged second remission (Healey *et al.*, 1993). Treatment following recurrence after primary chemotherapy is more difficult and the use of non-cross-resistant regimens compared with the initial therapy has been advocated. Indeed, there are reports that recurrence after MOPP chemotherapy responds to ABVD salvage therapy with good effect. Others have suggested that sensitivity to chemotherapy may be a better indicator of future response and that re-treatment with the same induction chemotherapy is possible providing that the first remission was longer than a year. Overall, 45 per cent of patients who achieve a complete or good partial second remission will remain alive and disease-free for more than 15 years on long-term follow-up.

Second and subsequent recurrence (Fig. 44.9) The survival of patients with recurrent disease is inferior to that of patients who remain in continuous remission, the median survival decreasing with subsequent recurrences. The single most important factor affecting survival appears to be response or sensitivity to chemotherapy. Sensitivity to conventional chemotherapy and response are also good prognostic factors for response following high-dose chemotherapy with haematological stem cell rescue. With a median duration of second remission of 12 years following successful 'salvage' treatment, it would seem that high-dose chemotherapy at first recurrence would be inappropriate unless conventional chemotherapy had demonstrably failed.

Resistant disease The prognosis of patients who have disease resistant to combination chemotherapy is very grave. Unfortunately, lack of response with conventional chemotherapy often correlates with poor response to high-dose chemotherapy, although some would disagree. Despite the use of chemotherapy and radiotherapy, remission is never achieved in a proportion of patients (20 per cent). There are also many patients with recurrent disease in whom a subsequent remission cannot be achieved and for whom the outlook is poor. However, persistent disease may not imply immediate death and patients may remain with indolent disease for months or even years. Palliative therapy can be used to control symptoms for as long as possible with the minimum of side-effects. Single-agent chemotherapy, given orally, can be particularly useful in this situation. Prednisolone is useful in controlling systemic symptoms including B symptoms, whilst CCNU (1-(2-chloroethyl)-3-cyclohexyl-1-nitrosurea; lomustine) every 4 weeks is excellent palliation.

HIGH-DOSE CHEMOTHERAPY (Table 44.4)

High-dose chemotherapy followed by autologous bone marrow or peripheral stem cell transplantation is becoming more frequently used in Hodgkin's disease, particularly in the setting of relapsed or refractory disease. The rationale is based on *in-vitro* and *in-vivo* studies, which suggest that clinical drug resistance can be overcome by using agents that have a 'steep' dose–response curve. Despite the large number of published series of patients treated with high-dose chemotherapy and autologous bone marrow or stem cell support, its long-term benefits over conventional salvage therapy still have not been tested in the setting of randomized trials. Although complete response rates of greater than 50 per cent have been achieved, with 30–65 per cent of these highly selected patients benefiting from prolonged disease-free periods, the follow-up in these trials is generally short. In addition, the various high-dose regimens and the heterogeneity of patients selected and treated makes it difficult for critical analysis and uniform criteria to be given.

The demonstration that the majority of patients can undergo high-dose chemotherapy safely with a mortality rate of less than 5 per cent has resulted in a shift of emphasis to try and define the patients for whom this potentially toxic procedure is of value in prolonging survival. Factors of favourable prognostic importance are good performance status at the time of treatment, low tumour bulk, less than two previous chemotherapy regimens and 'sensitive' disease. Reduction of disease with conventional chemotherapy prior to high-dose treatment allows selection of patients with 'sensitive' disease as well as reducing the amount of tumour. However, it has been

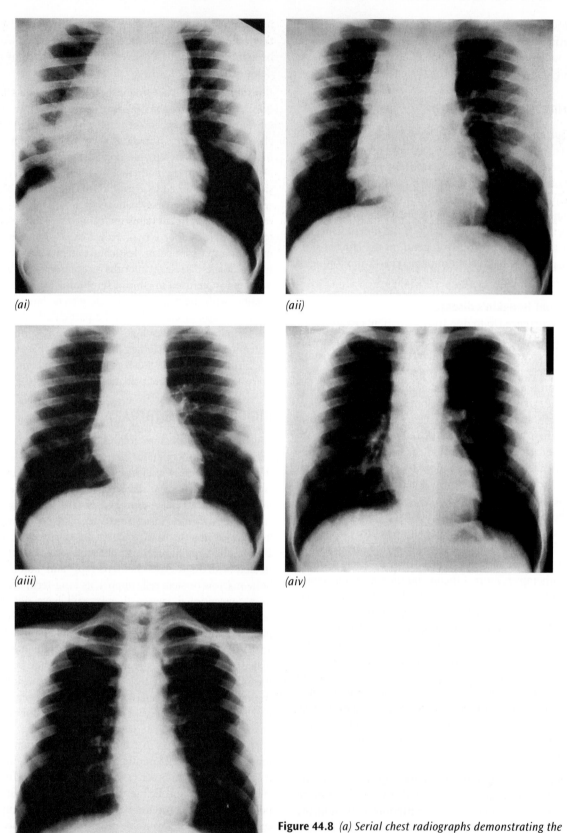

(ai)

(aii)

(aiii)

(aiv)

(av)

Figure 44.8 *(a) Serial chest radiographs demonstrating the response to successive cycles of chemotherapy in a young patient with CS IIAXE Hodgkin's disease. (i) At presentation. (ii) One week after starting chemotherapy. (iii) Following the cycle of chemotherapy. (iv) Following six cycles of chemotherapy. (v) Three months after consolidation with mantle field irradiation.*

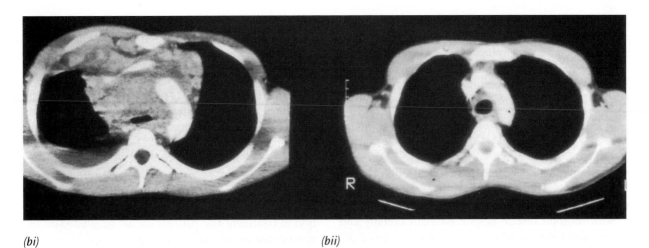

(bi)   *(bii)*

Figure 44.8 *(b) CT scans through the mediastinum prior to treatment and after all treatment in the same patient.*
(i) At presentation. (ii) Post-chemotherapy and radiotherapy.

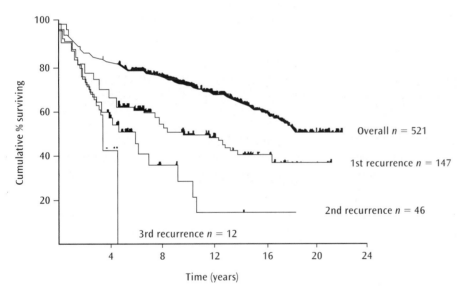

Overall *n* = 521

1st recurrence *n* = 147

2nd recurrence *n* = 46

3rd recurrence *n* = 12

Figure 44.9 *Survival of patients with recurrence of Hodgkin's disease, compared with overall survival of 521 patients treated at St Bartholomew's Hospital during the period 1968–84. (From Oza et al., 1993, with permission).*

Table 44.4 *Autologous bone marrow transplantation in Hodgkin's disease*

Regimen	No. patients	Toxic deaths	CR	Relapse (%)	Disease-free	Follow-up
CBV	104	11	57	33	35	max. 7 years
CBV	59	7	59	33	39	2–6 years
CBV	20	10	89	20	65	3–22 months
BEAM	44	5	50	9	45	1–4 years
Cyclophosphamide Cyclophosphamide + TBI	26	23	69	44	38	min. 3.5 years med. 4.5 years
Cyclophosphamide, etoposide + TNI	17	24	71	8	65	4–35 months
MBE	38	21	53	15	45	4–20 months
Total	*n* = 308;	χ = 12	59	28	42	

BEAM, BCNU, etoposide, Ara-C (cytarabine), melphalan; CBV, cyclophosphamide, BCNU (carmustine), etoposide; MBE, melphalan,
BCNU, etoposide; TBI, total body irradiation; TNI, total nodal irradiation.
From Kauftnan, D. and Longo, D.L. (1992), with permission.

shown that response to a high-dose regimen can occur in some patients even though the disease appears to be resistant to conventional chemotherapy.

The optimal timing for investigation or recommending high-dose treatment remains unclear (Desch *et al.*, 1992). It may be reasonable to consider such treatment for patients:

- with a short first remission, e.g. less than 12 months (Longo *et al.*, 1992);
- who have developed recurrent disease despite two different modalities of therapy;
- perhaps with systemic symptoms at recurrence; or
- with resistant disease despite standard therapy and therefore failure to achieve a remission (Chopra *et al.*, 1992).

It should be remembered, however, as mentioned earlier, that conventional chemotherapy can induce a durable second remission in about 50 per cent of patients with recurrent Hodgkin's disease. Despite advocates of high-dose treatment in poor risk patients at first remission, its role in this situation is still not clear.

COMPLICATIONS OF TREATMENT

Radiotherapy

Complications of treatment may be acute and delayed.

ACUTE EFFECTS

The acute effects of irradiation are those that occur during or within 8 weeks of completion of treatment. They reflect the effect of irradiation on renewing tissues, particularly the skin, gastrointestinal epithelium and bone marrow.

Fatigue
Fatigue usually improves 3–4 weeks after therapy is completed, though some patients experience continuing lassitude for some months after radiotherapy.

Xerostomia and dental problems
The upper border of the mantle field will encompass the sublingual, submaxillary and a large portion of the parotid glands. There is a reduction of saliva production and the saliva itself becomes more viscous, resulting in a dry mouth and altered taste sensation. The latter usually returns to normal within 3 months, although the symptoms of dry mouth may persist. Oral hygiene is essential before, during and after radiotherapy and dental work should be undertaken before the start of treatment.

Nausea, vomiting and weight loss
Anorexia is common following radiotherapy and may be associated with nausea and vomiting, which may be controlled by administration of simple anti-emetics. Nausea and vomiting are more common with subdiaphragmatic irradiation. Weight loss may occur during a standard course of treatment and attention should be paid to food intake.

Skin reaction
General skin reactions have been greatly reduced by the introduction of megavoltage irradiation. Erythema and sometimes moist desquamation may occur in skin folds, e.g. in the axilla. Washing should be kept to a minimum in the treated area, the use of E45 cream and avoidance of perfumed soaps, talc and deodorants is recommended during the course of radiotherapy. Direct exposure to sunlight is inadvisable for at least 6 months on completion of treatment and patients should be advised on the appropriate use of sunscreen preparations.

Dysphagia and mucositis
A pharyngeal reaction and dysphagia may accompany mantle field irradiation, usually from the second week of therapy. The use of an anterior larynx shield may reduce the reaction, but any discomfort is self-limiting and patients should be reassured that such symptoms will resolve within a few days after treatment.

Alopecia
Temporary hair loss from the area over the occiput and axilla is inevitable if these areas are included in the radiation field. Hair growth usually recommences within 3 months following completion of treatment. Similarly, loss of beard hair may occur and patients should be advised to dry shave during and for a period after treatment.

Haematological effects
Haematological depression is uncommon during mantle irradiation, although regular review of blood counts is essential. However, bone marrow suppression may occur in patients who have received prior radiation or chemotherapy or in those receiving subdiaphragmatic therapy post-mantle, for example, as part of TNI. A 4-week interval between the mantle and inverted Y fields helps to minimize the effects of haematological toxicity.

Diarrhoea
Subdiaphragmatic fields may produce gastrointestinal side-effects such as cramps, flatulence and occasionally diarrhoea. These symptoms can be minimized by the use of agents that reduce gut motility, e.g. codeine phosphate or loperamide, and appropriate dietary advice.

DELAYED EFFECTS

These occur after a period of months or years following radiotherapy and are usually permanent. Delayed effects reflect either changes to organs and tissues that renew slowly, or secondary to damage of the mesenchymal stroma.

Thyroid
Thyroid dysfunction is common following mantle irradiation; 50 per cent of patients treated with radiotherapy

followed up for 20 years will require thyroxine for compensated hypothyroidism [elevated thyroid stimulating hormone (TSH) and normal total thyroxine] but clinical hypothyroidism is rare. There is also an increased risk of Graves' disease and the development of single or multiple nodules. The risk of thyroid cancer is 15 times higher than the expected risk. This reinforces the need for continued clinical and biochemical evaluation and thyroxine replacement when indicated (Hancock *et al.*, 1991).

Respiratory

Pneumonitis is a rare complication following mantle irradiation unless large volumes of lung are included in the radiation field. This is particularly true of the treatment of bulky mediastinal disease or hilar lymphadenopathy when wide fields are employed. Acute pneumonitis may occur 2–4 months following treatment and is usually controlled symptomatically with corticosteroids (debatable). Pulmonary fibrosis will develop in areas of the lung included in the full treatment field over a period of 4–18 months. Although this rarely causes a clinical problem, paramediastinal and apical lung fibrosis are commonly seen on a chest X-ray. The prior or concurrent use of certain drugs, in particular bleomycin and doxorubicin, may accentuate pulmonary reactions. The radiotherapy fields and dose must be considered carefully in these circumstances.

Gastrointestinal

Upper abdominal irradiation rarely produces late intestinal damage except in those patients who had previously undergone staging laparotomy. Small bowel obstruction and peptic ulceration have been reported.

Neurological

The most common symptoms, i.e. numbness, tingling or an 'electric shock' sensation in the lumbar region or upper or lower limbs may occur 2–4 months after finishing mantle field irradiation. This is known as Lhermitte's syndrome and classically occurs with neck flexion and may last for up to 6 months but will settle without intervention. It is thought to be due to transient demyelination. Transverse myelitis is a potential risk when mantle and subdiaphragmatic fields are incorrectly matched and overdose occurs at the site overlap. Normal spinal cord tolerance should be taken into account when considering re-treatment with radiotherapy.

Cardiovascular

Delayed cardiac complications ranging from pericardial effusion to myocardial infarction have been reported in up to 30 per cent of cases following mantle radiotherapy. Importantly, this is now much less of a problem with an evenly weighted anterior-posterior opposed technique, thereby reducing the dose to the myocardium. Previously used anterior mantle field alone resulted in exposing the myocardium to a high dose of irradiation. The risk of damage increases with doses above 35 Gy in 20 fractions and with prior or concurrent drug therapy, particularly doxorubicin.

Renal

Subdiaphragmatic irradiation of the upper abdomen invariably includes the upper part of the left kidney, but patients treated in this manner show no clinical consequence on long-term follow-up. Radioisotope investigations will demonstrate reduced uptake and abnormal function in the upper pole of the left kidney due to cortical atrophy, although intravenous pyelogram (IVP) appearances should remain unchanged. Providing there is normal renal function before treatment, irradiation damage to 25 per cent of the total renal volume is usually without clinical sequelae.

Skeletal

In adults, irradiation to bones with the doses used in the treatment of Hodgkin's disease is usually harmless. However, in the developing bones of children it can potentially be a serious problem. The development of avascular necrosis in either the femoral or humeral heads has been reported following either radiotherapy or chemotherapy (or both).

Gonadal effects

Testis Gonadal dysfunction as evidenced by semen analysis may be present in 30 per cent of male patients with Hodgkin's disease at presentation. Radiation has a selective effect on the testis with potential damage to the seminiferous tubules, yet the Leydig cells that produce testosterone are radioresistant. Thus spermatogenesis can be affected at all stages whilst hormone levels remain unchanged. With a tumour dose of 35–40 Gy to an inverted Y field, the testicular dose may be as high as 3.5–4 Gy if no special blocking is used. This will produce prolonged or permanent azoospermia. The use of double thickness midline block and testicular shielding can reduce this dose to 0.75–3.0 per cent of the tumour dose, with a reasonable chance of recovering spermatogenesis. The opportunity to store sperm must be offered to all males who have suitable semen analysis provided a delay in commencing treatment would not be detrimental to the patient. However, many patients have abnormal spermatogenesis at the time of diagnosis of Hodgkin's disease.

Ovary The ovary differs in two fundamental ways from the male testis. First, there is a fixed population of oocytes in the postpubertal ovary and, second, the production of the hormones luteinizing hormone (LH) and follicle stimulating hormone (FSH) is directly related to the presence of viable ovarian follicles. The threshold dose of radiation to result in premature ovarian failure is not known although doses above 8 Gy must be anticipated to cause permanent amenorrhoea. It appears that ovarian function is more sensitive with age. Oophoropexy at the time of staging laparotomy, as mentioned earlier, has been relatively successful.

Chemotherapy

ACUTE EFFECTS (PRICE AND LISTER, 1991)

Nausea and vomiting

These are the most distressing side-effects of chemotherapy as reported by patients themselves. Most protocols used for the treatment of Hodgkin's disease are administered on an outpatient basis. Severe nausea and vomiting are uncommon and can be predicted for the particular drugs being given. Mustine and dacarbazine are powerful inducers of emesis, followed by cyclophosphamide and doxorubicin. However, the management of nausea is less of a problem with the availability of a wide variety of anti-emetics that can be used singly or in combination, orally or intravenously. The high efficacy of 5-hydroxytryptamine (5-HT) antagonists has made a dramatic impact on patients receiving chemotherapy.

Local tissue necrosis

The majority of patients with Hodgkin's disease will receive intermittent outpatient chemotherapy and therefore do not need continuous venous access, e.g. indwelling venous catheter. Treatment including vesicant drugs such as doxorubicin may result in local tissue necrosis ('chemotherapy burn') if inadvertent extravasation of the drug occurs. This is usually avoided by good clinical practice.

Hypersensitivity reactions

This is an uncommon problem. Bleomycin commonly produces fever, sometimes with rigors and hypertension, 2–4 hours after administration. Pre-treatment with hydrocortisone and chlorpheniramine (Piriton) may prevent this reaction in susceptible individuals. Anaphylactic reactions to doxorubicin have been reported as has sudden death, which is more likely to be due to cardiac arrhythmias.

Neurological

Vincristine can cause peripheral neuritis with patients experiencing paraesthesia in the tips of both fingers and toes and reduction of motor function if not recognized early. The majority of the symptoms will resolve following cessation of the course of treatment but may take several months; physiotherapy may be required.

Renal and metabolic

The tumour lysis syndrome is extremely rare in the setting of Hodgkin's disease. However, hyperuricaemia can occur in the absence of other manifestations of the tumour lysis syndrome during treatment. Routine testing of serum urate before initiation of therapy and the use of allopurinol, at least during the early weeks of therapy, are therefore recommended.

Haematological

Myelosuppression is the most important toxicity of a number of cytotoxic agents and is dose limiting in the majority of combination chemotherapy regimens. The degree of myelosuppression will depend upon several factors: the drugs used, their dose and route of administration, and host factors such as age, previous treatment with drugs or radiotherapy and bone marrow infiltration with tumour, which is usually seen in the advanced stages of recurrent Hodgkin's disease. A modest fall in the blood count will occur in most patients treated as outpatients, but not to a degree or duration that is likely to cause complications. However, as this is unpredictable, all patients should be warned carefully of the possible problems and risks involved. Urgent hospital admission may be necessary for the prompt treatment of neutropenic fever and possible sepsis.

Mucositis and stomatitis

These side-effects are a result of cytotoxic-induced failure of mucosal repair and local oral infections, usually fungal during the leucocyte nadir. Both doxorubicin and etoposide are particularly associated with this complication. Oral hygiene and the regular use of antifungal agents in the form of oral suspension and lozenges are important.

Gastrointestinal

Intestinal mucosa has a high proliferative index and is therefore a site for primary damage as a result of both chemotherapy and radiotherapy. However, with most chemotherapy regimens used in Hodgkin's disease, there is rarely any problem. Vincristine does affect gastrointestinal motility, resulting in constipation via its effects on the autonomic nerve supply to the bowel.

Alopecia

Hair loss caused by some cytotoxic agents, although reversible, causes anxiety and distress to many patients receiving such therapy. Reassurance that hair growth will occur once therapy has been completed should be given.

DELAYED

Cardiovascular

Doxorubicin is the most commonly used anthracycline in the treatment of Hodgkin's disease. The cardiotoxicity is dependent upon the cumulative dose with the possibility of cardiac failure being increasingly likely if the total dose exceeds $550 \, mg/m^2$. Providing a pre-treatment ECG is normal, it is probably unnecessary to perform routine ECGs during and after treatment. Cyclophosphamide has an appreciable effect but only at high doses used as part of myeloablative regimens.

Long-term complications

Immune deficiency and infections

Patients with Hodgkin's disease at presentation or even in remission have an increased incidence of infection with opportunistic pathogens as a consequence of a persistent defect in cellular immunity. Indeed, the cellular immune defect may precede the development of the disease and may well contribute to its pathogenesis. Natural killer cell-mediated cytotoxicity is depressed in untreated patients and humoral immune function is transiently reduced following treatment. Viral, fungal and *Pneumocystis carinii* infections are more prevalent complications in patients with Hodgkin's disease than in those with other forms of lymphoma. In particular, herpes zoster, cytomegalovirus and cryptococcus are significantly more common. There is also an increased incidence of disseminated herpes zoster in patients with Hodgkin's disease.

Patients who have had a splenectomy may be offered vaccination against pneumococcus. Prophylaxis with low-dose phenoxymethylpenicillin (penicillin V) should also be considered, particularly in children.

Infertility

As discussed earlier, active Hodgkin's disease may itself suppress fertility and chemotherapy and radiotherapy may also affect gonadal function. Certain combination chemotherapy regimens, e.g. MOPP, almost invariably result in sterility after six or more cycles. However, other regimens, e.g. ABVD, are associated with only temporary oligospermia and long-term infertility is unusual in men.

Premature ovarian failure is associated with both subdiaphragmatic irradiation and chemotherapy; however, it is age dependent with persistent ovarian failure occurring in older patients. The young patient may thus retain fertility after chemotherapy but have an early onset of the menopause. Advice and counselling should be given to patients with respect to the timing of any planned pregnancy in relation to their own prognosis and likely effects on the fetus. For those who have premature ovarian failure, early hormone replacement is advised in order to reduce such complications as bone demineralization, etc.

Second malignancy

The success in treatment for Hodgkin's disease has resulted in another potentially and indeed often fatal consequence, the risk of developing a second malignant disease. Several reports in the past few years with long-term follow-up on patients treated in the 1960s and 1970s has revealed that about one in every six patients with Hodgkin's disease is likely to develop a second malignancy within 15 years of treatment (Boivin *et al.*, 1984; Henry-Amar, 1992; Swerdlow *et al.*, 1992; Abrahamsen *et al.*, 1993; Rodriguez *et al.*, 1993).

Risk of acute myeloid leukaemia

The increased risk of myelodysplasia and acute leukaemia after chemotherapy containing alkylating agent(s) and also etoposide for Hodgkin's disease is well established. Whether radiotherapy alone is associated with an increased risk is not clear or, indeed, whether it adds to the risk of chemotherapy when used in combined modality regimens is also unclear. Thus, the cumulative risk of secondary leukaemia after MOPP in first remission is 1.5–3 per cent

at 10 years; the risk after ABVD alone is nil. There is some suggestion that the risk is related to advanced disease stage, splenectomy and age. Apparently, the risk peaks at 5–7 years after treatment but remains elevated even beyond 10 years. It seems that the excess risk of developing leukaemia relates to treatment rather than to Hodgkin's disease itself.

Non-Hodgkin's lymphoma

There is certainly an increased incidence of lymphoma which does not appear to be related to any particular form of therapy other than perhaps local radiotherapy and multiple alkylating agents. Therefore, it should not be an important consideration when considering the type of therapy. It is important to note whether re-biopsy was performed when analysing the reported incidence. It is possible that the occurrence of these lymphomas is part of the natural course of Hodgkin's disease or of its effects, such as immunosuppression.

Solid tumours

Unfortunately, the risk of developing a second malignancy of the solid tumour variety continues to increase with time, reaching a cumulative incidence rate of about 14 per cent at 20 years. The increased risk is associated particularly with radiotherapy, but also to a lesser extent with chemotherapy and other factors, including age and cigarette smoking. The most common tumours, including some in which radiation carcinogenesis has been established, are lung, breast (Hancock *et al.*, 1993), colon, stomach, prostate, thyroid (Hancock *et al.*, 1991) and melanoma.

Continued close regular follow-up of all patients treated for Hodgkin's disease is mandatory. For female patients, regular examination of the breasts and annual cervical smears should be advised. Exposure to direct sunlight and cigarette smoking should be strongly discouraged. Nevertheless, the benefits of curative treatment outweigh the risk of the late and sometimes fatal consequences (Boice, 1993).

Psychological and social consequences

The psychological aspects of the diagnosis of a malignant disease and its subsequent treatment, with its inherent mortality and possible morbidity, should be remembered. Many patients will be overwhelmed by having been told the diagnosis. Different emotions arise, including shock, fear, denial, anger, resentment, anxiety or depression. Although common at the time of diagnosis, some of these emotional problems continue after the commencement of treatment. Some reports suggest that many patients may experience substantial long-term problems such as chronic fatigue, marital, sexual and employment difficulties. Not surprisingly, the possibility of infertility, second malignancy and recurrence all have a psychosocial effect on patients who, in remission from Hodgkin's disease, are attempting to live a relatively normal life.

PROGNOSIS

The actuarial survival rate of patients with Hodgkin's disease has progressively increased from 1 per cent with no treatment to 23 per cent with kilovoltage radiotherapy and now is approaching 70 per cent using modern radiotherapy and chemotherapy (Fig. 44.10, Table 44.5). Thus, a patient with early-stage Hodgkin's disease has an excellent chance of achieving complete remission (95 per cent) and remaining disease-free, with a probability as high as 70 per cent at 5 years (Oza *et al.*, 1993). A patient with advanced disease also has a good chance of entering complete remission (70 per cent) and then a 65 per cent probability of being free of disease at 5 years (Oza *et al.*, 1992). The problems, however, are the deaths due to intercurrent diseases, particularly second malignancies and cardiac

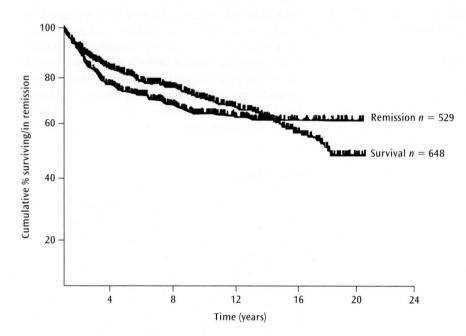

Figure 44.10 *Survival and remission duration for patients treated at St Bartholomew's Hospital. (From Oza* et al., *1991b, with permission.)*

Table 44.5 *Proportion of patients with Hodgkin's disease achieving complete remission, relapse-free survival (in complete responders), and survival at 5 and 15 years according to Ann Arbor stage*

Clinical stage	No. patients	% With complete remission	% With relapse-free survival at 5 years[a]	% With relapse-free survival at 10 years[a]	% Survival at 5 years	% Survival at 15 years
IA						
1970–79	1516	98	80	75	90	70
After 1980	949	98			90	
IIA						
1970–79	2488	95	74	70	88	70
After 1980	1511	94			90	
IB/IIB						
1970–79	1081	87	73	69	80	62
After 1980	721	83			81	
IIIA						
1970–79	940	87[b]	75	63	78	57
After 1980	510	87			83	
IIIB						
1970–79	1001	77[b]	65	61	64	42
After 1980	641	75			70	
IV						
1970–79	544	62	66	62	54	35
After 1980	752	63			62	

[a] In complete responders.
[b] All results for clinical stage III together.
From Carde, P. (1992), with permission.

and pulmonary disease, resulting in an overall mortality rate still twice that of the general population, demographically matched. The majority of deaths (64 per cent) due to second cancer occur in the 5–14-year interval after treatment. The distinction between Hodgkin's disease-related deaths and intercurrent deaths is of great importance and a major problem, especially in a disease that has a long expected survival after successful treatment.

FUTURE DEVELOPMENTS

Although advances have been made in Hodgkin's disease, both biologically and clinically, there remain areas for further developments (Rosenberg, 1991). Research into the biology of Hodgkin's disease is of major interest and advances in molecular biological techniques may allow the molecular dissection of the disease. It is essential to identify objective biological parameters that can be used to predict the progression of the disease and prognosis of an individual patient.

The development of new treatment regimens and chemotherapy combinations, which have a lower rate of long-term complications, is a major aim, without reducing the high rates of remission obtainable at the present time. Examples, which are already part of clinical trials, include continuing to push the lower limits of chemotherapy and radiotherapy dose in early-stage disease and, in advanced disease, the development of new drug combinations and ongoing investigation into the role of high-dose chemotherapy in first remissions.

Other more specific forms of therapy are under development for Hodgkin's disease. The use of radiolabelled antibodies such as yttrium-labelled ferritin immunoglobulin is an example and has been incorporated into chemotherapy regimens. Other antibodies against CD molecules on the surface of Sternberg–Reed cells are under investigation, e.g. anti-CD16 and anti-CD30 antibodies. The covalent linking of such antibodies with immunotoxins such as saporin has also started trials. The context in which these forms of therapies will be used is unclear, and may be limited to treating patients with minimal residual disease.

CHILDHOOD HODGKIN'S DISEASE

The biology and natural history of Hodgkin's disease in children (cases below the age of 16 years account for 7 per cent of the total) shows no apparent differences from the disease in adults (Donaldson, 1990). However, the management must take into account two important differences: the growing child and the potential longer lifespan. The clinical presentation and histological features are similar, apart from a small increase in lymphocyte predominant subtype of the disease.

Investigations are conducted as in adults, although staging laparotomy should be avoided. The radiological appearance of the thymus can cause difficulties in interpretation. Children with early-stage disease and no adverse prognostic factors may be treated with chemotherapy followed by involved field irradiation. If B symptoms or bulky disease are present, then six cycles of chemotherapy with involved field radiotherapy in certain situations is recommended. For advanced disease, treatment is principally combination chemotherapy. Complete remission and survival rates are in the order of 95 per cent at 5 years.

The main difference between children and adults relates to the long-term complications and sequelae of treatment. The initial manifestation of the effects of radiotherapy is impairment of soft tissue and bone growth due to high-dose extended field irradiation. It is evident that age under 13 years and a total dose of more than 25 Gy to the axial skeleton are associated with a greater likelihood of growth retardation. Other late effects such as gonadal dysfunction, thyroid dysfunction and cardiopulmonary complications are all major problems. However, the most serious of all potential problems following treatment in children is the development of a second malignancy. Radiotherapy alone appears to increase the risk of developing a solid tumour, whilst children treated with chemotherapy alone or in combination with radiotherapy have an increased risk of developing acute leukaemia or non-Hodgkin's lymphoma. The overall cumulative risk patterns for the different second malignancies is similar to that seen in adults with age at the time of treatment being a major risk factor.

The challenge in the management of Hodgkin's disease in children is therefore not only to continue improvements in therapy and maintain the high long-term remission rates, but also to minimize the unfortunate sequelae of treatments.

CONCLUSIONS

Hodgkin's disease is one of the forms of malignancy with the highest long-term survival. Developments in the 1960s and 1970s, both in the understanding of the natural history of the disease and the development of radiotherapy and combination chemotherapy have led to an excellent prognosis in an otherwise fatal condition. Biological and molecular studies have advanced the understanding of the disease, although the aetiology and the role of various agents including viruses remain obscure.

The situation is, however, far from satisfactory; long-term survival has not increased in the last two decades. Reduction in the mortality related to Hodgkin's disease may require more aggressive therapeutic manoeuvres earlier in the treatment programme, perhaps based on prognostic factors, both biological and clinical. High-dose chemotherapy with haematological stem cell rescue, immunotoxins and immunotherapy may all begin to play a larger role in the management of patients with recurrent disease. Mortality not related directly to Hodgkin's disease in potentially 'cured' patients is reflected by the fact that the probability of death is more than doubled. Thus, along with the more aggressive approach, there is also a trend to reduce the overall amount of treatment, perhaps using combined modality regimens including involved field radiotherapy in early-stage disease, thereby reducing long-term adverse events such as second malignancies and cardiopulmonary disease. The development of non-sterilizing chemotherapy combinations is also a challenge. It must, however, be remembered that such advances must not compromise the excellent remission rates that are currently achieved.

debate the identification of the most effective and safe drug regimen.

- The most common late complication of radiotherapy to the mantle region is hypothyroidism.
- The success in the treatment of Hodgkin's disease has resulted in another potentially and, indeed, often fatal consequence – the risk of developing a second malignant disease – with about one in six patients with Hodgkin's disease likely to develop a second malignancy within 15 years of treatment.

SIGNIFICANT POINTS

- Hodgkin's disease is uncommon, accounting for about 1 per cent of malignant diseases diagnosed in countries in the Western world each year and an annual incidence of 2.4 new cases per 100 000 population in the UK.
- Untreated Hodgkin's disease has a 5-year survival of less than 5 per cent.
- Hodgkin's disease is a histological diagnosis based on the recognition of neoplastic Sternberg–Reed cells in an appropriate background of essentially normal or reactive cells predominantly composed of helper T cells.
- Painless enlargement of superficial lymph nodes is the most common presentation of Hodgkin's disease and is evident at the time of diagnosis in at least 70 per cent of patients.
- Systemic symptoms, particularly low-grade fever and drenching night sweats, are present in about 40 per cent of patients at presentation, usually in those with more advanced disease.
- A patient with early-stage Hodgkin's disease has an excellent chance of achieving complete remission (95 per cent) and remaining disease free, with a probability as high as 70 per cent at 5 years.
- Radiotherapy remains the most effective single agent for the treatment of nodal Hodgkin's disease.
- Combination chemotherapy is the treatment of choice for advanced stage Hodgkin's disease; however, the current controversies

KEY REFERENCES

The 2nd International Symposium on Hodgkin's Disease, Cologne, Germany, 3–5 October 1991. *Ann. Oncol.* **4**, 1–133.

Carde, P. (1992) Hodgkin's disease. I: Identification and classification. *Br. Med. J.* **305**, 99–102.

Carde, P. (1992) Hodgkin's lymphoma. II: Treatment and delayed morbidity. *Br. Med. J.* **305**, 173–6.

DeVita, V. Jr and Hubbard, S.M. (1993) Hodgkin's disease. *N. Engl. J. Med.* **328**, 560–5.

Drexler, H.G. (1992) Recent results on the biology of Hodgkin and Reed–Sternberg cells. I. Biopsy material. *Leuk Lymphonia* **8**, 283–313.

Harris, N.L., Jaffe, E.S., Stein, H. *et al.* (1994) A revised European-American classification of lymphoid neoplasms: a proposal from the International Lymphoma Study Group [*see* comments]. *Blood* **84**, 1361–92.

Kaufman, D. and Longo, D.L. (1992) Hodgkin's disease. *Crit. Rev. Oncol. Hematol.* **13**, 135–87.

Urba, W.J. and Longo, D.L. (1992) Hodgkin's disease. *N. Engl. J. Med.* **326**, 678–87.

REFERENCES

Abrahamsen, J.F., Andersen, A., Hannisdal, E. *et al.* (1993) Second malignancies after treatment of Hodgkin's disease: the influence of treatment, follow-up time, and age. *J. Clin. Oncol.* **11**, 255–61.

Biti, G.P., Cimino, G., Cartoni, C. *et al.* (1992) Extended-field radiotherapy is superior to MOPP chemotherapy for the treatment of pathologic stage I-IIA Hodgkin's disease: eight-year update of an Italian prospective randomized study. *J. Clin. Oncol.* **10**, 378–82.

Boice, J.D. Jr (1993) Second cancer after Hodgkin's disease–the price of success? (editorial). *J. Natl Cancer Inst.* **85**, 4–5.

Boivin, L.F., Hutchison, G.B., Lyden, M. *et al.* (1984) Second primary cancers following treatment of Hodgkin's disease. *J. Natl Cancer Inst.* **72**, 233–41.

Bonadonna, G., Zucali, R., Monfardini, S., De-Lena, M. and Uslenghi, C. (1975) Combination chemotherapy of Hodgkin's disease with adriamycin, bleomycin, vinblastine, and imidazole carboxamide versus MOPP. *Cancer* **36**, 252–9.

Bonadonna, G., Santoro, A., Gianni, A.M. *et al.* (1991) Primary and salvage chemotherapy in advanced Hodgkin's disease: the Milan Cancer Institute experience. *Ann. Oncol.* **1**, 9–16.

Butler, J.J. (1992) The histologic diagnosis of Hodgkin's disease. *Semin. Diagn. Pathol.* **9**, 252–6.

Canellos, G.P., Anderson, J.R., Propert, K.J. *et al.* (1992) Chemotherapy of advanced Hodgkin's disease with MOPP, ABVD, or MOPP alternating with ABVD. *N. Engl. J. Med.* **327**, 1478–84.

Carde, P. (1992) Hodgkin's disease. I: Identification and classification. *Br. Med. J.* **305**, 99–102.

Carde, P., Hayat, M., Cosset, J.M. *et al.* (1988) Comparison of total nodal irradiation versus combined sequence of mantle irradiation with mechlorethamine, vincristine, procarbazine, and prednisone in clinical stages I and II Hodgkin's disease: experience of the European Organization for Research and Treatment of Cancer. *NCI Monogr* 303–10.

Chopra, R., Linch, D.C., McMillan, A.K. *et al. (1992)* Mini-BEAM followed by BEAM and ABMT for very poor risk Hodgkin's disease. *Br. J. Haematol.* **81**, 197–202.

Desch, C.E., Lasala, M.R., Smith, T.J. and Hillner, B.E. (1992) The optimal timing of autologous bone marrow transplantation in Hodgkin's disease patients after a chemotherapy relapse. *J. Clin. Oncol.* **10**, 200–9.

DeVita, V.T., Simon, R.M., Hubbard, S.M. *et al.* (1980) Curability of advanced Hodgkin's disease with chemotherapy. Long-term follow-up of MOPP-treated patients at the National Cancer Institute. *Ann. Intern. Med.* **92**, 587–95.

Diehl, V., Franklin, J., Hasenclever, D. *et al.* (1998) BEACOPP: a new regimen for advanced Hodgkin's disease. German Hodgkin's Lymphoma Study Group. *Ann. Oncol.* **9**(suppl. 5), S67–71.

Donaldson, S.S. (1990) Hodgkin's disease in children. *Semin. Oncol.* **17**, 736–48.

Ferry, L.A., Linggood, R.M., Convery, K.M. *et al.* (1993) Hodgkin disease, nodular sclerosis type. Implications of histologic subclassification. *Cancer* **71**, 457–63.

Ganesan, T.S., Oza, A., Perry, N. *et al.* (1992) Management of stage II Hodgkin's disease: 15 years experience at St. Bartholomew's Hospital. *Ann. Oncol.* **3**, 349–56.

Gilbert, R. (1939) Radiotherapy in Hodgkin's disease (malignant granulomatosis). Anatomic and clinical foundations: governing principles: results. *Am. J. Roentgenol.* **41**, 198–241.

Glatstein, E., Guernsey, J.M., Rosenberg, S.A. and Kaplan, H.S. (1969). The value of laparotomy and splenectomy in the staging of Hodgkin's disease. *Cancer* **24**, 709–18.

Hamilton Fairly, G., Patterson, M.I.L. and Bodley Scott, R. (1966) Chemotherapy of Hodgkin's disease with cyclophosphamide, vinblastine and procarbazine. *Br. Med. J.* **2**, 75–8.

Hancock, S.L., Cox, R.S. and McDougall, I.R. (1991) Thyroid diseases after treatment of Hodgkin's disease. *N. Engl. J. Med.* **325**, 599–605.

Hancock, S.L., Tucker, M.A. and Hoppe, R.T. (1993) Breast cancer after treatment of Hodgkin's disease. *J. Natl Cancer Inst.* **85**, 25–31.

Harris, N.L., Jaffe, E.S., Stein, H. *et al.* (1994) A revised European-American classification of lymphoid neoplasms: a proposal from the International Lymphoma Study Group [*see* comments]. *Blood* **84**, 1361–92.

Hasenclever, D. and Diehl, V. (1998) A prognostic score for advanced Hodgkin's disease. International Prognostic Factors Project on Advanced Hodgkin's Disease [*see* comments]. *N. Engl. J. Med.* **339**, 1506–14.

Healey, E.A., Tarbell, N.J., Kalish, L.A. *et al.* (1993) Prognostic factors for patients with Hodgkin's disease in first relapse. *Cancer* **71**, 2613–20.

Henry-Amar, M. (1992) Second cancer after the treatment for Hodgkin's disease: a report from the International Database on Hodgkin's disease. *Ann. Oncol.* **4**, 117–28.

Hoppe, R.T. (1990) Radiation therapy in the management of Hodgkin's disease. *Semin. Oncol.* **17**, 704–15.

Hoppe, R.T. (1991) Early-stage Hodgkin's disease: a choice of treatments or a treatment of choice? *J. Clin. Oncol.* **9**, 897–901.

Horning, S.J., Rosenberg, S.A. and Hoppe, R.T. (1996) Brief chemotherapy (Stanford V) and adjuvant radiotherapy for bulky or advanced Hodgkin's disease: an update. *Ann. Oncol.* **7**(suppl. 4), 105–8.

Jarrett, R.F. (1992) Hodgkin's disease. *Baillière's Clin. Haematol.* **5**, 57–79.

Kanzler, H., Kuppers, R., Hansmann, M.L. and Rajewsky, K. (1996) Hodgkin and Reed–Sternberg cells in Hodgkin's disease represent the outgrowth of a dominant tumor clone derived from (crippled) germinal center B cells. *J. Exp. Med.* **184**, 1495–1505.

Kaplan, H.S. (1966) Evidence for a tumoricidal dose level in the radiotherapy of Hodgkin's disease. *Cancer Res.* **26**, 1221–4.

Kaufman, D. and Longo, D.L. (1992) Hodgkin's disease. *Crit. Rev. Oncol. Hematol.* **13**, 135–87.

Lacher, M.J. and Durrant, J.R. (1965) Combined vinblastine and chlorambucil therapy of Hodgkin's disease. *Ann. Intern. Med.* **62**, 468–76.

Lister, T.A. and Crowther, D. (1990) Staging for Hodgkin's disease. *Semin. Oncol.* **17**, 696–703.

Lister, T.A., Crowther, D., Sutcliffe, S.B. *et al.* (1989) Report of a committee convened to discuss the evaluation and staging of patients with Hodgkin's disease: cotswolds meeting. *J. Clin. Oncol.* **7**, 1630–6.

Longo, D.L., Duffey, P.L., Young, R. C. *et al.* (1992) Conventional-dose salvage combination chemotherapy in patients relapsing with Hodgkin's disease after combination chemotherapy: the low probability for cure. *J. Clin. Oncol.* **10**, 210–18.

Longo, D.L., Young, R.C., Wesley, M. *et al.* (1986) Twenty years of MOPP therapy for Hodgkin's disease. *J. Clin. Oncol.* **4**, 1295–306.

Lukes, R.J., Craver, L.F., Hall, T.C., Rappaport, H. and Rubin, P. (1966) Report of the nomenclature committee. *Cancer Res.* **26**, 1311.

Mueller, N. (1991) An epidemiologist's view of the new molecular biology findings in Hodgkin's disease. *Ann. Oncol.* **2**, 23–8.

Oudejans, J.J., Jiwa, N.M., Kummer, J.A. *et al.* (1996) Analysis of major histocompatibility complex class I expression on Reed–Sternberg cells in relation to the cytotoxic T-cell response in Epstein–Barr virus-positive and -negative Hodgkin's disease. *Blood* **87**, 3844–51.

Oza, A.M., Leahy, M., Lim, J. *et al.* (1991a) The treatment of stage IIIA Hodgkin's disease – total nodal irradiation versus combination chemotherapy: either or neither (letter). *J. Clin. Oncol.* **9**, 1514–16.

Oza, A.M., Rohatiner, A.Z. and Lister, T.A. (1991b) Chemotherapy of Hodgkin's disease. *Baillière's Clin. Haematol.* **4**, 131–56.

Oza, A.M., Ganesan, T.S., Dorreen, M. *et al.* (1992) Patterns of survival in patients with advanced Hodgkin's disease (HD) treated in a single centre over *20* years. *Br. J. Cancer* **65**, 429–37.

Oza, A.M., Ganesan, T.S., Leahy, M. *et al.* (1993) Patterns of survival in patients with Hodgkin's disease: long follow up in a single centre. *Ann. Oncol.* **4**, 385–92.

Peters, M.V. and Middlemiss, K.C.H. (1958) A study of Hodgkin's disease treated by irradiation. *Am. J. Roentgenol.* **79**, 114–21.

Price, C.G.A. and Lister, T.A. (1991) Acute complications of treatment for adult malignancy. In Plowman, P.N., McElwain, T.J. and Meadows, A. (eds), *Complications of cancer management*. Oxford: Butterworth-Heinemann, 76–94.

Rodriguez, M.A., Fuller, L.M., Zimmerman, S.O. *et al.* (1993) Hodgkin's disease: study of treatment intensities and incidences of second malignancies. *Ann. Oncol.* **4**, 125–31.

Rosenberg, S.A. (1991) The continuing challenge of Hodgkin's disease. *Ann. Oncol.* **2**, 29–31.

Stein, H. and Hummel, M. (1999) Cellular origin and clonality of classic Hodgkin's lymphoma: immunophenotypic and molecular studies. *Semin. Hematol.* **36**, 233–41.

Strickler, J.G., Michie, S.A., Warnke, R.A. and Dorfman, R.F. (1986) The 'syncytial variant' of nodular sclerosing Hodgkin's disease. *Am. J. Surg. Pathol.* **10**, 470–7.

Swerdlow, X.L., Douglas, A.L., Hudson, G.V. *et al.* (1992) Risk of second primary cancers after Hodgkin's disease by type of treatment: analysis of 2846 patients in the British National Lymphoma Investigation. *Br. Med. J.* **304**, 1137–43.

Ultmann, L.E. (1992) Classification of Hodgkin's disease: yesterday, today and tomorrow. *Eur. J. Cancer* **12**, 2074–9.

Urba, W.J. and Longo, D.L. (1992) Hodgkin's disease. *N. Engl. J. Med.* **326**, 678–87.

Weiss, L.M. and Chang, K.L. (1992) Molecular biologic studies of Hodgkin's disease. *Semin. Diagn. Pathol.* **9**, 272–8.

45

Non-Hodgkin's lymphoma

CHRISTOPHER G.A. PRICE AND SRINIVASAN MADHUSUDAN

INTRODUCTION

Non-Hodgkin's lymphoma (NHL) is an umbrella term for what is in fact a heterogeneous group of malignant diseases arising from lymphoid tissue. NHL is increasing in incidence and now ranks just below the common 'solid' tumours of adulthood, i.e. lung, breast, colorectum, bladder and prostate. It occurs four times more frequently than Hodgkin's disease and accounts for 4 per cent of new cancer diagnoses and a similar proportion of cancer-related deaths in Western countries. The annual UK incidence is approximately one per 7500 population, so that a regional cancer centre covering a population of between 750 000 and 1.5 million will be referred 100–200 new cases each year; a general practitioner may expect the diagnosis to be made in one of his patients every 3 years. The age of onset of NHL is typically later than for Hodgkin's disease, with a peak incidence in the sixth and seventh decades. However, it is also the third most common cancer under the age of 15, accounting for 10 per cent of Caucasian childhood cancer deaths and, in comparison with the common epithelial cancers, affects a disproportionately large number of young adults.

NHL has a particular importance in clinical practice not only because of the diversity of its subtypes and their modes of presentation but also because of the range and relative efficacy of available treatment, which is curative in a significant minority of cases. A widening choice of therapeutic interventions has improved the outlook for some groups of patients in recent years and advances in the understanding of lymphoma biology allow that the future be viewed with cautious optimism.

EPIDEMIOLOGY

The incidence has been rising over the past two decades at >5 per cent per year (Groves *et al.*, 2000), although this rate may have slowed during the late 1990s. This striking rise, which has sometimes been described as an 'epidemic', is largely unexplained. A contribution has undoubtedly been made by more accurate reporting, for example through more vigorous investigation of elderly patients and better laboratory techniques for defining the true nature of 'undifferentiated' malignant lesions. The high incidence of lymphoma in association with human immunodeficiency virus (HIV) is another easily identified factor. These do not, however, account for the bulk of the increase, which is not confined to the elderly or indeed to any other specific patient group. There has been a disproportionate increase in the frequency of primary extranodal lymphomas.

Recent international co-operative studies have highlighted marked geographical and ethnic variation in the distribution of lymphoma subtypes (Anderson *et al.*, 1998). Follicular lymphoma, for example, is seen most frequently in the USA and is more common in the UK than in other European countries. There is a much lower incidence of this subtype in Asia. France, Switzerland and Kuwait record a particularly high incidence of extranodal lymphomas; in Kuwait, the increase is largely in upper gastrointestinal tract lymphomas. Although elsewhere an extremely rare entity, angiocentric nasal T/NK-cell lymphoma makes up approximately 8 per cent of all lymphomas seen in Hong Kong. There is also a slight and so far unexplained 'sun-belt' effect, such that in some regions the incidence of lymphoma is positively correlated with sunlight exposure, mirroring the distribution of malignant melanoma (McMichael *et al.*, 1996).

AETIOLOGY

The evolution of non-Hodgkin's lymphoma is multifactorial. Certain predisposing and causal factors for NHL are well established, including specific infections and congenital and acquired immunodeficiency states. There is also increasing interest in the possible role of environmental carcinogens. Aetiology nevertheless remains unknown in the large majority of cases arising in the general population.

Infections

VIRAL INFECTIONS

Epstein–Barr virus (EBV)

EBV is a double-stranded DNA virus. Infection is ubiquitous, such that in all geographical areas most of the population has been infected before reaching adulthood. Epstein–Barr virus infection is a causal factor in almost all cases of endemic (or African) Burkitt's lymphoma (Geser *et al.*, 1982), and in a high proportion of lymphomas seen in association with immunodeficiency or immunosuppression (see below). There is also evidence implicating EBV infection in the development of a variety of other lymphomas including Hodgkin's disease (nodular sclerosing and mixed cellularity subtypes), non-endemic Burkitt's lymphoma and some T-cell subtypes.

Lymphoma only develops in a very small proportion of those infected with EBV. Impaired T-cell immunity is the usual critical cofactor. Expression of EBV-associated antigens such as EBNA-1; EBNA- 2 and LMP-1 promotes B-lymphocyte proliferation and survival. Impaired T-cell immunity removes the T-cell control of B-cell proliferation. The consequence of these effects in combination can be progression to malignant lymphoma.

Other viruses

Human T-cell lymphotropic virus 1 (HTLV1) Adult T-cell leukaemia/lymphoma (ATL) is causally linked to infection with the HTLV1 retrovirus. HTLV1 virus infection is rare outside the Caribbean, south-eastern USA and Japan; in Japan, rates of infection with the virus may be as high as 1 per cent. Although the exact mechanisms of lymphomagenesis are unclear, viral latency and expression of two genes, *tax* and *rex*, in transformed T cell leads to overexpression of both interleukin-2 (IL-2) and the IL-2 receptor.

Hepatitis C virus Hepatitis C virus is a hepatotropic and lymphotropic RNA virus. There is increasing evidence suggesting an aetiological role for hepatitis C virus in some low-grade lymphoproliferative disorders (Kitay-Cohen *et al.*, 2000). There are marked regional differences in the

prevalence of hepatitis C viral infection in NHL; studies from Italy and Asia have shown this to be as high as 30 per cent. This is an area of ongoing research and may be important in developing new prevention and treatment strategies for NHL.

HHV-8 This virus has recently been shown to be associated with the rare primary effusion lymphoma (PEL) which typically arises within the pleural cavity.

OTHER INFECTIONS

Helicobacter pylori

There is now convincing clinical, epidemiological and experimental data to suggest an association between gastric lymphoma and *Helicobacter pylori* infection. Infection with *H. pylori* leads to polyclonal proliferation of gastric lymphoid tissue from which a clonal malignant lesion can eventually evolve.

Immunodeficiency

Immunodeficiency, whether genetic, viral or iatrogenic in origin, is an established risk factor for the development of lymphoma. Not all lymphomas developing in this context can be attributed to EBV or any other yet identified infectious agent. Suppression of T-cell-mediated immunity may permit uncontrolled B-cell proliferation resulting in expansion of the B-cell compartment, in turn increasing the risk of molecular genetic abnormalities. These may be sufficient to result in malignant transformation.

CONGENITAL IMMUNODEFICIENCY SYNDROMES

Congenital immunodeficiency syndromes associated with an increased risk of lymphoma include Wiskott–Aldrich syndrome, ataxia telangiectasia (A-T) and common variable hypogammaglobulinaemia. The risk of development of lymphoma for Wiskott–Aldrich sufferers is more than 100 times that for unaffected individuals. In A-T the underlying defect is in DNA repair. This results both in immunodeficiency with the associated secondary risk of development of B-cell neoplasia and also an increased risk of both T- and B-cell neoplasms as a direct consequence of aberrant genetic recombination. Approximately 10 per cent of individuals with A-T eventually develop lymphoma.

ACQUIRED IMMUNODEFICIENCY SYNDROME (AIDS)

Up to 3 per cent of AIDS patients present with NHL at diagnosis. The risk of NHL in this group is increasing, largely due to improved survival rates through more effective control of opportunistic infections and the use of antiretroviral agents.

HIV infection is particularly associated with Burkitt's lymphoma and diffuse large cell lymphoma. Elevated EBV titres and clonal EBV DNA integration can be demonstrated in many of these tumours, including 100 per cent with primary central nervous system (CNS) disease. In common with other immunodeficiency-associated lymphomas, there is frequent involvement of extranodal sites such as the CNS and gastrointestinal tract.

IATROGENIC IMMUNOSUPPRESSION

Recipients of solid organ transplants and bone marrow transplants have depressed cellular immunity due to iatrogenic immunosuppression. Reactivation of EBV under these circumstances may induce a spectrum of post-transplant lymphoproliferative disorders (PTLD) ranging from polyclonal lymphoproliferation to clonal malignant lymphomas. The intensity and type of immunosuppression are crucial risk factors for the development of these disorders; under some circumstances they may respond or remit on reversal or reduction in immunosuppression without any specific anti-lymphoma therapy (initially shown by Starzl et al., 1984). The risk varies with the type of transplant, so that an incidence of 9–20 per cent has been reported following heart and heart–lung transplants whereas the rate in renal transplant patients is only 1–3 per cent. In allogeneic bone marrow transplantation, T-cell depletion and use of unrelated or mismatched donors increases the risk, which may be as high as 18 per cent. Among the various immunosuppressive agents used in transplant recipients, OKT3, used in cardiac transplantation, is most strongly associated with PTLD.

AUTOIMMUNE DISORDERS

There is an increased incidence of lymphoma in association with autoimmune disorders such as rheumatoid arthritis, SLE, Sjögren's syndrome and Hashimoto's disease. It is likely that the basis for this association is multifactorial and includes the use of immunosuppressive therapy as well as the underlying deficiency of immune regulation characteristic of the primary disorder.

Environmental exposure

Epidemiological studies have demonstrated an increased incidence of lymphoma in farmers and other workers who have had heavy exposure to pesticides, particularly the phenoxy herbicides and organophosphate insecticides. Hair dyes, hair spray and industrial exposure to solvents have also been implicated as factors associated with increased risk.

PATHOLOGY

Lymphomas arise through clonal expansion of B or T lymphocytes whose normal maturation has been arrested and proliferation and apoptosis deregulated. The morphological appearance seen by the pathologist is the result of infiltration of normal structures with these malignant cells and the consequent reactive changes in surrounding normal cell populations. Histologically, they are a highly complex group of neoplasms. The appropriate clinical management in an individual case requires accurate interpretation of histology leading to correct categorization within a recognized subtype, the likely clinical course of which is clearly understood. This interpretation is increasingly regarded as the preserve of the designated specialist lymphoma pathologist who works closely with the clinical team. Conventional assessment of morphology is now usually supplemented by immunophenotypic and/or molecular genetic analysis.

Histopathological classification of NHL

Major advances in the histopathological classification of lymphomas have been made during the 1980s and 1990s which have greatly simplified and improved what was previously a source of confusion. Before then a variety of pathological classification systems had been developed but these were hampered by poor reproducibility, incomplete acceptance and had failed in some areas to provide the clinician with a reliable predictor of clinical behaviour.

The 'working formulation' was devised by Rosenberg et al. in 1982 as a means of translating between classifications then in use, including those of Rapaport, Lennert (Kiel) and Lukes and Collins. It was based on clinical data obtained from over 1000 well-documented cases from Europe and the USA and focused on histological features identifiable reproducibly by light microscopy. It divided lymphomas into 10 subtypes within the broad categories of low, intermediate and high grade, which related to the natural history of the diseases as modified by treatment then available. The original intention was that it should not be used as a substitute classification in its own right. In practice it was widely used as a classification for clinical use for over a decade and, despite a number of important limitations, proved a valuable tool.

The chief disadvantages were as follows: first, by failing to differentiate between B-cell and T-cell lymphomas it forced pathologists to lump the minority T-cell lymphomas into categories which, in reality, were of relevance only to B-cell tumours. The T-cell lymphomas remained a poorly understood group of diseases, which appeared to behave unpredictably. Further, by remaining exclusively based on light microscopy, it failed to absorb new information provided by immunophenotypic and genetic analysis and was thus impossible to adapt to encompass many of the new entities, developments and controversies in lymphoma pathology.

A new system devised by a group of European and North American pathologists as the REAL (Revised European-American Lymphoma) classification in 1994 (Harris et al., 1994) has proved to be a substantial advance. This is in fact no more than a list of all currently defined disease entities based on information available from morphological, phenotypic, cytogenetic and molecular genetic analysis. It has superseded other classifications because the entities described permit interpretation that is consistent between pathologists and because new information can rapidly be incorporated. Clinicians have found, possibly to their surprise, that an understanding of each of the listed diseases is feasible without the need to lump different entities together into crudely defined categories. Accumulation of correlative clinical data, which has followed the general acceptance of the new definitions, continues to increase the relevance of the new classification to clinical practice (Armitage *et al.*, 1998). The previously important clinical appreciation of 'low-', 'intermediate-' and 'high-grade' disease, not referred to in the REAL classification, is evolving into an understanding of the wider spectrum of lymphoma clinical behaviour. As the choice of treatments broadens from the short list available when the Working Formulation was devised almost 20 years ago, this will increasingly be found to be an advantage.

The REAL classification has been adopted by the World Health Organization and has been updated with relatively minor modifications as the WHO classification (Harris *et al.*, 1999). This classification is shown in Table 45.1.

Special techniques in pathological diagnosis

IMMUNOPHENOTYPING

A series of monoclonal antibodies have been raised against lymphoid cell markers over the past 15–20 years. The specific markers expressed by a lymphoma will indicate B- or T-cell lineage and may indicate the level of differentiation attained by its cell of origin during normal lymphocyte maturation. Immunophenotyping is used to distinguish between lymphomas and other tumours where the morphology is ambiguous and can augment morphological assessment in assigning a subtype.

The most basic differential lies between undifferentiated carcinoma and lymphoma. Antibodies to the leucocyte common antigen (LCA or CD45) react with the great majority of lymphomas and are particularly useful in this context. Conversely, lymphomas will not react with antibodies specific for epithelial tumour markers (e.g. cytokeratins, carcinoembryonic antigen). The diagnostic use of immunocytochemistry usually depends on examining reactions to a profile of antibodies chosen to support or exclude a diagnosis. Other commonly used antibodies are specific for B lymphocyte markers (e.g. CD10, CD19, CD20, CD79a) or T lymphocyte markers (CD2, CD3, CD4, CD8). Characteristic immunophenotypes are seen in some lymphomas such as anaplastic large cell lymphoma (ALCL). This latter entity stains positively with the CD30 antibody (Ki-1) originally found to react with Hodgkin and Reed–Sternberg cells (Schwab *et al.*, 1982). It may express one or more T-cell antigens, although some cases are of neither T- or B-cell phenotype (null cell type). ALCL is an important clinical entity, which, before the availability of anti-CD30 immunophenotyping, was often incorrectly diagnosed as undifferentiated carcinoma (Jaffe, 2001).

GENE REARRANGEMENT ANALYSIS

The majority of lymphomas are monoclonal and are derived from cells of either B or T lineage. Although clonality does not necessarily equate with malignancy,

Table 45.1 *Proposed World Health Organization classification of lymphomas (published 1999)[a]*

B-cell neoplasms	T-cell and NK cell neoplasms
Precursor B-cell neoplasm **B-lymphoblastic leukaemia/lymphoma**	*Precursor T-cell neoplasm* **T-lymphoblastic leukaemia/lymphoma**
Mature B-cell neoplasms **B-cell chronic lymphocytic leukaemia/small lymphocytic lymphoma** B-cell prolymphocytic leukaemia Lymphoplasmacytic lymphoma Splenic marginal zone B-cell lymphoma (±villous lymphocytes) **Hairy cell leukaemia** **Plasma cell myeloma**/plasmacytoma **Extranodal marginal zone lymphoma (of MALT type)** **Nodal marginal zone lymphoma** **Follicular lymphoma** **Mantle cell lymphoma** **Diffuse large B-cell lymphoma** Subtypes: **mediastinal (thymic)**, intravascular, primary effusion lymphoma **Burkitt's lymphoma/Burkitt cell leukaemia**	*Mature T-cell and NK-cell neoplasms* T-cell prolymphocytic leukaemia T-cell large granular cell lymphocytic leukaemia NK-cell leukaemia Adult T-cell leukaemia/lymphoma Extranodal NK-/T-cell lymphoma, nasal type Enteropathic-type intestinal T-cell lymphoma Hepatosplenic γ/δ T-cell lymphoma Subcutaneous panniculitis-like T-cell lymphoma **Mycosis fungoides**/Sézary syndrome Primary cutaneous anaplastic large cell lymphoma **Peripheral T-cell lymphoma, not otherwise characterized** Angioimmunoblastic T-cell lymphoma **Systemic anaplastic large cell lymphoma**

[a] More common entities are shown in bold type.

the demonstration of clonality is of particular value in differentiating between lymphoma and benign reactive lymphoid proliferation. Clonality in B-cell tumours was traditionally established by demonstrating that all cells express the same light chain (κ or λ). This technique will not, however, detect a small clonal population within a sample and can only be applied to tumours that express surface immunoglobulin. Antigen receptor gene rearrangement analysis can detect a clonal population of cells with identically rearranged immunoglobulin genes (in B cells) or T-cell receptor (TCR) genes (in T cells) even where they comprise only 1 per cent to 0.01 per cent of the sample, the sensitivity depending on the method employed. The efficacy of this approach does not depend on functional gene expression.

It is helpful to review the physiological process of antigen gene receptor rearrangement at this stage to explain better how this can be exploited diagnostically and also to highlight the plasticity of the antigen receptor genes. Aberration of antigen gene receptor rearrangement is a recurring theme in lymphomagenesis at the molecular level.

Physiological antigen receptor gene rearrangement during B-cell maturation

The normal rearrangement of the antigen receptor genes occurs early during B- and T-cell development and determines the antigen specificity of the immunoglobulin or TCR molecule carried by each specific cell. For immunoglobulin, heavy (IgH) and light chain (Igκ and Igλ) genes reside on different chromosomes and rearrange independently although, once expressed, heavy and light chain proteins associate to form the completed immunoglobulin molecule. There are two varieties of TCR, one containing α and β chains, the other γ and δ. α, β, γ and δ chains are the products of the four TCR genes which similarly undergo independent rearrangement.

IgH gene rearrangements can be used to illustrate the physiological mechanism of rearrangement, which is broadly similar in each of the genes involved. The *IgH* gene resides on chromosome 14q32 and contains discontinuous clusters of short gene segments, the variable (V_H), diversity (D_H) and joining (J_H) region genes. There are approximately 200 V genes, 30 D genes and six J genes on each allele. Rearrangement occurs sequentially through breakage, deletion and rejoining so that a unique VDJ segment is the result of joining of one D gene to a J gene and subsequent joining of the DJ segment so formed to a V gene. The DNA 'recombination signal' sequences that direct this process and the enzyme complex involved have been partially elucidated; many features are shared by TCR genes. Completion of VDJ joining usually occurs on only one of the heavy chain gene alleles. The resultant VDJ gene encodes the heavy chain component of the variable region of the immunoglobulin molecule (Tonegawa, 1983). The expression of antibody on the surface of the B cell is essential for the survival and development of the early B cell. Naïve B cells with surface immunoglobulins that recognize specific antigens move to the germinal centre of the lymph node. These germinal centre B cells multiply and during this phase their rearranged immunoglobulin genes undergo further modification by the process of somatic hypermutation, and class switching. In somatic hypermutation the V genes accumulate point mutations and deletion. This widens the repertoire of antigen recognition and enables B cells that produce antibodies with enhanced affinity to the antigen to be positively selected. These cells are then released into the circulation as plasma cells or memory B cells. The potential number of different antibodies that can be generated by this mechanism is greatly in excess of antigen variability.

Antigen receptor gene analysis by polymerase chain reaction (PCR)

The clonal IgH and TCR VDJ rearrangements can be exploited as specific B-cell or T-cell tumour markers (Arnold *et al.*, 1983). Such rearrangements can be detected within a population of cells by Southern blot analysis if the clone comprises >1–5 per cent of the sample. In many laboratories this cumbersome technique has been superseded by PCR which is quicker, cheaper, can be performed on smaller and less well preserved samples and can be refined to detect clonal populations of 0.1 per cent or less (Deane *et al.*, 1991). There are, however, important limitations to the PCR technique that limit its diagnostic sensitivity. This means that a negative result does not exclude clonality. In particular, standard PCR reactions will not detect every possible complete or any incomplete VDJ rearrangements, and in B-cell lymphomas may misinterpret as oligoclonal or polyclonal a malignant cell population in which there has been significant germinal centre processing of the *IgH* gene leading to subclones with different rearranged gene sequences. Positive results also need to be treated with caution. PCR is vulnerable to artefact as a consequence of contamination with the products of previous reactions and the amplification of non-specific target sequences. Furthermore, certain benign conditions, such as Sjögren's syndrome, can harbour clonal populations large enough to be detected by this technique.

CYTOGENETIC AND MOLECULAR GENETIC STUDIES IN LYMPHOMA

Non-random chromosomal abnormalities are a common feature of NHL subjected to karyotypic analysis. These are now understood to result in rearrangements of the genes flanking the breakpoint sites. Alterations in these genes contribute to the altered characteristics of the tumour cell. Analysis of these abnormalities can be a useful adjunct to diagnosis and classification since there they often correlate with a characteristic morphological appearance or pattern of behaviour. Fluorescent in-situ hybridization (FISH) can detect some rearrangements not detected by conventional karyotyping and, importantly, can be carried out on interphase cells. Common recurrent translocations currently recognized in NHL are listed in Table 45.2, together with the genes involved, where these have been identified.

The first described recurrent cytogenetic abnormality in lymphoma was the 14q+ marker chromosome seen in Burkitt's lymphoma. This was later shown to result from translocation t(8;14)(q24;q32). Molecular analysis demonstrates that the chromosome 8 breakpoint is within or adjacent to the *c-myc* oncogene, whereas the chromosome 14 breakpoint lies within the immunoglobulin heavy chain gene *(IgH)*. The translocation results in deregulation of c-myc as a consequence of its juxtaposition with immunoglobulin gene enhancer elements and simultaneous loss or mutation of part of its own regulatory region. c-myc plays an essential role in cell proliferation, and it appears that the translocation is important to the pathogenesis of Burkitt's lymphoma which is characteristically an aggressive tumour with high proliferative activity.

Other important B-cell-specific translocations also involve the *IgH* gene on chromosome band 14q32 and in most cases arise as a consequence of aberrant physiological

IgH gene rearrangement. Translocation t(14;18) (q32;q24) is the commonest recurring cytogenetic abnormality identified in non-Hodgkin's lymphoma. The overall frequency of t(14;18) in non-Hodgkin's lymphoma in some populations may be as high as 47 per cent, based on an Australian series of 147 cases successfully karyotyped at presentation (Juneja *et al.*, 1990). t(14;18) is most closely associated with follicular lymphoma, being present in 70–85 per cent of cases, but has also been described in 26–40 per cent of diffuse large cell lymphomas. Some of these tumours may represent histological transformation of an earlier follicular lymphoma. The translocation joins the *BCL2* gene from 18q21 with the *IgH* gene. A structurally normal BCL2 protein product is expressed in lymphoma cells as a consequence, but the level of expression is higher and shows no evidence of the physiological downregulation that is a feature of normal germinal centre B lymphocytes.

BCL2 enhances the survival of cells which normally die by apoptosis and results in an expanded population of long-lived B cells of low malignant potential. Their prolonged survival promotes the development of secondary

Table 45.2 *Recurrent chromosomal translocations in NHL subtypes resulting in oncogene deregulation*

Histology	Translocation	Alteration of gene function	Mechanism/Features of translocation	Frequency (%)
Follicular lymphoma	t(14;18)(q32;21)	Upregulation of BCL2 (inhibitor of apoptosis)	BCL2 relocates to IgH locus. Error in physiological IgH rearrangement. Seen rarely in normal B cells	80
Burkitt's lymphoma	t(8;14)(q24;q32); t(2;8)(p12;q24); t(8;22)(q24;q11)	Upregulation of c-*myc*; (transcription factor for cell cycle progression/ proliferation)	c-*myc* relocates to IgH locus or to one of the light chain gene loci	100
Mantle cell lymphoma	t(11;14)(q13;q32)	Upregulation of cyclin D1 (G1 cyclin)	Cyclin D1 relocates to IgH	>90
Diffuse large B cell lymphoma[a]	t(3;14)(q27;932) & several others involving 3q27	Deregulation of BCL6 (zinc finger transcription factor)	BCL6 relocates to IgH, IgL, IgK or one of many other non-Ig loci	30–40
Extranodal marginal zone lymphoma (MALT)	t(11;18)(q21;q21)	Gene fusion of AP12 and MLT/MALT1 genes (AP12 is inhibitor of apoptosis)	Gene fusion	20–35
Extranodal marginal zone lymphoma (MALT)	t(1;14)(q22;q32)	Deregulation of BCL10 (apoptosis regulatory protein)	BCL10 relocates to IgH locus	<5
Lymphaplasmacytic lymphoma	t(9;14)(q13;q32)	Deregulation of PAX5 (paired homeobox transcription factor)	PAX5 relocates to IgH locus	50
Anaplastic large cell lymphoma	t(2;5)(p23;q35) & others involving 2p23	Gene fusion of ALK (anaplastic lymphoma kinase, a receptor tyrosine kinase) and NPM (located at 5q35) or other gene Malignant transforming capacity *in vitro* & *in vivo*	Gene fusion	50 ALK-NPM; 15 others

[a] BCL2 (30%) and c-*myc* (10%) rearrangements are also frequently seen in diffuse large B-cell NHL.

molecular genetic changes, which propel the cell to malignancy. This putative sequence of events correlates with the clinical behaviour and histopathological characteristics of follicular lymphoma. Usually an indolent tumour which may be associated with prolonged survival, there is a risk of high-grade transformation which eventually occurs, albeit sometimes after as long as 10–18 years (Horning, 1994), in 40–60 per cent of those patients who do not succumb to other complications of the disease. However, it appears that the low-grade follicular lymphoma phenotype also requires molecular genetic abnormalities in addition to t(14;18). It has now repeatedly been shown that t(14;18) can be detected in occasional B cells in peripheral blood, bone marrow and reactive lymphoid tissue of normal individuals (Limpens *et al.*, 1995), indicating that lymphoma is not the inevitable consequence of this translocation but rather the translocation is an early event in a multistep pathway.

STAGING

Staging of NHL is important for the initial treatment planning, assessing prognosis and as a yardstick by which to monitor response to subsequent therapy. The Ann Arbor staging system designed for Hodgkin's disease is also used in NHL (Table 45.3). Since NHL does not tend to spread predictably to contiguous sites and frequently involves extranodal sites, staging has a lower prognostic value here than in Hodgkin's disease.

The initial question raised during the staging of NHL is whether the disease is limited in extent and thus potentially treatable with radiotherapy alone or combined radiotherapy and chemotherapy, or advanced, in which case systemic therapy is the mainstay.

Table 45.3 *Ann Arbor staging system for the classification of lymphomas*

Stage I	Single lymph-node region affected/single extralymphatic organ or site (stage IE)
Stage II	Two or more lymph-node sites affected on the same side of the diaphragm, with or without disease involving local extralymphatic site (IIE)
Stage III	Lymph-node regions affected on both sides of the diaphragm with or without involvement of spleen or local extralymphatic site (IIIE)
Stage IV	Disseminated disease involving one or more extralymphatic organs with or without lymph node involvement
Also record	*absence* (A) or *presence* (B) of constitutional symptoms, i.e. fever, night sweats or weight loss >10%

'Limited disease' usually refers to stage I or II disease without B symptoms and without sites of bulk disease >10 cm in diameter.

INVESTIGATIONS

Haematology

Bone marrow involvement is common in the low-grade lymphomas (50 per cent) and may be detected even in the presence of nodal disease of limited extent; it is generally less common (20 per cent) in intermediate-grade and high-grade lymphomas and then usually correlates with more extensive disease. Bone marrow involvement in lymphoma may be patchy and the pattern of infiltration varies with the histological type. Follicular lymphoma, for example, characteristically forms paratrabecular nodules. A generous trephine biopsy is required to assess this architectural variation and bone marrow involvement is very frequently missed if aspiration alone is performed.

Sometimes, in the presence of bone marrow infiltration, lymphoma cells may be detectable in the peripheral blood by light microscopy. This leukaemic component is most common in small lymphocytic, mantle cell and lymphoblastic lymphomas. A circulating clone is detectable in a much higher proportion of cases if specific immunological or molecular genetic techniques are used.

Anaemia is common at presentation in advanced-stage lymphoma and does not always indicate marrow infiltration; in some series it has been found to be significantly associated with a poor prognosis. Haemolysis is an important cause of anaemia, particularly in association with small lymphocytic lymphoma. Isolated thrombocytopenia may be the result of hypersplenism or immune-mediated platelet destruction. Pancytopenia at presentation usually correlates with extensive bone marrow replacement with lymphoma.

Biochemistry

A variety of biochemical abnormalities can be present at diagnosis in lymphoma and dictate that an extended biochemical profile be part of the initial assessment.

Abnormal liver function can result from organ infiltration or obstruction of the biliary tree by lymphadenopathy at the porta hepatis. Renal infiltration is relatively uncommon but ureteric obstruction leading to renal failure is an important reversible emergency in lymphoma management. Hyperuricaemia is associated with rapidly proliferative lesions, particularly Burkitt's and lymphoblastic lymphoma. This must be corrected and further uric acid production inhibited with allopurinol before chemotherapy is started if tumour lysis syndrome is to be avoided. Hypercalcaemia is seen in some cases of intermediate and high-grade lymphoma and is a characteristic feature of HTLV1-associated adult T-cell leukaemia/ lymphoma. Hypercalcaemia will usually respond to initiation of definitive therapy, although other corrective measures including hydration will often be necessary. Low serum albumin and particularly elevated levels of the enzyme lactate dehydrogenase (LDH) have important prognostic significance; LDH is incorporated in the International Prognostic Index for diffuse large cell lymphoma (International NHL Prognostic Factors Project, 1993; see below). Lymphoplasmacytic lymphoma and plasmacytoma may secrete immunoglobulin or free light chains which can be detected as a monoclonal band on serum protein electropheresis.

Imaging investigations

A chest X-ray may indicate mediastinal or hilar lymphadenopathy, pleural effusion or pulmonary infiltration. Mediastinal involvement is seen in virtually all cases of T-cell lymphoblastic lymphoma and sclerosing B-cell lymphoma of the mediastinum. In contrast to Hodgkin's disease, mediastinal involvement in advanced NHL is somewhat less common than abdominal nodal involvement.

A computed tomography (CT) scan of the thorax is routinely performed as this is more sensitive than X-ray in the detection of mediastinal lymphadenopathy and pulmonary infiltration. Abdominal imaging, usually with CT scan, is mandatory in all cases of lymphoma. This will assess the para-aortic, mesenteric and other lymph node areas as well as the liver, spleen, kidneys and pancreas. The scan should be extended into the pelvis; this will often provide additional information and, in the presence of disease clinically localized to the inguinal region, will indicate whether there is associated iliac disease, which may be too extensive for local irradiation.

Imaging with isotopic bone scans, skeletal X-rays, or magnetic resonance imaging (MRI) scans of the brain or spine will be indicated if there is clinical reason to suspect bone, intracranial or spinal involvement. For lymphoma primarily involving the gastrointestinal tract, scanning of the abdomen is an essential part of staging but is unlikely to provide adequately detailed information about gastrointestinal involvement *per se*. The diagnosis is most likely to be made at surgery or endoscopy but barium studies may be useful to demonstrate the extent of disease.

Other procedures

LAPAROTOMY

Laparotomy is no longer performed as part of the routine staging workup in non-Hodgkin's lymphoma. Laparoscopy or laparotomy may occasionally be required to obtain diagnostic tissue from an abdominal mass, but where lymphoma is suspected from the outset, percutaneous core biopsy under CT or ultrasound guidance should be performed if the mass is accessible to this approach.

LUMBAR PUNCTURE

The cerebrospinal fluid (CSF) should be examined cytologically for the presence of lymphoma cells in patients with neurological abnormalities (assuming there is no suspicion of raised intracranial pressure) and also in specific situations where there is a high risk of meningeal involvement. These include:

- high-risk histologies *per se*, i.e. lymphoblastic lymphoma and Burkitt's lymphoma; and
- large cell lymphomas with high-risk extranodal sites of disease, e.g. involvement of paranasal sinuses (associated with CNS involvement in up to 50 per cent of cases), testicular involvement or extensive bone marrow involvement.

INDOLENT LYMPHOMAS

Follicular lymphoma accounts for approximately 30 per cent of NHL in the UK and is the most important of the group of lymphomas which are characterised by indolent clinical behaviour and were previously classified within the working formulation as 'low grade'. The others are small lymphocytic, lymphaplasmacytic and the nodal and extranodal marginal zone lymphomas which together make up 10–15 per cent of NHL. In this chapter, follicular lymphoma is described in detail and the others are dealt with more briefly, highlighting the ways in which they differ from follicular lymphoma.

Follicular lymphoma

Pathology

The recognition of a follicular pattern in biopsies is highly reproducible. Within the malignant follicle is an admixture of benign T cells, small centrocytes (cleaved follicle centre cells) and large centroblasts (non-cleaved follicle centre cells). Centrocytes and centroblasts represent different developmental stages of the same malignant B-cell clone. The minority of cases (<10 per cent) in which a high proportion of centroblasts are seen (>25 per cent) arguably exhibit more aggressive behaviour and are sometimes treated differently, for example with protocols used for diffuse large B-cell lymphoma.

BIOLOGY

Proliferation and apoptotic indices
Typically the proliferative rate is low, indicated by infrequent mitosis and low staining with proliferation markers

such as the Ki-67 monoclonal antibody. As previously noted, the majority of follicular lymphomas express BCL2 which promotes cell survival by inhibiting apoptosis. Accordingly, there is a low apoptotic index compared with the physiological lymphoid follicle (Hollowood and Macartney, 1991).

Submicroscopic disease

The t(14;18) translocation can be detected at submicroscopic levels in blood, bone marrow and other tissues using PCR (Lee *et al.*, 1987). This type of analysis has demonstrated that:

- follicular lymphoma is virtually always a systemic disease even where conventional staging investigations indicate localized involvement; and
- the t(14;18) bearing clone may persist even where the clinical response has been complete and durable (Price *et al.*, 1991).

The clinical significance of systemic disease at this level remains unclear, however.

Histological transformation

Transformation to an intermediate-grade lymphoma (diffuse large cell) is a common feature in the natural history of follicular lymphoma; there is a continuous risk during the course of the disease so that the actuarial incidence approaches 50 per cent 18 years after diagnosis (Horning, 1994). A policy of performing repeat biopsies at relapse specifically to exclude this possibility is justified. The numerous genetic changes which may accompany histological transformation, for example mutations of the tumour supressor genes *p53* (Lo Coco *et al.*, 1993) and *p16* (Pinyol *et al.*, 1998), continue to be defined but as yet have not enabled prediction of future transformation or directly influenced clinical management policies.

CLINICAL PRESENTATION

The median age at diagnosis for follicular lymphoma is 55–60 years. It is rarely diagnosed below the age of 30 and extremely uncommon below 20. Presentation is most frequently with lymphadenopathy, often with a history of gradual or intermittent node enlargement. Symptomatic extranodal disease at presentation is unusual, although cytopenia due to marrow involvement and hepatosplenomegaly are seen in advanced cases. The majority of patients present with advanced disease.

TREATMENT

Localized disease

Only 10–15 per cent of follicular lymphomas present with localized disease (here referring to stage I, or stage II if confined to contiguous nodal sites). About 50 per cent of these patients can be cured with involved field radiotherapy alone. Although combined chemotherapy and radiotherapy can increase duration of remission (Seymour *et al.*, 1996), there is less evidence that this improves the long-term outlook for those patients destined to relapse after radiotherapy alone. Radiotherapy should therefore be used initially in this situation, with chemotherapy being reserved for those patients who develop systemic recurrence.

Initial management for advanced disease

The optimal treatment of advanced follicular lymphoma is currently far from clear. The median survival with conventional therapy has remained unchanged at 8–10 years for the past three decades. Accurately defining the role of each of a number of new approaches to treatment which have emerged at approximately the same time in a condition with a long natural history is clearly very difficult, although in many respects this is an enviable situation and there is emerging evidence that for the first time the natural history of the disease is being altered. Table 45.4 lists available approaches to treatment of advanced disease with some of their advantages and disadvantages. There are often several opportunities for therapeutic intervention in advanced follicular lymphoma during the course of the disease. The order in which treatments should be used and to what extent newer approaches should be used 'up front' ahead of manifestly inadequate standard treatments is currently the subject of controversy and, appropriately, clinical trial activity.

'Watch and wait' Follicular lymphoma is usually responsive to initial therapy but recurrence is expected. Despite being considered to be of 'favourable histology', and despite recent increases in the range of therapeutic options, advanced disease remains incurable with currently available treatment. The rate of progression is typically slow so that urgent initiation of therapy is not usually necessary and a 'watch and wait' approach, in which intervention is deferred until there are symptoms or evidence of compromise of organ function is a reasonable management option and the one most frequently adopted in middle-aged and elderly patients. There is, however, some concern that the 'watch and wait' approach allows patients with advanced disease to slide into a less favourable prognostic group before treatment is initiated. The comparisons which indicate that delays in starting therapy do not affect overall prognosis overlook the possibility that patients who present with good performance status, low volume disease and absence of systemic symptoms are those who may have done better if therapy was started earlier. This controversy remains unresolved. Nevertheless, 'watch and wait' is now used less frequently in young patients <40–50 years in whom a more active approach may now be justified.

Chemotherapy: single-agent chlorambucil For advanced disease, oral chlorambucil, either as a single agent or in combination with prednisolone, has been the most commonly used treatment in the UK. It is usual to give treatment intermittently rather than continuously, e.g. chlorambucil 10 mg daily for 2 weeks each month. This is usually very well tolerated, the most important side-effect

Table 45.4 *Some current treatment options for follicular lymphoma*

Treatment option	Positive aspects	Negative aspects
'Watch and wait'	No evidence for worse overall outcome	Risk of clinical deterioration before institution of therapy
Oral chlorambucil	Well tolerated oral therapy Minimal life-style disruption	Low rate of complete remission Bone marrow damage from repeated courses may hinder future autologous stem cell transplantation
Conventional dose combination chemotherapy, e.g. CHOP	Rapid response in ill patient or with organ compromise Moderate CR rate Widely available Effective if clinical suspicion of histological transformation Suitable for stem cell mobilization	More toxic than single agent Cardiotoxicity of anthracyclines
Fludarabine	Well tolerated without alopecia or cardiotoxicity	Expensive for short-term palliation Persisting immunosuppression
Fludarabine combinations, e.g. FMD	High CR rate Some 'molecular' CRs recorded	Immunosuppressive May hinder stem cell mobilization
Rituximab (anti-CD20 antibody)	Very well tolerated Non-cross-resistant with chemotherapy	Expensive for short-term palliation Role in combination uncertain
Radioimmuno-conjugates	High overall and complete response rate	Myelotoxic Not yet licensed in UK
High-dose therapy/autologous stem cell transplant	Long remissions in some poor prognosis patients May be curative within some subgroups	Uncertainty of survival benefit Optimal protocol unclear, including purging $\pm$ Toxic with mortality rate approx. 2–3% Risk of myelodysplasia/AML
Allogeneic transplantation (including non-myeloablative conditioning)	Graft-v-lymphoma effect Low relapse rate raises possibility of some cures Mini-allograft technique may be relatively safer	Only for fit, younger patients Primarily for patients with matched related donor High early mortality rate Only small numbers yet performed

being mild myelosuppression. The majority of patients will respond although only a minority will achieve complete remission. Prolonged or repeated use of alkylating agents causes long-term bone marrow damage and severely limits future lymphoma treatment strategies. For this reason it is becoming a less popular initial therapy for young patients.

Established combination chemotherapy such as CHOP
There is no direct evidence that a more intensive approach using a combination of cytotoxic agents is more effective in the long term, although partial and complete response rates are higher. However, if a rapid response is required in patients with severe symptoms from advanced disease, an established combination chemotherapy regimen such as CHOP (cyclophosphamide, doxorubicin, vincristine and prednisolone) can bring about disease control more rapidly. This would be recommended, for example, in patients with obstructive uropathy from bulky retroperitoneal lymphadenopathy. In young patients (<40–50) the attainment of complete remission (CR) to therapy is

now sometimes seen as a useful goal of in itself. Particularly if the bone marrow can be cleared, a wider range of treatment choices can then be considered, e.g. autologous stem cell harvesting. The higher CR rate with CHOP may justify the choice of this regimen at an early stage in this patient group.

MANAGEMENT OF RECURRENT DISEASE

Conventional dose salvage chemotherapy

Recurrence is to be anticipated in patients treated for advanced follicular grade lymphoma. Rebiopsy should be considered to exclude histological transformation. If the histology is unchanged, a further period of 'watchful waiting' may be appropriate since the pattern may still be one of waxing and waning of lymphadenopathy or slow asymptomatic progression for which immediate treatment is unnecessary. Radiotherapy can be a useful treatment for symptomatic localized sites of recurrent disease. Systemic retreatment with the same single agent or combination regimen as that used at induction can be effective in patients who responded well to initial treatment and who have enjoyed remission durations of more than 12–18 months. Although there is a general trend to progressively shorter remissions, many patients will respond repeatedly to courses of chemotherapy given for recurrences occurring at intervals over a prolonged time period. In one series the median survival of patients from the time of first recurrence was 6 years, and the median remission duration did not differ significantly for the first three courses of treatment given an average of 33 months apart (Gallagher *et al.*, 1986).

High-dose therapy

For younger patients, acceptance of the incurability of low-grade lymphoma, albeit with an extended disease course, is difficult for patient and physician alike. A possible role for high-dose treatment with autologous stem cell support has been investigated in the hope that this might permit some cures in patients with advanced disease. Several non-randomized studies of such treatment have been reported in patients with recurrent disease (Rohatiner *et al.*, 1994; Brice *et al.*, 2000). The high incidence of marrow infiltration has prompted investigation of techniques to purge the harvested bone marrow *in vitro* before reinfusion. At present the value of such treatment policies and the optimum technique still remains to be established. The picture that is emerging is one of longer-lasting remissions than with conventional therapy, but most patients nevertheless relapse and a survival advantage has not yet been demonstrated (Rohatiner *et al.*, 1994). The possibility that certain groups of patients benefit, for example those treated earlier in the course of their disease, those for whom *in-vitro* treatment of bone marrow successfully removes PCR evidence of infiltration (Gribben *et al.*, 1991) and those with histological transformation (Williams *et al.*, 2001), will require longer follow-up to confirm. A serious concern is the high incidence of myelodysplasia and myeloid leukaemia in patients so treated. The rate appears to be influenced to some extent by the previous therapy to which the patient has been exposed and the nature of the high-dose therapy used.

Newer agents

Fludarabine Fludarabine, a purine analogue, is active and generally well tolerated with response rates of 50–65 per cent (Hochster *et al.*, 1992). However, the CR rate is low and duration of response not consistently better than standard combination chemotherapy regimens. It causes a long-lasting immunosuppression due to an effect on T-cell function and there is therefore a risk of opportunistic infection. In combination with mitozantrone and dexamethasone (FMD, McLaughlin *et al.*, 1996) or with cyclophoshamide, however, CR rates ranging between 20 per cent and >80 per cent in previously treated and untreated patients have been recorded, with several patients achieving 'molecular remission', i.e. loss of cells carrying t(14;18) translocation as measured by PCR. These figures could represent a genuine improvement when compared to conventional therapy and so the FMD combination is now being tested in a UK national phase III trial in previously untreated patients. Fludarabine alone or in combination is currently most frequently considered as third-line therapy for patients who have relapsed after chlorambucil and also an anthracycline-based regimen such as CHOP.

Monoclonal antibodies as therapy Rituximab is a chimeric humanized monoclonal antibody directed against the pan-B-cell antigen CD20. Administered by intravenous infusion weekly for 4 weeks, it has been shown to have activity comparable to combination chemotherapy in previously treated follicular lymphoma with responses in the region of 50 per cent (McLaughlin *et al.*, 1998). The toxicity is very low and up to 50 per cent of initially responding patients may benefit from re-treatment. Although as a single agent it is a worthwhile addition to the list of active drugs in this condition, the cost (approximately UK£4000 for a course) may limit its use as a palliative treatment for heavily pre-treated patients. Much interest now focuses on other potential applications, for example in combination with chemotherapy (Czuczman *et al.*, 1999), as maintenance therapy and as a means of reducing the level of lymphomatous contamination of autologous stem cell collections through 'pre-emptive' administration of the antibody to patients being prepared for harvesting (Magni *et al.*, 2000).

Tositumomab is another anti-CD20 antibody but in this case the antibody is used as a means of targeting a therapeutic dose of radiation to the lymphoma. This is effected through labelling of the antibody with iodine-131. Response rates reported from the early trials in both treated and previously untreated patients have been very encouraging (Liu *et al.*, 1998) and the conjugate is now licensed for use in the USA but not yet in the UK.

Experimental approaches to therapy An array of experimental therapies are currently being evaluated. Examples include antisense therapy, patient-specific vaccines (Bendandi *et al.*, 1999) and immunotoxins. The overexpressed *BCL2* gene provides a natural target for antisense olignucleotide therapy. Switching off the gene may lead directly to apoptosis in lymphoma cells or may heighten their sensitivity to chemotherapy. A phase I clinical trial has already been reported from the Royal Marsden Hospital, London (Waters *et al.*, 2000).

Allogeneic transplantation Allogeneic bone marrow transplantation is a toxic treatment with a high early mortality. In follicular lymphoma few patients have been so treated but results are beginning to suggest that there may be an important graft-versus-lymphoma effect. Even though many of the transplanted patients have been very heavily pre-treated and with a poor prognosis, recurrent lymphoma has rarely been seen in patients surviving more than 2 years post-transplant (van Besian, 1998). A less toxic and hazardous method of harnessing the graft-versus-lymphoma effect may be provided by the 'mini-allograft' for which very intensive ablative preparative therapy is not required (Champlin *et al.*, 1999). Several units are now considering this for selected patients but it will be very difficult to subject this to randomized controlled trial. We await the freedom from recurrence and survival figures from the first groups of patients so treated with great interest.

Other indolent B-cell lymphomas

EXTRANODAL MARGINAL ZONE LYMPHOMA (PREVIOUSLY MALTOMA)

These relatively common tumours (8–10 per cent of NHL) have been increasingly recognized since their first description by Isaacson and Wright in 1983. The majority present with localized stage I or II extranodal disease involving glandular epithelium at various sites, most frequently stomach but also salivary glands, thyroid, lacrimal glands, breast, prostate, bladder and lung. There is an association with autoimmune disease such as Hashimoto's disease and Sjögren's syndrome and in the stomach with *Helicobacter pylori* infection. Gastric involvement can be shown to be antigen driven and successful eradication of *Helicobacter* can lead to regression of early lesions (Wotherspoon *et al.*, 1993; Papa *et al.*, 2000). Non-responding gastric lesions should be treated with simple chemotherapy initially but radiotherapy or resection may be required for persistent symptomatic disease. Transformation to large cell lymphoma can occur; standard combination chemotherapy, e.g. CHOP, is then required. At other sites the initial treatment is as for follicular lymphoma. Radiotherapy is frequently indicated in view of the tendency to remain localized. Bone marrow infiltration is unusual. The role of the newer therapies (as described for follicular lymphoma at relapse) are for the most part undefined.

SMALL LYMPHOCYTIC LYMPHOMA

This condition differs from chronic lymphocytic leukaemia (CLL) only in its presentation with predominantly nodal and other organ infiltration rather than with peripheral blood involvement. Bone marrow involvement is usual. Autoimmune haemolytic anaemia is an important cause for severe anaemia. High-grade transformation is less common than in follicular lymphoma. The treatment choices mirror those for follicular lymphoma closely, although complete responses are less common. The response rate with rituximab is lower and the early toxicity of this agent is highest in patients with a high circulating lymphocyte count.

HAIRY CELL LEUKAEMIA

This low-grade B-cell lymphoma typically involves spleen and bone marrow and presents with pancytopenia, splenomegaly and recurrent infections. The characteristic cell is a small lymphoid cell with 'hairy' projections seen on smear preparations, which is positive for B-cell antigens and surface immunoglobulin. The normal counterpart of this cell is unknown. Previously splenectomy was the treatment of choice and was often associated with significant clinical improvement. In recent years, however, interferon-α (IFNα), deoxycoformycin and 2-chlorodeoxyadenosine (2-CDA) have all been shown to be highly active, the latter agent being capable of bringing about complete remissions which may in some cases prove to be durable.

AGGRESSIVE LYMPHOMAS

Diffuse large B-cell lymphoma

Diffuse large B-cell lymphoma (DLBCL) is the most common NHL subtype. The REAL/WHO classification has not retained previous subdivisions of this type, such as immunoblastic lymphoma, since the distinctions were not universally accepted, reproducibility was low and there was no consistent distinction in clinical behaviour. Sclerosing B-cell lymphoma of the mediastinum and the rare intravascular and primary effusion lymphomas are the only entities given separate mention in the new classification. Together these entities comprise 50 per cent of all lymphomas. They are often referred to as lymphomas with 'unfavourable' or 'aggressive' histology but, despite these epithets, they are highly responsive to combination chemotherapy and approximately 40 per cent of patients with advanced disease can be cured with current treatment. Clinical presentation is typically with rapidly enlarging lymph-node masses, but extranodal sites are frequently involved and may include unusual sites such as soft tissue, testis, bone, lung and pancreas. The median age at presentation is 50–55, somewhat lower than for indolent lymphomas.

INITIAL TREATMENT

Radiotherapy
Radiotherapy given alone has a limited role in the primary management of diffuse large cell lymphoma. Combined chemotherapy and radiotherapy, however, has become established as the treatment of choice for localized disease and will produce long-term remission in approximately 80 per cent of patients (Miller *et al.*, 1998). An attenuated course of chemotherapy (for example CHOP × three cycles) is usual for non-bulky lesions. Radiotherapy alone may be used for unfit elderly patients or for disease confined to the skin, where the risk of systemic involvement is low.

Chemotherapy
Combination chemotherapy is required for the large majority of patients with intermediate-grade lymphoma.

Table 45.5 *CHOP chemotherapy regimen*

Drug	Dose (mg/m^2) and schedule
Cyclophosphamide	750 i.v. on day 1
Doxorubicin	50 i.v. on day 1
Vincristine	1.4 i.v. on day 1 (max 2 mg)
Prednisolone	50 orally on days 1–5

Treatment repeated every 21 days.
Usual total number of cycles = 6.

The CHOP regimen (Table 45.5) was introduced in the 1970s. It is a myelosuppressive regimen which is given every 21 days to allow haematopoietic recovery between cycles. In the majority of series, CHOP has a complete remission rate of approximately 60–65 per cent with long-term survival in about 60 per cent of these (35–40 per cent of all patients treated). A variety of modified regimens based on CHOP were developed in the early 1980s. These 'second-generation' regimens were then superseded by 'third-generation' weekly intensive chemotherapy regimens modelled on the MACOP-B regimen initially reported in 1985 from Vancouver (Klimo and Connors, 1985). An overall response rate of 100 per cent was achieved in the first 61 patients treated, 84 per cent achieving complete response. The actuarial 5-year survival for this group when reported in 1988 was 65 per cent. In 1993 a randomized trial comparing three dose-intensive regimens with CHOP was reported by the South-west Oncology Group (SWOG) in the USA. Their trial included 1138 patients (Fisher *et al.*, 1993); 3-year actuarial survival ranged from 41 per cent to 46 per cent for the four treatment arms with no significant difference between each. The figure of 41 per cent was identical for CHOP and MACOP-B. Toxic deaths were highest with MACOP-B (6 per cent) and lowest for CHOP (1 per cent). Subgroup analysis did not identify a particular group of patients who benefited from the more intensive approach. The implication of this was that the simple CHOP regimen could reasonably remain the standard treatment for the majority of patients outside clinical trials.

This result was seen as disappointing by clinicians treating patients with large cell lymphoma, since it suggested that no progress has been made in two decades of clinical research. In fact now, some 7 years after the publication of the SWOG trial, CHOP remains the standard treatment and the standard arm in ongoing randomized trials. None of the newer approaches, including dose-intense therapy supported by haematopoietic growth factors and 'upfront' high-dose therapy with autologous stem cell transplantation, has convincingly been shown to be superior. A UK trial comparing CHOP × six cycles with CHOP × three cycles, followed by high-dose therapy in poor prognosis DLBCL will soon complete and will contribute to this debate. Some optimism has been engendered by the good results obtained in a small trial of 'sequential high-dose therapy' devised by Gianni *et al.* (1997).

However, the pitfalls of enthusiastic adoption of new treatments based on limited data are now well recognized and a large-scale comparative trial is still awaited. In elderly patients, a French trial comparing CHOP with CHOP plus rituximab has recently completed and early analysis suggests an advantage for the combination. A number of trials examining the same combination in younger patients are currently open to recruitment.

SALVAGE THERAPY AT RELAPSE

Salvage therapy is required for the 60 per cent of patients with intermediate-grade lymphoma who either fail first-line therapy or who relapse after initial response. Numerous 'conventional dose' chemotherapy regimens have been assessed for efficacy in this context; these have not cured a significant number of patients or materially influenced the poor overall prognosis. Typically only 10–15 per cent of patients remain disease-free after 2 years. High-dose chemotherapy supported by autologous stem cells (where possible harvested from peripheral blood) is now established as the most effective salvage treatment. This has been demonstrated by the landmark Parma international trial (Philip *et al.*, 1995) in which DHAP (dexamethasone, cytosine arabinoside and cisplatin), one of the best conventional dose salvage regimens with a 34 per cent reported complete response rate (Velasquez *et al.*, 1988), was compared with the high-dose BEAC regimen (BCNU, etoposide, cytosine arabinoside and cyclophosphamide) in patients achieving a complete response to two initial cycles of DHAP. This trial confirmed the activity of DHAP, but there was a significant improvement in event-free survival (46 per cent versus 12 per cent at 5 years) and overall survival (53 per cent versus 32 per cent at 5 years, $P = 0.038$) in the patients in the high dose arm.

Patients with diffuse large cell lymphoma relapsing within 2 years of completion of initial therapy should now routinely be considered for high-dose salvage therapy. A short course of conventional dose salvage chemotherapy is used to reduce the bulk of disease and to assess chemosensitivity. There is no consensus on the optimal regimen for this, although DHAP or the related ESHAP regimen (cytosine arabinoside, cisplatin, etoposide and methylprednisolone) is frequently used. Patients who progress during initial chemotherapy (refractory disease) or who fail to respond to initial conventional dose salvage chemotherapy (resistant disease) have a markedly lower chance of benefiting from high-dose therapy; the outlook is very poor and supportive care may be a preferable alternative to aggressive therapy.

PROGNOSTIC FACTORS IN DIFFUSE LARGE CELL LYMPHOMA

International Prognostic Index (IPI)

The analysis of factors associated with favourable or unfavourable outcomes of treatment is of practical importance in the management of intermediate-grade lymphomas. These are manifestly a disparate group and include some patients who are unlikely to be cured by conventional chemotherapy. For these, new and possibly more intensive approaches are required; conversely, some patients with favourable disease may be adequately treated with less toxic regimens. A retrospective analysis of over 2000 patients from 16 centres in Europe and the USA was published in 1993 (International NHL Prognostic Factors Project, 1993). The factors identified as having greatest independent prognostic significance were age, stage, performance status, number of extranodal sites involved and serum LDH level. These were combined to subdivide patients into four risk groups according to number of adverse prognostic factors present. The 5-year survival for the best and worst groups was 73 per cent and 26 per cent, respectively. This simple prognostic index has been widely accepted and is used to stratify patients in clinical trials and to make comparisons between groups of patients treated in different trials.

New prognostic factors

New information provided by the pathologist and from molecular genetic analysis can give additional prognostic information. For example, many studies have now shown that BCL2 expression in DLBCL is associated with a lower probability of long-term disease-free survival. As technology and knowledge increase, more complex analyses are possible. 'Gene expression profiling' is the assessment of the expression of large numbers of genes simultaneously. This can be performed in an automated fashion using microarrays. Very early data suggests that subgrouping of DLBCL according to patterns of gene expression will identify patients with widely different prognoses even within the groups identified by the IPI (Alizadeh et al., 2000).

MEDIASTINAL (THYMIC) B-CELL LYMPHOMA

This subtype of diffuse large cell lymphoma appears to be a distinct clinicopathological entity. It usually involves the thymus and typically presents with a locally invasive mediastinal mass, frequently compressing the superior vena cava and large airways. With a median presentation in the fourth decade it affects a younger age group than is usual for large cell lymphoma and there is a female preponderance. The prognosis is relatively poor with standard combination chemotherapy but may be as good as, or better than, that for the majority of diffuse large cell lymphomas if a combination of chemotherapy and mediastinal radiotherapy is used.

Mantle cell lymphoma

Mantle cell lymphoma makes up 5–8 per cent of NHL. Most cases were previously included in the 'diffuse small cleaved' subtype of the working formulation. It is associated with translocation t(11;14) in the majority of cases; this leads to overexpression of cyclin D1 which can be detected by immunocytochemistry. There is marked male

predominance and the majority of patients present with advanced disease. There is a high incidence of bone marrow involvement. Optimal treatmant for this condition has not yet been established; responses to both single agent and combination chemotherapy tend to be incomplete and the median survival is only 3–4 years. Recently high complete response rate have been achieved with more aggressive initial therapy using drugs in addition to those included in CHOP (e.g. HyperCVAD; Khouri et al., 1998). The aim of this approach has been to enable up-front high-dose therapy with autologous stem cell support. The long-term benefits of this approach remain to be defined.

Lymphoblastic lymphoma

Lymphoblastic lymphoma can be considered to belong to a disease spectrum which includes acute lymphoblastic leukaemia but which is designated lymphoma when the infiltration predominantly involves nodal tissue and the degree of bone marrow involvement is low; the presence of less than 25 per cent lymphoblasts in the marrow is a typical arbitrary diagnostic cut-off level. Men are affected twice as often as women and the peak incidence is in the decade 15–25. The majority of cases are of T-cell phenotype and 60–70 per cent present with a mediastinal mass. B symptoms are common. CNS involvement is a particular risk; this should be sought by examination of the CSF at the time of diagnosis and specifically protected against by the use of CNS prophylaxis incorporated into the treatment regimen.

The majority of cases respond rapidly to standard combination chemotherapy of the type used in large cell lymphoma. Unfortunately, with conventional therapy the majority of patients relapse early either systemically or in the CNS; their disease is then usually refractory to further chemotherapy. This unsatisfactory remission duration and the overall poor prognosis of lymphoblastic lymphoma has prompted use of more aggressive induction regimens similar to those used in acute lymphoblastic leukaemia and trials of high-dose therapy supported by stem cell transplantation. Combined data from a number of small non-randomized European studies have suggested an advantage for this approach both as salvage therapy at relapse and for consolidation of first remission in poor-risk patients (Sweetenham et al., 1994). In a UK Lymphoma Group study, randomizing between either conventional dose maintenance chemotherapy or high-dose consolidation supported by stem cell transplantation in patients achieving remission after initial induction therapy is consistent with a benefit from high-dose therapy (Sweetenham et al., 2001), although the number of patients randomized in the trial was small.

Burkitt's lymphoma

Burkitt's lymphoma is characterized histologically by small non-cleaved cells with a very high proliferation rate; Ki-67 score approaches 100 per cent indicating that the large majority of cells are cycling. As previously discussed, the characteristic chromosomal abnormality is the t(8;14) translocation. 'Endemic' or 'African' Burkitt's lymphoma differs from the European/USA 'sporadic' type both clinically and at the genetic level since the translocation involves different regions of both the c-*myc* and immunoglobulin heavy chain gene in the two variants. African Burkitt's lymphoma presents typically with a localized tumour, often involving the jaw, in a young child, whereas sporadic Burkitt's frequently presents with a rapidly enlarging abdominal mass. Extranodal sites including the CNS are also commonly involved.

In Burkitt's lymphoma, low-volume localized disease, for example involving the ileocaecal region where it may present early and be macroscopically resected, has a good prognosis with consolidation chemotherapy. More advanced bulky or widespread disease characteristically responds very rapidly to initial treatment, but if standard CHOP-type regimens are used early relapse is the norm. The outlook for the disease has been transformed by the use of the short-duration highly intensive alternating combination regimen CODOX-M/IVAC which was developed by Magrath *et al.* (1996) at the US National Cancer Institute and is based on paediatric lymphoma protocols incorporating high-dose methotrexate. Patients treated with this regimen have a risk of recurrence of <25–30 per cent; this figure has recently been achieved in a UK national confirmatory phase II study. Burkitt's lymphoma is rare in the UK (1 per cent of NHL) so that most units will only see one or two cases annually. It has major clinical importance, however, because:

- the rapid clinical course mandates that the diagnosis should always be treated as a medical emergency. Patients should be transferred without delay to a specialist unit; and
- the very rapid response to the institution of therapy results in a high risk of tumour lysis syndrome which can be fatal if not correctly managed.

T-CELL LYMPHOMAS

Peripheral T-cell lymphomas

Peripheral T-cell lymphomas make up approximately 10–15 per cent of all NHL. They remain a rather poorly understood group, largely because they were not defined separately in the Working Formulation and thus for the most part clear clinical data have not been collected. They were usually included in the diffuse mixed, diffuse large cell, diffuse small cleaved and immunoblastic categories where, in each case, they are significantly outnumbered by B-cell tumours. Where the prognostic significance of T-cell phenotype has been assessed, a tendency to less favourable outcome emerges, but the finding is not consistent

between series. In most cases, combination chemotherapy such as CHOP is required. A particularly poor prognosis is seen with bulky or stage IV disease. As with DLBCL, a poor prognostic group can be defined using the IPI. Novel or more intensive treatment approaches may be appropriate for this group.

Mycosis fungoides/Sézary syndrome

Mycosis fungoides is a rare cutaneous T-cell lymphoma which characteristically involves the epidermis and initially presents with disseminated psoriatic-like lesions but progresses to plaque and tumour formation. The clinical course is usually slow, but ultimately regional node and distant organ involvement can occur. Cutaneous disease can often be controlled with electron-beam radiotherapy and photochemotherapy. Systemic chemotherapy may produce transient responses but is not the mainstay of treatment. Advanced disease is usually resistant to therapy and carries a poor prognosis. Sézary syndrome describes the association of T-cell chronic lymphocytic leukaemia and erythroderma. In fact, this occurs as part of the spectrum of mycosis fungoides since the malignant cell is the same in both conditions and the skin lesions may be identical histologically.

Enteropathy-associated T-cell lymphoma (EATL)

This aggressive T-cell lymphoma is usually confined to the small intestine and presents with abdominal pain due to obstruction or perforation of the jejunum or ileum. There may be a previous history of gluten-sensitive enteropathy and the condition is more common in areas where there is an increased incidence of coeliac disease. There may be features of villous atrophy in the bowel adjacent to sites of involvement. The initial management often involves surgery to relieve the acute abdomen. Most patients have been treated with CHOP or variants when chemotherapy has been required. The results are poor as a consequence of the relative chemoresistance of the disease, the tendency to early aggressive relapse and the poor nutritional status of the patient, particularly where the diagnosis has been delayed. A series of more than 30 patients treated at a single centre (Gale *et al.*, 2000) includes a small subset who have received high-dose therapy. Although these appear to have done better than those treated conventionally, the numbers are too small to estimate the true impact of this approach.

CNS LYMPHOMA

Lymphoma involving the CNS is considered separately since it presents unique management problems.

Primary cerebral lymphoma

Primary CNS lymphoma accounts for only 1 per cent of the total, although the incidence appears to be rising. Virtually all cases are either diffuse large B-cell lymphomas or Burkitt's lymphoma, the latter seen particularly in association with immunosuppression or HIV infection. Systemic disease is rare. The presentation is identical to that for other rapidly progressive intracranial tumours with progressive neurological signs, with or without features of raised intracranial pressure. The CT scan appearances may be of unifocal or multifocal disease. The standard treatment is corticosteroids and whole-brain irradiation (35–50 Gy). The majority of patients respond initially but early recurrence is the norm and the 2-year disease-free survival is only 10–20 per cent. Currently attempts are being made to improve the outlook with combined chemotherapy and radiotherapy. Results with the CHOD/BVAM regimen (Bessell *et al.*, 1996) are typical of those seen in a small number of phase II trials of CNS targeted chemotherapy given before radiotherapy. It appears that between 30 and 40 per cent of younger, fitter patients may enjoy long-term freedom from recurrence beyond 3 years, a significant improvement on the results with single modality therapy. Unfortunately, there is a high incidence of long-term neuropsychological impairment in survivors, which mandates continued attempts to improve on this. Since radiotherapy may be the chief cause of such damage, there is currently interest in limiting the amount of radiotherapy delivered to patients responding to chemotherapy.

Secondary CNS lymphoma

Meningeal (or less commonly parenchymal) involvement is most commonly seen in association with aggressive B-cell or T-cell lymphomas, where there is involvement of high-risk extranodal sites such as paranasal sinus, testis or bone marrow. Very high serum LDH is also a risk factor (Tomita *et al.*, 2000). Presentation is usually with headache or backache and cranial nerve or peripheral root palsies. Treatment is usually palliative and involves radiotherapy and/or instillation of the chemotherapeutic agents methotrexate (10–12.5 mg) and cytosine arabinoside (50–70 mg) into the CSF either by regular (twice-weekly) lumbar puncture or through an Ommaya reservoir into the lateral ventricle. Liposomal cytosine arabinoside (Depocyte) is a novel formulation of the drug recently licensed for use in the USA, although not yet in Europe. This has the advantage of better sustained levels of drug in the CSF and a reduction in the required frequency of instillation. The extent of radiotherapy is usually determined by the overall aims of treatment. Whole neuraxis irradiation is probably the most effective treatment but is debilitating and is not usually justified unless there is the potential for long-term disease eradication.

CNS prophylaxis is routinely given to patients with diffuse large cell lymphoma with involvement of high-risk extranodal sites such as testis and paranasal sinus. This either involves regular lumbar punctures with methotrexate and cytosine arabinoside instillation or the incorporation of high-dose intravenous methotrexate into the systemic chemotherapy schedule. The efficacy of these measures in preventing CNS relapse is uncertain.

SIGNIFICANT POINTS

- The WHO classification of lymphomas (1999) describes all currently recognized NHL subtypes and will be adapted to incorporate new information. Future reclassifications may be unnecessary.
- Advanced low-grade lymphoma remains incurable but the available treatment options have increased substantially. The optimal sequence of therapies remains to be defined.
- CHOP remains a standard therapy for diffuse large-cell lymphoma, the commonest NHL subtype. High-dose chemotherapy with autologous stem-cell transplantation is an effective salvage therapy in up to 50 per cent of those DLC patients who relapse after initial therapy.

KEY REFERENCES

Harris, N.L., Jaffe, E.S., Diebold, J. *et al.* (1999) World Health Organisation classification of neoplastic diseases of the haematopoietic and lymphoid tissues: report of the Clinical Advisory Committee Meeting, Airlie House Virginia November 1997. *J. Clin. Oncol.* **17**(12), 3835–49.

Johnson, P.W.M., Rohatiner, A.Z.S., Whelan, J.S. *et al.* (1995) Patterns of survival in patients with recurrent follicular lymphoma: a 20 year study from a single centre. *J. Clin. Oncol.* **13**, 140–7.

Willis, T.G. and Dyer, M.J.S. (2000) The role of immunoglobulin translocations in the pathogenesis of B-cell malignancies. *Blood* **96**(3), 808–22.

REFERENCES

Alizadeh, A.A., Eisen, M.B., Davis, R.E. *et al.* (2000) Distinct types of diffuse large B-cell lymphoma identified by gene expression profiling. *Nature* **403**, 503–11.

Anderson, J.R., Armitage, J.O. and Weisenburger, D.D. (1998) Epidemiology of the non-Hodgkin's lymphomas: distributions of the major subtypes differ by geographic locations. Non-Hodgkin's Lymphoma Classification Project. *Ann. Oncol.* **9**(7), 717–20.

Armitage, J.O. and Weisenburger, D.D. (1998) New approach to classifying non-Hodgkin's lymphomas: clinical features of the major histologic subtypes. Non-Hodgkin's Lymphoma Classification Project. *J. Clin. Oncol.* **16**(8), 2780–95.

Arnold, A., Cossman, J. Bakhshi, A. *et al.* (1983) Immunoglobulin gene rearrangements as unique clonal markers in human lymphoid neoplasms. *N. Engl. J. Med.* **309**, 1593–9.

Bendandi, M., Gocke, C.D., Kobrin, C.B. *et al.* (1999) Complete molecular remissions induced by patient-specific vaccination plus granulocyte-monocyte colony-stimulating factor against lymphoma. *Nat. Med.* **5**(10), 1171–7.

Bessell, E.M., Graus, F., Punt, J.A. *et al.* (1996) Primary non-Hodgkin's lymphoma of the CNS treated with BVAM or CHOD/BVAM chemotherapy before radiotherapy. *J. Clin. Oncol.* **14**(3), 945–54.

Brice, P., Simon, D., Bouabdallah, R. *et al.* (2000) High-dose therapy with autologous stem-cell transplantation (ASCT) after first progression: prolonged survival of follicular lymphoma patients included in the prospective GELF 86 protocol. *Ann. Oncol.* **11**(12), 1585–90.

Champlin, R.E., Khouri, I., Kornblau, S., Molidrem, J. and Giralt, S. (1999) Reinventing bone marrow transplantation: nonmyeloablative preparative regimens and induction of graft-vs-malignancy effects. *Oncology* **3**, 621–8.

Czuczman, M.S., Grillo-Lopez, A.J., White, C.A. *et al.* (1999) Treatment of patients with low-grade B-cell lymphoma with the combination of chimeric anti-CD20 antibody and CHOP chemotherapy. *J. Clin. Oncol.* **17**, 268–76.

Deane, M., McCarthy, K.P., Wiedermann, L.M. *et al.* (1991) An improved method for detection of B-lymphoid clonality by polymerase chain reaction. *Leukemia* **5**, 726–30.

Fisher, R.I., Gaynor, E.R., Daffiberg, S. *et al.* (1993) Comparison of a standard regimen (CHOP) with three intensive chemotherapy regimens for advanced non-Hodgkin's lymphoma. *N. Engl. J. Med.* **316**, 1493–8.

Gale, J., Simmonds, P.D., Mead, G.M., Sweetenham, J.W. and Wright, D.H. (2000) Enteropathy-type intestinal T-cell lymphoma: clinical features and treatment of 31 patients in a single center. *J. Clin. Oncol.* **18**(4), 795–803.

Gallagher, C.J., Gregory, W.M., Jones, A.E. *et al.* (1986) Follicular lymphoma: prognostic factors for response and survival. *J. Clin. Oncol.* **4**, 1470–80.

Geser, A., DeThe, G., Lenoir, G. *et al.* (1982) Final case reporting from the Uganda prospective study of the relationship between EBV and lymphoma. *Int. J. Cancer* **29**, 397–400.

Gianni, A.M., Bregni, M., Siena, S. *et al.* (1997) High-dose chemotherapy and autologous bone marrow transplantation compared with MACOP-B in aggressive B-cell lymphoma. *N. Engl. J. Med.* **336**(18), 1290–7.

Gribben, J.G., Freedman, A.F., Neuberg, D. *et al.* (1991) Immunologic purging of marrow assessed by PCR before autologous bone marrow transplantation for B-cell lymphoma. *N. Engl. J. Med.* **325**, 1525–33.

Groves, F.D., Linet, M.S., Travis, L.B. and Devesa, S.S. (2000) Cancer surveillance series: non-Hodgkin's lymphoma incidence by histologic subtype in the United States from 1978 through 1995. *J. Natl Cancer Inst.* **92**(15), 1240–51.

Harris, N.L., Jaffe, E.S., Stein, H. *et al.* (1994) A revised European-American Classification of lymphoid neoplasms: a proposal from the International Lymphoma Study Group. *Blood* **84**, 1361–92.

Hochster, H.S., Kim, K., Green, M.D. *et al.* (1992) Activity of fludarabine in previously treated non-Hodgkin's low grade lymphoma: results of an Eastern Cooperative Oncology Group study. *J. Clin. Oncol.* **10**, 28–32.

Hollowood, K. and Macartney, J.C. (1991) Reduced apoptotic cell death in follicular lymphoma. *J. Pathol.* **163**, 337–42.

Horning, S.J. (1994) Low grade lymphoma 1993: state of the art. *Ann. Oncol.* **5**(suppl. 2), S23–7.

International NHL Prognostic Factors Project (1993) Development of a predictive model for aggressive lymphoma: The International NHL Prognostic Factors Project. *N. Engl. J. Med.* **329**, 987–94.

Isaacson, P. and Wright, D. (1983) Malignant lymphoma of mucosal associated lymphoid tissue. A distinctive B cell lymphoma. *Cancer* **52**, 1410.

Jaffe, E.S. (2001) Anaplastic large cell lymphoma: the shifting sands of diagnostic hematopathology. *Mod. Pathol.* **14**(3), 219–28.

Juneja, S., Lukeis, R., Tan, L. *et al.* (1990) Cytogenetic analysis of 147 cases of non-Hodgkin's lymphoma: non-random chromosomal abnormalities and histological correlations. *Br. J. Haematol.* **76**, 231.

Khouri, I.F., Romaguera, J., Kantarjian, H. *et al.* (1998) Hyper-CVAD and high-dose methotrexate/cytarabine followed by stem-cell transplantation: an active regimen for aggressive mantle-cell lymphoma. *J. Clin. Oncol.* **16**(12), 3803–9.

Kitay-Cohen, Y., Amiel, A., Hilzenrat, N. *et al.* (2000) Bcl-2 rearrangement in patients with chronic hepatitis C associated with essential mixed cryoglobulinemia type II. *Blood* **96**(8), 2910–12.

Klimo, P. and Connors, J.M. (1985) MACOP-B chemotherapy for the treatment of diffuse large-cell lymphoma. *Ann. Intern. Med.* **102**, 596–602.

Lee, M.S., Chang, K.S., Cabanillas, F. *et al.* (1987) Detection of minimal residual cells carrying the t(14;18) by DNA sequence amplification. *Science* **237**, 175–8.

Limpens, J., Stad, R., Vos, C. *et al.* (1995) Lymphoma-associated translocation t(14;18) in blood B cells of normal individuals. *Blood* **85**(9), 2528–36.

Liu, S.Y., Eary, J.F., Petersdorf, S.H. *et al.* (1998) Follow up of relapsed B-cell lymphoma patients treated with iodine-131-labelled anti-CD20 antibody and autologous stem cell rescue. *J. Clin. Oncol.* **16**, 3628–33.

Lo Coco, F., Gaidano, G., Louie, D.C. *et al.* (1993) p53 mutations are associated with histologic transformation of follicular lymphoma. *Blood* **82**(8), 2289–95.

Magni, M., Di Nicola, M., Devizzi, L. *et al.* (2000) Successful in vivo purging of CD34-containing peripheral blood harvests in mantle cell and indolent lymphoma: evidence for a role of both chemotherapy and rituximab infusion. *Blood* **96**(3), 864–9.

Magrath, I., Adde, M., Shad, A. *et al.* (1996) Adults and children with small non-cleaved-cell lymphoma have a similar excellent outcome when treated with the same chemotherapy regimen. *J. Clin. Oncol.* **14**(3), 925–34.

McLaughlin, P., Hagemeister, F.B., Romaguera, J.E. *et al.* (1996) Fludarabine, mitoxantrone, and dexamethasone: an effective new regimen for indolent lymphoma. *J. Clin. Oncol.* **14**(4), 1262–8.

McLaughlin, P., Grillo-Lopez, A., Link, B. *et al.* (1998) Rituximab chimeric anti CD-20 monoclonal antibody therapy for relapsed indolent lymphoma: half of patients respond to a 4-dose treatment programme. *J. Clin. Oncol.* **16**, 2825–33.

McMichael, A.J. and Giles, G.G. (1996) Have increases in solar ultraviolet exposure contributed to the rise in incidence of non-Hodgkin's lymphoma? *Br. J. Cancer.* **73**(7), 945–50.

Miller, T.P., Dahlberg, S., Cassady, J.R. *et al.* (1998) Chemotherapy alone compared with chemotherapy plus radiotherapy for localized intermediate- and high-grade non-Hodgkin's lymphoma. *N. Engl. J. Med.* **339**(1), 21–6.

Papa, A., Cammarota, G., Tursi, A. *et al.* (2000) Helicobacter pylori eradication and remission of low-grade gastric mucosa-associated lymphoid tissue lymphoma: a long-term follow-up study. *J. Clin. Gastroenterol.* **31**(2), 169–71.

Philip, T., Guglielmi, C., Hagenbeek, A. *et al.* (1995) Autologous bone marrow transplantation as compared with salvage chemotherapy in relapses of chemotherapy-sensitive non-Hodgkin's lymphoma. *N. Engl. J. Med.* **333**(23), 1540–5.

Pinyol, M., Cobo, F., Bea, S. *et al.* (1998) p16(INK4a) gene inactivation by deletions, mutations, and hypermethylation is associated with transformed and aggressive variants of non-Hodgkin's lymphomas. *Blood* **91**(8), 2977–84.

Price, C.G.A., Meerabux, L., Murtagh, S. *et al.* (1991) The significance of circulating cells carrying t(14;18) in long remission from follicular lymphoma. *J. Clin. Oncol.* **9**, 1527–32.

Rohatiner, A.Z.S., Johnson, P.W.M., Price, C.G.A. *et al.* (1994) Myeloablative therapy with autologous bone marrow transplantation as consolidation therapy for recurrent follicular lymphoma. *J. Clin. Oncol.* **12**, 1177–84.

Rosenberg, S.A. and members of the Non-Hodgkin's Lymphoma Pathologic Classification Project (1982) National Cancer Institute sponsored study of classification of non-Hodgkin's lymphomas. Summary and description of a working formulation for clinical usage. *Cancer* **49**, 2112–35.

Schwab, U., Stein, H., Gerdes, J. *et al.* (1982) Production of a monoclonal antibody specific for Hodgkin and Sternberg–Reed cells of Hodgkin's disease and a subset of normal lymphoid cells. *Nature* **299**, 65–7.

Seymour, J.F., McLaughlin, P., Fuller, L.M. *et al.* (1996) High rate of prolonged remissions following combined modality therapy for patients with localized low-grade lymphoma. *Ann. Oncol.* **7**(2), 157–63.

Starzl, T.E., Nalesnik, M.A., Porter, K.A. *et al.* (1984) Reversibility of lymphoma and lymphoproliferative lesions developing under cyclosporin and steroid therapy. *Lancet* **323**, 583–7.

Sweetenham, L.W., Liberti, G., Pearce, R. *et al.* (1994) High-dose therapy and autologous bone marrow transplantation for adult patients with lymphoblastic lymphoma: results of the European Group for Bone Marrow Transplantation. *J. Clin. Oncol.* **12**, 1358–65.

Sweetenham, J.W., Santini, G., Qian, W. *et al.* (2001) High-dose therapy and autologous stem-cell transplantation versus conventional-dose consolidation/maintenance therapy as postremission therapy for adult patients with lymphoblastic lymphoma: results of a randomized trial of the European Group for Blood and Marrow Transplantation and the United Kingdom Lymphoma Group. *J. Clin. Oncol.* **19**(11), 2927–36.

Tomita, N., Kodama, F., Sakai, R. *et al.* (2000) Predictive factors for central nervous system involvement in non-Hodgkin's lymphoma: significance of very high serum LDH concentrations. *Leuk. Lymphoma* **38**(3–4), 335–43.

Tonegawa, S. (1983) Somatic generation of antibody diversity. *Nature* **302**, 575–81.

Van Besian, K., Sobocinski, K., Rowlings, P.A. *et al.* (1998) Allogeneic bone marrow transplantation for low-grade lymphoma. *Blood* **92**, 1832–6.

Velasquez, W.S., Cabanillas, F., Salvador, P. *et al.* (1988) Effective salvage therapy for lymphoma with cisplatin in combination with high dose Ara-C and dexamethasone (DHAP). *Blood* **71**, 117–22.

Waters, J.S., Webb, A., Cunningham, D. *et al.* (2000) Phase I clinical and pharmacokinetic study of *bcl-2* antisense oligonucleotide therapy in patients with non-Hodgkin's lymphoma. *J. Clin. Oncol.* **18**(9), 1812–23.

Williams, C.D., Harrison, C.N., Lister, T.A. *et al.* (2001) High-dose therapy and autologous stem-cell support for chemosensitive transformed low-grade follicular non-Hodgkin's lymphoma: a case-matched study from the European Bone Marrow Transplant Registry. *J. Clin. Oncol.* **19**(3), 727–35.

Wotherspoon, A., Doglioni, D.C., Diss, T. *et al.* (1993) Regression of primary low-grade B-cell gastric lymphoma of mucosal associated lymphoid tissue type after eradication of *Helicobacter pylori*. *Lancet* **342**, 575.

Multiple myeloma

DIANA SAMSON

INTRODUCTION

Multiple myeloma (MM) is a malignant disease of plasma cells in the bone marrow, which is characterized by the production of a monoclonal immunoglobulin (Ig) molecule and which is frequently associated with bone pain, anaemia and renal failure. In 80 per cent of patients there is a paraprotein in the serum, usually of the IgG or IgA class. The abnormal cells may also produce free light chains, which pass into the urine as Bence Jones protein (BJP), frequently causing tubular damage. In 20 per cent of patients, free light chains only are produced (Bence Jones only myeloma) and there is no paraprotein in the serum. The number of plasma cells in the bone marrow is focally increased and osteoclasts are activated in the region of plasma cell foci, causing bone resorption. The residual normal B-cell population is suppressed, leading to a reduction in polyclonal immunoglobulins and increased susceptibility to infection. The median survival is 3–4 years, although survival varies widely according to a number of prognostic factors, the most important of which are serum β_2-microglobulin and deletion of chromosome 13. Guidelines on the diagnosis and management of myeloma have recently been produced by the UK Myeloma Forum on behalf of the British Committee for Standards in Haematology (UK Myeloma Forum, 2001).

INCIDENCE AND AETIOLOGY

Incidence

Myeloma accounts for about 1 per cent of all cancers and 10 per cent of haematological malignancies. The annual incidence in the UK and North America is around 40 per million, and there are approximately 2500 new cases each year in the UK. The incidence increases with age; most patients are over the age of 60 and MM is very rare below the age of 40. It is more common in males, with a male : female ratio of around 1.5. In the USA the highest incidence rates have been reported for African-Americans, with an incidence 1.5–2.0 times that of Caucasian Americans. On the other hand, Asians living in the USA appear to have low incidence rates. In the UK the incidence in immigrants from West Africa and the Caribbean is 2–4 times that in native Britons.

There is some evidence to suggest that the incidence of myeloma has been increasing in recent years (Bray et al., 2001).

Radiation exposure

The only clearly defined risk factor for the development of myeloma is exposure to ionizing radiation, as in

Japanese survivors of the atomic bombs dropped on Hiroshima and Nagasaki in 1945, and in radiologists exposed to relatively large doses of irradiation over many years. There have subsequently been numerous studies of radiation-exposed workers at nuclear plants in the USA, the UK and other countries, which have generally shown an increased incidence of myeloma compared to the unexposed population, and also a direct relationship between radiation dose and mortality (Herrinton *et al.*, 1998). Some authors have observed a modest increase in myeloma incidence in patients who have received therapeutic irradiation or who have been exposed to numerous diagnostic X-ray procedures (Boice *et al.*, 1991), but evidence from a recent study in the US suggested that exposure to diagnostic X-rays does not increase the risk of developing MM (Hatcher *et al.*, 2001).

Other epidemiological risk factors

Numerous studies have been published looking at exposure to other chemical and physical agents, including solvents, pesticides and metals (Herrinton *et al.*, 1998; Speer *et al.*, 2002). The incidence of myeloma appears to be increased in persons exposed to benzene, petroleum refinery waste or pesticides. The use of pesticides may partly account for the increased risk of myeloma which has been observed in agricultural workers. The use of personal hair dyes has been reported in some (but not all) studies to be associated with an increased risk, although the incidence of myeloma in hairdressers is not increased (Herrinton *et al.*, 1998).

It is possible that chronic exposure to a given antigen could drive a particular plasma cell clone to proliferate. However, epidemiological studies in patients with allergic conditions and those undergoing immunization procedures do not suggest that immune stimulation increases myeloma risk. Similarly, there is no clear evidence for an increased risk in patients with autoimmune disease.

Monoclonal gammopathy of undetermined significance

Monoclonal gammopathy of undetermined significance (MGUS) is a condition where a patient is found by chance to have a paraprotein in the serum but with no other features to suggest myeloma. There are fewer than 10 per cent plasma cells in the marrow, no bone lesions, and normal haemoglobin and renal function. Although many patients with MGUS remain stable, long-term follow-up has shown that the annual risk of transformation to MM is around 1 per cent (Kyle *et al.*, 2002). Epidemiological studies have identified similar risk factors for MGUS and MM. The incidence of both conditions increases with age, is higher among males than females, and in African-Americans than in Caucasians, while MGUS and MM have been reported in the same family. The association

of MGUS and MM supports the concept of multi-step carcinogenesis in the development of myeloma, with a first oncogenic event causing MGUS and one or more subsequent events leading to malignant transformation.

Familial myeloma

There have been a small number of reports of myeloma and MGUS developing in two or more members of one family, but it is unclear whether this reflects genetic or environmental factors (Grosbois *et al.*, 1999; Lynch *et al.*, 2001).

PATHOGENESIS AND BIOLOGY

The cell of origin

Myeloma is essentially a tumour of the plasma cells in the bone marrow, but there are a number of lines of evidence suggesting that cells earlier in the B-cell lineage are also involved, such as the expression in some cases of immature B-cell antigens on the cell surface. However, recent studies of the immunoglobulin heavy chain (IgH) gene in myeloma marrow have demonstrated that the cell of origin is a post-germinal-centre B cell. Not only is there a consistent and unique IgH rearrangement in each individual patient, but the complementarity-determining regions of the IgH gene sequence show mutations from the germ-line sequence which are identical in all the cells of the clone (Bakkus *et al.*, 1994; Vescio *et al.*, 1995). This indicates that the malignant transformation must have occurred in a B cell which has already undergone somatic mutation, i.e. has been exposed to antigen in the germinal centre of the lymph node. IgH gene rearrangement studies have also shown that peripheral-blood B lymphocytes contain a proportion of cells belonging to the myeloma clone (Billadeau *et al.*, 1992). It is currently considered that the malignant transformation occurs in a post-germinal-centre B cell in the lymph node, whose progeny migrate to the marrow via the peripheral blood and develop there into plasma cell tumours. The expression of adhesion molecules, such as neural cell adhesion molecule (N-CAM; CD56), syndecan 1 (CD138) and platelet endothelial cell adhesion molecule (PECAM 1; CD31), on myeloma plasma cells is thought to facilitate homing to the marrow (van Riet *et al.*, 1998), while the production of interleukin-6 (IL-6) and other cytokines by the marrow stroma provides an optimal environment for the growth of the myeloma cells (Klein *et al.*, 1995).

Myeloma and the micro-environment

It has become apparent over the past few years that there is a close relationship between MM cells and the marrow

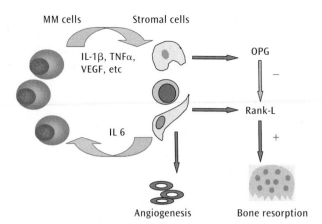

Figure 46.1 *Interactions between myeloma cells and the marrow micro-environment.*

micro-environment, which promotes tumour growth and also leads to the development of myeloma bone disease. Interactions between MM cells and stromal cells, including fibroblasts, macrophages and osteoclasts, are mediated by cell-to-cell contact, adhesion molecules and cytokines. The stromal cells are stimulated by the MM cells to produce IL-6, which is essential for the growth and survival of myelomatous plasma cells, and also RANK-L (the ligand for receptor activator of NFκB), which causes osteoclast activation. In turn, adhesion to stromal cells up-regulates secretion of VEGF (vascular endothelial growth factor) by the myeloma cells, leading to increased new vessel formation which promotes tumour growth. The interaction between MM cells and the micro-environment is therefore crucial both to the growth and survival of the malignant plasma cells and to the development of lytic bone disease (Fig. 46.1).

THE ROLE OF IL-6

IL-6 is responsible for the maturation of normal B cells into plasma cells, and is essential for the proliferation and the survival of myeloma plasma cells, which express specific receptors for IL-6 (Klein *et al.*, 1995). IL-6 is not only an important growth factor for myeloma plasma cells *in vitro* but there is also evidence that it is involved in the growth of myeloma *in vivo*. Disease responses have been reported in late-stage patients treated with monoclonal antibody to IL-6, while raised serum IL-6 levels in myeloma patients are associated with a poor prognosis (Bataille *et al.*, 1989). IL-6 and its receptor are potential targets for therapeutic intervention, as are intracellular pathways that are triggered by IL-6 activation.

MYELOMA BONE DISEASE

Numerous osteoclast-activating factors are released by the myeloma cells directly or by the normal marrow cells in response to the myeloma cells. These include IL-6, IL-1β, TNFα, hepatocyte growth factor and macrophage-inhibitory protein 1α (Callander and Roodman, 2001).

Recent evidence, however, suggests that the fundamental abnormality in myeloma bone disease is an altered balance between RANK-L and osteoprotegerin (OPG), which are the most important regulators of normal osteoclast activity. Both are produced by stromal cells in the marrow, including osteoblasts. RANK-L interacts with its receptor (RANK) on osteoclast precursors to promote differentiation, and on osteoclasts to stimulate resorption. OPG acts as a soluble decoy receptor: it binds with RANK-L, inhibiting its interaction with RANK and thus preventing bone resorption (Fig. 46.1). The expression of RANK-L by stromal cells in MM is increased (Roux *et al.*, 2002), while the expression of OPG is down-regulated (Giuliani *et al.*, 2001). Co-culture of MM cells with stromal cells up-regulates the production of RANK-L, probably as the result of secretion of osteoclast-activating factors like IL-1β and TNFα. In addition, myeloma cells themselves can produce RANK-L (Croucher *et al.*, 2001). The importance of RANK-L in MM bone disease has been confirmed in animal models, where infusion of RANK-L inhibitors including recombinant OPG prevents the development of lytic lesions and may also inhibit tumour growth (Croucher *et al.*, 2001; Yaccoby *et al.*, 2002). Similar compounds are currently undergoing clinical trial in myeloma patients.

ANGIOGENESIS

Increased microvessel formation has been noted in trephine biopsies from MM patients, and is associated with tumour growth. There is a high correlation between the extent of bone marrow angiogenesis, evaluated as microvessel density (MVD) and the proportion of MM cells in S-phase (Vacca *et al.*, 1994). Plasma cells from patients with myeloma express and secrete vascular endothelial growth factor (VEGF), and the expression of VEGF is up-regulated by adherence to marrow stroma (Bellamy, 2001; Gupta *et al.*, 2001) (Fig. 46.1). In addition to VEGF, other angiogenic factors have been identified in MM including basic FGF and tissue metalloproteinases (Bellamy, 2001). The finding of increased angiogenesis in MM provides a rationale for the use of antiangiogenic therapy, such as thalidomide (*see* below).

Cytogenetic abnormalities

Conventional cytogenetic analysis is often unsuccessful in myeloma, because of the low rate of mitosis of plasma cells. However, with improved methodology and the use of techniques such as fluorescence *in situ* hybridization (FISH), it has become clear that cytogenetic abnormalities are present in at least 75 per cent of cases and that these are often complex (Zandecki, 1996; Dalton *et al.*, 2001). In cases with an abnormal karyotype, translocations occur in 50 per cent, and these usually involve chromosome 14q, the site of the IgH gene (Bergsagel and Kuehl, 2001). A variety of partner chromosomes have been identified, including 11q, 4p and 8q. The breakpoints in these chromosomes are frequently near the site of cellular proto-oncogenes, e.g. cyclin D1 on 11q13, fibroblast growth factor receptor 3 on 4p16 and c-*myc* on 8q24. These translocations may lead to overexpression of important genes, such as the up-regulation of the FGFR3 receptor which occurs in cases with the 4;14 translocation. Multiple trisomies are also common, as are losses of all or part of a chromosome. Of particular importance is 13q−, involving loss of the *Rb* gene, which occurs in at least 35 per cent of cases and which is associated with a poor prognosis (Tricot *et al.*, 1995; Fonseca *et al.*, 2002). Other abnormalities reported include point mutations of *ras*, *p53* and *Fas*. Whether these cytogenetic abnormalities play a role in the origin or growth of the myeloma is as yet unclear. However, cytogenetic abnormalities are also common in MGUS. It appears that translocations of chromosome 14 are as common as in MM but chromosome 13 deletions are less frequent in MGUS and may predict for transformation to overt myeloma (Avet-Louiseau *et al.*, 1999). These observations are consistent with a multi-step pathogenesis for MM in which early dysregulation of oncogenes leads to immortalization of plasma cells and subsequent cytogenetic changes such as loss of *Rb* or activating *ras* mutations lead to tumour progression.

The role of HHV8

HHV8, or the Kaposi's sarcoma associated herpes virus, has been implicated in the pathogenesis of body-cavity lymphomas in HIV-positive patients, and in multicentric Castleman's disease. The viral genome codes for production of a viral IL-6 homologue, and in view of the role of IL-6 in myeloma growth (*see* above) it was possible that HHV8 might also play a role in the pathogenesis of myeloma. Said *et al.* (1997) detected HHV8 gene sequences in dendritic cells (DCs) from the bone marrow of myeloma patients, but not in marrow from healthy controls, and postulated that infection of the DCs led in some way to the growth of the malignant plasma cells. However, although similar results have been reported by some groups, several others have failed to detect HHV8 gene sequences in the marrow from myeloma patients and at present evidence for HHV8 involvement in myeloma remains controversial.

CLINICAL FEATURES AND COMPLICATIONS

Bone disease

Bone pain is the most common presenting symptom, affecting 60 per cent of patients. The back and ribs are the most frequent sites of pain. X-rays may show lytic lesions and generalized osteoporosis is also common. Some patients have osteoporosis without lytic lesions. Vertebral collapse is frequent in myeloma patients, leading to back pain, kyphosis and loss of height, and occasionally resulting in cord compression. Pathological fracture of a long bone may also occur. The bone destruction may result in hypercalcaemia, although serum alkaline phosphatase (ALP) is usually normal since bone ALP reflects osteoblast activity and in myeloma osteoblast activity is inhibited. For the same reason, radionuclide bone scans may be negative in myeloma and a radiological skeletal survey is a better method of detecting sites of tumour.

Renal failure

Renal failure is also a common problem in myeloma patients. Twenty-five to 30 per cent of patients have some degree of renal impairment and about 5 per cent will present with severe renal failure. This is most commonly due to BJP, which damages the tubules as it passes through the kidney. The classic histological features are of fractured distal tubular casts with a surrounding chronic inflammatory infiltrate including giant cells ('myeloma kidney'). Much less frequently, light-chain deposition may produce a form of glomerulonephritis (light-chain deposition disease). Other factors which can contribute to renal failure include hypercalcaemia, infection, dehydration, hyperuricaemia, amyloid deposition and non-steroidal anti-inflammatory drugs. Renal failure which results acutely from hypercalcaemia or dehydration is often reversible with appropriate management, but that due to BJP is less likely to recover. Renal failure is an adverse prognostic factor in myeloma but is less important than in the past because of the general availability of dialysis. Renal failure is more common in patients with a high tumour burden, and although impaired renal function does reduce life expectancy to some extent the outlook is much more closely related to that of the underlying myeloma (Iggo, 1998). Renal failure is reversible in about 50 per cent of cases (Knudsen *et al.*, 2000) and should certainly not be a contraindication to active management.

Other clinical features

Anaemia is another common presenting feature, with a haemoglobin below 120 g/L in 60 per cent of patients. Severe anaemia, neutropenia and thrombocytopenia are, however, rare at presentation and the anaemia appears to be mediated by cytokines rather than being directly due to marrow replacement (Silvestris, *et al.*, 2002). In some patients, renal failure may also contribute to the anaemia. There is impairment of both humoral and cell-mediated immunity, leading to an increased susceptibility to infection, both bacterial and viral. Chest infections are particularly common. About 10 per cent of patients with myeloma develop primary amyloidosis. The kidney is usually affected, with deposition of amyloid in the glomeruli leading to generalized proteinuria and the nephrotic syndrome. Peripheral neuropathy (particularly carpal tunnel syndrome), congestive cardiac failure and involvement of skin, muscle and joints may also occur. Peripheral neuropathy may also occur in myeloma patients without amyloidosis (Gawler, 1998). Very high Ig levels, particularly of IgA, may result in hyperviscosity syndrome, with headaches, visual disturbance and loss of concentration.

Asymptomatic patients

An increasing number of patients are being diagnosed as a result of finding a raised erythrocyte sedimentation rate (ESR) or abnormal protein electrophoresis on routine screening, or when being investigated for an unrelated problem.

INVESTIGATION, DIAGNOSIS AND STAGING

Appropriate investigations are summarized in Table 46.1.

Table 46.1 *Investigation of a patient with suspected myeloma*

Useful screening tests:
FBC: anaemia may be present; film may show
    rouleaux formation
ESR: raised in presence of a serum paraprotein
Biochemical profile: may indicate renal impairment
    and/or hypercalcaemia; may show raised total
    protein and/or low albumin
X-ray of any symptomatic areas

Diagnostic tests:
Electrophoresis of serum and concentrated urine to
    identify paraprotein
Immunofixation to confirm and type the paraprotein
Quantitation of serum non-paraprotein Igs to
    look for immunosuppression
Bone marrow examination
Skeletal survey to look for lytic lesions,
    if not already identified

Tests to establish tumour burden and prognosis:
FBC: degree of anaemia, any neutropenia or
    thrombocytopenia
Serum paraprotein level
24-hour urine for total BJP excretion, if applicable
Creatinine, calcium, uric acid and albumin
β_2-microglobulin
LDH and C-reactive protein
Skeletal survey, if not already performed

Tests that may be useful in some patients:
Creatinine clearance
24-hour total protein excretion
Amyloid scan or biopsy for amyloid
Plasma or whole-blood viscosity
CT scan and/or MRI

CT, computed tomography; FBC, full blood count;
ESR, erythrocyte sedimentation rate; LDH, lactate dehydrogenase;
MRI, magnetic resonance imaging.

Haematological investigations

The blood count commonly shows a normocytic normochromic anaemia. The blood film typically shows rouleaux formation. Plasma cells are not often seen in the peripheral blood film but may be present in patients with advanced or aggressive disease. A circulating plasma cell count of over 2×10^9/L is termed plasma cell leukaemia. The ESR is usually raised in myeloma as the result of the high serum Ig level, combined in many cases with a low albumin. However, the ESR is often normal in patients with Bence Jones only myeloma. A bone marrow examination is an essential diagnostic investigation. A marrow aspirate may be sufficient to confirm the diagnosis, but because of the patchy nature of the marrow involvement, a trephine biopsy will yield a more reliable estimate of plasma cell numbers. Immunocytochemistry to demonstrate monoclonality is useful where there is only a modest increase in plasma cell numbers. Cytogenetic analysis of the marrow plasma cells is now performed more widely because of the prognostic significance of abnormalities such as 13q−. The plasma cell labelling index (LI), may be determined using [^{3}H]thymidine or bromodeoxyuridine, but although this is also an important prognostic factor, the technique is not widely available.

Biochemical investigations

A routine biochemical profile may show abnormalities of urea, creatinine, calcium, uric acid, total protein and/or albumin. Serum ALP is usually normal (*see* above) but may be raised after a fracture. Electrophoresis of both serum and concentrated urine should be undertaken to look for the presence of a paraprotein. It is important to test the urine in all patients, since patients with Bence Jones only myeloma have no paraprotein in the serum, and patients with a serum paraprotein are more at risk of renal failure if they also produce BJP. The paraprotein in the serum and/or urine is then confirmed and identified by immuno-electrophoresis or immunofixation. Eighty per cent of patients have a paraprotein in the serum (IgG in 55–60 per cent of cases and IgA in 20–25 per cent), of whom two-thirds also have BJP in the urine. In rare patients, the paraprotein may be of IgD, IgE or IgM type. Overall two-thirds of paraproteins have κ light chains and one-third λ. In 20 per cent of cases, free light chains only are produced. In less than 1 per cent of patients (nonsecretory myeloma) no paraprotein is detectable in either serum or urine, although in most of these cases the plasma cells in the marrow can be shown to contain monoclonal immunoglobulin. The level of paraprotein in the serum and the 24-hour urinary excretion of BJP should be measured as a baseline against which to monitor the progress of the disease, and the levels of non-isotypic immunoglobulins should be measured to assess immune paresis. Serum β_2-microglobulin should be estimated in all patients at diagnosis because of its prognostic significance. C-reactive protein (CRP), lactate dehydrogenase (LDH) and serum thymidine kinase (TK) are also useful prognostic factors.

Radiology and imaging

A skeletal survey should be performed in all patients, even if the diagnosis has already been established, because it is important to document areas of bone destruction which could lead to pathological fracture. It should include cervical, thoracic, and lumbar spine, skull, chest and pelvis, the humeri and the femora, i.e. all the sites of active marrow in the adult. Deposits can occur outside these areas, but this is rare. The most common radiographic findings are a combination of osteoporosis, lytic lesions and fractures, the latter usually involving the vertebral bodies and the ribs. Soft-tissue extension may be noted on plain X-rays. Osteoporosis without lytic lesions occurs in 5–10 per cent of patients. Sclerotic lesions are very rare, except in the POEMS syndrome (*see* below). As already noted, radionuclide bone scans are less useful than X-rays for detecting sites of disease, but may occasionally be helpful in patients with pain at sites not easily visualized on X-ray, e.g. the sternum or scapulae. Computed tomography (CT) and magnetic resonance imaging (MRI) scans are also useful in such patients. MRI differs from other radiological techniques in that it visualizes the marrow directly, and does not visualize the cortical bone. Myelomatous deposits have a decreased signal intensity on T_1-weighted images compared to the normal marrow, and an increased signal on T_2 images (Healy and Armstrong, 1988). Marked enhancement is seen with gadolinium DTPA (diethylenetriaminepentaacetic acid). MRI is the most sensitive imaging method routinely available and is particularly valuable in patients with suspected cord compression, where there may be involvement at several vertebral levels. MRI scanning is also of prognostic significance in predicting which patients with asymptomatic myeloma are likely to progress in the near future (Mariette *et al.*, 1999). Fluoro-deoxyglucose positron emission tomography is useful for the detection of occult lesions (Orchard *et al.*, 2002).

Differential diagnosis

Confirmation of the diagnosis is usually based on the finding of a paraprotein in the serum or in the urine and/or lytic lesions on X-ray, together with over 10 per cent plasma cells in the bone marrow (Table 46.2). The principal differential diagnosis in a patient with paraproteinaemia but without the clinical features of myeloma is MGUS. Other conditions in which a paraprotein may be present include primary amyloidosis, B-cell non-Hodgkin's lymphoma and connective tissue disorders. Currently accepted criteria for distinguishing between myeloma and MGUS are shown in Table 46.3. It is important to realize that these

Table 46.2 *Diagnostic criteria for multiple myeloma*

1. More than 10% plasma cells in the bone marrow.
   Most patients present with >20% plasma cells in the marrow but in some cases only a slight elevation may be present. Trephine biopsy provides a better assessment of the degree of plasmacytosis than aspirate alone. Immunophenotyping to demonstrate light chain restriction is helpful in confirming monoclonality.
2. The presence of a paraprotein in serum and/or urine.
   There is no specific level of paraprotein or, BJP excretion that distinguishes myeloma from MGUS. If there is a strong suspicion of myeloma and routine electrophoresis is normal, immunofixation should also be performed. Note that a small proportion of patients with MM have no paraprotein in either serum or urine.
3. Osteolytic bone lesions.
   Some patients have osteoporosis without lytic lesions, but osteoporosis alone is not considered a diagnostic criterion.

Diagnosis is normally based on the finding of at least two of the above, but not all cases fulfil these criteria. Findings such as typical myeloma kidney on renal biopsy or the presence of tissue plasmacytomas would be additional factors to be taken into account in individual cases.

Table 46.3 *Criteria for distinguishing multiple myeloma (MM) and monoclonal gammopathy of undetermined significance (MGUS)*

	MM	MGUS
Bone marrow plasma cells	>10%	<10%
Serum paraprotein:		
IgG	Variable	Usually <35 g/L
IgA	Variable	Usually <20 g/L
Bence Jones protein	Often present	Rarely present
Immunosuppression	Often present	Rarely present
Lytic bone lesions	Often present	Absent
Symptoms		Absent
Hb, renal function, calcium		Normal

are to some extent arbitrary and the only way to be certain whether the disease will behave as myeloma, i.e. progress, or as MGUS, i.e. remain stable, is to monitor the patient carefully over time. Patients who fulfil the current diagnostic criteria for myeloma rather than MGUS but in whom the disease is asymptomatic and stable over the period of observation have variously been termed equivocal, indolent or smouldering myeloma, according to different criteria. These distinctions are, however, of limited value; the essential question is whether or not treatment for myeloma is required; this issue is discussed below.

Table 46.4 *The Durie–Salmon staging system. Patients are staged as I, II or III and as A or B*

	Stage I	Stage II	Stage III
Tumour cell mass	Low	Medium	High
	All of the following:	Not fitting stage I or III	One or more of the following:
Monoclonal IgG (g/L)	<50		>70
Monoclonal IgA (g/L)	<30		>50
BJP excretion (g/24 h)	<4		>12
Hb (g/dL)	>10		<8.5
Calcium (mmol/L)	<2.6		>2.6
Lytic lesions	None or one		Advanced

Stage A: Serum creatinine <175 μmol/L
Stage B: Serum creatinine >175 μmol/L

Prognostic factors and staging

The average survival in myeloma is 3–4 years with conventional treatment, but survival in individual patients varies widely, from a few months to over 10 years. The outlook depends on a number of prognostic factors, the most important of which are the level of β_2-microglobulin in the serum and the presence or absence of chromosome 13 deletion. Anaemia and hypercalcaemia are both adverse risk factors, as are a low albumin level and a raised LDH and C-reactive protein. A raised CRP and a low albumin both reflect raised IL-6. Other prognostic indices which are less widely available include cytogenetic abnormalities, plasma cell labelling index, and serum levels of thymidine kinase, IL-6 and sIL-6R. These various factors have been combined in a variety of ways to produce a number of staging systems, which reflect overall tumour burden and behaviour rather than anatomical spread. The most widely used staging system is that of Durie and Salmon (1975) (Table 46.4), which is based on a number of clinical and laboratory parameters that were shown to be correlated with myeloma cell mass. The advantage of this system is that the parameters are simple and available at diagnosis in all patients, and it is able to separate patients with poor, average and good prognosis. However, it does not include two of the most powerful prognostic factors, β_2-microglobulin or serum albumin, nor cytogenic data. A number of alternative staging systems have been proposed, but in practice the Durie–Salmon system is still the most widely used.

THE COURSE OF THE DISEASE

Multiple myeloma continues to present a therapeutic challenge. In spite of new approaches to treatment, MM at present remains incurable with a median survival of 3–4 years. Treatment produces a response in approximately two-thirds of patients, with a fall in paraprotein and improvement or resolution of clinical symptoms. However, complete remission (CR) or disappearance of the paraprotein is very rare, except after high-dose therapy and transplantation. In most patients the paraprotein falls but reaches a plateau after a few months of treatment. At this stage the patient is said to be in 'plateau phase' and treatment is stopped. Sooner or later the paraprotein starts to rise again, indicating relapse, or there may be a recurrence of symptoms. Further treatment at this stage, perhaps with a different drug or drug combination, may again produce a response, but the duration of response is usually shorter than that of the initial remission. Eventually the disease becomes refractory to treatment and the patient succumbs to infection, renal failure or other disease complication.

WHEN TO START TREATMENT

Patients with equivocal, indolent or smouldering myeloma, i.e. those with no symptoms, normal haemoglobin, calcium and renal function and no bone lesions (Durie–Salmon stage IA), can remain stable for a long period without treatment, and the consensus is that they should not be treated at this stage. Such patients should be followed carefully, and this should include periodic bone marrow examinations and skeletal X-rays, since the first sign of progression may be the development of bone disease. Patients who are asymptomatic, but in whom X-rays show evidence of bone disease, should be treated at diagnosis as they are likely to progress within 1 year (Dimopoulos *et al.*, 1993). Patients with normal X-rays but abnormal marrow appearance on MRI are also more likely to progress rapidly than those with normal MRI scans (Mariette *et al.*, 1999). If in doubt as to whether to start treatment, it is better to withhold therapy and reassess the situation in 2–3 months. In young patients with stage I myeloma, consideration should be given to storing stem cells at diagnosis, using granulocyte colony stimulating factor (G-CSF) for mobilization, and if there are features suggesting that the patient will soon progress, it may be appropriate to consider early treatment with a view to high-dose therapy.

GENERAL ASPECTS OF CARE

These include maintenance of good hydration, correction of hypercalcaemia, and pain control where relevant (Table 46.5).

Table 46.5 *General aspects of care in multiple myeloma*

Renal function	Maintain adequate hydration in all patients (fluid intake of at least 3 L/day) Avoid potentially nephrotoxic drugs.
Hypercalcaemia	Volume replacement with intravenous saline and an intravenous bisphosphonate. (A loop diuretic is not of additional benefit unless there is volume overload.)
Bone disease and pain management	*Analgesia:* A variety of analgesics may be used, including simple analgesics, opiates and fentanyl patches. NSAIDs should be avoided in patients with renal impairment and used with caution in other patients. *Chemotherapy and radiotherapy:* Response to chemotherapy is a major factor in reducing progression of bone disease. Local radiotherapy may be of benefit in patients with localized severe pain. *Orthopaedic surgery:* Fixation of long bones may be required to treat or prevent pathological fracture. Radiotherapy, if required, is better given post-operatively once healing has occurred rather than pre-operatively. *Bisphosphonates:* All patients should receive a bisphosphonate long-term. *General measures:* It is important to maintain mobility as immobility increases bone loss and the risk of infection, as well as impairing quality of life. Physiotherapy and aids such as spinal supports may be useful.
Hyperviscosity	Symptomatic patients should be treated urgently with plasma exchange; isovolaemic venesection may be used if plasma exchange facilities are not immediately available. If transfusion is essential exchange transfusion should be performed. Chemotherapy should be instituted promptly.
Spinal cord compression	Management requires emergency hospital admission and investigation with MRI scanning to define the site and extent of tumour. CT scanning may be used if MRI is unavailable or contra-indicated. Dexamethasone should be commenced immediately. Local radiotherapy is the treatment of choice; there is no advantage in outcome for surgical treatment in the absence of spinal instability. Spinal surgery in myeloma patients may be difficult because of osteoporosis but may be indicated for spinal instability.
Infection	Arrangements should be in place to ensure 24-hour access to specialist team advice. Admission for intravenous antibiotic therapy is usually needed for severe systemic infection. Influenza vaccination should be given to myeloma patients annually. Pneumococcal and haemophilus vaccinations may be given, although there is no evidence of their efficacy in multiple myeloma patients.
Anaemia	Transfuse as appropriate or consider erythropoietin.
Psychological problems	Depression and anxiety occur and should be actively managed with appropriate referral to psychiatric/psychological services.

Renal failure

Renal failure can often be prevented by maintaining a high fluid intake, correcting dehydration and treating hypercalcaemia. Patients with established renal failure may need dialysis. In some patients renal function recovers as the disease responds to treatment, but in other patients long-term dialysis may be needed. Early plasmapheresis may improve the chance of recovery of renal function (Johnson *et al.*, 1990).

Hypercalcaemia

An intravenous bisphosphonate is the most effective treatment for hypercalcaemia which is not rapidly corrected by rehydration. In addition, randomized trials have shown that long-term use of a bisphosphonate,

either intravenous or oral, can reduce the rate of progression of myeloma bone disease (*see* below).

Pain control

Localized painful bone lesions are best treated by radiotherapy, which usually improves the pain within a few days. Analgesia is obviously important. Non-steroidal anti-inflammatory drugs can be helpful, but caution is needed because of the risk of renal toxicity. Patients with progressive bone disease often require opiate analgesia.

Anaemia

Anaemia usually improves when the disease responds to treatment. Blood transfusions may be needed to improve the haemoglobin level if there is severe anaemia.

Table 46.6 *Treatment options in multiple myeloma*

Induction	Consolidation/maintenance	Relapsed/refractory disease
Simple alkylating agents: melphalan or cyclophosphamide ± prednisolone	High-dose therapy with stem-cell support (autograft)	Primarily refractory to alkylating agents: VAD or VAD-type regimen
Combination chemotherapy: e.g. ABCM, VMCP/VBAP	Allogeneic BMT in selected patients	Primarily refractory to VAD: intermediate or high-dose melphalan with stem-cell support
	Mini-allograft under trial	
VAD-type regimens: VAD, VAMP, C-VAMP, Z-Dex	Interferon maintenance	Relapsed disease: any regimen used for induction; thalidomide ± dexamethasone; steroids alone; DHBI
Dexamethasone alone	Thalidomide maintenance under trial	
	Vaccination strategies under trial	New approaches under trial: Thalidomide analogues; PS341; Other biological approaches Monoclonal antibodies

ABCM: Adriamycin (R), BCNU, cyclophosphamide, melphalan; VMCP/VBAP: vincristine, melphalan, cyclophosphamide, prednisolone/vincristine, BCNU, Adriamycin (R), prednisolone; VAD: infused vincristine and Adriamycin (R) with pulsed dexamethasone; VAMP: as VAD with methyl prednisolone in place of dexamethasone; C-VAMP: as VAMP with addition of weekly cyclophosphamide; Z-Dex: oral idarubicin with dexamethasone; DHBI: double hemi-body irradiation; PS341: proteasome inhibitor 341.

Erythropoietin injections can also improve anaemia and improve quality of life, even in the absence of renal failure (Dammacco *et al.*, 2001).

Infection

Any infection must be treated promptly and vigorously. Patients should be advised what to do in the event of symptoms of infection, and in some cases provision of standby antibiotics may be appropriate. Patients with recurrent infections may benefit from immunoglobulin replacement. All patients should receive influenza vaccine annually.

CHEMOTHERAPY

The available options are summarized in Table 46.6. Unfortunately there have been no real advances in terms of new active cytotoxic drugs. In particular, in contrast to their efficacy in Waldenstrom's disease, fludarabine and 2-chlorodeoxyadenosine have no significant activity in myeloma. However, there are a number of promising new biological approaches to treatment which are currently under investigation (*see* below).

Alkylating agents with steroids

Intermittent melphalan (M) and prednis(ol)one (P) has been the standard therapy for MM for many years (Alexanian and Dimopoulos, 1994), although there are some studies which do not support the conclusion that the addition of steroid improves long-term survival. M and P are usually given for 4 days every 4–6 weeks;

typical doses being M 7–8 mg/m^2 per day and P 40–60 mg/day. Oral or intravenous cyclophosphamide is also effective. A frequently used schedule is weekly intravenous cyclophosphamide (150–300 mg/m^2) with alternate-day prednisolone. An oral equivalent of the i.v. cyclophosphamide weekly schedule is cyclophosphamide 200–400 mg/m^2 weekly. Weekly cyclophosphamide is considerably less myelotoxic than melphalan, but causes more alopecia. Fifty to 60 per cent of patients will respond to this type of therapy, usually over a period of 3–6 months, and will reach a stable plateau phase, during which the paraprotein level does not continue to fall but remains steady. Response is usually defined as a fall in serum and/or urinary paraprotein by at least 50 per cent. Complete remission, i.e. disappearance of the paraprotein with a normal number of plasma cells in the bone marrow, is exceptional. Treatment is usually stopped when a stable plateau is reached, since giving further chemotherapy does not prolong the duration of the remission and may favour the development of drug resistance. The median duration of remission is around 18 months, with a median survival duration of around 3 years in most series.

Combination chemotherapy

A number of combination chemotherapy regimens have been developed with the hope of improving response rate and survival. Vincristine (V), Adriamycin® (A) and the nitrosoureas, especially carmustine (BCNU)(B), together with melphalan (M) and cyclophosphamide (C) have been the mainstay of combination chemotherapy schedules. Several regimens have been developed which incorporate some or all of these agents, usually together with prednis(ol)one (P). The most widely used have been the VBMCP regimen used by the Eastern Cooperative

Oncology Group (ECOG) and the VMCP/VBAP protocol developed by the South-west Oncology Group (SWOG). In the UK, the ABCM regimen (Adriamycin®, BCNU, cyclophosphamide and melphalan) is widely used.

There is little difference in long-term outcome between any of these regimens, and little evidence that they are more effective than single-agent therapy. Most of the published studies comparing combination chemotherapy regimens with oral melphalan and prednisolone (MP) have shown an improved response rate but no significant improvement in survival. One of the few studies to show a benefit for combination chemotherapy was the Medical Research Council's Myeloma V trial which compared ABCM with oral melphalan (without P), and although there was a significant survival benefit for ABCM in this study, the difference in median survival was only a few months (Maclennan et al., 1992). A recent meta-analysis reviewing the results of 27 published studies concluded that overall there was no difference in survival between combination chemotherapy and MP (Myeloma Trialists' Collaborative Group, 1998) (Fig. 46.2), and the current consensus is that combination chemotherapy has little advantage over simpler regimens.

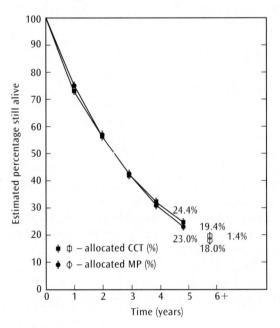

Deaths/person-years:

CCT 642/1999 392/1456 305/1044 196/724 133/506 255/1130
MP 576/1968 407/1423 294/983 194/652 130/444 215/839

Figure 46.2 *Overall survival of 6633 patients in 27 randomized trials comparing melphalan plus prednisolone (MP) and combination chemotherapy (CCT). Median survival in both groups was 29 months. (Reproduced with permission from Myeloma Trialists' Collaborative Group (1998) Combination chemotherapy versus melphalan plus prednisone as treatment for multiple myeloma: an overview of 6633 patients from 27 randomized trials. J. Clin. Oncol. 16, 3832–42.)*

VAD and other infusional regimens

The VAD regimen is a combination of vincristine (V), Adriamycin® (A) and dexamethasone (D), but differs from conventional regimens in that the V and A are given not as bolus injections but by continuous infusion over 4 days. Modifications of the regimen include VAMP, where methyl prednisolone replaces dexamethasone, and MOD, where mitoxantrone is substituted for Adriamycin®. The underlying rationale being that because myeloma cells are slowly dividing, usually with under 1 per cent in S-phase at any time, drugs which act only against cycling cells would be likely to kill more cells if given over a longer period. The VAD regimen was found to be more effective than any previously described regimen in relapsed and refractory patients (Barlogie et al., 1984). Subsequent studies in previously untreated patients showed that over 80 per cent of these patients respond, with 10–20 per cent achieving complete remission (CR). Unfortunately these remissions are not durable, lasting on average only 18 months, even in those patients who achieve CR. Nevertheless, the VAD regimen has advantages in certain situations. Since none of the drugs are excreted by the kidney, it can be given without dosage modification in patients in severe renal failure, including those on dialysis. It produces very little myelosuppression and so is particularly useful in patients presenting with neutropenia or thrombocytopenia, and is an ideal initial cytoreductive therapy for younger patients in whom it is planned to proceed to stem-cell harvest. The rate of response is dramatic, with most patients achieving 90 per cent of their maximum response within 6 weeks, an advantage in patients who require rapid tumour reduction, e.g. those with rapidly progressive bone disease or incipient renal failure. The main disadvantages are the necessity for a central venous line for administration, and the high incidence of steroid-related side-effects.

The introduction of oral idarubicin has allowed the development of anthracycline-based oral regimens which appear to be as effective as VAD in terms of inducing responses and avoid the need for a central line (Cook et al., 1996). Furthermore, it is recognized that the high-dose dexamethasone is responsible for much of the effect of the VAD regimen, and dexamethasone alone has been shown to be an effective agent for inducing remission (Alexanian et al., 1992).

Choice of initial chemotherapy

The choice of initial therapy will be governed largely by the patient's age and general fitness, particularly the level of renal function. It is also essential to take into account at diagnosis the possibility of future autologous transplantation, so as to avoid the use of stem-cell damaging drugs in patients where autografting is an option. Patients up to the age of at least 65 years should be considered as possible candidates for future autografting, even if performance status is initially poor or if they present with acute renal failure. In these patients, VAD or a VAD-type regimen should be used. Autografting can be safely performed in older patients with good performance status, but for most patients over 65 years, the choice lies between simple oral chemotherapy and standard combination regimens. Overall there is little difference in long-term outcome between these options and simple oral treatment therefore seems the most appropriate choice for older patients (UK Myeloma Forum, 2001). For patients presenting with renal failure, VAD is the obvious choice, and can be used in some older patients. Oral idarubicin and dexamethasone is an alternative but, as yet, there are insufficient data on its use in patients to recommend its use without dosage modification in patients with renal failure. Melphalan and cyclophosphamide are both difficult to use in patients with renal impairment, since myelosuppression is unpredictable even when the doses are reduced. Steroids alone, e.g. pulsed high-dose dexamethasone, are very useful initial therapy in patients where there is an urgency to treat but in whom it is difficult to decide immediately on appropriate chemotherapy, e.g. those presenting with pancytopenia or patients with renal failure who may be unsuitable for intravenous therapy.

Chemotherapy should be continued until the patient has reached plateau phase, i.e. observations have been stable for a period of 3 months, since there is no advantage to prolonging therapy once plateau has been reached. In patients who are proceeding to high-dose therapy and transplant as consolidation therapy, there is probably no advantage to continuing induction chemotherapy beyond the point of maximum response; this is usually no longer than 3–4 months when VAD-type regimens are used.

RADIOTHERAPY

Myeloma is a very radiosensitive tumour and the limitation of radiotherapy as a treatment modality is myelosuppression. Until recently the use of radiotherapy was confined mainly to treating local areas, but its role has now expanded to include whole-body treatment, either in the form of double hemi-body irradiation or as part of high-dose preparative regimens for bone-marrow or peripheral blood transplantation.

Local radiotherapy

Local radiotherapy is a very effective means of relieving bone pain, with improvement usually seen within a few days of starting treatment. This is more rapid than can be achieved with any form of chemotherapy, even the VAD regimen. Treatment may be given as a single fraction (usually 8 Gy) or as a fractionated course (usually 15–20 Gy in 7–10 fractions or 30–35 Gy in 10–15 fractions; Rowell and Tobias, 1991). A dose of 8–10 Gy is usually sufficient to provide pain relief, and above this dose there is no

evidence of a dose–response curve in relation to quality and duration of symptomatic control. However, higher doses (30–35 Gy) may be needed for a tumoricidal effect (Norin, 1957). In cases of fracture or impending fracture of a long bone, surgical fixation is required but radiation may be given immediately wound healing is complete. A randomized study of single-fraction versus fractionated radiotherapy for painful lesions showed no difference in rapidity of onset or duration of pain relief. However, fractionated radiotherapy is preferable for the relief of spinal-cord compression (30–35 Gy) because there is less risk of radiation-induced oedema, and dexamethasone should also be given (e.g. 4 mg four times daily) and continued to cover the period of radiation.

Double hemi-body irradiation and total body irradiation

TBI has been widely used as part of the myeloablative regimen prior to stem-cell transplantation in myeloma and other diseases. It forms an essential part of the standard conditioning regimen for allogeneic transplantation, TBI in combination with high-dose cyclophosphamide, because of its immunosuppressive effect. The detailed schedules of administration vary in different centres depending on the number of fractions and rate of delivery and whether or not lung shielding is used, but a total dose of 12 Gy in 6 fractions over 3 days is widely used (Apperley et al., 2000).

Following on from its use in allogeneic transplantation, TBI has also been widely used in autologous transplantation in myeloma, generally in combination with high-dose melphalan. However, recent data have indicated that the addition of TBI to high-dose melphalan increases toxicity without improving remission duration (Moreau et al., 2002) and the consensus view is that conditioning should be with chemotherapy alone (UK Myeloma Forum, 2001).

Radiotherapy may also be used to treat the whole body without stem-cell support by treating the upper and lower halves of the body at an interval sufficient to allow recovery of haematopoiesis between treatment fractions (double hemi-body irradiation, DHBI). Normally the upper half of the body is treated first and then the lower part, each usually being treated in a single fraction. Different centres vary in the exact technique employed, including dose, dose rate, exact field limits (i.e. whether the head and the lower legs are included) and the areas shielded (Rowell and Tobias, 1991). In addition to predictable myelosuppression, nausea, vomiting, mucositis and gastrointestinal toxicity are common. Radiation pneumonitis is the most serious potential complication and may occur up to 6 months after treatment. The risk of pneumonitis is correlated with radiation dose and dose rate, and the risk is higher in patients who have previously received nitrosureas and alkylating agents.

DHBI has been used most widely in patients with relapsed and refractory myeloma. Marked symptomatic relief is achieved in the majority of those who have bone pain. It is difficult to assess response rate and survival from these studies, since the patient group treated is very heterogeneous, but objective responses are reported in over 25 per cent of patients. These results are similar to those of second-line chemotherapy, but myelosuppression is significantly greater with DHBI. This form of therapy is therefore most useful in relapsed patients with generalized bone pain.

HIGH-DOSE THERAPY AND STEM-CELL TRANSPLANTATION

Autologous transplantation

Because of the disappointing results of conventional chemotherapy there has been increasing interest in high-dose therapy and stem-cell support. The most widely used regimens for high-dose therapy have been high-dose melphalan alone at a dosage of $200\,mg/m^2$ or high-dose melphalan $140\,mg/m^2$ with TBI, although as discussed above TBI is no longer recommended. It is now evident that autologous transplantation, using peripheral blood progenitor cells (PBPC) with or without post-transplant growth factors, is an extremely safe procedure for patients up to at least the age of 65 years. However, it is also evident that at present no patients are cured by autologous transplantation. The median duration of event-free survival (EFS) is around 2 years in most series and all patients ultimately relapse, although those who achieve CR post-transplant may have very long survival. Since autologous transplantation is not curative, it is important to establish whether or not it prolongs remission and/or survival as compared with conventional chemotherapy. The first randomized study comparing autologous transplantation with conventional chemotherapy was carried out by the Intergroupe Français du Myélome (IFM) (Attal *et al.*, 1996; Attal and Harousseau, 2001). Two hundred newly diagnosed patients were randomized to receive either two courses of combination chemotherapy (VMCP/VBAP) followed by autograft or 10 courses of VMCP/VBAP. There was a significant benefit in remission duration and survival for the autograft arm (Fig. 46.3), the probability of survival at 5 years from diagnosis being 52 per cent versus 12 per cent in the chemotherapy arm. There was also a significant difference in event-free survival (28 per cent versus 10 per cent at 5 years). A randomized study comparing transplant in first remission with standard chemotherapy followed by transplant at relapse has showed no difference in survival but an advantage in duration of first remission and quality of life for early autograft (Fermand *et al.*, 1998). An historical case-control study of patients undergoing high-dose therapy and standard-dose chemotherapy from the Nordic Myeloma Study Group also showed a survival advantage for HDT; median survival was 44 months in the standard-dose group but had

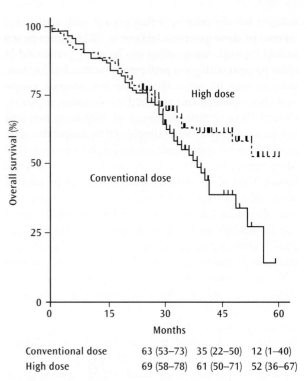

Conventional dose	63 (53–73)	35 (22–50)	12 (1–40)
High dose	69 (58–78)	61 (50–71)	52 (36–67)

Figure 46.3 *Overall survival of newly diagnosed patients randomized to combination chemotherapy or autologous transplantation. (Reproduced with permission from Attal* et al. *(1996) Autologous bone marrow transplantation versus conventional chemotherapy in multiple myeloma: a prospective, randomized trial. N. Eng. J. Med.* **335**, *91–7.* *Copyright 1996 Massachusetts Medical Society. All rights reserved.)*

not been reached in the high-dose group (Lenhoff *et al.*, 2000). Further randomized studies are in progress, but current evidence indicates that high-dose therapy prolongs remission and survival and should form part of the standard approach to initial treatment in younger patients (UK Myeloma Forum, 2001).

Contamination and purging of harvested peripheral blood progenitor cells

It is not known whether relapse results from residual disease in the patient or from reinfused myeloma cells. It was initially hoped that the use of PBPC, rather than marrow (BM), for autografting would result in a lower relapse risk, since plasma cells do not normally circulate in the peripheral blood. However, data comparing PBPC and BM as a source of stem cells failed to show any difference in relapse rate, and it is now clear from molecular studies that mobilized PBPC are in fact contaminated with cells belonging to the myeloma clone in the majority of patients, if not all. This has led to attempts to purge harvested stem cells, either by negative purging or, more recently, by the use of positive selection based on CD34 antigen expression. CD34 is expressed on normal stem cells but not on myeloma cells, and CD34-selection of harvested PBPC has been shown to reduce the level of contamination in the reinfused product. However, this has not led to a lower relapse risk (Stewart et al., 2001). The use of anti-B-cell monoclonal antibodies in addition to, or instead of, CD34+ selection may further reduce tumour cell contamination.

Double autologous transplantation

A double (tandem) autograft represents a means of attempting to deliver more effective eradication of endogenous disease. This approach has been pioneered by the Little Rock group (Barlogie et al., 1999). They have shown that the results are superior to standard therapy, but have not compared their results with those of single autografts either in a randomized trial or in a case-control study. The French IFM group has carried out a randomized study (IFM 94) comparing one high-dose procedure with two. Interim analysis showed a possible survival benefit for two procedures in a subgroup of patients receiving two transplants with peripheral blood stem cells as opposed to bone marrow, but there was no significant difference overall in outcome (Attal and Harousseau, 2001). Interim analysis of three other randomized studies from France, Italy and the Netherlands has also not so far shown an overall survival benefit for tandem transplants and at present this approach cannot be recommended as standard therapy (Vesole et al., 2001).

Allogeneic bone-marrow transplants

The largest body of data on allogeneic bone-marrow transplants (BMT) is that collected by the EBMT registry, now totalling some 800 patients transplanted at various stages of disease. Transplant-related mortality (TRM) is higher in myeloma patients than those with leukaemia and although TRM has been lower in recent years, probably due to better patient selection, overall TRM remains at around 30 per cent (Gahrton et al., 2001). This is due to a variety of causes including graft-versus-host disease, infection and idiopathic pneumonitis. Relapse also remains a major problem, occurring in over 50 per cent of patients who survive the transplant. Nevertheless, the survival curve approaches a plateau beyond 5 years, with a projected long-term overall survival for all patients of around 35 per cent (Gahrton et al., 1991). The two pre-transplant factors most strongly influencing survival are whether the transplant is undertaken after first-line therapy or later in the course of the disease (long-term survival 40 versus 20 per cent) and patient gender, TRM being significantly higher in male patients, for reasons which are not evident (Bjorkstrand et al., 1996). Overall, for a patient allografted in first remission, there is approximately a 30 per cent risk of transplant-related death, a 30 per cent chance of surviving with subsequent relapse, and a 30 per cent chance of long-term disease-free remission. The choice between allogeneic and autologous transplant in those patients who have the option is a difficult one and depends on assessment of the risks and benefits on an individual basis. Factors such as age and cytomegalovirus (CMV) status should be taken into account, particularly in male patients.

Graft versus myeloma

It is now apparent that donor lymphocyte infusions (DLI) given to patients not in remission after allogeneic BMT can produce a disease response, clearly demonstrating a graft-versus-myeloma effect (Lokhorst et al., 2000). At least 50 per cent of patients respond, but response is closely associated with the development of graft-versus-host disease and fatal marrow aplasia may also occur. Thus DLI is an effective treatment but can be associated with a high treatment-related mortality. This could potentially be reduced by using gradually escalating doses of T cells.

High-dose therapy: future directions

It is evident from the relapse rate after allogeneic BMT that the currently used preparative regimens do not eradicate disease in most patients. Given the existing high TRM after allografting and the age range of patients undergoing autologous transplantation, dose escalation is unlikely to be possible. Alternative approaches, such as the use of radiolabelled monoclonal antibodies directed against haemopoietic cells, are therefore worth exploring. The contribution of re-infused myeloma cells to relapse after autografting needs to be determined by gene-marking experiments, in order to determine whether attempts at improving purging efficacy are worthwhile, or whether efforts should be directed more towards disease eradication in the patient. The graft-versus-myeloma effect in the allogeneic situation could be exploited while also attempting to reduce transplant-related mortality by using non-myeloablative conditioning regimens (mini-allografts). There are currently a number of studies exploring the feasibility of autologous transplantation followed by a mini-allograft (Kroger et al., 2001; Maloney et al., 2001).

α-INTERFERON

α-Interferon (INF) has anti-myeloma activity and has been used as a single agent, in combination with induction chemotherapy, or as maintenance therapy after the patient has responded to initial chemotherapy. It appears that the addition of INF to induction chemotherapy can increase the proportion of patients meeting the criteria for response. However, there is no clear survival benefit and increased toxicity, so that INF is not widely used in this way. There have also been numerous trials addressing the issue of whether maintenance therapy with INF prolongs remission and/or survival. Some trials (but not all) have shown a benefit in terms of remission duration, but a survival benefit has been difficult to demonstrate. A meta-analysis of over 4000 patients in 24 different trials suggested that INF either during induction or maintenance prolongs remission by about 6 months and survival by about 3 months (Myeloma Trialists Collaborative Group, 2001). INF maintenance also appears to prolong remission after autologous transplantation (Cunningham et al., 1998). Overall, therefore, it appears that interferon confers a small benefit, which must be weighed up against the cost and side-effects.

BISPHOSPHONATES

Bisphosphonates, which act by inhibiting osteoclast-mediated bone resorption, are the treatment of choice for hypercalcaemia persisting after rehydration. The question of whether long-term use of bisphosphonates can arrest progression of bone disease in patient with MM has been addressed in a number of trials. Etidronate, the least potent bisphosphonate, was found to be without significant benefit, but both oral clodronate and intravenous pamidronate were found, in different studies, to reduce bone pain and the incidence of fractures (Lahtinen et al., 1992; Berenson et al., 1998; McCloskey et al., 1998). Zoledronate has been shown to be as effective as pamidronate in reducing skeletal-related events in patients with bone disease due to MM or breast cancer (Berenson et al., 2001) and is more convenient to administer. Patients with bone disease should therefore receive a bisphosphonate long term; there is also a convincing rationale for use in patients without radiological evidence of bone disease, since benefit in the above studies was not confined to patients with bone disease at the start of treatment. It is currently recommended that all patients who require treatment for their myeloma should receive a bisphosphonate long-term (UK Myeloma Forum, 2001; Djulbegovic et al., 2001). At present there is no evidence to support the use of bisphosphonates in asymptomatic patients. There are no data comparing the efficacy of clodronate with that of pamidronate or zoledronate; the absorption of bisphosphonates is poor and variable but there are practical advantages of prescribing an oral drug. It has been suggested that the use of bisphosphonates long-term may also improve survival (Berenson et al., 1998), but a meta-analysis of published data found no significant survival benefit (Djulbegovic et al., 2001).

REFRACTORY AND RELAPSED DISEASE

All patients with myeloma will relapse, and at this stage the disease may respond to the same chemotherapy as that used previously, to a different regimen, or prove refractory to treatment. Expression of increased levels of P-glycoprotein (the mdr phenotype) is a common cause of drug resistance in relapsed patients, being present in 43 per cent of previously treated patients (Grogan et al., 1993), and 83 per cent of those who had received over 340 mg of Adriamycin®.

Unless the relapse occurs soon after stopping treatment, it is worth trying the same regimen that induced the initial remission. Over 50 per cent of patients who initially responded to MP will respond again to MP at relapse (Belch et al., 1988). Patients refractory to MP may still respond to cyclophosphamide. In younger patients, VAD is generally preferred at relapse, although the oral anthracycline-based regimens, Z-Dex and CIDEX (Parameswaran et al., 2000) are suitable alternatives to VAD and other intravenous anthracycline-containing regimens. For patients not responding to VAD, combinations of VAD with drug-resistance modifiers such as cyclosporin have been used (Sonneveld et al., 1992), but with limited success.

Patients relapsing after, or refractory to, more than one chemotherapy regimen may do well on steroids alone, and double hemi-body irradiation can also be useful in this situation. Thalidomide, with or without dexamethasone, in very effective in relapsed disease and is being increasingly widely used in preference to further chemotherapy (see below).

Some patients also exhibit resistance to primary treatment. Patients who are refractory to initial VAD usually respond well to intermediate or high-dose melphalan, while those refractory to MP may respond to cyclophosphamide or an anthracycline-containing regimen. Thalidomide can also be effective in primary refractory disease.

NEW APPROACHES TO TREATMENT

The increased understanding of the biology of myeloma and the interaction between myeloma cells and the micro-environment has led to the recent development of a wide variety of new drugs aimed at targeting these interactions or specific intracellular signaling pathways (Anderson, 2001; Hideshima et al., 2001).

Thalidomide

Since the first observation by Singhal et al. (1999) on the successful use of thalidomide in MM, a large number of reports have confirmed the remarkable activity of this drug in patients with refractory and relapsed disease (Tosi and Cavo, 2002). Thalidomide alone in doses of 100–800 mg daily produces a response in 30 per cent of relapsed/refractory patients (Barlogie et al., 2001; Juliusson et al., 2000) and when combined with dexamethasone the response rate rises to over 50 per cent (Palumbo et al., 2001). Preliminary studies in newly diagnosed patients indicate similar rates of response. Trials of thalidomide in combination with cytotoxic drugs are in progress. Caution is required since an increased risk of venous thromboembolism has been observed in patients receiving thalidomide and chemotherapy (Zangari *et al.*, 2001).

Thalidomide probably does not act primarily by reducing angiogenesis, as there is no correlation between response and reduction in MVD. It has many other activities, including modulation of cytokine production and of the immune response, and the precise mechanism by which it acts in myeloma is unclear. Apart from the risk of birth defects, thalidomide has a number of important side effects including peripheral neuropathy and an increased risk of thrombosis, particularly when combined with chemotherapy (Zangari *et al.*, 2001). Analogues of thalidomide that are not teratogenic are currently undergoing Phase I/II trials.

Other new drugs

New drugs currently in clinical trial include inhibitors of receptor tyrosine kinases (including the VEGF receptor and the FGFR3 receptor), proteasome inhibitors, farnesyl transferase inhibitors and the antisense oligonucleotide to bcl2, which is overexpressed in most cases of MM.

Some of these drugs, particularly the proteasome inhibitor PS341, have already shown promising activity in relapsed and refractory patients. Arsenic trioxide is also undergoing clinical trial in MM (Anderson *et al.*, 2002).

Immunological approaches

Treatment with murine monoclonal antibody to IL-6 has produced transient responses, and trials with chimeric human–murine IL-6 antibodies, antibodies to the IL-6 receptor and new IL-6 inhibitors are under way. Another approach under evaluation is to use monoclonal antibodies directed against plasma cells to deliver either an immunotoxin or a radioactive agent to the tumour cells. There is considerable interest in vaccination strategies using either the idiotypic protein or the idiotypic DNA to induce immune responses. Such strategies would be most applicable to patients in remission after high-dose therapy with a low level of residual tumour.

OTHER RELATED CONDITIONS

Monoclonal gammopathy of undetermined significance

Patients with MGUS should be monitored regularly, measuring paraprotein levels every 3 months initially and then every 6 months if the levels are stable. Patients should be seen and examined at least once a year, and clinical and laboratory features re-evaluated to determine if there is any evidence of progression to myeloma or other related disorder. Consideration should also be given to repeating bone-marrow aspiration and radiological examinations. Treatment is not indicated in the absence of any features of progression, but in young patients it is appropriate to store stem cells at diagnosis, using G-CSF for mobilization.

Solitary plasmacytoma of bone

Solitary plasmacytoma of bone (SPB) may involve any bone but is most common in the axial skeleton. Pain and nerve root or cord compression are the most common modes of presentation. Biopsy of the lesion shows a monoclonal population of plasma cells. A serum and/or urinary paraprotein may be present, but the bone marrow and radiological skeletal survey are normal. Local radiotherapy (40–50 Gy over 3–5 weeks) achieves disease control in almost all patients (Greenberg *et al.*, 1987). However, patients should continue to be monitored carefully, because the risk of recurrence at a single site is around 25 per cent, and that of developing MM is around 50 per cent over a 15-year period (Dimopoulos *et al.*, 1992). It is evident, therefore, that the disease is not truly localized at diagnosis in many patients. Where a paraprotein is present, failure to disappear following completion of radiotherapy, or a fall followed by a rise, almost always indicates disease elsewhere (Wilder *et al.*, 2002). In 30 per cent of patients with SPB on standard criteria, MRI scans show abnormalities consistent with myeloma (Moulopoulos *et al.*, 1993) and thus a normal MRI scan of the spine and pelvis is required for the accurate diagnosis of SPB.

Extramedullary plasmacytoma

In contrast to SPB, extramedullary plasmacytoma (EMP) appears to be truly localized in the majority of cases and rarely progresses to MM (Greenberg *et al.*, 1987). It most commonly arises in the upper respiratory passages, but a wide variety of different organs may occasionally be involved. As with SPB, biopsy of the lesion shows a monoclonal population of plasma cells, and a serum and/or urinary paraprotein may be present, but the bone marrow and radiological skeletal survey are normal. Local radiotherapy (40–50 Gy over 3–5 weeks), rather than surgical removal, is the treatment of choice. The paraprotein should be monitored following completion of radiotherapy and will normally disappear within 6 months.

POEMS syndrome

This is a rare syndrome in which a serum paraprotein (M-component) is associated with polyneuropathy (P), organomegaly (O), endocrinopathy (E) and skin changes

(S). Approximately 50 per cent of cases are associated with multiple myeloma and the remainder with solitary plasmacytomas or more subtle plasma cell dyscrasias. The cardinal feature is a severe sensorimotor neuropathy with osteosclerotic bone lesions, hepatomegaly and lymphadenopathy, hormonal abnormalities and skin hyperpigmentation. The mechanism for these multisystem changes is unknown. Treatment is generally unsatisfactory, but local radiotherapy is used for localized plasmacytomas and chemotherapy or steroid therapy for more generalized disease (Gawler, 1998). Recently there have been a number of reports of improvement following high-dose therapy and stem-cell transplantation (Rovira et al., 2001).

SIGNIFICANT POINTS

- Myeloma is due to proliferation of a single clone of plasma cells, which originate from a post-germinal-centre B lymphocyte.
- Growth of myeloma in the bone marrow and consequent bone destruction is dependent on interactions between myeloma plasma cells and marrow stromal cells, including osteoclasts.
- The classical presenting features are bone pain, anaemia and renal impairment.
- A serum paraprotein is present in 80 per cent of cases, but in 20 per cent free light chains only are produced and there is no paraprotein in the serum. In <1 per cent of cases there is no paraprotein in serum or in urine.
- The most important prognostic factors are serum β_2-microglobulin and the presence of deletion of chromosome 13q. Other factors are serum albumin, serum calcium, haemoglobin and renal function.
- The combination of melphalan and prednisolone results in a 50 per cent response rate, a median response duration of 18 months and a median survival of 3–4 years. Combination chemotherapy regimens have not proven more effective.
- Autologous transplantation in younger patients results in a higher frequency of response, including up to 50 per cent complete remissions, a longer duration of response and a median survival of around 5 years.
- Patients who are potential candidates for autologous transplantation should receive initial chemotherapy with a regimen such as VAD that induces a rapid response without damaging normal marrow stem cells.
- Allogeneic transplantation has a high mortality but may be curative. This effect is mediated at least partly by a graft-versus-myeloma effect.
- Maintenance therapy with α-interferon in responding patients has been shown to prolong remission duration by approximately 6 months and survival by approximately 3 months.
- Thalidomide has proved remarkably effective in relapsed disease and its role at earlier stages is being explored.

KEY REFERENCES

Attal, M. and Harousseau, J. (2001) Randomized trial experience of the Intergroupe Francophone du Myelome. *Semin. Hematol.* **38**, 226–30.

Anderson, K.C. (2001) Multiple myeloma. Advances in disease biology: therapeutic implications. *Semin. Hematol.* **38**, 6–10.

Callander, N.S. and Roodman, G.D. (2001) Myeloma bone disease. *Semin. Hematol.* **38**, 276–85.

Dalton, W.S., Bergsagel, P.L., Kuehl, W.M., Anderson, K.C. and Harousseau, J.L. (2001) *Multiple myeloma. Hematology* (Am. Soc. Hematol. Educ. Program) 2001 Jan, 157–77 (available on line).

UK Myeloma Forum (2001) Guideline: diagnosis and treatment of multiple myeloma. *Br. J. Haematol.* **115**, 522–40.

REFERENCES

Alexanian, R. and Dimopoulos, M. (1994) The treatment of multiple myeloma. *N. Engl. J. Med.* **330**, 484–9.

Alexanian, R., Dimopoulos, M.A., Delasalle, K. and Barlogie, B. (1992) Primary dexamethasone treatment of multiple myeloma. *Blood* **80**, 887–90.

Anderson, K.C. (2001) Multiple myeloma. Advances in disease biology: therapeutic implications. *Semin. Hematol.* **38**, 6–10.

Anderson, K.C., Boise, L.H., Louie, R. and Waxman, S. (2002) Arsenic trioxide in multiple myeloma: rationale and future directions. *Cancer J.* **8**, 12–25.

Apperley, J.F., Bacigalupo, A., Friedrich, W. (2000) Principles of conditioning regimens. In Apperley, J.F., Gluckman, E. and Gratwohl, A. (eds), *The EBMT handbook: blood and marrow transplantation*, 2nd edition. Paris: European School of Haematology & Robert Arts Graphiques.

Attal, M. and Harousseau, J. (2001) Randomized trial experience of the Intergroupe Francophone du Myelome. *Semin. Hematol.* **38**, 226–30.

Attal, M., Harousseau, J.L., Stoppa, A.M. *et al.* (1996) Autologous bone marrow transplantation versus conventional chemotherapy in multiple myeloma: a prospective, randomized trial. *N. Engl. J. Med.* **335**, 91–7.

Avet-Loiseau, H., Li, J.Y., Morineau, N. *et al.* (1999) Monosomy 13 is associated with the transition of monoclonal gammopathy of undetermined significance to multiple myeloma. *Blood* **94**, 2583–9.

Bakkus, M.H., Heirman, C., van Riet, I. and van Camp, B. (1994) Evidence that the clonogenic cell in multiple myeloma originates from a pre-switched but somatically mutated B cell. *Blood* **80**, 2326–35.

Barlogie, B., Smith, L. and Alexanian, R. (1984) Effective treatment of advanced mutliple myeloma refractory to alkylating agents. *N. Engl. J. Med.* **310**, 1353–6.

Barlogie, B., Jagannath, S., Desikan, K.R. *et al.* (1999) Total therapy with tandem transplants for newly diagnosed multiple myeloma. *Blood* **93**, 55–65.

Barlogie, B., Zangari, M., Spencer, T. *et al.* (2001) Thalidomide in the management of multiple myeloma. *Semin. Hematol.* **38**, 250–9.

Bataille, R. and Harousseau, J.L. (1997) Multiple myeloma. *N. Engl. J. Med.* **336**, 1657–63.

Bataille, R., Jourdan, M., Zhang, X.G. and Klein, B. (1989) Serum levels of interleukin 6, a potent myeloma cell growth factor, as a reflection of disease severity in plasma cell dyscrasia. *J. Clin. Invest.* **84**, 2008–11.

Belch, A., Shelley, W., Bergsagel, D. *et al.* (1988) A randomized trial of maintenance versus no maintenance melphalan and prednisone in responding multiple myeloma patients. *Br. J. Cancer* **57**, 94–9.

Bellamy, W.T. (2001) Expression of vascular endothelial growth factor and its receptors in multiple myeloma and other hematopoietic malignancies. *Semin. Oncol.* **28**, 551–9.

Berenson, J., Lichtenstein, A., Porter, L. *et al.* (1998) Long-term pamidronate treatment of advanced multiple myeloma patients reduces skeletal events. Myeloma Aredia Study Group. *J. Clin. Oncol.* **16**, 593–602.

Berenson, J.R., Rosen, L.S., Howell, A. *et al.* (2001) Zoledronic acid reduces skeletal-related events in patients with osteolytic metastases. *Cancer* **91**, 1191–200.

Bergsagel, P.L. and Kuehl, W.M. (2001) Chromosome translocations in multiple myeloma. *Oncogene* **20**, 5611–22.

Billadeau, D., Quam, L., Thomas, W. *et al.* (1992) Detection and quantitation of malignant cells in the peripheral blood of multiple myeloma patients. *Blood* **80**, 1818–24.

Bjorkstrand, B., Ljungman, P., Svensson, H. *et al.* (1996) Allogeneic bone marrow transplantation versus autologous stem cell transplantation in multiple myeloma – a retrospective case-matched study from the European Group for Blood and Marrow Transplantation (EBMT). *Blood* **88**, 4711–18.

Boice, J.D., Morin, M.M., Glass, A.G. *et al.* (1991) Diagnostic X-ray procedures and the risk of leukaemia, lymphoma and multiple myeloma. *JAMA* **265**, 1290–4.

Bray, I., Brennan, P. and Boffetta, P. (2001) Current trends and future projections of lymphoid neoplasms – an age-period-cohort analysis. *Cancer Causes Control* **12**, 813–20.

Callander, N.S. and Roodman, G.D. (2001) Myeloma bone disease. *Semin. Hematol.* **38**, 276–85.

Cook, G., Sharp, R.A., Tansey, P. and Franklin, I.M. (1996) A phase I/II trial of Z-Dex (oral idarubicin and dexamethasone), an oral equivalent of VAD, as initial therapy at diagnosis or progression in multiple myeloma. *Br. J. Haematol.* **93**, 931–4.

Croucher, P.I., Shipman, C.M., Lippitt, J. *et al.* (2001) Osteoprotegerin inhibits the development of osteolytic bone disease in multiple myeloma. *Blood* **98**, 3534–40.

Cunningham, D., Powles, R., Malpas, J. *et al.* (1998) A randomised trial of maintenance interferon following high-dose therapy in multiple myeloma: long-term follow-up results. *Br. J. Haematol.* **102**, 495–502.

Dalton, W.S., Bergsagel, P.L., Kuehl, W.M., Anderson, K.C. and Harousseau, J.L. (2001) Multiple myeloma. Hematology (Am. Soc. Hematol. Educ. Program) 2001 Jan, 157–77 (available on line).

Dammacco, F., Castoldi, G. and Rodjer, S. (2001) Efficacy of epoietin alfa in the treatment of anaemia of multiple myeloma. *Br. J. Haematol.* **113**, 172–9.

Dimopoulos, M.A., Goldstein, J., Fuller, L, Delasalle, K. and Alexanian, R. (1992) Curability of solitary bone plasmacytoma. *J. Clin. Oncol.* **10**, 145–50.

Dimopoulos, M.A., Moulopoulos, L.A., Smith, T., Delasalle, K.B. and Alexanian, R. (1993) Risk of disease progression in asymptomatic multiple myeloma. *Am. J. Med.* **94**, 57–61.

Djulbegovic, B., Wheatley, K., Ross, J. *et al.* (2001) *Bisphosphonates in multiple myeloma* (Cochrane Review). Cochrane Database Syst. Rev.4:CD003188.

Durie, B.G.M. and Salmon, S.E. (1975) A clinical staging system for multiple myeloma. *Cancer* **36**, 842–54.

Fermand, J.P., Ravaud, P., Chevret. S. *et al.* (1998) High-dose therapy and autologous peripheral blood stem cell transplantation in multiple myeloma: up-front or rescue treatment? Results of a multicenter randomised trial. *Blood* **92**, 3131–6.

Fonseca, R., Harrington, D., Oken, M.M. *et al.* (2002) Biological and prognostic significance of interphase fluorescence *in situ* hybridization detection of chromosome 13 abnormalities (delta 13) in multiple myeloma: an Eastern Cooperative Oncology Group study. *Cancer Res.* **62**, 715–20.

Gahrton, G., Tura, S., Ljungman, P. *et al.* (1991) Allogeneic bone marrow transplantation in multiple myeloma. *N. Engl. J. Med.* **325**, 1267–73.

Gahrton, G., Svensson, H., Cavo, M. *et al.* (2001) Progress in allogeneic bone marrow and peripheral blood stem cell transplantation for multiple myeloma: a comparison between transplants performed 1983–93 and 1994–8 at European Group for Blood and Marrow Transplantation centres. *Br. J. Haematol.* **113**, 209–16.

Gawler, J. (1998) Neurological manifestations of myeloma and their management. In Malpas, J.S., Bergsagel, D.E., Kyle, R.A. and Anderson, K.C. (eds), *Myeloma: biology and management.* Oxford: Oxford University Press, 402–38.

Giuliani, N., Bataille, R., Mancini, C., Lazzaretti, M. and Barille, S. (2001) Myeloma cells induce imbalance in the osteoprotegerin/osteoprotegerin ligand system in the human bone marrow environment. *Blood* **98**, 3527–33.

Greenberg, P., Parker, R.G., Fu, Y.S. and Abemayor, E. (1987) The treatment of solitary plasmacytoma of bone and extramedullary plasmacytoma. *Am. J. Clin. Oncol.* **10**, 199–204.

Grogan, T.M., Spier, C.M., Salmon, S.E. *et al.* (1993) P-glycoprotein expression in human plasma cell myeloma: correlation with prior chemotherapy. *Blood* **72**, 219–23.

Grosbois, B., Jego, P., Attal, M. *et al.* (1999) Familial multiple myeloma: report of fifteen families. *Br. J. Haematol.* **105**, 768–70.

Gupta, D., Treon, S.P., Shima, Y. *et al.* (2001) Adherence of multiple myeloma cells to bone marrow stromal cells upregulates vascular endothelial growth factor secretion: therapeutic applications. *Leukemia* **15**, 1950–61.

Hatcher, J.L., Baris, D., Olshan, A.F. *et al.* (2001) Diagnostic radiation and the risk of multiple myeloma (United States). *Cancer Causes Control* **12**, 755–61.

Healy, J.C. and Armstrong, P. (1998) Radiological features of multiple myeloma. In Malpas, J.S., Bergsagel, D.E., Kyle, R.A. and Anderson, K.C. (eds), *Myeloma: biology and management.* Oxford: Oxford University Press, 235–65.

Herrinton, L.J., Weiss, N.S. and Olshan, A.F. (1998) Epidemiology of myeloma. In Malpas, J.S., Bergsagel, D.E., Kyle, R.A. and Anderson, K.C. (eds), *Myeloma: biology and management.* Oxford: Oxford University Press, 150–86.

Hideshima, T., Chauhan, D., Podar, K., Schlossman, R.L., Richardson, P. and Anderson, K.C. (2001) Novel therapies targeting the myeloma cell and its bone marrow microenvironment. *Semin. Oncol.* **28**, 607–12.

Iggo, N. (1998) Management of renal complications. In Malpas, J.S., Bergsagel, D.E., Kyle, R.A. and

Anderson, K.C. (eds), *Myeloma: biology and management.* Oxford: Oxford University Press, 381–401.

Johnson, W.J., Kyle, R.A., Pineda, A.A., O'Brien, P.C. and Holley, K.E. (1990) Treatment of renal failure associated with multiple myeloma. Plasmapheresis, hemodialysis and chemotherapy. *Arch. Int. Med.* **150**, 863–9.

Juliusson, G., Celsing, F., Turesson, I., Lenhoff, S., Andriansson, M. and Malm, C. (2000) Frequent good partial remissions with thalidomide including best response ever in patients with advanced refractory and relapsed myeloma. *Br. J. Haematol.* **109**, 89–96.

Klein, B., Zhang, X.G., Lu, Z.Y. and Bataille, R. (1995) Interleukin-6 in human multiple myeloma. *Blood* **85**, 863–72.

Knudsen, L.M., Hjorth, M. and Hippe, E. (2000) Renal failure in multiple myeloma: reversibility and impact on the prognosis. Nordic Myeloma Study Group. *Eur. J. Haematol.* **65**, 175–81.

Kroger, N., Kiehl, M., Schwerdtfeger, R. *et al.* (2001) Phase I/II trial of high-dose chemotherapy with autograft followed by dose-reduced allograft for multiple myeloma. *Blood* **98**(suppl. 1) 198a (abstr 830).

Kyle, P.A., Therneau, T.M., Rajkumar, S.V. *et al.* (2002) A long-term study of prognosis in monoclonal gammopathy of undetermined significance. *N. Engl. J. Med.* **346**, 564–9.

Lahtinen, R., Laakso, M., Palva, I. *et al.* (1992) Randomised placebo-controlled multicentre trial of clodronate in multiple myeloma. *Lancet* **340**, 1049–52.

Lenhoff, S., Hjorth, M., Homberg, E. *et al.* (2000) Impact on survival of high-dose therapy with autologous stem cell support in patients younger than 64 years with newly diagnosed multiple myeloma: a population based study. *Blood* **95**, 7–11.

Lokhorst, H.M., Schattenberg, A., Cornelissen, J.J. *et al.* (2000) Donor lymphocyte infusions for relapsed multiple myeloma after allogeneic stem cell transplantation: predictive factors for response and long-term outcome. *J. Clin. Oncol.* **18**, 3031–7.

Lynch, H.T., Sanger, W.G., Pirruccello, S., Quinn-Laquer, B. and Weisenburger, D.D. (2001) Familial multiple myeloma: a family study and review of the literature. *J. Natl Cancer Inst.* **93**, 1479–83.

Maclennan, I.C.M., Chapman, C., Dunn, J. and Kelly, K. (1992) Combined chemotherapy with ABCM versus melphalan for treatment of myelomatosis. *Lancet* **339**, 200–5.

Maloney, D.G., Sahebi, F., Stockerl-Goldstein, K. *et al.* (2001) Combining an allogeneic graft-v-myeloma effect with high-dose autologous stem cell rescue in the treatment of multiple myeloma. *Blood* **98**(suppl. 1) 434a (abstr 1822).

Mariette, X., Zagdanski, A.M., Guermazi, A. *et al.* (1999) Prognostic value of vertebral lesions detected by magnetic resonance imaging in patients with stage I multiple myeloma. *Br. J. Haematol.* **104**, 723–9.

McCloskey, E.V., Maclennan, I.C.M., Drayson, M.T. *et al.* (1998) A randomized trial of the effect of clodronate on skeletal morbidity in multiple myeloma. *Br. J. Haematol.* **103**, 902–10.

Moreau, P., Facon, T., Attal, M. *et al.* (2002) Comparison of 200 mg/m^2 melphalan and 8 Gy total body irradiation plus 140 mg/m^2 melphalan as conditioning regimens for peripheral blood stem cell transplantation in patients with newly diagnosed multiple myeloma: final analysis of the Intergroupe Francophone du Myelome 9502 randomized trial. *Blood* **99**, 731–5.

Moulopoulos, L.A., Dimopoulos, M.A., Weber, D. *et al.* (1993) Magnetic resonance imaging in the staging of solitary plasmacytoma of bone. *J. Clin. Oncol.* **11**, 1311–15.

Myeloma Trialists' Collaborative Group (1998) Combination chemotherapy versus melphalan plus prednisone as treatment for multiple myeloma: an overview of 6,633 patients from 27 randomized trials. *J. Clin. Oncol.* **16**, 3832–42.

Myeloma Trialists' Collaborative group (2001) Interferon as therapy for multiple myeloma: an individual patient data overview of 24 randomised trials and 4012 patients. *Br. J. Haematol.* **113**, 1020–34.

Nishida, K., Tamura, A., Nakazawa, N. *et al.* (1997) The Ig heavy chain gene is frequently involved in chromosomal translocations in multiple myeloma and plasma cel leukaemia as detected by *in situ* hybridisation. *Blood* **90**, 526–34.

Norin, T. (1957) Roentgen treatment of myeloma with special consideration to the dosage. *Acta Radiol.* **47**, 46–54.

Orchard, K., Barrington, S., Buscombe, J., Hilson, A., Prentice, H.G. and Mehta, A. (2002) Fluoro-deoxy glucose positron emission tomography imaging for the detection of occult disease in multiple myeloma. *Br. J. Haematol.* **117**, 133–7.

Palumbo, A., Giaccone, L., Bartola, A. *et al.* (2001) Low dose thalidomide plus dexamethasone is an effective salvage therapy for advanced myeloma. *Haematologica* **86**, 399–403.

Parameswaran, R., Giles, C., Kelsey, S.M. *et al.* (2000) Oral idarubicin, CCNU and dexamethasone (CIDEX) in patients with relapsed and refractory myeloma: an effective regimen with acceptable toxicity. *Br. J. Haematol.* **109**, 571–5.

Roux, S., Meignin, V. and Quillard, J. (2002) RANK (receptor activator of nuclear factor-kappa B) and RANKL expression in multiple myeloma. *Br. J. Haematol.* **117**, 86–92.

Rovira, M., Carreras, E. and Blade, J. (2001) Dramatic improvement of POEMS syndrome following autologous haematopoietic cell transplantation. *Br. J. Haematol.* **115**, 373–5.

Rowell, N.P. and Tobias, J.S. (1991) The role of radiotherapy in the management of multiple myeloma. *Blood Rev.* **5**, 801–4.

Said, J., Rettig, M., Heppner, K. *et al.* (1997) Localisation of Kaposi's sarcoma-associated herpes virus in bone marrow biopsy samples from patients with multiple myeloma. *Blood* **90**, 4278–82.

Silvestris, F., Cafforio, P., Tucci, M. and Dammacco, F. (2002) Negative regulation of erythroblast maturation by Fas-L + / TRAIL + highly malignant plasma cells: a major pathogenetic mechanism of anemia in multiple myeloma. *Blood* **99**, 1305–13.

Singhal, S., Mehta, J., Desikan, R. *et al.* (1999) Antitumor activity of thalidomide in refractory myeloma. *N. Engl. J. Med.* **341**, 1565–71.

Sonneveld, P., Durie, B.G., Lokhorst, H.M. *et al.* (1992) Modulation of multidrug resistant multiple myeloma by cyclosporin. The Leukaemia Group of the EORTC and the HOVON. *Lancet* **340**, 255–9.

Speer, S.A., Semenza, J.C., Kurosaki, T. and Anton-Culver, H. (2002) Risk factors for acute myeloid leukaemia and multiple myeloma: a combination of GIS and case-control studies. *J. Environ. Health* **64**, 9–16.

Stewart, A.K., Vescio, R., Schiller, G. *et al.* (2001) Purging of autologous peripheral-blood stem cells using CD34 does not improve overall or progression-free survival after high-dose chemotherapy for multiple myeloma: results of a multicenter controlled trial. *J. Clin. Oncol.* **19**, 3771–9.

Tosi, P. and Cavo, M. (2002) Thalidomide in myeloma: state of art. *Haematologica* **87**, 233–4.

Tricot, G., Barlogie, B., Jagganath, S. *et al.* (1995) Poor prognosis in multiple myeloma is asssociated only with partial or complete deletion of chromosome 13 or abnormalities involving 11q and not with other karyotypic abnormalities. *Blood* **86**, 4250–6.

UK Myeloma Forum (2001) Guideline: diagnosis and treatment of multiple myeloma. *Br. J. Haematol.* **115**, 522–40.

Vacca, A., Ribatti, D., Roncali, L. *et al.* (1994) Bone marrow angiogenesis and progression in multiple myeloma. *Br. J. Haematol.* **87**, 503–8.

Van Riet, I., Vanderkerken, K., de Greef, C. and Van Camp, B. (1998) Homing behaviour of the malignant cell clone in multiple myeloma. *Med. Oncol.* **15**, 154–64.

Vescio, R.A., Cao, J., Hong, C.H. *et al.* (1995) Myeloma Ig heavy chain V region sequences reveal prior antigenic selection and marked somatic mutation but no intraclonal diversity. *J. Immunol.* **155**, 2487–97.

Vesole, D., Simic, A. and Lazarus, H.M. (2001) Controversy in multiple myeloma transplants: tandem autotransplants and mini-allografts. *Bone Marrow Transplant* **28**, 725–35.

Wilder, R.B., Ha, C.S., Cox, J.D., Weber, D., Delasalle, K. and Alexanian, R. (2002) Persistence of myeloma protein for more than one year after radiotherapy is an adverse prognostic factor in solitary plasmacytoma of bone. *Cancer* **94**, 1323–37.

Yaccoby, S., Pearse, R.N., Johnson, C.L., Barlogie, B., Choi, Y. and Epstein, J. (2002) Myeloma interacts with the bone marrow microenvironment to induce osteoclastogenesis and is dependent on osteoclast activity. *Br. J. Haematol.* **116**, 278–90.

Zangari, M., Anaissie, E., Barlogie, B. *et al.* (2001) Increased risk of deep-vein thrombosis in patients with multiple myeloma receiving thalidomide and chemotherapy. *Blood* **98**, 1614–15.

Zandecki, M. (1996) Multiple myeloma: almost all patients are cytogenetically abnormal. *Br. J. Haematol.* **94**, 217–27.

47

Cancer in childhood

CORINNE HAYES, EDWARD J. ESTLIN, ANNABEL B.M. FOOT AND STEPHEN P. LOWIS

GENERAL INTRODUCTION

Paediatric tumours are all rare. Even the largest centre in the UK will see perhaps 150 new referrals each year, and many of these will have diverse histology. Even for the most common solid tumours – neuroblastoma, soft tissue and bone sarcomas, Wilms' tumour – the value of an individual centre adopting its own strategy is severely limited, and for this reason, combined, systematic treatment according to defined protocols has long been the aim in the UK, Europe and worldwide. The large majority of solid tumours have been treated according to national protocols for many years, and accurate data for survival has followed from these.

The ways in which a child or infant may present with a tumour may differ from adults, particularly for brain tumours. A suprasellar tumour, for example, may present with visual loss, but identification of this in an infant may prove difficult. Strabismus, abnormal ocular movements or being easily startled may be presenting features. Raised intracranial pressure may cause symptoms such as irritability and vomiting, but other effects include diencephalic syndrome, disturbance of sleep pattern and failing school achievement. These may go unrecognized.

Children differ greatly in their needs, developmental levels, and their physical and emotional maturity, and for this reason, a paediatric oncologist must be a paediatrician first: an understanding of the child must precede an understanding of their tumour. The majority of children with malignant disease will be cured, and for most, a long and relatively normal life can be expected. Follow-up of these patients should essentially be life long. The recognition of 'late' effects such as cardiac damage or second primary malignancy is dependent upon this.

To minimize the burden of survival, for the child and their family has long been important to paediatric oncologists, and an approach which differs from that needed for adult patients is sometimes evident. Delaying or sometimes omitting radiotherapy in young children with brain tumours or sarcomas is sometimes judged appropriate, even accepting a higher risk of relapse. Partly because of this, and because the majority of childhood tumours are chemosensitive, great reliance is placed upon chemotherapy. Children will often tolerate more intense chemotherapy than adults, and perhaps because consent for treatment comes from their parents, a greater degree of toxicity is often accepted. Chemotherapy regimens are often therefore intense, involving frequent or prolonged admission to hospital. Grades 3 and 4 toxicity to bone marrow in particular is commonplace.

Paediatric oncologists must work together with many other medical and non-medical individuals to act as a focus for the patient and co-ordinate services on their behalf (Table 47.1).

EPIDEMIOLOGY

The total incidence of childhood cancer (cancer in children less than 15 years of age) is about 1 per cent of that of the adult population. The total age-standardized annual incidence of childhood cancer in the UK has been measured at 118.3 per million children less than 15 years of age, with

Table 47.1 *Healthcare professionals involved with the paediatric oncology team*

Medical
Paediatric oncologist
Paediatrician in hospital or community
General practitioner and PHT
Surgeons – oncology, orthopaedic oncology,
    neurosurgeon, ENT, plastic, maxillo-facial as appropriate
Radiotherapist, supported by a team familiar with
    children, young people and their families
Pathologist, neuropathologist
Radiologist, supported by a team of radiographers
    familiar with children
Anaesthetist
Child psychiatrist
Endocrinologist
Other specialities (neurologist, cardiologist, respiratory
    paediatrician, ophthalmologist as appropriate)

Non-medical
Paediatric oncology, surgical and neurosurgical
    nursing teams
Specialist paediatric nursing teams in district hospitals
Paediatric oncology pharmacy support
Specialist social worker
Specialist play therapists
Specialist rehabilitation team – physiotherapists,
    occupational therapists
Paediatric dietitian
Audiometrist
Speech and language therapist
Clinical psychologist, educational psychologist or
    neuropsychologist

Adapted from 'Guidance for Services for Children and Young
People with Brain and Spinal Tumours' RCPCH, 1997
ISBN 1 900954 18 4.

Table 47.2 *Age-standardized incidence rates of the common childhood cancers*

Diagnostic group	Age-standardized incidence rates (per million per year)
Leukaemia	
Acute lymphoblastic	32.3
Acute non-lymphocytic	5.9
Lymphomas	
Hodgkin's disease	4.6
Non-Hodgkin's lymphoma	6.2
Central nervous system	
Astrocytoma	10.0
Primitive neuroectodermal tumour	6.0
Ependymoma	3.1
Sympathetic nervous system	
Neuroblastoma	8.1
Renal	
Wilms' tumour	7.6
Bone	
Osteogenic sarcoma	2.5
Ewing's tumour	2.3
Soft tissue sarcoma	
Rhabdomyosarcoma	5.2
Fibrosarcoma	1.0
Other tumours	
Retinoblastoma	3.7
Germ-cell tumours	3.6
Epithelial	3.0

Adapted from Stiller *et al.* (1995).

a risk of developing a malignancy in childhood of 1 in 581 (Stiller *et al.*, 1995). In the USA, there has been no substantial change in incidence for the major paediatric cancers since the mid-1980s, when modest increases, which probably reflected diagnostic improvements or reporting changes, were reported for central nervous system (CNS) tumours, leukaemia and infant neuroblastoma (Linet *et al.*, 1999). In the paediatric setting, the most frequently encountered diagnostic tumour groups are acute leukaemia, central nervous system tumours, lymphomas and soft tissue sarcomas (Table 47.2).

The incidence of overall and individual cancers can vary internationally. For example, the rate of childhood cancer in Ibadan, Nigeria is four times higher than that reported for the Indian population of Fiji (Robison, 1997). For acute lymphoblastic leukaemia, CNS tumours and neuroblastoma, higher rates are found in western Europe and the USA than Africa and Asia. Racial differences in the incidence of individual cancers within a single country are recognized, with acute leukaemia and Ewing's found more commonly in the white compared in the black

population of the USA. Overall, childhood cancer is more common in boys than girls (Robison, 1997).

Unlike cancer in adults, where the overwhelming majority of cancers are carcinomas which originate in epithelial surfaces, malignancy in children rarely takes the form of a carcinoma. In general, other than in leukaemia, most of the common forms of childhood cancer mimic developing or embryonal tissue development. For example, rhabdomyosarcoma and Wilms' tumour resemble developing myogenic mesenchyme and renal tissue, respectively. Moreover, certain childhood tumours, such as neuroblastoma and Wilms' tumour, are more common in the first 5 years of life (Stiller *et al.*, 1995), suggesting that many cases of childhood cancer represent gestation-related defects in tissue growth and differentiation. However, whereas CNS tumours and acute lymphoblastic leukaemia also have a higher incidence in early childhood, the peak incidence of Ewing's tumour, Hodgkin's disease and osteogenic sarcoma is found in early adolescence (Plon and Peterson, 1997).

Despite the histological features and age of onset of many childhood cancers, less than 5 per cent of cases are associated with a known genetic or cancer-predisposition syndrome. However, certain conditions are associated with an inherited predisposition to cancer (Plon and Peterson, 1997). For example, children with the constitutional chromosomal abnormality of Down's syndrome have a 20-fold increased risk of developing acute leukaemia during the first 10 years of life. Sex chromosomes abnormalities also confer a risk for developing certain malignancies. Any phenotypic female with part or all of a Y chromosome, such as testicular feminization syndrome and girls with mosaic 46 XO/XY Turner's syndrome, are at increased risk of gonadoblastoma. Similarly, males with Klinefelter's syndrome (47 XXY) are at risk of developing dysgerminomas.

The study of the genetic abnormalities found in childhood malignancies and the identification of certain cancer-predisposition genes is providing invaluable information for understanding of the pathogenesis of childhood cancer (Pritchard-Jones, 1996). For example, the inappropriate activation of normal growth promoting genes, or cellular proto-oncogenes, is increasingly recognized as playing a role in the pathogenesis of childhood cancers. An example of this is seen with the t(8,14) translocation found with Burkitt's lymphoma, where the c-*myc* gene is brought under the influence of immunoglobulin heavy chain enhancers at the breakpoint region on chromosome 14, which results in the inappropriate overexpression of this transcription factor. Alternatively, the functional inactivation of tumour suppressor genes can cause a cancer predisposition phenotype with autosomal recessive characteristics, and the example of the retinoblastoma tumour suppressor gene (*RB1*) on chromosome 13q14 has become a paradigm for the analysis of the inherited cancer-predisposition syndromes. For example, genetic predisposition to cancer is recognized in the Wilms'-aniridia-genitourinary abnormalities-retardation (WAGR) syndrome and the Beckwith–Wiedeman syndrome, where loss of the putative tumour suppressor genes *WT-1* (chromosome 11p13) and *WT-2* (chromosome 11p15), respectively, are associated with the development of Wilms' tumour. Similarly, the Li–Fraumeni syndrome, where there are germline mutations in the *p53* gene, is characterized by the familial clustering of multiple malignancies, including paediatric sarcomas, breast cancer, leukaemias, CNS tumours and adrenocortical carcinoma.

Other conditions that are known to predispose to childhood cancer include multiple endocrine neoplasia (MEN) 2, certain phakomatoses and disorders that are associated with defects in DNA replication or repair. Children with MEN 2A and the related MEN 2B are at risk of developing medullary thyroid carcinoma , and the molecular genetic studies suggest that these children may inherit a mutation of 10q11.2 which activates the *RET* oncogene (Plon and Peterson, 1997). Children with neurofibromatosis type 1 (NF-1) are at a risk of developing low-grade glioma, especially of the optic nerve/optic pathway, malignant peripheral nerve sheath tumours, rhabdomyosarcoma and acute myeloid leukaemia. Overall,

the incidence of NF-1 for children with cancer has been found to be six- to eightfold higher than the general population (Matsui *et al.*, 1993). Tuberous sclerosis, which is classically characterized by seizures, mental retardation and facial angiofibroma, is a phakomatous condition associated with the development of retinal hamartomas, giant cell astrocytomas, other CNS tumours and rhabdomyosarcoma (Narod *et al.*, 1991). Unlike tuberous sclerosis and NF-1, von Hippel–Lindau disease (VHL) is not associated with any specific dermatological or developmental abnormalities. Children with VHL are at increased risk of developing cerebellar haemangioblastoma, retinal haemangioma, renal cell carcinoma and phaeochromocytoma. Finally, children with DNA repair defects such as ataxia telangiectasia, Fanconi's anaemia and hereditary immunodeficiency diseases are known to be at increased risk for the development of leukaemia and lymphoma (Plon and Peterson, 1997).

Exogenous factors such as exposure to ultraviolet radiation and ionizing radiation are also associated with the development in malignancy in children. Most children with skin cancer are white and are genetically predisposed because of xeroderma pigmentosum, dysplastic naevoid syndrome or albinism. However, exposure to ultraviolet light in childhood is related to the development of malignant melanoma in later life (Plon and Peterson, 1997). Children are especially sensitive to ionizing radiation-induced leukaemia and thyroid cancer. At present, only weak evidence exists for an association between individual or paternal exposure to electromagnetic fields and various chemical carcinogens and cancer in childhood (Plon and Peterson, 1997).

In summary, epidemiological studies have played an important role in the clinical characterization of individual childhood cancers. Although the vast majority of childhood cancer occurs in children who do not have a predisposing factor, and the importance of environmental factors are largely uncertain, the identification of cancer predisposition syndromes has allowed the evolution of the molecular genetic characterization of diseases such as Wilms' tumour. Such information is providing an invaluable insight into the pathogenesis of childhood cancer.

SPECIFIC DISEASES

Childhood leukaemia

Childhood leukaemia is the commonest childhood malignancy accounting for around 35 per cent of all cases. Acute lymphoblastic leukaemia (ALL) is the commonest leukaemia in childhood, making up 75 per cent of cases. Acute myeloid leukaemia (AML) accounts for around 23 per cent of cases. The rest are mainly chronic myeloid leukaemia (CML) with chronic lymphocytic leukaemia (CLL) almost unheard of in children.

ACUTE LYMPHOBLASTIC LEUKAEMIA

Acute lymphoblastic leukaemia being the most common childhood leukaemia, has an annual incidence of 3.6 cases per 100 000. The peak incidence occurs between the ages of 2 and 6 years. As well as being the commonest childhood leukaemia, it also has the best outlook with more that 70 per cent of cases achieving sustained remission.

The French–American–British (FAB) classification of cell morphology describes three categories (LI, L2 and L3) but has limited clinical value. A number of factors have been postulated to have prognostic importance in childhood ALL. The current consensus from a number of clinical trials and working parties is that age, presenting white cell count, particular cytogenetic abnormalities and response to early treatment are the only reliable prognostic indicators (Table 47.3).

Treatment strategies for childhood ALL differ across the world. The BFM group pioneered the philosophy of 're-induction' (consolidation) showing emphatically that the increased toxicity was offset by better disease-free survival. There continues to be marked variation of drugs used, drug doses and timing of consolidation 'blocks'. Now that the survival figures are universally high, it is unlikely that in the context of a randomized trial any changes will produce significant improvement in outcome unless very large numbers of patients are amassed. To date there is no international consensus trial but a number of trials are attempting to answer the same questions. These questions include:

- Is dexamethasone superior to prednisolone? The Dutch Childhood Leukaemia Group substituted dexamethasone for prednisolone in a previous trial and found better event-free survival compared with their historical controls. Large randomized trials will

hopefully give greater clarity to this question particularly given concerns about the increased toxicity of dexamethasone.

- What is the best preparation and dose schedule of L-asparaginase. It is likely that both *in vivo* and *in vitro* studies will advocate change in practice.
- What is the role of cranial irradiation? Cranial radiotherapy was originally the standard approach, but because of its potential for damaging intellect and the hypothalamic-pituitary axis it is now reserved for children thought to be at highest risk. The best alternative CNS-directed therapy is still uncertain. Whether triple intrathecal therapy (adding cytarabine and hydrocortisone to methotrexate) rather than intrathecal methotrexate alone is beneficial is currently under evaluation in a number of studies.
- Is it possible to reduce toxicity without an adverse effect on outcome? Intensive re-induction schedules generally involve anthracyclines, alkylating agents and epidophyllotoxins. Whether particular drugs can be omitted to reduce toxicity without an adverse effect on outcome is being explored. In the first instance patients stratified as 'good risk' are targeted for reduced toxicity regimens. In the past this approach has failed, with high relapse rates, but the hope is that risk groups are now better defined.
- Is 6-thioguanine (6-TG) superior to 6-mercaptopurine (6-MP)? There is evidence from *in vitro* data that ALL cells are more sensitive to 6-TG than 6-MP. The differences in their metabolism mean that high concentrations of intracellular 6-TP nucleotides are more reliably achieved with 6-TG (Lennard *et al.*, 1993). The two drugs are currently under evaluation in a number of randomized trials.
- What is the role of minimal residual disease (MRD) studies? There are a number of molecular techniques for the detection of MRD in haematological malignancies with sensitivities of detection of the order of one malignant cell in 10^3–10^5. Further studies are required to compare differing methods with respect to sensitivity, specificity and reproducibility of results when processing large numbers of specimens. In addition, it is not clear what impact detection of MRD has on final outcome. The UK MRC ALL97 trial is collecting data on MRD prospectively with samples being collected at specified intervals to determine the significance of time of detection with respect to potential for intervention to alter outcome.
- What is optimal maintenance therapy? Maintenance treatment is based on oral antimetabolites and is more typical of an aggressive immunosuppressive programme than an antineoplastic chemotherapy schedule. Childhood ALL is unique among human cancers in requiring such an approach for its successful eradication but over the years all attempts to curtail maintenance have produced inferior results. Late relapses are often attributed to failed maintenance therapy.

Table 47.3 *Risk groups in childhood ALL*

Standard risk
>1, <10 years old; WBC <50 × 10^9/L; Absence of the Philadelphia chromosome, hypodiploidy (<45 chromosomes) or if 12–24 months old, an MLL gene rearrangement

Intermediate risk
>10 years old; WBC >50 × 10^9/L; Absence of the Philadelphia chromosome, hypodiploidy (<45 chromosomes) or if 12–24 months old, an MLL gene rearrangement

High risk
Presence of the Philadelphia chromosome, hypodiploidy (<45 chromosomes) or if 12–24 months old, an MLL gene rearrangement
All children irrespective of initial risk category who have a slow early response to treatment

MLL, mixed lineage leukaemia; WBC, white blood cells.

This may be due to developing resistance to anti-metabolites or problems with compliance. Given that treatment of childhood ALL takes up to 3 years it is understandable that compliance is a difficult area. Time needs to be spent with the child and their family explaining the rationale and importance of mainten-ance therapy (Chessells, 1995). Doctors need to be vigi-lant with regard to drug dosing and regular monitoring of blood counts.

Relapsed disease

The management of relapsed disease is dependent on the time of relapse. Relapses more than 48 months from the time of diagnosis can be salvaged with further chemother-apy and without the need for bone marrow transplant. There are more second relapses with conventional chemo-therapy but this is balanced out by the increased number of toxic deaths following bone-marrow transplantation (BMT). This may change in the future with the growing experience of paediatric BMT units resulting in better supportive care and reduced toxicity. Encouraging data from the Bristol paediatric BMT unit indicates that results are now comparable for matched sibling and unrelated donors (Oakhill *et al.*, 1996). Relapses earlier than 48 months from diagnosis are managed by consolidation with BMT but only after establishment of a second remission.

Summary

In general, the outlook for patients with childhood ALL is good. The aim is to cure the maximum number of patients with the minimum of toxicity. The number of survivors with unacceptable morbidity are far fewer than the number of children who relapse and cannot be salvaged. Whilst attempts are made to reduce toxicity, the major drive of current research is predicting those at risk of relapse and intensifying their treatment accordingly.

ACUTE MYELOID LEUKAEMIA

Overall the outlook is less optimistic for AML compared with ALL. There has, however, been marked improve-ment in outcome in the past two decades (R.F. Stevens *et al.*, 1998). Survival figures currently are nudging over 50 per cent. The morphology of childhood AML is similar to adult disease (Cline, 1994).

There are a number of predisposing factors for child-hood AML. Children with Down's syndrome have an approximately 20-fold increased risk of developing leukaemia. The types of leukaemia follow the usual dis-tribution of childhood leukaemia except that under the age of 3, M7 AML (megakaryoblastic) is the most com-mon. Neonates with trisomy 21 may develop a transient myeloproliferation which is morphologically identical to congenital leukaemia. Although this myeloproloferative syndrome regresses spontaneously within 1–3 months,

up to 30 per cent go on to develop true AML before the age of 3. Other syndromes associated with AML include Fanconi anaemia, Bloom syndrome, Kostmann syndrome, Li–Fraumeni syndrome and neurofibromatosis.

Prognostic indicators

There is no clear consensus as to the important prognos-tic indicators of childhood AML. The AML-BFM-83 allowed the identification of prognostic factors predict-ing relapse-free survival. Standard risk patients were those with the FAB types M1/M2 with Auer rods, M3 and M4 eo, responding to induction therapy; all other children (approximately 70 per cent) being high-risk patients. The UK AML-12 study defines three risk groups accord-ing to the results of the AML-10 study. Good risk patients are those with favourable karyotypic abnormalities. These are t(8;21), t(15;17) and inv(16) and these patients are good risk irrespective of their response to early treat-ment. Standard risk is any patient without a favourable karyotype but with not more than 20 per cent blasts in the marrow after first induction. Poor risk is determined by a poor response to early treatment.

Treatment

The introduction of cytosine arabinoside (Ara-C) in combination with anthracyclines for induction was a major breakthrough in the successful treatment of AML in children and adults (Creutzig *et al.*, 1990). Thereafter an increased disease-free survival has been observed in patients whose induction was intensified by early deliv-ery of a second induction 'block' (double induction) (Woods *et al.*, 1996).

The optimal intensity and duration of post-remission therapy is not clear. The use of high dose Ara-C with the goal of saturating cytarabine triphosphate (ara-CTP) formation and overcoming resistance of Ara-C has been explored in adults. It remains to be seen whether the increased remission rates outweigh the increased toxicity in children.

The duration of post-remission therapy varies con-siderably in different trials. In some studies maintenance therapy of up to 18 months is advocated. Others main-tain that the increased intensity of remission induction and post-remission induction makes long-term main-tenance less important (Wells *et al.*, 1994). It may be that certain groups will be selected for more or less treatment. Maintenance might be appropriate for those with slowly proliferating disease, responding slowly to treatment. The UK MRC AML-12 study compares four versus five courses of chemotherapy but patients with Down's syndrome who have a favourable outcome are not randomized and will only receive four courses.

CNS involvement occurs in only 5–10 per cent of patients with childhood AML. However, CNS-directed therapy is indicated in all paediatric AML patients. Early studies showed high (20–40 per cent) CNS relapse rates without CNS-directed therapy.

Daunorubicin is probably the most commonly used anthracycline in childhood AML. Cardiotoxicity is the major concern, particularly with higher cumulative doses. Reduced doses and alternative drugs such as mitoxantrone with less cardiotoxicity are currently under evaluation. Other drugs under scrutiny are 2-chlorodeoxyadenosine (2-CDA) and fludarabine. Fludarabine enhances ara-CTP formation given in combination with Ara-C and granulyte colony stimulating factor (G-CSF) in the FLAG regimen. These are other possible alternatives to the use of anthracyclines.

The indications for and appropriate timing of BMT are controversial in the treatment of childhood AML. BMT is not indicated for 'good risk' patients in first complete remission. The BFM group and the UK leukaemia working party both advocate BMT for higher risk groups in first complete remission only if there is a matched sibling donor. There is a clear indication for BMT in second complete remission and for those relapsing late (>18 months) there is a good outcome.

Detection of minimal residual disease (MRD) is an area of research in childhood AML as well as ALL. Early response to treatment can now be monitored by MRD studies. There is increasing evidence that slow early response to treatment as measured by MRD indicates a high probability of relapse. Future studies will evaluate the benefit of intensification of treatment in MRD-positive patients.

Summary

The improved outcome in childhood AML has arisen as a result of the intensification of treatment. This success has only been made possible by concomitant advances in supportive care. There is a high risk of tumour lysis at induction, of infections related to the long periods of bone marrow aplasia , bleeding and malnutrition. Accordingly, treatment should only be undertaken by specialist paediatric oncology units.

Hodgkin's disease

Hodgkin's Disease (HD) accounts for approximately 5 per cent of childhood malignancies with an incidence of 14 cases per 100 000 population aged less than 15 years. There is a male predominance more pronounced in the younger age group. HD is very unusual in under-5-year-olds in the Western world. In general it has a good prognosis and newer treatment strategies have the aim of maintaining the high cure rates with a reduction in toxicity.

Histologically paediatric HD is classified according to the Rye classification. Mixed cellularity type HD is more common in children than adults. Along with nodular sclerosing HD, these histological subtypes make up the majority of cases. The incidence of mixed cellularity HD decreases with higher socioeconomic class and has an association with Epstein–Barr Virus (EBV). Lymphocyte predominant HD carries a favourable prognosis compared with lymphocyte depleted, which has a poor prognosis. For these histological subtypes the differentiation from large cell anaplastic lymphoma can be difficult and raises concerns about appropriate treatment regimens. The European-American lymphoma classification (Harris et al., 1994) includes HD with immunological and genetic markers used to discriminate the various forms.

Currently all paediatric HD is treated in a similar manner until the impact of histology, genetics and immunophenotype is better understood.

Staging is according to the Ann Arbor classification. Standard staging investigations include chest X-ray and abdominal ultrasound. The additional value of magnetic resonance scanning (MRI) remains to be proven. Specific indications like extranodal spread into soft tissue seem to warrant MRI. The United Kingdom Children's Cancer Study Group currently recommends that the choice of computed tomography (CT)/MRI of chest and abdomen for each case be discussed with a paediatric radiologist.

Bone marrow aspirates and trephines are performed only on those patients with stage III/IV disease or B symptoms. In general though, paediatric patients are less likely to present with B symptoms compared with adult patients.

There is a differing relative emphasis on chemotherapy and radiotherapy amongst the international groups. The toxicity associated with radiotherapy has most impact in younger patient groups. They include soft tissue and bony undergrowth and thyroid impairment in neck disease. Chemotherapy-associated toxicity includes infertility in males and premature menopause in females, cardiac toxicity and the risk of secondary malignancy.

In the adult population, prognostic parameters are better defined for HD. The only factors verified in children are stage IV disease, B-type symptoms and the presence of a mediastinal mass or other bulky disease. Previously most groups stratified treatment into two groups, i.e. 'good risk' (stage I–IIIA) and 'poor risk' (stage IV or B symptoms with bulky disease). Now most groups are exploring criteria for stratification of an 'intermediate-risk' group. Stage IA disease is treated with radiotherapy alone in a number of protocols. The German approach is two cycles of chemotherapy and, if not in complete remission on re-evaluation, then radiotherapy is added. In the UK, additional chemotherapy is given to patients with bulky disease. Other groups are using B symptoms to direct treatment decisions.

Overall 5-year survival for stage I–IIIA disease is of the order of 90 per cent. Stage IV disease has a significantly poorer outcome. Survival figures from different groups using combination treatment vary from 60 to 79 per cent disease-free survival. Studies suggest that an initial poor response to treatment indicates an overall poor prognosis. Newer strategies are therefore directed according to early treatment response.

Treatment outcome data for relapsed or refractory HD are relatively limited due to the low number of treatment failures. There is a risk that this experience may grow as treatment for the better prognostic groups is reduced in an attempt to limit toxicity. In general, salvage treatments are alternative chemotherapeutic agents to those used in primary treatment with radiotherapy. High-dose chemotherapy with stem cell rescue is reserved for poor prognostic groups such as progressive disease on treatment and early second relapse.

Non-Hodgkin's lymphoma

Non Hodgkin's lymphoma (NHL) has an annual incidence of 7 cases per million children. There is a male predominance and the peak incidence between the ages of 7 and 10 years. The prognosis has improved dramatically in recent decades with the overall cure rate being more than 75 per cent. Burkitt's lymphoma is endemic in Africa and has an association with EBV. Certain immunodeficiency syndromes such as ataxia telangiectasia, Wiskott–Aldrich and acquired immunodeficiency secondary to acquired immunodeficiency syndrome (AIDS) or post-transplant procedures are associated with NHL.

There are various classifications of NHL. In 1994 the 'Revised European American classification of Lymphoid neoplasms' (REAL) was devised (Harris *et al.*, 1994) and has been accepted by the Société française d'Oncologie Pédiatrique (SFOP), the United Kingdom Children's Cancer Study Group (UKCCSG) and the United States Children's Cancer Group (USCCG) (Table 47.4). Classification takes account of morphology and immunophenotyping. Morphology alone is prone to marked variation (Armitage and Weisenburger, 1998).

In childhood NHL the commonest pathological subtypes are Burkitt's and lymphoblastic, accounting for 70–80 per cent of cases.

BURKITT'S LYMPHOMA

Burkitt's lymphoma is characterized by a translocation involving the long arm of chromosome 8. The oncogene c-*myc* moves from its normal position on chromosome 8 and is rearranged with the gene for heavy chain immunoglobulin. Transcriptional deregulation of the c-*myc* gene is thought to play a crucial role in the genesis of this malignancy (Croce and Nowell, 1985). Endemic Burkitt's frequently involves the face. Non-endemic Burkitt's is not associated with EBV and tends to present with abdominal disease with frequent bone marrow involvement. In general, Burkitt's lymphoma tends to disseminate early into both bone marrow and the CNS. In spite of this, the prognosis is excellent with overall cure rates of more than 90 per cent. Current protocols attempt to identify prognostic groups and limit treatment-associated toxicity to the good prognosis groups. Poor prognostic indicators are CNS disease, elevated lactate dehydrogenase (LDH) and poor response to early treatment. Treatment for these groups is with high-toxicity protocols, generally with grade IV haematological toxicity and severe mucositis. Success with these protocols is dependent on rigorous supportive care in specialist paediatric oncology units.

TREATMENT STRATEGIES FOR NHL

In general, treatment strategies are stratified into three groups, mature B-cell, T-cell and anaplastic large cell lymphoma (ALCL).

Burkitt's, Burkitt's-like and diffuse large cell B-cell lymphomas are all treated on CHOP-based (cyclophosphamide, doxorubicin, vincristine and prednisolone) regimens. Protocols give differing doses of alkylating agents, anthracyclines and differing CNS-directed treatment. There is concern that some patients with less advanced disease are being overtreated. The FAB collaboration (FAB 96) as a result advocate only two courses of chemotherapy (cyclophosphamide, prednisolone, doxorubicin and vincristine) for stage I or completely resected abdominal disease. In the same study, treatment has been reduced for unresected stage II and stage III disease by reducing the cumulative dose of cyclophosphamide. At the other end of the spectrum there is evidence that dose intensification improves outcome in stage IV B-cell disease (Patte *et al.*, 1986). The role of megatherapy in B-cell disease remains unclear. Relapsed stage I and II disease is salvageable with additional cycles of conventional chemotherapy. Megatherapy using BEAM (BCNU, etoposide, cytosine arabinoside and melphalan) is reserved for relapse of more advance disease or disease poorly responsive to conventional doses. Relapsed stage IV disease is virtually incurable except for isolated CNS relapse.

T-cell disease and precursor lymphoblastic B-cell disease are treated using leukaemia protocols. It is more difficult to identify prognostic groups in the same way as ALL. The majority of patients with T-cell disease have mediastinal involvement. If the chest X-ray is not normal after induction and early intensification, then this identifies a poor prognostic group and treatment thereafter is intensified. Relapsed disease follows a similar pattern to relapsed ALL. Early relapse (less than 24 months from diagnosis) is difficult to cure. Allogeneic BMT is advocated in these patients but only after a second remission has been achieved. Involved field radiotherapy is unlikely to be helpful.

Table 47.4 *REAL classification*

Burkitt's
High-grade B-cell, Burkitt's-like
Precursor B-lymphoblastic
Precursor T-lymphoblastic
Diffuse large B-cell
Anaplastic large cell
Peripheral T-cell, unspecified

Adapted from Harris *et al.* (1994).

Table 47.5 *Prognostic grouping in anaplastic large cell lymphoma*

Group A	Completely resected localized disease
Group B 'good risk'	No skin or mediastinal involvement Non-lymphohistiocytic variant
Group C 'poor risk'	Any one of the following: biopsy proven skin lesions (unless completely excised = group A); mediastinal or lung involvement; lymphohistiocytic variant
Group D	CNS involvement

Anaplastic large cell lymphoma (ALCL) only accounts for around 10 per cent of childhood NHL. The presence of CD30 and EMA (epithelial membrane antigen) positivity is characteristic of ALCL. In addition the t(2;5) translocation is specific to ALCL. Before these advances in immunophenotyping and cytogenetics, ALCL was commonly mistaken for tumours such as Hodgkin's disease, malignant histiocytosis and peripheral T-cell lymphoma. Localized tumours are rare and CNS disease is exceptional. B-type symptoms are common. Staging according to conventional systems is not helpful. Instead ALCL is stratified according to histology and site of disease (Table 47.5).

Given that CNS disease is rare, it is unclear whether CNS-directed treatment is necessary in groups A, B and C. Previous BFM and UKCCSG trials have included intrathecal therapy whereas the SFOP and Italian groups omitted it with no reported cases of CNS relapse. The combined UKCCSG/SFOP study includes high-dose methotrexate ($3 \, \text{g/m}^2$) in all treatment regimens whilst intrathecal therapy and higher-dose methotrexate ($8 \, \text{g/m}^2$) is reserved for patients with CNS involvement. The same study has included weekly vinblastine for one year in those patients in the poor risk group. This is based on the findings of the French group that 10 patients in relapse (some third and fourth relapses) achieved long periods of complete remission with weekly vinblastine for 6–24 months. The role of high-dose chemotherapy and radiotherapy in ALCL remain unclear.

Low-grade NHL is rare in children. There were only seven of a total of 447 childhood NHL cases in the UKCCSG national registry. It tends to present as localized disease whereby surgery alone may be curative. More advanced disease responds to both chemotherapy and radiotherapy with 94 per cent 5-year even-free survival (EFS) reported by the St Jude's series.

In summary, many advances have been made in the classification and treatment of childhood NHL. Improved outcomes have resulted from careful patient selection to avoid unnecessary toxicity and good supportive care

of those poor-risk patients undergoing more intensive regimens.

Tumours of the central nervous system

EPIDEMIOLOGY

As a group, CNS tumours represent the second most frequent malignancy in children under the age of 15 years, with an approximate annual incidence in the USA of 2.8 cases per 100 000 children per year (Heideman *et al.*, 1997). Within the first 10 years of life, a predominance of embryonal CNS neoplasms is found, with a relative absence of gliomas. After early adolescence there is an increase in the incidence of typically adult CNS tumours. The WHO classification for paediatric CNS tumours (Table 47.6) recognizes both traditional morphological entities and degree of anaplasia, as well as providing for the designation of location within the CNS (Rorke *et al.*, 1985).

CLINICAL PRESENTATION

The clinical presentation of children with CNS tumours varies considerably with age, development and the site of origin of the tumour. Infratentorial (brainstem and cerebellar) tumours may present with disturbances of truncal steadiness, upper extremity co-ordination and gait and cranial nerve function. Children with supratentorial tumours may present with features of raised intracranial pressure, irritability, seizures, regression of developmental milestones and upper motor neuron signs such as hemiparesis. Tumours of the optic chiasm may result in visual field defects such as a bitemporal hemianopia, nystagmus and head tilt. In addition, hypothalamic tumours may give rise to the diencephalic syndrome (failure to thrive, euphoria and hyperactivity), and endocrine disorders such as diabetes insipidus, hypogonadism and precocious puberty (Cokgor *et al.*, 1998). MRI scanning is now the investigation of choice for tumours of the central nervous system in childhood.

GLIAL TUMOURS

Glial tumours are classified as grade I (pilocytic astrocytoma), grade II (fibrillary astrocytoma), grade III (anaplastic astrocytoma) and grade IV (glioblastoma multiforme). The designation of a glial tumour as low grade (I and II) and high grade (II and IV) carries an important impact in terms of both treatment and prognosis (Cokgor *et al.*, 1998).

Low-grade gliomas

In their review of a decade of experience at St Jude Children's Research Hospital, Gajjar *et al.* (1997) found low-grade gliomas to arise from the cerebral hemispheres (20 per cent), cerebellar hemispheres (35 per cent), hypothalamus (12 per cent), thalamus (12 per cent), brainstem (12 per cent), spinal cord (4 per cent) and

Table 47.6 *WHO classification of paediatric CNS tumours*

Glial tumours	Neuronal tumours	Primitive neuroectodermal tumours (PNET)	Pineal cell tumours
Astrocytic astrocytoma	Gangliocytoma	PNET not otherwise specified	Pineocytoma
Anaplastic astrocytoma	Ganglioglioma	PNET with differentiation (astrocytic, ependymal, neuronal)	Pineoblastoma (PNET)
Subependymal giant cell tumour	Anaplastic ganglioglioma	Medulloepithelioma	
Giant cell glioma			
Oligodendroglioma			
Anaplastic oligodendroglioma			
Ependymoma			
Anaplastic ependymoma			
Myxopapillary ependymoma			
Choroid plexus papilloma			
Anaplastic choroid plexus tumour			
Mixed gliomas			
Glioblastoma multiforme			

optic nerve/chiasm (3 per cent). Although the median age at diagnosis was 7 years, 32 per cent of children were younger than 5 years at diagnosis. In addition, although the overall 4-year survival rate was 90 per cent at 4 years, children below the age of 5 years had a poorer progression-free survival (PFS) than those diagnosed after the age of 5 years, and this difference was most pronounced in children with hypothalamic or thalamic tumours.

Surgery is the mainstay of therapy for low-grade glioma of the cerebral hemispheres (Pollack *et al.*, 1995) or cerebellum (Gajjar *et al.*, 1997), with radiotherapy or chemotherapy being reserved for recurrent or progressive inoperable disease. Although there have been no randomized trials to compare radiotherapy and observation alone for residual tumours (Cokgor *et al.*, 1998), local field radiotherapy, at a dose of 54 Gy administered over 30 fractions is generally used for incompletely resected and progressive low-grade glioma.

For tumours of the optic chiasm/hypothalamus, curative surgery is not usually possible, and surgery is usually indicated to debulk symptomatic tumours, relieve obstruction at the foramen of Monro and to obtain a diagnostic biopsy. Fifty per cent of children with optic chiasm/hypothalamus tumours present before the age of 5 years, and although approximately 33 per cent of these children have NF-1 and a more indolent course, the majority of cases progress within 6 years of diagnosis (Janss *et al.*, 1995). Chemotherapy with vincristine and carboplatin been shown to be effective in controlling disease progression at this site, thereby postponing radiotherapy until after the age of 5 years in the majority of cases (Janss *et al.*, 1995).

High-grade gliomas
High-grade gliomas comprise 7–11 per cent of childhood CNS tumours (Heideman *et al.*, 1997). The vast majority are supratentorial, with 63 per cent occurring in the superficial cerebral hemisphere, 28 per cent in the midline cerebrum, and 8 per cent in the posterior fossa (Wishoff *et al.*, 1998). Unlike adult high-grade gliomas, very few of these tumours in children demonstrate *p53* mutation, loss of heterozygosity (LOH) for chromosome 10 and amplification of epidermal growth factor receptor (Cokgor *et al.*, 1998).

The prognosis for high-grade glioma has been shown to relate to the extent of surgical resection (Wishoff *et al.*, 1998). Thus, for children with anaplastic astrocytoma, 5-year PFS rates of 44 per cent and 22 per cent were observed for children achieving a radical resection and less extensive resection, respectively. Similarly, for children with glioblastoma multiforme (GBM), 5-year PFS rates of 26 per cent and 5 per cent were observed for children achieving a radical resection and less extensive resection, respectively.

The role of chemotherapy in the management of high-grade glioma in children is uncertain at present. Sposto *et al.* (1989) reported an increase in 5-year EFS for children with GBM who had been randomized to receive radiotherapy plus lomustine (CCNU), vincristine and prednisone (42 per cent) versus radiotherapy alone (6 per cent), provided the tumour had been at least partially resected. For the follow-on study, CCG-1945, no difference was found in the survival of children randomized to receive either chemotherapy with the eight-in-one regimen or CCNU, vincristine and prednisone as an adjunct to radiotherapy. However, the overall 5-year EFS rate of 36 per cent found with either regimen is thought to have been superior to historical controls treated with radiotherapy alone (Finlay *et al.*, 1995). Similarly, the benefit of high-dose chemotherapy with thiotepa and etoposide for the treatment of children with high-grade glioma at presentation or relapse remains uncertain, but may play a role where a complete remission is achieved prior to high-dose therapy (Cokgor *et al.*, 1998).

Tumours arising in the midbrain, pons and medulla oblongata account for 10–20 per cent of all childhood CNS tumours, and usually present in children between the ages of 5 and 9 years (Heideman *et al.*, 1997). High-grade gliomas of the brainstem are chemoresistant, and although clinical improvement is observed in the majority of children with 54 Gy radiotherapy, the tumours have an extremely poor prognosis (Cokgor *et al.*, 1998).

Ependymomas

Ependymoma accounts for 6–12 per cent of CNS tumours in childhood, with 50 per cent of cases occurring before the age of 5 years (Bouffet *et al.*, 1998b). Ependymomas develop from the neuroepithelial lining of the ventricles and central canal of the spinal cord and are classified as subependymoma and myxopapillary ependymoma (grade I tumour), low-grade ependymoma (grade II) and anaplastic ependymoma (grade III). However, the relationship between tumour anaplasia and prognosis is uncertain (Bouffet *et al.*, 1998b). The clinical presentation of ependymoma is usually due to the signs and symptoms of raised intracranial pressure (ICP), although posterior fossa ependymomas commonly adhere to and invade the brainstem, causing palsies of cranial nerves VI–X.

Surgical resection is the mainstay of therapy for ependymoma. For children with supratentorial tumours, a complete resection is possible for approximately 50 per cent of cases, which compares with only 30 per cent for children with infratentorial tumours (Bouffet *et al.*, 1998b). The extent of surgical resection has been found to be an important determinant of prognosis for children receiving postoperative local radiotherapy for ependymoma. For children with no imagable disease, postoperatively the 5-year PFS of 60–70 per cent compares with 5–10 per cent for children with residual disease (Perilongo *et al.*, 1997). Although no randomized study has been conducted to measure the benefit of radiotherapy in the treatment of ependymoma, local radiotherapy remains the standard postoperative treatment for this tumour (Bouffet *et al.*, 1998b).

The role of chemotherapy in the treatment of ependymomas remains unknown, and there are no reports that indicate a survival advantage for chemotherapy when compared with historical controls, or patients receiving radiotherapy alone (Bouffet *et al.*, 1998b). However, encouraging pilot results have been obtained with the use of carboplatin, vincristine, ifosfamide and etoposide in addition to radiotherapy (Needle *et al.*, 1997). As with high-grade glioma, there is no clear role for high-dose chemotherapy in the treatment of ependymoma (Bouffet *et al.*, 1998b).

Other glial tumours

Two recently described glial tumours include the dysembryoplastic neuroepithelial tumour and the desmoplastic

infantile ganglioglioma. These tumours have limited growth potential and tend to occur in infants and young children, and the tumours may cause intractable epilepsy if they arise in the frontal or temporal lobes (Cokgor *et al.*, 1998).

PRIMITIVE NEUROECTODERMAL TUMOUR (PNET)

Primitive neuroectodermal tumour (PNET) is the most common malignant primary brain tumour of childhood, comprising approximately 30–40 per cent of such tumours and affecting 0.5 per 100 000 children each year. The peak incidence is at the age of 7 years, although cases are reported up to late adult life. There is a slight male preponderance. The most common site is in the posterior fossa, and such tumours are referred to as medulloblastoma or PNET-MB. Biologically these are not different from supratentorial PNET or pineal parenchymal tumours (pineoblastoma), although the prognosis for medulloblastoma is generally better than at other sites.

Presentation

Clinical features relate to the site of the tumour and often include truncal ataxia and signs of raised intracranial pressure.

The majority of tumours are in the posterior fossa, involving the cerebellar vermis. Spread is by local invasion, to the cerebellar peduncle, floor of the fourth ventricle, and cervical spine. Occasionally, rostral extension is seen. Involvement of brainstem may give rise to cranial nerve palsies. Brainstem involvement has been reported to carry an adverse outcome, relating to the difficulty in attaining a complete surgical excision. Spread may also be through the CSF, and leptomeningeal deposits are seen in approximately 30 per cent of patients.

Assessment

The primary tumour may be imaged by CT or better, MRI, and appears as a solid, often homogeneously enhancing mass. All patients should have imaging of the spinal cord and whole brain by gadolinium-enhanced MRI: the entire spine must be imaged in at least two planes. Preoperative assessment is preferred to postoperative, but an interval of no more than 72 hours after operation is generally agreed to be acceptable in the assessment of metastatic disease. Lumbar puncture has been shown to have a higher diagnostic value than ventricular CSF sampling, and an attempt to obtain lumbar CSF should be made before treatment commences. Initial tumour assessment is of importance in stratification of patients into standard or high-risk groups, for which outcome is significantly different.

Dissemination is the most powerful adverse prognostic marker, but in addition, younger age at diagnosis, subtotal resection and a supratentorial tumour indicate a likely poor outcome (Packer *et al.*, 1985; Evans *et al.*, 1990). The prognostic importance of brainstem involvement is still being debated. Patients with poor risk are children younger than 3 years of age or those with metastatic disease and/or subtotal resection and/or non-posterior fossa location. As for all tumours, these prognostic variables must be evaluated in the context of the treatment received.

Pathology

PNET is a highly malignant embryonal tumour of the CNS, with the capacity for differentiation along diverse pathways. The cell of origin is debated, but may be subependymal. Cells appear as undifferentiated round cells, but may mark with antibodies to synaptophysin, vimentin, glial fibrillary acidic protein (GFAP), neural cell adhesion molecules (NCAMs), retinal S-antigen and the low-affinity (p75-) nerve growth factor (NGF) receptor.

Desmoplastic PNET is said to have a more favourable prognosis than classical PNET, possibly because it is more lobulated and therefore more readily removed, although this is not in itself used to stratify therapy.

Molecular and cytogenetics

Approximately 50 per cent of patients demonstrate isochromosome 17q, with a consequent loss of 17p. LOH 17p has been localized to the region 17p13.3, and a candidate gene affected is the hypermethylated in cancer (HIC)-1 gene, but this remains unproven. Other associated genes in medullobastoma include PAX5 and PAX6 and the PTCH genes.

Therapy

Standard therapy for PNET-MB involves initial stabilization of the patient, which may require external ventricular drainage, and surgical resection. Complete surgical resection is a positive feature, but aggressive resection is not recommended where this would lead to increased morbidity. Postoperative craniospinal radiotherapy is almost always recommended, and attempts to avoid radiotherapy completely in 'at-risk' groups such as infants have been associated with poor outcomes. Less than 10 per cent of PNET-MB will be cured with conventional chemotherapy, whereas long-term disease-free survival of between 55 and 70 per cent is reported with craniospinal radiotherapy and local tumour boost. In poor-risk disease, chemotherapy improves survival (Packer et al., 1985; Evans et al., 1990; Packer, 1990) and in recent years there has been increasing acceptance of chemotherapy for patients with metastatic disease.

The value of chemotherapy is less well defined for patients with localized, completely resected disease, although Packer reported 5-year disease-free survival of 90 per cent for such patients treated with standard radiotherapy and a prolonged (48-week) course of chemotherapy with cisplatin, CCNU and vincristine (Packer et al., 1994). By contrast, the Société Internationale Oncologie Pédiatrique (SIOP) first study (CCNU, vincristine) showed no benefit for localized disease, although a benefit for chemotherapy was seen for patients with partial or sub-total surgery ($P = 0.007$), brainstem involvement ($P = 0.001$), and stage T3 and T4 disease ($P = 0.002$) (Tait et al., 1990).

In the second SIOP study, no benefit from pre-radiotherapy chemotherapy (with vincristine, procarbazine and methotrexate given in a 6-week module) was seen for any group. In addition, a particularly poor outcome was seen for those children receiving chemotherapy and reduced-dose radiotherapy (Bailey et al., 1995).

The adverse long-term consequences of radiotherapy, particularly in young children, are potentially profound, and attempts have been made to reduce overall radiation doses used (Packer et al., 1985; Deutsch et al., 1991; Bailey et al., 1995; Goldwein et al., 1996; Packer, 1999). Whilst some studies have found non-significant differences when patients received reduced-dose radiotherapy, more generally, there is a trend towards increasing rates of relapse. A combined Children's Cancer Study Group/ Pediatric Oncology Group (CCSG/POG) study of craniospinal radiotherapy to a dose of 23.4 versus 36 Gy (without chemotherapy) was halted prematurely because of a statistically significant difference in early relapse of good prognosis patients. Reduced-dose radiotherapy with adjuvant chemotherapy may avoid an increased rate of relapse. This was not the case in the second SIOP study (Bailey et al., 1995), but encouraging results have been reported by others (Goldwein et al., 1996; Packer, 1999).

Infant PNET

The treatment of young children with PNET is more problematic than for older children, given the adverse consequences of craniospinal radiotherapy at this age. Attempts to eliminate radiotherapy have for the most part been unsuccessful, with relapse-free survival of 10 per cent at best, whilst survival of infants with metastatic PNET treated with craniospinal radiotherapy approaches 40 per cent. There is, therefore, an ethical dilemma in the choice of therapy, which the physician cannot make alone.

The chemosensitivity of PNET has lead to the development of high-dose and high-dose-intensity regimens, but as yet these include small patient numbers. Studies of high-dose therapy with busulphan and thiotepa are hopeful, albeit with severe toxicity (Dupuis-Girod et al., 1996).

Relapsed PNET

Recurrent PNET is rarely curable, and median survival is generally less than one year (Torres et al., 1994; Bouffet et al., 1998a). There does seem to be a role for high-dose therapy in such patients, however, provided tumour remission can be achieved (Graham et al., 1997; Dunkel et al., 1998).

The value of hyperfractionated radiotherapy remains unclear, but this approach will form at least part of the next SIOP study (Prados et al., 1999).

CHOROID PLEXUS PAPILLOMA AND CARCINOMA

Tumours of the choroid plexus epithelium are very rare, accounting for 0.5 per cent of all CNS tumours. The differentiation between papilloma and carcinoma is not clear cut, but papilloma is defined as grade I, carcinoma as grade III. Atypical tumours are described, and there is evidence of increasing malignancy with time (Chow *et al.*, 1999). There has been considerable interest in the possible role of SV40 virus in the development of choroid plexus carcinoma. SV40-like DNA was found in 10 of 20 tumours in the series of Bergsagel *et al.* (1992) and transgenic mice expressing the early region of SV40 develop choroid plexus tumours with high frequency (Brinster *et al.*, 1984; Cho *et al.*, 1989). Malignant atypical teratoid/rhabdoid tumours may show differentiation towards choroid plexus carcinoma, and there are reports of choroid plexus carcinoma in families with Li–Fraumeni syndrome, and with mutations in *hSNF5/INI1*.

Maximum surgical clearance is thought to be of prognostic value (Pierga *et al.*, 1993; Berger *et al.*, 1998). Radiotherapy is associated with improved survival (Wolff *et al.*, 1999), but for many patients diagnosed at a young age, this may be an unacceptable modality. Chemotherapy has been reported to be effective in small series, allowing delay or even omission of radiotherapy altogether (Duffner *et al.*, 1995). Potentially active agents include bleomycin, cisplatin, carboplatin, cyclophosphamide, etoposide, vincristine, procarbazine.

Overall survival in patients with completely resected choroid plexus papilloma is at least 80 per cent. For patients with carcinoma, Wolff reported survival of 68 per cent with radiotherapy, and 12 per cent without radiotherapy. Overall survival including patients without total surgical resection is approximately 25 per cent.

CRANIOPHARYNGIOMA

Craniopharyngioma is a benign tumour, believed to arise from epithelial remnants of Rathke's pouch and typically seen in the sellar and suprasellar region. They comprise approximately 6–9 per cent of primary brain tumours, most presenting before the age of 20 years. The median age of presentation is 8 years, and presentation below 2 years of age is rare.

Clinical presentation is usually with raised intracranial pressure, and approximately 50 per cent show hydrocephalus. Visual defects, hypothalamic dysfunction and pituitary hormone deficits, principally growth hormone and diabetes insipidus, are commonly found, and should be anticipated preoperatively. Craniopharyngioma is typically slow growing, and large tumours causing marked visual loss may be found.

MR imaging typically shows a mixed signal with T_1 weighting: hyperintense cystic components and isointense solid components. CT typically shows calcification and variable enhancement. The tumour is often lobulated, and may extend anteriorly, posteriorly or inferiorly.

Treatment of craniopharyngioma is primarily surgical, and complete surgical resection is associated with a low (10 per cent) local recurrence rate, and 70 per cent long-term disease-free survival (DFS). For residual disease

in excess of 5 cm in diameter, the prognosis is worse, with overall survival (OS) of less than 50 per cent at 10 years. The large majority of such tumours recur within 2–5 years unless radiotherapy is included in initial treatment. Radical attempts to remove tumours completely are never indicated, causing unacceptable neurological and endocrine sequelae.

The sequelae of craniopharyngioma may be severe, affecting not only vision and endocrine function (DeVile *et al.*, 1996), but behaviour and mood (Anderson *et al.*, 1997), memory (Cavazzuti *et al.*, 1983), control of thirst and hunger, and abilities to perform problem-solving tasks. To some extent these may be minimized with primary conservative surgery and radiotherapy (Cavazzuti *et al.*, 1983).

Atypical teratoid rhabdoid tumours (ATTRhT)

Atypical teratoid rhabdoid tumours are rare embryonal tumours showing some similarities to renal rhabdoid tumour of infancy. This is complicated by the fact that there is an association of renal rhabdoid tumours with other CNS embryonal tumours, e.g. PNET, and by the presence within ATTRhTs of areas showing differentiation towards neuroectodermal tumour, sarcoma or carcinoma (Rorke *et al.*, 1995). In addition, 60 per cent show an abnormality of chromosome 22, and more recently, mutations in the gene *hSNF5/INI1* have been identified in this and other tumours (Sevenet *et al.*, 1999). Familial cases have been reported, and Figure 47.1 was of an infant with ATTRhT who had siblings with choroid plexus carcinoma and a renal rhabdoid tumour.

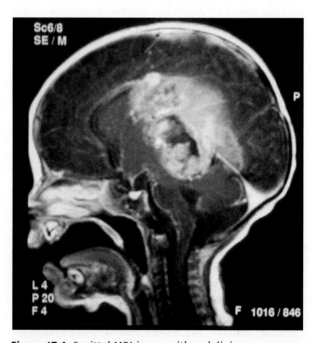

Figure 47.1 *Sagittal MRI image with gadolinium enhancement of a patient with a primary atypical teratoid rhabdoid tumour. The tumour appears to have arisen in the posterior fossa and eroded through the tentorium.*

Tumours arise in all parts of the CNS, and spread contiguously or by dissemination: approximately one-third are metastatic at diagnosis. These are highly malignant tumours, and can spread through dense fibrous structures such as tentorium.

ATTRhTs typically present in early childhood, median age 20 months, and show a preponderence of males (M : F; 1.6 : 1).

Prognosis

In the series reported by Rorke *et al.* (1996), median time to progression was 4.5 months, and median OS was 6 months. Occasional long-term survivors have been reported, although no systematic study of therapy has been reported.

CNS TUMOURS IN INFANTS AND YOUNG CHILDREN

Approximately 12–15 per cent of all childhood CNS tumours occur in children less than 2 years of age, and two-thirds of these are supratentorial in location (Heideman *et al.*, 1997). The predominant histological diagnoses are medulloblastoma-PNET (30–40 per cent), ependymoma (8–28 per cent) and low-grade gliomas (21–36 per cent) and malignant glioma (15 per cent). Because infants and very young children with CNS tumours are at risk of catastrophic long-term intellectual sequelae if radiotherapy is administered at such an early age, chemotherapy schedules have been investigated with the aim of delaying, or even avoiding, radiotherapy.

Duffner *et al.* (1993) described effective postoperative chemotherapy with cyclophosphamide/vincristine and cisplatin/etoposide that delayed the need for radiotherapy in a significant number of cases. The overall PFS was 33 per cent at 2 years, and children with medulloblastoma, ependymoma and malignant glioma fared better than children with supratentorial PNET. Moreover, a PFS of approximately 45 per cent has also been described for children with anaplastic astrocytoma who received treatment with the eight-in-one regimen prior to planned radiotherapy (Geyer *et al.*, 1995). This indicates that chemotherapy may confer considerable benefit for this group of patients even without radiotherapy. However, the survival of infants with medulloblastoma and PNET remains poor without radiotherapy.

Retinoblastoma

Retinoblastoma is the most common intraocular tumour of childhood with an incidence of approximately 1 in 20 000 live births. Presentation is before the age of 5 in 95 per cent of cases. The majority of cases are confined to the eye and have an excellent prognosis; spread outside the globe is associated with a dismal prognosis. Overall though, cure rates are in excess of 90 per cent. There are two forms: genetic (hereditary) and non-genetic (non-hereditary).

The genetic form is generally multi-focal and is associated with an increased incidence of other malignancies (osteosarcoma, small cell carcinoma of the lung, breast and bladder). The human retinoblastoma susceptibility gene (*Rb1*) is situated on the long arm of chromosome 13. The D-deletion syndrome in 5 per cent of patients with retinoblastoma is associated with a constitutional deletion of the long arm of chromosome 13. Features are retinoblastoma, mental retardation, failure to thrive and facial dysmorphism.

Presentation may be an abnormal white reflex (leucocoria), strabismus and more occasionally deteriorating vision. Staging investigations are not generally indicated for small intraocular tumours. For more extensive disease investigations include cytological examination of CSF, CT scan of head and orbits and cytogenetic studies to exclude defects of chromosome 13.

The aim of treatment is to preserve vision without compromising survival. In spite of retinoblastoma being a radiosensitive tumour, this modality of treatment is avoided in infancy unless it is felt to be the only option. A number of chemotherapy protocols are currently under evaluation. In view of its biological similarity to other neuroectodermal tumours, multi-drug combinations containing platinum have been used with some success. There are a number of techniques available for focal therapy. These include photocoagulation, cryotherapy, radioactive plaques and diode lasers. There is a risk of vitreous seeding with photocoagulation. External-beam radiotherapy is used for larger tumours where vitreous seeding has occurred. The late effects of radiotherapy include cataract formation, 'dry eye syndrome' and asymmetry of orbital growth. Enucleation is mandatory where there is involvement of the optic nerve, extrascleral extension or conservative treatment fails.

Neuroblastoma

Neuroblastoma, accounting for 6–8 per cent of all paediatric malignancy, is predominantly a disease of early childhood. It is the most common malignant disease of infancy, has a median age of presentation of 2 years, and is rarely encountered over the age of 10 years. There is a slight increased incidence in boys (M : F; 1.2 : 1) and up to 70 per cent of children present with metastatic disease.

The aetiology of the condition remains unknown. It has been associated with other neural crest lesions such as neurofibromatosis and Hirschsprung's disease, and familial cases are recognized although infrequent. A pertinent observation is the high incidence of neuroblastoma *in situ*, microscopic nodules of neuroblasts within the adrenals found exclusively in fetuses and infants. This may be a normal part of embryonic adrenal development which regresses in health but persists in disease, i.e. that a dysregulation of cellular differentiation plays a part in the aetiology.

There have undoubtedly been many advances in the understanding of various aspects of this disease over recent years, with the recognition of prognostic variables and moves towards stratification of treatment. This tumour group as a whole, however, ranging from the undifferentiated neuroblastoma to mature ganglioneuroma, continues to fascinate scientists and clinicians alike. On the one hand it demonstrates not only both spontaneous and induced maturation but also the ability to undergo spontaneous regression. On the other hand, however, it still has one of the poorest outcomes overall in the case of metastatic disease accounting for 15 per cent of all deaths in children from cancer.

CLINICAL FEATURES

Symptoms at presentation are extremely variable. The tumour arises from neural crest cells, which migrate to form the adrenal medulla and sympathetic chain, thus the primary can arise from cranium to pelvis. An adrenal (50 per cent) or abdominal (25 per cent) primary is more frequent in older children, whereas infants have a high incidence of thoracic (33 per cent) tumours. A common presentation is with obstructive symptoms such as respiratory embarrassment, and local invasion of neural foramina with spinal cord compression at any level is a well-recognized complication. As the disease is disseminated at presentation in over two-thirds of the cases, more generalized symptoms such as anorexia, bone pain, fever and anaemia from bone marrow infiltration are common, and periorbital ecchymoses and proptosis are frequent signs of retrobulbar metastases. In addition to haematogenous dissemination of tumour to bone and bone marrow, spread to lung and brain parenchyma is now increasingly recognized, and regional or distant lymphadenopathy may be present. In the particular case of stage 4S neuroblastoma confined to infants (*see* Table 47.1), disease commonly extends to the liver (massive hepatomegaly) and skin (subcutaneous nodules).

STAGING

There have been multiple staging systems utilized over the last few decades. In an attempt to rationalize these and permit accurate comparison of data, an International Neuroblastoma Staging System (INSS) has been proposed, which it is hoped will be adopted universally if validated (*see* Table 47.7).

INVESTIGATIONS

As a result of the complex nature of this disease, diagnostic workup and monitoring of treatment progress involves an elaborate schedule of investigations. Urinary catecholamines are raised in up to 90 per cent of tumours, providing a relatively simple diagnostic aid. However, confirmation of the disease requires additional pathological evidence. In the light of an increasing panel of

Table 47.7 *INSS staging*

Stage 1
Localized tumour with complete gross excision, with or without microscopic residual disease; representative ipsilateral lymph nodes negative for tumour microscopically (nodes attached to and removed with the primary tumour may be positive)

Stage 2A
Localized tumour with incomplete gross excision; representative ipsilateral non-adherent lymph nodes negative for tumour microscopically

Stage 2B
Localized tumour with or without gross excision, with ipsilateral non-adherent lymph nodes positive for tumour. Enlarged contralateral lymph nodes must be negative microscopically

Stage 3
Unresectable unilateral tumour, infiltrating across the midline,[a] with or without regional lymph node involvement; OR localized unilateral tumour with contralateral regional lymph node involvement; OR midline tumour with bilateral extension by infiltration or lymph node involvement

Stage 4
Any primary tumour with dissemination to distant lymph nodes, bone, bone marrow, liver and/or other organs (except as defined in stage 4s)

Stage 4s
Localized primary tumour (as defined for stage 1, 2A or 2B), with dissemination limited to liver, skin, and/or bone marrow[b] (limited to infants <1 year of age)

Notes
Multifocal primary tumours (e.g. bilateral adrenal primary tumours) should be staged according to the greatest extent of disease, as defined above, and be followed by a subscript 'M' (e.g. stage 3_M).

[a] The midline is defined as the vertebral column. Tumours originating on one side and crossing the midline must infiltrate to or beyond the opposite side of the vertebral column.
[b] Marrow involvement in stage 4s should be minimal, i.e. <10% nucleated cells on bone marrow biopsy or quantitive assessment of nucleated cells on marrow aspirate. More extensive bone marrow involvement should be considered stage 4. The MIBG scan (if done) should be negative in the marrow for stage 4s.

prognostic markers, biopsy material is necessary not only for light microscopy confirmation, but also recommended for tumour biology (MYCN, 1p deletion, ploidy). Since disseminated disease is a frequent finding at diagnosis, an extensive metastatic workup is recommended. This should incorporate bone marrow examination (aspirates/trephines) in addition to thorough radiological assessment which may include a combination of plain X-rays, ultrasound, CT/MRI scan, ^{131}I-labelled metaiodobenzylguanidine (MIBG) scan and technetium bone scan if MIBG scan unavailable or negative.

PROGNOSTIC FACTORS

Disease stage and patient age are the two most important clinical prognostic factors in this disease. Certainly excellent survival is reported for localized neuroblastoma, and, in the case of metastatic disease, infants fare much better than older children. Although various serum markers (ferritin, LDH, neuron-specific enolase) have been investigated for prognostic value, none is specific and probably reflect tumour burden rather than any strong relationship. Of far more import, it would seem, are the biological variables. The strongest of these is MYCN amplification, associated with a very poor survival and usually disseminated disease. Deletion of the short arm of chromosome 1 (1p) also appears to herald a poor outlook, although its power as an independent prognostic variable is uncertain as in many cases it occurs with MYCN amplification. More recently, gain of the long arm of 17 (17q) has been shown to be an independent factor (Bown et al., 1999). The DNA content of the tumour has also been evaluated – hyperdiploid status is of good prognostic portent, especially in infants.

TREATMENT

The three main treatment modalities all have their place in the management of this complex disease. Chemotherapy is certainly widely used for this chemosensitive tumour (vincristine, cyclophosphamide, cisplatin, doxorubicin, etoposide, carboplatin, melphalan, and ifosfamide all active as single agents) and surgery remains an important component of the treatment of this solid tumour. Although now much less frequently used for primary therapy, conventional radiotherapy remains a useful palliative option.

From observations clinically and biologically, Brodeur (1995) proposed classification of this disease into three main subtypes with excellent, intermediate and very poor outlook. These have been increasingly adopted, somewhat modified, and essentially form the basis of current broad treatment strategies.

Low risk

A low-risk group (localized tumours and infants with stage 4S, all with favourable biology) has an excellent prognosis (90–95 per cent PFS) and aims should therefore be avoidance of toxicity from treatment and minimal intervention. Surgery alone is recommended for localized tumours within this group. Although some children will have residual disease post-surgery, there appears to be no survival advantage documented with the routine use of adjuvant therapy (Evans et al., 1996), and this should be reserved for relapses. Because of the high rate of spontaneous regression, the majority of infants with stage 4S disease can be managed with supportive care alone. Limited chemotherapy should be reserved for those patients with life-threatening symptoms, the aim obviously being cure but avoiding long-term toxicity if at all possible.

Intermediate risk

This group includes stage III disease (all ages) and stage IV disease (infants), but only if biological factors are favourable. These patients are treated with conventional chemotherapy (number of courses variable) together with surgery. However, ultimately they still have a good chance of cure from their disease (70–85 per cent PFS).

High risk

High-risk patients (consisting mainly of children over 1 year of age with stage 4 disease, but also lower age and stage with unfavourable biology), evidently form the bulk of patients. Historically they have a very poor outlook (5–25 per cent PFS) and unfortunately little headway has been made in improving this in recent years. Although often responsive initially to conventional dose chemotherapy, early relapse is commonplace. Dose escalation and high-dose therapy procedures with autologous stem cell rescue have both been employed. These certainly appear to offer longer periods of remission in subsets of patients (Matthay et al., 1999) although the question as to whether this ultimately translates into long-term cure remains. Induction of differentiation with 13-cis-retinoic acid in the absence of progressive disease also improves EFS (Matthay et al., 1999). Other current alternative approaches to treatment of this aggressive disease include the use of therapeutic [131I]MIBG (either with or without conventional chemotherapy) and immunomodulatory therapy.

SCREENING

Mass screening of urinary catecholamines in infants was first carried out in Japan in the 1970s, and subsequently in Europe and North America, under the assumption that delayed clinical detection of low-stage disease ultimately evolves into high-risk disease and therefore earlier diagnosis could reduce mortality. This does not in reality appear to be the case – these screening programmes in infants have not, in fact, resulted in a reduction in either the incidence or mortality of older children with neuroblastoma. Indeed, there has probably been increased morbidity from higher detection of infants with favourable disease, which, if left undisturbed, might subsequently have regressed spontaneously. Ongoing programmes are currently investigating whether delaying the screening to 13 months confers any advantage, but otherwise present data do not support the value of neuroblastoma screening (Philip, 1999).

Rhabdomyosarcoma

Although rare in adults, rhabdomyosarcoma (RMS) is the most common soft tissue sarcoma of childhood, accounting for 4–5 per cent of paediatric malignancies overall. It is primarily a tumour of young children, with three out of four cases presenting under 10 years of age, although two peaks of incidence are generally recognized: a major one at pre-school age between 2 and 5 years, and a less marked one during adolescence. Although aetiology remains unknown, it has occasionally been associated with other anomalies (including congenital lung cysts, neurofibromatosis, Gorlin's syndrome) and it is one of the tumour types encountered in the Li–Fraumeni syndrome.

Being a tumour of embryonic mesenchymal origin, it can arise throughout the body. Common primary site areas include the head and neck area (40 per cent), genitourinary tract (20 per cent) and extremities (20 per cent). RMS is an aggressive tumour, locally invasive into surrounding organs and along tissue planes. Distant dissemination via lymphatic and haematogenous systems (commonly to lung, bone and bone marrow) is recognized in up to 20 per cent of patients at presentation. Overall, however, it is essentially a curable disease in up to two-thirds of children (Crist et al., 1995; Flamant et al., 1998).

HISTOPATHOLOGY

Several histological subsets of RMS are recognized, although microscopic distinction between them may prove extremely difficult. Embryonal RMS is the most common, accounting for about two-thirds and typically arising in head and neck/genitourinary sites. One variant of embryonal type is the botryoid form, where tumours arise under the mucosal surface (vagina, bladder and nares sites) and another is the spindle cell variant (paratesticular site). These subsets are associated with a more favourable outcome. Conversely, alveolar RMS, present in up to a quarter of cases, has a more sinister prognosis, and is usually encountered in older children and often at extremity sites. The pleomorphic variant of RMS is very rarely encountered in children.

Advances in molecular biology can certainly aid subtype distinction. Two characteristic chromosomal translocations are associated with alveolar subtype: t(2;13), t(1;13), involving the *FKHR* gene on chromosome 13 and either *PAX3* on chromosome 2 (approximately 70 per cent of alveolar RMS) or *PAX7* on chromosome 1 (approximately 20 per cent of alveolar RMS). A genetic marker for embryonal RMS is currently still elusive.

SYMPTOMS AND SIGNS

As site of origin is so varied, so too are presenting symptoms. The primary site often determines both timing and mode of presentation. Orbital tumours, for example, frequently have an early presentation with proptosis and diplopia. Nasopharyngeal tumours may cause nasal/airway obstruction, or a polypoid extrusion with discharge, as can also be found with lesions of the vagina. A painless mass may be the only finding, as with many paratesticular lesions. On the other hand, deep-seated pelvic masses may grow to considerable size before presentation, often with obstructive symptoms.

STAGING

Diagnostic workup should include accurate assessment of the primary lesion and lymph nodes with CT/MRI scan, and examination of potential metastatic sites (CT chest, bone marrow aspirate and trephine, bone scan, and consideration of brain CT/MRI in the case of limb primary and alveolar histology). Unfortunately, there is currently no universal staging system used in the management of RMS. Interpretation of the literature and valid comparisons are therefore hindered by differing terminology. The two major staging systems encountered are the North American (IRS) grouping system (based on initial surgery and resectability), and the European (SIOP) TNM-based system. It is hoped that increasing collaboration between the two groups towards a standard approach will resolve some of these difficulties in the near future.

PROGNOSTIC VARIABLES

As with many cancers, our knowledge of this tumour has advanced markedly over recent years. With the aid of national/international collaborative research, we are increasingly recognizing both clinical and biological factors, which appear to have important prognostic significance.

It is certainly possible in some cases to predict outcome based largely on clinical features alone. Site of primary, extent of disease and pathological subtype are all crucial factors (Crist et al., 1995; Flamant et al., 1998). They are also often frustratingly interconnected. Favourable sites include orbital and non-bladder/prostate genitourinary (GU) origin, with 5-year survivals of 80–90 per cent. This may well reflect a relatively short lag time to presentation with symptoms in these sites, although it is pertinent to note that metastatic disease and alveolar histology (both poor prognostic factors) are not commonly associated features. On the other hand, extremity primaries and the so-called 'other' sites (non-head and neck/non-GU origin) carry the worst prognosis and frequently are alveolar histology and/or metastatic at presentation.

Age is also a discerning factor. Poor prognostic variables (alveolar histology, limb primaries, metastatic disease) are much more frequent in the older child and certainly associated with a dismal outlook if all are present. On the other hand, metastatic disease in younger children (<10 years) with embryonal histology may be curable in up to 50 per cent of cases.

Recent advances relating to the biology of the tumour have helped to define prognosis further. Hyperdiploid tumours have a more favourable outcome (often embryonal histology), whereas diploid/tetraploid tumours fare worse (alveolar histology being associated with the latter) (DeZen et al., 1997). Obviously the characteristic translocations associated with alveolar histology can also assist. Even here, there appear to be subtle differences evolving, with t(1;13) tending to occur in younger children and possibly associated with a better prognosis than t(2;13) (Kelly et al., 1997).

TREATMENT

The treatment of RMS is very much multimodal. It is certainly a chemosensitive tumour and the importance of multi-agent chemotherapy has been clearly demonstrated. Many agents have been shown to be active (classically cyclophosphamide, vincristine, actinomycin D, but also including ifosfamide, doxorubicin, melphalan, etoposide, cisplatin, dacarbazine, carboplatin and epirubicin). Local control of the tumour, though, is essential if a realistic chance of cure is to be pursued and thus surgery and radiotherapy both have potentially significant roles to play. Debates and controversies exist, however, as to timing, extent and need for both these modalities. Certainly quality of life issues in survivors concerning the cosmetic and functional late effects of radiotherapy and mutilating surgery – that is, the burden of therapy – should be considered in any outcome measures. These issues, in fact, reflect the main philosophical differences between North American and European strategies, the latter adopting a more conservative approach to local treatment in good responders with the aim of gaining quality of life in survivors. The cost of this approach is the fact that local relapse rates in the SIOP studies are higher than those documented elsewhere (Flamant et al., 1998); however, not only can a significant number of these be salvaged with further therapy, but the majority of survivors overall have a reduced burden of therapy.

The outlook for children with metastatic disease unfortunately remains dismal. Effectively there has been little progress made in this small but significant group of patients over the last two decades, with current 5-year survival rates of around 20 per cent. Although clinical complete remission is achievable in up to two-thirds, early relapse is a frequent occurrence. High-dose therapy with autologous stem cell rescue following conventional treatment as a method of eliminating the assumed minimal residual disease has certainly been employed. Although it would appear to prolong the time interval to progression in comparison to conventional therapy, there is no apparent effect on overall survival (Carli et al., 1999). An alternative approach is to attempt to use dose escalation at a much earlier stage of treatment and this is being assessed in the current SIOP study.

Osteogenic sarcoma

Osteogenic sarcoma (OGS) is the most common primary tumour of bone. The incidence is reported to be between 6.2 and 7.2 cases per 100 000 population between the ages of 10 and 24 years. The incidence in black Afro-Caribbeans is substantially less. The peak incidence is seen between ages 15 and 20 years, and there is a male predominance of approximately 3:2. Overall, there are 100–130 new osteogenic sarcomas diagnosed in the UK annually (UKCCSG annual report).

The majority of cases of OGS are sporadic, but the tumour is recognized to be associated with a number of underlying disorders. The incidence of OGS is high in patients treated with radiotherapy for retinoblastoma. Whilst karyotypic abnormalities involving chromosome 13q14 (carrying the Rb gene) are seen in sporadic OGS, this is not typically the case. More recently however, evidence for a high incidence of LOH of the Rb gene has been reported (Feugeas et al., 1996).

OGS is also a component of the Li–Fraumeni syndrome. Karyotypic abnormalities involving 17q13 are also seen with sporadic OGS, but overall only a small proportion of OGS are likely to be attributable to a known underlying predisposition (Carnevale et al., 1997).

OGS is recognized as a second primary malignancy following prior treatment with radiotherapy (Newton et al., 1991).

CLINICAL PRESENTATION

The typical presentation of OGS is with pain and swelling of the affected limb or bone. OGS typically affects the most rapidly growing areas of the skeleton, the metaphyseal regions of the femur, tibia and proximal humerus (knees and elbows), although it is not known why this is the case. Possibly because of this pattern of disease, the delay between onset of symptoms and diagnosis tends to be less than for Ewing's tumour (6–10 weeks compared to 5–6 months for Ewing's), a smaller proportion of patients present with metastases – 10–20 per cent compared with 25 per cent for Ewing's – and patients have fewer systemic symptoms.

RADIOLOGICAL ASSESSMENT OF OGS

Plain radiographs may show a pathological fracture, elevation of the periosteum and new bone formation. Oedema and a variable amount of soft tissue may be associated.

MRI is the preferred investigation to assess primary disease, since this will allow definition of soft tissue, and more importantly marrow involvement.

Plain chest X-ray may demonstrate metastases, and CT, particularly spiral CT scanning, is likely to identify smaller deposits, causing an increase in identified metastatic patients. Migration between stages will presumably influence outcomes for those patients with no evidence of metastasis.

Technetium-99 bone scanning may show bony deposits. Skeletal metastasis carries a very poor prognosis, and any area of abnormality seen on bone scan should have a plain radiograph to confirm this.

DIAGNOSIS

The diagnosis of OGS is histological, supported by appropriate clinical and radiological evidence. A biopsy is necessary, and this should be done by the surgeon who will perform the subsequent definitive procedure. The biopsy track will need to be resected at definitive surgery, and must avoid the apex of the tumour. Failure to do so risks causing tumour ulceration and fungation.

Osteogenic sarcoma is characterized by the presence of bone or osteoid tissue by the tumour cells. A distinction between central (medullary) and surface (peripheral) tumours is made, although the majority of tumours fall into the central osteosarcoma subgroup.

The most common pathological subtype is conventional central osteosarcoma, which is characterized by areas of necrosis, atypical mitoses, and malignant cartilage (Schajowicz *et al.*, 1995). Subtypes of high-grade osteoblastic, chondroblastic and fibroblastic OGS are identified, but do not seem to carry significant prognostic value with the exception of chondroblastic osteosarcoma in one series (Bacci *et al.*, 1998c).

Occasionally, little or no osteoid may be seen, and differentiation from Ewing's tumour may be problematic. In this, as in the majority of paediatric tumours, the simultaneous processing of material for immunohistochemical and cytogenetic analysis is likely to allow an accurate diagnosis. Biopsy should not be performed by a surgeon who does not have appropriate pathological, immuno-histochemical and cytogenetic support.

STAGING

The Enneking system (Table 47.8) remains in use, although its value prognostically is limited (Enneking, 1986). The majority of patients fall into group IIb.

BIOLOGICAL MARKERS

Biological factors may offer prognostic value at diagnosis. Demonstration of LOH of the *Rb* gene in newly diagnosed patients with osteosarcoma has been reported to predict early treatment failure (Feugeas *et al.*, 1996). Event-free survival at 5 years was 100 per cent for patients without LOH, 43 per cent for all patients with *Rb* LOH, and 65 per cent for non-metastatic patients with *Rb* LOH. Similarly, LOH *p53* has been reported to correlate with lack of chemoresponsiveness *in vitro* (Asada *et al.*, 1999) and *in vivo* (Goto *et al.*, 1998).

TREATMENT

Surgery

Osteogenic sarcoma treated by surgical excision alone leads to an overall survival of at best, 20 per cent (Sweetnam, 1973). Pulmonary metastases develop in the large majority of patients so treated, indicating that control of metastatic disease is the major factor in determining survival. It is not surprising that intra-arterial therapies have produced no improvement in outcome (Winkler *et al.*, 1990; Bielack *et al.*, 1993). Local control is essential, however, and failure to remove the primary tumour completely is associated with a high risk of subsequent local and metastatic relapse even with adjuvant chemotherapy (Bacci *et al.*, 1998d). Local relapse is often associated with simultaneous metastatic recurrence (Bacci *et al.*, 1998b).

In centres where limb salvage is the expected approach, low rates of local recurrence, and favourable local and metastatic relapse rates are expected (Szendroi *et al.*, 2000), even where there is a pathological fracture, provided adequate surgical margin can be attained (Abudu *et al.*, 1996).

It is beyond the scope of this chapter to discuss the orthopaedic approaches taken for limb conservation surgery, but the patient and their family need to be aware of the benefits and drawbacks of a given procedure. For some, amputation may offer the best and most reliable chance of return to normal life. One particular approach worthy of consideration where an above-knee amputation might otherwise be necessary is the rotationplasty, for which excellent functional outcome may be obtained (Kawai *et al.*, 1995).

Chemotherapy

Single chemotherapy agents with activity against osteosarcoma include doxorubicin, methotrexate, cisplatin and ifosfamide, carboplatin and etoposide in combination with ifosfamide. A beneficial effect of melphalan in high-dose therapy has also been reported (Ohira, 1990).

The value of combination chemotherapy in addition to surgery has been demonstrated in the two major studies performed in the 1970s. In the MIOS study, using the T-10 regimen, EFS at 2 years was 66 per cent with chemotherapy and 17 per cent without chemotherapy (Link *et al.*, 1986). Overall survival, after patients who had relapsed had been treated with further surgery and chemotherapy, was 71 per cent for the initial chemotherapy group, and 51 per cent for the group with no initial chemotherapy (Link, 1993). Similar benefit of chemotherapy was reported by Eilber *et al.* (1987).

The first European Osteosarcoma Intergroup (EOI) study (EORTC 80831) compared the efficacy of a two-drug regimen (cisplatin and doxorubicin) with the same drugs, with the addition of methotrexate at a dose of $8 \, \text{g/m}^2$ (Bramwell *et al.*, 1992). Toxicities for both regimens did not differ, and overall survival was not significantly different (at 53 months: 64 per cent for two-drug, 50 per cent for three-drug), but disease-free survival for the two-drug arm was significantly greater (57 per cent versus 41 per cent).

The second European Osteosarcoma Intergroup study (EORTC 80861) compared the efficacy of this two-drug regimen (cisplatin and doxorubicin) with a multi-agent regimen similar to that used by Rosen in the T-10

Table 47.8 *Enneking staging system*

Stage		Grade	Site	Metastases
I	A	Low	Intracompartmental (T1)	None (M0)
	B	Low	Extracompartmental (T2)	None (M0)
II	A	High	Intracompartmental (T1)	None (M0)
	B	High	Extracompartmental (T2)	None (M0)
III	A	Low	Any	Any (M1)
	B	High	Any	Any (M1)

protocol (preoperative vincristine, high-dose methotrexate and doxorubicin; postoperative bleomycin, cyclophosphamide, dactinomycin, vincristine, methotrexate, doxorubicin, and cisplatin) (Souhami *et al.*, 1997). All patients receiving the multi-agent chemotherapy arm received cisplatin, rather than only those identified to have a poor histological response. A total of 407 patients were entered in this randomized study, and no benefit from the multi-drug arm over the two-drug arm was seen. At 5 years, overall survival was 55 per cent and progression-free survival was 44 per cent in both groups. The two-drug regimen was shorter in duration and better tolerated.

An analysis of the received dose intensity in these patients indicated that those patients who were treated at less than 50 per cent of the intended dose intensity had a 3-year overall survival of less than 50 per cent, compared to over 70 per cent for those treated at above 50 per cent of the intended dose intensity (Ian Lewis, personal communication). It was not possible to distinguish the relative effect of absolute dose or dose intensity from this study, but the importance of doxorubicin and methotrexate dose intensity has been reported elsewhere (Smith *et al.*, 1991; Bacci *et al.*, 1992; Delepine *et al.*, 1996). There is little evidence to support an effect of cisplatin dose intensity. Following a pilot study which demonstrated acceptable toxicity (Ornadel *et al.*, 1994), the current EOI study, EOI 931 involves a randomization to receive either 3-weekly or 2-weekly cisplatin and doxorubicin, with G-CSF support for the rapid schedule. This study is still recruiting.

Despite the negative results of the first EOI study, there is good evidence that cumulative dose and dose intensity of methotrexate treatment affects response, and by implication, outcome. The importance of dose intensity of methotrexate is reviewed by Delepine *et al.* (1996). First, there is a correlation between a pharmacokinetic parameter, methotrexate concentration at the end of infusion, and tumour response as measured by the degree of tumour necrosis (Graf *et al.*, 1994; Bacci *et al.*, 1998c). A concentration of methotrexate of 700 µM after a 6-hour infusion (Bacci *et al.*, 1998c), or 1000 µM at the end of a 4-hour infusion (Delepine *et al.*, 1988; Graf *et al.*, 1994) has been shown to be predictive of response, allowing stratification according to a surrogate end point early on in treatment. Second, dose adaptation based upon pharmacokinetic parameters has been performed, and a survival benefit seen (Delepine *et al.*, 1995).

For patients treated with a methotrexate dose of 8, 10 or 12 g/m^2, the proportion of patients attaining a methotrexate concentration in excess of 700 µM has been reported to be 44 per cent, 59 per cent and 85 per cent (Bacci, 1998) and one explanation for the variable reports of efficacy of methotrexate stems from this variability.

STRATIFICATION OF PATIENTS

The concept of stratification of patients based upon histological response of the resected tumour was introduced early in the history of chemotherapy, although it has yet to be proven whether modification of therapy affects overall prognosis (Bielack *et al.*, 1999; Meyers *et al.*, 1998; Bacci *et al.*, 2000). In the majority of series, the presence of more than 90 per cent necrosis in the resection specimen identifies a good prognostic group, for whom a high (>75 per cent) overall survival may be expected. In the EOI first study, OS for patients with >90 per cent necrosis was 85 per cent, compared with 40 per cent for those with less than 90 per cent. In the second EOI study only 30 per cent of patients had ≥90 per cent necrosis with the two-drug regimen and 27 per cent with multi-agent therapy (NS) (Souhami *et al.*, 1997). Higher good response rates have been seen by the Co-operative Osteosarcoma Study (COSS) and SFOP groups (Bielack *et al.*, 1999; Philip *et al.*, 1999).

A poor response to initial chemotherapy may be explained by the tumour itself, or by the type of therapy used. The tumour may be intrinsically more resistant to chemotherapy, because of underlying biological differences, or the chemotherapy used may be inadequate: the concentration of drug, total duration of exposure or some other parameter may be insufficient. Recent identification of adverse biological factors, such as LOF of the *Rb* gene, may allow an appropriate aggressive approach to be taken early in the course of treatment, and may in time point to novel therapeutic strategies. More immediately, the identification that dose intensity, and further, concentration of drug, correlates with response emphasizes the need to use chemotherapy optimally, and perhaps to individualize therapy to each patient. Strategies to include extra agents such as methotrexate have often led to reduction in dose intensity of all agents, with a consequent failure to improve outcome.

POOR PROGNOSIS DISEASE

Although the majority of tumours arise in peripheral long bones, at least 20 per cent of patients present with flat-bone, axial or metastatic disease at diagnosis. These patients have a mixed prognosis. Chemotherapy alone is unlikely to be curative, and for some, surgical resection is not possible. The prognosis for patients with primary metastatic disease is dependent upon site. In the study of Harris *et al.* (1998), patients with primary bone metastasis had a particularly poor outcome. Most patients will have pulmonary metastasis, and for this group, surgical resection seems to be of benefit (Carter *et al.*, 1991; van Rijk-Zwikker *et al.*, 1991; Tabone *et al.*, 1994). Bacci *et al.* (1998a) reported a 5-year OS of only 14 per cent with an aggressive regimen using methotrexate (8 g/m^2), cisplatin, doxorubicin, ifosfamide and etoposide. All patients who did not achieve a complete surgical or chemotherapeutic remission died. By contrast, patients in the series of Harris *et al.*, who presented with less than eight pulmonary nodules, had a relatively high chance of cure. Of 18, 12 were alive at 5 years, and patients with unilateral disease had a 5-year EFS of 75 per cent. These data are encouraging, and indicate that an aggressive, multimodality approach may overcome previously adverse prognostic factors.

Ewing's tumour

Ewing's tumour comprises 10–15 per cent of primary bone tumours in childhood and adolescence, affecting 0.6 people per million population, or 1.7 per million children. Ewing's tumour has a peak incidence at 10–15 years of age, affecting boys more than girls. It is rare below 5 years and after 30 years, and in black and oriental races.

Ewing's tumour will typically present as a bony lump, often with pain. There may be associated neurological deficit, and a fever, due either to tumour load or to superinfection. The majority of tumours arise (in order of frequency) in distal extremities, proximal limb, pelvis, chest wall, axial skeleton. Extra-osseous Ewing's tumour arises in the trunk, extremities, head and neck and retroperitoneum. Extra-osseous Ewing's tumours are likely to be larger and less amenable to definitive local surgery than bony Ewing's.

HISTOPATHOLOGY

Pathologically, the Ewing's tumour family fall within the group of malignancies referred to as the small round blue cell tumours of childhood, although microscopic, immuno-histochemical and molecular diagnostic techniques allow this group to be identified with accuracy.

The tumour arises within the medullary cavity of bone, but erodes the cortex and at presentation may have a highly variable soft tissue component. In the extreme, Ewing's tumour may have a barely identifiable or no recognizable bony component – so-called extra-osseous Ewing's tumour. The major differential diagnosis is of other primary bone tumours, osteogenic sarcoma, malignant fibrous histiocytoma and osteomyelitis. Where the soft tissue component predominates, other small round blue cell tumours must be distinguished. These include rhabdomyosarcoma and other non-rhabdomyomatous sarcomas, neuroblastoma and lymphoma. Ewing's tumour may show elements of neural differentiation, and in this, overlaps with PNETs. A third tumour, the Askin tumour, presents as a chest wall tumour in adolescence, and similarly shares many features.

All three tumours are characterized by translocations involving chromosome 22q12 and in the majority of cases, chromosome 11q24. The breakpoint region of this translocation has been cloned and the transcript has been sequenced (Delattre et al., 1994). The novel transcript includes the DNA-binding domain of the (human homologue of the) Fli-1 gene and the EWS gene, bringing the Fli-1 gene under the control of the EWS promotor and producing a transforming capacity not present in the wild-type Fli-1 gene product. In about 20 per cent

of cases, the EWS gene is translocated to the ERG region of chromosome 21. This is a similar DNA-binding protein to Fli-1. Many different fusion products are seen even within the EWS-Fli-1 rearrangements. The most common (type 1, 72 per cent) links Exon 6 of Fli-1 with Exon 7 of EWS, but at least eight other transcripts are known. Presence of the type 1 transcript seems to be an independent prognostic variable for localized tumours, with significant better relapse-free survival (de Alava et al., 1998). Approximately 30 per cent of tumours show a secondary change, trisomy 8, the significance of which is unclear.

Translocation of the EWS region to other chromosomes leads to other tumour types, such as desmoplastic small round cell tumour of adolescence, associated with an EWS-WT1 translocation.

Current clinical practice for PNETs is to treat according to either a Ewing's protocol, or a soft tissue sarcoma protocol. Whilst aspects of these therapies are similar, the importance of local therapy – radical surgery or radiotherapy – is emphasized more for Ewing's type strategies. Information regarding the comparative benefits of such approaches is not available at present.

Accurate diagnosis is essential for appropriate therapy to be instigated, and the importance of a combined approach by oncologist, surgeon, radiologist and pathologist cannot be overstated.

In his original reports of diffuse endothelioma of bone, Ewing described the radiosensitivity of the tumour (Ewing, 1921), although with radiotherapy alone, the large majority of patients relapsed with disseminated disease within 2–5 years. Numerous agents have been shown to have activity in Ewing's tumour including cyclophosphamide, doxorubicin, ifosfamide, vincristine, actinomycin D, melphalan, BCNU and 5-fluorouracil (5-FU). Etoposide and ifosfamide administered in combination have been reported to have high activity (Miser et al., 1987; Meyer et al., 1992). Combination chemotherapy has been used for many years, and overall survival has progressively increased. It is clear, however, that cure cannot be achieved by chemotherapy alone, and either radiotherapy or surgery is required to eradicate local disease (Thomas et al., 1984). The issues of chemotherapy, radiotherapy and surgery have been addressed in the major national and international trials.

THE US INTERGROUP EWING'S SARCOMA STUDY (IESS I AND II) TRIALS

IESS I randomized patients with localized disease to receive three-drug (vincristine, actinomycin D, cyclophosphamide, VAC) or four-drug chemotherapy (VAC + doxorubicin, VACA), or three drugs with pulmonary irradiation. A significant survival and relapse-free benefit was seen with four-drug therapy, with EFS at 5 years being 60 per cent, compared with 44 per cent with VAC + radiation, and 24 per cent after VAC alone.

The IESS II study (Burgert *et al.*, 1990) examined the effect of intensity of treatment on survival, comparing VACA given in high-dose intermittent schedule with a moderate-dose continuous schedule. Intensity of chemotherapy was important, and doxorubicin was believed to be the major factor in this. EFS at 5 years was 68 per cent in the high intensity, and 48 per cent in the moderate intensity arms.

THE CO-OPERATIVE EWING'S SARCOMA STUDY (CESS) TRIALS

The first Co-operative Ewing's Sarcoma Study, CESS 81 ran from 1981 to 1985, and enrolled 93 patients (Jurgens *et al.*, 1985). Patients were treated with four-drug chemotherapy (VACA) in four 9-week courses. Surgical resection of the primary tumour was performed if possible, and radiotherapy administered at a dose of 36 Gy for residual disease postoperatively. Where radiotherapy was the only local therapy, a dose of 46–60 Gy was administered, with a 5 cm safety margin. Whole compartment radiotherapy was also given, to a dose of 36 Gy. EFS at 10 years was 53 per cent, with greater survival in those patients who received both surgery and radiotherapy (69 per cent) than with radiotherapy (44 per cent) or surgery (48 per cent) alone.

CESS 81 also demonstrated the possibility of defining risk groups other than metastasis. Patients with small (<100 mL) tumours had EFS of 80 per cent, compared with 32 per cent for those with >100 mL tumours. In 54 patients, an assessment of histological response to surgery was made, and a good response (>90 per cent tumour cell kill) associated with a significantly better outcome (79 per cent versus 31 per cent for poor responders) (Jurgens *et al.*, 1985, 1988).

The rate of local relapse in CESS 81 was high, particularly in patients where radiotherapy alone was used (22 per cent), next where both used (14 per cent), lowest with surgery alone (3 per cent). This led to central radiotherapy planning such that radiation portals were subsequently planned according to X-rays defining disease at presentation. Failure rates have since fallen (Sauer *et al.*, 1987).

Following CESS 81, CESS 86 enrolled 177 patients with localized tumour between 1986 and 1991. Based on the results of CESS 81, treatment intensity was adapted to tumour volume and site, with high-risk patients (>100 mL volume at diagnosis) and all central tumours receiving four-drug chemotherapy using ifosfamide rather than cyclophosphamide. In addition, the preferred local therapy of larger tumours was surgery where possible, and local therapy was brought forward to week 9. A larger radiation dose was given postoperatively (45 Gy rather than 40) and for definitive therapy (60 Gy). In addition, patients received either conventional or hyperfractionated radiotherapy. With this approach, the prognostic significance of tumour volume was changed, such

that patients with a tumour volume of >100 mL did not differ in outcome from those with a smaller volume. Instead, a new stratification at 200 mL was produced (Ahrens *et al.*, 1999). Patients with tumour volume >200 mL had an EFS at 8 years of 42 per cent, which was significantly worse than those with a volume of 100–200 mL (70 per cent) or <100 mL (63 per cent). The greatest survival was seen in patients previously regarded as being at high risk, who received intensified therapy with ifosfamide. Age, gender, tumour site and the histological response to chemotherapy were no longer prognostic.

UK-ET TRIALS

The first UK Ewing's tumour (ET) study recruited 144 patients, of whom 15 per cent had metastases at diagnosis. All patients received local irradiation and four-drug therapy (VACA) for 1 year (Craft *et al.*, 1993). EFS at 10 years for patients with local disease at presentation was 41 per cent, but only 31 per cent for axial tumours.

The second UK trial enrolled 201 patients with localized tumour between 1987 and 1993 (Shankar *et al.*, 1999). ET-2 was identical to ET-1, except that ifosfamide replaced cyclophosphamide (VACA versus VAIA). The 5-year disease-free survival was 67 per cent. No significant difference was seen between patients receiving surgery alone, radiotherapy alone or both as local therapy, although dual therapy was again associated with the highest survival. Radiotherapy was clearly of benefit in the setting of incomplete surgical resection.

EICESS 92

EICESS 92 enrolled patients until January 2000, and a total of 631 patients were registered (Paulussen *et al.*, 1999). Patients were stratified according to the information available in 1992 into Standard risk (volume < 100 mL) or high risk (volume >100 mL ± metastatic disease). Standard risk patients received initial therapy with four drugs (VAIA), and were randomized to receive four-drug therapy with either cyclophosphamide or ifosfamide. High-risk patients received either four-drug (VAIA) or five-drug (VAIA and etoposide) therapy. Total therapy was for 14 cycles over 44 weeks. Patients were assessed after two cycles, and surgery performed after four cycles. Guidelines indicated surgery to be the preferred local therapy where response was slow, and for large tumours. Preoperative radiotherapy (45 Gy) was given to poor responders.

A total of 369 patients were randomized. Three-year EFS has been reported to be 66 per cent for patients with localized tumours, 43 per cent for patients with primary pulmonary/pleural metastases, and 29 per cent for patients with other metastases. Large tumour volume or pelvic site appear to be adverse prognostic factors.

Paulussen *et al.* (1998) has reported preliminary data for 171 patients with metastatic disease at diagnosis registered up to 1995. Thirty-six received myeloablative megatherapy with stem cell rescue following conventional treatment. Bilateral whole-lung irradiation was administered in 57 with pulmonary involvement. Event-free survival at 4 years from diagnosis for all 171 patients was 27 per cent. EFS for isolated lung metastases was 34 per cent, for bone/bone marrow metastases, 28 per cent, and for combined lung plus bone/bone marrow metastases, 14 per cent ($P < 0.005$). Whole-lung irradiation improved outcome in case of isolated pulmonary involvement (40 versus 19 per cent at 4 years, $P < 0.05$). In patients with combined pulmonary/skeletal metastases, intensification by megatherapy and/or whole-lung irradiation improved EFS from 0 to 27 per cent ($P = 0.0001$).

Whether intensification of therapy will lead to improved overall survival is as yet unclear. Doxorubicin dose intensity has been reported to be the most important parameter affecting outcome (Smith, 1991; Smith et al., 1991). A dose-intense regimen with escalating ifosfamide dose intensity to 2.5 times and cyclophosphamide dose intensity to 1.5 times previous protocols (Marina et al., 1999) reported good overall survival (localized disease 90 ± 6 per cent), although small numbers of patients were treated.

The role of high-dose chemotherapy with stem cell support is under investigation in the current European study of Ewing's tumour, EuroEWINGS 99. Patients with intermediate risk disease, defined by initial tumour volume and the presence of pulmonary metastases are randomized to receive a maintenance phase of chemotherapy VAI or high-dose therapy with busulphan and melphalan. Studies of high-dose chemotherapy ± radiotherapy in patients with high risk or relapsed disease have given promising results (Burdach et al., 1993; Stewart et al., 1996; Atra et al., 1997).

Histiocytosis

Langerhans cell histiocytosis (LCH), previously known as histiocytosis X, encompasses a broad range of clinical syndromes. It is rare with incidence rates quoted of three to seven cases per million. It is more common in males. The terminology of classification of the histiocytoses has changed over many decades, representing a better though still incomplete understanding of their pathogenesis. Terms such as Hand–Schüller–Christian, Lettere–Siwe and eosinophilic granuloma of bone are now redundant. The establishment of the International Histiocyte Society led to reclassification of these disorders in 1987 (Chu et al., 1987). This classification delineated Langerhans cell histiocytosis, non-Langerhans cell histiocytosis (haemophagocytic lymphohistiocytoses) and malignant histiocytoses. LCH is defined according to pathological criteria. Langerhans cells are mononuclear cells with a lobulated grooved nucleus, uneven chromatin and eosinophilic cytoplasm with positive CD1a staining by immunohistochemistry. The presence of Birbeck granules (racquet-shaped organelles) are seen on electron microscopy. LCH is characterized by the presence of these cells along with lymphocytes, eosinophils and normal histiocytes.

Langerhans cells in LCH have been shown to be clonal (Willman et al., 1994). Still LCH is not generally classified as a cancer although treatment options include cytotoxics. Arceci (1999) describes LCH as a 'clonal proliferative neoplasm with variable clinical manifestations'. These manifestations vary from self-limiting localized single-system disease to disseminated rapidly progressive fatal disease.

Single-system disease most often involves bone. Lesions are lytic on plain X-ray and may be found incidentally in asymptomatic patients. It is common practice to perform a skeletal survey rather then a bone scan to look for other lesions. If the patient is well with no anaemia, hepatosplenomegaly, skin lesions or symptoms, then no further investigations or treatment are necessary. Biopsy to confirm diagnosis with curettage may be curative. Painful lesions may be treated with intralesional steroids. If lesions involve vertebral bodies with associated neurological deficit, then low-dose radiotherapy may be necessary. Low doses are used due to the potential risk of secondary malignancy. Indomethacin and other non-steroidal drugs are used for relief of symptoms of pain or discomfort. Their use has been associated with subsequent resolution of lesions and healing of bone. This may be due to their inhibition of intralesional interleukin-2 (IL-2) or prostaglandin E2 (McLean and Pritchard, 1996).

Other systems involved include skin (typically a seborrhoeic rash), lymph nodes (often suppurative with sinus formation), lung (diffuse infiltration with fibrosis), liver, spleen, bone marrow and central nervous system. There may be associated diabetes insipidus due to involvement of the pituitary gland. Non-specific markers of disease activity include erythrocyte sedimentation rate and thrombocytosis (Claming and Henter, 1998).

Given the wide spectrum of disease states in this condition, treatment is designated according to defined risk groups. Low-risk patients are those aged >2 years without involvement of the liver, spleen, lungs or haematopoietic system. Patients with minimal involvement usually require minimal or no treatment. Patients with more extensive disease benefit from systemic cytotoxics and/or steroid. Agents commonly used include vinblastine, etoposide and 6-MP. Current trials are exploring the benefit of etoposide at induction and its use in continuation therapy. The initial response to treatment is a predictor of outcome (Ladisch and Gadner, 1994). Poor response to early therapy for patients with multi-system disease predicts a poor overall outcome for both morbidity and mortality. Treatment intensification for these higher-risk patients has not yet been proven to be beneficial. The role of autologous bone marrow transplant as well as various immunomodulatory approaches is currently under evaluation by the International Histiocyte Society.

Haemophagocytic lymphohistiocytosis (HLH) may be familial or non-familial. The non-familial HLH is usually induced by viruses such as adenovirus, herpes simplex virus (HSV), EBV or cytomegalovirus (CMV). HLH is characterized by infiltrates of non-clonal lymphocytes and macrophages. Macrophages appear activated and haemophagocytosis of all marrow elements as well as other organs such as the liver is observed. HLH is associated with a number of immune abnormalities and might be better classified as an immunodeficiency syndrome rather than a primary proliferative disorder like LCH. Presentation includes fever, splenomegaly, lymphadenopathy, rash, oedema and jaundice. CNS involvement is common. Laboratory investigations reveal pancytopenia, hypertriglyceridaemia, hyperferritinaemia and abnormal liver function tests including coagulopathy. Virus-induced HLH is usually self-limiting. Familial HLH is a progressive disease, which results in death by infection or bleeding. With the growing evidence that this is a disorder of immune function, treatment strategies have included immunosuppression and replacement of unknown defect in the immune system by allogeneic stem cell transplant.

Malignant germ cell tumours

Germ cell tumours account for approximately 3 per cent of all childhood malignancies in the UK, with an annual incidence of 2.4 per million children per year (Pinkerton, 1997). Malignant germ cell tumours (MGCT) usually arise in the midline structures, i.e. the sacrococcygeal region, retroperitoneum, mediastinum and midbrain. The morphological subtype of a MGCT reflects the differentiation pathway to which a cell becomes committed (Fig. 47.2).

An increased incidence of germ cell tumours is found for children with dysgenic gonads, Klinefelter's syndrome and defects in the urogenital tract such as cryptorchidism and sacral agenesis. The relative incidence of GCT according to age, sex and pathological subtype is shown in Table 47.9.

The cytogenetics of germ cell tumours differ with respect to age, sex and tumour location. For testicular or mediastinal tumours in adolescent boys, isochromosome 12p is a common finding, and deletion of 1p/gain of 1q and chromosome 3 are the most common abnormalities among the MGCTs from both sexes (Bussey et al., 1999). Staging of MGCT can be based on conventional TMN stage I–IV criteria, or on the basis of risk groupings (Pinkerton, 1997). Patients with surgically completely resected tumours, and in whom the tumour markers α-fetoprotein (AFP) and β-human chorionic gonadotrophin (β-hCG) rapidly normalize can be observed without further therapy, and children with metastatic disease require chemotherapy.

MGCT may present as an asymptomatic mass, or with symptoms due to compression/obstruction, i.e. respiratory distress due to a mediastinal tumour, and visual disturbances, diabetes insipidus and hypopituitarism in the case of intracranial germ cell tumours (Castleberry et al., 1997). Elevated serum levels of, or

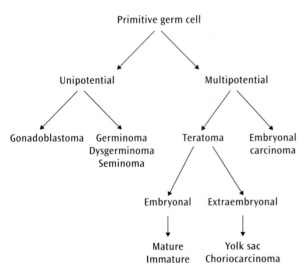

Figure 47.2 *Differentiation pathway for malignant germ cell tumours.*

Table 47.9 *Relative incidence of childhood germ cell tumours*

Site	Age	Relative incidence (%)	Pathology
Sacrococcyx	Neonate	35	Teratoma (malignant 10–30%)
Vagina	Infant	2	Yolk sac
Ovary	Adolescence	25	Teratoma (malignant 30%)
Testis	Infant and adolescent	20	Teratoma (malignant 80%)
Retroperitoneum	Infant	5	Teratoma (rarely malignant)
Mediastinum	Adolescent	5	Teratoma (malignant 20–40%)
Head and neck	Infant and neonate	3	Teratoma (rarely malignant)
Cranium	Infant	5	Germinoma, embryonal carcinoma, mature teratoma

positive immunohistochemical staining of, germ cell tumours for AFP indicates the presence of a malignant component, i.e. yolk-sac tumour or embryonal carcinoma. Elevations of β-hCG in patients with germ cell tumours occur with choriocarcinoma and germinomas (Castleberry *et al.*, 1997).

Whereas surgical resection is the treatment of choice for benign germ cell tumours, radical resection of malignant lesions is generally limited to gonadal sites (Pinkerton, 1997). With the exception of MGCT of the CNS, radiotherapy has little role in the management of MGCT, except in the treatment of residual tumour following second-line chemotherapy and surgery (Pinkerton, 1997). Chemotherapy with bleomycin, etoposide and cisplatin (BEP) has become the gold standard regimen for the therapy of MGCT (Pinkerton, 1997). However, chemotherapy based on bleomycin, carboplatin and etoposide (JEB) is undergoing evaluation, and preliminary results suggest that JEB has reduced long-term nephro- and ototoxicity more than BEP, without compromising efficacy (Pinkerton, 1997).

Whereas the majority of intracranial germinomas are cured by radiotherapy alone, secreting intracranial tumours such as yolk-sac tumour, embryonal carcinoma and choriocarcinoma have a poorer prognosis with radiotherapy alone. A combination of chemotherapy with cisplatin, ifosfamide and etoposide (PEI), followed by surgery and craniospinal radiotherapy has shown very promising results for these tumours, with an EFS of 80 per cent (Calaminus *et al.*, 1997).

For children with relapsed disease, a regimen such as ifosfamide, vincristine, and doxorubicin may be curative when combined with surgery (Pinkerton, 1997), and high-dose therapy with carboplatin and etoposide may be curative for patients with relapsed or resistant disease (Nichols *et al.*, 1992). In summary, although the current therapy for paediatric MGCT confers a high cure rate, further studies are needed to define, in relation to internationally agreed risk classifications, the minimal effective therapy for this group of childhood tumours.

Liver tumours

Primary malignant hepatic tumours represent 1.2 per cent of all cancers in children. There are two main types of malignant tumours, namely hepatoblastoma and hepatocellular carcinoma, plus the rarer mesenchymal tumours such as rhabdomyosarcoma and undifferentiated sarcoma (Perilongo and Shafford, 1999). Benign hepatic tumours include haemangioendothelioma, mesenchymal hamartoma and the rare hepatic adenoma and focal nodular hyperplasia.

HEPATOBLASTOMA

Hepatoblastoma is the most common liver tumour of childhood, with an incidence worldwide of 0.5–1.5 cases per million children (Perilongo and Shafford, 1999). Hepatoblastoma is essentially a disease of young children, with a median age of presentation of 16 months. Cytogenetic and LOH analyses have uncovered frequent deletions of 1p and 1q, which may suggest the location of putative tumour suppressor genes at these sites (Kraus *et al.*, 1996). Although most cases of hepatoblastoma appear to be sporadic, there are known associations with Beckwith–Wiedeman syndrome, familial adenomatous polyposis, Gardner's syndrome and extreme low birth weight (Perilongo and Shafford, 1999).

Hepatoblastoma may present as a symptomatic abdominal mass, although weight loss, anorexia, vomiting and abdominal pain are features of more advanced disease. Many patients are anaemic and thrombocytosis is common. An elevated level of serum AFP is found in >90 per cent of cases.

For the Liver Tumour Study Group of the International Society of Paediatric Oncology (SIOPEL), where therapeutic strategy is based on primary chemotherapy, the PRETEXT (pre-treatment extent of disease) system describes the site and size of the tumour, along with invasion of vessels and distant spread as defined by radiological evaluation. The system identifies four categories, which reflect the sections of the liver that are free of tumour, plus any extension of the disease beyond the liver into the inferior vena cava (IVC)/hepatic veins (V), portal vein (P), extra-hepatic abdomen (E) and distant metastases (M).

For hepatoblastoma, only complete resection of the tumour offers a chance of cure. However, surgery alone cures very few patients; >50 per cent of cases present with unresectable primary tumours or distant metastases, and a 30 per cent relapse rate is found for children treated with surgery alone (Feusner *et al.*, 1993). Therefore, several study groups prefer to defer surgery until after 2 or 3 months of chemotherapy as this may improve tumour resectability. For example, for the SIOPEL I study, 85 per cent of patients responded to preoperative chemotherapy with doxorubicin and cisplatin, and a complete tumour resection was achieved for 69 per cent of patients (Plaschkes *et al.*, 1996).

The extent of disease at diagnosis has been shown to relate to survival for children with hepatoblastoma. For the SIOPEL 1 study, children with PRETEXT I disease had a 100 per cent 3-year EFS, which compared to an EFS of 83, 59, and 44 per cent for patients with PRETEXT II–IV disease (Plaschkes *et al.*, 1995). Orthotopic liver transplantation is currently undergoing evaluation as a treatment modality for children with unresectable hepatoblastoma, and an overall 5-year survival rate of 62 per cent has been reported for children without extra-hepatic metastases (Al-Qabandi *et al.*, 1999).

HEPATOCELLULAR CARCINOMA

In most countries, hepatocellular carcinoma (HCC) is less common than hepatoblastoma. However, considerable geographic variation in incidence exists, with rates varying from 0.2 per million children in England and Wales to 2.1 per million children in Hong Kong. HCC is commoner in males and is associated with cirrhosis and other pre-existing parenchymal liver disorders, and more rarely for children with Gardner's syndrome or familial adenomatous polyposis (Perilongo and Shafford, 1999). In comparison to hepatoblastoma, HCC is a tumour of older children, with a peak incidence between 10 and 14 years. LOH on the distal part of chromosome 1p, which has been mapped to 1p35-1p36, may indicate that certain HCC and hepatoblastoma tumours share a molecular pathway in their pathogenesis (Kraus *et al.*, 1996).

HCC usually presents as an abdominal mass, with jaundice and abdominal pain and serum AFP is elevated in 60–90 per cent of cases. As with hepatoblastoma, treatment is primarily surgical. However, HCC does not appear to be as chemoresponsive as hepatoblastoma, with poorer resection rates achieved post-chemotherapy (Plaschkes *et al.*, 1996). Therefore, the outlook for HCC remains poor with only 20 per cent of children surviving 5 years (Haas *et al.*, 1989).

In summary, national and international collaboration has allowed for significant advances in the therapy of hepatoblastoma, such that studies can now begin to address reduction in the late effects of chemotherapy. For HCC, more effective chemotherapy is needed for children with disease that is unresectable at diagnosis.

Renal tumours

Renal tumours constitute 6–8 per cent of childhood cancer in the USA (Green *et al.*, 1997). Wilms' tumour, the most common renal tumour of childhood, is a paradigm for the multimodal treatment of a solid tumours in children.

WILMS' TUMOUR

The incidence of Wilms' tumour (WT) is 8.1 cases per million Caucasian children less than 15 years of age (Green, 1997). WT usually presents before 5 years of age, and is associated with congenital abnormalities such as aniridia, hemihypertrophy and hypospadias, and with the Denys–Drash, Beckwith–Weidemann and WAGR syndromes (Green, 1997). At least three genes are associated with Wilms' tumour and since the incidence of familial WT is less than 1 per cent, the genetics of WT do not always follow the simple two-hit model of tumour suppressor genes (Pritchard-Jones, 1996). Patients with the WAGR (hemihypertrophy, aniridia, genitourinary malformation and mental retardation) syndrome have a constitutional deletion of the Wilms' tumour suppressor gene, *WT-1*, which is located at 11p13 (Pritchard-Jones, 1996). Although constitutional mutations of *WT-1* are described for children with the rare Denys–Drash syndrome, specific mutations of *WT-1* have been found in

less than 10 per cent of sporadic Wilms' tumour (Li *et al.*, 1996). *WT-2* has been found to map to 11p15.5, which is also the location of the Beckwith–Weidemann gene abnormality, and familial WT genes are also located at 17q12 and 7p13 (Green, 1997b). Nephrogenic rests, which are small, usually microscopic, clusters of blastemal cells, tubules and stromal cells found at the periphery of the renal lobe, are thought to be precursor lesions for WT (Green *et al.*, 1997).

Most children present with a history of an abdominal mass or swelling. Abdominal pain, gross haematuria and pyrexia are frequently observed, and hypertension is encountered in 25 per cent of cases (Green *et al.*, 1997). Investigations performed at diagnosis include abdominal ultrasound and CT, with the aim of determining the extent of spread of tumour into adjacent organs such as the liver, the involvement of the inferior vena cava with tumour, and radiological abnormalities of the opposite kidney. A chest X-ray is also indicated to exclude pulmonary metastases. However, staging of WT also depends the involvement of regional lymph nodes and direct examination of the contralateral kidney by the surgeon. The presence of tumour cells in retroperitoneal lymph nodes is an important prognostic factor for children with WT, and lymph-node sampling forms part of the staging of WT according to the National Wilms' Tumour Study Group (NWTSG; Table 47.10).

Classically, Wilms' tumour is made up of varying proportions of three cell types, namely blastemal, stromal and epithelial. Wilms' tumour histology is designated favourable or anaplastic, depending on the presence of gigantic polypoid nuclei within the tumour sample in the latter case. The finding of diffuse or focal tumour anaplasia, which occurs in approximately 5 per cent of cases of Wilms' tumour, generally results in more aggressive treatment (Green *et al.*, 1997).

The therapy of Wilms' tumour comprises a combination of surgery, chemotherapy and radiotherapy that is dependent on the stage and histology of the tumour. Whereas in the USA, immediate nephrectomy is performed, followed by treatment with chemotherapy ± radiotherapy, more recent trials conducted by SIOP have employed pre-nephrectomy chemotherapy (Green, 1997). The use of pre-nephrectomy chemotherapy may confer an advantage both in terms of a lower tumour rupture rate at operation, therefore possibly reducing the risk of local relapse (Shamberger *et al.*, 1999), and the identification of good prognostic subgroups based on tumour response (Boccon-Gibod *et al.*, 2000). However, immediate nephrectomy is advocated by the NWTSG to avoid possible modification of tumour histology and staging, and the administration of chemotherapy to children with non-Wilms' malignancies or benign lesions (Green, 1997). Approximately 1 per cent of children with unilateral Wilms' tumour develop disease in the contralateral kidney, and as for children with bilateral Wilms' tumour at presentation, consideration is given to renal sparing surgery.

Table 47.10 *The staging of Wilms' tumour by the National Wilms' Tumour Study Group*

Stage I	Tumour limited to the kidney and completely excised. The renal capsule has an intact outer surface. The tumour is not ruptured or biopsied prior to removal (fine-needle aspiration allowed). Renal sinus vessels not involved. No evidence of tumour at or beyond the margins of resection.
Stage II	Tumour extends beyond the kidney, but was completely excised. There may be regional extension of tumour (i.e. penetration of the renal capsule or extensive invasion of the renal sinus). The blood vessels outside the renal parenchyma, including those of the renal sinus, may contain tumour. The tumour is biopsied (except for fine needle aspiration), or there is spillage of tumour before or during surgery that is contained to the flank, and does not involve the peritoneal surface. There must be no evidence of tumour at or beyond the margins of resection.
Stage III	Residual non-haematogenous tumour is present, and confined to the abdomen. (1) Lymph nodes within the abdomen or pelvis are found to be involved with tumour (renal hilar, para-aortic or beyond). (2) The tumour has penetrated the peritoneal surface. (3) Tumour implants are found in the peritoneal surface. (4) There is residual or microscopic tumour postoperatively. (5) The tumour is not completely resectable because of local infiltration into vital structures. (6) Tumour spill is not confined to the flank either before or during surgery.
Stage IV	Haematogenous metastases (lung, liver, bone, brain, etc.) or lymph node metastases outside the abdomino-pelvic region are present.
Stage V	Bilateral renal involvement is present at diagnosis. An attempt should be made to stage each side according to the above criteria on the basis of the extent of disease prior to biopsy or treatment.

The chemotherapy for European and NWTSG studies is largely based on combination therapy with vincristine, actinomycin D and doxorubicin, with radiotherapy generally being employed for stage III or stage IV disease. However, the excellent survival of approximately 80 per cent for children with advanced disease has led national collaborative groups devising studies to try to identify minimal necessary therapy for this disease. For example, for the National Wilms' Tumour Study-3 (NWTS-3), the 87 per cent relapse-free survival for stage II patients receiving 15 months of therapy with vincristine and actinomycin D was not improved by the addition of an anthracycline and/or addition of 20 Gy radiotherapy (D'Angio *et al.*, 1989).

For children with relapsed Wilms' tumour, high-dose chemotherapy with carboplatin, etoposide and melphalan has been reported to confer a prolonged disease-free survival in approximately 50 per cent of cases (Pein *et al.*, 1998).

OTHER RENAL TUMOURS

Clear cell sarcoma of the kidney is a primary renal tumour which has a significantly higher relapse rate and death rate than favourable histology Wilms' tumour (Green *et al.*, 1997). As with Wilms' tumour, clear cell sarcoma metastasizes most frequently to the lungs, and has a tendency to metastasize to bone and brain. The tumour is more common in boys, and presents at a median age of 1.5 years (Argani *et al.*, 2000). The overall survival for clear cell sarcoma is 69 per cent, and survival has been found to relate to stage, age at diagnosis and treatment with doxorubicin, with stage I patients having a 98 per cent EFS rate on NWTSG studies (Argani *et al.*, 2000). The rhabdoid tumour of the kidney is a distinctive and

highly malignant tumour which metastasizes to the lungs and CNS, is more common in males and presents at a median age of 13 months (Green *et al.*, 1997). Clear cell sarcoma and the rhabdoid tumour of the kidney are distinct entities, they are often treated as 'unfavourable' histological subtypes on Wilms' tumour protocols and receive triple chemotherapy and radiotherapy (Green, 1997).

In summary, for Wilms' tumour, current clinical research is directed towards reducing therapy for good-prognosis patients, and identifying groups of patients for whom more intensive treatment is necessary. For this end, possible biological prognostic factors, such as LOH of 16q (Grundy *et al.*, 1994), and response to pre-nephrectomy chemotherapy may identify children with a higher risk of relapse and a requirement for more intensive therapy.

LATE EFFECTS OF TREATMENT

The survival of children with cancer has shown dramatic improvements over the last few decades and currently there is no sign of this trend abating. We now expect over two-thirds of children treated to be cured of their malignancy, and present estimates are that 1 in 900 adults aged 16–34 years are survivors of cancer in childhood, with over 10 000 known adult survivors of childhood cancer within the UK. Consideration of the quality of life of survivors – medical, psychosocial and educational – is therefore an increasing issue. The younger the patient at the time of treatment, the greater the risk of long-term consequences. Many of these survivors have paid a significant price for their cure, and data suggest that about half experience at least one chronic medical condition.

(M.C.G. Stevens *et al.*, 1998) Some of these may well be acceptable, if unfortunate – others may not. Other less definable effects, such as social interaction and emotional status, should not be under-rated. Potential problems faced by these individuals into their adult lives are many-fold, and indeed an ever-changing spectrum in line with the varied treatment administered over the years. Although some effects are now well known, the most important of which are described below, it must be borne in mind that others may yet declare themselves as newer treatments are undertaken. It is vital that these children continue to be assessed regularly into adult life.

Second malignancies

The development of a second malignant neoplasm is undoubtedly one of the most serious problems encountered in survivors, with a lifetime risk 10–20 times that of age-matched controls. The overall estimated probability ranges from 2 to 12 per cent at 25 years, with a trend to increasing incidence over recent times. Important factors include the nature of the original tumour, the constitution of treatment initially received, an inherent predisposition, or an interaction of any or all three factors.

Certain tumour groups are recognized to have an increased predisposition to second malignancies. Survivors of Hodgkin's disease have a 20-year actuarial risk estimated between 12 and 20 per cent with acute myeloid leukaemia and non-Hodgkin's lymphoma encountered early and solid tumours much later. Children with a genetic risk imposed by the retinoblastoma gene have a high chance of future development of bone and soft tissue sarcomas in particular, which triples if radiation is part of their treatment.

Radiotherapy is certainly mutagenic. Sarcomas, carcinomas, and brain tumours are all acknowledged late events, 85 per cent arising within the radiation field. Of increasing importance, however, are chemotherapy-related myelodysplasia/leukaemia (tAML) syndromes, which appear to be dose dependent (Hawkins *et al.*, 1992). tAML associated with alkylating agents, for example, most frequently involves deletions of chromosomes 5 and/or 7 with a myelodysplastic presentation several years (peak 4–7 years) post-treatment. tAML associated with topoisomerase-II inhibitors, on the other hand, occurs much sooner and involves 11q23 rearrangements. With the trend towards dose-intensive treatment for poor-risk disease, this complication is increasingly seen.

Finally, an inherent risk towards developing tumours may be found in familial cancer syndromes, the most frequently recognized being the Li–Fraumeni syndrome (predisposition to soft tissue sarcomas, brain tumours, breast cancer, osteosarcoma and leukaemia). It is estimated that 0.7 per cent of childhood cancers are consequent to this syndrome, with survivors continuing to be at increased risk of developing a second malignancy.

Growth

Any child surviving malignancy and its treatment should be given every opportunity to grow and develop normally, but to achieve this, close vigilance is necessary. Both nutrition and growth hormone (GH) are necessary for a normal growth rate during childhood. Hormone replacement or manipulation is often necessary to influence the growth pattern beneficially in these survivors of childhood malignancy, and may well be advantageous through into adult life. Therefore close collaboration with endocrinology colleagues is paramount.

Certainly, GH insufficiency is the most common growth abnormality encountered after cancer treatment in children. Cranial irradiation is a prime cause, with GH insufficiency usually the first, and sometimes the only anterior pituitary function to be affected, and is dose- and to a lesser extent, age-related. All children who receive more than 30 Gy to the hypothalamus will exhibit subnormal GH responses by 2–5 years post-irradiation. Obviously, in some cases growth may be compromised from non-hormonal causes following treatment for malignancy. Radiation to both the spine and the long bones can certainly impact on final height, the more so the younger the child at age of treatment. Chemotherapy-induced growth failure is definitely encountered, with steroids and methotrexate implicated in particular, although mechanisms are poorly understood. The combined effect of all these factors is clearly seen following bone marrow transplant in children, particularly if heavily pre-treated for leukaemia or complicated by the need for continued immunosuppression.

Fertility and sex hormone function

Radiotherapy and chemotherapy may both influence gonadal function. Damage to germ cells is common with treatment – this will lead to loss of both endocrine function and fertility in females, but as Leydig cell failure is rare in males, endocrine function may be preserved. Prior to commencing treatment, consideration of both the potential to avoid damage to or actually preserve germ cells should be undertaken. Germ cell failure will certainly ensue if the gonads remain in a radiation field – consideration of shielding or repositioning should be contemplated before treatment whenever possible. Uterine dysfunction following radiotherapy may also jeopardize future pregnancies – a factor that should be borne in mind if *in vitro* fertilization programmes are contemplated.

Cytotoxic agents, particularly alkylating agents, may cause gonadal damage which is dose, sex and age dependent – chemotherapy is much less toxic to the germ cells of the ovary than the testis, and the ovaries of prepubertal girls, with their abundance of follicles, are more resistant to the effects of chemotherapy than adolescents and adults. With conventional alkylator-based chemotherapy regimens, Leydig cell dysfunction is usually subclinical with raised levels of luteinizing hormone (LH) but normal testosterone; in the female, transient ovarian dysfunction may occur. Even if females continue to menstruate regularly, they remain at risk of early menopause. Not only should they be advised accordingly if contemplating a family, but they will also be predisposed to developing osteoporosis and coronary heart disease and should be carefully monitored for both.

Finally, the health and well-being of their actual offspring is an understandable area of concern for survivors of childhood malignancy. As yet, there are few published mature data in this field, although it would appear that there is no current evidence of appreciable excess risk of either malignancy or congenital malformations (Hawkins, 1994).

Organ toxicity

Cardiotoxicity associated with anthracycline therapy has been well recognized for over 20 years (Shan et al., 1996). In addition to cumulative dose, other risk factors proposed include mediastinal irradiation, younger age, higher rates of drug administration and rate of infusion. It is salient to realize that three differing forms are recognized: acute toxicity (rare), chronic toxicity leading to cardiomyopathy (more common and clinically the most important) and late-onset ventricular dysfunction and arrhythmias (now increasingly recognized). Disturbingly, abnormalities would appear to increase with the period of follow-up. With the passage from childhood to adulthood, such factors need to be taken into account with such activities as vigorous exercise and weight lifting, and childbirth – certainly close links with the obstetrics team must be encouraged for the latter.

Surgery and radiotherapy can potentially cause renal dysfunction, although often minimal with nephrectomy alone, or radiotherapy restricted to less than 20 Gy. As in many other areas, our understanding of the long-term effects of chemotherapy is still evolving. Glomerular damage is certainly a well-known complication of cisplatin therapy. Ifosfamide, a relative newcomer to the cytotoxic scene and one now frequently used in childhood cancer, may cause significant tubular and glomerular damage and is an important potential factor in the development of chronic nephrotoxicity, particularly in children (Skinner et al., 1993).

Although limited in its use in the paediatric field, lung irradiation commonly results in pulmonary toxicity, not only by its effect on the lung directly but also impinging on the growth of the chest wall. BCNU and CCNU are not frequently applied in the field of childhood cancer but bleomycin is certainly a cause of lung toxicity. Damage from methotrexate is rare but may be linked to administration at a young age.

Educational

Childhood and adolescence is the most critical time of learning and acquisition of skills, and the potential insult to the learning capacity of a survivor of childhood malignancy at this time may therefore be considerable. School-related problems and impaired performance are especially common. The most obvious cause is actual time lost from schooling. However, the underlying condition (brain tumours) the use of neurotoxic therapy (cranial irradiation, systemic or intrathecal methotrexate), and the age at the time of treatment (especially <3 years) are also important physical factors. Thus problems are most frequently encountered in long-term survivors of brain tumours, childhood leukaemia and BMT, and may range from minor subtle changes through particularly specific learning difficulties with underlying deficits in essential cognitive processing systems to global mental retardation. Such high-risk groups should therefore undergo function-specific neuropsychological assessment at an early stage if possible, to identify specific problem areas and concentrate resources on improvement. This area obviously has a major impact on future employment and quality of life in general.

Quality of life

The survivor's perspective of the quality of his own life is an aspect that is so obviously of paramount importance, but until quite recently has been neglected certainly in the literature, largely because of inherent difficulties in definition. Adjusting any such measure to children and adolescents is even more complex. Child health has been defined as 'the ability to participate fully in developmentally appropriate activities and requires physical, psychological and social energy', but obviously changes with age; those major concerns of a 5-year-old (e.g. family relationships, physical activity) are very different from a teenager (e.g. body image, peer relationships). Although we can outline many of the late effects that may be encountered in the battle to survive cancer, only the patient can relate the importance of it to him/herself and therefore its impact on leading a normal life. It is reassuring to note, therefore that many clinical trials are building such quality of life issues into the studies, so that in the future we may better understand this so far rather neglected aspect of both paediatric and adult cancer care.

SUPPORTIVE CARE

The outcome of children diagnosed with cancer has improved steadily in recent decades. This is largely due to the success of more intensive treatment protocols. This progress has been achieved because of the advances in supportive care.

Infection

A major factor in the increased survival rates of childhood malignancy has been the increased vigilance in prevention and early treatment of infection in the immunocompromised child. The use of broad-spectrum antibiotics in febrile neutropenic patients post-chemotherapy has contributed greatly to the marked fall in mortality due to infection in the past two decades. Additional impact has been achieved from prophylaxis and early treatment of fungal infection, opportunistic infections such as pneumocystis and viral infections, in particular varicella zoster. It is important that the child and the family are well informed of the importance of compliance with prophylactic antibiotics and the early reporting of signs of infection. Children will be encouraged to attend school as much as possible whilst on treatment. In order to reduce their chance of exposure to infection, particularly chicken pox, the school body as a whole must be well informed of the risk. This is implemented by good communication between the school and the health-care team. Where contact has occurred passive immunization with zoster immunoglobulin (ZIG) is indicated as soon as possible after contact unless the child has previously been documented as immune. If any signs of infection appear, then intravenous high-dose aciclovir is indicated to avoid visceral dissemination to lung, liver and brain.

Nutrition

Children with cancer will present with nutritional problems either as a result of their disease or more commonly as a result of their treatment. As with all children, growth is monitored carefully as a marker of general well-being. Loss of more than 10–15 per cent of body weight is associated with a high mortality due to the increased risk of infection, metabolic disturbances and specific nutritional deficiencies. The child with cancer may have increased nutritional requirements and yet struggle to meet them due to decreased appetite, nausea and vomiting or mucositis. The incidence of protein energy malnutrition (PEM) is reported to be between 6 per cent and 50 per cent of children with cancer. Consideration is given to parenteral nutrition, gastrostomy feeding and nutritional supplements. The paediatric dietitian is another essential member of the team. Nutritional intervention should begin at diagnosis and continue throughout the course of treatment.

Central venous catheters (CVCs)

The routine practice of inserting indwelling central venous catheters (CVCs) has had an enormous impact on the management of children with cancer. Previously survivors of childhood malignancy would vividly remember the pain, discomfort and anguish associated with repeated puncture sites for blood sampling and administration of drugs. The current protocols for the treatment of acute lymphoblastic leukaemia necessitate that the first month of treatment is managed without a CVC due to the increased risk of thromboembolic events with asparaginase. This has served as a painful reminder. In general otherwise, the advantages of an indwelling CVC outweigh the risks such as infection and embolic events. The type of device used (e.g. single versus double lumen or porta-cath) depends on the treatment strategy and options will be discussed with the patient and their family by the surgeon and paediatric oncologist.

Control of emesis

Nausea and vomiting associated with both chemotherapy and radiotherapy are common and often severe. Adequate control is essential for the patient's overall well-being. Inadequate control may exacerbate problems with nutrition and impair the patient's ability to tolerate a given treatment protocol. Control of nausea and vomiting is better achieved by prevention than by increasing therapy after onset of symptoms. A number of drugs are available with 5-HT$_3$ antagonists generally being the most popular due to their efficacy and limited toxicity. Lorazepam is useful for anticipatory nausea and vomiting, particularly in the adolescent population. Given that it is often the least experienced members of the oncology team responsible for prescribing anti-emetics, a number of paediatric units have developed written protocols (Foot and Hayes, 1994).

Palliative care

Each medical decision must be based not just on available technology but also on the wishes of the child. The child and their family should be aware of options, including those for palliative care. One of the reasons palliative care is not offered to families of dying children is that the prospect of a child dying is not accepted by society – including the parents and the medical team.

The same modalities of treatment are available for both curative intent and palliation, i.e. surgery, chemotherapy and radiotherapy. Supportive care of the dying child includes pain control, control of emesis (which may be triggered by the disease itself, drugs and anxiety) and transfusion of blood products. Pain management includes drugs, in particular opiates as well as antidepressants and anxiolytics. Other strategies include local anaesthetic blocks and psychological approaches.

Self-esteem of the child with cancer is threatened by pain, change in body image, isolation and anxiety, particularly about the possibility of death. The involvement of the multidisciplinary team should ensure that all these issues are tackled in an ongoing manner. In this way it is often the child who most easily comes to terms with the prospect of death. The family, particularly parents and siblings, need extensive support. They need to be helped in allowing the child to die and support should continue after the death. Families will be used to the involvement of the various professionals in their lives during the child's illness and feel abandoned if that involvement is not continued after the child's death.

The majority of children will die at home. Children's hospices do exist in the UK but comparatively few children with cancer have been admitted. Their role differs from the adult model with the majority of patients having long-term problems from metabolic or neurodegenerative disease and many admissions being for respite rather than terminal care.

PSYCHOLOGICAL ASPECTS OF CHILDHOOD CANCER

The psychological impact of the diagnosis of cancer in a child is enormous. There will be feelings of fear, guilt, anxiety, anger, denial, hopelessness and depression. It is the responsibility of the health-care team to support the child and their family. The team necessary to provide such support should include doctors, nurses, psychologists, the clergy and social workers (*see* Table 47.1). The parents should be together, to support one another, when the doctor explains the diagnosis. Discussions with the family should be in the presence of an experienced nurse or social worker, who may later help them assimilate the information. Information should be repeated and reinforced where possible with written material. The initial response of parents will be grief, despair and helplessness. They may feel disempowered as parents and an experienced medical team needs to recognize their feelings, reassure them that they are appropriate, normal responses and help them see the importance of their role in the child's care.

Talking to the child

'It is difficult for children, and certainly adolescents, to handle emotions. As a child with cancer you try to be strong for your parents. You feel responsible for their grief. This painful situation prevents you from accepting and dealing with your disease.

As a parent you can avoid a lot of suffering for your child if you're able to talk to them.'

The above quote is an extract from a speech given by a childhood cancer survivor at the ICCCPO Conference 1999.

Talking to the child with cancer is difficult for parents and they look to the extended team for guidance. The approach will depend on the child's chronological age, their developmental age and their past experiences.

Children may be unable to express their feelings in words, so need to explore other means of communication such as art therapy, music therapy and play therapy.

Prior to 1970 most of those dealing with childhood cancer believed that unless a child was older than 10, they were incapable of understanding death and therefore did not experience anxiety about it. Subsequent research asking the children to tell a story depicted in standardized pictorial scenes demonstrates that even young pre-school age children have a concept of the seriousness of their illness. Those children who had not had the opportunity to express their feelings demonstrated a psychological distance from those around them, leaving them isolated.

Educating the child with cancer

Fortunately, with the increased incidence of childhood cancer is an increasing cohort of childhood cancer survivors. It is important that treatment allows those survivors to reach their full potential in life. Maintaining attendance at school allows the child to keep up with and maintain identity within their peer group. It presents an image of hope to teachers, classmates, parents and the child. In addition, continuing education not only advances cognitive skills, it also enhances social and coping skills to help the child better deal with their illness.

Teachers need to be supported in supporting the child. In the main, support is provided by the specialist nurses, psychologists and the staff of the hospital school. It is important to set the child realistic goals to prevent further loss of self-esteem through failure.

Classmates will also need counselling and ongoing support.

Preparing children for the death of a classmate needs careful management involving parents, teachers, the medical team and often the ill child.

Psychoneuroimmunology

'Make a Wish' organizations such as the Starlight Foundation propose that granting a wish may reduce stress and influence immunity, so favourably impacting on the course of the patient's illness. In the authors' own experience, the opportunity to facilitate such a wish caused a dramatic change in a particular teenage patient's compliance. It seemed to trigger in her a belief that the medical team was 'on her side'.

Parent support groups

There are a number of parent support groups in existence. Early in 1999 a National Alliance of Childhood Cancer Parents Organizations (NACCPO) was formed to model the International Confederation of Childhood Cancer Parent Organizations (ICCCPO). Such an organization will link parent groups in the same way professionals are linked through national and international organizations such as the United Kingdom Children's Cancer Study Group (UKCCSG) and Société Internationale Oncologie Pédiatrique (SIOP). In addition, NACCPO seeks to become the voice of parents and families of children affected by cancer at a national level through interactions with government, health authorities and social services, to communicate the issues and represent their needs.

Supporting siblings

The siblings of a child with cancer will be significantly affected. Again, according to their age and understanding, they should be kept well informed. There are likely to be repeated episodes where the affected child and one or both parents will be away from home. The sibling left behind will deal with this better if they are aware of why it is happening. There are a number of support groups for siblings. In general, the support available to the affected child is also extended to the siblings.

Ambulatory paediatrics

The multidisciplinary paediatric oncology team have been the pioneers of ambulatory paediatrics. Minimizing time spent in hospital has been for the psychological benefit of the child and their family rather than the economic benefit to the health service. In fact, the resources needed to provide such a service are enormous. Specialist domiciliary care nurses do far more than just travel to the child's home or school to take blood samples or administer treatment. Integral to the success of ambulatory care is extensive education of all those involved in caring for the child. This includes parents, teachers and general practitioners. In addition, the child and their family need to know that they have rapid and easy access to medical support.

The rights of the child

The child with cancer should be well informed at a level appropriate to their age and understanding. This is a legal requirement of care. The Children's Act of 1989 in the UK and the United Nations Convention on the Rights of the Child (also 1989) exhort those involved in the care of children to inform the child of their situation, to solicit their opinion and when appropriate to regard their opinion as determinative. Clearly this may seem a huge responsibility for the child. They will look for advocates such as their parents, nursing staff or a social worker to help support them with making decisions regarding their care. By not soliciting the child's opinion, their autonomy is violated and the natural pathway to emerging independence in adult life is interrupted.

SIGNIFICANT POINTS

- The majority of children with malignancy are cured (>65 per cent).
- Treatment is according to national/ international protocols in order to recruit significant numbers to assess response.
- Radiotherapy is often omitted or delayed due to the unacceptable morbidity associated with its use in young children.
- Treatment of childhood cancer depends on a multidisciplinary team to provide the best care to the child and their family.
- With more than one in 1000 adults currently survivors of childhood cancer, careful surveillance of the late effects of treatment is imperative.

KEY REFERENCES

Chessells, J.M. (1995) Maintenance treatment and shared care in lymphoblastic leukaemia. *Arch. Dis. Child.* **73**, 368–73.

Heideman, R.L., Packer, R.J., Albright, L.A. *et al.* (1997) Tumours of the central nervous system. In Pizzo, P.A. and Poplack, D.G. (eds), *Principles and practice of pediatric oncology.* Philadelphia: Lippincott-Raven, 633–97.

Stevens, M.C.G., Mahler, H. and Parkes, S. (1998) The health status of adult survivors of cancer in childhood. *Eur. J. Cancer* **34**, 694–8.

Thomas, P.R., Perez, C.A., Neff, J.R., Nesbit, M.E. and Evans, R.G. (1984) The management of Ewing's sarcoma: role of radiotherapy in local tumor control. *Cancer Treat. Rep.* **68**, 703–10.

Wishoff, J.H., Boyett, J.M., Berger, M.S. *et al.* (1998) Current neurosurgical management and the impact of the extent of resection in the treatment of malignant gliomas of childhood: a report of the Children's Cancer Group Trial No. CCG-1945. *J. Neurosurg.* **89**, 52–9.

REFERENCES

Abudu, A., Sferopoulos, N.K., Tillman, R.M., Carter, S.R. and Grimer, R.J. (1996) The surgical treatment and outcome of pathological fractures in localised osteosarcoma. *J. Bone Joint Surg. [Br]* **78**, 694–8.

Ahrens, S., Hoffmann, C., Jabar, S. *et al.* (1999) Evaluation of prognostic factors in a tumor volume-adapted treatment strategy for localized Ewing sarcoma of bone: the CESS 86 experience. Cooperative Ewing Sarcoma Study. *Med. Pediatr. Oncol.* **32**, 186–95.

Al-Qabandi, W., Jenkinson, H.C., Buckels, J.A. *et al.* (1999) Orthotopic liver transplantation for unresectable hepatoblastoma: a single centres experience. *J. Pediatr. Surg.* **34**, 1261–4.

Anderson, C.A., Wilkening, G.N., Filley, C.M., Reardon, M.S. and Kleinschmidt-DeMasters, B.K. (1997) Neurobehavioral outcome in pediatric craniopharyngioma. *Pediatr. Neurosurg.* **26**, 255–60.

Arceci, R.J. (1999) The histiocytoses: the fall of the Tower of Babel. *Eur. J. Cancer* **35**, 747–69.

Argani, P., Perlman, E.J., Breslow, N.E. *et al.* (2000) Clear cell sarcoma of the kidney: a review of 351 cases from the National Wilms' Tumour Study Group Pathology Center. *Am. J. Surg. Pathol.* B, 4–18.

Armitage, J.O. and Weisenburger, D.D. (1998) New approach to classifying non-Hodgkin's lymphoma: clinical features of the major histological subtypes. *J. Clin. Oncol.* **16**, 2780–95.

Asada, N., Tsuchiya, H. and Tomita, K. (1999) *De novo* deletions of p53 gene and wild-type p53 correlate with acquired cisplatin-resistance in human osteosarcoma OST cell line. *Anticancer Res.* **19**, 5131–7.

Atra, A., Whelan, J.S., Calvagna, V. *et al.* (1997) High-dose busulphan/melphalan with autologous stem cell rescue in Ewing's sarcoma. *Bone Marrow Transplant.* **20**, 843–6.

Bacci, G. (1998) Letter. *J. Clin. Oncol.* **16**, 2290–1.

Bacci, G., Picci, P., Ferrari, S. *et al.* (1993) Primary chemotherapy and delayed surgery for nonmetastatic osteosarcoma of the extremities. Results in 164 patients preoperatively treated with high doses of methotrexate followed by cisplatin and doxorubicin. *Cancer* **72**, 3227–38.

Bacci, G., Briccoli, A., Mercuri, M. *et al.* (1998a) Osteosarcoma of the extremities with synchronous lung metastases: long-term results in 44 patients treated with neoadjuvant chemotherapy. *J. Chemother.* **10**, 69–76.

Bacci, G., Donati, D., Manfrini, M. *et al.* (1998b) [Local recurrence after surgical or surgical-chemotherapeutic treatment of osteosarcoma of the limbs. Incidence, risk factors and prognosis]. *Minerva Chir.* **53**(7–8), 619–29.

Bacci, G., Ferrari, S., Delepine, N. *et al.* (1998c) Predictive factors of histologic response to primary chemotherapy in osteosarcoma of the extremity: study of 272 patients preoperatively treated with high-dose methotrexate, doxorubicin, and cisplatin [*see* comments]. *J. Clin. Oncol.* **16**, 658–63.

Bacci, G., Ferrari, S., Mercuri, M. *et al.* (1998d) Predictive factors for local recurrence in osteosarcoma: 540 patients with extremity tumors followed for minimum 2.5 years after neoadjuvant chemotherapy. *Acta Orthop. Scand.* **69**, 230–6.

Bacci, G., Briccoli, A., Ferrari, S. *et al.* (2000) Neoadjuvant chemotherapy for osteosarcoma of the extremities with synchronous lung metastases: treatment with cisplatin, adriamycin and high dose of methotrexate and ifosfamide. *Oncol. Rep.* **7**, 339–46.

Bailey, C.C., Gnekow, A., Wellek, S. *et al.* (1995) Prospective randomised trial of chemotherapy given before radiotherapy in childhood medulloblastoma. International Society of Paediatric Oncology (SIOP) and the (German) Society of Paediatric Oncology (GPO): SIOP II. *Med. Pediatr. Oncol.* **25**, 166–78.

Berger, C., Thiesse, P., Lellouch-Tubiana, A., Kalifa, C., Pierre-Kahn, A. and Bouffet, E. (1998) Choroid plexus carcinomas in childhood: clinical features and prognostic factors. *Neurosurgery* **42**, 470–5.

Bergsagel, D.J., Finegold, M.J., Butel, J.S., Kupsky, W.J. and Garcoa, R.L. (1992) DNA sequences similar to those of simian virus 40 in ependymomas and choroid plexus tumors of childhood. *N. Engl. J. Med.* **326**, 988–93.

Bielack, S.S., Bieling, P., Erttmann, R. and Winkler, K. (1993) Intraarterial chemotherapy for osteosarcoma: does the result really justify the effort? *Cancer Treat. Res.* **62**, 85–92.

Bielack, S., Kempf-Bielack, B., Schwenzer, D. *et al.* (1999) Neoadjuvant therapy for localized osteosarcoma of extremities. Results from the Cooperative osteosarcoma study group COSS of 925 patients. *Klin. Padiatr.* **211**, 260–70.

Boccon-Gibod, L., Rey, A., Sandstedt, B. *et al.* (2000) Complete necrosis induced by preoperative chemotherapy in Wilms' tumour as an indicator of low risk: report of three international society of paediatric oncology (SIOP) nephroblastoma trial and study 9. *Med. Pediatr. Oncol.* **34**, 183–90.

Bouffet, E., Doz, F., Demaille, M.C. *et al.* (1998a) Improving survival in recurrent medulloblastoma: earlier detection, better treatment or still an impasse? *Br. J. Cancer* **77**, 1321–6.

Bouffet, E., Perilongo, G., Canete, A. and Massimino, M. (1998b) Intracranial ependymomas in children: a critical review of prognostic factors and a plea for cooperation. *Med. Pediatr. Oncol.* **30**, 319–31.

Bown, N., Cotterill, S., Lastowska, M., *et al.* (1999) Gain of chromosome arm 17q and adverse outcome in patients with neuroblastoma. *N. Engl. J. Med.* **340**, 1954–61.

Bramwell, V.H., Burgers, M., Sneath, R. *et al.* (1992) A comparison of two short intensive adjuvant chemotherapy regimens in operable osteosarcoma of limbs in children and young adults: the first study of the European Osteosarcoma Intergroup. *J. Clin. Oncol.* **10**, 1579–91.

Brinster, R.L., Chen, H.Y., Messing, A., van Dyke, T., Levine, A.J. and Palmiter, R.D. (1984) Transgenic mice harboring SV40 T-antigen genes develop characteristic brain tumors. *Cell* **37**, 367–79.

Brodeur, G.M. (1995) Molecular basis for heterogeneity in human neuroblastomas. *Eur. J. Cancer* **31**, 505–10.

Burdach, S., Jurgens, H., Peters, C. *et al.* (1993) Myeloablative radiochemotherapy and hematopoietic stem-cell rescue in poor-prognosis Ewing's sarcoma. *J. Clin. Oncol.* **11**, 1482–8.

Burgert, E.O. Jr, Nesbit, M.E., Garnsey, L.A. *et al.* (1990) Multimodal therapy for the management of nonpelvic, localized Ewing's sarcoma of bone: intergroup study IESS-II [*see* comments]. *J. Clin. Oncol.* **8**, 1514–24.

Bussey, K.J., Lawce, H.J., Olson, S.B. *et al.* (1999) Chromosome abnormalities of eighty-one pediatric germ cell tumours: sex-, age-, site- and histopathology-related differences – a Children's Cancer Group Study. *Genes Chromosomes Cancer* **25**, 134–46.

Calaminus, G., Andreussi, L., Garre, M.L. *et al.* (1997) Secreting germ cell tumours of the central nervous system (CNS). First results of the cooperative German/Italian pilot study (CNS sGCT). *Klin. Padiatr.* **209**, 222–7.

Carli, M., Colombatti, R., Oberlin, O. *et al.* (1999) High-dose melphalan with autologous stem-cell rescue in metastatic rhabdomyosarcoma. *J. Clin. Oncol.* **17**, 2796–803.

Carnevale, A., Lieberman, E. and Cardenas, R. (1997) Li-Fraumeni syndrome in pediatric patients with soft tissue sarcoma or osteosarcoma. *Arch. Med. Res.* **28**, 383–6.

Carter, S.R., Grimer, R.J., Sneath, R.S. and Matthews, H.R. (1991) Results of thoracotomy in osteogenic sarcoma with pulmonary metastases. *Thorax* **46**, 727–31.

Castleberry, R.P., Cushing, B., Perlman, E. and Hawkins, E.P. (1997). Germ cell tumours. In Pizzo, P.A. and Poplack, D.G. (eds), *Principles and practice of pediatric oncology*. Philadelphia: Lippincott-Raven, 921–45.

Cavazzuti, V., Fischer, E.G., Welch, K., Belli, J.A. and Winston, K.R. (1983) Neurological and psychophysiological sequelae following different treatments of craniopharyngioma in children. *J. Neurosurg.* **59**, 409–17.

Chessells, J.M. (1995) Maintenance treatment and shared care in lymphoblastic leukaemia. *Arch. Dis. Child.* **73**, 368–73.

Cho, H.J., Seiberg, M., Georgoff, I., Teresky, A.K., Marks, J.R. and Levine, A.J. (1989) Impact of the genetic background of transgenic mice upon the formation and timing of choroid plexus papillomas. *J. Neurosci. Res.* **24**, 115–22.

Chow, E., Jenkins, J.J., Burger, P.C. *et al.* (1999) Malignant evolution of choroid plexus papilloma. *Pediatr. Neurosurg.* **31**, 127–30.

Chu, T., D'Angio, G.J., Favara, B. *et al.* (1987) Histiocytosis syndromes in children. *Lancet* **1**, 208–9.

Claming, U. and Henter, J.-I. (1998) Elevated ESR and thrombocytosis may be valuable markers of active disease in Langerhans cell histiocytosis. *Acta Pediatr.* **87**, 1085–7.

Cline, M.J. (1994) The molecular basis of leukaemia. *N. Engl. J. Med.* **330**, 328–36.

Cokgor, I., Friedman, A.H. and Friedman, H.S. (1998) Paediatric update: gliomas. *Eur. J. Cancer* **12**, 1910–18.

Craft, A., Cotterill, S. *et al.* (1993) Improvement in survival for Ewing's sarcoma by substitution of ifosfamide for cyclophosphamide. *Am. J. Pediatr. Hematol. Oncol.* **15**(suppl. A), 531–5.

Creutzig, U., Ritter, J. and Schelling, G. (1990) Identification of 2 risk groups in childhood acute myelogenous leukaemia after therapy intensification in the study AML-BFM-83 as compared with the study AML-BFM-78. *Blood* **75**, 1932–40.

Crist, W., Gehan, E.A., Ragab, A.H. *et al.* (1995) The third Intergroup Rhabdomyosarcoma Study. *J. Clin. Oncol.* **13**, 610–30.

Croce, C.M. and Nowell, P.C. (1985) Molecular basis of human B-cell neoplasia. *Blood* **65**, 1.

D'Angio, G.J., Breslow, N., Beckwith, J.B. *et al.* (1989) The treatment of Wilms' tumour: results of the Third National Wilms' Tumour Study. *Cancer* **64**, 349–60.

de Alava, E., Kawai, A., Healey, J.H. *et al.* (1998) EWS-FLI1 fusion transcript structure is an independent determinant of prognosis in Ewing's sarcoma [published erratum appears in *J. Clin. Oncol.* 1998; **16**(8): 2895] [*see* comments]. *J. Clin. Oncol.* **16**, 1248–55.

Delattre, O., Zucman, J., Melot, T. *et al.* (1994) The Ewing family of tumors – a subgroup of small-round-cell tumors defined by specific chimeric transcripts [*see* comments]. *N. Engl. J. Med.* **331**, 294–9.

Delepine, N., Delepine, G., Jasmin, C., Desbois, J.C., Cornille, H. and Mathe, G. (1988) Importance of age and methotrexate dosage: prognosis in children and young adults with high-grade osteosarcomas. *Biomed. Pharmacother.* **42**, 257–62.

Delepine, N., Cornille, D.G., Brion, H. *et al.* (1995) Dose escalation with pharmacokinetics monitoring in methotrexate chemotherapy of osteosarcoma. *Anticancer Res.* **15**, 489–94.

Delepine, N., Delepine, G., Bacci, G., Rosen, G. and Desbois, J.C. (1996) Influence of methotrexate dose intensity on outcome of patients with high grade osteogenic osteosarcoma. Analysis of the literature [*see* comments]. *Cancer* **78**, 2127–35.

DeVile, C.J., Grant, D.B., Hayward, R.D. and Stanhope, R. (1996) Growth and endocrine sequelae of craniopharyngioma. *Arch. Dis. Child.* **75**, 108–14.

Deutsch, M., Thomas, P., Boyett, J. *et al.* (1991) Low stage medullobastoma: a Children's Cancer Study Group (CCSG) and Pediatric Oncology Group (POG) randomized study of standard vs reduced neuraxis radiation. *Proc. ASCO* **10**, A363.

DeZen, L., Sommaggio, A., d'Amore, E. *et al.* (1997) Clinical relevance of DNA ploidy and proliferative activity in childhood rhabdomyosarcoma: a retrospective analysis of patients enrolled onto the Italian Cooperative Rhabdomyosarcoma Study RMS88. *J. Clin. Oncol.* **15**, 1198–205.

Duffner, P.K., Horowitz, M.E., Krischer, J.P. *et al.* (1993) Postoperative chemotherapy and delayed radiation in children less than three years of age with malignant brain tumours. *N. Engl. J. Med.* **328**, 1725–31.

Duffner, P.K., Kun, L.E., Burger, P.C. *et al.* (1995) Postoperative chemotherapy and delayed radiation in infants and very young children with choroid plexus carcinomas. The Pediatric Oncology Group. *Pediatr. Neurosurg.* **22**, 189–96.

Dunkel, I.J., Boyett, J.M., Yates, A. *et al.* (1998) High-dose carboplatin, thiotepa, and etoposide with autologous stem-cell rescue for patients with recurrent medulloblastoma. Children's Cancer Group. *J. Clin. Oncol.* **16**, 222–8.

Dupuis-Girod, S., Hartmann, O., Benhamou, E. *et al.* (1996) Will high dose chemotherapy followed by autologous bone marrow transplantation supplant cranio-spinal irradiation in young children treated for medulloblastoma? *J. Neurooncol.* **27**, 87–98.

Eilber, F., Giuliano, A., Eckardt, J., Patterson, K., Moseley, S. and Goodnight, J. (1987) Adjuvant chemotherapy for osteosarcoma: a randomized prospective trial. *J. Clin. Oncol.* **5**, 21–6.

Enneking, W.F. (1986) A system of staging musculoskeletal neoplasms. *Clin. Orthop.* **204**, 9–24.

Evans, A.E., Jenkin, R.D., Sposto, R. *et al.* (1990) The treatment of medulloblastoma. Results of a prospective randomized trial of radiation therapy with and without CCNU, vincristine, and prednisone. *J. Neurosurg.* **72**, 572–82.

Evans, A.E., Silber, J.H., Shpilsky, A. *et al.* (1996) Successful management of low stage neuroblastoma without adjuvant therapies: a comparison of two decades, 1972 through 1981 and 1982 through 1992, in a single institution. *J. Clin. Oncol.* **14**, 2504–10.

Ewing, J. (1921) Diffuse endothelioma of bone. *Proc. N. Y. Pathol. Soc.* **21**, 17–24.

Feugeas, O., Guriec, N., Babin-Boilletot, A. *et al.* (1996) Loss of heterozygosity of the RB gene is a poor prognostic factor in patients with osteosarcoma [published erratum appears in *J. Clin. Oncol.* 1996; **14**(8): 2411]. *J. Clin. Oncol.* **14**, 467–72.

Feusner, J.H., Krailo, M.D. and Haas, J.E. (1993) Treatment of pulmonary metastases of initial stage I hepatoblastoma in childhood. Report from the Children's Cancer Group. *Cancer* **71**, 859–64.

Finlay, J.L., Boyett, J.M., Yates, A.J. *et al.* (1995) Randomized phase III trial in childhood high-grade astrocytoma comparing vincristine, lomustine and prednisone with the eight-drugs-in-one day regimen. *J. Clin. Oncol.* **13**, 112–23.

Flamant, F., Rodary, C., Rey, A. *et al.* (1998) Treatment of non-metastatic rhabdomyosarcomas in childhood and adolescence. Results of the second study of the International Society of Paediatric Oncology: MMT84. *Eur. J. Cancer* **34**, 1050–62.

Foot, A.B.M. and Hayes, C. (1994) Audit of guidelines for effective control of chemotherapy induced emesis. *Arch. Dis. Child.* **71**, 475–7.

Gajjar, A., Sanford, R.A., Heideman, R. *et al.* (1997) Low-grade astrocytoma: a decade of experience at St. Jude Children's Research Hospital. *J. Clin. Oncol.* **15**, 2792–9.

Geyer, J.R., Finlay, J.L., Boyett, J.M. *et al.* (1995) Survival of infants with malignant astrocytomas. A report from the Children's Cancer Group. *Cancer* **75**, 1045–50.

Goldwein, J.W., Radcliffe, J., Johnson, J. *et al.* (1996) Updated results of a pilot study of low dose craniospinal irradiation plus chemotherapy for children under five with cerebellar primitive neuroectodermal tumors (medulloblastoma). *Int. J. Radiat. Oncol. Biol. Phys.* **34**, 899–904.

Goto, A., Kanda, H., Ishikawa, Y. *et al.* (1998) Association of loss of heterozygosity at the p53 locus with chemoresistance in osteosarcomas. *Jpn. J. Cancer Res.* **89**, 539–47.

Graf, N., Winkler, K., Betlemovic, M., Fuchs, N. and Bode, U. (1994) Methotrexate pharmacokinetics and prognosis in osteosarcoma. *J. Clin. Oncol.* **12**, 1443–51.

Graham, M.L., Herndon, J.E., Casey, J.R. *et al.* (1997) High-dose chemotherapy with autologous stem-cell rescue in patients with recurrent and high-risk pediatric brain tumors. *J. Clin. Oncol.* **15**, 1814–23.

Green, D.M. (1997) Wilms' tumour. *Eur. J. Cancer* **33**, 409–18.

Green, D.M., Coppes, M.J., Breslow, N.F. *et al.* (1997) Wilms' tumour. In Pizzo, P.A. and Poplack, D.G. (eds), *Principles and practice of pediatric oncology*. Philadelphia: Lippincott-Raven, 733–59.

Grundy, P.E., Telzerlow, P.E., Breslow, N. *et al.* (1994) Loss of heterozygosity for chromosomes 16q and 1p in Wilms' tumours predicts an adverse outcome. *Cancer Res.* **54**, 2331–3.

Haas, J.E., Muczynski, K.A., Krailo, M. *et al.* (1989) Histopathology and prognosis in childhood hepatoblastoma and hepatocellular carcinoma. *Cancer* **64**, 1082.

Harris, M.B., Gieser, P., Goorin, A.M. *et al.* (1998) Treatment of metastatic osteosarcoma at diagnosis: a Pediatric Oncology Group Study. *J. Clin. Oncol.* **16**, 3641–8.

Harris, N.L., Jaffe, E.S., Stein, H. *et al.* (1994) A revised European-American classification of lymphoid neoplasm: a proposal from the International Lymphoma Study Group. *Blood* **84**, 1361–92.

Hawkins, M.M. (1994) Pregnancy outcome and offspring after childhood cancer [editorial]. *Br. Med. J.* **309**, 1034.

Hawkins, M.M., Kinnier-Wilson, L.M., Stovall, M.A. *et al.* (1992) Epipodophyllotoxins, alkylating agents, and radiation and risk of secondary leukaemia after childhood cancer. *Br. Med. J.* **304**, 951–8.

Heideman, R.L., Packer, R.J., Albright, L.A. *et al.* (1997) Tumours of the central nervous system. In Pizzo, P.A.

and Poplack, D.G. (eds), *Principles and practice of pediatric oncology*. Philadelphia: Lippincott-Raven, 633–97.

Janss, A.J., Grundy, R., Cnaan, A. *et al.* (1995) Optic pathway and hypothalamic/chiasmatic gliomas in children younger than age 5 years with a 6-year follow up. *Cancer* **75**, 1051–9.

Jurgens, H., Gobel, V., Michaelis, J. *et al.* (1985) The Cooperative Ewing Sarcoma Study CESS 81 of the German Pediatric Oncology Society – analysis after 4 years. *Klin. Padiatr.* **197**, 225–32.

Jurgens, H., Exner, U., Gadner, H. *et al.* (1988) Multidisciplinary treatment of primary Ewing's sarcoma of bone. A 6-year experience of a European Cooperative Trial. *Cancer* **61**, 23–32.

Kawai, A., Hamada, M., Sugihara, S., Hashizume, H., Nagashima, H. and Inoue, H. (1995) Rotationplasty for patients with osteosarcoma around the knee joint. *Acta Med. Okayama* **49**, 221–6.

Kelly, K.M., Womer, R.B., Sorensen, P.H. *et al.* (1997) Common and variant gene fusions predict distinct clinical phenotypes in rhabdomyosarcoma. *J. Clin. Oncol.* **15**, 1831–6.

Kraus, J.A., Albrecht, S., Wiestler, O.D. *et al.* (1996) Loss of heterozygosity on chromosome 1 in hepatoblastoma. *Int. J. Cancer* **67**, 467–71.

Ladisch, S. and Gadner, H. (1994) Treatment of Langerhans cell histiocytosis – evolution and current approaches. *Br. J. Cancer* **70**(suppl. XXIII), S41–6.

Lennard, L., Davies, H.A. and Lilleyman, J.S. (1993) Is thioguanine more appropriate than 6-mercaptopurine for children with acute lymphoblastic leukaemia? *Br. J. Cancer* **68**, 186–90.

Li, F.P., Breslow, N.E., Morgan, J.M. *et al.* (1996) Germline WT1 mutations in Wilms' tumor patients: preliminary results. *Med. Pediatr. Oncol.* **27**, 404–7.

Linet, M.S., Ries, L.A., Smith, M.A. *et al.* (1999) Cancer surveillance series: recent trends in childhood cancer incidence and mortality in the United States. *J. Natl Cancer Inst.* **91**, 1051–8.

Link, M.P. (1993) The multi-institutional osteosarcoma study: an update. *Cancer Treat. Res.* **62**, 261–7.

Link, M.P., Goorin, A.M., Miser, A.W. *et al.* (1986) The effect of adjuvant chemotherapy on relapse-free survival in patients with osteosarcoma of the extremity. *N. Engl. J. Med.* **314**, 1600–6.

McLean, T.W. and Pritchard, J. (1996) Langerhans cell histiocytosis and hypercalcaemia: clinical response to indomethacin. *J. Pediatr. Hematol. Oncol.* **18**, 318–20.

Marina, N.M., Pappo, A.S., Parham, D.M. *et al.* (1999) Chemotherapy dose-intensification for pediatric patients with Ewing's family of tumors and desmoplastic small round-cell tumors: a feasibility study at St. Jude Children's Research Hospital. *J. Clin. Oncol.* **17**, 180–90.

Matthay, K.K., Villablanca, J.G., Seeger, R.C. *et al.* (1999) Treatment of high-risk neuroblastoma with intensive chemotherapy, radiotherapy, autologous bone marrow transplantation, and 13-cis-retinoic acid. *N. Engl. J. Med.* **341**, 1165–73.

Matsui, I., Tanimura, M., Kobayashi, N. *et al.* (1993) Neurofibromatosis type 1 and childhood cancer. *Cancer* **72**, 2746.

Meyer, W.H., Kun, L., Marina, N. *et al.* (1992) Ifosfamide plus etoposide in newly diagnosed Ewing's sarcoma of bone. *J. Clin. Oncol.* **10**, 1737–42.

Meyers, P.A., Gorlick, R., Heller, G. *et al.* (1998) Intensification of preoperative chemotherapy for osteogenic sarcoma: results of the Memorial Sloan-Kettering (T12) protocol. *J. Clin. Oncol.* **16**, 2452–8.

Miser, J.S., Kinsella, T.J., Triche, T.J. *et al.* (1987) Ifosfamide with mesna uroprotection and etoposide: an effective regimen in the treatment of recurrent sarcomas and other tumors of children and young adults. *J. Clin. Oncol.* **5**, 1191–8.

Narod, S., Stiller, C. and Lenior, G. (1991) An estimate of the heritable fraction of childhood cancer. *Br. J. Cancer* **63**, 993.

Needle, M.N., Goldwein, J.W., Grass, J. *et al.* (1997) Adjuvant chemotherapy for the treatment of intracranial ependymoma of childhood. *Cancer* **80**, 341–7.

Newton, W.A., Meadows, A., Shimada, H., Bunin, G.R., Vawter, G.F. and Newton, W.A. Jr (1991) Bone sarcomas as second malignant neoplasms following childhood cancer. *Cancer* **67**, 193–201.

Nichols, C.R., Anderson, J., Lazarus, H.M. *et al.* (1992) High dose carboplatin and etoposide with autologous bone marrow transplantation in refractory germ cell cancer: an Eastern Cooperative Oncology Group protocol. *J. Clin. Oncol.* **10**, 558.

Oakhill, A., Pamphilon, D.H., Potter, M.N. *et al.* (1996) Unrelated donor bone marrow transplantation for children with relapsed acute lymphoblastic leukaemia in second complete remission. *Br. J. Haematol.* **94**, 574–8.

Ohira, M. (1990) Autologous bone marrow transplantation in pediatric cancer. *Gan To Kagaku Ryoho* **17**, 2299–306.

Ornadel, D., Souhami, R.L., Whelan, J. *et al.* (1994) Doxorubicin and cisplatin with granulocyte colony-stimulating factor as adjuvant chemotherapy for osteosarcoma: phase II trial of the European Osteosarcoma Intergroup. *J. Clin. Oncol.* **12**, 1842–8.

Packer, R.J. (1990) Chemotherapy for medulloblastoma/ primitive neuroectodermal tumors of the posterior fossa. *Ann. Neurol.* **28**, 823–8.

Packer, R.J. (1999) Childhood medulloblastoma: progress and future challenges. *Brain Dev.* **21**, 75–81.

Packer, R.J., Sutton, L.N., D'Angio, G., Evans, A.E. and Schut, L. (1985) Management of children with primitive neuroectodermal tumors of the posterior fossa/medulloblastoma. *Pediatr. Neurosci.* **12**, 272–82.

Packer, R.J., Sutton, L.N., Elterman, R. *et al.* (1994) Outcome for children with medulloblastoma treated with radiation and cisplatin, CCNU, and vincristine chemotherapy. *J. Neurosurg.* **81**, 690–8.

Patte, C., Philip, T., Rodary, C. *et al.* (1986) Improved survival rate in children with stage III and IV B NHL and leukaemia using multi-agent chemotherapy: results of a study of 114 children from the French Pediatric Oncology Society *J. Clin. Oncol.* **4**, 1219–26.

Paulussen, M., Ahrens, S., Burdach, S. *et al.* (1998) Primary metastatic (stage IV) Ewing tumor: survival analysis of 171 patients from the EICESS studies. European Intergroup Cooperative Ewing Sarcoma Studies. *Ann. Oncol.* **9**, 275–81.

Paulussen, M., Ahrens, S., Braun-Munzinger, G. *et al.* (1999) EICESS 92 (European Intergroup Cooperative Ewing's Sarcoma Study) – preliminary results. *Klin. Padiatr.* **211**, 276–83.

Pein, F., Michon, J., Valteau-Couanet, D. *et al.* (1998) High-dose melphalan, etoposide and carboplatin followed by autologous stem-cell rescue in paediatric high-risk recurrent Wilms' tumour: a French Society of Pediatric Oncology study. *J. Clin. Oncol.* **16**, 3295–301.

Perilongo, G., Massimino, M., Sotti, G. *et al.* (1997) Analyses of prognostic factors in a retrospective review of 92 children with ependymoma: Italian Paediatric Neuro-Oncology Group. *Med. Pediatr. Oncol.* **29**, 79–85.

Perilongo, G. and Shafford, E.A. (1999) Liver tumours. *Eur. J. Cancer* **35**, 953–9.

Philip, T. (1999) Early detection of neuroblastoma in infants. Research? Yes. Routine screening? No. Report of the 1998 consensus conference on neuroblastoma screening. *Med. Pediatr. Oncol.* **33**, 355–9.

Philip, T., Iliescu, C., Demaille, M.C. *et al.* (1999) High-dose methotrexate and HELP [Holoxan (ifosfamide), eldesine (vindesine), platinum]–doxorubicin in non-metastatic osteosarcoma of the extremity: a French multicentre pilot study. Federation Nationale des Centres de Lutte contre le Cancer and Societe Francaise d'Oncologie Pediatrique. *Ann. Oncol.* **10**, 1065–71.

Pierga, J.Y., Kalifa, C., Terrier-Lacombe, M.J., Habrand, J.L. and Lemerle, J. (1993) Carcinoma of the choroid plexus: a pediatric experience. *Med. Pediatr. Oncol.* **21**, 480–7.

Pinkerton, C.R. (1997) Malignant germ cell tumours in childhood. *Eur. J. Cancer* **33**, 895–902.

Plaschkes, J., Perilongo, G. and Shafford, E. (1995) Childhood hepatoblastoma: an investigation into variables of prognostic relevance using data from the SIOP liver tumour study (SIOPEL 1). SIOP XXVII meeting abstract. *Med. Pediatr. Oncol.* **25**, 256.

Plaschkes, J., Perilongo, G. and Shafford, E. (1996) Pre-operative chemotherapy – cisplatin (PLA) and doxorubicin (DO) PLADO for the treatment of hepatoblastoma and hepatocellular carcinoma – results after 2 years' follow up. *Med. Pediatr. Oncol.* **27**, 256.

Plon, S.E. and Peterson, L.E. (1997) Childhood cancer, hereditary and the environment. In Pizzo, P.A. and Poplack, D.G. (eds), *Principles and practice of pediatric oncology*. Philadelphia: Lippincott-Raven, 11–36.

Pollack, I.F., Claassen, D., al-Shboul, Q. *et al.* (1995) Low-grade gliomas of the cerebral hemispheres in children: an analysis of 71 cases. *J. Neurosurg.* **82**, 536–47.

Prados, M.D., Edwards, M.S., Chang, S.M. *et al.* (1999) Hyperfractionated craniospinal radiation therapy for primitive neuroectodermal tumors: results of a Phase II study. *Int. J. Radiat. Oncol. Biol. Phys.* **43**, 279–85.

Pritchard-Jones, K. (1996) Genetics of childhood cancer. *Br. Med. Bull.* **52**, 704–23.

Robison, L.L. (1997) General principles of the epidemiology of childhood cancer. In Pizzo, P.A. and Poplack, D.G. (eds), *Principles and practice of pediatric oncology*. Philadelphia: Lippincott-Raven, 1–10.

Rorke, L.B., Gilles, F.H., Davis, R.L. and Becker, L.E. (1985) Revision of the World Health Organization classification of brain tumours for childhood brain tumours. *Cancer* **56**, 1869.

Rorke, L.B., Packer, R. and Biegel, J. (1995) Central nervous system atypical teratoid/rhabdoid tumors of infancy and childhood. *J. Neurooncol.* **24**, 21–8.

Rorke, L.B., Packer, R.J. and Biegel, J. (1996) Central nervous system atypical teratoid/rhabdoid tumors of infancy and childhood: definition of an entity. *J. Neurosurg.* **85**, 56–65.

Sauer, R., Jurgens, H., Burgers, J.M., Dunst, J., Hawlicek, R. and Michaelis, J. (1987) Prognostic factors in the treatment of Ewing's sarcoma. The Ewing's Sarcoma Study Group of the German Society of Paediatric Oncology CESS 81. *Radiother. Oncol.* **10**, 101–10.

Schajowicz, F., Sissons, H. and Sobin, L.H. (1995) The World Health Organization's histologic classification of bone tumors: a commentary on the second edition. *Cancer* **75**, 1208–14.

Sevenet, N., Sheridan, E., Amram, D., Schneider, P., Handgretinger, R. and Delattre, O. (1999) Constitutional mutations of the *hSNF5/INI1* gene predispose to a variety of cancers. *Am. J. Hum. Genet.* **65**, 1342–8.

Shamberger, R.C., Guthrie, K.A., Ritchey, M.L. *et al.* (1999) Surgery-related factors and local recurrence of Wilms' tumour in National Wilms' Tumour Study 4. *Ann. Surg.* **229**, 292–7.

Shan, K., Lincoff, M.A. and Young, J.B. (1996) Anthracycline-induced cardiotoxicity. *Ann. Intern. Med.* **125**, 47–58.

Shankar, A.G., Pinkerton, C.R., Atra, A. *et al.* (1999) Local therapy and other factors influencing site of relapse in patients with localised Ewing's sarcoma. United Kingdom Children's Cancer Study Group (UKCCSG). *Eur. J. Cancer* **35**, 1698–704.

Skinner, R., Sharkey, I.M., Pearson, A.D.J. *et al.* (1993) Ifosfamide, Mesna, and nephrotoxicity in children. *J. Clin. Oncol.* **11**, 173–90.

Smith, M.A. (1991) The impact of doxorubicin dose intensity on survival of patients with Ewing's sarcoma [letter; comment]. *J. Clin. Oncol.* **9**, 889–91.

Smith, M.A., Ungerleider, R.S., Horowitz, M.E. and Simon, R. (1991) Influence of doxorubicin dose intensity on response and outcome for patients with osteogenic sarcoma and Ewing's sarcoma [*see* comments]. *J. Natl Cancer Inst.* **83**, 1460–70.

Souhami, R.L., Craft, A.W., Van der Eijken, J.W. *et al.* (1997) Randomised trial of two regimens of chemotherapy in operable osteosarcoma: a study of the European Osteosarcoma Intergroup [*see* comments]. *Lancet* **350**, 911–17.

Sposto, R., Ertel, I.J., Jenkin, R.D.T. *et al.* (1989) The effectiveness of chemotherapy for treatment of high grade astrocytoma in children: results of a randomised trial. *J. Neurooncol.* **7**, 165–77.

Stevens, M.C.G., Mahler, H. and Parkes, S. (1998) The health status of adult survivors of cancer in childhood. *Eur. J. Cancer* **34**, 694–8.

Stevens, R.F., Hann, I.M., Wheatley, K., *et al.* (1998) Marked improvements in outcome with chemotherapy alone in paediatric acute myeloid leukaemia. Results of AML10. *Br. J. Haematol.* **100**, 130–40.

Stewart, D.A., Gyonyor, E., Patterson, A.H. *et al.* (1996) High-dose melphalan ± total body irradiation and autologous hematopoietic stem cell rescue for adult patients with Ewing's sarcoma or peripheral neuroectodermal tumor. *Bone Marrow Transplant.* **18**, 315–18.

Stiller, C.A., Allen, M.B. and Eatock, E.M. (1995) Childhood cancer in Britain: the national registry of childhood tumours and incidence rates 1978–1987. *Eur. J. Cancer* **31A**, 2028–34.

Sweetnam, R. (1973) Amputation in osteosarcoma. Disarticulation of the hip or high thigh amputation for lower femoral growths? *J. Bone Joint Surg. [Br]* **55**, 189–92.

Szendroi, M., Papai, Z., Koos, R. and Illes, T. (2000) Limb-saving surgery, survival, and prognostic factors for osteosarcoma: the Hungarian experience. *J. Surg. Oncol.* **73**, 87–94.

Tabone, M.D., Kalifa, C., Rodary, C., Raquin, M., Valteau-Casanet, D. and Lemerle, J. (1994) Osteosarcoma recurrences in pediatric patients previously treated with intensive chemotherapy. *J. Clin. Oncol.* **12**, 2614–20.

Tait, D.M., Thornton-Jones, H., Bloom, H.J., Lemerle, J. and Morris-Jones, P. (1990) Adjuvant chemotherapy for medulloblastoma: the first multi-centre control trial of the International Society of Paediatric Oncology (SIOP I). *Eur. J. Cancer* **26**, 464–9.

Thomas, P.R., Perez, C.A., Neff, J.R., Nesbit, M.E. and Evans, R.G. (1984) The management of Ewing's sarcoma: role of radiotherapy in local tumor control. *Cancer Treat. Rep.* **68**, 703–10.

Torres, C.F., Rebsamen, S., Silber, J.H. *et al.* (1994) Surveillance scanning of children with medulloblastoma [see comments]. *N. Engl. J. Med.* **330**, 892–5.

van Rijk-Zwikker, G.L., Nooy, M.A., Taminiau, A., Kappetein, A.P. and Huysmans, H.A. (1991) Pulmonary metastasectomy in patients with osteosarcoma. *Eur. J. Cardiothorac. Surg.* **5**, 406–9.

Wells, R.J., Wood, W.G., Buckley, J.D. *et al.* (1994) Treatment of newly diagnosed children and adolescents with AML: a CCG study. *J. Clin. Oncol.* **12**, 2367–77.

Willman, C.L., Busque, L., Griffith, B.B. *et al.* (1994) Langerhans cell histiocytosis (histiocytosis X) – a clonal proliferative disease. *N. Engl. J. Med.* **331**, 154–60.

Winkler, K., Bielack, S., Delling, G. *et al.* (1990) Effect of intraarterial versus intravenous cisplatin in addition to systemic doxorubicin, high-dose methotrexate, and ifosfamide on histologic tumor response in osteosarcoma (study COSS-86). *Cancer* **66**, 1703–10.

Wishoff, J.H., Boyett, J.M., Berger, M.S. *et al.* (1998) Current neurosurgical management and the impact of the extent of resection in the treatment of malignant gliomas of childhood: a report of the Children's Cancer Group Trial No. CCG-1945. *J. Neurosurg.* **89**, 52–9.

Wolff, J.E., Sajedi, M., Coppes, M.J., Anderson, R.A. and Egeler, R.M. (1999) Radiation therapy and survival in choroid plexus carcinoma [letter]. *Lancet* **353**, 2126.

Woods, W.G., Kobrinsky, N., Buckley, J.D. *et al.* (1996) Timed sequential induction therapy improves remission outcome in acute myeloid leukaemia: a report from the Children's Cancer Study Group. *Blood* **87**, 4979–89.

48

AIDS-related cancer

MARK BOWER AND KATE FIFE

INTRODUCTION

The human immunodeficiency virus (HIV) was recognized as a human pathogen less than 20 years ago, but in that time it has infected millions of people, resulting in a global pandemic. The consequence of HIV infection is a relentless destruction of the immune system, culminating in the diagnosis of acquired immunodeficiency syndrome (AIDS). The World Health Organization estimated that at the start of 2002, 40 million people were living with HIV. During 2001 there were an estimated 5 million people infected with HIV or 14 000 each day. Over 90 per cent of the new HIV infections occurred in developing countries, 10 per cent were children under 15 years old, >40 per cent were women and >50 per cent were aged 15–24 years old. In most of the established market economy countries the HIV infection rate peaked in the late 1980s and has declined. Furthermore, a significant reduction in the death rate for people with AIDS has been seen with the introduction of potent combination antiretroviral drugs. Thus in these countries there are increasing numbers of people living longer with their HIV infection.

Both primary congenital immunosuppression and iatrogenic secondary immunosuppression have long been recognized to predispose patients to particular malignancies and it was therefore not surprising that these malignancies occurred more frequently in people with HIV infection. Many of the malignancies associated with immunosuppression are thought to have a viral aetiology,

with herpesviruses (Kaposi's sarcoma, non-Hodgkin's lymphoma) and papillomaviruses (cervical cancer, anal cancer) implicated. It is of interest that some of the tumours (such as Burkitt's lymphoma and Hodgkin's disease) that occur more frequently in HIV are not associated with other forms of immunosuppression, and that some tumours in which viruses have been implicated (such as hepatocellular carcinoma) do not occur more frequently in HIV patients.

The development of effective antiretroviral therapies commenced in the mid-1980s with the introduction of zidovudine, and since that time there has been a rapid expansion of the therapeutic armamentarium to combat HIV. There are three classes of drugs currently licensed for the treatment of HIV: nucleoside analogue reverse transcriptase inhibitors, non-nucleoside analogue reverse transcriptase inhibitors and protease inhibitors. The introduction of the last two classes in the late 1990s led to the use of combination highly active antiretroviral treatment (HAART). This advance was associated with profound and sustained suppression of HIV viral replication, a dramatic reduction in opportunistic infections, AIDS-defining illnesses and mortality amongst HIV-infected persons. In addition to reducing the incidence of opportunistic infections, HAART has been associated with a reduction in the incidence of Kaposi's sarcoma and primary cerebral lymphoma, although there appears to be have been no major reduction in the incidence of systemic lymphoma.

KAPOSI'S SARCOMA

Epidemiology

The era of AIDS was heralded by the emergence of two previously uncommon diseases, *Pneumocystis carinii* pneumonia and Kaposi's sarcoma (KS). An aggressive form of KS emerged in homosexual men in the USA in 1981 (Friedman-Kien *et al.*, 1981). Prior to 1981, three different clinical expressions of the disease had been recognized. Classical KS is an indolent variant, predominantly affecting elderly men of Mediterranean and Jewish descent. A more severe form affects children and young adults in sub-Saharan Africa (endemic KS). Thirdly, KS comprises up to 5 per cent of malignancies in immunosuppressed allogeneic transplant recipients. AIDS-related Kaposi's sarcoma is the cancer most frequently seen in patients with HIV and develops in 10–15 per cent of people with AIDS during the course of the illness.

Evidence for co-infection by a second agent

The epidemiology of AIDS-KS points to an infectious agent transmitted independently of HIV. An analysis of 13 000 persons with AIDS reported to the Centre for Disease Control, Atlanta up to 1989 revealed that the incidence of KS in homosexual and bisexual men infected with HIV is 10 times greater than in other seropositive transmission groups (Beral *et al.*, 1990). The lifetime incidence in some cohorts of homosexual men with AIDS is 50 per cent. A study of the sexual behaviour of 65 homosexual or bisexual men with AIDS suggested that faeco-oral contact was likely to be the main route of transmission of a putative KS infectious agent in this risk group. However, blood transmission may also occur, as 4 per cent of HIV-seropositive patients infected by blood transfusion develop AIDS-KS. The risk of developing KS in haemophiliacs is lower (1 per cent), implying that blood transmission may be cell- rather than serum-related. KS has also been reported in HIV-negative homosexual men, in whom it follows the indolent course found in classical

KS. Furthermore, there is evidence that classical KS was increasing prior to the AIDS epidemic, with a doubling of incidence in Sweden over 25 years prior to 1982.

Human herpes virus-8 discovery

In 1994 Chang and Moore isolated unique DNA sequences from KS biopsies using representational difference analysis, a polymerase chain reaction (PCR)-based technique that enriches DNA fragments ('representations') present in the tumour but absent from normal unaffected skin from the same subject. The original sequences that were found were homologous to, but distinct from, capsid and tegument protein genes of the gammaherpes viruses *Herpesvirus saimiri* and Epstein–Barr virus (Chang *et al.*, 1994). Complete genomic sequencing of this novel herpes virus, initially named Kaposi sarcoma herpes virus (KSHV) and subsequently renamed human herpes virus-8 (HHV8) has been completed (Russo *et al.*, 1996). The sequence analysis confirms that HHV8 is most closely related to *Herpesvirus saimiri*, which induces lymphoid malignancies in New World primates, and Epstein–Barr virus, a human oncogenic herpes virus.

The HHV8 genome consists of a 140 kb unique coding region flanked by terminal repeat sequences. The unique region includes at least 81 open reading frames (ORFs) that potentially encode proteins. In addition to structural proteins and viral enzymes, HHV8 encodes several pirated eukaryotic cellular proteins which could maintain its latent state in B lymphocytes or in KS-associated spindle cells and contribute to tumour formation. These include homologues for a G-protein-coupled receptor, cyclin D, interleukin-6, bcl-2 and interferon regulatory factor (Fig. 48.1).

HHV8 has been demonstrated in KS lesions from patients with all forms of the disease including HIV-associated KS, endemic KS, classical KS, allograft recipients with KS and HIV-seronegative gay men with KS. In addition, HHV8 has been detected in two rare HIV-associated lymphoproliferative disorders, multicentric Castleman's disease and primary effusion lymphoma (Cesarman *et al.*, 1995; Soulier *et al.*, 1995).

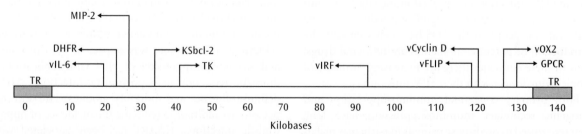

Figure 48.1 *HHV8 genome and location of pirated cellular homologues. TR, Terminal repeat; TK, thymidine kinase; vIL-6, viral interleukin-6; vIRF, viral interferon regulatory factor; DHFR, dihydrofolate reductase; vFLIP, viral FLICE inhibitory protein; MIP-2, macrophage inhibitory protein-2; GPRC, G-protein-coupled receptor; KSbcl2, Kaposi's sarcoma B-cell lymphoma 2.*

Molecular virology of human herpes virus-8

Molecular epidemiological studies and first-generation serological assays have demonstrated that HHV8 is not ubiquitous. The virus appears to be more prevalent in those populations at increased risk for developing KS, including homosexual men, Africans and certain populations in Mediterranean Europe, while the prevalence of HHV8 appears quite low (<5 per cent) in the general population of the US and UK.

The mode of transmission of HHV8 remains unclear. Initial studies suggested that the virus was present in semen; however, numerous investigators have failed to confirm this finding and the only frequent source of HHV8 from patients with KS is peripheral blood mononuclear cells and saliva. In a serial cohort study from New York that covers the period 1984–97, the annual HHV8 sero-conversion rate among 245 homosexual men was 6 per cent per annum, and was higher with increasing numbers of partners. Horizontal as well as vertical transmission of HHV8 is supported by immunofluorescence assay data from twin studies in Gambia. Eight per cent of twins under 2 years old are seropositive, suggesting vertical transmission. The seropositive rate rises with age, to 65 per cent in those aged 45–54 years, supporting horizontal transmission of HHV8.

The presence of HHV8 DNA in the peripheral blood of HIV-positive patients without KS has been shown to predict for the later development of clinical KS. KS lesions appeared in half the HHV8-positive men within 30 months of follow-up (Whitby et al., 1995). The risk of KS appears to be greater in those with a higher HHV8 antibody titre, in both HIV-negative and -positive subjects (Beral et al., 1999). Thus a group of patients at high risk of KS may be identified and could form the focus of preventative treatment strategies.

The evidence for a causal role for HHV8 in the pathogenesis of KS is accumulating. HHV8 infection precedes the clinical development of KS and the epidemiology and risk factors for HHV8 infection and KS overlap. HHV8 has been demonstrated in KS spindle cells and in the endothelial cells in KS lesions. Finally, HHV8 infects and transforms primary human endothelial cells, thought to be the precursor cells of malignant KS spindle cells.

Is Kaposi's sarcoma a malignancy?

All forms of KS have the same characteristic histology, comprising spindle-shaped stromal cells, abnormal proliferating endothelial cells and extravasated erythrocytes. The major component of KS lesions is composed of endothelial cells, fibroblasts and inflammatory cells, which form slit-like vascular channels to resemble neoangiogenesis. The cell of origin for KS remains controversial; mesenchymal cells, vascular and lymphatic endothelial cells and smooth muscle cells have all been proposed as potential spindle-cell precursors. It is uncertain whether KS is a polyclonal proliferation or a true malignancy. Spindle cells contain a normal chromosomal complement and lack nuclear atypia, which might favour a non-malignant process. There is, however, increasing evidence supporting the definition of KS as a true malignancy. KSY-1, a cell line derived from the pleural effusion of a man with AIDS-KS, has metastatic properties in animal models. In addition, tumour clonality has been shown in some human tumour biopsies by X-chromosome inactivation patterns in women patients with AIDS-KS (Rabkin et al., 1995).

Other pathogenetic factors

CYTOKINES

The expression of growth factors and their receptors by KS cells has been demonstrated by immunocytochemical staining and in culture. Amongst the many growth factors that are expressed by KS cells are basic fibroblast growth factor (bFGF), interleukin-1β, interleukin-6, interleukin-8, oncostatin-M and vascular endothelial growth factor (VEGF). These cytokines are mitogenic for KS cells in culture, suggesting that they may act as autocrine growth factors. In contrast, transforming growth factor-β (TGF-β), which is also expressed by KS cells, acts as an autocrine growth inhibitor. Moreover, bFGF acts not only as an autocrine growth factor for KS cells but also stimulates endothelial cell migration and proliferation. Antisense oligonucleotides to bFGF mRNA block KS cell growth and lesion formation in nude mice xenografts. Furthermore, subcutaneous injections of bFGF induce KS-like skin lesions in nude mice (Ensoli et al., 1994). Thus host cytokines appear to play an important role in the development of KS lesions and form a second potential target for novel therapeutic strategies.

HIV VIRAL FACTORS

The role of HIV itself in the pathogenesis of KS has been a focus of research since early in the AIDS epidemic. The tat gene product of HIV is a potent transactivator which upregulates viral gene expression by transcriptional and post-transcriptional enhancement and is necessary for viral replication. HIV Tat is released from HIV-infected T lymphocytes. In cell culture, Tat stimulates KS cell growth and promotes the migration and proliferation of cytokine-activated endothelial cells. When injected subcutaneously into nude mice, Tat causes KS-like lesions and there is a synergy between Tat and bFGF in this effect (Ensoli et al., 1994). Moreover, about 15 per cent of male transgenic mice overexpressing the tat gene developed skin tumours resembling KS at age 12–18 months (Vogel et al., 1988). These lesions were multifocal and contained spindle-shaped cells in the dermis and slit-like spaces with extravasated blood cells. The effect of Tat in KS is thought to be mediated by integrin receptors. These are receptors for extracellular matrix (ECM) proteins which induce cell adhesion and invasion, facilitating angiogenesis. The Tat protein contains an RGD domain which is the receptor-binding sequence for integrins and Tat is able to bind to the VEGF receptor Flk-1 and induce a mitogenic signal. It is believed that these actions of Tat may account for the rather aggressive course of AIDS-KS compared with the more indolent behaviour of KS in the HIV-seronegative population.

HUMAN CHORIONIC GONADOTROPHIN

The striking male predominance of classical KS was first noted in the nineteenth century by Kaposi in his original description of the disease, and has been observed in all forms of the disease. Men develop KS with a greater frequency than women in all HIV transmission groups (Beral et al., 1990). Case reports of complete regression of KS during and shortly after pregnancy in two women with AIDS (Lunardi-Iskandar et al., 1995) led to suggestions that human chorionic gonadotrophin (hCG) may have a role in the pathogenesis of KS. Immunohistochemical staining of biopsies of AIDS-KS lesions demonstrated the presence of hCG receptors, which are not expressed by normal human skin. Murine models of KS have revealed that a pregnancy-related molecule has anti-tumour activity. However, further studies have shown that full-length recombinant hCG heterodimer is inactive and the active element may be either a fragment of hCG or another molecule that co-purifies with hCG.

Clinical features and differential diagnosis

AIDS-related KS has a wide variety of clinical presentations. The earliest cutaneous lesions are frequently asymptomatic, innocuous-looking, macular, pigmented lesions, which vary in colour from faint pink to vivid purple. Larger plaques occur usually on the trunk as oblong lesions following the line of skin creases. Lesions may develop to form large plaques and nodules which can be associated with painful oedema. Lymphatic infiltration is a common feature in the limbs and causes lymphoedema and ulceration.

Oral lesions are a frequent accompaniment which may lead to ulceration, dysphagia and secondary infection. Gastrointestinal lesions are usually asymptomatic but may bleed. Pulmonary KS is a life-threatening complication that usually presents with dyspnoea, with or without fever and may cause haemoptysis. Chest X-ray typically reveals a diffuse reticulo-nodular infiltrate and pleural effusion. Visceral KS has been described in all organs at post-mortem examinations. In making the diagnosis of visceral KS the complications of biopsy (particularly haemorrhage) must be carefully weighed up against the benefits of confirming the diagnosis histologically.

The main differential diagnosis is bacillary angiomatosis or epitheloid angiomatosis, which is caused by a fastidious Gram-negative rikettsia-like organism Bartonella henselae (previously known as Rochalimea henselae). This infection can be treated effectively with erythromycin. These diagnoses can only be reliably distinguished histopathologically and so a biopsy is essential to confirm the diagnosis of KS.

Staging

The staging system described for AIDS-KS does not follow the standard TNM approach but instead includes an assessment of immune function as determined by the CD4 cell count. In the modified AIDS Clinical Trials Group staging classification, poor-risk tumour (T1) includes ulcerated KS, KS-associated oedema, nodular oral KS or KS involvement of any visceral organ. Poor immune status (I1) is defined as a CD4 T-lymphocyte count of $<150/\mu L$ (Krown et al., 1997) (Table 48.1).

Treatment options

The management of AIDS patients with KS must balance the benefits of tumour regression with the potential effects of treatment upon the patient's immunological and haematological status. For patients with symptomatic disease or life-threatening visceral disease prompt, effective therapy is usually merited, whereas for patients with asymptomatic indolent lesions, treatment will not prolong survival, although it can bring significant cosmetic and psychological benefits. Although the treatment of early cutaneous KS with systemic chemotherapy yields response

Table 48.1 *The modified AIDS Clinical Trials Group staging of Kaposi's sarcoma (KS) (Krown et al., 1997)*

	Good risk (all of the following)	Poor risk (any of the following)
Tumour (T)	Confined to skin, lymph nodes or minimal oral disease	Tumour-associated oedema or ulceration Extensive oral KS Gastrointestinal KS KS in other non-nodal viscera
Immune status (I)	CD4 count $>150/\mu L$	CD4 $<150/\mu L$

rates in excess of 40 per cent, these responses are not durable (Uthayakumar *et al.*, 1996) and the toxicity of chemotherapy in this patient population has led to a less aggressive approach to early disease where immune restoration by HAART is the mainstay.

Highly active antiretroviral therapies

Although there is epidemiological evidence for a reduction in the incidence of AIDS-related KS as a first AIDS diagnosis, this data is confused by the alterations to the definition of AIDS by the US Centers for Disease Control, most recently in 1993. None the less, the current data suggest that there is a genuine fall in the incidence of KS both as a first AIDS diagnosis and a subsequent manifestation in HIV seropositive cohorts from established market economies. This decline in KS coincides with the introduction of highly active antiretroviral therapies (HAART) and in some cohort studies the relative risk of developing KS is significantly lower amongst people receiving HAART regimens.

Furthermore, early in the AIDS epidemic it was recognized through anecdotal reports that regression of KS occasionally occurred on antiretroviral monotherapy with zidovudine. Moreover, response rates in KS improved when zidovudine was added to interferon-α. This led to speculation that immune reconstitution following the initiation of HAART therapy may lead to regression of KS, and a number of case reports and small studies documenting responses of KS to HAART have been published. A cohort study of 78 patients with established KS has demonstrated that the introduction of HAART therapy is associated with a prolongation of the time to treatment failure of KS (Bower *et al.*, 1999a) and this effect complements the reported reduction in the incidence of KS developing in patients on HAART. Thus HAART therapy has a major influence both on the epidemiology and clinical progression of KS without apparently having a direct effect upon the causative herpes virus, HHV8. The postulated mechanism of this effect is the immune reconstitution of cytotoxic T-lymphocyte responses to HHV8 which have been demonstrated (Osman *et al.*, 1999).

INTRALESIONAL CHEMOTHERAPY

Localized therapies are advocated for patients with limited cutaneous disease. Intralesional injection of a dilute solution of vinblastine (0.2 mg/mL), using volumes of up to 0.5 mL per lesion, is an effective easy and well-tolerated treatment for lesions under 1 cm in diameter. This treatment may cause pain at the site of injection and this may be reduced by prior use of local anaesthetic. There is frequently an initial flare reaction and lesions then regress, flatten and become fainter over the ensuing fortnight. However, post-treatment hyperpigmentation leaves brown spots at the sites and may be cosmetically unsatisfactory. Intralesional vinblastine has no significant systemic effects and injections may be repeated two or three times. This

approach is also valuable for small intra-oral lesions and gingival KS.

RADIOTHERAPY

Larger cutaneous or oral lesions may be treated with radiotherapy, and local control is generally achieved with doses above 8 Gy. For cutaneous lesions, either a single fraction of 8 Gy or 16 Gy in four daily fractions is routinely used. Although the response rate and duration of local control may be better with fractionated regimens compared with single-fraction treatment, toxicity and patient convenience are worse. Cosmetic improvement is usually achieved, although there may be a halo appearance on account of the margin around treated lesions. Severe mucositis and acute oedema may follow radiation treatment of the oral cavity and feet, and for this reason treatment is given in four fractions of 4 Gy each at weekly intervals. Recurrent tumour within radiation fields is common and therefore radiotherapy treatment is usually reserved for symptomatic and cosmetically disturbing lesions. Superficial X-rays (90 kV) or low-energy electrons (4–6 MeV) with skin bolus are adequate for most skin lesions. Conjunctival lesions may be amenable to strontium-90 applicators. Megavoltage photons (6 MeV) with a direct anterior 'Bermuda shorts' field and skin bolus may be required for the common clinical problem of gross inguinal lymphadenopathy with groin KS lesions. Sensitive areas such as the oral cavity, groins and the soles of the feet are best treated with fractionations of either 16 Gy in 4 fractions over 4 weeks or 20 Gy in 10 fractions over 2 weeks.

IMMUNOTHERAPY

Immunotherapy for good-risk disease has been advocated in patients with well-preserved immune function (generally CD4 counts >200/μL). Interferons inhibit HIV replication and angiogenesis and interferon-α (IFN-α) was the first agent licensed for use in AIDS-KS. Low-dose IFN-α (3–5 MU) produces response rates in KS of 10 per cent, whereas higher doses (>20 MU) yield response rates of 30 per cent. The response rates were highest in patients with higher CD4 levels, no B symptoms and no opportunistic infections. The response may take several weeks to achieve and there is considerable toxicity associated with this treatment, including myalgia, arthralgia, fevers, chills, anorexia, weight loss, nausea, diarrhoea, anaemia, neutropaenia and elevated liver enzymes. In combination with nucleoside analogues, interferon acts synergistically on KS cells *in vitro*. Initial studies have shown higher response rates for the combination of zidovudine and IFN-α, and lower IFN-α doses may be used. The combination causes considerable myelosuppression and granulocyte colony stimulating factor (G-CSF) may be needed to compensate for this. The considerable toxicity of immunotherapy and its lack of efficacy in patients with advanced immunosuppression severely limit the benefits of this strategy.

CHEMOTHERAPY

Chemotherapy is advocated for advanced cutaneous and visceral Kaposi's sarcoma, but is not merited for early disease in view of the brief response durations observed (Uthayakumar *et al.*, 1996). Early single-agent studies confirmed the activity of a number of cytotoxic agents. In particular, anthracyclines, vinca alkaloids, bleomycin and etoposide were found to have clinical activity, with observed response rates of 20–60 per cent. Although comparative studies assessing single-agent and combination chemotherapy have not generally been undertaken, combination chemotherapy schedules were designed for KS in an attempt to enhance efficacy without additive toxicity. The most frequently used combination chemotherapy for KS is bleomycin and vincristine, with or without doxorubicin®. Cohort studies of bleomycin and vincristine with or without doxorubicin have reported response rates between 23 and 88 per cent. However, the criteria for reporting responses in KS varied between studies until 1989, when recognized guidelines for evaluating responses were published (Krown *et al.*, 1989) (Table 48.2).

In Europe, bleomycin plus vincristine (BV) was the most frequently prescribed chemotherapy for KS until the mid-1990s. It is considered safe and effective, the main toxicity being peripheral neuropathy, although reduced transfer factor is seen with cumulative bleomycin doses in excess of 100 IU. The recommended maximum total bleomycin dosage is 300 IU and for doxorubicin is 450 mg/m^2. However, these limits are suggested to prevent the long-term toxicities associated with these agents and are generally inappropriate to this group of patients. The addition of doxorubicin was widely practised in America and may increase the response rate marginally but results in myelosuppression and alopecia.

Our standard first-line combination chemotherapy regimen for advanced KS in that era was bleomycin 15 IU i.v. bolus and vincristine 1 mg i.v. bolus every 2 weeks. This combination is generally well tolerated, causing little myelosuppression. Hypersensitivity reactions to bleomycin may be prevented by hydrocortisone 100 mg i.v. bolus, and anti-emetics are not routinely required. Vincristine-related peripheral neuropathy may develop, particularly in patients also prescribed zalcitabine (ddC), and for these patients vinblastine 5 mg i.v. bolus may be substituted for the vincristine, although this regimen is more myelosuppressive.

Liposomal anthracyclines

Liposome encapsulation of anthracyclines constitutes a considerable advance in the chemotherapy of KS. The advantages of liposomal formulation include increased tumour uptake and hence favourable pharmacokinetics. Moreover, the liposomal forms are less cardiotoxic than the parent anthracyclines. Both liposome-encapsulated

Table 48.2 *Response criteria for HIV-associated Kaposi's sarcoma (Krown et al., 1989)*

Complete response (CR)
The complete resolution of all KS with no new lesions, lasting for at least 4 weeks. A biopsy is required to confirm the absence of residual KS in flat lesions containing pigmentation. Endoscopies must be repeated to confirm the complete resolution of previously detected visceral disease

Clinical complete response (CCR)
Patients who have no detectable residual KS lesions for at least 4 weeks but whose response was not confirmed by biopsy and/or repeat endoscopy

Partial response (PR)
One or more of the following in the absence of
(i) new cutaneous lesions, (ii) new visceral/oral lesions, (iii) increasing KS-associated oedema, (iv) a 25% or more increase in the product of the bidimensional diameters of any index lesion:

1. A 50% or greater decrease in the number of measurable lesions on the skin and/or in the mouth or viscera
2. A 50% or greater decrease in the size of the lesions as defined by one of the following three criteria:
   (a) a 50% or more decrease in the sums of the products of the largest bidimensional diameters of the index lesions
   (b) a complete flattening of at least 50% of the lesions
   (c) where 75% or more of the nodular lesions become indurated plaques

Stable disease (SD)
Any response that does not meet the above criteria

Progressive disease (PD)
Any of the following:

1. A 25% or more increase in the product of the bidimensional diameters of any index lesion
2. The appearance of new lesions
3. Where 25% or more of previously flat lesions become raised
4. The appearance of new or increased KS-associated oedema

daunorubicin (DaunoXome®) and the pegylated liposomal doxorubicin (Caelyx®, Doxil®) have been shown to have good anti-tumour activity. The toxicity profile is better than for other anthracyclines, with no reported cardiotoxicity, even with high cumulative dosages, and rarely significant alopecia; however, there remains considerable myelosuppression and occasional emesis. In addition, infusion-related hypotension and hand/foot syndrome are novel side-effects seen with these liposomal formulations. In randomized comparisons of liposomal doxorubicin compared to both ABV (Northfelt *et al.*, 1995) and BV (Stewart *et al.*, 1998) as first-line therapy for KS, response rates were higher in the Caelyx® arms. A phase III randomized comparison of DaunoXome® and ABV demonstrated no improvement in response rate, time to treatment failure or survival duration, and there was

Table 48.3 *The results of phase III trials of liposomal anthracyclines for Kaposi's sarcoma*

Agent	Dose (mg/m²)	Schedule	Assessable patients	Response rates (%)	Median response duration (m)	References
DaunoXome®	40	Every 2 weeks	116	25	3.8	Gill *et al.* (1996)
Doxil®/Caelyx®	20	Every 2 weeks	133	46	3.0	Northfelt *et al.* (1995)
Doxil®/Caelyx®	20	Every 2 weeks	62	79	8.1	Mitsuyasu *et al.* (1997)
Doxil®/Caelyx®	20	Every 3 weeks	121	58	5.0	Stewart *et al.* (1998)

Table 48.4 *Table of experimental studies of pathogenesis-based therapy for Kaposi's sarcoma*

Agent	Mechanism	Phase	Reference
Thalidomide	Anti-angiogenesis	Phase II	Welles *et al.* (1997); Fife *et al.* (1998)
TNP-470 (fumagillin analogue)	Anti-angiogenesis	Phase I	Dezube *et al.* (1997)
Interleukin-12	Anti-angiogenesis	Phase I	Pluda *et al.* (1999)
IM-862	Anti-angiogenesis	Phase I/II	Gill *et al.* (1998)
Interleukin-4	Cytokine modulation	Phase I/II	Tulpule *et al.* (1997)
Pentosan polysulphate	Anti-angiogenesis	Phase II	Schwartsmann *et al.* (1995)
Tecogalan (SP-PG)	Anti-angiogenesis	Phase I	Eckhardt *et al.* (1996)
SU 5416	Anti-angiogenesis	Phase I	Rosen *et al.* (1998)
Recombinant platelet factor-4	Anti-angiogenesis	Phase I/II	Khan *et al.* (1993); Staddon *et al.* (1994)

significantly more neutropaenia with the liposomal daunorubicin (Gill *et al.*, 1996). Table 48.3 summarizes the results of phase III trials of liposomal anthracyclines for KS. These results may not be directly comparable, but it is unlikely that a head-to-head comparison of Caelyx® and DaunoXome® will be completed. Based on the response rates, median response durations and the toxicity profile, liposomal anthracyclines are considered first-line chemotherapy for advanced KS.

Paclitaxel

Paclitaxel has been shown to have single-agent activity against KS and has a valuable role in the management of refractory disease. The toxicities of paclitaxel are well recognized, although they appear to be no worse in patients with HIV than in other groups treated with equivalent dosages. Two studies of refractory KS have shown response rates of 53 and 71 per cent and median response durations of 7.4 and 10.4 months (Gill *et al.*, 1995; Saville *et al.*, 1995). These results have led to the rapid acceptance of paclitaxel as the treatment of choice for refractory KS.

NOVEL THERAPIES FOR KAPOSI'S SARCOMA

The importance of angiogenesis and host cytokine activity in the pathogenesis of KS lesions and the recently identified role of HHV8 has led to several novel approaches to the management of KS.

Topical retinoids

In vitro retinoids inhibit the proliferation of KS-derived spindle-cell lines and all-*trans* retinoic acid has been shown to induce apoptotic cell death in these lines. Moreover, retinoids downregulate the expression of interleukin-6 receptors, which are thought to play a role in the autocrine stimulation of KS cells. Systemic therapy with both all-*trans* retinoic acid and 13-*cis* retinoic acid has been disappointing. More promising results have been reported for the topical application (Duvic *et al.*, 1997) and oral administration (Friedman-Kien *et al.*, 1998) of 9-*cis* retinoic acid, which binds to both classes of retinoid receptors: retinoic acid receptors (RAR) and retinoid X-receptors (RXR).

Anti-angiogenic therapies

Kaposi's sarcoma is an easily accessible and evaluable tumour that is composed predominantly of proliferating endothelial cells and is a valuable model of tumour angiogenesis. For this reason a number of anti-angiogenic agents have been studied in Kaposi's sarcoma. Thalidomide inhibits bFGF-induced vascular proliferation, production of tumour necrosis factor-α (TNF-α), intercellular adhesion and vascular maturation. Two small studies of thalidomide in AIDS-related KS have documented regression of lesions (Welles *et al.*, 1997; Fife *et al.*, 1998). Other anti-angiogenic agents have been investigated in clinical trials in KS and are listed in Table 48.4.

Anti-human herpes virus-8 approaches

The discovery of HHV8 opens up a potential therapeutic target for the management and prevention of HHV8-associated malignancies. There are anecdotal reports of regression of KS with the anti-herpetic agent foscarnet and studies that demonstrate a reduced incidence of KS among patients previously treated with anti-herpes drugs (Mocroft *et al.*, 1996). These data suggest that inhibition of HHV8 could have a role in the treatment and prophylaxis of KS. *In vitro* the most effective antiviral agent tested has been cidofovir which, in addition, inhibits viral interleukin-6 (vIL-6) production by KS cells in culture. Furthermore, cidofovir inhibits the development of KS xenografts in nude mice. Although it is unlikely that

Table 48.5 *Frequency of HIV-NHL subtypes according to Working Formulation (WF) and Revised European American Lymphoma (REAL) classifications*

WF	REAL	Frequency (%)
Small non-cleaved cell: J		24–38
Burkitt's	Burkitt's	
non-Burkitt's	High-grade B-cell lymphoma Burkitt-like	
Large cell immunoblastic: H	Diffuse large B-cell lymphoma	18–31
Diffuse large cell: G	Diffuse large B-cell lymphoma	17–40

antiviral agents will be of significant benefit in established tumours, their role in cancer prophylaxis amongst HHV8-seropositive patients may prove valuable.

SYSTEMIC NON-HODGKIN'S LYMPHOMA

Epidemiology

The Center for Disease Control (CDC) included high-grade B-cell non-Hodgkin's lymphoma (NHL) as an AIDS-defining illness in 1985, following the description of NHL in 90 men from a population at risk for AIDS (Ziegler *et al.*, 1984). It is now recognized that NHL in HIV-positive patients is 60 times more common than in the general population (Beral *et al.*, 1991). NHL is the AIDS-defining diagnosis in 3.0–3.5 per cent of patients in Europe. The annual rate of developing NHL after a diagnosis of AIDS is 2.4 per cent per year, remaining constant over a 5-year period. An estimated 5–10 per cent of patients will therefore develop HIV-NHL at some time during their illness. HIV-associated NHL accounts for 12–16 per cent of all deaths attributable to AIDS. It appears to be slightly more common in haemophiliacs and less common in intravenous drug users than in other HIV transmission groups (Beral *et al.*, 1991). The age incidence is bimodal, with peaks in the 10–19-year and 50–59-year age groups, reflecting peaks in Burkitt's lymphoma and diffuse large-cell/immunoblastic lymphomas, respectively.

The incidence of HIV-NHL rises with progressive immunosuppression. The cumulative risk of NHL 3 years after commencing antiretroviral therapy was 19 per cent in one cohort. The introduction of HAART has been associated with a dramatic reduction in the incidence of Kaposi's sarcoma and a fall in the cases of primary cerebral lymphoma has also been found; however, there appears to be less change in the incidence of systemic lymphomas in cohort studies.

Biology

HIV-associated NHLs are B-cell aggressive lymphomas of high or intermediate grade. The most common histological types and their frequencies from three large series

are shown in Table 48.5 (Ioachim *et al.*, 1991; Raphael *et al.*, 1993; Carbone *et al.*, 1996). Approximately one-third are classified as small non-cleaved cell lymphomas (SNCCL; Burkitt or Burkitt-like lymphomas). The remaining two-thirds are diffuse large cell (DLC) lymphomas. These may be immunoblastic lymphomas or large non-cleaved cell lymphomas.

EPSTEIN–BARR VIRUS

Primary infection of epithelial cells by Epstein–Barr virus (EBV) is associated with the infection of some resting B lymphocytes via the CD3 receptor. Most infected B lymphocytes express EBV latently with a type 3 latency expression, producing up to six EBNAs (EBV nuclear antigens) as well as latent membrane proteins 1, 2A and 2B. These lymphocytes are destroyed by cytotoxic T lymphocytes. Some lymphocytes appear to switch to a latency 1 pattern, expressing only EBNA-1 (EBV nuclear antigen) and these cells persist and are believed to be the origin of EBV-positive reactivation and NHL. Indeed, EBV genomic terminal analysis has shown clonal EBV infection in HIV-associated NHL, implying that EBV infection precedes clonal expansion. HIV-associated diffuse large-cell and immunoblastic lymphomas are frequently associated with Epstein–Barr virus. The EBV genome in these lymphomas expresses latency type 3 antigens, including EBNA-2 and latent membrane protein (LMP)-1 and 2, which have transforming activity *in vitro*. However, the EBV genome can be detected in only 60 per cent of these HIV-associated large-cell lymphomas, compared to almost all cases of post-transplantation NHL. This implicates other factors in the aetiology of these malignancies associated with HIV infection, including polyclonal B-cell expansion and impaired T-cell immunosurveillance. In contrast, EBV is present in around 30 per cent of HIV-associated Burkitt's lymphoma, and in these tumours EBV is found in the latency type 1 profile expressing only EBNA-1.

c-myc

Burkitt's lymphoma (BL) is not associated with other forms of immunosuppression. The HIV-associated BL resembles sporadic BL in that only 30 per cent of tumours are EBV positive and c-*myc*/immunoglobulin gene translocations are found in most cases. The translocation breakpoints on chromosome 8 occur most frequently in exon 1 or intron 1 of the c-*myc* gene in AIDS-related NHL, rather than 5′ upstream of the gene. This pattern of translocation breakpoints on c-*myc* do not alter the peptide sequence, since exon 1 is not translated, and resemble the breakpoints observed in sporadic BL rather than endemic BL. The reciprocal breakpoint most often found lies in the Sμ portion of the immunoglobulin heavy chain gene on chromosome 14. This pattern, which is also found in sporadic BL, suggests that the mechanism of translocation is defective recombination during isotype class switching of the constant region of the heavy chain of immunoglobulin, which occurs late in B-lymphocyte ontogeny.

HUMAN HERPES VIRUS 8

Human herpes virus 8 (HHV8) has been demonstrated in both HIV-associated primary effusion lymphoma and Castleman's disease (Cesarman *et al.*, 1995; Soulier *et al.*, 1995).

p53

The tumour suppressor gene *p53* has a central role in cell-cycle control and hence regulates cell replication. About 40 per cent of HIV-associated NHL have been found to have mutations of *p53* gene. These mutations are found most commonly associated with the small non-cleaved cell or Burkitt-like variants, rather than the diffuse large-cell histologies. In contrast, mutations of the retinoblastoma gene which is also a cell-cycle regulator, have not been found in HIV-associated NHL.

bcl-6

Chromosome 3q27 translocations in diffuse large-cell lymphomas led to the identification of a novel oncogene *bcl-6*. This gene is rearranged in 30–40 per cent of diffuse large-cell lymphomas, and rearrangements have been found in 20 per cent of HIV-associated NHL, including mutations of the 5′ regulatory sequences. In contrast, rearrangements of *bcl-1* and *bcl-2* have not been demonstrated in AIDS-associated NHL.

Prognostic factors

The staging of HIV-associated lymphomas follows the Ann Arbor system and is identical to that employed for the staging of non-HIV-related NHL. The majority of patients present with advanced-stage, B symptoms and/or extranodal disease and these factors are therefore less discriminatory regarding prognosis. The most frequent extranodal sites of lymphoma are the gastrointestinal tract, liver and bone marrow. The most influential prognostic factors in patients with HIV-associated NHL relate to the severity of immunosuppression rather than lymphoma-related

Table 48.6 *Prognostic factors in HIV-NHL*

Major poor prognostic factors	Minor poor prognostic factors
Prior AIDS diagnosis	Bone marrow involvement
CD4 cells <100/mm³	Extranodal disease
ECOG performance status >2	Raised serum LDH
Primary cerebral origin	Age >35 years

factors. Table 48.6 shows major prognostic factors, which have been shown to be significant indicators of a poor prognosis in most series, and other variables which have been of prognostic significance in individual series (Gisselbrecht *et al.*, 1993; Kaplan *et al.*, 1989; Levine *et al.*, 1991b). An International Prognostic Index for lymphoma has been introduced for aggressive lymphomas and this scoring system has been evaluated in HIV-associated lymphomas. Elevated serum lactate dehydrogenase (LDH), age over 40 years and CD4 lymphocyte count <100/μL were confirmed as adverse prognostic variables. However, more recent prospective data, such as that provided by a recent AIDS Clinical Trials Group (ACTG) study, suggested that the prognostic variables in AIDS-related lymphoma closely resemble those in the International Prognostic Index for non-HIV associated non-Hodgkin's lymphoma.

In one series of 73 patients from Italy with HIV-associated lymphoma, a subgroup of 13 patients who achieved a durable complete remission of at least 2 years was identified. This group had higher CD4 lymphocyte counts and better prognostic scores at presentation than the remaining patients. However, there were no differences in the histological subtypes between the long-term survivors and the other patients (Tirelli *et al.*, 1996). This group reported in 1996 that the 2-year survival for good-prognosis patients treated with chemotherapy was 50 per cent compared with 24 per cent for poor-prognosis patients (Vaccher *et al.*, 1996). The good-prognosis patients in complete remission following chemotherapy had a median survival of 34.5 months. In an earlier series published in 1991, a similar group of patients was found to have a median survival of 18 months (Levine *et al.*, 1991b). The improvement in median survival in this group of patients is probably real and represents advances in the management of HIV, since many of these patients will succumb to HIV-related illness rather than the NHL.

Management

A biopsy is essential for the diagnosis of systemic lymphomas as they can be mimicked by many AIDS-related illnesses. Patients with systemic NHL should be staged with CT scan of chest/abdomen/pelvis, a bone-marrow biopsy and lumbar puncture. Patients with AIDS-related systemic NHL generally have disseminated disease and extranodal involvement and hence the optimal treatment is combination chemotherapy. However, early in the AIDS epidemic it was recognized that the complications and toxicities of standard chemotherapy in this group were greatly enhanced and the prognosis, particularly in the presence of adverse factors, was very short. This led to most centres adopting an approach where treatment is stratified according to prognostic factors. Generally, patients with the major poor-prognostic factors listed in Table 48.6 should undergo palliative treatment with low-toxicity chemotherapy, with the aim of improving or maintaining their quality of life. A suitable regimen is vincristine 1 mg i.v. bolus and bleomycin 30 mg i.v. bolus every 3 weeks, with prednisolone 25 mg orally on alternate days. No major studies have addressed the role of palliative chemotherapy in this context. Prophylaxis against both pneumocystis and mycobacterium infections are routinely prescribed. Radiotherapy may be of value for the relief of specific symptoms. The median survival of this group is 3–6 months, depending on their response to therapy.

Treatment for patients who fall into the good-prognostic group initially focused on the use of conventional standard-dose combination chemotherapy. However, it was soon recognized that the high infection rates complicating these schedules prevented the delivery of the planned doses. Initial studies used dose-modified chemotherapy such as the modified mBACOD schedule used by the ACTG (Levine et al., 1991a). The introduction of haematopoetic growth factors led to a randomized study in AIDS-related NHL that compared full-dose mBACOD with GM-CSF (granulocyte/macrophage colony stimulating factor) support and low-dose mBACOD. There was no significant difference in response rates or median survival between patients enrolled on the two arms, but there were significantly more episodes of neutropaenic sepsis in the full-dose arm, despite the growth factor support (Kaplan et al., 1995). A number of prospective trials of chemotherapy have been published which have employed standard or dose-modified schedules based upon treatments used for the management of lymphoma in the immunocompetent population (mBACOD, CHOP, MACOP-B, COMET A, LNH84). These have yielded complete remission rates of 33–63 per cent and median survivals of 5–11 months. These series are not comparable, as the case mix varies and the patient-selection criteria are rarely described. However, the complete response rate to chemotherapy (approximately 50 per cent in most large series) is lower than in a population not infected with HIV, as is the median survival – in the region of only 7–9 months. None the less, 30–40 per cent of good-prognosis patients may be cured and survive long term until other AIDS-related illnesses ensue. Recent series (Bower et al., 1999b) have reported higher median survivals without a change in the remission rates and these improvements reflect advances in antiretroviral therapy, prolonging survival amongst patients who do not relapse with NHL.

Recent reports have documented the role of infusional chemotherapy as an alternative in this group of patients. The combination of cyclophosphamide, doxorubicin and etoposide (CDE) has been administered as a 96-hour continuous infusion for up to six courses at 4 weekly intervals, together with G-CSF and didanosine. Initial reports in a selected group of 25 patients with a median CD4 count of 117/μL, produced an impressive median survival of 18.4 months (Sparano et al., 1996). More recently this schedule has been used in conjunction with protease inhibitor based HAART therapy, with similar results, although there was more mucositis with the protease inhibitor. Whether the impressive survival with CDE reflects a schedule which truly produces more durable responses on account of the steroid sparing or infusional schedule, or alternatively is due to recent improvements in the overall management of HIV disease, remains to be seen.

HAEMATOPOIETIC GROWTH FACTORS

Patients in the good prognostic category may be treated with conventional NHL chemotherapy regimens with the aim of cure. However, because of the underlying immunodeficiency and poor bone-marrow reserve, owing to HIV myelodysplasia and concomitant use of myelosuppressive agents such as zidovudine and ganciclovir, many patients develop opportunistic infections, neutropaenic sepsis or persisting neutropaenia, causing chemotherapy delays and hence suboptimal treatment. The use of bone-marrow stimulatory factors may facilitate giving chemotherapy, but improved survival has not been demonstrated. There is also concern that GM-CSF may enhance HIV replication in monocytes, although this does not appear to occur with G-CSF.

ANTIRETROVIRAL DRUGS

The concomitant use of antiretroviral agents with chemotherapy is generally acceptable practice, with the exception of zidovudine which significantly adds to the myelosuppression of combination chemotherapy, and didanosine which may worsen the peripheral neuropathy caused by vinca alkaloids. Little is known about the interactions of protease inhibitors and chemotherapy, although the inhibition of P450 may reduce hepatic metabolism of cyclophosphamide and the anthracyclines.

INTRATHECAL CHEMOTHERAPY

There is a high rate of meningeal involvement in HIV-associated systemic NHL, and it is not necessarily associated with bone-marrow involvement or a poor prognosis. Although the frequency of meningeal relapse can be reduced by the use of prophylactic intrathecal chemotherapy, this necessitates repeated lumbar punctures. Intrathecal chemotherapy (methotrexate or cytosine arabinoside) should therefore be given to patients with meningeal disease or at high risk of cranial disease by virtue of Burkitt's histology or extensive sinus and base of skull disease. Most centres also recommend prophylactic intrathecal chemotherapy for patients with bone-marrow involvement.

NEW DEVELOPMENTS

MGBG (methyl-glyoxal-*bis* guanylhydrazone), a relatively non-myelotoxic spermidine analogue which inhibits cellular polyamine synthesis, has been used with some success in both relapsed systemic NHL and in primary cerebral NHL (Levine *et al.*, 1996). Monoclonal antibodies to IL-6 have been evaluated in AIDS-related lymphoma, with limited success (Emilie *et al.*, 1993). In addition, antibody conjugates have been tested in refractory HIV-associated lymphoma. This conjugate was formed of ricin bound to a mouse-derived IgG1 monoclonal antibody B1 (antiCD19). CD19 is expressed on normal and malignant B lymphocytes. No significant toxicity was reported in a phase I dose-escalating study in nine patients, and the response rate was 22 per cent (Tulpule *et al.*, 1994). Following initial positive results, the ricin-blocked anti-CD19 antibody conjugate was used in combination with low-dose mBACOD chemotherapy. The complete remission rate was 67 per cent although the contribution of the immunoconjugate cannot be separated from that of the chemotherapy (Scadden *et al.*, 1993). Furthermore, studies of rituximab, a humanized monoclonal antibody to CD20, are under way in this group of patients.

Primary effusion lymphoma

Primary effusion lymphoma (PEL), or body-cavity-based lymphoma (BCBL), is a rare variant of HIV-associated lymphoma that is characterized by effusions in serosal cavities (pleura, pericardium and peritoneum) in the absence of solid nodal masses. PELs express an indeterminate immunophenotype with clonal immunoglobulin gene-rearrangements. All PELs are associated with HHV8 infection, and tumour cells carry a high HHV8 viral copy number per cell (Cesarman *et al.*, 1995). In addition, many PELs are co-infected with EBV. The clinical management of PEL does not differ from that of HIV-associated NHL. Patients present with a median CD4 count of 90/μL, and the median survival is 5 months.

PRIMARY CENTRAL NERVOUS SYSTEM LYMPHOMA

Epidemiology

Primary central nervous system lymphoma (PCNSL) is defined as non-Hodgkin's lymphoma (NHL) that is confined to the cranio-spinal axis without systemic involvement. This diagnosis is rare in immunocompetent patients but occurs more frequently in patients with both congenital and acquired immunodeficiency. Since 1985 high-grade B-cell NHL, including PCNSL, has been an AIDS-defining diagnosis. AIDS-related PCNSL occurs equally frequently across all ages and transmission risk groups. The incidence of systemic NHL in HIV patients is increasing now that prevention of opportunistic infections and treatment with highly affective antiretroviral therapy (HAART) have prolonged survival, although this is not the case for PCNSL.

Pathogenesis

The presence of EBV is a universal feature of HIV-associated primary cerebral NHLs, which are monoclonal immunoblastic lymphomas, but is not found in other primary cerebral lymphomas (MacMahon *et al.*, 1991; Cinque *et al.*, 1993). EBV may be detected by immuno-cytochemical staining of biopsy tissue or by polymerase chain reaction (PCR) amplification of cerebrospinal fluid (CSF) using EBV-specific oligonucleotide primers.

Differential diagnosis

Toxoplasmosis and lymphoma are the most common causes of cerebral mass lesions in HIV-seropositive patients, and the differential diagnosis often proves difficult. Both diagnoses occur in patients with advanced immunodeficiency (CD4 count <50/μL) and present with headaches and focal neurological deficits. Clinical features that favour a diagnosis of PCNSL include a more gradual onset over 2–8 weeks and the absence of a fever. CT and MRI scanning usually reveal solitary or multiple ring enhancing lesions with prominent mass effect and oedema. Again these features occur in both diagnoses, although PCNSL lesions are usually periventricular whereas toxoplasmosis more often affects the basal ganglia. Thus even the combination of clinical findings and standard radiological investigations rarely provide a definitive diagnosis. Moreover, toxoplasma serology (IgG) is falsely negative in 10–15 per cent of patients with cerebral toxoplasmosis. More than 85 per cent of patients with cerebral toxoplasmosis will respond clinically and radiologically to 2 weeks of anti-toxoplasma therapy, and this has become the cornerstone of the diagnostic algorithm for cerebral masses in severely immunodeficient patients. In these patients it has been standard practice to commence empirical anti-toxoplasmosis treatment for 2 weeks' duration, and resort to a brain biopsy if there is no clinical or radiological improvement. This strategy avoids the routine use of brain biopsy in these patients, who frequently have a very poor performance status and prognosis (Fig. 48.2).

Although the algorithm shown in Figure 48.2 avoids early surgical intervention, it is relatively ineffective in diagnosing PCNSL early, and may compromise the outcome

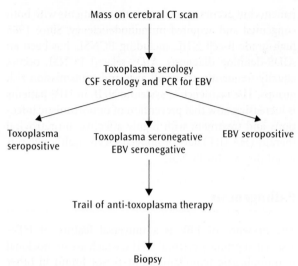

Mass on cerebral CT scan

Toxoplasma serology
CSF serology and PCR for EBV

Toxoplasma seropositive

Toxoplasma seronegative
EBV seronegative

EBV seropositive

Trail of anti-toxoplasma therapy

Biopsy

Figure 48.2 *Diagnostic algorithm for primary cerebral non-Hodgkin's lymphoma.*

of therapy in these patients. In addition, there is a disinclination to treat patients with radiotherapy or chemotherapy based exclusively on the failure of anti-toxoplasmosis treatment without a definitive histological diagnosis.

The discovery that all HIV-associated PCNSLs which histologically are diffuse high-grade B-cell NHLs are associated with Epstein–Barr virus infection has led to the development of a PCR method that can detect EBV DNA in the cerebrospinal fluid. The detection of EBV DNA in the cerebrospinal fluid (CSF) by PCR in patients with PCNSL has become established as a diagnostic test with a high sensitivity (83–100 per cent) and specificity (>90 per cent) (Cinque *et al.*, 1993; Arribas *et al.*, 1995; De Luca *et al.*, 1995).

Radionuclide imaging by thallium-201 single positron emission computed tomography (^{201}Th-SPECT) or [^{18}F]fluorodeoxyglucose positron emission tomography (FDG-PET) is able to differentiate between PCNSL and cerebral toxoplasmosis. PCNSLs are thallium avid and demonstrate increased uptake on PET scanning; however, although both techniques have high specificity for PCNSL, neither are highly sensitive and thus cannot be used as single test, but in combination with PCR are emerging as a diagnostic alternative to brain biopsy. The application of PCR and ^{201}Th-SPECT in the diagnosis of contrast-enhancing brain lesions in 27 patients was shown to result in a positive and a negative predictive value of 100 per cent and 88 per cent, respectively, which supports their combined value as an alternative to brain biopsy (Castagna *et al.*, 1997). Further studies are now required to compare the effectiveness of PCR with ^{201}Th-SPECT or FDG-PET.

Treatment

The standard treatment modality for PCNSL in HIV patients is whole-brain irradiation with 20 Gy in 5 fractions over 1 week. This treatment is associated with

progressive impairment of cognitive function and neurological status, secondary to chronic encephalopathy, and the median survival time is just 2.5 months. The use of chemotherapy for PCNSL is limited by the poor penetration of cytotoxics into brain parenchyma on account of the blood–brain barrier, and the toxicity, especially myelosuppression, of these agents in patients with advanced immunosuppression and poor performance status. Combination chemotherapy regimens may prolong the median survival of PCNSL in immunocompetent patients, but at the cost of severe myelotoxicity. Single-agent chemotherapy with intravenous high-dose methotrexate and folinic acid rescue was recently studied in AIDS patients with PCNSL in the context of a prospective uncontrolled study which included 15 patients. The results showed a complete response in 47 per cent of patients, a median survival of 19 months; a low relapse rate of approximately 14 per cent, and no evidence of neurological impairment nor treatment-limiting myelotoxicity (Jacomet *et al.*, 1997). A controlled trial of intravenous methotrexate versus whole-brain irradiation is needed to confirm these encouraging results. Now that antiretroviral therapies are improving survival, it is necessary to reassess currently available diagnostic and treatment modalities aiming to cure HIV-associated brain lymphomas.

CASTLEMAN'S DISEASE

Castleman's disease is a rare lymphoproliferative disorder, originally described in 1956 and characterized by angio-follicular lymphoid hyperplasia (Castleman *et al.*, 1956). Two histological variants are recognized: a hyaline vascular variant and a less common plasma cell variant. Castleman's disease has germinal centre hyalinization or atrophy surrounded by concentric layers of lymphocytes with prominent vascular hyperplasia, hyalinization of small vessels and interfollicular sheets of plasma cells and immunoblasts. An association between HIV infection, Kaposi's sarcoma and multicentric plasma cell type Castleman's disease has been noted, and HHV8 has been found in these lesions (Soulier *et al.*, 1995). Patients present with constitutional symptoms, including fever, weight loss and night sweats. Clinical findings include lymphadenopathy, hepatosplenomegaly and rashes. Investigations frequently reveal microcytic anaemia, hypoalbuminaemia and polyclonal hypergammaglobulinaemia. Ultimately the diagnosis is made histologically.

The optimum treatment for Castleman's disease remains uncertain. Early reports of multicentric Castleman's disease in seropositive patients suggested a median survival of less than 6 months. However, earlier recognition of the diagnosis and treatment with splenectomy followed by single-agent chemotherapy may prolong survival. In the largest reported series, from Paris, of 20 patients treated

Table 48.7 *Comparison of Hodgkin's disease in HIV-negative and -positive patients*

HIV-associated HD	Non-HIV-associated HD
High incidence of EBV in HD tissues	Low incidence of EBV in HD tissues
Mixed cellularity and lymphocyte-depleted histologies predominate	Nodular sclerosis histology predominates
Advanced stage at presentation (75–85% stage III/IV)	Earlier stage at presentation
B symptoms common	B symptoms less common
Extranodal disease common	Extranodal disease less common
Lower CR rate (45–60%)	Higher CR rate (80–95%)
High relapse rate	Low relapse rate
Median survival 8–18 months	Median survival >12 years

with splenectomy and vinblastine, the median survival was 14 months (Oksenhendler *et al.*, 1996).

HODGKIN'S DISEASE

Epidemiology

The incidence of Hodgkin's disease (HD) appears to be higher in individuals with HIV, although there remains controversy around this issue and, indeed, HD is not an AIDS-defining diagnosis. Some, but not all, clinical epidemiological studies have identified an increase in the risk of HD in HIV-seropositive patients. No significantly increased incidence of HD was detected in the earliest large study from San Francisco in 1984 of single men aged 20–49, or in the New York cancer registry data of the same era. However, subgroup analysis of the latter data revealed an increased incidence of HD amongst HIV patients who were intravenous drug users (IVDU). In contrast, in 1988 the Italian Co-operative Group for AIDS-related Tumours described a cohort of 35 HIV patients with HD, almost all of whom were IVDUs (Tirelli *et al.*, 1988).

More recent studies have included larger numbers of patients and suggest an increased incidence of HD, but the number of reported cases remains small and therefore the confidence intervals are wide. The San Francisco City Clinic reported eight cases amongst a cohort of 6704 homosexual HIV-positive men, giving an excess risk of 19/100 000 person-years (Hessol *et al.*, 1992), whereas the MACS study (Multicentre AIDS Cohort Study) of 1199 homosexual men reported two cases from 1984 to 1993, giving a rate of 85/100 000 person-years and a relative risk compared to that of an age-adjusted general population of 19.8 times (95 per cent confidence interval 2.4–71, $P < 0.005$) (Lyter *et al.*, 1995).

As with other malignancies associated with HIV, a virus (in this case Epstein–Barr virus) has been implicated in the pathogenesis, and there appears to be a higher incidence of EBV detected in HIV-associated HD tissues than in HD samples from HIV-seronegative patients.

In addition, the natural history and treatment outcomes in HIV-associated HD may differ from those in general population. This may, in part, reflect the less favourable histology and advanced stage at presentation, as well as the high incidence of opportunistic infection in HIV-associated HD (Table 48.7).

Treatment

The optimal chemotherapy schedule for HIV-associated HD has not been determined. However, nitrogen mustard, vincristine, procarbazine and prednisolone (MOPP), adriamycin, bleomycin, vinblastine and dacarbazine (ABVD) and hybrid regimens combining both have been used in a number of series. In general, the complete remission rates are 45–60 per cent and the median survivals range from 8 to 18 months (Rubio, 1994; Levy *et al.*, 1995; Tirelli *et al.*, 1995). The causes of death in these patients are as frequently due to opportunist infections as Hodgkin's disease, and the high incidence of opportunist infections occurs not only during the chemotherapy but persists following its completion.

ANAL CANCER

Epidemiology

There is a strikingly increased incidence of anal carcinoma amongst HIV-positive patients (Melbye *et al.*, 1994), but it has been shown that homosexual men were at increased risk of this malignancy before the onset of the AIDS epidemic. Indeed, the incidence of anal cancer amongst gay men in the pre-AIDS era was estimated to be 35/100 000, which resembles the incidence of cervical cancer before the introduction of routine Papanicolaou (Pap) smear screening. None the less, anal cancer is twice as common in HIV-positive gay men as it is in HIV-negative gay men (Palefsky *et al.*, 1998), although, unlike invasive cervical cancer, invasive anal cancer is not an AIDS-defining diagnosis.

Pathogenesis

Anal cancer shares many features with cervical cancer, including a strong association with human papillomavirus (HPV) infection and similar histology. High-grade squamous intra-epithelial lesion (HSIL) or anal intra-epithelial neoplasia (AIN) of the anus is believed to progress to invasive anal cancer in a fashion analogous to the progression from cervical high-grade squamous intra-epithelial lesion (HSIL) or cervical intraepithelial neoplasia (CIN) to invasive cervical cancer.

Effects of highly active antiretroviral therapy on pre-invasive anal lesions

Cohort studies of men with anal HSIL have demonstrated that these lesions do not regress with highly active anti-retroviral therapy (HAART), despite the established benefit of HAART on other viral infections and associated diseases in HIV-infected patients (Palefsky *et al.*, 1999b). The optimal management of anal HSIL remains unclear. The therapeutic options for anal HSIL include surgical excision and laser ablation. These procedures are performed under general anaesthesia and, although complications are uncommon, postoperative pain may persist for several days or weeks. Anal HSIL appears to be a field effect and hence recurrence is frequent, suggesting the need for medical therapies, although none have proved so far to be very effective. The prolonged survival of HIV-infected people in the era of HAART and the lack of regression of anal HSIL suggests that the incidence of invasive anal cancer will increase in this population.

Management of invasive anal cancer

The standard approach to anal cancer in immunocompetent patients was surgery until the report in 1974 that combined-modality therapy (CMT) of chemotherapy (5-fluorouracil (5-FU) and Mitomycin C®) with radiation treatment could result in microscopic and histological tumour ablation with sphincter preservation (Nigro *et al.*, 1974). Subsequently it was demonstrated that the resulting survival rates were at least as good as those achieved with surgery alone, most centres reporting that 85 per cent of tumours can be controlled locally with 5-year survival rates in the range of 65–85 per cent. The superiority of CMT over radiation alone was later confirmed by two large multicentre, randomized trials. Both the UKCCCR (United Kingdom Co-ordinating Committee for Cancer Research) and EORTC (European Organization for the Research and Treatment of Cancer) trials reported superior local control rates with CMT, without an overall survival advantage. HIV-infected people tolerate both chemotherapy and radiotherapy poorly. For this reason, coupled with the limited prognosis of patients with HIV prior to the introduction of more active antiretroviral

regimens, there was some reluctance to treat anal carcinoma in the setting of HIV with standard-dose CMT. However, more recently CMT has been adopted for the management of HIV-associated anal cancer with high response rates and documented durable remissions, although the toxicity appears to be greater than in the HIV-negative population (Chadha *et al.*, 1994; Holland and Swift, 1994; Hoffman *et al.*, 1999).

Future

The future of anal cancer in HIV-seropositive people may lie with effective screening of the at-risk population and early intervention. Anoscopic cytology has been found to be an effective method of screening for AIN and, if therapeutic interventions could be shown to reduce progression and mortality, this would be an attractive strategy.

CERVICAL CANCER

Epidemiology

Invasive cervical cancer was included as an AIDS-defining diagnosis in 1993, although the incidence of cervical cancer is not increased significantly in HIV-seropositive women. None the less, there is good epidemiological evidence that the precursor lesions, cervical intra-epithelial neoplasia (CIN) or squamous intra-epithelial lesion (SIL), occur more frequently in women with HIV. The prolonged incubation between CIN and invasive cervical cancer of over 10 years may account for the low incidence of invasive cervical cancer in HIV-seropositive women, whose life expectancy in many parts of the world will be shorter than this. Human papillomavirus (HPV) has a central role in the pathogenesis of both CIN and invasive cervical cancer. In the US, 30 per cent of female college students have cervical HPV infection, and the modes of transmission of HIV and HPV are similar. Two oncoproteins present in HPV are believed to be responsible for the oncogenic properties of this virus, E6 and E7. E6 transforms cells by binding to the host cellular regulatory protein p53, forming a complex of p53, E6 and E6-associated protein. This complex is degraded rapidly in cellular proteosomes, resulting in depletion of p53, which leads to loss of the G_1 checkpoint of cell-cycle control. E7 binds the retinoblastoma protein Rb, releasing E2F transcription factor and this overcomes the G_2/M checkpoint, resulting in the activation of mitosis.

The Women's Interagency HIV Study (WIHS) case-control cohort has studied 2015 HIV-positive women and 577 matched HIV-negative women. An increased rate of HPV infection, often with multiple HPV genotypes, and a higher rate of cytological and histological precursor lesion has been found in the cases (Table 48.8). Within this study the risk of SIL was greatest amongst women with CD4 cell

Table 48.8 *Table of findings of WIHS study of cervical screening for human papillomavirus and CIN in HIV-seropositive women and matched controls*

	HIV+ cases	HIV− controls
Number	2015	577
HVP detected in cervical lavage by PCR (%)	58	26
Multiple HPV genotypes present in lavage (%)	42	16
Abnormal Pap smear (%)	49	17
Cervical SIL on biopsy (%)	30	7

HPV, human papillomavirus; PCR, polymerase chain reaction; CIN, cervical intra-epithelial neoplasia; Pap smear, Papanicolaou smear; SIL, squamous intra-epithelial lesion; WIHS, Women's Interagency HIV Study.

counts <200/μL, where HPV was detected in cervical lavage specimens by PCR amplification, when multiple HPV genotypes were present and where HPV genotypes 16, 18, 31, 33 and 35 were detected (Palefsky *et al.*, 1999a).

HIV is associated not only with a higher prevalence of HPV in the cervix, a high frequency of multiple HPV genotypes and persistence of HPV in the cervix, but also a higher prevalence of CIN/SIL, a higher progression from low-grade SIL to high-grade SIL and a greater likelihood of relapse of CIN II/III after therapy. These findings mandate continuing close colposcopic surveillance.

Effects of highly active antiretroviral treatment on pre-invasive cervical cancer

The effect of HAART on the natural history of CIN has been addressed in 49 women with advanced HIV. Five months after starting HAART the prevalence of CIN fell from 66 per cent to 49 per cent, regression of high-grade SIL to low-grade SIL occurred in 23 per cent, and from low-grade SIL to normal in 43 per cent. These changes occurred without a significant change in the level of HPV DNA in cervical tissue (Heard *et al.*, 1998). These findings suggest that frequent (at least annual) cervical smears should be offered to all HIV-positive women. CIN II/III should be treated and followed up by frequent (at least 6-monthly) colposcopic surveillance and should be considered an indication for starting HAART therapy.

Invasive cervical cancer management

It is perhaps surprising that epidemiological evidence fails to demonstrate an increased incidence of invasive cervical cancer in HIV-positive women, even in areas of the world where Pap screening is not routine practice. This fact may be related to the prolonged latency between HPV infection and the development of invasive cervical cancer, which may exceed the life span of women with

Table 48.9 *Comparison of HIV− and HIV+ women with invasive cervical cancer from one centre (Maiman et al., 1993)*

	HIV+	HIV−
Number	16	68
Stage III/IV	70%	28%
Relapsed after definitive therapy	100%	49%
Median survival	9 months	28 months

HIV. In most centres HIV-seropositive women with invasive cervical cancer are treated using the same protocols as for immunocompetent women. One retrospective series compared 16 HIV-positive women with 68 HIV-seronegative women treated at the same institution during the same time period. The results demonstrated that women with HIV had more advanced cervical cancer at presentation, relapsed more frequently and had a worse median survival (Table 48.9) (Maiman *et al.*, 1993).

Future

The most attractive strategies aimed at reducing the mortality of cervical cancer are focused on vaccination against HPV, both as prophylaxis and potential treatment; although the multiple genotypes of HPV, which include more than 85 well-characterized genotypes, greatly complicates this approach. Virus-like particles (VLPs) are formed of HPV capsid proteins which autoassemble in the absence of viral DNA, and these may be manipulated to incorporate additional proteins. These modified VLPs have been shown to be efficient inducers of neutralizing antibodies to HPV, and may form part of an effective therapy against HPV-induced neoplasia.

LEIOMYOSARCOMA IN CHILDREN

Smooth-muscle tumours, including leiomyomas and leiomyosarcomas, are very uncommon tumours in childhood, but are found more frequently in children with HIV (Granovsky *et al.*, 1998), where they are the second most common tumour and are an AIDS-defining diagnosis. Leiomyosarcomas are also rarely reported in young adults and may be associated with Epstein–Barr virus (McClain *et al.*, 1995).

SQUAMOUS CELL CARCINOMAS OF CONJUNCTIVA

Squamous cell carcinoma of the conjunctiva typically presents with ocular-surface epithelial dysplasia, most frequently on the nasal aspect of the eye. Metastases are very rare and the prognosis with local excision is good.

These tumours occur more frequently in sub-Saharan Africa, where the incidence is up to $12/10^6$ per year, and have been thought to relate to exposure to UV light. A number of case-control studies have been conducted in Africa, demonstrating an increased incidence of these tumours in HIV-positive people, with a relative risk of around 10 (Goedert and Cote, 1995). In a cattle model for squamous cell carcinoma of the conjunctiva, an association has been found with bovine papillomavirus, suggesting that HPV might have a role in the pathogenesis of this malignancy in humans.

OTHER SKIN TUMOURS

The risk for development of skin tumours other than KS appears to be greater in HIV-positive persons. The second most common skin tumour is basal cell carcinoma, which frequently occurs on the trunk, is superficial and multicentric. There is no correlation between basal cell cancers and degree of immunosuppression (Wang *et al.*, 1995; Remick, 1996). Similarly dysplastic naevi and melanoma have been reported with HIV and may occur more frequently than expected. The lesions are frequently thicker and metastasise early compared to non HIV-infected persons, particularly when the CD4 count is low (Wang *et al.*, 1995; Remick, 1996).

TESTICULAR GERM-CELL TUMOURS

Testicular tumours, including lymphoma, non-seminomatous germ-cell tumours (NSGCT) and seminoma, have been reported to occur more frequently in HIV-positive men than in the general population. Wilson *et al.* (1992) reported an incidence of 0.2 per cent of testis tumours in 3015 HIV-positive men seen over a 2-year period, which was 57 times greater than in the general population. Similarly, within the MACS cohort of homosexual men with HIV an increased incidence of testicular seminoma has been noted (Lyter *et al.*, 1995).

OTHER TUMOURS

Rates of other cancers appear to be marginally increased in HIV-positive patients, including myeloma, melanoma and adenocarcinoma of the lung (Gunthel and Northfelt, 1994; Lyter *et al.*, 1998; Speck *et al.*, 1998).

CONCLUSION

The management of people with AIDS-related cancer is most effective in a multidisciplinary setting including oncologists, HIV physicians and access to specific counselling and social services. The underlying immuno-suppression has a major influence on both the treatment and prognosis for these individuals. For Kaposi's sarcoma, the maintenance of quality of life is of utmost importance, as a 'cure' cannot be achieved. Modulation of systemic HIV treatment (HAART) should always be considered in conjunction with HIV physicians. For NHL, patients with relatively preserved immune function and good performance status should be treated aggressively as a cure rate of around 50 per cent may be achieved.

The psychological impact of a second life-threatening and/or cosmetically disfiguring diagnosis on the background of HIV infection cannot be underestimated. Our patients need sensitive management and often require psychological support. However, recent rapid advances in the fields of basic science have been translated into improvements in HIV medicine, oncology and infectious disease. The new and improved treatment options available are leading to guarded optimism in the complex field of AIDS-related cancers.

SIGNIFICANT POINTS

- Worldwide at the start of 2002 over 40 million are living with HIV.
- HIV infection is associated with an increased incidence of virus-associated malignancies, particularly Kaposi's sarcoma, high-grade B-cell non-Hodgkin's lymphoma, cervical and anal cancer.
- Kaposi's sarcoma is treated with HAART and local therapies, including radiation and intralesional chemotherapy, or with systemic chemotherapy. It is a model system for numerous studies of novel anti-angiogenic agents.
- AIDS-associated NHL treatment should be stratified according to prognostic factors, and patients with very advanced HIV disease are usually better treated with palliative rather than curative intent.
- Primary cerebral lymphoma is an important differential diagnosis in HIV-positive patients with cerebral space-occupying lesions, and has a particularly poor prognosis.

KEY REFERENCES

Beral, V., Peterman, T.A., Berkelman, R.L. and Jaffe, H.W. (1990) Kaposi's sarcoma among persons with AIDS: a sexually transmitted infection? *Lancet* **335**, 123–8.

Beral, V., Peterman, T., Berkelman, R. and Jaffe, H. (1991) AIDS-associated non-Hodgkin lymphoma. *Lancet* **337**, 805–9.

Chang, Y., Cesarman, E., Pessin, M. *et al.* (1994) Identification of herpesvirus-like DNA sequences in AIDS-associated Kaposi's sarcoma. *Science* **266**, 1865–9.

Krown, S.E, Metroka, C. and Wernz, J.C. (1989) Kaposi's sarcoma in the acquired immune deficiency syndrome: a proposal for uniform evaluation, response, and staging criteria. AIDS Clinical Trials Group Oncology Committee. *J. Clin. Oncol.* **7**, 1201–7.

Krown, S.E., Testa, M.A., Huang, J. for the AIDS Clinical Trials Group (1997) AIDS-related Kaposi's sarcoma: prospective validation of the AIDS Clinical Trials Group Staging Classification. *J. Clin. Oncol.* **15**, 3085–92.

REFERENCES

Arribas, J., Clifford, D., Fichtenbaum, C. *et al.* (1995) Detection of Epstein–Barr virus DNA in cerebrospinal fluid for diagnosis of AIDS-related central nervous system lymphoma. *J. Clin. Microbiol.* **33**, 1580–3.

Beral, V., Peterman, T.A., Berkelman, R.L. and Jaffe, H.W. (1990) Kaposi's sarcoma among persons with AIDS: a sexually transmitted infection? *Lancet* **335**, 123–8.

Beral, V., Peterman, T., Berkelman, R. and Jaffe, H. (1991) AIDS-associated non-Hodgkin lymphoma. *Lancet* **337**, 805–9.

Beral, V., Newton, R. and Sitas, F. (1999) Human Herpesvirus 8 and cancer. *J. Natl Cancer Inst.* **91**, 1440–1.

Bower, M., Fox, P., Fife, K., Gill, J., Nelson, M. and Gazzard, B.G. (1999a) HAART prolongs time to treatment failure (TTF) in Kaposi's sarcoma. *AIDS* **13**, 2105–11.

Bower, M., Stern, S., Fife, K., Nelson, M. and Gazzard, B.G. (1999b) Weekly alternating combination chemotherapy for good prognosis AIDS related lymphoma. *Eur. J. Cancer* **36**, 363–7.

Carbone, A., Dolcetti, R., Gloghini, A. *et al.* (1996) Immunophenotypic and molecular analyses of acquired immune deficiency syndrome-related and Epstein–Barr virus-associated lymphomas: a comparative study. *Hum. Pathol.* **27**, 133–46.

Castagna, A., Cinque, P., d'Amico, A. *et al.* (1997) Evaluation of contrast-enhancing brain lesions in AIDS patients by means of Epstein–Barr virus detection in cerebrospinal fluid and 201-thallium single photon emission tomography. *AIDS* **11**, 1522–3.

Castleman, B., Iverson, L. and Menendez, V. (1956) Localized mediastinal lymph-node hyperplasia resembling thymoma. *Cancer* **9**, 822–30.

Cesarman, E., Chang, Y., Moore, P.S., Said, J.W. and Knowles, D.M. (1995) Kaposi's sarcoma-associated herpesvirus-like DNA sequences in AIDS-related body-cavity-based lymphomas *N. Engl. J. Med.* **332**, 1186–91.

Chadha, M., Rosenblatt, E.A., Malamud, S., Pisch, J. and Berson, A. (1994) Squamous-cell carcinoma of the anus in HIV-positive patients. *Dis. Colon Rectum* **37**, 861–5.

Chang, Y., Cesarman, E., Pessin, M. *et al.* (1994) Identification of herpesvirus-like DNA sequences in AIDS-associated Kaposi's sarcoma. *Science* **266**, 1865–9.

Cinque, P., Brytting, M., Vago, L. *et al.* (1993) Epstein–Barr virus DNA in cerebrospinal fluid from patients with AIDS-related primary lymphoma of the central nervous system. *Lancet* **342**, 398–401.

De Luca, A., Antinori, A., Cingolani, A. *et al.* (1995) Evaluation of cerebrospinal fluid EBV-DNA and IL-10 as markers for *in vivo* diagnosis of AIDS-related primary central nervous system lymphoma. *Br. J. Haematol.* **90**, 844–9.

Dezube, B., von Roenn, J., Holden-Wiltse, J. *et al.* (1997) Fumagillin analogue (TNP-470) in the treatment of Kaposi's sarcoma: a phase I AIDS Clinical Trials Group study. *J. Immune Deficiency Syndr. Hum. Retrovirol.* **14**, A35.

Duvic, M., Friedman-Kien, A., Miles, S. *et al.* (1997) Phase I/II evaluation of Panretin (ALRT 1057; LGD 1057; AGN 192013; 9-*cis*-retinoic acid) topical gel for AIDS-related Kaposi's sarcoma. *Proc. Am. Soc. Clin. Oncol.* **16**, 46a.

Eckhardt, S., Burris, H., Eckhardt, J. *et al.* (1996) A phase I clinical and pharmacokinetic study of the angiogenesis inhibitor, tecogalan sodium. *Ann. Oncol.* **7**, 491–6.

Emilie, D., Marfaing, A., Merrien, D. *et al.* (1993) Treatment of AIDS-lymphomas with an anti-IL-6 monoclonal antibody. *Blood* **82**, 387a.

Ensoli, B., Gendelman, R., Markham, P. *et al.* (1994) Synergy between basic fibroblast growth factor and HIV-1 Tat protein in induction of Kaposi's sarcoma. *Nature* **371**, 674–80.

Fife, K., Howard, M.R., Gracie, F., Phillips, R.H. and Bower, M. (1998) Activity of thalidomide in AIDS-related Kaposi's sarcoma and correlation with HHV8 titre. *Int. J. STD AIDS* **9**, 751–5.

Friedman-Kien, A., Laubenstein, L., Marmor, M. *et al.* (1981) Kaposi's sarcoma and pneumocystis pneumonia among homosexual men – New York and California. *Morbid. Mortal. Weekly Rep.* **30**, 250–4.

Friedman-Kien, A., Dezube, B., Lee, J. *et al.* (1998) Oral 9-*cis* retinoic acid is active in AIDS-related Kaposi's sarcoma: AIDS Malignancy Consortium Study. *J. Immune Deficiency Syndr. Hum. Retrovirol.* **17**, A25.

Gill, P.S., Hadjenberg, J., Espina, B.M. et al. (1995) Low dose paclitaxel (Taxol) every two weeks over 3 hours is safe and effective in the treatment of advanced AIDS-related Kaposi's sarcoma. *Blood* **382a**, 1516.

Gill, P., Wernz, J., Scadden, D. et al. (1996) Randomized phase III trial of liposomal daunorubicin (Daunoxome) versus doxorubicin, bleomycin, vincristine (ABV) in AIDS-related Kaposi's sarcoma. *J. Clin. Oncol.* **14**, 2353–64.

Gill, P.S., Scadden, D.T., Tulpule, A. et al. (1998) Preliminary results of IM-862 nasal solution in the treatment of patients with AIDS-related Kaposi's sarcoma. *J. Immune Deficiency Syndr. Hum. Retrovirol.* **17**, A16.

Gisselbrecht, C., Oksenhendler, E., Tirelli, U. et al. (1993) Human immunodeficiency virus-related lymphoma treatment with intensive combination chemotherapy. French–Italian Cooperative Group. *Am. J. Med.* **95**, 188–96.

Goedert, J. and Cote, T. (1995) Conjunctival malignant disease with AIDS in USA. *Lancet* **346**, 257–8.

Granovsky, M., Mueller, B., Nicholson, H., Rosenberg, P. and Rabkin, C. (1998) Cancer in human immunodeficiency virus-infected children: a case series from the children's cancer group and the National Cancer Institute. *J. Clin. Oncol.* **16**, 1729–35.

Gunthel, C. and Northfelt, D. (1994) Cancers not associated with immunodeficiency in HIV infected persons. *Oncology* **8**, 59–68.

Heard, I., Schmitz, V., Costagliola, D. et al. (1998) Early regression of cervical lesions in HIV-seropositive women receiving highly active antiretroviral therapy. *AIDS* **12**, 1459–64.

Hessol, N., Katz, M., Liu, J. et al. (1992) Increased incidence of Hodgkin's disease in homosexual men with HIV infection. *Ann. Intern. Med.* **117**, 309–11.

Hoffman, R., Welton, M.L., Klencke, B., Weinberg, V. and Kreig, R. (1999) The significance of pretreatment CD4 count on the outcome and treatment tolerance of HIV-positive patients with anal cancer. *Int. J. Radiat. Oncol. Biol. Phys.* **44**, 127–31.

Holland, J.M. and Swift, P.S. (1994) Tolerance of patients with human immunodeficiency virus and anal carcinoma to treatment with combined chemotherapy and radiation treatment. *Radiology* **193**, 251–4.

Ioachim, H.L., Dorsett, B., Cronin, W., Maya, M. and Wahl, S. (1991) Acquired immunodeficiency syndrome-associated lymphomas: clinical, pathologic, immunologic, and viral characteristics of 111 cases. *Hum. Pathol.* **22**, 659–73.

Jacomet, C., Girard, P., Lebrette, M., Farese, V., Monfort, L. and Rozenbaum, W. (1997) Intravenous methotrexate for primary central nervous system non-Hodgkin's lymphoma in AIDS. *AIDS* **11**, 1725–30.

Kaplan, L.D., Abrams, D.I., Feigal, E. et al. (1989) AIDS-associated non-Hodgkin's lymphoma in San Francisco. *JAMA* **261**, 719–24.

Kaplan, L., Straus, D., Testa, M. and Levine, A. (1995) Randomized trial of standard dose mBACOD with GM-CSF vs. reduced dose mBACOD for systemic HIV-associated lymphoma: ACTG 142. *Proc. Am. Soc. Clin. Oncol.* **14**, 288.

Khan, J., Ruiz, R., Kerschman, R. et al. (1993) A phase I/II study of recombinant platelet factor 4 (rPF4) in patients with AIDS-related Kaposi's sarcoma. *Proc. Am. Soc. Clin. Oncol.* **12**, 50.

Krown, S.E., Metroka, C. and Wernz, J.C. (1989) Kaposi's sarcoma in the acquired immune deficiency syndrome: a proposal for uniform evaluation, response, and staging criteria. AIDS Clinical Trials Group Oncology Committee. *J. Clin. Oncol.* **7**, 1201–7.

Krown, S.E., Testa, M.A., Huang, J. for the AIDS Clinical Trials Group (1997) AIDS-related Kaposi's sarcoma: prospective validation of the AIDS Clinical Trials Group Staging Classification. *J. Clin. Oncol.* **15**, 3085–92.

Levine, A.M., Wernz, J.C., Kaplan, L. et al. (1991a) Low dose chemotherapy with central nervous system prophylaxis and zidovudine maintenance in AIDS-related lymphoma. *JAMA* **266**, 84–8.

Levine, A.M., Sullivan Halley, J., Pike, M.C. et al. (1991b) Human immunodeficiency virus-related lymphoma. Prognostic factors predictive of survival. *Cancer* **68**, 2466–72.

Levine, A., Tulpule, A., Espina, B., Von Hoff, D. and Tessman, D. (1996) Mitoguazone (MGBG) with radiation therapy in AIDS-related primary CNS-lymphoma. *Proceedings of the XI International Conference on AIDS* **2**, 222.

Levy, R., Colonna, P., Tourani, J.-M. et al. (1995) Human immunodeficiency virus associated Hodgkin's disease: report of 45 cases from the French Registry of HIV-associated tumours. *Leuk. Lymphoma* **16**, 451–6.

Lunardi-Iskandar, Y., Bryant, J., Zeeman, R. et al. (1995) Tumorigenesis and metastasis of neoplastic Kaposi's sarcoma cell line in immunodeficient mice blocked by a human pregnancy hormone. *Nature* **375**, 64–8.

Lyter, D., Bryant, J., Thackeray, R. et al. (1995) Incidence of human immunodeficiency virus related and non related malignancies in a large cohort of homosexual men. *J. Clin. Oncol.* **13**, 2540–6.

Lyter, D., Bryant, J., Thackeray, R. et al. (1998) Non-AIDS defining malignancies in the Multicentre AIDS Cohort Study, 1984–1996. *J. Acquired Immune Deficiency Syndr. Hum. Retrovirol.* **17**, A13.

MacMahon, E., Glass, J., Hayward, S. et al. (1991) Epstein–Barr virus in AIDS-related primary central nervous system lymphoma. *Lancet* **338**, 969–73.

Maiman, M., Fruchter, R., Guy, L., Cuthill, S., Levine, P. and Serur, E. (1993) Human immunodeficiency virus infection and invasive cervical carcinoma. *Cancer* **71**, 402–6.

McClain, K., Leach, C., Jemson, H. *et al.* (1995) Association of Epstein–Barr virus with leiomyosarcomas in young people with AIDS. *N. Engl. J. Med.* **332**, 12–18.

Melbye, M., Cote, T.R., Kessler, L., Gail, M., Biggar, R.J. and AIDS/Cancer working group (1994) High incidence of anal cancer among AIDS patients. *Lancet* **343**, 636–9.

Mitsuyasu, R., Von Roenn, J., Krown, S. *et al.* (1997) Comparison study of liposomal doxorubicin alone or with bleomycin and vincristine for treatment of advanced AIDS-associated Kaposi's sarcoma (AIDS-KS): AIDS Clinical Trial Group (ACTG) protocol 286. *Proc. Am. Soc. Clin. Oncol.* **16**, 55a.

Mocroft, A., Youle, M., Gazzard, B.G., Morcinek, J., Halai, R. and Phillips, A.N. (1996) Antiherpesvirus treatment and risk of Kaposi's sarcoma in HIV infection. Royal Free/Chelsea and Westminster Hospitals Collaborative Group. *AIDS* **10**, 1101–5.

Nigro, N.D., Vaitkevicius, V.K. and Considine, B. (1974) Combined therapy for cancer of the anal canal. A preliminary report. *Dis. Colon Rectum*, **17**, 354–6.

Northfelt, D.W., Dezube, B., Miller, B. *et al.* (1995) Randomized comparative trial of Doxil vs Adriamycin, bleomycin, and vincristine (ABV) in the treatment of severe AIDS-related Kaposi's sarcoma. *Blood* **86**, 382a.

Oksenhendler, E., Duarte, M., Soulier, J. *et al.* (1996) Multicentric Castleman's disease in HIV infection: a clinical and pathological study of 20 patients. *AIDS* **10**, 61–7.

Osman, M., Kubo, R., Gill, J. *et al.* (1999) Identification of HHV-8 specific cytotoxic T cell responses. *J. Virol.* **73**, 6136–40.

Palefsky, J.M., Holly, E.A., Ralston, M. *et al.* (1998) High incidence of anal high-grade squamous intra-epithelial lesions among HIV-positive and HIV-negative homosexual and bisexual men. *AIDS* **12**, 495–503.

Palefsky, J., Minkoff, H., Kalish, L.A. *et al.* (1999a) Cervicovaginal human papillomavirus infection in human immunodeficiency virus-1 positive and high risk HIV-negative women. *J. Natl Cancer Inst.* **91**, 226–36.

Palefsky, J.M., Holly, E.A., Ralston, M.L., Darragh, T., Jay, N. and Berry, M. (1999b) The effect of HAART on the natural history of anal squamous intraepithelial lesion in HIV+ men. *JAIDS* **21**, A13.

Pluda, J., Wyvill, K., Little, R. *et al.* (1999) Administration of interleukin 12 (IL-12) to patients with AIDS-associated Kaposi's sarcoma: preliminary results of a pilot study. *JAIDS* **21**, A29.

Rabkin, C., Bedi, G., Musaba, E. *et al.* (1995) AIDS-related Kaposi's sarcoma is a clonal neoplasm. *Clin. Cancer Res.* **1**, 257–60.

Raphael, M., Audouin, J., Tulliez, M. *et al.* (1993) Anatomic and histologic distribution of 448 cases of AIDS-related non-Hodgkin's lymphoma. Proceedings of the Annual Meeting of the American Society of Haematology. *Blood* **82**(suppl. 1), 386a.

Remick, S. (1996) Non-AIDS defining cancers. *Hematol. Oncol. Clin. North Am.* **10**, 1203–13.

Rosen, L., Kabbinavir, F., Rosen, P. *et al.* (1998) Phase I trial of SU5416, a novel angiogenesis inhibitor in patients with advanced malignancies. *Proc. Am. Soc. Clin. Oncol.* **17**, 218a.

Rubio, R. (1994) Hodgkin's disease associated with HIV: a clinical study of 46 cases. *Cancer* **73**, 2400–7.

Russo, J.J., Bohenzky, R.A., Chien, M.C. *et al.* (1996) Nucleotide sequence of the Kaposi sarcoma-associated herpesvirus (HHV8). *Proc. Natl Acad. Sci. USA* **93**, 14862–7.

Saville, M.W., Lietzau, J., Pluda, J.M. *et al.* (1995) Treatment of HIV-associated Kaposi's sarcoma with paclitaxel. *Lancet* **346**, 26–8.

Scadden, D.T., Doweiko, J., Schenkein, D. *et al.* (1993) A phase I/II trial of combined immunoconjugate and chemotherapy for AIDS-related lymphoma. *Blood* **82**, 386a.

Schwartsmann, G., Mans, D., Machado, V., Sander, E., Sprinz, E. and Kalakun, L. (1995) Phase II study of the basic fibroblast growth factor (b-FGF) inhibiting agent pentosan polysulphate (PPS) in patients with AIDS-related Kaposi's sarcoma. *Proc. Am. Soc. Clin. Oncol.* **14**, 290.

Soulier, J., Grollet, L., Oksenhendlder, E. *et al.* (1995) Kaposi's sarcoma-associated Herpesvirus-like DNA sequences in multicentric Castleman's disease. *Blood* **86**, 1276–80.

Sparano, J.A., Wiernik, P.H., Hu, X. *et al.* (1996) Pilot trial of infusional cyclophosphamide, doxorubicin and etoposide plus didanosine and filgrastim in patients with HIV associated non-Hodgkin's lymphoma. *J. Clin. Oncol.* **14**, 3026–35.

Speck, C., Levine, A., Carter, N. and Enger, S. (1998) Non-AIDS defining malignancies among 5,574 HIV seropositive members of a large managed care-based cohort. *J. Acquired Immune Deficiency Syndr. Hum. Retrovirol.* **17**, A14.

Staddon, A., Henry, D., Bonnem, E. *et al.* (1994) A randomised dose finding study of recombinant platelet factor 4 (rPF4) in cutaneous AIDS-related Kaposi's sarcoma. *Proc. Am. Soc. Clin. Oncol.* **13**, 50.

Stewart, S., Jablonowski, H., Goebel, F.D. *et al.* (1998) Randomised comparative trial of pegylated liposomal doxorubicin versus bleomycin and vincristine in the treatment of AIDS-related Kaposi's sarcoma. *J. Clin. Oncol.* **16**, 683–91.

Tirelli, U., Vaccher, E., Rezza, G. *et al.* (1988) Hodgkin's disease and infection with the human immunodeficiency virus in Italy. *Ann. Intern. Med.* **108**, 309–10.

Tirelli, U., Errante, D., Dolcetti, R. *et al.* (1995) Hodgkin's disease and HIV infection: clinicopathologic and virologic features of 114 patients from the Italian cooperative group on AIDS and tumors. *J. Clin. Oncol.* **13**, 1758–67.

Tirelli, U., Errante, D., Spina, M. *et al.* (1996) Long-term survival of patients with HIV-related systemic non-Hodgkin's lymphomas. *Hematol. Oncol.* **14**, 7–15.

Tulpule, A., Anderson, L.J.J., Levine, A.M. *et al.* (1994) Anti-B4 (CD19) monoclonal antibody conjugated with ricin (B4-blocked ricin) in refractory AIDS-lymphoma. *Proc. Am. Soc. Clin. Oncol.* **13**, 52.

Tulpule, A., Joshi, B., DeGuzman, N. *et al.* (1997) Interleukin-4 in the treatment of AIDS-related Kaposi's sarcoma. *Ann. Oncol.* **8**, 79–83.

Uthayakumar, S., Bower, M., Money-Kyrle, J. *et al.* (1996) Randomised cross-over comparison of liposomal daunorubicin versus observation for early Kaposi's sarcoma. *AIDS* **10**, 515–19.

Vaccher, E., Tirelli, U., Spina, M. *et al.* (1996) Age and serum lactate dehydrogenase level are independent prognostic factors in Human Immunodeficiency Virus-related Non-Hodgkin's lymphomas: a single-institute study of 96 patients. *J. Clin. Oncol.* **14**, 2217–23.

Vogel, J., Hinrichs, S., Reynolds, R., Luciw, P. and Jay, G. (1988) The HIV tat gene induces dermal lesions resembling Kaposi's sarcoma in transgenic mice. *Nature* **335**, 606–11.

Wang, C., Brodland, D. and Su, W. (1995) Skin cancers associated with acquired immunodeficiency syndrome. *Proc. Mayo Clin.* **70**, 766–72.

Welles, L., Little, R., Wyvill, K. *et al.* (1997) Preliminary results of a phase II study of oral thalidomide in patients with HIV infection and Kaposi's sarcoma (KS). *J. Acquired Immune Deficiency Syndr. Hum. Retrovirol.* **14**, A21.

Whitby, D., Howard, M.R., Tenant Flowers, M. *et al.* (1995) Detection of Kaposi sarcoma associated herpesvirus in peripheral blood of HIV-infected individuals and progression to Kaposi's sarcoma. *Lancet* **346**, 799–802.

Wilson, W., Frenkel, E., Vuitch, F. *et al.* (1992) Testicular tumors in men with human immunodeficiency virus. *J. Urol.* **147**, 1038–40.

Ziegler, J.L., Beckstead, J.A., Volberding, P.A. *et al.* (1984) Non-Hodgkin's lymphoma in 90 homosexual men. Relation to generalized lymphadenopathy and the acquired immunodeficiency syndrome. *N. Engl. J. Med.* **311**, 565–70.

Management

49

Medical care

DAVID CHAO AND RICHARD H.J. BEGENT

Management of a patient with cancer requires an holistic approach, including the characterization of the tumour, its eradication or control and attention to the full range of personal, family, psychological and general medical issues. Study of patients with cancer shows us that there is a whole range of medical problems which are more or less peculiar to these diseases. Particular patterns of the development of the disease and of disruption of normal functions caused by malignant infiltration and the paraneoplastic phenomena are sufficiently complex to be a specialist subject in their own right. The oncologist is in a crucial position to develop expertise in the recognition and management of these syndromes and must accept responsibility for co-ordinating with other specialists who, of course, play important roles as well.

This chapter will review the more important syndromes and problems of management. Paraneoplastic syndromes which are an integral part of the presentations of particular malignancies are covered in the separate chapters relating to these tumour types. Others, relevant to several tumour types, are dealt with here. Improved understanding of the nature of paraneoplastic phenomena must improve our comprehension of the underlying nature of cancer. Recognition of their often subtle features in the face of symptoms and signs caused more directly by the tumour may be demanding, but if diagnosed, many can be treated with benefit to the patient. Other syndromes produced directly by tumour involvement in various systems present major problems in management and deserve special consideration of the way in which they affect the patient with cancer and of the best means of treating them in the presence of the underlying disease.

PLAN OF TREATMENT

A patient with cancer may expect cure, prolonged survival without cure or only palliation. The choice of management of his general medical problems will often depend on these broader issues. Everything that follows needs to be considered in this light. The knowledge and experience of the oncologist are tested particularly by the patient whose tumour can be expected to respond, probably with some prolongation of survival, but in whom cure is extremely unlikely. As chemotherapy improves in effectiveness and can be given with less toxicity, the case for treating such patients becomes stronger. In these cases, the patient and his family need to be involved in the decision of whether to treat in order to prolong survival. However, the onus is on the oncologist to advise whether the duration and quality of life that may be expected is sufficient to justify the anticipated toxicity of therapy and nuisance associated with hospital visits. Whatever decision is taken, time must be given to ensure that medical and nursing staff, as well as the patient and family, understand the reasons for the course of action chosen and know that the policy may be changed if circumstances alter.

RESPIRATORY SYSTEM

Respiratory failure

BRONCHIAL OBSTRUCTION

Management depends on the site, the pathology and the aims of the treatment. Early endoscopy and biopsy of the obstructing lesion is nearly always essential. Occasionally the obstruction will be found to be caused by a non-malignant lesion. Tumours arising in the bronchial tree tend to present at an early stage and may cause obstruction, which may present as an emergency. The treatment of choice is bronchoscopy, when the obstruction may be relieved with neodymium yttrium–aluminium–garnet (Nd-YAG) laser therapy (Turner and Wang, 1999), or possibly with electrocautery, cryotherapy or placement of airway stents (Becker *et al.*, 1995; Prakash, 1999). Radiotherapy is often effective in relieving obstruction of a bronchus caused by a variety of tumour types, and may be combined with bronchoscopy to be delivered intrabronchially as brachytherapy (Prakash, 1999). Bronchoscopic procedures are invaluable both as emergency treatment and in palliation so that definitive treatment can be planned and given after the immediate distress has been relieved.

Surgical resection of a primary pulmonary tumour may give a 10-year survival in 10–20 per cent of patients, and should always be considered if disease appears to be localized. Chemosensitive tumours, such as small cell carcinoma of the bronchus, lymphomas and testicular germ-cell tumours, are best treated with cytotoxic drugs, which will often give a rapid response and also deal with disease at distant sites, as is commonly present with these tumour types (Fig. 49.1).

PARENCHYMAL LUNG DISEASE

Diffuse lung infiltration in a patient with cancer may be caused by tumour, infection, drugs, radiation, various other causes or a mixture of pathologies. Patients are frequently so ill that full investigation is not possible. Where biopsy material cannot be obtained, serum tumour markers can be valuable in making a diagnosis of choriocarcinoma or a germ-cell tumour. Trends in serum carcinoembryonic antigen (CEA) and other markers of common epithelial malignancies will also indicate whether there is tumour progression at some site.

A systematic search for infection is important, but it is often necessary to start treatment for infection before a microbiological diagnosis is made. Multiple tumour deposits can predispose to areas of pulmonary infection

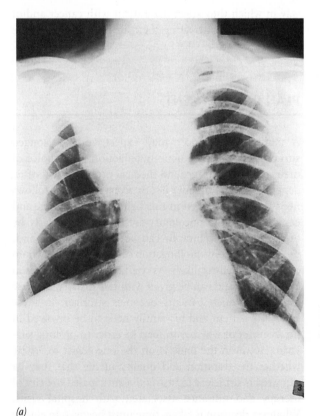

(a)

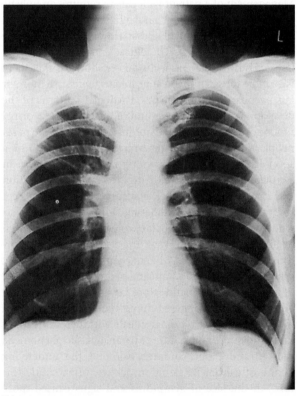

(b)

Figure 49.1 *(a) Chest X-ray, showing collapse of the right upper lobe in a patient with a malignant germ-cell tumour of the testis. Biopsy of a tumour obstructing the left upper-lobe bronchus contained metastatic germ-cell tumour, and cytotoxic chemotherapy was given. (b) After chemotherapy as the only treatment, the tumour resolved completely, leading to re-expansion of the lobe.*

distal to obstruction. Therefore, patients in severe respiratory failure who have a known widespread lung tumour are best given a broad-spectrum antibiotic as well as anti-tumour therapy, even though it may be impossible to prove infection. Opportunistic infection, particularly with *Pneumocystis carinii* and tuberculosis should be considered. When cytotoxic chemotherapy is begun for a drug-sensitive tumour such as choriocarcinoma or a germ-cell tumour, the respiratory failure may deteriorate for the first few days (Fig. 49.2). This is thought to be caused by oedema and inflammation around necrotic tumour cells. In patients with dyspnoea at rest, chemotherapy should be started less intensively than usual. Arterial Po_2 should be monitored from the start of treatment to detect such deterioration as early as possible. Oxygen is often helpful and, although ventilation is occasionally successful in supporting a patient until the lungs improve, in our experience most patients who are ventilated die. It can often be difficult to discriminate between tumour progression, infection and drug-induced lung fibrosis (Fig. 49.3). However, the clinician may be alerted by a careful history and knowledge of the types of allergic lesion seen with bleomycin, methotrexate, Mitomycin C® and procarbazine and the diffuse interstitial pneumonitis with fibrosis which may result from bleomycin, cyclophosphamide, chlorambucil, busulfan, BCNU (1, 3-*bis* (2-chloroethyl)-1-nitrosurea), and methotrexate (Weiss and Muggia, 1980; Batist and Andrews, 1981). Combination chemotherapy often makes it difficult to be certain of the causative drug. Lung biopsy may discriminate between drug-induced, infective and neoplastic causes of diffuse interstitial pneumonitis. It is unclear if the concomitant use of oxygen, itself toxic to the lung, may exacerbate bleomycin toxicity. There is anecdotal evidence that high-dose corticosteroids may prevent or reverse the pulmonary toxicity (Maher and Daly, 1993), but there have been no formal trials, and the use of cyto-protectants such as amifostine remains experimental (Santini and Giles, 1999).

Radiation-induced lung disease (Fig. 49.4) is characterized by dry cough, low-grade fever and dyspnoea occurring 2–3 months after radiation. A diffuse pulmonary opacity closely corresponding to the radiation field, with straight margins, is typical. This may be followed at 9–12 months by fibrosis with loss of lung volume. The picture may easily be complicated by the presence of recurrent tumour or drug-induced fibrosis. Although its efficacy has not been proved, it is customary to give a course of corticosteroids for the acute reaction.

Pleural effusion

Rational management of a pleural effusion requires an understanding of the cause. At one level, it is important to exclude non-malignant conditions causing effusions in patients with cancer. At another level, management will depend on whether the malignant effusion is a transudate caused by venous or lymphatic obstruction in the lung or mediastinum, an exudate from malignant infiltration of the pleura or a chylous effusion from rupture of the thoracic duct by tumour.

Examination of the pleural fluid by culture and cytology is important. The presence of malignant cells in the pleural fluid is generally a clear indication of direct pleural involvement. However, the pleura may be infiltrated without cells being detectable. Here, evidence of an exudate is in favour of pleural infiltration. The level of tumour markers in the pleural fluid compared to serum may also be helpful (Begent and Rustin, 1989).

Although different criteria for an exudate have been used, those of Light *et al.* (1972) have been widely cited. They are: a ratio of pleural fluid to serum protein of greater than 0.5, a ratio of pleural fluid to serum lactate dehydrogenase (LDH) of greater than 0.6 and pleural fluid LDH of greater than 200 mg/dL. The presence of opaque white pleural fluid strongly suggests a chylothorax. However, a similar appearance can occur with desquamating pleural and tumour cells. It is prudent, therefore, to confirm the chylous nature of the fluid by staining for fat with Sudan III.

When a pleural effusion is a manifestation of a disseminated malignancy for which there is an effective systemic therapy and it is not causing dyspnoea, systemic treatment alone is often the best management. The effusion will provide a valuable means for evaluating the effectiveness of treatment. When the therapy includes methotrexate, toxicity may be increased by the presence of the effusion. Methotrexate diffuses into the pleural fluid when serum concentrations are high but is then cleared more slowly than the drug in the circulation. The result is a depot effect, methotrexate being released into the circulation over several days. If possible, methotrexate therapy should be avoided, particularly in high doses, and even prolonged folinic acid rescue may not be protective.

In the absence of effective systemic therapy, palliation can often be given by local means. Aspiration of the effusion close to dryness at an early stage usually gives immediate relief of symptoms while the results of investigations are obtained, the rate of re-accumulation observed and definite treatment planned. When there is also solid tumour in the thorax, aspiration under ultrasound control can assist in optimal location of fluid for removal. In a minority, the rate of re-accumulation is very slow and occasional aspirations give adequate palliation. Generally, however, measures are required to prevent or slow down fluid formation. The standard therapy is drainage of the pleural cavity to dryness with an intercostal drain followed by instillation of either bleomycin (60 mg) or tetracycline (1000 mg), although historically other cytotoxic drugs and sclerosants have been used. The response rate varies from 30 to 70 per cent (Moores, 1991; Hartman *et al.*, 1993; Martinez-Moragon *et al.*, 1997) with some studies showing a clear superiority of bleomycin over tetracycline and others showing no

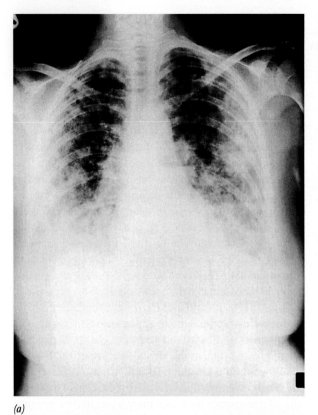

(a)

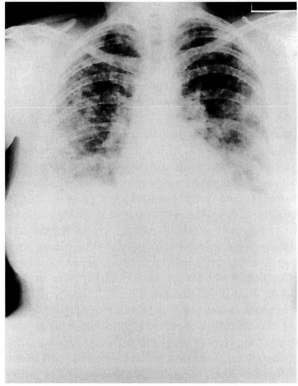

(b)

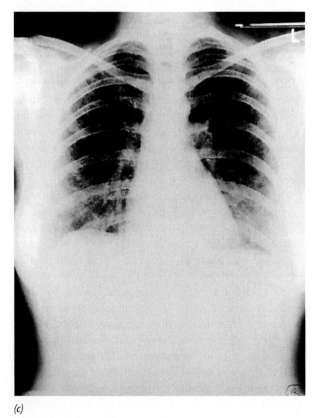

(c)

Figure 49.2 *(a) Chest X-ray, showing diffuse pulmonary shadowing caused by metastases of gestational choriocarcinomas. Dyspnoea and arterial P_{O_2} deteriorated 2 days after starting a shortened course of chemotherapy. (b) Thirteen days after starting chemotherapy there was no improvement in the radiograph nor in the patient's dyspnoea. (c) The metastases did eventually resolve. The patient is tumour-free 3 years later.*

significant differences. Bleomycin tends to cause more fevers, whereas tetracycline is associated with more chest pain requiring morphine as analgesia. There is evidence to suggest that insufflated talc under thoracoscopic guidance may give the best results (Hartman *et al.*, 1993). Patients who fail standard chemical pleurodesis may be referred to the cardiothoracic service for either talc pleurodesis or pleurectomy.

Transudates caused by pulmonary or mediastinal tumour invasion of veins or lymphatics are best treated

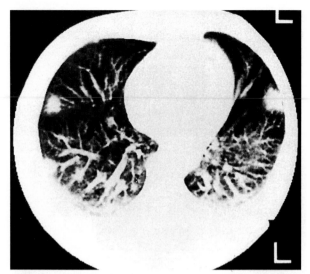

Figure 49.3 *Computed tomographic scan of the lungs in a patient receiving chemotherapy, including bleomycin, for a malignant germ-cell tumour of the testis. Multiple opacities are present in the parenchyma of the lungs. The differential diagnosis was between progressing tumour, bleomycin-induced lung fibrosis and infection. The blurred edges of the lesions are atypical for tumour metastases, and after a rise in antibody titres to cytomegalovirus was shown, the changes were attributed to infection with this virus. The changes resolved and did not recur when chemotherapy was resumed.*

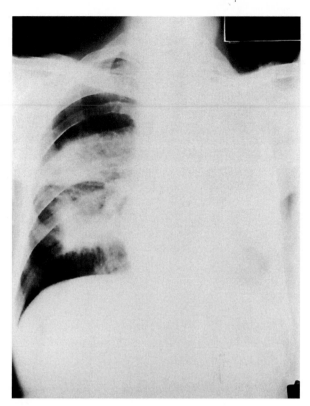

Figure 49.4 *Chest X-ray of a patient who had a pneumonectomy for carcinoma of the left lung. A recurrence at the right hilum was treated with radiation and an area of radiation fibrosis corresponding to the field is shown. The straight edges of the opacity are typical.*

by radiotherapy or systemic chemotherapy. Chylothorax will sometimes resolve after mediastinal radiotherapy or successful chemotherapy.

Hypertrophic pulmonary osteoarthropathy

This paraneoplastic syndrome characterized by clubbing, periostitis of long bones and, sometimes, a polyarthropathy occurs not uncommonly with non-small cell carcinoma of the lung and various other primary and secondary neoplasms in the thorax. Polyarthropathy may be the presenting feature without clubbing and can give a positive bone scan. Hypertrophic pulmonary osteoarthropathy (HPOA) can be associated with severe pain, and treatment of the underlying malignancy will often control the pain, but where this fails or is not possible, radiotherapy can be given to the affected bony site (Yeo *et al.*, 1996).

CARDIOVASCULAR SYSTEM

Superior vena caval obstruction (SVCO)

The syndrome of non-pulsatile distention of cervical and thoracic veins with facial, cervical and upper thoracic

oedema and dyspnoea is well known. Sometimes there is conjunctival oedema and oral mucosal engorgement in addition (Perez *et al.*, 1978). Central nervous system features such as headache, papilloedema and altered consciousness are attributed to raised intracranial pressure resulting from venous distension. A histological diagnosis is important since benign goitres, aortic aneurysms, thrombotic syndromes and idiopathic sclerosing mediastinitis may cause superior vena caval obstruction (SVCO) in about 3 per cent of cases (Lokich and Goodman, 1975). The first case described by William Hunter in 1757 was caused by a syphilitic aortic aneurysm, but infective causes were much more common before antibiotics were available. Bronchial carcinoma is the most common causative malignancy (80 per cent) with small cell carcinoma more frequent than squamous cell carcinoma, followed by lymphoma (17 per cent), with non-Hodgkin's lymphoma as the most frequent type (Perez *et al.*, 1978).

Treatment should be started urgently and it may be justifiable to do this without a histological diagnosis if the patient is very unwell. Under these circumstances stenting is the treatment of choice as it gives prompt relief and preserves tumour tissue for biopsy before definitive treatment. If this is not available or possible then radiotherapy should be given and a biopsy obtained as soon as possible.

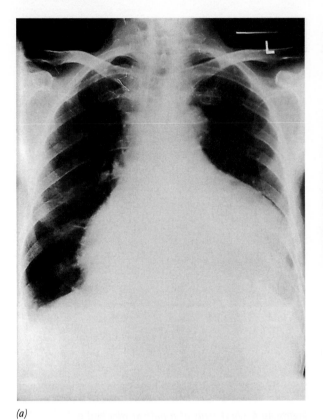
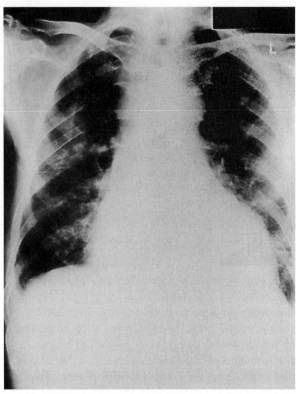

(a)   (b)

Figure 49.5 *(a) Chest X-ray, showing a large pericardial effusion which caused cardiac tamponade in a patient with pericardial metastases of hypernephroma. Fenestration was performed and 7 months later (b) the effusion had not reaccumulated and there was no recurrence of the tamponade.*

Radiotherapy produces symptomatic relief in up to 85 per cent of patients (Davenport *et al.*, 1978) and is the treatment of choice for squamous cell carcinoma of the bronchus. However, small cell carcinoma and non-Hodgkin's lymphoma make up half of all the malignant causes of SVCO, and for these tumour types chemotherapy should be strongly considered as the primary therapy because of the chemosensitivity of the tumour types and because these are essentially systemic diseases. If the tumour fails to respond to treatment, or if treatment cannot be given, stenting may give good palliation (Zollikofer *et al.*, 1995). When SVCO fails to respond to treatment, venous thrombosis rather than persistent tumour should also be considered.

Pericardial tumour

The frequent involvement of the pericardium by metastatic tumour, familiar in the post-mortem room, is now a common incidental finding with CT or ultrasound examinations. It is unusual for symptoms to occur, but cardiac tamponade produced either by effusion or constrictive pericardial tumour may have an insidious onset and easily be missed in a patient with disseminated malignancy. Emergency treatment of tamponade by aspiration of pericardial fluid is followed by chemotherapy or radiotherapy

if the tumour is likely to respond. Intrapericardial mustine, thiotepa, 5-fluorouracil, tetracycline and radioactive colloidal gold or phosphorus have been used historically. In chronic recurring effusions, fenestration of the pericardium into the pleural cavity is worth considering (Hankins *et al.*, 1980). This is a relatively simple procedure with little morbidity and a high probability of preventing re-accummulation of the effusion. An example is shown in Figure 49.5.

Cardiac toxicity

This may occur with anthracycline therapy, cardiac radiotherapy, cyclophosphamide and iron overload from repeated transfusion. The most important and common cardiotoxicity follows anthracycline chemotherapy (Singal and Iliskovic, 1998). Acute toxicity after doxorubicin most commonly takes the form of arrhythmias or conduction defects. An acute myocarditis–pericarditis syndrome has also been described. Chronic toxicity dependent upon the cumulative dose was clinically evident in 1–10 per cent of patients who received a cumulative dose of $550\,\mathrm{mg/m^2}$ (Von Hoff and Layard, 1979). Cardiomyopathy followed by congestive cardiac failure is the principal manifestation, and once it has developed the prospects for improvement are poor. Therefore prevention of cardiac toxicity is vital. Cardiac dysfunction can be measured at an earlier stage by echocardiography or radionuclide imaging, where the first sign is a decrease in left ventricular ejection fraction, particularly with exercise stress testing. Cardiotoxicity may be reduced by using infusional doxorubicin, or doxorubicin analogues, such as epirubicin and mitoxantrone, although these have varying degrees of cardiotoxicity (Ewer and Benjamin, 1996). Mitoxantrone is one of the least cardiac toxic analogues but its anti-tumour effect may not always be comparable. There has been interest in the cytoprotectant dexrazoxane which, when co-administered with doxorubicin, appears to reduce the incidence of cardiac toxicity, but dexrazoxane may potentiate doxorubicin-induced myelosuppression and it is not clear if it interferes with the activity of chemotherapy or will protect against late cardiac toxicity (Hensley *et al.*, 1999). Taxol can cause bradycardia, heart block or other arrhythmias during or shortly after infusion (Ewer and Benjamin, 1996). 5-Fluorouracil may cause precordial pain, S-T and T wave changes on ECG, atrial or ventricular arrhythmias or sudden death. The incidence of significant effects may reach 5 per cent in patients with previous heart disease.

UROGENITAL SYSTEM

Obstructive uropathy

Renal failure caused by ureteric obstruction in gynaecological, urinary and gastrointestinal malignancy and lymphoma has, in the past, been welcomed as a relatively gentle way for the patient to die. Modern chemotherapy, particularly for carcinoma of the cervix and urinary bladder, lymphoma and germ-cell tumours has changed this so that many patients may be offered several months of good-quality life or even cure. Good renal function is essential for effective chemotherapy and optimal management of the ureteric obstruction becomes crucial for success. Ultrasound is the best method for demonstrating the hydronephrosis. When obstruction is not complete, an isotope renogram is useful to show the extent of the renal obstruction and the degree of impairment to each kidney.

After correcting hypercalaemia, ureteric stenting or percutaneous nephrostomy is the most satisfactory emergency measure to relieve obstruction (Sing *et al.*, 1979; Fallon *et al.*, 1980; Ho *et al.*, 1980). Chemotherapy or radiotherapy may then be given in safety provided that the glomerular filtration rate recovers. If there is a good tumour response but persisting obstruction due to fibrosis, a permanent urinary diversion may be considered at a later stage. This is sometimes valuable for long-standing urinary fistulas as well.

When the obstruction is incomplete and the response rate to drugs or radiation is high, obstruction may be

rapidly relieved by these means. Drugs metabolized by the kidneys must be used with great care or, particularly in the case of methotrexate, avoided altogether. Etoposide and low-dose cisplatin have proved useful for treatment of germ-cell tumours in this context (Newlands *et al.*, 1983). The full range and dose of drugs may then be given as soon as renal function has improved.

Renal parenchymal disease

Renal impairment is infrequently caused by direct tumour involvement, but lymphoma and chronic lymphocytic leukaemia can occasionally have this effect (Fig. 49.6). The renal failure of myeloma is complex; direct damage by immunoglobulin light chains, amyloid and hypercalcaemia may contribute. Amyloid has been reported in hypernephroma and Hodgkin's disease.

Nephrotic syndrome is a rare complaint of a wide range of malignancies. Hodgkin's disease is the most common and is usually associated with minimal change or lipoid nephropathy (Zimmerman, 1982). Membranous glomerulitis is the more common type of lesion in carcinomas and non-Hodgkin's lymphoma. Deposition of immune complexes containing tumour-associated antigens has been shown in some instances of carcinomas. Resolution of nephrotic syndrome has been reported when the causative tumour is successfully treated. Disseminated intravascular coagulation in malignancy is associated with renal impairment in 25 per cent of cases (Siegal *et al.*, 1978). Like the nephrotic syndrome, it may resolve when a causative malignancy is treated successfully.

Urate nephropathy results from release of purines by necrosing tumour cells and consequent precipitation of urate in the renal tubules. It occurs in myeloproliferative

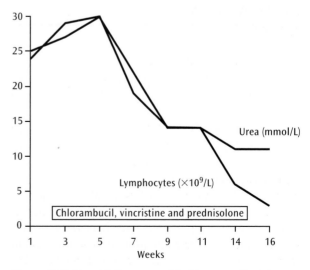

Figure 49.6 *Renal failure caused by biopsy-confirmed infiltration of the kidney by chronic lymphocytic leukaemia. Treatment with chlorambucil, vincristine and prednisolone led to a fall in the lymphocyte count, with a corresponding fall of plasma urea.*

disorders but most strikingly after treatment of tumours, such as leukaemias and lymphomas, which respond rapidly to chemotherapy. It is prevented by good hydration during chemotherapy, administration of allopurinol and ensuring an alkaline urine (Crittenden and Ackerman, 1977).

Tumour lysis syndrome occurs when rapid tumour destruction leads to hyperkalaemia, hyperphosphataemia with hypocalcaemia, lactic acidosis and urate nephropathy, and may be fatal. It occurs after the start of treatment of tumours such as Burkitt's lymphoma and lymphoblastic leukaemia in which response may be dramatic. With care to ensure good hydration, alkaline urine and allopurinol prophylaxis, it should be a manageable problem (Warrell, 1993). However, where there is pre-existing renal impairment, peritoneal or haemodialysis may be necessary.

Hepatorenal syndrome is a progressive oliguric renal failure due to renal hypoperfusion secondary to liver failure. In the oncological setting it may be caused by a coexisting medical condition, commonly advanced cirrhosis, or as a complication of treatment, such as chemoembolization of liver lesions. The prognosis is grave as the only effective treatment is liver transplantation, for which oncology patients are nearly always contraindicated. Treatments such as transjugular intrahepatic portosystemic shunts and renal vasodilators may temporarily improve renal function and should be considered (Gentilni *et al.*, 1999).

The nephrotoxicity of radiation, cytotoxic drugs, such as cisplatinum, methotrexate and nitrosources, and antibiotics, such as the aminoglycosides, is dealt with elsewhere.

ALIMENTARY SYSTEM

Nutrition

Weight loss is so clearly a stigmata of cancer that the whole topic of nutrition easily arouses confusion and strong feelings in the patient and those caring for the patient. The weight loss may be due to gastrointestinal tract involvement with subsequent difficulties in eating, or it may be due to the anorexia–cachexia syndrome, or both. The anorexia–cachexia syndrome is a major clinical problem and is not the same as simple starvation, as discussed further below. Therefore it is not surprising that ensuring an adequate diet alone rarely reverses the syndrome, although successful treatment of the tumour commonly does. The patient's nutritional status must be assessed before treatment to decide whether there are sufficient reserves to prevent the patient becoming severely, or even fatally, malnourished during surgery, radiotherapy or chemotherapy. The criteria for making such an assessment are not well defined. Weight is influenced by

hydration, and plasma albumin by hepatic function and renal loss. Other parameters, such as creatinine/height ratio, are similarly unreliable. This is not an excuse for not considering malnutrition when they are abnormal. A period of observation by nurses and dieticians in hospital will identify patients ingesting less than 1000–1500 calories daily. Such patients will need nutritional support if intensive therapy is to be given over a prolonged period. Those who can be helped by simple dietary advice, mouth care or a liquid diet will also have been identified.

A clear idea of the aims of treatment is essential before deciding on nutritional support, and, where possible, nutrition should always be supplied in the least invasive and most physiological way. If therapy is palliative, total parenteral nutrition or forced enteral nutrition are usually inappropriate and the patient and his family can be reassured that it is not necessary to eat if to do so is distressing. However, measures to relieve the discomfort of oral ulceration or infection and relief of oesophageal obstruction may be of great benefit in palliation.

If the patient is undergoing active treatment, then nutritional support appears logical, but in fact has been difficult to prove in clinical trials (Body, 1999). Nevertheless, if patients are temporarily unable to swallow, it is justifiable to insert a nasogastric tube for feeding. Patients who cannot tolerate a nasogastric tube, or in whom one cannot be passed, can be satisfactorily fed through a percutaneous gastrostomy or gastrojejunostomy tube (Larson *et al.*, 1987). Total parenteral nutrition can also be justified in selected patients with intestinal obstruction from ovarian or other carcinomas in which there is a reasonable chance of a remission of some months if the patient can be supported for the first few weeks. The decision to start such support should be made early if it is going to be undertaken, and it is certainly not appropriate for all. Nevertheless, for some patients the chance of a few extra months of life out of hospital will be of great worth.

Causes of catabolic states

The anorexia–cachexia syndrome has a complex pathophysiology which is only now being appreciated (Body, 1999). There is suppression of hunger in the face of weight loss, and one of the key features is equal mobilization of fat and muscle, whereas in simple starvation there is preferential mobilization of fat. Cytokines are now thought to play a major role in the syndrome, but extrapolating from animal models to patients has not proved straightforward. Tumour necrosis factor-α (cachectin, TNF-α) induces cachexia in animal tumour models in which anti-TNF antibodies reduce cachexia, but there is no clear association between serum TNF levels and cachexia in humans. Interleukin-6 correlates best with the development of cachexia in patients, but by itself interleukin-6 does not induce cachexia in animal models.

Insulin resistance and decreased insulin : glucagon ratio are commonly documented, but the cause of these changes is not clear, and attempts to correct them by insulin therapy have not been successful. The most common agents in clinical use for anorexia–cachexia syndrome are corticosteroids and progestogens. Clinical studies suggest that they are of equal efficacy but have different toxicity profiles, with progestogens having more thromboembolic and oedema problems, and corticosteroids having classical corticosteroid toxicities (Ottery et al., 1998; Loprinzi et al., 1999). Doses commonly used in studies have been dexamethasone (4 mg once daily), megestrol acetate (800 mg once daily) and medroxyprogesterone acetate (500 mg twice daily). There is clearly a need for new agents, which will come from our increasing understanding of this distressing condition.

Malabsorption

Tumour infiltration, particularly by lymphoma, surgery and radiotherapy may contribute to malabsorption. Some patients with a variety of malignancies appear to have a paraneoplastic type of malabsorption characterized by a flat mucosa or, less often, subtotal villous atrophy. The syndrome usually resolves with successful treatment of the tumour.

Diets with putative anti-tumour effect

The many claims for therapeutic effect on tumours of particular diets appear to lack satisfactory scientific support, although with the renewed interest in alternative medicine we may expect more properly conducted clinical trials (Fugh-Berman, 1997). Where the diet is innocuous and the patient has faith in it, there seems little to gain by discouraging its use. However, there are a number of alternative medicine diets which clearly do not maintain an adequate nutritional intake and in these situations it may be appropriate for encouragement to resume a more nutritional diet, particularly if the patient is undergoing active treatment.

Obstruction of the gastrointestinal tract

Management is generally by well-established surgical principles. It is salutary occasionally to see patients with intestinal obstruction who are being given antiemetics for their vomiting in the mistaken belief that their symptoms are caused by cytotoxic drugs or abdominal radiotherapy. Also it is easy to overlook common non-malignant causes of intestinal obstruction, such as strangulated hernia, in patients with cancer. Obstruction by malignant disease is, of course, best treated by definitive therapy of the tumour. When this is not possible, surgical bypass of biliary, duodenal, small intestinal and large

bowel obstruction can often be achieved at the initial operation. However, where surgery is not possible, good palliation may still be achieved by either using the Nd-YAG laser through an endoscope or by the placement of stents, either endoscopically or radiologically (see Fig. 49.7; Zollikofer et al., 2000). Laser endoscopy has the advantage that it may be repeated as often as required, although there is a risk of bowel perforation (Bown, 1998). Stenting is particularly suitable for short-term palliation due to life expectancy or expected response to active treatment because in the longer term the tumour tends to overgrow and obstruct the stent. Biliary stenting is reviewed below.

If the obstruction is not bypassable by surgery or stenting, and response to chemotherapy unlikely, then conservative management to palliate symptoms is appropriate. This situation is particularly common with advanced ovarian and gastrointestinal malignancies and is highly distressing to the patient. The initial management involves nasogastric tube suction and intravenous fluids. A trial of dexamethasone (16 mg daily intravenously for up to a week) may help to relieve the obstruction, presumably by reducing inflammation and possibly a direct anti-tumour effect, but should be discontinued if the obstruction persists (Feuer and Broadley, 1999). Octreotide is a long-acting analogue of somatostatin, and, amongst its other effects, it reduces intestinal secretions and promotes absorption. There is good evidence that it may improve nausea and vomiting associated with intestinal obstruction, probably by these mechanisms (Khoo et al., 1994), but it is less clear if octreotide actually helps to relieve the obstruction itself. Patients in whom these pharmacological approaches fail are often forced to retain their nasogastric tubes, although percutaneous endoscopic gastrostomy has been used safely for decompression in unresolving intestinal obstruction and allows the removal of the nasogastric tube (Campagnutta et al., 1996).

Vomiting induced by cytotoxic drugs

Mild nausea and vomiting are often prevented with meto-clopramide (10–20 mg, 6-hourly orally or intramuscularly). At these doses metoclopramide acts as a dopamine receptor antagonist. Vomiting in anticipation of chemotherapy can sometimes be prevented with lorazepam (1–2 mg orally). For severe vomiting, as may occur with cisplatin, hydration and electrolyte balance must be maintained to minimize renal damage, or with methotrexate to avoid toxicity from delayed renal excretion of the drug.

Emesis from cisplatin or other highly emetic drugs should be treated with a 5-hydroxytryptamine 3 (5-HT$_3$) receptor antagonist, such as ondansetron or granisetron. Cisplatin-induced emesis has an acute and delayed phase. There is good evidence that the 5-HT$_3$ antagonists are more effective in controlling acute emesis when combined with corticosteroids. However, the evidence is less clear for delayed emesis, where corticosteroids appear to be the most important anti-emetic drug and the addition of 5-HT$_3$ antagonists has had varying effect (Latreille *et al.*, 1998). Nevertheless, it remains common practice to give both a corticosteroid and a 5-HT$_3$ antagonist for 48 hours after cisplatin chemotherapy. 5-HT$_3$ antagonists are associated with significant constipation, headaches and alteration in liver enzymes.

Jaundice

The various causes of jaundice in patients with cancer are well covered in standard medical texts. Awareness of hepatic dysfunction is important because of enhanced toxicity of drugs metabolized in the liver.

Obstructive jaundice in patients with cancer is worthy of special mention because it is common with primary and metastatic tumours of the liver and bile ducts. Pruritis can be distressing and obstruction probably accelerates the progress of renal failure. Relief of obstruction is often worthwhile, therefore, even if little anti-tumour therapy is possible. Biliary diversion when the diagnostic laparotomy shows an unresectable tumour causing obstruction will usually relieve symptoms and give a time of improved quality of life. When the diagnosis is known, laparotomy is rarely justified to relieve obstructive jaundice. However, biliary stents can be placed either endoscopically or percutaneously, and can be made of either plastic or metal (Fig. 49.7; Zollikofer *et al.*, 2000). Endoscopic insertion is preferred, where possible, as there is a higher success rate with fewer complications (Speer *et al.*, 1987). Plastic stents are cheaper but may require changing every 3–6 months due to blockage. Metal stents are more costly but last longer because of their wider bore and lower tendency to migrate.

Ascites

Non-malignant causes for ascites should always be considered in patients with cancer. The presence of malignant cells on cytology should always be sought. A protein content over 2.5 g/100 mL or a raised CEA value (Begent and Rustin, 1989) also supports a diagnosis of malignancy, although the former may, of course, be a feature of inflammatory ascites, tuberculous ascites being particularly difficult to discriminate from malignancy on clinical grounds. A diagnosis of chylous ascites, with a typical milky appearance of the fluid, should be confirmed by staining fluid with Sudan III to show the presence of lipid. Repeat aspiration leads to protein and fluid loss.

Treatment of the tumour with systemic therapy is the most satisfactory solution and is often applicable, for instance in breast and ovarian cancer. Intraperitoneal

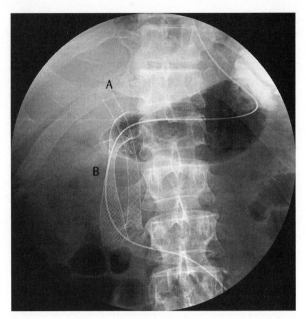

Figure 49.7 *This patient had a pancreatic cancer causing both biliary and gastric outlet obstruction. Stent A is a mesh metal stent in the biliary tree. Stent B is a mesh metal stent through the gastric outlet and extending into the duodenum; a guide-wire is still in place in the duodenum.*

cytotoxic chemotherapy and radionuclide therapy have a long history and there is an attraction as these deliver a high dose of therapy locally. However, this route of administration is not in common usage outside clinical trials because of difficulties with the administration and distribution of the agent within the peritoneal cavity. If systemic therapy is not possible, then the ascites may be tapped and spironolactone started (Greenway *et al.*, 1982). If there is re-accumulation, then subsequent management depends upon the rate of re-accumulation and the prognosis of the patient. If there is a slow rate of re-accumulation, then ascitic taps as required may provide good palliation. If there is rapid re-accumulation with a relatively long prognosis, then a LeVeen shunt should be considered. The LeVeen shunt drains fluid from the peritoneal cavity into the superior vena cava via subcutaneously tunnelled catheter. A pressure-sensitive one-way valve permits flow when the pressure intraperitoneally exceeds that in the superior vena cava by 2–3 cm water. It is simply inserted and appears satisfactory for chylous ascites and for malignant ascites which relapse chronically. When the ascites are bloodstained or particularly rich in malignant cells or protein then clotting is apt to occur, making the shunt unusable. Disseminated intravascular coagulation has been reported with LeVeen shunts but this appears to be unusual in the absence of pre-existing hepatic dysfunction. For carefully selected patients this technique can give excellent palliation (Straus *et al.*, 1977).

CENTRAL NERVOUS SYSTEM

Spinal cord compression

Epidural metastases, usually with adjacent bony involvement, are the most common cause of spinal-cord compression, which may be the presenting feature of malignancy. Radiation myelitis should be remembered in the differential diagnosis. Most patients have previously known bone metastases and there is an association between cerebral metastasis and spinal-cord compression in small cell lung carcinoma (Goldman *et al.*, 1989). In a representative recent series the most common presenting symptoms were motor weakness (96 per cent), pain (94 per cent), sensory disturbance (79 per cent) and sphincter disturbance (61 per cent). Ninety-one per cent of patients had had symptoms for at least 1 week (Hill *et al.*, 1993). Early diagnosis is critical because patients who are ambulatory at the time when treatment is started have a higher chance of remaining ambulatory. Patients with known bony metastasis should be warned to report pain, weakness or sensory disturbance urgently.

Magnetic resonance imaging (MRI) is now the imaging modality of choice, and myelography, with or without CT scanning, is rarely required. MRI is safer, faster and gives additional anatomical information which can be used for planning of surgery and radiotherapy. The initial treatment is with steroids, typically dexamethasone 16 mg once daily, which are thought to reduce oedema at the site of compression. However, the benefits of steroids at these doses have not been proven in randomized trials. The only positive data is for much higher doses of dexamethasone (96 mg once daily) but the benefit was countered by significant side effects (Sorenson *et al.*, 1994). It is critical to involve both the radiotherapist and neurosurgeon at an early stage, as one or both specialities may be required. Generally, if there is spinal instability, compression of the cord by bone, previous radiotherapy or if the histology is unknown, then surgery is indicated. Tumours arising posteriorly may be suitable for laminectomy, but 85 per cent of epidural tumours arise anteriorly in the vertebral body, and the operation of choice is vertebral body resection and stabilization, which gives better results than the more traditional laminectomy which was supposed to decompress the spinal cord but often led to further destabilization (Siegal and Siegal, 1985; Sundaresan *et al.*, 1985). The response to radiotherapy is well established. Early clinical trials showed that radiotherapy alone gave comparable results to laminectomy plus radiotherapy (Gilbert *et al.*, 1978), although later studies suggest that vertebral body resection may give better results in selected patients (Siegal and Siegal, 1985). The optimal dose and schedule for radiotherapy remains unclear, although cord tolerance is the limiting factor. The indications for radiotherapy include known radiosensitive tumour with no spinal instability, and following surgery.

Chemotherapy has a place in the management of spinal cord compression of drug-sensitive tumours. Friedman *et al.* (1986) have reviewed reports of 51 such patients. Improvement in spinal-cord function occurred after chemotherapy with or without radiotherapy in nearly all patients with lymphomas, Hodgkin's disease, myeloma, neuroblastoma and testicular germ-cell tumours. Choriocarcinoma is also successfully treated by chemotherapy. Moderate success was reported with carcinoma of the breast and prostate. The advantage of chemotherapy is that it is treating the disease systemically, and indeed a disadvantage of radiotherapy is that by ablating part of the bone marrow it can make subsequent chemotherapy more difficult to give by making the patient more sensitive to myelosuppression.

Raised intracranial pressure

When a cerebral tumour meant almost certain death this topic was of little relevance, except for the palliation which could be achieved with dexamethasone. However, advances in neurosurgery, chemotherapy and radiotherapy have changed this, and in selected patients more aggressive treatment is indicated. Death is usually caused by raised intracranial pressure which results in herniation of the cerebral hemispheres and presents as headache and vomiting. Palsies of the third and sixth cranial nerves are particularly suggestive of imminent cerebral herniation. Dexamethasone (16–32 mg daily) should be commenced immediately and an MRI or CT scan performed. The subsequent optimal management depends upon the mode of presentation and the prognosis for the tumour type (Vecht, 1998).

If the presentation is *de novo*, then surgery is indicated or, if not possible, a biopsy should be attempted, because the histology is crucial to subsequent treatment. In certain primary brain tumours, such as medulloblastoma, surgery may be curative. If the presentation is of cerebral metastases from a known primary tumour, then the appropriate treatment depends upon the tumour type and condition of the patient. In potentially curable tumours such as choriocarcinoma, germ-cell tumours and lymphomas, one aim of surgery is to protect against raised intracranial pressure by ventriculo-peritoneal shunting, craniotomy or resection of the metastasis to allow further treatment with chemotherapy and radiotherapy. Chemotherapy may actually exacerbate raised intracranial pressure by causing necrosis and bleeding into cerebral metastases, and there should be a low threshold for neurosurgical intervention. For example, choriocarcinoma with cerebral metastases has a mortality rate of 25 per cent in the first 2 weeks, with most deaths due to raised intracranial pressure and herniation, and survivors have a high chance of cure (Athanassiou *et al.*, 1983).

In patients with less drug-sensitive tumour types, the appropriate treatment depends upon the condition of the patient. If there is progressive systemic disease, or where surgery is not possible, such as the presence of multiple metastases, then whole-brain radiotherapy (WBRT) is indicated. If the cerebral metastases are the only manifestation of disease or the systemic disease is stable, then consideration should be given to surgery followed by WBRT, and in selected patients this gives superior results in terms of quality of life and survival. There is some evidence that stereotactic radiosurgery may be equivalent to surgery plus WBRT and superior to WBRT alone, and in centres with access to stereotactic radiosurgery this should be considered (Young, 1998). There is also accumulating evidence that chemotherapy combined with radiotherapy may be superior to radiotherapy alone, and clearly more clinical trials are needed to evaluate this (Postmus and Smit, 1999).

Paraneoplastic syndromes of the nervous system

These are listed in Table 49.1 and a full discussion of them is beyond the scope of this text. The reader is referred to the review by Bunn and Ridgway (1993). Advances in tumour immunology have recently shown that paraneoplastic neurological disorders may be due to neural antigens being expressed by tumours and targeted by the immune system (Voltz et al., 1999). Paraneoplastic syndromes often precede other manifestations of tumours, and therefore one practical application is that diagnostic tests may define malignancy, and even the

Table 49.1 *Paraneoplastic syndromes of the nervous system (modified from Bunn and Minna, 1985)*

Syndrome	Main tumour type
Brain	
Subacute cerebellar degeneration	Common epithelial
Dementia	Lung
Limbic encephalitis	Lung, Hodgkin's
Spinal cord	
Amyotrophic lateral sclerosis	
Subacute necrotic myelopathy	Lung, kidney
Subacute motor neuropathy	Lymphoma
Peripheral nerves	
Sensory neuropathy	Lung
Sensorimotor peripheral neuropathy	Common epithelial
Guillain–Barré syndrome	Lymphoma
Autonomic and gastrointestinal neuropathy	Small cell bronchus
Neuromuscular junction and muscle	
Dermatomyositis and polymyositis	Common epithelial
Eaton–Lambert syndrome	Small cell bronchus
Myasthenia gravis	Thymoma

type of tumour, early on as the cause of the neurological disorder.

ENDOCRINE SYSTEM

Eutopic hormone production

Tumours of many endocrine glands are characterized by secretion of their eutopic hormones. The associated syndromes often produced the presenting features of such tumours. Their investigations and therapy is dealt with elsewhere under the separate tumour types. Very high levels of human chorionic gonadotrophin (hCG) are worthy of special mention for the hyperthyroidism with which they are associated. This is believed to be caused by a cross-reaction between hCG and thyroid stimulating hormone (Nisula and Taliadouras, 1980).

Ectopic hormone production: ectopic ACTH syndrome

Some 5 per cent of patients with small cell lung cancer have clinical features of Cushing's syndrome (Lokich, 1982). Carcinoid, medullary thyroid carcinoma, neuroblastoma and phaechromocytomas are also associated with the syndrome, which is also seen occasionally with a variety of other tumour types. Production of 'big ACTH' by the tumour produces the effect through adrenocortical stimulation. Other derivatives of this hormone may function as melanocyte stimulating hormone or opiate-like hormones.

The ectopic ACTH syndrome is characterized by oedema, muscle weakness, hypertension, hypokalaemia, alkalosis and hyperglycaemia. Moon facies, striae and buffalo hump may be seen in patients with rapidly progressing tumours. The syndrome may be the presenting feature of a malignancy. The measurement of 24-hour urinary free cortisol is the most sensitive and specific test to confirm Cushing's syndrome. Serum ACTH levels usually exceed 200 pg/mL. A high-dose dexamethasone suppression test will distinguish between pituitary and ectopic ACTH secretion. Treatment of the tumour is the most effective means of control. Where this is not possible, medical means of suppression of the adrenal cortex should be tried first. The steroid biosynthesis inhibitors aminoglutethamide, metyrapone and ketoconazole have been used effectively (Engelhardt and Weber, 1994), or the adrenal cortex may be ablated with mitotane (o',p'-DDD). If these fail, then surgery should be considered. Replacement of the physiological requirements of corticosteroid is required if the adrenal cortex is successfully suppressed or ablated.

Ectopic secretion of hCG is worthy of mention here, not because it causes troublesome clinical features, but because measurements of serum hCG concentration can be used as a tumour marker (Crawford *et al.*, 1986). Ectopic hormone secretion in relation to hypercalcaemia and hyponatraemia is dealt with below.

Metabolic syndromes with more than one cause

HYPERCALCAEMIA

Hypercalcaemia occurs in about 10 per cent of patients with cancer at some stage in their disease, and is more common with breast cancer, myeloma and squamous cell carcinomas. Although bony metastases are present in the majority of cases of hypercalcaemia, this is not invariably the case, and there is no correlation between hypercalcaemia and the extent of skeletal involvement. Hypercalcaemia is caused by humoral agents released by the tumour, such as parathyroid hormone-related peptide which binds to the parathyroid hormone receptor but is not detected by standard parathyroid hormone assays. In assessing hypercalcaemia, correction of the serum value according to serum protein levels is important because the effects of calcium are dependent on the ionized fraction and can be calculated from the formula:

Corrected calcium (mmol/L) = measured
calcium + [0.02(47 − serum albumin (g/L))]

Malaise, nausea, vomiting, polydipsia, polyuria, hyporeflexia, weight loss and constipation are common presenting features. Hypovolaemia from the loss of sodium and water associated with excess calcium excretion is followed by renal failure. Excretion of calcium is decreased at this stage and the progression of hypercalcaemia accelerates. Confusion, psychosis, seizures and death may ensue.

Therapy depends on the severity of hypercalcaemia. If mild, without dehydration and detected at the outset of a treatable malignancy, therapy of the tumour with attention to good hydration will suffice. With dehydration, renal impairment or markedly raised serum calcium levels, a more intensive approach is required. Correction of hypovolaemia is the first step, with 3–4 L/day of 0.9 per cent sodium chloride with potassium supplementation as required. Frusemide should only be used to prevent or treat heart failure. Fluid therapy alone will improve patients, but will not control the hypercalcaemia in the long term. Effective chemotherapy is required, but in many patients this will not be available or will not act sufficiently quickly.

The bisphosphonates inhibit osteoclast-mediated bone resorption and are highly effective in the treatment of hypercalcaemia (Body *et al.*, 1998). Two are currently commonly used in the treatment of malignant hypercalcaemia: disodium pamidronate and sodium clodronate, and both should only be used once the dehydration and renal impairment have been corrected. Disodium pamidronate is given as a single infusion of 30–90 mg, dependent upon serum calcium concentration, at a rate of 1 mg/min. Sodium clodronate is given as a single infusion of 1.5 g over 4 hours. The serum calcium concentration falls and reaches a nadir between 3 and 5 days. Side-effects are few, although fever and bone pain have been reported with pamidronate, and mild gastrointestinal upsets with clodronate. Hypercalcaemia tends to recur within a few weeks unless the underlying tumour has been treated, and if this is not possible, then infusions of pamidronate or clodronate may be given every 3–4 weeks, or else oral clodronate 1.6 g to 3.2 g/day can be started once the acute episode has been treated. Bisphosphonates are also valuable in relieving pain from bony metastases and may delay the development of bony metastases in breast and prostatic carcinoma and multiple myeloma (Body *et al.*, 1998; Coleman, 1998).

Other drugs that have been used to control hypercalcaemia include mithramycin (Mundy *et al.*, 1983) and calcitonin (Ralston *et al.*, 1986), but these have greater side-effects and are rarely required now. Corticosteroids are only partially effective and work better with haematological malignancies (Thallasionos and Joplin, 1968; Mundy *et al.*, 1983).

HYPONATRAEMIA

Hyponatraemia is a common problem in patients with cancer. Its causes are diverse and a systematic approach to investigation is crucial. Figure 49.8 gives a scheme of points to consider for this purpose.

The syndrome of inappropriate antidiuretic hormone (ADH) secretion deserves special mention because the hormone responsible may be secreted by tumours, particularly small cell carcinoma of the bronchus and head and neck cancers (Sorensen *et al.*, 1995). Caution

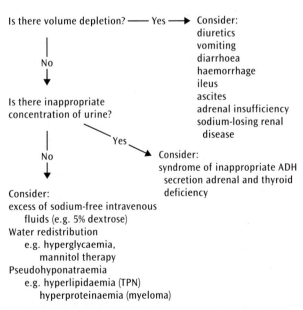

Figure 49.8 *The causes of hyponatraemia. TPN, total parenteral nutrition.*

must be exercised in making an assumption of this cause because there are a large number of non-malignant causes, e.g. infection and drugs, including cytotoxics such as vincristine and cyclophosphamide (DeFronzo and Thier, 1980). The selective retention of water under the influence of ADH results in hyponatraemia and low plasma osmolarity with inappropriate concentration and high osmolarity of urine. The retained water is principally intracellular so that oedema or raised venous pressure are unusual. The intracellular hypo-osmolarity presents the chief danger, causing seizures and death if extreme.

Removal of the cause by therapy of the tumour or other causative factor is central to management. However, when the serum sodium is very low other direct measures to control this are important. Water restriction to 500 mL daily will usually bring improvement. The tetracycline derivative, demeclocycline (600–1200 mg daily) is also effective and has been found to be superior to lithium (Forrest *et al.*, 1978). If a patient is comatose or having convulsions, more rapid means of increasing the plasma sodium are imperative. The problem here is that rapid correction of hyponatraemia appears to be capable of causing permanent brain damage (Swales, 1987). The best course appears to be only to use a minimum of isotonic or hypertonic (308–462 mmol/L) saline, with care not to cause a rapid rise of plasma sodium (more than 12 mmol/L a day). Frusemide is usually required if hypertonic saline is given. It is very unusual, however, for intravenous saline to be justifiable and the other measures given are usually adequate.

HYPOGLYCAEMIA

Although classically associated with insulinomas, hypoglycaemia is occasionally seen with almost any type of malignancy, particularly when there is a large tumour mass. Weakness, fatigue, confusion and occasionally focal neurological signs, most marked after fasting, are presenting features. Oversecretion of insulin is classically associated with insulinomas and very occasionally other non-islet cell tumours (Seckl *et al.*, 1999), but otherwise hypoglycaemia is caused by incompletely processed insulin-like growth factor-II (IGF-II), which binds to and activates the insulin receptor (Le Roith, 1999). In addition, it also binds to IGF-I receptors in the pituitary, downregulating growth hormone secretion, which further exacerbates the hypoglycaemia by reducing gluconeogenesis in the liver.

Treatment in emergency is by infusion of 50 per cent dextrose. Therapy should then be directed at tumour control. When this is not rapidly possible, frequent meals will often prevent symptoms and it is occasionally necessary for a patient to be wakened to eat in the early hours to avoid hypoglycaemia at the normal waking time. Glucocorticoids and growth hormone may also be effective if these measures are not sufficient.

HYPOMAGNESAEMIA

This came to light as a frequent problem with the use of cisplatin, which causes impairment of renal absorptive capacity for magnesium (Schlinsky and Anderson, 1979). The renal loss can be compensated for with an adequate diet, but in anorexic patients hypomagnaesemia could cause muscular twitching, tetany and convulsions. The condition was often compounded by hypocalcaemia. Macaulay *et al.* (1982) showed that the problem could effectively be eliminated by giving magnesium sulphate (3 g in 3 litres of 154 mmol saline) as part of the intravenous infusion accompanying cisplatin therapy.

SKIN

Many skin lesions have been proposed as paraneoplastic phenomena. For some, the association has not been proved, while others are so strongly associated that their recognition should be followed by a systematic search for malignancy. The subject has been well reviewed (Helm and Helm, 1979; Callen, 1985). Tables 49.2 and 49.3 summarize these different categories.

HAEMATOLOGICAL MANIFESTATIONS OF MALIGNANCY

Anaemia

Tumours commonly cause anaemia by direct blood loss from the tumour, bone marrow infiltration or tumours can be associated with an 'anaemia of chronic disorders', which is characterized by normal iron stores. Blood transfusion remains the mainstay of treatment for anaemia. However, clinical trials have shown that recombinant human erythropoietin (EPO) can reduce the degree of anaemia and the transfusion requirements in cancer patients, both on treatment with chemotherapy or not being treated, with a concomitant improvement in quality of life assessments (Thatcher, 1998; Groopman and Itri, 1999). The use of EPO has been limited because it is only effective in a proportion of cancer patients (47 per cent of those with solid tumours) and for economic considerations. This may change as better predictors of response become available and the cost of blood transfusions rises, but for now the use of EPO tends to be limited to certain subgroups of patients, including those with the chronic anaemia secondary to renal cell carcinoma or myeloma and those who cannot receive blood transfusions, such as Jehovah's Witnesses.

Red cell aplasia is reported with thymomas and a variety of other malignancies (Jacobs *et al.*, 1959; Guthrie and Thornton, 1983). Megaloblastic anaemias are associated with cytotoxic chemotherapy in the absence of

Table 49.2 *Cutaneous conditions frequently associated with malignancy*

Condition	Description	Associated malignancy
Acanthosis nigricans	Pigmented hyperkeratosis in skin folds	Gastric and other GI carcinomas
Weber–Christian disease	Crops of tender, erythematous subcutaneous areas of fat necrosis	Pancreatic carcinoma
Gardner's syndrome	Epidermal and sebaceous cysts, dermoid tumours, lipomas, fibromas	Colonic carcinoma and polyposis (hereditary)
Tylosis	Hyperkeratosis of palms and soles after age of 10	Oesophageal cancer (hereditary)
Necrolytic migratory erythema	Blistering and erosive erythema on limbs, mucositis	Glucagonoma
Erythema gyratum repens	Rapidly changing gyri	Breast, lung
Paget's disease of nipple	Keratotic erythematous patch on or near nipple	Breast
Bowen's disease	Non-elevated, scaly squamous carcinoma	Internal malignancy
Hypertrichosis lanuginosa (malignant down)	Rapidly growing long hair on ears, forehead and other parts	Internal malignancy
Dermatomyositis	Purplish erythema of face and hands	Various malignancies
Fanconi's anaemia	Patchy hyperpigmentation	Leukaemia (hereditary)
Chediak–Higashi syndrome	Recurrent pyoderma dilution of skin and hair colour	Lymphoma (hereditary)

Table 49.3 *Cutaneous conditions occasionally associated with malignancy*

Condition	Associated malignancy
Generalized melanosis	Melanoma or chronic liver disease
Pigmentation of Addison's disease	Infiltration of adrenals
Striae of Cushing's syndrome	Ectopic ACTH, adrenal tumours
Porphyria cutanea tarda	Liver tumours
Dermatitis herpetiformis	Lymphomas and others
Flushing	Carcinoid tumours
Herpes zoster	Lymphomas, immunosuppressive therapy
Multiple seborrhoeic keratoses	Lymphomas, gastrointestinal tumours
Exfoliative dermatitis	Lymphomas
Hirsutism	Adrenal tumours
Pruritis	Lymphoma and others
Peutz–Jeghers syndrome (pigmentation of lips, face, oral mucosa and digits) (hereditary)	Gastrointestinal
Neurofibromatosis	Phaeochromocytoma

vitamin B_{12} deficiency. When folate deficiency is shown in patients with cancer, it is customary not to treat it for fear that folate will permit more rapid tumour growth. Autoimmune haemolytic anaemias are associated particularly with B-cell lymphomas but occur with many other malignancies and occasionally with cytotoxic drugs. When caused by tumour, they are usually refractory to treatment with corticosteroids but tend to resolve if the tumour is successfully treated.

Venous thrombosis

The high incidence of venous thrombosis in cancer was recognized by Trousseau in the nineteenth century (Rickles and Edwards, 1983). Prophylactic anticoagulation has generally not been given because of concern about haemorrhage, but a study of low-dose warfarin (starting dose 1 mg daily), in which international normalized ratio (INR) was maintained at 1.3–1.9 after the first 6 weeks, showed a relative risk reduction of 85 per cent by comparison with placebo-treated controls (Levine *et al.*, 1994). The cause of thromboembolism may not be evident but disseminated intravascular coagulation (DIC) is often implicated.

MICROANGIOPATHIC HAEMOLYTIC ANAEMIA

This comprises a diverse group of coagulopathies, including thrombocytopenic thrombotic purpura, haemolytic–uraemic syndrome and chemotherapy-induced microangiopathic haemolytic anaemia. The triggering event may differ but the common pathological pathway is endothelial damage with the formation of thrombin and end-organ damage, particularly renal, through thrombosis. Fragmented erythrocytes (schistocytes) are an invariable finding. Supportive therapy is the mainstay of treatment (Gordon and Kwaan, 1999). Plasmapheresis may be helpful, although dialysis may still be required.

DISSEMINATED INTRAVASCULAR COAGULATION

DIC is characterized by widespread coagulation resulting in end-organ failure by thrombosis, and simultaneously the resultant thrombocytopenia and coagulopathy can result in severe bleeding (Levi and ten Cate, 1999).

There is no single diagnostic test for DIC. Clinically it can be diagnosed by a low or falling platelet count, coagulopathy and presence of fibrin degradation products. DIC is associated with a wide variety of conditions, including septicaemia. Laboratory features of the condition without clinical manifestations may occur in up to 15 per cent of patients with cancer (Rickles and Edwards, 1983). The cause of DIC in malignancy has not been clearly defined but is thought to be due to the expression of tissue factor on the tumour cells. Management depends upon treatment of the underlying malignancy and supportive therapy for the complications. Theoretically, interruption of the coagulation pathway should stop further thrombin deposition and end-organ damage, and patients with overt thromboembolic phenomenon should probably be treated with heparin (Sack *et al.*, 1977), although trial data are lacking. Other active treatments, such as anti-thrombin III and tissue factor inhibitors, are still the subject of clinical trials.

THROMBOCYTHAEMIA WITHOUT DISSEMINATED INTRAVASCULAR COAGULATION, GRANULOCYTHAEMIA, EOSINOPHILIA, POLYCYTHAEMIA

Thrombocythaemia without DIC, granulocythaemia, eosinophilia or polycythaemia are all associated with malignancy or various types. So, too, are an idiopathic thrombocytopenia-like syndrome, granulocytopenia and red cell aplasia.

INFECTION

Patients with cancer are immunocompromised, either directly due to the disease or indirectly from treatment, and the basis for the increased risk and examples of the results are listed in Table 49.4. Infections are common in this population and the most common manifestation is fever, although fever can be absent in the profoundly immunosuppressed or as a result of drugs such as steroids. Fever in such patients can also have non-infectious causes and, unfortunately, there is no pattern of fever which is pathognomonic of infections. The most important decisions regarding fever in the immunocompromised patient are the urgency of evaluation and empirical antibiotic therapy. For example, patients who are neutropenic from chemotherapy require urgent evaluation. The majority of patients (60 per cent) will not have an identifiable focus of infection, and while there are no definitive guidelines, the likely organisms can be identified from the type, degree and duration of immunosuppression as well as other factors, such as the presence of indwelling intravenous access catheters. For most chemotherapy regimens the period of neutropenia lasts less than 1 week, and bacteria are the most common organism, with coagulase-negative staphylococci as the leading cause of acute

Table 49.4 *Factors predisposing to infection*

Impairment of mechanical barriers to infection
Epithelial surface breached by:
  Tumour infiltration
  Chemotherapy, e.g. oral ulceration
  Radiotherapy
  Surgery
  Intravenous catheters
Consequences:
  Bacterial or fungal infections with endogenous
    organisms, e.g. systemic infection with bowel
    organisms including anaerobes; *Staphylococcus
    epidermidis* in venous access catheters

Granulocyte/macrophage phagocytosis
Reduced cell counts by:
  Tumour infiltration of bone marrow
  Chemotherapy
  Radiotherapy
Impaired phagocytic function by:
  Reduced opsonization after splenectomy
  Reduced phagocytosis, chemotaxis and bactericidal
    activity in haematological malignancies
Consequences:
  Bacterial or fungal infections with endogenous or
    exogenous organisms, e.g. Gram-negative
    septicaemia, aspergillus and candida infections

T- and B-cell-mediated immunity
Reduced in:
  Lymphoid malignancies
  Advanced malignancy of other types
  Cytotoxic chemotherapy
  Radiotherapy
  Corticosteroid therapy
  Malnutrition
Consequences:
  Bacterial, fungal, viral and protozoal infections,
    e.g. pyogenic bacterial, cryptococcus, herpes
    simplex, varicella zoster, cytomegalovirus,
    toxoplasma, pneumocystis

Exceptional exposure to pathogenic organisms
Resistant organisms in hospitals
Change in endogenous flora after antibiotic therapy
Cross-infection from other patients
Consequences:
  e.g. infection with resistant staphylococci,
    pseudomembranous colitis, spread of
    varicella and enteric infections

bacterial infections in this population. The increasing use of indwelling intravenous access catheters may be partly responsible for the dominance of coagulase-negative staphylococci. Patients with bone-marrow transplants in the immediate post-transplant period have the same risk profile, but in the late post-transplant period (more than 100 days) become more susceptible to encapsulated bacteria such as *Streptococcus pneumoniae*. Treatment regimens must be dependent upon an institution's own guidelines, but, in general, broad-spectrum antibiotic therapy with intravenous combination antibiotics or monotherapy with third-generation cephalosporins, such as ceftazidime, is started while awaiting the results of the septic screen. There is also evidence that in selected patients treatment with oral antibiotics on an outpatient basis may be safe (Finberg and Talcott, 1999).

The use of recombinant human granulocyte colony stimulating factor (G-CSF) has become routine in oncology where there is proven benefit in prophylaxis to prevent neutropenic sepsis (American Society of Clinical Oncology, 1996). During an episode of neutropenic sepsis there is evidence that G-CSF may shorten the duration of the neutropenic episode, but there is no evidence that there is any clinical benefit (Hartmann et al., 1997). However, in a severely ill neutropenic patient administration of G-CSF remains common clinical practice, although there is a lack of clinical trial data to support this, largely due to difficulties in conducting trials in these situations.

Description of the presentation and treatment of the many different types and manifestations of infections in patients with cancer is beyond the scope of this text. The reader is referred to specific reviews (Rosenberg and Brown, 1993; Pizzo, 1999).

PAIN

Pain is commonly associated with terminal cancer and is one of the most feared symptoms. Pain can be controlled in the vast majority of patients and patients should be reassured that they will be rendered pain-free. Patients may also have fears about taking morphine and should be reassured that they will not become addicted or that taking morphine necessarily heralds imminent death. It should be remembered that often effective treatment of the tumour by chemotherapy, radiotherapy or surgery gives the best pain relief, and therefore morphine may be a temporary measure. It is beyond the scope of this review to discuss pain management and readers are referred to reviews (Portenoy, 1995; Ahmedzai, 1997). Pain management is now often a subspeciality undertaken by anaesthetics or palliative care medicine, and further referral should made if the pain control is not adequate.

CONCLUSIONS

The medical manifestations of cancer have a fascinating diversity and include many syndromes which are more or less exclusive to patients with cancer. Recognition of the condition calls for considerable clinical acumen in patients who may have a range of other symptoms directly attributable to the malignancy. Our understanding of these conditions is increasing at the cellular and molecular level, and will doubtless lead to better therapies that will improve the symptoms and save the lives of patients through appropriate diagnosis and treatment.

SIGNIFICANT POINTS

- Cancer is a multisystem disease.
- Medical aspects of care contribute significantly to quality of life.
- Medical aspects of care contribute significantly to the prospects of giving effective anti-tumour therapy.

KEY REFERENCES

Body, J.J., Bartl, R., Burckhardt, P. et al. (1998) Current use of bisphosphonates in oncology: International Bone and Cancer Study Group. J. Clin. Oncol. 16, 3890–9.

Bunn, P.A. and Ridgway, E.C. (1993) Paraneoplastic syndromes. In DeVita, V.T., Hellman, S. and Rosenberg, S.A. (eds), Cancer: principles and practice of oncology (4th edn). Philadelphia: Lippincott, 2026–71.

Pizzo, P.A. (1999) Current concepts: fever in immunocompromised patients. N. Engl. J. Med. 341, 893–900.

Vecht, C.J. (1998) Clinical management of brain metastasis. J. Neurol. 245, 127–31.

REFERENCES

Ahmedzai, S. (1997) Current strategies for pain control. Ann. Oncol. 8 (suppl. 3), S21–24.

American Society of Clinical Oncology (1996) Update of recommendations for the use of hematopoietic colony-stimulating factors: evidence-based, clinical practice guidelines. J. Clin. Oncol. 14, 1957–60.

Athanassiou, A., Begent, R.H.J., Newlands, E.S. et al. (1983) Central nervous system metastases of choriocarcinoma: 23 years experience at Charing Cross Hospital. Cancer 52, 1728–35.

Batist, G. and Andrews, J.L. (1981). Pulmonary toxicity of antineoplastic drugs. JAMA 246, 1449–53.

Becker, H.D., Wagner, B., Lierman, D. et al. (1995) Stenting of the central airways. In Liermann, D.D. (ed.), Stents – State of the art and future developments. Boston: Boston Scientific Corporation, 249–55.

Begent, R.H.J. and Rustin, G.J.S. (1989) Tumour markers: from carcinoembryonic antigen to products of hybridoma technology. Cancer Surv. 8, 107–21.

Body, J.J. (1999) The syndrome of anorexia–cachexia. *Curr. Opin. Oncol.* **11**, 255–60.

Body, J.J., Bartl, R., Burckhardt, P. *et al.* (1998) Current use of bisphosphonates in oncology: International Bone and Cancer Study Group. *J. Clin. Oncol.* **16**, 3890–9.

Bown, S.G. (1998) New techniques in laser therapy. *BMJ* **316**, 754–7.

Bunn, P.A. and Minna, J.D. (1985) Paraneoplastic syndromes. In DeVita, D.T., Hellman, S. and Rosenberg, S.A. (eds), *Cancer: principles and practice of oncology* (2nd edn). Philadelphia: J.B. Lippincott, 1811–16.

Bunn, P.A. and Ridgway, E.C. (1993) Paraneoplastic syndromes. In DeVita, V.T., Hellman, S. and Rosenberg, S.A. (eds), *Cancer: principles and practice of oncology* (4th edn). Philadelphia: Lippincott, 2026–71.

Callen, J.P. (1985) Cutaneous complications of cancer. In Calabresi, P., Schein, P. and Rosenberg, S.A. (eds), *Medical oncology. Basic principles and clinical management.* New York: Macmillan, 223–34.

Campagnutta, E., Cannizzaro, R., Gallo, A. *et al.* (1996) Palliative treatment of upper intestinal obstruction by gynecological malignancy: the usefulness of percutaneous endoscopic gastrostomy. *Gynecol. Oncol.* **62**, 103–5.

Coleman, R.E. (1998) How can we improve the treatment of bone metastases further? *Curr. Opin. Oncol.* **10**(suppl. 1), S7–13.

Crawford, S.M., Ledermann, J.A., Turkie, W. *et al.* (1986) Is production of ectopic human chorionic gonadotrophin (hCG) and alpha fetoprotein (AFP) by tumours a marker of chemosensitivity? *Eur. J. Cancer Clin. Oncol.* **22**, 1483–7.

Crittenden, D.R. and Akerman, G.L. (1977) Hyperuricaemia acute renal failure in disseminated carcinoma. *Arch. Intern. Med.* **137**, 97–9.

Davenport, D., Ferree, C. and Blake, D. (1978) Radiation therapy in the treatment of superior vena cava obstruction. *Cancer* **42**, 2600–3.

DeFronzo, R.A. and Thier, S.O. (1980) A pathophysiologic approach to hyponatraemia. *Arch. Intern. Med.* **147**, 897–902.

Engelhardt, D. and Weber, M.M. (1994) Therapy of Cushing's syndrome with steroid biosynthesis inhibitors. *J. Steroid Biochem. Mol. Biol.* **49**, 261–7.

Ewer, M.S. and Benjamin, R.S. (1996) Cardiotoxicity of chemotherapeutic drugs. In Perry, M.C. (ed.), *The chemotherapy source book* (2nd edn). Baltimore: Williams and Wilkins, 649–64.

Fallon, B., Olney, L. and Culp, D.A. (1980) Nephrostomy in cancer patients: to do or not to do. *Br. J. Urol.* **52**, 237–42.

Feuer, D.J. and Broadley, K.E. (1999) Systematic review and meta-analysis of corticosteroids for the resolution of malignant bowel obstruction in advanced gynaecological and gastrointestinal cancers. *Ann. Oncol.* **10**, 1035–41.

Finberg, R.W. and Talcott, J.A. (1999) Fever and neutropenia – How to use a new treatment strategy. *N. Engl. J. Med.* **341**, 362–3.

Forrest, J.N., Cox, M., Hong, C. *et al.* (1978) Superiority of demeclocycline over lithium in treatment of chronic syndrome of inappropriate secretion of antidiurectic hormone. *N. Engl. J. Med.* **298**, 173–7.

Friedman, H.M., Sheetz, S., Levine, H.L. *et al.* (1986) Combination chemotherapy and radiotherapy: the medical management of epidural spinal cord compression. *Arch. Intern. Med.* **146**, 509–12.

Fugh-Berman, A. (1997) *Alternative medicine: what works.* Baltimore: Lippincott Williams and Wilkins.

Gentilni, P., La Villa, G., Casini-Raggi, V. *et al.* (1999) Hepatorenal syndrome and its treatment today. *Eur. J. Gastroent. Hepatol.* **11**, 1061–5.

Gilbert, R.W., Kim, J.H. and Posner, J.B. (1978) Epidural spinal cord compression from metastatic tumour: diagnosis and treatment. *Ann. Neurol.* **3**, 40–51.

Goldman, J.M., Ash, C.M., Souhami, R.L. *et al.* (1989) Spinal cord compression in small cell lung cancer: a retrospective study of 610 patients. *Br. J. Cancer* **59**, 591–3.

Gordon, L.I. and Kwaan, H.C. (1999) Thrombotic microangiopathy manifesting as thrombotic thrombocytopenic purpura/hemolytic uremic syndrome in the cancer patient. *Semin. Thromb. Hemost.* **25**, 217–21.

Greenway, B., Johnson, P.J. and Williams, R. (1982) Control of malignant ascites with spironolactone. *Br. J. Surg.* **69**, 441–2.

Groopman, J.E. and Itri, L.M. (1999) Chemotherapy-induced anemia in adults: incidence and treatment. *J. Natl Cancer Inst.* **91**, 1616–34.

Guthrie, T.H. and Thornton, R.M. (1983) Pure red cell aplasia obscured by a diagnosis of carcinoma. *South. Med. J.* **76**, 632–4.

Hankins, J.R., Satterfield, J.R., Aisner, J. *et al.* (1980) Pericardial window for malignant pericardial effusion. *Ann. Thorac. Surg.* **30**, 465.

Hartman, D.L., Gaither, J.M., Kesler, K.A. *et al.* (1993) Comparison of insufflated talc under thorascopic guidance with standard tetracycline and bleomycin pleurodesis for control of malignant of pleural effusions. *J. Thorac. Cardiovasc. Surg.* **105**, 743–7.

Hartmann, L.C., Tschetter, L.K., Habermann, T.M. *et al.* (1997) Granulocyte colony-stimulating factor in severe chemotherapy-induced afebrile neutropenia. *N. Engl. J. Med.* **336**, 1776–80.

Helm, F. and Helm, J. (1979) Cutaneous markers of internal malignancies. In Helm, F. (ed.), *Cancer dermatology.* Philadelphia: Lea and Febiger, 247–83.

Hensley, M.L., Schucter, L.M., Lindley, C. *et al.* (1999) American Society of Clinical Oncology clinical practice guidelines for the use of chemotherapy and radiotherapy protectants. *J. Clin. Oncol.* **17**, 3333–5.

Hill, M.E., Richards, M.A., Gregory, W.M. *et al.* (1993) Spinal cord compression in breast cancer: a review of 70 cases. *Br. J. Cancer* **68**, 969–73.

Ho, P.C., Talner, L.B., Parsons, C.L. and Schmidt, J.D. (1980) Percutaneous nephrostomy: experience in 107 kidneys. *Urology* **16**, 532–5.

Jacobs, E.M., Hutter, R.V.P., Pool, J.L. and Ley, A.B. (1959) Benign thymoma and selective erythroid aplasia of the bone marrow. *Cancer* **12**, 47–57.

Khoo, D., Hall, E., Motson, R. *et al.* (1994) Palliation of malignant intestinal obstruction using octreotide. *Eur. J. Cancer* **30**, 28–30.

Larson, D.E., Burton, D.D., Schroder, K.W. and DiMagno, E.P. (1987) Percutaneous endoscopic gastrostomy. *Gastroenterology* **93**, 48–52.

Latreille, J., Johnston, D., Pater, J. *et al.* (1998) Use of dexamethasone and granisetron in the control of delayed emesis for patients who receive highly emetogenic chemotherapy. National Cancer Institute of Canada Clinical Trials Group. *J. Clin. Oncol.* **16**, 1174–8.

Le Roith, D. (1999) Tumour-induced hypoglycaemia. *N. Engl. J. Med.* **341**, 757–9.

Levi, M. and ten Cate, H. (1999) Current concepts: disseminated intravascular coagulation. *N. Engl. J. Med.* **341**, 586–92.

Levine, M., Hirsh, J., Gent, M. *et al.* (1994) Double blind randomised trial of very low dose warfarin for prevention of thromboembolism in stage IV breast cancer. *Lancet* **343**, 886–9.

Light, R.W., MacGregor, M.I., Luchsinger, P.C. and Ball, W.C. (1972) Pleural effusions: the diagnostic separation of transudates and exudates. *Ann. Int. Med.* **77**, 507–13.

Lokich, J.J. (1982) The frequency and clinical biology of the ectopic ACTH syndromes of small cell carcinoma. *Cancer* **50**, 2111–14.

Lokich, J.J. and Goodman, R.L. (1975) Superior vena cava syndrome. *JAMA* **231**, 58–71.

Loprinzi, C.L., Kugler, J.W., Sloan, J.A. *et al.* (1999) Randomised comparision of megestrol acetate versus dexamethasone versus fluoxymesterone for the treatment of cancer anorexia/cachexia. *J. Clin. Oncol.* **17**, 3299–306.

Macaulay, V.M., Begent, R.H.J., Philip, M.E. and Newlands, E.S. (1982) Prophylaxis against hypomagnesaemia induced by cisplatinum combination chemotherapy. *Cancer Chemother. Pharmacol.* **9**, 179–81.

Maher, J. and Daly, P.A. (1993) Severe bleomycin lung toxicity: reversal with high dose corticosteroids. *Thorax* **48**, 92–4.

Martinez-Moragon, E., Aparicio, J., Rogado, M.C. *et al.* (1997) Pleurodesis in malignant pleural effusions: a randomised study of tetracycline versus bleomycin. *Eur. Resp. J.* **10**, 2380–3.

Moores, D.W. (1991) Malignant pleural effusion. *Semin. Oncol.* **18**(1 suppl. 2), 59–61.

Mundy, G.R., Wilkinson, R. and Heath, D.A. (1983) Comparative study of available medical therapy for hypercalcaemia of malignancy. *Am. J. Med.* **74**, 421–32.

Newlands, E.S., Begent, R.H.J., Rustin, G.J.S. *et al.* (1983) Further advances in the management of malignant teratomas of the testis and other sites. *Lancet* **i**, 948–51.

Nisula, B.C. and Taliadouros, G.S. (1980) Thyroid function in gestational trophoblastic neoplasia: evidence that the thyrotrophic activity of chorionic gonadotophin mediates the thyrotoxicosis of choriocarcinoma. *Am. J. Obstet. Gynecol.* **138**, 77.

Ottery, F.D., Walsh, D. and Strawford, A. (1998) Pharmacologic management of anorexia–cachexia. *Semin. Oncol.* **25**(suppl. 6), 35–44.

Perez, C.A., Presant, C.A. and Amburg, A.L. (1978) Management of superior vena cava syndrome. *Semin. Oncol.* **5**, 123–34.

Pizzo, P.A. (1999) Current concepts: fever in immunocompromised patients. *N. Engl. J. Med.* **341**, 893–900.

Portenoy, R.K. (1995) Pharmacologic management of cancer pain. *Semin. Oncol.* **22**(2 suppl. 3), 112–20.

Postmus, P.E. and Smit, E.F. (1999) Chemotherapy for brain metastases of lung cancer: a review. *Ann. Oncol.* **10**, 753–9.

Prakash, U.B. (1999) Advances in bronchoscopic procedures. *Chest* **116**, 1403–8.

Ralston, S.H., Alzait, A.A., Gardner, M.D. and Boyle, I.T. (1986) Treatment of cancer associated hypercalcaemia with combined diphosponate and calcitonin. *BMJ* **292**, 1549–50.

Rickles, F.R. and Edwards, R.L. (1983) Activation of blood coagulation in cancer: Trousseau's syndrome revisited. *Blood* **63**, 14–31.

Rosenberg, A.S. and Brown, A.E. (1993) Infection in the cancer patient. *Disease a Month* **39**, 505–69.

Sack, G.H., Leven, J. and Bell, W.R. (1977) Trousseau's syndrome and other manifestations of chronic disseminated coagulopathy in patients with neoplasms. *Medicine* **56**, 1–37.

Santini, V. and Giles, F.J. (1999) The potential of amifostine: from cytoprotectant to therapeutic agent. *Haematologica* **84**, 1035–42.

Schlinsky, R.L. and Anderson, T. (1979) Hypomagnesaemia and renal magnesium wasting in patients receiving cisplatin. *Ann. Intern. Med.* **90**, 929–31.

Seckl, M.J., Mulholland, P.J., Bishop, A.E. *et al.* (1999) Hypoglycaemia due to an insulin-secreting small cell carcinoma of the cervix. *N. Engl. J. Med.* **341**, 733–7.

Siegal, T. and Siegal, T. (1985) Treatment of malignancy epidural cord and cauda equina compression. *Prog. Exp. Tumor Res.* **29**, 225–34.

Siegal, T., Seligsohn, U., Aghai, E. and Modan, M. (1978) Clinical and laboratory aspects of disseminated intravascular coagulation (DIC), a study of 118 cases. *Thromb. Haemost.* **39**, 122.

Sing, B., Kim, H. and Wax, S.J. (1979) Stent versus nephrostomy: is there a choice? *J. Urol.* **121**, 268–70.

Singal, P.K. and Iliskovic, N. (1998) Current concepts: doxorubicin-induced cardiomyopathy. *N. Engl. J. Med.* **339**, 900–5.

Sorensen, J.B., Andersen, M.K. and Hansen, H.H. (1995) Syndrome of inappropriate secretion of antidiuretic hormone in malignant disease. *J. Int. Med.* **238**, 97–110.

Sorenson, S., Helweg-Larsen, S., Mouridsen, H. and Hansen, H.H. (1994) Effect of high-dose dexamethasone in carcinomatous metastatic spinal cord compression treated with radiotherapy: a randomized trial. *Eur. J. Cancer* **30A**, 22–7.

Speer, A.G., Cotton, P.B., Russell, R.C.G. *et al.* (1987) Randomised trial of endoscopic versus percutaneous stent insertion in malignant obstructive jaundice. *Lancet* **ii**, 57–62.

Strauss, A.K., Roseman, D.L. and Shapiro, T.M. (1977) Peritoneovenous shunting in the management of malignant ascites. *Arch. Surg.* **114**, 489–91.

Sundaresan, N., Galicich, J.H., Lane, J.M. *et al.* (1985) Treatment of neoplastic epidural spinal cord compression by vertebral body resection and stabilisation. *J. Neurosurg.* **63**, 676–84.

Swales, J.D. (1987) Dangers in treating hyponatraemia. *BMJ* **294**, 261–2.

Thallasionos, N. and Joplin, G.F. (1968) Phosphate treatment of hypercalcaemia due to carcinoma. *BMJ* **4**, 14–19.

Thatcher, N. (1998) Management of chemotherapy-induced anaemia. *Semin. Oncol.* **25**(3 suppl. 7), 23–6.

Turner, J.F. and Wang, K.P. (1999) Endobronchial laser therapy. *Clin. Chest Med.* **20**, 107–22.

Vecht, C.J. (1998) Clinical management of brain metastasis. *J. Neurol.* **245**, 127–31.

Voltz, R., Gultekin, H., Rosenfeld, M.R. *et al.* (1999) A serologic marker of paraneoplastic limbic and brain stem encephalitis in patients with testicular cancer. *N. Engl. J. Med.* **340**, 1788–95.

Von Hoff, D. and Layard, D. (1979) Risk factors for doxorubicin induced congestive cardiac failure. *Ann. Int. Med.* **91**, 710–17.

Warrell, R.P. (1993) Metabolic emergencies. In DeVita, V.T., Hellman, S. and Rosenberg, S.A. (eds), *Cancer: principles and practice of oncology* (4th edn). Philadelphia: Lippincott, 2128–37.

Weiss, R.B. and Muggia, F.M. (1980) Cytotoxic drug-induced pulmonary disease: update 1980. *Am. J. Med.* **68**, 259–66.

Yeo, W., Leung, S.F., Chan, A.T. and Chiu, K.W. (1996) Radiotherapy for extreme hypertrophic pulmonary osteoarthropathy associated with malignancy. *Clin. Oncol.* **8**, 195–7.

Young, R.F. (1998) Radiosurgery for the treatment of brain metastases. *Semin. Surg. Oncol.* **14**, 70–8.

Zimmerman, S.W. (1982) Glomerulopathies associated with malignant disease. In Garnick, M.B. and Rieselbach, R.E. (eds), *Cancer and the kidney*. Philadelphia: Lea and Febiger.

Zollikofer, C.L., Anonucci, F., Stuckman, G. *et al.* (1995) The use of stents in venous vessels. In Liermann, D.D. (ed.), *Stents – state of the art and future developments*. Boston: Boston Scientific Corporation, 73–8.

Zollikofer, C.L., Jost, R., Schoch, E. and Decurtins, M. (2000) Gastrointestinal stenting. *Eur. Radiol.* **10**, 329–41.

50

Anti-emetic therapy

R. KATE GREGORY AND MARY E.R. O'BRIEN

INTRODUCTION

There has been an exponential increase in the use of cytotoxic drugs to treat malignancy over recent years. Patients previously not being treated with chemotherapy are now routinely receiving cytotoxic drugs, e.g. Dukes' C carcinoma of the colon and postmenopausal women with node-negative breast cancer. Drugs are also being administered in different forms, e.g. ambulatory (infusional) chemotherapy and chemotherapy given in the community to children receiving the maintenance phase of treatment of leukaemia. An increasing number of oral agents is also available now, e.g. oral Navelbine® and 5-fluorouracil (5-FU) formulations. All of these factors are increasing both the burden and the budget on anti-emetics.

Cytotoxic drugs have a variety of side-effects, some of which are closely linked to a particular class or compound, such as cardiomyopathy with the anthracyclines and peripheral neuropathy with the vinca alkaloids. However, nausea and vomiting may be induced by virtually any cytotoxic agent and also by radiotherapy. From the patient's point of view, emesis is ranked as the worst side-effect of chemotherapy (Coates *et al.*, 1983); indeed, some patients fear vomiting so much that they are reluctant to undergo chemotherapy. Therefore, whether cytotoxic drugs are given as a curative treatment, as, for example, in lymphoma or teratoma, or as palliative treatment, control of emesis must be a priority for all involved clinicians. In addition, with the increasing availability of oral preparations of cytotoxic agents, emetic control is essential in ensuring adequate dose delivery.

NEUROPATHOPHYSIOLOGY

The neurophysiology of vomiting is a complex process that involves the co-ordination of a number of somatic and autonomic events (Table 50.1). Wang and Borison (1950) demonstrated that electrical stimulation of the mid-brain of dogs and cats produced vomiting, and they called this area the vomiting centre (VC). Although the concept of the VC has been a useful one, it may not exist as a distinct entity but as a series of separate nuclei (Davis *et al.*, 1986). There are several inputs to the VC, as illustrated in Figure 50.1.

The neuronal afferent inputs from the gut are thought to be mainly derived from the vagus nerve. This can be stimulated by the release of polypeptides such as serotonin (5-HT), substance P or cholecystokinin (CCK) from enterochromaffin cells (EC cells) in the gut mucosa (Mei, 1983). Also, the peptides released by these cells leach into the systemic circulation via the portal vein (Andrews and

Table 50.1 *Autonomic and somatic events associated with vomiting*

Autonomic	Somatic
Salivation	Licking
Tachycardia	Opening of the mouth
Pallor	Contraction of:
Relaxation of proximal stomach	intercostal muscles
Retrograde peristalsis	abdominal muscles diaphragm

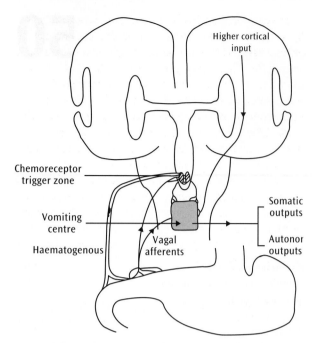

Figure 50.1 *Schematic diagram of the pathways involved in chemotherapy-induced vomiting.*

Orback, 1973) and may therefore have an indirect effect on the VC. Stretch receptors in the antrum and duodenal mucosa may also trigger vomiting: this may be particularly relevant to organic obstruction of the gut but also to chemotherapy-induced emesis because it is known that *cis*-platinum causes disordered gastric motility. Spectral analysis on electrogastric activity during a 15-second period 2 hours before reported nausea and during nausea have shown that gastric tachyarrhythmia is significantly increased during nausea, a situation analogous to that seen in motion sickness (Morrow and Morrell, 1982).

Another important input to the VC is the area postrema (AP). Ablation of this area prevents amorphine-induced emesis and, in view of this, it has been termed the chemoreceptor trigger zone (CTZ) (Borison and Wang, 1953). This is thought to be an important area for the detection of toxic substances in the blood and, therefore, it has logically been implicated in chemotherapy-induced emesis. The CTZ derives its blood supply from the vertebral artery and therefore lies outside the blood–brain barrier. However, its ependymal surface is permeable, thereby permitting the detection of toxins or chemicals in the cerebrospinal fluid. Stimulation of the gut vagal afferents increases metabolism in the CTZ, supporting a direct input from peripheral afferents to the CTZ (Andrews *et al.*, 1987).

It is thought that free-radical generation is probably the key step by which cytotoxic drugs evoke the calcium-dependent exocytic release of serotonin by enterochromaffin cells in the proximal gut (Matsuki *et al.*, 1993). Serotonin then acts locally on the 5-HT$_3$ receptors on vagal afferents or systemically on the 5-HT$_3$ receptors which have been found close to the CTZ in the nucleus tractus

solitarius (NTS). Recently there has been increasing recognition of the significance of the NTS, with the discovery that dendrites from this area invade the AP. In man cisplatin has been shown to increase 5-hydroxyindole-acetic acid (5-HIAA), which is one of the metabolites of serotonin (Cubeddu *et al.*, 1990). Vagotomy in ferrets delays, but does not prevent, *cis*-platinum emesis and therefore, although the vagal input is important, it is not the exclusive means by which emesis is induced (Andrews and Hawthorn, 1987). Indeed, clinical experience with patients receiving chemotherapy who have had vagotomy shows that they are still responsive to the noxious stimuli of cytotoxic drugs. There are also important inputs from higher cortical centres, which may be particularly relevant to anticipatory vomiting, and there are other inputs from the vestibular apparatus.

Within the area postrema and the VC there are a number of potential transmitters, receptors and degrading enzymes. Dopamine, 5-HT, noradrenaline, vasoactive intestinal polypeptide (VIP), [Leu]- and [Met]enkephalins have been identified, along with other polypeptides. Traditionally, anti-emetic therapy has been directed against the dopamine receptors, using dopamine antagonists, but the 5-HT$_3$ receptor antagonists are now firmly established in the prevention of cytotoxin-induced emesis. However, even when the emetic response is blocked with 5-HT$_3$ receptor antagonists, activation still occurs in some brainstem regions, especially the AP, possibly accounting for some of the other deleterious effects of cytotoxics, e.g. nausea and reduced appetite (Andrews *et al.*, 1998). Nausea is usually associated with vomiting, but relatively little is known about the neurophysiology because it has been extremely difficult to investigate in animal models.

In view of the complex nature of the pathways we have described for the induction of vomiting, it is clear that there are many possible mechanisms by which cytotoxic drugs may promote emesis. Inhibition of degrading enzymes in the medulla (Harris, 1982) or in the gastrointestinal tract is one possibility. Enzyme inhibition would possibly account for the delay, usually 4–8 hours, between the administration of chemotherapy and the onset of vomiting. Damage to the gastrointestinal tract may also lead to the release of a variety of hormones and peptides, which could then act locally or centrally. We have shown significant ultrastructural changes to the small bowel enterocyte following chemotherapy (Cunningham *et al.*, 1985b). The vestibular apparatus may also be relevant to cytotoxic drug-induced emesis (Money and Cheung, 1983) and, certainly, it is known that changes in posture may precipitate emesis in patients who have had *cis*-platinum. The mechanism of delayed emesis is poorly understood and it is possible that different pathways and receptors are involved. Selective non-peptide antagonists for the NK1 (neurokinin-1) receptor have the ability to prevent emesis associated with a wide variety of emetic stimuli. It has been postulated that these drugs block responses to peripheral and central stimuli and antagonize substance

P at the NTS, and, because of this, it is thought that the stimulation of the NK1 receptor may be central to the phenomenon of delayed emesis (Watson *et al.*, 1995). In reality, it is obvious that candidate mechanisms are not mutually exclusive and may interact with each other, providing several different lines of defence against naturally occurring ingested and blood-borne toxins, and, in the same way, protect against the effects of cytotoxic drugs.

CLINICAL FEATURES

The acute phase of vomiting usually develops within 4–8 hours of the administration of chemotherapy. The range of severity of these symptoms is extremely variable and is related to a number of factors. These include the dose and number of cytotoxic drugs, the reaction to previous chemotherapy and also the premorbid personality of the patient. Anxious, introverted individuals tend to experience more severe symptoms.

Patients with large, compared to minimal, tumour burden also appear to have more acute and delayed nausea (Hursti *et al.*, 1996). The authors defined large tumour burden as >2 cm, and found that these patients were more likely to have delayed nausea on days 2–7 and more acute nausea. The effect of tumour burden on nausea seemed to be more marked in patients over the age of 55.

However, the most important factor is the cytotoxic drug that is used; in Table 50.2 the degree of emetogenicity of commonly used cytotoxic drugs is shown. The acute phase of vomiting may persist for 12–24 hours, at which

Table 50.2 *Emetogenicity of chemotherapy agents in current use*

High emetic risk	Low emetic risk
Cisplatin	Bleomycin
Actinomycin D	Busulphan
Carboplatin	Chlorambucil
Carmustine (BCNU)	Fludarabine
Cyclophosphamide	Flurouracil
Cytarabine	Melphalan
Dacarbazine (DTIC)	Methotrexate
Daunorubicin	Thioguanine
Doxorubicin	Vinblastine
Epirubicin	Vincristine
Idarubicin	Vinorelbine
Ifosfamide	
Streptozocin	
Intermediate emetic risk	
Docetaxel	
Etoposide	
Gemcitibine	
Irinotecan	
Mitomycin C	
Mitozantrone	
Paclitaxel	

stage symptoms gradually resolve. This may be followed by a more chronic phase, where the patient experiences nausea with only occasional episodes of vomiting, symptoms which may persist for as long as 14 days, even after chemotherapy regimens without cisplatinum (Cunningham *et al.*, 1987a). Delayed emesis has also been reported in relation to *cis*-platinum treatment (Kris *et al.*, 1985). It is characterized by complete control of emesis during the first 24-hour period but if anti-emetic therapy is not continued, up to 80 per cent of patients will develop nausea or vomiting during the following 4 days. In view of these findings, anti-emetic treatment is given for 3–5 days after chemotherapy, but the problem of delayed emesis remains, with 50 per cent of patients experiencing prolonged nausea and vomiting despite prophylactic anti-emetics.

ANTICIPATORY NAUSEA AND VOMITING

Anticipatory nausea and vomiting may develop in up to 26 per cent of patients receiving chemotherapy (Devlen *et al.*, 1987). It is analogous to the Pavlovian conditioned reflex in that nausea and vomiting is precipitated by an event or events associated with the administration of chemotherapy in patients who have had chemotherapy-induced emesis in the past. For example, the smell of the hospital or the sight of a needle may be sufficent to trigger vomiting. Anxiolytic therapy with lorazepam has been useful in some cases and, in addition, the semi-synthetic cannabinoid, nabilone, may also be beneficial because of its anxiolytic properties. Relaxation therapy may also be helpful and has been used with some success (Lyles *et al.*, 1982). Anticipatory nausea and vomiting is extremely difficult to treat effectively and illustrates the importance of acheiving good control of emesis in the first place.

ANTI-EMETICS

5-Hydroxytryptamine M-receptor (5-HT$_3$) antagonists

These compounds have revolutionized the management of cytotoxic-induced emesis. They are most commonly used in combination with corticosteroids (*see* below) for the prevention of acute emesis.

Metoclopramide, a dopamine antagonist (*see* below), is an effective anti-emetic at a high dose but a poor anti-emetic at lower doses. At low dose it is a potent dopamine antagonist and therefore it was not entirely clear why escalating the dose improved its anti-emetic efficacy. However, at high dose metoclopramide antagonizes the 5-HT$_3$ receptor (Fozard and Mobarok, 1978), therefore suggesting that this is the mechanism by which it is anti-emetic. In animal models, 5-HT$_3$-receptor antagonists have successfully controlled the nausea and vomiting induced by cytotoxic drugs (Miner and Sanger, 1986). Furthermore, in a pilot study of GR28032F (Glaxo Group Research Ltd., Ware, UK), a 5-HT$_3$-receptor antagonist, it proved possible to completely control emesis in 14/15 patients who were receiving chemotherapy that had produced emesis refractory to conventional anti-nauseant treatment, such as dexamethasone or domperidone (Cunningham et al., 1987b).

Three randomized controlled trials have been compared ondansetron to high-dose metoclopramide in patients receiving cisplatin doses of >50 mg/m^2. Ondansetron was superior in the control of emesis and had fewer side-effects (De Mulder et al., 1990; Marty et al., 1990; Hainsworth et al., 1991).

In moderately emetogenic regimens, only one of four randomized studies comparing ondansetron to other anti-emetics has shown a significant improvement in complete control of emesis (Bonneterre et al., 1990; Kaasa et al., 1990; Jones et al., 1991; Marschner et al., 1991). Ondansetron was equal to dexamethasone both in the control of acute and delayed emesis, with no difference in the number of adverse events. Ondansetron was superior to placebo and superior to the other anti-emetics in the control of emesis induced by hemi-body radiotherapy, suggesting that serotonin and its receptors may also have a role in this form of emesis (Scarantino et al., 1992).

Granisetron (BRL 43694A) – a pure 5-HT$_3$ antagonist – has been compared to high-dose metoclopramide and dexamethasone in patients receiving high-dose cisplatin, and showed equal efficacy. In patients receiving moderately emetogenic chemotherapy, granisetron was superior to chlorpromazine in combination with dexamethasone – complete control 70 per cent versus 50 per cent, respectively, $P < 0.001$ (Chevallier, 1993). Tropisetron (ICS 205-930) – a weak antagonist at the 5-HT$_4$ receptor, like ondansetron – has been compared to dexamethasone and high-dose metoclopramide. Among patients who received tropisetron, 34 per cent experienced no emesis, compared to 53 per cent who received the standard therapy, $P = 0.04$ (Kris and Tyson, 1993). These latter 5-HT$_3$ receptor antagonists have a half-life 2–3 times that for ondansetron, conferring the advantage of less frequent dosing. However, in the majority of studies, superior efficacy with these newer agents has not been demonstrated (Martoni et al., 1998; Roila et al., 1997; Gregory and Ettinger, 1998).

The most recent addition to the group is itasetron, an oral agent with a potency 10 times that of ondansetron in animal models of chemotherapy-induced emesis. In a multi-centred double blind study, oral ondansetron controlled emesis in only 65 per cent of patients, compared to control in 88 per cent of patients receiving >1 mg of itasetron (Goldschmidt et al., 1997). The newer drugs have similar side-effects of sedation to ondansetron, albeit in a small percentage of patients: headaches can occur in about 14 per cent of patients, constipation in 4 per cent and raised liver enzymes have been described – extrapyramidal reaction (EPR) side-effects do not occur.

Various groups have looked at different ways of administering these agents to try to maximize their anti-emetic potential. One study investigated the role of a continuous infusion of granisetron or ondansetron following high-dose chemotherapy. No advantage was found to this regime, and no difference between the granisetron or ondansetron arm (Kalaycio et al., 1998). The oral route of administration appears to confer comparable control to the i.v. route. In a study of patients receiving moderately anti-emetic chemotherapy, oral ondansetron gave emetic control in 72.9 per cent of patients compared to 76.6 per cent with i.v. granisetron (Park et al., 1997). Ondansetron is also available in suppository form; in a randomized study of patients receiving cyclophosphamide-based chemotherapy, the suppository form proved equivalent to the oral formulation in the control of nausea (73 per cent versus 81 per cent) (Davidson et al., 1997).

Three double-blind trials have addressed the issue of ondansetron in delayed emesis. Ondansetron was better than placebo in the control of vomiting, but equal in the control of nausea (Gandara, 1991); it was equal to metoclopramide in the control of vomiting but inferior in the control of nausea (De Mulder et al., 1990) and no better than dexamethasone in another study (Jones et al., 1991). While the 5-HT$_3$ receptor antagonists are very effective in treating emesis in the first 24 hours following chemotherapy, they appear to be less effective in the treatment of delayed emesis.

Corticosteroids

The glucocorticoids are established as effective anti-emetics against cytotoxic drugs and are considered to be the most useful of any agent in the prevention of delayed emesis. It has been postulated that anti-emesis is achieved by stabilization of lysosomal membranes, which thereby reduces serum prostaglandins. This is highly speculative and as yet unconfirmed. Methylprednisolone (Rich et al., 1980) and dexamethasone are equally effective against a broad spectrum of cytotoxic drugs. In randomized trials, dexamethasone has been shown to be superior to prochlorperazine, domperidone and intermediate-dose metoclopramide in controlling acute emesis (Markman et al., 1984; Cunningham et al., 1987a).

There is still no fixed regimen for the administration of dexamethasone, many regimens being effective. A single-blind study has addressed this question specifically; dexamethasone was given intravenously, starting at 8 mg and increasing by 8 mg increments to 40 mg. Prochloperazine was given with each cycle. In 17/22 patients there was no apparent improvement from doses of dexamethasone above 8 mg, while for 5/22 patients a dose of more than 8 mg was optimal, suggesting that some patients can be rescued by a higher dose (Drapkin et al., 1982). A recent randomized study demonstrated improved efficacy without worsened side-effects with dexamethasone (in addition to a 5-HT₃ antagonist) given at 20 mg compared to 4 mg (Gralla *et al.*, 1999).

Control of delayed emesis has been addressed in two double-blind crossover studies. Oral dexamethasone alone was as effective as an oral dexamethasone/metoclopramide combination when assessed over a 3-week period (O'Brien *et al.*, 1989), whereas the combination of metoclopramide/ dexamethasone was superior to dexamethasone alone in another trial where patients were assessed for 4 days after chemotherapy (Kris *et al.*, 1989).

The side-effects of dexamethasone are generally reported as infrequent and relatively easy for patient and doctor to cope with. However, with increasing use of dexamethasone the complete spectrum of steroid side-effects is seen and at times is disturbing, they include insomnia, euphoria, dysphoria, dyspepsia and raised blood sugar with deterioration in diabetic control.

Dopamine antagonists

Chlorpromazine has been used widely and may be given parenterally at a dose of 25 mg intramuscularly (i.m.) every 4–6 hours. It does however, cause sedation, dryness of the mouth and extrapyramidal reactions (EPR). Using this dose schedule it will control emesis in approximately 50 per cent of patients receiving regimens without *cis*-platinum, but is not very effective against *cis*-platinum-induced emesis, and i.m. injections are unpleasant for the patient (Cunningham *et al.*, 1985c).

Another phenothiazine, prochlorperazine 5 mg three times daily orally (or 12.5 mg i.m.), is also commonly used, but is not very effective against the more emetogenic chemotherapy. The butyrophenones, haloperidol and droperidol, have similar anti-emetic potency to chlor-promazine. Optimally, droperidol should be given as an intravenous infusion of 1–1.5 mg/h over 8 hours because it has a short intravenous half-life.

Metoclopramide is a substituted benzamide which, at a conventional dose (10–20 mg three times daily orally) has limited use against cisplatin-induced emesis. At higher doses (2 mg/kg as a loading dose and then 0.4 mg/kg per hour for 8–12 hours) metoclopramide has useful anti-emetic efficacy against a variety of cytotoxic drugs, includ-ing *cis*-platinum (Gralla *et al.*, 1981; Cunningham *et al.*, 1985c). Using either intermittent (2 mg/kg given over 15 min every 2–3 hours) or continuous intravenous infu-sion schedules (loading dose of 2 mg/kg followed by a continuous infusion of 0.4 mg/kg per hour for 8–12 hours) it is possible to completely control nausea and vomiting in 30–45 per cent of patients receiving *cis*-platinum or *cis*-platinum combinations, and in 70–80 per cent of patients receiving regimens without *cis*-platinum. The usual side-effects associated with high-dose metoclopramide are sedation (60 per cent), diarrhoea (15–30 per cent) and EPR, which may develop in up to 20 per cent of patients (Cunningham *et al.*, 1988). EPRs are more likely to occur

in patients under the age of 30 and are seen in up to 30 per cent of children. Diphenhydramine (30 mg i.v.), procyclidine (5 mg i.v.) or benzatropine (1 mg i.v.) may be given prophylactically to prevent EPR. Once established, EPR can be terminated by using the above drugs.

Domperidone is a benzimadazole derivative which has poor penetration of the blood–brain barrier and, because of this, is associated with a lower incidence of EPR than metoclopramide. Given orally at a dose of 20 mg three times daily, it is useful for prevention of emesis induced by chemotherapy regimens, including those containing *cis*-platinum, and is also available in suppository form which may be useful for controlling established vomiting. It is not available for intravenous use because of reports of cardiac dysrhythmias with this route of administration.

Less used routinely in the management of cytotoxin-induced emesis is the dopamine-2 antagonist, metho-trimeprazine (levomepromazine). This is a sedative, antipsychotic phenothiazine with 5-HT antagonist actions. In a study of 113 patients who were refractory to other anti-emetics and receiving a variety of cytotoxics, includ-ing cisplatin, 62 per cent were fully protected from nausea and vomiting and a further 34 per cent showed consider-able improvement in their symptoms (Higi *et al.*, 1980). Methotrimeprazine can be administered orally or by subcutaneous infusion (e.g. in patients with obstruction) and may have a role to play in the management of patients not controlled on standard regimens.

Cannabinoids

9-Tetra-hydrocannabinol (THC), which is derived from the Indian hemp plant, was investigated as an anti-emetic subsequent to anecdotal reports that the smoking of mari-juana protected against cytotoxic drug-induced emesis. It is undoubtedly useful in preventing cytotoxin-induced emesis (Sallan *et al.*, 1980) but the best anti-emetic control is only experienced in those patients who develop a 'high' on treatment. Side-effects include sedation, hypotension and dizziness, although the drug's anxiolytic properties may be useful. Because of the problems of oral absorption with THC and its abuse potential, a semi-synthetic can-nabinoid, nabilone, was developed which is less likely to promote hypotension or tachycardia. However, it still pro-duces euphoria or dysphoria in approximately 30 per cent of patients. When it is combined with prochlorperazine the incidence of adverse effects on the CNS is reduced sig-nificantly, by a mechanism which has yet to be elucidated (Cunningham *et al.*, 1985a). Because the cannabinoids and nabilone are lipid soluble, they have a long biological half-life and therefore repeated oral dosing leads to accu-mulation of the drug. Therefore, a maximum of three doses of nabilone is recommended. Using a combination of nabilone 1 mg twice daily, given at the same time as prochlorperazine 5 mg twice daily, nausea and vomiting were completely controlled in 80 per cent of patients receiving chemotherapy regimens without *cis*-platinum (Cunningham *et al.*, 1985a). However, it is not a very effective treatment against *cis*-platinum-induced emesis, although it has been successful in controlling carboplatin-induced emesis (Cunningham *et al.*, 1988).

Lorazepam

Lorazepam has proved a useful addition to the more conventional anti-emetic drugs (*see* above), particularly in patients where anticipatory nausea is a problem (Maher, 1981). In one randomized trial, it was shown to have similar anti-emetic efficacy to high-dose metoclopramide (Bowcock *et al.*, 1984). However, the major drawback is drowsiness, and virtually all patients experience some degree of somnolence on therapy. Patients also develop amnesia for the period during which they receive chemotherapy and this may occasionally be helpful, particularly for those patients who have anticipatory vomiting. Sedation generally means that the agent is not useful for outpatient administration. It can be given as a slow intravenous injection of 1–2 mg/m^2 prior to chemotherapy, or orally at a dose of 1–2 mg 2 hours before chemotherapy. An alternative, which we have found useful in our practice, is to administer the dose sublingually for more rapid onset of action.

Cyclizine

Cyclizine is a histamine H$_1$-receptor antagonist of the piperazine class. The exact mechanism by which it can prevent or reduce nausea and vomiting is unknown. However, it acts to increase lower oesophageal tone and decrease the sensitivity of the labyrinthine apparatus (Wood *et al.*, 1979). Cyclizine can be given i.v., i.m. or orally at a dose of 50 mg three times daily or as a s.c. or i.v. infusion at a rate of 75–150 mg over 24 hours. Oral cyclizine was found to be only marginally effective in controlling nausea and vomiting following radiotherapy (Rowlands and Currie, 1976), and comparable to placebo in treating nausea and vomiting due to chemotherapy (Williams *et al.*, 1980). From the literature cyclizine appears, therefore, to be relatively inactive in the prevention of emesis, but we have found it to be an effective anti-emetic in the management of patients not controlled by standard anti-emetic regimens.

Neurokinin-1 (NK1) receptor antagonists

Selective non-peptide antagonists for the NK1 receptor have the ability to block the retching and vomiting response to a wide variety of emetic stimuli, including cisplatin, radiotherapy, apomorphine and motion. It has been postulated that these drugs block responses to peripheral and central stimuli, antagonize substance P at the NTS and, because of this, may have a role in the prevention of delayed emesis (Watson *et al.*, 1995). The NK1

receptor antagonists are now in clinical trial. In a double-blind randomized study of patients receiving cisplatin chemotherapy for a variety of solid tumours, the NK1 receptor antagonist L-758,298 showed anti-emetic activity almost equal to that of ondansetron in acute emesis, and superior activity in the control of delayed emesis (Van Belle *et al.*, 1998). The potential for control of delayed emesis raises the possibility of using this new class of drugs in combination. A recent study investigated the potential role of the NK1 antagonist CJ-11,974 in combination with granisetron and dexamethasone in patients receiving cisplatin. In group 1 (G1) patients received granisetron, dexamethasone and the NK1 antagonist; patients in group 2 (G2) received granisetron and dexamethasone only. The emesis rates on day 1 were 85.7 per cent (G1) and 63.3 per cent (G2); the emesis rates for days 2–5 were 67.8 per cent (G1) and 36.1 per cent (G2), $P = 0.04$. The authors concluded that the NK1 antagonist CJ-11,974 may have a role to play in improving the prevention of acute and delayed emesis after cisplatin (Hesketh *et al.*, 1998).

PHARMACO-ECONOMICS

Cost and effectiveness are important issues in any treatment evaluation. In the treatment of emesis this is of relevance in the prescription of the 5-HT$_3$ receptor antagonists and newer agents under development, as most of the other anti-emetics are of low cost. However, with the increasing use of cytotoxic drugs the total quantity of anti-emetics being used is increasing and this obviously has cost implications. In the economic evaluation of the comparison of two drug regimens where outcome is equal then the preparation, administration, duration of hospital stay, nursing and medical time and the consequences of failed first-line treatment, in addition to the actual cost of the drug, must be considered.

Ondansetron has been compared to high-dose metoclopramide and costed over a 24-hour period. The higher drug price was compensated by its superior efficacy and associated lower administration costs, to give an overall difference of £3 – ondansetron £95.20, metoclopramide £92.20 (Cunningham *et al.*, 1993). Adding dexamethasone to both drugs in another comparative study showed that the combination of ondansetron and dexamethasone was superior to metoclopramide, dexamethasone and lorazepam in terms of control of emesis (93 per cent versus 76 per cent) and, in addition, for drugs alone the ondansetron/dexamethasone combination was cheaper (£16.25 versus £17.35) because of the added expense of rescue medication in patients who failed treatment (Sands *et al.*, 1992).

Another more recent study costed ondansetron versus other anti-emetic regimens. The authors found no cost differences between the drug regimens but there was a significant reduction of emesis management costs overall in the group who had received ondansetron (Stewart *et al.*, 1999).

COMBINATIONS OF ANTI-EMETICS

In clinical practice, combinations of anti-emetics with different modes of action are now commonly used. For inpatient regimens, such as those that include *cis*-platinum,

Table 50.3 *Anti-emetic schedules suitable for patients receiving chemotherapy regimens without* cis-*platinum on an outpatient basis*

Drug	Dose schedule
Dexamethasone	8 mg i.v. with chemotherapy, then 4 mg orally three times daily for 3 days +
Metoclopramide	20 mg four times daily for 3 days
For patients who vomit despite the above:	
Granisetron	3 mg i.v. with chemotherapy +
Dexamethasone	8 mg i.v. with chemotherapy, then 4 mg orally three times daily for 3 days +
Cyclizine	50 mg three times daily orally for 3 days +
Lorazepam	1–2 mg sublingual, orally or i.v. pre-chemotherapy (particularly if anticipatory nausea a problem)

Table 50.4 *Anti-emetic schedules suitable for patients receiving* cis-*platinum-based chemotherapy*

Drug	Dose schedule
Granisetron	3 mg i.v. with chemotherapy +
Dexamethasone	8 mg i.v. with chemotherapy, then 4 mg orally three times daily for 3 days +
Metoclopramide	20 mg four times daily for 3 days
For patients who vomit despite the above:	
Granisetron	3 mg i.v. with chemotherapy, then 3 mg i.v. 12 hours post chemotherapy; consider 1 mg orally twice daily for 3 days +
Dexamethasone	8 mg i.v. with chemotherapy, then 4 mg orally three times daily for 3 days +
Cyclizine	50 mg three times daily i.v. while an inpatient, then orally for 3 days +
Lorazepam	1–2 mg sublingual, orally or i.v. pre-chemotherapy (particularly if anticipatory nausea is a problem)
For patients continuing to vomit, consider:	
Cyclizine	75–150 mg subcutaneously over 24 hours or
Haloperidol	1–3 mg subcutaneously over 24 hours

an intravenous anti-emetic treatment is clearly appropriate, but for outpatient regimens oral treatments are more satisfactory. Outlines of recommended regimens are given in Tables 50.3 and 50.4.

The combination of dexamethasone and high-dose metoclopramide is better than either agent alone in the control of acute emesis in patients receiving high-dose *cis*-platinum (Allan *et al.*, 1984; O'Brien *et al.*, 1989). The addition of diphendramine to this combination minimizes the risks of EPRs. The anti-emetic effects of ondansetron can be potentiated by the addition of dexamethasone (Roila *et al.*, 1991; Smith *et al.*, 1991; Smyth *et al.*, 1991) and this combination has now been compared to the standard regimen (Roila *et al.*, 1992). Complete control of emesis was acheived in 79 per cent (ondansetron and dexamethasone) and 60 per cent (high-dose metoclopramide, dexamethasone, diphenhydramine) of patients on day 1 after chemotherapy. The ondansetron/dexamethasone combination continued to give superior control of delayed emesis on days 2 and 3 when compared to high-dose metoclopramide, dexamethasone and diphenhydramine. However, these combinations appear to lose their efficacy over multiple cycles of chemotherapy, with one study reporting control in 66 per cent of patients in the first course reducing to 30 per cent in later courses (De Wit *et al.*, 1996).

SIGNIFICANT POINTS

- The pathophysiology of emesis is incompletely understood and each drug may have a different promotion pathway.
- The most important factor is the emetogenic potential of the cytotoxic drug.
- Acute emesis is best controlled by a combination of a 5-HT$_3$ antagonist and dexamethasone.
- Dexamethasone is the single most effective agent in the control of delayed emesis, the role of 5-HT$_3$ antagonists in this setting is uncertain, but newer agents, e.g. the NK1 antagonists, may have a role to play.
- Anticipatory nausea and vomiting may develop in up to 25 per cent of patients and is very difficult to treat. Anxiolytics and cannabinoids may be helpful in this setting, but the most important factor in preventing the development of this complication is optimal control of emesis during the first cycle of treatment.

KEY REFERENCES

Andrews, P.L.R., Naylor, R.J. and Joss, R.A. (1998) Neuropharmacology of emesis and its relevance to anti-emetic therapy. *Support Care Cancer* **6**, 197–203.

Antiemetic Subcommittee of the Multinational Association of Supportive Care in Cancer (1998) Prevention of chemotherapy and radiotherapy induced emesis: results of the Perugia Consensus Conference. *Ann. Oncol.* **9**, 811–19.

Gralla, R.J., Osoba, D., Kris, M.G. *et al.* (1999) Recommendations for the use of anti-emetics: evidence-based, Clinical Practice Guidelines. *J. Clin. Oncol.* **17**(9), 2971–94.

Kris, M.G., Roila, F., De Mulder, P.H.M. *et al.* (1998) Delayed emesis following anticancer chemotherapy. *Support Care Cancer* **6**, 228–32.

REFERENCES

Allan, S.G., Cornbleet, M.A., Warrington, P.S. *et al.* (1984) Dexamethasone and high dose metoclopramide: efficacy in controlling cisplatin induced nausea and vomiting. *BMJ* **289**, 878–9.

Andrews, P.L.R. and Hawthorn, J. (1987) Evidence for an extra-abdominal site of action for the 5-HT$_3$ receptor antagonist BRL 24924 in the inhibition of radiation-evoked emesis in the ferret. *Neuropharmacology* **26**, 1367–70.

Andrews, P.L.R. and Orback, J. (1973) A study of compounds which initiate and block nerve impulses in the perfused liver. *Br. J. Pharmacol.* **49**, 192–204.

Andrews, P.L.R., Davis, C.J., Grahame-Smith, D.G. and Leslie, R.A. (1987) Increase in 3 (H)-2-deoxyglucose uptake in the ferret area postrema produced by apomorphine administration or electrical stimulation of the abdominal vagus. *J. Physiol.* **382**,188 [abstract].

Andrews, P.L.R., Naylor, R.J. and Joss, R.A. (1998) Neuropharmacology of emesis and its relevance to anti-emetic therapy. *Support Care Cancer* **6**, 197–203.

Bonneterre, J., Chevallier, B., Metz, R. *et al.* (1990) A randomised double-blind comparison of ondansetron and metoclopramide in the prophylaxis of emesis induced by cyclophosphamide, fluorouracil and doxorubicin or epirubicin chemotherapy. *J. Clin. Oncol.* **8**, 1063–9.

Borison, H.L. and Wang, S.C. (1953) Physiology and pharmacology of vomiting. *Pharmacol. Rev.* **5**, 193–230.

Bowcock, S.J., Stockdale, A.D., Bolton, J.A.R. *et al.* (1984) Antiemetic prophylaxis with high dose metoclopramide or lorazepam and vomiting induced by chemotherapy. *BMJ* **288**, 1879.

Chevallier, B. (1993) The control of acute cisplatin-induced emesis – a comparative study of granisetron and a combination regimen of high-dose metoclopramide and dexamethosone. *Br. J. Cancer* **68**, 176–80.

Coates, A., Abraham, S., Kaye, S.B. *et al.* (1983) On the receiving end-patient perception of the side-effects of cancer chemotherapy. *Eur. J. Cancer Clin. Oncol.* **19**, 203–8.

Cocquyt, V., Van-Belle, S., Reinhardt, R.R. *et al.* (2001) Comparison of L-758,298, a prodrug for the selective neurokinin-1 antagonist, L-754,030, with ondansetron for the prevention of cisplatin-induced emesis. *Eur. J. Cancer* **37**, 835–42.

Cubeddu, L.X., Hoffmann, I.S., Fuenmayor, N.T. and Finn, A.L. (1990) Efficacy of ondansetron (GR38032F) and the role of serotonin in cisplatin-induced nausea and vomiting. *N. Engl. J. Med.* **332**, 810–16.

Cunningham, D., Forrest, G.J., Soukop, M. *et al.* (1985a) Nabilone and prochlorperazine: a useful combination for emesis induced by cytotoxic drugs. *BMJ* **291**, 864–5.

Cunningham, D., Morgan, R.J., Mills, P.R. *et al.* (1985b) Functional and structural changes of the proximal small intestine after cytotoxic therapy. *J. Clin. Pathol.* **38**, 265–70.

Cunningham, D., Soukop, M., Gilchrist, N.L. *et al.* (1985c) Randomised trial of intravenous high dose metoclopramide and intramuscular chlorpromazine in controlling nausea and vomiting induced by cytotoxic drugs. *BMJ* **290**, 604–5.

Cunningham, D., Evans, C., Gazet, J.C. *et al.* (1987a) Comparison of antiemetic efficacy of domperidone, metoclopramide, and dexamethasone in patients receiving outpatient chemotherapy regimens. *BMJ* **265**, 250.

Cunningham, D., Hawthorn, J., Pople, A. *et al.* (1987b) Prevention of emesis in patients receiving cytotoxic drugs by GR38032F, a selective 5HT3 receptor antagonist. *Lancet* **I**, 1461–2.

Cunningham, D., Bradley, C.J., Forrest, G.J. *et al.* (1988) A randomised trial of oral nabilone and prochloperazine compared to intravenous metoclopramide and dexamethasone in treatment of emesis induced by chemotherapy regimens containing cisplatin analogues. *Eur. J. Cancer* **24**, 685–9.

Cunningham, D., Gore, M., Davidson, N., Miocevich, M., Manchanda, M. and Wells, N. (1993) The real costs of emesis – an economic analysis of ondansetron vs metoclopramide in controlling emesis in patients receiving chemotherapy for cancer. *Eur. J. Cancer* **29A**, 303–6.

Davidson, N.G., Paska, W., Van-Belle, S. *et al.* (1997) Ondansetron suppository: a randomised, double-blind, double-dummy, parallel group comparison with oral ondansetron for the prevention of cyclophosphamide induced emesis and nausea. *Oncology* **54**(5), 380–6.

Davis, C.J., Harding, R.K., Leslie, R.A. and Andrews, P.L.R. (1986) The organisation of vomiting as a protective reflex: a commentary on the first days discussions. In Davis, C.J., Lake-Bakaar, G.V. and Grahame-Smith, D.G. (eds), *Nausea and vomiting: mechanisms and treatment*. Berlin: Springer-Verlag, 280–7.

De Mulder, P.H.M., Seynaeve, C., Vermoken, J.B. *et al.* (1990) Ondansetron compared with high dose metoclopramide in prophylaxis of acute and delayed cisplatin-induced nausea and vomiting. A multi-centre, randomised, double-blind crossover study. *Ann. Intern. Med.* **113**, 834–40.

Devlen, J., Maguire, P., Phillips, P. *et al.* (1987) Psychological problems associated with diagnosis and treatment of lymphomas II: prospective study. *BMJ* **295**, 955–7.

De Wit, R., Berg, H., Burghouts, J. *et al.* (1996) Despite initial high anti-emetic efficacy of granisetron/dexamethasone combination for highly anti-emetogenic chemotherapy: this effect is not maintained over multiple cycles. *Proc. Ann. Meet. Am. Soc. Clin. Oncol.* **15**, A1734.

Drapkin, R.L., Sokol, G.H., Paladine, W.J. *et al.* (1982) The antiemetic effect and dose response of dexamethason in patients receiving cisplatinum. *Proc. Am. Soc. Clin. Oncol.* C236.

Fozard, J.R. and Mobarok Ali, A.T.M. (1978) Blockade of neuronal tryptamine receptors by metoclopramide. *Eur. J. Pharmacol.* **49**, 109–12.

Gandara, D.R. (1991) Progress in the control of acute and delayed emesis induced by cisplatin. *Eur. J. Cancer* **27**(suppl. 1), S9–11.

Goldschmidt, H., Salwender, H., Egerer, G. *et al.* (1997) Oral itasetron hydrochloride: a long-acting highly bioavailable alternative to ondansetron. *Proc. Am. Soc. Clin. Oncol.* **16**, A172.

Gralla, R.J., Itri, L.M., Pisko, S.E. *et al.* (1981) Antiemetic efficacy of high-dose metoclopramide: randomised trials with placebo and prochlorperazine in patients with chemotherapy-induced nausea and vomiting. *N. Engl. J. Med.* **305**, 905–9.

Gralla, R.J., Osoba, D., Kris, M.G. *et al.* (1999) Recommendations for the use of anti-emetics: evidence-based, Clinical Practice Guidelines. *J. Clin. Oncol.* **17**(9), 2971–94.

Gregroy, R.E. and Ettinger, D.S. (1998) 5HT$_3$ receptor antagonists for the prevention of chemotherapy induced nausea and vomiting. A comparison of their pharmacology and clinical efficacy. *Drugs* **55**, 173–89.

Hainsworth, J., Harvey, W., Pendergrass, K. *et al.* (1991) A single-blind antagonist, with intravenous metoclopramide in the prevention of nausea and vomiting associated with high-dose cisplatin chemotherapy. *J. Clin. Oncol.* **9**, 721–8.

Harris, A.L. (1982) Cytotoxic therapy induced vomiting is mediated via enkephalin pathways. *Lancet* **I**, 714–16.

Hesketh, P.J., Gralla, R.J., Webb, R.T. *et al.* (1998) Randomised phase II trial of the neurokinin-1 antagonist CJ-11,974 for the control of cisplatin-induced emesis. *Proc. Am. Soc. Clin. Oncol.* **17**, A199.

Higi, M., Niederle, N., Bierbaum, W. *et al.* (1980) Pronounced antiemetic activity of the antipsychotic drug levomepromacine in patients receiving cancer chemotherapy. *J. Cancer Res. Clin. Oncol.* **97**(1), 81–6.

Hursti, T.J., Avall-Lundqvist, E., Borjeson, S. *et al.* (1996) Impact of tumour burden on chemotherapy induced nausea and vomiting. *Br. J. Cancer* **74**(7), 1114–19.

Jones, A.L., Hill, A.S., Soukop, M. *et al.* (1991) Comparison of dexamethasone in the prophylaxis of emesis induced by moderately emetogenic chemotherapy. *Lancet* **388**, 483–7.

Kaasa, S., Kvaloy, S., Dicato, M.A. *et al.* (1990) A comparison of ondansetron with metoclopramide in the prophylaxis of chemotherapy-induced nausea and vomiting: a randomised, double-blind study. *Eur. J. Cancer* **26**, 311–14.

Kalaycio, M., Mendez, Z., Pahiman, B. *et al.* (1998) Continuous infusion granisetron compared to ondansetron for the prevention of nausea and vomiting after high dose chemotherapy. *J. Cancer Res. Clin. Oncol.* **124/5**, 265–9.

Kris, M.G. and Tyson, L.B. (1993) Tropisetron ICS (205-930): a selective 5-hydroxytryptamine antagonist. *Eur. J. Cancer* **29A**(suppl. 1), S30–32.

Kris, M.G., Gralla, R.J., Clark, R.A. *et al.* (1985) Incidence, course and severity of delayed nausea and vomiting following the administration of high dose cisplatin. *J. Clin. Oncol.* **3**, 1379–83.

Kris, M.G., Gralla, R.J., Tyson, L.B. *et al.* (1989) Controlling delayed vomiting: double-blind, randomised trial comparing placebo, dexamethasone alone and metoclopramide plus dexamethasone in patients receiving cisplatin. *J. Clin. Oncol.* **7**, 108.

Lyles, J.N., Burish, T.G., Krozely, M.G. and Oldham, R.K. (1982) Efficacy of relaxation training and guided imagery in reducing the aversiveness of cancer chemotherapy. *J. Cons. Clin. Psychol.* **50**, 509–24.

Maher, J. (1981) Intravenous lorazepam to prevent nausea and vomiting associated with cancer chemotherapy. *Lancet* **I**, 91–2.

Markman, M., Sheilder, V., Ettinger, D.S. *et al.* (1984) Antiemetic efficacy of dexamethasone. Randomised, double-blind, crossover study with prochloperazine in patients receiving cancer chemotherapy. *N. Engl. J. Med.* **311**, 549–52.

Marschner, N.W., Adler, M., Nagel, G.A. *et al.* (1991) Doule-blind randomised trial of the antiemetic efficacy and safety of ondansetron and metoclopramide in advanced breast cancer patients treated with epirubicinand cyclophosphamide. *Eur. J. Cancer* **27**, 1137–40.

Martoni, A., Angelli, L.B., Gvaraldi, L.M. *et al.* (1998) An open randomised cross-over study on granisetron versus ondansetron in the prevention of acute emesis induced by moderate dose cisplatin containing regimens. *Eur. J. Cancer Part A* **32**, 82–5.

Marty, M., Pouillart, P., Scholl, S. *et al.* (1990) Comparison of the 5-hydroxytryptamine (serotonin) antagonist ondansetron (GR38032F) with high-dose metoclopramide in the control of cisplatin-induced emesis. *N. Engl. J. Med.* **322**, 816–21.

Matsuki, N., Torri, Y., Saito, H. *et al.* (1993) Effects of iron and desferrioxamine on cisplatin-induced emesis: further evidence for the role of free radicals. *Eur. J. Pharmacol.* **248**, 329–31.

Mei, N. (1983) Sensory structures in the viscera. In Ottoson, D. (ed.), *Sensory physiology*, vol. 4. New York: Springer-Verlag, 1–42.

Miner, W.D. and Sanger, G.J. (1986) Inhibition of cisplatin induced vomiting by selective 5-hydroxytryptamine M-receptor antagonism. *Br. J. Pharmacol.* **88**, 497–9.

Money, K.E. and Cheung, B.S. (1983) Another function of the inner ear: facilitation of the emetic response to poisons. *Aviation Space Environ. Med.* **22**, 1476–80.

Morrow, G.R. and Morrell, C. (1982) Behavioural treatment for the anticipatory nausea and vomiting induced by cancer chemotherapy. *N. Engl. J. Med.* **307**, 1476–80.

O'Brien, M.E.R., Cullen, M.H., Woodroffe, C. *et al.* (1989) The role of metoclopramide in acute and delayed chemotherapy induced emesis: a randomised double blind trial. *Br. J. Cancer* **60**, 759–63.

Park, J.O., Rha, S.Y., Yoo, N.C. *et al.* (1997) A comparitive study of IV granisetron versus IV and oral ondansetron in the prevention of nausea and vomiting associated with moderately emetogenic chemotherapy. *Am. J. Clin. Oncol.* **20**, 569–72.

Rich, W.M., Yoglu, G.U. and DiSala, P.J. (1980) Methylprednisolone as an antiemetic during cancer chemotherapy – a pilot study. *Gynecol. Oncol.* **9**, 193–8.

Roila, F., Tonato, M., Cognetti, F. *et al.* (1991) Prevention of cisplatin-induced emesis: a double-blind multicentre randomised cross-over study comparing ondansetron and ondansetron plus dexamethasone. *J. Clin. Oncol.* **9**, 675–8.

Roila, F., Tonato, M., Favalli, G. *et al.* (1992) A multicentre double-blind study comparing the antiemetic efficacy and safety of ondansetron plus dexamethasone vs metoclopramide plus DEX and diphenhydramine in cisplatin treated cancer patients. *Proc. Am. Soc. Clin. Oncol.* **11**, 394.

Roila, F., Ballatoil, E., Tonata, M. *et al.* (1997) 5HT₃ receptor antagonists, differences and similarities. *Eur. J. Cancer* **33**(a), 1364–70.

Rowlands, G. and Currie, C.J. (1976) A trial of valoid tablets in the control of nausea and vomiting associated with radiotherapy. *Br. J. Clin. Pract.* **30**,197–9.

Sallan, S.E., Zinberg, N.E. and Frei, E. (1980) Antiemetic effect of delta-9-tetrahydrocannabinol and prochlorperazine. *N. Engl. J. Med.* **302**, 135–8.

Sands, R., Roberts, J.T., Marsh, M. *et al.* (1992) Low dose ondansetron and dexamethasone; a cost effective alternative to high dose metoclopramide/ dexamethasone/lorazepam in the prevention of acute cisplatin induced emesis. *Clin. Oncol. Lett.* **4**(1), 67.

Scaratino, C.W., Ornitz, R.D., Hoffman, L.G. *et al.* (1992) Radiation induced emesis: effects of ondansetron. *Semin. Oncol.* **19**(suppl. 15), 38–43.

Smith, D.B., Newlands, E.S., Rustin, G.J.S. *et al.* (1991) Comparison of ondansetron and ondansetron plus dexamethasone as antiemetic prophylaxis during cisplatin-containing chemotherapy. *Lancet* **388**, 487–90.

Smyth, J.F., Coleman, R.E., Nicholson, N. *et al.* (1991) Does dexamethasone enhance control of acute cisplatin induced emesis by ondansetron? *BMJ* **303**, 1423–6.

Stewart, D.J., Dahrouge, S., Coyle, D. and Evans, W.K. (1999) Costs of treating and preventing nausea and vomiting in patients receiving chemotherapy. *J. Clin. Oncol.* **17**(1), 344–51.

Wang, S.C. and Borison, H.L. (1950) The vomiting centre. *Arch. Neurol. Psychiat.* **63**, 928–41.

Watson, J.W., Gonsalves, S.F., Fossa, A.A. *et al.* (1995) The anti-emetic effects of CP-99,994 in the ferret and the dog: the role of the NK1 receptor. *Br. J. Pharmacol.* **115**, 84–94.

Williams, C.J., Bolton, A., De Pemberton, R. *et al.* (1980) Anti-emetics for patients treated with anti-tumour chemotherapy. *Cancer Clin. Trials* **3**, 363–7.

Wood, C.D. (1979) Antimotion sickness and anti-emetic drugs. *Drugs* **17**, 471–9.

51

Brachytherapy

J. ROGER OWEN

HISTORICAL INTRODUCTION

The story of brachytherapy begins in 1898 when Marie and Pierre Curie, working in their laboratory in Paris, succeeded in isolating radium from pitchblende. Within a few years Robert Abbe, an American surgeon, had used radium, with an afterloading technique, to treat cancer. The first English-language textbook of radium therapy, by Wickham and Degrais, was published in 1910.

Between the end of the First World War and the early 1930s, the major developmental work was carried out in Paris. Basic implantation techniques and clinical indications were defined. Clinical studies in patients with cervix cancer led to an optimization of the radiation dose and dose rate.

A little later, a major development took place in England where painstakingly careful measurement of exposure rates in air, at certain distances from radiation sources, by Meredith in the early 1930s led to the development of the 'Manchester system' (Paterson and Parker, 1934). This didactic set of rules rid brachytherapy of empiricism and permitted implants to be performed according to a pre-determined plan. The importance of this system, which became universally accepted, cannot be overemphasized. For the first time it set limits within which an implant would be safe, but outside of which the risks to the patient were too high. This principle holds true today with other more modern systems, such as the 'Paris system'.

The advent of megavoltage machinery resulted in a decline in brachytherapy during the 1950s and 1960s. However, the development of artificial radioactive isotopes brought new possibilities. Afterloading was developed using smaller, flexible sources. In Europe it was again the Parisians who took a leading role, particularly at the Institut Gustav Roussy where Bernard Pierquin, following his father and godfather before him, Andrée Dutreix and Daniel Chassagne, opened new possibilities for brachytherapy, using iridium-192 wire with afterloading techniques (Pierquin *et al.*, 1964).

These methods, and the accompanying Paris system of dosimetry, form the basis for this chapter, which will deal only with low-dose-rate implants.

GENERAL CONSIDERATIONS

There are two essential characteristics of interstitial brachytherapy, the first of which is probably the more important:

1 Physical: by placing the radioactive sources directly into the tumour-bearing tissue, very high and localized doses are achieved. The rapid fall-off of dose with distance ensures that surrounding normal tissues are relatively spared and that the irradiated volume is precisely tailored to the tumour-bearing tissues.
2 Biological: low, continuous dose-rate treatment and short overall treatment time. Radical doses can be given over a few days only.

Brachytherapy techniques tend to be time-consuming and therefore relatively costly when compared with a short course of external irradiation. Their use in palliation is therefore seldom justified. The primary indication is the radical treatment of relatively small, well-circumscribed tumours in accessible sites. Radical doses may be given by the implant alone, or the implant may be used to boost the dose locally after external irradiation. Evidence is accumulating, although not from randomized clinical trials, that the chances of cure are highest when the total dose is given by the implant. The mean dose within an implanted volume may be in the region of twice the dose prescribed to the reference isodose. Thus, a radical implant delivering 60 Gy to the treatment isodose could result in a mean tumour dose of 120 Gy or more. In comparison, an implant boost of 25 Gy after 50 Gy external irradiation to the same tumour leads to an estimated total tumour dose of only 100 Gy (with no allowance for the different dose rates).

In cases where a tumour is fairly large and there is a significant risk of subclinical lymph-node metastases, external irradiation may be given first, in sufficient doses to give a high chance of sterilizing these small-volume tumour deposits. In general, the volume of tissue implanted to give the 'boost' in these circumstances is substantially the same volume as would have been implanted had no external irradiation been given. However, the implant dose is lower, thus reducing the risk of normal tissue necrosis, but at the same time risking a reduced chance of local cure.

Another way of maximizing the benefits of brachytherapy is to perform a perioperative implant. Thus, the bulk of the tumour is removed surgically and the excision margins can be implanted under direct vision.

Although high doses can be given by implantation techniques, there is inevitably a rapid fall-off and cases where the tumour margin is poorly defined or very irregular may not be suitable because of the risk of underdosing the tumour edge. Very large-volume implants are poorly tolerated and also there will be significantly higher doses in the central part of the volume compared to the periphery.

Some normal tissues have a poor tolerance of implantation (e.g. bone and skin at pressure points or of the lower leg). The risk of normal tissue necrosis at such sites may be high. Inevitably some tumour sites are poorly accessible and geometrically satisfactory implants in these regions are difficult to achieve.

RADIATION SAFETY

Each radiotherapist engaged in brachytherapy must develop, with his physicists and radiographers, a system of safe practice to minimize the chances of preventable errors.

Monitoring the patient

A system for checking the position and number of sources at regular intervals during the implant must be established and a record sheet maintained by nursing staff.

Loading and unloading the implant

1 Implants should only be loaded or unloaded by experienced trained staff – it is not a job for an inexperienced or unsupervised junior doctor.
2 Loading and unloading must take place under strictly controlled conditions. The following are essential:
   (a) a relaxed, pain-free patient;
   (b) the operator should not be working alone as he/she would be unable to leave the patient to call for help if necessary;
   (c) some local anaesthetic and catgut on a round-bodied needle should be immediately available in case of haemorrhage that does not respond to pressure (rare);
   (d) a good light and the correct equipment;
   (e) as far as possible these procedures should be timed to occur during normal working hours;
   (f) radiation monitoring of the patient and room after removal of sources to ensure that no source, or part of a source, is left in the patient or protected room.

DOSIMETRY

The dose received at a point in the vicinity of a brachytherapy source diminishes rapidly with distance. This is because of the inverse square law, which dominates the dosimetry of interstitial therapy. A dosimetry system is similar in principle to the 'Highway Code', which does not tell you how to drive a car, but does set boundaries beyond which it is unsafe to stray. Similarly, dosimetry systems set the parameters within which it is safe to work, where the risks of causing necrosis due to very high doses, or of tumour recurrence as a result of underdosing, are minimized. All dosimetry systems consist of two parts: (1) the rules of implantation; and (2) the method of calculating the time the sources must remain in place to deliver the prescribed dose to the intended volume of tissue.

Table 51.1 *Physical properties of iridium-192*

Production	^{191}Ir (n·γ) → ^{192}Ir
Half-life of ^{192}Ir	74 days
Decay	16 gamma-ray energies, 4 with an abundance of greater than 10%
	Weighted mean energy = 0.370 MeV
Iridium-192 wire	Iridium/platinum alloy in platinum sheath
	Overall diameter = 0.3 mm for wire; 0.5 or 0.6 mm for 'hairpins'
	A range of linear activities is available
	The wire is springy but easily bent
Protection	Half-value thickness = 3 mm lead

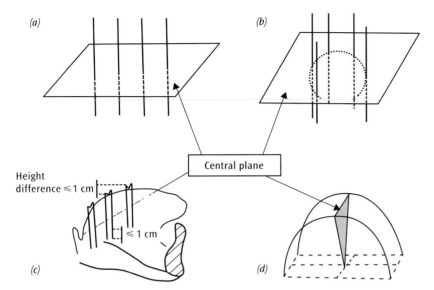

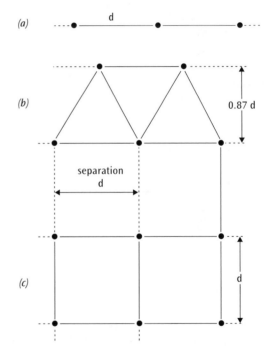

Figure 51.1 *Definition of the central plane with examples. (a) Single plane of wires, e.g. skin implant; (b) curved plane of wires, e.g. anal canal implant; (c) hairpins in tongue; (d) curved wires, e.g. soft palate implant. Adapted from Pierquin and Marinello (1992).*

Although other dosimetry systems exist, the Paris system is best adapted to interstitial brachytherapy using iridium wire (Table 51.1) (Pierquin *et al.*, 1987). This system was born of the twin needs to extend the indications of brachytherapy by using newly available miniaturized sources, but at the same time basing the dosimetry calculations on the dose at certain fixed points *within* the implanted volume. The system can be used for straight or curved wires, loops or hairpins. It is flexible and allows the separation between sources to be varied, within limits, to suit the volume being treated. Above all, the Paris system allows the brachytherapist to rapidly pre-plan his implant without needing to resort to complicated calculations or tables.

Principles of the Paris system

1 The radioactive sources must be parallel and arranged so that their centres lie in the same plane, called the 'central plane'. This plane is the perpendicular bisector of straight radioactive source wires, or passes through the centres of curved wires or the legs of hairpins and loops (Fig. 51.1).
2 The linear activity of each source wire must be uniform along its length and identical for all the sources. However, seed ribbons are permitted within the system provided the distance between adjacent seeds is equal or less than 1.5 times the active length of the seed and, similarly, a mobile stepping source is permitted as long as the steps and dwell time in each position are identical for each of the vectors.
3 The radioactive sources must be equidistant. When more than one plane of sources is required, these are positioned so that their pattern as they cross the central plane is either equilateral triangles or squares (Fig. 51.2).

Figure 51.2 *The principle of equidistance. (a) Single plane of wires; (b) wires arranged 'in triangles'; (c) wires arranged 'in squares'. Adapted from Pierquin and Marinello (1992).*

Dose specification

In the Paris system dosimetry calculations are always made in the central plane. Around each linear source wire lies a high-dose zone or sleeve; midway between adjacent sources there will lie a minimum dose-rate point (basal dose rate) and surrounding the implant as a whole there are continuous isodose lines or envelopes (Fig. 51.3).

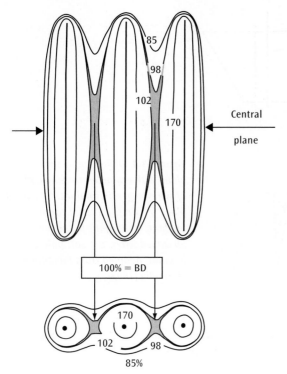

Figure 51.3 *Dose distribution in the central plane for three linear coplanar sources. BD, basal dose. Adapted from Pierquin and Marinello (1992).*

The system enables the radiotherapist to perform an implant that has the following characteristics:

1 The reference isodose line (to which the treatment prescription is applied) is a fixed percentage (85 per cent) of the basal dose rate, and its position coincides with the borders of the target volume.
2 The diameter of the high-dose sleeve around each source wire is not allowed to become too large. If it were to do so, there would be an unacceptable risk of necrosis.

By these means, the tumour receives the intended dose but, at the same time, the risk of necrosis is controlled.

Definitions

- The *central plane* is the plane at right angles to the plane of the wires and passes through their mid points. In practice, the mid points of each wire seldom lie exactly in one plane and a mean central plane is used (Fig. 51.4).
- *Basal dose rate* within the implant: between the sources are points where the dose rate is minimal. These are elementary minimal dose rates. The basal dose rate of the implant is the arithmetic mean of these individual dose rates, which should not vary from the mean by >10 per cent. Examples of basal dose rates are shown in Figures 51.5 and 51.6.

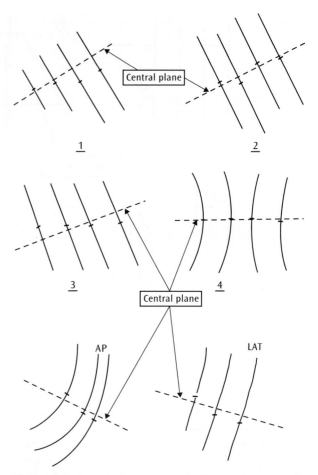

Figure 51.4 *Central plane – examples from radiographs of implants.*

- *Reference isodose:* the prescribed dose is applied to the reference isodose line, which is defined as 85 per cent of the mean basal dose rate, thus inextricably linking the prescribed dose to the minimal doses in the interior of the implant.
- *Tumour volume* is that volume known to be occupied by tumour and it may be estimated by direct measurement or radiography.
- *Target volume* is the known tumour volume with a surrounding margin of tissue, which may contain tumour cells at the microscopic level.
- *Treated volume* is that volume encompassed by the reference isodose. This can be defined by its thickness, length and width. An appreciation of these parameters and their relation to the positions of the sources is the central concept of the Paris system. Figures 51.7–51.11 show how the thickness treated, length treated and width treated are defined.
- *Thickness treated* (T) is the average thickness of tissue encompassed by the reference isodose (Figs 51.7, 51.9–51.11).
- *Length treated* (L) is the average length of tissue covered by the reference isodose, midway between wires for single-plane and midway between the planes for multi-plane implants (Figs 51.9 and 51.10).

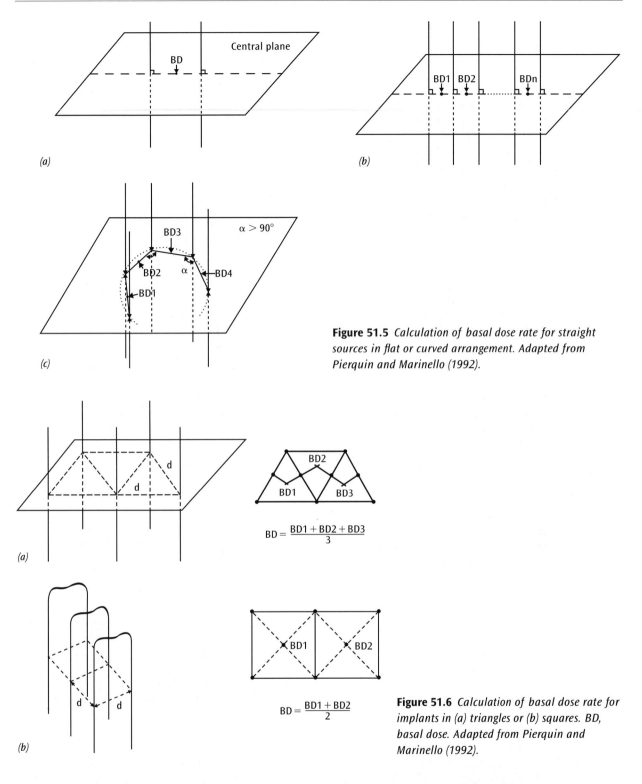

Figure 51.5 *Calculation of basal dose rate for straight sources in flat or curved arrangement. Adapted from Pierquin and Marinello (1992).*

$$BD = \frac{BD1 + BD2 + BD3}{3}$$

$$BD = \frac{BD1 + BD2}{2}$$

Figure 51.6 *Calculation of basal dose rate for implants in (a) triangles or (b) squares. BD, basal dose. Adapted from Pierquin and Marinello (1992).*

- *High-dose volume* is the volume around each source wire that is encompassed by the isodose that is twice the reference isodose, i.e. 170 per cent of the basal dose rate (Figs 51.7–51.10).
- *Lateral safety margin* is the distance, measured in the central plane of the implant and midway between the planes of wires for multi-plane implants, from the outmost source wire to the position of the reference isodose (Figs 51.7, 51.9 and 51.10).

How to find the central plane

As the Paris system allows the sources to be of different lengths, this gives rise to some difficulties in finding the central plane. In practice, a mean central plane is normally used. Figure 51.4 gives some examples.

For hairpins, the central plane is that plane passing through the mid points or the straight 'legs' of each hairpin (Fig. 51.6). Similarly, loops have to be divided into a curved bridge piece and straight legs, and the central plane passes through the mid points of the legs. A loop must correspond to certain criteria before it can be used for volume implants (Fig. 51.12).

Although the central plane is ideally perpendicular to the wires, situations arise when this is not the case, e.g. when hairpins are placed in the tongue and there is a difference in their heights (Fig. 51.1). The plane used to reconstruct the implant and for dosimetry must not be more than 10° beyond the perpendicular, or the reconstruction will make it appear that the hairpins are significantly further apart than they are in reality and the patient will be overdosed as a result.

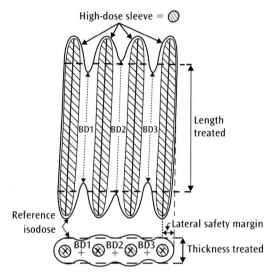

Figure 51.7 *Definition of the volume treated and the high-dose sleeve for implants of several co-planar lines. BD, basal dose. Adapted from Pierquin and Marinello (1992).*

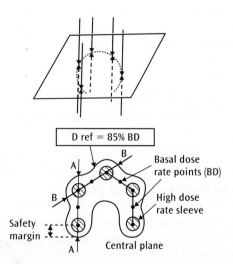

Figure 51.8 *Definition of treated volume and high-dose sleeve for straight sources arranged around a curve. BD, basal dose. Adapted from Pierquin and Marinello (1992).*

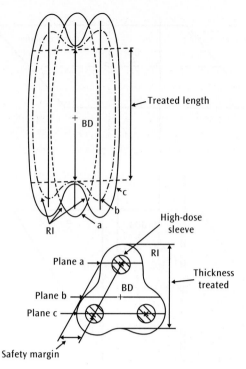

Figure 51.9 *Definition of dimensions of volume treated and high-dose sleeve for implantation of triangles. BD, basal dose; RI, reference isodose. Adapted from Pierquin and Marinello (1992).*

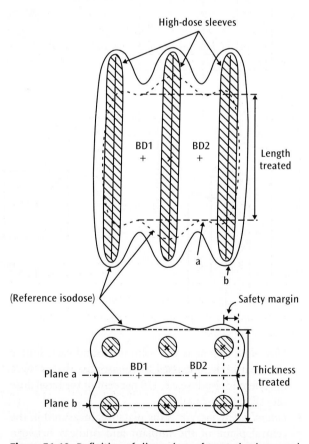

Figure 51.10 *Definition of dimensions of treated volume and high-dose sleeves in cases of implantation in squares. BD, basal dose. Adapted from Pierquin and Marinello (1992).*

Relation between source positions and reference isodose

In the Paris system the prescribed dose is applied to the reference isodose, which has a fixed relationship to the average basal dose rate within the radioactive set-up. In their turn, the basal dose rates depend upon the distances between each source and the basal dose rate points, the linear activity of the sources and the radioisotope used.

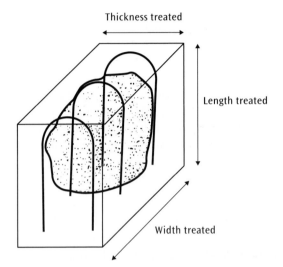

Figure 51.11 *Definition of dimensions of treated volume in the case of hairpins or loops. The 'thickness' is the dimension parallel to the bridge of the loop. Adapted from Pierquin and Marinello (1992).*

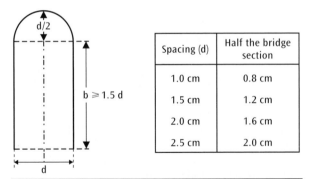

Spacing (d)	Half the bridge section
1.0 cm	0.8 cm
1.5 cm	1.2 cm
2.0 cm	1.6 cm
2.5 cm	2.0 cm

Half the active length = half the bridge section + length of one leg (b)

Figure 51.12 *Conditions that need to be satisfied for a loop to be used for a 'volume implant'. Adapted from Pierquin and Marinello (1992).*

Thus, given ^{192}Ir wire of uniform activity, there are easily definable relationships between the wire positions and the treated volume, as described by the reference isodose. These are summarized in Table 51.2.

Relationship between source positions and high-dose volume

Figure 51.13 shows that, as the distance between adjacent source wires increases, the diameter of each sleeve of high dose around the sources also becomes progressively greater; the relationship is non-linear. Clinical experience over 30 years has led to the understanding that, when this high-dose sleeve is more than 8 mm in diameter, there is a significantly higher risk of necrosis. The graph shows that this critical point is reached at a separation of 22 mm for wires of 10 cm length but at about 20 mm for 5 cm wires. For wires of less than 5 cm length it is reached when their separation is 15–16 mm.

Practical constraints on the wire separation

Just as the excess risk of necrosis occurring when wires are placed far apart limits their maximum spacing, so there are limitations that govern how close the sources may be placed. These are partly practical and partly dosimetric. First, it is, in practice, very difficult to achieve a good geometry when implanting many wires very close together. Secondly, if the wires are too near, then minor deviations from parallelism will produce major variations in dose. Table 51.3 shows the practical safe ranges for wire separation.

PRE-PLANNING AN IMPLANT

Faced with a patient whose tumour is suitable for implantation, the brachytherapist must pre-plan how the desired dose distribution will be achieved and which implant technique will be used.

Steps in achieving a correct dose distribution

1 Careful clinical evaluation of the tumour volume.
2 Evaluation of the desired tumour margin around the tumour that is to be treated to the prescribed dose,

Table 51.2 *Relationships between wire positions and treated volume (adapted from Pierquin and Marinello, 1992)*

Arrangement	Treated length/ active length	Thickness treated/ separation	Lateral safety margin separation	Safety margin/ separation
2 lines	0.7	0.5	0.37	–
'n' lines in one plane	0.7	0.6	0.33	–
'n' lines in squares	0.7	1.55–1.60	–	0.27
'n' lines in triangles	0.7	1.3	–	0.20

i.e. the target volume. Measurement of the thickness, width and length of this target volume.

3 Determination of the number of planes to be used. Using the information in Tables 51.2 and 51.3, it is clear that, with a maximum safe separation of source wires of 20 mm, the maximum thickness of tissue that can be irradiated by a single plane implant is

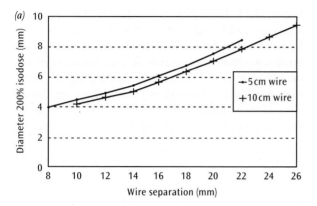

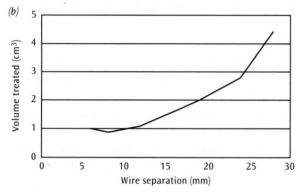

Figure 51.13 (a) Diameter of 200% isodose around central wires (four-wire, single-plane implant); (b) volume enclosed by 170% for four wires 5 cm long at different separations.

Table 51.3 Minimum and maximum source spacing

	Source spacing	
Source length (cm)	Minimum (cm)	Maximum (cm)
Short (1–4)	0.8	1.5
Long (10+)	1.5	2.2

$20 \times 0.6 = 12$ mm. Target volumes thicker than 12 mm require two or more planes of wires.

4 If a multi-plane implant is to be used, a decision must be made whether to implant the sources 'in triangles' or 'in squares'. This is determined by the shape of the target volume and also by the tumour site.

5 With the aid of the ratio of thickness treated to source separation (Table 51.2) corresponding to the source arrangement chosen, determination of the minimal separation to adhere to and the number of sources needed.

6 Calculation of the length of each wire by multiplying the target volume length by 1.4 and multiplying this length by the number of wires to obtain the total amount of wire needed.

Thus, by relatively simple calculations the brachytherapist now knows the position and length of each wire which, when implanted, will produce a reference isodose envelope that exactly covers the intended target volume.

Choice of implant technique

The tumour site and size will determine which technique is used.

MINIATURE PLASTIC-TUBE TECHNIQUE

The iridium wire is loaded inside plastic tubes of external diameter 0.8 mm. This technique is admirably suited to superficial tumours, particularly where the surface is irregular and there are advantages to allowing the sources to conform to the shape of the tissues, e.g. basal cell carcinoma of the nose.

HYPODERMIC NEEDLE TECHNIQUE

Simple hypodermic needles or spinal needles of diameter 0.8 mm are used as the vector. Bare iridium wire may be slid inside the needles, which then need to be blocked at both ends. Small tumours in soft parts of the body are particularly suitable, e.g. lip, ear and penile tumours. By using rigid needles the geometry of the implant is maintained.

GUIDE-NEEDLE TECHNIQUE

Needles of internal diameter 1.2 mm are used, left in the tissue and usually connected to templates to maintain

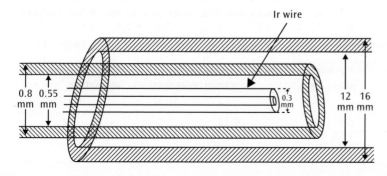

Figure 51.14 Diagram of outer and inner plastic tubes. Adapted from Pierquin et al. (1987).

the geometry. This is suitable for large tumour volumes in soft tissue, e.g. breast, anal canal.

PLASTIC-TUBE TECHNIQUE

This is the most suitable technique for larger tumours or intra-operative brachytherapy. The vector plastic tube has an external diameter of ʟ6 mm; through this is afterloaded the smaller plastic tube of 0.8 mm external diameter, which is preloaded with iridium wire (Fig. 51.14).

PLASTIC-TUBE LOOPS

The same system can be formed into loops. This has the effect of crossing one end of the implant and is particularly useful in positions where there is limited access or where it is impossible to exit the wire internally (with its necessary extra length to allow for the 'uncrossed' end), e.g. base of tongue, floor of mouth.

GUIDE GUTTER TECHNIQUE

These metal guides are commonly used for implanting smaller tumours of the tongue or tonsil. They carry wire pins, either single or double 'hairpins'. It is normal to remove the metal guide leaving bare iridium wire in the tissues. The hairpins have a fixed separation between their legs of 12 mm. This means that they can only be used to treat target volumes of 18 mm thickness or less.

Iridium wire for hairpins and single pins is manufactured in diameters of 0.5 or 0.6 mm so is stiffer than the usual wire, which is 0.3 mm external diameter.

Ordering the wire

The following steps need to be done before ordering the iridium wire:

1 Construction on graph paper of the central plane of the proposed implant.
2 Measurement of the distance between each wire and each basal dose rate point.
3 Determination of the dose rate contribution from each wire to each dose rate point. This is done by using tables or graphs of the absorbed dose rate as a function of distance, assuming wire of reference linear activity (Table 51.4).

Table 51.4 Absorbed dose rate as a function of the distance to ^{192}Ir wires of different lengths and 0.3 mm in diameter (from Pierquin et al. (1987) with permission)

Source length (cm)	Distance to the source (cm)										
	0.2	0.3	0.4	0.5	0.6	0.7	0.8	0.9	1.0	1.1	1.2
1	13.1	7.63	5.00	3.52	2.60	1.99	1.57	1.27	1.05	0.875	0.743
2	14.8	9.30	6.55	4.90	3.82	3.06	2.50	2.09	1.76	1.51	1.30
3	15.3	9.86	7.13	5.48	4.37	3.59	3.00	2.55	2.19	1.91	1.67
4	15.5	10.1	7.40	5.76	4.66	3.87	3.28	2.82	2.46	2.16	1.91
5	15.6	10.3	7.55	5.92	4.83	4.04	3.45	2.99	2.63	2.33	2.08
6	15.7	10.3	7.65	6.02	4.94	4.16	3.57	3.11	2.74	2.44	2.19
7	15.8	10.4	7.71	6.09	5.01	4.23	3.65	3.19	2.82	2.52	2.27
8	15.8	10.4	7.76	6.14	5.06	4.29	3.70	3.25	2.88	2.58	2.33
10	15.8	10.5	7.82	6.21	5.13	4.36	3.78	3.33	2.96	2.67	2.42
12	15.9	10.5	7.86	6.25	5.17	4.41	3.83	3.38	3.01	2.72	2.47
14	16.0	10.6	7.88	6.28	5.20	4.44	3.86	3.41	3.05	2.75	2.50

Source length (cm)	Distance to the source (cm)										
	1	2	3	4	5	6	7	8	10	12	15
1	1.05	0.278	0.125	0.070	0.045	0.031	0.022	0.017	0.010	0.007	0.004
2	1.76	0.523	0.242	0.138	0.088	0.061	0.044	0.033	0.020	0.013	0.008
3	2.19	0.725	0.348	0.202	0.130	0.090	0.066	0.050	0.030	0.020	0.012
4	2.46	0.882	0.441	0.260	0.170	0.118	0.087	0.066	0.040	0.026	0.016
5	2.63	1.003	0.520	0.313	0.206	0.145	0.107	0.081	0.049	0.033	0.020
6	2.74	1.096	0.587	0.360	0.240	0.170	0.126	0.096	0.059	0.039	0.023
7	2.82	1.170	0.642	0.401	0.271	0.194	0.144	0.110	0.068	0.045	0.027
8	2.88	1.228	0.689	0.437	0.299	0.215	0.161	0.124	0.076	0.051	0.031
10	2.96	1.312	0.762	0.496	0.347	0.253	0.191	0.148	0.093	0.063	0.038
12	3.01	1.368	0.814	0.542	0.385	0.285	0.218	0.170	0.108	0.074	0.045
14	3.05	1.408	0.853	0.577	0.415	0.311	0.240	0.189	0.122	0.084	0.052

Absorbed dose rate in cGy/h in water at the mid-plane of iridium-192 wires 0.3 mm in diameter with a reference linear kerma rate in air equal to 1 μGy/h/m²/cm, taking into account oblique filtration of the γ radiations by the platinum sheath and the attenuation and diffusion of the γ in the water.

4 Calculation of the average basal dose rate.

5 Calculation of reference dose rate by multiplying by 0.85.

6 Allowance for filtration of source vectors, e.g. metal needles if left *in situ* may reduce the dose rate by approximately 2 per cent.

7 Calculation of activity of wire at mid-implant by the fraction:

$$\frac{\text{required reference dose rate}}{\left(\begin{array}{c}\text{reference dose rate for}\\ \text{unit wire activity}\end{array}\right)} = \text{activity required}.$$

8 Adjustment of mid-implant wire activity to activity on the day that the iridium is calibrated and despatched by the manufacturers. This is necessary because ^{192}Ir decays with half-life of 74 days. Mid-implant activity should be increased by approximately 1 per cent/day for every day between the date the manufacturer specifies the activity and the mid-implant date.

9 Allowance for the fact that 10–20 per cent of the wire may be wasted during the process of cutting and loading into the inner plastic tubes.

10 Order for total required length of iridium wire of activity that corresponds most closely to that required.

PREPARATION OF IMPLANT PATIENTS AND MANAGEMENT OF COMPLICATIONS

General preparation

General preparation is both psychological and physical. Implant techniques are not commonly understood by the general public or even by non-specialist colleagues, so a full explanation of the process must be given to each patient. Alternative methods of treatment, where such exist, should be explained. Patients are often frightened about being isolated in a hospital room, sometimes without windows, where they cannot have visits from family or friends. Some are not prepared to give up smoking even for the short period of hospitalization. Dietary factors are important. Implants in the oral cavity prevent normal eating and the patient should be allowed to get accustomed to a liquid or semi-solid diet before admission. If the anal canal is the site of brachytherapy, then a low-residue diet needs to be started 5–6 days before the procedure is carried out.

In general, skin care is uncomplicated and no special precautions are necessary. Any patient with valvular disease of the heart requires suitable antibiotic cover to prevent the risk of subacute bacterial endocarditis.

Patients undergoing implant for tumours of the rectum or anal canal need full bowel preparation and oral constipants, e.g. codeine phosphate 60 mg three times daily, as they will be unable to defecate for 3–4 days.

Preoperative

Preoperative investigations should include chest X-ray, electrocardiogram, full blood count and clotting screen.

Premedication

Atropine (or scopolamine) is very helpful in preventing excessive viscous salivation, which can hinder an oral cavity implantation.

Operation

At the time of the operation skin cleaning with aqueous chlorhexidine is sufficient. Parenteral analgesia should be commenced towards the end of the anaesthetic and prescribed routinely for the first 12 hours or so postoperatively.

Postoperative

In the postoperative period adequate analgesia must be maintained. Reactive oedema may occur and is treatable by dexamethasone or non-steroidal anti-inflammatory drugs. Oral hygiene of a high standard needs to be maintained; patients with implants in the oral cavity may be unable to brush their teeth for 4–5 weeks overall and will need to use a mild antiseptic mouthwash several times daily.

The hospital dietician is a very important member of the team. Careful attention to the individual patient's dietary needs is essential for their general comfort and well-being. Normal hospital food is often totally unsatisfactory for these patients.

Complications

Complications can be categorized as acute, delayed and radiation safety.

ACUTE

Haemorrhage
Haemorrhage due to puncturing a vessel during the implant procedure causes concern but is seldom dangerous. The needle should be withdrawn and pressure applied. Venous bleeds stop within 1–2 min but pressure on an artery should be maintained for a full 5 min.

Oedema
Reactive oedema takes some hours to develop and may last for the majority of the implant duration. Sources may become moved apart as the tissues swell up, significantly altering the dosimetry. If this is not checked and

allowed for, the tumour may be underdosed. It is often advantageous to repeat check X-rays 24 hours after implantation.

Infection

Infection is remarkable by its absence during the acute phase. However, an acute radiation reaction may develop surface infection. Systemic antibiotics are seldom, if ever, required.

DELAYED

Fibrosis

One of the characteristics of an implant treatment is the relative lack of post-radiation fibrosis compared to external-beam radiotherapy. It is minimized by careful dosimetry, selection of the appropriate dose and dose rate, and by accurately conforming the high-dose volume to the tumour-bearing tissue.

Delayed haemorrhage

Delayed haemorrhage due to necrosis of a vessel wall is a rare complication. When it occurs the usual cause is recurrent tumour in association with the poor vascularity secondary to radiation-induced small-vessel damage. Immediate surgical management is required.

Infection

Infection is only a significant problem if it accompanies a mucosal skin or bone necrosis. Under these circumstances adequate doses of systemic antibiotics are essential, both to control pain and also to set the conditions under which the necrosis may heal.

Necrosis

A degree of normal tissue necrosis commonly occurs. If this is in the centre of an area of breast tissue, e.g., it is usually asymptomatic and undetectable. A mucosal necrosis in the oral cavity may be acutely painful, requiring some strong analgesics as well as measures to promote healing. All mucosal necroses of 1 cm or less have a good chance of healing with conservative management. The important measures are to abolish surface infection, prevent the patient from smoking and prevent the patient from drinking wines or spirits. Necroses of more than 1 cm seldom heal and should be referred for surgical management.

Bone necrosis of the mandible is a potential complication of implants to the floor of the mouth or alveolus. The risk is directly proportional to the number of wires placed within 2–3 mm of the periosteum, so careful attention to the exact placing of sources is critically important. Bone necrosis is a serious complication, which causes the patient several months of severe pain. For this reason, although small tongue tumours are optimally treated by an implant, equally small and curable floor of mouth tumours may be better dealt with by primary surgical excision. This is particularly true with the modern techniques of microvascular anastamosis

that have so improved surgery to this area. The other factor that may predispose to bone necrosis, is poor dental hygiene.

Dental care and prevention of necrosis

Prior to brachytherapy patients must be examined by an experienced dentist or stomatologist to determine the risk of developing bone exposure or full-blown osteoradionecrosis. The areas of highest risk are points of underlying bone having sharp bony exostoses or a sharp ridge covered by a thin layer of mucosa, such as the mylohyoid ridge.

Pre-treatment evaluation includes clinical and radiological assessment. A dental treatment programme should include considerations of the patient's socio-economic situation, general health status, degree of motivation and oral hygiene.

Patients who have all or most of their natural teeth present in reasonably good condition should not normally be considered for extractions. They should be motivated to raise their level of oral hygiene to prevent any further loss of teeth. In patients with teeth in poor condition or with many missing teeth several factors must be evaluated. A dentition in poor periodontal condition presents a greater risk than one with many carious lesions but with an acceptable periodontal state. Lower molars in the radiation field present a high-risk area. Any infection located in the bifurcation area is particularly difficult to eradicate.

The factors to be considered in decision making are:

1 the general condition of the mouth and teeth as well as the specific condition of each individual tooth, with particular attention to teeth that will be in the radiation field;
2 the patient's level of oral hygiene and the degree of compliance to oral hygiene measures that is to be expected;
3 mandibular teeth should be scrutinized more closely than maxillary teeth;
4 factors relating to the tumour, such as its rate of growth, the prognosis, the size of the radiation field, and the dosage and the mode of application of the radiation.

If the tumour is rapidly growing, delay for dental treatment may not be in the patient's best interest. The technical factors in the treatment determine the severity of the changes in the oral environment.

Preventative protocol If the teeth are to be maintained, a preventative protocol is started. The patient must be educated and trained to maintain excellent oral hygiene. Daily application of fluoride gel to the teeth is mandatory in order to reduce the occurrence of 'radiation caries'. The method of preference is a daily, 5-minute, self-application by the patient using a custom-made fluoride carrier. The fluoride treatment is started during the radiation therapy and is ideally continued for the rest of the patient's life. When mucositis is at its worst during treatment the use of carriers and gel may be temporarily replaced by a fluoride mouth-rinsing solution.

Special considerations in interstitial therapy Special custom-made protection devices may be made that may keep the dentition out of the radiation field, e.g. in the case of the lower lip implantation or a tongue lesion. These consist of individually made acrylic protectors embedded with lead foil. A 2 mm foil reduces the transmitted dose by 50 per cent, while the extra spacing will further reduce the dose considerably. Critical aspects in this management procedure are the vulnerable area of the mylohyoid ridge, which should be entirely covered, as well as making sure of the patient's compliance in maintaining the device in place during the treatment time. It is advisable to prepare a second acrylic protector having an identical shape but without lead shielding.

DOSE AND DOSE-RATE CONSIDERATIONS

Dose and dose rate

Empirical experiments by Regaud and his team at the Foundation Curie during the early 1920s led to standardization in the filtration of radium sources and, compromising between tumoricidal effects and normal tissue tolerance, an 'optimal' dose was established. This was described in terms of 'millicuries equivalent destroyed'. With the establishment of the Manchester system this dose became described as 7000 roëntgens (approximately 60 Gy) in 7 days at the reference isodose. Excellent results were achieved using this prescription, but inevitably clinicians sought to modify and refine their experience, mainly in an effort to reduce the long overall treatment times which were difficult for patients to tolerate.

In 1952 Paterson recommended a dose reduction for treatment times of less than 7 days (e.g. 46 Gy for a treatment time of 3 days) and a dose increase for treatment times of greater than 7 days (e.g. 62 Gy for 9 days). His model was used extensively for more than 20 years.

Pierquin *et al.* (1973), on the other hand, found no apparent effects on local control and necrosis rates when a dose of 70 Gy was given to oropharyngeal tumours with overall treatment times that varied between 3 and 8 days, (0.9–0.3 Gy/hour approximately). He advised against dose adjustment that might lead to underdosing of tumours.

During the 1970s other authors studying a variety of tumour sites confirmed that it was difficult to demonstrate a significant effect of dose rate on tumour control or necrosis rates in the clinical setting (Barklay and Fletcher, 1976; Larra *et al.*, 1977). However, in recent years several reports have appeared that have demonstrated just such effects. Larger numbers of cases treated in the same hospital by closely controlled methods and the modern statistical tools of univariate and multivariate analyses may be responsible for bringing a greater

degree of precision (Fontanesi *et al.*, 1989; Mazeron *et al.*, 1991a, b). For example, the study of Mazeron *et al.* (1991b) on T1 and T2 squamous carcinomas of the anterior two-thirds of the tongue and floor of the mouth was able to recommend a dose prescription that, in their hands, gave the optimum results as:

- dose: 65 Gy to reference isodose (Paris system)
- dose rate: 0.4–0.5 Gy/h at reference isodose
- source spacing: 12–15 mm.

Quality measures

To be able to compare one implant with another, internationally agreed rules for describing dose and volume need to be developed. Such a set of recommendations has been published by the International Commission on Radiation Units (ICRU). However, the presence of significant 'hot spots' or lack of equality in source spacing – to mention just two parameters – are quality measures that are difficult to standardize. Dose–volume histograms represent an attempt to describe implants in such a way as to enable further analysis and comparison. A dose–volume histogram which suppresses the inverse square law effects has been developed by Anderson (1986) and is called the 'natural' dose–volume histogram (DVH).

Figure 51.15 shows two such dose–volume histograms, which should demonstrate a clear peak. Greater dose uniformity is implied by higher narrower peaks. The prescribed dose rate is lower than the DVH maximum since, in this region, the volume treated by particular dose rates changes very rapidly.

Radiobiological aspects of brachytherapy

Irradiation from a source or sources implanted within a tumour has a distinct geometrical advantage as it inevitably spares the surrounding normal tissues, which receive a lower dose. The non-uniformity of radiation dose and dose rate around an implant has important radiobiological consequences. Close to the sources the dose rate is high and the degree of cell killing will be close to that indicated by the acute radiation survival curve. As you move away, however, two changes will occur. First, cells will be less sensitive at the lower dose rates and, secondly, within the given period of implantation the accumulated dose will be less. Close to sources the level of cell killing is so high that cells of any radiosensitivity will be killed. Further out, the effects will be so slight that even the most radiosensitive cells will all survive. Between these two extremes there is a critical zone where, over a very short distance, the probability of local cure will pass from nearly 100 per cent to virtually zero. Steel *et al.* (1989) described this change from high to low local cure probability as being like a cliff-face. The

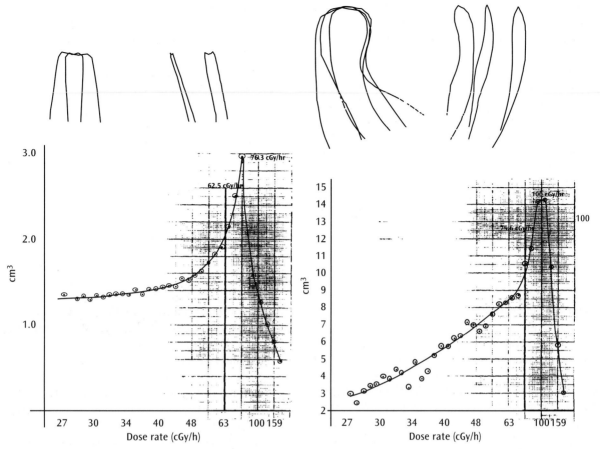

Figure 51.15 *Two clinical examples of natural dose–volume histograms. (a) Two 'hairpins' in tongue; (b) three loops of wire in anal canal/rectum.*

distance from the source to the cliff edge is determined by the radiosensitivity of the cells at low dose rate, being further for radiosensitive cells and nearer for those more radioresistant. Systems of implant rules such as the Manchester or Paris systems must therefore function by enabling the brachytherapist to place his sources in such a way that these 'cliffs' lie beyond the edges of the tumour.

Apart from geometrical optimization of dose, the other clear advantage for brachytherapy in radiobiological terms is that the overall treatment time is very short – a radical dose is given over just a few days. Tumour cell repopulation is therefore minimized. This will confer a therapeutic advantage for the treatment of the more rapidly repopulating tumour types, such as squamous tumours of the oropharynx.

DOSIMETRY *IN VIVO*

The dose distribution of a completed implant can be determined from knowing the source positions, geometry and source strengths.

Localization of source positions

Source positions may be determined by several different methods:

1 Direct measurement from the implanted wires or vector material.
2 Tomography (including CT scanning) through the central plane of the implant.
3 Orthogonal radiographs.
4 Isocentric radiographs, i.e. two radiographs separated by an angle not equal to 90°.

Direct measurement is suitable only for wires in a superficial location, offering easy access for accurate measurement. The wires must also be straight and parallel so that the measurements in one plane are representative of the wire separation along their whole length.

Tomography is most suitable for wires, which are known to be straight and parallel, since information is obtained in the central plane only. Care must be taken to ensure that the tomographic slice is taken perpendicular to the wires, since if it is taken at an angle, the wire separations appear to be larger than their true separations. Angles of up to 10° from the perpendicular will not introduce a serious error.

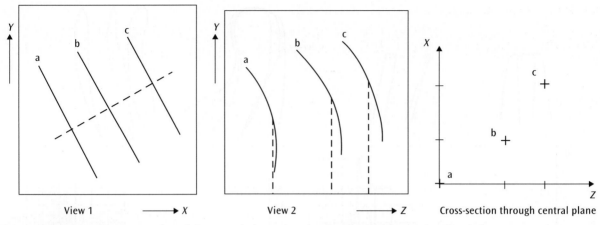

Figure 51.16 *Manual reconstruction of the central plane of an implant from orthogonal radiographs.*

Pairs of radiographs, whether orthogonal or not, can be used to provide full three-dimensional coordinate information of the wires along their full length. Orthogonal and isocentric radiographs must be used if the wires are not parallel or are curved. Whenever pairs of films are used for dosimetry purposes, a few simple rules must be followed to achieve accurate results:

1 The patient must not move or be moved between radiographs.

2 A magnification marker must be placed close to the implants so that the radiograph magnification at the position of the implant can be determined on each film. If the radiographs are taken on a radiotherapy simulator, the implant can be set at the isocentre of the machine and the field-defining wires are used to determine the magnification.

3 If possible, the patient should be radiographed in a position which is likely to be representative of his or her position throughout the treatment time.

4 When using an afterloading technique it is often helpful to load the vectors with dummy sources of different design. This will assist with the identification of individual wires on the two views. For example, one dummy source may consist of 10 mm of lead wire alternating with 10 mm of plastic tube, and another may be 20 mm of lead wire alternating with 10 mm of plastic tube.

If there is difficulty in identification of the individual wires on the two radiographs it may be helpful to adopt the following technique on a radiotherapy simulator. The patient is screened while rotating the simulator from one required view to the other. Each person present is allocated one wire on the initial image and observes it carefully as the simulator is rotated. By observing only one wire as the simulator rotates the observers are able to identify the position of 'their' wire on the final image.

Manual reconstruction of the central plane of the implant from orthogonal radiographs

A three-dimensional object can be represented by the coordinates x, y and z measured along orthogonal axes. One of the orthogonal pair of radiographs can be considered to provide the x and y coordinates, and the second provides the z and y coordinates. Work will be facilitated if the films are placed side by side with the common y axes parallel.

Before starting the reconstruction, each wire must be clearly identifiable from the others. Then, on one view, a line is drawn through the approximate centre of the implant perpendicular to the average wire direction. This line represents the central plane. The points at which the central plane intersects the wires can then be marked on view 2. This may most easily be done by calculating the y coordinate of the intersection point on view 1 and then marking a point with the calculated y coordinate on the same wire on view 2 (Fig. 51.16). This is repeated for all the wires. It is generally most convenient to use one end of the wire marked as the coordinate origin when carrying out this procedure. If the films have different magnifications, this must be taken into account when calculating the y coordinates.

A reconstruction of the central plane may then be carried out by measuring the distances to the wires on view 1 along the marked plane from an arbitrary origin, and marking these distances along one axis of a piece of graph paper. It is usually convenient to use one of the wire positions as the origin. On view 2 the marked intersections should then be projected down onto the z axis. (This will be a line parallel to the patient couch). The distances between the projected marks should then be transferred to the second axis of the graph paper using the same origin as for view 1. Using these points, the positions of each wire may then be marked. A plot is thus obtained of the marked central plane, which is approximately at right angles to the

Table 51.5 *Dose rates for unit source strength*

Wire number and length	Distance to DB1 (mm)	Dose rate to DB1 (Gy/h)	Distance to DB2 (mm)	Dose rate to DB2 (Gy/h)	Distance to DB3 (mm)	Dose Rate to DB3 (Gy/h)
1 (70 mm)	6	0.497	18	0.120	30	0.063
2 (70 mm)	6	0.497	6	0.497	18	0.12
3 (70 mm)	18	0.120	6	0.497	6	0.497
4 (50 mm)	30	0.051	18	0.111	6	0.493
Total		1.165		1.225		1.173

average wire direction. The described method may be inaccurate if the wires on at least one view are not approximately parallel to the common axis designated y.

Calculation of the dose rate

The dose distribution around a particular source is a function of the source geometry, i.e. its diameter construction material and length. Data of dose rate against perpendicular distance from the wire for ^{192}Ir wires of different lengths are available in tabular form (Pierquin *et al.*, 1987) and graphical form (Welsh *et al.*, 1983) for unit source strength.

To calculate the dose rate at a particular point in the central plane, the distance from each wire to the dose point is measured on the cross-section of the implant. The data appropriate for each length of wire are then selected. From the table or graph for the required wire length the measured distances are used to read off the dose rate that a wire of unit source strength will give at that distance. This process is repeated for all the wires in the implant and the contributions from each wire are summed to find the total dose rate at the point required for unit source strength wire. This calculation is best presented in the form of a table.

The dose rate is finally modified to allow for the source strength actually used. Iridium-192 has a half-life of 74 days and decays by just under 1 per cent/day. To obtain a dose rate that is representative of the implant throughout its entire insertion time, it is necessary to use the mid-implant activity:

> Dose rate = dose rate for unit source strength
> × mid-implant source strength

To calculate the treatment time in the Paris system the dose rate at each of the basal dose rate points is calculated as described above. The average basal dose rate is calculated and the reference dose rate which is 85 per cent of the average basal dose rate if found. The treatment time is then calculated by dividing the prescribed dose by the true reference dose rate.

When the calculation has been completed it must be independently checked by a second qualified person. Particular attention must be paid to the accuracy of the reconstruction since small changes in wire position result in large differences in dose rate to the patient.

SUMMARY

> Basal dose = basal dose rate for unit source strength
> rate (BDR) × mid-implant source strength

$$\text{Average basal dose rate} = \frac{(\text{BDR1} + \text{BDR2} + \cdots + \text{BDR}n)}{n}$$

> Reference dose rate = 0.85 × average basal dose rate

$$\text{Treatment time} = \frac{\text{prescribed dose}}{\text{reference dose rate}}$$

EXAMPLE

Four wires are implanted, each separated by 12 mm. The most lateral wire is 50 mm long and the others are 70 mm in length. The wire used has a source strength per mm of 587 nGy/h per mm at 1 m on 15 April. The implant will deliver 60 Gy to the reference isodose and the wires will be inserted on 19 April. How long must it be left in place?

The dose rates for unit source strength are given in Table 51.5.

Actual source strength 15 April = 587 nGy/h per mm at 1 m.

Unit source strength = 1000 nGy/h per mm at 1 m.

Average basal dose rate = (1.165 + 1.225 + 1.173)/3
= 1.188 Gy/h.

Expected mid-implant date 22 April.

1 week decay factor = 0.937.

Basal dose rate corrected for activity at mid-implant = 1.189 × 0.937 × 587/1000 = 0.65 Gy/h.

Reference dose rate = 0.85 × 0.65 = 0.56 Gy/h.

Time for 60 Gy = 60/0.56 = 107 h = 4 days 11 hours.

Source strength specification

The recommended quantity for source strength specifications is air kerma rate at 1 m/mm; the units are mGy/h per mm at 1 m. There are many other ways in which source strength has been specified in the past, e.g. milligrams radium equivalent, millicuries, exposure rate at 1 m/mm. To convert from one quantity to another requires the use of a conversion factor, and care must be taken in their application as not all the published values of these factors are in agreement. Ideally one would specify source strengths only in air kerma rate to prevent any possible confusion but, unfortunately, some computer programs do not have the facility to accept source strengths in this way, so it is inevitable that a variety of units will continue to be used for some time.

Use of computers

Calculations of the dose distribution are frequently carried out by computer. The computed dose distributions are usually obtained by regarding the iridium wires as a very large number of point sources. As with any computer dosimetry system, extensive checking should be carried out by the user at the commissioning of the system before it is used for the calculation of any patient treatment times. The simplest way of carrying out these checks maybe to compare the computer results with the results of the hand calculations made by methods similar to those described above. Even when computers are used for patient dosimetry, an entirely independent check must still be made of the reconstruction of the implant and the other data entered by the operator, to ensure that no error has been made.

Checking of the wire prior to use

It is the user's responsibility to ensure that the wire supplied is of the correct activity and satisfactory uniformity. To achieve this it is necessary not only to measure the total source strength of the delivered source but also to check that the expected length of wire has been received and to make some other check of the source strength per unit length. It is recommended that the following checks are carried out:

1 Compare the order, delivery note and measurement certificate to check that they agree.
2 Measure the source strength in a radionuclide calibrator with a calibration traceable to the national standard. Allowing for radioactive decay. This measurement should agree with the manufacturer's measurement prior to despatch.
3 Make a check to ensure that not only is the total activity of the source correct; but that the source strength per unit length is as expected. This can be done by:
   (a) measuring the strength of individual sources cut from the wire to see that the total strength of the individual wires is in agreement with that expected from the source strength per unitlength; or
   (b) weighing the wires after the total source strength has been measured. The weight of the wire is accurately proportional to its length and so this measurement will confirm that the expected

length of wire has been delivered. This may not detect whether a small length of the active core is missing, since the radioactive core of the 0.3 mm diameter wire contributes only 10 per cent of the weight of the wire; or
   (c) autoradiograph the entire length of the newly delivered source. This is likely to be possible for hairpins and loops but is difficult to achieve for long, coiled wires.

CLINICAL INDICATIONS

The principal reasons for choosing interstitial radiotherapy in preference to external-beam treatment relate to dose delivery and dose distribution. Suitable sites clearly need to be easily accessible and the tumourbearing normal tissue needs to be one that tolerates radiation well.

The following is a brief and by no means exhaustive list of tumour sites that are particularly well suited to treatment by interstitial brachytherapy. For more detailed description of techniques and results the reader should consult a textbook on brachytherapy (e.g. Pierquin *et al.*, 1987; Pierquin and Marinello, 1992).

Cancer of the tongue

Squamous carcinoma usually occurs on the lateral borders and ventral surfaces. Tumours of 3 cm maximum diameter or less are suitable for implanting, with a very high chance of local cure. The 'thickness' dimension of the target volume is its lateral dimension. Target volumes of 18 mm 'thickness' or less can be implanted using hairpins: thicker lesions need the wider separation that can be obtained with loops of iridium wire in plastic tubes. When this technique is used, the plastic tubes enter and exit in the submental area, with the apex of the loop arching over the dorsum of the tongue. Spacing between the legs of the loop of more than 15 mm is not recommended, which means in effect that target volumes 'thicker' than 24 mm are not ideally suited for radical treatment by interstitial implantation. They may, however, be boosted by brachytherapy after some external irradiation.

There is a general view, however, that although this combination of external radiotherapy with a brachytherapy boost probably does reduce the risk of necrosis, it also reduces the chance of local control. Pernot *et al.* (1988) have shown that the local control rate of T2N0 cases treated by implant alone (70 cases) was 89 per cent at 5 years, whereas 72 cases of T2N0 tumours treated by external radiotherapy with ^{192}Ir boost was 50 per cent only. Published local control rates for T1N0 tumours are in the range of 95–100 per cent at 5 years for patients treated by initial iridium implant and surgery for salvage (Mazeron *et al.*, 1989; Pernot *et al.*, 1990).

These excellent figures, coupled with the superb functional result seen after brachytherapy, suggest strongly that the optimum management for smaller squamous carcinomas of the tongue is interstitial implant to dose of 65 Gy followed by surgery to salvage the few recurrences that occur. Radiotherapists not practised in performing good implants should refer such cases on to a colleague who sub-specializes in brachytherapy.

Treatment by external radiotherapy alone is definitely associated with poorer results. In areas where implantation techniques are not available, patients may be better managed by primary surgical excision and reconstruction, followed by external irradiation in the postoperative period if appropriate, even though the functional result is less satisfactory. All patients with T2N0 tumours should be considered for prophylactic treatment to the upper neck nodes. If the T2 group is subdivided into those <3 cm diameter and those >3 cm, a significant difference in local control and locoregional control emerges in the majority of published series. Although these differences may be partly due to tumour biological factors, many brachytherapists believe that the higher doses achievable by radical dose implant treatment of the 'smaller' tumours is largely responsible.

Cancer of the floor of the mouth

Similar indications and techniques apply for floor of the mouth tumours as for tongue lesions. The floor of the mouth is a horseshoe shape but narrower posteriorly than anteriorly. This leads to some difficulties in placing the hairpins or loops of ^{192}Ir parallel. The one significant problem is the proximity of the mandible. When a tumour is fixed to and/or involving bone, surgery is recommended. In cases where more than three iridium wires lie close (3 mm or nearer) to the mandible there is a significant risk of causing an area of osteoradionecrosis, and surgical treatment may well be the better option. Small tumours, however, are very curable, with local control rates of 92 per cent when the lesion is small enough to be treated by a radical dose implant. For larger tumours, where a combination of external-beam radiation and implant was used, the control rates fell to 55 per cent (Owen *et al.*, 1981).

Cancer of the lip

The lip tolerates low dose-rate irradiation extremely well and the functional and cosmetic results of brachytherapy are usually excellent. The implant is done transversely and it may be necessary to leave one of the radioactive wires 'in air' in order to pull the treatment isodose upwards to cover an exophytic tumour. This is achieved by using rigid afterloading needles held in place at each end by small perspex templates to maintain the correct spacing. The teeth and gingiva may be protected by putting some

distance between them and the source wires. Simply inserting a roll of cotton wool in the anterior gingival sulcus achieves the desired effect. Results of treatment show local control rates of 95 per cent (Mazeron and Richaud, 1984). Locoregional control rates are similar because lymph-node involvement is rare in this tumour.

Skin cancers

Skin cancers in some sites are well adapted to treatment by brachytherapy techniques. Tumours that site over the bridge of the nose, like a saddle on a horse's back, and those on the free edge of the pinna are two good examples as they are difficult to treat by external irradiation. Furthermore there appears to be no significant risk of cartilagenous necrosis with low dose-rate radiation. The miniature plastic tube technique or hypodermic needle technique is used. Basal cell carcinomas respond well to 60 Gy to the reference isodose, but 65 Gy is prefered for squamous cell lesions.

Cancers of anal canal and lower rectum

The use of brachytherapy to boost the dose to the anal canal or lower rectum after chemoradiation is associated with high rates of local control (and thus low rates of abdominoperineal resection for salvage). After a dose of 45 Gy external irradiation (25 treatments over 5 weeks) the patient is allowed a significantly long rest period of 6 weeks before being given the implant. Afterloading rigid needles are implanted along the axis of the anal canal at least 3–4 mm deep to the mucosal surface and are held in place by a perspex template, which is sutured to the perineum. Not more than 50 per cent of the circumference of the anal canal should be implanted, to reduce the risk of post-radiation stricture formation. It should be remembered that the ends of these implants are 'uncrossed' and the active wire must be implanted far enough up into the rectal wall to cover the target volume. A dose of 20–25 Gy is prescribed.

Cancer of the penis

Smaller tumours of the glans penis can be treated by a volume implant with local control rates of >90 per cent (Daly *et al.*, 1982). After adequate prior circumcision, the implant is performed using rigid afterloading needles held in place by two perspex templates placed dorsally and ventrally. Care must be taken not to insert any needle through the urethra (patient catheterized). The skin and mucosal reaction that occurs after 65 Gy is sometimes prolonged. Patients must be aware of this beforehand and should be well motivated to tolerate it. Conservation of the penis is achieved in more than 80 per cent of cases. The majority of sexually active patients retain their potency.

Cancer of the breast

The breast tolerates low dose-rate radiation well and up to one-third of its volume may be implanted safely. Indications vary. Commonly, a boost dose to the site of an excised tumour is given after external irradiation to the whole breast. Alternatively, brachytherapy may be used in patients who will not accept any surgical excision or as salvage therapy for local recurrence. Its main advantage is the ability to deliver high doses without causing unsightly skin changes. This gives the combination of good cosmetic appearance and high rate of tumour control. It must be said, however, that external radiation with an electron field boost gives good results for most patients who have undergone a complete surgical excision with accurate histological control of the margins. Implant techniques should, however, be considered for those cases where the radiotherapist feels that a higher dose is required, for example, in cases where there has been no tumour excision or incomplete tumour excision, in high-grade tumours and in young patients with a high risk of local recurrence who will not accept a mastectomy.

Rigid afterloading needles are used, together with pre-drilled perspex templates to maintain the separation of the wires. These volume implants can be large, with two or sometimes three planes and commonly 7–9 radio-active lines. After 45–50 Gy external irradiation a boost dose of 25–30 Gy to the reference isodose gives local control rates of 97 per cent for T1 tumours at 15 years (Leung *et al.*, 1986; Pierquin *et al.*, 1991).

Prostate cancer

In recent years there has been a resurgence of interest in prostate brachytherapy as a means of treating localized prostate cancers. The basis for this is the development of trans-rectal ultrasound with template guidance to permit accurate placing of needles within the prostate. Small, low-activity permanent sources, usually iodine 125 or palladium-103 can be fed down these hollow needles to achieve accurate placement of 30–100 'seeds'. These sources deliver their dose over a period of weeks or months.

The implant procedure is a three-step process, as follows:

1 An ultrasound prostate volume study is undertaken. From the data received, the number and position of the seeds to be implanted are calculated by computer program. The seeds are ordered.
2 For the implant, the ultrasound 'picture' of the prostate is reproduced and the seeds are then implanted transperineally. The position of each needle is carefully checked against the plan prior to emptying it of seeds as the needles are withdrawn. The patient stays in hospital overnight.
3 Post-implant dosimetry for quality assurance purposes.

The advantages of brachytherapy over radical surgery or external-beam radiotherapy are:

- The practicality of a single 24-hour admission, and most patients are back to normal activities within a week.
- Low morbidity. The implanted volume is exactly conformal with the prostate itself plus a margin of 2–3 mm beyond the capsule. The irradiated volume is therefore much smaller than with external irradiation. There is a correspondingly low incidence of rectal complications or incontinence.
- Cost. Comparative figures from American Health Insurers suggest that the brachytherapy option may be 25 per cent cheaper than external irradiation and 50 per cent cheaper than radical surgery.
- Effectiveness. No direct comparisons within the context of prospective, controlled, randomized clinical trials are available. When results are stratified according to the presenting prostate-specific antigen (PSA) level, brachytherapy appears to be equivalent to radical prostatectomy, but long-term (>10 years) comparisons are not yet available.

Patients are selected according to age, PSA, the Gleason Score of the tumour, the tumour volume and clinical stage:

- ideally the PSA should be less than 10, but no more than 30;
- the implant volume should not exceed 50 mL.
- clinical stage T1–T2c, i.e. organ-confined disease.

This selection process will give a group of patients with a probability of involved pelvic nodes of approximately 10 per cent, which is similar to the selection often made for radical prostatectomy.

It is usual to prescribe a minimum dose of 160 Gy to the prostate capsule plus a margin of 2–3 mm. The urethral dose should not exceed 300 Gy and normally receives somewhat less. Contraindications include disease beyond the prostate, a previous transurethral resection of the prostate (TURP) and a life expectancy significantly shortened by intercurrent illness or thought to be less than 10 years.

SIGNIFICANT POINTS

- Brachytherapy is an essential technique for the clinical oncologist.
- Physical optimization of dose leads to high cure rates in suitable tumours.
- The clinician must understand the dosimetry system so that he can adapt each implant to the individual tumour being treated.
- Computers save time but cannot be used without the brachytherapist also having a good understanding of the dosimetry system being used.

- Good clinical indications for interstitial brachytherapy include tumours of the tongue, floor of the mouth, lip, breast, anal canal and prostate.
- Pre-planning the implant is essential.
- Above all, meticulous attention to detail is needed for best results.

KEY REFERENCES

Pierquin, B. and Marinello, G. (1992) *Manuel practique de Curietherapy*. Paris: Hermann, Editeurs des Sciences at des Arts.

Pierquin, B. and Marinello, G. (1997) *A practical manual of brachytherapy*. Madison, WI: Medical Physics Publishing.

Pierquin, B., Wilson, J.-F. and Chassagne, D. (1987) *Modern brachytherapy*. New York: Mason Publishing Inc.

Steel, G.G. (ed.) (1993) *Basic clinical radiobiology*. London: Edward Arnold.

REFERENCES

Anderson, L.L. (1986) A 'natural' dose–volume histogram for brachytherapy. *Med. Phys.* **13**, 898–903.

Barklay, H.Y. and Fletcher, G. (1976) Volume and time factors in interstitial gamma-ray therapy. *Am. J. Roentgenol.* **126**, 163–70.

Daly, N.J., Douchez, J. and Coombes, P.F. (1982) Treating carcinoma of the penis by iridium 192 wire implant. *Int. J. Radiat. Oncol. Biol. Phys.* **8**, 1239–43.

Fontanesi, M.D., Hetzler, D. and Ross, J. (1989) Effects of dose rate on local control and complications in the re-irradiation of head and neck tumours with interstitial 192-iridium. *Int. J. Radiat. Oncol. Biol. Phys.* **17**, 365–9.

Larra, F., Dixon, B., Couette, J.E. *et al.* (1977) Facteur temps en curietherapie. *J. Radiol. Electrol.* **58**, 329–33.

Leung, S., Otmezguine, Y., Calitchi, E. *et al.* (1986) Locoregional recurrences following radical external beam irradiation and interstitial implantation for operable breast cancer. A twenty-three year experience. *Radiother. Oncol.* **5**, 1–10.

Mazeron, J.J. and Richaud, P. (1984) Compte-rendu de la 18e reunion du Groupe Européen de Curie-thérapie. Session consacrée aux cancers de la lèvre. Padoue (Italie). *J. Eur. Radiother.* **5**, 50–6.

Mazeron, J.J., Crook, J., Beuk, V., Walop, W. and Pierquin, B. (1989) Iridium 192 implantation for T1 T2 epidermoid carcinomas of the mobile tongue: the Creteil experience. *Int. J. Radiat. Oncol. Biol. Phys.* **17** (suppl. 1), 225.

Mazeron, J.J., Simon, J.M., Crook, J. *et al.* (1991a) Influence of dose rate on local control of breast carcinoma treated by external beam irradiation plus 192-iridium implant. *Int. J. Radiat. Oncol. Biol. Phys.* **21**, 1173–7.

Mazeron, J.J., Simon, J.M., Le Péchoux, C. *et al.* (1991b) Effect of dose rate on local control of T1–T2 squamous cell carcinomas of mobile tongue and floor of mouth with interstitial 192-iridium. *Radiother. Oncol.* **21**, 39–47.

Owen, J.R., Maylin, C., Le Bourgeois, J.P. *et al.* (1981) 192 Iridium implantation of tumours of the anterior two-thirds of tongue and floor of mouth. A retrospective analysis of treatment results and sites and causes of failures. *J. Eur. Radiother.* **2**, 93–102.

Paterson, R. (1952) Studies in optimum dosage. *Br. J. Radiol.* **25**, 505–16.

Paterson, R. and Parker, H.M. (1934) A dosage system for gammaray therapy. *Br. J. Radiol.* **7**, 592.

Pernot, M., Malissard, L., Hoffstetter, S. *et al.* (1988) 455 cases of carcinoma of the tongue: results of different modes of treatment. *Abstracts of ESTRO* (Den Haag), p. 468.

Pernot, M., Mallisard, L., Aletti, P. *et al.* (1990) Brachytherapy in the management of 147 T2N0 oral tongue carcinoma treated with irradiation alone. *Int. J. Radiat. Oncol. Biol. Phys.* **19**(suppl. 1), 139–40.

Pierquin, B. and Marinello, G. (1992) *Manuel pratique de Curietherapy*. Paris: Hermann, Editeurs des Sciences et des Arts.

Pierquin, B., Chassagne, D. and Perez, R. (1964) *Precis de Curietherapie*. Paris: Masson and Co.

Pierquin, B., Chassagne, D., Baillet, F. and Paine, C. (1973) Clinical observations on the time factor in interstitial radiotherapy using 192-iridium. *Clin. Radiol.* **24**, 506–9.

Pierquin, B., Wilson, J.F. and Chassagne, D. (1987) *Modern brachytherapy*. New York: Masson Publishing Inc.

Pierquin, B., Huart, M., Raynal, M. *et al.* (1991) Conservative treatment for breast cancer: long term results (15 years). *Radiother. Oncol.* **20**, 16–23.

Steel, G.G., Kelland, L.R. and Peacock, J.H. (1989) The radiobiological basis of low dose-rate radiotherapy. In Mould, R.F. (ed.), *Brachytherapy 2, Proceedings of the 5th International Selectron Users' Meeting 1988*. Leersum, The Netherlands: Nucietron International B.V., 15–25.

Welsh, A., Dixon-Brown, A. and Stedeford, B. (1983) Calculation of dose distributions for iridium 192 implants. *Acta Radiol. Oncol.* **22**, 331.

Wickham, L. and Degrais, P. (1910) *Radium therapy*. New York: Funk and Wagnalls.

52

Planning techniques

H. JANE DOBBS

OUTLINE OF THE RADIOTHERAPY PLANNING PROCESS

The decision to use radiotherapy as a treatment modality is that of the radiation oncologist after a thorough clinical assessment of the whole patient, including an accurate histological diagnosis and definition of the site, size and extent of tumour. All patients undergoing radiotherapy should have the tumour classified according to a recognized staging system, such as TNM, FIGO, AJCCS, as this is essential in order to define the aim of local treatment as being either radical or palliative. The decision to treat is the first in a series of a large number of steps which make up the radiotherapy procedure and lead from the treatment prescription through treatment preparation to treatment delivery. This process demands close liaison between all members of the team, including physicists, radiographers, planning technicians and diagnostic radiologists as well as radiation oncologists, in order to ensure the highest standard of care. The roles of surgery and chemotherapy in relation to a course of radiotherapy should be considered at the start of treatment, as they may influence the site and size of the target volume as well as the radiation dose to be delivered.

The transfer of data during each step of the procedure is critical and human errors of transcription or of data interpretation or data input at any stage can lead to the creation of systematic errors. (Bel *et al.*, 1994). A quality assurance programme to ensure accurate treatment outcome should be set up as part of the radiotherapy procedure and is necessary in order to achieve optimum treatment in terms of maximizing tumour control probability and minimizing normal tissue complication.

Figure 52.1 illustrates the different steps that have to be taken successively during the radiotherapy planning process, and there should be a continuous feedback between all the different steps so that new information can be integrated into the final treatment policy. It is essential that at each step there is recording of information and full

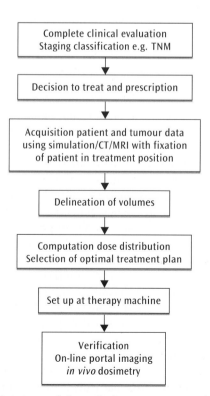

Figure 52.1 *Steps of the radiotherapy treatment planning process.*

documentation. When the final decision to use radiotherapy is made, the treatment prescription is given, including a statement of the aim of therapy, the definition of target volume to be treated and the specification of dose, fractionation, overall time and other treatment parameters, as described in ICRU Report 50 (Landberg *et al.*, 1993) and ICRU Report 62 (Landberg *et al.*, 1999).

This chapter will describe the importance of patient positioning and immobilization, the acquisition of patient and tumour data using different imaging modalities, definitions of tumour and target volume, use of computerized dose planning and verification of treatment in order to obtain the high standards of radiotherapy treatment planning.

ACQUISITION OF PATIENT AND TUMOUR DATA

Traditionally, clinical data for radiotherapy treatment planning have been collected in the cross-sectional plane. The conventional method of tumour localization involves the use of antero-posterior (AP) and lateral radiographs, often with the use of contrast media to define the target volume, usually obtained with the use of a simulator. A transverse outline of the patient at the centre of the target volume is then taken and the tumour and anatomical data transferred to the cross-sectional map. However, this method of localization fails to visualize the tumour itself in most cases, as orthogonal radiographs merely show bony landmarks with contrast outlining hollow viscera. Tumours such as those of the bladder, oesophagus, prostate, rectum and vagina may be outlined directly, but in most cases the contrast media outlines anatomical structures only. The advent of X-ray computed tomography (CT) scanners in the late 1970s provided a method of obtaining the required tumour information accurately, rapidly and in a transverse axial plane ideal for radiotherapy planning. In almost all cases, the primary tumour and its extensions can be visualized, together with the precise positions of sensitive organs such as kidneys, lungs and spinal cord and the patient's external body contour. In the past decade computed tomography scanning has become truly three dimensional, not only for graphic visualization but also for three-dimensional dosimetric calculations. This enables both visualization and localization of the tumour, target volume and normal organs as a three-dimensional display with subsequent three-dimensional planning. This has led to more complex treatment field arrangements with detailed field shaping and the ability to perform conformal therapy (*see* Chapter 53).

The increased use of magnetic resonance imaging (MRI) in the staging of malignant disease (Husband *et al.*, 1999) has shown it to be particularly useful for tumours of the central nervous system (CNS), head and neck, musculoskeletal tumours, and prostate and cervical cancer,

where it provides new information about the site and extent of the gross tumour. Additional information may be obtained from ultrasound examination, positron emission tomography (PET) or single positron emission computed tomography (SPECT), scanning. Image registration methods are being developed to combine these data from different modalities using a variety of algorithms. However, it should be remembered that all available information must be used when performing localization of the target volume, including clinical examination (under general anaesthesia in some instances) and surgical and histopathological details which, for some tumour sites, may provide the most important data.

PATIENT POSITIONING AND FIXATION DEVICES

The position of the patient for treatment must be comfortable, easily reproducible and suitable for acquisition of images using localization equipment and for delivering treatment. The extent of day-to-day variation in position of the patient differs from one part of the anatomy to another. This is illustrated by a wealth of studies in the literature recording the accuracy of reproducibility of patient positioning during a course of treatment for a variety of different tumour sites. Care given to the immobilization of the patient and development of innovative fixation devices is essential. It has also been clearly shown that displacement of tumour and normal organs occurs with variation in the position of the patient (Dutreix, 1984). Examples of organ movement are displacement of the larynx on swallowing, cardiac pulsation, movement of the lungs and the kidneys on respiration, variation in position of the prostate, seminal vesicles and bladder with change in bladder and rectal filling.

Close liaison is necessary with mould room technicians preparing fixation devices, so that details of the position of the patient and tumour site to be treated are all defined; the most relevant device can then be made and, wherever possible, markings made on the fixation device rather than the patient's skin. Full use must be made of immobilization devices, lasers and placing permanent skin markers, such as tattoos, at optimum sites. All of these details must be carefully documented to ensure accurate transfer of data from localization through all the stages of the planning process and subsequent treatment. A Polaroid photograph of the patient at the time of localization in the simulator or CT scanner aids in recording the set-up parameters.

Head and neck

Rosenthal *et al.* (1992) reported a comparative study of simulator and treatment portal films in 51 patients with head and neck malignancy who were immobilized using

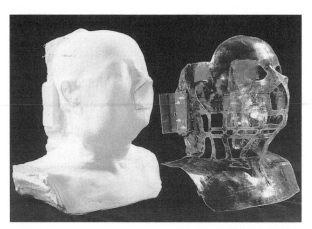

Figure 52.2 *Vacuum-moulded Perspex shell with plaster-cast impression.*

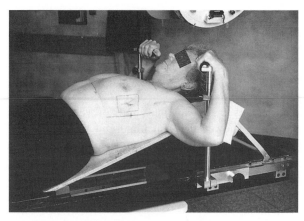

Figure 52.3 *Immobilization device for breast irradiation with variable wedge angle and adjustable arm poles suitable for localization using a simulator.*

a bite and block technique. They showed a total median uncertainty of 7 mm, with 21 per cent of portal films showing an uncertainty of more than 10 mm. In contrast, Graham *et al.* (1991) looked at immobilization of four patients using a Perspex shell system, with a similar number immobilized using a stereotactic frame. The main displacement of the lateral fields using a Perspex shell was 1.8 mm compared with 1 mm for the stereotactic frame. These studies clearly show that the development of more sophisticated immobilization systems for treatment of patients with head and neck malignancy reduces the risk of error due to movement of the patient during treatment. For most radiotherapy treatments the Perspex shell system (with an uncertainty of 1–2 mm) would make this the optimum fixation device, as it is relatively comfortable for the patient and has the advantage of being transparent and provides a vehicle for field centre and portal delineation marks to aid with set-up of the treatment (Fig. 52.2). Sections can be removed from the shell to allow for skin sparing and to reduce the extent of erythema.

Thorax

The accuracy of set-up for breast irradiation has been addressed in many publications (Van Tienhoven *et al.*, 1991; Holmberg *et al.*, 1994). Mitine *et al.* (1991) looked at 376 portal films performed on 14 patients undergoing tangential breast radiotherapy with tangential fields. The study showed that the standard deviation in a cranio-caudal direction between portal films and simulator films decreased from 5.8 mm to 3.7 mm with a new technique using fixation of one arm to an arm pole. This study provides objective data to show that fixation of the patient during breast radiotherapy is essential to improve accuracy of field reproducibility. A variety of immobilization techniques are used, depending on whether localization is performed on a simulator or CT scanner.

If localization for breast irradiation is to be performed on a CT scanner, then the patient needs to be supine with one or both arms raised and secured above the head in order to pass through the aperture of the scanner. Gagliardi *et al.* (1992) presented an analysis of their treatment techniques of patients with node-negative breast cancer using three-dimensional CT treatment planning. The patient was immobilized supine with one arm above the head using a vacuum-moulded polystyrene bag. They analysed the shift on a grid drawn on the skin of the patient's breast according to movement in the position of the ipsilateral arm. When the arm was abducted to 130°, as for entry through a CT scanner for planning, the central mammillary plane was shifted upwards by 2 cm and the displacement was up to 4 cm in the axilla. If the arm was abducted to 90°, the displacement in the cranio-caudal direction was small over the breast, but in the region of the shoulder joint there was a difference of 2 cm between the grids. This illustrates that, if the arm position is varied between localization in a CT scanner and treatment on a therapy unit, there will be an error in set-up. It also shows that the use of skin tattoos as landmarks for setting up treatment fields is highly dependent on the arm position and that fixation of the arm(s) is essential.

Location of the breast for radiotherapy can also be performed on the simulator using an isocentric technique and manual or automatic contouring at multiple levels. A breast board with a wedge can then be used to bring the sternum horizontal, so obviating the need for collimator angle on the tangential fields and reducing the complexity of dosimetric calculations. Figure 52.3 shows a patient on a purpose-built wedge with two arm poles for symmetry, each of which has a full range of movement in all directions to maximize the comfort of individual patients. A foot board ensures support for the patient in the cranio-caudal plane and the angle of the wedge is fully adjustable to allow for individual patient variation.

Abdomen

Immobilization of patients for abdominal and pelvic radiotherapy is unsatisfactory and no ideal technique has yet been devised. Griffiths *et al.* (1991) reported a study of pelvic radiotherapy which showed that errors in movement were greatest in the cranio-caudal direction and that the use of lasers improved lateral shift errors, particularly in prone patients. All patients should have lateral tattoos which should be aligned with lasers as a minimum requirement to prevent lateral rotation (Fig. 52.4). The study also showed that it is important to examine the type of mattress used on the treatment couch as, if these vary between simulator and treatment unit, they can introduce error, as can the use of a 'tennis racquet' and other couch windows necessary for under-couch treatments. The use of carbon-fibre couch inserts on both simulator and treatment units has largely eliminated this type of variation.

For treatment of prostate cancer, some centres used to treat patients with a full bladder in order to distend the bladder mucosa away from the prostate target volume and to displace small bowel from the irradiated area. However, Ten Haken *et al.* (1991) showed that by filling the bladder or rectum using catheters, to simulate treatment conditions of urine or stool contents, the prostate gland moved 0–2 cm (mean 0.5 cm). This displacement of the prostate gland was shown to occur out of the high dose radiation zone, leading to inadequate dosage of the tumour. Other studies (Balter *et al.*, 1995; Van Herk *et al.*, 1995; Beard *et al.*, 1996) have confirmed and quantified the movement of the prostate gland and seminal vesicles during radiotherapy. Zelefsky *et al.* (1999) evaluated 50 patients with serial CT scans and showed that prostatic and seminal vesicle displacement during radiotherapy was more pronounced amongst patients whose initial planning scans had large rectal and bladder volumes. Patients in their study were in the prone position with an empty bladder. They showed that prostatic displacement was more common in the AP and cranio-caudal directions and less so laterally. It would appear from these studies that asking patients to open their bowels and empty their bladders before both planning CT scan and treatment each day, reduces movement of the prostate and seminal vesicles.

The impact of patient immobilization on set-up accuracy for prostate irradiation is controversial (Fiorino *et al.*, 1998). Soffen *et al.* (1991) are among those convinced that rigid immobilization is necessary. However, equally good results have been reported by Catton *et al.* (1997) and Dearnaley *et al.* (1999), who advocate using supports for the legs or feet position only. Song *et al.* (1996) compared the set-up accuracy of four immobilization devices versus none, and concluded that laser-aligned multiple tattoos with meticulous patient positioning by trained radiographers was as good as the use of formal immobilization devices.

Several studies have evaluated changes in bladder volume and position during radiotherapy for bladder cancer (Dobbs, 1993; Sur *et al.*, 1993; Turner *et al.*, 1997; Harris and Buchanan, 1998). The most significant directions for bladder movement were in the AP and cranio-caudal directions and appeared to be random in time and direction. Turner *et al.* (1997) found that bladder movement occurred in up to 60 per cent of patients as a displacement greater than 1.5 cm between the bladder wall and 95 per cent isodose, and they recommend a margin of 2 cm, at least for tumour-bearing regions of the bladder. Most centres require patients to empty the bladder by voluntary micturition just before CT scanning and each day before radiotherapy for treatment of bladder cancer. It is important to avoid large volumes of oral contrast media during scanning as these lead to distension of the bladder, causing inappropriately enlarged volumes.

A recent review of set-up error verification using portal imaging describes a 'state of the art' set-up accuracy of 2 mm for head and neck treatments (one standard deviation of the random and systematic set-up error), 2.5 mm for prostate, 3.0 mm for pelvis and 3.5 mm for lung treatments (Hurkmans *et al.*, 2001).

METHODS OF TUMOUR LOCALIZATION

In any particular radiotherapy department, the choice of equipment used for localization will depend on the workload and range of patients and tumour sites to be treated, the techniques employed in planning and irradiation and the resources available (Dobbs and Parker, 1984). For most tumour sites, CT planning scans should be performed in order to localize both the gross tumour and critical normal organs as accurately as possible. For malignancies of the central nervous system, head and neck region, musculo-skeletal tumours, prostate and cervix, additional diagnostic information is gained from MRI scans and this should be incorporated into the localization procedure. Current methods of tumour and target localization include the use of the simulator, CT scanning and simulator CT and CT simulator facilities.

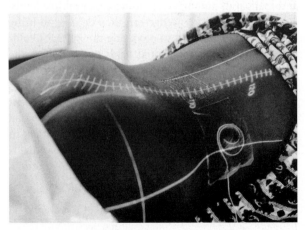

Figure 52.4 *Patient positioning using laser lights to align midline and lateral skin tattoos.*

CT planning

It has been shown that CT scanning information alters the radiation fields used in approximately 30 per cent of patients receiving radical radiotherapy treatment (Goitein, 1982; Dobbs *et al.*, 1983). These studies compared conventional planning with CT scanning as used for localization of the target volume, and showed that in around 30 per cent of cases a change in the margins of the target volumes was necessary in order to ensure coverage of the tumour and avoid geographical miss. Two studies have addressed the difficult question of whether this improvement in accuracy of targeting radiotherapy translates into an improvement in survival, although there is as yet no randomized study in the literature looking at improvement in local tumour control. Rothwell *et al.* (1985) made a retrospective comparison of the survival rate of patients whose bladder tumours were included within a 90 per cent treatment isodose with those who, by CT criteria, had tumour lying outside the 90 per cent isodose, i.e. a geographical miss. Although CT scans were obtained before radiotherapy treatment was given, the comparison was made following treatment which had been delivered using the conventional plan. A significant difference was found in survival rate in favour of those whose tumours lay within the 90 per cent isodose. Overall the study predicted a 4–5 per cent increase in survival of the whole group of patients with bladder cancer at 3 years, if all tumours were included in all patients. However, the histopathological staging of the two groups of patients was found to be different. The incidence of positive lymphadenopathy was 73 per cent in the group treated to less than the 90 per cent isodose, compared with 21 per cent in the group with adequate tumour coverage, suggesting that the survival difference might be due to this prognostic factor rather than to the volume irradiated.

Tsujii *et al.* (1989) reported a study of patients with post-nasal sinus tumours in which those treated with the use of Perspex shell before 1979 were compared with those treated after 1979 with the addition of CT planning – approximately 80 patients in each group. A significant difference in survival rate was reported in favour of the patients with CT planning, particularly for supra-structure tumours. The study also showed a reduction in field sizes and complication rates with the use of CT planning. There is no doubt that CT information improves localization of the target volume for many tumour sites, even though the translation of this accuracy into improved survival rates may be modest (Goitein, 1979).

CT scans taken for radiotherapy treatment planning require different considerations from those taken for diagnostic use, where the prime object is to detect the presence of malignant disease. The radiation oncologist must determine the exact position of the tumour, its extent in all directions, the site of adjacent structures and the relationship between the organs, and the tumour and external landmarks which are to be used for setting up the patient on the therapy unit. The acquisition of tumour data involves the use of optimum imaging modalities defined in tumour site protocols and developed in collaboration with diagnostic radiologists (Husband and Reznek, 1998). Interpretation of data by an expert in oncological diagnostic imaging is essential for ensuring accurate tumour delineation.

The patient position and set-up and immobilization must be identical for CT scanning as for the treatment. The reproducibility of the patient's position on the CT scanner can best be ensured by the presence of a therapy radiographer assisting the diagnostic team in the positioning of the patient on the CT couch. Exactly the same immobilization devices e.g. Perspex shell, vacuum bag, arm pole must be used on the CT scanner and a record made of these devices and any polystyrene head or knee pads or pillows used. Sagittal and lateral lasers should be available in the CT scanning room to align the patient and permanent skin markers are placed on the skin over the nearest immobile bony landmark to the tumour site. Lateral tattoos are also made to prevent lateral rotation of the patient. All of these support devices should be radiolucent, so as not to produce artefacts. Skin markers should be covered with either radiopaque catheters or barium paste, in order that their site is recorded on both topogram and CT scans (Fig. 52.5).

There must be a flat insert on the CT scanner couch and good quality control of the image and spatial resolution. It must be remembered that even though the aperture size of the CT scanner may be up to 80 cm, the reconstructed diameter, which describes the area over which an image can be obtained or a scan reconstructed, may be smaller than this and limit the information that can be gained. The topogram (scanogram) produced by CT scanners is a digital radiograph obtained by moving the patient on the couch through the stationary fan beam of the machine. This is used to localize the anatomical position of the resulting CT slices (Fig. 52.6), but it must be remembered that the image is distorted laterally due to fan

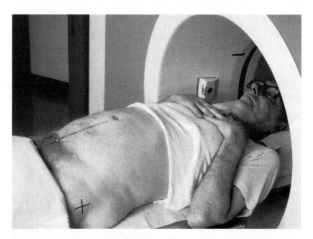

Figure 52.5 *Polaroid photographic record of patient in treatment position on CT scanner. Tattoo over pubic symphysis marked with barium paste, midline radiopaque catheter and lateral tattoos are all illustrated.*

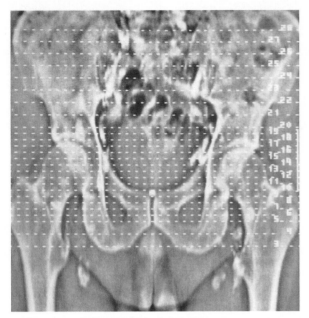

Figure 52.6 *Topogram (scanogram) of the pelvis with CT sections recorded. Barium paste landmarks skin tattoo over pubic symphysis.*

beam geometry and that the geometrical representation is not the same as that of the treatment beam as it is not divergent in all directions. Contrast media are used orally to outline small bowel and oesophagus, but can affect dose calculations if these are based on CT density data. For treatment of bladder cancer, patients should empty the bladder before CT scanning and treatment. For prostate tumours, it has been shown that excess gas or faeces in the rectum causes variation in position of the prostate, and a repeat CT scan should be performed on another day if this occurs. Use of contrast in a rectal catheter should be avoided, in view of the fact that it distorts the anatomy for planning and will not be used during the treatment. It is important to mark structures such as the introitus, anal margin, vagina and any tumour masses or operative scar with barium or radiopaque catheters, so that they are visualized both on the scan and topograms.

With modern multi-slice CT scanners, images are taken very rapidly in a fraction of a respiratory cycle. First, a topogram is obtained over the part of the body of interest and then CT scans taken at 2–10 mm intervals using a slice thickness of 2–10 mm. It is important that close liaison is made with the diagnostic radiologist to make sure that the CT scans obtained have the maximum amount of diagnostic information, as well as full body contour necessary for treatment planning. Misinterpretation of CT data can be a source of error in the delineation of the target volume (Denham *et al.*, 1992) due, for example, to erroneous evaluation of vascular structures, unopacified bowel and the partial volume edge effect. It is usual now for diagnostic scans to already have been taken as part of the initial staging procedure and subsequent additional CT scans for treatment planning are then performed (Fig. 52.7a, b).

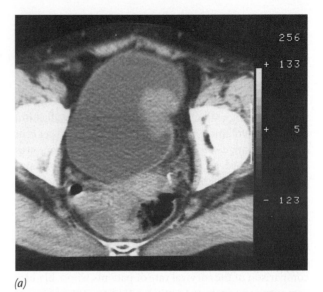

(a)

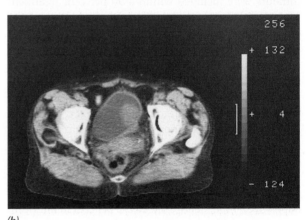

(b)

Figure 52.7 *CT scans of carcinoma of the bladder: (a) bladder full, diagnostic images, (b) after micturition, CT planning images taken under treatment conditions, showing full body contour.*

This is because of the necessity of having the patient under conditions for therapy with accurate external markers on the skin and to obtain data, not only of the tumour itself, but also in relation to external landmarks (Ash *et al.*, 1983).

The CT scanner and treatment planning computer should be networked to allow for direct transfer of CT images. Outlining of body contour, tumour, clinical target volume (CTV), planning target volume (PTV) (Fig. 52.8) and normal organs, takes place at the planning computer on each individual CT slice with an interactive software programme. For three-dimensional treatment planning, multiple slices must be taken using contiguous thin (2–4 mm) slices in order to obtain the maximum amount of information, as this is necessary to permit accurate three-dimensional dose calculations and for the formation of good quality digitally reconstructed radiographs (DRRs). An automatic facility allows the body contour to be drawn rapidly, but all other structures have to be outlined by the clinician. This is a time-consuming procedure

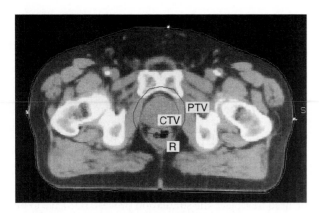

Figure 52.8 *CT image of the pelvis for prostate tumour irradiation showing clinical target volume (CTV), planning target volume (PTV) and rectum (R), and midline and lateral skin tattoos.*

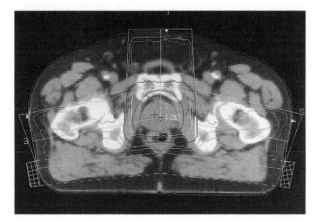

Figure 52.9 *Dose distribution using three fields produced by integrated CT planning system on the central slice for two-dimensional planning.*

as well as one which is prone to inter-clinician variability (Urie *et al.*, 1991; Perez *et al.*, 1995).

For two-dimensional planning, a dose distribution is calculated on the CT image corresponding to the centre of the proposed target volume (Fig. 52.9). Off-axis beam data can be used to determine the dose distribution at other levels within the target volume, in order to record the homogeneity of the dose throughout the entire volume. A beam's eye view facility may help in the choice of beam configuration. Three-dimensional graphic display and dose volume histograms give additional information for the comparison of three-dimensional treatment plans. Immobilization techniques become critical and quality assurance studies are essential to verify patient and organ movement when using three-dimensional planning and conformal therapy.

Simulator

The simulator is an isocentrically mounted diagnostic X-ray machine which can reproduce treatment parameters

and has the facility for screening by the use of an image intensifier. It has a couch which is flat and capable of all the movements of the therapy unit and a gantry which can be rotated through 360°. The patient is set up on the simulator in the treatment position and any tumour masses are marked with wire and contrast medium placed in the bladder, rectum, vagina or oesophagus. A skin tattoo is placed over the nearest immobile bony landmark to the tumour, such as the pubic symphysis in the pelvis or the xiphisternum in the chest, to act as a reference point. Lateral tattoos should also be placed on the skin at fixed distances up from the couch on each side and laser lights are needed in the simulator to align the patient and prevent rotation. Therapy machines may operate at a fixed distance between the source and the skin (SSD). Alternatively, the machine may rotate around the patient on an axis centred on a fixed point called the isocentre, which is 100 cm from the source and is usually placed at the centre of the target volume. The position of the isocentre can either be measured below the skin and called a pin depth or located by reference to the couch top by using the couch height scale, to measure the distance from the isocentre to the couch. For many patients this distance may be less variable than the pin depth measurement, because of obesity of the anterior abdominal wall and variability of abdominal contents. If field sizes are defined using the simulator guide wires on the skin surface, they will appear larger than the target volume at depth because of the inward bowing of the isodose curves. Sufficient margin around the planning target volume must be allowed in order to give the required dose at depth. Alternatively, the simulator can be used to take a radiograph of the relevant area of the body and the target volume defined on the simulator film, and a dose plan made so that the correct field size can be chosen to give the required dose at the target volume. Similarly, when an isocentric treatment plan is verified on the simulator, the field sizes on the skin will appear larger than the target volume in order to ensure adequate dose at depth, and this should be remembered and no adjustment made.

When opposing fields are used, the doses are calculated at the mid point between the fields. When more than two fields are used, then a dose plan is computed and the target volume and normal organs are transferred from a simulator radiograph to a transverse outline of the body contour taken through the centre of the target volume (Dobbs *et al.*, 1999). Contouring devices may be simple use of plaster of Paris or wire or a more sophisticated variety of automated contouring systems. By convention, outlines are orientated looking up from feet to the head in exactly the same way as CT scans. It is important that midline and lateral skin reference marks are located on this contour, and the separation between two fixed points is measured with callipers on the patient and marked on to the sheet of paper. The length of the perpendicular line through the midline should correspond to the separation measured on the patient. For single or opposing fields, an AP film is taken as a record of the treatment fields that have been localized. For three or more fields, an AP film is taken with rulers, magnification rings or a simulator graticule rule to indicate the magnification factor. For the lateral film, a ruler is placed on the midline of the patient over the centre of the tumour. It should be remembered that if the target volume is offset antero-posteriorly or laterally, then this should be taken into account when calculating the magnification factor. The position of important adjacent normal organs, such as the lens, spinal cord, lungs and kidneys, should be marked on the outline along with the target volume. These details and the proposed treatment technique should be discussed with the planning technician or physicist prior to a computerized dose plan being constructed.

Simulator CT

A CT modality attached to the gantry of a simulator can be used to produce images with a relatively limited resolution but at the same time as the simulation process (Verellen *et al.*, 1999). Simulator CT scanners therefore have a larger aperture size than CT scanners, but still have a limited reconstruction diameter. The scan time is much slower than the CT scanner and the spatial resolution reduced (Dobbs and Webb, 1988). However, they combine the facilities available on the simulator with a limited CT facility which can provide body contour and outline of structures such as the lungs, heart and bone contour, and can be used for simple inhomogeneity corrections. Images do not produce detailed tumour information or accurate CT numbers. However, the cost is low compared with that of the CT scanner and is particularly appropriate for techniques such as tangential breast irradiation, where it provides CT slices at the central, superior and inferior axes of the target volume. A recent study has shown that 80 per cent of plans for tangential breast irradiation using three level outlines are as good as those using an entire three-dimensional data set in terms of dose inhomogeneity assessment (Vincent *et al.*, 1999). It is possible to use multiple level outlines not only to improve breast dose homogeneity but also to localize the position of the lungs for tissue inhomogeneity corrections. Bornstein *et al.* (1990) and Neal and Yarnold (1995) showed that the central lung distance (CLD) on a simulator film was the most useful predictor of ipsilateral lung volume included in tangential fields of breast radiotherapy, and correlated well with the lung volume measured on CT scanning. Hurkmans *et al.* (2000) have shown that the maximum heart distance (MHD) on a simulator film of tangential breast fields correlates well with normal tissue control probability (NTCP) values for excess cardiac mortality from breast radiotherapy. Hence CLD and MHD, which are relatively easy to measure on the simulator film and portal image, can be used as good predictors of normal tissue toxicity. The spatial resolution of a simulator CT is not satisfactory in

the pelvis or abdomen at present for either normal organ or tumour localization, and it is not possible to use this equipment to produce fully three-dimensional computerized plans.

CT simulator

CT scanners which provide state-of-the-art imaging can be combined with software to produce virtual simulation from a beam's eye perspective with images which are equivalent to conventional simulator images. These can be used to replace the simulation process, but have to be related to an internal isocentre within the patient, anchoring data to external landmarks. A multi-image display system and three-dimensional treatment-planning computer are linked with a portal imaging system to verify the dosimetric plan. The ability to derive CT scans and to provide target volume definition with margin generation, dose calculation and simulation all on one work station is a major advance. The CT simulator provides maximum tumour information as well as full three-dimensional planning capabilities. Although equipment is costly and localization rather time consuming, this is likely to improve very rapidly. The major use of the CT simulator is for three-dimensional computerized treatment planning and conformal therapy in the development of innovative treatment techniques.

Magnetic resonance imaging

The main advantage of MRI is that it gives additional diagnostic information, particularly in tumours of the central nervous system (Fig. 52.10), head and neck region, musculoskeletal tumours, cervix and prostate tumours. These data are available in multiple planes, including those not directly imaged by CT, and also give superior soft-tissue contrast. However, there is no bone signal, making comparison with conventional X-rays difficult. There is a geometric distortion inherent in MRI scans which is in the region of up to 3 mm and this inaccuracy has, until now, limited the direct use of MRI for delineation of the target volume. At the moment, scan times are relatively long and the small aperture often noisy and uncomfortable for patients. There is no direct correlation between MRI and electron density of tissue and so the data cannot be used directly for dose computation. However, integration of CT and MRI data into a single workstation using image registration is now possible in the CNS, and is likely to become available at other anatomical sites too.

Ultrasound

The main use of ultrasound for treatment planning is in the localization of superficial tumour masses. For instance, in patients who present with stage 3 carcinoma of the

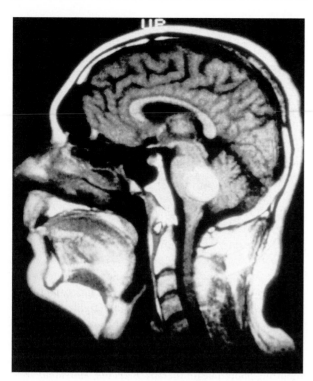

Figure 52.10 *Magnetic resonance image of tumour of the fourth ventricle.*

breast there may be an excellent response to chemotherapy and this may be followed by subsequent radical radiotherapy. Clinical examination may then fail to detect an abnormality but ultrasound can be used to localize any small residual tumour masses within the breast and mark the skin for targeting the booster dose of irradiation. Ultrasound has also been useful in the choice of electron energy for adjuvant radiotherapy to the breast tumour bed (Helyer *et al.*, 1999).

Image registration

At present, CT remains the mainstay for acquisition of anatomical and tumour data for radiotherapy treatment planning, partly because correlation of CT numbers with electron densities makes it ideal. However, for many tumour sites MRI, PET, ultrasound or SPECT may provide optimum tumour information, rather than CT. It has therefore become imperative to find methods of combining optimum tumour imaging data with CT data for radiotherapy treatment planning. This correlation is difficult because of differences in patient positioning, geometric distortions of magnetic resonance images, varying anatomical boundaries and differences in spatial resolution. Image registration methods can be used to transform the position point in an image to the corresponding physical point in the patient and to find a match between two image sets from different modalities. Extrinsic landmarks can be matched using reference points, which may be located using fiducial markers or systems such as

stereotactic frames, Perspex helmets, dental moulds or ear plugs for the brain. Markers can be glued to the skin, but the accuracy of this technique is limited by skin movement. Currently most work is being carried out on CNS tumours looking at image registration between CT, MRI, PET and SPECT (Studholme *et al.*, 1997; Rosenman *et al.*, 1998). However, it has been shown that prostate tumours are better defined on MRI than CT (Rasch *et al.*, 1999), and image registration studies are also going ahead in the pelvis for prostate tumours (Van Herk and Kooy, 1994; Van Herk *et al.*, 1995).

DEFINITIONS OF TUMOUR AND TARGET VOLUME

The next step in the planning process is to define the extent of gross tumour as delineated by clinical examination and optimum imaging, and then to decide on the target volume, which is designed to receive a radical dose of radiotherapy aimed at eradicating the tumour. The process of determining these volumes for treatment of malignant disease consists of several distinct steps which have been well described in the ICRU Report 50 and ICRU Report 62.

The first volume is that of the gross tumour volume (GTV), which is the palpable or visible extent of malignant tumour and corresponds to the site where the tumour cell concentration is at its maximum. Staging systems such as the TNM and FIGO classifications describe the site, size and extent of GTV; however, delineation of the GTV is very dependent on imaging. The UICC TNM staging classification states that imaging should be used to define the T stage, but there are no guidelines as to which is the best imaging modality for each primary tumour site. Expert advice from a diagnostic radiologist is essential to gain maximum information from any imaging modality, such as CT and MRI, which is used to locate the site and extent of the tumour (Husband and Reznek, 1998).

A margin is then added around the GTV in order to include direct local subclinical microscopic spread. This margin usually has a decreasing malignant cell density towards the periphery, where it should reach zero, and, with the GTV, constitutes the clinical target volume (CTV). The size of the clinical margin chosen for subclinical disease depends primarily on tumour characteristics such as histological type, grade and features such as lymphatic, vascular and perineural infiltration. The size of this margin appears to vary widely, depending on the clinician's experience and interpretation of the histological features of the tumour and its projected natural history. Data for defining this margin are sparse, and it is the most subjective step in the planning process. Knowledge from surgical and post-mortem specimens, patterns of tumour recurrence, as well as from clinical experience are used to quantify the margin.

Urie *et al.* (1991) revealed marked differences in the size and site of the clinical target volume for treatment of the same nasopharyngeal tumour prescribed by two different clinicians. Denham *et al.* (1992) have reported a study of patients planned for radiotherapy for non-small cell lung cancer, in which they showed a wide interclinician variation in the choice of tumour and target volumes, even with the use of CT scanning. The main causes of interclinician variation were found to be radiological interpretation, margin described for microscopic disease, and margin allowed for geometric variables. Studies of interclinician variation in delineation of the target volume for central nervous system tumours (Leunens *et al.*, 1993) and prostate tumours (Seddon *et al.*, 2000) show that for some tumours it has to be accepted that the GTV cannot be drawn as a well-demarcated volume with precise borders. There may remain a zone of uncertainty around the GTV due to inherent limitations of the imaging technique, inexperience or interpretation of imaging data and this should be expressed in a qualitative or quantitative way.

If the tumour has been removed prior to radiotherapy (e.g. operable breast cancer), then no GTV can be defined, and the volume of subclinical disease constitutes a CTV. If treatment is planned to a primary tumour and lymph node areas too, then there may be two clinical target volumes in a patient. The next step is to add a margin around the CTV to account for variation in size and position of tissues relative to the treatment beams due to organ movement, patient movement and variation in daily set up, i.e. physiological or technical factors. For instance, swallowing causes movement of a laryngeal tumour, respiration leads to movement of bronchial tumours and the breast during irradiation. Variations in bladder or rectal filling can cause movement of bladder and prostate tumours.

Verification studies have shown organ motion varying from 1 mm for the brain, 3 mm for the breast, 8 mm for the prostate, and 15 mm for bladder wall, as two standard deviations from the mean. ICRU Report 62 defines an internal margin (IM) to allow for the physiological variations in the shape, position, and size of the organ, therefore defining an internal target volume (ITV) when added to the CTV.

Intrafractional and interfractional variations occur in patient position and in alignment of the beams with external marks. To account for these changes, a set-up margin (SM) can be defined for each technique, using verification studies or a quality assurance programme. For example, set-up variations of 10 mm for the pelvis, 13 mm for the breast, and 2–4 mm for the head and neck have been reported as two standard deviations from the mean. Combining the internal margin for physiological changes and the set-up margin for technical variations with the CTV leads to the planning target volume (PTV) (Fig. 52.11). The PTV is a geometrical concept used for planning treatment, selection of appropriate beam sizes and arrangements, and should ensure that the prescribed

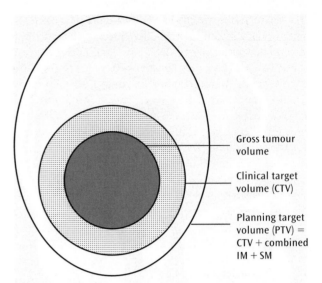

Figure 52.11 *Definitions of volumes according to ICRU Reports 50 and 62. IM, internal margin; SM, set-up margin. (Reproduced with permission from International Commission on Radiation Units 1993, ICRU Report 50; and 1999, ICRU Report 62. Prescribing, Recording and reporting photon beam therapy. Bethesda, Maryland: International Commission on Radiation Units.)*

dose is actually delivered to the CTV when variations are taken into account.

It is not usually practical to add up all of the uncertainties linearly, because of normal tissue tolerances which may influence the maximum volume considered to be appropriate for treatment. Where random uncertainties (class A) are probability distributed, and systematic uncertainties (class B) are estimated by approximate standard deviations, then their combined effect can be estimated. The total standard deviation is then the root of the sum of the squares of all class A and B uncertainties. This final choice of margin will mean that the CTV is located within the enveloping isodose with a confidence interval of 70 per cent (or 90 per cent with two standard deviations). In practice, there is a tendency to use standard margins added to the CTV to define the PTV, and much work is in progress (McKenzie *et al.*, 2000). The margins may be asymmetrical. For instance, for a lung tumour the margin may be 11 mm in the transverse plane and 15 mm in the cranio-caudal direction, due to the effect of respiration (Ekberg *et al.*, 1998). McKenzie (2000) examines the issue of breathing-induced motion and suggests that the margin to allow for respiration should be added linearly to the quadrature sum of the other contributing errors. It is recommended that each institution should evaluate local variations and uncertainties (which are dependent on immobilization, set-up, technique, etc.) and define a reasonable level of probability for the different components.

In 1976, ICRU Report 24 considered that ±5 per cent accuracy was required in the delivery of absorbed dose. Brahme *et al.* (1988) and Mijnheer *et al.* (1987) suggested that the requirement for accuracy should be 3.5 per cent, one standard deviation, in the dose value at the specification point in the target volume. This requirement is based on the sigmoid shape and steepness of dose–response curves for both tumour control and normal tissue complications. These curves show that a small variation in dose level can have a considerable influence on the probability of tumour control and also on the likelihood of normal tissue complications. However, within the target volume, there is a variation in tumour cell density. There also exists heterogeneity of cell type and radiosensitivity as well as distribution within the cell cycle, so that clinical dose–effect data curves have a reduced steepness. A clinical study reported from the Institut Gustave Roussy suggested that an increase in dose of 7–10 per cent resulted in clinically detectable reactions (Chassagne *et al.*, 1976; Dutreix, 1984). These studies show that accuracy is important, and a multidisciplinary team effort with a careful quality assurance programme is essential to ensure optimum quality throughout the whole radiotherapy process and so achieve a successful treatment outcome.

COMPUTERIZED DOSE PLANNING

Data are transferred from the CT scanner or simulator via a direct line, magnetic tape or via a digitizer to the computerized planning system. Quality control measures are essential for both the method of transfer and the planning system, in order to guard against systematic errors being introduced at this stage. Discussion then follows between clinician and physicist or planning technician on the following:

1 Choice of treatment machine
2 Possible configuration of beams for treatment planning
3 Dose specification point
4 Prescribed target dose, maximum and minimum doses acceptable, maximum permissible doses to vital organs outlined on the plan
5 Need for bolus (e.g. to maximise skin dose)
6 Need for compensators, beam shaping.

Treatment machines

Megavoltage treatment machines include cobalt-60 machines producing 1.25 MV gamma irradiation and linear accelerators operating between 4 and 25 MV. These vary in their build-up depth (D_{max}) and percentage depth dose characteristics, as well as other features such as availability of half-beam blocking, or multileaf collimators, ease of lead shielding, rotational facility, effect of penumbra on beam definition and couch attachments. Cobalt units produce beams of less penetration than linear accelerators, have less skin sparing and a greater penumbra, longer treatment times but require less maintenance.

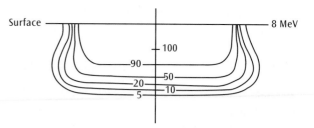

Figure 52.12 *Isodose curves for an 8 MeV electron beam 10 cm × 10 cm.*

Electron therapy may be useful for single-field treatments of superficial tumours, particularly where sparing of underlying cartilage or bone is important (e.g. nose, ear). High-energy electron beams (15–25 MeV) are used in the treatment of head and neck tumours, such as cervical lymph nodes, thyroid carcinomas and parotid tumours, to avoid dose to the underlying spinal cord. Electron beams have a sharp fall off in dose beyond the 90 per cent isodose and so the energy of the electron is chosen to encompass the target volume by the 90–95 per cent isodose. The effective treatment depth in centimetres is approximately one-third of the beam energy in MeV, and total range about half, dependent on field size (Fig. 52.12).

Electron beams provide a small amount of skin sparing and if this is not required, then bolus material must be used to increase dose to the skin surface. The volume included by the 90 per cent isodose is less than the field size on the surface, and hence wider margins must be allowed when delineating the target volume. However, at depth, the 40 per cent isodoses and below tend to bow outwards so increasing dose laterally. If the target volume is near a critical structure such as the eye, shielding against lateral scatter must be applied or an alternative modality of treatment be considered. Doses beyond cavities may be higher than expected even after density corrections, e.g. when using electron therapy to treat the chest wall after mastectomy where there is lung beneath the ribs.

Configuration of beams

SINGLE FIELD

A single megavoltage field may be used for palliative treatment, e.g. bone metastases, for ease of set-up and convenience to the patient. The fall off of dose across the target volume produces an inhomogeneous effect, but this is adequate for achieving pain relief. However, the site of the lesion, e.g. vertebral metastasis, must be considered when specifying the dose, as well as the dose-limiting structure, e.g. spinal cord. Table 52.1 shows the variations in the depth of the spinal cord along with the vertebral column and differences in percentage depth dose from different megavoltage machines. If the dose is prescribed as an 'applied dose', i.e. 100 per cent at the D_{max}, then the dose to the anterior vertebral body may be inadequate.

Table 52.1 *Variation in depth of spinal cord along the vertebral column and differences in percentage depth doses from treatment machines*

Structure	Depth (cm)	Percentage depth dose	
		Cobalt-60	6 MV
Cervical canal	5	75–80	83–88
Thoracic canal	6	70–75	81
Lumbar canal	7	65–70	79
Lumbar vertebral body	10	52–57	64

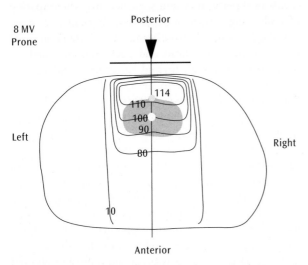

Figure 52.13 *Isodose distribution from an 8 MV single direct posterior beam. Centre of target volume (100 per cent) is ICRU dose specification point, maximum dose = 114 per cent, minimum dose = 90 per cent.*

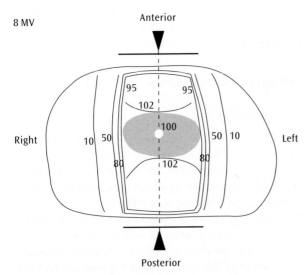

Figure 52.14 *Isodose distribution from 8 MV opposing anterior and posterior beams. Centre of target volume (100 per cent), maximum dose = 102 per cent, minimum dose = 95 per cent.*

For megavoltage irradiation the ICRU dose specification point, which lies at the centre of the target volume, is therefore chosen and the maximum and minimum doses carefully recorded (Fig. 52.13).

OPPOSING FIELDS

The isodose distribution from two parallel opposing fields (Fig. 52.14) is not homogeneous, does not conform well to the target volume and irradiates much normal tissue to the same dose or greater than the tumour. Hence this technique is more commonly used for palliative treatments. However, for tumours such as the larynx and hypopharynx, opposing lateral fields with the use of wedges often give a satisfactory distribution for the target volume and may be ideal for radical treatment. Doses are prescribed at the midplane point on the central axis of the beam. It must be remembered that there is narrowing of the isodoses in the centre of the volume and hence a larger field size on the skin must be chosen to adequately treat a central volume. The maximum dose occurs peripherally due to the build-up effects, and care must be taken to ensure that this dose is calculated as it may lie over a vital structure, e.g. spinal cord. ICRU Report 50 requires the midplane dose and maximum and minimum doses as specified doses for opposing fields.

The applied dose to each field is determined from depth dose charts, which are available for each field size for each treatment machine and are normalized to 100 per cent at the depth of maximum build-up for a $10 \times 10\,cm$ field at the standard SSD. When irregular or rectangular fields are used, the contribution from scattered irradiation is different from that from square fields, and tables must therefore be consulted to obtain equivalent square fields.

Sample calculation for parallel opposing fields treated on 6 MV linear accelerator, using an isocentric technique

Field size $= 12 \times 17\,cm$
Equivalent square $= 14\,cm^2$
Interplanar distance (separation of patient) $= 18\,cm$
Depth of midpoint $= 9\,cm$
Midpoint corresponds to centre of target volume (ICRU point) and is therefore placed at the isocentre.

$$SSD = 100 - 9 = 91\,cm$$

Output factor for a $14\,cm^2$ field at $9\,cm = 0.86$.
For 2 Gy per fraction at ICRU dose specification point

$$\text{monitor units per field} = \frac{100}{0.86} = 116.$$

MULTIPLE FIELDS

Combinations of two, three or more fields are commonly used for most radical treatments (Fig. 52.15). Wedges are used to alter the dose distribution to compensate for missing tissue due to body contour (Figs 52.16a, b) and to avoid high dose areas when beams are combined. Wedges attenuate the beam and hence, for the same incident dose, a greater number of monitor units are set compared with when an open field is used. In order to concentrate dose at the target volume and reduce dose to critical organs, 'weighting' may be used so that different amounts of radiation are given by each of the beams. Compensators may be designed individually and placed in the beam to correct dose inhomogeneity due to obliquity of body contour and varying depth of the target volume in the patient (e.g. oesophagus). Compensators are often made of aluminium alloy as this makes them easy to handle.

BEAM SHAPING

Conventional shielding is achieved by cerrobend blocks which may be standard shapes or individually designed

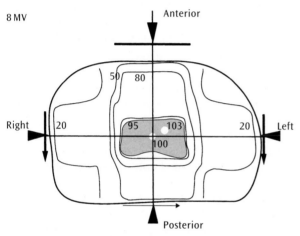

Figure 52.15 *Isodose distribution from 8 MV linear accelerator, anterior, posterior and two lateral beams. Centre of target volume ICRU dose specification point = 100 per cent, maximum target volume = 103 per cent, minimum target volume = 95 per cent.*

for each patient. For the mantle technique, blocks are made to allow for beam divergence to improve the accuracy of shielding at the interface between beam and block (Dobbs *et al.*, 1999). Half-beam blocking can be achieved with independent collimator jaws, eliminating divergence so that a straight beam edge can be used. Multileaf collimators provide detailed and dynamic beam shaping and, if available, can be used instead of cerrobend blocks with reduction in treatment delivery times. The beam's eye view facility may improve selection of field configurations and provides detailed information about the projection of the beam in relation to normal organs. However, the use of field shaping to match the target volume is dependent on the reliability of CT interpretation and the accuracy of definition of margins around the tumour. Great care must be used to ensure that elaborate shielding does not inadvertently obscure dose to the tumour.

HETEROGENEITY CORRECTIONS

Lung tissue attenuates the radiation beam less than other soft tissues and this factor alters both the shape of the dose distribution and the value of the isodoses. For irradiation of tumours of the breast, chest wall, lung, oesophagus, etc. in the thorax it is recommended that the lung tissue is localized on to the outline with the target volume. Either a correction factor of 0.25–0.3 can be applied or, using CT planning, a pixel by pixel correction can be made, taking into account the presence of pleural fluid, atelectasis and other abnormal as well as normal lung densities. It is not usually necessary to make similar corrections in the pelvis, as differences may be variable, e.g. gas in the bowel and rectum. If iodinated contrast medium has been used for CT planning scans (e.g. to outline small bowel or bladder), this may affect heterogeneity corrections if they are applied automatically, thereby introducing an error.

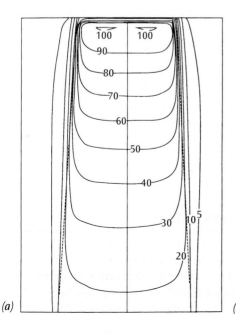

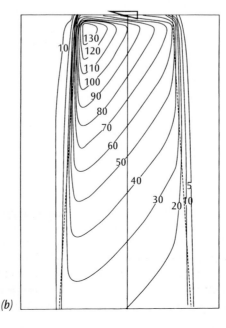

(a)   *(b)*

Figure 52.16 *(a) 12 cm × 12 cm 6 MV open field; (b) same field with 60° wedge.*

Choice of dose specification

The International Commission for Radiation Units and Measurements (ICRU) published Report 50 in 1993 (Landberg *et al.*, 1993) to encourage a common international language for the reporting and recording of radiation dose. The ICRU dose specification point is chosen at the centre of the target volume because it is easy to determine, is representative of the dose distribution and does not lie in a peripheral steep dose gradient. This point frequently lies on the central axis of the beam or intersection of the beams, where the dose is more accurately defined. It is essential that the dose at the dose specification point is accompanied by the maximum and minimum target doses in order to describe the homogeneity of the irradiation throughout the target volume. Ideally this variation should be limited to ±5 per cent, depending on the clinical situation. The minimum target dose is an important parameter because it correlates with the probability of tumour control. However, there is heterogeneity of tumour cell population throughout the target volume, commonly with the highest cell density at the centre of the GTV and the lowest cell density at the periphery of the clinical target volume. Although it is difficult to predict the biological effect of a given dose because of these variations, it is important to have an internationally accepted method of dose specification in order to assess effectiveness of treatment and to allow intercomparison between radiotherapy centres.

Traditionally, many centres use the minimum isodose around the target volume as a dose specification point. However, this has several disadvantages. The minimum isodose frequently lies in a region of steep dose gradient at the periphery of the volume and it also lies at the edge of the beam, where calculation of dose is less accurate than on the central axis of the beam. The minimum isodose lies on the periphery of the target volume where there is great interclinician variability as to its site and size and where the cell density is believed to be lowest. The minimum isodose may also be 10–15 per cent lower than the maximum isodose and, as such, is not a good description of the entire target volume. The use of the ICRU dose specification point is therefore recommended for prescribing doses, as well as reporting and recording to allow comparison between treatment centres.

If changes are made in a radiotherapy department from specifying dose at the minimum isodose to the new ICRU point, then for each treatment technique, dose plans should be normalized both to the old and new specification point and a clinical decision made as to whether there needs to be a change in the prescribed dose. For example, if a dose of 50 Gy has hitherto been given to the minimum or 90 per cent isodose, this will have given a dose of 55 Gy to the 100 per cent isodose. If the dose specification point is changed to the intersection of the beams, and this lies on or near the 100 per cent isodose, then a decision has to be made as to whether the dose prescription is changed

to 55 Gy to the new dose specification point, which will give the same clinical result. For three-dimensional treatment plans it is recommended that the dose at the ICRU point, maximum and minimum doses and, in addition, the mean dose and dose-volume histograms are all recorded in order to describe the treatment in three dimensions.

VERIFICATION OF TREATMENT

On the first day of treatment all the treatment planning parameters are checked and the patient is positioned on the treatment couch according to the instructions on the treatment prescription sheet, which includes details of immobilization, fixation devices, position of the arms, full or empty bladder, and a photograph as a helpful visual record. Laser beams are used to align the patient according to permanent skin tattoos in both the midline and lateral planes in order to ensure reproducibility of the treatment set-up. Machine parameters are checked and treatment verified, both for geometry and for dose delivered. Geometric verification can be achieved with a radiograph taken on the treatment unit (portal film) or by real-time visualization of the patient using an on-line electronic portal imaging device. Local guidelines must be drawn up as to acceptable limits of variation, as these should correlate with the margin around the clinical target volume which has been chosen to ensure that the planning target volume allows for day-to-day variability. *In vivo* dosimetry can be performed using either lithium fluoride thermoluminescent dosimetry or silicon diodes, and this provides a final check of the overall accuracy of the dose delivered.

A quality assurance programme for therapy equipment and simulators includes check of geometry, dosimetry, beam data, wedges and other accessories. National and regional dosimetry intercomparison studies between centres ensure the validity of output measurements. Quality-control protocols for computerized planning systems should be adhered to, in order to provide accurate dose planning calculations. Radiographers are instructed in the importance of daily checks on patient positioning using laser alignment, measurement of patient separation, fitting the immobilization devices and attention to detailed instructions for individual patients. The aim of an ongoing quality assurance programme is to eliminate any errors during the multiple steps in the planning and delivery of radiation treatment and is an essential part of the work of a radiation oncology department.

SIGNIFICANT POINTS

- The choice of equipment used for localization will depend on the workload and range of patients and tumour sites to be treated, the techniques employed in planning and irradiation and the resources available.

- It has been shown that CT scanning information alters the radiation fields used in approximately 30 per cent of patients receiving radical radiotherapy treatment.
- The process of determining tumour and target volumes for treatment of malignant disease consists of several distinct steps, which have been well described in ICRU Report 50 (Landberg et al., 1993) and ICRU Report 62 (Landberg et al., 1999).
- Integration of CT, MRI and SPECT/PET data using image registration may revolutionize the acquisition of clinical and tumour data.
- Brahme et al. (1988) and Mijnheer et al. (1987) suggested that the requirement for accuracy should be 3.5 per cent, one standard deviation, in the dose value at the specification point in the target volume.
- The ICRU dose specification point is chosen at the centre of the target volume because it is easy to determine, representative of the dose distribution and does not lie in a peripheral steep dose gradient.
- It is essential that the dose at the dose specification point is accompanied by the maximum and minimum target doses in order to describe the homogeneity of the irradiation throughout the target volume.
- For three-dimensional treatment plans, it is recommended that the dose at the ICRU point, maximum and minimum doses and, in addition, the mean dose and dose-volume histogram are all recorded.
- The aim of an ongoing quality assurance programme is to eliminate any errors during the multiple steps in the planning and delivery of radiation treatment and is an essential part of a radiation oncology department.

KEY REFERENCES

Dobbs, J., Barrett, A. and Ash, D. (1999) Basic principles of treatment planning. In Dobbs, J., Barrett, A. and Ash, D. (eds), *Practical radiotherapy planning* (3rd edn). London: Arnold.

Hurkmans, C.W., Remeijer, P., Lebesque, J.V. and Mijnheer, B.J. (2001) Set-up verification using portal imaging: review of current clinical practice. *Radiother. Oncol.* **58**, 105–20.

Husband, J.E.S. and Reznek, R.H. (eds) (1998) *Imaging in oncology* vols I and II. Oxford: Isis Medical Media.

Landberg, T., Chavaudra, J., Dobbs, H.J. et al. (1999) International Commission on Radiation Units and Measurements, ICRU Report 62, Supplement to ICRU Report 50. *Prescribing, recording, and reporting photon beam therapy*. Bethesda, Maryland: ICRU.

REFERENCES

Ash, D.V., Andrews, B. and Stubbs, B. (1983) A method for integrating a CT scanner into radiotherapy planning and treatment. *Clin. Radiol.* **34**, 99–101.

Balter, J.M., Sandler, H.M., Lam, K. et al. (1995) Measurement of prostate movement over the course of routine radiotherapy using implanted markers. *Int. J. Radiat. Oncol. Biol. Phys.* **31**, 113–18.

Beard, C.J., Kijewski, P., Bussiere, M. et al. (1996) Analysis of prostate and seminal vesicle motion: implications for treatment planning. *Int. J. Radiat. Oncol. Biol. Phys.* **34**, 451–8.

Bel, A., Bartelink, H., Vijlbrief, R.E. and Lebesque, J. (1994) Transfer errors of planning CT to simulator: a possible source of set-up inaccuracies? *Radiother. Oncol.* **31**, 176–80.

Bornstein, B.A., Cheng, C.W., Rhodes, L.M. et al. (1990) Can simulation measurements be used to predict the irradiated lung volume in the tangential fields in patients treated for breast cancer? *Int. J. Radiat. Oncol. Biol. Phys.* **18**, 181–7.

Brahme, A., Chavaudra, J. and Landberg, T. et al. (1988) Accuracy requirements and quality assurance of external beam therapy with photons and electrons. *Acta Oncol.* **27**(suppl. 1).

Catton, C., Lebar, L., Warde, P. et al. (1997) Improvement in total positioning error for lateral prostatic fields using a soft immobilisation device. *Radiother. Oncol.* **44**(3), 265–70.

Chassagne, D., Dutreix, J. and Dutreix, A. (1976) Report on a systematic overdosage of patients in 1970 and 1971. Internal report, Institut Gustave Roussy, Villejuif.

Dearnaley, D., Shoo, V., Norman, A. et al. (1999) Comparison of radiation side-effects of conformal and conventional radiotherapy in prostate cancer: a randomised trial. *Lancet* **353**, 267–71.

Denham, J.W., Hamilton, C.S., Joseph, D.J. et al. (1992) The use of simulator and CT information in the planning of radiotherapy for non-small cell lung cancer: Australasian patterns of practice study. *Lung Cancer* **8**, 275–84.

Dobbs, H.J. (1993) From GTV (Gross Tumour Volume) to PTV (Planning Tumour Volume). In Minet, P. (ed.), *Three dimensional treatment planning*. Proceedings of 5th Workshop organized by Commission Informatique, European Association of Radiology, Liège.

Dobbs, H.J. and Parker, R.P. (1984) The respective roles of the simulator and computed tomography in radiotherapy planning: a review. *Clin. Radiol.* **35**, 433–9.

Dobbs, H.J. and Webb, S. (1988) Clinical applications of X-ray computed tomography in radiotherapy planning. In Webb, S. (ed.), *The physics of medical imaging*. Bristol: Adam Hilger.

Dobbs, J., Barrett, A. and Ash, D. (1999) Basic principles of treatment planning. In Dobbs, J., Barrett, A. and Ash, D. (eds), *Practical Radiotherapy Planning* (3rd edn). London: Arnold.

Dobbs, H.J., Parker, R.P., Hodson, N.J. *et al.* (1983) The use of CT in radiotherapy treatment planning. *Radiother. Oncol.* **1**, 133–41.

Dutreix, A. (1984) When and how can we improve precision in radiotherapy? *Radiother. Oncol.* **2**, 275–92.

Ekberg, L., Holmberg, O., Wittgren, L. *et al.* (1998) What margins should be added to the clinical target volume in radiotherapy treatment planning for lung cancer? *Radiother. Oncol.* **48**, 71–7.

Fiorino, C., Reni, M., Bolognesi, A. *et al.* (1998) Set-up error in supine positioned patients immobilised with two different modalities during conformal radiotherapy of prostate cancer. *Radiother. Oncol.* **49**, 133–41.

Gagliardi, G., Lax, I. and Rutqvist, L.E. (1992) Radiation therapy of stage 1 breast cancer: analysis of treatment technique accuracy using three dimensional treatment planning tools. *Radiother. Oncol.* **24**, 94–101.

Goitein, M. (1979) The utility of computed tomography in radiation therapy: an estimate of outcome. *Int. J. Radiat. Oncol. Biol. Phys.* **5**, 1799–807.

Goitein, M. (1982) Applications of computed tomography in radiotherapy treatment planning. *Progr. Med. Radiat. Phys.* New York: Plenum Press, 195–287.

Graham, J.D., Warrington, A.P., Gill, S.S. and Brada, M. (1991) A non invasive, relocatable sterotactic frame for fractionated radiotherapy and multiple imaging. *Radiother. Oncol.* **21**, 60–2.

Griffiths, S.E., Khoury, G.G. and Eddy, A. (1991) Quality control of radiotherapy during pelvic irradiation. *Radiother. Oncol.* **20**, 203–6.

Harris, S.J. and Buchanan, R.B. (1998) An audit and evaluation of bladder movements during radical radiotherapy. *Clin. Oncol.* **10**, 262–4.

Helyer, S.J., Moskovic, E., Ashley, S. *et al.* (1999) A study testing the routine use of ultrasound measurements when selecting the electron energy for breast boost radiotherapy. *Clin. Oncol.* **11**(3), 164–8.

Holmberg, O., Huizenga, H., Idzes, M.H.M. *et al.* (1994) *In vivo* determination of the accuracy of field matching in breast cancer irradiation using an electronic portal imaging device. *Radiother. Oncol.* **33**, 157–66.

Hurkmans, C.W., Borger, J.H., Bos, L.J. *et al.* (2000) Cardiac and lung complication probabilities after breast cancer irradiation. *Radiother. Oncol.* **55**, 145–51.

Hurkmans, C.W., Remeijer, P., Lebesque, J.V. and Mijnheer, B.J. (2001) Set-up verification using portal imaging: review of current clinical practice. *Radiother. Oncol.* **58**, 105–20.

Husband, J.E.S. and Reznek, R.H. (eds) (1998) *Imaging in oncology* vols I and II. Oxford: Isis Medical Media.

Husband, J.E.S., Johnson, R.J. and Reznek, R.H. (1999) *A guide to the practical use of MRI in oncology*. Board of the Faculty of Clinical Radiology, The Royal College of Radiologists, London.

Landberg, T., Chavaudra, J., Dobbs, H.J. *et al.* (1993) International Commission on Radiation Units and Measurements ICRU Report 50. *Prescribing, recording, and reporting photon beam therapy*. Bethesda, Maryland: ICRU.

Landberg, T., Chavaudra, J., Dobbs, H.J. *et al.* (1999) International Commission on Radiation Units and Measurements, ICRU Report 62, Supplement to ICRU Report 50. *Prescribing, recording, and reporting photon beam therapy*. Bethesda, Maryland: ICTU.

Leunens, G., Menten, J., Weltens, C., Verstraete, J. and Van der Scheuren, E. (1993) Quality assessment of medical decision making in radiation oncology: variability in target volume delineation for brain tumours. *Radiother. Oncol.* **29**, 169–75.

McKenzie, A.L. (2000) How should breathing motion be combined with other errors when drawing margins around clinical target volumes? *Br. J. Radiol.* **73**, 973–7.

McKenzie, A.L., Van Herk, M. and Mijnheer, B. (2000) The width of margins in radiotherapy treatment plans. *Phys. Med. Biol.* **45**(11), 3331–42.

Mijnheer, B.J., Battermann, J.J. and Wambersie, A. (1987) What degree of accuracy is required and can be achieved in photon and neutron therapy? *Radiother. Oncol.* **8**, 237–52.

Mitine, C., Dutreix, A. and Van der Schueren, E. (1991) Tangential breast irradiation: influence of technique of set up on transfer errors and reproducibility. *Radiother. Oncol.* **22**, 308–10.

Neal, A.J. and Yarnold, J.R. (1995) Estimating the volume of lung irradiated during tangential breast irradiation using the central lung distance. *Br. J. Radiol.* **68**, 1004–8.

Perez, C.A., Purdy, J.A., Harris, W. *et al.* (1995) Three-dimensional treatment planning and conformal radiation therapy: preliminary evaluation. *Radiother. Oncol.* **36**, 32–43.

Rasch, C., Barillot, I., Remeijer, P. *et al.* (1999) Definition of the prostate in CT and MRI: a multi-observer study. *Int. J. Radiat. Oncol. Biol. Phys.* **43**(1), 57–66.

Rosenman, J.G., Miller, E.P., Tracton, G. and Cullip, T.J. (1998) Image registration: an essential part of radiation therapy treatment planning. *Int. J. Radiat. Oncol. Biol. Phys.* **40**(1), 197–205.

Rosenthal, S.A., Galvin, J.M., Goldwein, J.W. *et al.* (1992) Improved methods for determination of variability in patient positioning for radiation therapy using simulation and serial portal film measurements. *Int. J. Radiat. Oncol. Biol. Phys.* **23**, 621–5.

Rothwell, R.I., Ash, D.V. and Thorogood, J. (1985) An analysis of the contribution of computed tomography to the treatment outcome in bladder cancer. *Clin. Radiol.* **36**, 369–72.

Seddon, B., Bidmead, M., Wilson, J., Khoo, V. and Dearnaley, D. (2000) Target volume definition in conformal radiotherapy for prostate cancer: quality assurance in the MRC RT-01 trial. *Radiother. Oncol.* **56**, 73–83.

Soffen, D., Hanks, G., Huang, C. and Chu, J. (1991) Conformal static field therapy for low volume low grade prostate cancer with rigid immobilisation. *Int. J. Radiat. Oncol. Biol. Phys.* **20**, 141–6.

Song, P., Washington, M. and Vaida, F. (1996) A comparison of four patients immobilisation devices and the treatment of prostate cancer patients with three-dimensional conformal radiotherapy. *Int. J. Radiat. Oncol. Biol. Phys.* **34**, 213–19.

Studholme, C., Hill, D.L. and Hawkes, D.J. (1997) Automated three-dimensional registration of magnetic resonance and positron emission tomography brain images by multi-resolution optimisation of voxel similarity measures. *Med. Phys.* **24**(1), 25–35.

Sur, R.K., Clinkard, J., Jones, W.G. *et al.* (1993) Changes in target volume during radiotherapy treatment of invasive bladder carcinoma. *Clin. Oncol.* **5**, 30–3.

Ten Haken, R.K., Former, J.D., Heimberger, D.K. *et al.* (1991) Treatment planning issues related to prostate movement in response to differential filling of the rectum and bladder. *Int. J. Radiat. Oncol. Biol. Phys.* **20**, 1317–24.

Tsujii, H., Kamada, T., Matsuoka, Y. *et al.* (1989). The value of treatment planning using CT and an immobilising shell in radiotherapy for paranasal sinus carcinomas. *Int. J. Radiat. Oncol. Biol. Phys.* **16**, 243–9.

Turner, S.L., Swindell, R., Bowl, N. *et al.* (1997) Bladder movement during radiation therapy for bladder cancer: implications for treatment planning. *Int. J. Radiat. Oncol. Biol. Phys.* **39**(2), 355–60.

Urie, M.M., Goitein, M., Doppke, K. *et al.* (1991) The role of uncertainty analysis in treatment planning. *Int. J. Radiat. Oncol. Biol. Phys.* **21**, 91–107.

Van Herk, M. and Kooy, H.M. (1994) Automatic three-dimensional correlation of CT-CT, CT-MRI and CT-SPECT using chamfer matching. *Med. Phys.* **21**, 1163–78.

Van Herk, M., Bruce, A., Krocs, A.P.G. *et al.* (1995) Quantification of organ motion during conformal radiotherapy of the prostate by three dimensional (3D) image registration. *Int. J. Radiat. Oncol. Biol. Phys.* **33**, 1311–20.

Van Tienhoven, G., Lanson, J.H., Crabeels, D. *et al.* (1991) Accuracy in tangential breast treatment set-up: a portal imaging study. *Radiother. Oncol.* **22**, 317–22.

Verellen, D., Vinh-Hung, V., Bijdekerke, P. *et al.* (1999) Characteristics and clinical application of a treatment simulator with CT-option. *Radiother. Oncol.* **50**, 355–66.

Vincent, D., Beckham, W. and Delaney, G. (1999) An assessment of the number of CT slices necessary to plan breast radiotherapy. *Radiother. Oncol.* **52**, 179–83.

Zelefsky, M.J., Crean, D., Mageras, G.S. *et al.* (1999) Quantification and predictors of prostate position variability in 50 patients evaluated with multiple CT scans during conformal radiotherapy. *Radiother. Oncol.* **50**, 225–34.

Conformal therapy

DIANA M. TAIT

INTRODUCTION

Radiotherapy practice has always strived to use available technology to ensure that the high-dose volume conforms as closely as possible to the target volume. Until relatively recently efforts were limited by the constraints of two-dimensional treatment planning and coplanar, isocentric, static treatment fields. The application of computer technology to radiotherapy planning and treatment delivery has, however, revolutionized traditional concepts and capabilities in this area, the practical application of which has become known as conformal therapy. This is a generic term which does not describe a specific technique or approach, but one which encompasses a series of variable complementary components. In general, and as far as external-beam radiotherapy is concerned, the constituents of conformal therapy can be considered under three main headings: three-dimensional planning, treatment execution and treatment verification. The technical section of this chapter will deal with each of these components in turn.

As a treatment modality, radiotherapy can be considered to have failed whenever tumour is not controlled locally or when normal tissue toxicity is 'unacceptable'. Unfortunately there is an inextricable relationship between these two, so that increasing tumour control generally leads to increased toxicity. Ideally, developments should aim to separate the two and provide both an improvement in local control rates, while, at the same time, decreasing toxicity. In theory, conformal radiotherapy offers the possibility to achieve this. Provided sufficient normal tissue can be spared to permit the target dose to be escalated, then local tumour control rates might be expected to improve and, at the same time, be accompanied either

by equivalent, or reduced, toxicity when compared with conventional treatments. This is an exciting scenario in itself, but its significance becomes emphasized when considering the impact that improving local control would have for certain tumour sites where such an outcome might also be accompanied by improved survival (Suit and Westgate, 1986; Lawton *et al.*, 1991; Armstrong *et al.*, 1997). For these potential benefits to become a reality there are two essential prerequisites: a volume effect for normal tissue toxicity, and a dose–response effect for tumour control. The biological section of this chapter will discuss these two components.

BIOLOGICAL BACKGROUND

Volume effect for normal tissues

The radiation dose that can be delivered to tumours is generally determined by the radiation tolerance of the adjacent normal tissues. Only for very radiosensitive tumours, such as Hodgkin's lymphoma and seminoma, is the effective dose range such that normal tissues rarely influence the dose prescribed. For the majority of tumours, radiation doses above those currently used in standard practice cannot safely be delivered unless normal tissues can be protected or excluded in some way. Reliable clinical dose–response information for normal tissues is difficult to establish. The only certain way to avoid radiation to normal tissues is to avoid radiation altogether. However, the limited data available suggest that dose–response curves are steep within the dose range employed for curative radiotherapy (Dearnaley *et al.*, 1997; Nguyen *et al.*, 1998). This makes it very likely that any increase in target dose will be accompanied by a significant increase in normal tissue toxicity. Radiotherapists tend to have a working code for the tolerance dose of individual normal tissues and organs, which is based on collective and personal experience. A number of variables such as fractionation, patient age, concurrent chemotherapy and the volume of normal tissue irradiated are known to have some influence on these values. For example, the tolerance dose for many organs appears to increase as the irradiated volume of that organ decreases, although there are few good clinical data to support this clinical impression. However, the available data in the radiotherapy literature with regard to tolerance dose for uniform whole or partial organ irradiation have been compiled for 28 critical normal tissues (Emami et al., 1991). Unfortunately, in practice, treatment plans rarely involve uniform irradiation of critical organs. Algorithms have therefore been developed which transform dose–volume histogram information into equivalent uniform partial organ irradiation data.

The mechanisms underlying normal tissue damage are not fully understood. However, it has been suggested that tissue architecture may be important in determining tolerance dose for partially irradiated structures (Withers et al., 1988). It is envisaged that individual cells within an organ may be arranged in functional subunits (FSUs) and it is the integrity of a sufficient number of these subunits that determines functional capacity of that organ. It is hypothesized that, for some organs, FSUs are structurally defined so that, for example, in the kidney the FSU would be the nephron and in the lung the acinus. For organs such as skin and mucosae the FSU is structurally undefined but can be considered as the area or volume that can be repopulated from a single surviving clonogen. Using this model, the number of clonogenic cells in an FSU, whether it be structurally defined or not, has an important influence on the tolerance dose of that organ or tissue.

The model has been developed further in terms of a volume effect on the dose–response curves for normal tissue by considering the arrangement of FSUs within a particular tissue. It is envisaged that, for certain end points in some organs, FSUs are arranged 'in series' and consequently damage to a single FSU is sufficient to produce functional failure. Myelitis of the spinal cord and stricture of the bowel are examples of complications that are thought to result from the arrangement of FSUs in series (Schultheiss et al., 1983; Wolbarst, 1984; Niemierko and Goitein, 1993). The alternative arrangement for FSUs is that they be 'in parallel'. This is thought to be the case for organs such as lung, kidney and liver, where it is hypothesized that the complications of pneumonitis, nephritis and liver failure will only occur if a sufficient number of FSUs are damaged (Wolbarst et al., 1982; Jackson et al., 1993; Niemierko and Goitein, 1993; Yorke et al., 1993). At present there is considerable interest and activity in using these, and other hypotheses, to perform modelling exercises. A model may be thought of as a means of defining a synthetic system which, hopefully, closely mimics the true situation. In conformal therapy, models are currently being applied to investigate the two major outcomes of treatment; probability of tumour control (TCP) and probability of normal tissue complication (NTCP). Some of the work on modelling in this area is summarized later in this chapter.

Reliable clinical data supporting a volume effect, or describing a dose–response relationship for normal tissue complications, are few. A number of older studies, using field size as an indicator of normal tissue inclusion, support the suggestion that volume does have an effect. However, these studies provide a very crude measure of normal tissue volumes and it is only with the introduction of three-dimensional planning that it has been possible to make a more accurate assessment. For example, in a study of small bowel tolerance, computed tomography (CT) was used to measure small bowel volumes which were then correlated with late side-effects. A volume effect was, in fact, demonstrated and was of the order of magnitude such that, if the small bowel volume was increased by a factor of two, the total dose had to be reduced by 17 per cent in order to maintain the same incidence of small bowel complications (Letschert et al., 1990). More recently, a randomized trial in prostate cancer demonstrated less proctitis and rectal bleeding in patients treated in the conformal arm of the trial which excluded significant rectal volume from the target (Dearnaley et al., 1999).

The increasing use of three-dimensional planning will hopefully provide more data of this sort for all sites of treatment, but its reliability will depend upon a number of factors, probably, most importantly, the accurate documentation of side-effects of treatment.

Dose–response effect for tumour control

The rationale behind attempting to escalate tumour dose lies in the assumption that the dose–response curve for human tumours is steep, as indicated by theoretical modelling based on random cell killing. For obvious ethical reasons reliable clinical dose–response data are scanty. However, for those human tumours on which data are available, the slope of the tumour control probability curve is shallower than might be expected (Williams et al., 1984), although these and similar data currently available are crude, on two accounts. First, in any individual study the tumours included are heterogeneous with respect to a number of biological parameters which, at present, are difficult to identify and select for. Secondly, the dose information used in these analyses has, by necessity, been extremely limited. It will not be until large groups of patients have been studied, with the sort of detailed dose information available from three-dimensional planning, that the question of a dose–response can be truly addressed. As a result of the patient, tumour and dosimetry mix, any benefit from a 10 per cent dose escalation is unlikely to be detected by current clinical investigations. Reviewing published data on human tumours, it was estimated that up to 300 patients would be required per dose level in order to detect any benefit from a 10 per cent dose escalation in tumours controlled at the 50 per cent level by conventional doses (Thames *et al.*, 1992). In the same review, a mathematical model was used to see what effect selecting tumours on the basis of radiosensitivity, as measured by SF_2 (surviving fraction at 2 Gy), would have on the steepness of the dose–response curve. The model predicts that selecting a more homogeneous tumour population in this way would allow the benefit of dose escalation to be demonstrated with far fewer patients. This, in conjunction with selection of more homogeneous patient groups with respect to dose, as is now available in three-dimensional planning, should provide much purer data on dose response. The question of tumour heterogeneity is currently under scrutiny and better understanding of this issue should improve the robustness, and hence clinical usefulness, of the models (Brahme and Agren, 1987; Fenwick, 1998).

Biological modelling for probability of outcome

The outcome of radiotherapy is generally measured in terms of the probability of controlling tumour (tumour control probability: TCP) and the probability of inducing a complication in the normal tissues (probability of normal tissue complication: NTCP). In accepting a treatment plan and prescribing a radiation dose the aim is to maximize TCP while, at the same time, keeping the NTCP at or below some defined 'acceptable' level. With conventional single-plane dosimetry it is relatively easy to compare and rank plans which offer different beam parameters, however inadequate this information obviously is. With the availability of three-dimensional dosimetry, the process of evaluation and optimization of treatment plans has become an enormously complex issue. The rationale for developing models based on radiobiological parameters is to allow this evaluation and scoring of treatment plans to be done in a more quantitative and clinically relevant manner, taking into account clinical and laboratory experience.

Modelling is currently a fashionable area of activity which is becoming increasingly sophisticated in mathematical terms (Caudry *et al.*, 1993; Niemierko and Goitein, 1993; Sanchez-Nieto and Nahum, 1999). However, in many respects models must be considered crude, and it is important to be aware of the consequent limitations. Any model is only as valid as the accuracy of the available data relating to the biological parameters on which it is based. For example, for the spinal cord, α/β ratio values from 1 to more than 5 Gy have been reported, a difference that could determine safety or disaster, depending on the value applied to the model (Withers and Taylor, 1993).

At the present time, models cannot be used for precise quantitative prediction of complication rates, either on an individual or population basis, because of the incorporation of a number of untested assumptions. However, they do perform a function; they highlight the sort of information that is needed to quantify the effects of inhomogeneous distributions of fractionated doses in various body structures. They have also facilitated a very exciting interaction between biology and physics which has the potential to improve the practice of radiotherapy.

TECHNICAL COMPONENTS

Three-dimensional planning

Computer technology has revolutionized the way in which, first, computed tomography (CT) and, more recently, magnetic resonance (MR) data can be assimilated for radiotherapy planning. The ability to reconstruct transaxial CT data and display the information in any chosen plane, gave rise to the concept of three-dimensional planning (Cook, 1981). Three-dimensional reconstruction of tumour, target volume and normal tissues in this way allows a far more complex appreciation of anatomical relationships (Plate 11). Despite these impressive advances, there is an inherent limitation in the process because of the current resolution of imaging techniques and their consequent inability to identify absolute boundaries between tumour and normal tissue. However, steady improvement is being made in this area and further information with regard to tumour extent may be reliably provided by techniques such as positron emission tomography (PET) and magnetic resonance spectroscopy (MRS). In the foreseeable future, however, it is unlikely that any single technique, or indeed combinations of technique, will provide an absolute distinction between malignant and non-malignant tissue, and radiotherapy planning must therefore continue to take into account histopathological and clinical data regarding the potential extent of tumour spread.

The adequate planning and treatment of individual patients, and also the reliable comparison of data between different centres, requires a clear understanding and universal application of the terms tumour volume, target volume and treatment volume for the successful development of conformal therapy (Fig. 53.1). These have been established definitely in the ICRU report 50 (1993) and ICRU report 62 (1999). Gross tumour volume (GTV) denotes tumour demonstrable either by palpation or imaging, and represents the highest density of clonogenic cells. Clinical target volume (CTV) denotes this demonstrable tumour (when present) but also includes volumes with suspected (subclinical) tumour, for example the margin around the GTV and regional lymph nodes, (N0 according to the TNM Classification (UICC, 1997)),

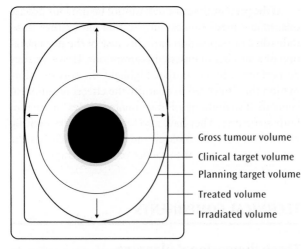

Figure 53.1 *Schematic representation of planning volumes as defined by ICRU 95 (reproduced with kind permission from ICRU).*

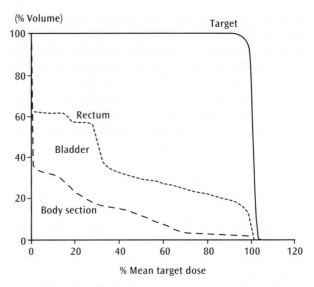

Figure 53.2 *Cumulative dose–volume diagram (dose–volume histogram, DVH). The ideal average of the target volume should be represented by a perfectly horizontal line falling to zero within a few per cent of the dose range around the 100 per cent target dose point. By comparison, organs at risk should be separated as far as possible from this line, with a rapid fall in percentage volume over the low target dose range, and with none, or only a very small percentage volume receiving 100 per cent of the target dose.*

considered to be at risk for microscopic disease spread and to need treatment. The requirements for inclusion of tissue in the CTV will vary, depending on the tumour type and its patterns of spread. Where the tumour has been removed surgically, there is no identifiable GTV and radiotherapy is based on the subclinical disease occupying a volume of tissue at risk, the CTV. Planning target volume (PTV) consists of the CTV and a margin to account for variations in size, shape and position of this target relative to the treatment beams. In the most recent ICRU report (ICRU 62, 1999) an attempt has been made to distinguish between the two components, physiological and technical, of the PTV. An internal margin (IM) is described, which allows for physiological variation in the shape, size and position of an organ. When added to the CTV, this margin describes the internal target volume (ITV). Typical organ movements include those caused by respiration, bladder filling and rectal distension, and are generally quite hard to measure. Technical variations are accommodated by a set-up margin (SM) and, ideally, these should be calculated locally for each treatment site and technique. This margin is easier to calculate but does require systematic verification studies which should form part of the quality assurance programme. By combining the IM and the SM, the appropriate margin can be added to the CTV to establish the PTV.

The PTV is thus a geometrical concept used to ensure that the CTV receives the prescribed dose despite unavoidable physiological and technical variations, and it is defined in relation to a fixed coordinate system. Note that in the example shown (Fig. 53.1) the magnitude of foreseen movements of the CTV is different in different directions. Treated volume is the volume that receives a dose that is considered important for local cure or palliation. Irradiated volume is the volume that receives a dose that is considered important for normal tissue tolerance (other than those specifically defined for organs at risk).

The challenge of conformal therapy is to be able to execute treatment plans that arrange for the high-dose volume to conform as closely as possible, in terms of shape and size, to the ideal target volume. In addition, dose variations throughout the high-dose volume, resulting from factors such as body contouring and tissue inhomogeneity, must be minimized to produce as uniform a dose distribution as possible. Conventional radiotherapy techniques are usually co-planar, isocentric and stationary. Three-dimensional treatment planning and computer control of treatment machines open up a range of possibilities with regard to technique. As a result, noncoplanar or dynamic treatments, or a combination of both features, are becoming used increasingly in conformal therapy. Also, because of the ability to develop complex therapies without operator intervention, there is now no practical or technical reason why 10, or even 20, fields at different gantry angles cannot be delivered under computer control. This greater flexibility of beam delivery has led to a revived interest in mathematical methods of planning the best treatment. Novel and interesting work has shown that combining several beams with a non-uniform profile can result in dose distributions that conform to high-dose volumes of virtually any shape, including concave volumes that wrap round, and even totally encircle, sensitive structures (Brahme, 1987; Webb, 1989). Dose–volume histograms (DVH) provide a means of describing, assessing and comparing individual treatment plans (Fig. 53.2). They allow a comparison of the radiation effect on different structures, including tumour and defined normal tissues. The correlation of dose–volume histogram data with acute and late normal tissue toxicity data is an important part of the process of defining a volume effect for normal tissues.

Treatment execution

The range of conformal treatment facilities and techniques under evaluation and in routine use is wide and cannot be covered comprehensively in this chapter. This section will therefore concentrate on those techniques that are already in clinical use and which are likely to become relatively widely available or which offer exciting possibilities.

FIELD SHAPING

Customized blocks

To produce the shapely treatment volumes required of conformal therapy, some form of field shaping is necessary. Standard collimator design limits radiation beams to square or rectangular shapes, but these can be modified by the insertion of custom-designed blocks within the path of the beam. Customized blocks of this kind have been in use for a long time, for example to protect the lungs in mantle irradiation, but it is only relatively recently that their construction has been based on three-dimensional CT information. This can be assimilated using a beam's-eye view (BEV) facility to appreciate the three-dimensional relationship between target and normal tissue structures within the trajectory of any single beam (Fig. 53.3). Customized blocks have the appeal that virtually all radiotherapy departments have block-making facilities which, if linked to a three-dimensional planning system, can form the basis of a conformal

technique. Although the availability of automatic block-cutting machines now makes the process less time consuming, shielding blocks are heavy and unwieldy and, in practice, are really limited to three or four-field plans.

Multileaf collimation

Optimized conformal radiotherapy may require the delivery of complex treatment plans incorporating multiple (more than four) shaped fields, non-coplanar fields and dynamically delivered arcs and rotations. To achieve this, a computer-controlled and -monitored treatment machine becomes a necessity and the multileaf collimator (MLC) provides such a capacity (Kallman *et al.*, 1988; Webb, 1992; Galvin *et al.*, 1993). This facility consists of many (typically 80) narrow blades or leaves of thickness sufficient to transmit only a small percentage of the incident radiation. The position of each leaf is controlled by a small motor and thus an irregular field outline can be achieved by remote control, removing the need to manually position heavy shielding in the beam path (Fernandez *et al.*, 1995) (Fig. 53.4). Manufacturers of linear accelerators now incorporate multileaf collimators as standard in their machines, but continue to refine the design. It seems likely that MLC beam shaping will become the most widely available means of delivering conformal therapy over the next 10 years.

Before an MLC is applied in clinical practice, consideration must be given as to whether the dose distribution produced by MLC-shaped fields is acceptable relative to that achieved with custom-designed blocks. The most important difference between these two forms of field shaping is the dosimetry of the penumbral region. The 'stepped' field edge produced by an MLC could be a significant disadvantage compared with the smoothly varying contour of a customized block. The isodose contours of an MLC field show a corresponding 'scalloping' effect with a periodicity that is a function of leaf width and the distance between adjacent leaves. A number of preclinical planning studies have addressed this concern (Galvin *et al.*, 1993; LoSasso *et al.*, 1993) and indicate

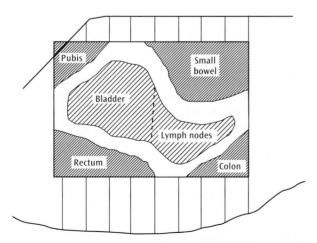

Figure 53.3 *Beam's-eye view of lateral field used to treat a target volume of bladder and lymph nodes. The customized blocks are shown and the normal tissue structure they protect is indicated in each case.*

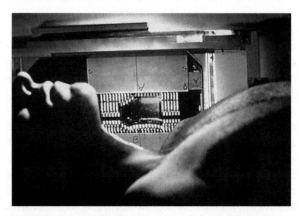

Figure 53.4 *A multileaf collimator (MLC) providing a shaped field for treatment of the neck.*

that, when multiple-field irradiation techniques are used, there is a negligible difference in dose distribution between traditional customized blocking and multileaf collimation for the same target volume. In addition, any differences between the two are generally smaller when more fields are used, because of the strong influence of the irradiation technique on the delivered dose distribution (Webb, 1992).

DYNAMIC THERAPY

The term, 'dynamic therapy' has been coined to describe treatment set-ups that incorporate adjustment of machine parameters while the radiation beam is turned on. To this extent rotation therapy is a form of dynamic therapy, but computer control of all machine parameters will allow far greater versatility. At the present time there are a number of 'simple' applications of dynamic therapy in clinical practice. For example, software control can allow independent movement of the collimator pairs to produce the equivalent of a wedged field. In practice, this is done by moving the appropriate single collimator across the field so that the beam intensity varies as it would by the introduction of a manual wedge. However, as more than one collimator can be adjusted at the same time, the effect can simulate those of a customized compensator. The independent collimator action can also be used to produce shaped fields (Thiel *et al.*, 1988). This is achieved by considering the target volume as a series of consecutive segments, for each of which the collimators can be adjusted to give adequate coverage. Segments can either be treated by a series of static fields or the collimators can be adjusted while the beam is being swept along the length of the target volume. At the present time the software required to perform the latter is not available for clinical use.

The tracking cobalt unit provides another example of dynamic therapy, and this has been most applied to improve dosimetry in treatment of the spinal cord (Tate and Shentall, 1989). By moving the couch in the horizontal plane the cobalt beam can be made to follow the length of the spinal cord, removing the necessity for junctioning adjacent fields and the consequent dose uncertainties that this introduces. At the same time, the couch can be moved in the vertical plane so that the target volume is kept at a fixed distance from the source, thus improving the dose uniformity without having to construct a tissue compensator.

At the other end of the spectrum, in terms of complexity of dynamic therapy, is the race-track microtron. This development combines a multileaf collimator with a magnetically scanned electron beam with a maximum energy of 50 MeV (Brahme, 1987). A novel feature in this exciting development is the use of helium in the sealed treatment head to reduce air scattering of electrons, thereby making it possible to shape electrons and photon beams with the multileaf collimator. This equipment

might make it a practical proposition to deliver several deliberately non-uniform beams under software control of the scanning pattern, provided that the elementary beams were sufficiently narrow.

INTENSITY MODULATED RADIATION THERAPY (IMRT)

The ability to vary the intensity of the radiation beam, or beams, offers potential both in terms of target shaping and dose uniformity, and planned dose heterogeneity. Often, these two functions are related as, for example, when there is a concavity in the target surface. Clinically, this most often arises where tumour lies close to the spinal cord or brainstem. Although these normal tissue structures can tolerate about 75 per cent of the necessary target dose, they must be protected from the full dose. The most simple way to achieve this is to divide each beam into two parts, with one part covering the entire target, including normal tissue, and the other part excluding the sensitive normal tissue (Webb, 1992). The weighting given to each of the two parts can be adjusted to minimize normal tissue dose. However, more can be achieved by dividing each field into a number of segments and, by varying the intensity of each, tighter conformation to the target volume, with compensation for tissue density inhomogeneity, can be secured (Derycke *et al.*, 1997).

A micro-multileaf collimator, with 2 mm wide jaws, has been developed to irradiate small target volumes (Shiu *et al.*, 1997). Movement of the jaws, while the beam is turned on, can vary the intensity such that a beam profile of almost any specification can be produced. Combined with other beams, this can either provide uniform dose distribution within almost any target volume or provide planned non-uniformity.

STEREOTACTIC RADIOTHERAPY

Stereotactic radiotherapy or radiosurgery is a type of conformal therapy that is currently being evaluated clinically. The essence of the technique is technical and anatomical precision and, in order to achieve this, the patient's head is positioned during treatment in the same stereotactic frame as is used for CT examination, planning and biopsy. The defined target volume is then irradiated, by multiple small circular fields, typically 20–30 mm in diameter. The technique is being refined by incorporating complexities such as non-coplanar arcs (Graham *et al.*, 1991). These techniques produce small, spherical, high-dose volumes surrounded by rapid dose fall-off, but further development and clinical application lies in the ability to produce irregular-shaped high-dose volumes.

PROTON THERAPY

In theory, protons provide an ideal tool for conformal therapy because of their well-defined range in tissue. To be practically useful, high energies are required, such as can be achieved by the Harvard cyclotron, which accelerates protons to 160 MeV, giving a range of penetration in tissue of up to 15.9 cm. However, in order to reach deep-seated tumours, beam energies of 200–250 MeV are required. Proton therapy is being investigated clinically at around 20 facilities worldwide, with the first purpose-built, hospital-based proton-beam treatment centre being at Loma Linda in California, USA, where treatment commenced in 1990. This facility has a maximum energy of 250 MeV and three treatment rooms with moveable gantries enabling fields to be delivered isocentrically at different angles. The worldwide proton facilities, and their potential to contribute to conformal therapy, has been reviewed (Webb et al., 1997). Protons obviously have significant potential in terms of being able to deliver dose distributions that 'conform' to a much higher degree than do photons. However, what is much less certain is the balance of clinical benefits with high treatment costs.

Quality control

Quality control in the planning and delivery of radiotherapy treatment has become a major issue. The planning process and the daily delivery of complex treatment set-ups involves a series of technical procedures, each of which needs to be monitored. Small errors at individual steps may be cumulative and responsible for treatment failure. In conformal radiotherapy the requirements for accuracy are maximized. The close conformation of the high-dose volume to the target volume means that the average distance between the boundary of the target volume and the edge of the high-dose volume is far less than when larger, box-shaped, volumes typical of conventional techniques are employed. As a result the problems of patient movement and/or beam malalignment, shifting some region of the target volume into a zone of lower dose, is correspondingly greater, with a consequent increased risk of failure to control tumours.

The importance of patient set-up inaccuracies has recently attracted considerable attention. A number of clinical studies have now quantified these errors and investigated the nature and size of the constituent parts (Rabinowitz et al., 1985; Griffiths et al., 1987; Huizenga et al., 1988; Huddart et al., 1996; Hanley et al., 1997; Mubata et al., 1998). Frequently quoted indicators of error include: random error, a measure of the deviation of all port films from the average port film position; systematic error, a measure of the difference between the average port film and the simulator film; and total uncertainty, a measure of the overall deviation, including both random and systematic uncertainties.

PATIENT IMMOBILIZATION

Fixation masks have long been standard practice for brain and head and neck radiotherapy, where the close approximation of critical normal tissue structures demands high precision. In addition, fixation devices provide a better surface for the accurate maintenance of 'skin' marks over a long course of treatment. As a result, and with the precision required for conformal techniques, there is increased interest in using such devices for other treatment sites and in assessing their value (Creutzberg et al., 1993). With prostate being the most common site for conformal therapy, the value of an immobilization device has been investigated for this setting and reports are generally of reduced patient positioning error (Soffen et al., 1991; Hanley et al., 1997; Mubata et al., 1998).

INTERNAL ANATOMY

Physiological organ movements occur due to respiration, circulation, peristalsis and organ filling. For the most part these changes are non-avoidable, non-controllable and, to some extent, unpredictable. As a result of these movements, the position, shape, size and integral density of structures will vary. An appreciation and measure of these changes is critical for conformal therapy. Ignoring these variables is likely to have important implications, especially when escalating the target dose, and may lead to poorer local control rates and enhanced toxicity.

In pelvic radiotherapy, patients are treated on a daily basis with variable filling of the rectum and bladder, even when some crude attempt is made to standardize bladder volume. The effect of bladder and rectal filling on the position of the prostate has been measured in a series of patients and the dosimetry implications discussed (Ten Haken et al., 1991; Althof et al., 1996; Melain et al., 1997). The range of prostate movements demonstrated under different conditions of rectal and bladder filling is in the order of 0–2 cm, with an average of 0.5 cm. Similarly, kidney position varies with respiration and there are obvious unavoidable cardiac and thoracic movements. Consideration needs to be given to potential movements at any site where conformal radiotherapy is contemplated, and target volumes need to be defined taking these movements into account.

PORTAL IMAGING

Traditionally the accuracy and reproducibility of radiotherapy treatment set-ups has been assessed by portal films with reference to bony landmarks (Rabinowitz et al., 1985; Griffiths et al., 1987; Huizenga et al., 1988). However, these films are developed off-line and are therefore not available for review until after that day's treatment. Since the mid-1980s there have been major developments in what has become termed 'on-line megavoltage imaging', which involves the use of a variety of electronic devices to produce images using the actual treatment beam, which can be viewed virtually instantaneously (Wade and Nicholas, 1991; Boyer et al., 1992) (Fig. 53.5). As a result, these devices can be used interventionally by immediate evaluation of the portal image, followed by corrective measures, before the major part of that fraction is

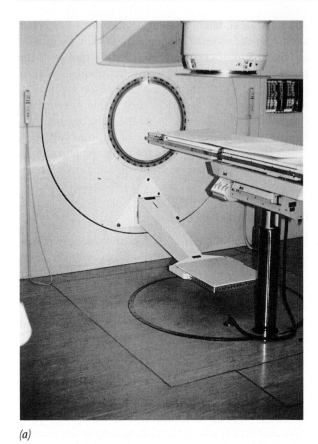

(a)

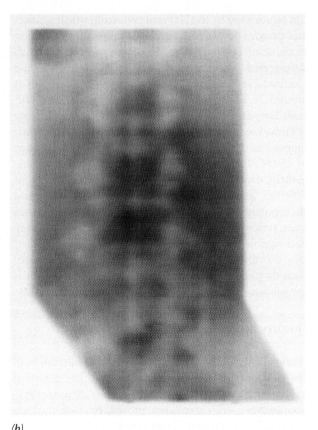

(b)

Figure 53.5 *(a) The Royal Marsden Hospital/Institute of Cancer Research megavoltage portal imaging system attached to the gantry of a Philips SL25 linear accelerator. (b) A megavoltage image of a dog-leg field taking during an actual treatment fraction. The imager has a 19 × 19 cm field of view at the isocentre and hence the top and bottom margins of the field are outside this field of view.*

delivered. Additionally, the image quality has greatly improved. Several groups are currently working on ways of fast automatic comparison between the on-line megavoltage image and that obtained from the simulator or, alternatively, from one digitally reconstructed from the CT planning images.

Interactive studies are less common, but it has been shown that by intervention in pelvic radiotherapy, based on images from a scanning detector, it is possible to reduce the mean field placement error from 4.3 mm to 2 mm (Gildersleve *et al.*, 1992). Studies such as this will enable clinicians to judge better the appropriate treatment margins for any particular treatment site, in order to ensure that underdosing does not occur as a result of the change from conventional to conformal technique. However, routine use of interventionalist techniques will have significant implications for departments, with an estimated average of a 36 per cent increase in treatment time when using such a facility (De Neve *et al.*, 1993).

The contribution of accurate patient set-up to overall treatment outcome has rarely been assessed. However, in a patterns of care survey in 181 patients with Hodgkin's disease treated at various institutions, review of portal films defined 36 per cent of treatment as inadequate. In these patients there was a 50 per cent relapse rate,

compared with a 15 per cent relapse rate for those whose treatments were judged as adequate by a portal film review. This difference was significant at the $P = 0.0001$ level and emphasizes the importance of precise alignment of the treatment field (Kinzie *et al.*, 1983).

EVALUATION OF CONFORMAL THERAPY

Requirements of evaluation

Because conformal therapy is a composite entity its evaluation is an extremely complex issue. In addition, for each of its constituent parts there are now a large number of variables in terms of hardware systems and computer software, and in terms of the technical and clinical application of such. It is essential that each component is evaluated individually and there is already a considerable literature describing and assessing these technical innovations. However, in terms of improving patient care, it is the entire conformal treatment package and its impact on outcome that must be evaluated. Where can conformal therapy make a significant contribution in terms of overall oncology practice?

Developments in conformal therapy tend to be polarized and driven by different forces accordingly. On the one hand is sophisticated, state of the art, high technology development, often tackling theoretical or unusual and complicated clinical problems. This type of activity is often inspired by science and technology and is obviously limited to specialist centres with a research and development remit. On the other hand is the very pragmatic approach of using relatively 'low-tech' equipment which is more widely available and has immediate practical application to common treatment situations. Development of the latter arises from wider clinical needs. Both aspects are important, but good communication between the two is essential in order to optimize developments to meet clinical requirements.

Technical developments and evaluation

Technical developments related to conformal radiotherapy are numerous and diverse. The physics involved is complicated and sophisticated and beyond the scope of this chapter. However, an attempt has been made here to outline some of the main areas and process of development and to describe their interaction.

COMPUTER OPTIMIZATION OF TREATMENT PLANNING

The introduction of computers to treatment planning has already had a profound impact in terms of radiotherapy practice and potential. Current developments aim to optimize the process and provide far greater flexibility in terms of treatment possibilities. One such development has been termed 'inverse planning' and, as the name implies, involves a reversal of the usual procedure. This means that instead of the selection of beams being the primary move, with subsequent scrutiny of the resultant dose distribution, the starting point is the selection of the optimum dose distribution and, based on these requirements, beam and machine parameters are selected by computer (Reinstein et al., 1998). Another approach to improving dose distribution is the removal of the constraints imposed by uniform beam profiles. Computer variance of beam intensity (IMRT) has the potential to produce concave dose distributions, a planning goal in those situations where the target volume wraps itself around a critical normal tissue structure. Means of producing intensity-modulated beams has become a very active research area and this has been reviewed recently (Webb et al., 1997). One system developed for this function, called 'Peacock', claims to be adaptable to most linear accelerators and to be capable of creating and implementing a three-dimensional conformal plan for target volumes of almost any shape and in almost any anatomical location (Carol et al., 1993; Kalnicki et al., 1994; Woo et al., 1994). This is an exciting area of work, although, in practice, the system still requires fine tuning

and careful validation. Ongoing development of beam models makes an important contribution to optimizing treatment planning in conformal therapy. Current models are often primitive and fail to fully take into account issues such as scatter, tissue inhomogeneity and disequilibrium. Further refining of the models will provide 'truer' dose distributions, an absolute requirement for the development of reliable conformal therapy and its evaluation.

RADIOTHERAPY EQUIPMENT

The development of radiotherapy hardware systems relies on collaboration between industry and radiotherapy physics. The usual process is for a prototype to be designed and undergo initial development and testing in the factory, and for it subsequently to be assessed within a clinical radiotherapy department. This is the way in which MLC systems have been developed and accepted as judged by technical performance. Further technical development will involve dynamic movement of individual leaves, initially with static, and subsequently with dynamic, fields.

Radiotherapy networking systems are a recent commercial development which are now in clinical use and undergoing further refinement. By computer facilitation these systems allow the transfer of radiotherapy treatment details between the simulator and treatment machines, and from one treatment machine to another. This has obvious implications for conformal therapy in that it allows the rapid and precise transfer of the more complicated details inherent in more sophisticated radiotherapy.

Simulator systems also undergo constant development. One aspect is the incorporation of a CT facility from which verification, or simulator, images can be produced by computer projection through the CT density matrix with an appropriately divergent beam simulating the field. This produces a digitally reconstructed radiograph (DRR), the process having become known as CT, or virtual, simulation (Sherouse et al., 1990). Appealing as this facility is to the conformal therapy process, there are shortcomings. Amongst these, the most restricting is the fact that it may not be possible to scan the patient in the required treatment position as, for example, with some breast treatment techniques. However, machine design and treatment technique modification are likely to overcome such difficulties. Other disadvantages are long scanning times and poor image quality. These are important considerations for patient throughput and conformal planning, but it is obviously an exciting development which, in the future, is likely to integrate with CT verification systems.

TREATMENT VERIFICATION

The two main components of treatment verification are:

1 ensuring that the position of the patient relative to the radiotherapy field is reproducibly accurate; and
2 confirming that the dose delivered corresponds with that accepted in the planning process.

Both areas are a source of much activity at the current time and, as part of the overall issue of quality assurance, are of enormous relevance to conformal therapy.

As far as verification of patient position is concerned, megavoltage imaging is an important development, the benefits of which have been outlined on pp. 1151–2. A further potential advance in this area of 'on-line verification' is the megavoltage CT device (Swindell *et al.*, 1983; Brahme *et al.*, 1987). This, used in conjunction with CT simulation, will allow all aspects of treatment planning and verification to be based on CT data. Networking systems should allow rapid transfer of this information and permit automatic comparison of proposed and actual treatment set-ups.

In-vivo verification of dose delivery has traditionally been confined to surface measurements using TLD (thermoluminescent dosimeter) chips. The introduction of semiconductor diodes allows a more immediate assessment but still generally restricts measurement to surface sites or body cavities. However, it does provide a means of checking planning algorithms and detecting errors along the dosimetric chain (WHO, 1988; Burman *et al.*, 1997). Transit dosimetry is an innovative technique providing non-invasive, *in-vivo*, dosimetry based on an electronic portal imaging device. This device measures the exit radiation from a small test dose of megavoltage X-rays delivered via the treatment fields with the patient in the treatment position. The electronic image of the transmitted radiation is converted into a map representing density and internal anatomy. A further development of the approach is to link the transit dosimetry data to the automatic design, and cutting of a customized tissue compensator. This process, and particularly its clinical outcome, is currently being validated in a randomized study involving breast irradiation at the Royal Marsden Hospital, which has completed accrual.

Clinical evaluation

Philosophically, three-dimensional planning and conformal radiotherapy are advances that ought to imply better treatment. However there are at least two caveats that need consideration. First, any potential benefit is only likely to be translated into realistic gain if there is high precision and accuracy for each of the component parts. This must be assessed on an individual centre basis so that the specifications for conformal therapy can be defined to accommodate the limits on accuracy in that system. Secondly, the size of the clinical benefit needs to be quantified in order to make rational decisions regarding cost-effectiveness and resource allocation. It seems likely that, at certain treatment sites, conformal therapy will permit a useful dose escalation and therefore be a valuable approach. However, it is equally likely that, at other sites, and for certain types of patient, it will be inappropriate, and these areas need to be defined. In order

to do this in a reliable fashion and eliminate selection bias, randomized trials need to be designed which compare conventional treatment with conformal techniques and conformal techniques comparing different doses. So far, assessment of conformal therapy has not taken this direction in a major way and there is a grave danger that the single-arm studies being performed will fail to address the broader issues of the role of conformal therapy in a radiotherapy practice.

IMPACT ON TOXICITY

One of the fundamental tests of the likely impact of conformal techniques lies in being able to demonstrate that a reduction in the volume of normal tissue included within the high-dose volume will, in fact, lead to a reduction in normal tissue toxicity. Such an effect would provide a sound basis for embarking on dose-escalation studies. Carcinoma of the prostate is an area in which conformal therapy theoretically looks promising and has therefore attracted considerable interest for studies. A number of groups have attempted to demonstrate a reduction in toxicity when applying a conformal technique compared with standard approaches; in other words, they have tried to demonstrate a volume effect for bowel toxicity. In one such study, a group of 20 patients treated with a variety of non-conformal techniques were compared with 26 patients treated conformally. In both patient groups the prescribed median dose was 68 Gy given in either 1.8 Gy or 2 Gy daily fractions (Soffen *et al.*, 1992). The conformal technique allowed an average of 14 per cent bladder and 14 per cent rectal volume receiving a given dose to be eliminated compared with staged-matched controls treated conventionally. Although the documented frequency of acute urinary and rectal symptoms was similar in the two groups, only 31 per cent of those treated conformally, compared with 60 per cent treated conventionally, experienced symptoms that warranted physician intervention in terms of prescribing medication or interrupting treatment. In addition, symptoms persisted for an average of 2.5 weeks, compared with 3.5 weeks in the conventionally treated group. Although not a randomized study, these results suggest that the reduction of volume of critical structures of the order achieved here produces a detectable difference in the severity and duration of acute symptoms. However, care needs to be exercised in undertaking this type of study as there are pitfalls. A further study also attempted to correlate acute toxicity with radiotherapy technique in localized prostate cancer (Vijayakumar *et al.*, 1993). In this retrospective study, patients planned conventionally were compared with a CT-planned group and with a beam's-eye view (BEV) planned group, in terms of documented acute toxicity. The conclusion drawn was that BEV treatment resulted in fewer symptoms than either CT-based or conventional fields. This result is slightly difficult to reconcile with the fact that the 'true volumes' with the

BEV technique were larger than with the CT technique. Unfortunately, the results were not accompanied by dose–volume histograms for the three techniques, a deficiency which emphasis the necessity for collecting such information in order to make sense of this type of analysis.

The Royal Marsden Hospital undertook a randomized trial comparing a standard pelvic treatment technique with one employing BEV-designed customized blocks, in terms of acute toxicity (Tait *et al.*, 1993). Comparing the standard with the conformal technique, the mean percentage sparing of tissue at the 90 per cent dose level was 54 per cent for rectum, 45 per cent for large bowel and 57 per cent for small bowel. Despite this, it was not possible to demonstrate any statistically significant difference between the two arms of the trial in terms of level of symptoms from side-effects or medication requirements to counteract these symptoms (Tait *et al.*, 1997). The trial continued to accrue, in terms of prostate patients, such that a comparison of late effects was possible for this group. This analysis revealed a significant reduction in the development of radiation-induced proctitis and bleeding in those patients treated conformally (Dearnaley *et al.*, 1999). Similar benefits were demonstrated in a recent European randomized trial (Koper *et al.*, 1999). It has now, therefore, been established that the implementation of conformal radiotherapy can reduce radiation-related morbidity.

Aspects of acute toxicity offer attractive end points because of the frequency with which they occur, whereas with currently employed dose levels late toxic events are relatively rare. However, there are drawbacks. Acute toxicity is very much more under the influence of other factors with, for example, diet and coincidental medication playing an important part in bowel toxicity in abdominal and pelvic radiation. Additionally, physician intervention in terms of medication and treatment interruption, or dose fractionation modification, will have a profound effect and needs to be taken into account in any analysis. The Royal Marsden trial clearly demonstrated the limitations of acute end points, although the precise reason for this remains speculative.

DOSE ESCALATION

Several centres have embarked upon single-arm phase II dose-escalation studies to determine what target dose a conformal technique will permit for the same level of normal tissue injury that is normally considered acceptable with conventional techniques. Again, prostate cancer is the dominant area of activity at present, and doses have been escalated to more than 80 Gy, a dose level which, when delivered by conventional techniques, would be associated with substantial morbidity. At the Netherlands Cancer Institute, customized, partial transmission blocks are being used to deliver 1.5 Gy daily fractions to the whole pelvis, with 2 Gy daily fractions to the prostate itself. Using this approach, the dose was first escalated to 70 Gy and subsequently to 80 and 85 Gy. A similar study at the University of Michigan delivered 76 Gy to the prostate, using customized blocks, with an acceptable normal tissue reaction (Lichter, 1991). This centre is now treating patients to a dose of 80 Gy and assessing the resultant toxicity of this further dose escalation. A recent report of prostate dose escalation included 743 patients and provided good evidence for a dose response (Zelefsky *et al.*, 1998). Furthermore, it has been demonstrated that after 5 years the hazard of biochemical failure decreases by 8 per cent for each additional 1 Gy delivered (Hanks *et al.*, 1998).

At the present time, studies of this sort apply an increase in dose to a group of patients without consideration of their individual dose–volume characteristics. However, in an analysis of normal tissue-sparing achievable by a simple blocking technique for pelvic tumours there was considerable variation in dose distribution in the rectum between different patients (Tait *et al.*, 1988). Dose–volume histograms demonstrate this clearly and could provide the basis for selection of patients for dose escalation. In one study the potential for increased tumour control probability by customized dose prescription in pelvic malignancies was investigated by applying the Kutcher–Burman normal tissue complication probability model to dose–volume histogram data for 51 patients (Nahum and Tait, 1992). This exercise demonstrated considerable variation between patients and indicated that, even with current techniques, there is a group of patients in which there is potential for increasing the tumour control probability by customizing the target dose. Selecting optimized treatment, both in physical and biological terms, for individual patients is an attractive approach currently being explored. This has already been applied to patients in a study of intra-arterial 5-fluorouracil and focal radiotherapy in primary and metastatic liver tumours. Dose–volume histograms were used as a basis on which to determine the prescribed dose. For example, depending upon the percentage volume of normal liver spared, as defined by the 50 per cent isodose, the prescribed dose was either 36, 48 or 66 Gy. This is one of the first studies to utilize dose–volume histograms of individual patients to determine dose, and is an exciting approach in that it allows the new technology to select patients at various levels of risk of toxicity.

SIGNIFICANT POINTS

- Conformal therapy offers the opportunity to deliver higher doses, improve local control and, consequently, survival in certain tumour sites.
- It has the potential to reduce normal tissue toxicity.

- For its effectiveness, it depends on the existence of a dose response for tumour control and a volume effect for normal tissues.
- Conformal therapy requires high-precision radiotherapy in terms of planning, treatment execution and verification.
- Identification of appropriate planning margins is required.
- Conformal therapy warrants careful clinical evaluation, including cost-effectiveness analysis.

KEY REFERENCES

Leibel, S.A., Ling, C.C., Kutcher, G.I. *et al.* (1991) The biological basis for conformal three-dimensional radiation therapy. *Int. J. Radiat. Oncol. Biol. Phys.* **21**, 805–11.

Lyman, J.T. and Wolbarst, A.B. (1987) Optimization of radiation therapy. III. A method of assessing complication probabilities from dose–volume histograms. *Int. J. Radiat. Oncol. Biol. Phys.* **12**, 103–9.

Suit, H.D. and Bois, D.W. (1991) The importance of optimal treatment planning in radiation therapy. *Int. J. Radiat. Oncol. Biol. Phys.* **21**, 1471–8.

Suit, H.D., Becht, L., Leong, J. *et al.* (1988) Potential for improvement in radiation therapy. *Int. J. Radiat. Oncol. Biol. Phys.* **14**, 777–86.

Urie, M.M., Goitein, M., Koppke, K. *et al.* (1991) The role of uncertainty analysis in treatment planning. *Int. J. Radiat. Oncol. Biol. Phys.* **21**, 91–107.

REFERENCES

Althof, V.G., Hoekstra, C.J. and te Loo, H.J. (1996) Variation in prostate position relative to adjacent bony anatomy. *Int. J. Radiat. Oncol. Biol. Phys.* **34**(3), 709–15.

Armstrong, J., Raben, A., Zelefsky, M. *et al.* (1997) Promising survival with three-dimensional conformal radiation therapy for non-small cell lung cancer. *Radiother. Oncol.* **44**(1), 17–22.

Boyer, A.L., Antonuk, L., Fenster, A. *et al.* (1992) A review of electronic portal imaging devices (EPIDs). *Med. Phys.* **19**, 1–16.

Brahme, A. (1987) Design principles and clinical possibilities with a new generation of radiation therapy equipment. *Acta Oncol.* **26**, 403–12.

Brahme, A. and Agren, A.K. (1987) Optimal dose distribution for eradication of heterogeneous tumours. *Acta Oncol.* **26**, 377–85.

Brahme, A., Lind, B. and Nfstadius, P. (1987) Radiotherapeutic computed tomography with scanned photon beams. *Int. J. Radiat. Oncol. Biol. Phys.* **13**(1), 95–101.

Burman, C., Chui, C.S., Kutcher, G. *et al.* (1997) Planning, delivery, and quality assurance of intensity-modulated radiotherapy using dynamic multileaf collimator: a strategy for large-scale implementation for the treatment of carcinoma of the prostate. *Int. J. Radiat. Oncol. Biol. Phys.* **39**(4), 863–73.

Carol, M.P., Targovnik, H., Campbell, C. *et al.* (1993) An automatic 3D treatment planning and implementation system for optimized conformal therapy. In Minet, P. (ed.), *Three-dimensional treatment planning.* Belgium: Etienne Riga, 173–87.

Caudry, J.M., Causse, N., Trouette, R. *et al.* (1993) Radiotoxic model for three-dimensional treatment planning. Part 1: theoretical basis. *Int. J. Radiat. Oncol. Biol. Phys.* **25**, 907–19.

Cook, P.N. (1981) A study of three-dimensional reconstruction algorithms. *Orthop. Med.* **4**, 3–12.

Creutzberg, C.L., Althof, V.G.M., Huizenga, H., Visser, A.G. and Levendag, P.C. (1993) Quality assurance using portal imaging: the accuracy of patient positioning in irradiation of breast cancer. *Int. J. Radiat. Oncol. Biol. Phys.* **25**, 529–39.

Dearnaley, D.P., Shearer, R.J., Ellingham, L., Gadd, J. and Horwich, A. (1997) Basic principles and initial results of adjuvant hormone therapy and irradiation of prostatic carcinoma. *Schweiz. Rundsch. Med. Prax.* **86**(48), 1895–901.

Dearnaley, D.P., Khoo, V.S., Norman, A.R. *et al.* (1999) Comparison of radiation side-effects of conformal and conventional radiotherapy in prostate cancer: a randomised trial. *Lancet* **353**(9149), 267–72.

DeNeve, W., Van den Heuvel, F., Coghe, M. *et al.* (1993) Interactive use of on-line portal imaging in pelvic radiation. *Int. J. Radiat. Oncol. Biol. Phys.* **25**, 517–24.

Derycke, S., Van Duyse, B., De Gersem, W., De Wagter, C. and De Neve, W. (1997) Non-coplanar beam intensity modulation allows large dose escalation in stage III lung cancer. *Radiother. Oncol.* **45**(3), 253–61.

Emami, B., Lyman, I., Brown, A. *et al.* (1991) Tolerance of normal tissue to therapeutic irradiation. *Int. J. Radiat. Oncol. Biol. Phys.* **21**, 109–22.

Fenwick, J.D. (1998) Predicting the radiation control probability of heterogeneous tumour ensembles: data analysis and parameter estimation using a closed-form expression. *Phys. Med. Biol.* **43**(8), 2159–78.

Fernandez, E.M., Shentall, G.S., Mayles, W.P. and Dearnaley, D.P. (1995) The acceptability of a multileaf collimator as a replacement for conventional blocks. *Radiother. Oncol.* **36**(1), 65–74.

Galvin, J.M., Smith, A.R. and Lally, B. (1993) Characterization of a multileaf collimator system. *Int. J. Radiat. Oncol. Biol. Phys.* **25**, 181–92.

Gildersleve, J., Swindell, M., Evans, P. *et al.* (1992) Verification of patient positioning during radiotherapy using an integrated megavoltage imaging system. In Breit, A. (ed.), *Advanced radiation therapy – tumor response monitoring and treatment planning*. Heidelberg: Springer-Verlag, 693–5.

Graham, I.D., Nahum, A.E. and Brada, M. (1991) Optimum technique for stereotactic radiotherapy by linear accelerator based on 3-dimensional dose distributions. *Radiother. Oncol.* **22**, 29–35.

Griffiths, S.E., Pearcey, R.G. and Thorogood, J. (1987) Quality control in radiotherapy: the reduction of field placement errors. *Int. J. Radiat. Oncol. Biol. Phys.* **13**, 1583–8.

Hanks, G.E., Hanlon, A.L., Schultheiss, T.E. *et al.* (1998) Dose escalation with 3D conformal treatment: five year outcomes, treatment optimization, and future directions. *Int. J. Radiat. Oncol. Biol. Phys.* **41**(3), 501–10.

Hanley, J., Lumley, M.A., Mageras, G.S. *et al.* (1997) Measurement of patient positioning errors in three-dimensional conformal radiotherapy of the prostate. *Int. J. Radiat. Oncol. Biol. Phys.* **7**(2), 435–44.

Huddart, R.A., Nahum, A., Neal, A. *et al.* (1996) Accuracy of pelvic radiotherapy: prospective analysis of 90 patients in a randomised trial of blocked versus standard radiotherapy. *Radiother. Oncol.* **39**(1), 19–29.

Huizenga, H., Levendag, P.C., De-Poore, P.M. and Visser, A.G. (1988) Accuracy in radiation field alignment in head and neck cancer: a prospective study. *Radiother. Oncol.* **11**, 181–7.

ICRU (1993) *Prescribing, recording and reporting photon beam therapy*. International Commission on Radiological Units and Measurements, Report No. 50. ICRU, Bethesda, Maryland, USA.

ICRU (1999) *Prescribing, recording and reporting photon beam therapy*. Supplement to ICRU Report 50 Report 62. ICRU, Bethesda, Maryland, USA.

Jackson, A., Kutcher, G.J. and Yorke E.D. (1993) Probability of radiation induced complications for normal tissues with parallel architecture subject to non-uniform irradiation. *Med. Phys.* **20**, 613–25.

Kallman, P., Lind, B., Elkof, A. and Brahme, A. (1988) Shaping of arbitrary dose distribution by dynamic multileaf collimation. *Phys. Med. Biol.* **33**, 1291–300.

Kalnicki, S., Wu, A., Berta, C., Targovnik, H., Chen, A. and Carol, M. (1994) Illustrations of Peacock treatment plans for patients with localised diseases (Proceedings of the World Congress on Medical Physics and Biomedical Engineering, Rio de Janeiro, 1994). *Phys. Med. Biol.* **39A**, 517.

Kinzie, I.I., Hanks, G.E., MacLean, C.I. and Kramer, S. (1983) Patterns of care study: Hodgkin's disease relapse rates and adequacy of portals. *Cancer* **52**, 2223–6.

Koper, P.C., Stroom, J.C., van Putten, W.L. *et al.* (1999) Acute morbidity reduction using 3DCRT for prostate carcinoma: a randomized study. *Int. J. Radiat. Oncol. Biol. Phys.* **43**(4), 727–34.

Lawton, C.A., Won, M., Pilepi, M.V. *et al.* (1991) Long-term treatment sequelae following external beam irradiation for adenocarcinoma of the prostate: analysis of RTOG studies 7506 and 7706. *Int. J. Radiat. Oncol. Biol. Phys.* **21**, 935–9.

Letschert, I.G.J., Lebesque, J.V., de Boer, R.W., Hart, A.A.M. and Bartelink, H. (1990) Dose–volume correlation in radiation-related late small bowel complications: a clinical study. *Radiother. Oncol.* **18**, 307–20.

Lichter, A.S. (1991) Three-dimensional conformal radiation therapy: a testable hypothesis. *Int. J. Radiat. Oncol. Biol. Phys.* **21**, 853–5.

LoSasso, T., Chui, C.S., Kutcher, G. *et al.* (1993) The use of multi-leaf collimator for conformal radiotherapy of carcinomas of the prostate and nasopharynx. *Int. J. Radiat. Oncol. Biol. Phys.* **25**, 161–70.

Melian, E., Mageras, G.S., Fuks, Z. *et al.* (1997) Variation in prostate position quantitation and implications for three-dimensional conformal treatment planning. *Int. J. Radiat. Oncol. Biol. Phys.* **38**(1), 73–81.

Mubata, C.D., Bidmead, A.M., Ellingham, L.M., Thompson, V. and Dearnaley, D.P. (1998) Portal imaging protocol for radical dose-escalated radiotherapy treatment of prostate cancer. *Int. J. Radiat. Oncol. Biol. Phys.* **40**(1), 221–31.

Nahum, A.E. and Tait, D.M. (1992) Maximizing local control by customized dose prescription for pelvic tumours. In Breit, A. (ed.), *Advanced radiation therapy tumor response monitoring and treatment planning*. Heidelberg: Springer-Verlag, 425–31.

Niemierko, A. and Goitein, M. (1993) Modeling of normal tissue response to radiation: the critical volume model. *Int. J. Radiat. Oncol. Biol. Phys.* **25**, 135–45.

Nguyen, L.N., Pollack, A. and Zagars, G.K. (1998) Late effects after radiotherapy for prostate cancer in a randomized dose–response study: results of a self-assessment questionnaire. *Urology* **51**(6), 991–7.

Rabinowitz, I., Broomberg, J., Coitein, M., McCarthy, K. and Leong, J. (1985) Accuracy of radiation field alignment in clinical practice. *Int. J. Radiat. Oncol. Biol. Phys.* **11**, 1857–67.

Reinstein, L.E., Wang, X.H., Burman, C.M. *et al.* (1998) A feasibility study of automated inverse treatment planning for cancer of the prostate. *Int. J. Radiat. Oncol. Biol. Phys.* **40**(1), 207–14.

Sanchez-Nieto, B. and Nahum, A.E. (1999) The Delta-TCP concept: a clinically useful measure of tumour control probability. *Int. J. Radiat. Oncol. Biol. Phys.* **44**, 369–80.

Schultheiss, T.E., Orton, C.G. and Peck, R.A. (1983) Models in radiation therapy: volume effects. *Med. Phys.* **10**, 410–15.

Sherouse, G.W., Novins, K. and Chaney, E.L. (1990) Computation of digitally reconstructed radiographs for use in radiotherapy treatment design. *Int. J. Radiat. Oncol. Biol. Phys.* **18**(3), 651–8.

Shiu, A.S., Kooy, H.M., Ewton, J.R. *et al.* (1997) Stereotactic treatment. *Int. J. Radiat. Oncol. Biol. Phys.* **37**(3), 679–88.

Soffen, E.M., Hanks, G.E., Hwang, C.C. and Chu, J.C.H. (1991) Conformal static field therapy for low volume low grade prostate cancer with rigid immobilization. *Int. J. Radiat. Oncol. Biol. Phys.* **20**, 141–6.

Soffen, E.M., Hanks, G.E., Hunt, M.A. and Epstein, B.E. (1992) Conformal static field radiation therapy treatment of early prostate cancer versus non-conformal techniques: a reduction in acute morbidity. *Int. J. Radiat. Oncol. Biol. Phys.* **24**(3), 485–8.

Suit, H.D. and Westgate, S.J. (1986) Impact of improved local control on survival. *J. Rad. Oncol. Biol. Phys.* **12**, 453–8.

Swindell, W., Simpson, R.G., Oleson, J.R., Chen, C.T. and Grubbs, E.A. (1983) Computer tomography with a linear accelerator with radiotherapy applications. *Med. Phys.* **10**, 416–20.

Tait, D.M., Nahum, A.E., Southall, C. *et al.* (1988) Benefits expected from simple conformal radiotherapy in the treatment of pelvic tumours. *J. Eur. Soc. Ther. Rad. Oncol.* **13**, 23–30.

Tait, D., Nahum, A.E., Rigby, L. *et al.* (1993) Conformal radiotherapy of the pelvis: assessment of acute toxicity. *Radiother. Oncol.* **29**(2), 117–26.

Tait, D.M., Nahum, A.E., Meyer, L.C. *et al.* (1997) Acute toxicity in pelvic radiotherapy: a randomised trial of conformal versus conventional treatment. *Radiother. Oncol.* **42**(2), 121–36.

Tate, T. and Shental, G. (1989) Conformation therapy to improve the irradiation to the spinal axis. *Int. J. Radiat. Oncol. Biol. Phys.* **16**(2), 502–10.

Tattoo, T. and Shentall, G. (1989) Conformation therapy to improve the irradiation of the spinal axis. *Int. J. Radiat. Oncol. Biol. Phys.* **16**, 505–10.

Ten Haken, R.K., Forman, J.D., Heimburger, D.K. *et al.* (1991) Treatment planning issues related to prostate movement in response to differential filling of the rectum and bladder. *Int. J. Radiat. Oncol. Biol. Phys.* **20**, 1317–24.

Thames, H.D., Schultheiss, T.E., Hendry, J.H. *et al.* (1992) Can modest escalations of dose be detected as increased tumour control? *Int. J. Radiat. Oncol. Biol. Phys.* **22**, 241–6.

Thiel, H.J., Muller, R.G., Lux, J. *et al.* (1988) Individualkollimatoren also Hilfsmittel zur Verbes-serung det Einstellgenaliigkeit und Reproduzierbarkeit det Bestrahlung und zur Schon. *Strahlenther. Onkol.* **164**, 734–45.

UICC (1997) *TNM classification of malignant tumors*, 5th edn. L.H. Sobin and Ch. Wittekind.

Vijayakumar, S., Awan, A., Karrison, T. *et al.* (1993) Acute toxicity during external-beam radiotherapy for localized prostate cancer: comparison of different techniques. *Int. J. Radiat. Oncol. Biol. Phys.* **25**, 359–71.

Wade, J.P. and Nicholas, D.N. (1991) Clinical application of an electronic imaging device for assisting patients set-up radiotherapy. *Br. J. Radiol.* **64**, 596–602.

Webb, S. (1989) Optimisation of conformal radiotherapy dose distributions by simulated annealing. *Phys. Med. Biol.* **34**, 1349–70.

Webb, S. (1992) Optimization by simulated annealing of three-dimensional confirmed treatment planning for radiation fields defined by a multileaf collimator. II. Inclusion of two-dimensional modulation of the X-ray intensity. *Phys. Med. Biol.* **37**, 1689–704.

Webb, S., Bortfeld, T., Stein, J. and Convery, D. (1997) The effect of stair–step leaf transmission on the 'tongue-and-groove problem' in dynamic radiotherapy with a multileaf collimator. *Phys. Med. Biol.* **42**(3), 595–602.

WHO (World Health Organisation) (1988) *Quality assurance in radiotherapy*. Geneva: World Health Organisation.

Williams, M.V., Denekamp, J. and Fowler, J.F. (1984) Dose–response relationships for human tumors: implications for clinical trials of dose modifying agents. *Int. J. Radiat. Oncol. Biol. Phys.* **10**, 1703–7.

Withers, H.R. and Taylor, J.M.G. (1993) Critical volume model. *Int. J. Radiat. Oncol. Biol. Phys.* **25**, 151–2.

Withers, H.R., Taylor, J.M.G. and Maciejewski, B. (1988) Treatment volume and tissue tolerance. *Int. J. Radiat. Oncol. Biol. Phys.* **14**, 751–9.

Wolbarst, A.B. (1984) Optimization of radiation therapy. II. The critical voxel model. *Int. J. Radiat. Oncol. Biol. Phys.* **10**, 741–5.

Wolbarst, A.B., Chin, L.M. and Svensson, G.K. (1982) Optimization of radiation therapy: integral-response of a model biological system. *Int. J. Radiat. Oncol. Biol. Phys.* **8**, 1761–9.

Woo, S.Y., Saunders, M., Grant, W. and Butler, E.B. (1994) Does the 'Peacock' have anything to do with radiotherapy. *Int. J. Radiat. Oncol. Biol. Phys.* **29**, 213–14.

Yorke, E.D., Kutcher, G.J., Jackson, A. and Ling, C.C. (1993) Probability of radiation-induced complications in normal tissues with parallel architecture under conditions of uniform whole or partial organ irradiation. *Radiother. Oncol.* **26**(3), 226–37.

Zelefsky, M.J., Leibel, S.A., Gaudin, P.B. *et al.* (1998) Dose escalation with three-dimensional conformal radiation therapy affects the outcome in prostate cancer. *Int. J. Radiat. Oncol. Biol. Phys.* **41**(3), 491–500.

54

Palliative care

ANNE NAYSMITH

INTRODUCTION

Palliative care is the active total care of patients and their families by a multi-professional team when the patient's disease is no longer responsive to curative treatment (World Health Organization, 1990). Many patients with cancer can benefit from the palliative care approach, which aims to relieve symptoms and promote physical and psychosocial well-being (National Council for Hospice and Specialist Palliative Care Services, 1995), even if cure is the goal of their anti-tumour treatment. Cancer patients at all stages of the illness should have access to palliative care, and referral to specialist palliative care services if appropriate. All clinicians working with cancer patients need the basic skills to deal with the issues described in this chapter.

Specialist palliative care

Specialist palliative care services in the UK are multi-professional and involve clinicians with appropriate specialist training and experience. There are four core service structures: hospital support teams, community support teams (which also cover residential and nursing homes), specialist day care and specialist inpatient care. The majority of inpatient beds are provided by voluntary hospices.

Similar models of care, with structures developed in line with the local health care system, exist in many other countries.

Patients may be referred to a specialist palliative care service at any stage of their illness, if there is a clinical need for specialist advice or care. Access to specialist services should be solely on the basis of clinical need. There must be equity of access for all patients, irrespective of their ethnic or cultural background or the presence of other problems, such as severe psychiatric illness. Referral should not be on the basis of prognosis, particularly as it is rarely possible to estimate this with any accuracy (Viganò et al., 2000).

In general, specialist palliative care services for children are separate from adult services. Many of the needs of children with a terminal disease are specific to the paediatric setting, and require appropriately trained staff.

PLANNING MANAGEMENT

When disease is advanced and progressive, there should be a clear overall management plan for the final phases of the illness. Although flexibility is essential, and the plan may need to be developed over a period of time, it should be agreed between the patient and family and the multi-professional team involved in the care. The goals of management should be negotiated with the patient, and be focused on quality of life. The management plan, and any later amendments, including what information has been given to the patient and the family, must be shared with all the professionals involved in the patient's care. This is particularly important when planning the discharge from hospital of terminally ill patients.

Preferred place of death

Not all patients can acknowledge that death is inevitable. But many do, at some stage in their illness. The majority would prefer to die at home, if sufficient support is available. Some prefer to die in a hospice, rather than an acute hospital. If the patient has made a choice (or revised an earlier choice), it is important that this is communicated to everyone involved in the patient's care, so that inappropriate and unnecessary hospital admissions can be avoided.

Communication with patient and family

Good communication is an essential part of the care of all cancer patients. For many patients, there is a succession of disappointments and setbacks along their cancer pathway. Whilst it is important that patients are given truthful information, it is also essential that they remain aware that they are important and cared about, and that they will not be abandoned, even after all attempts at anti-cancer treatment have ended. Most people need to feel that they retain some element of control over their illness, and that they are valued partners in treatment, even in very late stages of the illness.

PHYSICAL SYMPTOMS

The majority of patients with advanced and progressive cancer have multiple physical symptoms. Pain is often the most feared, although only two-thirds of cancer patients experience significant pain. Breathlessness, anorexia and weakness are also common. Although good palliative care involves the whole person, their psychological, spiritual and social needs as well as their physical ones, good symptom control is essential if the patient is to have a reasonable quality of life.

PAIN

Good pain control can only be achieved if there is a thorough, preferably multidisciplinary assessment of the patient's pain. The assessment should include the patient's own description of the severity of the pain. It should also document the type, site, radiation and timing of each pain, any precipitating or relieving factors and the response to previous analgesia, both regular and rescue medication. The assessment should be repeated regularly and should form the basis of changes in therapy.

Barriers to pain control

The principles of analgesia are well known to most clinicians. Nevertheless, a significant proportion of patients with advanced cancer continue to have poorly controlled pain. Barriers to good pain control are created by the beliefs and behaviours both of clinicians, and of patients and their carers.

Clinicians often underestimate the severity of cancer pain. Although effective rating scales have been described (Bruera and Pereira, 1998), they are seldom used (Pargeon and Hailey, 1999). Doctors and patients share unrealistic fears about treatment with opioids, particularly morphine, and may be reluctant to start treatment, or to increase it to an effective dose. Morphine is associated with the terminal phase, so that starting morphine seems equivalent to a death sentence.

WHO analgesic ladder

Although criticized for its lack of a basis in randomized controlled trials, the World Health Organization 'analgesic ladder' has stood the test of time and clinical experience, and is the most straightforward way to consider control of chronic pain. The principles are:

- Analgesics are given by mouth wherever possible.
- Analgesia for chronic pain should be given regularly, at intervals corresponding to the drug's duration of action.
- Extra medication should be available for breakthrough pain.
- Side-effects should be actively managed, so that the analgesic can be titrated upwards until the pain is controlled.
- Simple analgesics are tried initially (the 'first step' of the ladder).
- If inadequate, opioids such as dihydrocodeine are given in low doses (the 'second step' of the ladder).
- Finally, opioids such as morphine are given regularly and titrated upwards to achieve pain control (the 'third step' of the ladder)
- Adjuvant drugs such as non-steroidal anti-inflammatory drugs (NSAIDs), or drugs for neuropathic pain, may be needed at any point for pain which is not fully opioid responsive.

Simple analgesics, NSAIDs and coxibs

Mild pain may be adequately treated with paracetamol 1 g q.d.s. Drugs with anti-inflammatory activity, the traditional NSAIDs and the newer COX-2 inhibitors (coxibs), are useful alone for mild pain, and as adjuvant drugs for pain arising from bones, joints or an inflammatory process such as hepatic metastases. There are many NSAIDs available. Most patients find more potent drugs, such as diclofenac, more helpful than ibuprofen. For oral use, a drug which can be used once or twice daily should be selected, e.g. piroxicam, diclofenac m/r (modified release). Ketorolac is a potent NSAID which can be used parenterally, including by continuous subcutaneous infusion. Some NSAIDs are also available in suppository form. They can be helpful to relieve muscular stiffness and the discomfort of immobility in the last hours or days of life.

Low-dose opioids

If moderate pain is not controlled by a simple analgesic alone, an opioid is given in low dose, often together with an anti-inflammatory adjuvant drug. Although combinations of paracetamol and an opioid, such as codeine or dihydrocodeine, are often used, this is seldom a logical approach, particularly if the patient is also taking an NSAID. The paracetamol content becomes dose limiting, and the combination has to be given four times a day because of the short plasma half-life of paracetamol. It is usually preferable to use an opioid alone, together with an NSAID if appropriate. Modified-release dihydrocodeine can be helpful.

Tramadol, an atypical opioid which is both a μ-opioid receptor agonist and also inhibits noradrenaline and serotonin reuptake, can be given orally in doses of 200–400 mg/day. Normal-release and modified-release formulations are available, allowing its use for baseline and rescue analgesia.

Higher-dose opioids

Morphine is the gold standard drug in the management of severe cancer pain. It should be given regularly by mouth, titrated upwards as necessary to achieve adequate pain relief. Common side-effects, such as nausea and constipation, must be treated effectively to allow effective analgesic doses to be given. The dose requirement should be established using normal-release morphine before changing to a modified-release preparation. Unless patients have previously taken another opioid analgesic, 5–10 mg 4-hourly is a normal starting dose.

Oral morphine undergoes considerable first-pass metabolism, so that its systemic availability is 20–30 per cent (Hanks and Hawkins, 2000). The main active metabolite is morphine-6-glucuronide (M6G), which is renally excreted. Both morphine and M6G bind to the μ-opioid receptor. M6G accumulates in renal failure and is the main contributor to morphine toxicity in this situation. Morphine should be used extremely cautiously in patients with renal failure.

There is clinically no ceiling to the effective dose of morphine. As the dose increases, either pain relief is achieved or side-effects become dose limiting. Neither respiratory depression nor dependence is significant in the management of cancer pain. Sedation, confusion and ultimately delirium are the major dose-limiting side-effects.

Breakthrough pain

It is rare for patients to remain pain free over 24 hours as a result of their baseline analgesia only. The majority of patients with severe pain will experience some breakthrough pain from time to time, and all patients who have chronic pain need to be prescribed appropriate rescue analgesia.

Breakthrough pain can be assigned to one of three categories. End-of-dose pain occurs when the next dose of baseline analgesia is almost due. It is an indicator that the dose of baseline analgesia is too low and should be increased.

Incident pain is provoked in a predictable way by certain stimuli, which may be physical, such as movement or weight bearing, or psychological, such as anxiety. The pain can be reduced by modifying the behaviour that provokes the pain. Increasing the dose of baseline analgesia may produce only an increase in side-effects, such as sedation, when the incident pain is not present. Bone metastases are a frequent cause of incident pain. Adjuvant drugs, radiation therapy, nerve blocks or spinal analgesia may be helpful.

True breakthrough pain arises spontaneously and unpredictably. It is typically of rapid onset, may be severe, and often lasts less than 30 minutes. The reported prevalence in hospice patients varies from 40 per cent to 86 per cent (Zeppetella et al., 2000). The brevity of many episodes of breakthrough pain means that rescue medication needs to have a rapid onset and short duration of action, to minimize side-effects, and to be readily available to the patient, with no delay in administration. Rescue medication should be the normal-release equivalent of the baseline analgesia, and usually the same drug is used. The next regular dose of analgesia should not be delayed. If the baseline analgesic dose is changed, the dose of the rescue medication also needs to be adjusted so that it remains equivalent.

Opioid switching

Some patients experience severe adverse effects with morphine. Although in some cases this may be due to dehydration, renal impairment and the accumulation of morphine metabolites, this does not seem an adequate explanation in all cases. Sometimes, reducing the opioid dose relieves the adverse effects without loss of analgesia. Changing to a different strong opioid may reduce the side-effects, so that the patient can take an effective analgesic dose. This is known as opioid switching. The explanation is not clear. There seems to be incomplete cross-tolerance between opioid agonists. Also, there are differences between the drugs in their affinity for different opioid receptors (Hanks and Hawkins, 2000).

A number of strong opioid drugs are available. Hydromorphone and oxycodone are used orally in ways similar to morphine. Fentanyl is available as a transdermal preparation for baseline analgesia and a buccal lozenge for rescue medication. This may be useful in patients intolerant of oral medication or poorly compliant. Methadone has been claimed to be more useful than other opioids for neuropathic pain and other difficult pain problems. However, this is not at present supported by data from clinical trials. The long elimination half-life, leading to accumulation, makes methadone a more hazardous drug to use in routine clinical practice, particularly in the elderly. When switching from one opioid to another, caution should be used in selecting the equivalent dose, because of the likelihood of incomplete cross-tolerance.

Adjuvant therapy

It is often not possible to control cancer pain using opioids alone. Incident pain, bone pain, neuropathic pain, gut colic and other non-nociceptive pain syndromes may contain a component of pain which is poorly responsive to opioids by oral or parenteral administration. In this situation, adjuvant drugs are commonly used both to improve pain control and to minimize the side-effects of the high doses of opioids that might otherwise be required. There is little randomized controlled trial data for the use of adjuvant drugs in cancer patients. Drug selection is based mainly on evidence from non-malignant pain patients and clinical experience.

BONE PAIN

Bone pain is the major cause of incident pain, one of the factors that predict a poorer response to standard opioid analgesia.

Anti-inflammatory drugs

Despite a lack of evidence from controlled trials in cancer patients, anti-inflammatory drugs are widely believed to be a useful adjuvant to opioid therapy for bone pain. NSAIDs are usually thought to act peripherally, but there is evidence that they also produce effects centrally (Byrne, 2000). In small studies they have been shown to be effective for cancer pain, with efficacy comparable to 5–10 mg of intramuscular morphine in single-dose studies but fewer side-effects. The published trials are too small to confirm whether or not NSAIDs are particularly useful for bone pain.

The side-effects of NSAIDs are broadly similar. Gastric erosions or peptic ulceration can lead to perforation or life-threatening haemorrhage. Risk factors for gastrointestinal problems include age >60, past history of peptic ulceration and significant ill-health. Most cancer patients are at increased risk of gastrointestinal problems and should be given prophylaxis with either misoprostol 200 μg twice daily or a proton pump inhibitor. The simultaneous administration of NSAIDs and corticosteroids is particularly risky. Neither aspirin nor anticoagulant therapy should be given concomitantly. It is not yet clear that coxibs offer significantly safer treatment for patients with major gastrointestinal risk factors.

Both NSAIDs and coxibs have an equal risk of causing renal impairment in chronic use. Elderly patients are at particular risk. In general, anti-inflammatory drugs should be avoided in patients with pre-existing renal impairment.

Adjuvant radiotherapy

Radiotherapy is the single most effective treatment for a painful bone metastasis (Hoskin, 1995). The form of irradiation, the radiation dose and the primary tumour type seem not to influence significantly the likelihood of response. Improvement in localized bone pain has been reported after radiotherapy in 70–80 per cent of patients, although pain relief is rarely complete. Pain may recur after a few months, and re-treatment may be indicated.

Scattered bone pain can be treated with wide-field irradiation or systemic treatment with a radioisotope. Both are effective. The latter causes fewer side-effects. Neither is commonly used.

Bisphosphonates for bone pain

In patients with bone metastases, treatment with bisphosphonates reduces both pain and pathological fractures, and leads to improved functional status (Mannix et al., 2000). The evidence is best for multiple myeloma and breast cancer. It is less good for other cancers, and there is little evidence to suggest effectiveness in cancer of the prostate.

For rapid management of metastatic bone pain, 50–60 per cent of patients will get significant reduction in pain within 14 days after the first dose of a bisphosphonate. A quarter of the remainder may respond after a second course. Patients who do not respond after two courses are unlikely to do so. Both pamidronate and clodronate are effective. Intravenous treatment is better tolerated and more effective than oral. A dose response has been demonstrated for pamidronate. An intravenous infusion of pamidronate 90–120 mg or clodronate 600–1500 mg is therefore recommended. A new biphosphonate, zoledronic acid, may supersede these because it is more convenient to administer.

NEUROPATHIC PAIN

A variety of neuropathic pain syndromes occurs in patients with advanced cancer. Opioid therapy can be effective. Trials in patients with non-malignant neuropathic pain have shown benefit from tramadol, oxycodone and fentanyl. Methadone, because it is a non-competitive NMDA (N-methyl D-asparatate) receptor antagonist, has also been recommended, but the supporting clinical evidence is lacking. Opioids should be titrated to maximum effectiveness before considering adjuvant medication.

The majority of drugs used as adjuvants for neuropathic pain are unlicensed, but many have a supporting evidence base in non-malignant neuropathic pain. Tricyclic antidepressants are the most effective group. Amitriptyline is commonly used, starting with a small dose and titrating up to 75 mg at night. Response may be seen within 5 days of starting treatment. Comparative trials suggest selective serotonin reuptake inhibitors (SSRIs) are less effective (Quigley, 2000).

Anticonvulsants have been used for neuropathic pain on the basis of experience with trigeminal neuralgia. There is insufficient evidence to determine whether antidepressants or anticonvulsants are more effective, or whether the response rate would be higher if both were combined. Gabapentin, a recently introduced anticonvulsant, has been licensed for the treatment of neuropathic pain, but trials suggest it is no more effective than amitriptyline. Dizziness is the major side-effect, and the drug is better tolerated if upward titration is done slowly to a dose of 900–1800 mg/day, or sometimes more.

Systemically administered local anaesthetic-type drugs have been evaluated, including systemic lignocaine and oral mexiletine. Although they are effective in non-malignant pain, the small number of studies reported so far in cancer-related neuropathic pain has failed to show benefit. Drugs antagonistic at the NMDA receptor might theoretically be expected to be helpful, and ketamine has been shown to be effective in a variety of non-malignant pain states. Ketamine may be used parenterally or orally. Early studies suggest NMDA receptor antagonists may be more useful in combination with morphine than used alone.

The drugs currently used for neuropathic pain are at best partly effective, and cancer-related neuropathic pain remains a difficult management problem. A number of new agents are being studied, and the situation may improve in the near future.

INTERVENTIONAL PAIN TREATMENTS

Improvements in drug treatment have reduced the number of patients for whom invasive therapies are indicated. Nevertheless, for the small proportion of cancer patients with intractable pain syndromes, these therapies should be considered. Local anaesthetic and steroid injections usually have only a transient effect. Neurolytic coeliac plexus block has been reported to have a high success rate, but is rarely performed; serious side-effects may occur.

The most useful technique is epidural or spinal infusion, either of opioids alone or of a mixture of opioid and other drugs, frequently bupivacaine. Implantable pump systems have been used very successfully, but side-effects and complications have been reported in 15–25 per cent of patients (Williams, 2000). These techniques are probably indicated in fewer than 2 per cent of patients with advanced cancer. They will often be offered near the end of life, when the patient is unfit for an implantable pump, and the infusion will be maintained via a tunnelled catheter.

Tenesmus

Tenesmus is defined as 'ineffectual, painful straining' and may arise from rectum or bladder. Some patients have spasms of excruciating pain, and may constantly feel that they need to defaecate or urinate. It is associated with a tumour mass, usually from a rectal primary, in the pelvis. Local radiotherapy or endoscopic or laser resection may provide symptomatic relief.

Corticosteroids may relieve the pressure caused by the tumour mass. There have been reports of responses to antidepressants and anticonvulsants, as in neuropathic pain, and to calcium channel blocking agents, such as diltiazem and nifedipine. Some patients need intraspinal treatment, either with a local anaesthetic infusion or a neurolytic block. There is little good evidence to guide further treatment, although a small study of lumbar sympathectomy in 12 patients reported pain relief in 10 (Rich and Ellershaw, 2000).

RESPIRATORY SYMPTOMS

Patients with advanced cancer may have a variety of respiratory symptoms, including breathlessness, wheeze, cough, haemoptysis and stridor. The rapid onset of new respiratory symptoms may indicate a complication such as bronchial obstruction, superior vena caval obstruction, infection or pulmonary embolism.

Dyspnoea

Breathlessness is common in patients with advanced cancer. The prevalence varies with the underlying primary site and with prognosis. Dyspnoea becomes commoner as death approaches, and the overall reported incidence rises to 70 per cent in patients in the last 6 weeks of life. Risk factors include primary or secondary lung cancer, pleural metastases and pre-existing respiratory or cardiac disease (Rawlinson, 2000).

Dyspnoea is usually multifactorial (LeGrand and Walsh, 1999), and in advanced cancer respiratory muscle weakness may be a major contributing factor. Anxiety is rarely the sole cause, but may worsen the subjective sensation of dyspnoea and lead to panic attacks, when the patient is afraid of choking to death.

Subjective improvement may follow treatment of any reversible factors, good nursing care and physiotherapy. Although patients often use oxygen, if they are not hypoxaemic there is little evidence that it helps. The mainstay of management is drug treatment. Low-dose morphine

(2–4 mg 4-hourly or as required) is the most effective agent for relieving the sensation of breathlessness. The dose can be titrated upwards as for pain, but lower doses and smaller increments are likely to be needed. Placebo-controlled trials have not shown either slow-release morphine or nebulized morphine to be beneficial (LeGrand and Walsh, 1999).

Benzodiazepines do not directly improve dyspnoea, but many patients benefit from relief of anxiety. Lorazepam 0.5–1 mg sublingually can help acute episodes of breathlessness. Regular diazepam (5–10 mg daily) may be needed if chronic anxiety is a symptom (Davis, 1997).

Corticosteroids may be useful in lymphangitis carcinomatosis and in superior vena caval obstruction (LeGrand and Walsh, 1999). If sputum retention is a problem, nebulized saline may help to produce an increased volume of more fluid sputum, or nebulized bronchodilators if there is bronchoconstriction.

Cough

Cough in patients with advanced cancer may be productive or non-productive. Productive cough is usually a problem only if the patient is too weak, or the sputum too thick and viscid, for the cough to be effective. Persistent coughing can disturb sleep (of the family as well as the patient), and can cause chest pain, vomiting, rib fractures and exhaustion.

If the productive cough is due to underlying infection, it may be appropriate to give antibiotics even in very ill patients in order to control the very distressing symptoms, but each situation has to be managed individually and in discussion with the patient and family.

Nebulized saline can be used to thin sputum, in order to help patients expectorate effectively. However, this should not be done if the patient is completely unable to produce an effective cough, as it can produce very large volumes of sputum, which add to the patient's distress.

Cough suppressants are appropriate for chronic, unproductive cough. Although codeine is traditionally used, it is not an effective cough suppressant (Herbert, 2000). Strong opioids such as morphine do seem to be useful. Methadone at night can be helpful because it has a long half-life. Nebulized local anaesthetics, e.g. lidocaine (up to 5 mL of 2 per cent solution every 6 hours) or bupivacaine (up to 5 mL of 0.25 per cent solution every 8 hours), can relieve intractable unproductive cough. They may cause bronchospasm, and a nebulized bronchodilator should be available. They also reduce the sensitivity of the gag reflex, and patients should not eat or drink for an hour afterwards.

Haemoptysis

Minor haemoptysis is a common symptom of primary, and sometimes secondary, tumours of the lung. If radiotherapy of the tumour is not indicated, an oral haemostatic drug such as tranexamic acid or etamsylate is often helpful.

Stridor

Stridor results from obstruction of the larynx or major airways. It is frightening both for the patient and for his family. The patient's position should be adjusted to minimize the obstruction. If relief of the obstruction with radiotherapy or stenting is not possible, high-dose corticosteroid therapy, such as dexamethasone 16 mg daily, can give temporary relief. Breathing a mixture of helium and oxygen (in a ratio of 4:1) reduces the work of breathing and may be symptomatically helpful (Davis, 1997).

GASTROINTESTINAL PROBLEMS

Mouth problems

A dry, dirty or painful mouth is common in advanced cancer, and can reduce the patient's oral intake. If the mouth is not infected, local measures including brushing the teeth and tongue, using a mouthwash, chewing chunks of fresh or tinned pineapple (which contains the proteolytic enzyme annanase) or dissolving effervescent vitamin C (0.5 g) on the tongue can all help.

Ulceration may be due to mucositis from recent antitumour treatment, aphthous ulceration or infection. Regular use of a benzydamine mouthwash or benzocaine lozenges may make the mouth less painful, but benzocaine must be avoided before eating. Severe pain may require opioid analgesia. Bacterial infection can be improved with regular mouthwashes of chlorhexidine or tetracycline (Sweeney and Bagg, 1995). Herpes simplex may be difficult to diagnose, and requires specific antiviral treatment. Aphthous ulceration may respond to a short course of thalidomide.

ORAL CANDIDOSIS

This is common in patients with advanced cancer. It may present as the typical white plaques, erythema or angular cheilitis. Patients find nystatin suspension difficult to comply with; it is only effective if used four times daily for more than 5 days. Ketoconazole 200 mg once daily for 5 days is easier for patients and more cost-effective, but interacts with a number of commonly prescribed drugs. Fluconazole 150 mg orally as a single dose (Regnard, 1994) is equally effective though more expensive. Dentures must be cleaned and sterilized to prevent re-infection.

DRY MOUTH

Dry mouth (xerostomia) is a common and distressing symptom. It has been reported in 30 per cent of patients receiving palliative care and 77 per cent of patients admitted to a hospice. It is often assumed to be a sign of dehydration, but the correlation between xerostomia and the patient's state of hydration is very poor. It is much more often due to drug treatment or to the effects of previous surgery or radiotherapy. Drugs commonly implicated include analgesics (e.g. morphine), antidepressants (e.g. amitriptyline) and hypnotics (e.g. temazepam).

Most patients find frequent sips of water or semi-frozen drinks as effective as any other treatment. Artificial saliva sprays are widely prescribed. Mucin-based artificial salivas are more effective than carboxymethylcellulose-based ones, but the effect lasts only minutes. Offered artificial saliva or a low-tack, sugar-free chewing gum, patients found the gum acceptable and more effective than artificial saliva (Davies, 2000). In a comparative study, pilocarpine 5 mg t.d.s. was more effective than artificial saliva (Davies *et al.*, 1998) but produced a higher incidence of side-effects. The side-effects of pilocarpine are dose related, and patients with drug-induced xerostomia may respond to a lower dose. After a dose of pilocarpine, saliva flow peaks at 1 hour and remains increased for up to 4 hours.

DROOLING

Unlike xerostomia, drooling is fairly uncommon but can occur either following head and neck tumours or as a result of primary or secondary brain tumours. A normal amount of saliva is produced, but inability to manage the saliva interferes with eating, and can lead to irritation of the lips and chin, angular cheilitis or bacterial infection. The saliva may also be aspirated, leading to choking.

Treatment aims to reduce the amount of saliva. Inhibition of salivation can be produced with very low doses of anticholinergic drugs. Hyoscine hydrobromide is given either sublingually or transdermally (1 mg/72 hours). Glycopyrrolate does not cause central side-effects. It can be administered orally or via percutaneous gastrostomy tubes (Lucas and Schofield, 2000) and is absorbed sufficiently to reduce saliva production for up to 6 hours. Low dose amitriptyline (10–25 mg at night) is often effective.

Dysphagia

Dysphagia may arise as a result of intrinsic or extrinsic tumour compression. If stenting or other intervention is not possible in very ill patients, corticosteroids may temporarily reduce the volume of the tumour and relieve the dysphagia slightly.

Some patients experience severe pain on swallowing, not always associated with dysphagia. The pain may be due to oesophageal spasm, infection or benign ulceration in the oesophagus. Endoscopy is useful for accurate diagnosis. Infection is most commonly candidiasis, and responds to an imidazole or triazole antifungal. Ulceration may be due to reflux or corticosteroid therapy, best treated with a proton pump inhibitor. Nifedipine m/r

(10–20 mg twice daily) has been used as a smooth muscle relaxant to relieve oesophageal spasm. Hypotension is the dose-limiting side-effect.

Nausea and vomiting

Nausea and vomiting are common in advanced cancer, affecting 40–70 per cent of patients. Good initial assessment and frequent reassessment are essential. Vomiting is mediated via the vomiting centre in the brain, which receives and integrates input from various sources and generates the stimulus to the act of vomiting. Input to the vomiting centre comes from:

- the chemoreceptor trigger zone, stimulated by drugs or chemicals in plasma such as opioids, urea or calcium;
- the vagus and vestibular apparatus;
- mechanoreceptors and chemoreceptors in gut, liver and other organs, mainly via $5-HT_3$ and dopamine receptors;
- higher centres, which are involved both in conditioned vomiting and in stress-induced delay in gastric emptying.

It is important to identify the likely underlying mechanism(s) and the route through which they are provoking vomiting. An anti-emetic with the appropriate site of action can then be prescribed. Any treatable underlying cause, such as raised intracerebral pressure or hypercalcaemia, should be treated effectively if possible. Nausea has to be assessed separately. A patient who remains nauseated, despite control of vomiting, will still be extremely symptomatic and distressed.

Common causes of nausea and vomiting in advanced cancer include:

- disease or obstruction within the gastrointestinal tract, including delayed gastric emptying due to opioids, hepatomegaly or the anorexia-cachexia syndrome;
- drugs, e.g. opioids, NSAIDs, digoxin, metronidazole;
- metabolic causes, e.g. hypercalcaemia, renal failure;
- anti-tumour therapy, e.g. chemotherapy, radiotherapy to the abdomen;
- raised intracerebral pressure, or brain metastases affecting the vestibular system;
- pharyngeal irritation due to chronic cough or sputum.

There is a wide range of anti-emetic drugs. They can be grouped according to their main site or mechanism of action. A recent consensus statement from the European Association for Palliative Care (Twycross and Back, 1998) offers helpful guidelines for anti-emetic selection. Good first-line drugs:

- are *prokinetic* (gastric stasis, opioid-induced ileus) – metoclopramide 10 mg t.d.s./q.d.s. orally or 30–100 mg/ 24 hours by subcutaneous infusion;
- act on the *chemoreceptor trigger zone* (opioids, hypercalcaemia, renal failure) – haloperidol 1.5–5 mg nocte orally or 5–10 mg/24 hours by subcutaneous infusion;

- act on the *vomiting centre* (mechanical bowel obstruction, raised intracranial pressure, pharyngeal irritation, movement induced nausea) – cyclizine 50 mg t.d.s. orally or 150 mg/24 hours by subcutaneous infusion.

Since prokinetic drugs act through cholinergic receptors, they should not be prescribed at the same time as anticholinergic drugs such as cyclizine or hyoscine. The route of administration is important. Nauseated patients may have very poor absorption via the oral route, and may require rectal or parenteral administration until the nausea and vomiting are controlled.

The patient should be regularly reassessed. If the underlying mechanism seems to have been wrongly identified, the anti-emetic should be changed. If the patient has more than one underlying cause for vomiting (30 per cent of patients) a second anti-emetic, such as haloperidol added to metoclopramide, may be needed.

If first-line anti-emetics are not effective, adding dexamethasone may be helpful. Alternatively, therapy can be changed to levomepromazine (methotrimeprazine), a very broad-spectrum anti-emetic. It has a long half-life and can usually be given as a single oral dose of 6.25–25 mg at night or as a subcutaneous infusion. In intractable nausea or vomiting, 5-HT$_3$ antagonists, e.g. granisetron, may be tried, but in view of their cost should be rapidly discontinued if not effective. Young patients with chemotherapy-induced vomiting often find cannabinoids helpful; large studies in advanced cancer have not been carried out.

Constipation

Decreased oral intake, increasing immobility and drug therapy, especially with opioids and anticholinergic drugs, are the major contributory factors to constipation in cancer patients. But confused or immobile patients also have difficulty reaching a toilet or commode, and may be embarrassed to ask for help. In severe constipation, the clinical findings may mimic intestinal obstruction. Plain X-ray of the abdomen is diagnostic if there is any doubt about the diagnosis of constipation.

Laxatives can be classified as either predominantly softening or predominantly peristalsis stimulating. Most patients require both a softener, such as lactulose or docusate, and a stimulant, such as senna or bisacodyl. Co-danthramer and co-danthrusate suspensions and capsules are convenient combinations of a softener and the stimulant, dantron, and are licensed for the terminally ill. Hydrophylic bulk-forming agents should be avoided. Patients can rarely drink the volume of fluid required with these agents, and they may precipitate obstruction. If possible, the patient should be encouraged to increase their fibre and fluid intake; some sip-feeds are enriched with fibre.

True diarrhoea is relatively rare in patients with advanced cancer, and the commonest cause is over-use of laxatives, although infective and antibiotic-induced diarrhoea also occur. Once overflow diarrhoea and infection have been ruled out, if an anti-diarrhoeal agent is required loperamide is safe and effective.

Intestinal obstruction

Patients presenting with signs of intestinal obstruction must be carefully assessed to distinguish malignant obstruction from drug-induced ileus, faecal impaction or obstruction secondary to benign pathology such as adhesions. Few patients with advanced cancer and malignant obstruction have a localized site of blockage and are fit enough to be considered for surgery. Mortality of palliative surgery is high (12–30 per cent), average survival is short and there is a high incidence of postoperative complications such as fistula formation (Baines, 1997). There is limited evidence that malignant obstruction, particularly if it is high in the gastrointestinal tract, may be more likely to resolve after corticosteroids. Dexamethasone has been given parenterally in doses of 6–16 mg daily. There is no evidence on which to select a suitable dose (Feuer and Broadley, 2000).

Most patients are best managed medically. Oral drugs are poorly absorbed, and treatment should be given parenterally, preferably by continuous subcutaneous infusion. The major symptoms are continuous abdominal pain, colic and vomiting. Patients usually require diamorphine for analgesia, and either haloperidol or cyclizine, or both, for control of nausea. Hyoscine butylbromide (60 mg/24 hours), titrated upwards as required, is used to control colic and reduce the volume of intestinal secretions. If the patient continues to have large volume vomits, octreotide (300–600 µg/24 hours) can be substituted for the hyoscine. It is effective in reducing the volume of fluid in the obstructed bowel and also reduces peristalsis.

Dry mouth and thirst may be major problems. Patients whose nausea is controlled can drink at will, and regular mouth care is helpful. A few patients, not in the terminal stage of their disease but with intractable obstruction, may need parenteral hydration for symptom control. Patients rarely find a nasogastric tube helpful, unless their large volume vomiting cannot be controlled by any other means; if drainage is needed for more than a few days, the possibility of a venting gastrostomy should be considered. If drugs and fluids are both given by subcutaneous infusion, it is often possible to keep the patient at home despite the obstruction.

Ascites

Ascites is commonest in tumours of the breast, ovary or gastrointestinal tract. Progressive abdominal distension produces a tight discomfort. In addition, there is early satiety, and splinting of the diaphragms can cause respiratory embarrassment. Although the ascites can be drained percutaneously, it usually re-accumulates relatively quickly; repeated drainage leads to a progressive fall in the serum albumin. Diuretic therapy with spironolactone (100–400 mg/day), usually combined with a small dose of furosemide, has been used to slow down the re-accumulation of fluid. It is unlikely to be effective if the ascites is due solely to peritoneal tumour deposits. Peritoneo-venous shunts can be inserted to drain the ascites continuously back into a central vein. This prevents the fall in serum albumin seen with external drainage. Malignant effusions usually contain tumour cells and have a high protein content, so that blockage of the shunt is common. Shunt insertion is associated with significant morbidity and should only be considered in patients who are still quite fit.

CACHEXIA-ANOREXIA SYNDROME

This poorly understood symptom complex is common in patients with advanced cancer. Eighty per cent of patients have developed it by the time of death, although the disease burden is not correlated with the degree of cachexia. Cachexia is used to describe the wasting of body tissues, both fat and lean mass. Whereas in normal starvation, fat is lost preferentially and there is relative preservation of muscle tissue, in cancer cachexia there is equal loss of both tissue types and the overall wasting is out of proportion to the degree of anorexia. Parenteral nutrition or supplemental oral feeding does not reverse the weight loss (Nelson, 2000). Cancer cachexia is due to major metabolic abnormalities, caused mainly by cytokines and other products released by the tumour (Bruera, 1997). In most patients, these tumour products are the main cause of the anorexia.

Cachectic patients have poorer survival, and higher complication rates after anti-tumour treatment. Cachexia aggravates the fatigue and chronic weakness seen in advanced cancer. It often causes severe psychological distress both to patients and their families. Because people often assume the patient is starving to death, families may put great pressure on the patient to eat, leading to anxiety and conflict. Weight loss occurs earlier and is more severe in patients with dysphagia, pain on swallowing, abnormalities of taste or chronic nausea. Management therefore involves controlling nausea and other swallowing problems, as well as providing the patient with small quantities of appetizing food and removing any pressure, from staff or families, to eat more than can be managed. Drug treatment has limited effectiveness.

Corticosteroids

Corticosteroids improve appetite in many cancer patients. They also have a beneficial effect on well-being. Improvement is rapid, so that a short trial of 5–7 days is sufficient to establish if the drug is useful. The appetite stimulation is not translated into weight gain in most patients, and is often short-lived (3–6 weeks). There are no trial data to indicate the most useful dose. Dexamethasone is usually used in doses of 4–8 mg daily.

Progestational agents

Both megestrol acetate and medroxyprogesterone have been shown to stimulate appetite, food intake, energy level and weight gain in controlled trials. The weight gain is mainly fat. The optimal dose of megestrol acetate is reported to be 800 mg/day, although effects are seen with doses as low as 160 mg. Medroxyprogesterone should be given in a dose of 500 mg twice daily. Oedema and an increased tendency to thromboembolism are the main side-effects. The onset of benefit is slower than after corticosteroids.

Prokinetic agents

Chronic nausea and early satiety are common components of the anorexia-cachexia syndrome. The regular administration of a prokinetic anti-emetic, metoclopramide or domperidone, is helpful in reducing both symptoms.

Other drugs

Although the anorexia-cachexia syndrome is believed to be produced by the release of cytokines, trials of antagonists to various cytokines have so far been disappointing. However, positive results have been reported from trials of thalidomide in patients with human immunodeficiency virus (HIV) disease, and studies of cannabinoids are also in progress.

Chronic anaemia

Chronic anaemia in advanced cancer often coexists with weakness and fatigue, but is not always the cause. Chronic blood loss from lung or gastrointestinal tract may be reduced by regular tranexamic acid 1 g three times daily. Etamsylate 500 mg four times daily is safe when bleeding is from the kidney or bladder. The benefit of transfusion should be regularly reassessed, and transfusion only continued if the patient is symptomatically improved. In other countries, patients have been maintained on erythropoietin, but the high cost limits use of this drug in the UK.

Fatigue

Fatigue is associated with more advanced cancer, radiotherapy and chemotherapy. No specific treatment is effective. Corticosteroids are often prescribed, and some patients seem to find them helpful, but there is no supporting trial data. Patients should be advised about adjusting their lifestyle and pacing their activity. Any associated depression should be treated.

Magnesium deficiency is probably commoner in advanced cancer than is generally realized (Crosby *et al.*, 2000). It may present as generalized weakness, possibly with hypokalaemia and a variety of other symptoms and signs. It may follow platinum chemotherapy. The serum magnesium is maintained within the normal range until there is severe whole-body depletion, so that a normal serum magnesium does not rule out the diagnosis. Intravenous repletion followed by oral maintenance treatment reverses the symptoms.

LYMPHOEDEMA

Lymphoedema may follow anti-cancer treatment or disease recurrence. It is worsened by infection. The skin in a lymphoedematous limb should be cared for meticulously and kept moisturized to reduce the risk of skin breaks and cellulitis. Any infection that develops should be treated promptly. Light superficial massage and compression bandaging usually improve the swelling and reduce any leakage, although the benefits are only apparent after several weeks of treatment (Regnard *et al.*, 1997).

A lymphoedematous limb may feel heavy and stiff, but lymphoedema itself is not painful. Nor does it cause nerve damage. Pain or neurological signs indicate that there is another underlying pathology, often progressive tumour.

SWEATS

The prevalence of abnormal sweating in advanced cancer has been reported to be 16–28 per cent. Some patients have sweating of hormonal origin because of a menopause (natural or treatment-induced) in women, or anti-androgen therapy in men with prostate cancer. Low-dose megestrol acetate (40 mg/day) has been shown to be effective and safe in both groups; benefit is seen after 2–3 weeks.

More commonly, sweating is assumed to represent a paraneoplastic phenomenon. Simple measures such as cool surroundings and fresh air or a fan may make the sweating tolerable. Unless there is associated fever, antipyretics are not indicated. The main symptomatic agents used are not supported by a large volume of evidence (Hami and Trotman, 1999), and thioridazine, the drug with the highest reported rate of success, has been withdrawn from general clinical use. Hyoscine has been used successfully in opioid-induced sweating, and the use of cimetidine 400–800 mg daily has also been reported. In one case report, thalidomide 200 mg at night was used successfully; the side-effects of teratogenicity (though rarely a problem in palliative care patients) and peripheral neuropathy have to be remembered.

SKIN PROBLEMS

Pruritus

About 5 per cent of palliative care patients have troublesome itch. The commonest causes are cholestasis and renal failure. Itch is also common in lymphomas and haematological malignancies. If possible, the underlying cause should be relieved, e.g. by stenting of the common bile duct. Otherwise, treatment is symptomatic. The itch is usually exacerbated by heat and by dry skin; cool temperatures, light cotton clothes or bedclothes and emulsifying ointment or aqueous cream instead of soap should be advised.

There is little evidence to support the topical treatments commonly used. Of the systemic treatments available, antihistamines rarely relieve itch in uraemia, cholestasis or lymphoma, although their sedating effects may reduce associated anxiety and promote sleep. Placebo-controlled trials in cholestasis, and case reports in uraemia and opioid-induced pruritus, suggest that 5-HT_3 antagonists such as granisetron in normal antiemetic doses can be effective (Thorns and Edmonds, 2000). Small studies suggest that paroxetene, opioid antagonists and thalidomide may also be worth trying; there is a risk of opioid withdrawal effects with opioid antagonists, especially naloxone.

Fungating wounds

Fungating wounds cause psychological distress. Odour is the most distressing symptom; the wounds can produce a profuse exudate, which requires repeated dressings, may bleed and may be painful and itchy. The pain may be poorly responsive to opioids. Bacterial infection should be treated with a topical preparation such as metronidazole gel to reduce the odour. If the surrounding skin is inflamed and itchy, corticosteroid cream may be helpful. Bleeding can be controlled by a topical application of sucralfate (the suspension is placed on a non-adherent dressing) or of tranexamic acid (using the parenteral preparation) (Regnard *et al.*, 1997). Very absorbent dressings, such as alginate, reduce both the bulk and the frequency of dressings. Pain during dressings may be reduced by using diluted bupivacaine rather than saline to wash the wound, or teaching the patient to breathe a mixture of oxygen and nitrous oxide (Entonox). A top layer of a carbon-impregnated dressing, to absorb any remaining odour, may then make the situation more tolerable and manageable both for the patient and for the family.

EMERGENCY SITUATIONS

Not all acute problems are reversible in patients with advanced cancer. The adverse effects of treatment may outweigh a benefit which may be short-lived. If the patient is too ill to make his wishes clear, the situation should be discussed with those close to him so that agreement can be reached on the best course of action.

Severe infections

Infection may follow treatment, e.g. after chemotherapy, or arise as a consequence of the underlying illness. It is often difficult in the emergency situation to be clear whether the patient or his family would want aggressive treatment of the infection. Sometimes, when chemotherapy has been entirely palliative, the oncologist's judgement may be that it is better not to treat aggressively, but this can be psychologically very difficult to accept when active anti-tumour treatment is still being given. If possible, it is helpful to discuss with the patient in advance what his wishes would be in this situation. Some patients write Advance Directives, and their existence should be communicated to all the clinicians caring for the patient.

Hypercalcaemia

Treatment should be considered if the corrected serum calcium is >3 mmol/L, the patient is symptomatic or the serum calcium is rising very rapidly. Patients may present with confusion and vomiting, and are also likely to have thirst, polyuria, dehydration and constipation.

Intravenous bisphosphonates are the treatment of choice. After initial intravenous rehydration, a biphosphonate such as intravenous disodium pamidronate 90 mg or sodium clodronate 1500 mg is infused over 2–4 hours, followed if necessary by further intravenous fluids. The serum calcium begins to fall 3–5 days after treatment, and 80 per cent of patients will have a normal serum calcium within a week. Benefit is often transient. Oral clodronate may delay recurrence of hypercalcaemia. Further intravenous bisphosphonates can be given regularly or as required, depending on the speed with which the serum calcium rises again.

Alternative treatments are rarely required. Calcitonin acts very quickly, but tolerance usually develops within days or a very few weeks. Its only role is probably in the patient with life-threatening hypercalcaemia, who cannot wait 3 days for bisphosphonates to be effective. Gallium nitrate has been shown to be as effective as bisphosphonates, but is less well tolerated and rarely used. Corticosteroids are probably only effective when they have an anti-tumour effect, e.g. in lymphomas.

Superior vena caval obstruction (SVCO)

Most cases of SVCO are due to tumour within the mediastinum, usually from a primary cancer of the bronchus.

If the obstruction cannot be relieved, patients need symptomatic relief of breathlessness. High-dose corticosteroids are often helpful. Low-dose oral morphine can reduce the dyspnoea. Patients may also need a benzodiazepine for anxiety.

Massive haemorrhage

Those most at risk of massive haemorrhage include patients with carcinomas of the bronchus and haemoptysis, patients with a tumour which is eroding a major artery (usually in the neck or groin) and patients with a primary tumour of the upper gastrointestinal tract. It is rarely possible to stop a torrential haemorrhage, although some patients, as the massive blood loss results in hypotension, will stop bleeding spontaneously. If bleeding is from the lung, the patient should be positioned on his side with the diseased lung downwards, to reduce the chance that he will drown in his own blood. If the bleeding can be stopped, resuscitation measures can be considered, but may not always be appropriate, particularly if further bleeding is likely and cannot be prevented.

If a major haemorrhage can be anticipated, it may be helpful to warn the patient's family, especially if he is at home. However, it can be difficult to do this without causing panic. In a hospital or hospice situation, patients at risk of major haemorrhage should have on their drug charts a single large dose of sedative which can be injected if there is a major haemorrhage, to reduce the patient's distress and fear.

REHABILITATION

Patients with advanced cancer are often perceived to be progressing along a trajectory of deterioration which ends inevitably in death. This is an oversimplification. Despite progressive cancer, many patients can be helped to maximize their functional ability and independence by individualized programmes of rehabilitation, often involving physiotherapy, occupational therapy and psychological support. Rehabilitation is particularly important after events such as a pathological fracture or spinal cord compression, but often appropriate after radiotherapy or chemotherapy if there have been major side-effects. Good links between oncologists and palliative care or other rehabilitation facilities help to ensure patients achieve the best possible level of independence.

PSYCHOLOGICAL CARE

Cancer patients and their families need good psychological care throughout their illness. As the disease progresses, patients may have to deal with repeated sharing of information, much of it bad news, and may have to deal with a great deal of uncertainty, particularly regarding prognosis. Psychiatric disorders, particularly adjustment reactions, are common, and up to 80 per cent of this morbidity is unrecognized and untreated (Lloyd-Williams, 1999). Clinical psychiatric disease, particularly depression, is also common, but its prevalence is difficult to determine from published studies, as it varies markedly according to the methods and criteria used for assessment.

Depression

Depression is often unrecognized in an outpatient population. Among patients admitted to specialist palliative care units, estimates of prevalence range from 25 to 37 per cent (Lloyd-Williams, 1999). As somatic symptoms may be due to the physical illness, the diagnosis has to be established solely on psychological symptoms, including suicidal ideation, which should always be asked about.

Tricyclic antidepressants and SSRIs can both be used selectively in patients with advanced cancer, provided they are likely to live for the 2–4 weeks needed to see benefit. Tricyclic drugs tend to be used where patients are having difficulty sleeping. A long-acting SSRI such as fluoxetine may be preferable to a short-acting one, to avoid a withdrawal syndrome in the dying phase when the patient can no longer swallow. Response rates are difficult to assess, but have been reported to be lower than in patients without physical illness, and psychiatric help may be needed. If the patient's prognosis is very short, a psychostimulant such as methylphenidate may be considered.

Severe anxiety is often associated with depression. But if it is diagnosed independently, or does not respond to a sedating antidepressant, benzodiazepines are safe and effective.

Organic confusional states

An organic confusional state (delirium) may develop at any time, but becomes more prevalent as patients approach death. Common causes include brain tumours, infection, metabolic disturbances (including renal failure) and drugs, particularly opioids and psychotropic drugs. If possible, an underlying cause should be treated. No active management may be needed if the patient is not distressed by the confusion. But many patients become agitated, and require sedation.

Delirium may be accompanied by hallucinations and/or delusions. A neuroleptic such as haloperidol or, if more sedation is needed, levomepromazine, can be given orally or by subcutaneous infusion. If only sedation is required, a subcutaneous infusion of midazolam can be

titrated to give the patient comfort, and can be rapidly withdrawn if the underlying cause resolves.

SPIRITUAL SUPPORT

Being brought face to face with impending death often makes people want to explore existential and spiritual issues. These need not necessarily involve any formal religion, or even a faith in any God. People may wonder why they have been singled out for such an unfair punishment, or question the value of their life. They may feel guilty for deeds in the past, particularly if quarrels or problems have not been resolved. They may even feel their cancer is a punishment for living an evil life.

Those who have a religious faith may find it a source of comfort, but may conversely question the existence of a God who allows these things to happen. They may have tremendous fear and doubt about what is on the other side of death. Sometimes, well-meaning friends or fellow church members express the belief that the cancer will be cured if the sufferer has enough faith and prays enough. When the cancer is not cured, the patients are often left feeling guilty that they have not had sufficient faith, an unnecessary additional burden.

We live in a society in which people come from many cultural backgrounds and follow a wide variety of religions. As part of caring for the whole person, and their family, it is essential to respect religious beliefs and practices, even if that means adapting the normal routine of a hospital ward. In some religions, illness and death are seen as determined by fate, rather than the patient's deeds. This can be helpful in absolving the patient from any sense of personal guilt.

Spiritual issues are often left for a chaplain or trained counsellor to explore. Clinicians often feel out of their depth in such conversations. This is not necessarily helpful for the patient, who may prefer to discuss things with someone he knows well rather than with an unfamiliar professional, particularly if he does not have an identifiable religious faith. It is important for everyone to remain open to such conversations.

SOCIAL CARE

People rarely exist in isolation. They often have close family, and usually a social network. These carers also need support, and should be involved in the patient's care if that is what they and the patient want. Families cope better with death if they have been kept well informed as the patient's condition deteriorates, and can contribute to the discussions around management.

This is particularly important if the patient wants to spend his last period of life at home, as he will be dependent on family for much of the care, no matter how good a package of community care is organized.

THE DYING PHASE

Death from cancer is rarely sudden, unless it is precipitated by an event such as a pulmonary embolus. In the majority of patients there is a dying phase, which may last for hours or days. It is characterized by increasing sleepiness (and often finally loss of consciousness), confusion, weakness, difficulty in coughing and inability to swallow. It is essential that control of symptoms such as pain and vomiting is maintained, even when the patient is unable to swallow his usual medication. But other medication, particularly that for long-term conditions such as hypertension, should be discontinued.

Cancer sufferers come from a variety of cultural and religious backgrounds. While it is helpful to be familiar with the basic customs of the major religions around death, there is considerable individual variation in how, or whether, these are observed. Staff should always ask, as sensitively as possible, either the patient or a relative what they would like done during the dying period and also immediately after death. If a relative wants to take part in laying out the body, or the family needs to take over this function, this should be encouraged.

Assessment

Careful, preferably multi-professional assessment is essential, and should be regularly repeated. The situation may change very rapidly. The focus should be on the patient's problems. However, by this stage many patients are too weak to take part in discussions. Relatives often speak for them. There is evidence that both professionals and relatives may have views that differ from those of the patient (Working Party on Clinical Guidelines in Palliative Care, 1997). Relatives in particular may transfer their own distress to the patient, and describe his pain as worse than it actually is.

Maintaining symptom control by non-oral routes

Dying patients commonly lose the ability to swallow medication. All non-essential medication should be stopped. This will include replacement hormones, and often corticosteroids too. Some drugs can be given by the transdermal or rectal route, or by subcutaneous injection. Repeated injections should be avoided in cachectic patients. Many patients need a parenteral analgesic, such as diamorphine, together with additional drugs, to maintain symptom control over the dying phase. The simplest way to administer these is as a continuous subcutaneous infusion, using a small, battery-driven infusion pump. Pharmacists can advise on compatibilities when mixing drugs in one syringe.

Terminal agitation

Dying patients may experience overwhelming distress, or fear of impending death. This may be associated with their severe weakness, and a sense of being helpless and out of control. Sometimes it is related to unresolved conflict or to guilt over real or imagined past sins, or reflects their sadness at leaving behind a loved and dependent family. As confusion is common at this stage of life, agitated patients may not be able to express their anguish verbally, or be comforted or reassured.

The subcutaneous route can be used for sedation, either with a benzodiazepine such as midazolam (10 mg/24 hours titrated upwards as required) or, if an anti-emetic effect is also needed, with the phenothiazine, levomepromazine (12.5–25 mg/24 hours titrated upwards as required). Either can be mixed with diamorphine for infusion.

Death rattle

Noisy breathing, with a rattling sound in the throat or chest, may develop in the last hours or days. It mainly reflects the patient's inability to cough effectively. Fluid overload, particularly in hypoalbuminaemic patients, or bronchopneumonia may worsen it. Either glycopyrronium (0.6–1.2 mg/24 hours) or hyoscine given subcutaneously, by injection or infusion, can reduce the secretions. Hyoscine is given as the butylbromide in a dose of 20–40 mg/24 hours, or as the hydrobromide in a dose of 1.2–2.4 mg/24 hours.

Fluid needs

Dying patients are rarely able or willing to drink. Staff and relatives often worry that the patient's death will be accelerated, or made more uncomfortable, by dehydration. The expected symptoms of dehydration are a dry mouth and thirst. Research does not show any correlation between a dry mouth and biochemical indicators of dehydration (Ellershaw et al., 1995). Instead, a dry mouth is associated with treatment with particular drugs, such as opioids or tricyclic antidepressants. Water requirements are decreased at the end of life, and there is a risk that parenteral rehydration may cause increased pulmonary oedema, particularly in patients with hypoalbuminaemia (Steiner and Bruera, 1998).

It may be very difficult to convince relatives that the patient is not dying as a result of lack of food and water. A great deal of explanation and reassurance is often needed.

SUPPORT FOR STAFF

Caring for cancer patients who are terminally ill can be very stressful for professional staff. They may see their role as curative, and feel guilty about failing to cure particular patients, especially if the primary tumour was one with a high cure rate. Caring for a dying patient may also cause staff to consider their own future death, and this may lead to considerable anxiety. Staff are often particularly distressed if the dying patient is young, or has a very young family, or if in some other way they identify with the particular patient.

It is essential not to deny the reality of these feelings. They can sometimes lead professionals to avoid patients who are dying, or to deny that the patient's prognosis is short. Inappropriate management decisions may then be made. If staff are to continue to work well with all cancer patients, and not merely those in the early stages of the disease, they need support in dealing with their feelings of grief, anger, guilt and bereavement when patients are dying, and with their feelings of personal vulnerability.

BEREAVEMENT

Because the care of the terminally ill patient includes the care of his family, involvement should not end with the death of the patient. It is important to ensure that those who have been bereaved are grieving normally, and that help is available for those in whom there is a high risk of an abnormal or exceptionally severe grief reaction, such as parents who have lost a child, and those with a previous history of alcohol misuse or depressive illness.

In addition to feelings of numbness, disbelief and loss, many bereaved people feel strong anger. This may be displaced on to staff who were involved in the patient's care. This is particularly difficult to deal with if there is some basis for it, such as a delay in diagnosis. Grieving may also involve inappropriate feelings of guilt, whether for imagined failings in caring for the dead person or for estrangements which were not healed before death. It is helpful if it is made easier for the family to have an interview with a member of staff who knew the patient and the circumstances of the death. If the anger can be dealt with in an understanding way, rather than by confrontation, and honest explanations given for anything that is worrying the family, these difficult reactions will usually come to a natural end.

Families should be given information about community resources which offer support in bereavement, including the primary care team and voluntary organizations. Specialist help may be needed for children who have lost a parent, who need counselling appropriate to their age group.

SIGNIFICANT POINTS

- The majority of cancer patients will need palliative care, which should run alongside anti-cancer therapy.
- Palliative care is multi-professional and involves caring for the family as well as the patient.
- Good communication, both with the patient and among the clinical team, is essential.
- The management plan should reflect the goals of the patient and family, and should be shared with all the professionals involved.
- Good palliative care demands meticulous symptom control and requires a thorough knowledge of the pharmacology of analgesics, anti-emetics and drugs for the terminal phase.
- The patient's autonomy must be respected. This involves his right to information and to make choices, including the choice of where to die.

KEY REFERENCES

Bruera, E. and Higginson, I. (eds) (1996) *Cachexia-anorexia in cancer patients.* Oxford: Oxford University Press.

Doyle, D., Hanks, G.W.C. and MacDonald, N. (eds) (1998) *Oxford textbook of palliative medicine*, 2nd edn. Oxford: Oxford University Press.

Fallon, M. and O'Neill, W.M. (eds) (1998) *ABC of palliative care.* London: BMA Publishing.

Hillier, R., Finlay, I., Welsh, J. and Miles, A. (eds) (2000) *The effective management of cancer pain.* London: Aesculapius Medical Press.

Working Party on Clinical Guidelines in Palliative Care (1997) *Changing gear – guidelines for managing the last days of life in adults.* London: National Council for Hospice and Specialist Palliative Care Services.

REFERENCES

Baines, M. (1997) ABC of palliative care: nausea, vomiting and intestinal obstruction. *Br. Med. J.* **315**, 1148–50.

Bruera, E. (1997) ABC of palliative care: anorexia, cachexia and nutrition. *Br. Med. J.* **315**, 1219–22.

Bruera, E. and Pereira, J. (1998) Recent developments in palliative cancer care. *Acta Oncol.* **37**, 749–57.

Byrne, A. (2000) Recent progress in the use of non-steroidal analgesia: the place of old and new NSAIDs. In Hillier, R., Finlay, I., Welsh, J. and Miles, A. (eds), *The effective management of cancer pain*. London: Aesculapius Medical Press, 79–91.

Crosby, V., Wilcock, A., Lawson, N. and Corcoran, R. (2000) The importance of low magnesium in palliative care. *Palliat. Med.* **14**, 544.

Davies, A.N. (2000) A comparison of artificial saliva and chewing gum in the management of xerostomia in patients with advanced cancer. *Palliat. Med.* **14**, 197–203.

Davies, A.N., Daniels, C., Pugh, R. and Sharma, K. (1998) A comparison of artificial saliva and pilocarpine in the management of xerostomia in patients with advanced cancer. *Palliat. Med.* **12**, 105–11.

Davis, C.L. (1997) ABC of palliative care: breathlessness, cough and other respiratory symptoms. *Br. Med. J.* **315**, 931–4.

Ellershaw, J.E., Sutcliffe, J.M. and Saunders, C.M. (1995) Dehydration and the dying patient. *J. Pain Sympt. Manage.* **10**, 192–7.

Feuer, D.J. and Broadley, K.E. (2000) Corticosteroids for the resolution of malignant bowel obstruction in advanced gynaecological and gastrointestinal cancer (Cochrane review). *Cochrane Database Syst. Rev.* **2**, CD001219.

Hami, F. and Trotman, I. (1999) The treatment of sweating. *Eur. J. Palliat. Care* **6**, 184–7.

Hanks, G. and Hawkins, C. (2000) Agreeing a gold standard in the management of cancer pain: the role of opioids. In Hillier, R., Finlay, I., Welsh, J. and Miles, A. (eds), *The effective management of cancer pain*. London: Aesculapius Medical Press, 57–77.

Herbert, M.E. (2000) Myth: codeine is an effective cough suppressant for upper respiratory tract infections. *West. J. Med.* **173**, 283.

Hoskin, P.J. (1995) Radiotherapy for bone pain. *Pain* **63**, 137–9.

LeGrand, S.B. and Walsh, D. (1999) Palliative management of dyspnea in advanced cancer. *Curr. Opin. Oncol.* **11**, 250–4.

Lloyd-Williams, M. (1999) The assessment of depression in palliative care patients. *Eur. J. Palliat. Care* **6**, 150–3.

Lucas, V. and Schofield, L. (2000) Treatment of drooling. *Eur. J. Palliat. Care* **7**, 5–7.

Mannix, K., Ahmedzai, S.H., Anderson, H. *et al.* (2000) Using bisphosphonates to control the pain of bone metastases: evidence-based guidelines for palliative care. *Palliat. Med.* **14**, 455–61.

National Council for Hospice and Specialist Palliative Care Services (1995) *Specialist palliative care: a statement of definitions*, Occasional Paper 8. London: National Council for Hospice and Specialist Palliative Care Services.

Nelson, K.A. (2000) The cancer anorexia-cachexia syndrome. *Semin. Oncol.* **27**, 64–8.

Pargeon, K.L. and Hailey, B.J. (1999) Barriers to effective pain management: a review of the literature. *J. Pain Sympt. Manage.* **18**, 358–68.

Quigley, C. (2000) New approaches to the management of neuropathic pain. *CME Bull. Palliat. Med.* **2**, 35–40.

Rawlinson, F. (2000) Dyspnoea and cough. *Eur. J. Palliat. Care* **7**, 161–4.

Regnard, C. (1994) Single dose fluconazole versus five day ketoconazole in oral candidosis. *Palliat. Med.* **8**, 72–3.

Regnard, C., Allport, S. and Stephenson, L. (1997) ABC of palliative care: mouth care, skin care and lymphoedema. *Br. Med. J.* **315**, 1002–5.

Rich, A. and Ellershaw, J. (2000) Tenesmus/rectal pain – how is it best managed? *CME Bull. Palliat. Med.* **2**, 41–4.

Steiner, N. and Bruera, E. (1998) Methods of hydration in palliative care patients. *J. Palliat. Care* **14**, 6–13.

Sweeney, M.P. and Bagg, J. (1995) Oral care for hospice patients with advanced cancer. *Dent. Update* **22**, 424–7.

Thorns, A. and Edmonds, P. (2000) The management of pruritus in palliative care patients. *Eur. J. Palliat. Care* **7**, 9–12.

Twycross, R. and Back, I. (1998) Nausea and vomiting in advanced cancer. *Eur. J. Palliat. Care* **5**, 39–45.

Viganò, A., Dorgan, M., Buckingham, J. *et al.* (2000) Survival prediction in terminal cancer patients: a systematic review of the medical literature. *Palliat. Med.* **14**, 363–74.

Williams, J. (2000) Critical appraisal of invasive therapies used to treat chronic pain and cancer pain. *Eur. J. Palliat. Care* **7**, 121–5.

Working Party on Clinical Guidelines in Palliative Care (1997) *Changing gear – guidelines for managing the last days of life in adults*. London: National Council for Hospice and Specialist Palliative Care Services.

World Health Organization (1990) Cancer pain relief and palliative care. Report of a WHO Expert Committee. *WHO Tech. Rep. Series* **804**, 1–75.

Zeppetella, G., O'Doherty, C.A. and Collins, S. (2000) Prevalence and characteristics of breakthrough pain in cancer patients admitted to a hospice. *J. Pain Sympt. Manage.* **20**, 87–92.

55

The holistic approach to cancer

ROSY DANIEL

INTRODUCTION

The origins of the holistic health movement in Britain can be traced to the 1960s, when, along with the Beatles, the environmental movement and the quest for 'alternative lifestyles', came a strong alternative medical movement. This was influenced by Oriental philosophy and medical practice, which placed key emphasis on the natural rather than the high-tech. The inter-relationship between body, mind, spirit and environment in the aetiology, treatment and prevention of disease began to be of widespread public interest. There was a gradual re-introduction of traditional therapies such as homeopathy, herbalism and acupuncture, and encouragement of individuals to take responsibility for their health through attention to whole-food diets and self-help practices such as yoga, tai chi and meditation.

These times were also characterized by a general rejection of the materialism and repression of post-war Britain in favour of both libertarian and spiritually based values – a concept often referred to as 'New Age'. This alternative health movement grew strongly throughout the 1970s and 1980s with the development of health-food shops and natural therapy centres. These promoted the idea that individuals could play a very significant role in their own healing, growth and recovery through the use of complementary, nutritional, self-help, psychotherapeutic and spiritual therapies. Conventional practitioners were sceptical and there was almost no dialogue or encouragement from either general practices or hospitals. The two approaches became increasingly antagonistic. Until 1980 complementary therapies were rarely offered to cancer

patients in the UK, despite the plethora of unconventional approaches sought by patients in North America, France and Germany. This changed with the opening of the Bristol Cancer Help Centre, founded in 1980 by a cancer patient, Penny Brohn. The concept was to offer 'the gentle way with cancer' rather than the 'burning, cutting and poisoning' of cancer with orthodox medicine. These extreme paradigms did little to bring harmony between professionals. Some of the more extreme alternative cancer medicines, bizarre diets, fasts, detoxification regimens and the exaggerated claims made for their success, led to great concern amongst oncologists. There were also examples of patients being dissuaded from taking potentially curative medical treatment by alternative hard-liners.

Despite the extensive misgivings of the medical profession, dialogue continued throughout the 1980s, and a new model of complementarity emerged. The increasing academic interest in the psychological aspects of cancer led to more and better research in this difficult area. Enabling patients to get the best of both worlds – conventional and complementary – seemed a reasonable solution. With this shift came a stronger emphasis on the psycho-spiritual aspects of care, with the introduction of relaxation, massage, reflexology, counselling and yoga in hospitals. At that time a study revealed that 37 per cent of cancer patients were actually using complementary therapies of some sort, and found them helpful (Burke and Sikora, 1992). Several UK cancer centres introduced complementary programmes alongside conventional care, including the Hammersmith, Clatterbridge, Lancaster and Shrewsbury hospitals. Hospices were already using such techniques for patients at the end of their lives. The efforts of these teams demonstrated that not only could the holistic approach to cancer be complementary to mainstream medicine, but it could be integrated within conventional oncology services. In 1993, the first state-of-the-art integrated cancer support centre was purpose-built by the Cancer Relief Macmillan Fund at Mount Vernon Hospital.

The move towards the integration of holistic approaches into mainstream medicine has been fuelled during the 1990s by the development of the Foundation for Integrated Medicine (email: fimed@compuserve.com) established at the instigation of HRH The Prince of Wales. It must be noted that it is mainly the supportive care and symptom-control elements that have been integrated into cancer centres; the patient self-help approach still being viewed as questionable, although times are changing – a recent Canadian study (Montbriand, 1998) showed that 81 per cent of 300 lung cancer patients were using unconventional cancer treatments (UCTs) and a US study (Van de Creek *et al.*, 1999) showed that 76 per cent of breast cancer patients were using UCTs.

THE PATIENT'S PERSPECTIVE

In an attempt to understand the needs of people with cancer for support, self-management and complementary help, a collaborative team from Bristol Oncology Centre, Bristol Cancer Help Centre and the University of Warwick performed a focus group study in 1997 (Tritter *et al.*, 1998) to determine how people with cancer, and their supporters, reacted to the diagnosis of cancer (Fig. 55.1), and what steps they had taken as a result of their reactions.

Key emotions experienced by cancer patients

- Intense shock – disbelief, grief, the feeling of 'why me?', terror and occasionally paradoxical excitement at the time of diagnosis.
- Fear – of knowing more about the cancer, of recurrence and symptoms of the cancer, of death and dying, of hospitals, tests and doctors, and what would happen to their families who would probably survive them.
- Loss – of physical confidence, of a sense of an assured future, or emotional balance, of a sense of control and certainty in their lives, and of the continuity of care after treatment.
- Isolation – feeling cut off from others, as if the threat to their lives had moved them through an invisible social barrier, and a heightened sense of loneliness that this created.
- Confusion – about the complexity of medical options and different protocols available for the treatment of similar cancers, and the vast array of complementary self-help and support options.
- A complex set of feelings towards others – including a sense of failure, jealousy, distrust, resentment, guilt, gratitude and concern.

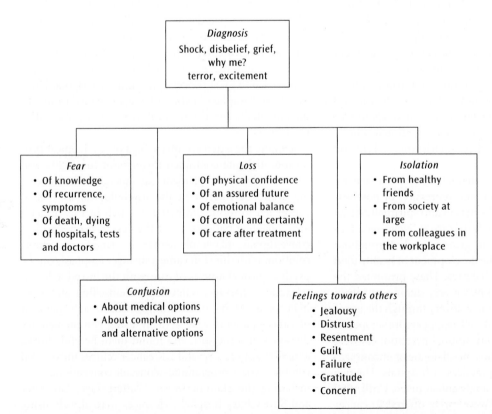

Figure 55.1 *The emotions of cancer patients following diagnosis.*

Reactions to the diagnosis of cancer

In response to the diagnosis of cancer, there were three common reactions (Fig. 55.2). The first was to go into avoidance or denial; the second to collapse completely; and the third, and most frequent, was to exert some form of control. Those who took control usually went into a period of information gathering in order to seek help to mitigate the emotional and spiritual impact of diagnosis, cope with their symptoms and treatment and attempt to survive cancer.

Mitigation of the emotional and spiritual impact included:

- 'normalization' and re-engagement with life;
- talking to others in groups;
- finding hope;
- getting the best out of life;
- facing death, uncertainty and cancer;
- getting life and cancer into perspective;
- finding peace of mind;
- exploring their own spirituality;
- helping others.

Coping with symptoms and treatment was achieved by finding ways of:

- managing anxiety;

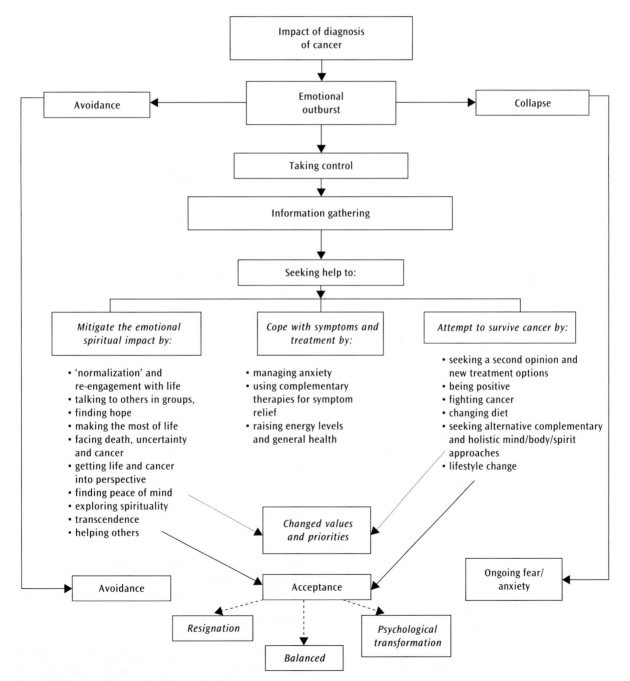

Figure 55.2 *Reactions to the diagnosis of cancer.*

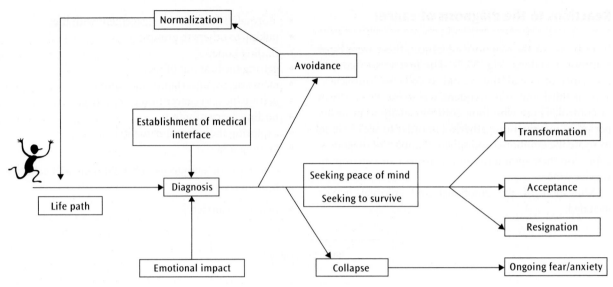

Figure 55.3 *The emotional cancer journey.*

- using complementary therapies for symptom relief;
- raising energy levels;
- improving general health through diet and exercise.

Attempts to survive cancer were made by:

- seeking second opinions and new treatment options;
- seeking alternative, complementary and holistic mind/body/spirit approaches;
- being positive;
- fighting cancer;
- changing diets;
- lifestyle changes.

When asked the reasons given for the use of complementary therapies and other self-help approaches, the views included that these therapies and techniques:

- provided high-quality supportive care by virtue of the therapist's skills, the emphasis placed on the empathic therapeutic relationship, the time given, and the engendering of feelings of security;
- provided help in facing orthodox treatment due to relief of side-effects, symptom control, improved state of mind and increased energy levels;
- enabled people to feel that they are being treated as individuals, helping them to focus on themselves and their needs;
- empowered people to take an active role, thereby bringing about a sense of control and involvement;
- gave practical ways of improving health;
- gave messages that individuals can play a role in restoring their health and well-being, however ill they are;
- focused on 'natural' rather than 'chemical' or 'high-tech' medicine.

It is interesting to note that none of the participants interviewed in this study talked about the intrinsic medical benefits of the therapies or practice, but concentrated on the psychological benefits they derived from their use.

The emotional cancer journey

It is clear that, for most people with cancer, early strategies revolve around the desire for normalization of life, either as a result of avoidance, or finding the psychological support to enable the threat of cancer to recede (Fig. 55.3). However, for many this cannot be achieved, with resulting ongoing fear, depression and loss of quality of life. Later in the journey, when either debilitating long-term symptoms or the advancement of the disease make normalization impossible, more serious attempts are often made to fight the illness or come to terms with it.

Although the Bristol Study was not quantitative, the impression gained was that those who had received supportive care, or who become involved in self-management strategies, were much more likely to make the transition into acceptance. In almost all cases participants had found their own way into supportive care and self-help. There was widespread criticism that cancer service provision did not routinely include encouragement of, and routine access to, supportive care and self-help activity or information about local and national services.

THE HOLISTIC MODEL AND ITS IMPLEMENTATION

The holistic model

The purist holistic model is a health-based model in which individuals and therapists work in partnership to achieve the best levels of health, energy, emotional and spiritual well-being, in the presence of illness. The holistic model is integrative, with a central theme that the states of mind, body and spirit are inextricably linked. This means that the state of an individual's spirit or will to live, mental state, stress, self-expression, lifestyle, physical and emotional state are all seen as relevant in terms of the aetiology of illness and the potential improvement of health within the context of illness. Within the holistic model the factors primarily affecting an individual's state and health are seen as:

- the state of the individual's 'spirit', purpose in living and will to live;
- the emotional state, both current and chronic;
- the underlying beliefs and past experiences which determine behaviour and relationship to oneself;
- the physical state – nutrition, fitness, posture and breathing patterns;
- the environment – socially and physically;
- lifestyle – particularly the balance of work with recreation and busy-ness with stillness and regenerative time.

STATE OF THE SPIRIT

It is often observed that if an individual has lost his or her will to live, then no medicine, orthodox or complementary, will help them. Similarly, if individuals have become dispirited or had their spirit crushed by hurt, loss, disappointment, abuse, social disadvantage, grief or continual stress, the body's ability to heal is severely compromised. The accent within the holistic approach is therefore placed strongly on helping to revive the individual's spirit through holistic therapies and individual and group psychotherapeutic processes. These aim to help the individual to rediscover a sense of purpose and meaning in life, to identify their core values and sources of uplift for their spirit. These processes may range from enjoying the beauty of nature, art and music, to engaging in spiritual practices, following a religion or helping others.

Another common reason for depression of the spirit is loneliness, and here the need is to connect individuals to others, either socially, in learning situations, community initiatives or support groups. It is also important to help individuals learn how to make good relationships and to communicate their needs clearly. This may require assertiveness training. The overall aim is to enable individuals to re-find their joy in living, a sense of purpose and belonging, and an outlet for authentic self-expression, and caring connections to other people and the community.

Commonly, times of extreme adversity are when individuals discover their spiritual nature and develop their own spirituality in very personal ways. This profoundly enriching process can be so important that there is sometimes a feeling that the illness has served to awaken the person to the real essence of life, 'transforming them' and enabling them to live a far happier life based on spiritual rather than material or fear-based values.

EMOTIONAL AND MENTAL STATE

In the holistic model great attention is paid to the emotional state, both current (particularly relating to the diagnosis of cancer) and chronic, especially in the way the individual handles their emotions. Because of the potentially deleterious effects of fear and repressed emotion on the body and immune system, strong efforts are made to help individuals learn how to relax and to feel safe to express their emotions, helping them to identify and meet their emotional need. At a deeper level, efforts are made to help individuals identify the beliefs and attitudes they hold, which in turn dictate the relationship they have to themselves and with others. Often those who have not been well cared for as children, and who do not have strong, positive self-images, will base a great deal of their behaviour on the desire to win approval and affection, often stressing and exhausting themselves severely in the process. Simultaneously, they may be alienating those whose affections they are trying to win.

Individuals are asked the fundamental questions: What is their relationship to themselves? How are they looking after themselves? Do they nourish, care for and protect themselves from destructive influences? Do they chronically abandon, neglect or even abuse themselves? The establishment of a new, loving and nurturing relationship to one's self is one of the most important themes within the holistic model, and individuals are enabled, through the holistic therapies, to learn to identify their needs and care for themselves properly. They can then go on to model their new relationship to themselves on the therapeutic relationships they have developed, through self-help practices and the development of more nurturing lifestyles.

PHYSICAL STATE

Here the key issues are getting individuals to examine their eating habits, their exercise patterns, their body posture and way of breathing. In the West most of us eat a very processed diet which is high in fat, sugar and protein, with too few fruits and overcooked vegetables, denatured and deficient in vitamins and minerals. This results in us becoming simultaneously overfed and undernourished, with too little fibre in our digestive tracts.

Individuals are also encouraged to exercise and stretch daily, even if they have to do this on a chair or in bed. Avoiding 'stagnation' of the lymphatic system and body energies is seen as an important part of many holistic therapies, and the achieving of a good posture is also encouraged. This has become increasingly relevant due to the very sedentary office and computer-based lifestyles many people in the West are living. Attention is also directed to breathing patterns. The combination of sedentary lifestyle, poor posture and emotional tension or depression leads to very shallow breathing. This in turn affects the mental state, leaving the individual feeling sluggish, depressed or anxious. Through relaxation and exercise it is possible to deepen breathing.

ENVIRONMENT

Socially one's environment may be dominated by difficult, demanding relationships, or by interpersonal pressures in the workplace or home. Many have discovered, through their holistic explorations, that they never had the chance to find out 'who they are' or what their own needs are because of having lived around extremely dominant family members, partners or colleagues whose needs were always prioritized. Re-establishing health and well-being may depend upon renegotiating boundaries and commitments; identifying and meeting personal needs and desires.

LIFESTYLE

The lifestyle of an individual is usually a very clear reflection of the nature of their relationship to themselves, and it is usually necessary for the relationship to the self to change before changes in lifestyle become possible and sustainable. The overall aim is to get the lifestyle into balance, helping people who have become workaholic to learn again how to play and relax; enabling individuals who have become addicted to being busy and constantly stimulated to learn how to become still. This process, which also enables the development of a rewarding inner life, can be helped by spiritual healing and learning the self-help techniques of relaxation and meditation. This, in turn, can help to break the cycle of individuals requiring more and more stimulation and ever higher achievement and excitement in order to have any sense of satisfaction. In relaxing and becoming more open, individuals regain their sensitivity and have an enhanced ability to experience pleasure and the more subtle dimensions of life.

The energy model

Another key concept within the holistic approach is to think in terms of the effect than an individual's behaviour, lifestyle and mental state has on their energy levels or vitality. In all the old traditional holistic systems there is a concept for this energy. It is called the vital force in homeopathy, chi in acupuncture, *prana* in yoga and *ki* in shiatsu. Once the energy has returned, the second key is for people to learn the importance of putting themselves first by reorganizing their priorities and values in life and by becoming involved with that which really excites and inspires them. We can look at this energy equation like an energy budget, getting clients to ask themselves 'How am I spending my energy, where is it all going, and is this right for me now?' And the second, even more important question 'How do I build my energy and am I spending more than I am generating?'

The holistic model of illness and therapy

In the holistic model, illness is seen to arise when the body's ability to resist disease has broken down due to a state of disharmony or imbalance between mind, body, spirit and the individual's environment. All holistic therapies and self-help techniques are therefore designed to strengthen and rebalance the body, increasing the individual's ability to stabilize the disease process and recover from illness. The therapies aimed at any of the levels of mind, body and spirit are seen as being able to affect all other levels because of the integrated nature of the system. After an initial exploratory assessment with the holistic doctor, nurse or practitioner, first a therapeutic and then a self-help plan is negotiated which feels most appropriate to the individual.

Implementation

In cancer medicine aspects of this approach are implemented in three settings:

- Psychosocial care given within hospitals, hospices, voluntary sector support groups, or within the community via health visitors, social workers or the Church, to ease psychological distress and the existential angst caused by the diagnosis, and to give spiritual comfort and guidance.
- The supportive care setting, used in hospitals, hospices and the community where there is increasing use of complementary therapies, particularly by nurses for symptom control, comfort and palliative care.
- The patient self-help movement, where a mixture of self-help approaches, complementary and alternative therapies, nutrition and psychological approaches are used with the aim of improving health, well-being and prognosis.

The guiding ethos or goals of practitioners in these different settings affects the patient's experience greatly. In all these settings there is likely to be help provided to:

- recover from the shock and trauma of diagnosis;
- receive rehabilitation back into life after treatment;
- receive help with symptom control and treatment side-effects.

However, it is usually only within the patient self-help movement that patients will receive the following messages:

- It is possible for them to work to improve their health, energy and possibly even improve prognosis.
- It is possible to transform the crisis of illness into the opportunity to find new meaning and personal fulfilment in life through application of the holistic approach.
- Help is available to work consciously with the personal issues around death and the process of dying.

The crucial difference for the patients in making this 'holistic paradigm shift' is that patients have their hope rekindled. Patients regain an all-important inner locus of control, have a positive course of action which greatly reduces anxiety and quickly produces positive benefits such as enhanced well-being, energy and increased personal fulfilment.

Components of the holistic model

The component parts of the holistic model (Fig. 55.4) are:

- complementary therapy
- alternative therapy
- self-help approaches
- nutrition
- counselling, psychotherapy and group work
- spiritual healing
- general support.

Implementation of the model is in two phases: therapeutic and self-help. During the therapeutic phase, help is sought from:

- Holistic doctors and nurses who provide medical counselling, lifestyle assessment, guidance on the use of complementary and alternative medicines, symptom control with stress reduction and natural remedies (herbal and homeopathic), and specific nutritional advice.
- Counselling, psychotherapy and group work, often using the transpersonal or the psychosynthesis model, aimed at promoting emotional expression, examination of lifestyle, stress and self-stressing attitudes, re-orientation and rehabilitation of individuals towards more authentic and meaningful personal values and goals, and learning self-help techniques of visualization or imagery, meditation and relaxation (Bridge *et al.*, 1988; Bindemann *et al.*, 1991) and the promotion of creative self-expression (Fig. 55.5). Richardson *et al.* (1997) showed that imagery reduced stress,

improved life vigour and most functional quality-of-life measures after a 6-week intervention.

- Support groups, where the accent is placed on effective implementation of the holistic approach and the building of personal support networks.
- Use of creative therapies, including art, music, dance and drama therapies.
- Complementary therapies, which at this stage should be the 'energy medicines' of acupuncture, shiatsu and homeopathy, which are helpful in increasing the patient's underlying energy, improving well-being and providing symptom control; or bodywork, such as massage and aromatherapy, which help greatly to reduce fear, tension, isolation and the alienation felt by cancer patients towards their diseased or disfigured bodies.
- Spiritual healing, which again lifts underlying energy, improves coping, is calming and has emotional and spiritual benefits.
- Support groups, aimed to give encouragement, social contact and support.

A point will come when, through the application of holistic therapies, the patient feels sufficiently strong to embark upon self-help approaches at home (Fig. 55.6). It is important not to encourage patients to take up self-help approaches before they are strong enough to do so, because if they are unable to implement this advice they will blame themselves and feel they have failed. Key self-help approaches include:

- Mind/body techniques, aimed at calming the mind, inducing states of well-being and happiness (e.g. the regular practice of relaxation and meditation). Another key practice is visualization, where positive mental focus is achieved through pictures or words (affirmation) in an attempt to affect disease outcome and

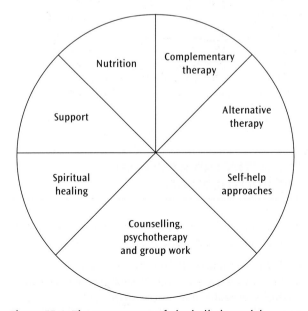

Figure 55.4 *The components of the holistic model.*

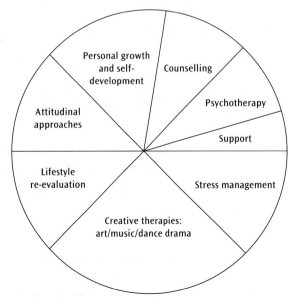

Figure 55.5 *Psychological approaches.*

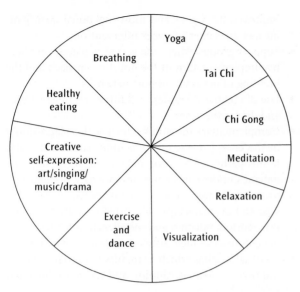

Figure 55.6 *The self-help approaches.*

morale. Visualization is divided into guided imagery, where therapists guide individuals or groups with sequential use of pleasant visual images into happier states of mind, or personal imaging where a cancer patient creates images of their cancer being eliminated from the body, or images of themselves as completely recovered. Use of visualization during chemotherapy by breast cancer patients has been found to confer a 17.5 per cent survival benefit (Walker *et al.*, 1999).

- Exercise. Cancer patients are encouraged to take up holistic forms of exercise such as yoga, tai chi or chi gong to the extent of their ability, which again promote emotional, physical and spiritual well-being.
- Healthy eating. Once the patient has been taught and guided through dietary changes, healthy eating can become incorporated into his or her lifestyle.
- Creative self-expression. Patients are encouraged to live more balanced, creative lifestyles where far more emphasis is placed on time spent in recreation, self-expression and the fulfilment of personal goals and ambitions.

Complementary therapies in the clinical setting

The main use of complementary therapies in the clinical setting is for supportive care and symptom management. The goal is either to use therapies or remedies that will reduce symptoms directly, or to teach techniques to the individual which will help them to alleviate symptoms as they arise.

Invariably, symptoms have three components: the physical level of the symptom, the fear and anxiety created by the symptom (which usually exacerbates it), and the emotional response to the symptom (which is very often repressed and can also exacerbate the symptom).

Holistic or complementary symptom management is therefore usually directed at addressing each of these levels independently.

First, attempts are made to relieve anxiety and fear by allowing the individual to talk about their fears as well as by learning relaxation techniques. Methods used to relax patients include massage, aromatherapy, talking patients down into a relaxed state, hypnotherapy, as well as soothing breathing techniques. Second, during this process it is often possible to facilitate emotional expression or catharsis if a sufficiently empathic bond has been made between the carer and the patient, who is given permission to 'let go'. Very often the symptom reduction as a result of relaxation and emotional expression is so great that either the symptom is manageable by the patient or can be controlled by smaller levels of conventional drugs or by natural medicines.

Managing the physical aspect of the symptom can involve specific therapies, such as acupuncture, reflexology, shiatsu, or remedies from the disciplines of homeopathy, herbalism or the Bach Flower remedies.

Another approach can be to use the mind itself to either change or transcend the symptom. In the former approach, conscious attention is focused directly on the symptom. While this may, in the short term, exacerbate the problem, giving the symptom full attention can often change it very significantly, especially once the additional fear and emotion raised by this exercise are expressed. By working directly with the symptom in a transpersonal counselling mode with a nurse or counsellor, the symptoms can be given meaning and perhaps a colour, shape or voice, and it is often surprising how bringing consciousness to symptoms in this way can transform or improve them, often providing extremely relevant, meaningful insight at the same time.

Promotion of emotional catharsis has also been shown to have survival benefits. Spiegel (1989) demonstrated a doubling of survival time for women with breast cancer who received 1fi hours of psychological support once a week for a year, and this result was repeated by Fawzy *et al.* (1993), in Los Angeles, who prolonged 5-year survival in a group of melanoma patients who received psychological support. In both cases the intervention was to help promote the expression of grief, anger and fear created by the diagnosis of cancer.

STRENGTHS AND WEAKNESSES OF THE HOLISTIC MODEL

Individually, patients report very significant benefits from the use of the holistic approach in:

- Reduction in fear, anxiety and isolation.
- Achieving a sense of control, involvement and partnership with healthcare professionals.
- Improvement in physical state, energy levels and sleep.

- Improved symptom control and tolerance of treatments.
- Greatly improved quality of life, enabling the crisis of cancer to be turned into an opportunity for learning, increased self-understanding, and greater personal fulfilment and happiness.
- Spiritual growth and transformation.
- Help to face consciously the issues of death and dying.

The weaknesses of the holistic approach include:

- Great confusion amongst individuals as to the right therapeutic or self-help path to take, especially in the light of the overwhelming amount of information now available through the internet and other directories and information services, and the lack of provision of supportive guidance in the use of these approaches in clinical oncology settings.
- The urging of patients towards self-help approaches when they are too weak or vulnerable to undertake them, which can create feelings of failure.
- The great cost of many of the therapies, diets and nutritional supplements.
- The implication by some holistic practitioners that all individuals have the power to heal themselves, which can lead to misplaced feelings of guilt, responsibility and blame if individuals do not recover.
- The possibility of exaggerated claims for effectiveness without adequate substantive proof.

As with all forms of medicine, the holistic approach can be practised well or badly, and in a balanced professional setting the effect of an individual's state on their health and the potential of their own efforts to improve their situation can be placed within the context of the multi-factorial nature of the aetiology of cancer, and the multi-disciplinary nature of its treatment. In this way the efforts of the individual can be given value and importance without too great a responsibility, and seen as one part of a team approach to getting optimum health management outcomes.

In essence, the focus of the holistic approach should be to improve the patient's quality of life, health and, when the time is right, dying. The goal is to lighten the load of the individual physically, emotionally and spiritually, and to ensure that the great benefits that can be gained from the holistic approach are not outweighed by neurotic adherence to complex, overdemanding, expensive alternative protocols, which may promise much and give little.

IMPLICATIONS OF THE HOLISTIC APPROACH

Implications for service delivery

In 1995 the Calman–Hine Policy Framework For Commissioning Cancer Services stated, as one of two most important aims, that 'The needs of patients and their carers should be the primary concern of purchasers, planners and professionals involved in cancer care' (Calman and Hine, 1995). It also urged that 'health care professionals take account of the views and preferences of patients and their carers as well as their own', pointing out that 'Individuals' perception of their needs may differ from those of the professional, meaning that good communication between the patients and the professional is especially important'.

Sadly, very little new money was made available for the implementation of these and the many other excellent recommendations of the report, and those interviewed in the Bristol focus group study (Tritter *et al.*, 1998) felt dismayed that 'currently information about support and self-help approaches is available by chance or coincidence' and that many healthcare professionals were dismissive or even rude about their efforts to find ways of helping themselves. It was felt that supportive care and complementary services which exist currently had developed around charismatic individuals within and without the health service, and that as yet there was no national policy for the provision of supportive care and access to self-help.

Concern was expressed about the current disparity in practice; some doctors tending to discourage the use of complementary therapies and self-help techniques, while others actively supported and encouraged their use, very few basing their response on what the patient thought was important. The feeling was that access and information should be given routinely, regardless of the personal attitudes of the health professionals, along with guidance on the use of supportive and self-help options from those who had studied their use.

The need for the following services was expressed:

- Information centres providing skilled help with the interpretation of all levels of information about cancer, its treatment and the range of options available.
- The provision of complementary therapies either free of charge or at low cost within the hospital setting.
- Self-help centres to teach and reinforce the learning of self-help skills, to help develop inner strength, peace of mind, positive coping styles and for symptom control.
- Counselling and support services for people with cancer and their carers, with appropriately trained supervised and supported staff.
- Access to support via permanent drop-in centres and, if possible, 24-hour helplines, as the point was made repeatedly that it was impossible to know when emotional crises will occur.
- Link workers to co-ordinate all aspects of supportive care for patients and to facilitate inter-agency communication.

Implications for medical practice

It is clear from the list of reasons given by participants in the Bristol Study for their use of complementary and self-help approaches that a great deal of the benefits they ascribe to these approaches came from the intimate and trusting nature of the therapeutic relationship which was developed with the practitioners (Tritter *et al.*, 1998). Many participants were distressed that they had not received the special help and awareness that was needed from their health professionals during diagnosis and treatment. Because of the intensely shocking, frightening and confusing nature of the news and information they were being given, all requested that healthcare professionals involved in their management should recognize that:

- the diagnosis of cancer is associated with a state of shock and a great need for sensitivity, patience, support, and the frequent repetition of important medical information, which they felt was particularly vital to ensure that they were able to give truly informed consent to medical procedures which may affect them for the rest of their lives;
- efforts should be made to reduce the wait for test results and to ensure that support was on hand during and after the delivery of bad news;
- there should be recognition that the trauma associated with diagnosis and treatment could be made much worse by poor communication and the passive patient role, which led to feelings of loss of control;
- far greater emphasis should be placed on communication skills and the development of the therapeutic relationship in the training of healthcare professionals, in order to establish good caring rapport and trust between doctors and people with cancer;
- ideally care must be taken to assess emotional state prior to embarking upon treatments; the process being modified or postponed if the person with cancer is too psychologically vulnerable; and
- the needs of carers must also be recognized and provided for.

Those involved in cancer service provision should learn how to communicate well with patients, develop good therapeutic relationships and elicit the values and beliefs of patients in order to make their experience of illness, its treatment and their recovery process as congruent, helpful and meaningful as possible. They should also study the values, theory and practice associated with the use of psychosocial, complementary, self-help and spiritual approaches.

It must also be recognized, however, that working more closely with the patient's emotional needs is also likely to be far more demanding on healthcare professionals. In order to provide this level of care, support and encouragement, it is vital to provide regular ongoing support and supervision for those caring for and treating people with cancer. Better still, it is advised that healthcare professionals themselves adopt an holistic approach to their own health, taking regular stock of their emotional and spiritual state, energy levels and the maintenance of the correct balance between work, rest and recreation.

RESEARCH PRIORITIES

To take the implementation of the holistic approach to cancer further it will be necessary to have additional high-quality research to evaluate which elements of the approach produce the best benefits for which patients under which circumstances. Research into the holistic approach to cancer has been slow, because of:

- the financial limitations historically of most holistic cancer centres, which have been mainly charitably based, making the setting up of research activity difficult;
- the difficulty of randomizing individuals into approaches which rely on personal commitment (and often financial outlay) by the patient;
- the lack of good holistic outcome measures;
- the integral nature of the effect of the practitioners and the therapeutic relationship on outcomes; and
- the multi-disciplinary nature of the holistic approach, which makes it hard and unethical to research the effects of its individual elements.

This has led to a situation where a very high level of usage of these approaches is taking place purely on the basis of anecdotal and patient-to-patient recommendation, rather than on the basis of evaluation. It is vital therefore that work continues to:

- develop qualitative and quantitative outcome measures to assess the benefits of the holistic approach to cancer;
- evaluate the effect of single-modality and multi-disciplinary holistic interventions on cancer symptom control, disease progression, and survival; psychological morbidity, spiritual growth and the quality of life and death of people with cancer;
- study the effect of these interventions on the change in usage and costs of conventional medical services.

It is hypothesized that use of holistic, complementary and self-help approaches makes a marked difference to the medical management of people with cancer. This is because the patient's levels of inner strength and ability to accept the reality of their situation improves greatly. This often enables patients to achieve an enhanced state of aliveness and spiritual awareness in which the fear of death diminishes. In this state the existing quality of life becomes more important than a potentially small increase in quality of life. It is also noted that patients who are less anxious and more involved in self-help activity are far less dependent on healthcare practitioners than those who are not. They are also far easier to 'look after' by both professional healthcarers and their supporters. It is therefore likely that widespread introduction of holistic self-help services would reduce rather than increase the cost of service provision.

SIGNIFICANT POINTS

- The holistic approach to cancer care has evolved rapidly in the UK since the opening of the Bristol Cancer Help Centre in 1980. There are now supportive complementary care units in several oncology centres, with widespread use of complementary therapies (CTs) by cancer nurses in hospital, community and hospice settings.
- Usage of CTs by cancer patients is estimated to be *c.* 40 per cent in the UK, and as high as 81 per cent in the US.
- Patients say they need complementary therapies and self-management approaches to:
  - find peace of mind, regain a sense of control and improve their quality of life;
  - relieve the symptoms of cancer and its treatment;
  - fight for their lives.
- The holistic approach to cancer help is divided into therapeutic and self-help levels. The therapeutic level is aimed at helping patients to recover from their diagnosis and treatment. Once strong enough, they are encouraged to enter the self-help phase to promote their health, albeit in the presence of illness. In addition to this, some cancer patients will also seek alternative cancer treatment, often outside the UK.
- Cancer patients want healthcare professionals to realize that the emotional impact of cancer is as great, if not greater, than the physical problems they suffer, and want their need for psychological and self-help approaches to be both supported and catered for. Scientific research has shown:
  - *survival benefits* in cancer patients in association with positive coping styles and the improvement of coping style in those who are vulnerable; with relaxation and visualization of positive treatment outcomes; supportive group therapy; adjuvant healthy diet and food supplementation and through the use of some unconventional cancer treatments;
  - *quality of life benefits* in association with counselling, group therapy, relaxation, meditation, visualization, breathing techniques, massage, healing and hypnotherapy;
  - *symptomatic relief* in association with herbal medicines, homeopathic remedies, massage, breathing techniques, relaxation, visualization and meditation.
- There is a great need for further research on the value of both individual complementary and alternative cancer treatments, and of the multiple interventions used in many complementary cancer centres.
- Meanwhile, there is an urgent need for the training of cancer healthcare professionals in the values, theory and science underpinning the use of complementary cancer care, and comprehensive policy change to provide routinely for the psycho-spiritual and self-management needs of people with cancer.

KEY REFERENCES

Fawzy, F. *et al.* (1990) A structured psychiatric intervention for cancer patients. II. Changes over time in immunological measures. *Arch. Gen. Psychiatry* **47**(8), 729.

Greer, S. (1992) Adjuvant psychological therapy for patients with cancer: a prospective randomised controlled trial. *BMJ* **304**, 675–80.

Greer, S. *et al.* (1990) Psychological response to breast cancer and 15 year outcome. *Lancet* **335**, 49.

Walker, L.G. (1999) Psychological interventions, host defences and survival. *Adv. Mind–body Med.* **15**, 236–81.

Walker, L. *et al.* (1997) Guided imagery and relaxation therapy can modify host defences in women receiving treatment for locally advanced breast cancer. *Br. J. Surg.* **84**(suppl. 1).

Walker, L.G., Walker, M.B., Ogstonn, K. *et al.* (1999) Psychological, clinical and pathological effects of relaxation training and guided imagery during primary chemotherapy. *Br. J. Cancer* **80**, 262–8.

Walker, L.G., Ratcliffe, M.A. and Dawson, A.A. (2000) Relaxation and hypnotherapy: long term effects on the survival of patients with lymphoma. *Psycho-oncology* **9**, 355–6.

REFERENCES

Bindemann, S., Sankop, M. and Kaye, S.B. (1991) Randomised controlled study of relaxation training. *Eur. J. Cancer* **27**(2), 170–4.

Bridge, L.R., Benson, P., Pietrone, P.C. and Purnest, R.G. (1988) Relaxation and imagery in the treatment of breast cancer. *BMJ* **297**(6657), 1169–72.

Burke, C. and Sikora, S. (1992) The dual approach. *Nursing Times* **88**(38).

Calman, K. and Hine, D. (1995) *A policy framework for commissioning cancer services: a report of the expert advisory group on cancer to the Chief Medical Officers of England and Wales.* London: Department of Health and Welsh Office.

Fawzy, I. *et al.* (1993) Malignant melanoma, effects of an early structured psychiatric intervention, coping and affective state on recurrence and survival six years later. *Arch. Gen. Psychiatry* **50**(a), 681.

Montbriand, M.J. (1998) Abandoning biomedicine for alternative therapies: oncology patients' stories. *Cancer Nurse* **21**, 36–45.

Richardson, M.A., Post-White, J., Grimm, E.A., Moye, L.A., Singleton, S.E. and Justice, B. (1997) Coping, life attitudes, and immune responses to imagery and group support after breast cancer treatment. *Alt. Ther. Health Med.* **3**(5), 62–70.

Spiegel, D. (1989) Effect of psychosocial treatment on survival of patients with metastatic breast cancer. *Lancet* **2**, 888.

Tritter, J., Daniel, R., Barley, Baldwin, S. and Cooke, H. (1998) *Meeting the needs of people with cancer for support and self management.* Bristol Cancer Help Centre.

Van de Creek, L., Rogers, E. and Lester, J. (1999) Use of alternative therapies amongst breast cancer outpatients compared with the general population. *Altern. Ther. Health Med.* **5**, 71–6.

Walker, L.G., Walker, M.B., Ogstonn, K. *et al.* (1999) Psychological, clinical and pathological effects of relaxation training and guided imagery during primary chemotherapy. *Br. J. Cancer* **80**, 262–8.

56

Communication with the cancer patient

RICHARD T. PENSON AND MAURICE L. SLEVIN

INTRODUCTION

Communication is often defined as 'to impart' or 'make known', but its Latin derivation is helpful in emphasizing the 'sharing' of information. 'Communis' means 'in common' and although the main aim remains to elicit and impart information (Spence, 1953), the way that this is accomplished can have a profound effect on the relationship between the doctor and the patient, and on the patient's approach to his or her disease and treatment.

This chapter is arranged in two parts: first, a review of the various aspects relating to effective communication with cancer patients and, secondly, communication issues that relate particularly to the practice of cancer medicine.

COMMUNICATION SKILLS

How important is communication?

Many aspects of communication are obscured by myths and moralizing, but communication is one of the most important influences on the quality of medical practice. The General Medical Council has stated that communication skills are fundamental to patient care (General Medical Council, 1987). Sir William Osler reputedly penned 'listen to the patient, he is telling you the diagnosis'. The history is still, justifiably, regarded as the most important part of the consultation (Short, 1993).

Good communication improves the accuracy of diagnosis, enables better management decisions and reduces unnecessary investigations and inappropriate treatment. For the doctor it is professionally rewarding and personally satisfying. For the patient it reduces anxiety (Fallowfield et al., 1986) and uncertainty. There is evidence that good communication improves compliance (Davis and Fallowfield, 1991) and that improving doctor–patient communication may be the most effective way of reducing the incidence of litigation (Shapiro et al., 1989).

Positive adjustment to the diagnosis of cancer has been cited as an independent prognostic factor (Greer and Watson, 1987) and it is even suggested from a

---

BOX 56.1 GENERAL MEDICAL COUNSEL

The General Medical Counsel requires that doctors make the care of their patient their primary concern, and treat every patient politely and considerately, with respect given to patient's dignity and privacy. The patients should be listened to, and respect be given to their views with information delivered in a way that they can understand. The patients should be fully involved in decisions about their care. Doctors have a responsibility to keep their professional knowledge and skills up to date, to recognize the limitations of their professional competence, and to be honest and trustworthy. Doctors should respect patients' confidentiality, and make sure that their personal beliefs should not prejudice their patients' care. They should act quickly to protect patients from risks if they have good reason to believe that they themselves, or a colleague, may not be fit to practice. Because of their particular responsibility, doctors should avoid abusing their position, and work with their colleagues to best serve a patient's interest.

randomized trial, as yet unconfirmed, that counselling for cancer patients may improve survival (Speigel *et al.*, 1989).

The current situation

In the past decade the swing from protective paternalism towards unsolicited candour (Novack *et al.*, 1979) has continued, though with more calls for a practice marked by congruent sharing of information (Schain, 1990). Galen described a 'confidence and hope that do more good than Physic'. Good medical practice should embrace both that high ideal and the technical quality of modern medicine. Yet dissatisfaction is high. Ley, in a review of hospital-based surveys, found a median 38 per cent (11–65 per cent) of patients dissatisfied with their consultations with doctors (Ley, 1988). Patients most common complaints continue to revolve around communication. The two most common criticisms of hospital practice being: 'doctors don't listen' (Blau, 1989), and 'not being told what's wrong' (Fletcher, 1980). Patients can relate a history without interruption in less than 2 minutes if allowed to talk (Blau, 1989) and yet are, in the main, interrupted within 18 seconds (Beckman and Frankel, 1984). With the rather sobering suggestion that policemen may break bad news better than doctors (Finlay and Dallimore, 1991) and that up to one-quarter of junior doctors fail to elicit the main problem in taking a history (Maguire *et al.*, 1986b), criticisms conspire to overwhelm the medical profession.

There has been a boom in the teaching of communication skills as it has been incorporated increasingly into the undergraduate medical curriculum, with the inclusion of role-play and video feedback to facilitate learning. In 1983 one-third of British medical schools offered no communication skills training. In 1992 this figure had fallen to only 3 of the 28 medical schools (McManus *et al.*, 1993). For many doctors practising today, however, there was little undergraduate training in communication skills. For physicians in practice, the Cancer Research Campaign (CRC) supports Professor Fallowfield's communication skills courses (Fallowfield *et al.*, 1998), and a number of other courses are available (Baile *et al.*, 1997).

Although there is presently a relatively small literature on the subject, this is increasing. Research in communication is severely hampered by the lack of a systematic and accepted model of psychological functioning, and the need for accurate controls to reduce bias.

What limits communication?

In this section the most important factors that limit effective communication will be considered. Areas that doctors and patients wish to leave uncharted will always be present and are discussed on p. 1191.

FROM THE DOCTOR'S PERSPECTIVE

Communication is stressful

Communication, particularly face to face interaction, is fundamental to the art of medicine, and yet arguably the biggest source of stress for both doctors (Firth-Cozens, 1987) and patients (McLaughlan, 1990). The scars of previous bad experiences, the fear of future wounds or the attrition of the work of the caring profession can create a significant aversion to communicating at any more than a superficial level and inhibit self-awareness.

The stigma of death

Although it is easy to graciously accept the credit for cures and remissions, the sting of the blame for failure is bitter. In an age marked by high expectations of modern technology, outcomes short of cure are very reasonably perceived as failure, and death still remains a taboo subject in our society. Few are comfortable with their own mortality (Feifel, 1976). Doctors, as well as patients, are uncertain, or even fearful, of feelings about such emotive issues, and this naturally limits the freedom with which they can be discussed.

The innate limits to good advice

Treatment almost always involves advice, either explanation or exhortation. Brief advice with the aim of changing behaviour has been shown to be effective, although with rather limited success. A meta-analysis of 39 controlled smoking cessation trials showed that success was most likely when individualized advice was repeated in different forms by several sources on multiple occasions, and yet success rates were found to most frequently be in the range of 5–10 per cent (Kottke *et al.*, 1988). It is becoming apparent that in circumstances when such 'lifestyle advice' is given there is considerable ambivalence. Taking too dictatorial a stance is risky in two ways. First, patients may tend to side with what they see as the other side of the coin, the alternative argument in their conflict of interests. Secondly, motivation varies, with a wide spectrum of readiness to change. Success may come by using a negotiation method in which the patient, rather than the doctor, articulates the benefits and costs involved, even if all that is achieved is movement toward the goal, in terms of pre-motivation (Rollnick *et al.*, 1993).

Words

In recent times considerable emphasis has been put on non-verbal communication. A media experiment serves to show the power of the words themselves. During the 'Mega-lab' week (25 March 1994), in which science was advertised, Sir Robin Day gave accounts of why *Gone with the wind* and *Some like it hot* were his favourite films, one account true and one account fictitious. These were broadcast on TV and radio and published in a daily newspaper. Those with the 'benefit' of the non-verbal clues, because of seeing the interview on television, guessed correctly less frequently (TV, 52 per cent; newspaper, 64 per cent; and radio, 73 per cent), perhaps because such non-verbal behaviour can add to what is actually said in an unhelpful way (R. Wiseman, personal communication).

Words themselves can, however, be a snare. For many the word 'cancer' equates with death and it is often important to explain that there are over 200 common varieties of cancer which all behave differently and have different treatments. Words do not mean the same to all people. 'Sorry' is a word dangerously contaminated with ambiguity. It can suggest sympathy or guilt. A lot of cancer- and treatment-related issues are very complex. Medical jargon can leave patients unable to understand or retain information on which important decisions are based.

Time

A lack of time is often blamed for limiting good communication, and rightly so. However, Richard Asher helpfully commented that '… to give the patient the impression that you could spare him an hour and yet make him satisfied with five minutes is an invaluable gift, and of much more use than spending half an hour with him during every minute of which he is made to feel he is encroaching on your time' (Asher, 1972).

Privacy

The lack of privacy may so militate against the safe disclosure by patients of difficult issues and important information that arranging another time and another place may be the only constructive way to proceed. For example, 'business' or 'teaching' ward rounds are not the place to dabble in emotionally charged issues.

FROM THE PATIENT'S PERSPECTIVE

Emotional chaos

Insensitive communication skill teaching can be de-skilling, leaving competent doctors vulnerable and embarrassed. This can happen particularly during role-play sessions, because of critical feedback. This, however, pales into insignificance beside the degree to which reversing roles and truly becoming a patient leaves members of the medical profession bereft of their insight and equanimity (Ingelfinger, 1980). At times of severe stress, taking in a mountain of facts and making important decisions can become impossible, and sensitivity to this can prevent it becoming a barrier to effective communication.

Denial and collusion

Most barriers to open communication are genuine attempts at damage limitation. Denial and collusion in cancer patients are often very reasonably founded, but with a high emotional cost. Dense denial of psychiatric proportions is rare and, to an extent, partial denial is universal – the hope for optimistic goals. Collusion is the attempt by the patient, or more commonly the family or friends, to protect others by denying reality. This can be challenged, to enable the transition from fighting cancer apart to fighting it together.

Depression

Depression in cancer patients should not be dismissed as an understandable reaction (Maguire et al., 1985). In patients with cancer, where the diagnosis is complicated by organic symptoms and the effects of treatment, a clear and persistent change in mood, hopelessness and an inability to enjoy anything are helpful symptoms that distinguish depression from fatigue. Active treatment often proves to be effective. In situations where there is not only anhedonia but also impaired concentration, feelings of worthlessness or inertia, the role of psychotherapy should await improvement with antidepressants (Goldberg and Cullen, 1986).

Age

Older patients want less information and less involvement in decision making (Cassileth et al., 1980). Particular account of this should be taken, both in offering to go into more detail with younger patients and in offering 'escape clauses' to older patients. Such escape clauses could be in terms of euphemisms or a positive response to the request to 'Do what you think is right, doctor'. Though this older group may offer fewer 'signposts' to the doctor hoping to steer a successful course through difficult issues, they tend to be more easily satisfied (Blanchard et al., 1986).

Improving communication skills

Communication is aided by an appropriate knowledge base, skills and attitude. Being a doctor is not instant accreditation in effective communication. Editorials and consensus statements are continual reminders that experience is insufficient as the sole qualification of a communicator (Simpson et al., 1991). We must practice what we preach (Roter et al., 2000).

There is evidence that how a diagnosis is delivered influences the impact of bad news. Cunningham reported five times as many parents satisfied with the way news that their child had Down's syndrome was broken, when staff had been trained to be unhurried, honest, balanced and empathic (Cunningham et al., 1984). Ensuring that such studies are well controlled is very difficult. The ability to establish rapport with patients and to find out what it is that they are really asking can be taught effectively in a relatively short period of time (Maguire, 1990). Maguire has shown, with medical students, that teaching by feedback through audio- and videotape is significantly superior to teaching by the apprenticeship method, although the students need an experienced tutor. A subgroup of 36 were followed up 4–6 years later. All had improved, but the group who had received feedback training maintained their superiority in a number of key skills, notably precision and the exploring of verbal and non-verbal cues (Maguire et al., 1986a).

Although skills can be learned, that does not ensure that they are used. Fear of patients' reactions or the

BOX 56.2 IMPROVED COMMUNICATION SKILLS

1 Improve the accuracy of diagnosis and quality of management.
2 Improve the eliciting and imparting of information.
3 Improve patients' understanding, retention of information and compliance.
4 Reduce anxiety, uncertainty and litigation.
5 Improve doctor and patient satisfaction.
6 Can be learned.

perception that elicited concerns would not be addressed creates a reluctance to apply learned skills (Maguire, 1990).

As with cardio-pulmonary resuscitation (CPR), having done it, and even doing it, does not guarantee high standards and, without attention, communication skills deteriorate. Courses in communication skills are available, such as those run by the Medical Interview Teaching Association and the Cancer Research Campaign (Fallowfield et al., 1998). There is no regulating authority, and most are recommended by word of mouth.

Good communication: essential elements

NON-VERBAL COMMUNICATION

Introductions should be courteous and orientate the patient with respect to who you are and how this consultation fits in to their management. Privacy, eye contact, posture, tone of voice, pauses and nods facilitate communication. Sensitivity to the patient's needs and expectations, careful negotiation of time and topic, and a responsive style prevent avoidable mistakes. Note-taking needs to be unobtrusive and interruptions prevented or kept to a minimum. As a nation, the British probably have the worst reputation for disquiet about touch (Heylings, 1973), although even this is now being taught in medical schools.

EMPATHY

Empathy is essentially making a connection with someone and experiencing their emotions as an extension of your own and communicating an understanding of their position and feelings. It can be as simple as tailoring how you proceed to how the patient responds to your questions, or as profound as the unspoken understanding of friends. A breadth of experience is an invaluable mentor (Albom, 1997).

VERBAL COMMUNICATION

An invitation to talk and when to move on can be negotiated with the patient. Open questions that invite an explanation enable patients to explain what is important to them. When it comes to what the patient thinks and feels, the patient is the expert. However, wide-open questions can be confusing or invite rambling responses. It is important to have clear objectives and to anchor open questions by being specific or directing the patient to the particular area of interest. Encouraging the expression of feelings early on in the consultation gives the message that it is all right to talk about them. Leading questions, value judgements and premature advice or reassurance tend to limit what patients feel able to say. Responding to verbal or non-verbal cues that there are other un-voiced issues that patients wish to discuss is important if the patient is to be given the opportunity to disclose all of his or her concerns. The use of excess in adjectives – '… devastated, furious, can you bear?' – communicates a genuine attempt to understand, rather than risking positive reinforcement of the distress.

There are three particularly helpful ways to proceed when difficult or distressing things are being discussed: reflection, clarification and summarizing.

Reflection

The repetition of the last few words, or word, that the patient said can give the patient the opportunity to say more if they wish. It is especially helpful in emotionally charged interviews, but risks confronting the patient with strong emotions. Sufficient control of the interview needs to be maintained to enable the patient to be moved on through to other matters if they appear to be wallowing in misery.

Clarifying

Checking that you understand correctly what has been said aids precision and avoids errors. Gut feelings that you have about the link between a particular cause and effect or the underlying emotion, should be explored: 'so you felt … because of the …?'.

Summarizing

Summarizing what has been said fundamentally improves understanding while giving the opportunity to order some of the chaos that cancer causes. There may be a lot to be gained in asking the patient to summarize.

ASSESSMENT

It remains the case that in the assessment of any symptom, the essentials of character, severity, frequency, duration and impact, as well as exacerbating and relieving factors, have to be established. However, in communicating, the goal is not simply a precise transcription. The aim, once the patient feels genuinely understood, is to establish that you are aware of all the problems and to prioritize them. Encouraging the patient to prioritize the problems and generate solutions, and talking through these strategies and goals can be very valuable.

COPING WITH REACTIONS

Patients exhibit the full spectrum of reaction, from anger and fear to depression and anxiety or denial. It is necessary

BOX 56.3 REACTIONS

1 Anger
2 Denial
3 Depression
4 Anxiety and fear
5 Resolution.

BOX 56.4 BASIC COMMUNICATION SKILLS

1 Have clear objectives.
2 Introduce yourself and establish some rapport.
3 Establish how much they know, want to know and what they were expecting.
4 Use open-ended, directive questions.
5 Assume nothing and be flexible.
6 Go at an appropriate pace.
7 Feedback what they say and possibly what they can't say.
8 Ask questions. Do they understand you? Do you understand them?
9 Summarize and ask if there are any other concerns.

to acknowledge distressing emotions and to try to understand their impact. If you don't understand why a patient has reacted in a particular way, then ask. Expressing strong emotions verbally is very therapeutic, and distancing tactics are more likely to exacerbate the problem.

CONTINUITY OF CARE

Patients frequently complain that they never see the same doctor. Improving this may be difficult, but rewarding. If consistent personal attention is not possible, then communication with colleagues about patients and accurate recording in the notes of assessments, plans and what patients have been told serves to promote good continuity of care.

SURVIVING COMMUNICATION AND BURN-OUT

Successfully engaging in the task of accompanying people through one of the most threatening of life events carries with it an inevitable cost in terms of time and emotions. Believing in what you do, positive feedback, confronting or even avoiding one's own reactions and planning rewarding elements to daily practice can help prevent 'burnout'. Burn-out is typically identified as emotional exhaustion, depersonalization and a sense of low personal accomplishment. Ramirez *et al.* (1996) investigated burn-out and psychiatric morbidity among gastroenterologists, surgeons, radiologists and oncologists in the UK, using a

questionnaire-based survey. Psychiatric morbidity was estimated using the General Health Questionnaire and the Maslach Burnout Inventory. Questionnaires were returned by 882 of 1133 consultants. The estimated prevalence of psychiatric morbidity was 27 per cent. Burn-out appeared to be associated with feeling overloaded and poorly managed and dealing with patients' suffering. Better training in communication and management skills was identified as potentially important in protecting against burn-out. A number of organizations, including the British Medical Association (BMA; Tel.: 020 7387 4499) offer anonymity and support to health professionals who find themselves in a position of intolerable strain.

ISSUES RELATING TO CANCER MEDICINE

How much talk is too much?

There is a lot of talk about cancer, with high-profile media coverage of celebrity cases. For most people, this anxious preoccupation remains at arm's length, but for individuals who develop cancer, for whom it becomes all too real, how much talk is too much? (Slevin, 1987).

It is an oversimplification to say that there are 'tellers' and 'non-tellers'. The majority of doctors will, to an extent, tailor what is said despite favourite allegories and familiar personalized patter.

For those who 'tell' there are three particular dangers. First, that they dwell on the morbid, not offering practical and positive advice. Secondly, that they tell patients what they already know but do not want to hear, or hear again; and, thirdly, that they fail to appreciate that, for some, considerable time is needed to adjust to bad news.

For 'non-tellers', who may very compassionately maintain that 'the truth but not the whole truth' is important, there are also risks. Patients may be left with half truths, irrational fears and negative previous experience to colour what information they do have. The Hippocratic practice of telling the family the stark truth while presenting a rosy interpretation to the patient invites collusion. Although this can remain a tenet of good practice at times of intolerable strain, this policy should be continually reviewed, and the option for patients to explore more of the 'whole truth' should given at a later date. Patients very reasonably overestimate their prognosis and yet can be bitter at being denied medium-term goals by unexpected deteriorations in their health. Being forewarned with respect to treatment side-effects is being forearmed, and to an extent this is also true of the effects of the illness.

There is no gold-standard answer to the question of how much is too much. It varies between doctors, between patients and often, for any one patient, varies with time. Patients are amazingly long suffering, they should be trusted to guide doctors in difficult interpersonal areas and we should apologize to them when mistakes are made.

Breaking bad news

There are many advocates of a right way to break bad news. However, common to each school of thought, there are a number of helpful essential elements (Maguire and Faulkner, 1988; Faulkner, 1992; Fallowfield, 1993; Baile et al., 2000). Breaking bad news is painful. Successfully approximating expectations and reality almost always takes more than one consultation.

Although the presence of friends and relatives can inhibit the disclosure of difficult things that patients may wish to discuss, the person may retain little information and may benefit from subsequently going over what was said again, with the spouse, friend or relative who was present (Fallowfield et al., 1987). Recall and adjustment may be helped by a tape if the interview was recorded (Hogbin and Fallowfield, 1989) or by written information and illustrations.

Patients often fear the worst about symptoms or investigations, and asking for their thoughts on the matter can help to establish how much the patient knows and wants to know. It also creates the opportunity to confirm bad news, rather than delivering bad news, unprepared for possible reactions. Rarely is someone's reaction to bad news purely dependant on the news itself. Everyone has 'personal baggage' that colours how they respond. By giving the patient the opportunity to explain their particular situation in advance, useful information may be made available that enables the interview to be structured to pre-empt problems.

The person needs to be prepared, if not, he or she needs to be warned that there is serious news. Giving the details about the diagnosis, stage and prognosis in a sequence of acceptably small packets offers the opportunity to tailor the information to the individual's needs. What the patient says, asks and how he or she reacts should determine how much is said at any one time. The danger with giving information in a 'ladder' like this is that patients may be reluctant to ask questions. One study, although not in the specific context of breaking bad news, found that 42 per cent of patients did not ask the questions about their diagnosis that they had planned to ask (Ley, 1988).

The patient needs to be informed of the facts and assessed with respect to consequent emotions and problems. Reinforce the elements that they perceive correctly and gently educate in areas of ignorance or error. Continually check for understanding. Have the confidence to ask them to help you understand how they feel. If they feel that you do understand their distress, then reassurance will be effective. Only if they want to move on can you succeed in making progress. The options have to be clearly explained. What can be, and what might not be, achieved.

Bad news inevitably brings a considerable number of problems. Establishing how the patient prioritizes these ensures that these are addressed in an appropriate order. It may be more productive to tackle most of them on another occasion. However, the first opportunity may be the best opportunity to hear all of the issues (Haven and Maguire, 1997).

It can be very helpful to ensure that it is not only the doctor who is available to pick up the pieces. Nurses and nurse specialists provide invaluable support. Patients need to be orientated with respect to what happens next, both with reference to the medical agenda and to their agenda. Establishing the point of next contact and the ground rules of how discussions might proceed, giving a telephone number through which you can be contacted and fostering realistic hopefulness is investing towards success.

Hope

SOURCES OF HOPE

It is often not the case that the diagnosis of cancer can be softened in the same breath with talk of cure. Honest information, not unduly negative or falsely reassuring, offers the safest path for patients to establish their own hopes. There is an obvious aversion to saying that there is no hope. Such statements should be clearly focused '… there is no chance of X, Y or Z but, yes, a very real chance of …'.

Very much as the profession reports response rates rather than failure rates, patients also wish to minimize the impact of 'failure': the half-full rather than half-empty glass. Patients consistently overestimate prognosis and are keen to opt for radical treatment with minimal chance of benefit (Slevin et al., 1990). The chance that new treatments might become available, however unlikely this may be, is an extremely common source of hope. Keeping the 'options open' is a very constructive way of coping for patients, and a common practice for doctors. It offers uncommitted hope and supports patients who often live 'a day at a time'. Perhaps all that separates hope from denial in some situations is that the latter is destructive or obstructive. Many realize that hopes for a cure are not

---

BOX 56.5 BREAKING BAD NEWS

Ideally, confirm bad news.

1. Be prepared, what do they know and want to know.
2. Warn that you have serious news.
3. Be simple and clear. Tailor the information to the patient.
4. Has the message been understood? If not check how much more information the patient wishes to know.
5. Pause to let it sink in, then respond to their reactions and to difficult questions.
6. Pick up the threads so that there is a plan for how to continue discussions at the next meeting.

realistic and yet they remain optimistic and appear to find meaning and value in life. In the palliative setting, patients consistently do realize short-term goals. Things that provide enjoyment, or at the least distraction, continuing support, and the fact that they will not be abandoned by their doctors contribute to a hopeful attitude.

It maybe helpful to conclude with the description by the psychiatrist, Victor Frankl, of his experience of the concentration camps of the Second World War (Frankl, 1946). He observed that people who felt that life had real purpose and meaning coped with the atrocities and the almost certain threat of death, while others, for whom life had lost all meaning, quickly succumbed to malnutrition and infection. The latter could be helped to regain the meaning in their lives, with a consequent improvement in its quality.

ENGENDERING HOPE

The way that we communicate can engender hope or minimize the risk of hopelessness.

Information and order

Information fills voids that can otherwise get filled with despair. Positive and practical information banishes fear of the unknown. Simply categorizing issues can chop up overwhelming distress into manageable worries.

A new perspective

Patients are often faced with what initially appear to be insurmountable problems. By bringing some objectivity, difficult issues can be divorced from the imagination, which so easily fuels despair. This also gives the patient the opportunity of a little distance from reality and the possibility of establishing a new perspective and positive readjustment.

Patients' fears often centre around symptoms that can be well controlled, such as pain. Reassurance can dispel unreasonable fears. Very reasonable fears about death are often not addressed and giving the opportunity to voice these may be constructive.

Confidence

Patients should be encouraged to take some control through involvement in decisions about major or minor matters, if this promotes confidence. There is a tremendous encouragement in not being alone. Patients need the support of friends and relatives and medical, psychological, social and spiritual support. They may find valuable support in an organized support group. At the very least, patients can be encouraged that many have faced the same fears and yet coped in the absence of other sources of confidence. Sadly, this is a well-trodden path.

To get in and out of emotionally laden issues and move people on through such distress is undoubtedly a skill to be cherished. Leaving the patient knowing that their concerns have been understood enables the sharing of painful issues to be a therapeutic manoeuvre.

BOX 56.6 THERAPEUTIC DIALOGUE

1 Listen, and ask open, but directive, questions.
2 Question and summarize until you have the whole picture.
3 Acknowledge and address issues.
4 Reinforce realistic hopefulness.

Spirituality

Frequently a distinction is drawn between religion (an organized system of beliefs with (an) authority figure(s), rules, rituals and traditions) and spirituality (a personal belief system related to the transcendent, to a search for meaning in one's life, and to that which gives one hope, joy, peace, contentment and energy).

The diagnosis of cancer can precipitate a search for meaning in the patient's life. Questions such as 'Why me?', 'Why this?' and 'Why now?' are common. Such existential questions can also reflect specifically spiritual concerns, such as 'What is the quality of my relationship to myself, others and God?' In addition to patients' spiritual beliefs, many have religious practices from which they derive comfort, e.g. prayer, or that enforce constraints, e.g. blood transfusions prohibited. Given the potential depth and breadth of spiritual and religious issues with which patients may be grappling, it may be very helpful to have an understanding of patient's ideas of their worth, their philosophy and their faith. Simply inquiring of a patient, 'What does this illness mean for you?' or 'What aspects of your religion or spirituality would be helpful for me to know?' can access important information for a therapeutic relationship.

Talking about prognosis

How many cancer patients wish to know about prognosis? In a national survey, 85 per cent of Americans wanted a 'realistic estimate' of how long they had to live if their type of cancer 'usually leads to death in less than a year' (President's Commission for the Study of Ethical Problems in Medicine and Biomedical and Behavioral Research, 1982). It is not known whether this figure falls when detached reasoning is challenged by imminent threat, or by crossing the Atlantic.

The prognosis of all cancer patients is uncertain. Statistics apply to populations, not individuals, and cannot predict survival for an individual patient. Fixed life expectancies can discolour remaining time and it has been suggested that uncertainty as to when life ends is a prerequisite for life to have meaning and value (Harris, 1985). It is common practice to say in response to questions about prognosis that it is genuinely not known, while checking that the patient's hopes are not completely unrealistic. Informing a patient is a continuous process. Although the first time may be the best time to tackle issues that patients wish to discuss, there are often other opportunities for patients to ask difficult questions. Some doctors respond to such questions by asking patients if they wish to know of signs of deterioration. Others give rough estimates, while explaining that overestimates risk procrastination on important issues and bitterness at unexpected deterioration, and that underestimates risk leaving the patient with a death sentence hanging over them once they exceed the deadline.

The Californian Supreme Court has debated traditional medical paternalism versus information sharing and patient-centred decision making with respect to information about prognosis. The family of a patient who had received chemotherapy after the incidental discovery of carcinoma of the pancreas at a laparotomy for a non-functioning kidney successfully sued after his death because the patient was not specifically told that he had a less than 5 per cent chance of surviving 5 years (Annas, 1994). The court challenged the aphorism that if patients don't ask they don't want to know. The court ruling was that patients have to specifically state that they do not want to be told of the prognosis to be denied information about actuarial survival statistics. The ruling affirmed information sharing and patient-centred decision making in the context of a fiduciary (based on trust) physician–patient relationship, and clearly stated that the weighing of the impact of distressing news against a patient's individual hopes and fears was a non-medical judgement reserved for the patient alone. This ruling was in line with other American legislation, for example with respect to withholding CPR. Such legislation has been criticized for ignoring medical issues in favour of legal considerations (Snider, 1991).

Ethics is, to an extent, the codification of the will of the people. We live in an age increasingly dominated by autonomy. However, patient-centred ethics has to be balanced with benevolence, non-malevolence and justice. Constructing healthcare to mirror patients and their needs doesn't always work. Dr Solomon Papper tells an amusing story of an unkempt drug addict who refused to be seen by a particular medical student who looked rather like him, complaining that he was a 'slob'. He wanted a starchy doctor in a tie (Papper, 1983).

Talking with children

Being told that your child has cancer is one of the hardest things for parents to face. Children generally suspect that there is something seriously wrong despite being shielded from the diagnosis. They have florid imaginations and often feel guilty that the illness is a punishment. Explanations, by necessity, are age dependent. The

illness can be explained in terms of cells that are 'good guys' and 'bad guys'. Cartoons or talking to other patients can help. Keeping in touch with schooling and school friends is important. Parents should be encouraged to tell their children that it is alright to feel sad and cry, to ask questions and to talk with the child about the child's thoughts and feelings. Letting them have some control over things that don't interfere with their health can be helpful, but setting limits is important. 'Bending the rules' tends to provoke the anxiety that things are worse than they seem (US Department of Health and Human Services, 1994).

Informed consent

NHS Management Executive guidelines have been a reminder of the legal requirement to obtain informed consent from patients undergoing treatment (Delamothe, 1990). One paper purporting to investigate whether the British patients or their doctors are afraid of informed consent, compared a simple and a detailed information sheet about complications of elective inguinal hernia repair. The latter was eight times as long, giving the statistical risk of discomfort, failure and permanent damage as well as stating unlikely complications, including death. No increase in anxiety was documented in the group who received the detailed information sheet. However, nearly a quarter (8/33) of these patients felt that they had been given 'too much' information. The subgroup of patients who were more anxious prior to the study appeared to be significantly less anxious when given the simpler information ($P = 0.05$) (Kerrigan et al., 1993).

Fully informed consent can be 'needlessly cruel' (Tobias and Souhami, 1993) and intolerable indecision in anxious patients can be immobilizing, even when the patient is the editor of the New England Journal of Medicine (Ingelfinger, 1980). After being diagnosed as having cancer, Dr Franz Ingelfinger was inundated with well intentioned but contradictory advice. He benefited enormously from a wise physician, whom he trusted, who took responsibility for the medical decisions.

The extent to which patients wish to participate in the decision making process is highly variable, as found in a much quoted study, where at least one-third of patients preferred to leave decision making to the doctor alone (Cassileth et al., 1980). The injudicious involvement of all patients in medical decisions is likely to heighten anxiety in an already fraught situation. In clinical practice it is wise to be guided by the patient's verbal and non-verbal cues.

Accrual to randomized trials and phase I and II studies

Randomized trials, though rightly hailed as the only solution to many medical problems, generate significant problems themselves, not only in workload. The trust that patients give doctors is grounded on the expectation that the doctors motive is to make them better. When secondary motives, such as 'learning something', become priorities this needs to be clearly justified and the significant benefits of external audit, attention and advancing the science of medicine explained. Tackling uncertainty in such a detached way needs to be tempered with information, assurances and reassurance. In one study of patients with inoperable lung cancer, more depression was found in the observation group, with many of those who were not formally depressed appearing 'puzzled and unhappy'. Those in the treatment groups expressed appreciation of radiotherapy and chemotherapy even if obtaining little symptomatic benefit and suffering unpleasant side-effects (Hughes, 1985). Good research is difficult. Balancing the need for randomized trials so that 'the most' can benefit, forwarding science, making wise individualized judgements and containing uncertainty while being the patient's advocate is obviously extremely difficult. Collins *et al.* (1992) draw attention to the fact that the ISIS-2 trial of aspirin and streptokinase in myocardial infarction was delayed by poor recruitment in the United States because of 'humanly inappropriate' written informed consent procedures, compared with the UK, where consent was obtained in the manner considered to be in the best interests of individual patients. The authors highlight the thousands of deaths that may have resulted worldwide from the unnecessary delay in completing the study. The expeditious neglect of the ethical imperative to inform patients is still hotly debated (Kiebert and Kaasa, 1996).

Many patients in whom cure is considered highly unlikely and the chance of palliation and prolongation of life is unknown are eligible for entry to phase I and II studies of new drugs. Toxic treatments known to have some anti-cancer activity, yet which may have a negative impact on quality of life with an unknown chance of remission, are weighed against manoeuvres aimed at symptom relief. Treatment may be extremely inappropriate for some, yet reluctance to treat these people may in some cases lead to disappointment, resentment and perhaps despair (Cody and Slevin, 1989).

Assessing quality of life

The constituents of quality of life (QOL) are personal and will always remain immutably subjective. In palliative oncology, QOL is rightly paramount when considering the worth of treatment. It may be helpful to make patients aware that not only does more effective treatment improve QOL, but that side-effects may be less important than control of disease and that QOL often improves despite the absence of an objective response, possibly due to minimal shrinkage of the tumour (Slevin *et al.*, 1988).

There are devotees of questionnaires to support history taking (Short, 1993), they may not increase objectivity but improve completeness and precision. There are now very well-validated measures of QOL (Maguire and Selby, 1989; Kiebert and Kaasa, 1996). Asking patients to fill in such questionnaires outside the context of clinical trials may improve the detection of unspoken emotional distress, functional limitation or social deprivation. These may be things that should be addressed or treated.

Communication issues and screening for cancer

Screening potentially offers a fairly rapid and important impact on cancer mortality. Although screening provokes considerable anxiety it offers the hope of cure with less radical treatment to some who would have died. The majority eventually find screening reassuring. Effective communication may improve accrual to screening programmes. The potential impact of screening on cures, the procedure and likelihood of a positive and false-positive results, lag and lead time and the overtreatment of borderline abnormalities need to be clearly explained.

Sexuality

Sexual dysfunction is common among cancer patients because of anxiety, ill health and organic causes. It is difficult to treat because of the large psychogenic element. However, sexual counselling has been shown to be effective in reducing long-term morbidity (Capone *et al.*, 1980). The message has been aptly put: talk about it (Crowther *et al.*, 1994). Patients do not volunteer sexual problems and specific enquiry should be made of sexual function beyond broader issues such as 'Who are the most important people in your life?' This is often met with relief rather than embarrassment, particularly in those with problems (Tomlinson, 1998).

Multidisciplinary teams, the general practitioner and support organizations

Ensuring discussion about patients' cases between different specialists can contribute greatly to good standards of care. Working alongside colleagues in a structured way offers a safety net against error and enables continuing education as well as support. Timely, clear and, perhaps, structured correspondence with the general practitioner can avoid distancing the family doctor during a crucial illness. The general practitioner needs clear information about treatment, side-effects, prognosis and what the patient has been told.

There are many useful organizations that offer information, advice and emotional support. Patients feel less anxious through the anonymity of the telephone and can benefit from talking to an independent cancer nurse (Cancer BACUP, Tel.: 0808-800-1234).

CONCLUSION

Good communication potentially offers the most reward-ing aspect of total patient care, but at not inconsiderable cost. Patients have a very important and valid contribu-tion to their ongoing care. The way in which they are involved and the way in which information is elicited and imparted can maximize the quality of their treatment. With sensitivity and a readiness to learn we should not be afraid to say 'I don't know' (Buckman, 1988), but never leave it there.

SIGNIFICANT POINTS

- Have clear objectives, assume nothing and be flexible.
- Introduce yourself and establish some rapport.
- Listen and ask open, but directive, questions.
- Question and summarize until you have the whole picture.
- Acknowledge and address issues.
- Summarize and screen for other issues.
- Be simple and clear, tailor the information to the patient.
- Reinforce realistic hopefulness.

KEY REFERENCES

Buckman, R. (1992) *I don't know what to say.* Vancouver, WA: Vintage books.

Davis, H. and Fallowfield, L. (1991) *Counselling and communication in health care.* Chichester: John Wiley and Sons.

Faulkner, A. (1992) *Effective interaction with patients.* Edinburgh: Churchill Livingstone.

Simpson, M. *et al.* (1991) Doctor–patient communication: the Toronto consensus statement. *BMJ* **303**, 1385–7.

Slevin, M.L. (1987) Talking about cancer: how much is too much? *Br. J. Hosp. Med.* **38**, 58–9.

REFERENCES

Albom, M. (1997) *Tuesdays with Morrie.* New York: Doubleday.

Annas, G.J. (1994) Informed consent, cancer and truth in prognosis. *N. Engl. J. Med.* **330**(3), 223–5.

Asher, R. (1972) *Talking sense.* Tunbridge Wells: Pitman.

Baile, W.F., Lenzi, R., Kudelka, A.P. *et al.* (1997) Improving physician–patient communication in cancer care: outcome of a workshop for oncologists. *J. Cancer Educ.* **12**, 166–73.

Baile, W.F., Buckman, R., Lenzi, R. *et al.* (2000) SPIKES – A six-step protocol for delivering bad news: application to the patient with cancer. *Oncologist* **5**(4), 302–11.

Beckman, H. and Frankel, R. (1984) The effect of physician behaviour on the collection of data. *Ann. Intern. Med.* **101**, 692–6.

Blanchard, C., Ruckeschel, M.D. and Fletcher, B.A. (1986) The impact of oncologists' behaviour on patient satisfaction with morning rounds. *Cancer* **58**, 387–93.

Blau, J. (1989) Time to let the patient speak. *BMJ* **298**, 39.

Buckman, R. (1988) *I don't know what to say.* London: Papermac.

Capone, M., Good, R.S., Wentie, K.S. *et al.* (1980) Psychosocial rehabilitation of gynaecologic oncology patients. *Arch. Phys. Med. Rehabil.* **61**, 128–32.

Cassileth, B., Zupkis, R.V., Sutton-Smith, K. *et al.* (1980) Information and participation preferences among cancer patients. *Ann. Intern. Med.* **92**, 832–6.

Cody, M. and Slevin, M. (1989) Treatment decisions in advanced ovarian cancer. *Br. J. Cancer* **60**, 155–6.

Collins, R., Doll, R. and Peto, R. (1992) Ethics in clinical trials. In Williams, C.J. (ed.), *Introducing new treatments of cancer: practical, ethical and legal problems.* Chichester: Wiley, 49–65.

Crowther, M., Corney, R. and Shepherd, J. (1994) Psychosexual implications of gynaecological cancer: talk about it. *BMJ* **308**, 869–70.

Cunningham, C., Morgan, P. and McGucken, R. (1984) Down's syndrome: is dissatisfaction with disclosure of diagnosis inevitable? *Dev. Med. Child. Neurol.* **26**, 33–9.

Davis, H. and Fallowfield, L. (1991) *Counselling and communication in health care.* Chichester: John Wiley and Sons.

Delamothe, A. (1990) Consenting patients. *BMJ* **301**, 510.

Fallowfield, L. (1993) Giving sad and bad news. *Lancet* **341**(8843), 476–8.

Fallowfield, L.J., Baum, M. and Maguire, G.P. (1986) Effects of breast conservation on psychological morbidity associated with diagnosis and treatment of early breast cancer. *BMJ* **293**, 1331–4.

Fallowfield, L., Baum, M., Maguire, G.P. *et al.* (1987) Addressing the psychological needs of the conservatively treated cancer patient. *J. R. Soc. Med.* **80**, 696–700.

Fallowfield, L., Lipkin, M. and Hall, A. (1998) Teaching senior oncologists communication skills: results from phase I of a comprehensive longitudinal program in the United Kingdom. *J. Clin. Oncol.* **16**, 1961–8.

Faulkner, A. (1992) *Effective interaction with patients.* Edinburgh: Churchill Livingstone.

Feifel, H. (1976) Toward death: a psychological perspective. In Schneidmen, E.S. (ed.), *Death: current perspectives.* Palo Alto, California: Mayfield Publishing.

Finlay, I. and Dallimore, D. (1991) Your child is dead. *BMJ* **302**, 1524–5.

Firth-Cozens, J. (1987) Emotional distress in junior house officers. *BMJ* **295**, 533–6.

Fletcher, C. (1980) Listening and talking to patients. *BMJ* **281**, 994.

Frankl, V.E. (1946) *Man's searching for meaning.* Washington DC: Washington Square Press.

General Medical Council (1987) *Recommendations on general clinical training.* London: GMC.

Goldberg, R. and Cullen, L. (1986) Use of psychotropics in cancer patients. *Psychosomatics* **27**, 687–700.

Greer, S. and Watson, M. (1987) Mental adjustment to cancer; its measurement and prognostic importance. *Cancer Surv.* **6**, 439–53.

Harris, J. (1985) *The value of life – an introduction to medical ethics.* London: Routledge and Kegan Paul, 87–110.

Haven, C.M. and Maguire, P. (1997) Disclosure of concerns by hospice patients and their identification by nurses. *Palliat. Med.* **11**, 283–90.

Heylings, P. (1973) The no touch epidemic – an English disease. *BMJ* **2**, 111.

Hogbin, B. and Fallowfield, L. (1989) Getting it taped: the 'bad news' consultation with cancer patients. *Br. J. Hosp. Med.* **41**, 330–33.

Hughes, J. (1985) Depressive illness and lung cancer. II. Follow-up of inoperable patients. *Eur. J. Surg. Oncol.* **11**, 21.

Ingelfinger, F. (1980) Arrogance. *N. Engl. J. Med.* **303**, 1507–11.

Kerrigan, D., Thevasagayam, R.S., Woods, T.O. *et al.* (1993) Who's afraid of informed consent? *BMJ* **306**, 298–300.

Kiebert, G.M. and Kaasa, S. (1996) Quality of life in clinical cancer trials: experience and perspective of the European Organization for Research and Treatment of Cancer. *J. Natl Cancer Inst. Monographs* **20**, 91–5.

Kottke, T., Battista, R.N., De Grise, G. *et al.* (1988) Attributes of successful smoking cessation interventions in medical practice. A meta analysis of 39 controlled trials. *JAMA* **259**, 2882–9.

Ley, P. (1988) *Communicating with patients.* London: Croom Helm.

Maguire, P. (1990) Can communication skills be taught? *Br. J. Hosp. Med.* **43**, 215–16.

Maguire, P. and Faulkner, A. (1988) Communicate with cancer patients: 1. Handling bad news and difficult questions. *BMJ* **297**, 907–9.

Maguire, P. and Selby, P. (1989) Assessing quality of life in cancer patients. *Br. J. Cancer* **60**, 437–40.

Maguire, P., Hopwood, P., Tarlier, N. *et al.* (1985) Treatment of depression in cancer patients. *Acta Psychiatr. Scand. Suppl.* **320**(81), 81–4.

Maguire, P., Fairbairn, S. and Fletcher, C. (1986a) Consultation skills of young doctors: I – benefits of feedback training in interviewing as students persist. *BMJ* **292**, 1573–6.

Maguire, P., Fairbairn, S. and Fletcher, C. (1986b) Consultation skills of young doctors: II – most young doctors are bad at giving information. *BMJ* **292**, 1576–8.

McLaughlan, C. (1990) Handling distressed relatives and breaking bad news. *BMJ* **301**, 1145–9.

McManus, I., Vincent, C.A., Thom, S. *et al.* (1993) Teaching communication skills to clinical students. *BMJ* **306**, 1322–7.

Novack, D., Plumber, R., Smith, R.L. *et al.* (1979) Changes in physicians' attitudes towards telling the cancer patient. *JAMA* **241**, 897.

Papper, S. (1983) *Doing right. Everyday medical ethics.* Boston: Little, Brown and Co, 125.

President's Commission for the Study of Ethical Problems in Medicine and Biomedical and Behavioral Research (1982) *Making health care decisions: the ethical and legal implications of informed consent in the patient-practitioner relationship*, vol. 2, Appendices. Washington DC: Government Printing Office, 245–6.

Ramirez, A.J., Graham, J., Richards, M.A. *et al.* (1996) Mental health of hospital consultants: the effects of stress and satisfaction at work. *Lancet* **347**, 724–8.

Rollnick, S., Kinnersley, P. and Stott, N. (1993) Methods of helping patients with behaviour change. *BMJ* **307**, 188–90.

Roter, D.L., Larson, S., Fischer, G.S., Arnold, R.M. and Tulsky, J.A. (2000) Experts practice what they preach: a descriptive study of best and normative practices in end-of-life discussions. *Arch. Intern. Med.* **160**(22), 3477–85.

Schain, W.S. (1990) Physician–patient communication about breast cancer. A challenge for the 1990s. *Surg. Clin. North Am.* **70**(4), 917–36.

Shapiro, R., Simpson, D.E., Lawrence, S.L. *et al.* (1989) A survey of sued and nonsued physicians and suing patients. *Arch. Intern. Med.* **149**, 2190–6.

Short, D. (1993) History taking. *Br. J. Hosp. Med.* **50**, 337–9.

Simpson, M., Buckman, R., Stewart, M. *et al.* (1991) Doctor–patient communication: the Toronto consensus statement. *BMJ* **303**, 1385–7.

Slevin, M.L. (1987) Talking about cancer: how much is too much? *Br. J. Hosp. Med.* **38**, 56, 58–9.

Slevin, M., Plaut, H.J., Lynch, D. (1988) Who should measure quality of life, the doctor or the patient? *Br. J. Cancer* **57**, 109–12.

Slevin, M., Stubbs, L., Plaut, H.J. *et al.* (1990) Attitudes to chemotherapy: comparing views of patients with cancer with those of doctors, nurses and general public. *BMJ* **300**, 1458–60.

Snider, G. (1991) The do not resuscitate order – ethical and legal imperative or medical decision? *Am. Rev. Respir. Dis.* **143**, 665–74.

Spence, J. (1953) Function of the hospital out-patient department. *Lancet* **261**, 275.

Spiegel, D., Bloom, J.R., Kraemer, H.C. *et al.* (1989) Effects of psychological treatment on survival of patients with metastatic breast cancer. *Lancet* **ii**, 888–91.

Tobias, J. and Souhami, R. (1993) Fully informed consent can be needlessly cruel. *BMJ* **307**, 1199–201.

Tomlinson, J. (1998) ABC of sexual health: taking a sexual history. *BMJ* **317**, 1573–6.

US Department of Health and Human Services (1994) *Talking with your child about cancer*. Bethesda, Maryland: National Institutes of Health.

57

Clinical cancer genetics

GILLIAN MITCHELL AND ROS A. EELES

INTRODUCTION

Cancer is a common disease, affecting up to a third of the population at some time in their lives. All cancer can be termed 'genetic' as cancer is caused by genetic mutations (alterations in the DNA code), which result in abnormal cellular growth and/or proliferation. The majority of cancers are sporadic (the mutations only occur in the cancer cell) and only a small proportion of cancers (approximately 5–10 per cent) (Easton and Peto, 1990) is due to the inheritance of a mutation in a cancer predisposition gene. This mutation is present in every somatic cell and, on average, half the gametes (a gamete only contains half the total genes) and therefore can be passed onto a proportion of the offspring. These mutated cancer predisposition genes have a well-defined pattern of inheritance. Approximately, a further 20 per cent of cancer cases can be described as familial, i.e. there is a clustering of cancer cases within the family but they do not show a well-defined pattern of inheritance. These families may be due to the chance clustering of common cancers, the inheritance of genes that are associated with only a slightly increased cancer risk, the sharing of common environmental influences or be of multifactorial origin, possibly as a result of the inheritance of genes which render an individual more susceptible to environmental influences. This chapter focuses on cancer predisposition genes, cancer risks associated with these genes and the management of suspected gene carriers.

CANCER PREDISPOSITION GENES: INHERITANCE AND MECHANISMS OF ACTION

Cancer predisposition genes are mutated genes, the normal function of which is to regulate cell growth or the detection and/or repair of DNA damage. These are germline mutations and are present in all nucleated cells, including, on average, half the germ cells. The risk that a cancer predisposition gene gives rise to the development of cancer is designated the penetrance, and the fact that many of these genes do not universally result in cancer development is termed incomplete penetrance.

Familial clustering of the same type of cancer may be due to more than one type of cancer predisposition gene. This is termed 'genetic heterogeneity'. For example, familial breast cancer, in which there are clusters of ≥ 4 cases of breast cancer at ≤ 60 years of age in the same lineage, may be due to mutations in either *BRCA1* or *BRCA2* genes (breast cancer genes 1 and 2). However, calculations from the breast Cancer Linkage Consortium (Ford *et al.*, 1998), which collates international data from breast cancer families, have suggested that 63 per cent of such families be due to either *BRCA1* or *BRCA2*. The remaining 37 per cent of families are likely to be due to gene(s) that remain to be discovered.

Cancer predisposition genes can be associated with syndromes that predominantly consist of clustering of cancers at either one or multiple associated sites (Table 57.1).

Table 57.1 *Syndromes associated with increased risk of malignancy where the major feature associated with the syndrome is the development of cancer*

Syndrome name	Malignancies	Risk (%)[a]	Mode[b]	Chromosomal location[c]	Gene name	Reference
Melanoma	Melanoma	53	D	9p	*CDKN* (*P16*)	Cannon-Albright *et al.* (1994)
Familial polyposis coli	Large bowel cancer	≈100	D	5q	*APC*	Bodmer *et al.* (1987)
	Cancer of upper gastrointestinal tract		5			
	Desmoid tumour	20				
Breast/ovary cancer syndrome	Breast (female)	85	D	17q	*BRCA1*	Miki *et al.* (1994); Ford *et al.* (1998)
	Ovary	60				
	Colon	6				
	Prostate	6				
Site-specific breast cancer	Breast (female)	85	D	13q	*BRCA2*	Wooster *et al.* (1995); Ford *et al.* (1998)
	Ovary	27				
	Prostate	14				
	Breast (male)	5				
	Pancreas	4				
	Other cancers e.g. cutaneous and ocular melanoma, gall bladder, bile duct, fallopian tube, stomach	? <1				
HNPCC						
Lynch type 1	Site-specific colon only	70 (some studies suggest a lower penetrance in women)	D	2p	*hMSH2*	Lynch and Lynch (1994)
Lynch type 2	Colon	70–80	D	3p	*HMLH1*	Lynch and Lynch (1994)
	Endometrium	43		2p	*hMLH6*	Papadopoulos *et al.* (1995)
	Ovary	9–19		3p	*TGF-β*	Markowitz *et al.* (1995)
	Gastric/biliary tract; transitional cell carcinoma of the renal pelvis; melanoma; head and neck; brain; small bowel	<10		2q	*PMS1*	Nicolaides *et al.* (1994)
				7q	*PMS2*	
Muir–Torré syndrome	As HNPCC with skin lesions; keratoacanthoma/ sebaceous cysts		D	2p	*hMSH2*	Hall *et al.* (1994)

Table 57.1 (*continued*)

Syndrome name	Malignancies	Risk (%)[a]	Mode[b]	Chromosomal location[c]	Gene name	Reference
Turcot's syndrome	Brain tumour; very early onset colon cancer (<20 years) with *café-au-lait* patches	?	?	D/R	*hMSH2* *hMLH1* *APC* *PMS2*	Itoh *et al.* (1993)
Hereditary prostate cancer	Prostate	85	D/R/X-linked	?1q ?1p Xq	?	Eeles (1999)
Li–Fraumeni syndrome	Sarcoma Early-onset breast cancer Brain tumour Leukaemia Adrenocortical tumour Other cancers	24 childhood cancer Overall cancer risk, 74 in men, 95 in women	D	17p	*TP53*	Malkin *et al.* (1990)
Multiple endocrine neoplasia type I	Parathyroid, endocrine pancreas, pituitary	70–90		11q	*MEN 1*	Thakker *et al.* (1989)
Multiple endocrine neoplasia type II	Medullary carcinoma of thyroid Phaeochromocytoma (type 2A)	70 50	D	10q	*RET*	Ponder and Smith (1996)
Retinoblastoma	Retinoblastoma Osteosarcoma Other cancers	90 6 8	D	13q	*RB1*	Draper *et al.* (1992)

[a] The risk is either the 'lifetime risk', as quoted in the reference articles, or the 'risk to age 70 years' in those studies which have performed detailed age-specific calculations. Where possible, risks by set ages or a 'per site' risk is given; in the absence of such figures a 'syndrome' penetrance estimate (risk of cancer development) is provided. These risks are approximate and may vary between different populations with different mutation profiles.

[b] Mode of inheritance is classified as 'autosomal dominant' (D) or 'autosomal recessive' (R).

[c] Chromosomal arms: 'q', long arm; 'p', short arm.

For example, *BRCA1/2* genes predispose to both breast and ovarian cancer and hereditary non-polyposis colon cancer (HNPCC) syndrome mismatch repair genes predispose to gastrointestinal, gynaecological, urinary and other cancers. Other genetic syndromes are associated with an increased risk of cancer in addition to other, non-malignant, features of a syndrome such as neurofibromatosis, multiple endocrine neoplasia (MEN) 1 and 2 and ataxia telangiectasia syndromes (Table 57.2). The ability to recognize clustering of cancers at different sites as being part of a syndrome is an important part of recognizing the possible presence of a cancer predisposition gene in a family.

Inheritance of cancer predisposition genes

Inheritance of germline mutations in cancer predisposition genes may be either dominant or recessive at the genetic level or X-linked. We all carry two copies (alleles) of every gene, one copy from each parent, and as only one allele can be passed down to the next generation, there is a 50:50 chance as to which allele is inherited (Plate 12). In dominant inheritance, the presence of a single mutated allele is usually sufficient to cause the associated disease and approximately 50 per cent of all offspring develop the disease. In recessive inheritance, the presence of a single mutated allele is not usually sufficient for disease

Table 57.2 *Some of the 'rare' genetic syndromes associated with an increased risk of malignancy*

Syndrome	Neoplasia or malignancy	Risk (%)[a]	Mode[b]	Chromosomal location[c]	Gene name	Reference
Neurofibromatosis type 1	Plexiform neurofibroma, optic glioma, neurofibrosarcoma	4–5	D	17q	NF1	Huson *et al.* (1989)
Neurofibromatosis type 2	Acoustic neuroma (vestibular schwannoma)		D	22q	NF2	Evans (1999)
	bilateral	85				
	unilateral	6				
	Meningioma	45				
	Spinal tumours	26				
	Astrocytomas	4				
	Ependymomas	3				
von Hippel–Lindau	Cerebellar haemangioblastoma	35–84	D	3p	VHL	Maher *et al.* (1995)
	Retinal angioma	41–70				
	Renal cell carcinoma	25–69				
	Phaeochromocytoma	15				
	Renal, liver and pancreatic cysts	16–50				
Ataxia telangiectasia	Lymphoma	60	R	11q	ATM	Johnson (1989)
	Leukaemia	27				
Bloom syndrome	Many sites Immunodeficiency	40	R	15q	BLM	Ellis and German (1996)
Cowden syndrome	Breast cancer (female)	30–50[d]	D	10q	PTEN	Eng (1998)
	Thyroid cancer	15				
	Bowel cancer	?3				
	Multiple hamartomas of skin, tongue and bowel	100				
Basal cell naevus/ Gorlin's sydrome	Basal cell carcinoma	80	D	9q	PTCH	Kimonis *et al.* (1997)
	Ovarian fibroma	17				
	Medulloblastoma	4				
	Falx calcification, bifid ribs, macrocephaly	85				

[a] Lifetime risk of neoplasia or cancer.
[b] Mode of inheritance is classified as 'autosomal dominant' (D) or 'autosomal recessive' (R).
[c] Chromosomal arms: p, short arm; q, long arm.
[d] Risk by age 50 years.

expression and requires two mutated alleles for disease expression. Usually both parents have to carry the mutated allele for the creation of an offspring affected by disease, for example in the inheritance of cystic fibrosis or β-thalassaemia disease. The majority of cancer predisposition genes are recessively inherited at the genetic level. In X-linked inheritance, the mutated gene is carried on the X chromosome; for example, X-linked familial prostate cancer has been observed in a small number of families although the exact gene has not yet been identified (Xu et al., 1998).

Mechanisms of action

Cancer predisposition genes can be oncogenes, tumour suppressor genes or mismatch repair genes. Oncogenes are mutated normal genes (proto-oncogenes) in which mutation tends to cause a 'gain in function' effect resulting in increased growth or proliferation of the affected cells. Most oncogenes tend to act in a dominant manner and include the RET oncogene in the MEN 2A syndrome or MET oncogene in familial papillary renal cancer. Tumour suppressor genes are normal genes in which mutation tends to cause a 'loss of function' effect in the control mechanisms of growth and/or cellular proliferation pathways. Most cancer predisposition genes are tumour suppressor genes and are recessively inherited at the genetic level. However, they tend to express a dominant phenotype (the physical or biochemical effect of the genotype, such as the development of cancer) as a sporadic mutation of the remaining normal allele frequently occurs in a somatic cell during the lifetime of the germline mutation carrier. Mismatch repair genes (HNPCC syndrome) maintain the integrity of the genome and mutations in them permit acquired genetic damage to accumulate, resulting in the creation of a cancer cell. They are inherited as recessive genes requiring a somatic mutation for phenotypic expression.

RESEARCH APPROACHES FOR THE IDENTIFICATION OF CANCER PREDISPOSITION GENES

When a cancer predisposition gene is thought to be the cause of familial clustering of cancer cases, there are several approaches to locate the gene. Once located and characterized (cloned), genetic testing can then be offered in the clinical setting.

Cytogenetic alterations

Gross chromosomal changes can be seen on cytogenetic analysis. Rarely, a study of a constitutional chromosomal alteration seen on cytogenetic analysis in an individual who has an unusually early onset of cancer and other unusual phenotypic features can indicate the location of a cancer predisposition gene. The chromosomal study of a man with mental retardation and polyposis led to the finding of a loss of part of chromosome 5, subsequently found to be the location of the polyposis gene, APC (Bodmer et al., 1987).

Linkage analysis

The concept of genetic linkage was first recognized by Gregor Mendel, who noted that certain characteristics of his experimental plants tended to be co-inherited. The explanation for this became clear once it was recognized that chromosomes contain the genetic material and two traits are linked only if the corresponding genes for them reside close together on the same chromosome. The search for cancer predisposition genes using linkage relies on collections of families with numerous cancer cases of the same cancer type. Co-inheritance of specific genetic markers with the disease is said to show evidence of linkage if the co-inheritance is greater than would be expected by chance. This is expressed as a 'LOD score' (logarithm to base 10 of the odds). A LOD score is similar to a P value in clinical trials, and a LOD score of >3 is statistically significant and equivalent to odds of linkage of 1000 to 1 ($\log_{10}1000 = 3$).

Phenotypic features

A physical characteristic associated with a cancer predisposition syndrome may give a clue as to the location of the cancer predisposition gene.

Association studies

A number of disease susceptibility loci have been identified through direct testing of candidate genes, looking for associations between particular alleles and disease, by comparing allele frequencies in affected individuals and controls. A candidate gene can be identified by a number of methods, including knowledge of the natural history of specific cancers; for example, in prostate cancer androgen receptor gene polymorphisms (variants in the genetic code) are associated with prostate cancer risk in some studies (Platz et al., 1998).

CANCER RISKS ASSOCIATED WITH CANCER PREDISPOSITION GENES

Cancer risks depend on the exact cancer predisposition gene and its penetrance. Penetrance may be affected by a number of external factors such as lifestyle and may also depend on the ethnic origin of an individual due to population-specific mutation risks. Furthermore, the estimate of penetrance can be confounded by the presence of phenocopies when research into the identification of a cancer predisposition gene is undertaken. Phenocopies are people who have developed the disease of interest but are found not to carry the disease predisposition gene, therefore the disease occurred by chance alone. Phenocopies are a particular problem in syndromes associated with common cancers such as breast or prostate cancer.

Different ethnic populations may have a different gene penetrance, which is illustrated by the breast cancer penetrance estimates for *BRCA1/2* mutation carriers. Using data from the Breast Cancer Linkage Consortium based on breast and ovarian cancer families identified from a worldwide population of high-risk families with breast cancer, the risk of breast cancer is estimated to be 85 per cent by 80 years (Ford *et al.*, 1998). In contrast, certain ethnic populations have specific founder mutations, which are a limited range of mutations attributed to a common ancestor, or 'founder'. Estimates based on the Ashkenazim are 60 per cent by 70 years (Struewing *et al.*, 1997) and for the Icelandic founder mutation carriers to be 37 per cent by 80 years (Thorlacius *et al.*, 1998), in contrast to a general population risk of breast cancer of 10 per cent by 80 years (Marsh, 1993). The ethnic population differences may be due to a founder mutation-dependent risk, the effect of other modifying genes in a population or the added effect of environmental influences, which may be shared within specific populations. It is therefore extremely important to ascertain the genetic origin of the patient before formal genetic counselling is initiated. Tables 57.1 and 57.2 summarize the current penetrance/risk estimates associated with known cancer predisposition genes.

Risk assessment

This is arguably the most difficult part of cancer genetic counselling, first to arrive at a number of risk estimates and second, to convey this information in the most appropriate manner to the individual so that they can understand and retain this information and are not made unduly anxious about their risks.

The first risk estimation is the chance that a familial cluster is due to genetic predisposition. This is called the prior probability of a genetic predisposition gene being present in a family. This estimation can be based upon published data or clinical experiences when published data are lacking, which unfortunately is often the case with rare genetic conditions. In the case of breast cancer families, we are in the fortunate position of having risk estimates available from the Cancer and Steroid Hormone ('CASH' or 'Claus') study (Claus *et al.*, 1991). This was a study of 4700 women with breast cancer who had their family history taken. A statistical model (Claus model,

named after the author of the study) was developed which estimated the chance a cancer predisposition gene was present in a family. This model can be used to generate the curves in Figure 57.1, which can be used easily in a genetics clinic to estimate risk. For example, if an individual has two first-degree relatives with breast cancer at 45 years (Fig. 57.2), there is a 60 per cent chance that there is a breast cancer predisposition gene present.

The second estimation is the chance the individual has inherited a particular gene based upon their position in the family tree, if they are affected by cancer and their current age. This is termed the posterior probability. The risk that the individual in Figure 57.2 may have inherited this gene is therefore half of 60 per cent (the chance there is a cancer predisposition gene in the family), i.e. 30 per cent.

The final calculation is the chance that cancer will develop. Penetrance estimates are essential to calculate this risk. Using breast cancer as an example again, penetrance curves for *BRCA1* have been derived from the Breast

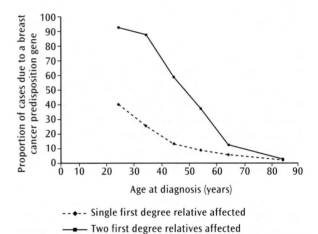

Figure 57.1 *Graph showing the probability that breast cancer is due to a predisposition gene by age at diagnosis of breast cancer (from Claus* et al., *1991). Graph courtesy of Prof. D.T. Bishop.*

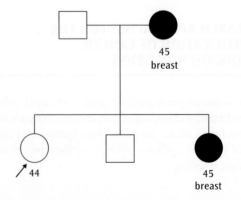

Figure 57.2 *A sample family tree demonstrating a family history of breast cancer in two individuals. Key: unaffected by cancer,* □, ○; *affected by cancer (site specified),* ●; *consultand,* ↗; *Numbers are ages at death, cancer diagnosis or current age.*

Cancer Linkage Consortium data set (Ford *et al.*, 1998) (Fig. 57.3). These calculations can be complex, particularly if there are multiple generations to consider and there may be intervening unaffected individuals between affected individuals as demonstrated in Figure 57.4. Laptop computer software packages (e.g. Cyrillic version 3.0, Cherwell Scientific, UK) are now available to do these calculations; however, they are very model-dependent and knowledge of the inadequacies of the various models is very important to determine whether risks are being over- or underestimated.

Risk perception

Expressing these risks in a form that is meaningful for the individual seaking advice is difficult. The uptake of preventive strategies may depend upon an individual's

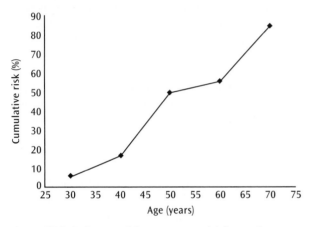

Figure 57.3 *Estimates of breast cancer risk by age in carriers of germline mutations BRCA1/2 genes (from Breast Cancer Linkage Consortium, Ford* et al., *1998).*

perception of risk; for example Croyle *et al.* (1993) have shown that individuals who perceive themselves to be at increased risk of heart disease were more likely to express their intentions to modify their lifestyle than those at perceived population risk. Therefore, the understanding and retention of this information is important and may depend upon the format in which it is presented and the individual's attitudes to risk.

As discussed, risk estimation is complex; the expression of this risk can be delivered in a number of formats (Table 57.3). The optimal format for conveying risk information is unknown. Currently, risk estimates tend to be given as a percentage risk or a '1 in *x*' value and followed up with a written summary, incorporating this risk estimate, to the individual attending the genetics consultation. Unfortunately, there are data that suggest that women prefer not to have, or remember, numerical information. For example, 98 per cent of women attending a cancer family clinic because of a family history of breast cancer could not remember their percentage annual risk, even when this was given both verbally in the clinic, and by follow-up letter. They were somewhat better at remembering their own lifetime risk, but 35 per cent still gave an incorrect figure. More importantly though, they were able to report the qualitative category of their risk (low, medium, high) with reasonable accuracy, but this did not relate to their perception that they were more or less likely to get cancer (Lloyd *et al.*, 1996). This suggests that consultands have a poor understanding of the risk information being given. Green and Brown (1978) have

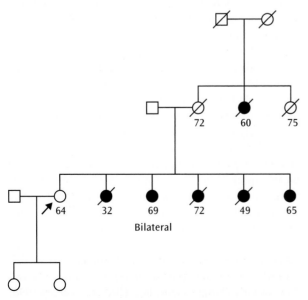

Figure 57.4 *A sample family tree demonstrating a complex family history of breast cancer. Key:* ●, *breast cancer.*

Table 57.3 *Methods of presentation of cancer risk estimates*

Method of presentation	Expression of risk
Numerical	Risk per year
	Risk by certain age
	1 in *x* value or percentage format
	Relative risk corrected for age
General categorization	High/moderate/low risk
Situation analogy	A situation carrying an equivalent risk without any numerical information, e.g. the chances of picking an ace if one card is chosen blind from a card pack
The risk figure measure	Risk of developing cancer
	Risk of not developing cancer
Risk of death from cancer (this is rarely given in clinics as it is perceived as too distressing)	

suggested that the qualitative aspect of risk is more important than the quantitative aspect. However, this finding contrasts with that of Josten *et al.* (1985) who report from a cancer family clinic in Wisconsin, USA that 'clients say that a number gives them boundaries rather than having an ambiguous sense of being high risk'. The main problem with the quantitative approach is that one person's high risk is another's moderate risk.

The individual's background information, sociodemographic factors (e.g. educational level) and psychological profile could conceivably alter the optimal method of risk presentation since these can act as barriers to adequate information content (Lerman *et al.*, 1994). Furthermore, in cancer families, it is possible that a larger cancer burden (the number, age at diagnosis, and closeness of relationship of the cancer cases) may distort the perceived risk above the true level (Ardern-Jones, 1998). Many people in cancer families think erroneously that their risk of developing cancer is 100 per cent, and the only uncertainty is the point in time when the disease will occur. Lerman *et al.* (1994) have reported that members of cancer families distort their risk, even when their family history consists of only one affected relative.

The points above have been summarized by Vlek (1987) who claims that there are five factors underlying perception of risk. These are:

1 the potential degree of harm or lethality associated with the risk;
2 the controllability through safety/rescue measures (i.e. prevention/early detection);
3 the number of people exposed (this would equate to the cancer burden in the family);
4 the familiarity with the effects of the risk; and
5 the degree of voluntariness of exposure to the risk.

There are reports which suggest that those at highest risk have a lower rate of adoption of health preventive measures due to avoidance behaviours instigated by high levels of anxiety (Kash *et al.*, 1991). If cancer family clinics are to provide a useful service, it is important to ensure that those counselled understand the risk information and advice they are given. Lack of understanding of their risk could impact on their ability to use this information when making decisions about the future management of their health and may also affect their mental health if cancer-related worries are increased through misunderstanding of information given in the clinic.

MANAGEMENT OF A KNOWN OR SUSPECTED CANCER PREDISPOSITION GENE MUTATION CARRIER

Identification of an at-risk family

A family at genetic risk of cancer must first be identified. There are many potential sources of identification, for example, through consultation with a general practitioner (GP) or a hospital clinic while under treatment for an associated disease, through conversation with an associated professional such a practice or clinic nurse, radiographer or doctor or through an individual's own perception of a potential genetic problem in their family precipitating contact with a health-care professional. Unless an individual directly expresses concern about their perceived risk, then the only way an at-risk family will be identified is by systematic questioning of all patients about a family history of cancer while eliciting a general medical history, in addition to a general professional knowledge about cancer predisposition genes and disease patterns which may be associated with them. As a quick guideline, taking a history of all first-degree relatives only (parents, siblings and children) and then asking if there are any other cancers in the family will detect 95 per cent of familial syndromes. Due to the limited time available during most consultations, it would not be appropriate to spend a prolonged consultation deriving a detailed family history from the patient as we have found that many patients have poor immediate recall of their extended family structure and health. From this quick family history it should be possible to make an assessment whether the family history warrants further investigation. Further information can be obtained by asking the consultand to complete a full family history out to third-degree relatives. Often help from other family members has to be requested by the consultand in order to complete this, so this is best undertaken by the consultand in their own time.

It is neither currently possible, nor appropriate, to see all individuals with a family history of cancer in a cancer genetics clinic due to the limited availability of resources; therefore it is important that the local cancer genetics clinics provide guidelines for referral (*see* Table 57.4 for an example of the Royal Marsden Hospital NHS Trust genetics clinic referral guidelines for 1999), which will depend upon local resources for genetic and cancer services and current medical practice. The genetics clinic should also suggest appropriate management plans for individuals at increased risk of cancer but not sufficiently high as to warrant referral to a specialist centre. This is particularly true for breast cancer, which is a common disease, associated with a high level of public anxiety, particularly regarding familial clustering of the disease. Referrals to genetics clinics could then be precipitated by anxious women with only a moderately increased risk of breast cancer. Using the family tree, a doctor may be able to reassure an individual, suggest an increased cancer screening schedule, or initiate referral to a genetics clinic for the minority of patients who may benefit from the specialist services of such a genetics clinic. Taking breast cancer as an example, a number of women may qualify for earlier mammographic screening according to British Association of Surgical Oncology (BASO) (Blamey, 1998) and Cancer Family Study Group (CFSG) guidelines (Eccles *et al.*, 2000), but do not require specialist genetic

Table 57.4 *Suggested referral guidelines to the Royal Marsden NHS Trust familial cancer clinic*[a]

Breast cancer families
Single case <40 years if of Ashkenazi Jewish origin
Two cases of breast cancer diagnosed under the age of 50
Three cases of breast cancer diagnosed under the age of 60
Four or more cases of breast cancer diagnosed at any age
Breast cancer and ovarian cancer. This includes the case where a patient develops both cancers
Any male breast cancer cases with a relative affected with breast cancer (male or female)

Ovarian cancer families
Any family with two or more cases of ovarian cancer
Any family with ovarian cancer and any of colorectal, endometrial or breast cancer diagnosed under the age of 50

Colon cancer families
Families with three or more cases of the following: colorectal cancer ± endometrial cancer and/or ovarian cancer and/or breast cancer
Single cases of colorectal cancer diagnosed under the age of 45
Two cases of colorectal cancer under the age of 45 years

Prostate cancer families
Any family with two cases with prostate cancer where one is diagnosed under the age of 65
Families with three or more cases of prostate cancer at any age

Li–Fraumeni families/Li–Fraumeni-like families
Childhood cancer or sarcoma/brain tumour/adrenocortical cancer diagnosed under 45 years with first- or second-degree relative with sarcoma/breast cancer/ brain tumour/leukaemia/adrenocortical cancer at any age and another first- or second-degree relative with cancer diagnosed under 60 years
Sarcoma at any age with two of the following in first- or second-degree relatives: breast or stomach cancer diagnosed under 50 years or brain tumour/ adrenocortical cancer/prostate cancer/melanoma/germ cell tumour/leukaemia diagnosed under 60 years or sarcoma at any age.

Other families
Any other families with an unusual pattern of cancer in the family or rare syndromes, e.g. testicular cancer in two or more relatives at any age, MEN, von Hippel–Lindau, etc.

[a] The family history should be in the same lineage.

services due to the limited family history. A woman with a single first-degree relative with breast cancer diagnosed under the age of 40 or two relatives diagnosed with breast cancer under the age of 60 (but not 50 years) would be at increased risk of breast cancer (nearly 4 × population risk) but not at high enough risk to consider genetic testing. The main difficulty for the non-geneticist is making an assessment of the level of genetic risk. Guidelines are helpful, but a number of computer software packages are now available to aid risk assessment (Emery *et al.*, 1999). There are a number of potential problems with these packages so trials are currently in progress to assess their role in the primary care setting.

Genetics clinics

Following the identification of an at-risk individual, referral to a specialist clinic should occur for formal assessment of the individual or family risk, screening and management strategies and the possibility of genetic testing.

AIM OF GENETICS CLINICS

Cancer genetics counselling aims to provide an explanation of how cancer develops (most commonly as a result of somatic mutation), the principles of genetic inheritance, an estimation of the chance that a familial cluster is due to genetic predisposition, information about the likely specific predisposition gene present, an estimation of cancer risk, options for managing the risk and the opportunity for genetic testing.

STRUCTURE OF THE GENETICS CLINIC

As in many other areas of oncology, the multidisciplinary approach is being increasingly used in cancer genetic counselling clinics. Most of these clinics are located within, or in close association with, the regional clinical genetics service; however, it is desirable that cancer genetic counselling personnel have training in both genetics and oncology. In the UK, genetic counsellors/clinical nurse specialists in cancer genetics counselling are starting to conduct a lot of the routine counselling, working closely with medical personnel who provide the medical back-up and formal risk assessment.

Medical history and examination

It must be established from the history and examination whether the patient is an affected or an at-risk member of the family, and the consultand should be questioned on any symptoms indicative of cancer or congenital abnormalities. It is extremely important to ascertain the genetic origin of the patient as mutations in some cancer genes are more common in certain populations, particularly those from less out-bred ethnic groups.

The taking of a full family history is central to the practice of the management of familial cancer. The individuals with cancer should be noted in a family tree (*see* Fig. 57.5).

Standard notation is:

- Male: square (□)
- Female: circle (○)

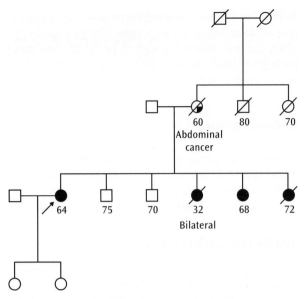

Figure 57.5 *A sample family tree demonstrating a family history of cancer. The chance that this family has a cancer predisposition gene is >95 per cent. Tracing of the diagnosis of the abdominal cancer, via the cancer registry or medical records, verified that this was ovarian cancer indicating that the family has breast/ovarian cancer syndrome. Key: ●, breast cancer; ◐, any other type of cancer, specified.*

- Deceased: diagonal line through symbol (⊘).
- Proband: arrow indicates consultand who is giving the family history (↗).

There is variation in notation of the shading of the symbols between clinics and, as the shading is not standardized, a legend should be attached to a family tree if referring to a family history in a medical report.

Studies have shown that recall of family history is superior for first-degree relatives as compared to more distant relatives and recall of breast cancer family history is approximately 90 per cent accurate (Douglas *et al.*, 1999). However, accuracy falls for cancer at more indeterminate sites such as ovarian cancer which is often reported as 'abdominal' or 'stomach' (Douglas *et al.*, 1999); this has approximately a 17 per cent miscall rate. Verification of diagnosis would therefore be important in individuals such as that with 'abdominal cancer' in Figure 57.5 since if this were shown to be ovarian cancer, the family in Figure 57.5 would have breast/ovarian cancer syndrome.

Not all cancer genetics clinics verify all breast cancer cases because of the high accuracy of recall and the fact that recall is more likely to be an over-recall, since mastectomy may have been performed for benign disease. This would result in an over-screening of only 5–10 per cent of patients and it is often not cost-effective to verify all breast cancer cases. An exception would be if an individual wishes to undertake more extreme measures such as prophylactic surgery since cases of Münchhausen's syndrome by proxy (individuals passing on to other family members

a fictitious family history of cancer in order to provoke them to take preventive measures) have been reported, although these are rare (<1 per cent) (Douglas *et al.*, 1999). Douglas *et al.* (1999) showed that verification of all family histories in their cancer genetics clinic resulted in an 11 per cent change in recommendations for management and most of the changes were related to verification of cancers at abdominal sites.

Initial clinical examination involves looking for any dysmorphic features and congenital anomalies. The skin should be carefully examined, as many cancer syndromes are associated with dermatological features, such as pigmentary abnormalities, e.g. freckles on the lip in Peutz–Jeghers syndrome, *café au lait* patches in neurofibromatosis I or Turcot's syndrome, basal cell naevi in Gorlin's syndrome. Skin tumours, such as the epidermoid cysts seen in FAP (familial adenomatous polyposis), keratoacanthomas seen in Muir–Torré syndrome, or tricholemmomas of Cowden's syndrome can be indicators that the individual is very likely to be a gene carrier before confirmation by formal DNA genetic testing.

Throughout the consultation, it is important to be sensitive to potential psychopathology. Frequently there will have been bereavement due to the premature death of close relatives, particularly a parent or child. Unresolved bereavement may make it difficult for people to accept their own risks and make decisions about their own management. In addition, patients are sometimes unable to cope with their worries. Referral for formal psychological counselling may resolve these problems. Of particular concern are those individuals who have prophylactic surgery because of excess anxiety but who, while being temporarily relieved, could return at a later date with further cancer phobic symptoms. A psychological assessment and counselling should be strongly suggested before prophylactic surgery.

Clinical management

The subsequent management of an individual and their family will depend upon the final risk estimates regarding the inheritance of a cancer predisposition gene and the potential cancer risks associated with this. In general, management strategies fall into four categories: cancer screening, lifestyle changes, preventive strategies and genetic testing.

CANCER SCREENING

Cancer screening strategies can be advised for many individuals at increased risk of developing cancer. Table 57.5 outlines guidance protocols for screening in individuals with a high probability of mutations in cancer predisposition genes. Not all of the screening schedules described have been proven to reduce mortality from the relevant cancer, but these schedules represent a pragmatic approach to the management of individuals at risk.

Table 57.5 *Screening protocols (for guidance only as different clinics may have alterations for this schema)*

Disease	Screen	Age (years) at start of screen/range for screening
von Hippel–Lindau Affected	Annual: physical examination Urine testing Direct ophthalmoscopy Fluorescein angiography 24-h urinary VMA Renal ultrasound 3-yearly: MRI brain CT kidneys (more frequent if multiple cysts)	
von Hippel–Lindau At-risk relatives	Annual: physical examination Urine testing Direct ophthalmoscopy Fluorescein angiography 24-h urinary VMA Renal ultrasound 3-yearly: MRI brain CT kidneys (more frequent if multiple cysts) 5-yearly: MRI brain	5 upwards 5 upwards 10 until 60 20 until 65 15 until 40 20 until 65 40 until 60
Familial polyposis Affected	Offer total colectomy with ileorectal anastomosis Annual rectal stump screening (if conserved in surgery) Upper gastrointestinal endoscopy 3-yearly (annually if polyps found)	Teenager (*see* below) 20 upwards
Familial polyposis At-risk relatives	Offer genetic analysis if possible Annual sigmoidoscopy Perform colonoscopy when polyps found on sigmoidoscopy and arrange colectomy	 11 (polyps are rare before this age) until 40
Gorlin's syndrome Affected (at-risk children usually have abnormal skull or spine X-rays by 5 years)	Annual dermatological examination Yearly orthopantomogram for jaw cysts Examination of infants for signs of medulloblatoma (some advocate MRI but not CT due to radiosensitivity)	Infants upwards
MEN II	Offer genetic screening if possible – if positive perform prophylactic thyroidectomy Annual: plasma calcium, phosphate and parathormone Pentagastrin test Thyroid ultrasound Abdominal ultrasound and CT 24-h urinary VMA/blood catecholamines	5 8 until 70
MEN I	Annual: symptom enquiry (dyspepsia, diarrhoea, renal colic, fits, amenorrhoea, galactorrhoea) Examination Serum calcium Parathormone Renal function Pituitary hormones (PL, GH, ACTH, FSH, TSH) Pancreatic hormones (gastrin, VIP, glucagon, neurotensin, somatostatin, pancreatic polypeptide) Lateral skull X-ray for pituitary size or MRI for pituitary adenomas	5
Wilms' tumour At-risk individuals	3-monthly: renal ultrasound 6-monthly: renal ultrasound	Birth–8 years 8 until 12
Retinoblastoma (siblings and offspring of affected)	Offer genetic screening if possible Monthly retinal examination without anaesthetic 3-monthly retinal examination under anaesthetic	 Birth–3 months 3 months until 2 years

Table 57.5 (*continued*)

Disease	Screen	Age (years) at start of screen/range for screening
Retinoblastoma (contd.) (siblings and offspring of affected)	4-monthly retinal examination under anaesthetic	2–3 years
	6-monthly retinal examination without anaesthetic	3–5 years
	Annual retinal examination without anaesthetic	5–11 years
	Annual examination for sarcoma	Early teens for life
Li–Fraumeni	Annual breast examination	18 until 60
	?MRI (under investigation)	
	Annual examination	Lifelong
NF1 Affected	Annual examination	Lifelong
		Visual field assessment
NF2 At-risk relatives	Offer genetic screening if possible	
	Annual examination	Childhood
	Ophthalmoscopy for congenital cataracts	
	Annual audiometry	10 until 40
	Brainstem auditory-evoked potentials	
	3-yearly MRI brain	
Lynch I syndrome	2-yearly colonoscopy	25 upwards
Lynch II syndrome	2-yearly colonoscopy	25 upwards
	Annual ovarian and endometrial ultrasound and CA 125	30 upwards
	Some screen for other cancers in kindred such as skin and urothelial malignancy (annual urine cytology and dermatological examination)	35 upwards
	Annual mammography	35 upwards. Its use depends on incidence of breast cancer in family
Muir–Torré syndrome	2-yearly colonoscopy	25 upwards
Turcot's syndrome	2-yearly colonoscopy	20 upwards
Colon cancer in a single relative aged <45 years	5-yearly colonoscopy (3-yearly if polyps are found)	35 upwards
Familial melanoma	Annual skin examination	Teenager upwards
	General sun avoidance advice	
Breast/ovarian syndrome	Annual mammography	35 upwards or 5 years younger than youngest case (not less than 25–30) 35 upwards (30 if young ovarian cancer case in family)
	Transvaginal ultrasound	
	CA125	
Familial breast cancer	Annual mammography	35 upwards or 5 years younger than youngest case (not less than 25)
Familial ovarian cancer	Transvaginal ultrasound	30–35 upwards
	CA 125	
Familial prostate cancer	Annual serum prostate-specific antigen	50 upwards or 5 years younger than youngest case (minimum age 40)
	Digital rectal examination	
Familial testicular cancer	Regular testicular self-examination	Late teens–50

LIFESTYLE CHANGES

Lifestyle changes may take many forms such as the avoidance of known cancer causing factors such as sunlight in xeroderma pigmentosum and X-ray exposure in the Li–Fraumeni syndrome. Other lifestyle changes are less well established in the prevention of cancer but have been suggested based upon current understanding of tumour biology and a small number of epidemiologically based studies. Although lifestyle changes may have a greater role in the prevention of sporadic cancers, they may still be of benefit in cancers associated with a genetic predisposition. For example, a diet rich in plant phytoestrogens

Table 57.6 *Location of and status of testing for cancer predisposition genes in 1999*

Disease	Location	Mutation analysis available
Breast/ovarian	17q21	BRCA1
Familial breast cancer/male breast cancer	13q12	BRCA2
von Hippel–Lindau	3p25	VHL (research only)
Familial adenomatous polyposis	5q21	APC
Gorlin's syndrome	9q22	PTCH (research only)
Multiple endocrine neoplasia type 2	10q11	RET
Multiple endocrine neoplasia type 1	11q13	MEN I (research only)
Wilms' tumour	11p13	WT1 (research only)
Retinoblastoma	13q14	RB1
Li–Fraumeni syndrome	17p13	TP53
Neurofibromatosis I	17q11	NF1 (research only)
Neurofibromatosis II	22q12	NF2
Lynch syndrome I	2p22	hMLH1
Lynch syndrome II	3p21	hMSH2

may protect against the development of breast cancer (Ingram *et al.*, 1997) or the avoidance of excessive exposure to ovarian hormones may reduce the risk of breast cancer in genetically predisposed individuals (Ursin *et al.*, 1997). A high-fibre diet may reduce the risk of colorectal cancer (Howe *et al.*, 1992).

PREVENTIVE STRATEGIES

Preventive strategies can take many forms including prophylactic surgery and chemoprevention. The evidence in support of the efficacy of these measures is variable, mainly due to rarity of the genetic mutation making clinical trials difficult to perform. Established measures include total colectomy in the FAP syndrome (Nyam *et al.*, 1997) and total thyroidectomy in the MEN II syndrome (Lallier *et al.*, 1998). More contentious roles for prophylactic surgery include mastectomy or oophorectomy in patients with known or suspected *BRCA1/2* mutations. Limited retrospective data suggest that the risk of breast cancer is reduced following prophylactic mastectomy, although there is still a residual risk of breast cancer due to the inability to remove all breast epithelial cells at mastectomy (Hartmann, 1999). Prophylactic oophorectomy has been shown to reduce ovarian cancer risk (Struewing *et al.*, 1995), in addition to a reduction in breast cancer risk (Rebbeck *et al.*, 1999). A risk of peritoneal carcinomatosis remains due to the shared embryonic origin of both peritoneum and ovarian epithelium (Kemp *et al.*, 1992).

The role of chemoprevention is much less certain, but includes a reduction of ovarian cancer risk in users of the combined oral contraceptive pill (Narod *et al.*, 1998). Data on the role of tamoxifen in the prevention of breast cancer in high-risk women are conflicting. A large American study, NSAB-P1, has suggested a 45 per cent reduction in breast cancer risk in women at increased risk who took tamoxifen chemoprevention (Fisher *et al.*, 1998). However, the effect was not replicated by two European studies (Powles *et al.*, 1998; Veronesi *et al.*, 1998). Of current interest is the demonstration of a reduction in incidence of colonic cancer in long-term users of non-steroidal anti-inflammatory drugs and has led to the current study (CAPP2) of aspirin prevention of colonic cancer in HNPCC families.

GENETIC TESTING

Genetic testing is possible for some cancer predisposition genes (Table 57.6) and is performed on DNA from venous blood. Genetic testing may either be diagnostic (the detection of a mutation in an individual affected by cancer) or predictive (the detection of a mutation in a clinically unaffected individual). Mutations in cancer predisposition genes often occur throughout the gene and the vast majority of mutations so far have only been observed in limited numbers of families except in specific ethnic groups with known founder mutations such as the Icelandic (Thorlacius *et al.*, 1997) and Ashkenazi (Tonin *et al.*, 1996) populations with *BRCA1/2* mutations. Hence, unless an individual is a member of such a group, the specific mutation for that family must first be identified. An affected family member is tested first because they are the family member most likely to have the cancer-predisposing mutation. Once a mutation is suspected, one has to check it is likely to be cancer causing and not a rare normal variant of the gene (polymorphism). Predictive testing may then be offered to unaffected family members for the identified mutation. Misleading results may occur if an unaffected individual has a genetic test in order to identify a mutation without first identifying it in an affected relative.

A negative diagnostic test result (i.e. no mutation is identified in the cancer predisposition gene tested) may not be a true negative for several reasons:

- the family history is due to a gene other than that being tested;

- the mutation may be regulatory which means that it controls how the gene is expressed but the gene itself (and therefore the test which looks at the gene code) is normal;
- the genetic test sensitivity is not 100 per cent for the genetic coding mutations and may therefore have missed mutations.

When the specific mutation has been identified in an affected individual, if it is not found in an unaffected relative, this is then a truly negative result.

Unfortunately, due to the high penetrance of certain predisposition genes, for example *BRCA1/2*, it is not uncommon to be presented with a family with multiple cases of cancer and all affected individuals have died from their cancer. In this difficult situation it is not currently possible to offer mutation testing to unaffected cases and their future clinical management will depend upon their probability of having inherited a mutation. An exception is the rare circumstance of a closed ethnic group (e.g. the Ashkenazi) with known founder mutations.

Genetic testing should only take place following full genetic counselling to outline the implications of genetic testing. A recognized counselling schedule allows at least a month of reflection between two counselling sessions prior to taking blood for mutation analysis. The personal and wider social implications of positive and negative results are issues discussed during these sessions. A positive result could have psychological implications as well as widespread repercussions involving the rest of the family.

The social implications of the ability to purchase life and medical insurance, mortgages and a possible effect on employment opportunities may be just as, if not more important than, the personal and familial implications. At present, effects on employment are theoretical. Currently, any results of genetic tests have to be declared when applying for a new insurance policy. Following a recent statement from the Association of British Insurers in 1997, genetic test results are not taken into account if they are detrimental to a person's insurance position if they are applying for an insurance policy for life coverage for a mortgage of £300 000 or less (Association of British Insurers, 2001). This is currently under review. A negative test result may have psychological consequences due to the recognized 'survivor guilt syndrome', which has been documented in the setting of Huntington's disease (Demyttenaere *et al.*, 1992).

For genes predisposing to adult-onset cancers, testing of young children is not advised as the age of cancer onset permits the individual to make their own decision to have genetic testing once they have reached adulthood following full genetic counselling. Children tend to be offered genetic testing when it may alter management, for example, in MEN IIA syndrome when thyroidectomy is offered at 5–15 years for gene carriers as it is totally protective against medullary thyroid cancer or in familial polyposis where regular colonoscopies or colectomy may be avoided.

SUMMARY

Cancer is a common disease but only a small proportion of cases can be attributed to the inheritance of specific cancer predisposition genes. However, in absolute terms, this represents a significant number of families or individuals due to the high population frequency of cancer. Only a few cancer predisposition genes have been identified, although the existence of many more is suspected. Currently we can offer limited advice regarding risks, genetic testing and general management of suspected gene carriers but cancer genetics is one of the most rapidly expanding areas of oncological knowledge. Any advice given regarding cancer predisposition genes may be liable to change with advances in research and knowledge and specialists in the field of cancer genetics should facilitate the dissemination of any changes in advice to other colleagues likely to be in contact with individuals at risk.

SIGNIFICANT POINTS

- The majority of cancer cases are sporadic and not related to the inheritance of a cancer predisposition gene.
- Most cancer families who may benefit from referral to a specialist cancer genetics unit can be detected by taking a limited family history. This should include all first-degree relatives (parents/siblings/children) and any other cancer cases in other relatives.
- Cancer site and age of onset are important.
- Early cancer screening may be available for specific cancer predisposition syndromes.
- Genetic testing for the presence of a familial cancer predisposition gene can usually only be performed by direct DNA analysis using venous blood from a living relative affected by cancer.

KEY REFERENCES

Eeles, R.A., Ponder, B.A.J., Easton, D.F. and Horwich, A. (eds) 1996 *Genetic predisposition to cancer*. London: Chapman and Hall Medical.

Ford, D., Easton, D.F., Stratton, M. *et al.* (1998) Genetic heterogeneity and penetrance analysis of the *BRCA*1 and *BRCA*2 genes in breast cancer families. The Breast Cancer Linkage Consortium. *Am. J. Hum. Genet.* **62**, 676–89.

Lynch, H.T. and Lynch, J.F. (1994) 25 years of HNPCC. *Anticancer Res.* **14**, 1617–24.

Malkin, D., Li, F.P., Strong, L.C. *et al.* (1990) Germ line p53 mutations in a familial syndrome of breast cancer, sarcomas and other neoplasms. *Science* **250**, 1233–8.

REFERENCES

Ardern-Jones, A. (1998) Living with a cancer legacy: the experience of hereditary cancer in the family. Institute of Cancer Research, London University, MSc dissertation.

Association of British Insurers (1997) Genetic Tests and Insurance. *Declaration by Association of British Insurers, December 1997.*

Blamey, R.W. (1998) The British Association of Surgical Oncology Guidelines for surgeons in the management of symptomatic breast disease in the UK (1998 revision). BASO Speciality Group. *Eur. J. Surg. Oncol.* **24**, 464–76.

Bodmer, W.F., Bailey, C.J., Bodmer, J. *et al.* (1987) Localization of the gene for familial adenomatous polyposis on chromosome 5. *Nature* **328**, 614–16.

Cannon-Albright, L.A., Meyer, L.J., Goldgar, D.E. *et al.* (1994) Penetrance and expressivity of the chromosome 9p melanoma susceptibility locus (MLM). *Cancer Res.* **54**, 6041–4.

Claus, E.B., Risch, N.J. and Thompson, W.D. (1991) Genetic analysis of breast cancer in the cancer and steroid hormone study. *Am. J. Hum. Genet.* **48**, 232–42.

Croyle, R.T., Sun, Y.C. and Louie, D.H. (1993) Psychological minimization of cholesterol test results: moderators of appraisal in college students and community residents. *Health Psychol.* **12**, 503–7.

Demyttenaere, K., Evers-Kiehooms, G. and Decruyenaere, M. (1992) Pitfalls in counselling for predictive testing in Huntington's disease. *Birth Defects* **28**, 105–11.

Douglas, F.S., O'Dair, L.C., Robinson, M. *et al.* (1999) The accuracy of diagnoses as reported in families with cancer: a retrospective study. *J. Med. Genet.* **36**, 309–12.

Draper, G.J., Sanders, B.M., Brownbill, P.A. and Hawkins, M.M. (1992) Patterns of risk of hereditary retinoblastoma and applications to genetic counselling. *Br. J. Cancer* **66**, 211–19.

Easton, D.F. and Peto, J. (1990) The contribution of inherited predisposition to cancer incidence. *Cancer Surv.* **9**, 395–416.

Eccles, D.M., Evans, D.G.R. and McKay, J. (2000) Guidelines for a genetic risk based approach to screening women with a family history of breast cancer. UK Cancer Family Study Group. *J. Med. Genet.* **37**, 203–9.

Eeles, R.A. (1999) Genetic predisposition to prostate cancer. *Prostate Cancer Prostat. Dis.* **2**, 9–15.

Ellis, N.A. and German, J. (1996) Molecular genetics of Bloom's syndrome. *Hum. Mol. Genet.* **5**, 1457–63.

Emery, J., Walton, R., Coulson, A. *et al.* (1999) Computer support for recording and interpreting family histories of breast and ovarian cancer in primary care (RAGs): qualitative evaluation with simulated patients. *Br. Med. J.* **319**, 32–6.

Eng, C. (1998) Genetics of Cowden's syndrome: through the looking glass of oncology. *Int. J. Cancer* **12**, 701–10.

Evans, D.G.R. (1999) Neurofibromatosis type 2: genetic and clinical features. *Ear Nose Throat J.* **78**, 97–100.

Fisher, B., Costantino, J.P., Wickerham, D.L. *et al.* (1998) Tamoxifen for prevention of breast cancer: report of the National Surgical Adjuvant Breast and Bowel Project P-1 Study. *J. Natl Cancer Inst.* **90**, 1371–88.

Ford, D., Easton, D.F., Stratton, M. *et al.* (1998) Genetic heterogeneity and penetrance analysis of the *BRCA*1 and *BRCA*2 genes in breast cancer families. The Breast Cancer Linkage Consortium. *Am. J. Hum. Genet.* **62**, 676–89.

Green, H. and Brown, R.A. (1978) Counting lives. *J. Occup. Accid.* **2**, 55.

Hall, N.R., Murday, V.A., Chapman, P. *et al.* (1994) Genetic linkage in Muir–Torre syndrome to the same chromosomal region as cancer family syndrome. *Eur. J. Cancer* **30A**, 180–2.

Hartmann, L.C. (1999) Efficacy of bilateral prophylactic mastectomy in women with a family history of breast cancer. *N. Engl. J. Med.* **340**, 77–84.

Howe, G.R., Benito, E., Castelleto, R. *et al.* (1992) Dietary intake of fiber and decreased risk of cancers of the colon and rectum: evidence from the combined analysis of 13 case-control studies. *J. Natl Cancer Inst.* **84**, 1887–96.

Huson, S.M., Compston, D.A. and Harper, P.S. (1989) A genetic study of von Recklinghausen neurofibromatosis in south east Wales. *J. Med. Genet.* **26**, 712–21.

Ingram, D., Sanders, K., Kolybaba, M. and Lopez, D. (1997) Case-control study of phyto-oestrogens and breast cancer. *Lancet* **350**, 990–4.

Itoh, H., Hirata, K. and Ohsato, K. (1993) Turcot's syndrome and familial adenomatous polyposis associated with brain tumour: review of related literature. *Int. J. Colorectal Dis.* **8**, 87–94.

Johnson, J.A. (1989) Ataxia telangiectasia and other alpha-fetoprotein-associated disorders. In Lynch, H.T. and Hirayama, T. (eds), *Genetic epidemiology of cancer*. Boca Raton: CRC Press, 145–147.

Josten, D.M., Evans, A.M. and Love, R.R. (1985) The cancer prevention clinic: a service program for cancer-prone families. *J. Psychosoc. Oncol.* **3**, 5–20.

Kash, K.M., Holland, J.C., Halper, M.S. and Miller, D.G. (1991) Psychological distress and surveillance behaviours of women with a family history of breast cancer. *J. Natl Cancer Inst.* **84**, 24–30.

Kemp, G.M., Hsiu, J.G. and Andrews, M.C. (1992) Papillary peritoneal carcinomatosis after prophylactic oophorectomy. *Gynecol. Oncol.* **47**, 395–7.

Kimonis, V.E., Goldstein, A.M., Pastakia, B. *et al.* (1997) Clinical manifestations in 105 persons with nevoid basal cell carcinoma syndrome. *Am. J. Med. Genet.* **69**, 299–308.

Lallier, M., St-Vil, D., Giroux, M. *et al.* (1998) Prophylactic thyroidectomy for medullary thyroid cancer in gene carriers of MEN2 syndrome. *J. Pediatr. Surg.* **33**, 846–8.

Lerman, C., Daly, M., Masny, A. and Balshem, A. (1994) Attitudes about genetic testing for breast-ovarian cancer susceptibility. *J. Clin. Oncol.* **12**, 843–50.

Lloyd, S., Watson, M., Waites, B. *et al.* (1996) Familial breast cancer: a controlled study of risk perception, psychological morbidity and health beliefs in women attending for genetic counselling. *Br. J. Cancer* **74**, 482–7.

Lynch, H.T. and Lynch, J.F. (1994) 25 years of HNPCC. *Anticancer Res.* **14**, 1617–24.

Maher, E.R., Webster, A.R. and Moore, A.T. (1995) Clincial features and molecular genetics of von Hippel-Lindau disease. *Ophthal. Genet.* **16**, 79–84.

Malkin, D., Li, F.P., Strong, L.C. *et al.* (1990) Germ line p53 mutations in a familial syndrome of breast cancer, sarcomas and other neoplasms. *Science* **250**, 1233–8.

Markowitz, S., Wang, J., Myeroff, L. *et al.* (1995) Inactivation of the type II TGF-β receptor in colon cancer cells with microsatellite instability. *Science* **268**, 1336–8.

Marsh, E. (1993) Search for a killer: focus shifts from fat to hormones. *Science* **259**, 618–21.

Miki, Y., Swensen, J., Shattuck-Eidens, D. *et al.* (1994) Isolation of *BRCA*1, the 17q-linked breast and ovarian cancer susceptibility gene. *Science* **266**, 66–71.

Narod, S.A., Risch, H., Moslchi, R. *et al.* (1998) Oral contraceptives and the risk of hereditary ovarian cancer. Hereditary Ovarian Cancer Clinical Study Group. *N. Engl. J. Med.* **339**, 424–8.

Nicolaides, N.C., Papadopoulos, N., Liu, B. *et al.* (1994) Mutations of two *PMS* homologues in heriditary nonpolyposis colon cancer. *Nature* **371**, 75–80.

Nyam, D.C., Brillant, P.T., Dozois, R.R. *et al.* (1997) Ileal pouch-anal canal anastomosis for familial adenomatous polyposis: early and late results. *Ann. Surg.* **226**, 514–19.

Papadopoulos, N., Nicolaides, N.C., Liu, B. *et al.* (1995) Mutations of GTBP in genetically unstable cells. *Science* **268**, 1915–17.

Platz, E.A., Giovannucci, E., Dahl, D.M. *et al.* (1998) The androgen receptor gene GGN microsatellite and prostate cancer risk. *Cancer Epidemiol. Biomarkers Prev.* **7**, 379–84.

Ponder, B.A.J. and Smith, D. (1996) the MEN2 syndromes and the role of the ret proto-oncogene. *Adv. Cancer Res.* **70**, 179–222.

Powles, T., Eeles, R., Ashley, S. *et al.* (1998) Interim analysis of the incidence of breast cancer in the Royal Marsden Hospital tamoxifen randomised chemoprevention trial. *Lancet* **352**, 98–101.

Rebbeck, T.R., Levin, A.M., Eisen, A. *et al.* (1999) Breast cancer risk after bilateral prophylactic oophorectomy in *BRCA*1 mutation carriers. *J. Natl Cancer Inst.* **91**, 1475–9.

Struewing, J.P., Watson, P., Easton, D.F. *et al.* (1995) Prophylactic oophorectomy in inherited breast/ovarian cancer families. *J. Natl Cancer Inst. Monogr.* **17**, 33–5.

Struewing, J.P., Hartge, P., Wacholder, S. *et al.* (1997) The risk of cancer associated with specific mutations of *BRCA*1 and *BRCA*2 among Ashkenazi Jews. *N. Engl. J. Med.* **336**, 1401–8.

Thakker, R.V., Bouloux, P., Wooding, C. *et al.* (1989) Association of parathyroid tumours in multiple endocrine neoplasia type 1 with loss of alleles on chromosome 11. *N. Engl. J. Med.* **321**, 218–24.

Thorlacius, S., Sigurdsson, S., Bjarnadottir, H. *et al.* (1997) Study of a single *BRCA*2 mutation with high carrier frequency in a small population. *Am. J. Hum. Genet.* **60**, 1079–84.

Thorlacius, S., Struewing, J.P., Hartge, P. *et al.* (1998) Population based study of risk of breast cancer in carriers of *BRCA*2 mutations. *Lancet* **352**, 1337–9.

Tonin, P., Weber, B.L., Offit, K. *et al.* (1996) Frequency of recurrent *BRCA*1 and *BRCA*2 mutations in Ashkenazi Jewish breast cancer families. *Nat. Med.* **2**, 1179–83.

Ursin, G., Henderson, B.E., Haile, R.W. *et al.* (1997) Does oral contraceptive use increase the risk of breast cancer in women with *BRCA*1/*BRCA*2 mutations more than in other women? *Cancer Res.* **57**, 3678–81.

Veronesi, U., Maisonneuve, P., Costa, A. *et al.* (1998) Prevention of breast cancer with tamoxifen: preliminary findings from the Italian randomised trial among hysterectomised women. *Lancet* **352**, 93–7.

Vlek, C. (1987) Risk assessment, risk perception and decision making about courses of action involving genetic risk: an overview of concepts and methods. *Birth Defects* **23**, 171–207.

Wooster, R., Bignell, G., Lancaster, J. *et al.* (1995) Identification of the breast cancer susceptibility gene, *BRCA*2. *Nature* **378**, 789–92.

Xu, J., Meyers, D., Freije, D. *et al.* (1998) Evidence for a prostate cancer susceptibility locus on the x-chromosome. *Nat. Genet.* **20**, 175–9.

58

Large-scale randomized evidence: trials and overviews[1]

RICHARD GRAY, RORY COLLINS, RICHARD PETO AND KEITH WHEATLEY

INTRODUCTION AND SUMMARY

This chapter is intended principally for those who want to know why some types of evidence are much more reliable than others. It is concerned with treatments that might improve survival (or some other really major aspect of long-term disease outcome), and its chief point is that as long as doctors start with a healthy scepticism about the many apparently striking claims that appear in the medical literature, large-scale trials do make sense. The main enemy of common sense is overoptimism: there are a few striking exceptions of treatments for serious disease that really do turn out to work extremely well, but in general most of the claims of vast improvements from new therapies turn out to be evanescent. *Hence, clinical trials need to be able to detect or to refute really reliably the more moderate differences in long-term outcome that it is medically realistic to expect.* Once this common-sense idea is explicitly recognized, the rest follows naturally, and it becomes fairly obvious what types of evidence can and cannot be trusted. Although this chapter may also be of some interest or encouragement to doctors who are considering participating in (or even planning) some large trial, its main intended audience is the practising clinician. For, even the most definite results from large-scale randomized evidence cannot save lives unless practising clinicians accept and apply them. The chapter does not go into a lot of statistical details: instead, it tries to communicate the spirit that underlies the increasing emphasis over the past decade or so on large-scale randomized evidence.

Unrealistic hopes about the chances of discovering big treatment effects can be a serious obstacle, not only to appropriate patient care but also to good clinical research. For, such hopes may misleadingly suggest to some research workers or funding agencies that small, or even non-randomized, studies may suffice. In contrast, realistically moderate expectations of what treatment might achieve (or, if one treatment is to be compared with another, realistically moderate expectations of how large any difference between those treatments is likely to be) should, in contrast, tend to foster the design of studies that aim to discriminate reliably between (1) differences in outcome that are realistically *moderate but still worthwhile*, and (2) differences in outcome that are *too small to be of any material importance* (Yusuf *et al.*, 1984). Studies with this particular aim must guarantee

[1] Adapted from Collins, R., Peto, R., Gray, R. and Parish, S. (1996) Large-scale randomised evidence: trials and overviews. In Weatherall, D., Ledingham, J.G.G. and Warrell, D.A. (eds), *Oxford Textbook of Medicine*, Vol. 1. Oxford: Oxford University Press.

strict control of bias (which, in general, requires proper randomization and appropriate statistical analysis, with no unduly 'data-dependent' emphasis on specific parts of the overall evidence), and must guarantee strict control of the play of chance (which, in general, requires large numbers rather than a lot of detail). The conclusion is obvious: moderate biases and moderate random errors must both be avoided if moderate benefits are to be assessed or refuted reliably. This leads to the need for large numbers of properly randomized patients, which in turn leads both to large simple randomized trials (or 'mega-trials') and to large systematic overviews (or 'meta-analyses') of related randomized trials (Collins et al., 1987).

Non-randomized evidence, unduly small randomized trials or unduly small overviews of trials are all much inferior as sources of evidence about current patient management or as foundations for future research strategies. For they cannot discriminate reliably between moderate (but worthwhile) differences and negligible differences in outcome, and the mistaken clinical conclusions that they engender could well result in the worldwide under-treatment, overtreatment or other mismanagement of millions of future patients. In contrast, hundreds of thousands of premature deaths a year could be avoided by seeking appropriately large-scale randomized evidence about various widely practicable treatments for the common causes of death, and by disseminating such evidence appropriately. Likewise, appropriately large-scale randomized evidence could substantially improve the management of many important, but non-fatal, medical problems.

The value of large-scale randomized evidence is illustrated in this chapter by the trials of fibrinolytic therapy for acute myocardial infarction, of antiplatelet therapy for a wide range of vascular conditions, and of hormonal therapy for early breast cancer. In these examples, proof of benefit that could not have been achieved either by small-scale randomized evidence or by non-randomized evidence has led to widespread changes in practice that are now preventing tens of thousands of premature deaths each year.

Moderate (but worthwhile) effects on major outcomes are generally more plausible than large effects

Some treatments do have large, and hence obvious, effects on survival – for example, it is clear without randomized trials that insulin treatment of diabetic coma or surgery for breast and colorectal cancer saves lives. But, perhaps in part due to these striking successes, in the past few decades the hopes of large treatment effects on mortality and major morbidity in other serious diseases have been unrealistically high. Of course, treatments do quite commonly have large effects on various less fundamental

measures: for example, many tumours can be shrunk temporarily by radiotherapy or chemotherapy; giving 5-fluorouracil by continuous infusion rather than bolus, or in combination with folinic acid, can double the number of responding patients; in acute myocardial infarction, tissue plasminogen activator dissolves coronary thrombi more rapidly than streptokinase; drugs readily reduce blood pressure, blood lipids and blood glucose. But, although all of these effects are large, any effects on mortality are much more modest – indeed, there is still dispute as to whether any net improvement in survival results from any of these interventions.

In general, if substantial uncertainty remains about the efficacy of a practicable treatment, its effects on major end points are probably either negligibly small, or only moderate, rather than large. Indirect support for this rather pessimistic conclusion comes from many sources, including:

1 the previous few decades of disappointingly slow progress in the curative treatment of cancer and the common chronic diseases of middle age;
2 the heterogeneity of each single disease, as evidenced by the unpredictability of survival duration even when apparently similar patients are compared with each other;
3 the variety of different mechanisms in certain diseases that can lead to death, only one of which may be appreciably influenced by any one particular therapy; and
4 the modest effects often suggested by systematic overviews (or 'meta-analyses'; see later) of various therapies.

Having accepted that, with many currently available interventions, only *moderate* reductions in mortality are plausible, how worthwhile might such effects be, if they could be detected reliably? To some clinicians, reducing the risk of death from breast cancer from 50 per 100 women down to 45 per 100 women treated may not seem particularly worthwhile – and, indeed, if such a reduction was only transient, or involved an extremely expensive or toxic treatment, this might well be an appropriate view. Worldwide, however, 800 000 women a year are diagnosed with breast cancer, and if just half of these women were to be given a simple, non-toxic, widely practicable treatment that reduced the risk of death from 50 per cent down to 45 per cent (i.e. a 10 per cent proportional reduction), then this would avoid 10 000 or 20 000 deaths. For example, more than two million women worldwide are currently taking tamoxifen as adjuvant therapy of breast cancer, and this must be avoiding tens of thousands of deaths each year (see below). Such absolute gains are substantial – and might, indeed, considerably exceed the numbers of lives that could be saved by a much more effective treatment for a less common disease.

Table 58.1 *Requirements for reliable assessment of MODERATE effects: negligible biases and small random errors*

Negligible biases (i.e. guaranteed avoidance of MODERATE biases)

Proper RANDOMIZATION (non-randomized methods might suffer moderate biases)

Analysis by ALLOCATED treatment (including all randomized patients: 'intention-to-treat' analysis)

Chief emphasis on OVERALL results (no unduly data-dependent emphasis on particular subgroups)

Systematic OVERVIEW of all relevant randomized trials (no unduly data-dependent emphasis on particular studies)

Small random errors (i.e. guaranteed avoidance of MODERATE random errors)

LARGE NUMBERS in any new trials (to be really large, trials should be 'streamlined')

Systematic OVERVIEWS of all relevant randomized trials (which yields the largest possible total numbers)

Reliable detection or refutation of moderate differences requires avoidance of BOTH moderate biases and moderate random errors

If realistically moderate differences in outcome are to be reliably detected or reliably refuted, then the errors in comparative assessments of the effects of treatment need to be much smaller than the difference between a moderate but worthwhile effect on the one hand, and, on the other, an effect that is too small to be of any material importance. This, in turn, implies that moderate biases cannot be tolerated, and that moderate random errors cannot be tolerated. The only way to guarantee very small random errors is to study really large numbers, and this can be achieved in two main ways: make individual studies large, and combine information from as many relevant studies as possible in systematic overviews (Table 58.1). But, it is not much use having very small random errors if there may well be moderate biases, so even the large sizes of some non-randomized analyses of computerized hospital records cannot guarantee medically reliable comparisons between the effects of different treatments.

AVOIDING MODERATE BIASES

Proper randomization avoids systematic differences between the types of patient in different treatment groups

The fundamental reason for randomization is to make possible the avoidance of moderate biases by ensuring that each type of patient can be expected to have been allocated in similar proportions to the different treatment strategies that are to be compared, so that only random differences should affect the final comparisons of outcome. Non-randomized methods, by contrast, cannot in general guarantee that the types of patient given the study treatment do not differ systematically in any important ways from the types of patient given other treatment(s) with which the study treatment is to be compared. For example, moderate biases might arise if the study treatment was novel and doctors were afraid to use it for the most seriously ill patients – or, conversely, if they were more ready to try it out on those who were desperately ill. There may also be other ways in which the severity of the condition differentially affects the likelihood of being assigned to different treatments by the doctor's choice (or by any other non-random procedure).

It might at first sight appear that by collecting enough information about various prognostic features it would be possible to make some mathematical adjustments that would correct for any such differences between the types of patients who, in a non-randomized study, actually get given the different treatments that are to be compared. The hope is that such methods (which are sometimes called 'outcomes analyses') might achieve comparability between those entering the different treatment groups, but in general they cannot be guaranteed to do so. For some important prognostic factors may be unrecorded, while some other prognostic features may be difficult to assess exactly, and hence difficult to adjust for properly. There are two reasons for this difficulty. First, it is often not realized that, even if there are no systematic differences between one treatment group and another in the accuracy with which prognostic factors are recorded, purely random errors in assessing prognostic factors can introduce systematic biases into the statistically adjusted comparison between treatments in a non-randomized study. Second, in a non-randomized comparison the care with which prognostic factors are recorded may differ between one treatment group and another. Doctors studying a novel treatment may investigate their patients particularly carefully, and, perhaps surprisingly, this extra accuracy can introduce a moderate bias. For example, an unusually careful search of the axilla among women with early breast cancer will sometimes result in the discovery of tiny deposits of cancer cells that would normally have been overlooked, and hence some women who would have been classified as 'stage I' will be reclassified as 'stage II'. The prognosis of these 'down-staged' women is worse than that of those who remain as stage I, but better than that of those already classified as stage II by less intensive investigation. Paradoxically, therefore, such down-staging not only improves the average prognosis of 'stage I' breast cancer but also improves the average prognosis of 'stage II' breast cancer, biasing any non-randomized comparison with other women with stage I or stage II disease for whom the staging was less careful.

The machinery of a properly randomized trial: no foreknowledge of treatment allocation, no bias in patient management, unbiased outcome assessment and no post-randomization exclusions

NO FOREKNOWLEDGE OF WHAT THE NEXT TREATMENT WILL BE

In a properly randomized trial, the decision to enter a patient is made irreversibly, in ignorance of which of the trial treatments that patient will be allocated. The treatment allocation is made after trial entry has been decided upon. (The purpose of this sequence is to ensure that foreknowledge of what the next treatment is going to be cannot affect the decision to enter the patient: if it did, then those allocated one treatment might differ systematically from those allocated another.) Ideally, any major prognostic features should also be irreversibly recorded before the treatment is revealed, especially if these are to be used in any analyses of treatment. For, if the recorded value of some prognostic factor might be affected by knowledge of the trial treatment allocation, then treatment comparisons within subgroups that are defined by that factor might be moderately biased. In particular, treatment comparisons just among 'responders' or just among 'non-responders' can be extremely misleading, unless the response is assessed before treatment allocation.

NO BIAS IN PATIENT MANAGEMENT OR IN OUTCOME ASSESSMENT

An additional difficulty, both in randomized and in non-randomized comparisons of various treatments, is that there might be systematic differences in the use of other treatments (including general supportive care), or in the assessment of major outcomes. A non-randomized comparison, especially if it merely involves retrospective review of medical records, may well suffer uncorrectably from moderate biases due to such systematic differences in ancillary care or assessment. In the context of a randomized comparison, however, it is generally possible to devise ways to keep any such biases small. For example, placebo tablets may be given to control-allocated patients and certain subjective assessments may be 'blinded' (although this is less important in studies assessing mortality).

'INTENTION-TO-TREAT' ANALYSES WITH NO POST-RANDOMIZATION EXCLUSIONS

Even in a properly randomized trial, unnecessary biases could be introduced by inappropriate statistical analysis. One of the most important sources of bias in the analysis is undue concentration on just one part of the evidence (i.e. on 'data-derived subgroup analyses': *see* below) instead of on the totality of the evidence. Another bias, which is easily avoided, is caused by post-randomization

exclusion of patients, especially if the type (and prognosis) of those excluded from one treatment group differs from that of those excluded from another. The fundamental statistical analysis of a trial should, therefore, generally compare all those originally allocated one treatment (even though some of them may not have actually received it) with all those allocated the other treatment (i.e. it should be an 'intention-to-treat' analysis). Additional analyses can also be reported: for example, in describing the frequency of some very specific side-effect it may be preferable to describe its incidence only among those who actually received the treatment. (This is because strictly randomized comparisons may not be needed to assess extreme relative risks.) But, in assessing the overall outcome, such 'on-treatment' analyses can be misleading, and 'intention-to-treat' analyses are generally a more trustworthy guide as to whether there is any real difference between the trial treatments in their effects on long-term outcome (for further discussion, *see* Peto *et al.*, 1976, 1977, Section 13).

Problems produced by unduly data-dependent emphasis on particular results

The treatment that is appropriate for one patient may be inappropriate for another. Ideally, therefore, what is wanted is not only an answer to the question 'Is this treatment helpful on average for a wide range of patients?', but also an answer to the question 'For which recognizable categories of patient is this treatment helpful?'. This ideal is, however, difficult to attain directly because the direct use of clinical trial results in particular subgroups of patients is surprisingly unreliable. Even if the real sizes of the effects of treatment in specific subgroups are importantly different, standard subgroup analyses are so statistically insensitive that they may well fail to demonstrate these differences. Conversely, even if there is a highly significant 'interaction' (i.e. an apparent difference between the *sizes* of the therapeutic effects in different subgroups) and the results seem to suggest that treatment works in some subgroups but not in others (thereby giving the appearance of a 'qualitative interaction'), this may still not be good evidence for subgroup-specific treatment preferences.

Questions about such 'interactions' between patient characteristics and the effects of treatment are easy to ask, but surprisingly difficult to answer reliably. Apparent interactions can often be produced just by the play of chance and, in particular subgroups, can mimic or obscure some of the moderate treatment effects that might realistically be expected. To demonstrate this, a subgroup analysis was performed based on the astrological birth signs of patients randomized in the very large ISIS-2 trial of the treatment of acute myocardial infarction (ISIS-2 Collaborative Group, 1988). Overall in this trial, the one-month

Table 58.2 *False negative mortality effect in a subgroup defined only by the astrological 'birth sign': the ISIS-2 trial of aspirin among over 17 000 acute myocardial infarction patients*

Astrological 'birth sign'	No. of 1-month deaths (aspirin versus placebo)	Statistical significance
Libra or Gemini	150 versus 147	NS
All other signs	654 versus 869	$2P < 0.000001$
Any birth sign[a]	804 (9.4%) versus 1016 (11.8%)	$2P < 0.000001$

[a] Appropriate overall analysis for assessing the true effect in all subgroups.

survival advantage produced by aspirin was particularly clearly demonstrated (804 vascular deaths among 8587 patients allocated aspirin versus 1016 among 8600 allocated control; 23 per cent reduction; $P < 0.000001$). But, when these aspirin analyses were subdivided by the patients' astrological 'birth signs', to illustrate the unreliability of subgroup analyses, aspirin appeared to be totally ineffective for those born under Libra or Gemini (Table 58.2). It would obviously be unwise to conclude from such a result that patients born under the sign of Libra or Gemini should not be given this particular treatment. Yet, similar conclusions based on 'exploratory' data-derived subgroup analyses that, from a purely statistical viewpoint, are no more reliable than these, are often reported and believed, with inappropriate effects on practice.

There are three main remedies for this unavoidable conflict between the reliable subgroup-specific conclusions that doctors want and the unreliable findings that direct subgroup analyses can usually offer. But, the extent to which these remedies are helpful in particular instances is one on which informed judgements differ.

First, where there are good a priori reasons for anticipating that the effect of treatment might be different in different circumstances, then a limited number of subgroup analyses may be pre-specified in the study protocol, along with a prediction of the direction of such proposed interactions. For example, it was expected that the benefits of tamoxifen would be greater for women with hormone-sensitive (oestrogen-receptor positive) breast tumours; and that the benefits of fibrinolytic therapy for acute myocardial infarction would be greater the earlier patients were treated (and so some studies pre-specified analyses subdivided by time from onset of symptoms to treatment: see later). These pre-specified subgroup-specific analyses are then to be taken much more seriously than other subgroup analyses.

The second approach is to emphasize chiefly the overall results of a trial (or, better still, of all such trials) for particular outcomes as a guide – or at least a context for speculation – as to the qualitative results in various specific subgroups of patients, and to give less weight to the actual results in each separate subgroup. This is clearly the right way to interpret the findings in Table 58.2, but it is also likely in many other circumstances to provide the best assessment of whether one treatment is better than the other in particular subgroups. Of course, the extrapolation needs to be done in a medically sensible way. For example, if one treatment has substantial side-effects then it may be inappropriate for low-risk patients. (In this case, the side-effects in a particular subgroup and the proportional benefit in that subgroup should be estimated separately, but the estimation for both might be more reliable if based on an appropriate extrapolation from the overall results rather than on the results in that one subgroup alone.)

The third approach is to be influenced, in discussing the likely effects on mortality in specific subgroups, not only by the mortality analyses in these subgroups but also by the analyses of recurrence-free interval or some other major 'surrogate' outcome. For, if the overall results are similar but much more highly significant for recurrence-free interval than for mortality, subgroup analyses with respect to the former may be more stable and may provide a better guide as to whether there are any big differences between subgroups in the effects of treatment (particularly if such subgroup analyses were specified before results were available).

AVOIDING MODERATE RANDOM ERRORS

The need for large-scale randomization

To distinguish reliably between the two alternatives either that there is no worthwhile difference in survival, or that treatment confers a moderate, but worthwhile, benefit (e.g. 10 or 20 per cent fewer deaths), not only must systematic errors be guaranteed to be small (*see* above) compared with such a moderate risk reduction, but so too must any of the purely random errors that are produced just by chance. Random errors can be reliably avoided only by studying large enough numbers of patients. It is not, however, sufficiently widely appreciated just how large clinical trials really need to be, in order to detect moderate differences reliably. This can be illustrated by a hypothetical trial that is actually quite inadequate – even though by previous standards it is moderately large – in which a 20 per cent reduction in mortality (from 50 per cent down to 40 per cent) is supposed to be detected among 400 cancer patients (200 treated and 200 controls). In this case, one might predict finding about 100 deaths (50 per cent) in the control group and 80 (40 per cent) in the treated group. Even if exactly this difference were to be observed, however, it would not be conventionally significant (P-value = 0.1; indicating that even if there is no real difference between the effects of the trial treatments, it would still be relatively easy for a result at least as extreme as this to arise by chance alone). Although the play of chance might well increase the difference enough to make it conventionally significant (e.g. to 110 deaths versus 70 deaths; $P < 0.001$), it might equally well dilute, obliterate (e.g. to 90 deaths versus 90 deaths) or even reverse it. The situation in real life is often even worse, as the average trial size may be only several dozen patients, rather than the several thousand that would ideally be needed.

Mega-trials: how to randomize large numbers

One of the chief techniques for obtaining appropriately large-scale randomized evidence is to make trials extremely simple, and then to invite hundreds of hospitals to collaborate. The first of these large simple trials (or 'mega-trials') were the ISIS and GISSI studies (GISSI, 1986; ISIS-2 Collaborative Group, 1988) in heart attack treatment, and a few mega-trials have now been undertaken in cancer, such as the QUASAR ('Quick And Simple And Reliable') study of colorectal cancer chemotherapy (QUASAR Collaborative Group, 2000). But, in terms of medically significant findings, what has been achieved so far is only a fraction of what could quite readily be achieved by the wholehearted pursuit of such research strategies. Any obstacle to simplicity is an obstacle to large size, so it is worth making enormous efforts at the design stage to simplify and streamline the process of entering, treating and assessing patients. Many trials would be of much greater scientific value if they collected 10 times less data, both at entry and during follow-up, on 10 times more patients. It is particularly necessary to simplify the entry of patients, for if this is not done then rapid recruitment may be difficult. The current fashions for unduly complicated eligibility criteria, overly detailed 'informed' consent, extensive auditing of data, and excessive quality-of-life assessments and measurements of the economic costs of treatment are often inappropriate (Yusuf *et al.*, 1984; Collins *et al.*, 1992).

Simplification of economic and 'quality-of-life' assessments

Often, the effectiveness of various treatments needs to be balanced against the costs, but that does not necessarily imply that costs should be assessed in the same studies in which effectiveness is to be assessed, especially if attempts to assess costs seriously damage attempts to assess the effects on mortality and major morbidity sufficiently reliably. Moreover, what really matters is the cost of a treatment in routine practice, not its cost when given in the particular circumstances of a randomized trial. For this reason, it is better to measure differences in resource usage between treatments rather than differences in costs.

Likewise, of course, any important ways in which treatments affect the quality of life need to be understood, but again that does not necessarily imply that 'quality-of-life' indices should be assessed in the same trials that assess the main effects of treatment. In particular, although several thousand patients may be required for reliable assessment of the effects of treatment on mortality and major morbidity, only a few hundred are likely to be needed for sufficiently reliable assessment of the effects of treatment on quality-of-life measures (or on costs of treatment). Because of these different sample size requirements, if such assessments are to be incorporated within a large mortality study, then they can be included as small sub-studies. Also, as for clinical outcome data, the work involved in collecting economic and quality-of-life data should be kept to a minimum so recruitment is not compromised. But, even this may be difficult in practice, and there are many instances where what should be a large, simple trial of clinical efficacy should not be jeopardized by the measurement of such factors. Moreover, the effects of a treatment on quality of life in a trial when both the doctors and the patients are uncertain about any clinical benefits of the treatment may differ substantially from its effects on quality of life after the treatment has been shown to improve survival. Hence, it may be better to assess these other outcome measures only after having determined whether the treatment has any worthwhile effects on mortality and major morbidity, and if (as is often the case) it does not, then any costs and adverse effects on quality of life may be largely irrelevant.

Simplification of entry procedures for trials: the 'uncertainty principle'

For ethical reasons, patients cannot have their treatment chosen at random if either they or their doctor are already reasonably certain what treatment to prefer. Hence, randomization can be offered only if both doctor and patient feel substantially uncertain as to which of the trial treatments is best. The question then arises: of those about whose treatment there is such uncertainty, which categories should be offered randomization? The obvious answer is all of them, welcoming the heterogeneity that this will produce. (For example, either the treatment of choice will turn out to be the same for men and women, in which case the trial might as well include both, or it will be different, in which case it is particularly important to study both sexes.)

This approach of randomizing a wide range of patients in whom there is substantial uncertainty as to which treatment option is best was used in the MRC's European Carotid Surgery Trial (ECST), which compared a policy of immediate carotid endarterectomy versus a policy of 'watchful waiting' in patients with partial carotid artery stenosis and a recent minor stroke in the part of the brain supplied by that carotid artery (European Carotid Surgery Trialists' Collaborative Group, 1991). If a patient was prepared at least to consider surgery then the neurologist and surgeon responsible for that individual patient's care considered in their own way whatever medical, personal or other factors seemed to them to be relevant (Fig. 58.1), including, of course, the patient's own preferences and values:

1 If they were then reasonably certain, for any reasons, that they did wish to recommend immediate surgery for that particular individual, then the patient was ineligible and was not part of the ECST.
2 Conversely, if they were reasonably certain, for any reason, that they did not wish to recommend immediate surgery, then that patient was likewise ineligible.

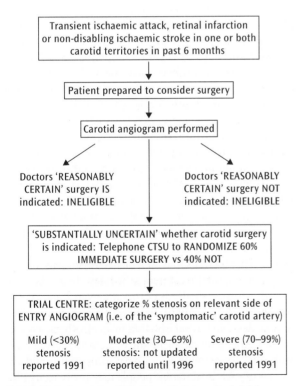

Figure 58.1 *Example of the 'uncertainty principle' for trial entry: the chief eligibility criterion for the European Carotid Surgery Trial (ECST) was that the doctors and patient should be substantially uncertain whether to risk immediate or deferred surgery. (Partly because this criterion was appropriately flexible, ECST became the largest ever trial of vascular surgery.)*

3 If, but only if, they were substantially uncertain what to recommend, then that individual patient was automatically eligible for randomization between immediate versus no immediate surgery (with all patients receiving whatever their doctors judged to be the best available medical care – which generally included advice to stop smoking, treatment of any hypertension, and the use of aspirin as an antithrombotic drug).

There were substantial differences between individual doctors in the types of patients they were uncertain about (in terms of the severity of carotid stenosis, as well as in various other characteristics). This guaranteed that no category – mild, moderate or severe stenosis – would be wholly excluded, and hence that the trial would yield at least some direct evidence in each. As a result of the wide and simple entry criteria adopted by ECST, 3000 patients were randomized and the study was therefore able to provide some clear answers about who needed carotid endarterectomy. For patients with only mild (0–29 per cent) carotid artery stenosis on their pre-randomization angiogram, there was little risk of ipsilateral ischaemic stroke, even in the absence of surgery, so the benefits of surgery over the next few years were small and outweighed by its early risks. Conversely, for patients with severe (70–99 per cent) stenosis, the risks of surgery were significantly outweighed by its later benefits over the next few years. For both of these categories the trial stopped early, but for the intermediate category of patients with moderate (30–69 per cent) stenosis, the balance of surgical risk and eventual benefit remained uncertain, so recruitment into the study continued, with entry still governed by the 'uncertainty principle' as before (European Carotid Surgery Trialists' Collaborative Group, 1996).

In large trials, homogeneity of patients is generally a defect, while heterogeneity is generally a strength. Consider, for example, the trials of fibrinolytic therapy for acute myocardial infarction: if the coronary artery has been occluded for long enough, then the heart muscle that it supplies will have been irreversibly destroyed: how late after the heart attack starts is fibrinolytic treatment still worth risking – 3 hours? 6 hours? 12 hours? 24 hours? Before the large trials of fibrinolysis, it was forcefully, but mistakenly, argued that such treatments could not possibly be of any worthwhile benefit if given more than a few hours after the onset of symptoms. Consequently, some trials had restrictive entry criteria that allowed inclusion of only those patients who presented 0–6 hours after pain onset, so those trials contributed almost nothing to the key question of how late such treatment can still be useful. In contrast, trials with wider, more heterogeneous entry criteria that included some patients with longer delays between pain onset and randomization assessed this question prospectively, and were able to show that fibrinolytic therapy can have definite protective effects when given not only 0–6 but also

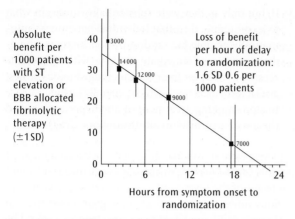

Figure 58.2 *Benefit versus delay (0–1, 2–3, 4–6, 7–12, or 13–24 hours) in the nine largest randomized trials of fibrinolytic therapy versus control in patients with acute myocardial infarction. One-month mortality results for 45 000 patients with ST elevation or bundle branch block (BBB) when randomized, showing the definite net benefit even for the 9000 randomized 7–12 hours after the onset of pain. (Fibrinolytic Therapy Trialists' Collaboration, 1994.)*

7–12 hours after pain onset (Fibrinolytic Therapy Trialists' Collaborative Group, 1991) (*see* below).

The longer that fibrinolytic treatment for such patients was delayed, however, the less benefit it seemed to produce. The benefit was greatest (about 30 lives saved per 1000) among those randomized 0–6 hours after the onset of pain (Fig. 58.2). But, the mortality reduction was still substantial and significant (about 20 per 1000, $2P < 0.003$) when such patients were randomized 7–12 hours after pain onset. Indeed, if they were randomized 13–18 hours after pain onset there still appeared to be some net reduction in mortality (about 10 per 1000, but not statistically definite). The regression line in Figure 58.2 reinforces, in a more reliable way, these separate subgroup analyses.

The 'uncertainty principle' meets simultaneously the requirements of ethicality, heterogeneity, simplicity and maximal trial size. It states that the fundamental eligibility criterion is that both patient and doctor should be substantially uncertain about the appropriateness for this particular patient of each of the trial treatments. With such uncertainty as the fundamental principle of eligibility, informed consent can also be simplified. For, the degree of 'informed consent' that is humanly appropriate in a randomized comparison of different treatments that is governed by the 'uncertainty principle' should probably not differ greatly from that which is humanly appropriate in routine practice outside of trials, where treatment is being chosen haphazardly – or, to put it another way, 'double standards' between trial and non-trial situations are not appropriate. The haphazard nature of many non-randomized treatment choices is reflected in the wide variations in practice between and within countries (and, even when practice is similar,

it may be similarly wrong: for example, before the ISIS-2 results became available [see later], almost all doctors around the world were not using fibrinolytic therapy for acute myocardial infarction). Provided that trials are governed by the 'uncertainty principle', there is an approximate parallelism between good science and good ethics. Indeed, in such circumstances, excessively detailed consent procedures (which can be distressing and inhumane, and so would not be considered appropriate in routine practice) would not be either scientifically or ethically appropriate (for further discussion, *see* Collins *et al.*, 1992).

This 'uncertainty principle' is just one of many ways to simplify trials, and thereby help them to avoid becoming enmeshed in a mass of wholly unnecessary traditional complexity. If randomized trials can be vastly simplified, as has already been achieved in a few major diseases, and thereby made vastly larger, then they will play an appropriately central role in the development of rational criteria for the planning of healthcare throughout the world.

MINIMIZING BOTH BIAS AND RANDOM ERROR: SYSTEMATIC OVERVIEWS ('META-ANALYSES') OF RANDOMIZED TRIALS

When several trials have all addressed much the same therapeutic question, then the traditional procedure of choosing only a few of them for emphasis and fame may be a source of serious bias, since chance fluctuations for or against treatment may affect which trials become famous. To avoid this, it is appropriate to base inference chiefly on a systematic overview (or 'meta-analysis') of all the results from all the trials that have addressed a particular type of question (or on an unbiased subset of such trials), and not on some potentially biased subset of the trials (Collins *et al.*, 1987; Chalmers, 1994). Such overviews will also minimize random errors in the assessment of treatment, since, in general, far more patients are involved in an overview than in any individual trial that contributes to it.

The separate trials may well be heterogeneous in their entry criteria, their treatment schedules, their follow-up procedures, their methods of treating relapse, etc. At one extreme, each trial might, in view of this heterogeneity, be considered in virtual isolation from all others, while at the opposite extreme all might be considered together. Both of these extreme views have some merit, and the pursuit of each by different people may prove more illuminating than too definite an insistence on any one particular approach. The heterogeneity of the different trials, however, merely argues for careful interpretation of any overviews of different trial results, rather than arguing against any such overviews. For, whatever the difficulties of interpretation of overviews may be, without systematic overviews moderate biases and random errors that may obscure any moderate treatment effects (or, conversely, may imply effects where none exists) cannot reliably be avoided.

Which overviews are trustworthy?

Over the past decade or two, a large (and rapidly increasing) number of meta-analyses of randomized trial results have been reported, not all of which are trustworthy. The two fundamental questions are how carefully the meta-analysis has been done, and how large it is. The simplest approach is merely to have collected and tabulated the published data from whatever randomized trial reports can be found easily in the literature, and sometimes this may suffice. At the opposite extreme, extensive efforts may have been made by those organizing the overview to locate every potentially relevant randomized trial, to collaborate closely with the trialists to seek individual data on each patient ever randomized into those trials, and then (after extensive checks and corrections of such data) to produce, in collaboration with those trialists, agreed analyses and publications. The results of some of the largest such collaborations will be described later: the Antiplatelet Trialists' (APT) Collaborative Group (1994), the Fibrinolytic Trialists' (FTT) Collaborative Group (1994), the Early Breast Cancer Trialists' Collaborative Group (EBCTCG) (1992) and the Colorectal Cancer Collaborative Group (2001). Collaboration of the original trialists in the overview process, with collection of individual patient data, can help to avoid or minimize the biases that could be produced by missing trials (e.g. due to the greater likelihood of extremely good, or extremely bad, results being particularly widely known about and published), by inappropriate post-randomization withdrawals or by failure to allocate treatment properly at random. If randomization was done properly in the first place, then post-randomization withdrawals can often be followed up and restored to the study for an appropriate 'intention-to-treat' analysis. Knowledge of the exact methods of treatment allocation (backed up by checks on whether the main prognostic factors recorded are non-randomly distributed between the treatment groups in a particular trial) may help to identify trials that were not, in fact, properly randomized, and that should therefore be excluded from an overview of randomized trials. Overviews based on individual patient data may also provide more information about treatment effects than the more usual overviews of grouped data, for they allow more detailed analyses – indeed, if they are really large then they may actually yield statistically reliable subgroup analyses of the effects of treatment in particular types of patient.

Conversely, however, even a perfectly conducted overview may not be large enough to be reliable. An overview that brings together complete data from all the trials that have ever been done of a certain treatment but still (because the trials were all small) includes a total of only 100 deaths will have random errors that are no smaller than those for a single trial with 100 deaths among such patients. Small-scale evidence, whether from an overview or from one trial, is often unreliable, and will often be found in retrospect to have yielded wrong answers. What is needed is large-scale randomized evidence; it does not matter much whether that evidence comes from a properly conducted overview or a properly conducted trial. The practical medical value of such evidence will now be illustrated by a few recent examples.

SOME EXAMPLES OF IMPORTANT RESULTS IN THE TREATMENT OF VASCULAR AND OF NEOPLASTIC DISEASE THAT COULD HAVE BEEN RELIABLY ESTABLISHED ONLY BY LARGE-SCALE RANDOMIZED EVIDENCE

Definite result from a single very large trial: benefit from medium-dose aspirin for patients with suspected acute myocardial infarction (and benefits among other groups of patients indicated by overviews of trials)

In the ISIS-2 trial, half of 17 000 patients with suspected acute myocardial infarction were allocated aspirin tablets (162 mg/day for 1 month, which virtually completely inhibits cyclo-oxygenase-dependent platelet inhibition), and half were allocated placebo (i.e. dummy) tablets (ISIS-2 Collaborative Group, 1988). Before 1988, when the ISIS-2 results were published, aspirin was not routinely used in acute myocardial infarction, and no other major trial had (or has subsequently) assessed aspirin in suspected acute myocardial infarction. But, the effects of 1 month of aspirin were so definite in ISIS-2 (804/8587 vascular deaths among those allocated aspirin versus 1016/8600 among those not) that even the lower 99 per cent confidence limit would have represented a worthwhile benefit from so simple and inexpensive a treatment (Fig. 58.3).

As a result, worldwide treatment patterns changed sharply when the ISIS-2 results emerged, and aspirin is now routinely used in many different countries for the majority of emergency hospital admissions with suspected acute myocardial infarction. In the UK, for example, two British Heart Foundation surveys found cardiologists reporting that routine aspirin use in acute coronary care had increased from under 10 per cent in 1987 to over 90 per cent in 1989 (Collins and Julian, 1991). Worldwide, the annual number of patients with suspected myocardial infarction who would nowadays be given such treatment must be well over a million a year, suggesting that in this clinical context alone aspirin is already preventing tens of thousands of premature deaths each year.

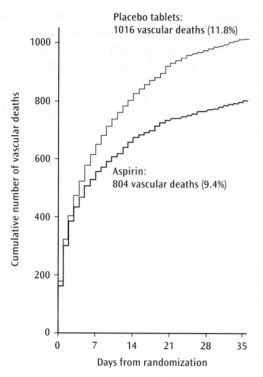

Figure 58.3 *Effect of administration of aspirin for 1 month on 35-day mortality in the ISIS-2 trial among over 17 000 acute myocardial infarction patients. (Absolute survival advantage: 24 [SD 5] lives saved per 1000 allocated aspirin; 2P < 0.00001.)*

But, if the ISIS-2 trial had been 10 times smaller (i.e. 1700 instead of 17 000 patients), then exactly the same proportional reduction in mortality as in Figure 58.3 would not have been conventionally significant, and therefore would have been much less likely to influence medical practice – indeed, the result might by chance have appeared exactly flat, greatly damaging future research on aspirin in this context. Likewise, if the ISIS-2 trial had been non-randomized, then it might well have got the wrong answer (since in a non-randomized study doctors might tend to give active treatment to patients who were particularly ill, or who were in various other ways somewhat different from those not given active treatment). And, even if a non-randomized study did happen to get an unbiasedly correct answer, it would be impossible to be sure that it had actually done so, and hence again a non-randomized study might have had much less influence on medical practice than did ISIS-2.

In the ISIS-2 trial, aspirin significantly reduced the 1-month mortality, but it also significantly reduced the number of non-fatal strokes and of non-fatal reinfarctions that were recorded in hospital. Combining all these three outcomes into 'vascular events' (stroke, death or reinfarction), 13 per cent of those allocated aspirin, and 17 per cent of those who were not, were known to have suffered a vascular event in the month after randomization (Table 58.3: an absolute difference of 40 events per

1000 treated – or, perhaps more relevantly, of 40 000 per million) (Antiplatelet Trialists' Collaboration, 1994). The randomized trials of aspirin, or of other antiplatelet regimens, in other types of high-risk patients (e.g. a few years of aspirin for those who have survived a myocardial infarction or stroke) have not been as large as ISIS-2, and so, taken separately, most have yielded false negative results. But, when the results from many such trials are combined, statistically definite reductions in 'vascular events' are seen (Table 58.3). Since such treatments do not appear to increase non-vascular mortality, all-cause mortality is also significantly reduced.

In principle these findings could, if appropriately widely exploited, prevent about 100 000 premature vascular deaths a year in developed countries alone, and there are probably at least as many vascular deaths in less-developed as in developed countries. So, with realistically achievable levels of use of 'medium-dose' aspirin (75–325 mg/day) for the secondary prevention of vascular disease, it might well be possible in practice to ensure that aspirin is used in enough high-risk patients to prevent, or substantially delay, at least 100 000 vascular deaths a year worldwide, and such use of aspirin would, in addition, prevent a comparable number of non-fatal strokes or heart attacks. (Medium-dose aspirin was the least expensive and most widely tested antiplatelet regimen: it is of proven efficacy and, on review of all the antiplatelet trials, no other antiplatelet regimen has been shown to be of greater efficacy in preventing vascular events: *see* notes to Table 58.3.) This large-scale randomized evidence about medium-dose aspirin is now changing worldwide clinical practice in ways that will, at low cost, prevent much death and disability in high-risk patients. But, small trials, small overviews or non-randomized studies (however large) could not possibly have provided appropriately reliable evidence about such moderate risk reductions.

Definite result from a very large overview of trials: benefit from 'adjuvant' hormonal therapy with tamoxifen for patients with 'early' breast cancer (and further benefits with ovarian ablation in younger women)

By definition, in 'early' breast cancer all detectable deposits of disease are limited to the breast and the loco-regional lymph nodes, and can be removed surgically. But, experience shows that undetectably small deposits may remain elsewhere that eventually, perhaps after a delay of several years, cause clinical recurrence at a distant site, which is then usually followed by death from the disease. These micrometastatic deposits may have been stimulated by the body's own hormones during the years before recurrence became detectable. So, among women who have had the detectable deposits of breast cancer removed by surgery (or by surgery with radiotherapy) there have

Table 58.3 *Summary of overall results in trials of aspirin (or other antiplatelet drugs)[a] for the prevention of vascular events: the Antiplatelet Trialists' Collaboration, involving a total of about 100 000 randomized patients in over 100 trials*

Type of patient studied	Average scheduled treatment duration (and approximate numbers of patients randomized)	Proportions who suffered a non-fatal stroke, non-fatal heart attack or vascular death during the trials		
		Antiplatelet (%)	Control (%)	Events avoided in these trials
High risk:				
Suspected acute heart attack	1 month (20 000)	10	14	40 per 1000 ($2P < 0.00001$)
Previous history of heart attack	2 years (20 000)	13	17	40 per 1000 ($2P < 0.00001$)
Previous history of stroke or TIA	3 years (10 000)	18	22	40 per 1000 ($2P < 0.00001$)
Other vascular disease[b]	1 year (20 000)	7	9	20 per 1000 ($2P < 0.00001$)
Low risk:				
Primary prevention in low-risk people	5 years (30 000)	4.4	4.8	4 per 1000 ($2P > 0.05$)

[a] The most widely tested regimen was medium-dose aspirin, involving an average daily dose of 75–325 mg, and no other antiplatelet regimen appeared to be significantly more or less effective than this at preventing such vascular events.

[b] For example, angina, peripheral vascular disease, arterial surgery or angioplasty, etc.

been many trials of 'adjuvant' treatments that either reduce the production of endogenous oestrogens (e.g. various forms of ovarian ablation), or that block the access of those oestrogens to the tumour cells (e.g. tamoxifen, which blocks the oestrogen receptor protein in some breast cancer cells).

Taken separately, most of these adjuvant trials have been too small to provide reliable evidence about long-term survival (Early Breast Cancer Trialists' Collaborative Group, 1992). But, if the results of all of them are combined, then some very definite differences in 10-year survival do emerge (Fig. 58.4). Among women with stage II disease who were less than 50 years old (and, therefore, generally pre- or peri-menopausal), ovarian ablation appears to produce about a 10 per cent absolute difference in 10-year survival (e.g. 50 per cent versus 40 per cent). This finding is based on the analysis of only a few hundred deaths, so it is still not as reliable as might ideally be wished, and, because substantial uncertainty remains, much larger trials are now in progress. Among older stage II women, ovarian ablation is unlikely to be of much relevance (since most of the endogenous oestrogen at older ages comes from sources other than the ovaries) but, in aggregate, the randomized trials among such women have shown very definitely that a few years of tamoxifen likewise produces about a 10 per cent absolute difference in 10-year survival. A smaller, but still highly significant, reduction in mortality by tamoxifen is also seen among the 10 000 randomized women with stage I disease. Taken separately, however, 37 of the 42 tamoxifen trials were too small to have yielded statistically reliable evidence on their own ($2P > 0.01$) – and, the five other trials were significant only because, by chance, they had results that were too good to be true.

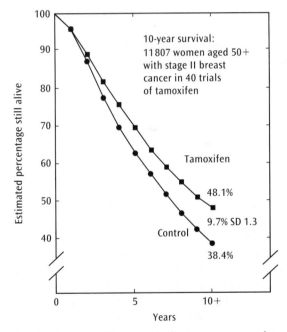

Figure 58.4 *Effects of hormonal adjuvant treatments for early breast cancer on 10-year survival in a worldwide overview of randomized trials. (Early Breast Cancer Trialists' Collaborative Group, 1992.)*

These tamoxifen overview results have already changed clinical practice substantially, and have re-directed research towards large randomized trials (e.g. ATLAS and aTTom) of the effects of different durations of tamoxifen: should tamoxifen in asymptomatic women continue for 2 years, for 5 years, or indefinitely? Large randomized studies of the primary prevention of breast cancer among high-risk women by tamoxifen have also been undertaken, encouraged by the results from the tamoxifen trials overview. In 30 000 women with established cancer (stage I or stage II) in one breast, there was a highly significant reduction of one-third in the likelihood of development of contralateral breast cancer, but a small absolute increase in endometrial cancer. Again, this degree of trustworthy detail would not have been attained without large-scale randomized evidence.

Factorial (2 × 2) trial designs: separate assessment of more than one treatment in the same trial

In ISIS-2, not only were patients randomly allocated to receive aspirin or placebo tablets (as described above: Fig. 58.3), but they were also separately allocated to receive intravenous streptokinase or a placebo infusion (ISIS-2 Collaborative Group, 1988). In this 'factorial' design (which allows the separate assessment of more than one treatment without any material loss in the statistical reliability of each comparison), one-quarter of patients were allocated aspirin alone, one-quarter were allocated streptokinase alone, one-quarter were allocated both streptokinase and aspirin, and one-quarter were allocated neither (i.e. placebo tablets and placebo infusion). Streptokinase, like aspirin, produced a highly significant reduction in mortality (and the combination of streptokinase and aspirin was highly significantly better than either aspirin or streptokinase alone: Fig. 58.5).

It might appear, from Figure 58.5, that there was no need for any more randomized evidence about fibrinolytic therapy, but this ignores the potential hazards of such treatment and the heterogeneity of patients. Taken separately, even ISIS-2, the largest of these trials, was not big enough for statistically reliable subgroup analyses, but when the nine largest trials were all taken together they included a total of about 60 000 patients, half of whom were randomly allocated fibrinolytic. Those entering a coronary care unit with a diagnosis of suspected or definite acute myocardial infarction range from patients who are already in cardiogenic shock, with low blood pressure and a fast pulse (half of whom will die rapidly) to those who have merely got a history of chest pain and no very definite changes on their ECG (of whom 'only' a small percentage will die before discharge). Fibrinolytic therapy often causes a frightening blood pressure drop: should it be used in patients who are already dangerously hypotensive? It occasionally causes serious strokes: should it be used in patients who are elderly or hypertensive, and therefore already have an above-average risk of stroke (or who have only slight changes on their ECG, and therefore have only a low risk of cardiac death)?

These questions needed to be answered reliably before appropriate and generally accepted indications for, and against, such an immediately hazardous but potentially effective therapy could be devised. To address them, all

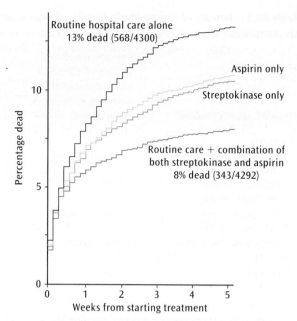

Figure 58.5 *Effects of one-hour streptokinase infusion (and of 1 month of aspirin) on 35-day mortality in ISIS-2 among 17 187 acute myocardial infarction patients who would not normally have received streptokinase or aspirin, divided at random into four similar groups to receive aspirin only, streptokinase only, both, or neither. (Any doctor who believed that a particular patient should be given either treatment gave it, and did not include that patient in ISIS-2.)*

fibrinolytic therapy trialists have collaborated in a systematic overview of the randomized evidence (Fibrinolytic Therapy Trialists' Collaborative Group, 1994). On review of the 60 000 patients randomized between fibrinolytic therapy and control in trials of more than 1000 patients, some of the therapeutic questions were relatively easy to answer satisfactorily. For example, it appeared that most of those whose ECG was still fairly normal (or showed some other pattern that indicated only a low risk of death) might as well be left untreated, leaving open the option of starting fibrinolytic treatment urgently if their ECG changes suddenly for the worse in the following few hours. Conversely, among those who already had 'high-risk' ECG changes when they were randomized, the absolute benefit of immediate fibrinolytic therapy was, if anything, slightly greater than is indicated by Figure 58.5, and age, sex, blood pressure, heart rate, diabetes and previous history of myocardial infarction could not identify reliably any group that would not, on average, have their chances of survival appreciably increased by treatment.

Such detailed inferences are difficult enough with large-scale, properly randomized evidence, and would be impossible without it; because of their unknowable biases (*see* above), non-randomized database analyses are simply not a viable alternative to large-scale randomized evidence. Nor would randomization of 'only' several thousand patients have been sufficient. Indeed, in several important respects what is still needed is more, rather than less, randomized evidence about the effects of fibrinolytic therapy in various particular types of patient. For example, it is still not clear whether patients who present 12–18, or even 18–24, hours after pain onset should be treated: more randomized evidence is still needed (Fig. 58.2). Nevertheless, substantial progress has been made by the past decade of mega-trials of fibrinolytic agents. Worldwide, in the mid-1990s, about half a million patients per year were given fibrinolytic therapy, avoiding about 10 000 early deaths each year.

Small trials refuted by a mega-trial: lack of significant benefit from magnesium infusion in suspected acute myocardial infarction

It had been suggested that, in patients with suspected acute myocardial infarction, an infusion of a magnesium salt might reduce early mortality. Several small trials, involving between them a total of only about 1500 patients, had addressed this question by 1990, and their aggregated results indicated a statistically significant, but implausibly large, benefit (42/754 deaths among those allocated magnesium versus 86/740 among the controls; $2P < 0.001$) (ISIS-4 Collaborative Group, 1995). Some argued that such results constituted proof beyond reasonable doubt that magnesium was of sufficient value to justify widespread usage without seeking further randomized evidence, but others remained sceptical, arguing that the apparent results were far too good to be true.

Two trials, one (LIMIT-2; Woods *et al.*, 1992) involving 2000 patients and one (ISIS-4; ISIS-4 Collaborative Group, 1995) involving 58 000, were therefore set up to test more reliably the possible effects of magnesium. The former yielded a moderately promising result (Table 58.4) indicating avoidance of about one-quarter of the early deaths, but because of its small size this result was statistically compatible with a true benefit that ranged from about zero to about a halving of early mortality. The much larger ISIS-4 trial, however, yielded a completely

unpromising result, so the overall evidence, based on about 60 000 randomized patients, is now non-significantly adverse (ISIS-4 Collaborative Group, 1995).

In view of the striking disparity between the apparent effects of magnesium before and after ISIS-4 had provided large-scale randomized evidence, it is of interest to recall some of the expert views that were expressed while ISIS-4 was in progress. Some felt so strongly that magnesium was already of proven benefit (and hence that further randomization was unethical) that the data monitoring committee of ISIS-4 was lobbied to try to have the study stopped early and all future patients given magnesium. In contrast, the ISIS-4 steering committee was sufficiently sceptical to want large-scale randomized evidence. They believed that the available evidence was consistent with a negligible benefit, or even a small net hazard – although they all thought it more likely that at least some net benefit would be seen. Even after the LIMIT-2 result was available, they continued to hold these opinions, and thought that if there was any real benefit then this was likely to be less than LIMIT-2 had suggested (and hence very much less than the other small trials had suggested).

Those who had trusted the implausibly extreme results from the previous small trials may well have been disappointed by the results of the ISIS-4 mega-trial, which now provide strong evidence that the routine use of magnesium has little or no effect on mortality in acute myocardial infarction. But, in a world where moderate benefits are much more plausible than large benefits, it will commonly happen that striking results in small-scale trials, in small-scale overviews or in small subgroups prove evanescent. The medical assumption that both a moderate mortality difference or a zero mortality difference may be plausible, but that an extreme mortality difference is much less so, has surprisingly strong consequences for the interpretation of randomized evidence. In particular, it implies that even quite highly significant (e.g. $2P = 0.001$) mortality differences that are based on only relatively small numbers of deaths may provide untrustworthy evidence of the existence of any real difference (ISIS-4 Collaborative Group, 1995).

Table 58.4 *Magnesium in acute myocardial infarction: contrast between the results of the smaller and the larger randomized trials*

	Number of patients randomized	1-month mortality	
		Allocated magnesium	Allocated control
9 small trials	1500	42/754 (5.6%)	86/740 (11.6%)
LIMIT-2 trial	2300	90/1159 (7.8%)	118/1157 (10.2%)
ISIS-4 trial	58 000	2216/29 011 (7.6%)	2103/29 039 (7.2%)
All trials	62 000	2348/30 924 (7.59%)	2307/30 936 (7.46%)

There is highly significant heterogeneity ($P < 0.001$) between the group of small trials, the 'hypothesis-generating' results of which led to the testing of magnesium in ISIS-4, and the pair of larger trials (ISIS-4 and LIMIT-2), the results of which tested that hypothesis.

RESULTS FROM LARGE, ANONYMOUS TRIALS ARE RELEVANT TO REAL CLINICAL PRACTICE

A clinician is used to dealing with individual patients, and may feel that the results of large trials somehow deny the individuality of each patient. This is almost the opposite of the truth, for one of the main reasons why trials have to be large is just because patients are so different from one another. Two apparently similar patients may run entirely different clinical courses, one remaining stable and the other progressing rapidly to severe disability or early death. Consequently, it is only when really large groups of patients are compared that the proportion of truly good and bad prognosis patients in each can be relied on to be reasonably similar. One commonly hears statements such as: 'If a treatment effect isn't obvious in a couple of hundred patients then it isn't worth knowing about.' As the previous examples demonstrate, such statements may reveal not clinical wisdom but statistical naïvety.

It is also said that what is really wanted is not a blanket recommendation for everybody, but rather some means of identifying those few individuals who really stand to benefit from therapy. If any criteria (e.g. short-term response to a non-placebo-controlled course of some disease-modifying agent) can be proposed that are likely to discriminate between people who will and who will not benefit, then these can, of course, be recorded prospectively at entry and the eventual trial results sub-divided with respect to them. There is, however, a danger in too detailed an analysis of the apparent response of small subgroups chosen for separate emphasis because of the apparently remarkable effects of treatment in those subgroups. Even if an agent brought no benefit, it would have to be acutely poisonous for it not to appear beneficial in one or two such subgroups! Conversely, if an intervention really avoids an approximately similar proportion of the risk in each category of patient, it will, by chance alone, appear not to do so in some category or other. The surprising extent to which this happens is evident from the example in Table 58.2. A large, anonymous trial will at least still help answer the practical question of whether on average a policy of widespread treatment (except where clearly contraindicated) is preferable to a general policy of no immediate use of the treatment (except where clearly indicated). Moreover, without a few really large trials it is difficult to see how else many such questions could be resolved over the next few years. For example, digitalis has already been in use for over two centuries, and there is still no reliable consensus as to its net long-term effects on mortality. Trials are at least a practical way of making some solid progress, and it would be unfortunate if desire for the perfect (i.e. knowledge of exactly who will benefit from treatment) were to become the enemy of the possible (i.e. knowledge of the direction and approximate size of the effects of the treatment of many large categories of patient).

SIGNIFICANT POINTS

- Proper randomization avoids systematic differences between different types of patient in different treatment groups.
- Randomized control trials have resulted in changes in cancer care which have prevented tens of thousands of premature deaths.
- Non-randomized evidence is far inferior as a source of evidence.
- Moderate benefits of major outcomes are more plausible than large effects.

KEY REFERENCES

Chalmers, I. (1994) The Cochrane Collaboration: preparing, maintaining and disseminating systematic reviews of the effects of health care. *Ann. NY Acad. Sci.* **703**, 156–63.

Collins, R., Doll, R. and Peto, R. (1992) Ethics of clinical trials. In Williams, C.J. (ed.), *Introducing new treatments for cancer: practical, ethical and legal problems*. Chichester: John Wiley & Sons, 49.

Peto, R., Pike, M.C., Armitage, P. *et al.* (1976) Design and analysis of randomized clinical trials requiring prolonged observation of each patient. Part I: Introduction and design. *Br. J. Cancer* **34**, 585–612.

Peto, R., Pike, M.C., Armitage, P. *et al.* (1977) Design and analysis of randomized clinical trials requiring prolonged observation of each patient. Part II: Analysis and examples. *Br. J. Cancer* **35**, 1–39.

Yusuf, S., Collins, R. and Peto, R. (1984) Why do we need some large, simple randomized trials? *Stat. Med.* **3**, 409–20.

REFERENCES

Antiplatelet Trialists' Collaboration (1994) Collaborative overview of randomised trials of antiplatelet therapy. I: Prevention of death, myocardial infarction, and stroke by prolonged antiplatelet therapy in various categories of patients. *BMJ* **308**, 81–106.

Chalmers, I. (1994) The Cochrane Collaboration: preparing, maintaining and disseminating systematic reviews of the effects of health care. *Ann. NY Acad. Sci.* **703**, 156–63.

Collins, R. and Julian, D. (1991) British Heart Foundation Surveys (1987 and 1989) of United Kingdom: policies for acute myocardial infarction. *Br. Heart J.* **66**, 250–5.

Collins, R., Gray, R., Godwin, J. and Peto, R. (1987) Avoidance of large biases and large random errors in the assessment of moderate treatment effects: the need for systematic overviews. *Stat. Med.* **6**, 245–50.

Collins, R., Doll, R. and Peto, R. (1992) Ethics of clinical trials. In Williams, C.J. (ed.), *Introducing new treatments for cancer: practical, ethical and legal problems.* Chichester: John Wiley & Sons, 49.

Colorectal Cancer Collaborative Group (2001) Adjuvant radiotherapy for rectal cancer: a systematic overview of 8507 patients from 22 randomized trials. *Lancet* **358**, 1291–304.

Early Breast Cancer Trialists' Collaborative Group (1992) Systemic treatment of early breast cancer by hormonal, cytotoxic, or immune therapy: 133 randomised trials involving 31,000 recurrences and 24,000 deaths among 75,000 women. *Lancet* **339**, 1–15 and 71–85.

European Carotid Surgery Trialists' Collaborative Group (1991) MRC European Carotid Surgery Trial: interim results for symptomatic patients with severe (70–99%) or with mild (0–29%) carotid stenosis. *Lancet* **337**, 1235–43.

European Carotid Surgery Trialists' Collaborative Group (1996) Endarterectomy for moderate symptomatic carotid sterosis: interim results from the MRC European Carotid Surgery Trial. *Lancet* **347**, 1591–3.

Fibrinolytic Therapy Trialists' Collaborative Group (1994) Indications for fibrinolytic therapy in suspected acute myocardial infarction: collaborative overview of early mortality and major morbidity results from all randomised trials of more than 1000 patients. *Lancet* **343**, 311–22.

Gruppo Italiano per lo Studio della Streptochinasi nell'infarto miocardico (GISSI) (1986) Effectiveness of intravenous thrombolytic treatment in acute myocardial infarction. *Lancet* **i**, 397–402.

ISIS-2 (Second International Study of Infarct Survival) Collaborative Group (1988) Randomised trial of intravenous streptokinase, oral aspirin, both, or neither among 17,187 cases of suspected acute myocardial infarction: ISIS-2. *Lancet* **ii**, 349–60.

ISIS-4 (Fourth International Study of Infarct Survival) Collaborative Group (1995) ISIS-4: A randomised factorial trial assessing early oral captopril, oral mononitrate, and intravenous magnesium sulphate in 58,050 patients with suspected acute myocardial infarction. *Lancet* **345**, 669–85.

Peto, R., Pike, M.C., Armitage, P. *et al.* (1976) Design and analysis of randomized clinical trials requiring prolonged observation of each patient. Part I: Introduction and design. *Br. J. Cancer* **34**, 585–612.

Peto, R., Pike, M.C., Armitage, P. *et al.* (1977) Design and analysis of randomized clinical trials requiring prolonged observation of each patient. Part II: Analysis and examples. *Br. J. Cancer* **35**, 1–39.

QUASAR Collaborative Group (2000) Comparison of fluorouracil with additional levamisole, higher-dose folinic acid, or both, as adjuvant chemotherapy for colorectal cancer: a randomised trial. *Lancet* **355**, 1588–96.

Woods, K.L., Fletcher, S., Roffe, C. and Haider, Y. (1992) Intravenous magnesium sulphate in suspected acute myocardial infarction: results of the second Leicester Intravenous Magnesium Intervention Trial (LIMIT-2). *Lancet* **339**, 1553–8.

Yusuf, S., Collins, R. and Peto, R. (1984) Why do we need some large, simple randomized trials? *Stat. Med.* **3**, 409–20.

59

Costs of non-surgical cancer treatment: the UK perspective

E. JANE MAHER AND GRAHAM READ

INTRODUCTION

The organization of cancer services, resources available and methods of measuring cost and outcome of cancer therapy vary both between and within different countries (Lawton and Maher, 1991; Maher, 1991; Coia *et al.*, 1992; Maher *et al.*, 1992; Duncan *et al.*, 1993). These differences influence both the selection of patients for different therapies and the type of therapy delivered. This is particularly the case when cure is not possible. A few particularly important variables are shown in Table 59.1.

This chapter will focus only on non-surgical oncology practice in the UK, to illustrate some of the important issues in this area, remembering that cost/benefit data from one country are not applicable to another. Specifically both surgery and palliative care are not included.

The current context in the UK is as follows. Following a White Paper (Secretaries of State, 1989) a major review of the National Health Service in Great Britain split District Health Authorities (DHAs) in 1991 into purchaser units – which purchase services for patients from their own hospitals, other authorities' hospitals, self-governing trust hospitals or from the private sector – and provider units – usually representing their district general hospitals (DGHs), which provided patient services. A further innovation was the creation of fund holding general practices which, with money top-sliced from the

DHAs, were able to buy services from those provider units which, in their view, offered the best services. With a change of government in 1997 a further major revision has been initiated (HMG, 1997). Fund holding

Table 59.1 *Influential factors affecting interpretation of cost/benefit data between countries*

- System of referral to specialist cancer services (self, family practitioners via other specialists)
- Location of specialist services (office outside a hospital, non-specialist hospital, cancer centre)
- Role of staff narrow or broadly defined (e.g. specialists prescribe *either* chemotherapy or radiotherapy *or* involved in giving both; radiographers *only* involved in giving treatment, or also in counselling, patient care or treatment planning)
- Inpatient beds under direct supervision (and in budget of) oncologists or admitted under the care of other specialists
- Source of funds (e.g. private, university, local government, central government or capitation)
- Unit of account (e.g. per patient, per course of treatment, per injection/fraction of chemotherapy/radiotherapy, per patient weighted for complexity of therapy (e.g. HRG), completed consultant episode)
- Availability of other services under other budgets, e.g. hospices, palliative care specialists, community nurses with expertise in symptom control

HRG, Healthcare resource group.

by general practitioners has been abolished and, in England, 481 primary-care groups (PCGs), each serving approximately 100 000 people (range 46 000–257 000), have been created. Similar arrangements will exist in Wales and Northern Ireland, but in Scotland all forms of GP commissioning will end (Secretary of State for Scotland, 1997). Four possible levels of function of PCGs are currently envisaged, with the highest being a primary care trust (PCT), having total purchasing power for its population. Certain services, such as specialist cancer services, may again be purchased by Regional Health Authorities (RHAs), restoring some functions that had previously been eroded – indeed, they had been merged into eight units in 1994 and complete abolition had been scheduled for 1996. Despite these reforms, the basic purchaser/provider division has been retained.

Oncological services in the UK have undergone a fundamental change following the report of the chief medical officers of England and Wales (Calman, 1995). This was provoked by the recognition of considerable inequalities in cancer care, and recommended the creation of cancer units in DGHs linked to a cancer centre. The stated aim was that 'all patients should have access to a uniformly high quality of care in the community or hospital wherever they may live to ensure the maximum possible cure rates and best quality of life'. Accreditation of the cancer units has begun to ensure that they are functioning appropriately. With the recognition of the importance of primary care in cancer management, there is a developing concept of managed clinical networks following whole-care pathways, rather than hub–spoke arrangements, looking only at acute trusts. This has developed furthest in Scotland, but concepts of management, joint accountability and financial flows across such networks are embryonic as yet.

UK government policy has reflected the move towards a greater use of evidence-based medicine with the setting up of the National Institute for Clinical Effectiveness (NICE), which is intended to produce 30–50 definitive guidelines per year, and the Commission for Health Improvement (CHI) which is a statutory regulatory body. There will also be a greater use of performance indicators (NHS Consultation Document, 1997). Thus all specialized cancer therapy units will be obliged to examine their practices and outcomes in order to achieve the most efficient way of providing services. Although the need to carry out an economic evaluation of guidelines before their acceptance into widespread use is generally acknowledged (Dent and Hawke, 1997), there is little evidence that this is being done. One barrier is the relatively large number of economic variables which can significantly increase the required sample sizes in randomized trials, thus increasing their cost. There is a growing literature on the challenges to implementing guidelines in an NHS in a state of accelerating change, and the recognition that the hidden costs limiting doctors' discretion and the autonomy

of local commissioners can lead to a distortion in decision making which may not be in the best interests of patients (Haycox et al., 1999).

RESOURCE ALLOCATION

The problem of the level of funding in the UK remains as keen as ever. The Eurocare Study has highlighted differences in outcomes (almost always unfavourable) between the UK and the rest of Europe, and attention is frequently drawn to the lower proportion of the gross domestic product devoted to health care – 6.9 per cent, compared to Germany (9.5 per cent) and the US (14.3 per cent) (Abbasi, 1997). The creation of the Welsh and Scottish assemblies may further exacerbate existing differences in funding between the constituent parts of the UK (Dixon et al., 1999).

The need for more consistent methods of funding (Orme, 1991) has long been recognized. Discussion now centres not only around the funding of new agents but also the variable ability to fund treatments regarded as standard in Europe and the US. Using an evidence-based approach may still lead to inconsistencies as health authorities contrive to use a variable threshold, depending upon their financial position (Foy et al., 1999).

COST COMPARISONS

There are several analytical methods relating to the costs and consequences of healthcare programmes. Terms such as cost effectiveness or cost benefit are often loosely used, but the more precise definitions defined below are generally accepted. The rising costs of healthcare have led to increasing numbers of cost analyses, most particularly in medical oncology because of the high costs (Smith et al., 1993). Indeed, it has been suggested that an economic analysis should be included routinely in all newly devised randomized controlled trials (Drummond and Coyle, 1998). However, it is also recognized that trials involving economic analysing may involve a large number of variables and very large sample sizes.

Cost minimization

The method compares the total costs of two different strategies which have the same outcome. Unfortunately, in clinical practice it is rare to find two significantly differing modalities (and therefore significantly differing costs) in which there is general agreement that the outcomes are the same. In general, comparisons of modalities in the literature have focused on survival and side-effects, and only in recent years has the specific issue of cost comparison been addressed. Recent examples include the relief of bone pain and the management of early glottic cancer (Foote *et al.*, 1997; Macklis *et al.*, 1998).

Cost effectiveness

This form of analysis relates the cost of a treatment to its outcome. Two or more treatments can be compared provided there is a common unit of outcome or effectiveness, such as 'life years gained', 'pain-free days' or 'positive cases detected'. Thus in a cost-effectiveness analysis a ratio of benefit to cost is derived for each option. The most cost-effective option, therefore, can be defined either as that which maximizes benefits for a fixed cost or minimizes costs for a fixed benefit (Sugden and Williams, 1978). It should be noted that it is not necessarily the largest net benefit which represents the optimum choice. In assessing the benefits of a particular treatment, the question arises as to how to deal with costs which occur at different points in time. This is clearly of importance when considering the immediate benefits of a particular treatment versus its long-term risks, a common problem in the treatment of malignant disease. Traditionally, benefits have been discounted in a manner similar to that described below for dealing with costs, for example the 6 per cent per annum used in public sector projects (HM Treasury, 1997), which has the effect of weighting the short-term benefits. Adopting a zero discount rate, while it may be appropriate for areas such as neonatal care, would lead in cancer to an undue preoccupation with late effects in preference to immediate gains and may not, therefore, be appropriate. Currently the UK Department of Health recommends that benefit measures, such as quality-adjusted life years (QALYs), are discounted at a rate of 1.5–2.0 per cent (Department of Health, 1995).

Simple outcome measures may, however, be of limited value in the context of incurable disease, and may reflect selection criteria and referral policy more than results of particular therapy. Reviews suggest that over three-quarters of chemotherapy treatments and half of radiotherapy treatments aim not to cure but to palliate symptoms of the disease and improve quality of life (Maher *et al.*, 1990). Many palliative treatments are more expensive than those aimed at cure (Rees, 1985). Analysis of cost and benefit in the UK is further hampered by the fact that three-quarters of British clinical oncologists do not have access to the information technology required to obtain comprehensive data on survival of their patients after different therapies, without laborious retrospective examination of case notes (Maher *et al.*, 1993).

Economic evaluation of cancer treatments should involve comparison with relevant alternatives. It is important that all aspects of the alternative treatment are considered; for example, if this is a 'wait and see' policy,

then the costs of treatment of the later symptomatic disease should be included. The perspective for the analysis should be considered as this may range from a limited consideration of costs to a provider of a department in a hospital providing a service, the hospital in which the department is situated, the patient, or even society as a whole. Goddard and Drummond have suggested a list of questions to ask of any published study (Goddard and Drummond, 1991).

A number of studies have shown that, in general, radiotherapy is remarkably cost effective. For example, Glazebrook was able to show that for external-beam radiotherapy the cost of a year of life gained was C$_{1992}$ 661 (C$_{1992}$ 1.82 per day – which he compared to the cost of a city bus ride!). This was one or more orders of magnitude different from the costs of a year gained by, for example, coronary bypass (C$_{1992}$ 6698), renal dialysis (C$_{1992}$ 67 345) or school testing for tuberculosis (C$_{1992}$ 69 634) (Glazebrook, 1992).

Cost utility

Although cost-effectiveness analyses may be very useful, they are unable to compare different diseases or strategies where the outcomes cannot be measured in a common unit. This may arise where, for example, a healthcare purchaser wishes to decide between, say, allocating money to cataract surgery or cancer chemotherapy. Cost utility relates the cost of different medical procedures to the increased utility, 'the amount of well being', they produce in terms of improved quantity and quality of life. Approaches to evaluation of the duration of benefit include concepts such as the notional patient benefit year cost (Rees, 1985):

$$\text{mean total cost} \times \left(\frac{100}{\text{Response rate}} \right) \times \left(\frac{12}{\text{Mean duration of response}} \right),$$

or the fraction of normal remaining life span (Vaidya and Mittra, 1997). Particular health states may be assessed through health state preference values, that is the value which a healthy person would place hypothetically on a particular deterioration in health, or a sick person on their return to health. Methods such as rating scale, time trade off or standard gamble measurements have been used to assign such values. The quality-adjusted life year can then be calculated by multiplying the preference value with the time a patient is likely spend in that state. However, the use of QALYs and other measures remains controversial (for a summary of quality of life measures, *see* Hopkins, 1992).

Quality of life rating scales (e.g. EORTC QLQ-C30 global quality of life rating scale) tend to be lower than utilities obtained by asking a person to theoretically rate their present health by the extent to which they would trade time in present health for a shorter length of time in perfect health (time trade off) or the extent to which they would accept the theoretical risk of death to avoid a particular health state (standard gamble) (Read et al., 1984). QL scales have been transformed to an estimate of utility using published transformation factors to compensate for the lower utility obtained when a person describes quality of life without risking possible loss to that individual (O'Leary et al., 1995), e.g. using EORTC QLQ-C30 utility $= 1.07 \times$ QL rating scale for $R < 0.95$; utility $= 100 \times$ QL rating scale for $R > 0.95$ (Bloomfield et al., 1998). In theory, retrospective economic analysis can be applied to any trials incorporating a global QL measuring EORTC QLQ-C30 (Osoba et al., 1996).

Problems remain in interpreting the relationship between a health-related QL approach, relating utility to the presence of symptoms, level of function and other attributes, and an assessment based on a preference for a health state made under conditions of uncertainty (Revicki and Kaplan, 1993). Furthermore, not only will different values of utility be obtained from a rating scale compared to time trade-off or standard gamble, they will also depend on whether the subject is the patient, the spouse or the general public (Torrance, 1986; Slevin et al., 1988). There is an ongoing debate as to the appropriate group from whom to elicit utilities: the patient suffering the illness or the tax payer.

The attraction of a utility related to a health state is that one unit of outcome, e.g. cost per quality of life adjusted years (QALY), is a universal yardstick incorporating additional costs and additional benefits in one measure applicable across health states. The difficulty with the QALY concept is the variability in how QALYs are calculated in terms of cost and utility, which makes justification of a health intervention based on ranking of cost per QALY tenuous (Naylor et al., 1993).

There is now a wide range of questionnaires that have been developed in an attempt to measure overall health status, such as the Nottingham health profile (Hunt et al., 1981), the SF-36 general health index and the McMaster health utilities index questionnaire (Patrick and Erikson, 1993). Disease-specific measures may be more appropriate in some circumstances (Fallowfield, 1995). However, even with apparently 'objective' scales, assessments made by doctors, patients and their relatives will differ (Slevin et al., 1988) and scepticism remains as to what extent any of them truly measures quality of life (Muldoon et al., 1998).

In the UK, most patients, particularly those with a poor prognosis, will not be followed in a specialist centre, but in conjunction with several different local physicians or surgeons, or by the primary healthcare team, depending on the site of the disease and available local expertise. Formal measurement of outcome involving multi-dimensional self-assessment questionnaires then needs the co-operation of a variety of different staff, based in multiple locations with no clear management link. Inevitably, this will have associated administrative and financial implications. As a result of such difficulties, authors have resorted to a variety of 'estimated' outcomes. For example, bone metastases, primary lung cancer and brain metastases are the most common areas treated with palliative radiotherapy. Published studies demonstrate that the most common aim of treatment is to relieve symptoms (Maher et al., 1990; Maher, 1991). Previous studies have identified specific tumour-related symptoms which are both particularly distressing (i.e. can be shown to affect quality of life) and respond to palliative radiotherapy in a majority of cases. Examples include haemoptysis associated with bronchial cancer (Saunders et al., 1984) and bone pain associated with bone metastases (Maher, 1992). Given such a known response rate, the presence of such symptoms in a treatment population has been used both as a measure for appropriate selection of treatment and a surrogate measure of outcome where collection of prospective data is associated with costs disproportionate to their eventual value (Crellin et al., 1989; Goddard et al., 1991).

Cost benefit

This form of analysis, in many ways the most difficult, seeks to determine whether the benefits of using a given therapy outweigh its costs. A monetary value has, therefore, to be assigned to each strategy or treatment, which may amount to deciding how much it costs to save a life or to enable a person live a pain free-one life. Some people have an ethical objection to putting a monetary value on a human life, but such decisions are regularly made in economic planning even if they are not implicitly stated. In fact, for many years, cost–benefit analysis has been used regularly in the analysis of economic and social policy in the public sector. Roberts estimated in 1985 that the NHS could not afford more than $£_{1984}$ 14 000 to save a life (Roberts et al., 1985) and Rees felt that treatments costing less than $£_{1991}$ 1000 for an improvement in benefit were excellent value, whereas those costing $£_{1991}$ 10 000 probably represented an unfair distribution of resources (Rees, 1991).

Various approaches have been adopted in benefit evaluation. Initial approaches were based on the loss of income incurred by illness, but this clearly does not take into account benefits in the retired or unemployed. Another approach is to evaluate whether we are willing to pay the stated cost for a particular procedure or service. This is often expressed as a proportion of average income as an alternative to a straight monetary cost. Thus, in one study, Thompson found that patients with rheumatoid arthritis were willing to pay 22 per cent for a hypothetical cure of the disease.

RADIOTHERAPY

Unit of accounting

Existing evidence on the costs of radiotherapy has previously been summarized (Goddard and Hutton, 1988). Much of the published data comes from outside the UK. Reviews have concentrated either on the cost per fraction (or attendance) of radiotherapy, with estimates[1] varying from £10.46 to £70.56 per fraction/attendance, or, alternatively, estimates of the cost of a course of treatment varying from £505 to £4529. Despite widespread acceptance of their limitations, returns of clinical activity to central government in the UK have, up until 1999, been made using OPCS-4[2] and ICD-10[3] codes, based on finished consultant episodes (FCEs). Oncology is particularly disadvantaged by this system as much of its activity is performed on an outpatient basis, which may not be recorded, and ICD-10 contains a marked paucity of codes in relation to radiotherapy. Alternatives such as Read Version 3 have still not been implemented.

The reasons for such marked variations can be shown to include the size and limitation of the department, whether the radiotherapy department is part of a specialist hospital or a general hospital, workload and throughput of the department, and the type and age of equipment (Goddard and Hutton, 1988). A crucial influence is the clinical policy of a centre with regard to treatment of particular types of patient. These have been shown to differ significantly, both between centres in the same country (Priestman et al., 1989) as well as between countries (Lawton and Maher, 1991; Maher, 1991; Maher et al., 1992; Duncan et al., 1993). Finally, costs will also depend on what is included in the costing process.

UK estimates of radiotherapy costs

As a result of the purchaser/provider concept, hospital accountants have been obliged to prepare estimates of the cost of radiotherapy. These have usually been made by a 'top down' approach (Fig. 59.1), that is by taking the known total costs, including overheads, reserves and capital charges, allocating them to specialities including radiotherapy and calculating a cost based on the number of consultant episodes. The principal cost areas are shown in Table 59.2.

Three detailed UK studies have considered costs calculated from the components of treatment (bottom up). Greene (1983) estimated the cost of a radiotherapy treatment on a linear accelerator, with a separate estimate for

those treatments employing beam-direction shells, on the basis of a department which had four linear accelerators. In a reply, Atherton (1984) provided a further estimate of the cost, based upon calculations made by Philips Medical Systems but in the context of a department having two linear accelerators. Some aspects of the papers were inconsistent or incomplete, and in order to

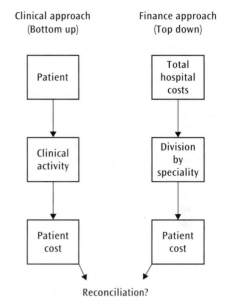

Figure 59.1 *Top down and bottom up approaches.*

Table 59.2 *Principal cost areas in radiotherapy*

Capital	Main equipment	Linear accelerators
		Cobalt units
		Superficial units
		Afterloading units
	Auxiliary machines	Simulator
		CT scanner/ MRI scanner
		Planning computer
	Other facilities	Mould room
		Sealed sources store
	Building and installation	
	Capital interest and depreciation	
Staff	Radiotherapists	
	Radiographers	
	Nurses	
	Physicists	
	Engineering technicians	
	Clerical and reception	
	Portering	
	Cleaning	
	Administration	
Maintenance	Equipment maintenance and parts	
	Building maintenance, electricity and heating	

---

[1] For clarity all costs have been converted to 1993 £UK, based on the UK retail price index.
[2] Office of Population Censuses and Surveys (1986) *Classification of surgical operations* (4th edn). London: OPCS.
[3] International Classification of Diseases, Version 10.

make a comparison possible, they were reworked by Goddard and Hutton (1988). A study of costs at Mount Vernon Hospital in 1991 made particular reference to the costs of palliative treatments and did not therefore take into account the costs of more complicated planning, such as the use of the mould room and computer planning. Using the costs per fraction from the three series, one can derive costs for various fractionation schedules as shown in Table 59.3. However, simple multiplication from the cost of a single fraction to obtain the costs of radical treatments of various lengths is unlikely to give a correct result. Individually costing each treatment is laborious and is unlikely to be feasible. An alternative approach has been to identify the 'core' elements of the costs of delivering a particular type of therapy to defined groups of patients, e.g. for palliative radiotherapy given to relieve the symptoms of incurable cancer (Goddard et al., 1991), at the same time identifying some 'non-essential' factors involved, e.g. mode of transport, outpatient or inpatient care, point from which drugs are obtained, which might have a varying influence on unit costs, depending on local circumstances.

Healthcare resource groups

A second alternative is to establish iso-resource or health-care resource groups (HRGs). They are intended to

represent groups of patients who are both clinically relevant and who consume a similar level of resources (National Casemix Office, 1993a, 1993b). The HRGs developed for oncology differ from those of other specialities in that they contain groups which are procedure orientated rather than being related to the patient's diagnosis. The reason for this is that whereas a diagnosis of, say, appendicitis carries some implications of what resources might be required for treatment, a patient with diagnosis of breast cancer might have treatment varying from a single consultation to many courses of chemotherapy, radiotherapy and surgery over a number of years.

Radiotherapy HRGs

In the UK a series of workshops were convened by the National Casemix Office between 1990 and 1992. As a result, provisional groupings were developed for radiotherapy and piloted at 12 centres. Within external-beam radiotherapy two activities contribute to the use of resources – the resource used to plan the treatment, which may vary from nothing more than a skin marker pen to the full use of a dedicated mould room, and the resource used to deliver the treatment, which can be estimated simply by counting the number of fractions. Hence external-beam treatments can be displayed on a two-dimensional matrix. For brachytherapy or sealed-source work the relevant factors are the use of general anaesthesia, the mould room and remote afterloading. These groups were brought into general use in April 2000.

Table 59.3 *Cost per course of radiotherapy in three studies* ($£_{1993}$)

	Greene[a]	Atherton[a]	Goddard[b]
Single fraction	27	35	46
Radical, 5 fractions	134	176	231
Radical, 15 fractions	401	529	693
Radical, 30 fractions	803	1058	1387

[a] Estimate based on 800 treatments at 12 fractions.
[b] Based on 40 316 attendances in 1988.

Application of radiotherapy HRGs

Using these groups, one can easily display the work of a radiotherapy department for any desired time period. Figure 59.2 illustrates the groups applied to the Christie Hospital, Manchester, using data collected by a clinical computer system (Read and Swindell, 1991). In this

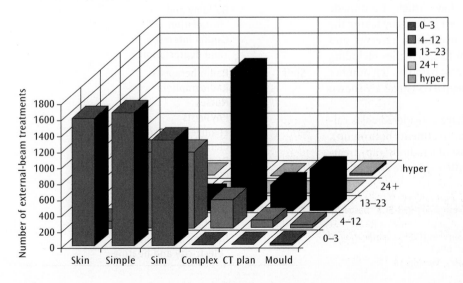

Figure 59.2 *Christie Hospital: external-beam treatments in 1 year.*

department it can be seen that single and simple palliative treatments predominate. However, these groups do not represent the major costs in terms of resources and staff time and, in order to use these data, a system of weighting the treatments has to be devised for costing. This is necessary to allow for the considerably greater resources needed, for example, to plan a mould-room treatment, and the longer time required to deliver them. An arbitrary weighting system is shown in Table 59.4, and applying this to the data in Figure 59.2 shows the relative costs of the various groups (Fig. 59.3). It will be seen that, in this department, the complex (mainly breast), CT planning and mould-room treatments are responsible for the greater proportion of the costs.

Average and marginal costs

Although estimates of average costs have frequently been used in healthcare accounting, it may be more useful to estimate the marginal costs, that is those costs associated with a small change in healthcare activity (Goddard and Hutton, 1991). The marginal costs, incurred in delivering, for example, a few extra fractions of radiotherapy or, conversely, the offset costs from reducing the number of fractions, cannot be measured accurately using average cost estimates. Some elements of costs will remain fixed over relatively large changes in workload. There will be a negligible rise in cost from machine use or staff if a

patient received four rather than three fractions of palliative radiotherapy. This only becomes important if there is a substantial change affecting many patients treated in a department, which might necessitate the employment of a new staff member or the purchase of a new machine. Conversely, reducing the numbers of fractions may potentially allow the release of such resources only if practice changes substantially for a significant number of patients. Although machines and staff are unlikely to become laid off as a result of such reduction, treatment for other patients can be substituted in order to take advantage of such savings. Additionally, increasing demands for quality assurance may mean that less machine time is available for treatment, and release of resources may facilitate this.

Staff costs

Many previous studies of radiotherapy considered only some of the staff involved in treatment; for example, Greene excluded radiotherapy staff costs (Greene, 1983). Others do not state explicitly whether they include all radiography staff. In addition, some other important staff associated with radiotherapy and chemotherapy treatment are located in medical physics, bioengineering, nursing, pharmacy, haematology and administration. Indeed, such costs might actually fall into another budget, but cannot be excluded if the true costs of services are to be estimated. The estimation of accurate staff costs causes particular

Table 59.4 *Possible weightings for radiotherapy HRG groups*

HRG planning resource	Possible cost weighting	
	Planning	**Treatment**
Superficial: <160 kV machine	1	1
Simple: megavoltage single field or parallel pair planned without simulation	1	1
Simulator: simple treatment planned using a planning simulator	3	1
Complex: more complex field arrangement using multiple beams	4	2
Imaging: requires treatment-planning computer, usually with CT imaging	10	4
Technical support: requires mould-room facilities	20	4

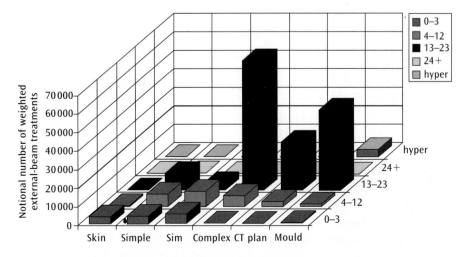

Figure 59.3 *Christie Hospital: external-beam treatments in 1 year adjusted by possible cost weightings.*

difficulties, as it is obvious that many staff will also be involved in the care of patients who do not receive radiotherapy and chemotherapy but who do pass through a cancer centre. The care of such patients uses resources in terms of staff time, but without undertaking a prospective analysis it is not possible to estimate accurately the proportion spent only on radiotherapy or chemotherapy treatment. This difficulty relates to the problems of separating therapy from cancer care in general. In the UK, consultant clinical oncologists and nursing staff do not deal just with radiotherapy patients, or chemotherapy patients, but with cancer patients in general, who may receive counselling, support, analgesia, etc.

In the absence of such information, various assumptions can be made. In the Mount Vernon palliative radiotherapy study the assumptions made were as follows: first, all radiographer time and a proportion of physics and bioengineering staff allocated for radiotherapy, were apportioned to radiotherapy; second, 70 per cent of the costs associated with the consultant, radiotherapists, nursing, other medical staff and administration and clerical staff in the department were allocated to the radiotherapy department. The rationale for this was based on the fact that consultants, nursing and other medical staff within the department also spent part of their time with chemotherapy patients and with those receiving no specific treatment. On the basis of the numbers of radiotherapy and chemotherapy patients seen annually in this unit, the relevant split on the basis of activity was approximately 86 per cent radiotherapy and 14 per cent chemotherapy. However, this excludes those who received no specific treatment, but still consumed resources such as staff time. Most radiotherapy centres do not keep systematic records of the numbers of such patients and, thus, in the absence of firm data, it was assumed that such patients would comprise a total of about a fifth the total workload in the department. This implies that overall the relevant apportionment for radiotherapy activity versus other activity was 70 per cent to 30 per cent. This provided only a very broad estimate and highlights an additional problem, that is the distinction between activity and resource use: apportioning the resource on the basis of patient numbers is not accurate as, for example, it often takes more time to explain that no treatment is available than to explain the details of a treatment that is. Again, the most satisfactory solution is a detailed prospective, patient-based survey, logging the treatment received and time spent. This has, until recently, been beyond the scope of most departments.

Capital costs

The most obvious items of capital equipment used in radiotherapy are the machines that actually deliver the irradiation. Planning involves other items of equipment, such as simulators, planning computers and, in some departments, CT scanners. Such machines, although expensive, will last for some years, and the calculation of equivalent annual cost (EAC) makes allowance for the depreciation of machinery over time and for the opportunity cost incurred in the purchase of the items. Many existing studies of radiotherapy costs use historical costs in the calculation of capital costs (Hughes and McEvedy, 1981) and in many of the others, the force of the capital costs is unstated (Friedlander and Tattersall, 1982). However, in order to allow the variations in the time of purchase of equipment it is necessary to consider the replacement costs, rather than the historical cost of the item. It is important to note that, for some items of equipment, particularly older machines, it would be inappropriate to assume that they would be replaced by a similar piece of equipment and, in such cases, replacement costs of a preferred item should be used. Similarly, in discounting the costs over time, the discount period should be set at the useful life of the equipment, and the discounting should not be undertaken using simple interest rates, as in some studies (Greene, 1983), but an appropriate discount rate, such as 6 per cent, should be used, which is the test discount rate for the public sector. The method of dealing with the revenue costs of capital equipment have been defined in the UK by Treasury rates (HM Treasury, 1982). An EAC is calculated based on depreciation over 15 years (10 for computer equipment), interest on its capital value, and indexation at Health Services Prices Index (HSPI) rates. Additional revenue costs arise from the use of the buildings that house the radiotherapy department and equipment. Again, these represent an opportunity cost and their replacement value should ideally be discounted over the useful life of the buildings, which by convention is taken as 60 years (Drummond, 1980). However, a further complication arises when considering the treatment rooms used to house the radiotherapy machines, because they are very specialized and have little chance for alternative use. It might therefore be more appropriate to use a shorter expected useful life of these areas of the buildings. The revenue costs in Greene's study were not calculated according to Treasury rules and were reworked by Goddard and Hutton. The annual revenue costs for the three studies are shown in Table 59.5.

Table 59.5 *Annual costs of radiotherapy in three studies*

	Greene 4 linaccs	Atherton 2 linaccs	Goddard 5 linaccs
Capital	323 452	179 307	259 236
Buildings			298 267
Staff	573 913	441 600	1 040 226
Maintenance and power	60 108	38 615	
General overheads	57 533	32 690	215 992
Total	1 015 005	692 172	1 813 721

linaccs, Linear accelerators.

CHEMOTHERAPY

Radiotherapy, which has high capital costs and relatively low running costs, contrasts with chemotherapy, in which capital costs are low, except in the case of purpose-built high-dependency units, such as those for the treatment of acute leukaemia. In consideration of the costs of chemotherapy, emphasis is often placed on the cost of the chemotherapy drugs, yet Richards found that only 8 per cent of the cost of cancer management was due to chemotherapy (Richards *et al.*, 1993). In the UK in 1993 the budget for all cytotoxic drugs was £58 million, whereas the budget for omeprazole alone was £250 million (Leonard *et al.*, 1997). More important cost drivers include the number of inpatient days, day cases and consultant visits. Thus in 1991 carboplatin was more expensive than *cis*-platinum, but because it is administered to outpatients its use avoids the cost of an inpatient stay and the associated need for fluid hydration, leading to an overall cheaper cost (Calvert and Urie, 1991). Furthermore, the cost of treating the complications of chemotherapy, such as septicaemia, may be more expensive than the chemotherapy drugs themselves, due to the cost of inpatient stay, antibiotics and fluids. In addition, the cost of a drug may be subject to considerable variation, particularly when its patent life expires. A high percentage of chemotherapy is given in the palliative situation. Most studies demonstrate a characteristic pattern of cumulative cost profile, with an initial shallow increase in periods of outpatient treatment and a steep use in cumulative costs at the end of life. The dominant cost (about 60 per cent in many studies) will always be inpatient care for uncontrolled symptom management (Bloomfield *et al.*, 1998) (*see* Tables 59.6 and 59.7).

Chemotherapy HRGs

The HRGs which are currently being developed for chemotherapy aim to reflect these difficulties. These are likely to be based upon the cost of a complete chemotherapy programme rather than cycles or courses, which are difficult to define in a consistent manner.

SUMMARY

Costing of non-surgical cancer treatment represents a complex challenge in the UK. It involves contributions from services based at non-specialist hospitals and in the community as well as specialist centres. It is often difficult to identify and measure and apportion costs for all the different elements of care. The most satisfactory approach is to cost the whole package of care provided, including initial consultation, investigations, treatment and follow-up. No region currently has sufficient data from all relevant sectors of the healthcare and non-healthcare systems to provide this information.

Table 59.6 *Wrexham peripheral clinic study (1985) – Wrexham Hospital costs*

	Total costs (£$_{1993}$)
XRT	N/A
Drugs	13 245
Surgery	N/A
Radiology	6446
Biochemistry	3379
Outpatient	22 511
Inpatient	N/A
Total	45 581

N/A, Not available.

Table 59.7 *Wrexham peripheral clinic study (1984) – Christie Hospital costs*

	Total costs (1993)
XRT	68 221
Drugs	6 409
Surgery	5 306
Radiology	5 962
Biochemistry	9 963
Outpatient	2 629
Inpatient	306 105
Total	404 595

SIGNIFICANT POINTS

- Costing of non-surgical cancer treatment in the UK is carried out poorly at the present time.
- It is important to try to estimate the entire package of care provided.
- Data systems are lacking in the UK and require urgent improvement.

KEY REFERENCES

Abbasi, K. (1997) United Kingdom spends less than average on health care. *BMJ* **315**, 568.

Haycox, A., Bagust, A. and Walley, T. (1999) Clinical guidelines – the hidden costs. *BMJ* **318**, 391–3.

Macklis, R.M., Cornelli, H. and Lasher, J. (1998) Brief courses of palliative radiotherapy for metastatic bone pain: a pilot cost-minimization analysis. *Am. J. Clin. Oncol.* **21**(6), 617–22.

Smith, T., Hillner, B.E. and Desch, C.E. (1993) Efficacy and cost-effectiveness of cancer treatment: Rational allocation of resources based on decision analysis. *J. Natl Cancer Inst.* **85**, 1460–74.

REFERENCES

Abbasi, K. (1997) United Kingdom spends less than average on health care. *BMJ* **315**, 568.

Atherton, L. (1984) The cost of radiotherapy treatments on a linear accelerator. *Br. J. Radiol.* **57**, 106–7.

Bloomfield, D.J., Krahn, M.D., Neogi, T. *et al.* (1998) Economic evaluation of chemotherapy with Mitoxantrone plus Prednisone for symptomatic hormone-resistant prostate cancer: based on a Canadian randomized trial with palliative end points. *J. Clin. Oncol.* **16**(6), 2272–9.

Calman, K.C. (1995) *A policy framework for commissioning cancer services.* A report by the expert advisory group on cancer to the Chief Medical Officers of England and Wales. Department of Health, HMSO.

Calvert, A.H. and Urie, J. (1991) The costs of carboplatin treatment. *Semin. Oncol.* **18**(1 suppl. 2), 28–31.

Coia, L.R., Owen, J.B., Maher, E.J. and Hanks, G.E. (1992) Factors affecting treatment patterns of radiation oncologists in the United States in the palliative treatment of cancer. *Clin. Oncol.* **4**, 6–10.

Crellin, A.M., Marks, A. and Maher, E.J. (1989) Why don't British radiotherapists give single fractions of radiotherapy for bone metastases? *Clin. Oncol.* **1**, 63–6.

Dent, T.H. and Hawke, S. (1997) Too soon to market. *BMJ* **315**, 1248–9.

Department of Health (1995) *Policy appraisal and health.* A guide from the Department of Health. London.

Dixon, J., Inglis, S. and Klein, R. (1999) Is the English NHS underfunded? *BMJ* **318**, 522–6.

Drummond, M.F. (1980) *Principles of economic appraisals in health care.* Oxford: Oxford University Press.

Drummond, M.F. and Coyle, D. (1998) The role of pilot studies in the economic evaluation of health technologies. *Int. J. Technol. Assess. Health Care* **14**(3), 405–18.

Duncan, G., Duncan, W. and Maher, E.J. (1993) Patterns of palliative radiotherapy in Canada. *Clin. Oncol.* **5**, 92–7.

Fallowfield, L.J. (1995) Assessment of quality of life in breast cancer. *Acta Oncol.* **34**, 689–94.

Foote, R.L., Buskirk, S.J., Grado, G.L. and Bonner, J.A. (1997) Has radiotherapy become too expensive to be considered a treatment option for early glottic cancer? *Head Neck* **19**(8), 692–700.

Foy, R., So, J., Rous, E. and Scarffe, H. (1999) Perspectives of commissioners and cancer specialists in prioritising new cancer drugs: impact of the evidence threshold. *BMJ* **318**, 456–9.

Friedlander, M.L. and Tattersall, M.H.N. (1982) Counting the costs of cancer therapy. *Eur. J. Cancer Clin. Oncol.* **18**, 1237–41.

Glazebrook, G.A. (1992) Radiation therapy: a long term cost benefit analysis in a North American Region. *Clin. Oncol.* **4**, 302–5.

Goddard, M.F. and Drummond, M.F. (1991) The economic evaluation of cancer treatment programs. *Eur. J. Cancer* **27** (10), 1191–6.

Goddard, M. and Hutton, J. (1988) *The costs of radiotherapy in cancer treatment.* Centre for Health Economics Discussion paper 48, University of York, UK.

Goddard, M. and Hutton, J. (1991) Economic evaluation of trends in cancer therapy. Marginal or average costs? *Int. J. Technol. Assess. Health Care* **7**(4), 594–603.

Goddard, M., Maher, E.J. Hutton, J. and Shah, D. (1991) Palliative radiotherapy counting the costs of changing practice. *Health Policy* **17**, 243–56.

Greene, D. (1983) The cost of radiotherapy treatments on a linear accelerator. *Br. J. Radiol.* **56**, 189–91.

HMG White paper (1997) *The new NHS – modern, dependable.* London: HMSO.

HM Treasury (1982) *Investment appraisal in the public sector.* London: HMSO.

HM Treasury (1997) *Appraisal and evaluation in central government. Treasury guidance.* London: HMSO.

Haycox, A., Bagust, A. and Walley, T. (1999) Clinical guidelines – the hidden costs. *BMJ* **318**, 391–3.

Hopkins, A. (ed.) (1992) *Measures of quality of life.* London: Royal College of General Practitioners.

Hughes, D. and McEvedy, M. (1981) The effective cost of medical treatment. *Management Account*, February, 38–96.

Hunt, S.M., McKenna, S.P., McEwen, J., Williams, J. and Papp, E. (1981) The Nottingham Health Profile: subjective health status and medical consultation. *Soc. Sci. Med.* **19**, 787–805.

Lawton, P.A. and Maher, E.J. (1991) Treatment strategies for advanced and metastatic cancer in Europe. *Radiother. Oncol.* **22**, 1–6.

Leonard, R.C.F., on behalf of members of the executive committee of the Association of Cancer Physicians (1997) More money is need to care for patients with cancer. *BMJ* **315**, 811–12.

Macklis, R.M., Cornelli, H. and Lasher, J. (1998) Brief courses of palliative radiotherapy for metastatic bone pain: a pilot cost-minimization analysis. *Am. J. Clin. Oncol.* **21**(6), 617–22.

Maher, E.J. (1991) The influence of national attitudes on the use of radiotherapy in advanced and metastatic cancer, with particular reference to differences between the United Kingdom and the United States of America: Implications for future studies. *Int. J. Radiat. Oncol. Biol. Phys.* **20**, 1369–73.

Maher, E.J. (1992) The use of palliative radiotherapy in the management of breast cancer. *Eur. J. Cancer* **28**, 706–10.

Maher, E.J., Dische, S., Grosch, E. *et al.* (1990) Who gets radiotherapy? *Health Trends* **2**, 78–83.

Maher, E.J., Coia, L., Duncan,G. and Lawton, P.A. (1992) Treatment strategies in advanced and metastatic cancer in Canada, Europe and the USA. *Int. J. Radiat. Oncol. Biol. Phys.* **23**, 239–44.

Maher, E.J., Timothy, A., Squire, C.J. *et al.* The Audit Group on behalf of the Faculty of Oncology, The Royal College of Radiologists (1993) Audit: the use of radiotherapy for NSCLC in the UK. *Clin. Oncol.* **5**, 72–9.

Muldoon, M.F., Barger, S.D., Flory, J.D. and Manuck, S.B. (1998) What are quality of life measurements measuring? *BMJ* **316**, 542–5.

National Casemix Office (1993a) *HRG definitions manual*, Version 1.0. IMG(ME)G, HMSO.

National Casemix Office (1993b) *What are healthcare resource groups?* IMG(ME), HMSO.

Naylor, D.C., Williams, I.J., Basinski, A. *et al.* (1993) Technology assessment and cost-effectiveness analysis: misguided guidelines? *Can. Med. Assoc. J.* **148**, 921–4.

NHS Consultation Document (1997) *A First Class Service.* London: HMSO.

O'Leary, J.F., Fairclough, D.L., Jankowski, M.K. *et al.* (1995) Comparison of time-tradeoff utilities and rating scale values of cancer patients and their relatives: evidence for a plateau relationship. *Med. Decis. Making* **15**, 132–7.

Orme, M. (1991) How to pay for expensive drugs. *BMJ* **303**, 593–4.

Osoba, D., Dancey, J., Zees, B. *et al.* (1996) Health-related quality of life studies of the National Cancer Institute of Canada Clinical Trials Group. *J. Natl Cancer Inst. Monogr.* **20**, 107–11.

Patrick, D.L. and Erikson, P. (1993) *Health Status and Health Policy.* New York: Oxford University Press.

Priestman, T.J., Bullimore, J.A., Godden, T.P. and Deutsch, G.P. (1989) The Royal College of Radiologists's fractionation survey. *Clin. Oncol.* **1**, 39–46.

Read, G. and Swindell, R. (1991) A computerised system for radiotherapy. *Clin. Oncol.* **3**, 230–2.

Read, J.L., Quinn, R.J., Berwick, D.M. *et al.* (1984) Preferences for health outcomes comparison of assessment methods. *Med. Decis. Making* **4**, 315–29.

Rees, G.J.G. (1985) Cost effectiveness in oncology. *Lancet* **ii**, 1405–8.

Rees, G. (1991) Cancer treatment: deciding what we can afford. *BMJ* **302**, 799–800.

Revicki, D.A. and Kaplan, R.M. (1993) Relationship between psychometric and utility-based approaches to the measurement of health-related quality of life. *Qual. Life Res.* **2**, 477–87.

Richards, M.A., Braysher, S., Gregory, W.M. and Rubens, R.D. (1993) Advanced breast cancer: use of resources and cost implications. *Br. J. Cancer* **76**, 856–60.

Roberts, C.J., Farrow, S.C. and Charny, M.C. (1985) How much can the NHS afford to spend. *Lancet* **i**, 89–91.

Saunders, M.I., Bennett, M.H., Dische, S. and Anderson, P.J. (1984) Primary tumour control after radiotherapy for cancer of the bronchus. *Int. J. Radiat. Oncol. Biol. Phys.* **10**, 499–501.

Secretaries of State for Health, Wales, Northern Ireland and Scotland (1989) *Working for patients.* London: HMSO.

Secretary of State for Scotland (1997) *Designed to care: renewing the National health service in Scotland.* Edinburgh: Stationery Office.

Slevin, M.L., Plant, H., Lynch, D., Drinkwater, J. and Gregory, W.M. (1988) Who should measure quality of life, the doctor or the patient? *Br. J. Cancer* **57**, 109–12.

Smith, T., Hillner, B.E. and Desch, C.E. (1993) Efficacy and cost-effectiveness of cancer treatment: Rational allocation of resources based on decision analysis. *J. Natl Cancer Inst.* **85**, 1460–74.

Sugden, R. and Williams, A. (1978) *The principles of practical cost benefit analysis.* Oxford: Oxford University Press.

Torrance, G.W. (1986) Measurement of health state utilities for economic appraisal. *J. Health Econ.* **5**, 1–30.

Vaidya, J.S. and Mittra, I. (1997) Fraction of remaining normal life span: a new method for expressing survival in cancer. *BMJ* **314**, 1682–4.

APPENDIX A: GLOSSARY OF TERMS

Bottom-up costing: calculation based on an aggregation of individual cost elements.

Direct costs: costs that can be attributed to a particular activity.

Fixed costs: costs that do not vary with changes in activity levels over a given time span.

Indirect costs: costs that cannot be directly attributed to a particular activity but can be shared over a number of them.

Marginal costs: costs incurred by a small increase in treatment activity, such as one additional patient.

Overhead costs: costs of support services which are not directly related to the volume of activity.

Ring fenced: protected money.

Semi-variable (semi-fixed) or 'step' costs: costs that are fixed for a given level of activity but may change if the activity rises or falls beyond a certain 'step'.

Top down costing: calculation based on an apportioning of total expenditure.

Top sliced: money removed at each NHS tier before allocation.

Variable costs: costs that vary in proportion to activity levels.

For a more detailed explanation see NHS(ME) Costing for Contracting. EL(93)26 Annex A.

60

Medical audit

AMIT K. BAHL AND GARETH J.G. REES

INTRODUCTION

Sporadic audit has always been part of medical practice, observations of the results of interventions leading to improvements in care for future patients. In recent years there has been a growing recognition of the importance of devoting adequate time to audit, and of doing it in an organized, systematic and cost-effective way. Regular participation in audit is now a contractual requirement for doctors working in the National Health Service. The climate for the assurance of standards has moved on considerably from the early 1990s. Far more external inspection of the performance of individual consultants is now envisaged and no anonymity is likely to be permitted. Under clinical governance, consultants will be required to demonstrate audit of their performance and results (Department of Health, 1998).

Medical audit of radiotherapy dates back to 1898 when the Roentgen Society appointed a committee to collect data on the effects of X-rays. A report of the results of treatment was a condition of the loan of radioactive material to hospitals in the late 1920s by the National Radium Commission, and this led to the establishment of national cancer registration. Radiotherapists can therefore be regarded as being among the leaders of medical audit in the UK (Hong *et al.*, 1990).

Audit of a business involves preparing a profit and loss account, which enables assessment of its success or failure, and identification of which elements of the business are fruitful and which are not. Audit in medicine has essentially the same objectives. It is an examination of activity that attempts to measure success or failure, and to identify remediable shortcomings. Improving care is dependent to a large extent on discovering what is being achieved at present. Most providers of cancer care have little or no objective quantitative information on what they are achieving for most of their patients in terms of quantity or quality of life. This degree of ignorance about achievement would be surprising in any other area of human endeavour utilizing comparable resources.

Medical audit has been defined as:

1 'The systematic, critical analysis of the quality of medical care, including procedures used for diagnosis and treatment, the use of resources and the resulting outcome and quality of life for the patients.'
2 'The sharing by a group of peers of information gained from personal experience and/or medical records in order to assess the care provided to their patients, to improve their own learning and to contribute to medical knowledge.'

Medical audit is different from clinical audit. The former is concerned with the quality of care provided and supervised by doctors. The latter involves assessment of the service provided by the healthcare system as a whole and is a multidisciplinary activity. The purpose of medical audit is to improve the quality of care by striving to ensure that individual doctors practise medicine to the highest standard which can reasonably be achieved with the resources available, and that they use those resources most effectively. Audit should be regarded principally as an educational process, mainly through promoting discussion between colleagues about clinical practice. The quality of medical work can, to a large extent, only be reviewed by a doctor's peers. Medical audit is an activity which is done by doctors and led by doctors.

Attempts are often made to draw a clear dividing line between medical audit and research. The quest for discovering new and better ways of caring for patients is research. Audit is concerned with analysing how effectively the knowledge gained from research is applied, with assessing and changing routine medical practice and improving standards. However, much of what has been described hitherto as clinical research has involved retrospective or prospective studies of groups of patients, their management and how they fared, with the aim of acquiring new knowledge which might help the management of future patients. This is essentially the first stage of medical audit. Clinical research and medical audit merge into one another. Indeed, the entry of patients into some types of prospective clinical trials, particularly those that involve already well-established treatments, should be viewed as an especially effective form of audit. Sitting somewhere in between the two disciplines of audit and research (although admittedly closer to research), health technology assessment (HTA) evaluates whether a piece of medical technology which has worked in a laboratory setting is actually effective in general use.

Audit is central to any programme to enhance the quality of care. An effective programme of audit will help to provide reassurance to patients, doctors and managers that the best possible care is being offered with the resources available. While the primary purpose of medical audit is clinical rather than managerial, and its focus is the process and results of medical care rather than resources, the results of audit may have implications for strategic decision-making by administrators and politicians on the allocation of resources and on the organization of services.

METHODOLOGY

General

Many techniques can be used for audit. These include such different activities as informal discussion of individual cases, large surveys of the management of groups of patients or the use of particular treatments and healthcare systems, comparative studies of the services provided by different doctors, departments, hospitals or even national healthcare systems.

Audit can be concerned with examining the resources provided and the way in which they are used for patients, in the belief that these – 'structure' and 'process' – will have a bearing on the result, or 'outcome' of care. However, for cancer patients what matters most is the outcome – are they being given the maximum chance of both quantity and quality of life? Outcome is the ideal indicator of the quality of patient care. Some measurements of outcome, e.g. survival, can be fairly easy to measure, while others, such as symptom relief or quality of life, are more difficult to quantify.

Audit of structure involves examination of the quantity and quality of resources, including both staff and equipment. Structure is not in itself an indicator of the quality of care and should only be used in conjunction with assessments of process and outcome. It can be helpful to identify significant variations in the provision of resources to examine whether they do affect results. Surveys of provision of oncologists and radiotherapy equipment have identified substantial intranational and international variations. In some instances, it is self-evident or already established, as a result of previous clinical research or medical audit, that certain structures and processes do influence outcome. However, the relationship between structure and process and outcomes is often more a matter of belief than science.

Effective audit will establish areas where outcome, process or structure is unsatisfactory, identify causal relationships between process/structure and outcome, and set in train alterations in management aimed at improving the care for future patients. However, audit is only truly successful if it goes on to establish that the improvements hoped for have been achieved. In audit jargon this is known as 'closing the loop'.

There are few aspects of care that might not benefit from critical review. Audit can involve analysis at many different levels of organization, from examining the care given to a single patient to comparisons of outcomes for patients treated in different continents. In most instances, medical audit is primarily of local value, but sometimes the methods and findings are relevant to a wider audience and suitable for presentation at meetings or for publication. However, the extent to which published audits have impact elsewhere is probably overestimated. Someone else's audit results are usually less powerful than one's own as an incentive to alter clinical practice.

Medical audit is principally an educational process for doctors. It is important that all doctors working within a department, including those in training, are fully involved. From time to time it will be helpful to involve paramedical staff in meetings devoted to clinical audit, e.g. nurses, radiographers and physicists, when particular topics of interdisciplinary interest are discussed.

Medical audit must be conducted within a clearly defined organizational framework if it is to be fully effective. It is best led by senior doctors. It will be more successful if there is maximum and enthusiastic participation. This is substantially dependent on the provision of adequate amounts of time and support. The latter includes personnel and appropriate computer hardware and software to facilitate the gathering and processing of statistical information. Enthusiasm also depends on the participants having freedom to decide those areas of medical care worth examining.

Confidentiality is extremely important for participation as well as for medico-legal reasons. Peer review findings concerning individual cases and doctors should usually be absolutely confidential, but it is often desirable for the more general or aggregated results of medical audit to be made more widely available. There should also be mechanisms for remedial action where mistakes are made repeatedly by individuals or groups.

The knowledge that errors will be discussed may, in itself, be a stimulus to improve quality of care, but it is difficult to maintain high levels of attendance if audit meetings are not stimulating and enjoyable. The atmosphere at meetings should not be threatening or adversarial. Criticism should be constructive and it should be acknowledged that everyone makes mistakes and that many variations in medical practice are acceptable. It is also important that audit should not be allowed to discourage doctors from undertaking difficult clinical work just because there is an element of risk involved.

The data for medical audit should ideally be readily accessible, timely, accurate, clinically relevant and as complete as possible. The quality of information produced by analysis of data is directly related to the quality of the data provided. The quality may be enhanced by involving clinicians in selecting the data to be collected and by collecting it as close to the activity that generates it as possible. It also helps to have regular involvement of those involved in data recording and collection in the audit process, and by keeping data collection within a realistic range. It is easy for medical audit to be over-ambitious. It is usually more sensible to audit particular aspects of care thoroughly and sequentially, rather than to try to examine several different areas simultaneously.

Good audit is a continuous cycle. This involves observing practice, setting desirable standards, comparing practice with standards, implementing change and observing the new practice. Ascertaining what has been or is being achieved is really only the beginning of audit. Audit is not just about measuring where you are – it is about measuring how far away you are from where you want to be.

Doctors could spend so long auditing themselves or other people that there would no longer be time to do the work that they are really meant to be doing. It makes sense to concentrate on those aspects that need looking at and to examine them in detail. If the time and resources made available for audit are to be used most effectively, the purpose of the audit should be made clear to all involved and topics for analysis should be chosen carefully, reflecting genuine interest and relevance. It is easy to waste large amounts of time and money on audit through a lack of clarity of purpose, unfocused data collection and inadequate motivation. Lasting change is usually very difficult to achieve and is greatly dependent on motivation.

The topics most suitable for audit will be those concerned with activities that are common, risky or expensive, or with areas where there are wide variations in management. Audit should provide an important means for the review and development of departmental treatment policies. Ideally a rolling programme should be established, enabling the sequential review of the management of particular conditions. It is important that no major area of care is excluded from audit. Ideally audit should be concerned not only with process and outcome, but with cost as well. Inequitably high expenditure on some patients will deprive a larger number of other patients of their entitlement, thereby reducing the average quality of care.

The management of individual patients or groups of patients should ideally be judged against predetermined guidelines, which may have been established locally or nationally. There is an increasing trend towards the development of clinical management guidelines at consensus development conferences, but such guidelines are often not very effective in promoting change without locally developed motivation and incentives.

Medical audit may reveal deficiencies in care that involve a few patients at random, deficiencies which are confined to those patients treated under particular circumstances, e.g. by a particular doctor or unit or at particular times, or deficiencies involving the care of all patients. The cause of deficiencies must be discovered before they can be remedied. Most instances of deficient care will be caused by a lack of one or more of the following:

1 feedback (doctors do not know how their performance compares with what can be achieved);
2 knowledge or skill;
3 motivation (e.g. discouraging working environment, personal health or emotional problems);
4 appropriate procedures (e.g. insufficient clarity about agreed clinical management policies or protocols, inadequate communications or documentation);
5 sufficient resources (equipment, drugs, staffing).

It is important to keep written records of audit meetings. Records should include lists of those attending and some broad information on the topics discussed, and the resulting conclusions and recommendations. These must be strictly confidential and the identity of patients and clinicians and other hospital staff must not be entered or be capable of being traced. A strict code of confidentiality must be established and maintained for all staff involved in audit, medical and non-medical.

Audit of audit

Not all audit studies are as effective as they could be. Completed audit studies should themselves be audited. An assessment of any audit study should involve asking *why* it was done, *how* it was done, and *what* it found.

The question asked should be simple and the methodology straightforward. All audit studies should have a clearly stated purpose. Ideally, the topic chosen should concern routine medical practice, be well defined and amenable to standard setting. This means the establishment of a consensus on what constitutes acceptable care and on the proportion of cases (which may be all of them) in which the care given should be at least as good as this. Such clear statements about the desired standard of care facilitate objective and quantitative comparison of the care actually given with that standard. This, where possible, is preferable to subjective assessment of the quality of care, dependent as it is on the vagaries of individual clinical judgement.

Meaningful conclusions from audit studies are as dependent on sample size as research studies. There is little point in trying to form conclusions about clinical management policies and quality on the basis of comparisons of the outcome for different groups of patients if the observed differences could easily have come about by chance. In drawing conclusions it is important to remember possible causes of bias in the study, such as case mix, non-response from sending questionnaires, the failure of some patients to attend for follow-up, and the unavailability of certain types of case notes (e.g. those of dead patients).

An ideal audit study will place emphasis on the implementation of change. It should not only identify room for improvement in the quality of care but should lead to recommendations, preferably specific, on how to remedy deficiencies, and then demonstrate that the recommendations have successfully been put into practice, thus completing the 'audit cycle'.

Computers

Computers are not needed for some types of audit, e.g. for case reviews and peer discussion of clinical practice, but systematic audit often requires the generation, storage and manipulation of large volumes of clinical information. Computerized clinical information systems are usually essential to support this type of activity.

It is important to decide what is wanted from a computer before buying one. Present and future uses must be taken into account. The production of information for audit is likely to be only part of its function. Collection and storage of data on patients and their management may also be required for resource management or research. Other functions, such as the automatic production of discharge summaries, may also be desirable. The types and amounts of data to be stored and processed, linkages with other systems and possible future extensions all need to be considered.

Many different software packages have been developed to support audit. Most have been designed to run on personal computers, but others have been developed for multi-user operation as part of, or integrating with, hospital or regional information systems. Such multi-user systems can offer a more cost-effective approach to audit, particularly as medical audit and hospital administration have some common information requirements. However, it is essential that linkages between systems be such that access to audit information is strictly controlled.

Several features may be important in choosing software. These include the flexibility to tailor the programme to individual requirements; a word processing facility; the ability to select cases against precept criteria indicating unexpected or adverse events and to identify cases falling outside a defined range of values; the potential for review of a particular topic (e.g. by diagnosis, complication or procedure). The system should be capable of simple data analysis or designed to be used with a statistical package. The mode of presentation of information is also important and a graphics facility is usually desirable. It is essential to take advice from appropriate experts before choosing a system but, where possible, it makes sense to use a system that has already been proven successful. Benghiat et al. (1999) have described a PC-based computer network that caters for the clinical information needs of a cancer centre, crossing speciality boundaries and involving all members of the multidisciplinary team. Data are captured at all stages of patients' progress, from diagnosis through to treatment and follow-up. Office automation is integral to the system, which produces workload and processes audit information as well as clinical outcomes. Data are entered prospectively at the point of care by healthcare professionals, ensuring a high degree of clinical confidence.

A dedicated computer information system for use in British oncological departments was developed through the Audit Office of the Royal College of Radiologists (Karp, 1994). Known as the Clinical Oncology Information Network (COIN), this system could computerize clinical records, facilitate patient management through monitoring progress through the various processes of care, summarize treatments and store data for audit. In addition, the system can facilitate recording of tumour stage using a graphical interface and could be used to prescribe chemotherapy and prevent errors. All clinical information, including details of radiotherapy and chemotherapy, could be entered via workstations situated in appropriate places. This departmental system will communicate with the hospital information system. The advantages of such a system for systematic medical audit in oncology are obvious and the use of a common system with agreed uniform standards for record keeping would facilitate the comparison of data between different centres.

The COIN workstation development represents a system that would support the clinician and evidence-based patient management (Rosalki and Karp, 1999). The successful deployment of a workstation as envisaged in COIN would permit audit on a remarkably complex scale, hopefully with all audit proving to be a by-product of the day-to-day management of patients (Karp, 1999).

Oncological audit

Much of the management of cancer patients, particularly non-surgical treatment, is centralized in regional cancer centres. Oncological audit should not be confined merely to what goes on in the cancer centre. It should embrace the wider geographical perspective and also the multidisciplinary nature of the total management of cancer patients.

Collaboration with general practitioners and with clinical and non-clinical hospital colleagues can be very fruitful. Useful audit can also be conducted through collaboration between centres, looking particularly at variations in process and outcome, and possible justifications and reasons for them. National and supranational societies and Royal Colleges can play a useful co-ordinating role. Wide variations still exist in the UK in the management of common cancers in adults. Development of, and adherence to, nationally agreed treatment protocols is a key measure in reducing variations in treatment and in outcomes for patients with cancer (Kunkler, 1997). The RCR COIN project was created in 1994 on behalf of the Faculty of Clinical Oncology and the Joint Council for Clinical Oncology, to co-ordinate the production of evidence-based clinical practice guidelines in oncology and to identify data sets to audit compliance with the guidelines. The guidelines for prostate, lung and breast cancer and generic radiotherapy have been published in *Clinical Oncology*. These are available on the website of the Royal College of Radiologists, UK.

INDIVIDUAL CASE REVIEW

This is one of the simplest types of audit. Cases are selected for discussion at regular meetings. They may be chosen at random but some selection helps to avoid repeated similar discussion about the management of patients with common conditions. For example, it may be useful to select patients with complications, or those who have died unexpectedly. Discussion on such cases is different from traditional 'staff rounds' in that the cases are selected and the discussion led by someone not involved in the patient's management. A structured approach to case review is often helpful.

Cases may be chosen for discussion on the basis of a list of pre-set well-defined criteria. Examples of such criteria are listed in Table 60.1. Large numbers of case notes may be screened by a non-medically qualified audit assistant, thereby making most effective use of doctors' time for audit.

The management of many of the cases selected for discussion on the basis of such criteria will not be found to have been deficient – often there will be acceptable reasons for what did or did not happen. However, such a process can highlight individual and systematic deficiencies in the service, and it can also illuminate areas where available resources are not being used effectively.

Necropsies can be a fruitful component of individual case review. Many studies have showed that about 1 in 10 cases coming to necropsy have pathological lesions that would have materially altered clinical management if they had been identified before death. There has been a decline in hospital necropsies in the UK.

Table 60.1 *Examples of criteria for selecting cases for discussion*

Delay of more than a specified duration between referral and clinic appointment

Delay of more than a specified duration between clinic consultation and start of treatment

Delay of more than a specified duration between consultation and letter to GP

Histology report not filed in notes

Lack of specification in notes of TNM stage for patients receiving radical treatment

Target symptom(s) not specified for patients receiving palliative treatment

Lack of documentation of information given to patient and/or relatives

No up-to-date serum haemoglobin estimation for patients embarking on radical radiotherapy

Treatment not completed as planned

Lack of documentation of termination or alteration of systemic treatment following evidence of tumour progression

Death within a short time of completing radiotherapy or cytotoxic chemotherapy

Duration of palliative radiotherapy more than 10% of remaining survival

Death within 6 months of radical treatment

Lack of documentation of contact with general practitioner following death in hospital

---

Communication of results of necropsies to hospital doctors, general practitioners and relatives is often inadequate. A joint working party of the Royal Colleges of Pathologists, Physicians and Surgeons recommended in 1991 that the relevant clinicians should receive a summary of the significant findings within a couple of days of the necropsy and a complete report within 3 weeks, but these standards are frequently not attained. The negative effect of poor communication to clinicians may have contributed to the general decline in necropsy rates. In a study of lay perceptions of the results of necropsy, 88 per cent of relatives were reassured about the adequacy of medical care and benefited from explanations of their deceased relative's illness. It is often not practical for doctors to attend necropsies, but there is scope for increasing considerably the use of photographic and video material at clinicopathological conferences.

It is important that necropsies are themselves properly performed and audited. The working party recommended that histological examination should be part of every examination. It also recommended that, as well as necropsies performed for specific reasons such as verifying the cause of death, a necropsy rate of at least 10 per cent of other general hospital deaths should be the target. These two categories might together amount to a total of about a third of all hospital deaths. Discrepancies between ante-mortem and post-mortem diagnoses should be monitored and made available to consultants on an individual basis.

ANALYSIS OF GROUPS OF PATIENTS

Quantitative measurement of the process or outcome of care for defined groups of patients is a particularly important type of audit. The findings are often very illuminating in themselves, but sometimes they may also usefully be compared with results obtained elsewhere, and perhaps with consensus opinions on what are the optimal achievable standards of care.

Variations in process tend to be greater than variations in outcome. The identification of substantial variations in the use of resources, e.g. radiotherapy fractionation, can lead to more cost-effective management. However, where there is variation in resource usage it is important to relate this to outcome before concluding that the cheapest policy is the most cost effective.

The simplest and most important example of auditing outcome in oncology is the calculation of survival figures for patients with given tumours, stage by stage. The measurement of survival is particularly appropriate for cancer patients treated with curative intent and this long-established tradition accounts for oncological practice being in the vanguard of audit in twentieth-century medicine. Several cancer centres around the world now publish survival figures routinely.

It is important that survival figures are evaluated critically. It may not be reasonable to expect figures quoted

Table 60.2 *Examples of subjects for systematic audit in oncology*

Survival, stage by stage, for patients treated radically
Intervals between presentation, diagnosis and treatment
Waiting time in hospital departments
Usefulness of investigations
Adequacy of histopathological reports
Frequency of on-treatment review of patients receiving
  radiotherapy
Adequacy of excision margins
Incidence and severity of complications of treatment,
  including iatrogenic death
Prevention, management and outcome of complications
Success in relieving target symptom(s) with palliative
  treatment
Comparison of frequency of particular treatments,
  duration of treatment and hospital stay and policies of
  follow-up between different doctors, institutions and
  geographical areas
Conformity of investigations, drug usage and radiotherapy
  with agreed protocols
Costs and cost-effectiveness of care
Patient satisfaction with total service provided, and with
  particular aspects such as the provision of information
  and involvement in decisions
General practitioner satisfaction with service provided

in clinical research publications to be achieved in routine management elsewhere. There may have been deliberate or unwitting case selection, different staging procedures and publication bias. In comparing the results between different institutions, it is important to be satisfied that, as far as is possible, one is comparing like with like. Such studies must be particularly rigorous in their methodology and subject to monitoring by external assessors. Examples of other types of systematic analysis are shown in Table 60.2.

EXAMPLES OF PUBLISHED AUDITS

Structure and process

RESOURCE ALLOCATION

The Board of the Faculty of Clinical Oncology of the Royal College of Radiologists (1991) conducted a survey of medical manpower and workload in clinical oncology in the UK. There were 240 consultants in post, no more than a decade before, despite an increase of 20 per cent in the number of new patients referred during the decade and increased complexity of clinical management. On average each consultant saw 560 new patients per year, 2–3 times as many as their counterparts in the USA and Europe. On average each consultant had 2000 patients under his care at any one time, of which approximately half would be receiving active medical care.

The provision of facilities for radiotherapy in the USA, Europe and a single large British centre were compared by Maher *et al.* (1990). The mean annual numbers of patients per simulator in the American and European hospitals were 619 and 1185 respectively, compared with 3345 in the British centre. The corresponding figures for numbers of patients per megavoltage treatment machine were 210, 501 and 1100. There is also marked geographical variation in radiotherapeutic intent. For example, radiotherapy is given with radical intent for carcinoma of the bronchus to a far greater extent in Italy, Holland and the USA than in the UK.

A survey of clinical oncology services to district general hospitals in the UK revealed that the average total weekly commitment of cancer specialists at these hospitals was just under two sessions per week (Rees *et al.*, 1991). Many cancer patients were not being referred for a specialized oncological opinion. The authors identified a need for a substantial increase in sessional commitment by visiting oncologists to cope with the number of patients, the increased demands for more complex treatments and the need for better communication with patients.

Finlay *et al.* (1992) audited the use of, and satisfaction with, local services for the care of the dying in South Glamorgan. In general, there was a high level of satisfaction but inadequacies were perceived in the provision of inpatient and domiciliary nursing support and in services for patients without cancer. The survey was presented to the Health Authority and the recommendations aimed at remedying the inadequacies were implemented. The authors planned a further audit to evaluate the effectiveness of the implementations.

ORGANIZATION OF SERVICES

Earlam (1984) audited the management of oesophageal cancer in the North-East Thames Region. Hospital activity analysis data were used to examine the care given to 444 patients admitted with oesophageal cancer: 80 were intubated without a thoracotomy or laparotomy, 73 underwent surgery (66 per cent radical, 33 per cent palliative), with an overall mortality of 33 per cent; 55 were documented to have received radiotherapy and 179 patients had no recorded operation or investigation. These inpatients had been looked after by 177 different consultants, mostly general surgeons. Only five consultants looked after 10 or more patients each year. The audit underestimated the use of radiotherapy because radiotherapy given to outpatients was not included in the inpatient analysis. Nevertheless, there were strong arguments in favour of surgical specialization and it appeared that far too many patients were not receiving adequate palliation for their dysphagia. One hundred and nine patients died in hospital without any therapeutic procedure being recorded. Many acute hospital beds were being used inappropriately for terminal care, incurring a waste of large amounts of money. Earlam concluded that it would be more humane for more patients to die at home or in a hospice.

Junor et al. (1992) audited the travel and waiting times for outpatients receiving radiotherapy at a single centre. They found unacceptable treatment waiting times for many patients and concluded that the service might be improved by the provision of hostel or hotel accomodation and a computerized appointment system which would take into account the treatment machine, mode of transport and geographical area in which the patient lived.

Jones and Dudgeon (1992) investigated the time between a person presenting to a general practitioner with a symptom of cancer and that person starting treatment. They analysed retrospectively the records of 1465 cancer patients registered with 245 general practitioners, assuring confidentiality by using a coding system. They discovered considerable variation in processing, particularly in the time taken in different (unnamed) hospitals from hospital appointment to treatment. The authors believed that their study highlighted the need for general practitioners to review their diagnostic procedures on a regular basis and for hospital staff to review their own work.

DIAGNOSIS

MacKie and Hole (1992) evaluated a public campaign to encourage earlier referral and treatment of primary cutaneous melanoma in the west of Scotland. Following the distribution of educational material, the referrals to the pigmented lesion clinic increased almost fourfold and the numbers of newly diagnosed melanomas more than doubled. The percentage of tumours detected that were less than 1.5 mm thick rose significantly from 38 per cent to 54 per cent. Three years after the campaign started there was a decline in mortality from melanoma in women.

Schmidt et al. (1998) audited the reporting of 26 711 diagnostic breast-imaging studies performed over a period of 5 years. Within the first 18 months, several general radiologists reported mammograms, whereas during the rest of the evaluated period only one radiologist was responsible for all mammography reporting. In the first 2 years the percentages of small cancers detected (Tis or T1a, b) were 27.2 per cent and 25.7 per cent, respectively. In the third, fourth and fifth years, the percentages increased to 38.8 per cent, 34.5 per cent and 38.8 per cent, respectively. The authors concluded that the detection of curable early stage breast carcinomas requires the dedication and commitment of a small group of radiologists who are willing to spend most of their time on this single subject. This will increase considerably the number of early stage cancers found and reduce the number of false-positive diagnoses.

Many groups have studied delay in the diagnosis of cancer. It can be easy for hospital specialists to underestimate the difficulties faced by general practitioners. The major reason for delay attributable to the doctor is the low predictive value of most symptoms, which are far more likely to be caused by common benign conditions than malignancy. However, while Dixon et al. (1990) found that 70 per cent of patients with left-sided colorectal tumours and 87 per cent with right-sided tumours were referred by their GP urgently and with the correct diagnosis, 12 per cent of patients with easily palpable rectal tumours were referred for treatment of haemorrhoids without a rectal examination.

PATHOLOGY REPORTING

Blenkinsopp et al. (1981) reviewed the histopathology reports on 2046 patients from 22 histopathology departments. They found considerable observer variation in histological grading, Dukes' staging and in lymph-node harvesting. Most avoidable errors lay not in the assessment of microscopical appearances but in the macroscopic observations. This suggested that some histopathologists were not giving sufficient time or care to the 'cut-up' and morbid anatomical examination of surgical specimens. There was a need for more co-operation between surgeons and pathologists. The authors felt that cancer of the large bowel was sufficiently common for consistent and reliable reports to be obtainable with relatively little effort.

Dey et al. (1997) conducted a regional survey on the completeness of reporting on prognostic factors for breast cancer. The study population was 885 cases of invasive breast cancer diagnosed in NHS laboratories in Lancashire and Greater Manchester. Histological type, tumour size, presence or absence of tumour in vascular channels, and adequacy of excision were recorded for 843 (95 per cent), 803 (91 per cent), 436 (49 per cent) and 761 (86 per cent) cases, respectively. The authors concluded that non-screening and low throughput laboratories were significantly less likely to record certain histopathological features.

RADIOTHERAPY FRACTIONATION

A survey of British radiotherapeutic practice undertaken by Priestman *et al.* (1989) on behalf of the Royal College of Radiologists discovered a wide variety of dose/fractionation regimens. In only one situation – the palliative treatment of carcinoma of the bronchus – did more than 25 per cent of oncologists use the same treatment schedule. Training and established local policies, rather than the results of clinical trials, emerged as the major influences on practice. While the degree of therapeutic variation in radiobiological terms was far less marked, the survey did identify a need for critical appraisal of treatment schedules to ensure the most cost-effective use of resources.

Dodwell *et al.* (1993), in Leeds, studied the effect of medical audit on prescription of palliative radiotherapy. They reviewed the case notes of patients given palliative radiotherapy for bone metastases and for inoperable lung cancer over a 2-week period and presented their findings at two medical audit meetings to all consultants and junior staff. After discussion of two published prospective studies showing that shorter palliative regimens were as effective as longer ones for these two conditions, local consensus guidelines were established, suggesting that in most cases patients with painful bone metastases should be given a single fraction and those with inoperable lung cancer two fractions a week apart. A year later they reviewed the case notes of patients who had recently been treated for the same indications. The percentage of patients receiving courses of five or more fractions of palliative radiotherapy for painful bone metastases fell from 62 per cent (95 per cent confidence interval 50–74 per cent) to 27 per cent (18–38 per cent), and for lung cancer from 79 per cent (65–93 per cent) to 52 per cent (40–64 per cent). However, although there had been a statistically significant reduction overall in the number of fractions used for both indications, there was still a considerable difference between the local consensus guidelines and actual clinical practice, variations in practice between clinicians and a lack of entry in case notes of reasons for departure from consensus guidelines. Maher *et al.* (1990) also documented that consecutive audits conducted at Mount Vernon Hospital had demonstrated a reduction in the number of fractions used in palliative radiotherapy.

Process and outcome

MALIGNANT MELANOMA

Herd *et al.* (1992) conducted a study of patients who had had malignant melanomas excised by general practitioners. Completeness of excision was doubtful or incomplete in 23 per cent, compared with 4 per cent of hospital excisions, and melanoma had only been mentioned as a possible diagnosis in 15 per cent of the accompanying pathology request forms, indicating both a need for general practitioners to think more often of melanoma when they excise pigmented lesions and to excise such lesions with a lateral clearance of at least 2 mm.

GASTROINTESTINAL CANCER

Sue-Ling *et al.* (1993) described a prospective audit of all cases of gastric cancer treated in Leeds during 1970–89. Over this 20-year period the introduction of open-access endoscopy had resulted in a fourfold increase in its use. The proportion of patients undergoing potentially curative resection rose from 31 per cent in the first 5-year period to 53 per cent in the last 5-year period, reflecting an increase in the proportion of patients with stage I disease from 4 per cent to 26 per cent. Surgical resections were more radical in the 1980s than in the 1970s. More recent departmental policy was to perform wide gastric resection and a lymphadenectomy involving removal of the second tier of nodes beyond the perigastric nodes. Despite this, operative mortality decreased from 9 per cent in the 1970s to 5 per cent in the 1980s, and the incidence of serious postoperative complications fell from 33 per cent to 17 per cent.

By the late 1980s 5-year survival after operation was about 70 per cent. The authors concluded that an increasing proportion of patients with gastric cancer could be diagnosed at a relatively early pathological stage when about two-thirds are curable by radical surgery.

The incidence of anastomotic leakage after surgery for large bowel cancer varied from 0.5 per cent to 30 per cent in a study involving 84 surgeons (Fielding *et al.*, 1980). The Wessex Cancer Intelligence Unit (1990) studied the cost-effectiveness of treatment for colorectal cancer in three health districts. District 1 had the highest mean cost of surgical treatment for rectal cancer, largely attributable to longer inpatient stay and theatre time. However, the permanent colostomy rate was lower in district 1 and the mean survival of rectal cancer patients in this district was 3 years, compared with an average of 2.5 years in the other districts. The apparent advantages of treatment in this district persisted after stage standardization. In district 1, colorectal cancer was being treated primarily by one surgeon who had developed a specialized technique for rectal cancer, involving a lower than average anastomosis and total excision of the mesorectum. Although the cost of treatment was increased by this technique, the cost per life year gained was lower than in the other districts.

OVARIAN CANCER

In an audit of surgery for 908 patients treated in the North-East Thames Region for primary ovarian cancer and followed up to death or a minimum of 5 years, the full traditional procedure of total hysterectomy together with removal of the omentum, in addition to bilateral oophorectomy, was only recorded in 12 per cent of cases with FIGO stage III disease (Hudson *et al.*, 1991). In stages III and IV disease, optimal cytoreduction with minimal residual disease had been achieved in 85 of 372 cases (24 per cent). This contrasted with the achievement of optimal cytoreduction in about 85 per cent of cases operated on by specialist gynaecological oncologists. The overall survival of these patients was worse than most reports in the literature, and the authors concluded that there was a need for an enhanced provision of specialist gynaecological oncological expertise. While exclusive oncological subspecialization would not be feasible in many hospitals in the foreseeable future, it was argued that existing resources could be used with greater effect by improved preoperative investigation, consequent enablement of the optimal disposition of resources for an elective procedure, not allowing patients with potentially malignant ovarian masses to be left to unsupported trainee surgeons and enhanced collaboration between colleagues.

The 10-year survival of patients treated for early stage ovarian cancer in the west of Scotland in 1974 was significantly higher in teaching than in non-teaching hospitals (Gillis *et al.*, 1991). The 'curative' resection rate was higher in teaching hospitals. The overall survival rate in the west of Scotland for ovarian cancer improved by 6 per cent between 1975 and 1987, but the improvement in women under the age of 55 was significantly greater in teaching than in non-teaching hospitals, consistent with their having received more aggressive therapy.

CARCINOMA OF THE CERVIX

The Patterns of Care Study is designed to provide valid national average figures for the process and outcome of radiotherapy in the USA. Detailed analysis is performed of patient records from a random selection of treatment facilities. The findings of the second National Practice Survey of 565 patients with carcinoma of the cervix treated in 1978 were published in 1990 and a final report of the 1973 and 1978 studies was published in 1991 (Lanciano *et al.*, 1991). The use of intracavitary irradiation significantly improved survival and reduced local failures. The results were better for patients with unilateral rather than bilateral parametrial involvement, suggesting a possible justification for subdividing stage IIb disease. National USA benchmarks were established with respect to survival, pelvic control and complications.

A retrospective analysis of 140 patients with stage Ib cervical carcinoma treated by either surgery or radiotherapy demonstrated the two modalities to have equivalent efficacy, but there was increased late morbidity in irradiated patients (Gaze *et al.*, 1992). The audit resulted in increased multidisciplinary collaboration, agreed protocols for staging, treatment and follow-up and prospective recording of clinical data, investigations, full treatment details and assessment at follow-up, including standardized documentation of bowel, bladder and sexual function. The authors considered that these implementations would help to ensure that future audits would be more reliable.

TESTICULAR CANCER

The care of 429 patients with malignant teratoma treated in five different units in the west of Scotland was audited by Harding *et al.* (1993). The proportion of men receiving nationally agreed protocol treatment was higher in the authors' unit than elsewhere. Their unit treated the largest number of patients. The survival of patients treated at this unit, adjusted for other important prognostic variables, was also better than in the other units and the benefit seemed to be additional to any advantage resulting from protocol treatment. These patients had been treated over a 14-year period beginning 18 years earlier. The findings suggested strongly that centralization of treatment for malignant teratoma improves outcome. The authors concluded that the cumulative expertise in pathology, radiology, biochemistry and surgery, in addition to that of the oncology staff, contributed to the improved survival.

HEAD AND NECK CANCER

Audit of handicap after radical neck dissection in 46 patients showed that half had to give up work because of problems with the shoulder due to sacrifice of the accessory nerve (Shone and Yardley, 1991). Appreciable pain was experienced by one-third of patients. The authors believed that accessory nerve function should be preserved whenever possible.

Hong *et al.* (1990) at Mount Vernon Hospital audited the treatment and outcome of all 545 patients with head and neck cancer during the 8-year period from 1980 to 1987. Their local control and survival rates compared favourably with results reported from other institutions. The authors drew attention to the resources necessary to perform such an audit. Medical staff, data managers, cancer registry staff and statisticians together spent almost 1 hour for each patient. The increasing prospective computerization of patient data, treatment details and outcome would make similar audits much less labour intensive in future.

Robertson *et al.* (1998) audited the effect of the length and position of unplanned gaps in radiotherapy treatment schedules on 5-year local control of laryngeal cancer and the disease-free period. They reported that unplanned gaps in treatment were associated with poorer local control rates and an increased hazard of a local recurrence through extending the treatment time. A gap of 1 day was potentially damaging but the greatest effect was with treatment extensions of 3 or more days. The treatment extension as a result of the gap was more important than the position of the gap in the schedule. The authors concluded that gaps in the treatment schedule have a detrimental effect on the disease-free period and any gap in the treatment is potentially damaging.

BREAST CANCER

Basnett et al. (1992) compared the management and outcome of almost 1000 women with breast cancer presenting between 1982 and 1986 at two centres in a region, one of which was a teaching hospital. Patients treated in the teaching hospital were more likely to have isotopic bone scans, liver scans, ultrasound breast scans and mammography, but the diagnostic yield was lower, e.g. 1 in 10 bone scans was positive compared with 1 in 4 in the non-teaching hospital. Completeness of excision was mentioned in 79 per cent of the histopathology reports in the teaching hospital, but only in 11 per cent in the non-teaching hospital. Axillary sampling or clearance, radiotherapy, adjuvant chemotherapy and chemotherapy on relapse were all given more frequently in the teaching hospital. In both hospitals there was a decline in mean inpatient stay from 1982 to 1986. In 1982 the mean inpatient stay was almost twice as high in the teaching hospital, but by 1986 it was almost twice as high in the non-teaching hospital. There was no difference in local recurrence between the two hospitals, but survival, adjusted for age and stage, was significantly longer in patients treated at the teaching hospital. The authors urged caution in concluding that the increased survival was attributable to particular features of management. Staging was not done in a standard fashion in both centres and the study was retrospective and non-randomized. However, management was determined as much by where patients were referred as by the scientific evidence. The variations in management were difficult to justify and had substantial resource implications. The authors concluded that the study indicated a need to establish greater uniformity of care through the use of protocols based on consensus development.

The impetus for optimizing outpatient provision of breast-care services has come both from the patient and management in order to reduce anxiety and make full use of scarce resources. The one-stop diagnostic clinic for the investigation of symptomatic breast lesions is a relatively recent concept with well-known service benefits. Berry et al. (1998) audited patient acceptance of one-stop diagnosis for symptomatic breast disease and concluded that there was a high level of patient satisfaction.

MULTIPLE MYELOMA

A study of survival of patients with multiple myeloma in Finland showed that patients treated within clinical trials survived better than those treated outside trials (Karjalainen and Palva, 1989). The effect appeared to be unattributable to variations in prognostic variables, diagnostic procedures and the use of more effective regimens, suggesting that the use of a treatment protocol (giving rules on how to deal with relapses and side-effects) improved the end result of treatment. The authors postulated that physicians committed to the trials might have become more experienced.

SOFT-TISSUE SARCOMA

Clasby et al. (1997) audited the management of soft-tissue sarcoma by retrieving the records of 377 patients with primary soft-tissue sarcoma treated in the South-East Thames region between 1986 and 1992. Most patients (53.6 per cent) were treated by general surgeons, irrespective of tumour location. Overall only 21.3 per cent were investigated optimally, with wide variation among specialities. Only 60.0 per cent were treated adequately (wide excision or surgery with radiotherapy). Uptake of adjunctive therapy and follow-up were variable, and outcome was poorer, in patients having a marginal excision and recurrence. The authors concluded that investigation and management of many patients with soft-tissue sarcoma was both variable and suboptimal, having implications for patient care, resource uptake and costs, and they recommended that patients with sarcoma are more appropriately managed in specialist centres.

PAEDIATRIC CANCER

Stiller (1988) found that survival was higher at paediatric oncology centres than elsewhere for children with non-Hodgkin's lymphoma, Ewing's tumour, rhabdomyosarcoma and osteosarcoma. No differences were found for Hodgkin's disease, Wilms' tumour or neuroblastoma, but the paediatric centres had a considerably higher proportion of patients with advanced neuroblastoma.

Pritchard et al. (1989) found evidence of overtreatment of children with Wilms' tumour outside paediatric oncology centres. This study assessed the treatment of British children in centres that were not in the UK Children's Cancer Study Group (which had developed agreed protocols) over a 3-year period. Ten of the 20 children studied had received more treatment with radiotherapy or chemotherapy than recommended, and their survival rate was less than that for children treated contemporaneously in the UKCCSG first trial, although the difference was not statistically significant.

PALLIATIVE CARE

A clinical audit of the treatment of cancer-related pain, ordered by Stockholm County Council and the

Karolinska Institute, was performed at two Stockholm hospitals (Arner *et al.*, 1999). Of 153 consecutive cancer patients, 93 (61 per cent) reported pain, varying in intensity from 2.4 to 6.6 on a 10-point visual analogue scale. The pain was cancer related in 20 patients, treatment related in 28 patients, and associated with disease in 40 patients (e.g. post-herpetic neuralgia, urethritis, decubital ulcer or constipation). Nine patients had undetected neuropathic pain components, and 18 patients reported both significant pain intensity and dissatisfaction with the treatment. The auditors found these patients to have persistent pain problems despite the availability of time and opportunity to resolve them. The hospital departments were all found to be characterized by similar problems: lack of pain analysis or diagnosis, failure to detect neuropathic pain components, and underdosing of opioid analgesics irrespective of pain intensity. The auditors' conclusions included a need for pain education, particularly for doctors, as fewer doctors than nurses had attended pain courses.

EFFECTIVENESS OF FOLLOW-UP

Rathmell *et al.* (1993) examined the effectiveness of follow-up examinations and investigations for 29 patients who had relapsed following treatment for metastatic germ-cell tumours of the testis. The analysis showed that routine estimation of serum tumour markers was the single most important follow-up procedure, even in patients who were previously marker negative. It was the first indicator of relapse in 55 per cent of the patients. Regular clinical examinations and chest radiography in asymptomatic patients were of little value. Chest radiography gave the first evidence of relapse in only two patients, but computed tomographic (CT) scanning of the chest and abdomen was the first abnormal investigation in seven patients. The authors also undertook a cost analysis. The costs per relapse detected by tumour marker assay and by CT scanning were £1800 and £12 880, respectively. With such a large discrepancy in cost effectiveness it was concluded that the CT scan interval could be extended with a large cost saving, and to the potential detriment of only the few patients with marker-negative relapse.

GEOGRAPHICAL AND SOCIAL INFLUENCES

Marked variations in disease-specific mortality rates were observed among the 98 area health authorities in Wales and England (Charlton *et al.*, 1983). The differences persisted after standardization for social factors. There was a statistically significant fourfold difference in mortality from carcinoma of the cervix. Large sociodemographic differences in cancer survival have also been discovered (Kogevinas, 1990). Statistically significant regional differences in survival were found for bladder, breast and colon cancer, survival being better in the south and east regions of England and worse in the north of England and in Wales. For cancers of poor prognosis,

survival differences between socio-economic groups were small, but in some good-prognosis cancers the differences were wide, e.g. more than 2 years between owner-occupiers and council tenants for cancer of the corpus uteri. For the majority of cancers, people in better socio-economic circumstances had a greater probability of surviving their cancer than those in poorer circumstances, once account was taken of sex and age.

Marked international variations in cancer survival in Europe have been demonstrated in an analysis based on data from 33 cancer registries in 17 countries, covering the period 1978–89 (Coerbergh *et al.*, 1998). For all the common cancers – lung, breast, colorectal and prostate – the British survival figures are well below the European average. It seems likely that this reflects an inferior quality of care and the need for increased resources (Sikora, 1999).

SIGNIFICANT POINTS

- Good audit addresses important clinical activities (e.g. those that are common, high risk or high cost).
- It has a clearly stated purpose, is simple in design and uses resources efficiently.
- It assesses quality of care using objective criteria.
- It aims to bring about an improvement in outcome through a change in structure and/or process.
- It should be free of significant bias and be statistically sound.
- It requires regular and enthusiastic participation by all those involved.
- It stimulates the development and review of protocols for clinical management.

KEY REFERENCES

Crombie, I.K., Davies, H.T.O., Abraham, S.C.S. and Florey, C. du V. (1993) *The audit handbook.* Chichester: Wiley.

Pollock, A. and Evans, M. (1993) *Surgical audit.* Oxford: Butterworth-Heinemann.

Royal College of Physicians of London (1989) *Medical audit – a first report: what, why and how?* London: RCP.

Shaw, C. (1992) *Speciality medical audit.* London: King's Fund Centre.

Working Party of the Royal College of Radiologists (1991) *Medical audit in clinical oncology.* London: RCR.

REFERENCES

Arner, S., Killander, E. and Westerberg, H. (1999) Poor leadership behind poor pain relief. Medical audit of cancer-related pain treatment. *Lakartidningen* **96**(1–2), 33–6.

Basnett, I., Gill, M. and Tobias, J.S. (1992) Variations in breast cancer management between a teaching and a non-teaching district. *Eur. J. Cancer* **28A**, 1945–50.

Benghiat, A., Saunders, V. and Steele, W.V. (1999) Computerizing the cancer centre. *Clin. Oncol.* **11**(1), 33–9.

Berry, M.G., Chan, S.Y., Engledow, A. *et al.* (1998) An audit of patient acceptance of one-stop diagnosis for symptomatic breast disease. *Eur. J. Surg. Oncol.* **24**(6), 492–5.

Blenkinsopp, W.K., Stewart-Brown, S., Blesovsky, L. *et al.* (1981) Histopathology reporting in large bowel cancer. *J. Clin. Pathol.* **34**, 509–13.

Board of the Faculty of Clinical Oncology (1991) *Medical manpower and workload in clinical oncology in the United Kingdom.* London: The Royal College of Radiologists.

Charlton, J.R.H., Hartley, R.M., Silver, R. and Holland, W.W. (1983) Geographical variation in mortality from conditions amenable to medical intervention in England and Wales. *Lancet* **i**, 691–6.

Clasby, R., Tilling, K., Smith, M.A. and Fletcher, C.D. (1997) Variable management of soft tissue sarcoma: regional audit with implications for specialist care. *Br. J. Surg.* **84**(12), 1692–6.

Coebergh, J., Sant, M., Berrino, F. and Verdecchia, A. (1998) Survival of adult cancer patients in Europe diagnosed from 1978–1989: the Eurocare II study. *Eur. J. Cancer* **34**, 2137–278.

Department of Health (1998) *The new NHS: modern, dependable.* London: Department of Health.

Dey, P., Woodman, C.B., Gibbs, A. and Coyne, J. (1997) Completeness of reporting on prognostic factors for breast cancer: a regional survey. *J. Clin. Pathol.* **50**(10), 829–31.

Dixon, A.R., Thornton-Holmes, J. and Cheetham, N.M. (1990) General practitioners' awareness of colorectal cancer: a 10-year review. *BMJ* **301**, 152–3.

Dodwell, D., Bond, M., Elwell, C. *et al.* (1993) Effect of medical audit on prescription of palliative radiotherapy. *BMJ* **307**, 24–5.

Earlam, R. (1984) Oesophageal cancer treatment in North-East Thames region, 1981: medical audit using hospital activity analysis data. *BMJ* **288**, 1892–4.

Fielding, L.P., Stewart-Brown, S., Blesovsky, L. and Kearney, G. (1980) Anastomotic integrity after operations for large bowel cancer. A multicentre study. *BMJ* **281**, 411–14.

Finlay, I., Wilkinson, C. and Gibbs, C. (1992) Planning palliative care services. *Health Trends* **24**,139–41.

Gaze, M.N., Kelly, C.G., Dunlop, P.R.C. *et al.* (1992) Stage IB cervical carcinoma: a clinical audit. *Br. J. Radiol.* **65**, 1018–24.

Gillis, C.R., Hole, D.J., Still, R.M. *et al.* (1991) Medical audit, cancer registration, and survival in ovarian cancer. *Lancet* **337**, 611–12.

Harding, J.M., Paul, J., Gillis, C.R. and Kaye, S.B. (1993) Management of malignant teratoma: does referral to a specialist unit matter? *Lancet* **341**, 999–1002.

Herd, R.M., Hunter, J.A.A., McLaren, K.M. *et al.* (1992) Excision biopsy of malignant melanoma by general practitioners in south east Scotland 1982–91. *BMJ* **305**, 1476–8.

Hong, A., Saunders, M.I., Dische, S. *et al.* (1990) An audit of head and neck cancer treatment in a regional centre for radiotherapy and oncology. *Clin. Oncol.* **2**, 130–7.

Hudson, C.N., Potsides, P. and Curling, O.M. (1991) An audit of surgical treatment of ovarian cancer in a metropolitan health region. *J. R. Soc. Med.* **84**, 206–9.

Jones, R.V.H. and Dudgeon, T.A. (1992) Time between presentation and treatment of six common cancers: a study in Devon. *Br. J. Gen. Pract.* **42**, 419–22.

Junor, E.J., Macbeth, F.R. and Barrett, A. (1992) An audit of travel and waiting times for outpatient radiotherapy. *Clin. Oncol.* **4**, 174–6.

Karjalainen, S. and Palva, I. (1989) Do treatment protocols improve end results? A study of survival of patients with multiple myeloma in Finland. *BMJ* **299**, 1069–72.

Karp, S.J. (1994) Clinical Oncology Information Network. *BMJ* **308**, 147–8.

Karp, S.J. (1999) Clinical Oncology Information Network: from drawing board to reality. *Clin. Oncol.* **11**, 2–3.

Kogevinas, M. (1990) *Longitudinal study: sociodemographic differences in cancer survival.* Office of Population Censuses and Surveys. London: HMSO.

Kunkler, I.H. (1997) Variations in the management of cancer in the NHS: a legitimate cause for concern? *J. Eval. Clin. Pract.* **3**(3), 173–7.

Lanciano, R.M., Won, M., Coia, L.R. and Hanks, G.E. (1991) Pretreatment and treatment factors associated with improved outcome in squamous cell carcinoma of the uterine cervix: a final report of the 1973 and 1978 patterns of care studies. *Int. J. Radiat. Oncol. Biol. Phys.* **20**, 667–76.

MacKie, R.M. and Hole, D. (1992) Audit of public education campaign to encourage earlier detection of malignant melanoma. *BMJ* **304**, 1012–15.

Maher, E.J., Dische, S., Grosch, E. *et al.* (1990) Who gets radiotherapy? *Health Trends* **2**, 78–83.

Priestman, T.J., Bullimore, J.A., Godden, T.P. and Deutsch, G.P. (1989) The Royal College of Radiologists' fractionation survey. *Clin. Oncol.* **1**, 39–46.

Pritchard, J., Stiller, C.A. and Lennox, E.L. (1989) Overtreatment of children with Wilms' tumour outside paediatric oncology centres. *BMJ* **299**, 835–6.

Rathmell, A.J., Brand, I.R., Carey, B.M. and Jones, W.G. (1993) Early detection of relapse after treatment for metastatic germ cell tumour of the testis: an exercise in medical audit. *Clin. Oncol.* **5**, 34–8.

Rees, G.J.G., Deutsch, G.P., Dunlop, P.R.C. and Priestman, T.J. (1991) Clinical oncology services to district general hospitals: report of a working party of the Royal College of Radiologists. *Clin. Oncol.* **3**, 41–5.

Robertson, A.G., Robertson, C., Perone, C. *et al.* (1998) Effect of gap length and position on results of treatment of cancer of the larynx in Scotland by radiotherapy: a linear quadratic analysis. *Radiother. Oncol.* **48**(2), 165–73.

Rosalki, J.R. and Karp, S.J. (1999) The COIN workstation: state of the future art. *Clin. Oncol.* **11**, 15–27.

Schmidt, F., Hartwagner, K.A., Spork, E.B. and Groell, R. (1998) Medical Audit after 26 711 breast imaging studies: improved rate of detection of small breast carcinomas (classified as Tis or T1a,b). *Cancer* **83**(12), 2516–20.

Shone, G.R. and Yardley, M.P. (1991) An audit into the incidence of handicap after unilateral radical neck dissection. *J. Laryngol. Otol.* **105**, 760–2.

Sikora, K. (1999) Cancer survival in Britain is poorer than that of her comparable European neighbours. *BMJ* **7208**, 461–2.

Stiller, C.A. (1988) Centralisation of treatment and survival rates for cancer. *Arch. Dis. Child.* **63**, 23–30.

Sue-Ling, H.M., Johnston, D., Martin, I.G. *et al.* (1993) Gastric cancer: a curable disease in Britain. *BMJ* **307**, 591–6.

Wessex Cancer Intelligence Unit (1990). *Report on the cost-effectiveness of treatment for colorectal cancer in three health districts*. Winchester: Wessex Cancer Intelligence Unit.

61

The organization of cancer services: a UK perspective

JILL A. BULLIMORE

INTRODUCTION

People want to know that if they get cancer they can obtain effective care quickly. In every country, patients, the public in general, doctors, nurses and the government want a good cancer service. What, then, prevents good cancer care being available to all?

The main factors are the limits set by resources, both financial and human. Too few suitably trained staff and poor communication between the numerous groups who care for patients with cancer result in fragmented and inefficient care. Public ignorance of health matters in general, and of cancer in particular, compounds the problem.

The public want an efficient and effective service with an emphasis on screening and prevention, as well the assurance, that if 'the worst' should happen, proper care will be at hand. When members of the public become patients, their emphasis changes. Speedy referral to a specialist, rapid investigation and proper treatment become of prime importance. Patients expect be able to discuss the diagnosis and treatment options with the doctor who will be treating them and they want to know they are going to have 'the best treatment'.

Those who work in all parts of the service, from screening, through diagnosis, therapy and palliative care, need the satisfaction of doing a good job well; essential if morale and effectiveness are to be maintained.

The government consists of men and women who are also members of the public, some may be, or have been, patients. All will have relatives or friends who have cancer or have suffered from it. There will even be a few doctors and nurses and other healthcare professionals who have become members of parliament. So the individuals who make up the government will have similar aspirations to the people of the country as a whole. However, the government has the difficult task of funding the greater part of the cancer service, particularly in a country such as the UK, which is committed to providing a national health service and where only a small proportion of healthcare is provided privately.

Cancer services are expensive and have no finite limits as far as cost is concerned. Government is faced with the difficulty of providing funds for a service that will always be less than perfect, making ammunition for the news-hungry media. The battlefield of the National Health Service (NHS) in Britain has been, and will continue to be, fought over by politicians, both in government and out. The government of the day has to decide how much of its budget will be spent on healthcare and hence on cancer services. Comparisons of the proportion of gross national product spent on health in the countries of the developed world reveal differences that make uncomfortable reading in Great Britain. The public's anxiety about illness ensures that healthcare will remain a major factor in any political party's manifesto. Much political mileage is made out of what this party or that will do, or have done, to improve the service. The harsh realities remain the same for a government of any persuasion: cancer care is expensive and it is the government that is responsible for setting the limits on healthcare spending and has to carry the can for the shortcomings of the service it funds.

In 1993, the Chief Medical Officers for England and Wales gathered together an advisory group of healthcare professionals, expert in the various aspects of cancer treatment. This was in response to concern amongst healthcare professionals that there was apparent variation in the outcomes of treatment in different parts of the UK, and the public outcry, fuelled by reports in the media, that patients with apparently similar cancers received differing treatments.

The unanimous view of the group was that although excellent treatment was available in the UK, there was inequality of access to it. This inequality resulted, in part, from a lack of funds but also from the lack of agreed policies for managing the differing types of cancer. The delivery of the service differed across the country, with wide variations in the resources and priority health authorities gave to it. The service had developed in a piecemeal way over the preceding years, so that each region differed from the next in how, and to what extent, it made provision for cancer care. At that time, England and Wales were divided into 12 regions, later reduced to eight. Each regional health authority, outposts of the NHS executive, received money allocated by central government, with which it had the responsibility of securing all healthcare for the population it served. This is not the place to discuss the complex formulae by which the size of the allocation to each individual region was calculated. Suffice it to say that variation in the size of the allocation, in itself, gave rise to inequality of cancer services.

THE EXPERT ADVISORY GROUP ON CANCER (EAGC)

The task of the group was to study the problems and consider what changes would be necessary to improve the clinical and structural management of the service. They were to make recommendations that would lead to a nationally accepted policy for commissioning cancer services that would lead to a high-quality service accessible to all in the UK.

The group, which numbered 14, including the two Chief Medical Officers, consisted of doctors and nurses whose main clinical interest was the treatment of patients with cancer, a public health doctor, two general practitioners (GPs) and experts in the planning and delivering of cancer services.

A policy framework for commissioning cancer services (EAGC, 1995), the advisory group's recommendations, were accepted by the government and published in 1995. This report is also known as the Calman Hine report. Since that time, each health authority has been attempting to implement the recommendations, adapting them to fit the particular requirements of the people for whom they have the responsibility of providing cancer services.

This chapter is based mainly on the recommendations of *A policy framework for commissioning cancer services* and the ways in which efforts to implement them continue to be carried out.

THE PROBLEM

Cancer is a common disease much feared by the public. One in three people suffer from cancer and one in four die of it. Cancer is predominantly a disease of the elderly. The number of people living to an old age has risen, with a consequent increase in cancer incidence. Major improvements in surgery and radiotherapy techniques have reduced the morbidity suffered by patients and, together with cytotoxic chemotherapy, have resulted in greatly improved outcomes in some of the less common tumours, particularly in childhood cancer. Improvements in outcome have been less marked in cancer of the breast, lung and lower bowel which, if non-melanomatous skin cancers are excluded, account for more than half of all cancers. Over the past decade, advances in potentially curative treatment, developments in palliative care and greater emphasis given to the quality of life of patients throughout their illness, have benefited many patients. Unfortunately, these benefits have not been available to all the citizens of the UK.

The provision of healthcare takes up about 6 per cent of the NHS budget. It is not possible to identify the cost of providing treatment for cancer as a separate entity. It comes out of the government funding the health service as a whole. Patients and their families also bear hidden but extensive costs following a diagnosis of cancer. The advisory group recognized that, independent of the size of the NHS budget, the best and fairest use must be made of it in order to remove inequality.

A national framework for the provision of cancer services would provide a basis from which comparisons of service provision between the regions might be made. It would facilitate removal of inequalities and lead to improved care and outcomes of treatment. Regions where the standard of care is good would be identified and other regions have pressure exerted on them to bring their service up to the level of the best.

GENERAL PRINCIPLES

The principles that should govern the provision of cancer care were set out in *A policy framework for commissioning cancer services* as follows (EAGC, 1995):

1 All patients should have access to a uniformly high quality of care in the community or hospital wherever they may live, to ensure the maximum possible cure rates and best quality of life. Care should be provided as close to the patient's home as is compatible with high quality, safe and effective treatment.
2 Public and professional education to help early recognition of symptoms of cancer and the availability of national screening programmes are vital parts of any comprehensive programme of cancer care.
3 Patients, families and carers should be given clear information and assistance in a form they can understand about treatment options and outcomes available to them at all stages of treatment from diagnosis onwards.
4 The development of cancer services should be patient centred and should take account of patients', families' and carers' views and preferences, as well as those of professionals involved in cancer care. Individuals' perceptions of their needs may differ from those of the professional. Good communication between professionals and patients is especially important.
5 The primary care team is a central and continuing element in cancer care for both the patient and his or her family, from primary prevention, pre-symptomatic screening, initial diagnosis, through to care and follow-up or, in some cases, death and bereavement. Effective communication between sectors is imperative in achieving the best possible care.
6 In recognition of the impact that screening, diagnosis and treatment of cancer have on patients, families and their carers, psychosocial aspects of cancer should be considered at all stages.
7 Cancer registration and careful monitoring of treatment and outcomes is essential.

THE STRUCTURE OF CANCER SERVICES

The structure should consist of a network into which all the different aspects of cancer care fit. Primary care, secondary care provided at cancer units in district general hospitals and tertiary care at cancer centres in larger hospitals, form the basis of the structure. The network should have close links with hospices and care in the community, thus creating a comprehensive cancer service.

Wherever possible, cancer treatment and care should be given near to the patient's home, provided that the local expertise and facilities enable this to be done with safety, using treatment most likely to cure the patient. There will be some treatments too complex to be undertaken locally and for these, the patient will need to travel to the cancer centre. The needs of patients and their families must receive special consideration in these circumstances and long periods away from home minimized. Ideally, a continuum of care from screening, diagnosis, active treatment and palliation should be achieved.

THE ELEMENTS OF THE STRUCTURE

Primary care, secondary care and tertiary care

The primary care team is important to the patient not only at the time of presentation, but throughout treatment and aftercare. The GP knows the members of the patient's family and is best placed to ensure that they receive support.

Patients with cancer make up only a small part of the work that general practitioners and their primary care teams undertake; yet the role of the GP is crucial to the care of the patient. A visit to the GP is usually the first port of call for a patient who has symptoms or signs of a cancer. Having visited the doctor once, many patients are loath to make an early repeat visit, particularly if reassurance has been given on the first visit. This delay, if prolonged, may have an adverse effect on the outcome of treatment. General practitioners should encourage patients with new unexplained symptoms to seek another appointment if they do not resolve in a few weeks.

A network has existed for many years in the UK where specialists from major hospitals providing tertiary cancer care visit district general hospitals. Specialists in clinical oncology served numerous local hospitals in this way. Regular clinics were held at which new patients referred by surgeons and other clinicians were seen, as well as patients in need of post-treatment follow-up. The service was limited due to the small number of oncologists to carry out this work. In 1993, the total number of non-surgical oncologists in the UK was less than 400. This number had to provide a vital part of the cancer service for the whole country. Inadequate as this system was, it was realized that, with an expansion of trained staff and improved facilities at the district general hospitals (DGHs), it could form the basis for a non-surgical oncology network throughout the country.

The EAGC proposed a structure in which secondary care, including most of the diagnostic and surgical procedures for the common cancers, would be provided locally at DGHs designated cancer units. Cancer centres in large hospitals would provide treatment for the rare cancers and for those common cancers requiring particular treatment regimens that are too specialized, too technically demanding or too costly to be provided in a DGH. These would include specialized surgical techniques, complex cytotoxic chemotherapy and radiotherapy, together with expert specialized knowledge in radiology, pathology and other support services for cancer treatment. The cancer centre, as well as acting as a tertiary referral centre for rare cancers or those requiring particular specialized services, would act as a cancer unit for the population in its neighbourhood. This simple hub-and-spoke structure was intended to be flexible in order to meet the needs of the different types of populations and the varied terrain in which they live (Figs 61.1 and 61.2).

In order to achieve and maintain high standards of expertise in any of the clinical specialities, it is necessary for each specialist to treat enough patients with that type of disease. Clearly, many more clinicians will have this opportunity in the common cancers than in the less common ones. Specializing in particular areas of clinical practice is now actively encouraged; this was not universally the case in 1993. Surgeons have focused their work on cancers of particular sites or systems, rather than being general surgeons. Clinical oncologists have become similarly site specialized. It is important to maintain knowledge and practical ability in general surgery and oncology, but the bulk of a clinician's work should cover only a relatively narrow range of cancers, if expertise and up-to-date knowledge is to be maintained.

In order to provide sufficient clinical experience in the common cancers, a cancer unit should serve a population of about 250 000. A cancer centre ideally should serve a population of between two-thirds of a million and 1 million (Royal College of Radiologists, 1991; Independent Review of Specialist Services, 1993). A cancer centre serving less than 600 000 would be unlikely to treat enough patients to maintain the comprehensive clinical experience needed. In these circumstances, links should be made with a neighbouring centre, even if at a considerable distance, to treat those patients for whom expert specialized treatment cannot be provided. Similarly, DGHs, serving too small a population to achieve the necessary clinical experience to be designated a cancer unit treating all common cancers, should combine with a neighbouring DGH. In some instances, this will mean amalgamation of small neighbouring DGHs to form a larger unit that fulfils the criteria, and occasionally it will lead to cessation of elective treatment of cancer at some hospitals. Alternatively, agreement may be reached by two or more DGHs to enter a partnership, to jointly treat the common cancers, those of some sites being treated at one hospital and the rest at another. Recognition as a cancer unit for the treatment of particular sites or systems would be accorded to the appropriate hospital.

The key to a good cancer service is collaboration between the differing groups who, in turn, carry the main responsibility of caring for the patient. The surgical teams and the non-surgical oncology teams must work closely together. The primary care team and carers in the community must receive timely information from the hospital about the patient's diagnosis, current state of health, the treatment and what side-effects to expect. If the patient needs admission to a hospice, full information must be available promptly. Communication must be good in all directions, from the GP and hospice to the hospitals and from the hospitals back to the hospice and GP.

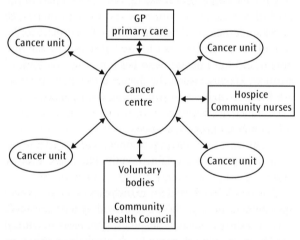

Figure 61.1 *Cancer centre as hub for its links in the cancer network.*

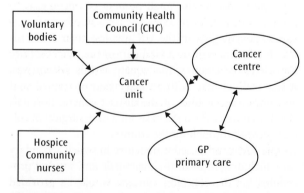

Figure 61.2 *Cancer unit as hub for its links in the cancer network.*

THE CANCER UNIT

A cancer unit is normally a large DGH providing secondary care to its surrounding population. The cancer unit is not a separate physical entity within the hospital but rather an association of the services for cancer within the hospital with a recognized combined identity. It is part of the DGH service provision and is supported by the general services of the hospital.

Surgeons most commonly manage the diagnosis and initial treatment of patients with cancer. It is recognized that subspecialization amongst surgeons and physicians in DGHs is necessary to concentrate clinical experience and expertise. Large DGHs provide specialist clinics in a number of specialities, including gastroenterology, diseases of the breast, respiratory disease, genitourinary disease, gynaecology and ENT. These clinics manage patients with benign as well as malignant disease, and it is to these clinics that patients in whom cancer is suspected should be referred.

The non-surgical oncology needs of a cancer unit are provided by clinical oncologists (accredited by the Royal College of Radiologists) or medical oncologists (accredited by the Royal College of Physicians). These clinicians ideally hold posts at the cancer centre as well as the cancer unit. The pattern of provision will vary according to the needs of the cancer unit. At present, clinical oncologists provide most of the non-surgical oncology service, as they have knowledge of radiotherapy and chemotherapy. Most large DGHs have a haematology service that treats some patients with malignant disease of the haematopoetic and lymphoid systems. The amount of such work and its complexity is variable. Where such a service is provided, it should be within the framework of the cancer unit and closely integrated with the clinical oncology department providing cytotoxic chemotherapy to patients with 'solid cancers'.

The cancer unit must work in close collaboration with the primary care and hospice services. Local guidelines for GPs on the recognition of sinister symptoms and agreed protocols for swift referral of patients in whom a GP suspects cancer should be developed. Arrangements must be in place for prompt transfer, whenever clinically indicated, of patients who present as emergencies to a hospital not providing cancer unit facilities.

Joint consultations between surgeons and physicians of the cancer unit and clinical oncologists must take place and multidisciplinary management, in accordance with agreed protocols, carried out. Joint clinics should be established between surgeons and oncologists whenever possible. Agreed protocols of management should be used for the management of each cancer and each stage of the cancer. They should include not only the appropriate investigations, type of surgery and radiotherapy to be undertaken, but also the place of cytotoxic chemotherapy or other therapies. Regular clinico-pathological conferences should be held, which include diagnostic radiology and pathology expertise as well as the relevant surgeons, physicians and oncologists. These meetings should be able to call on the advice of specialized palliative care nurses and doctors when needed. These conferences provide the base for teaching, training and clinical audit within the cancer unit.

In order that there is sufficient non-surgical oncology input into the cancer services of the cancer unit, the number of non-surgical oncology sessions per week recommended in *A policy framework for commissioning cancer services* is a minimum of five, even for the smallest of units. A large DGH serving a population of 250 000 or more will probably be providing care for all the common cancers and some of the less common ones. This level of service would require subspecialization in non-surgical oncology, provided by more than one oncologist. To allow non-surgical oncologists to play a proper part in multidisciplinary meetings, hold outpatient clinics and conduct inpatient consultations, 10 clinical sessions or more per week would be appropriate, and this has been achieved in some cancer units.

The cancer unit must have close links with the cancer centre (or centres in densely populated areas) in the region in which it is located. There should be shared protocols of management and clarity regarding those areas of clinical practice that are carried out at the cancer unit and those that are appropriately referred to the cancer centre. The range of surgical and non-surgical oncology procedures carried out at the cancer unit will vary with the expertise available there and the patient numbers concerned. These limits of practice should be agreed and joint protocols of management developed.

Many cytotoxic chemotherapy protocols for common cancers may be administered safely at the cancer unit, provided the necessary resources of oncology-trained clinical staff and suitable facilities are available. This proximity of the service renders it more accessible to patients. The chemotherapy service for clinical oncology should be combined with that established for malignant haematology, to ensure economic use of expensive facilities and the best use of oncology-trained nurses and other staff essential to both services.

Complex chemotherapy regimens requiring peripheral blood stem cell (PBSC) support should normally be administered at the cancer centre. Chemotherapy at the cancer unit should be given only in a special outpatient unit or on specially designated wards by specialist staff. It is hazardous if given on general wards by inexperienced staff from different disciplines with little or no oncology knowledge (Joint Council for Clinical Oncology, 1994).

Radiotherapy should be confined to cancer centres due to its complexity, the scarcity of trained staff and the high cost of the service. In some remote areas it may be necessary to provide a limited radiotherapy service at a cancer unit in close collaboration with a cancer centre. When this is necessary, the cancer unit's service must be regarded as a branch of the cancer centre's radiotherapy service, follow the same protocols and be subject to the same quality controls and audit.

Lead clinician

A clinician experienced in cancer care should be appointed to be responsible for the organization and co-ordination of the range of cancer services provided in the cancer unit and for ensuring that high-quality care is given. This clinician is called the lead clinician and should hold the post for a period specified by the hospital management. The lead clinician should be paid for specific sessions to enable his or her duties to be properly carried out. These duties include:

- supervision of the facilities for cancer care;
- ensuring there is adequate non-surgical support;
- supervising arrangements for audit and for continuing medical education;
- meeting regularly with colleagues from other cancer units, cancer centres and general practice, to guarantee uniform standards;
- developing protocols between primary care, cancer units and cancer centres to ensure an effective network of high standard care.

Cancer services are affected by, and affect all, the services of a hospital. The role of the lead clinician is crucial to the effectiveness of the cancer unit. He or she must have access to the management of the hospital and must have the benefit of information technology (IT) and secretarial help.

Each cancer unit has the potential to become the focus of care for the community it serves. It is where most surgery, chemotherapy and follow-up of patients take place. It has links to GP practices, community services, the local hospice and the cancer centre. It should be able to give current information about the progress of treatment and condition of patients to other professionals clinically involved. It should provide education about cancer and its treatment to patients and their families, as well as to GPs and community nurses. The cancer unit should host patient self-help groups and welcome input from the Community Health Council and voluntary bodies. All this can not be achieved without funding, but even a relatively small investment in senior secretarial staff with data management skills, working closely with oncology nurses, may reap rich rewards in the way of benefit to the patients.

THE CANCER CENTRE

The cancer centre should ideally be part of a large general hospital providing a full range of cancer treatments. A high degree of specialization in all the disciplines concerned in the treatment of cancer should be available. The centre must provide treatment for rare and less common tumours, together with specialized surgery and non-surgical oncology. A cancer centre must be in a general hospital dealing with all types of illness, in order that the patients with cancer may benefit from a full range of clinical support, including intensive care. Links with specialists in other clinical spheres is important to enable clinicians and nurses working in oncology specialities to

be aware of new techniques and to adopt and use them in the treatment of cancer.

The cancer centre must serve a population large enough to ensure an adequate number of patients to maintain expertise in clinical practice in the common and rare cancers. It should be properly equipped, with staff specialized in all the disciplines involved in care, together with sufficient non-clinical staff, including medical secretaries, managers, and IT personnel, to run an efficient service.

The special services provided at the cancer centre include:

- particular expertise and facilities for cancer surgery;
- specialized surgical services of plastic and reconstructive surgery;
- expert radiotherapy personnel and a full range of radiotherapy facilities;
- medical oncology;
- intensive chemotherapy and support techniques such as bone marrow transplantation or peripheral blood stem cell rescue;
- specialized haematological oncology, including facilities for autologous and autoimmune bone marrow transplantation;
- specialized radio-diagnostic and pathology services;
- paediatric and adolescent oncology services;
- specialised pharmacy provision;
- specialized palliative care and rehabilitation;
- research facilities – both for clinical and basic scientific research;
- facilities for teaching, training and professional development of staff.

Nurses working at a cancer centre should ideally hold a post-registration qualification in oncology and possess special knowledge of acute radiation reactions and chemotherapy side-effects. Oncology nurses fulfil many roles; they play a central role in the care of patients with cancer. Some specialize in the giving of cytotoxic chemotherapy; others become skilled in stoma care, breast care, lymphoedema management and palliative care. Some are especially skilled in psychosocial counselling.

Radiotherapy must be provided at the cancer centre. It is a speciality that uses complex technology and expensive machines. In order to give high-quality treatment the centre must have sufficient numbers of therapy machines and a range of equipment that allows appropriate choices to be made when planning radiotherapy for patients. Skilled physicists, mechanics and technicians are essential for the safe delivery of radiotherapy. Therapy radiographers are trained to deliver treatment to patients. This demands a high degree of expertise to work the equipment, management and administrative skills to make efficient use of the machines and the skill to support patients through what is always a stressful and sometimes physically uncomfortable time. Safety is of paramount importance and each radiotherapy department must have a system of verifiable quality control (Department of Health, 1991). Suitably trained staff members, essential to the safe running of an efficient and effective radiotherapy department, are in short supply and their skills should be concentrated in large centres.

The proximity of experts in all aspects of cancer treatment allows multidisciplinary consultation to be available in the planning and delivery of treatment, ensuring an accessible high quality of care.

Education, training and research are important aspects of the work of a cancer centre. It is responsible for training junior medical staff, nurses and other healthcare professionals and the continuing education of senior staff. Cancer units should be encouraged to share in many aspects of this work. The whole cancer network should be actively encouraged to participate in controlled clinical trials.

It is likely that many cancer centres will be in major hospitals that are part of a university medical school and undertake the teaching of medical students. The ethos of seeking to provide excellence in the treatment of patients with cancer should permeate the cancer centre, influencing the new generations of future workers.

The lead clinician in a cancer centre

The lead clinician should be responsible, like his or her counterpart in a cancer unit, for supervising the facilities for cancer care, ensuring there is adequate non-surgical oncology support and supervising arrangements for audit and continuing education. Creating and maintaining links between the cancer units and the cancer centre are important functions of the role. The clinical guidelines and protocols developed between site-specialized clinicians in the centre and the units, and the centre and primary care, are the responsibility of the specialists concerned, but the lead clinician is responsible for ensuring that they comply with national guidelines and are updated and audited. The lead clinician should meet regularly with colleagues in cancer units and general practice to ensure uniformity of care.

Frequently, the cancer centre is not all housed at one site. Some specialized services, such as neurosurgery, orthopaedic surgery and paediatric oncology, may be provided at hospitals distant from the hospital where the bulk of the services, including radiotherapy, are provided. Co-ordinating the parts of the specialized services at differing hospitals may present difficulties unless the protocols of management are fully understood by the clinical staff and by the management of the individual hospitals. The lead clinician has a vital role to play in these arrangements. The duties involved take considerable time and hard work. It has been found that in some cancer centres consisting of a group of hospitals serving numerous cancer units, the post requires whole-time commitment.

Lead clinician for a specific site or system

The clinicians within cancer centres and cancer units, specializing in treating cancer of particular sites or systems, are responsible for producing clinical guidelines for their speciality that reflect national guidelines. In order to maintain consistency of therapy, regional speciality groups should be formed with a chairman or lead clinician who will ensure that protocols are developed and audit carried out.

THE RELATIONSHIP BETWEEN CANCER UNITS AND CANCER CENTRE

A relationship of mutual trust and collaboration must be established between each cancer unit and the cancer centre. This is best fostered by face-to-face contact between staff members working at the two hospitals. Personal contact is likely to create bonds of friendship and respect. Both cancer centres and cancer units are involved in education, training, research and audit. Co-operation in research, in particular in the conduct of controlled clinical trials, strengthens their union by the desire to improve cancer care. Protocols of management for each cancer should be agreed between cancer centre and cancer unit. Cytotoxic chemotherapy regimens used at the cancer unit must be the same as those employed at the cancer centre. Compliance with the agreed protocols at each hospital should be audited.

PALLIATIVE CARE

Palliative care, that is, care to relieve suffering, is part of the role of all those who work with patients and tend to their various needs. It should come into the care given by doctors and nurses across the spectrum of specialities. It is also part of the work of radiographers, ambulance drivers, receptionists and even car park attendants at hospitals treating cancer. Kindness, consideration, respect are all part of palliation of distress, both physical and mental.

Palliative medicine and palliative nursing have become specialities in their own right, with official and academic institutions of their own. The skills of palliative care specialists should be available to all patients with cancer. Newly diagnosed patients, who may have a high chance of being cured, need relief of suffering as well as those who are terminally ill. Hospices are associated in the public's mind with terminal disease and death. This leads to reluctance to accept offers of early help from them. 'Counselling' has become acceptable to the public; this is one of the palliative care team's skills. Members of the palliative care team possessing the gift of good communication may be identified as counsellors rather than hospice or palliative care nurses, thereby helping to overcome patients' reticence.

Hospital-based palliative care teams give invaluable help to staff and patients in need of control of severe symptoms. Their knowledge is called upon to help patients, who do not have cancer but who have pain or other symptoms, for example, postoperatively. This integration of palliative care into the everyday work of a hospital helps not only patients but also the staff, who have skilled people to whom to turn for advice and, at the same time, from whom to learn.

The palliative care team in a cancer unit is often small; but its size may be augmented by co-operating with colleagues whose principal function is more active cancer treatment, such as doctors and nurses working in the oncology department.

A palliative care unit in a cancer centre should perform similar duties to those in a cancer unit and, in addition, must lead in research and teaching. It should foster joint research, particularly controlled clinical trials, across the whole cancer service network of which it is a part, and undertake collaborative work with services in other regions. It should develop links with the service in the cancer units it serves, and with primary care and community services.

Much palliative care is already given in the community, supporting patients and helping relatives and friends with the day-to-day care of terminally ill patients. In an ideal world, all those who wish to die at home should be able to do so. The majority of people still die in hospitals, some in hospices. When family, primary care, hospice, community services and hospitals succeed in collaborating closely and share firm links, more patients are enabled to spend the last part of their illness at home. Such an ideal system is inaccessible to many, at present, but in spite of money shortages it is for this ideal that the service should aim.

A palliative care team in a hospital or in the community should be multidisciplinary. It should have doctors, nurses, physiotherapists and access to special services such as dietetics and breast and stoma care nurses. The teams should link with the other parts of the cancer service and, where necessary, call on clinicians and nurses from other disciplines to supplement the care they provide.

Patients and their families need privacy. This should be provided for consultations, for counselling sessions and, especially, when a patient is dying. Single rooms should be made available for those dying in hospitals and hospices. Relatives should be able to remain with very ill patients and suitable arrangements for this must be made.

The spiritual needs of patients must be considered and spiritual care should be available to those who wish it.

Many hospices and some community palliative nursing care services were developed in response to local needs by fund-raising. Health authorities were slow to recognize the importance of palliative care and were understandably relieved that money for these developments was found from voluntary sources. The result of this is that palliative care evolved in an *ad hoc* manner, with great variability both in quantity and quality. Health authorities now recognize the value of palliative care and partially fund the service, but not in a uniform manner across the country. National bodies such as the Royal College of Nursing and the medical Royal Colleges, together with the National Council for Hospice and Specialist Palliative Care Services have developed quality standards and guidelines on service provision. These should be adopted to ensure greater uniformity of access to care of a high standard (National Council for Hospice and Specialist Palliative Care Services, 1998).

Charities and voluntary organizations play an important role in supporting the valuable work of hospices and palliative care teams. Without them, many services would not have developed and could not provide the comforts that they do. The involvement of the local community is an asset and provides many voluntary workers. As the service has developed, the need for close collaboration between the voluntary bodies and the NHS has become obvious. The place of palliative care in the overall cancer service has to be clearly defined and gaps recognized and filled; this can only be done by charities, voluntary bodies and the NHS working closely together, recognizing deficits and sharing ideas for future developments.

PRIMARY CARE AND THE CANCER SERVICES

It is widely acknowledged that GPs and others who work in primary care have a crucial impact on the course of events that happen to a patient with cancer. It is the GP who is most likely to recognize sinister symptoms, undertake preliminary tests and refer to a specialist, most commonly a consultant surgeon, to enable a diagnosis to be made and treatment started.

The number of people per year who develop cancer, in a practice of 2000, is in the region of six to eight. Inevitably, care of cancer patients represents a small part of the duties of primary care. A GP will probably not have been involved directly in diagnosing and treating patients with cancer since leaving hospital practice. Many therefore feel unsure of their ground when explaining new and complex therapies unfamiliar to them.

Patients need the help and support of their GP. They need to be confident that their doctor will recognize cancer in its early stages, will refer them to a specialist urgently and will continue to care for them during and after treatment. They need to feel that their GP knows more about their disease than they do and that, if a complication occurs when they are at home, the 'right thing' will be done.

A GP is at a disadvantage without timely information from those investigating and treating a patient in a cancer unit or cancer centre. Without easy and prompt access to an appropriate hospital clinic for patients in whom a practitioner suspects cancer, delays in diagnosis are inevitable.

Understanding between hospital consultants and GPs must be reached on significant signs and symptoms, preliminary tests to be undertaken in general practice and fast track referral paths to relevant clinics. Local guidelines, to aid identification of which patients to refer and to where they should be referred, benefit the patient, the GP and the hospital. Such guidelines should be drawn up, taking into account nationally agreed standards, and be updated regularly to comply with changing medical practice and patterns of service delivery. They will help to achieve the government's aim that all patients suspected of having cancer are seen by a consultant within 2 weeks. The even more important aim of starting treatment promptly following the diagnosis having been made, is being pressed by clinicians. Some standards have been developed for waiting times for radiotherapy and a national audit of these standards revealed wide discrepancies in waiting times in the UK, clearly related to resources (Board of Faculty of Clinical Oncology, 1998; Department of Health, 2000a).

The GP also needs to be kept informed during investigation and treatment. The diagnosis, stage of disease, proposed treatment and what the patient has been told should be made known to the GP before the patient or anxious relatives next consult him or her following the making of these decisions. This enables the patient to retain confidence in the primary care team's knowledge about his or her illness, and lessens the inevitable anxiety that accompanies the diagnosis of cancer. In turn, it is essential that the GP provide the hospital specialist with proper patient information. During treatment and follow-up the hospital specialist responsible for the patient's care should be told of any changes that have occurred between hospital visits. Throughout treatment, follow-up, relapse and terminal care the GP is a key figure, the patient's advocate and supporter.

COMMUNICATION

Communication between the parts of the service caring for the same patient is often sparse, and patients and their relatives are left confused and anxious. Poor communication leads to gaps in care when support is most needed. Modern means of communication, in particular the use of faxes, the development of patient-held records and access by recognized carers to hospital and GP notes would ease this problem. The use of modern information technology, however, is beset with problems concerning confidentiality. Safeguards must be built into the system to allow access only to those who are authorized. The increased use of e-mail would seem an obvious way of speeding information, but the lack of confidentiality often renders this too insecure a method of communication.

All parts of the cancer service must ensure that they develop IT and modern communication systems that are compatible. Passing of current relevant information between hospitals, primary care practices, hospices and community care workers is the key to a patient's smooth transition between the different parts of the service. This cannot be achieved without cost, but so important is the need for good communication that such systems should attract considerable priority in health authority and hospital budgets.

Patients need to retain control over their own lives. Their confidence is boosted when a member of the team caring for them is in possession of current relevant facts about their case. Patient-held records are a useful and effective means of supplementing communication between the parts of the cancer service. They give patients a sense of ownership over the events that happen to them and are helpful during treatment, both curative and palliative.

Cancer services start with public information about cancer. In particular, advice on screening and prevention should be made available to the public. Education at schools and establishments of higher education should be encouraged. It has proved difficult to interest the public at large in education of this kind. There is, however, educational benefit from the numerous articles in the press and on radio and television, some of which are of a high standard. Those reports that are inaccurate give the opportunity to refute the claims, so increasing the public's awareness. Information on the World Wide Web is freely available but is of variable quality. This medium is an ideal way of disseminating information about cancer and it is incumbent on the NHS, via its own internet site (www.nhs.uk) and other authorities, to make good use of it by publishing clear and accurate information.

MONITORING THE CANCER SERVICE

The policy document outlining the proposed structure was published in 1995. The NHS Executive (NHS(E)) was given the task by the government of implementing it nationally. The EAGC had outlined the aims of the proposed cancer service and described a broad structure within which these aims could be achieved. The recommendations were firm but the means of achieving them were left flexible, in order that each regional health authority (RHA) and district health authority (DHA) would be able to tailor the service to meet the needs of its own population.

The success in achieving the principal goals of the service, i.e. improved access to high-quality service and better clinical outcomes, has to be assessed in order that it may be monitored.

The Clinical Outcomes Group (COG) of the NHS(E) undertook to study the medical literature and, with recognized experts in all the disciplines involved in cancer care, to produce a series of evidence-based clinical guidelines on best practice, each devoted to cancer of a specific site or system. Those for the common cancers were produced first, followed by those for the less common.

The site specialist teams in the cancer units and cancer centres write their own protocols of clinical management, ensuring that they comply with accepted best practice. Co-operation in protocol development between the units and centres of a region should take place to facilitate audit of clinical outcomes and protocol compliance.

ACCREDITATION OF CANCER UNITS AND CANCER CENTRES

The health authorities were given the task of assisting clinicians and hospital managers to set up the structure of the local and regional cancer services. The regional health authority has the duty to decide which hospitals receive cancer centre status, taking into consideration the size of the population served, the density of population, the facilities and services in place, and access by road and rail. Each RHA set its own criteria for designation of centres and its own method of accreditation. DHAs undertake a similar task with respect to designation of cancer units. The cancer centres and cancer units thus accredited are re-accredited at regular intervals set by the health authorities.

The aim of the service is to improve outcomes. The effectiveness of the success of the cancer service will be measured by patient satisfaction, the fall in the annual incidence and mortality rates for cancer. These cannot be gauged without accurate and timely data.

THE CANCER REGISTRIES

Cancer registries record and analyse the number of new cases and the number of deaths from cancer per year. They have an essential part to play in improving and maintaining good standards of care. In 1993, there was considerable variation in the funding of cancer registries, and hence in the completeness and timeliness of their records. This inequality was, in part, due to the way the registries were financed. Depending on the importance the regional health authority placed on the collection of cancer statistics, the registry was well or poorly funded. It was recognized by the advisory group that, without reliable data on incidence and treatment outcomes for cancer, comparison of performance between districts, regions and countries would not be possible.

A national policy for cancer registration and funds to improve and expand the work of the registries would help the accurate, appropriate and speedy collection and analysis of cancer data, allowing valid comparison to be made across regions and countries.

THE PROGRESS OF THE ESTABLISHMENT OF THE NATIONAL CANCER SERVICE

A great deal has been achieved towards establishing the new structure of the cancer service throughout the UK, but there is still wide regional variation. This is due partially to the initial variability in resources allocated to cancer services in each region, and also to each health authority adopting its own criteria for accreditation of cancer centres or units.

The establishment of cancer units and cancer centres has been hampered in some parts of the country by managerial problems. The process of accreditation identified DGHs serving too small a population to be recognized as a cancer unit. In order to fulfil the criteria, some hospitals have had to combine their services for particular common cancers. This resulted in some small hospitals closing or ceasing to undertake acute surgery, as the loss of the cancer service had a major impact on their overall service provision. The accreditation of cancer centres often resulted in hospitals needing to combine their specialized services so that together they would fulfil the criteria without duplicating expensive services. Hospital trusts had to negotiate with the help of their health authorities and reach a satisfactory solution; sometimes this could be achieved only by merging into a single trust.

Funding for cancer is part of the budgets of many departments within a trust, and the difficulty of identifying specific funding for cancer hinders compliance with the EAGC's recommendations.

The need for the setting of national standards for accreditation of hospitals and the uniformity of standards adopted by the health authorities for the quality of the service for which they are responsible has become clear. The Manual of Cancer Services Standards attempts to meet this need (Department of Health, 2000b).

THE FUTURE OF CANCER SERVICES

It is incumbent on the government, whatever system it adopts to provide cancer services, not only to ensure that they are available to all its citizens, but that they are of a high and consistent quality. It is reasonable that it should seek value for its money. The National Institute for Clinical Excellence (NICE) (which has absorbed the role of COG) has the responsibility for advising on the clinical and cost-effectiveness of therapies.

In 2000, the UK government published The NHS Cancer Plan (Department of Health, 2000b), in which it states its commitment to implementing the recommendations of the Calman Hine report. The Cancer

Taskforce, which includes patient representatives, clinicians and managers, was formed in 2001, it is led by the National Cancer Director, a professional cancer doctor. The Taskforce has the responsibility for monitoring the implementation of the Cancer Plan.

There has been a firm commitment by the government to provide much greater funding for cancer services so that the number of cancer doctors, nurses and other professionals will be substantially increased. There will inevitably be a considerable time lag before sufficient numbers can be recruited and trained, e.g. a new medical student would take at least 10 years training before becoming a consultant oncologist. In the meantime, an improvement in the infrastructure of the service, in particular an increase in medical secretaries and IT support, will help doctors and other workers to cope with heavy workloads as efficiently and humanely as possible. It is to be hoped that the political will to improve cancer services will continue and sufficient funding to achieve this will be provided.

The health of the nation is heavily influenced by social factors, which it is the duty of the government to try to influence for the better. When social improvements, cancer prevention measures and public education succeed in altering cancer incidence, cancer is still likely to remain a significant cause of morbidity and death. The care given to those who develop cancer will continue to depend on the doctors, nurses, and others who are trained to look after them. An effective and efficient service is what health professionals want to provide, they must be given the resources to enable them to give to each patient the time and care he or she deserves.

SIGNIFICANT POINTS

- A national cancer service must be founded on agreed principles and must guarantee people equal access to high quality care throughout the country.
- The views of patients and those of the public must be allowed to influence the service.
- There must be agreed national standards for the service, which are reviewed and updated on a regular basis.
- Reliable data must be collected in order that the standards may be monitored and comparison between regions made. By these means equality of provision may be achieved.
- In each region cancer networks should be set up consisting of the cancer centres, cancer units, primary care, hospices and care in the community.

- Each network should enable swift and accurate clinical information to be exchanged between its various parts.
- Information on clinical and strategic management should be exchanged between networks to encourage the spread of good practice.
- There must be sufficient numbers of doctors, nurses and other professionals trained in the treatment of patients with cancer in each region to provide a high quality service for the population of that region.
- The facilities in which patients and their relatives are cared for must be suitable.
- Those who work with people with cancer need time to give each patient individual attention. Without proper support from secretaries and information technology the efficiency of the doctors and others is impaired and time that should be given to the patient is curtailed.
- It is essential that the funding provided by the government is sufficient to ensure that there are enough trained personnel and specialized equipment.

KEY REFERENCES

Department of Health (2000a) *The survey of radiotherapy provision.* www.doh.gov.uk/cancer

Department of Health (2000b) *The NHS Cancer Plan. A plan for investment. A plan for reform.* London: Department of Health.

Expert Advisory Group on Cancer (1995) *A policy framework for commissioning cancer services: A Report by the Expert Advisory Group on Cancer to the Chief Medical Officers of England and Wales.* London: Department of Health.

REFERENCES

Board of Faculty of Clinical Oncology, Royal College of Radiologists (1998) *A national audit of waiting times for radiotherapy.* London: Royal College of Radiologists.

Department of Health (1991) *Quality assurance in radiotherapy: a quality management system for radiotherapy.* London: Department of Health.

Department of Health (2000a) *The survey of radiotherapy provision.* www.doh.gov.uk/cancer

Department of Health (2000b) *The NHS Cancer Plan. A plan for investment. A plan for reform.* London: Department of Health.

Expert Advisory Group on Cancer (1995) *A policy framework for commissioning cancer services: A Report by the Expert Advisory Group on Cancer to the Chief Medical Officers of England and Wales.* London: Department of Health.

Independent Review of Specialist Services (1993) *Report of an Independent Review of Specialist Services (Cancer) in London.* London: HMSO.

Joint Council for Clinical Oncology (1994) *Quality control in cancer chemotherapy: managerial and procedural aspects.* London: Royal College of Physicians and Royal College of Radiologists.

National Council for Hospice and Specialist Palliative Care Services (1998) *Managing cancer pain.* London: Royal College of Physicians.

Royal College of Radiologists (1991) *Cancer care and treatment services: advice for purchasers and providers.* London: Royal College of Radiologists.

Index